Skin Cancer

Skin Cancer

KEYVAN NOURI, MD

Professor of Dermatology and Otolaryngology
Director of Mohs, Dermatologic and Laser Surgery
Director of Surgical Training
Department of Dermatology and Cutaneous Surgery
University of Miami Miller School of Medicine
Miami, Florida

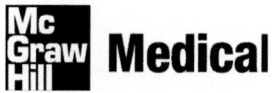

New York   Chicago   San Francisco   Lisbon   London
Madrid   Mexico City   Milan   New Delhi   San Juan
Scoul   Singapore   Sydney   Toronto

Skin Cancer

1 2 3 4 5 6 7 8 9 0 CTP/CTP 0 9 8

ISBN 978-0-07-147256-2
MHID 0-07-147256-8

This book was set in StempelSchneidler by Aptara.
The editors were Anne M. Sydor and Kim J. Davis.
The production supervisor was Sherri Souffrance.
Project management was provided by Aptara.
The interior designer was Alan Barnett.
The cover designer was Kelly Parr.
The index was prepared by Aptara.
China Translation & Printing, Inc. was printer and binder.

This book is printed on acid-free paper.

Library of Congress Cataloging-in-Publication Data

Skin cancer / [edited by] Keyvan Nouri.
    p. ; cm.
    Includes bibliographical references and index.
    ISBN-13: 978-0-07-147256-2 (hardcover : alk. paper)
    ISBN-10: 0-07-147256-8 (hardcover : alk. paper) 1. Skin–Cancer. I. Nouri, Keyvan.
    [DNLM: 1. Skin Neoplasms. WR 500 S6259 2008]
RC280.S5S572 2008
616.99'477–dc22

                       2007005746

I would like to dedicate this book to my wife Dr. Firouzeh Miremadi, my son Kian Nouri, my mother Zohreh Khajavi-Noori, my father Dr. Ali Nouri, my sister Dr. Mahnaz Nouri, my uncle Dr. Farrokh Khajavi-Noori, my grandparents, and my entire family and friends. Thank you for all your love and support throughout the years.

—*Keyvan Nouri, MD*

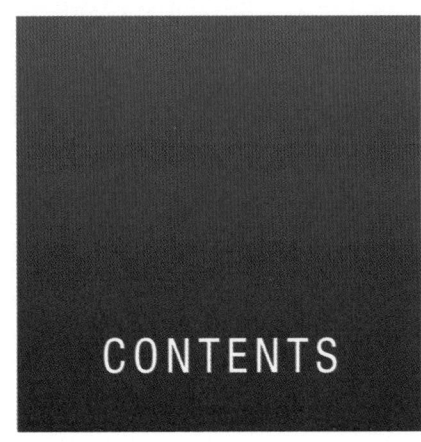

CONTENTS

CONTENTS

ix

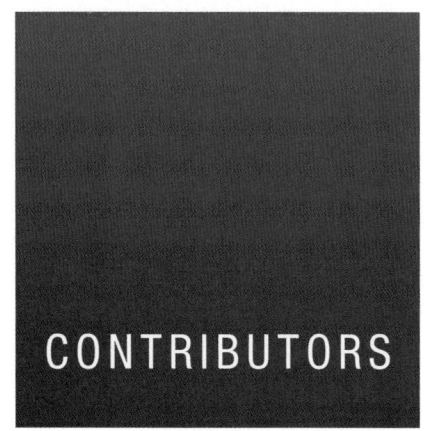

CONTRIBUTORS

Cheryl Aber, MD, FAAP
Fellow of Pediatric Dermatology
Department of Dermatology and
    Cutaneous Surgery
University of Miami Miller School
    of Medicine
Miami, Florida

Ammar M. Ahmed, MD
Baylor College of Medicine
Houston, Texas

Murad Alam, MD
Chief
Section of Cutaneous and Aesthetic
    Surgery
Department of Dermatology
Northwestern University
Chicago, Illinois

Samir K. Amin, BA
Medical Student
Baylor College of Medicine
Houston, Texas

Rana Anadolu-Brasie, MD
Professor of Dermatology and
    Venerology
Ankara University, School of Medicine
Ankara, Turkey

David L. Appert, MD
Dermatologic Surgery Fellow
Department of Dermatology
Mayo Clinic
Rochester, Minnesota

Rajesh Balkrishnan, MD
Merell Dow Professor
Pharmacy Practice and
    Administration
Associate Professor
Dermatology
The Ohio State University College
    of Medicine
Columbus, Ohio

Christopher J. Ballard, MD
Department of Dermatology and
    Cutaneous Surgery
University of Miami Miller School
    of Medicine
Miami, Florida

Raymond L. Barnhill, MD
Clinical Professor of Dermatology and
    Pathology
Senior Consultant for Melanoma
University of Miami Miller School
    of Medicine
Miami, Florida

Rueven Bergman, MD
Chairman
Dermatology
Rambam Medical Center and The
    Bruce Rappaport Faculty of Medicine,
    Technion Institute of Technology
Haifa, Israel

Brian Berman, MD, PhD
Professor
Department of Dermatology and
    Cutaneous Surgery and Internal
    Medicine
University of Miami Miller School
    of Medicine
Miami, Florida

Cindy Berthelot, MD
Medical Student
University of Texas Southwestern
    Medical School
Dallas, Texas

Marianne Berwick, PhD, MPH
Professor
Department of Internal Medicine
University of New Mexico
Albuquerque, New Mexico

Ashish Bhatia, MD
Assistant Professor of Clinical
    Dermatology
Mohs Micrographic Surgery, Laser &
    Cosmetic Surgery
Northwestern University School
    of Medicine
Chicago, Illinois

Norman Block, MD
Professor
Department of Urology
University of Miami Miller School
    of Medicine
Miami, Florida

Navid Bouzari, MD
Resident of Dermatology
Department of Dermatology and
    Cutaneous Surgery
University of Miami Miller School
    of Medicine
Miami, Florida

Carol P.R. Bowen-Wells, MD
Fellow
Surgical Oncology
University of Miami Miller School
    of Medicine
Miami, Florida

Ralph P. Braun, MD
Assistant Professor
Department of Dermatology
Hopitaux Universitaires
    de Geneve
Geneva Switzerland

Jerry D. Brewer, MD
Resident in Dermatology
Mayo Clinic, Graduate School
    of Medicine
Rochester, Minnesota

Walter HC Burgdorf, MD
Clinical Lecturer
Department of Dermatology
Ludwig Maximilian University
Munich, Germany

Jean-Claude Bystryn, MD
Professor
Department of Dermatology
New York University School of Medicine
New York, New York

Jeffrey Callen, MD
Professor and Chief
Division of Dermatology
University of Louisville School
of Medicine
Louisville, Kentucky

Ivan D. Camacho, MD
Internal Medicine Resident
Jackson Memorial Hospital
University of Miami Miller School
of Medicine
Miami, Florida

Piero Campolmi, MD
University Unit of Dermatology and
Physiotherapy
University of Florence
Florence, Italy

Caroline Caperton, MSPH
Research Fellow
Transdermal Delivery/Cutaneous
Biology Research Department of
Dermatology & Cutaneous Surgery
University of Miami Miller School
of Medicine
Miami, Florida

John Carucci, MD PhD
Director of Mohs Micrographic and
Dermatologic Surgery
Cornell University
New York, New York

Wolfgang H. Cerwinka, MD
Urology
Emory University
Atlanta, Georgia

Elbert H. Chen, MD
Fellow
Dermatology
Columbia University College
of Physicians and Surgeons
New York, New York

Brenda Chrastil, MD
Resident Physician
Dermatology
University of Texas Health Science Center
Houston, Texas

Francisco J. Civantos, MD
Director
Division of Head and Neck Surgery
Department of Otolaryngology
University of Miami Miller School
of Medicine
Miami, Florida

Philip R. Cohen, MD
Clinical Associate Professor
University of Texas
Houston Medical School
Houston, Texas

Elizabeth Alvarez Connelly, MD
Assistant Clinical Professor
Department of Dermatology and
Cutaneous Surgery
Department of Pediatrics

Assistant Director
Division of Pediatric Dermatology
University of Miami Miller School
of Medicine
Miami, Florida

Jesús Cuevas-Santos, MD
Pathology Service
Hospital General Guadalajara
Alcalá University
Madrid, Spain

Elena De las Heras, MD
Dermatology Service
Hospital Ramón y Cajal
Alcalá University
Madrid, Spain

Karen E. Edison, MD
Philip C. Anderson Professor and
Chairman
Department of Dermatology

Medical Director
Missouri Telehealth Network
University of Missouri Health Care
Columbia, Missouri

George W. Elgart, MD
Professor of Dermatology and
Cutaneous Surgery
Chief of Dermatopathology
University of Miami Miller School
of Medicine
Miami, Florida

Esther Erdei, PhD, MSc Hons.
Immunologist
Health Scientist
Division of Epidemiology and
Biostatistics
Department of Internal Medicine
University of New Mexico
Albuquerque, New Mexico

Steven Fakharzadeh, MD PhD
Department of Dermatology
Hospital of the University
of Pennsylvania
Philadelphia, Pennsylvania

Daniel Federman, MD
Professor of Medicine
Internal Medicine
Yale University School of Medicine
New Haven, Connecticut

Firm Chief
Internal Medicine
West Haven VA Medical Center
West Haven, Connecticut

Steven R. Feldman, MD, PhD
Professor
Dermatology, Pathology and Public
Health Sciences
Wake Forest University School
of Medicine
Winston-Salem, North Carolina

Manuel Fernández-Lorente, MD
Dermatology Service
Hospital Ramón y Cajal
Alcalá University
Madrid, Spain

Lynn Feun, MD
Professor of Medicine
University of Miami School of Medicine
Sylvester Comprehensive Cancer
Center
Miami, Florida

L.E. French, MD
Department of Dermatology
Geneva University Hospital
Geneva, Switzerland

Olivier Gaide, MD, PhD
Chef de Clinique Scientifique
Dermatologie et Vénéréologie
Hôpitaux Universitaire de Genève
Genève, Switzerland

Hassan I. Galadari, MD
Resident
Boston University/Tufts University
Dermatology Residency Program
Boston, Massachusetts

A. Gewirtzman, MD
Skin and Cancer Associates
Plantation, Florida

Lawrence Gibson, MD
Consultant in Dermatology
Mayo Clinic
Professor of Dermatology
Mayo College of Medicine
Rochester, Minnesota

Yolanda Gilaberte-Calzada, MD
Department of Dermatology
Hospital General San Jorge
Huesca, Spain

Barbara A. Gilchrest, MD
Professor and Chairman
Deptment of Dermatology
Boston University School
  of Medicine

Chief of Dermatology
Boston Medical Center
Boston, Massachusetts

David J. Goldberg, MD, JD
Clinical Professor of Dermatology
Mount Sinai School of Medicine
New York, New York

Melissa Gonzales, PhD
Assistant Professor
Division of Epidemiology
Department of Internal Medicine
University of New Mexico Health
  Sciences Center
Albuquerque, New Mexico

Mercedes E. Gonzalez, MD
Resident
Pediatrics
New York Presbyterian Hospital -
  Columbia University Medical
  Center
New York, New York

Salvador González, MD, PhD
Assistant Professor of Dermatology
Memorial Sloan-Kettering Cancer
  Center
New York, New York
Assistant Professor of Dermatology
Ramon y Cajal Hospital
Madrid, Spain

Gloria F. Graham, MD
Clinical Associate Professor
Department of Dermatology
Wake Forest University Baptist Medical
  School
Winston-Salem, North Carolina

Emma Guttmann-Yassky, MD, MSc
Instructor in Clinical Investigation
Laboratory for Investigative
  Dermatology
Rockefeller University
New York, New York

Physician
Rambam Medical Center
Department of Dermatology
Haifa, Israel

Matthew E. Halpern, MD
Mohs Surgery Fellow
Department of Dermatology
Columbia University College
  of Physicians and Surgeons
New York, New York

Anne Han, BA
Columbia University College
  of Physicians and Surgeons
New York, New York

Peter W. Heald, MD
Professor of Dermatology
Yale University School of Medicine
New Haven, Connecticut

Sung-Lan Hsia, MD
Professor
Department of Dermatology and
  Cutaneous Surgery
University of Miami Miller School
  of Medicine
Miami, Florida

Shasa Hu, MD
Dermatology Resident
Department of Dermatology and
  Cutaneous Surgery
University of Miami Miller School
  of Medicine
Miami, Florida

Jennifer I. Hui, MD
Lecturer
Bascom Palmer Eye Institute
Miami, Florida

Khoozan Irani, MD
Pedro Jaén-Olasolo, MD
Dermatology Service
Hospital Ramón y Cajal
Alcalá University
Madrid, Spain

M. Baris Karakullukcu, MD
Head and Neck Surgery Fellow
Departmet of Otolaryngology
University of Miami Miller School
  of Medicine
Miami, Florida

Julie K. Karen, MD
Instructor
Ronald O. Perelman Department of
  Dermatology
New York University School of Medicine
New York, New York

Robert S. Kirsner, MD, PhD
Professor and Vice-Chairman
Department of Dermatology and
  Cutaneous Surgery
University of Miami Miller School
  of Medicine
Miami, Florida

John YM Koo, MD
San Francisco Psoriasis Treatment Center
Vice Chair, Department of Dermatology
University of California, San Francisco
  Medical Center
San Francisco, California

Alfred W. Kopf, MD
Head
Oncology Section
Skin and Cancer Unit
New York University Medical Center

Head
New York University Melanoma
  Clinical Cooperative Group
New York University
New York, New York

Olympia I. Kovich, MD
Assistant Professor
New York University
New York, New York

Jeffrey Kravetz, MD
Assistant Professor of Medicine
Internal Medicine
Yale University School of Medicine
New Haven, Connecticut

Staff Physician
Internal Medicine
VA Connecticult Health Care System
West Haven, Connecticut

Vidhya A. Kunnathur, MD
Medical Student
Northeastern Ohio Universities College
  of Medicine
Rootstown, Ohio

Sena J. Lee, MD
Resident Physician
Dermatology
University of Pennsylvania
Philadelphia, Pennsylvania

Ken Lee, MD
Director of Dermatologic and Laser
  Surgery
Associate Professor of Dermatology,
  Surgery, Otolarynogology-Head and
  Neck Surgery
Oregon Health and Science University
Portland, Oregon

FA LeGal, MD
Pigmented Skin Lesion Unit
Department of Dermatology
University Hospital Geneva
Switzerland

Stephanie W. Liu, BA
Department of Dermatology and
  Department of Cutaneous and
  Aesthetic Surgery

Northwestern University Feinberg
   School of Medicine
Chicago, Illinois

Torello Lotti, MD
Professor and Chairman
U.O. Complessa di Fisioterapia
   Dermatologica
University of Florence
Florence, Italy

Vandana Madkan, MD
Clinical Research Fellow
Dermatology and Clinical Studies
Center for Clinical Studies
Houston, Texas

A Marghoob, MD
Associate Professor of Dermatology
Memorial Sloan-Kettering Cancer
   Center at Suffolk
Hauppauge New York

Paul T. Martinelli, MD
Fellow
Mohs Micrographic Surgery and
   Cutaneous Oncology
Dermatologic Surgery Center of
   Houston
Houston, Texas

Darius Mehregan, MD
Hermann Pinkus Chairman
Associate Professor
Department of Dermatology
Wayne State University
Detroit, Michigan

Dermatopathologist
Pinkus Dermatopathology Laboratory
Detroit, Michigan

David A. Mehregan, MD
Associate Professor
Department of Dermatology
Wayne State University School
   of Medicine
Detroit, Michigan

Clinical Associate Professor
Department of Pathology
Medical University of Ohio
Toledo, Ohio

Martin C. Mihm, Jr., MD, FACP
Senior Dermatopathologist
Massachusetts General Hospital
Boston, Massachusetts

Wendy Long Mitchell, MD
Instructor
Ronald O. Perelman Department
   of Dermatology
New York University School
   of Medicine
New York, New York

Frederick L. Moffat, Jr., MD
Professor of Surgery
Surgical Oncology
Sylvester Comprehensive Cancer Center
Miami, Florida

Niven Narain,
Director of Transdermal
   Delivery/Cutaneous Cancer Research
Department of Dermatology and
   Cutaneous Surgery
University of Miami Miller School
   of Medicine
Miami, Florida

Bruce R. Nelson, MD
Director
Dermatologic Surgery Center at Houston
Houston, Texas

Keyvan Nouri, MD
Professor of Dermatology and
   Otolaryngology
Director of Mohs, Dermatologic and
   Laser Surgery
Director of Surgical Training
Department of Dermatology and
   Cutaneous Surgery
University of Miami Miller School
   of Medicine
Miami, Florida

Mahnaz Nouri, MD
Assistant in Ophthalmology
Massachusetts Eye and Ear Infirmary
Boston, Massachusetts

Consultant Staff
Ophthalmology
Children's Hospital Boston
Boston, Massachusetts

Margaret Oliviero, ARNP
Dermatolgy
Skin and Cancer Associates
Ft. Lauderdale, Florida

Robert A. Ord, DDS, MD, FRCS, FACS
Professor and Chair
Oral and Maxillofacial Surgery
University of Maryland Medical Center
Marlene and Stuart Greenebaum
   Cancer Center
Baltimore, Maryland

Cindy England Owen, MD
Resident
Department of Dermatology
University of Louisville School
   of Medicine City
Louisville, Kentucky

Shalu S. Patel, BS
University of Miami Miller School
   of Medicine
Miami, Florida

Asha R. Patel, BS
Department of Dermatology and
   Cutaneous Surgery
University of Miami Miller School
   of Medicine
Miami, Florida

Daniel J. Pearce, MD
Dermatology Resident
Department of Dermatology
Wake Forest University School
   of Medicine
Winston-Salem, North Carolina

Oliver A. Perez, MD
Clinical Research Fellow
Department of Dermatology and
   Cutaneous Surgery
University of Miami Miller School
   of Medicine
Miami, Florida

Indushekhar Persaud, MD
Chief Bioengineer for Drug Delivery
   Therapeutics
Department of Dermatology and
   Cutaneous Surgery
University of Miami
Miami, Florida

Adriano Piris, MD
Dermatopathology Fellow
Pathology
Beth Israel Deaconess Medical Center-
   Harvard Medical School

Clinical Fellow in Pathology
Dermatopathology
Massachusetts General Hospital-
   Harvard Medical School
Boston, Massachusetts

Varee N. Poochareon, MD
Resident
Department of Dermatology and
   Cutaneous Surgery
University of Miami Miller School
   of Medicine
Miami, Florida

Harold Rabinovitz, MD
Voluntary Professor of Dermatology
University of Miami Miller School
   of Medicine
Miami, Florida

Claudia C. Ramirez, MD
Resident
Departamento de Dermatologia
Universidad de Chile
Santiago, Chile

RM Rashid, MD, PhD
MD PhD Program
Loyola Stritch School of Medicine
Maywood, Illinois

Desiree Ratner, MD
George Henry Fox Associate Clinical
  Professor of Dermatology
Director of Dermatologic Surgery
Department of Dermatology
Columbia University Medical Center of
  the New York Presbyterian Hospital
New York, New York

Douglas Roach, MD
Director of Medical Photography
Department of Biomedical
  Communications
University of Miami Miller School
  of Medicine
Miami, Florida

Perry Robins, MD
Professor of Dermatology
Department of Dermatology
New York University School of Medicine
New York, New York

Randall K. Roenigk, MD
Professor and Chair
Department of Dermatology
Mayo Clinic College of Medicine
Rochester, Minnesota

Thomas E. Rohrer, MD
Clinical Associate Professor
Dermatology
Boston University School of Medicine
Boston, Massachusetts

Ricardo Rossi, MD
University Unit of Dermatology and
  Physiotherapy
University of Florence
Florence, Italy

Jerry Rothenberg, MD
Associate Clinical Professor
Dermatology
New Jersey Medical School
Newark, New Jersey

Medical Director
New Jersey Dermatopathology
West Orange, New Jersey

Panta Rouhani, MPH
Department of Epidemiology and
  Public Health
Department of Dermatology and
  Cutaneous Surgery
University of Miami Miller School
  of Medicine
Miami, Florida

Andrew R. Salama, DDS, MD
Fellow
Oral and Maxillofacial Oncology
  and Reconstruction
University of Maryland Medical
  Systems Office
Baltimore, Maryland

Miguel Sanchez, MD
Associate Professor
Ronald O. Perelman Department
  of Dermatology
New York University School of Medicine
New York, New York

Daniel J. Santa Cruz, MD
Dermatopathologist
Cutaneous Pathology
WCP Laboratories, Inc
St Louis, Missouri

Ronit Sarid, PhD
The Mina and Everard Goodman
  Faculty of Life Sciences
Bar Ilan University
Ramat-Gan, Israel

J-H Saurat, MD
Professor and Chairman
Department of Dermatology
Hôpital cantonal universitaire
Genève, Switzerland

Niramol Savaraj, MD
Staff Physician
Medicine
VA. Medical Center

Research Professor
Medicine
University of Miami Miller School
  of Medicine
Miami, Florida

Lawrence A. Schachner, MD
Chairman and Harvey Blank Professor
Department of Dermatology and
  Cutaneous Surgery
University of Miami

Director
Division of Pediatric Dermatology
University of Miami Milller School
  of Medicine
Miama, Florida

Richard K. Scher, MD, FACP
Professor of Clinical Dermatology
Colubmia University
New York, New York

Keith E. Schulze, MD
Co-Director
Dermatologic Surgery Center of Houston
Houston, Texas

Robert A. Schwartz, MD, MPH
Professor and Head
Department of Dermatology
Professor of Pathology, Medicine,
  Pediatrics and Preventive Medicine
  and Community Health
New Jersey Medical School
Newark, New Jersey

Christopher Scott, MD
Chief Resident
Division of Dermatology
Department of Internal Medicine
The Brody School of Medicine at East
  Carolina University
Greenville, North Carolina

Anita Singh, MS
Department of Dermatology and
  Cutaneous Surgery
University of Miami Miller School
  of Medicine
Miami, Florida

Christopher J. Steen, MD
Chief Resident
Dermatology
New Jersey Medical School
Newark, New Jersey

Neil Swanson, MD
Professor and Chair
Department of Dermatology
Oregon Health and Science
  University
Portland, Oregon

Zeina Tannous, MD
Director
Mohs/Dermatologic Surgery
VA Medical Center

Instructor in Dermatology
Faculty Director for Resident Training
  in Dermatopathology
Harvard Medical School
Boston, Massachusetts

Jens Thiele, MD, PhD
Department of Dermatology
Boston University School of Medicine
Boston, Massachusetts

Valencia Thomas, MD
Clinical Instructor
Department of Dermatology
Oregon Health and Science
  University
Portland, Oregon

Whitney D. Tope, MPhil, MD
Dermatologist and Dermatologic
  Surgeon
Metropolitan Dermatology and
  Cutaneous Surgery, Pennsylvania
Wayzata, Minnesota

Jaime A. Tschen, MD
Associate Clinical Professor
Baylor College of Medicine

Director
St. Joseph Dermatopathology
Houston, Texas

David T. Tse, MD, FACS
Professor
Ophthalmic Plastic, Orbital Surgery
 and Oncology Service
Ophthalmology
Bascom Palmer Eye Institute
University of Miami Miller School
 of Medicine
Miami, Florida

Stephen Tyring, MD, PhD
Professor
Department of Dermatology
University of Texas Health Science Center
Houston, Texas

Voraphol Vejjabhinanta, MD
Clinical Research Fellow in
 Dermatologic Surgery
Mohs and Laser Unit
Department of Dermatology and
 Cutaneous Surgery
University of Miami Miller School
 of Medicine
Miami, Florida

Daniel I. Wasserman, MD
Resident
Boston University-Tufts Univesity
Boston, Massachusetts

Roger H. Weenig, MD, MPH
Assistant Professor
Dermatopathology Division
Department of Dermatology
Mayo Clinic
Rochester, Minnesota

Phillip Williford, MD, FACP
Associate Professor of Dermatology
Director of Dermatologic Surgery
Wake Forest University School
 of Medicine
Winston-Salem, North Carolina

Aaron H. Wolfson, MD
Professor and Vice Chairman
Department of Radiation Oncology
University of Miami Miller School
 of Medicine
Attending Physician
University of Miami Affiliated Hospitals
Miami, Florida

Bernhard Zelger, MD, MSc
Professor of Dermatology
Clinical Department of Dermatology &
 Venereology
Medical University Innsbruck
Innsbruck, Austria

Deborah Zell, MD
Resident
Department of Dermatology and
 Cutaneous Surgery
University of Miami Miller School
 of Medicine
Miami, Florida

Viktor Goncharuk, MD
Clinical Assistant Professor
Department of Dermatology
Wayne State University School of
 Medicine
Detroit, Michigan

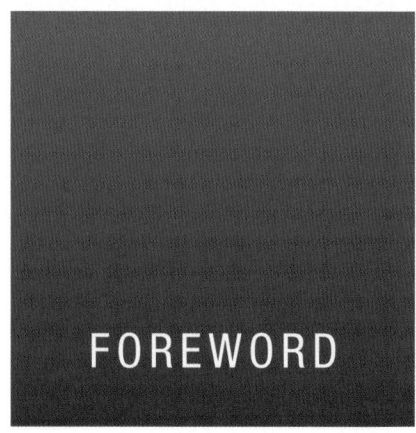

FOREWORD

Skin cancer is a growing concern worldwide. It is important that not only dermatologists, but also plastic surgeons, ENT surgeons, ophthalmologists, dentists, and even primary care physicians be aware of the basics of skin cancer. As the incidence and prevalence of skin cancer continue to increase, patients will expect that their physicians be capable of accurately diagnosing and managing their disease, as well as discussing preventive measures.

Skin Cancer edited by Dr. Keyvan Nouri is the latest, most comprehensive reference of cutaneous malignancies with many descriptive color illustrations. It takes the reader through all the cancers and tumors from their pathogenesis to their diagnosis and management to related frontiers in this area. This 65-chapter text provides a thorough resource for practitioners of all levels. This book can become the main reference for other specialists to learn about various aspects of cutaneous oncology. The first section provides an introduction to cancers and tumors encountered by dermatologists and other medical professionals. Because such a wide range of these lesions are discussed, the book truly appeals to and provides great value to all medical professionals. The second section focuses on various techniques and treatments used in cutaneous oncology. As patients are becoming more active in the management of their illnesses, it is even more crucial that all physicians understand treatment options and can relay the latest information to their patients. Finally, the text closes with a collection of issues emerging in the management and prevention of skin cancers. Economic and legal influences as well as technological advancements in imaging are included due to their growing impact in medicine.

This text is considered not only very comprehensive but also very user-friendly. Each chapter includes overview and summary boxes to cover the major points of each section. This makes each chapter appealing for readers of all levels, and for those who are pressed for time and would like to glance at the highlights of the chapter quickly.

This book is comprised of experts from across the globe contributing chapters in their field of specialty. This all-inclusive textbook contains the most comprehensive, up-to-date and detailed information on any topic related to skin cancer. I congratulate the editor for assembling such an all-encompassing, cutting-edge yet readable textbook. It could serve as the main resource for any physician for years to come.

Perry Robins, MD
President, Skin Cancer Foundation

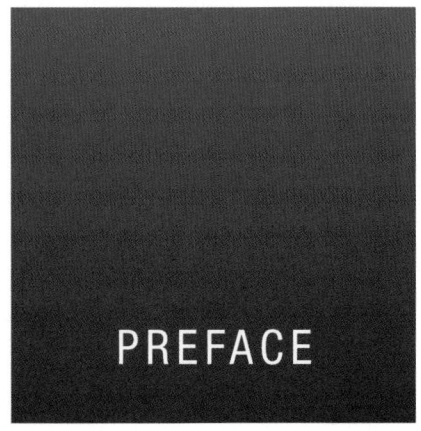

PREFACE

Skin cancer is a growing concern for populations worldwide. In fact, more than 50% of all cancers that occur are skin cancers, thereby creating a significant public health issue. While the incidence has significantly increased over the past decade, the dynamic field of cutaneous oncology has also grown equally through various advancements, both in our understanding of the disease and the technology to diagnose and treat it.

This comprehensive book includes a complete list of topics tailored to suit a wide range of readers. Because skin cancers are so prevalent, it is crucial that not only dermatologists, but also physicians be able to identify lesions accurately and design appropriate treatment plans. The textbook is structured into three major sections: Cancers and Tumors, Techniques and Treatments, and Related Issues and Frontiers. Overview and summary boxes are included in each chapter to cover the major points of each section.

The first section of the book contains common tumors such as basal cell carcinoma (BCC), squamous cell carcinoma (SCC), and melanoma, as well as rare tumors including dermatofibrosarcoma protuberans, sebaceous carcinoma, and Merkel cell carcinoma. Tumors that commonly occur within a specific subtype of patients such as children, HIV patients, organ transplant patients, and ethnic populations are also covered in this section.

The second section of the book describes common techniques and treatments. These techniques include surgical excision, Mohs micrographic surgery, and curettage and electrodessication among others. Treatments discussed include topical and systemic therapies, such as immunomodulators, NSAIDS, and other chemotherapeutic agents. Adjuvant therapies and vaccines are covered, along with reconstructive surgery for post-treatment of skin cancer.

Finally, the third section discusses factors relating to skin cancer, such as prevention, indoor tanning, teledermatology, and new approaches in the diagnosis of skin cancer. It also includes general concerns created by the growing prevalence of skin cancer and the importance of public education and awareness for prevention.

Our goal is that Skin Cancer will soon become the main reference book for senior medical students, residents, and physicians wanting to continue their education and discover the advancements emerging in this field. This all-inclusive textbook is unique in that it not only discusses the medical and scientific aspects of skin cancer and its treatments, but also incorporates economic relevance, legal issues, psychosocial aspects, and technological breakthroughs.

The contributors, who are renowned in their respective areas, are passionate about sharing their expertise in their respective fields with the readers. I sincerely hope that with this knowledge, we can improve treatment and survival, and reduce the incidence and prevalence of skin cancer.

Keyvan Nouri, MD

ACKNOWLEDGMENTS

First of all, I would like to thank my entire family for a lifetime of caring, encouragement and support. In addition, I would like to thank my friends and colleagues for making my world a wonderful place.

Dr. Lawrence A. Schachner, Chairman of the Department of Dermatology and Cutaneous Surgery at the University of Miami Miller School of Medicine. I thank him for his support, mentorship and guidance throughout my professional career. He has been a great role model and a very close friend for over 10 years, and many years to come. He has always been very encouraging, kind and willing to go an extra mile in support of my career.

Dr. William H. Eaglstein, former Chairman of Dermatology at the University of Miami School of Medicine, for launching my great journey into this wonderful world of dermatology. I would like to thank him for all of his support and friendship.

Dr. Perry Robins, Chief of Mohs Surgery at NYU Medical Center, for introducing me to the field of dermatologic surgery. He imparted not only his technical expertise but also his warm, kind ways of dealing with his patients, staff, colleagues, and students.

I would like to also acknowledge Dr. Robin Ashinoff, Dr. Vicki Levine for an excellent training in Mohs, Lasers, and cosmetic aspects of dermatologic surgery. I thank Dr. Seth Orlow, Dr. Irvin Freedberg and the entire faculty, residents, and staff at New York University School of Medicine Department of Dermatology for a wonderful experience during my dermatologic surgery fellowship. Dr. Hideko Kamino for her teaching in dermatopathology.

I thank the entire faculty at the University of Miami Miller School of Medicine, many of whom are contributing authors for this textbook, for all of their support, teaching, and camaraderie. I would like to acknowledge my administrative assistant Maria D. Garcia, who has not only helped with this textbook but also on a daily basis. I would also like to thank the great staff at UM Mohs/Laser center (Cathy Mamas, Juana Alonso, Tania Garcia, Alicia Rodriguez and Rosa Rook) for making my job a great pleasure. The residents at the University of Miami, whom I take pride in training in the field of dermatologic surgery, are an extremely talented group from whom I have learned more than I could have taught. My research fellows and medical students have been exceptional, and I offer them my greatest gratitude.

Dr. Anne Sydor and McGraw-Hill, for all of their hard work and effort towards the making of this book.

Shalu Patel, one of the kindest, brightest, and most dedicated and organized medical students I have worked with, for all of her contributions and effort towards this book.

Anita Singh, a kind, hardworking, intelligent medical student who has demonstrated her organizational skills and scholastic abilities in her contribution and assistance in the preparation of this book.

Chris Ballard, a hard-working former fellow, for his creativity and energy in the early stages of this project and his continuous work with our team.

Dr. Voraphol Vejjabhinanta, clinical research fellow in Dermatologic Surgery, for his hard work, dedication, expertise and contributing with many chapters in this book.

The authors of this textbook are world-renowned, and their expertise has made this book into one the most comprehensive and up-to-date sources of all the basic science, clinical relevance, and treatments in the field of cutaneous oncology. I truly appreciate all of their efforts.

Keyvan Nouri, MD

CHAPTER 1

Normal Skin

Rana Anadolu-Brasie, M.D.
Samir K. Amin, B.S.
Khoozan Irani, B.S.
Anita Singh, M.S.
Keyvan Nouri, M.D.

BOX 1-1 Overview

- The human skin is the largest organ in the body and helps maintain our internal homeostasis.
- There are seven important functions of the human skin. It functions as a barrier, a sensory organ, a site of transport, is involved in immune function, thermoregulation, protection against UV radiation, and secretion of pheromones.
- The skin consists of three primary layers—the epidermis, dermis, and hypodermis.
- The skin epithelium can be squamous, cuboidal, or columnar in shape.
- There are three types of junctional complexes in the human skin—desmosomes, focal contacts, and hemidesmosomes.
- There are five layers in the epidermis—the stratum corneum, stratum lucidum, stratum granulosum, stratum spinosum, and stratum germinativum (stratum basale).
- The epidermis contains keratinocytes, merkel cells, melanocytes, Langerhans cells, and intraepidermal T-lymphocytes.
- The dermis is the thickest part of the skin and differentiated into two parts: the superficial papillary dermis and the deeper reticular dermis
- The dermis contains blood vessels, nerves, pilosebaceous units, sweat glands, lymphatic system, muscles, and subcutaneous tissue.
- The major cells of the dermis are the fibroblasts, mast cells, macrophages, dendritic cells, and dermal T lymphocytes.
- There are two arterial plexuses in the dermis, the superficial, and deep plexus. Venules follow the arterioles in these areas.
- The lymphatic system follows arterioles and venules, and is arranged into an upper and lower plexus. It maintains plasma volume and prevents increased tissue pressure.
- Eccrine sweat glands produce sweat, which helps cool the body. They are never associated with hair follicles and are functional from birth.
- Apocrine sweat glands develop at puberty and produce pheromones that drain into a hair follicle.
- The pilosebaceous unit has the capacity to differentiate into either a terminal hair follicle or a sebaceous follicle. It is composed of a hair follicle and sebaceous glands.
- Muscles of hair erection are smooth muscles and associated with the hair follicles. They are innervated by the autonomic nervous system.
- The skin has both terminally myelinated sensory and autonomic innervation, as well as free and specialized nerve endings.
- Subcutaneous tissue functions mainly in insulation, cushioning of deeper tissues against injury, and fat storage.
- The cutaneous innate immune system controls the initial pathogenic assault, while more specific recognition and destruction of the pathogen occurs via the acquired immune system.

INTRODUCTION

The skin is our body's largest and most versatile organ. Adult human skin has an average surface area of 21 square feet, weighs 7 lbs. and comprises over 300 million cells.[1] There are about 10 hairs, 15 sebaceous glands, 100 sweat glands, and 3.2 feet of tiny blood vessels in each 0.5 square inch of the skin.[1] These numbers may seem at first excessive, but considering the number of skin cells that is shed everyday, these amounts become a necessity for replacing the lost cells and for the constant regeneration of the skin.

As a dynamic interface between our body and its environment, the skin provides many distinct functions. It serves as a protective barrier preventing internal tissues from exposure to trauma, ultraviolet radiation, temperature extremes, toxins, and bacteria. Other important functions include sensory perception, immunologic surveillance, thermoregulation, and control of fluid loss. These multifaceted functions of the skin are afforded by the minimal yet efficient organization of the skin's anatomy. The human skin consists of two mutually dependent layers, the epidermis, and dermis, which rest on a fatty subcutaneous layer, the hypodermis. The epidermis houses the pigment-containing melanocytes, antigen-processing Langerhans cells, and pressure-sensing Merkel cells. The dermis contains collagen, elastic fibers, blood vessels, sensory structures, and fibroblasts.[1] This chapter will provide an overview of the structure and function of healthy human skin.

FUNCTION

BOX 1-2 Summary

- A barrier to the environment radicals
- Secretion of pheromones
- Transport of elements and nutrients
- The body's largest sensory organ
- Immune function
- Thermoregulation
- Protection against UV radiation and oxygen free radicals

There are seven major functions of the skin, the most obvious of which is as the one of being barrier to infections, water loss, and friction. The skin is also a site of transport, that allows not only oxygen, nitrogen, and carbon dioxide to diffuse into the epidermis in small amounts but also tonically applied substances, such as medicines and ointments. The skin is the body's largest sensory organ. It contains free nerve endings in the three superficial layers that sense heat and cold, pain, and vibratory stimuli. There is also a nerve network around each hair follicle, in addition to Merkel cells, Meissner's corpuscles, and Pacinian corpuscles that sense touch and pressure. The skin also provides an immune function. It is considered a secondary lymphoid organ, and termed skin-associated lymphoid tissue (SALT). SALT includes keratinocytes, which secrete factors needed in T lymphocyte maturation and Langerhans cells, which are antigen-presenting cells that protect the body from bacteria. The skin also plays an active role in thermoregulation through eccrine sweat glands of the dermis, muscles of hair erection, and capillary beds in the dermal papillae. The adipose tissue in the underlying hypodermis insulates the body. Through the use of melanocytes that produce the pigment melanin, the skin also protects us from ultraviolet radiation and free oxygen radicals. Lastly, and certainly not the least important, the skin empowers us with sexuality with the use of apocrine and sebaceous glands in the dermis that secrete protein and lipid pheromones, respectively.[2–7]

LAYERS

BOX 1-3   Summary

- Three layers—from the most superficial to the least superficial
- Epidermis
- Dermis
- Hypodermis

The skin consists of two primary layers that encompass a fatty subcutaneous layer called the hypodermis. The most superficial layer is called the epidermis while the underlying layer is the dermis (Fig. 1-1).

EPITHELIUM

BOX 1-4   Summary

- There are three shapes, each of which is either simple or stratified
- Squamous—flat cells with nucleus in the middle
  - Simple squamous—lining vessels and good for nutrient exchange
  - Stratified squamous—either keratinized as on skin or nonkeratinized as in mucosal epithelium
- Cuboidal—same height and width with nucleus in the middle
  - Simple cuboidal—generally secretory and lines glands and ducts
  - Stratified cuboidal—thick and found in ducts that are exposed to mechanical stress such as the skin and salivary glands
- Columnar—cells that are tall and have a basal nucleus
  - Simple columnar—found in the lining of the gut; serves as a good water barrier, but does a poor job against abrasion.
  - Stratified columnar—thick and found in ducts that are exposed to mechanical stress such as in the skin and salivary glands

The epidermis is the uppermost epithelial layer of the skin, which is composed of layers of cells that rest on a basement membrane. The cells of the epidermis are called keratinocytes. They are attached to one another and to the basement

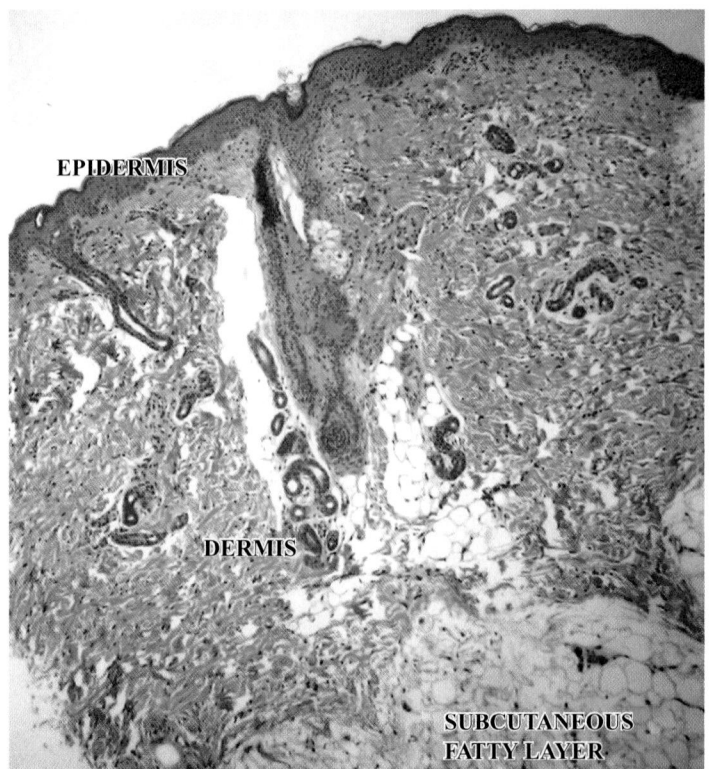

▲ **FIGURE 1-1** The layers of the skin: epidermis, dermis, and subcutaneous fatty layer.

membrane through junctional complexes. The type and amount of complexes depends on the function of that particular epithelium. The type of epithelium is determined by the underlying dermis in response to the immediate environment. An epithelium can be squamous, cuboidal, or columnar in shape, and either simple or stratified.[8]

Squamous epithelium contains cells that are each flat with its nucleus in the middle. Therefore, it is very thin and efficient for nutrient exchange. Simple squamous epithelium is usually found lining vessels. Each cell in cuboidal epithelium has the same dimensions in both height and width and have a central nucleus. Simple cuboidal epithelium is generally secretory, and therefore lines glands and ducts. Lastly, columnar epithelium contains cells that are each very tall and predominantly have a basal nucleus. Simple columnar epithelium serves well as a water barrier, but is a poor barrier against abrasion. Therefore, simple columnar epithelium is found in the lining of the gut.[8]

Stratified cuboidal and columnar epithelium are thick and thus are found in ducts that are exposed to mechanical stress, such as in the outer layer of skin and salivary glands. The multiple layers help prevent the ducts from collapsing.

Stratified squamous epithelium can either be found keratinized as on outer skin or nonkeratizined as in mucosal epithelium such as the oral cavity, glans penis, and the vagina. Keratinization is not a random phenomena. It is an environmentally induced process that is identified histologically by the absence of nuclei in the superficial cell layer of the epithelium. Keratinized epithelium has the advantage over nonkeratinized epithelium of providing a better barrier against infection.[8]

JUNCTIONAL COMPLEXES

BOX 1-5   Summary

- Three types of junctional complexes that are used to attach epidermal cells to each other and the basement membrane
- Desmosomes—connects cells laterally
- Focal contacts—connects cells basally to the basement membrane
- Hemidesmosomes—connects cells basally to the basement membrane

The skin has three types of junctional complexes: desmosomes, focal contacts, and hemidesmosomes. Desmosomes connect adjacent cells laterally using a class of transmembrane proteins called cadherins. They connect the intermediate filaments of one cell to those of another. A linker protein called desmoplakin connects to desmoglien; a cadherin, which interacts with desmogliens of adjacent cells.[9–11]

Hemidesmosomes and focal contacts connect cells basally to the basement membrane using a class of transmembrane proteins called integrins. Hemidesmosomes connect the intermediate filaments of a cell to the basement membrane. This is accomplished by intermediate filaments within the cell connecting to desmoplakin, a linker protein that binds to desmopenetrin. Desmopenetrin is an integrin that has a high affinity for type IV collagen in the basement membrane. The type IV collagen in the basement membrane is connected to type I collagen in the underlying connective tissue by reticular fibers (type VII collagen), providing the basement membrane with adhesion to layers above and below it.[9–11]

Focal contacts connect the actin filaments of a cell to the underlying basement membrane. Actin filaments bind to alpha-actinin, which binds to vinculin. Vinculin binds to talin, which binds to an integrin. Talin is present only in focal contacts of the skin, and therefore can serve as a histological marker for epithelial derived cells. Integrin has binding sites for laminin, fibronectin, heparin sulfate, and elastin fibers, in addition to type IV collagen.[9–11]

The epidermis, the outermost and thinnest layer, is a tough, avascular, and multilayered structure that continually repairs itself due to wear and tear from water, dust, infectious organisms, and ultraviolet rays. This renewal process occurs by cell division of keratinocytes in the basal layers of the epidermis, which migrate towards the surface layer, a process known as keratinization.

Keratinocytes are thought to have three different clonal subpopulations, with a different frequency in which they give rise to terminal cells. The three clonal subpopulations are the holoclones, paraclones, and meroclones.[12] The holoclone subpopulation was found to have the greatest growth potential, with fewer than 5% of the colonies formed by the holoclone subpopulation terminally differentiating and aborting.[12,13] The paraclone subpopulation mainly contains cells with a short replicative lifecycle, with no more than 15 generations.[12] These cells may grow rapidly at first, but after 15 generations these cells abort and become terminally differentiated. The meroclone subpopulation contains a combination of cells with different growth potentials.[12,13] It is considered as a transitional stage between the holoclone and paraclone subpopulations.[12,13]

The basal layer of the skin contains both stem and transient amplifying (TA) keratinocytes.[14] p63 has been used to differentiate between these two cell types. p63 is essential for regenerative proliferation and is a homologue of p53.[14] It is believed that the keratinocyte stem cells are from the holoclone subpopulation of cells, which is abundant in p63, and the transient amplifying cells are from the paraclone subpopulation, which does not contain p63.[14] According to the way the basal layer is patterned, it seems that the transient amplifying cells move over the basement membrane away from the stem cells.[15] Another population that has been found is the transient amplifying keratinocytes immediately after they leave the stem cell compartment. These cells have greatly reduced p63 concentrations and are thought to be from the meroclone subpopulation.[14]

The epidermis is very thick in nonglabrous skin such as in palms and soles, and thin in certain glabrous skin areas, such as eyelids. The epidermis is divided into five layers. From the bottom upwards these layers are; the stratum basale or germinativum, stratum spinosum, stratum granulosum, stratum lucidum, and the stratum corneum (Fig. 1-2). The stratum basale, commonly called the basal cell layer, consists of single columnar cells that are anchored to a basement membrane, separating the epidermis from the dermis. The basal cells in this layer are stem cells that are mitotically active, giving rise to the keratinocytes that compose the upper layers of the epidermis. The mitotic rate of the

■ EPIDERMIS

BOX 1-6 Summary

- Epidermis—the outermost and thinnest layer: there are five layers of the epidermis from the most superficial to the least superficial
  - Stratum corneum—the outermost layer composed mainly of dead cells
  - Stratum lucidum—a clear thin layer of dead skin cells
  - Stratum granulosum—two to three layers of nonmitotic flattened keratinocytes
  - Stratum spinosum—multilayered cuboidal cells which help provide structural support.
  - Stratum germinativum (stratum basale)—single columnar cells anchored to a basement membrane which separates the epidermis from the dermis.

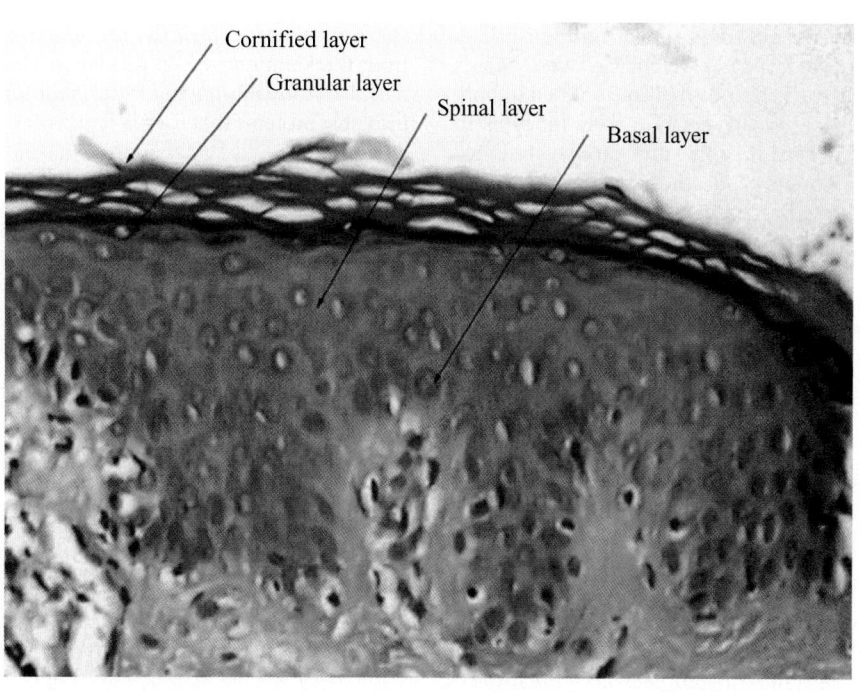

▲ **FIGURE 1-2** The epidermis and its layers.

Cornified layer
Granular layer
Spinal layer
Basal layer

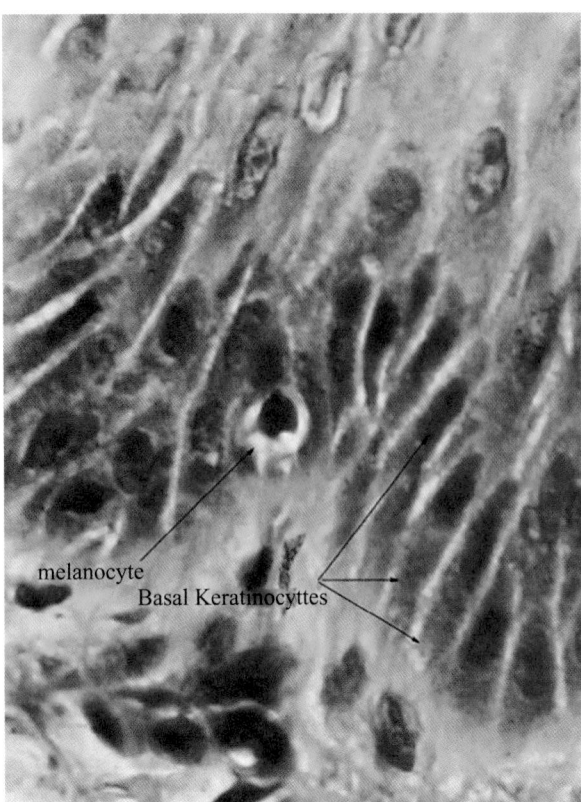

▲ **FIGURE 1-3** The basal layer of the epidermis.

ing due to aggregation and have anti-proteases, which defend the body against proteases released by bacteria trying to gain entry into the skin. These cells are flattened with dark, abundant intracellular keratohyaline granules. In addition to the intracellular keratohyaline, keratinocytes contain a soluble protein called involucrin. These two intracellular products are released during the pivotal event when keratinocytes undergo lysosomal rupture (Fig. 1-5).[2,3,5,16]

The stratum lucidum appears translucent and therefore is not histologically evident. This layer marks the point at which lysosomal rupture occurs releasing the intracellular products made in the granulosum. This programmed event induced by the environment in this layer is necessary for the progession of the proper keratinization process, triggering various events: the dissolution of nucleus and organelles in the keratinocytes, and precipitation of intracellular proteins including involucrin and keratohyalin. Involucrin precipitates around the inside of the plasma membrane and keratohyalin precipitates in and around the tonofibril bundles, gluing the strands together, and is composed of densely packed cells. By the end of these events, the keratinocyte has transformed into a dead product that remains as a flattened cell devoid of nuclei and organelles, whose protoplasm has transformed into a horny material or fibrous protein called keratin with only the desmosomes still intact.[2,3,16]

The stratum corneum (the horny layer) is composed of densely packed dead keratinocytes held together by desmosomes to form a barrier against abrasion and infection. This layer varies in thickness depending on its location on the body. It can be as thin as a few cells

basal cells is controlled by growth factors and hormones such as thyroid hormones, estrogen, testosterone, and feedback signals from keratinocytes in the stratum granulosum and stratum corneum. The basal cells hold on to one another through desmosomes and attach to the basement membrane via focal contacts and hemidesmosomes (Fig. 1-3).[2,3]

The stratum basale along with the overlying stratum spinosum are collectively called the Malphigian layer. Mitoses of the keratinocytes are confined to only these two layers. The keratinocytes in the stratum spinosum produce massive amounts of desmosomes in this layer, providing secure cell–cell cohesion and forming a barrier against friction and abrasion. The term "spinosum" comes from the spiny appearance of the cells in this layer because of the intercellular bridges formed in between the desmosomes and the keratinocytes (Fig. 1-4). In addition to the proliferation of desmosomes, the production of filaggrin also occurs in this layer. Filaggrin bundles tonofilaments into tonofibrils, providing the skin with tensile strength. Interspersed within this cell layer are Langerhans cells—dendritic cells that stem from the bone marrow and acquire an antigen-presenting capability. Once the differentiated cells accumulate and become denser in the stratum spinosum,

they then ascend to the overlying layer, the stratum granulosum.[2,3,5,16,17]

The stratum granulosum consists of two or three layers of synthetically active, nonmitotic keratinocytes that appear flattened. The keratinocytes produce lamellar granules (Odland bodies), keratohyalin, involucrin, and lysosomes. Lamellar granules are vesicles filled with phospholipid components that form the skin's water barrier once they are secreted from the keratinocytes in this layer. The dark keratohyalin granules are made of insoluble proteins that form a hard encas-

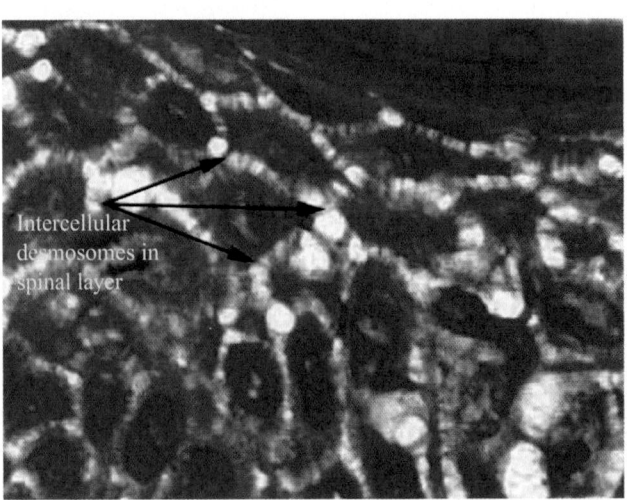

▲ **FIGURE 1-4** Desmosomal junctions in spinal layer in the epidermis.

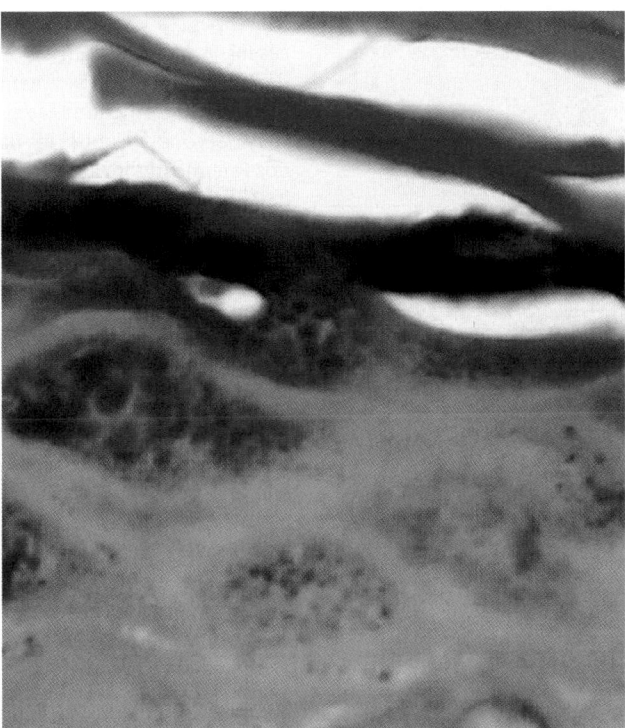

▲ FIGURE 1-5 The granular layer and the cornified layer of epidermis.

Haarscheiben clusters or touch domes.[18] The Merkel cell and the sensory axon form a Merkel cell—neurite complex. These complexes transmit slowly adapting type I mechanoreception.[18] These complexes can also be found in hair follicles and the oral mucosa. Merkel cells are highly modified pressure sensors. When deformed by pressure, they release neurotransmitters basally, which diffuse to neurons that sit on the basement membrane.[2,3]

Merkel cells are of epithelial origin and therefore have cytokeratin filaments. They possess dense-core granules, plasma membrane spines, and dendrites, as well as a loosely arranged cytoskeleton.[19] In addition, they possess focal contacts (with talin), hemidesmosomes, and desmosomes. They are nonmitotic and are not involved in the keratinization process.[2,3] The lifespan of Merkel cells is unknown at this time, but it is known that there is a denervation-sensitive subpopulation of Merkel cells that may die unless they become reinnervated.[18]

or as thick as 50 or more cells. Most of this layer is the stratum compactum. These layers of dead keratinocytes are the endpoint of the differentiation and migration of the basal cells. Each of these cells is enclosed within an envelope of insoluble proteins and lipids. It is at this stage, after cell death, where they can confer their structural properties to provide the skin with elasticity, impermeability, stability, and toughness. These cells are consistently renewed by terminally differentiated, dead keratinocytes as a layer of live keratinocytes from the stratum lucidum is pushed upwards into the stratum corneum. As these cells reach the surface, the "old" keratinocytes are shed, providing a place in the corneum for the new cells. The level at which the desmosomes are oxidized and the dead cells desquamate (the most superficial part of the corneum) is called the corneum disjunctum. This desquamation process occurs about 30 days after the birth of a keratinocyte.[2,3,16]

NONKERATINOCYTES IN THE EPIDERMIS

BOX 1-7 Summary

- Four nonkeratinocytes in the epidermis
  - Merkel cells—highly modified pressure sensors
  - Melanocyte—synthesize melanin in vesicles
  - Langerhans cells—highly specialized antigen-presenting cells
  - Intraepidermal T-lymphocytes—function unknown at this time

There are four important cell types that reside in the epidermis that are not keratinocytes: Merkel cells, Melanocytes, Langerhans cells, and Intraepidermal T lymphocytes.[2,3]

Merkel Cell

BOX 1-8 Summary

- Merkel cells are epithelial in origin and have cytokeratin filaments, dense-core granules, plasma membrane spines, dendrites, and a cytoskeleton.
- The main function of Merkel cells is sensory mechanoreception.
- A Merkel cell along with a sensory axon form a Merkel cell–neurite complex that transmit slowly adapting type I mechanoreception. These can be found in hair follicles and the oral mucosa.

Merkel cells function as sensory mechanoreceptors in the epidermis. They are found in association with sensory axons in the basal epidermal layer either independently or in clusters, known as

Melanocyte

BOX 1-9 Summary

- Melanocytes are dendritic cells of neural crest origin and are mostly found within the stratum basale.
- Melanocytes synthesize melanin in melanosomes, which are then delivered to keratinocytes through cytoplasmic processes. There is one melanocyte for every 5 to 10 basal keratinocyte.
- There are two major types of melanin—the brownish black eumelanin and the reddish yellow pheomelanin.
- The density of melanocytes remains the same in both light and dark skins.

Melanocytes are dendritic cells of neural crest origin and therefore have vimentin filaments in their cytoplasms (Fig. 1-6A). They are mostly found within the stratum basale. Although their density among the basal keratinocytes varies in different body regions, there is one melanocyte among every 5 to 10 basal keratinocyte.[20] Melanocytes synthesize melanin in vesicles called melanosomes that are delivered to keratinocytes through cytoplasmic processes extending from the melanocytes in a process known as cytocrine secretion. These processes fuse melanocytes with nearby keratinocytes by active phagocytoses to permit the passage of the melanosome from the cytoplasm of the melanocyte

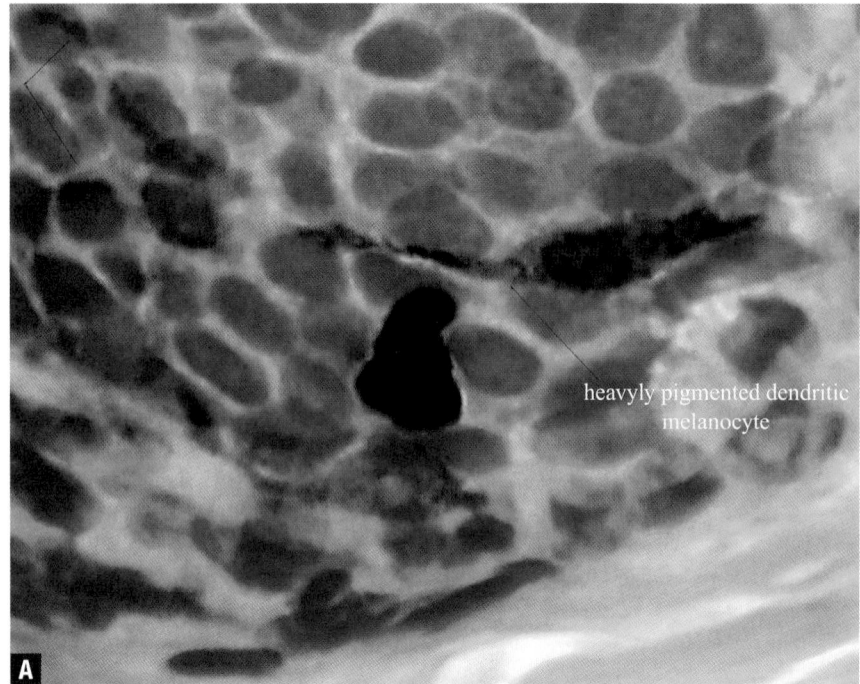

heavyly pigmented dendritic melanocyte

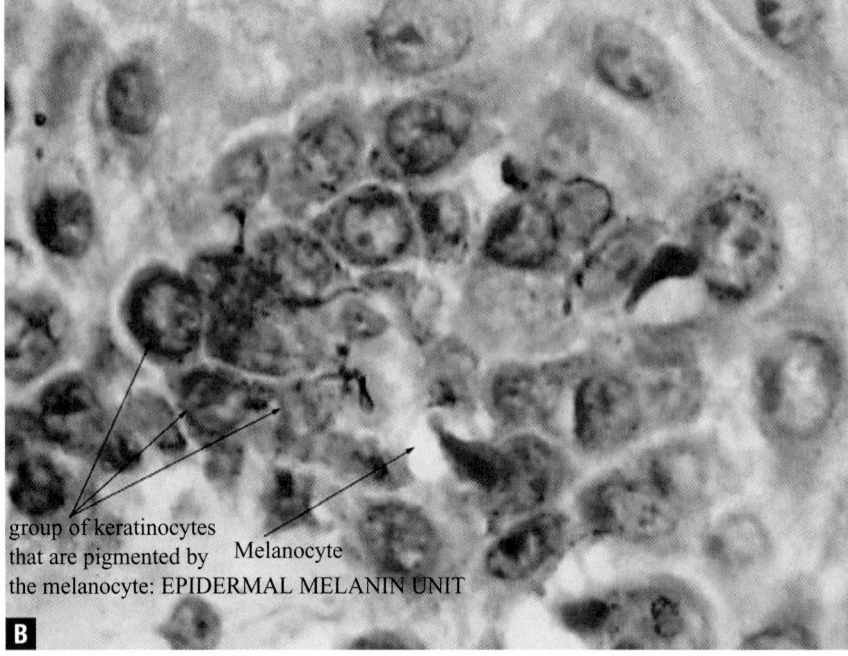

group of keratinocytes that are pigmented by the melanocyte: EPIDERMAL MELANIN UNIT

Melanocyte

▲ **FIGURE 1-6 A.** Melanocyte in the hair follicle. **B.** The epidermal melanin unit.

to that of the keratinocyte. One melanocyte and the surrounding keratinocytes that are being pigmented by it, is known as an epidermal melanin unit (Fig. 1-6B). Once phagocytosed by the keratinocyte, melanin then aggregates above the cell nucleus forming a "melanin cap" that protects the nuclear DNA from ultraviolet radiation. There are four classes of melanosomes:

- Stage I: contains only tyrosinase
- Stage II: contains mostly tyrosinase and some melanin

- Stage III: contains mostly melanin with some tyrosinase
- Stage IV: contains only melanin

Melanin is made sequentially—starting with tyrosine, which is converted to L-dopa, which is transformed into dopaquinone, which finally becomes melanin.[2,13,21,22]

One key point to mention is that the density of melanocytes (epidermal melanin unit) remains the same in both light and dark skins. The coloration of skin is due to three key differences.

Melanocytes extend cytoplasmic processes to the stratum granulosum in darker skins, but extend them only to the basale and spinosum layers in lighter skins. Secondly, light skins contain melanosome mostly in stages II and III, while darker skins contain melanosomes mainly in stages III and IV. Thirdly, lysosomes fuse with melanosomes in light skins, which eventually degrades the melanin.[2,3]

There are two major types of melanin—the brownish black eumelanin and the reddish yellow pheomelanin. Pheomelanin is synthesized by adding cysteine to dopaquinone. Eumelanin and pheomelanin are both present in human hair and in the epidermis. Both pheomelanin and eumelanin pigments protect skin from UV damage; however, pheomelanin also is a potent UV photosensitizer, possibly contributing to increased susceptibility of fair-skinned individuals with yellow or red hair to premature aging and melanoma.[22,23]

The regulation of the production of eumelanin versus pheomelanin involves the interaction of the melanocortin 1 receptor (MC1R) on the surface of the melanocyte with a variety of soluble factors. The most significant ones include proopiomelanocortin (POMC) derivatives, the melanocyte-stimulating hormone (MSH), and the agouti-signaling protein. The binding of MSH to MC1R results in the formation of eumelanin while the binding of the agouti protein to MC1R leads to the switch to pheomelanin production.[2,3,21,22]

Langerhans Cells

BOX 1-10 Summary

- Langerhans cells are apart of the innate immune response and the major histocompatibility class II (MHC II) dendritic cell subset.
- Langerhans cells are highly specialized antigen-presenting cells to T and B cells.
- Langerhans cells are located throughout the epidermis, but the highest concentration is in the upper spinosum layer.
- Langerhans cells and intraepidermal T lymphocytes together compose the cutaneous immune system.

Langerhans cells are a part of the innate immune response, capturing antigens entering through the skin and carrying them to nearby lymph nodes via lymphatic vessels upon stimulation by proinflammatory cytokines. These cells are bone marrow-derived cells that comprise approximately 5% of epidermal cells, and are a part of the major histocompatibility class II (MHC II) dendritic cell subset.[24] These cells are highly specialized antigen-presenting cells (APCs) to T and B cells. They are basically dendritic macrophages with numerous processes, which contain a unique organelle called a Birbeck granule, resembling a tennis racquet.

Langerhans cells are located throughout the epidermis forming a meshwork barrier; however, the highest concentration is found in the upper spinosum layer. Their highly dendritic structure allows antigen sampling of essentially the entire surface of the skin. The density of Langerhans cells varies over the surface of the body, with the face containing the most cells, at 600 to 1000 Langerhans cells per square millimeter.[25,26] The antigen-presentation capabilities of Langerhans cells become apparent only after cytokines like interleukin-1β (IL-1β) and tumor necrosis factor-α (TNF-α) induce migration of the Langerhans cells toward the lymph node.[27] After this migration, Langerhans cells can prime naïve T cells in the lymph node and initiate antigen-specific T cell immunity, as well as possibly present antigen intracutaneously to previously activated effector or memory T cells.[26,28] Epidermal Langerhans cells are assisted by intraepidermal T lymphocytes to monitor the skin for antigens, together composing the cutaneous immune system.[2,5]

Intraepidermal T Lymphocytes

BOX 1-11   Summary

- Intraepidermal T lymphocytes comprise less than 1% of epidermal cells and only about 2% of all normal skin T cells.
- The functions intraepidermal T cells of normal skin are not known at this time.

Intraepidermal T lymphocytes comprise less than 1% of epidermal cells and only about 2% of all normal skin T cells.[29] They are irregularly distributed, and reside within the basal and suprabasal layers of the epidermis. A majority of intraepidermal T cells in normal human skin are CLA+ and CD8+/CD45RO+. CLA expression is indicative of prior activation via cutaneous antigen exposure and CD45RO is indicative of a memory cell phenotype.[29] This suggests that intraepidermal T lymphocytes are not naïve T cells. The functions of these and other intraepidermal T cells of normal skin are not known at this time.

DERMIS

BOX 1-12   Summary

- Second layer of the skin under the epidermis
- Usually the thickest part of the skin; thickness varying by location
- Composed of extracellular matrix rather than cells
- Provides skin with elasticity and strength
- Structures contained in the dermis include
  - Blood vessels
  - Lymphatic system
  - Eccrine sweat glands
  - Apocrine sweat glands
  - Pilosebaceous unit
  - Muscles
  - Nerves and specialized nerve endings
  - Subcutaneous tissue
- Differentiated into two parts
  - The superficial papillary dermis
  - Deeper reticular dermis

The dermis is the second layer of skin underneath the epidermis. It is a layer of connective tissue that anchors the epidermis and binds it to the underlying hypodermis (Fig. 1-7). The dermal layer is usually the thickest part of the skin; however, it varies in thickness depending on the location of the skin, ranging from a tenth of a millimeter to a few millimeters.

In contrast to epithelium and many other tissues, the dermis as well as other types of connective tissue is made of mostly extracellular matrix rather than cells. Extracellular matrix is composed of protein fibers that are embedded in "hydrophilic gel" called intercellular ground substance that is made of anionic macromolecules (glycosaminoglycans and proteoglycans) and multi-adhesive glycoproteins (laminin and fibronectin). These fibers can be categorized into three types: collagen, reticular, and elastic fibers. Collagen and reticular fibers are formed by the protein collagen while elastic fibers are formed from the protein elastin. These fibers impart the skin with strength, flexibility, and elasticity while the ground substance acts as a base and a lubricant for shock absorption.[2,3]

In addition to providing skin with its elasticity and strength, the dermis also plays an important role in: thermoregulation; blood supply to the outer epidermal layer; sensory perception of touch, temperature, and pain; induction of the turnover pattern of the epidermis and the hair follicle; and defense against disease and injury. Structures found in the dermis are more complex and variable than those found in the epidermis, and include nerve endings, glands, hair follicles, and blood vessels. These structures are dispersed in different concentrations over different parts of the body.

The dermis itself is differentiated into two parts: the superficial papillary dermis and the deeper reticular dermis. The papillary dermis is made of loose (areolar) connective tissue, which consists of many cells, such as macrophages, fibroblasts, mast cells, and extravasated leukocytes, in addition to small bundles of type I collagen running in a random pattern. The reticular dermis is made of a network of connective tissue, consisting of a few cells, blood vessels, and large bundles of type I collagen running in a random pattern (Fig. 1-8).[2,3]

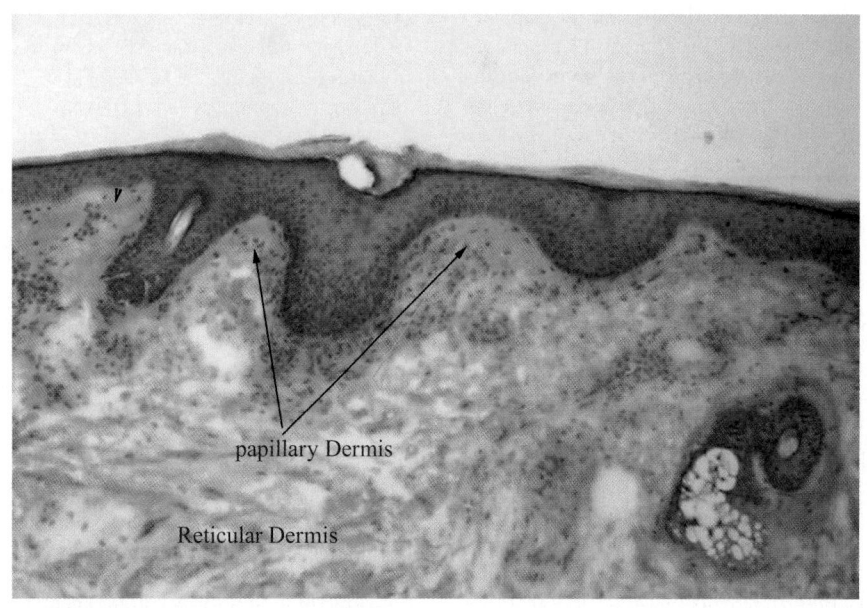

papillary Dermis

Reticular Dermis

▲ **FIGURE 1-7** Papillary and reticular dermis.

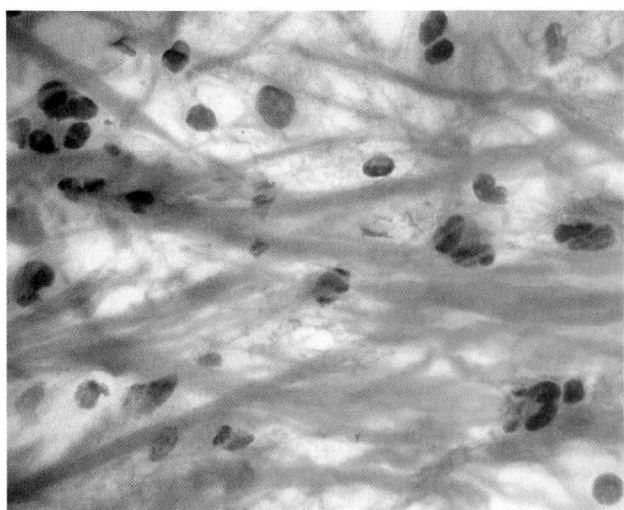

▲ **FIGURE 1-8** Reticular dermis collagen bundle network.

The papillary dermis is named so because it sends finger-like projections called dermal papillae into the overlying epidermis, which interdigitate with epidermal pegs to form a dermal–epidermal junction. This design of the dermal surface provides the skin with protection against pressure by preventing the two layers of the skin from sliding past each other due to friction. Therefore, dermal papillae are seen in higher quantities in locations that are more subject to frequent pressure, such as on the palms and the soles of the feet. The dermal papillae house free sensory nerve endings, Meissner's corpuscles for sensation (Fig. 1-9C), and capillary beds for thermoregulation and delivery of nutrients to the epidermis.[2]

The integrity of the dermal–epidermal junction is maintained by the basal lamina, which is found between the stratum basale of the epidermis and the papillary dermis (Fig. 1-10). The basal lamina consists of an electron-dense layer (lamina densa) sandwiched between two electron-lucid layers (lamina lucida). The lamina densa is composed of type IV collagen secreted by the epithelial cells while the lamina lucida is composed of a glycoprotein called laminin. The basal lamina is anchored to the connective tissue of the reticular dermis via type VII collagen fibrils that traverse the lamina reticularis. There is also a layer of type III collagen (reticular fibers) that lies beneath the basal lamina. Type VII collagen is formed, anchoring fibrils that bind type IV collagen in the lamina densa to type I collagen in the reticular dermis, thereby holding the epidermis to the dermis of the skin.[2,3]

The reticular dermis is denser than the papillary dermis because it has more type I collagen fibers that are thicker and houses an expansive network of elastic fibers. Consequently, the reticular layer strengthens the skin and provides much of the structure and elasticity, and also acts as a foundation of the skin structure. It also supports other parts of the skin, such as the blood vessels, hair follicles, sweat glands, and sebaceous glands.

CELLS OF THE DERMIS

BOX 1-13   Summary

- Fibroblasts—synthesize and degrade extracellular matrix proteins, and secrete mediators involved in immune responses
- Mast cells—mediate inflammation, and synthesize and release the growth factors, cytokines, and lipid mediators
- Macrophages—phagocytic cells that are apart of the innate immune system
- Dendritic cells—express markers common to other antigen-presenting cells, whose function is not exactly known at this time
- Dermal T lymphocytes—function is not exactly known at this time

The majority of cells in the dermis include fibroblasts, mast cells, macrophages, dendritic cells, and dermal T lymphocytes (Fig. 1-9A). Mesenchyme-derived dermal fibroblasts synthesize and degrade extracellular matrix proteins (collagen, elastin, proteoglycans, and fibronectin).[30] Their activity is increased during wound healing. In addition, fibroblasts also secrete several soluble mediators involved in immune responses when stimulated by cytokines.[31] Stem cell factor expression by fibroblasts may also contribute to normal cutaneous mast cell development (Fig. 1-9B).[32]

Mast cells are mediators of inflammation in response to stimuli, such as microorganisms and allergens, leading to the production of cytokines. They occur in normal skin at a density of approximately 7000 to 10,000/mm^3 and are often found near cutaneous appendages, blood vessels, and nerves.[33,34] Cutaneous mast cells have granules containing both tryptase and chymase. Mast cell involvement in the immediate allergic reaction is carried out via its stores of histamine, heparin, and IgE, in addition to various other mediators.[2,35] Mast cells also synthesize and release growth factors, cytokines, and lipid mediators such as leukotrienes, prostaglandins, and platelet-activating factors.[33] Furthermore, mast cells probably also participate in microbial defense against parasites and bacteria, control of vascular tone and permeability via histamine and leukotriene release; tissue repair and angiogenesis, and sensation of and response to a variety of immunologic and nonimmunologic stimuli.[33,36,37]

Dermal macrophages are phagocytic cells, derived from the bone marrow, that differentiate from blood monocytes after entering peripheral tissues.[38] Macrophages—components of the innate immune system—are involved in the phagocytosis of foreign substances, such as bacteria, particulates, damaged cells, various pigments, and extracellular debris. Their other functions in the skin include antigen processing and presentation, wound healing, microbicidal/tumoricidal activity, and general phagocytic and secretory activities.[39]

Dermal dendritic cells, which include dermal dendrocytes, are another cell population of the normal dermis. Dermal dendrocytes often are present near the mast cells and blood vessels.[40] These cells, similar to other dermal dendritic cells, express markers common to antigenpresenting cells.[40] The functions of the various dermal dendritic cells and their relationships to cutaneous macrophages are still unknown at this time.

Dermal T lymphocytes, normally located near post-capillary venules, make up approximately 90% of T cells found in the normal dermis.[30] On the other hand, B lymphocytes and natural killer cells are almost absent from the normal skin. Dermal T lymphocytes typically have equal number of CD4+ helper and CD8+ cytotoxic cells.[29] As in the case of intraepidermal T lymphocytes, little is known about the role of dermal T lymphocytes in cutaneous homeostasis and immunity.

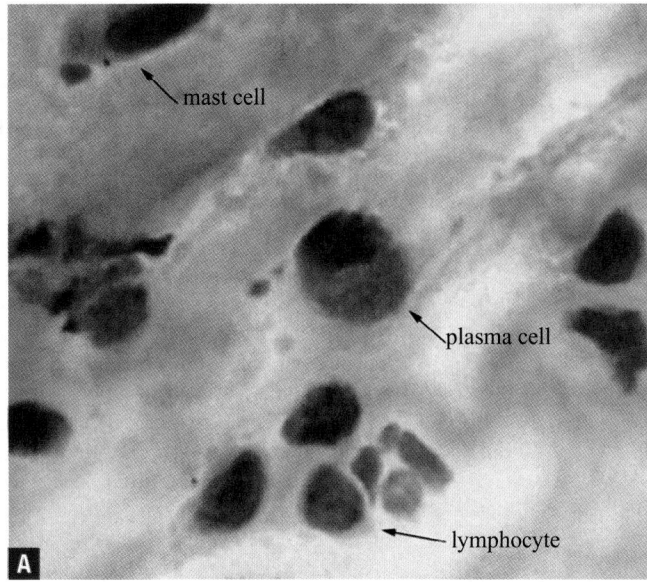

mast cell

plasma cell

lymphocyte

A

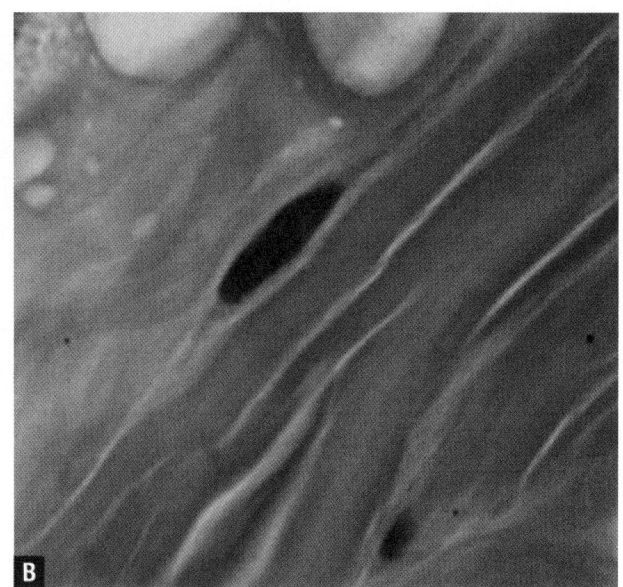

B

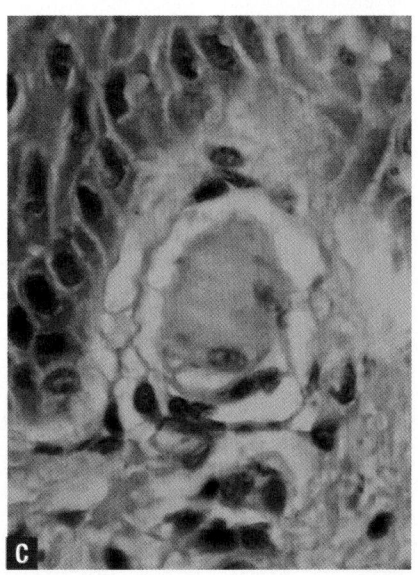

C

▲ FIGURE 1-9 A. Cells of the dermis. B. Fibroblast among collagen fibers. C. Meissner's corpuscle in the papillary dermis.

■ STRUCTURES IN THE DERMIS

BOX 1-14   Summary

- Blood vessels
- Lymphatic system
- Eccrine sweat glands
- Apocrine sweat glands
- Pilosebaceous unit
- Muscles
- Nerves and specialized nerve endings
- Subcutaneous tissue

Blood Vessels

BOX 1-15   Summary

- There are two arterial plexuses in the dermis, the superficial and deep plexus.

- Venules follow arterioles and form small plexuses around the hair follicles and eccrine glands
- Capillary lumens are lined by a simple layer of endothelial cells, pericytes, and a PAS (+) basement membrane
- A glomus body is a microscopic arterio-venular anastomosis in the reticular dermis. It is responsible for heat regulation and blood pressure by controlling the blood flow in between arterial and venous system

There are two microcirculations located in the skin, arranged in two horizontal arterial plexuses. In the dermal layer there is the superficial plexus and the deep plexus.[41] The superficial plexus is located 1 to 1.5 mm below the skin surface,[41] beneath the papillary dermis

and between the two layers of the dermis. The arterial capillaries from this layer form the dermal papillary loops that provide the nourishing component of the skin circulation.[41] The deep plexus is at the dermal-subcutaneous junction.[20,41] At this junction, there are collecting veins that contain valves that prevent the backflow of blood.[41]

Communicating arterioles connect the two main plexuses. Venules follow arterioles and together form small plexuses around the hair follicles and eccrine glands. Each dermal papilla has one main capillary loop, which connects to post-capillary venules. The venules of the superficial plexus and intercommunicating venous system reach the veins of the deep subcutaneous plexus.[20]

The capillary lumen is lined by a simple layer of endothelial cells, pericytes

9

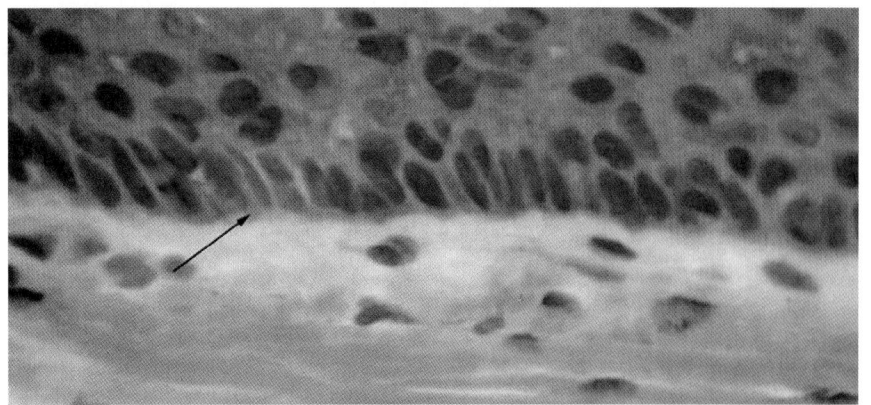

▲ **FIGURE 1-10** Dermal–epidermal junction.

and a PAS (+) basement membrane. Pericytes are undifferentiated mesenchymal cells. The arterioles of the superficial plexus and the arteries of the deep plexus have thicker vessel walls, which are composed of intima, media, and adventitial layers (Fig. 1-11A).[20] The innermost layer, the intima, is formed by endothelial cells lining the internal elastic lamina. The media layer is composed of muscle cells and the adventitia is basically supportive connective tissue immediately surrounding the vasculature. Postcapillary venules have a lining similar that of these capillaries, whereas, large venules and veins have true internal elastic lamina, as well as interluminal valves (Fig. 1-11B and C).[20]

A glomus body is a microscopic arteriovenular anastomosis in the reticular dermis, generally found in acral skin.[20] Glomus bodies regulate heat and blood pressure by controlling the blood flow in between arterial and venous system.[20] Blood flow is controlled by constriction and expansion, much like the vascular systems throughout the body, allowing heat to be released or conserved depending on the temperature. Low temperatures make the blood vessels constrict, allowing heat retention, while elevated temperatures make

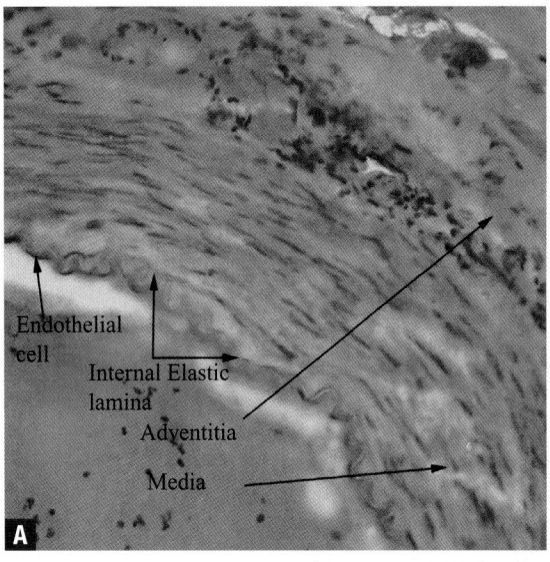

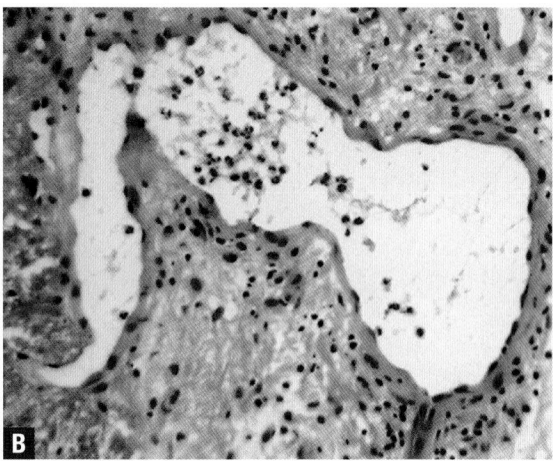

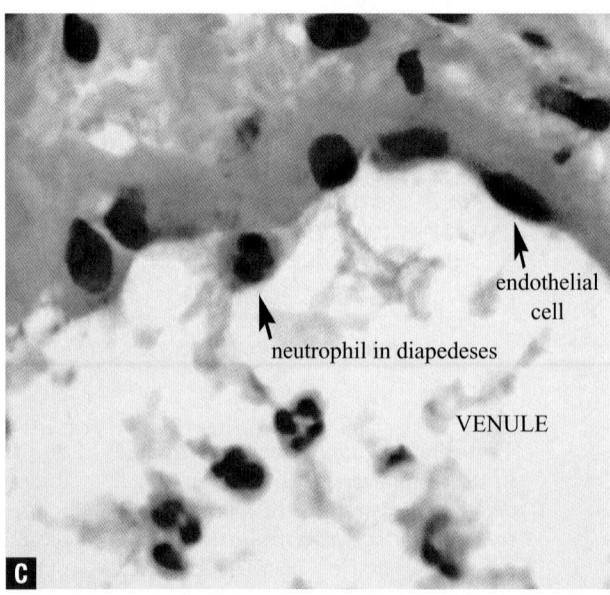

▲ **FIGURE 1-11** **A.** Vascular wall and deep cutaneous plexus. **B.** Large venule with valve. **C.** Neutrophil diapedesis via venule wall.

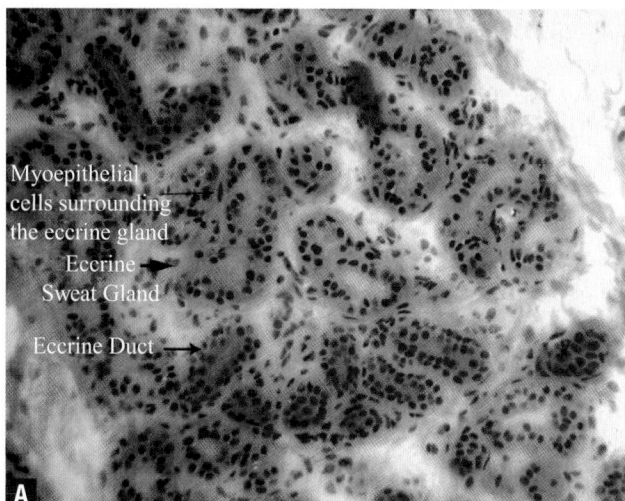

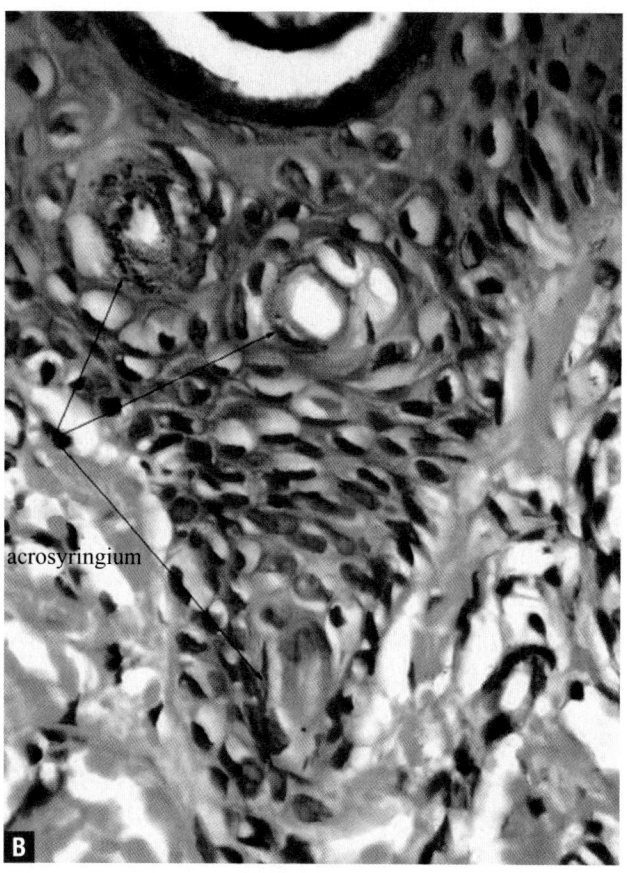

Myoepithelial cells surrounding the eccrine gland

Eccrine Sweat Gland

Eccrine Duct

acrosyringium

▲ **FIGURE 1-12** **A.** Eccrine unit situated in deep dermis. **B.** Acrosyringium: intraepidermal portion of the eccrine duct.

the blood vessels dilate, allowing for more blood to come to the surface and release excess heat.[2,3]

Lympathic System

> **BOX 1-16 Summary**
>
> • Follows arterioles and venules
> • Arranged into upper and lower plexus
> • Lymphatic capillaries lined only by endothelial cells and are devoid of pericytes and PAS (+) basement membrane
> • Maintains plasma volume and prevents increased tissue pressure

The lympathic system of the skin basically follows the arterioles and venules. In general, lymphatic vessels tend to be less densely distributed, have wider and more irregular lumens, and have thinner vessel walls.[42] Lymphatic vessels are arranged into upper and lower plexus, with deeper open-ended lymphatic vessels extending into the dermal papillae.[42] Vessels extending vertically connect the upper and lower plexus vessels of the lymphatic vasculature.[42] Lymphatic capillaries are lined only by endothelial cells and are devoid of pericytes and PAS (+) basement membrane.

Each day, half of the total circulating protein escapes from blood vessels. The lymphatic vessels return the fluid that was forced out of the macromolecules into the bloodstream, thus maintaining plasma volume and preventing increased tissue pressure.[42] Although larger lymphatic vessels have valves and thicker vessel walls, in general, cutaneous lymphatics are not readily observed in routine skin specimens under normal conditions.[20]

Eccrine Sweat Glands

> **BOX 1-17 Summary**
>
> • Produces sweat that helps cool the body
> • Controlled indirectly by a center in the hypothalamus that controls sympathetic cholinergic nerves
> • Are never associated with hair follicles and are functional from birth

In response to heat, the skin is cooled and regulated by sweat glands through the release of sweat, a solution made primarily of water and salt. The released sweat evaporates off the surface of the skin and helps cool the body. The light cells of these glands pump ions (ammonium, chloride, potassium, sodium, and

urea) and the dark cells secrete protein by merocrine secretion. The products of the light cells are pushed from the small lumen in these glands up into a duct by the contraction of surrounding myoepithelial cells arising from the dermis. The stratified cuboidal duct has a coiled tubular architecture, which starts in the dermis and pierces through the epidermis when secretion is needed. Sweat glands are controlled indirectly by a center in the hypothalamus that controls sympathetic cholinergic nerves, which innervate myoepithelial cells. It is estimated that the typical human has between two and five million sweat glands and can produce up to 10 liters of sweat per day. Eccrine sweat glands are never associated with hair follicles and are functional from birth (Fig. 1-12A and B).[2,20,43]

Apocrine Sweat Glands

> **BOX 1-18 Summary**
>
> • Composed of a secretory gland, proximal intradermal duct, and peripheral intraepidermal/intrafollicular duct
> • Produce pheromones by merocrine secretion
> • Drain their secretion into a hair follicle to reach the skin surface
> • Develops at puberty

These glands also possess a coiled tubular structure, but with a large lumen. An apocrine unit is also composed of a secretory gland, a proximal intradermal duct, and a peripheral intraepidermal/intrafollicular duct. The secretory portion is composed of a single ductal portion made of double cell layers. The cells of the glands produce proteinaceous pheromones by merocrine secretion, which is also called decapitation secretion, that are pushed up into a simple cuboidal or simple columnar duct when the surrounding myoepithelial cells contract upon sympathetic stimulation. They are similar to eccrine sweat glands in many respects, but drain their secretion into a hair follicle to reach the skin surface and develop at puberty. These glands always are associated with hair follicles, but only in the following places: the circumanal region, the areola of the breasts, and the axillae (Fig. 1-13).[2,20,43]

Pilosebaceous Unit

BOX 1-19   Summary

- Composed of a hair follicle and sebaceous glands
- Has the capacity to differentiate into either a terminal hair follicle or a sebaceous follicle
- Hair follicle stem cell (HFSC) is responsible for the restoration of the hair and sebaceous glands, as well as the long term replacement of the interfollicular epidermis
- Two basic types of hair follicles: vellus and terminal
- The hair follicle is a dynamic structure with three main stages: anagen, catagen, and telogen
- Hair follicles provide nourishment to their individual hair
- Sebaceous glands secrete lipid pheromones by holocrine secretion
- One of the main functions of sebaceous glands is secreting sebum, which in turn keeps the skin moist and soft
- Sebaceous glands develop and increase in size during adolescence in response to increased hormone levels

Pilosebaceous unit is composed of a hair follicle and sebaceous glands. These units are widely present throughout the skin, excluding the volar skin of the distal extremities (Fig. 1-14). Each pilosebaceous unit has the capacity to differentiate into either a terminal hair follicle or a sebaceous follicle. The terminal hair follicle has a large medullated hair that becomes the prominent structure. In a sebaceous follicle, the sebaceous gland becomes prominent and the hair remains vellus. Androgens play a key role in the development of the pilosebaceous unit in most areas of the body.[44]

HAIR FOLLICLES The structure of the hair follicle is shown in Fig. 1-15A and B. The infundibulum is the uppermost part of the follicle. It extends in between the follicular opening and the entrance of the sebaceous duct. This part of the follicular epithelium can easily be distinguished by the presence of the granular layer and keratinization.[20] The isthmus is the middle part of the follicle, which extends in between the entrance of the sebaceous duct and the insertion of the muscles of hair erection. This part of the follicular epithelium is similar to the epithelium of the distal sebaceous duct and keratinize, amorphously, without the granular layer.[20] The lower part of the hair follicle is in between the muscles of hair erection insertion and the base of the follicle. This part of the follicle is not only the most dynamic, but also functionally the most important in terms of hair production. The hair bulb is the bulbous, hair follicle base where the hair matrix cells reside and form hair. The mesenchymal cells and connective tissue invaginates at the base in the form of dermal hair papilla.[20]

The hair follicle stem cell (HFSC) is found in the bulge (outer region of the root sheath). It is responsible for the restoration of the hair and sebaceous glands, as well as the long-term replacement of the interfollicular epidermis.[45] The hair follicle structure is complex and multilayered. It is an appendage of the

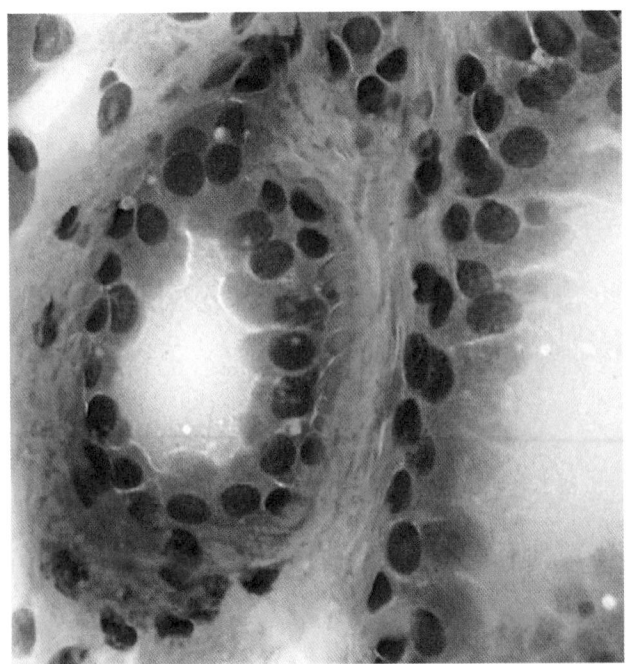

▲ **FIGURE 1-13** Apocrine unit. Apocrine glands with decapitation secretion.

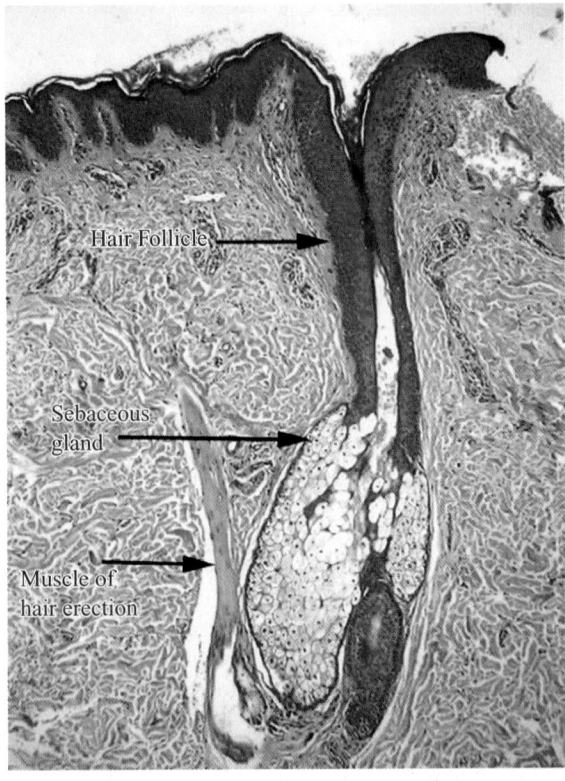

▲ **FIGURE 1-14** Pilosebaceous unit.

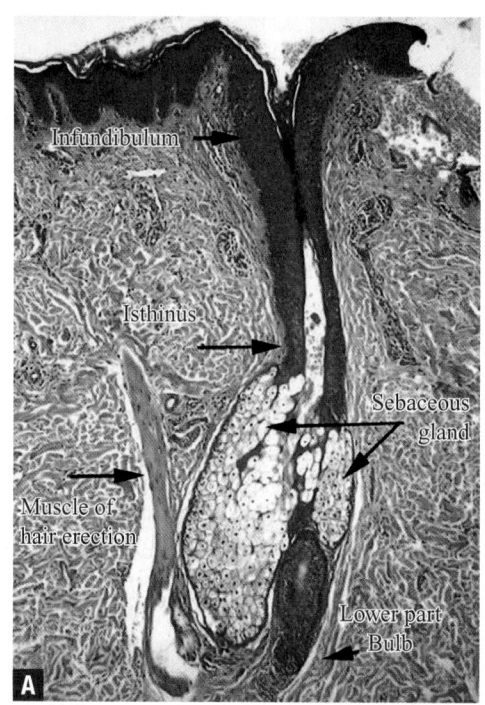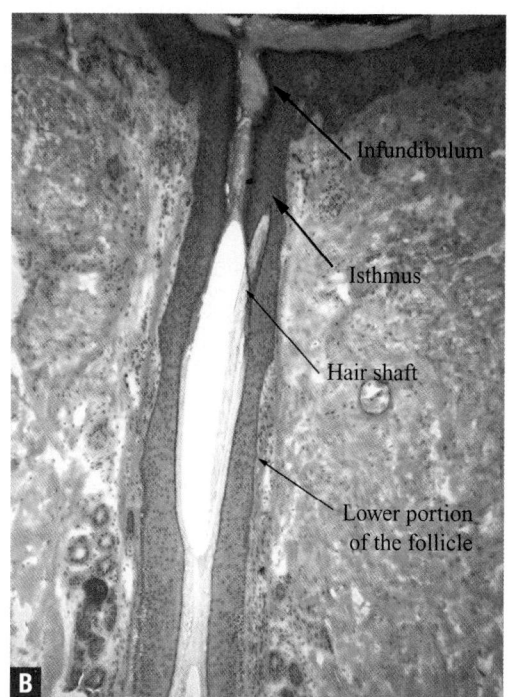

▲ **FIGURE 1-15** (**A** and **B**) Parts of the hair follicle.

skin and composed of follicular epithelial cells. Cells of the dermis surround and lie beneath the epidermal cells and are most likely the source of many hair follicle stem cell regulatory signals.[45] Depending upon the type of hair follicle and hair cycle phase, a hair follicle can extend from subcutaneous fat, which is found throughout the dermis. Reaching the epidermis, follicular epithelium joins with the surface epithelium in the form of a follicular orifice and the epithelial lining continues as epidermis.

Morphologically, there are two basic types of hair follicles, vellus, and terminal. Terminal hair follicles are situated in the subcutaneous fat and terminal hairs are thick, long, and darkly pigmented. On the other hand, vellus hair follicles are much smaller and situated in the dermis, bearing fine, short, thin, and light-colored vellus hair. During puberty, some vellus hair follicles transform into terminal hair follicles under hormonal influence in specific body sites.[20] In androgen-sensitive areas before puberty, the hair is vellus and the sebaceous glands are small.[44] In response to rising levels of androgens, pilosebaceous units become large terminal hair follicles in sexual hair areas or they become sebaceous follicles in sebaceous areas.[44] Androgens appear to promote sexual hair growth by recruiting a population of pilosebaceous units to switch from producing vellus hairs to initiating terminal hair growth.[44]

The hair follicle is a dynamic structure with three main stages. The anagen phase is the active hair growing stage. This is also the longest phase of the follicle. The catagen phase is the short regression stage of the follicle, when there is no longer hair growth in the bulb and the lower portion of the follicle retracts upward. The telogen phase is the dormant follicular stage, which eventually is followed by another anagen phase.[20]

Follicles provide nourishment to their individual hair with blood flow being concentrated at the dermal papilla—the base of the hair bulb. The cell layers of the anagen hair follicle from the center to the periphery are: medulla, cortex, hair cuticle, internal root sheath, and external root sheath.[20] The hair follicle is separated from the dermis by a glassy membrane, formed by the thickening of the basal lamina. Attached to this membrane are muscles of hair erection, which are smooth muscle bundles. They change the angle of the hair to a vertical alignment when they contract and help thermoregulation as well as when responding to neural stimulus. The melanocytes located in the bulb are responsible for the pigmentation of the hair.[20]

SEBACEOUS GLANDS These glands have an acinar structure. The cells of these glands secrete lipid pheromones by holocrine secretion and therefore possess no lumen. The secretions travel to the skin surface via stratified squamous ducts. These glands occur alongside every hair follicle as a tiny teardrop appendage and without hair follicles in the following four places: the areola of the breasts, glans penis, glans clitoris, and lips. One of the main functions of sebaceous glands is secreting oil, known as sebum, which in turn keeps the skin moist and soft. The oil also provides a barrier against foreign substances, lubricates hair and also facilitates sweating in the follicle. During adolescence, in response to increased hormone levels—namely androgen—sebaceous glands develop and increase in size and also secrete more sebum, playing an important role in the development of acne.[2,43,46]

Muscles

BOX 1-20 Summary

- Muscles of hair erection are smooth muscles and associated with hair follicles
- They are innervated by the autonomic nervous system
- External genitalia and areola have nonstriated smooth muscles, and have sympathetic innervation
- The head and neck region have striated voluntary muscles in the dermis

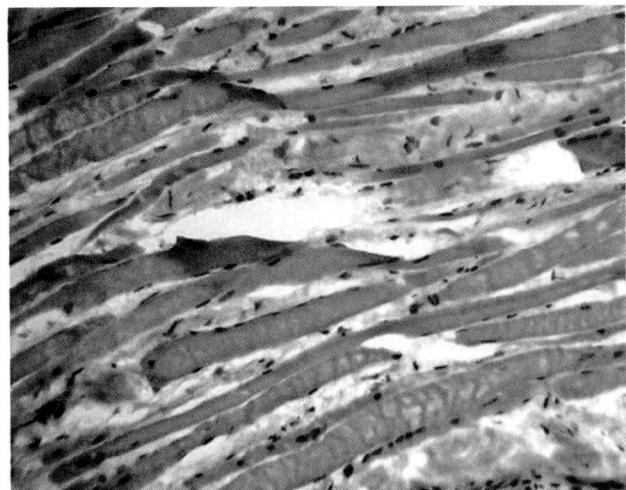

▲ **FIGURE 1-16** Striated voluntary muscles.

Muscles of hair erection are smooth muscles associated with the hair follicles in the dermis. The muscle of hair erection is a small band of smooth muscle that attaches to the bulge area of hair follicles deep in the reticular dermis and extends at an acute angle toward the epidermis.[47] The muscle is innervated by the autonomic nervous system and reacts to sympathetic stimuli by contracting and elevating the hair shaft.[47] Nonstriated smooth muscles are also present in external genitalia and areola. These muscles have sympathetic innervation. Striated voluntary muscles are situated in the lower dermis and subcutaneous fatty tissue, especially in the head and neck (Fig. 1-16).[20]

Nerves and Specialized Nerve Endings

BOX 1-21 Summary

- The skin has both terminally myelinated sensory and autonomic innervation as well as free and specialized nerve endings
- Autonomic nerves innervate involuntary vascular smooth muscle, muscles of hair erection, sweat glands, and sebaceous glands
- Afferent sensory nerves perceive the external environment
- Meissner's corpuscles are responsible for the touch sensation, whereas the Vater-Pacini corpuscles relay deep pressure

The skin is very rich in both terminally myelinated sensory and autonomic innervation, as well as free and specialized nerve endings (Fig. 1-17). Autonomic nerves innervate involun-

tary vascular smooth muscle, muscles of hair erection, sweat glands, and sebaceous glands.[48,49] Autonomic activities in the skin appear to be mediated by nonmyelinated postganglionic C-fibers. These autonomic fibers are classified as adrenergic, cholinergic, or purinergic.[48,49] All three subclasses of autonomic C-fibers innervate the microcirculation, with adrenergic fibers mediating vasoconstriction and cholinergic fibers mediating vasodilation.[20,48,49]

Afferent sensory nerves perceive the external environment. Terminal sensory nerve structures are called the free nerve endings. These nerve fibers are sheathed by Schwann cells and a basal lamina. They are present in the dermis and are particularly abundant in the papillary dermis. However, they lose much of their protective sheath upon penetrating the epidermis, thus acquiring the designation of free nerve endings.[48,49]

Sensory nerves form plexuses around the hair follicles, and free nerve endings extend through papillary dermis towards epidermis. Specialized nerve endings, such as Meissner's corpuscles and Vater-Pacini corpuscles, are situated at the papillary dermis and subcutaneous fat concomitantly (Fig. 1-18). Meissner's corpuscles are abundant in the volar skin and responsible for the touch sensation, whereas the Vater-Pacini corpuscles are mechanoreceptors with myelinated axons relaying deep pressure.[20]

Subcutaneous Tissue

BOX 1-22 Summary

- Located below the dermis and composed of loose connective tissue, elastic fibers, fibroblasts, and adipose tissue
- Functions mainly in insulation, cushioning of deeper tissues against injury, and fat storage

The subcutaneous tissue or the hypodermis is the layer directly under the dermis and is composed of loose connective tissue, elastic fibers, fibroblasts, and adipose tissue. However, adipose

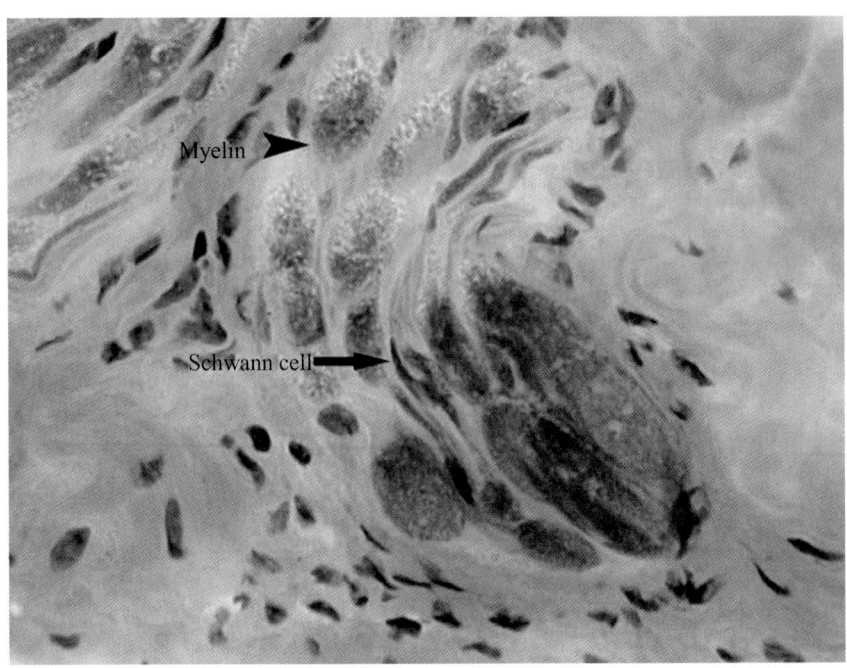

▲ **FIGURE 1-17** Myelinated peripheral sensory nerve in the skin.

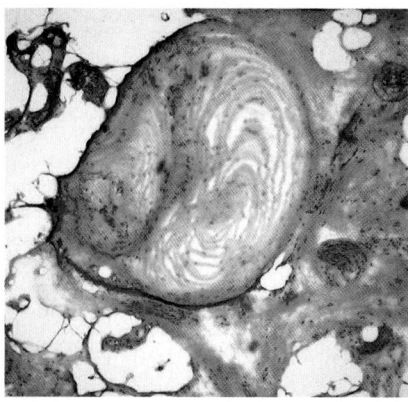

▲ **FIGURE 1-18** Vater-Pacini corpuscle in the subcutaneous fat.

tissue is absent in some areas, such as the eyelids, scrotum, penis, and the auricle of the ear pinna. This layer functions mainly as insulation, cushion for deeper tissues against injury, as well as a fat storage facility. The fat is organized into fat lobules separated by type III collagen matrix. In comparison with the dermis, the subcutaneous layer contains larger blood vessels, lymphatics, less nerve endings, and Pacinian corpuscles, which are mechanoreceptors with myelinated axons for deep pressure. The subcutaneous tissue is anchored to the deep fascia of underlying muscle via fibrous bands of connective tissue.[2]

CUTANEOUS IMMUNOLOGY

BOX 1-23 Summary

- Innate immunity of the skin can be divided into constitutive innate immunity, and inducible innate immunity.
- Constitutive innate immunity involves the skin as an anatomic and physiologic barrier
- Inducible innate immunity involves the acute inflammation that occurs after an insult and the cellular infiltration barrier that forms
- Acquired immunity may be activated by a variety of ways by the innate immune system
- The cutaneous innate immune system controls an initial pathogenic assault, while directing the more specific recognition and destruction of the pathogen via the acquired immune system

A vital function of the cutaneous immune system is to defend against pathogenic organisms. The first line of defense is the innate immune system. Innate immunity of the skin can be divided into constitutive innate immunity and in-

ducible innate immunity. Constitutive innate immunity involves the skin as an anatomic and physiologic barrier. Cutaneous constitutive innate immunity consists of the normal skin flora, cornified keratinocytes, constitutively expressed antimicrobial polypeptides and lipids, low pH, and normal body temperature.[43,48–50]

Inducible innate immunity involves the acute inflammation that occurs after an insult and the cellular infiltration barrier that forms. It is initiated by preformed IL-1α, stored in the cytoplasm of keratinocytes. IL-1α is released into the skin if the skin integrity is disturbed by stimulations of epidermal keratinocytes.[51] Mechanical deformation also appears to be sufficient to release IL-1α.[52] This may contribute to the itch/scratch-associated changes that often occur along with allergic skin disease.[52] Release of IL-1α appears to be a key factor in initiating a cascade of events that contribute to the classic signs of acute inflammation: redness, heat, swelling, and pain. Other important inducible soluble innate immunity molecules of the skin include inducible antimicrobial polypeptides, complement-activating and/or opsonin proteins, and complement proteins.[51]

Acquired immunity may be activated by a variety of ways by the innate immune system. Activation of acquired immunity requires that Langerhans cells, that have endocytosed antigen, exit the skin via lymph vessels and proceed to the draining lymph node.[53] In the initial step to develop acquired immunity, Langerhans cells process and present antigenic peptide to naïve T cells. The resulting activated antigen-specific effector or memory T cell expressing CLA (a modified form of P-selectin glycoprotein ligand-1) are targeted to infiltrate the inflammatory site.[54] In addition to T cells, B cells are the other key cells of acquired immunity. Differentiated B cells derived antigen-specific antibodies, particularly those of the IgE isotype, have a strong association with allergic diseases of the skin.[55] B cells can also recognize relatively intact antigens.[55]

A primary acquired immune response, which is the encounter of an antigen for the first time, requires several days for fully functional antigen-specific T and B cells to develop.[48,49] On the other hand, a secondary acquired immune response, which is an immune response to a previously encountered antigen, takes approximately one day to fully mobilize memory T cells.[48,49] The reaction is more vigorous, with significantly increased antigen-specific antibody titers produced by memory B cells.[48,49] In conclusion, the

cutaneous innate immune system controls an initial pathogenic assault while directing the more specific recognition and destruction of the pathogen via the acquired immune system.

FINAL THOUGHTS

The skin is a very versatile organ with many important functions. It is composed of many interdependent cells and structures that provide protection from the external environment. The skin is structured to prevent loss of essential body fluids, and to protect the body against the entry of toxic environmental chemicals and microorganisms. It is a vital part of the body's temperature regulation system, is also a huge sensory receptor for temperature, pain, and touch stimuli. In addition, it plays a role in innate and acquired immunity. Imbalances in factors affecting the delicate homeostasis that exists among skin cells may result in a variety of conditions such as wrinkles and hair loss, blisters, and rashes, and even life-threatening cancers and disorders of the immune regulation system.

REFERENCES

1. Murphy GF, Sellheyer K, Mihm MC. The Skin. Kumar: Robbins and Cotran In: *Pathologic Basis of Disease.* 7th ed. Pennsylvania: Elsevier Saunders; 2005;1228.
2. Junqueria, LC and Carneiro J. Skin. In: *Basic Histology: Text and Atlas.* 11th ed. Junqueria LC, Carneiro J, eds. New York: McGraw-Hill; 2005;260–372.
3. Kamel, MN. Anatomy of the Skin. In: *The Electronic Textbook of Dermatology.* Drugge R, ed. New York, NY: 2000; http://www.telemedicine. org/stamford. htm
4. Bouwstra, JA, Honeywell-Nguyen PL, Gooris GS, et al. Structure of the skin barrier and its modulation by vesicular formulations. *Prog Lipid Res.* 2003;42:1–36.
5. Edelson RL, Fink JM. The immunologic function of the skin. *Sci Am.* 1985;252:46.
6. Forslind B. A domain mosaic model of the skin barrier. *Acta Derm.* 1994;74:1–6.
7. Landmann L. The epidermal permeability barrier. *Anat Embryol.* 1988;178:1–13.
8. Abrahamsohn, PA. Epithelial tissue. In: *Basic Histology: Text and Atlas.* 11th ed. Junqueria LC, Carneiro J, eds. New York: McGraw-Hill; 2005;66–89.
9. Hentula M, J Peltonen, S Peltonen. Expression profiles of cell-cell and cell-matrix junction proteins developing human epidermis. *Arch Dermatol Res.* 2001;293:259.
10. Zorn T, TM. Connective tissue. In: Junqueria LC, Carneiro J, eds. *Basic Histology: Text and Atlas,* 11th ed. New York: McGraw-Hill, 2005;91–122.
11. Krypta, R, Bernfield M, Burridge K, et al. Cell junctions, cell adhesion, and the extracellular matrix. In: Alberts B, Johnson A, Lewis J, Raff M, Roberts K, Walter P, eds. *Molecular Biology of the Cell,*

4th ed. New York: Garland and Science Publishing; 2002:1065–1124.

12. Barrandon Y, Green H. Three clonal types of keratinocyte with different capacities for multiplication. *Proc Natl Acad Sci USA.* 1987;84(8):2302–2306.

13. Potten CS, Booth C. Keratinocyte stem cells: A commentary. *J Invest Dermatol.* 2002;119(4):888–899.

14. Pellegrini G, Dellambra E, Golisano O, et al. p63 identifies keratinocyte stem cells. *Proc Natl Acad Sci USA.* 2001;98(6):3156–3161.

15. Jensen UB, Lowell S, Watt FM. The spatial relationship between stem cells and their progeny in the basal layer of human epidermis: a new view based on whole-mount labeling and lineage analysis. *Development.* 1999;126(11):2409–2418.

16. Edwars, P, Enver T, Hughes S, et al. Histology: The lives and deaths of cells in tissues. In: Alberts B, Johnson A, Lewis J, Raff M, Roberts K, Walter P, eds. *Molecular Biology of the Cell.* 4th ed. New York: Garland and Science Publishing; 2002:1259–1311.

17. Candi E, Schmidt R, Melino G. The cornified envelope: a model of cell death in the skin. *Nat Rev Mol Cell Biol.* 2005;6(4):328–340.

18. Sidhu GS, Chandra P, Cassai ND. Merkel cells, normal and neoplastica: an update. *Ultrastruct Pathol.* 2005;29(3–4):287–294.

19. Moll I, Roessler M, Brandner JM, et al. Human Merkel cells—aspects of cell biology, distribution and functions. *Eur J Cell Biol.* 2005;84(2–3):259–271.

20. Elder D, Elenitsas R, Jaworsky C, Johnson B. *Lever's Histopathology of the Skin,* 8th ed. Philadelphia, PA: Lippincott-Raven Publishers; 1997:12–41.

21. Wood JM, Gibbons NC, Schallreuter KU. Melanocortins in human melanocytes. *Cell Mol Biol.* 2006;52(2):75–78. Review.

22. Sulaimon SS, Kitchell BE. The biology of melanocytes. *Vet Dermatol* 2003;14(2):57–65. Review.

23. Duval C, Smit NP, Kolb AM, et al. Keratinocytes control the pheo/eumelanin ratio in cultured normal human melanocytes. *Pigment Cell Res* 2002;15(6):440–446.

24. Strobl H, Riedl E, Bello-Fernandez C, et al. Epidermal Langerhans cell development and differentiation. *Immunobiology.* 1998;198:588.

25. Chen H, Yuan J, Wang Y, et al. Distribution of ATPase-positive Langerhans cells in normal adult human skin. *Br J Dermatol.* 1985;113:707.

26. Stingl G, Maurer D, Hauser C, et al. The epidermis: an immunologic microenvironment. In: Freedberg IM, Eisen AZ, Wolff K, et al, eds. *Fitzpatrick's Dermatology in General Medicine,* 5th ed. New York: McGraw-Hill; 1999:343.

27. Cumberbatch M, Dearman RJ, Kimber I. Langerhans cells require signals from both tumor necrosis factor-alpha and interleukin-1 beta for migration. *Immunology.* 1997;92:388.

28. Robert C, Kupper TS: Inflammatory skin diseases, T cells, and immune surveillance. *N Engl J Med.* 1999;341:1817.

29. Foster CA, Elbe A. Lymphocyte subpopulations of the skin. Bos JD, ed. *Skin Immune System.* 2nd ed. Boca Raton: CRC Press LLC; 1997:85.

30. Haake AR, Holbrook K. The structure and development of skin. In: Freedberg IM, Eisen AZ, Wolff K, et al, eds. *Fitzpatrick's Dermatology in General Medicine.* 5th ed. New York: McGraw-Hill; 1999:70.

31. Boxman IL, Ruwhof C, Boerman OC, et al. Role of fibroblasts in the regulation of pro-inflammatory interleukin IL-1, IL-6, and IL-8 levels induced by keratinocyte-derived IL-1. *Arch Dermatol Res.* 1996;288:391.

32. Yamamoto T, Hartmann K, Eckes B, et al. Role of stem cell factor and monocyte chemoattractant protein-1 in the interaction between fibroblasts and mast cells in fibrosis. *J Dermatol Sci.* 2001;26:106.

33. Tharp MD. Skin mast cells. In: Freinkel RK, Woodley DT, eds. *The Biology of the Skin.* New York: Parthenon; 2001:265.

34. Mikhail GR, Miller-Milinska A. Mast cell population in skin. *J Invest Dermatol* 1964;43:249.

35. Robert C, Kupper TS. Inflammatory skin diseases, T cells, and immune surveillance. *N Eng J Med.* 1999;341(24):1817–1828.

36. Henz BM, Maurer M, Lippert U, et al: Mast cells as initiators of immunity and host defense. *Exp Dermatol.* 2001;10:1.

37. Ribatti D, Crivellato E, Candussio L, et al. Mast cells and their secretory granules are angiogenic in the chick embryo chorioallantoic membrane. *Clin Exp Allergy.* 2001;31:602.

38. Rowden G. Macrophages and dendritic cells in the skin. Bos JD, ed. *Skin Immune System.* 2nd ed. Boca Raton: CRC Press LLC; 1997:109.

39. Nickoloff BJ, ed. *Dermal Immune System.* Boca Raton: CRC Press LLC; 1993.

40. Headington JT. The dermal dendrocyte. *Adv Dermatol.* 1986;1:159.

41. Braverman IM. The cutaneous microcirculation: Ultrastructure and microanatomical organization. *Microcirculation.* 1997;4(3):329–340.

42. Skobe M, Detmar M. Structure, function, and molecular control of the skin lymphatic system. *J Investig Dermatol Symp Proc.* 2000;5:14.

43. Schaller M, Plewig G. Structure and function of eccrine, apocrine, apoeccrine and sebaceous glands. In: *Dermatology.* Bolognia JL, Jorizzo JL, Rapini RP, et al, eds. Philadelphia: Mosby; 2003:525–530.

44. Deplewski D, Rosenfield RL. Role of hormones in pilosebaceous unit development. *Endocr Rev.* 2000;21(4):363–392.

45. Moore KA, Lemischka IR. Stem cells and their niches. *Science.* 2006;311(5769):1880–1885. Review.

46. Strauss JS, Pochi PE, Downing DT. The sebaceous glands: twenty-five years of progress. *J Invest Dermatol.* 1976;67(1):90–91.

47. Mendelson JK, Smoller BR, et al. The microanatomy of the distal arrector pili: Possible role for alpha1beta1 and alpha5beta1 integrins in mediating cell-cell adhesion and anchorage to the extracellular matrix. *J Cutan Pathol.* 2000;27(2):61–66.

48. Metze D, Luger T. Nervous system in the skin. In: Freinkel RK, Woodley DT, eds. *The Biology of the Skin,* New York: Parthenon; 2001:153.

49. Debenedictis C, Joubeh S, Zhang G, et al. *Immune functions of the skin. Clin Dermatol.* 2001;19:573.

50. Dahl MV. *Clinical Immunodermatology,* 3rd ed. St. Louis, 1996.

51. Murphy JE, Robert C, Kupper TS. Interleukin-1 and cutaneous inflammation: a crucial link between innate and acquired immunity. *J Invest Dermatol.* 2000;114:602.

52. Lee RT, Briggs WH, Cheng GC, et al. Mechanical deformation promotes secretion of IL-1 alpha and IL-1 receptor antagonist. *J Immunol.* 1997;159:5084.

53. Kimber I, Cumberbatch M, Dearman RJ, et al. Cytokines and chemokines in the initiation and regulation of epidermal Langerhans cell mobilization. *Br J Dermatol.* 2000;142:401.

54. Groves RW, Ross E, Barker JN, et al. Effect of in vivo interleukin-1 on adhesion molecule expression in normal human skin. *J Invest Dermatol.* 1992;98:384.

55. Goldsby RA, Kindt TJ, Osborne BA. *Kuby Immunology,* 4th ed. New York: WH Freeman; 2000.

CHAPTER 2

Aging Skin

Jens J. Thiele, M.D., Ph.D.
Barbara A. Gilchrest, M.D.

BOX 2-1 Overview

- The number and proportion of older people are increasing worldwide at an unprecedented rate.
- Skin aging is the interactive result of both a genetic program and cumulative wear and tear during the lifespan caused by endogenous and exogenous factors.
- Telomere shortening resulting in cellular senescence is thought to be a cancer prevention mechanism.
- Oxidative modifications of DNA, lipids, carbohydrates, and proteins caused by an imbalance of reactive oxygen species and antioxidant defense have been linked to skin aging.
- Loss of immunocompetent cells and immunosurveillance functions have been observed in aging skin and may contribute to age-associated development of skin cancer.
- Human skin provides an instructive contrast between intrinsic aging, changes attributable to the passage of time alone, and the superimposed additional changes that result from environmental damage, mainly due to solar UV irradiation and termed photoaging.
- Prevention of photodamage by use of adequate sun protection and sunscreens is considered the most effective strategy against photoaging.
- The beneficial effects of topical retinoids are clinically modest but have been well documented.
- The ability of topically applied or oral antioxidants to prevent or reduce skin aging has not yet been demonstrated in controlled human trials, although experimental evidence points to potential benefits in the prevention of both skin aging and carcinogenesis.

INTRODUCTION

The number and proportion of older people are increasing worldwide at an unprecedented rate,[1] and recent U.S. Census Bureau statistics detail an ever-increasing American life expectancy.[2] The number of people aged 65 years

and over in the United States alone was 36.3 million on July 1, 2004, which is 12% of the total population. Between 2003 and 2004, 351,000 people moved into this age group. Remarkably, the projected percentage increase in this segment of the population between 2000 and 2050 is 147%. By comparison, the population as a whole would have increased by only 49% over the same period.[2]

The incidence of skin cancer increases exponentially with age.[3] Potentially fatal skin malignancies, such as melanoma and cutaneous T-cell lymphoma, as well as numerous skin conditions that rarely threaten life but compromise its quality, are dramatically increasing in the geriatric population. At the same time, a rapidly increasing number of people are seeking dermatologic care for the prevention and treatment of the effects of aging skin. Although such therapies may well reduce the prevalence of dermatologic diseases, including skin cancer among older people, it is the demand for cosmetic improvement that is growing most rapidly.[4]

Aging is universal among eukaryotic organisms, but the molecular mechanisms underlying aging are only beginning to be elucidated.[5] This chapter reviews the underlying mechanisms, ultrastructural manifestations, and topical treatments of aging skin, with an emphasis on its relationship to the pathophysiology of skin cancers.

THEORIES OF AGING

BOX 2-2 Summary

- There are two fundamental and not mutually exclusive theories of aging: the programmatic theory and the stochastic theory.
- Many mutations affecting longevity pathways delay age-related diseases, and the molecular analysis of these pathways is leading to a mechanistic understanding of the linkage between aging and susceptibility to disease.
- Age-associated changes in gene expression pattern and cellular proliferative capacity appear to be largely under the control of the telomeres.
- Mammalian cells can undergo only a limited number of cell divisions and then arrest irreversibly in a state known as

replicative senescence, after which they are refractory to mitogenic stimuli.
- Critical shortening or experimental telomere disruption triggers multiple DNA damage responses that include cellular senescence.
- Senescence is thought to be a cancer prevention mechanism, since it prevents the unlimited and possibly unregulated growth of cells whose DNA has been progressively damaged over their organism's lifespan.
- The free radical theory of aging proposes that endogenously and exogenously generated reactive oxygen species eventually overwhelm cellular antioxidant defenses, leading to oxidative damage of biomolecules and the functional decline of organ systems.

In the past century, a multitude of theories of aging have been articulated, based on molecular, cellular, organismal, and evolutionary perspectives. There are two fundamental, and not mutually exclusive, theories of aging.[6] The programmatic theory states that aging, like development, is a preordained process due to an inherent genetic program that is played out at a rate characteristic of each species. The stochastic theory states that random cumulative environmental damage to genes and proteins ultimately produces aging and homeostatic failure.

Today, available data suggest that aging is in fact the interactive result of both a genetic program and cumulative wear and tear during the lifespan. Mutations in genes affecting DNA repair, endocrine signaling, stress responses, metabolism, and telomere maintenance can all increase or decrease the lifespan of model organisms. Specific evolutionarily conserved pathways have been described for aging, some of which appear to modulate the lifespan in response to environmental factors, such as caloric restriction or stress.[7] Importantly, many mutations affecting longevity pathways delay age-related diseases, and the molecular analysis of these pathways is leading to a mechanistic understanding of the linkage between aging and susceptibility to disease.

The Programmatic Theory

TELOMERE SHORTENING Age-associated changes in pattern of gene expression and cellular proliferative capacity appear largely under the control of the telomeres.[8]

17

Telomeres, the terminal portions of eukaryotic chromosomes, consist of up to many hundreds of tandem short sequence repeats (TTAGGG) (Fig. 2-1). During mitosis of somatic cells, DNA polymerase cannot replicate the final base pairs of each chromosome, resulting in progressive shortening with each round of cell division. A special reverse transcriptase, telomerase, can replicate these chromosomal ends but with few exceptions the enzyme is expressed normally only in germline cells. Human telomere length shortens more than 30% during adulthood even in relatively quiescent skin fibroblasts, and telomeres of patients with premature aging syndromes such as Werner's syndrome and progeria are shorter than those of age-matched controls.[9] Critical shortening or experimental telomere disruption triggers multiple DNA damage responses that include cellular senescence (Fig. 2-2). The specific initiating event is likely exposure of the otherwise concealed single-stranded 3 overhang, tandem repeats of TTAGGG, a signal that can be provided to cells in the absence of DNA damage by exogenously provided oligonucleotides homologous to the telomere overhang sequence (T-oligos).[8] Tissue-specific telomore shortening rates in the normal sun-protected human epidermis were reported to be relatively slow despite the very rapid turnover rate, suggesting that the epidermis contains telomerase activity or other mechanisms to lengthen telomerase without telomerase.[10] While elevated telomerase was reported in sun-exposed epidermis, a recent study found similar telomerase activity in aged and young human epidermis obtained from sun-protected sites.[11]

CELLULAR SENESCENCE Mammalian cells can undergo only a limited number of cell divisions and then arrest irreversibly in a state known as replicative senescence, after which they are refractory to mitogenic stimuli. This fact has led to the perception that aging evolved in multicellular organisms as a cancer prevention mechanism, since it prevents the unlimited and possibly unregulated growth of cells whose DNA has been progressively damaged over their organisms's lifespan.[12] This response, also referred to as cellular senescence, is under the control of the p53 and retinoblastoma (Rb) tumor-suppressor proteins and thus constitutes a potent anticancer mechanism. Senescent cells display critically short telomeres, irreversible growth arrest, resistance to apoptosis, and altered differentiation. The majority of genes overexpressed during *in vitro* cellular senescence contribute to blocking the cells in the G_1 phase of the cell cycle. Some encode DNA-binding proteins that act as gene regulators. Other relevant overex-

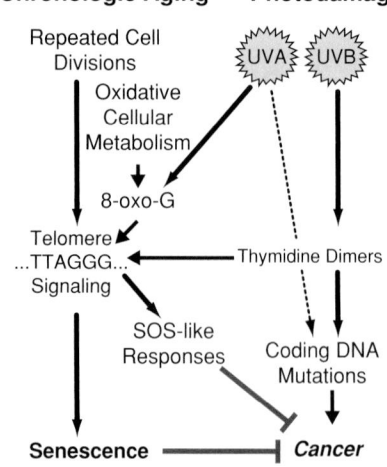

Chronologic Aging   Photodamage

▲ **FIGURE 2-2** Hypothetical common mechanism for chronological aging and photoaging. Photodamage leads to thymine dimers and ROS that damage genomic DNA and give rise to mutations in coding or regulatory DNA sequences of critical genes that may lead to cancer development. UV radiation also damages telomeres, indeed disproportionately, due to their greater proportion of target TT and G bases compared to the chromosome overall. Such damage is postulated to disrupt the telomere loop, expose the TTAGGG overhang, and promote "aging." Intrinsic aging is accompanied in most cases by repeated cell divisions that shorten telomeres. Aerobic cellular metabolism during the organism's lifespan also damages the telomeres at guanine residues, a further overlap between mechanisms of aging and photoaging. Exposure of the TTAGGG overhang sequence appears to initiate signaling leading to SOS-like responses, proliferative senescence or apoptosis, all of which interfere with carcinogenesis. (Modified from Halachmi et al.[127])

pressed or suppressed genes have been recently reviewed.[9] The former encode inhibitors of cell cycle regulatory nuclear proteins such as statin and the cyclin-dependent kinase inhibitors p21 and p16; the latter include genes that are required for progression through the G_1 phase of the cell cycle, including c-fos and certain helix-loop-helix transcription factors (Id1H and Id2H). Perhaps surprisingly, other overexpressed senescence-associated genes encoded products are involved in modulation of the extracellular matrix. These include structural proteins such as fibronectin, and matrix metalloproteinases (MMPs) such as collagenase and stromelysin. In contrast, the level of certain tissue inhibitors of matrix metalloproteinases (TIMPs) is decreased.[13] Thus, it is believed that senescent cells acquire phenotypic changes that may contribute to aging and certain age-related

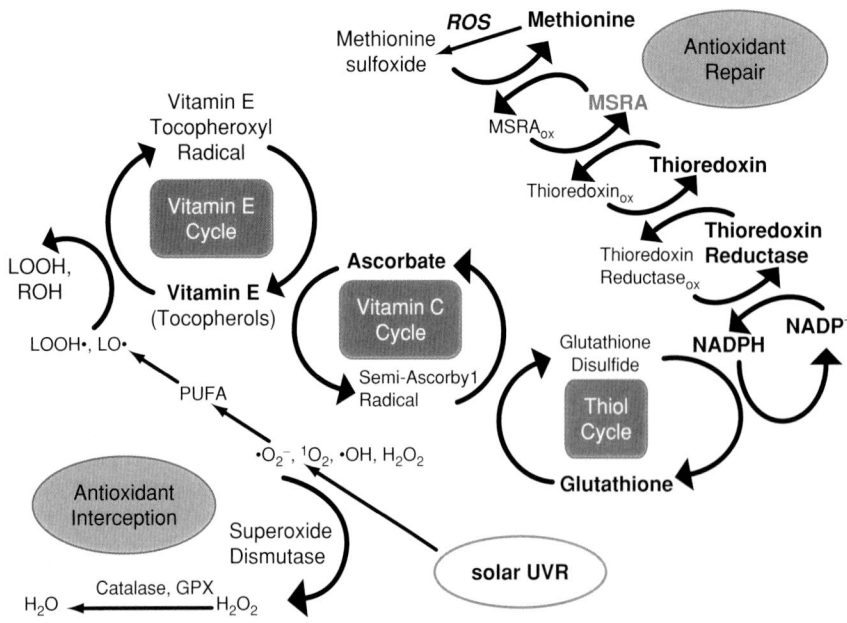

▲ **FIGURE 2-1** The antioxidant network of the skin and free radical interception and antioxidant repair. ROS: reactive oxygen species; $\cdot O_2^-$: superoxide anion; $^1O_2$: singlet oxygen; $\cdot OH$: hydroxyl radical; H_2O_2: hydrogen peroxide; LOOH: lipid hydroperoxides; LOO$\cdot$: lipid peroxyl radical; GPX: glutathione peroxidases; MSRA: methionine sulfoxide reductase.

diseases, ironically including late-life cancer.[14]

The Stochastic Theory

THE "FREE RADICAL THEORY OF AGING" AND OXIDATIVE STRESS A causative role for reactive oxygen species (ROS) in aging processes, referred to as the free radical theory of aging,[15] proposes that ROS in biological systems attack molecules and cause the functional decline of organ systems that eventually leads to death. Numerous cell culture, invertebrate, and mammalian models exist that lend support to this half-century-old hypothesis. The free radical theory is based on the observation that many age-related pathologies are the result of damage to macromolecules by ROS. In fact, the level of oxidative damage and the rate of aging of cells, tissues, and individuals correlate very well.[16] The identification and study of long-lived mutant animals has provided valuable insights into the mechanisms that limit the lifespan of organisms. Recent investigations on lifespan determination in *C. elegans* suggest that ROS, which are an inevitable consequence of life in an oxygen-rich world, are a leading proximal cause of aging. Studies of mutant strains of *C. elegans*, in particular daf-2, clk-1, and isp-1 mutants, suggest that the biology of reactive oxygen species in the mitochondria and elsewhere might be the main determinant of lifespan in this organism.[17]

ROS are generated in large part from single electrons escaping the mitochondrial respiratory chain and reducing the molecular oxygen to form the superoxide anion ($^{\cdot}O_2^-$) and, subsequently, other ROS including hydroxyl radicals, hydrogen peroxide, nitric oxide, and others. In addition to this erratic, but constant flux of endogenously generated ROS, cells and tissues face oxidative attack from inflammatory cell infiltrates capable of oxidative bursts, as well as from exogenous stressors such as ultraviolet radiation (UV). Both UVA (320 to 400 nm) and UVB (280 to 320 nm) have been shown to rapidly generate significant amounts of ROS in the epidermal and upper dermal layers of human skin (reviewed in [18]). The cascade of ROS formation is initiated when UV-photons (predominantly UVA) are absorbed by endogenous or exogenous chromophores in the skin. Of the many skin constituents absorbing UVA, *trans*-urocanic acid, melanins, flavins, porphyrins, quinones, protein-bound tryptophan, and advanced glycation end products are believed to be relevant photosensitizers initiating the ROS formation cascade. Following UV absorption, the activated chromophore may react in two ways. In type I photoreactions, the excited chromophore directly reacts with a substrate molecule via electron or hydrogen atom transfer and gives rise to free radical formation. In the presence of molecular oxygen (minor type II reaction), this reaction may lead to the formation of the superoxide anion radical ($^{\cdot}O_2^-$). Subsequently, $^{\cdot}O_2^-$ generates hydrogen peroxide (H_2O_2) by a dismutation reaction either spontaneously or catalyzed by cutaneous superoxide dismutase. Furthermore, in the presence of metal ions such as Fe(II) or Cu(II), H_2O_2 can be converted to the highly reactive hydroxyl radical ($^{\cdot}OH$). Otherwise (major type II reaction), electronically excited and reactive singlet oxygen ($^1O_2$) is formed by photoenergy transfer from UV-excited chromophores in the presence of triplet oxygen $^3O_2$ (molecular oxygen in its ground state). Following their formation, ROS species including $^1O_2$, $^{\cdot}O_2^-$, $^{\cdot}OH$, and H_2O_2 react with an array of skin biomolecules including lipids, proteins, carbohydrates, and DNA. Unsaturated lipids react with ROS forming lipid peroxyl ($LOO^{\cdot}$) and alkoxyl radicals ($LO^{\cdot}$), which may initiate a chain-propagating autocatalytic reaction ("lipid peroxidation"). Lipid peroxidation end products, such as malondialdehyde (MDA) or 4-hydroxy-nonenal (4-HNE), induce a number of cellular stress responses and, at higher concentrations, are cytotoxic. To counteract oxidative injury, human skin is equipped with a network of enzymatic and nonenzymatic antioxidant systems (Fig. 2-1; reviewed in [18]). An imbalance between oxidative attack by ROS and antioxidant defense systems results in specific oxidative modifications of macromolecules, which is generally referred to as "oxidative stress". Longer lived species generally show higher cellular oxidative stress resistance and lower levels of mitochondrial ROS production than shorter lived species. Caloric restriction, an intervention that extends lifespan in many species, is thought to decrease ROS production and thus oxidative damage.[19]

OXIDATIVE PROTEIN MODIFICATIONS A variety of proteins are important targets for oxidative modifications. Oxygen radicals and other activated oxygen species generated as by-products of cellular metabolism or from environmental sources cause modifications of the amino acids of proteins that generally result in functional changes in structural or enzymatic proteins. In addition to modification of amino acid side-chains, oxidation reactions can also mediate fragmentation of polypeptide chains and both intra- and intermolecular crosslinking of peptides and proteins.[20] Protein carbonyls may be formed either by oxidative cleavage of proteins, or by direct oxidation of lysine, arginine, proline, and threonine residues. In addition, carbonyl groups may be introduced into proteins by reactions with aldehydes (4-hydroxy-2-nonenal, malondialdehyde) produced during lipid peroxidation or with reactive carbonyl derivatives generated as a consequence of the reaction of reducing sugars or their oxidation products with lysine residues of proteins.[21] The presence of carbonyl groups in proteins has therefore been used as a marker of reactive oxygen-mediated protein oxidation. As measured by the introduction of carbonyl groups, protein oxidation has been associated with aging, oxidative stress, and a number of diseases, such as the premature aging diseases, progeria, and Werner's syndrome.[22] In human skin, oxidatively modified proteins are most pronounced in the papillary dermis and accumulate with age, and particularly, with chronic sun exposure.[23] Importantly, ROS may cause specific "fingerprint" modifications of amino acids resulting in functional changes of structural or enzymic proteins. In particular, methionine residues in proteins are easily oxidized to methionine sulfoxide (MetO) and the repair of this damage appears to be essential for tissues to survive in the presence of ROS.[24]

Besides "interceptive" antioxidant systems that intercept free radical accumulation and thus prevent oxidative damage, such as catalase, superoxide dismutases, and glutathione peroxidases, many cells are equipped with "repair enzymes" that are able to reverse and thus control protein oxidative damage. Mice lacking the well-characterized antioxidant repair enzyme, methionine sulfoxide reductase (MsrA), exhibit an increased sensitivity to oxidative stress challenges, leading to accumulation of higher tissue levels of oxidized proteins as well as a shorter lifespan.[25]

MsrA was recently detected in human skin, where it is most strongly expressed in basal and suprabasal epidermis and upregulated by UVA.[26] MsrA reverses the inactivation of many proteins due to oxidation of critical methionine (Met) residues by reducing methionine sulfoxide (MetO) to Met (Fig. 2-1). Initial studies in human skin point to an inverse correlation between MsrA expression and the levels of oxidative protein damage, pointing to an involvement in the cutaneous aging process.[26]

DNA DAMAGE The accurate maintenance of nuclear DNA is critical to cellular function, and therefore, numerous DNA repair systems have evolved. The efficiency of cellular DNA repair machinery itself appears to decline with age.[5] Unless precisely repaired, nuclear DNA damage can lead to mutation and/or other deleterious cellular and organismal consequences. Damage to both nuclear DNA, which encodes the vast majority of cellular RNA and proteins, and mitochondrial DNA has been proposed to contribute to aging.[27] In mice, levels of 8-oxoguanine, a major product of oxidative DNA damage, increase with age and can be inhibited by caloric restriction.[19] In humans, the only genes implicated in the rate of aging are those in which mutations are responsible for premature aging syndromes. For example, Cockayne syndrome patients display mutations in the DNA helicases encoded by the ERCC6 or ERCC8 genes leading to increased photosensitivity due to impaired DNA repair. Ataxia telangiectasia is caused by a mutation in the ATM gene, encoding a kinase that senses DNA damage and thus is crucial in DNA repair. Werner's syndrome, caused by a mutation in RECQL2, a gene encoding a DNA helicase, leads to increased frequency of recombination with a predisposition toward accelerated aging and cancer.[28] These findings suggest that decreased DNA repair capacity is associated with accelerated aging and that cumulative DNA damage plays a major role in the aging process. Still, the role of these genes in normal aging is not established, since patients with so-called premature aging syndromes display some manifestations of aging at an accelerated rate but lack other features of normal aging and have some other characteristic findings that differ greatly from those of normal aging.[9] In some species, so-called longevity genes have been identified whose mutation or overexpression increases lifespan. These mutations have revealed evolutionary conserved pathways for aging, some of which appear to extend the lifespan in response to sensory cues, caloric restriction, or stress.[7] The hypothesis that nuclear DNA is an important target of age-related change is supported by ample experimental evidence that nuclear DNA damage and mutations accumulate with age (recently reviewed in [5]). While ROS are likely to be one important source of this damage, there are numerous other cellular and environmental sources of damage, and

the impact of such lesions may be enhanced by age-related compromise of DNA repair. Possible mechanisms by which compromised DNA repair could contribute to aging include accumulation of damage in critical genes, p53-mediated senescence, and DNA damage induced apoptosis. Various lines of evidence suggest that p53 plays opposing roles in the aging process. While p53 suppresses the onset of malignancy and thereby extends the lifespan, at the same time it promotes cellular senescence and apoptosis in response to DNA damage, potentially contributing to the clinical changes of aging.[5]

A recent hypothesis links telomere shortening and acute DNA damage to a common cellular signaling pathway that, depending on both the cell type and signal intensity, mediates adaptive differentiation, apoptosis, or senescence.[29–31] Indirect experimental evidence suggests that exposure of the telomere 3′ overhang (repeats of TTAGGG approximately 100–400 bases in length) stimulates DNA damage signaling and plays a role in both chronological (intrinsic) aging and acute or chronic photodamage (photoaging; Fig. 2-2).[32] In the context of the present chapter, this hypothesis is especially notable in that the response may also be viewed as an evolutionarily conserved cancer-prevention mechanism.[30]

NONENZYMATIC GYCOSYLATION AND ADVANCED GLYCATION END PRODUCTS Glycation is a slow, nonenzymatic reaction that takes place between free amino groups in proteins, primarily between lysine and a reducing sugar such as glucose or ribose. In skin, this reaction creates new residues or formations of crosslinks [advanced glycation end products (AGEs)] in the extracellular matrix of the dermis. This process leads to brown discoloration, loss of function and altered degradation of affected protein. The formation of these bridges between dermal molecules has been suggested to be responsible for loss of elasticity or other properties of the dermis observed during aging. Glycation may therefore play an important role in chronologic aging. In skin, AGEs were reported to accumulate with age in dermal elastin and collagens and are thought to be responsible for loss of cutaneous elasticity.[33]

One study found that the average onset of AGEs accumulation in the dermis is around 35 years of age, and thereafter AGEs accumulate rapidly.[34] Enhanced dermal accumulation of AGEs was found in samples from UV-exposed

skin, with highest levels localizing to the elastic fiber network of solar elastosis.[34] Recently, the AGE receptor RAGE was demonstrated in skin,[35] where it was strongly expressed in fibroblasts, suggesting that AGE–RAGE interactions may influence the process of skin aging through mild stimulation of extracellular matrix gene expression.[35]

▌ IMMUNE SYSTEM

BOX 2-3   Summary

- While age-dependent defects in T- and B-cell functions are frequently observed in elderly patients, the essential elements of innate immunity appear to be remarkably well preserved.
- In both intrinsic aging and photoaging, Langerhans cells are reduced in density within the epidermis and display an atrophic morphology with fewer dendrites and Birbeck granules.
- Loss of immunosurveillance function in aging skin is thought to contribute to age-associated development of skin cancer.
- Age-related alterations in the adaptive immune system are associated with a loss of ability to recognize "self" and "foreign" antigens, which may result in the production of autoantibodies and an increased incidence of autoimmune diseases in the elderly.
- Clinical observations of decreased or variable contact hypersensitivity reactions among elderly patients have been linked to alterations in Langerhans cell frequency and function in aging skin.

Age-dependent alterations affecting both the defense against external insults and internal immunologic surveillance have been investigated in both the adaptive and innate parts of the immune system. Evidence for aging changes is strongest for adaptive immunity: alterations of the distribution of lymphocyte subsets, decline of T-cell functions including cytokine production, cell migration and an impaired reaction towards mitogens have all been described (reviewed in [36]). In contrast, little is known regarding defects of the innate immune system in aging. While age-dependent defects in T- and B-cell functions are frequently observed in elderly patients, the essential elements of innate immunity appear to be remarkably well preserved.[37]

There are significant differences between young and old skin with respect to both resting Langerhans cell numbers and their response to TNF-alpha. These age-related changes in Langerhans cell frequency and function have been suggested to contribute to the altered cutaneous immune function observed in the elderly.[38] In both intrinsic aging and photoaging Langerhans cells are reduced in density within the epidermis and display an atrophic morphology with fewer dendrites and Birbeck granules. It has been speculated that these morphological changes are associated with loss of dendritic cell functions, and that this contributes to age-associated development of skin cancer.[36] Furthermore, age-related alterations in the adaptive immune system have been shown to be accompanied by a loss of ability to recognize "self" and "foreign" antigens, which is thought to result in the production of autoantibodies and an increased incidence of autoimmune diseases.[39]

Compared to young adult controls, healthy older subjects are less able to manifest skin sensitivity to dinitrochlorobenzene (DNCB) or standard recall antigens,[40] reflecting the well-documented decrease in total number of circulating thymus-derived lymphocytes and in their responsiveness to standard mitogens, as well as the above-mentioned local cutaneous changes. The response patterns to patch testing in 1444 elderly subjects (>65 years) were recently compared with those of a control group of individuals aged between 20 and 40 years, both with suspected allergic contact dermatitis.[40] The data revealed an age-dependent decline of overall positive patch test reactions, but a higher sensitization rate to some allergens frequently used in the composition of topical treatments.[40] Furthermore, the frequency of fragrance allergy was found to be low in the first two decades of life (2.5 to 3.4%) and to gradually increase in females after the age of 20 years to peak in their 60s at 14.4%, then with a decline to 11.6% in their 80s. The prevalence in males rose more slowly and peaked at 13.7% in their 70s, declining to 10.8% in their 80s.[41] These findings support the hypothesis that allergy to fragrance results from a combination of repeated environmental exposure and age-related susceptibility factors including changes in the T-cell-mediated immune response. Since the development of an allergic response to patch testing was found to be delayed in elderly patients, an additional reading after 7 days and adjusted threshold for even weak reactions as valid positive patch test reactions was recently suggested.[40] The clinical observations of decreased or variable contact hypersensitivity reactions among elderly patients may be a reflection of the above-mentioned alterations in Langerhans cell frequency and function in aging skin. Furthermore, the frequently observed decrease in wound healing capability in the elderly has been linked to immunological factors. Studies in animal models and human skin indicate age-related shifts in both macrophage and T cell infiltration into wounds, alterations in chemokine content, and a concurrent decline in wound macrophage phagocytic function.[42] These alterations are likely to contribute to the delayed repair response of injured aging skin.

■ INTRINSIC SKIN AGING

BOX 2-4   Summary

- Intrinsic aging is manifested primarily by physiologic alterations with subtle but important consequences for both healthy and diseased skin.
- The most striking histological features of intrinsically aged dermis are considerable decreases in dermal thickness and vascularity, associated with a flat epidermal–dermal interface with loss of the dermal papillae.
- The age-associated loss of vascular bed, especially of the vertical capillary loops that occupy the dermal papillae in young skin, is felt to underlie many of the physiologic alterations in old skin, including palor, decreased skin temperature, and the dramatic reductions in cutaneous blood flow.
- Paradoxically, while papillary vascularization declines with age, aging skin exhibits a striking increase in vascular dysplasias, such as senile angiomata, angiokeratomata, purpura, palor, venous lake formation, and teleangiectasias.
- Aged skin exhibits a global reduction in stratum corneum lipids to about two-thirds that of young skin, resulting in a functional deficit of skin barrier function and repair.
- The appearance of rough, dry and flaky skin in the elderly, especially over the lower extremities, has been linked to a remarkable age-associated decrease in the content of epidermal filaggrin.
- Collagen I predominates in the reticular dermis and type III collagen in the papillary dermis as well as at sites of new collagen deposition. Diminished collagen synthesis found in intrinsically aged skin is believed to correlate with dermal atrophy and decreased wound healing ability.
- The skin of postmenopausal women exhibits decreased amounts of types I and III collagen compared to that of the premenopausal women.

Human skin provides an instructive contrast between intrinsic aging (elsewhere also referred to as "programmed," "chronological," "natural" or "genetic" aging), changes attributable to the passage of time alone, and the superimposed additional changes that result from environmental damage,[8] due mainly to solar UV irradiation and termed photoaging (also referred to as or "accelerated" or "extrinsic" aging). Photoaging has major morphologic as well as physiologic manifestations and corresponds more closely to the popular notion of old skin, while intrinsic aging is manifested primarily by physiologic alterations with subtle but undoubtedly important consequences for both healthy and diseased skin.[9]

Clinical, Histologic, and Ultrastructural Changes

STRATUM CORNEUM AND SKIN BARRIER

Age-related changes in the skin barrier, the stratum corneum (SC), have been recently reviewed.[43] Reduced content and synthesis of ceramides,[44] as well as reduced levels of cholesterol and free fatty acids[45] are found in aged SC. This global reduction in SC lipids to about two-thirds that of young SC explains the paucity of membrane structures in aged SC that underlie its functional barrier deficit. Reduced activities of the key rate-limiting enzymes for each of these lipids (serine palmitoyl transferase, HMGCoA reductase, and acetyl CoA carboxylase, sphingomyelinase, ceramide synthase) are in turn responsible.[46,47] The most profound abnormality is in cholesterol synthesis, and topical cholesterol-dominant lipid mixtures appear to normalize barrier function in aged epidermis.[43]

Although calcium levels are low in the basilar epidermis, extracellular and intracellular calcium levels peak in the outer stratum granulosum in young epidermis.[48] The epidermal calcium gradient serves at least two key functions: induction of terminal differentiation and regulation of exocytosis of lamellar bodies.[43] In aged epidermis, however, the calcium gradient is largely lost with calcium distributed more evenly throughout the epidermis,[49] due to either a decreased number or activity of ion pumps, ion channels, and/or ionotropic receptors in aged skin. This altered calcium gradient in aged epidermis has been postulated to account for the barrier abnormality.[49]

Few data are available on the presence and activity of enzymatic antioxidants such as catalase, superoxide dismutases (present in human skin as manganese and copper as well as zinc-dependent forms), and glutathione peroxidases in the SC. In most tissues, the highest catalase activities are found in the peroxisomes, where it constitutes about 50% of the peroxisomal protein. Remarkably high levels of catalase activity appear to persist in human SC[50] and protein levels of catalase of young adult SC are significantly higher than in SC of individuals 60 years and older.[23] These results were confirmed by Hellemans et al on the level of the enzyme activity of catalase.[51] While these studies suggest an increased vulnerability of the skin barrier with age, it remains to be investigated whether oral or topical supplementation with antioxidants can improve skin barrier function in aging skin.

EPIDERMIS Intrinsically aged skin is finely wrinkled, lax, dry, and rough, reflecting a loss of dermal cells and thus their secreted matrix proteins, in combination with subtle abnormalities of epidermal differentiation.[8] The most striking and consistent histological change in intrinsically aged skin is a flattening of the dermal–epidermal (DE) junction with effacement of both the dermal papillae and epidermal rete pegs (Table 2-1).[52] This is accompanied by >50% reduction in the number of DE interdigitations per unit skin surface length between the third and ninth decades of life. This results in a considerably smaller surface between the epidermis and dermis and presumably less communication and nutrient transfer. Dermal–epidermal separation has been demonstrated to occur more readily in old skin, undoubtedly explaining the propensity of the elderly to torn skin and superficial abrasions following minor trauma such as bandage removal and to bulla formation in edematous sites.[9]

Analysis of 96 abdominal skin samples using "mathematical morphology"[53] revealed that elderly subjects had a 36.3% decrease in rete peg-related roughness index when compared with younger subjects. For females, an abrupt descent occurs between 40 and 60 years of age, presumably in the perimenopausal period. In contrast, males show an almost monotonical decay. Epidermal thickness measured between rete pegs showed the same exponential decline for both sexes, with values from 22.6 to 11.4 μm.

More recently, histometric measurements by *in vivo* confocal laser scanning microscopy have been introduced as a very sensitive and noninvasive tool to characterize and quantify age-related histological changes of the epidermis and papillary dermis (Table 2-1).[54] Using this technique in volar forearm skin of young adults (18 to 25 years) and in individuals >65 years of age, the most dramatic age-related changes were observed in the number of papillae per area. As this parameter is closely linked to its function of supplying the epidermis with water and nutrients via the dermal vasculature, it was suggested as a more sensitive measure for qualitative evaluation of the epidermal junction than the measurement of height in histological sections. Less dramatic but still significant decreases were found for the thickness of the basal layer, while the size of cells in the granular layer, as well as, the size of corneocytes increases with age.[54] Measurements of skin surface topography using analysis of optical 3D measurements by mathematical algorithms (Fourier analysis) confirmed earlier findings using skin replica preparations on age-associated changes of the skin surface patterns, including increased furrow depth and overall

roughness.[55] The skin surface topography represents a patchwork of fine lines and furrows that is thought to be influenced by muscle and joint movements, as well as environmental factors.[56] Age effects on percutaneous absorption depend in part on drug structure, with hydrophilic substances such as hydrocortisone and benzoic acid being less well absorbed through the skin of old versus young individuals but with hydrophobic substances such as testosterone and estradiol being equally well absorbed.[57]

The appearance of rough, dry and flaky skin in the elderly, especially over the lower extremities, has been linked to a remarkable age-associated decrease in the content of epidermal filaggrin (Table 2-1). Filaggrin, required for binding of keratin filaments into macrofibrils, is also decreased in the skin of patients with ichthyosis vulgaris, and lack of filaggrin has been postulated to cause the increased scaliness in both conditions. Age-associated xerosis is thought to be caused by a decrease in the stratum corneum free amino acids, natural moisturizing factors derived from filaggrin. Since the expression of filaggrin mRNA in aged skin appears to be similar to that in young skin, the immunohistochemical decrease in filaggrin demonstrated in aged skin is thought to be caused by promotion of filaggrin proteolysis in the upper epidermal layers.[58] Epidermal turnover rate and thymidine-labeling index decrease approximately 30 to 50% between the third and eighth decades of life, with a corresponding prolongation in stratum corneum replacement rate. Linear growth rates also decrease for hair and nails, and the epidermal repair rate after wounding likewise declines with age.[9]

Table 2-1

Histologic and Ultrastructural Features of Aging Human Skin (Adapted From [9])

EPIDERMIS	DERMIS	APPENDAGES
Flattened dermal–epidermal junction	Atrophy (loss of dermal volume; most pronounced after seventh decade of life)	Depigmented hair
Variable thickness	Fewer fibroblasts	Conversion of terminal to vellus hair
Fewer Langerhans cells	Fewer mast cells	Loss of hair
Occasional nuclear atypia	Fewer blood vessels	Reduction in vascular network surrounding hair bulbs and glands
Fewer melanocytes	Shortened capillary loops	Atrophy and fibrosis of glands
Increased furrow depth	Abnormal nerve endings	Fewer total number of glands
Decrease in fillagrin	Decrease in subepidermal elastin in sun-protected and increase in sun-exposed skin	Abnormal nail plates
Decreased thickness of basal layer, increased size of corneocytes and cells in granular layer	Decrease of collagen types I and III in sun-exposed and sun-protected skin	

A decrease in the number of enzymatically active melanocytes per unit surface area of the skin, approximately 10 to 20% of the remaining cell population each decade of life, has been documented repeatedly, presumably reducing the body's protective barrier against UV radiation. The number of melanocytic nevi also decreases progressively with age, from a peak of 15 to 40 in the third and fourth decades of life to an average of four per person in the fifth decade of life; such nevi are rarely observed in persons beyond the age of 80 years.[9]

DERMIS Compared to photodamaged skin, sun-protected aged skin appears thinner, more evenly pigmented, laxer, and more finely lined.[59] The most striking histological features of intrinsically aged skin are considerable decreases in dermal thickness and vascularity,[60] associated with a flat epidermal–dermal interface with loss of the dermal papillae (Table 2-1). However, cellular polarity and normal epidermal differentiation appear to be maintained.[61] Using morphometric analysis on skin biopsies obtained from the upper inner arm, the age-dependent decrease of the total dermal thickness was found to decrease by 6% per decade of life, in both men and women.[62] Noninvasive ultrasound imaging of volar mid-forearm skin of 142 women revealed that the total skin thickness remains constant until the seventh decade of life, but diminishes thereafter.[63] Age-related changes in ultrasound studies appear to be dependent on body site as well as on the layer of the dermis. A progressive, age-related decrease in echogenicity of the upper dermis was found in sun-exposed regions (dorsal forearm, forehead), but not in moderately exposed regions (ventral forearm, ankle). However, the echogenicity of the lower dermis increased with age in all examined sites, including sun-protected sites.[64]

Key changes in cutaneous aging are thought to be related to changes in the extracellular dermal matrix. Deep expression lines, such as facial frown lines, most likely result from contractions of connective tissue septa within the subcutaneous fat. Hypodermal trabeculae of the retinacula cutis are broader and much shorter in wrinkled than in the surrounding skin. These trabeculae contain striated muscle cells. The hypertrophy of the extracellular matrix of the hypodermal septae is thought to be related to repetitive mechanical stimuli generated by the muscle cells.[65]

The striking age-associated loss of vascular bed, especially of the vertical capillary loops that occupy the dermal papillae in young skin, is felt to underlie many of the physiologic alterations in old skin, including palor, decreased skin temperature, and the approximately 60% reductions in basal and peak induced cutaneous blood flow.[66] Furthermore, reduction in the vascular network surrounding hair bulbs and eccrine, apocrine, and sebaceous glands may contribute to their gradual atrophy and fibrosis with age.[9]

Videocapillaroscopy analysis of human skin revealed that while the capillary loops in the dermal papillae decrease, the subpapillary plexus actually increases with age.[67]

Thermoregulatory cutaneous vasodilatation is attenuated in aged skin and thus predisposes the elderly to sometimes fatal heat stroke or hypothermia. The latter might be due to reduced vasoactivity of dermal arterioles, as well as to loss of subcutaneous fat.[9] In general, acetylcholine plays a role in thermally mediated vasodilation via nitric oxide (NO) and prostanoid-mediated pathways. There is an age-related shift toward cyclooxygenase vasoconstrictors contributing to basal cutaneous vasomotor tone. Older subjects have a diminished prostanoid contribution to acetylcholine-mediated vasodilatation.[68] Furthermore, cutaneous vasoconstriction in response to cooling is attenuated in older individuals. While cutaneous vasoconstriction in young skin is mediated by both noradrenaline and sympathetic cotransmitters, reflex vasoconstriction in aged skin is overall attenuated compared to young and appears to be mediated solely by noradrenaline.[69]

Impaired angiogenesis in aging is associated with a complex interplay of alterations in vessel density, matrix composition, inflammatory response, and growth factor expression.[70] Defects in the activation of nitric oxide synthases result in decreased nitric oxide production in aged skin relative to young skin. The subsequent lack of nitric oxide levels is thought to contribute to impaired angiogenesis in aging.[71] Paradoxically, while angiogenesis in the elderly is generally thought to decline with age (Tables 2-1 and 2-2), aging skin exhibits a striking increase in vascular dysplasias such as senile angiomata, angiokeratomata, purpura, palor, venous lake formation, and teleangiectasias. This might be due to local compensatory mechanisms, such as an age-related decreased expression of potent angiogenesis inhibitors, such as early population doubling level cDNA-1 (EPC-1).[72] A local pro-angiogenetic environment is likely to be involved in the development of cutaneous vascular diseases, as well as increased tumor growth and metastasis developing in the elderly. On a cellular level, endothelial cell aging and survival have been linked to proliferation, quiescence, apoptosis, and senescence as the four principal cytologic states that set the cutaneous microvasculature in a dynamic balance between maintenance and remodeling.[73]

Age-associated decreases in wheal resorption and dermal clearance of transepidermally absorbed materials have been reported,[74] probably due to alterations in both the vascular bed and the extracellular matrix. Conversely, the time required for development of a tense blister after topical ammonium hydroxide application is nearly twice as long in older individuals, suggesting a decreased transudation rate with age in injured skin.[74]

Collagen is a main constituent of the skin and provides the major support for skin resistance. The most abundant type, collagen I, predominates in the reticular dermis and type III collagen in the papillary dermis as well as at sites of new collagen deposition. Diminished collagen synthesis found in intrinsically aged skin is believed to correlate with

Table 2-2

Functions of Human Skin That Decline With Age (Adapted From [9])

- Cell replacement/turnover
- Barrier repair
- Chemical clearance
- Sensory perception
- Mechanical protection
- Wound healing
- Antioxidant protection
- Immune responsiveness
- Thermoregulation
- Sweat production
- Sebum production
- Vitamin D production
- DNA repair

dermal atrophy and decreased wound healing ability.[61] The elastic tissue is lost primarily in the fine subepidermal elaunin network. However, within the reticular dermis, the elastic network is irregularly thickened, fragmented, and disorganized. Immunohistochemical analysis of elastin and collagen types I and III in skin biopsies obtained from all age groups (first through ninth decade of life; all phototype IV) showed that there is gradual accumulation of elastin in sun-exposed skin and its loss and fragmentation in protected skin (Table 2-1). This is accompanied by a gradual reduction in the amount of collagen fibers in both sun-exposed and protected skin. In all age groups, the amount of elastin is higher in facial skin than in abdominal skin.[61] In contrast, the amount of both type I and type III collagen in older individuals was significantly lower in facial skin than in the abdominal skin.

Biochemical changes in collagen, elastin, and dermal ground substance during fetal and early postnatal development are far greater than those described with advancing age, but collagen content per unit area of skin surface decreases approximately 1% per year throughout adult life[75] and the remaining collagen fibrils appear disorganized, more compact, and granular.[76] Collagen damage is believed to be due, at least in part, to degradation by matrix metalloproteinases (MMP) released from epidermal keratinocytes and dermal fibroblasts, as MMP levels in skin increase as a function of age.[77] In addition to increased expression of enzymes that degrade collagen, decreased synthesis of procollagen also contributes to intrinsic skin aging. There is a sustained reduction in collagen synthesis in naturally aged skin as compared to young skin, which is considered a reflection of an intrinsic reduction in the capacity of old fibroblasts to synthesize collagen.[77] There is experimental evidence suggesting that MMP-mediated collagen damage could be responsible, at least in part, for the reduction in collagen production seen in both aged and, to an even greater degree, in photodamaged skin.[78]

Although many studies have been devoted to the age-related changes affecting collagen and elastin, little is known about other main components of the extracellular matrix, such as glycosaminoglycans (GAG) and proteoglycans. Small leucine-rich proteoglycans (SLURPs) belong to the family of proteoglycans and are strongly implicated in cell regulation. The major proteoglycans detected in extracts of human skin are decorin and versican.[79] In addition, adult human skin contains a truncated form of decorin, whereas fetal skin contains virtually undetectable levels of this truncated decorin. The detection of a catabolic fragment of decorin suggests the existence of a specific catabolic pathway for this proteoglycan. Because of the capacity of decorin to influence collagen fibrillogenesis, catabolism of decorin may have important functional implications with respect to the dermal collagen network.[79] Although total GAG synthesis and the expression of another SLURP, lumican, is decreased in aged skin, the rate of hyaloran synthesized by human skin fibroblasts increases during aging.[80] The total hyaluronan content of the dermis may be decreased in aged skin, however, since the activity of hyaluran degrading enzymes, hyaluronidases, appears to be increased, leading to a more rapid degradation of neosynthesized hyaluronan in the dermis.[80] These changes may adversely influence skin turgor because proteoglycans bind up to 1000 times their own weight in water.

The skin of postmenopausal women exhibits decreased amount of types I and III collagen as well as a decreased type III/I ratio in comparison with premenopausal women. Several controlled studies have demonstrated beneficial effects of estrogen replacement therapies on skin collagen content or skin thickness (reviewed in [81]). After menopause, skin elasticity was calculated to decline by 0.55% per year, while 12 months of hormone replacement therapy increased elasticity by 5.2%.[82] In addition to the occurrence of signs of aging skin such as wrinkles, such changes likely contribute to impaired wound healing in the elderly.

Changes in the mechanical properties of the skin during adulthood include progressive loss of elastic recovery, consistent with gradual destruction of the dermal elastic network, and marked prolongation of the time required for excised skin to return to its original thickness after compression (Table 2-2).[9] In vivo studies of ventral forearm skin of 133 volunteers in each decade of life revealed linear declines during adulthood of approximately 25% in both men and women for elasticity and extensibility.[83] Loss of elasticity began in childhood and continued through the ninth decade of life, whereas extensibility was constant through the sixth decade of life and then declined more rapidly thereafter. In another study in healthy women of various age groups, clinical wrinkling grades were related to measurements of the mechanical and ultrastructural properties of the skin using in vivo confocal microscopy and ultrasound imaging.[84] Skin elasticity, extensibility and echogenicity decreased with age. Wrinkling appeared to correlate well with loss of both elasticity and echogenicity in the upper dermis, which is thought to reflect structural tissue weakening.[84] Overall, a picture emerges of aging dermis as an increasingly rigid, inelastic, and unresponsive tissue that is less capable of undergoing modifications in response to stress.[9]

■ PHOTOAGING

BOX 2-5   Summary

- Solar ultraviolet radiation (UVR) is by far the most important environmental factor in premature skin aging, a process accordingly also termed photoaging.

- Photoaging exhibits features that are found exclusively in sun-exposed skin, making it an independent entity with its own pathophysiology.

- The most prominent dermal feature of photoaged skin is elastosis, which generally begins at the junction of the papillary and reticular dermis and is characterized histologically by tangled masses of degraded elastic fibers that further deteriorate to form an amorphous mass.

- Other prominent features are the replacement of mature collagen fibers by collagen with a distinct basophilic appearance, called basophilic degeneration, and increased deposition of glycosaminoglycans.

- The finding of increased inflammatory cells, including mast cells, histiocytes, and other mononuclear cells in chronically sun-exposed skin gave rise to the term *heliodermatitis*.

- Exposure of human skin to solar UVR initiates a complex sequence of specific molecular responses involving cell surface receptors, protein kinase signal transduction pathways, transcription factors, and enzymes that synthesize and degrade structural dermal proteins.

- Photochemical generation of ROS activates signaling pathways involved in remodeling of the extracellular matrix and causes accumulation of oxidatively damaged DNA, lipids and proteins in photoaging skin.

- The number of UVR induced mitochondrial DNA deletions correlates well with the patient age and may thus serve as biomarker for photoaged skin.

Among all environmental factors that human skin is exposed to, solar ultraviolet radiation (UVR) is by far the most important in premature skin aging, a process accordingly also termed photoaging.[32] Photoaged, chronically sun-exposed skin has a number of characteristics in common with sun-protected, chronologically aged skin. However, it exhibits features that are found exclusively in photoaged skin, making it an independent entity with its own pathophysiology. Both UVB (290–320 nm) and UVA (320–400 nm) radiation contribute to photoaging. The shorter wavelengths of UVB radiation cause erythema and sunburn, as well as DNA damage and skin cancer. UVA radiation can also cause erythema, but at levels about 1000 times higher than those required for UVB.[60] While photoaging preferentially affects individuals with lighter skin color[59] (skin phototypes I and II), photoaging also affects individuals with darker skin types (III and IV) with a history of ample past sun exposure.[9]

Photoaged skin by definition is present in areas that are habitually exposed to the sun and may appear not only dry but "coarse" and, depending on the individual's genetic endowment, also permanently "bronzed" with freckles and/or lentigines. Darker-skinned severely photodamaged individuals may have deep furrows, in addition to fine wrinkling, while fair-skinned comparably sun-exposed individuals tend to present with atrophic skin, multiple telangiectases and a variety of premalignant and malignant lesions.[8]

Modern techniques employing objective image processing and the precise and automatic calculation of skin topography parameters (roughness, developed surface area and peak-trough amplitude) and anisotropy (level of anisotropy and furrow density) were recently developed and studied on the forearms and temples of 40 men and 40 women including subjects in two age groups, 25–35 years and 50–65 years. The roughness of both sites increases with age, independent of sex, but to a lesser extent in women than in men. The developed surface area and the peak–trough amplitude increase significantly with age irrespective of the site and the sex. The level of anisotropy increases with age, in both men and women, on the forearm and the temple, the site more exposed to light being more affected. The density of the furrows decreases with age in both sexes and both sites but with a greater increase for the sun-exposed temple.[85]

Histologically, the stratum corneum may be thickened but is usually normal appearing. In contrast with the frequently atrophic epidermis in intrinsically aged skin, photodamaged skin frequently displays acanthosis and increased thickness of the basal membrane, with an irregular distribution of melanocytes that vary widely in size, dendricity, and pigmentation.[86] The most prominent dermal feature of photoaged skin is elastosis, often referred to as solar elastosis. Elastosis generally begins at the junction of the papillary and reticular dermis[87] and is characterized histologically by tangled masses of degraded elastic fibers that further deteriorate to form an amorphous mass.[86] Other prominent features are the replacement of mature collagen fibers by collagen with a distinct basophilic appearance, called basophilic degeneration, and increased deposition of glycosaminoglycans. Solar elastosis is primarily derived from elastic fibers and not from preexisting or newly synthesized collagens.[88] The finding of increased inflammatory cells, including mast cells, histiocytes, and other mononuclear cells in chronically sun-exposed skin gave rise to the term *heliodermatitis*.[9]

The clinical and histological characteristics of photoaged skin have been known for some time, but the underlying molecular mechanisms, although not yet fully understood, began to be elucidated only during the past decade of life. Exposure of human skin to solar UVR initiates a complex sequence of specific molecular responses involving cell surface receptors, protein kinase signal transduction pathways, transcription factors, and enzymes that synthesize and degrade structural dermal proteins.[59] Photochemical generation of ROS leads to cellular responses that alter skin connective tissue by direct oxidative modification of cellular components (i.e., DNA, proteins, and lipids),[23] ultimately contributing to photoaging.[43,59] The ROS thought to initiate molecular responses in human skin include superoxide anion radicals, hydrogen peroxide, and singlet oxygen.[32,59,89] The mechanisms of receptor activation by UV irradiation are not completely understood, but well documented.[90] In keratinocytes, NADPH oxidase activity is induced within 20 minutes following UV exposure, and pharmacological inhibition of UV-induced NADPH oxidase abrogates UV-induced hydrogen peroxide generation.[59] Thus, NADPH oxidase is a major enzymatic source of hydrogen peroxide production following UV irradiation in human keratinocytes.[59]

Within one hour of exposure, UVR activates protein kinase-mediated signaling pathways that up-regulate expression and functional activation of the nuclear transcription factor AP-1 (composed of Jun and Fos proteins) that subsequently stimulates transcription of genes for matrix-degrading enzymes, such as metalloproteinase (MMP)-1 (collagenase), MMP-3 (stromelysin 1), and MMP-9 (92-kDa gelatinase).[90] MMP-1 initiates cleavage of fibrillar collagen (type I and III in skin) at a single site within its central triple helix. Remarkably, UV-induction of metalloproteinase proteins and activities occurs at doses well below those that cause erythema; and all-*trans* retinoic acid, which transrepresses AP-1, applied before irradiation with UVB, substantially reduces AP-1 and metalloproteinase induction.[91] Once cleaved by MMP-1, collagen can be further degraded by elevated levels of MMP-3 and MMP-9. UVR-induced MMPs degrade skin collagen and thereby impair the structural integrity of the dermis. The TGF-beta/SMAD pathway is another major AP-1 dependent regulator of collagen production in connective tissue that has recently been shown to be relevant for photoaging.[92] Interestingly, major critical mediators of photoaging, such as the transcription factor AP-1 and AP-1–regulated MMPs both play critical roles in tumor formation, inflammation, and fibrosis.[59] The level of matrix metalloproteinase-1 protein and the activity of matrix metalloproteinase-2 are higher in the dermis of photoaged skin than in naturally aged skin.[93] These findings suggest that the natural aging process decreases collagen synthesis and increases the expression of matrix metalloproteinases, whereas photoaging results in an increase of collagen synthesis and greater matrix metalloproteinase expression in human skin *in vivo*.[93]

Collagen fragmentation and clumping is found in aged skin, but clearly more pronounced in photoaged skin. There is experimental evidence suggesting that damaged collagen, presumably caused by matrix metalloproteinases, may be responsible for the reduction in collagen production seen in photoaged skin.[78] Since photoaging correlates well with loss of endogenous dermal antioxidant protection and severe oxidative protein damage,[23] oxidatively modified proteins of the extracellular dermal matrix may also play a role in decreased collagen production. In biopsies from individuals with histologically confirmed solar elastosis, an accumulation of oxidatively modified proteins was found specifically within the upper dermis. Protein oxidation in photoaged skin is most likely due to UV irradiation because repetitive exposure of human buttock skin over 10 days to increasing UV doses, as well as *in vitro* irradiation of cultured dermal fibroblasts with UVB or UVA has been shown to cause protein oxidation.[23] The functional relevance of increased protein oxidation in the pathogenesis of photoaging is not yet understood. However, there is some recent experimental evidence that increased protein oxidation resulting from a single exposure of cultured human fibroblasts to UVA radiation inhibits proteasomal function and thereby affects intracellular signaling pathways involved in MMP-1 expression.[32]

Most if not all age-accelerating environmental factors damage DNA either directly or indirectly.[5] UVR directly affects DNA forming pyrimidine dimers (mostly caused by UVB) and indirectly via UV-generated ROS that cause oxidative DNA lesions (mostly UVA). Both mechanisms of DNA damage have been linked to carcinogenesis and are also thought to play a role in photoaging (see Fig. 2-2). The unique characteristics of photoaged skin, including its predisposition to cancer, reflect superimposed UV-induced DNA mutations in key regulatory genes that accumulate during the telomere-driven aging process.[8] Besides nuclear DNA, UVR also damages mitochondrial DNA (mtDNA), through ROS either generated by "electron leaks" in the mitochondrial electron-transport chain (intrinsic aging) or by UVA exposure. The latter mechanism, which is superimposed on the former, has been shown to be mediated largely by singlet oxygen and to occur in repetitively UVA irradiated skin in an experimental setting, as well as in photoaged human skin (reviewed in [32]).

AGING AND SKIN CANCER

BOX 2-6   Summary

- The incidence of both melanoma and nonmelanoma skin cancers increases exponentially with age.
- Despite recent trends showing improved survival and stabilization of incidence rates in younger Americans, melanoma incidence and mortality continue to rise unabated in older individuals, particularly in men over age 55.
- The capacity of DNA damage repair mechanisms decreases, while oncogene activation and the frequency of defects in tumor suppressor genes increases with aging.

The incidence of both melanoma and nonmelanoma skin cancers increases exponentially with age.[94] During the aging process, many biologic factors contribute to the increased risk of developing cancer, including increasing cumulative carcinogenic exposure and increased cellular susceptibility to DNA damage induced by carcinogens. The latter is thought to be due to an age-related decrease in cellular DNA repair capacity (Table 2-2).[95,96] Secondary to this decrease in DNA damage repair associated with aging, oncogene activation and amplification also occur, as does the frequency of defects in tumor suppressor genes. Population studies using peripheral blood lymphocytes, transformed lymphoblastoid cells, and primary skin fibroblasts have shown that human DNA repair capacity decreases with increasing age.[96,97] Reduced DNA repair capacity was a particularly important risk factor for young individuals with basal cell cancer (BCC; see Chapter 6) and for those individuals with a family history of skin cancer. Interestingly, young individuals (first two decades of life) with BCC repaired DNA damage poorly when compared with age-matched controls. Patients with reduced DNA repair capacities and overexposure to sunlight had an estimated risk of BCC, which is fivefold greater than the control group. Such a risk was even greater (10-fold) in female subjects.[97] In a more recent study in Japanese individuals of various age groups, the mRNA expression of DNA repair synthesis-related genes (DNA polymerase δ, replication factor C, and proliferating cell nuclear antigen) were markedly decreased in cells obtained from multiple elderly subjects compared to those from young subjects.[98] Therefore, it was concluded that the reduced post-UV DNA repair capacity in aging results from an impairment in the latter step of nucleotide excision repair by the decreased expression of factors in DNA repair synthesis.[98]

A recent study analyzed the number of mtDNA deletions in excised nonmelanoma skin cancers, as well as in the photodamaged tumor-free margins.[99] The number of mtDNA deletions correlated well with the patient's age and may thus serve as a biomarker for photoaged skin. However, significantly fewer deletions were detected in the tumors than in the tumor-free margins and the tumors often had no deletions, implying a potential selection for full-length mtDNA or perhaps even a protective role for mtDNA deletions in the process of tumorigenesis.[99]

Melanoma (see Chapter 11) accounts for the majority of skin cancer deaths worldwide and has dramatically increased in incidence over the past half-century.[100] Despite recent trends showing improved survival, and stabilization of incidence rates in younger Americans, melanoma incidence and mortality continue to rise unabated in older individuals, particularly in men over age 55.[100] Elderly men present with melanomas that are thicker than those of young adults, presumably in part because of difficulties or disinterest in properly examining their skin.[9] Other skin cancers with a high mean age of onset are discussed in detail in other chapters (see Chapters 13 and 15).

PREVENTION AND TREATMENT

BOX 2-7   Summary

- Prevention of photodamage by the use of adequate sun protection and sunscreens is considered the most effective strategy against photoaging.
- Inadequate use and incomplete protection from larger UV wavelengths may compromise the benefit from sunscreen use more than previously expected.
- The beneficial effects of topical retinoids are clinically modest but have been well documented in several double-blind, vehicle-controlled trials involving large number of subjects. The antiaging effects of topical retinoids are dose-dependent and increase with duration of therapy for at least 10 to 12 months.
- While many *in vitro* and *in vivo* studies have convincingly demonstrated that oxidative stress is increased in skin aging, the ability of topically applied antioxidants to prevent or reduce skin aging has not yet been demonstrated in large, controlled human studies.
- Considering the many common pathways of photoaging and photocarcinogenesis, it is conceivable that improvement or prevention of skin aging by means of sunscreens in combination with retinoids and antioxidants will go hand in hand with skin cancer prevention.

PHOTOPROTECTION Protection from the sun is critical to the prevention of both melanoma and nonmelanoma skin cancers, and protection is most effective when it is begun in early childhood. It is especially important to protect against intermittent sun exposures, in order to reduce genomic damage at a time of maximal cellular vulnerability and to reduce the risk of melanoma.[94] In addition to staying out of the sun, good protection strategies include wearing hats and other clothing. Sunscreen active ingredients now are incorporated into cosmetics products such as facial moisturizers to minimize photoaging changes. With the advances in technologies, several new UV filters with improved efficacy and safety have been developed recently (reviewed in [101]; see Chapter 55). In animals, the use of sunscreens has allowed repair of preexisting damage and prevented further damage caused by exposure to UVR. In a randomized trial of photodamaged adults, the use of a sunscreen with an SPF of 29 for two years stabilized histologic changes to the skin, whereas such photoaging increased in the placebo group (reviewed in [102]). Similar findings were noted in a 6-month randomized prospective trial of retinoic acid as a treatment for photoaged skin, in which the placebo (sunscreen only) group showed statistically significant modest improvement in objective measures of photoaging from their baseline status, albeit less improvement than the retinoic acid plus sunscreen group.[103] These data suggest an intrinsic repair capacity for photoaging and a central role for photoprotection in any treatment regimen. It should be noted, however, that several studies show that inadequate use and incomplete protection from larger UV wavelengths efficacy may compromise benefit from sunscreen use more than previously expected.[104]

All-*trans*-Retinoic Acids/Retinoids (See Also Chapters 53 and 55)

Although topical retinoids (vitamin A derivatives) were initially controversial, it is now accepted that they reduce the severity of photoaging.[102] The ability of topical retinoic acid, also termed tretinoin, to improve photoaging changes in skin was first suggested by studies in the rhino mouse model[105] and later confirmed in photoaged human skin.[106] Clinically modest but highly statistically significant improvements in global appearance, surface roughness, fine and coarse wrinkling, mottled pigmentation, and sallowness were shown subsequently in several double-blind, vehicle-controlled trials involving more than 700 subjects (reviewed in [60]). The beneficial effects are dose-dependent and increase with duration of therapy for at least 10 to 12 months. Reduction and redistribution of epidermal melanin

parallel improvement in mottled hyperpigmentation and lentigines.[60,107] Daily treatment of photodamaged skin with a 0.1% tretinoin cream for 10–12 months produced an 80% increase in collagen I formation in the papillary dermis, as compared to a 14% decrease in collagen formation with the use of vehicle alone.[108] In a recent 2-year placebo-controlled study to assess the safety and efficacy of long-term use of a 0.05% tretinoin cream for facial photodamage,[109] tretinoin significantly improved several clinical signs of photodamage (fine and coarse wrinkling, mottled hyperpigmentation, lentigines, and sallowness). Histologic evaluation did not show any increase in keratinocytic or melanocytic atypia, or negative effects on the stratum corneum, suggesting long term use of 0.05% tretinoin cream is effective and safe.[109]

Tretinoin effects on photoaged skin are presumed to be mediated through binding to the nuclear retinoic acid receptors (RARs) with subsequent binding of retinoic acid–RAR complexes to specific response elements in regulated genes.[59] In addition to reversing photoaging changes, it has been shown that tretinoin therapy blocks dermal matrix degradation following sun exposure.[108] Pretreatment of human skin with tretinoin inhibited induction of the AP-1 transcription factor and AP-1-regulated matrix-degrading metalloproteinases that otherwise followed even suberythemogenic UV exposures.[110] Tretinoin did not interfere with UV-induced upregulation of TIMP, the tissue inhibitor of metalloproteinases, thus favoring collagen preservation.[110]

In addition to tretinoin, another topical retinoid, tazarotene, has been approved by the Food and Drug Administration (FDA) for the treatment of the fine wrinkles and irregular pigmentation of photoaging.[102] A recent multicenter, randomized, double-blind trial of tazarotene 0.1% cream for the treatment of photodamage demonstrated that tazarotene cream was a significantly more effective than vehicle in reducing fine wrinkles, mottled hyperpigmentation, lentigines, irregular depigmentation, apparent pore size, elastosis, tactile roughness, and an overall integrated assessment of photodamage.[111] In this study, significance was achieved as early as week 2 for some parameters and had not plateaued by week 24. The majority of patients reported improvements in their photodamage as early as week 4. Adverse events were predominantly mild or moderate signs or symptoms of skin irritation.

It remains to be investigated in future studies whether tazarotene is more efficacious and/or less irritating than tretinoin.

Barrier Lipids

Although unperturbed aged epidermis displays normal barrier function, barrier recovery kinetics is delayed after acute insults, with a further delay in photoaged skin (Table 2-2). Based on the lipid biochemical abnormalities found in aged epidermis, it was investigated which type of SC lipid mixtures could correct this functional abnormality (reviewed in [43]). In young murine or human skin, any incomplete mixture of one or two of the three major lipid species (cholesterol, ceramides, and free fatty acids) worsens barrier function. In contrast, equimolar mixtures of the three key lipids allow normal rates of barrier recovery in young skin. Further adjustment of the three-component mixtures to 3:1:1 molar ratio actually accelerates barrier recovery significantly, and in young skin, each of the three key species can predominate. In contrast, in aged epidermis, with its global decline in lipid synthesis and profound abnormality in cholesterol synthesis, the requirements for barrier repair are quite different. Topical cholesterol alone, which delays barrier recovery in young skin, accelerates barrier recovery in aged murine and human skin.[46] These results underscore the selective abnormality in cholesterol synthesis that characterizes the aged epidermal permeability barrier. This concept has led to commercially available products addressing repair of the aged skin barrier, the efficacy of which is currently being tested in controlled studies.

Antioxidants

As outlined in this chapter, many fundamental pathophysiological mechanisms (e.g., DNA damage, regulation of longevity genes, protein oxidation, regulation of MMP-mediated collagen damage) underlying both intrinsic aging and photoaging are mediated at least in part by ROS.

While many *in vitro* and *in vivo* studies have convincingly demonstrated that ROS generated oxidative stress is increased in skin aging (reviewed in [18]), the ability of topically applied antioxidants to prevent or treat skin aging has not yet been demonstrated in large, controlled human studies.

Despite the fact that the sunscreen effect of most topical antioxidants is very modest, it has been suggested to improve the efficacy and stability of sunscreens by combination with synergistically acting antioxidants.[112] Interestingly, an *in vivo* electron spin resonance spectroscopy in Caucasian individuals was carried out to test the protection against ROS formation afforded by three high factor sunscreens that claim ultraviolet A (UVA) protection.[113] A "free-radical protection factor" calculated on the basis of these results was only 2 at the recommended application level, which contrasts strongly with the erythema-based sun protection factors (mainly indicative of ultraviolet B (UVB) protection) quoted by the manufacturers (20+).[113] Since ROS have been linked to carcinogenesis and aging, this study has sparked a debate about the safety of sunscreen use and the adequacy of currently available methods for testing the sun-protection factor. Another similar study found that sunscreens reduced the amount of ROS induced in the viable epidermis by a factor that correlated with the SPF.[114] The addition of the bioconvertible antioxidants vitamin E acetate and sodium ascorbyl phosphate improved photoprotection by converting to vitamins E and C, respectively, within the skin. The bioconversion apparently forms an antioxidant reservoir that deactivates the ROS generated within the strata granulosum, spinosum, and basale by the UV photons that sunscreens do not block or absorb.[114]

A significant body of research supports the use of cosmeceuticals containing vitamin C. Cutaneous benefits include the promotion of collagen synthesis, photoprotection from UVB and UVA, lightening hyperpigmentation, and reduction of inflammation (recently reviewed in [115] and [18]). A double-blind, half-face study compared the effects of topical vitamin C (10% water soluble ascorbic acid and 7% tetrahexyldecyl ascorbate (lipid soluble) in an anhydrous polysilicone gel base to one-half of the face and the vehicle polysilicone gel base to the other half. Clinically visible and statistically significant improvement in wrinkling was reported when used topically for 12 weeks, correlating with biopsy evidence of new collagen formation.[116] In a similar study, repeated topical application in facial skin (twice daily for 6 months) of a preparation containing both retinol and vitamin C was shown to reverse, at least in part, skin changes induced by both chronologic aging and photoaging and was suggested to be superior to the individual components.[117] In pig skin, a stable aqueous solution of 15% L-ascorbic acid (vitamin C) and 1% alpha-tocopherol (vitamin E) was tested against the vehicle for photoprotection against solar simulated irradiation. The combination of 15% L-ascorbic acid and 1% alpha-tocopherol provided significant protection against erythema and sunburn cell formation; either L-ascorbic acid or 1% alpha-tocopherol alone also was protective but the combination was superior. Application during 4 days provided progressive protection that yielded an "antioxidant protection factor" of 4. In addition, the combination of vitamins C and E provided protection against thymine dimer formation.[118] In a similar experimental setting, the antioxidant alpha-lipoic acid, which has been marketed as an antiaging compound, proved ineffective as a topical antioxidant for photoprotection of skin.[119] However, ferulic acid, a highly abundant phenolic phytochemical with antioxidant properties, when incorporated into a topical solution of 15% L-ascorbic acid and 1% alpha-tocopherol improved the chemical stability of the vitamin C and vitamin E, and doubled photoprotection against solar-simulated irradiation of skin from fourfold to approximately eightfold, as measured by both erythema and sunburn cell formation and efficiently reduced thymine dimer formation.[120] The combination of low molecular weight antioxidants appears to provide meaningful synergistic protection against oxidative stress in skin and may also be useful for protection against photoaging and skin cancer.

Pretreatment of human skin with the soy isoflavone genistein, known to have both antioxidant and estrogenic properties, inhibits ultraviolet-induced epidermal growth factor receptor tyrosine kinase activity as well as ultraviolet induction of both extracellular signal-regulated kinase and cJun N-terminal protein kinase activities.[121] Pretreatment of human skin with the water-soluble low-molecular antioxidant N-acetyl cysteine (NAC) inhibits extracellular signal-regulated kinase but not cJun N-terminal protein kinase activation. Both genistein and N-acetyl cysteine were shown to prevent ultraviolet induction of cJun protein. Consistent with this, genistein and N-acetyl cysteine blocked ultraviolet induction of cJun-driven enzyme collagenase. Neither genistein nor N-acetyl cysteine acted as sunscreens, as they had no effect on ultraviolet-induced erythema. These data indicate that compounds similar to genistein and N-acetyl cysteine, which possess tyrosine kinase inhibitory and/or antioxidant activities, may prevent photoaging.[121] However, confirmation in larger controlled human studies is needed. Specific squalene monohydroperoxide isomers were identified as highly ultraviolet A sensitive skin surface lipid breakdown products that may serve as a marker for photooxidative stress *in vitro* and *in vivo*.[122] In animal models, squalene hydroperoxides have been shown to induce comedogenesis and wrinkling.[123,124] Topical treatment with products containing natural vitamin E significantly inhibited photooxidation of squalene and thus may help to maintain the integrity of the skin barrier by providing protection against photooxidative stress at the level of skin surface lipids.[125] Again, while numerous small animal and human studies provide evidence for a photoprotective role of topical vitamin E formulations (reviewed in [126]), larger controlled human trials are lacking.

Many other natural, plant derived and synthetic antioxidants have been reported to exhibit photoprotective and anticarcinogenic properties (reviewed in [18]). In contrast to evidence provided for the efficacy of topical retinoids as antiaging compounds, there are no large, placebo controlled, double-blinded studies confirming the efficacy of many compounds with antioxidative properties.[126] Recent work in this field is based on a better understanding of the physiologic antioxidant network (Fig. 2-1), and focuses on increased efficacy of antioxidant combinations, adjunctive sunscreens, and combination of topical and oral antioxidant intake. Considering the many common pathways of photoaging and photocarcinogenesis addressed in this chapter, as well as the promising anticarcinogenic effects described for many topical and oral antioxidants (see Chapters 53 and 54) it is conceivable that improvement or prevention of skin aging by means of retinoids and antioxidants will go hand in hand with skin cancer prevention.

FINAL THOUGHTS

Skin aging results from a genetically determined program with superimposed environmental injuries, cumulated over a lifetime. Photoaging, the combination of chronic photodamage and intrinsic aging, is a large component of perceived skin aging. Direct UV damage and indirect oxidative damage to DNA and other cellular constituents drive the skin-aging processes. As a corollary, sun protection and optimizing antioxidant defenses are logical steps to reduce or delay unwanted age-associated changes. In addition to preventive measures, effective therapies for aged skin are theoretically possible, but the field is in its infancy.

REFERENCES

1. Yancik R. Population aging and cancer: a cross-national concern. *Cancer J.* 2005; 11:437–441.
2. U.S. Census Bureau, 2005, pp. http://www.census.gov/Press-Release/www/releases/archives/cb05-ff.07.pdf
3. Diepgen TL, Mahler V. The epidemiology of skin cancer. *Br J Dermatol.* 2002;146(suppl 61):1–6.
4. Kosmadaki MG, Gilchrest BA. The demographics of aging in the United States: implications for dermatology. *Arch Dermatol.* 2002;138:1427–1428.
5. Lombard DB, et al. DNA repair, genome stability, and aging. *Cell* 2005; 120:497–512.
6. Masoro EJ. Aging. In: Masoro EJ, ed. *Current Concepts in Aging.* Oxford, UK: University Press; 1995:3–24.
7. Kenyon C. The plasticity of aging: insights from long-lived mutants. *Cell.* 2005;120:449–460.
8. Kosmadaki MG, Gilchrest BA. The role of telomeres in skin aging/photoaging. *Micron* 2004;35:155–159.
9. Yaar M, Gilchrest BA. Aging of skin. In: Freedberg IM, et al, eds. Fitzpatrick's *Dermatology in General Medicine.* New York: McGraw-Hill; 2003:1386–1398.
10. Nakamura K, et al. Comparative analysis of telomere lengths and erosion with age in human epidermis and lingual epithelium. *J Invest Dermatol.* 2002;119: 1014–1019.
11. Gilhar A, et al. Ageing of human epidermis: the role of apoptosis, Fas and telomerase. *Br J Dermatol.* 2004;150: 56–63.
12. Campisi J. Replicative senescence: an old lives' tale? *Cell.* 1996;84:497–500.
13. Khorramizadeh MR, et al. Aging differentially modulates the expression of collagen and collagenase in dermal fibroblasts. *Mol Cell Biochem.* 1999;194:99–108.
14. Campisi J. Senescent cells, tumor suppression, and organismal aging: good citizens, bad neighbors. *Cell.* 2005;120: 513–522.
15. Harman D. Aging: a theory based on free radical and radiation chemistry. *J Gerontol.* 1956;11:298–300.
16. Beckman KB, Ames BN. The free radical theory of aging matures. *Physiol Rev.* 1998;78:547–581.
17. Hekimi S, Guarente L. Genetics and the specificity of the aging process. *Science.* 2003;299:1351–1354.
18. Thiele JJ, Dreher F. Antioxidant defense systems in skin. In: Elsner P, Maibach H, eds. *Cosmeceuticals and Active Cosmetics.* New York: Taylor & Francis; 2005:37–87.
19. Hamilton IM, et al. Interactions between vitamins C and E in human subjects. *Br J Nutr.* 2000;84(3):261–267.
20. Stadtman ER. Protein oxidation and aging. *Science.* 1992;257:1220–1224.
21. Berlett BS, Stadtman ER. Protein oxidation in aging, disease, and oxidative stress. *J Biol Chem.* 1997;272:20313–20316.
22. Oliver CN, et al. Age-related changes in oxidized proteins. *J Biol Chem.* 1987; 262:5488.
23. Sander CS, et al. Photoaging is associated with protein oxidation in human skin in vivo. *J Invest Dermatol.* 2002;118: 618–625.
24. Stadtman ER. Protein oxidation in aging and age-related diseases. *Ann N Y Acad Sci.* 2001;928:22–38.
25. Moskovitz J, et al. Methionine sulfoxide reductase (MsrA) is a regulator of antioxidant defense and lifespan in mammals. *Proc Natl Acad Sci USA.* 2001;98:12920–12925.
26. Ogawa F, et al. The repair enzyme peptide methionine-S-sulfoxide reductase is expressed in human epidermis and upregulated by UVA radiation. *J Invest Dermatol.* 2006;126:1128–1134.
27. Balaban RS, Nemoto S, Finkel T. Mitochondria, oxidants, and aging. *Cell.* 2005; 120:483–495.
28. Hickson ID. RecQ helicases: caretakers of the genome. *Nat Rev Cancer.* 2003;3: 169–178.
29. Li GZ, Eller MS, Firoozabadi R, Gilchrest BA. Evidence that exposure of the telomere 3′ overhang sequence induces senescence. *Proc Natl Acad Sci USA.* 2003;100:527–531.
30. Gilchrest BA, Eller MS. The tale of the telomere: implications for prevention and treatment of skin cancers. *J Investig Dermatol Symp Proc.* 2005;10:124–130.
31. Eller MS, et al. Induction of apoptosis by telomere 3′ overhang-specific DNA. *Exp Cell Res.* 2002;276:185–193.
32. Krutmann J, Gilchrest B. Photoaging of Skin. In: Krutmann J, Gilchrest B, eds. *Skin Ageing.* Berlin/Heidelberg: Springer; 2006.
33. Pageon H, Asselineau D. An in vitro approach to the chronological aging of skin by glycation of the collagen: the biological effect of glycation on the reconstructed skin model. *Ann N Y Acad Sci.* 2005;1043:529–532.
34. Jeanmaire C, Danoux L, Pauly G. Glycation during human dermal intrinsic and actinic ageing: an in vivo and in vitro model study. *Br J Dermatol.* 2001;145:10–18.
35. Lohwasser C, et al. The receptor for advanced glycation end products is highly expressed in the skin and upregulated by advanced glycation end products and tumor necrosis factor-alpha. *J Invest Dermatol.* 2006;126:291–299.
36. Grewe M. Chronological ageing and photoageing of dendritic cells. *Clin Exp Dermatol.* 2001;26:608–612.
37. Opal SM, Girard TD, Ely EW. The immunopathogenesis of sepsis in elderly patients. *Clin Infect Dis.* 2005;41(suppl 7):S504–S512.
38. Bhushan M, et al. Tumour necrosis factor-alpha-induced migration of human Langerhans cells: the influence of ageing. *Br J Dermatol.* 2002;146:32–40.
39. Prelog M. Aging of the immune system: a risk factor for autoimmunity? *Autoimmun Rev.* 2006;5:136–139.
40. Piaserico S, et al. Allergic contact sensitivity in elderly patients. *Aging Clin Exp Res.* 2004;16:221–225.
41. Buckley DA, Rycroft RJ, White IR, McFadden JP. The frequency of fragrance allergy in patch-tested patients increases with their age. *Br J Dermatol.* 2003;149:986–989.
42. Swift ME, Burns AL, Gray KL, DiPietro LA. Age-related alterations in the inflammatory response to dermal injury. *J Invest Dermatol.* 2001;117: 1027–1035.
43. Thiele JJ, Barland CO, Ghadially R, Elias PM. Permeability and antioxidant barriers in aged epidermis. In: Krutmann J, Gilchrest B, eds. *Skin Ageing.* Berlin/Heidelberg: Springer. 2006;65–80.
44. Denda M, et al. Age- and sex-dependent change in stratum corneum sphingolipids. *Arch Dermatol Res* 1993;285: 415–417.
45. Ghadially R, et al. The aged epidermal permeability barrier: structural, functional, and lipid biochemical abnormalities in humans and a senescent murine model. *J Clin Invest.* 1995;95:2281–2290.
46. Ghadially R, et al. Decreased epidermal lipid synthesis accounts for altered barrier function in aged mice. *J Invest Dermatol.* 1996;106:1064–1069.
47. Jensen JM, et al. Acid and neutral sphingomyelinase, ceramide synthase, and acid ceramidase activities in cutaneous aging. *Exp Dermatol.* 2005;14:609–618.
48. Mauro T, et al. Acute barrier perturbation abolishes the Ca^{2+} and K^+ gradients in murine epidermis: quantitative measurement using PIXE. *J Invest Dermatol.*1998;111:1198–1201.
49. Denda M, Tomitaka A, Akamatsu H, Matsunaga K. Altered distribution of calcium in facial epidermis of aged adults. *J Invest Dermatol.* 2003;121:1557–1558.
50. Guarrera M, Ferrari P, Rebora A. Catalase in the stratum corneum of patients with polymorphic light eruption. *Acta Derm Venereol.* 1998;78:335–336.
51. Hellemans L, et al. Antioxidant enzyme activity in human stratum corneum shows seasonal variation with an age-dependent recovery. *J Invest Dermatol.* 2003;120:434–439.
52. Kurban RS, Bhawan J. Histologic changes in skin associated with aging. *J Dermatol. Surg Oncol.* 1990;16:908–914.
53. Moragas A, Castells C, Sans M. Mathematical morphologic analysis of aging-related epidermal changes. *Anal Quant Cytol Histol.* 1993;15:75–82.
54. Sauermann K, et al. Age-related changes of human skin investigated with histometric measurements by confocal laser scanning microscopy in vivo. *Skin Res Technol.* 2002;8:52–56.
55. Ladenheim D, et al. The effect of a dermatological patch on stratum corneum hydration and percutaneous absorption. *Proceedings of the International Symposium on Controlled Release of Bioactive Materials, Orlando, FL, July 1992*;19:460–461.
56. De Paepe K, et al. Microrelief of the skin using a light transmission method. *Arch Dermatol Res.* 2000;292:500–510.
57. Roskos KV, Maibach HI, Guy RH. The effect of aging on percutaneous absorption in man. *J Pharmacokinet Biopharm.* 1989;17:617–630.
58. Takahashi M, Tezuka T. The content of free amino acids in the stratum corneum is increased in senile xerosis. *Arch Dermatol Res.* 2004;295:448–452.
59. Fisher GJ, et al. Mechanisms of photoaging and chronological skin aging. *Arch Dermato.l* 2002;138:1462–1470.
60. Gilchrest BA. A review of skin ageing and its medical therapy. *Br J Dermatol.* 1996;135:867–875.
61. El-Domyati M, et al. Intrinsic aging vs. photoaging: a comparative histopathological, immunohistochemical, and

ultrastructural study of skin. *Exp Dermatol.* 2002;11:398–405.

62. Branchet MC, Boisnic S, Frances C, Robert AM. Skin thickness changes in normal aging skin. *Gerontology.* 1990;36:28–35.

63. de Rigal J, et al. Assessment of aging of the human skin by in vivo ultrasonic imaging. *J Invest Dermatol.* 1989;93:621–625.

64. Gniadecka M, Jemec GB. Quantitative evaluation of chronological ageing and photoageing in vivo: studies on skin echogenicity and thickness. *Br J Dermatol.* 1998;139:815–821.

65. Pierard GE, Lapiere CM. The microanatomical basis of facial frown lines. *Arch Dermatol.* 1989;125:1090–1092.

66. Tsuchida Y. The effect of aging and arteriosclerosis on human skin blood flow. *J Dermatol Sci.* 1993;5:175–181.

67. Li L, et al. Age-related changes in skin topography and microcirculation. *Arch Dermatol Res.* 2005:1–5.

68. Holowatz LA, Thompson CS, Minson CT, Kenney WL. Mechanisms of acetylcholine-mediated vasodilatation in young and aged human skin. *J Physiol.* 2005;563:965–973.

69. Thompson CS, Kenney WL. Altered neurotransmitter control of reflex vasoconstriction in aged human skin. *J Physiol.* 2004;558:697–704.

70. Sadoun E, Reed MJ. Impaired angiogenesis in aging is associated with alterations in vessel density, matrix composition, inflammatory response, and growth factor expression. *J Histochem Cytochem.* 2003;51:1119–1130.

71. Bach MH, Sadoun E, Reed MJ. Defects in activation of nitric oxide synthases occur during delayed angiogenesis in aging. *Mech Ageing Dev.* 2005;126:467–473.

72. Francis MK, et al. Loss of EPC-1/PEDF expression during skin aging in vivo. *J Invest Dermatol.* 2004;122:1096–1105.

73. Chang E, Yang J, Nagavarapu U, Herron GS. Aging and survival of cutaneous microvasculature. *J Invest Dermatol.* 2002;118:752–758.

74. Roskos KV, Bircher AJ, Maibach HI, Guy RH. Pharmacodynamic measurements of methyl nicotinate percutaneous absorption: the effect of aging on microcirculation. *Br J Dermatol.* 1990;122:165–171.

75. Shuster S, Black MM, McVitie E. The influence of age and sex on skin thickness, skin collagen and density. *Br J Dermatol.* 1975;93:639–643.

76. Bernstein EF, et al. Long-term sun exposure alters the collagen of the papillary dermis. Comparison of sun-protected and photoaged skin by Northern analysis, immunohistochemical staining, and confocal laser scanning microscopy. *J Am Acad Dermatol.* 1996;34:209–218.

77. Varani J, et al. Vitamin A antagonizes decreased cell growth and elevated collagen-degrading matrix metalloproteinases and stimulates collagen accumulation in naturally aged human skin. *J Invest Dermatol.* 2000;114:480–486.

78. Fligiel SE, et al. Collagen degradation in aged/photodamaged skin in vivo and after exposure to matrix metalloproteinase-1 in vitro. *J Invest Dermatol.* 2003;120:842–848.

79. Carrino DA, et al. Age-related changes in the proteoglycans of human skin. Specific cleavage of decorin to yield a major catabolic fragment in adult skin. *J Biol Chem.* 2003;278:17566–17572.

80. Vuillermoz B, et al. Influence of aging on glycosaminoglycans and small leucine-rich proteoglycans production by skin fibroblasts. *Mol Cell Biochem.* 2005;277:63–72.

81. Verdier-Sevrain S, Bonte F, Gilchrest B. Biology of estrogens in skin: implications for skin aging. *Exp Dermatol.* 2006;15:83–94.

82. Sumino H, et al. Effects of aging, menopause, and hormone replacement therapy on forearm skin elasticity in women. *J Am Geriatr Soc.* 2004;52:945–949.

83. Escoffier C, et al. Age-related mechanical properties of human skin: an in vivo study. *J Invest Dermatol.* 1989;93:353–357.

84. Batisse D, et al. Influence of age on the wrinkling capacities of skin. *Skin Res Technol.* 2002;8:148–154.

85. Lagarde JM, Rouvrais C, Black D. Topography and anisotropy of the skin surface with ageing. *Skin Res Technol.* 2005;11:110–119.

86. Gilchrest BA, Blog FB, Szabo G. Effects of aging and chronic sun exposure on melanocytes in human skin. *J Invest Dermatol.* 1979;73:141–143.

87. Kligman AM. Early destructive effect of sunlight on human skin. *JAMA.* 1969;210:2377–2380.

88. Chen VL, et al. Immunochemistry of elastotic material in sun-damaged skin. *J Invest Dermatol.* 1986;87:334–337.

89. Chang H, Oehrl W, Elsner P, Thiele JJ. The role of H_2O_2 as a mediator of UVB-induced apoptosis in keratinocytes. *Free Radic Res.* 2003;37:655–663.

90. Shaulian E, Karin M. AP-1 as a regulator of cell life and death. *Nat Cell Biol.* 2002;4:E131–E136.

91. Fisher GJ, et al. Molecular basis of sun-induced premature skin ageing and retinoid antagonism. *Nature.* 1996;379:335–339.

92. Quan T, He T, Voorhees JJ, Fisher GJ. Ultraviolet irradiation induces Smad7 via induction of transcription factor AP-1 in human skin fibroblasts. *J Biol Chem.* 2005;280:8079–8085.

93. Chung JH, et al. Modulation of skin collagen metabolism in aged and photoaged human skin in vivo. *J Invest Dermatol.* 2001;117:1218–1224.

94. Gilchrest BA, Eller MS, Geller AC, Yaar M. The pathogenesis of melanoma induced by ultraviolet radiation. *N Engl J Med.* 1999;340:1341–1348.

95. Wei Q. Effect of aging on DNA repair and skin carcinogenesis: a minireview of population-based studies. *J Investig Dermatol Symp Proc.* 1998;3:19–22.

96. Goukassian D, et al. Mechanisms and implications of the age–associated decrease in DNA repair capacity. *FASEB J.* 2000;14:1325–1334.

97. Wei Q, et al. DNA repair and aging in basal cell carcinoma: a molecular epidemiology study. *Proc Natl Acad Sci USA.* 1993;90:1614–1618.

98. Takahashi Y, et al. Decreased gene expression responsible for post-ultraviolet DNA repair synthesis in aging: a possible mechanism of age-related reduction in DNA repair capacity. *J Invest Dermatol.* 2005;124:435–442.

99. Eshaghian A, et al. Mitochondrial DNA deletions serve as biomarkers of aging in the skin, but are typically absent in nonmelanoma skin cancers. *J Invest Dermatol* 2006;126:336–344.

100. Swetter SM, Geller AC, Kirkwood JM. Melanoma in the older person. *Oncology.* (Williston Park) 2004;18:1187–1196; discussion 1196–1187.

101. Tuchinda C, Lim HW, Osterwalder U, Rougier A. Novel emerging sunscreen technologies. *Dermatol Clin.* 2006;24:105–117.

102. Stern RS. Clinical practice. Treatment of photoaging. *N Engl J Med.* 2004;350:1526–1534.

103. Gilchrest BA. At last! A medical treatment for skin aging. *J Am Med Assoc.* 1988;259:569–570.

104. Maier T, Korting HC. Sunscreens—which and what for? *Skin Pharmacol Physiol.* 2005;18:253–262.

105. Kligman LH, Duo CH, Kligman AM. Topical retinoic acid enhances the repair of ultraviolet damaged dermal connective tissue. *Connect Tissue Res.* 1984;12:139–150.

106. Olsen EA, et al. Sustained improvement in photodamaged skin with reduced tretinoin emollient cream treatment regimen: effect of once-weekly and three-times-weekly applications. *J Am Acad Dermatol.* 1997;37:227–230.

107. Bhawan J, et al. Histologic evaluation of the long-term effects of tretinoin on photodamaged skin. *J Dermatol Sci.* 1996;11:177–182.

108. Griffiths CE, et al. Restoration of collagen formation in photodamaged human skin by tretinoin (retinoic acid). *N Engl J Med.* 1993;329:530–535.

109. Kang S, et al. Long-term efficacy and safety of tretinoin emollient cream 0.05% in the treatment of photodamaged facial skin: a two-year, randomized, placebo-controlled trial. *Am J Clin Dermatol.* 2005;6:245–253.

110. Fisher GJ, et al. Pathophysiology of premature skin aging induced by ultraviolet light. *N Engl J Med.* 1997;337:1419–1428.

111. Kang S, et al. A multicenter, randomized, double-blind trial of tazarotene 0.1% cream in the treatment of photodamage. *J Am Acad Dermatol.* 2005;52:268–274.

112. Thiele JJ. Oxidative targets in the stratum corneum: a new basis for antioxidative strategies. *Skin Pharmacol Appl Skin Physiol.* 2001;14(suppl 1):87–91.

113. Haywood R, Wardman P, Sanders R, Linge C. Sunscreens inadequately protect against ultraviolet-A-induced free radicals in skin: implications for skin aging and melanoma? *J Invest Dermatol.* 2003;121:862–868.

114. Hanson KM, Clegg RM. Bioconvertible vitamin antioxidants improve sunscreen photoprotection against UV-induced reactive oxygen species. *J Cosmet Sci.* 2003;54:589–598.

115. Farris PK. Topical vitamin C: a useful agent for treating photoaging and other

dermatologic conditions. *Dermatol Surg.* 2005;31:814–817; discussion 818.

116. Fitzpatrick RE, Rostan EF. Double-blind, half-face study comparing topical vitamin C and vehicle for rejuvenation of photodamage. *Dermatol Surg.* 2002; 28:231–236.

117. Seite S, et al. Histological evaluation of a topically applied retinol-vitamin C combination. *Skin Pharmacol Physiol.* 2005;18:81–87.

118. Lin JY, et al. UV photoprotection by combination topical antioxidants vitamin C and vitamin E. *J Am Acad Dermatol.* 2003;48:866–874.

119. Lin JY, et al. Alpha-lipoic acid is ineffective as a topical antioxidant for photoprotection of skin. *J Invest Dermatol.* 2004;123:996–998.

120. Lin FH, et al. Ferulic acid stabilizes a solution of vitamins C and E and dou-bles its photoprotection of skin. *J Invest Dermatol.* 2005;125:826–832.

121. Kang S, et al. Topical N-acetyl cysteine and genistein prevent ultraviolet-light-induced signaling that leads to photoaging in human skin in vivo. *J Invest Dermatol.* 2003;120:835–841.

122. Ekanayake Mudiyanselage S, Hamburger M, Elsner P, Thiele JJ. Ultraviolet A induces generation of squalene monohydroperoxide isomers in human sebum and skin surface lipids in vitro and in vivo. *J Invest Dermatol.* 2003;120: 915–922.

123. Chiba K, Kawakami K, Sone T, Onoue M. Characteristics of skin wrinkling and dermal changes induced by repeated application of squalene mono-hydroperoxide to hairless mouse skin. *Skin Pharmacol Appl Skin Physiol.* 2003;16:242–251.

124. Chiba K, Sone T, Kawakami K, Onoue M. Skin roughness and wrinkle formation induced by repeated application of squalene monohydroperoxide to the hairless mouse. *Exp Dermatol.* 1999;8(6): 471–479.

125. Ekanayake-Mudiyanselage S, et al. Vitamin E delivery to human skin by a rinse-off product: penetration of alpha-tocopherol versus wash-out effects of skin surface lipids. *Skin Pharmacol Physiol.* 2005;18:20–26.

126. Thiele JJ, Hsieh SN, Ekanayake-Mudiyanselage S. Vitamin E: critical review of its current use in cosmetic and clinical dermatology. *Dermatol Surg.* 2005;31:805–813; discussion 813.

127. Halachmi S, Yaar M, Gilchrest BA. Advances in skin aging/photoaging: theoretical and practical implications. *Ann Dermatol Venereol.* 2005;132:362–367.

CHAPTER 3

Epidemiology of Skin Cancer

Melissa Gonzales, Ph.D.
Esther Erdei, Ph.D.
Marianne Berwick, Ph.D.

BOX 3-1   Overview

- Skin cancer is the most common disease among Caucasians throughout the world.
- There are three major types of skin cancer: basal cell carcinoma, squamous cell carcinoma, and cutaneous malignant melanoma.
- Ultraviolet radiation is the major environmental risk factor for all three types of skin cancer.
- Metal exposures may play a role in the development of skin cancer, particularly in the interaction with ultraviolet radiation.
- Pigmentary characteristics are the most important host risk factors for skin cancer and are important in the response to ultraviolet radiation.
- The incidence of all three types of skin cancers appears to be increasing throughout the world among Caucasians.
- The mortality of nonmelanoma skin cancers (basal cell carcinoma and squamous cell carcinoma) appears to have declined.
- Immunologic factors are clearly important in the development of skin cancers, but elucidating their specific role has been elusive, to date.
- Human papilloma virus is a risk factor for nonmelanoma skin cancer.
- Multiple or atypical nevi are important risk factors for cutaneous malignant melanoma.

INTRODUCTION

Skin cancer is the most common cancer in the United States, estimated at over 1 million newly diagnosed cases each year, close to the total new cases of all other cancer combined.[1] It has been estimated that every year 2.75 million new cases of nonmelanoma skin cancer (NMSC) will be diagnosed worldwide.[2] In Australia, estimates for melanoma incidence range from 0.59 per 100,000 in dark-skinned populations to 40.5 per 100,000 in light-skinned populations (World Standard Rates). Although skin cancer is generally considered to be benign, deaths from melanoma are the most rapidly growing of cancer deaths in the United States.[3] It should be noted, however, that this growth is greatly due to the very low starting point, so that even a small increase is *proportionately* large. Most skin cancer has a higher incidence among light-skinned individuals and is less common among dark-skinned individuals. In addition, each skin cancer seems to develop from different patterns of sun exposure, with squamous cell carcinoma developing after a high level of continuous sun exposure, melanoma after intermittent sun exposure, and basal cell carcinoma somewhere in between.

TYPES OF SKIN CANCERS

BOX 3-2   Summary

- The three most common types of skin cancer are basal cell carcinoma (BCC), squamous cell carcinoma (SCC), and cutaneous malignant melanoma (CMM).
- BCC and SCC, otherwise known as "non-melanoma skin cancer" (NMSC), develop in keratinocytes and CMM develops in melanocytes.
- More than 1 million NMSC occur in the US each year and more than 56,000 CMMs.

The three most common types of skin cancer are basal cell carcinoma (BCC), squamous cell carcinoma (SCC), and cutaneous malignant melanoma (CMM). Basal cell carcinoma and squamous cell carcinoma are often referred to together as "nonmelanoma" skin cancer (NMSC).

Basal Cell Carcinoma

Basal cell carcinoma develops from epithelial keratinocytes in the basal layer of the skin. This is the most common skin cancer and has a very low rate of metastasis. It generally appears on the head, neck, arms or the back. There is no known "precursor" lesion for BCC, so new molecular discoveries are important for clarifying its etiology and thus preventing BCC.

Squamous Cell Carcinoma

Squamous cell carcinoma also develops from keratinocytes and certain pathological alterations, such as actinic or solar keratoses, are considered "precursor" lesions. These lesions frequently occur on the face, hands, and forearms, and are very commonly detected among individuals older than 40 years of age. It has been estimated that much of the time, actinic keratoses spontaneously regress, and only a few develop further to squamous cell carcinoma.[4]

Cutaneous Malignant Melanoma

Cutaneous malignant melanoma arises from melanocytes, and approximately 40% of the incidence is associated with common nevi (moles). A large proportion of melanomas appear to evolve through a slow-growing, radial growth phase that can develop into a vertical growth phase, when it then has the capacity for developing metastases. Other melanomas can arise rapidly and without nevus involvement. Breslow thickness is the depth of a melanoma lesion measured from the basement membrane of the epidermis to the deepest identified melanoma tumor cells. This thickness is the most important prognostic factor for melanoma[2] as deeper melanomas metastasize more easily as they can reach the blood and lymph systems.

EFFECTS OF SOLAR ULTRAVIOLET RADIATION ON THE SKIN

BOX 3-3   Summary

- Exposure to UVR is the major cause of most skin cancers.
- The pattern of exposure that leads to skin cancer differs for SCC and CMM.
- SCC develops with a cumulative high dose of UVR.
- CMM develops with an intermittent type of exposure, such as vacation exposure or beach exposure.
- BCC has a pattern that is somewhat mixed between SCC and CMM.

Exposure to ultraviolet radiation (UVR) is the main cause of melanoma and nonmelanoma skin cancers.[5] UVR induces skin cancers by three mechanisms: direct DNA damage leading to mutation; production of activated oxygen molecules that in turn damage DNA and other cellular structures; and localized immunosuppression blocking the body's natural anticancer defenses.[6,7] The UVR wavelengths primarily responsible for skin cancers are in the UVB (280 to 320 nm) and UVA (320 to 400 nm) range. The effects of these wavelengths are summarized in Table 3-1. Early research focused on UVB, in the

Table 3-1
Important Characteristics of UVA and UVB Radiation[a]

	WAVELENGTH	
	UVB (280–320 nm)	UVA (32–400 nm)
Relative occurrence[b]	~5%	~95%
Sunburn induction	+++	++
Pigmentation induction	+++	++
Epidermal thickening	+++	−
Skin aging (solar elastosis, keratoses)	+++	++
Stimulation of vitamin D synthesis	+++	+++
Types of DNA lesions	Pyrimidine dimers and pyrimidone photoproducts[c]	Primarily oxidative (as understood to date)[d]
Immunosuppression	+[e]	+[f]

[a]Data from [97–99].
[b]At the surface of the earth. Value is approximate and varies with latitude and zenith angle.
[c][16–18].
[d][10–14].
[e][96].
[f][94–95].

belief that this component of natural light was more important in carcinogenesis.[8,9] Recent work recognizes the role of UVA as well[10–14] (Table 3-1).

Far more UVA reaches melanocytes than UVB. On average, the epidermal layers overlaying the basal layer in Caucasian skin absorb 56% of the UVB and only 27% of UVA.[15] As UVB is absorbed in the epidermis by various molecules such as the keratins and DNA, it can suppress immune reactions, induce tolerance to antigens, upregulate gene expression, and induce mutations.[6] UVB directly mutates DNA[16–18] (Table 3-1) and is demonstrated to initiate cutaneous malignant melanoma in genetically engineered mice.[19] However, UVB also plays an important role in stimulating photoprotective adaptation of the skin. UVB-induced mutations (thymidine dinucleotides) in the epidermis are believed to stimulate a photoprotective response (PER), which includes the synthesis and release of melanosomes by melanocytes.[20–23] This in turn reduces the penetration of UV radiation to the basal epidermis and melanocytes. PER also includes the proliferation of keratinocytes, leading to a thickening of the stratum corneum, improved scattering of UV radiation, and reduced UV penetration of the skin. Under certain conditions, such as at high latitudes (where UVB flux is low) or when UVB blocking sunscreens are used, the natural protective epidermal response from UVB exposure is reduced and the basal epithelium, including the melanocytes, is exposed to a relatively large flux of UVA photons. These UVA photons in turn can cause oxidative damage to the guanine bases of DNA, which may ultimately result in mutation and melanoma promotion.[24–26]

PUVA Therapy

European and U.S. studies have shown that psoralen plus ultraviolet A (PUVA) therapy results in a significant, dose-dependent increased risk of squamous cell carcinoma, and a less clear risk of increase in the occurrence of basal cell carcinoma, as well as melanoma.[27] In another analysis with 4294 PUVA patients from five ethnically different, dark-skinned (Asians and Arabian-African) populations; the patients appeared not to be at increased risk in developing NMSC followed by long-term (at least 5 years) PUVA therapy.[28]

EPIDEMIOLOGY OF NONMELANOMA SKIN CANCERS (NMSC)

BOX 3-4 Summary

- There has been an increase in NMSC incidence during the last several decades.
- Incidence of NMSC is particularly difficult to evaluate as few registries routinely collect these data.
- Mortality is generally low in NMSC, but does occur among the relatively few aggressive SCCs.

- Risk factors include sun sensitive phenotype, immunologic factors, UV radiation, arsenic exposure and some viral exposures, such as HPV.

Incidence

The incidence of nonmelanoma skin cancer (BCC, SCC) is difficult to estimate accurately because they are often not counted by tumor registries due to their large number and the difficulty of consistent and reliable ascertainment from outpatient units where they are usually diagnosed. Estimates are that in the United States over 1 million cases of basal cell and squamous cell skin cancer will be diagnosed in 2006.[1]

Some data are available on the time trends for nonmelanoma skin cancer incidence. The U.S. National Cancer Institute sponsored a population-based skin cancer survey in 1977–1978 that found noticeable geographic variability in the NMSC incidence rates within the United States.[29] In 1998–1999, a follow-up NMSC survey in New Mexico, one of the original sites, showed that the incidence rate of basal cell carcinoma had increased by 50% in males and 20% in females and the incidence rate of squamous cell carcinoma roughly doubled in both genders.[30] These results are in accord with reports from various other populations.[31] Among US veterans, NMSC is being diagnosed at an earlier age than it was 30 years ago and appears more commonly on the extremities than before.[32] It is also noted[31] that the average age of NMSC development is 65, but lately more patients younger than 40 years have been diagnosed with NMSC.[33] Trends in Canada have shown an annual percent change of basal cell and squamous cell carcinoma of 2.4% from the early 1970s to 2000.[34] Although most analyses report an increase in incidence, some have reported a decline in SCC rates.[35] Very high incidence rates have been reported from Australia (1170/100,000), where increases in BCC and SCC are the greatest for people aged 60 years and older.[36] The public health importance of these trends in NMSC will produce increased treatment costs over the $426 million that Medicare currently spends on NMSC in the USA.[37]

An increased risk of second primary cancer after a diagnosis of NMSC has been observed in the first four years after diagnosis and the elevated risk remained higher in all age groups up to 75 years.[38] Among dark-skinned individuals the incidence rates of BCC and SCC are much lower than among light-skinned Caucasians.[39–41]

Mortality

The difficulty in accessing reliable epidemiological data on nonmelanoma skin cancer mortality is similar to the problems encountered in obtaining reliable incidence data. Basal cell carcinoma mortality is lower than squamous cell carcinoma mortality, which is 12 times as likely to be fatal, particularly among males and with increasing age.[42] Adults over 85 years age are experiencing death caused by skin cancer mostly because of squamous cell carcinoma progression.[31] Although many registries report an increased incidence, surprisingly, declines have been shown in mortality from NMSC in many areas such as Rhode Island,[43] Germany,[44] and Finland.[45] However, several misclassification issues shadow the accuracy of these data. All these problems argue for population-based epidemiological studies of nonmelanoma skin cancer.

Host Factors

Nonmelanoma skin cancers are strongly associated with interactions between host susceptibility and sunlight exposure. Individuals with light skin that does not tan easily are at risk for squamous cell carcinoma and at slightly less risk for basal cell carcinoma.[46] The odds ratio for developing SCC for individuals who do not tan is 6.9 compared to those who tan easily and the odds ratio for developing BCC for individuals who do not tan is 3.7 compared to those who tan easily.[46]

Immunologic Factors

Our knowledge of immunologic factors influencing NMSC and melanoma development is limited. Most information about the immunologic aspects of skin cancer is based on UV radiation-induced mouse models. A number of investigators have observed increases in NMSC among patients who have undergone solid organ transplantation or childhood cancer therapy. The considerable morbidity and long-term mortality due to NMSC can be explained by the patients' prolonged survival after transplantation and successful chemo- or radiation therapy.[47] The risk for invasive SCC increased 82-fold among kidney recipients compared with the non-transplanted population.[48] SCC occurs more frequently in transplant patients; even though BCC is approximately 4 times more frequent than SCC[47–50] in the general population. It seems that disturbance of host's cell-mediated immunity is

the dominant factor responsible for allowing NMSC growth. Normal skin contains a high level of major histocompatibility complex (MHC) class I molecules, while BCC shows complete absence or heterogeneous expression of these molecules. Furthermore, class I-negative BCC tumors were pathologically proven to be aggressive, whereas all nonaggressive BCC were class I-positive.[51]

 EXPOSURES (OTHER THAN ULTRAVIOLET RADIATION)

Metals

The most important metal exposure associated with skin cancer is arsenic. In different geographic areas, where arsenic exposure is chronic via water, soil, and food contamination (Bangladesh, India, Pakistan, Mexico, Chile, Argentina, etc.), arsenic exposure alone has been found to be responsible for a higher risk of skin cancer.[52] Other studies have found a higher risk among men occupationally exposed to arsenic.[53] Occupational skin cancers are often similar to those in nonoccupationally exposed patients, but some lesions, arsenical keratoses for example, directly point to an occupational exposure.[53] Increased risk for all types of skin cancer, including melanoma, was observed among Dutch men, who reported lifetime arsenic exposure.[54] Basal cell carcinoma (BCC) development is strongly associated with environmental factors and arsenic exposure is part of the complex exposure patterns.[55] Basal cell carcinoma also was related, though not statistically significant, to occupational arsenic exposure in the southeastern Arizona Health Study-2.[56]

The molecular mechanisms responsible for arsenic carcinogenesis are still under investigations as arsenic is not a "classical" genotoxic chemical or mutagen such as cadmium or chromium.[57] Inorganic arsenic is likely to be involved in molecular signaling pathways responsible for cell growth control and in DNA repair processes,[58,59] and might have the ability to modify p53 and p16 tumor suppressor genes' methylation patterns.[60] Others have suggested that arsenic in drinking water might need another carcinogenic effect such as ultraviolet radiation.[52] UV- and arsenic-induced oxidative stresses are also possible mechanisms leading to DNA damage and carcinogenic transformation.[61,62] Single nucleotide polymorphisms of certain oxidative stress enzymes (catalase, myeloperoxidase) were reported to be connected to susceptibility to arsenic-induced hyper-

keratosis in the Bangladesh population.[63] Arsenic together with human papilloma virus infection (tested as HPV seropositivity) was associated with a highly increased risk for NMSC in a Mexican clinic-based case-control study.[64]

Human Papilloma Virus Infections

Human papilloma viruses (HPVs) are small DNA viruses that infect epithelial cell and can induce proliferative lesions, such as warts, laryngeal papillomas, and cervical carcinoma.[65,66] HPVs are highly prevalent among humans and so far more than 90 different genotypes of them have been characterized. The papilloma viruses that commensally live in all people are activated by sunlight (UV) exposure, by immunosuppression, and/or specific genetic susceptibility of the host.

The causative involvement of HPV in human skin cancer has been described first in patients with the rare hereditary autosomal disease epidermodysplasia verruciformis (EV). This condition is characterized by widespread HPV infection in the form of flat warts and gradual development of multiple SCCs, mostly on sun-exposed sites.[66] The etiological connection for HPVs with keratinocyte cancer, such as squamous cell carcinoma (SCC) and basal cell carcinoma (BCC) of the skin, is still unknown.[67] HPVs found in macular lesions are commonly referred to as EV-HPV types (HPV 5, 8, 9, 12, 14, 15, 17, and 19).[43] HPV viral DNA usually persists extra-chromosomally in high copy numbers, but only in few carcinoma cells in the skin tumor, supporting the role of viral infections in the initiation and progression of the carcinogenesis.[68] The amount of HPV DNA was higher in skin tumors of immunosuppressed patients than in those of the general population.[68] One recent study detected HPV antibodies more frequently in SCC patients than in controls (OR = 1.6; 95% CI = 1.2 to 2.3), but did not find a difference in HPV seropositivity between BCC cases and controls.[67]

■ **MELANOMA**

BOX 3-5 Summary

- The incidence of CMM has increased among light-skinned individuals worldwide.
- Mortality rates have increased among older males, but have plateaued or declined among some age groups.
- Risk factors include multiple nevi, atypical nevi, immune factors, intermittent sun exposure, and possibly metal exposures.

- Genetic factors are under intensive investigation, and seem to be important in the development of melanoma.

Incidence

The incidence of melanoma is increasing worldwide[69–71] and UV radiation from sunlight has been implicated as the main environmental agent responsible for the initial transformation of benign melanocytes into melanoma.[72] Epidemiological studies have repeatedly shown that exposure to sunlight is the major risk factor for the development of melanoma in individuals with a fair-skinned complexion.[73] However, the association between sun exposure and melanoma is complex in terms of a lack of clear dose–response association, latent period, body site, distribution of cutaneous melanoma, histogenetic melanoma types, and many other factors.[74–76] For example, indoor workers often suffer higher rates of melanoma than outdoor workers,[77,78] and melanoma tumors often develop on areas of the body usually covered by clothing and only intermittently exposed to the sun.[79,80] In addition to sun exposure, pigmentary traits (hair color, eye color, and sun sensitivity), the presence and number of melanocytic and atypical nevi, as well as variants in DNA repair genes and tumor suppressor genes, have also been shown to increase melanoma risk in susceptible populations.

Mortality

Mortality rates for melanoma are more than five-fold lower than incidence rates throughout the world and have plateaued or declined among some age groups. Although New Zealand and Australia have the highest mortality rates among males, the mortality rate among females in Norway is slightly higher than in Australia. Overall, however, females seem to have better survival than males once melanoma has been diagnosed. There is little convincing evidence as to whether this is due to behavior, such as early detection, or biology, such as less aggressive tumors among women.

Host Factors

NEVI Numerous studies have shown a relationship between UV exposure and the development of nevi, which are a key risk factor for the later development of melanoma.[81–83] There is an apparent interaction between sun exposure and nevus density with regard to the site of the melanoma. For

example, in Australia, sex differences in nevus density on the back and lower extremities are similar to sex differences for melanoma—men having higher rates on the back, women having higher rates on the legs—areas that are not chronically exposed to the sun.[76] Whiteman et al[84] have proposed a model for cutaneous melanoma in which two pathways—chronic exposure to the sun and melanocyte instability—represent divergent pathways for developing melanoma. Under this

model, people with an inherently low propensity for melanocyte proliferation require chronic sun exposure to drive clonal expansion of transformed epidermal melanocytes. Melanomas arising in this group of people would occur on habitually sun-exposed body sites, such as the face. In contrast, the model would predict that in individuals with an inherently high propensity for melanocyte proliferation (e.g., high nevus counts), exposure to sunlight early in life would be required to start the process of

Odds Ratios for Occupational Sun Exposure

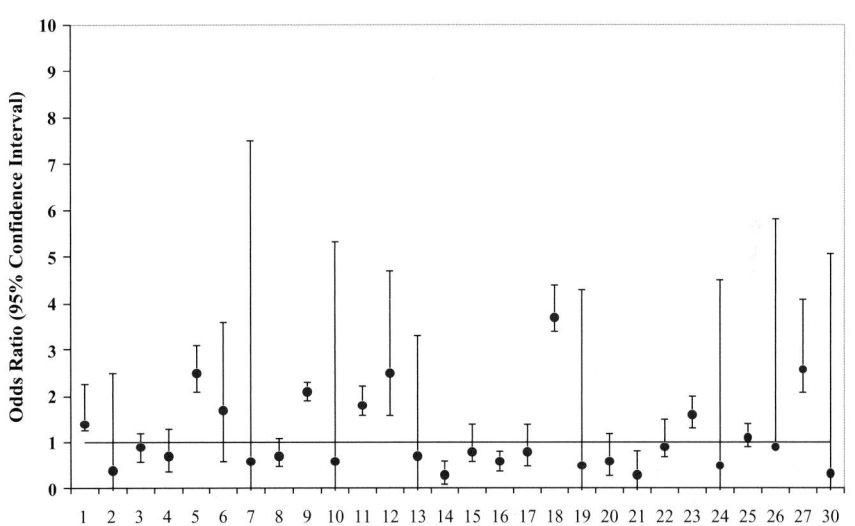

Odds Ratios for Intermitent Sun Exposure

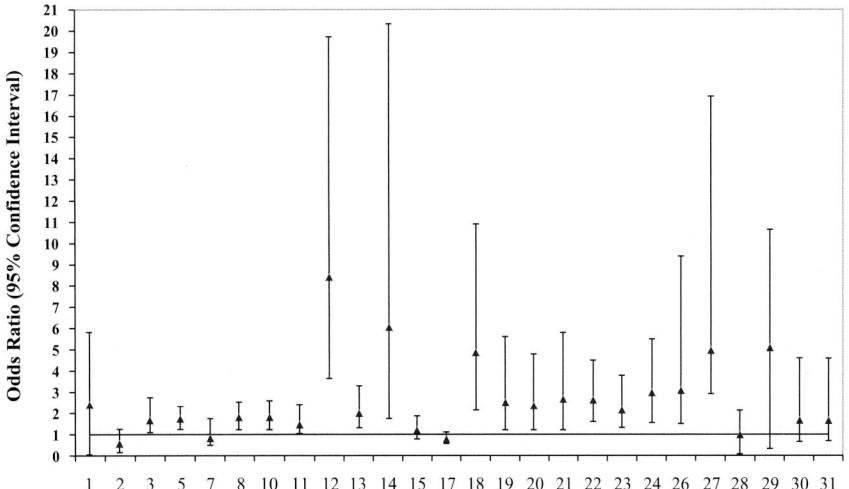

▲ **FIGURE 3-1** Results of case–control studies of intermittent (outdoor recreational activities, vacation exposure or sunburn history) and occupational sun exposure and melanoma. 1—Klepp and Magnus[100]; 2—Mackie and Aitchison[101]; 3—Elwood et al[102]; 4—Graham et al[103]; 5—Dubin et al[104]; 6—Elwood et al[105]; 7—Cristofolini et al[106]; 8—Østerlind et al[107]; 9—Zanetti et al[108]; 10—Beitner et al[109]; 11—Dubin et al[110]; 12—Grob et al[111]; 13—Herzfeld et al[112]; 14—Autier et al[113]; 15—Westerdahl et al[114]; 16—White et al[115]; 17—Holly et al (females)[116]; 18—Rodenas et al[117]; 19—Chen et al (head/neck)[118]; 20—Chen et al (upper limb)[118]; 21—Chen et al (lower limb)[118]; 22—Chen et al (trunk)[118]; 23—Espinosa Arranz et al[91]; 24—Espinosa Arranz et al[91]; 25—Settimi et al[119]; 26—Loria et al[120]; 27—Fargnoli et al[121]; 28—Lasithitakis et al[122]; 29—Chaudru et al[123]; 30—Nijsten et al[124]; 31—Naldi et al.[125]

carcinogenesis. These individuals would be expected to develop tumors on body sites with unstable melanocyte populations such as the trunk.

Immunologic Factors

The risk of malignant melanoma was also elevated among transplant patients.[48,49] One study also noticed that there was a trend for patients who experienced at least one acute rejection episode to develop melanoma,[50] which might be explained by immunosuppression related to melanoma disease development.

Exposures

SUN EXPOSURE Fig. 3-1 shows the odds ratios and confidence intervals from 31 case-control studies of melanoma conducted in North America and Europe examining occupational sun exposure and/or intermittent sun exposure (e.g., recreational, vacation exposures or sunburns). Among these studies there is a general trend for neutral to slightly protective associations between occupational sun exposure and melanoma (OR ≤ 1.0); but elevated, and more often statistically significant risk for melanoma with intermittent exposure (OR > 1.0). The reasons for the differing trends in melanoma risk between occupational and intermittent sun exposure are not well understood. Analyses of melanoma time trends from Canada,[85] New Zealand,[86] Germany,[87] Australia,[88,89] and Denmark[90] indicate that changes in lifestyle factors, such as sun exposure behaviors and fashion, correlate strongly with increases in melanoma on skin areas exposed intermittently to the sun (trunk, upper arms, and upper legs). With regard to chronic occupational sun exposure, it is also possible that additional phenotypic differences among workforce members may be influencing the direction and intensity of melanoma risk. In a study of occupational melanoma from Spain,[91] higher melanoma risk was observed among construction workers than among farmers. The melanoma risk in construction workers became more significant when adjusted for skin type, age, freckle count (OR = 4.3; 95% CI = 1.8 to 9.9), and number of nevi (OR = 2.8; 95% CI = 1.4 to 5.8), while the risk in farmers remained protective even with these adjustments.

Metal Exposure

Metal exposure may be quite important to the development of melanoma and has been very little studied. Occupational arsenic and mercury exposure have been associated with an increased risk for cutaneous melanoma among Swedish women who were members of an occupational cohort.[92] The Iowa Agricultural Workers Study found an increased risk for melanoma associated with arsenic exposure.[93]

FINAL THOUGHTS

New discoveries in genetic modifiers of risk for melanoma, as well as, advances in techniques for measuring UV exposure should lead to a clearer understanding of the important differences in patterns of occurrence of skin cancer, and thus help to develop new opportunities for prevention.

REFERENCES

1. Jemal A, Siegel R, Ward, et al. *Cancer Statistics, 2006. CA: A Cancer Journal for Clinicians*, xxx: ACS Publication; 2006.
2. Armstrong BK, Kricker A. Skin cancer. *Dermatoepidemiology*. 1995;13:583–xxx.
3. Abdulla FR, Feldman SR, Williford PM, et al. Tanning and skin cancer *Pediatr Dermatol*. 2005;22:501–512.
4. Harvey I, Frankel S, Marks R, et al. Nonmelanoma skin cancer and solar keratoses, II: analytical results of the South Wales skin cancer study *Br J Cancer*. 1996;74:1308–1312.
5. Armstrong BK, Kricker A. How much melanoma is caused by sun exposure? *Melanoma Res*. 1993;3:395–401.
6. Ichihashi M, Ueda M, Budiyanto A, et al. UV-induced skin damage. *Toxicology* 2003;189:21–39.
7. Owens DM, Watt FM. Contribution of stem cells and differentiated cells to epidermal tumours. *Nat Rev Cancer*. 2003;3: 444–451.
8. Knox J, Griffin A, Hakim H. Protection from ultraviolet carcinogenesis. *J Invest Dermatol*. 1960;34:51–57.
9. Kligman L, Akin F, Kligman A. Sunscreens prevent ultraviolet carcinogenesis. *J Am Acad Dermatol*. 1980;3:30–35.
10. Moan J, Dahlback A, Setlow RB. Epidemiological support for an hypothesis for melanoma induction indicating a role for UV-A radiation. *Photochem Photobiol*. 1999;70:243–247.
11. Wang SQ, Setlow R, Berwick M, Polsky D, Marghoob AA, Kopf AW, et al. Ultraviolet A and melanoma: a review. *J Am Acad Dermatol*. 2001;44:837–846.
12. Diffey BL. A quantitative estimate of melanoma mortality from ultraviolet A sunbed use in the UK. *Br J Dermatol*. 2003;149:578–581.
13. Kvam E, Tyrrell RM. The role of melanin in the induction of oxidative DNA base damage by ultraviolet A irradiation of DNA or melanoma cells. *J Invest Dermatol*. 1999;113:209–13.
14. Marrot L, Belaidi JP, Meunier JR. The human melanocyte as a particular target for UVA radiation and an endpoint for photoprotection assessment. *Photochem Photobiol*. 1999;69:686–93.
15. Kaidbey K, Agin O, Sayre R, et al. Photoprotection by melanin–a comparison of black and Caucasian skin. *J Am Acad Dermatol*. 1979;1:249–260.
16. Wikonkal NM, Brash DE. Ultraviolet radiation induced signature mutations in photocarcinogenesis. *J Investig Dermatol Symp Proc*. 1999;4:6–10.
17. Clingen PH, Arlett CF, Roza L, et al. Induction of cyclobutane pyrimidine dimers, pyrimidine (6-4) pyrimidone photoproducts, and Dewar valence isomers by natural sunlight in normal mononuclear cells. *Cancer Res*. 1995;55: 2245–48.
18. Young AR, Potten CS, Nikaido O, et al. Human melanocytes and keratinocytes exposed to UVA or UVB in vivo show comparable levels of thymine dimmers. *J Invest Dermatol*. 1998;111:936–940.
19. De Fabo EC, Noonan FP, Fears T, et al. Ultraviolet B but not ultraviolet A radiation initiates melanoma. *Cancer Res*. 2004;64:6372–6376.
20. Eller M, Maeda T, Magnini C, et al. Enhancement of DNA repair in human skin cells by thymidine dinucleotides: evidence for a p53-mediated mammalian SOS response. *Proc Natl Acad Sci USA*. 1997;94:12627–12632.
21. Hadshiew I, Eller M, Moll I, et al. Photoprotective mechanisms of human skin: Modulation by oligonucleotides. *Hautarzt*. 2002;52:167–173.
22. Agar N, Young AR. Melanogenesis: a photoprotective response to DNA damage? *Mutat Res*. 2005;571:121–132.
23. Bataille V, Bykov VJ, Sasieni P, et al. Photoadaptation to ultraviolet (UV) radiation in vivo: Photoproducts in epidermal cells following UVB therapy for psoriasis. *Br J Dermatol*. 2000;143:477–483.
24. Wang SQ, Setlow R, Berwick M, et al. Ultraviolet A and melanoma: a review. *J Am Acad Dermatol*. 2001;44:837–846.
25. Lim HW, Naylor M, Hönigsman H, et al. American Academy of Dermatology Consensus Conference on UVA protection of sunscreens: Summary and recommendations. *J Am Acad Dermatol*. 2001;44:505–508.
26. Wood SR, Berwick M, Ley RD, et al. UV causation of melanoma in Xiphophorus is dominated by melanin photosensitized oxidant production. *Proc Natl Acad Sci*. 2006;103:4111–4115.
27. Lindelof B, Sigurgeirsson B, Tegner E, et al. PUVA and cancer: a large-scale epidemiological study *Lancet*. 1991;338:91–93.
28. Murase J, Lee EE, Koo J Effect of ethnicity on the risk of developing nonmelanoma skin cancer following long-term PUVA therapy. *Int J Dermatol*. 2005;44:1016–1021.
29. Scotto J, Fears TR, Fraumeni JR. Incidence of nonmelanoma skin cancer in the United States. Publication No. NIH 82-2433. Washington DC: United States Department of Health and Human Services, 1981.
30. Athas WF, Hunt WC, Key CR. Changes in nonmelanoma skin cancer incidence between 1977–1978 and 1998–1999 in northcentral New Mexico. *Cancer Epid Biomarker Prev*. 2003;12:1105–1108.
31. Rigel DS, Friedman RJ, Dzubow LM, Reintgen DS, Bystryn J-C, Marks R, eds. *Cancer of the Skin*. Philadelphia: Elsevier Sanders; 2005.

32. Collins GL, Nickoonahand N, Morgan MB. Changing demographics and pathology of nonmelanoma skin cancer in the last 30 years. *Semin Cutan Med Surg.* 2004:23(1):80–83.

33. Christenson LJ, Borrowman TA, Vachon CM, et al. Incidence of basal cell and squamous cell carcinomas in a population younger than 40 years *JAMA.* 2005:294:681–690.

34. Demers AA, Nugent Z, Mihalcioiu C, et al. Trends of nonmelanoma skin cancer from 1960 through 2000 in Canadian population. *J Am Acad Dermatol.* 2005;53:320–328.

35. Stern RS: The mysteries of geographic variability in nonmelanoma skin cancer incidence. *Arch Dermatol.* 1999;135:843–844.

36. Staples MP, Elwood M, Burton RC, et al. Non-melanoma skin cancer in Australia: the 2002 national survey and trends since 1985. *Med J Aust.* 2006;184:6–10.

37. Chen JG, Fleischer AB Jr, Smith ED, et al. Cost of nonmelanoma skin cancer treatment in the United States. *Dermatol Surg.* 2001;27:1035–1038.

38. Nugent Z, Demers AA, Wiseman MC, et al. Risk of secondary primary cancer and death following a diagnosis of nonmelanoma skin cancer. *Cancer Epidemiol. Biomarkers Prev.* 2005;14:2584–2590.

39. Ceylan C, Ozturk G, Alper S. Nonmelanoma skin cancers between the years of 1990 and 1999 in Izmir, Turkey: demographic and clinicopathological characteristics *J Dermatol.* 2002;30:123–131.

40. Omari AK, Khammash MR, Matalka I. Skin cancer trends in northern Jordan *Inter J Dermatol.* 2006;45:384–388.

41. Koh D, Wang H, Lee J, et al. Basal cell carcinoma, squamous cell carcinoma and melanoma of the skin: analysis of the Singapore Cancer Registry data 1968–1997. *Br J Dermatol.* 2003;148:1161–1166.

42. Weinstock MA, Bogaars HA, Ashley M, et al. Non-melanoma skin cancer mortality. *Arch Dermatol.* 1991;127:1194–1197.

43. Lewis KG, Weinstock MA. Nonmelanoma skin cancer mortality (1988–2000): the Rhode Island follow-back study. *Arch Dermatol.* 2004;40:837–842.

44. Stang A, Jockel KH. Declining mortality rates for nonmelanoma skin cancers in West Germany, 1968–99. *Br J Dermatol.* 2004;150:517–522.

45. Hannuksela-Svahn A, Pukkala E, et al. Basal cell skin carcinoma and other nonmelanoma skin cancers in Finland from 1956 through 1995. *Arch Dermatol.* 1999;135:781–786.

46. Armstrong BK, Kricker A. The epidemiology of UV-induced skin cancer. *J Photochem Photobiol B: Biol.* 2001;63:8–18.

47. Perkins JL, Liu Y, Mitby PA, et al. Nonmelanoma skin cancer in survivors of childhood and adolescent cancer: a report from the Childhood Cancer Survivor Study. *J Clin Oncol.* 2005;23:3733–3741.

48. Moloney FJ, Comber H, O'Lorcain P, et al. A population-based study of skin cancer incidence and prevalence in renal transplant recipients. *Br J Dermatol.* 2006;154:498–504.

49. Hollenbeak CS, Todd MM, Billingsley EM, et al. Increased incidence of melanoma in renal transplantation recipients. *Cancer.* 2005;104:1962–1967.

50. Ulrich C, Schook T, Sachse MM, et al. Comparative epidemiology and pathogenic factors for nonmelanoma skin cancer in organ transplant patients. *Dermatol Surg.* 2004;30:622–627.

51. Cabrera T, Garrido V, Concha A, et al. HLA molecules in basal cell carcinoma of the skin *Immunobiol.* 1992;185:440–452.

52. Rossman TG, Uddin AN, Burns FJ, et al. Arsenite is a cocarcinogen with solar ultraviolet radiation for mouse skin: an animal model for arsenic carcinogenesis *Toxicol Appl Pharmacol.* 2001;176:64–71.

53. Gawkrodger DJ. Occupational skin cancers. *Occup Med.* 2004;54:458–463.

54. Kennedy C, Bajdik CD, Bouwes Bavinck JN. Chemical exposures other than arsenic are probably not important risk factors for squamous cell carcinoma, basal cell carcinoma and malignant melanoma of the skin *Br J Dermatol.* 2005;152:176–198.

55. Zak-Prelich M, Narbutt J, Sysa-Jedrzejowska A. Environmental risk factors predisposing to the development of basal call carcinoma. *Dermatol Surg.* 2004;30:248–252.

56. Mitropoulos P, Norman R. Occupational nonsolar risk factors of squamous cell carcinoma of the skin: a population-based case-controlled study. *Dermatol Online J.* 2005;11:5.

57. Simeonova PP, Luster MI. Mechanisms of arsenic carcinogenicity: genetic or epigenetic mechanisms? *J Environ Pathol Toxicol Oncol.* 2000:19(3);281–286.

58. Rossman TG, Uddin AN, Burns FJ. Evidence that arsenite acts as a cocarcinogen in skin cancer. *Toxicol Appl Pharmacol.* 2004;198:394–404.

59. Ding W, Hudson LG, Liu KJ. Inorganic arsenic compounds cause oxidative damage to DNA and protein by inducing ROS and RNS generation in human keratinocytes. *Mol Cell Biochem.* 2005;279:105–112.

60. Chanda S, Dasgupta UB, Guhamazumder D, et al. DNA hypermethylation of promoter of gene p53 and p16 in arsenic-exposed people with and without malignancy. *Toxicol Sci.* 2006;89:431–437.

61. Pi J, He Y, Bortner C, et al. Low level, long-term inorganic arsenite exposure causes generalized resistance to apoptosis in cultured human keratinocytes: potential role in skin co-carcinogenesis. *Int J Cancer.* 2005;116:20–26.

62. Graham-Evans B, Cohly HH, Yu H, et al. Arsenic-induced genotoxic and cytotoxic effects in human keratinocytes, melanocytes and dendritic cell. *Int J Environ Res Public Health.* 2004;1:83–89.

63. Ahsan H, Chen Y, Kibriaya MG, et al. Susceptibility to arsenic-induced hyperkeratosis and oxidative stress genes myeloperoxidase and catalase. *Cancer Lett.* 2003;201:57–65.

64. Rosales-Castillo JA, Acosta-Saavedra LC, Torres R, et al. Arsenic exposure and human papillomavirus response in nonmelanoma skin cancer Mexican patients: a pilot study. *Int Arch Occup Environ Health.* 2004;77:418–423.

65. Alani RM, Munger K. Human papillomaviruses and associated malignancies *J Clin Oncol.* 1998;16:330–337.

66. International Agency for Research on Cancer (IARC). Human papilloma viruses. IARC Monographs on the Evaluation of Carcinogenic Risks to Humans. Vol. 64, Lyon, France. 1995.

67. Karagas MR, Nelson HH, Sehr P, et al. Human papillomavirus infection and incidence of squamous cell and basal cell carcinomas of the skin. *J Natl Cancer Inst.* 2006;98:389–395.

68. Pfister H. Chapter 8: Human papillomavirus and skin cancer. *JNCI Monogr.* 2003;31:52–56.

69. Bevona C, Sober AJ. Melanoma incidence trends. *Dermatol Clin.* 2002;20:589–595.

70. Lends MB, Dawes M. Global perspectives of contemporary epidemiological trends of cutaneous malignant melanoma. *Br J Dermatol.* 2004;150:179–185.

71. Globocan 2000: *Cancer Incidence, Mortality and Prevalence Worldwide*, Version 1.0. IARC Cancer Base No. 5. Lyon: IARC Press; 2001.

72. Elwood JM. Melanoma and sun exposure. *Semin Oncol.* 1996;23:650–666.

73. Lee JA. The relationship between malignant melanoma of skin and exposure to sunlight. *Photochem Photobiol.* 1989;50:493–496.

74. Gilchrest BA, Eller MS, Geller AC, et al. The pathogenesis of melanoma induced by ultraviolet radiation. *N Engl J Med.* 1999;340:1341–1348.

75. Purdue MP, From L, Armstrong BK, et al. Etiologic and other factors predicting nevus-associated cutaneous malignant melanoma. *Cancer Epidemiol Biomarkers Prev.* 2005;14:2015–2022.

76. Green A. A theory of the site distribution of melanomas: Queensland, Australia. *Cancer Causes Control.* 1992;3:513–516.

77. Beral V, Robinson N. The relationship of malignant melanoma, basal and squamous skin cancers to outdoor and indoor work. *Br J Cancer.* 1981;44:886–8891.

78. Goodman KJ, Bible ML, London S, et al. Proportional melanoma incidence and occupation among white males in Los Angeles County (California, United States). *Cancer Causes Control.* 1995;6:451–459.

79. Green A, MacLennan R, You P, et al. Site distribution of cutaneous melanoma in Queensland. *Intl J Cancer.* 1993;53:232–236.

80. Bulliard JL, Cox B. Elwood JM. Comparison of the site distribution of melanoma in New Zealand and Canada. *Int J Cancer.* 1997;72:231–5.

81. Mackie RM, Marks R, Green A. The melanoma epidemic. Excess exposure to ultraviolet sunlight is established as a major risk factor. *BMJ.* 1996;321:1362–1363.

82. Tucker MA, Halpern A, Holly EA, et al. Clinically recognized dysplastic nevi. A central risk factor for cutaneous melanoma. *JAMA.* 1997;227:1439–1444.

83. Kelly JW, Rivers JK, Maclennan R, et al. Sunlight: a major factor associated with the development of melanocytic nevi in Australian schoolchildren. *J Am Acad Dermatol.* 1994;30:40–48.

84. Whiteman DC, Watt P, Purdie DM, et al. Melanocytic nevi, solar keratoses, and divergent pathways to cutaneous melanoma. *J Natl Cancer Inst.* 2003;95:806–812.

85. Bulliard J, Cox B. Trends by anatomical site in Incidence of cutaneous malignant melanoma in Canada: 1963–1993. *Cancer Causes Control.* 1999;10:407–416.

86. Bulliard J, Cox B. Incidence of cutaneous malignant melanoma in New Zealand by anatomical site: 1963–1993. *Inl J Epidemiol.* 2000;29:416–423.

87. Garbe C, Buettner PG, Weiss J, et al. Risk factors for developing cutaneous melanoma and criteria for identifying persons at risk: multicenter case-control study of Central Malignant Melanoma Registry of the German Dermatological Society. *J Invest Dermatol.* 1994;102: 695–699.

88. Garbe C, McLeod GR, Buettner PG. Time Trends in Cutaneous Melanoma in Queensland, Australia and Central Europe. *Cancer.* 2000;89:1269–1278.

89. Marrett LD, Nguyen HL, Armstrong BK. Trends in the incidence of cutaneous malignant melanoma in New South Wales, 1983–1996. *Int J Cancer.* 2001;92: 457–462.

90. Osterlind A, Engholm G, Jensen OM. Trends in cutaneous malignant melanoma in Denmark 1943–1982 by anatomical site. *APMIS.* 1988;96:953–63.

91. Espinosa Arranz J, Sanchez Hernandez JJ, Bravo Fernandez P, et al. Cutaneous malignant melanoma and sun exposure in Spain. *Melanoma Res.* 1999;2:199–205.

92. Perez-Gomez B, Aragones N, Gustavsson, P, et al. Cutaneous melanoma in Swedish women: occupational risk by anatomic site. *Am J Ind Med.* 2005;48(4):270–281.

93. Beane Freeman LE, Dennis LK, Lynch CF, et al. Toenail arsenic content and cutaneous melanoma in Iowa. *Am J Epidemiol.* 2004;160:679–687.

94. LeVee GL, Oberhelman L, Anderson T, et al. UVA II exposure of human skin results in decreased immunization capacity, increased induction of tolerance and a unique pattern of epidermal antigen-presenting cell alteration. *Photochem Photobiol.* 1997;65:622–629.

95. Damian D., Barnetson RS, Halliday GM. Low-dose UVA and UVB have different time courses for suppression of contact hypersensitivity to al recall antigen in humans. *J Invest Dermatol.* 1999;112: 939–944.

96. Sjovall P, Christensen OB. Local and systemic effect of ultraviolet irradiation (UVA and UVB) on human allergic contact dermatitis. *Acta Derm Venereol.* 1986;66:290–294.

97. deVries E, Coebergh JW. Cutaneous malignant melanoma in Europe. *Eur J Cancer.* 2004;40:2355–2366.

98. Geller AC, Annas GD. Epidemiology of melanoma and nonmelanoma skin cancer. *Semin Oncol Nursing.* 2003;19:2–11.

99. van Steeg H, Kraemer IH. Xeroderma pigmentosum and the role of UV-induced DNA damage in skin cancer. *Molecular Med Today.* 1992;5:86–94.

100. Klepp O, Magnus K. Some environmental and bodily characteristics of melanoma patients. A case-control study. *Int J Cancer.* 1979;23:482–486.

101. Mackie RM, Aitchison T. Severe sunburn and subsequent risk of primary cutaneous malignant melanoma in Scotland. *Br J Cancer.* 1982;46:955–960.

102. Elwood JM, Gallagher RP, Hill GB, et al. Cutaneous melanoma in relation to intermittent and constant sun exposure: the Western Canada Melanoma Study. *Int J Cancer.* 1985;35:427–443.

103. Graham S, Marshall J, Haughey B, et al. An inquiry into the epidemiology of melanoma. *Am J Epidemiol.* 1985;122: 606–619.

104. Dubin N, Moseson M, Pasternack BS. Epidemiology of malignant melanoma: pigmentary traits, ultraviolet radiation, and the identification of high risk populations. In: Gallagher RP, ed. *Epidemiology of Malignant Melanoma: Recent Results in Cancer Research.* Berlin: Springer-Verlag; 1986:56–75.

105. Elwood J, Williamson C, Stapleton PJ. Malignant melanoma in relation to moles, pigmentation, and exposure to fluorescent and other lighting sources. *Br J Cancer.* 1986;53:65–74.

106. Cristofolini, M, Franceschi S, Tasin L, et al. Risk factors for cutaneous malignant melanoma in a northern Italian population. *Int J Cancer.* 1987;39:150–54.

107. Østerlind A, Tucker MA, Stone BJ: The Danish case-control study of cutaneous malignant melanoma. II. Importance of UV-light exposure. *Int J Cancer.* 1988;42: 319–324.

108. Zanetti R, Rosso S, Faggiano, F, et al. Etude castémoins sur le melanome de la peau dans la province de Torino, Italie. *Rev. Epidemiol. Santé Publ.* 1988;36: 309–317.

109. Beitner H, Norell, SE, Ringborg U, et al. Malignant melanoma: aetiological importance of individual pigmentation and sun exposure. *Br J Dermatol.* 1990; 122:43–51.

110. Dubin, N, Pasternack, BS, Moseson M. Simultaneous assessment of risk factors for malignant melanoma and non-melanoma skin lesions, with emphasis on sun exposure and related variables. *Int J Epidemiol.* 1990;19:811–819.

111. Grob JJ, Gouvernet J, Aymar, D, et al. Count of benign melanocytic nevi as a major indicator of risk for nonfamilial nodular and superficial spreading melanoma. *Cancer.* 1990;66:387–395.

112. Herzfeld PM, Fitzgerald EF, Hwang S, et al. A case control study of malignant melanoma of the trunk among white males in upstate New York. *Cancer Detect. Prev.* 1993;17:601–608.

113. Autier P, et al. Recreational exposure to sunlight and lack of information as risk factors for cutaneous malignant melanoma. Results of a European Organization for Research and Treatment of Cancer (EORTC) case-control study in Belgium, France and Germany. *Melanoma Res.* 1994;4:79–85.

114. Westerdahl J, Olsson H, Ingvar C. At what age do sunburn episodes play a crucial role for the development of malignant melanoma? *Eur J Cancer.* 1994;30A;1647–1654.

115. White E, Kirkpatrick CS, Lee JH. Case-control study of malignant melanoma in Washington State. 1. Constitutional factors and sun exposure. *Am J Epidemiol.* 1994;139:857–868.

116. Holly EA, Aston DA, Cress RD, et al. Cutaneous melanoma in women. I. Exposure to sunlight, ability to tan, and other risk factors related to ultraviolet light. *Am J Epidemiol.* 1995;141:923–933.

117. Rodenas JM, Delgado-Rodriguez M, Herranz MT, et al. Sun exposure, pigmentary traits, and risk of cutaneous malignant melanoma: a case-control study in a Mediterranean population. *Cancer Causes Control.* 1996;7:275–283.

118. Chen Y, Dubro R, Holford TR, et al. Malignant melanoma risk factors by anatomic site: a case-control study and polychotomous logistic regression analysis. *Int J Cancer.* 1996;7:636–643.

119. Settimi L, Comba P, Bosia S, Ciapini C, et al. Cancer risk among male farmers: a multi-site case-control study. *Int J Occ Med Environ Health.* 2001;14:339–348.

120. Loria D, Matos E. Risk factors for cutaneous melanoma: a case-control study in Argentina. *Int J Dermatol.* 2001;40: 108–114.

121. Fargnoli MC, Piccolo D, Altobelli E, et al. Constitutional and environmental risk factors for cutaneous melanoma in an Italian population. A case-control study. *Melanoma Res.* 2004;14:151–7.

122. Lasithiotakis K, Kruger-Krasagakis S, et al. Epidemiological differences for cutaneous melanoma in a relatively dark-skinned Caucasian population with chronic sun exposure. *Eur J Cancer.* 2004;40:2502–2507.

123. Chaudru V, Chompret A, Bressac-de Paillerets B, et al. Influence of genes, nevi, and sun sensitivity on melanoma risk in a family sample unselected by family history and in melanoma-prone families. *J Natl Cancer Inst.* 2004;96:785–795.

124. Nijsten T, Leys C, Verbruggen K, et al. Case-control study to identify melanoma risk factors in the Belgian population: the significance of clinical examination. *J Eur Acad Dermatol Venerol.* 2005;19: 332–339.

125. Naldi L, Altieri A, Imberti GL, et al. Oncology Study Group of the Italian Group for Epidemiologic Research in Dermatology. Sun exposure, phenotypic characteristics, and cutaneous malignant melanoma. An analysis according to different clinico-pathological variants and anatomic locations (Italy). *Cancer Causes Control.* 2005;16:893–839.

CHAPTER 4

Etiology of Skin Cancer

Keyvan Nouri, M.D.
Shalu S. Patel, B.S.
Anita Singh, M.S.

BOX 4-1   Overview

- The widespread prevalence of skin cancer is matched by a variety of etiologic factors, including genetic predisposition, other diseases and disorders, and chemical and environmental carcinogens.
- Natural skin and hair color, presence of freckles and moles, age and gender all have corresponding risk levels for melanoma and nonmelanoma skin cancers.
- Diseases such as xeroderma pigmentosum, Gorlin syndrome, familial atypical multiple mole melanoma syndrome, albinism, epidermodysplasia verruciformis, bowenoid papulosis, discoid lupus erythematosus, and chronic inflammation have been associated with skin cancer.
- Chemical carcinogens such as arsenic, creosote, cigarette smoke, and PUVA lead to an increased chance of developing skin cancer.
- Environmental and artificial exposure to UV radiation is a leading cause of skin cancer.

INTRODUCTION

The incidence of skin cancer has increased dramatically during the past two decades. The National Cancer Institute warns that from 40 to 50% of all Americans who live to age 65 years will develop at least one skin cancer, if the current trend continues. As the incidence of skin cancers increase every year, it is now more important than ever to define an accurate etiology of skin cancer to pave the way for appropriate preventative measures to be taken.

This chapter aims to review the commonly known etiologies of both nonmelanoma skin cancers (NMSC) and melanoma. It also introduces new ideas that may play a role in causing skin cancer.

PREDISPOSITIONS

BOX 4-2   Summary

- People with light colored skin, hair and eyes are at a greater risk for skin cancer due to decreased melanin production.
- Age and gender also can influence the risk for skin cancer. Typically, men and the elderly are at the highest risk, although people of all ages can develop the disease.
- Having a family history of skin cancer is another predisposing factor for the disease.

Skin cancer develops in people of all colors, from the palest to the darkest. However, skin cancer is most likely to occur in individuals who have fair skin, blonde or red hair, a tendency to burn or freckle when exposed to the sun, multiple moles, a history of sun exposure,[1] and light colored eyes.[2] These individuals are at an increased risk due to the fact that they have less melanin production.[3] Melanin is manufactured in melanocytes (found in the stratum basale of the epidermis) from the amino acid tyrosin, using the enzyme tyrosinase. UV light stimulates the production of melanin in the form of insoluble melanosomes. These surround the epidermal cells, which move up to the surface of the skin and eventually result in a tan. More melanin is produced in the skin of dark-skinned individuals even in the absence of sunlight, and their type of melanin, eumelanin, is more effective at blocking UV rays. On the other hand, melanin (pheomelanin) is produced in the skin of light-skinned individuals only in the presence of sunlight and after the UV rays have penetrated the lower portion of the epidermis and have caused skin damage.[4–6]

Due to the fact that African Americans have more melanin produced in their skin,[3] the incidence of skin cancers within this population remains relatively low, but is not absent.[7]

Anatomic distribution of basal cell carcinomas may be similar to that seen in Caucasians but not for other skin cancers. In this population, melanoma most often develops on nonsun-exposed areas, such as the foot, underneath nails, and on the mucous membranes of the mouth, nasal passages, or genitals.[7] In addition, African Americans do not fare as well in terms of mortality as Caucasians for squamous cell carcinoma and melanoma. This difference probably

is due to the fact that either African Americans have more advanced stages of disease at diagnosis than do Caucasians and less accessibility to medical care and disease preventative screenings because of socioeconomic and cultural factors,[8] or because the course of the disease is more aggressive in African Americans for reasons yet unknown. Factors thought to be important in the pathogenesis of skin cancers in this group of patients include exposure to sunlight, scars from burns, X-rays, chronic inflammation, preexisting pigmented lesions, albinism, and chronic discoid lupus erythematosus, in addition to others.[9]

A second risk factor for development of skin cancer is age. Elderly individuals are more susceptible to the development of skin cancers than younger individuals. The risk of developing skin cancer increases with age, primarily because many skin cancers develop slowly. The damage that occurs during childhood or adolescence may not become apparent until middle age.[10] Still, skin cancer is not limited to older people. Basal cell and squamous cell carcinomas are increasing most quickly among women younger than 40 years of age.[11]

Thirdly, men are at 2 to 3 times greater risk than women for developing skin cancer. According to the Skin Cancer Foundation, the majority of individuals diagnosed with melanoma are white men over the age of 50 years and is currently the leading cancer in men over the age of 50 years. This is thought to be due to higher sun exposure. Men over the age of 40 years spend the most time outdoors and in fact have the highest yearly exposure to ultraviolet radiation. In addition, men over age 50 years do not regularly perform monthly skin self-examinations and do not visit their dermatologist regularly. Because of these factors this age group of men are the least likely to detect skin cancers in the early stages.

Finally, a personal or family history of skin cancer portends a greater risk of developing skin cancer. Patients having two or more close relatives with melanoma or have been treated for melanoma in the past are at a higher risk.[12] Additionally, patients with a history of basal or squamous cell carcinoma are at increased risk of getting additional basal and squamous cell carcinomas, as well as, melanomas. It has been found that about 50% of patients treated for nonmelanoma skin cancer have another skin cancer within 5 years.[13–16]

BOX 4-3   Summary

- Xeroderma pigmentosum is a genetic DNA repair disorder that fails to fix the damage caused by UV radiation, in particular the thymine dimers.
- Gorlin syndrome is caused by a gene mutation leading to an increased risk for basal cell carcinoma.
- Familial atypical multiple mole melanoma syndrome, as the name suggests, is a genetic disorder characterized by patients with an extensive family history of malignant melanoma.
- Albinism is a genetic disease caused by a lack of melanin production or distribution, leading to a complete or patchy lack of pigment in the skin.
- Epidermodysplasia verruciformis is a disease which renders patients immunocompromised and susceptible to HPV and squamous cell carcinoma.
- Bowenoid papulosis, also called squamous cell carcinoma *in situ*, is induced by HPV.
- Discoid lupus erythematosus is a chronic and recurrent disorder that can cause persistent inflammation and may eventually lead to the development of skin cancers.
- Chronic inflammation has been shown to be tumor promoting due to the effects of NF-κB.

Xeroderma Pigmentosum (XP)

Xeroderma pigmentosum is a rare autosomal recessive disorder characterized by skin malignancies, premature skin aging, photosensitivity, and pigmentary changes. It is a multisystem disorder, but sun-exposed skin and eyes (i.e., eyelids, conjunctivae) are the most affected tissues.[17] These manifestations are due to a cellular hypersensitivity to ultraviolet (UV) radiation resulting from a defect in nucleotide excision repair, this leads to deficient repair of DNA damaged by UV radiation. UV radiation induces dimerization between thymine nucleotides. After exposure to UV light, normal cells identify and excise the UV-induced thymine dimers and insert undamaged nucleotides after DNA synthesis and ligation. This repair process is deficient in XP.[18]

Individuals with this disease develop multiple skin neoplasms at a young age. The mean age of skin cancer development is 8 years in patients with XP compared to 60 years in the healthy population. Metastatic malignant melanoma and squamous cell carcinoma are the two most important causes of mortality in these patients. In fact, patients younger than 20 years of age have a 1000-fold increase in the incidence of nonmelanoma skin cancer and melanoma.[19]

XP typically passes through three stages. Stage one, which begins about 6 months after birth, is characterized by diffuse redness, scaling, and freckle-like areas over sun-exposed areas and later progressing to other parts. The second stage is characterized by poikiloderma. This stage consists of telangiectasias, skin atrophy, and areas of pigmentary changes. The third stage is where the appearance of numerous skin malignancies occurs in sun-exposed areas and may occur as early as 4 to 5 years of age.[20]

Gorlin Syndrome (Basal Cell Nevus Syndrome)

Gorlin syndrome is an autosomal dominant disorder characterized by extreme sensitivity to ionizing radiation. Very rarely, it can appear in a family with no past history of the condition because of a random gene mutation. These patients have a higher risk of developing multiple neoplasms, especially basal cell carcinomas and medulloblastoma. This syndrome can affect multiple organs, but the involvement is usually very minimal. Affected individuals may also have abnormalities of the jaw and other bones, eyes, and nervous tissue. This disorder is thought to be caused by germline mutations in the patched gene (PTCH). Currently, there have been more than 50 different germline mutations in PTCH described.[21]

Incidence of Gorlin syndrome is estimated to be 1 in 56,000 in the general population and may vary by region.[21] The main cause of early death from Gorlin syndrome is due to the effects of medulloblastoma, but this occurs rarely. Further, there is a very small chance of death from very aggressive invasive basal cell carcinomas after treatment with irradiation.[21] The irradiation used to treat the basal cell carcinoma can cause further damage and carcinogenesis. A diagnosis of Gorlin syndrome should be considered in any patient who presents with basal cell carcinomas at an early age (<30 years), especially if the tumors occur in skin with minimal sun exposure.

Familial Atypical Multiple Mole Melanoma Syndrome (FAMMM)

Familial atypical multiple mole and melanoma (FAMMM) syndrome, also sometimes called the familial dysplastic nevus syndrome (DNS), is an autosomal dominant disorder with variable incomplete penetrance of the clinical phenotypes. This condition is marked by the following: (1) one or more first- or second-degree relatives with malignant melanoma, (2) many moles (over 50), some of which are atypical (asymmetrical, raised, and/or different shades of tan, brown, black, or red) and often of different sizes, and (3) younger age of diagnosis of melanoma (usually by the age of 33 years).[22]

This disorder is believed to be caused by an increased rate of germline CDKN2A mutations (usually missense or nonsense changes) that impair the function of p16. The p16 protein is a negative regulator of cell cycle progression at the G1/S checkpoint.[23,24] It interacts with the cyclin-dependent kinases (CDK4 or CDK6), enzymes that control early events in the cell cycle, to catalyze phosphorylation of the retinoblastoma family of proteins.[23,24] The p16 protein binds to and inhibits CDK4, and thus serves as a brake on cell cycle progression. Inactivating mutations of p16 disrupt its inhibitory function on CDK4, thereby permitting inappropriate progression through the cell cycle and confers susceptibility to melanoma.[23,24]

Patients with FAMMM have an overall lifetime risk of melanoma of 100%.[25,26] Affected subjects may have over 100 nevi, with lesions that are predominantly truncal and in sun-exposed areas. However, they can also occur on the scalp, feet, and genitalia. Most lesions develop during childhood, and the result is a relatively stable number of nevi by the end of puberty. The median age at diagnosis is 33 years, well below that in patients with sporadic melanomas.[25,26] For this reason these patients should be followed carefully.

Albinism

Albinism is a group of hereditary disorders that involve an abnormality of melanin synthesis or distribution.[27] It can present as a pigmentation abnormality of the skin, hair, and/or eyes and can be divided into two categories: oculocutaneous albinism and ocular albinism. Oculocutaneous albinism involves both the skin and eyes, whereas, ocular albinism mainly affects the eyes with minimal-to-no skin involvement. Oculocutaneous albinism is mostly an autosomal recessive disorder.[28]

This disorder is caused by a defect in melanin metabolism, and the defect can lie with either melanin synthesis or distribution. Melanin is synthesized in melanocytes from the amino acid tyrosine; this process takes place in the melanosomes.[4-6] The pathophysiology of oculocutaneous albinism involves a reduction in the amount of melanin present in each of the melanosomes. These patients can present with either an absence of pigment from the hair, skin, or iris; patchy absence of pigment; or lighter than normal skin and hair.[29-31] In addition, they may have nystagmus, strabismus, photophobia, and decreased visual acuity or even functional blindness.[29-31] Because melanin protects the skin from the sun, people with albinism are very prone to sunburn and, therefore, to skin cancer. Even a few minutes of bright sunlight can cause serious burns. Individuals with albinism must protect themselves from sunlight, or they risk the early development of both cutaneous squamous cell carcinoma and basal cell carcinoma.[32]

Epidermodysplasia Verruciformis (EV)

Epidermodysplasia verruciformis (EV) is a rare, autosomal recessive hereditary disorder characterized by extreme susceptibility to cutaneous human papillomavirus (HPV) infection and squamous cell carcinoma (SCC). Lesions develop in childhood with malignant transformation during adulthood in 50% of the patients. The lesions are polymorphic, usually having a flat wart-like appearance on the dorsum of the hands and extremities, and pityriasis versicolor-like lesions located on the trunk, pubic area, neck, and face. The skin cancers initially appear on sun-exposed areas, such as the face and the ear lobes.[33,34]

Patients with epidermodysplasia verruciformis have a defective cell-mediated immune response to HPV infection.[35] It has been found that many of the HPV types found in EV lesions are nonpathogenic to the general population. The exact mechanisms involved in the malignant transformation of keratinocytes in skin lesions of patients with EV are still unclear. It is believed that interactions occur between oncogenic HPVs and antioncogene proteins, such as p53, in cell cycle regulation, DNA repair, and the activation of apoptosis.[35]

Malignant transformation of skin lesions has been observed in more than one half of the patients followed up for 20 to 30 years. Squamous cell carcinomas are typically found after age 30 years, usually during the fourth and fifth decades of life.[36] These tumors are numerous and initially progress as non-invasive, *in situ* carcinomas. Most squamous cell carcinomas remain local, and metastasis is extremely uncommon. Tumors are locally destructive without treatment.[36] The diagnosis of EV should be suspected in the clinical setting of numerous verrucous lesions or when lesions are resistant to appropriate therapy.

Bowenoid Papulosis

Bowenoid papulosis is a focal epidermal hyperplasia and dysplasia induced by human papillomavirus (HPV) infection (most commonly by HPV 16). The result is a papule demonstrating scattered atypical cells or full-thickness epidermal atypia (bowenoid dysplasia) that is thought to be the same as squamous cell carcinoma *in situ*. Bowenoid papulosis can be found on the genitalia of both sexes in sexually active individuals. Many of the lesions remain benign; however, there is a 2.6% chance of malignant invasive transformation.[37,38]

Bowenoid papulosis usually presents as solitary or multiple, small, pigmented (red, brown, or flesh-colored) papules with a flat-to-verrucous surface.[38] The lesions can combine into larger plaques and occur most commonly on the shaft of the penis or the external genitalia of females, however, they can occur anywhere on the genitalia and in the perianal region.[39] This disease occurs primarily in young, sexually active adults, with a mean age of 31 years. The male-to-female ratio is equal and affects all races equally.[40] It is recommended that the lesions be examined every 3 to 6 months because of the possibility of transformation to Bowen disease (squamous cell carcinoma *in situ*) or invasive squamous cell carcinoma. The risk of transformation is higher in patients who are immunocompromised and in the elderly.

Discoid Lupus Erythematosus

Discoid Lupus Erythematosus (DLE) is a chronic and recurrent disorder primarily affecting the skin and characterized by sharply circumscribed macules and plaques displaying erythema, follicular plugging, scales, telangiectasia, and atrophy.[41] Discoid lesions are most often seen on the face, neck, and scalp, but also occur on the ears, and infrequently on the upper torso. They tend to slowly expand with active inflammation at the periphery, and then to heal, leaving depressed central scars, atrophy, telangiectasias, and hyperpigmentation/depigmentation.[41]

DLE may occur in patients with systemic lupus erythematosus (SLE), and some patients (5 to 10%) with DLE progress to SLE.[42] The pathophysiology and genetic predisposition of DLE is not well understood. It has been suggested that a heat shock protein is induced in the keratinocyte following ultraviolet (UV) light exposure or stress, and this protein may act as a target for T-cell mediated epidermal cell cytotoxicity.[43]

DLE is slightly more common in African Americans than in Caucasians or Asians. The male-to-female ratio of DLE is 1:2. This disorder may occur at any age but most often occurs in persons aged 20 to 40 years, the mean age is approximately 38 years.[44] Patients with DLE rarely have clinically significant systemic disease. However, lesions may produce scarring or atrophy. Malignant degeneration of chronic lesions of DLE is possible, although rare, leading to nonmelanoma skin cancer. Dark-skinned individuals may be more prone to skin cancer because of the lack of pigmentation within the chronic lesion, combined with chronic inflammation and continued sun damage.[45]

Chronic Inflammation

Inflammation is an essential function of the innate immune system. It serves to protect us by initiating specific and long-term immunity, destroying infectious agents, and repairing damaged tissue.[46] However, it has been shown that there is a tumor-promoting role of inflammation in the development and progression of epithelial skin cancer.[46] Chronic inflammation due to burns, scars, sinus tracts infections, chronic ulcers, as well as others, has an increased risk of cutaneous squamous cell carcinoma (SCC). When a cutaneous SCC occurs in a chronic wound, it is also known as Marjolin's ulcer.[47]

It is now believed that NF-κB is the cause of the cancer-promoting action of inflammatory cells. NF-κB is very active in both inflammatory cells and in other cells of inflamed tissues. This protein may also be abnormally active in some cancers.[48] The cancer-promoting action of NF-κB may be due to the fact that its activity leads to the inhibition of apoptosis that removes defective cells, thereby, contributing to cancer development.[48] Approximately 1% of skin cancers arise in chronically inflamed skin and about 95% of these are SCCs.[49] The time between the initial skin damage and appearance of a tumor is very variable, with SCC appearing as early as 6 weeks or as many as 60 years after the inflammatory event.[47,50,51]

CHEMICAL CARCINOGENS AND OCCUPATIONAL SKIN CANCERS

BOX 4-4 Summary

- Arsenic exposure through drinking water or occupationally has been linked to causing a variety of cancers, nonmelanoma skin cancers included.
- Creosote, found in coal tar used for road paving and insecticides, can lead to skin cancer.
- Smokers are at an increased risk for developing squamous cell carcinoma perhaps due to its immunosuppressive effects.
- PUVA may induce skin cancer by: photomutagenicity, photoinduced immunosuppression, use of other immunosuppressive agents along with PUVA, and possible human papilloma virus (HPV) infection.
- Occupational skin cancers affect workers in a variety of workplace settings and can be caused by a wide range of substances.

Arsenic Exposure

Arsenic is a natural element found in many types of rocks, however, inorganic arsenicals are known to be chemical carcinogens. Arsenic compounds are used in many substances including industrial, agricultural, and medicinal substances. Additionally, it is found to be an environmental contaminant in drinking water, mostly well water, and an occupational hazard for miners and glass workers.[52,53] Chronic exposure to arsenic is associated with a variety of cancers. Consumption of contaminated drinking water and occupational exposure are associated with cutaneous squamous cell carcinomas and basal cell carcinomas.[52,53] Lesions commonly described are multiple squamous cell carcinomas, arising from the arsenic hyperkeratotic warts, as well as basal cell carcinomas arising from cells not associated with hyperkeratinization.[52,53]

The mechanism of carcinogenicity is not well understood. It is believed that the high affinity of arsenic for sulfhydryl groups makes keratin-rich cells, like keratinocytes, a target for arsenic-induced toxicity.[53] Arsenic has been shown to alter the epidermal keratinocyte differentiation processes, induce overexpression of growth factors, and enhance proliferation of human keratinocytes.[52,53]

Arsenical keratoses may remain benign and some may develop into invasive squamous cell carcinoma. Metastatic arsenic squamous cell carcinoma and arsenic-induced visceral malignancies may result in mortality.[52,53] Arsenic-induced skin cancers are very rare in the United States, only isolated incidences of cutaneous toxicity from environmental or medicinal exposure have been reported. However, arsenic-induced skin lesions have been noticed in some endemic regions, mainly due to long-term exposure to high levels of arsenic in drinking water.[52,53]

Creosote Exposure

The term "creosote" is often used to describe polycyclic aromatic hydrocarbons (PAH) rich products of combustion, and their distillates. It includes such products as wood creosote (from the combustion of beech and other woods), coal tar creosote (from the combustion of coal or coal tar), and coal tar pitch volatiles.[54] Wood creosote is rarely used today, but in the past has been used as a disinfectant, a laxative, and a cough treatment. The most widely used creosote in the United States is coal tar, which can be used in roofing, road paving, and aluminum smelting. In addition, coal tar products are used to treat skin diseases (i.e., psoriasis) but may be also used as repellents, insecticides, pesticides, and fungicides.[54]

Entry of PAHs into the body occurs through the airways, skin and digestive tract.[55] Metabolic activation of PAHs occurs primarily in the liver, but also in many other tissues, including the epithelial barriers. Although distribution through the circulatory system is widespread, slow absorption through most epithelia results in higher levels of enzymes that activate PAH substrates at the site of entry.[56] This uneven distribution of dose is a factor that may contribute to the high propensity of PAHs to act as carcinogens at the sites where they enter the body. Long-term exposure, especially direct contact with skin during wood treatment or manufacture of coal tar creosote-treated products has resulted in skin cancer.[56]

Smoking

Cigarette smoking is the most important preventable cause of death in the USA.[57,58] It is strongly associated with diseases such as cancer, lung disease, and heart disease; however, it also has cutaneous manifestations as well. It has been

found that smokers are at 3.3 times increased risk for developing squamous cell carcinoma (SCC) of the skin compared to nonsmokers.[57,58] Risk of cutaneous SCC increases with the number of packs smoked daily and the duration of the smoking habit.[57,58] The increased risk for SCC may be a result of the immunosuppressive effects of smoking.[59]

There has been no clear association between smoking and basal cell carcinoma (BCC), as well as, melanoma.[57,58] It has been suggested that when compared to nonsmokers, melanoma patients who are smokers are more likely to have metastases on initial presentation; have lower disease-free survival rates after diagnosis; are more likely to have visceral metastases; and are more likely to die from the melanoma than nonsmokers.[57,58] Smokers probably have a poorer prognosis because of the adverse effects of smoking on the immune system, including impaired immunosurveillance and a lowered capacity to mount an immune response.[59]

PUVA

PUVA photochemotherapy is a type of ultraviolet radiation treatment used for severe skin diseases. It is a combination treatment which consists of psoralens (P) and then exposing the skin to long wave ultraviolet radiation (UVA). It has been used to treat psoriasis, eczema, mycosis fungoides, vitiligo, and polymorphic light eruption.

The mechanism of PUVA induced skin cancer includes photomutagenicity, photoinduced immunosuppression, use of other immunosuppressive agents along with PUVA, and possible human papilloma virus (HPV) infection.[60] The occurrence of PUVA nonmelanoma skin cancers is dose related. In fact, patients receiving more than 200 treatments have 30 times increased risk of nonmelanoma skin cancer more than the general population.[61] Typically, patients receiving PUVA treatments consisting of more than 1000 J/cm^2 are at an increased risk of nonmelanoma skin cancer.[62-64] It is also reported that there is an increased incidence of malignant melanoma in patients treated with PUVA,[65,66] possibly due to the photomutagenicity and immunosuppressive effects.

Occupational Skin Cancers

Occupational skin diseases affect workers of all ages in a wide variety of work settings. Skin tumors can result from exposure to ionizing radiation, inorganic metals, arsenicals, polycyclic hydrocarbons, sunlight, as well as other substances. Ionizing radiation is a well-recognized cause of nonmelanoma skin cancer. It induces genomic instability in cells, including chromosomal abnormalities and hyperrecombination.[67] Workers who are affected by this are usually medical personnel, welders, airline flight personnel, those involved in the nuclear energy industry, etc.

Metals such as inorganic arsenic are well recognized as skin carcinogens. Metal workers are susceptible to the effects of these materials because there is evidence that early formulations of metalworking fluids and metal machining are carcinogenic to the skin.[68] Wood workers are susceptible to the exposure to creosotes used as wood preservatives. Creosotes are an established cause of nonmelanoma skin cancer, in addition to exposure to polycyclic hydrocarbons and coal tars.[68]

Individuals who work outdoors, such as telephone-line workers, sailors, postal workers, landscapers and construction workers are at an increased risk for developing basal cell carcinomas, squamous cell carcinomas and melanomas due to the fact that they have more exposure to sunlight.[69]

ENVIRONMENTAL AND LIFESTYLE CONCERNS

BOX 4-5 Summary

- Ozone layer depletion has allowed an increased penetrance to UVB, thereby increasing its chance for causing harmful sunburns.
- UV radiation damages DNA and disables it from repair, thereby permitting uncontrolled cell growth and allowing the development of skin cancer.
- Indoor tanning and sunlamp usage, though meant to provide an alternative to natural UV exposure, is also harmful due to overusage and disregard for regulations.

Exposure to Sun and Ultraviolet Radiation

Some speculate that the continuously increasing incidence may be partly due to the depleting stratospheric ozone layer. This has caused an increase in penetration of UVB, primarily responsible for sunburns, to the earth's surface.[70] Exposure to ultraviolet radiation also depends on geographical location and altitude.

Sunburn is an acute inflammatory reaction caused by over-exposure to ultraviolet radiation. When the skin is exposed to excessive radiation in the ultraviolet range, harmful effects may occur. Most commonly seen is acute sunburn or solar erythema, which is associated with changes in the skin.[71–73] The most characteristic changes in the skin include: thickening of the stratum corneum, formation of epidermal sunburn cells, damaged keratinocytes with hyaline cytoplasm and pyknotic nuclei, and a decrease in Langerhans cell and mast cell numbers. In addition, blood vessels show endothelial swelling, perivenular edema, and a mixed perivascular infiltrate.[71–73]

At a molecular level, exposure to ultraviolet radiation particularly ultraviolet B (wavelength 280 to 315 nm) is known to induce DNA mutagenesis.[74] Resultant induction of the p53 pathway then leads to either growth arrest and DNA repair or apoptosis.[74] Apoptosis serves a protective role by eliminating cells with damaged DNA and malignant potential. The balance between survival and apoptogenic factors determines the final cell fate, and growing evidence suggests that the deregulation of this balance by chronic UVB stress, results in the development of skin malignancy.[74]

Increased susceptibility can be expected in individuals with fair skin, light-colored hair, and history of sunburn with limited exposures to sunlight.[1,2] The long-term consequences of years of overexposure to the sun are significant. One blistering sunburn increases the likelihood of developing malignant melanoma.[75] In addition, cumulative sun exposure is also considered a significant risk factor for nonmelanoma skin cancer. There is evidence suggesting that early, intense exposure causing blistering sunburn in childhood may also play an important role in the cause of nonmelanoma skin cancer.[76]

Indoor Tanning and Sunlamps

The indoor tanning industry is booming now more than ever because many consumers consider it a safe alternative to real sun tanning. However, some do not abide by the regulations and actually exceed recommended UV exposures. In fact, 95% of people who use indoor tanning and sunlamps exceed these limits, and one-third start their sessions at the maximum dose.[77] Recent studies have sought to correlate sunbed use with an increased risk for melanoma, but many of these studies have yielded opposing results.[77] There is also varying evidence regarding the effects of indoor tanning

and sunlamps on nonmelanoma skin cancers.

For a further discussion on this topic, refer to the chapter entitled "Indoor Tanning".

FINAL THOUGHTS

The etiology of skin cancer encompasses a broad spectrum of genetic and environmental factors, some of which are still unknown to this day. However, knowing these is essential for a proper diagnosis, treatment and prevention of this ever-prevalent global disease.

REFERENCES

1. Han J, Colditz GA, Hunter DJ. Risk factors for skin cancers: a nested case–control study within the nurses' health study. *Int. J. Epidemiol.* August 2006 [Epub ahead of print].
2. Dwyer T, Blizzard L, Ashbolt R, et al. Cutaneous melanin density of Caucasians measured by spectrophotometry and risk of malignant melanoma, basal cell carcinoma, and squamous cell carcinoma of the skin. *Am J Epidemiol.* April 2002;155(7): 614–621.
3. Rijken F, Bruijnzeel PL, et al. Responses of black and white skin to solar-simulating radiation: differences in DNA photodamage, infiltrating neutrophils, proteolytic enzymes induced, keratinocyte activation, and IL-10 expression. *J Invest Dermatol.* June 2004;122(6):1448–1455.
4. Tadokoro T, Yamaguchi Y, et al. Mechanisms of skin tanning in different racial/ethnic groups in response to ultraviolet radiation. *J Invest Dermatol.* June 2005;124(6):1326–1332.
5. Van Den Bossche K, Naevaert JM, Lambert J. The quest for the mechanism of melanin transfer. *Traffic.* July 2006;7(7):769–778.
6. Westerhof W. The discovery of the human melanocyte. *Pigment Cell Res.* June 2006;19(3):183–193.
7. Byrd KM, Wilson DC, et al. Advanced presentation of melanoma in African Americans. *J Am Acad Dermatol.* January 2004;50(1):21–24. discussion 142-3.
8. Hu S, Soza-Vento RM, et al. Comparison of stage at diagnosis of melanoma among hispanic, black and white patients in Miami-Dade County, Florida. *Arch Dermatol.* June 2006;142(6):704–708.
9. Halder RM, Bridgeman-Shah S. Skin cancer in African Americans. *Cancer.* January 1995;75(2 suppl):667–673.
10. Desai A, Krathen R, et al. The age of skin cancers. *Sci Aging Knowl. Environ.* May 2006;2006(9):13.
11. Christenson LJ, Borrowman TA, et al. Incidence of basal cell and squamous cell carcinomas in a population younger than 40 years. *JAMA.* August 2005;294(6): 681–690.
12. Azzarello LM, Dessureault S, Jacobsen PB. Sun-protective behavior among individuals with a family history of melanoma. *Cancer Epidemiol Biomarkers Prev.* January 2006;15(1):142–145.

13. Marghoob AA, Kopf AW, Bart RS, et al. Risk of another basal cell carcinoma developing after treatment of a basal cell carcinoma. *J Am Acad Dermatol*. 1993; 28(1):22–28.

14. Marghoob AA, Slade J, Salopek TG, et al. Basal cell and squamous cell carcinomas are important risk factors for cutaneous malignant melanoma: screening implications. *Cancer*. 1995;75(2 suppl):707–714.

15. Frankel DH, Hanusa BH, Zitelli JA. New primary nonmelanoma skin cancer in patients with a history of squamous cell carcinoma of the skin: implications and recommendations for follow-up. *J Am Acad Dermatol*. 1992;26(5 pt 1):720–726.

16. Skin Cancer Prevention Study Group. Risk of subsequent basal cell carcinoma and squamous cell carcinoma of the skin among patients with prior skin cancer. *JAMA*. 1992;267(24):3305–3310.

17. Lambert WC, Kuo HR, Lambert MW. Xerderma pigmentosum. *Dermatol Clin*. January 1995;13(1):169–209.

18. de Laat WL, Jaspers NG, Hoeijmakers JH. Molecular mechanism of nucleotide excision repair. *Genes Dev*. April 1999;13(7): 768–785.

19. Kraemer KH, Lee MM, et al. The role of sunlight and DNA repair in melanoma and nonmelanoma skin cancer. The xeroderma pigmentosum paradigm. *Arch Dermatol*. August 1994;130(8):1018–1021.

20. Pradhan E, Padhye SB, et al. Case of xeroderma pigmentosum with well differentiated squamous cell carcinoma in the eye. Kathmandu Univ Med J. 2003;1(4): 278–283.

21. Taylor SF, Cook AE, Leatherbarrow B. Review of patients with basal cell nevus syndrome. *Ophthal Plast Reconstr Surg*. July/August 2006;22(4):259–265.

22. Czajkowski R, Placek W, et al. FAMMM syndrome: pathogenesis and management. *Dermatol Surg*. February 2004;30(2 pt 2):291–296.

23. Serrano M, Hannon GJ, Beach D. A new regulatory motif in cell-cycle control causing specific inhibition of cyclin D/CDK4. *Nature*. December 1993;366 (6456):704–707.

24. Ohtani N, Zebedee Z, et al. Opposing effects of Ets and Id proteins on p16INK4a expression during cellular senescence. *Nature*. February 2001;409(6823):1067–1070.

25. Clark WH Jr, Reimer RR, et al. Origin of familial malignant melanomas from heritable melanocytic lesions. 'The B-K mole syndrome'. *Arch Dermatol*. May 1978; 114(5):732–738.

26. Lynch HT, Frichot BC 3rd, Lynch JF. Familial atypical multiple mole-melanoma syndrome. *J Med Genet*. October 1978; 15(5):352–356.

27. King RA, Summers CG. Albinism. *Dermatol Clin*. April 1988;6(2):217–228.

28. Spritz, RA. Molecular genetics of oculocutaneous albinism. *Hum Mol Genet*. 1994;3: 1469–1475.

29. Gahl WA, Brantly M, et al. Genetic defects and clinical characteristics of patients with a form of oculocutaneous albinism (Hermansky-Pudlak syndrome). *N Engl J Med*. April 1998;338(18):1258–1264.

30. Oetting, WS. Albinism. *Curr Opin Pediatr*. December 1999;11(6):565–571.

31. Dorey SE, Neveu MM, et al. The clinical features of albinism and their correlation with visual evoked potentials. *Br J Ophthalmol*. June 2003;87(6):767–772.

32. Perry PK, Silverberg NB. Cutaneous malignancy in albinism. *Cutis*. May 2001;67(5): 427–430.

33. Fazel N, Wilczynski S, et al. Clinical, histopathologic, and molecular aspects of cutaneous human papillomavirus infections. *Dermatol Clin*. July1999;17(3): 521–536, viii.

34. Beutner KR. Nongenital human papillomavirus infections. *Clin Lab Med*. June 2000;20(2):423–430.

35. Akgül B, Cooke JC, Storey A. HPV-associated skin disease. *J Pathol*. January 2006;208(2):165–175.

36. Pfister, H. Chapter 8: Human papillomavirus and skin cancer. *J Natl Cancer Inst Monogr*. 2003;(31):52–56.

37. Bonnekoh B, Mahrle G, Steigleder GK. Transition to cutaneous squamous cell carcinoma in 2 patients with bowenoid papulomatosis. *Z Hautkr*. May 1987; 62(10):773–776; 780–784.

38. LaVoo, JW. Bowenoid papulosis. *Dis Colon Rectum*. January 1987;30(1):62–64.

39. Yoneta A, Yamashita T, et al. Development of squamous cell carcinoma by two high-risk human papillomaviruses (HPVs), a novel HPV-67 and HPV-31 from bowenoid papulosis. *Br J Dermatol*. September 2000; 143(3):604–608.

40. Schwartz RA, Janniger CK. Bowenoid papulosis. *J Am Acad Dermatol*. February 1991;24(2 pt 1):261–264.

41. Rowell, NR. Laboratory abnormalities in the diagnosis and management of lupus erythematosus. *Br J Dermatol*. 1971;84: 210.

42. Callen JP. Management of skin disease in patients with lupus erythematosus. *Best Pract Res Clin Rheumatol*. April 2002; 16(2):245–264.

43. Ghoreishi M, Katayama I, et al. Analysis of 70 kDa heat shock protein (HSP70) in the lesional skin of lupus erythematosus (LE) and LE related diseases. *J Dermatol*. July 1993;20(7):400–405.

44. Zamolo G, Coklo M, et al. Expression of p53 and apoptosis in discoid lupus erythematosus. *Croat Med J*. August 2005; 46(4):678–684.

45. Caruso WR, Stewart ML, et al. Squamous cell carcinoma of the skin in black patients with discoid lupus erythematosus. *J Rheumatol*. February 1987;14(1):156–159.

46. Balkwill E., Charles KA, Mantovani A. Smoldering and polarized inflammation in the initiation and promotion of malignant disease. *Cancer Cell*. March 2005; 7(3):211–217.

47. Akguner M, Barutcu A, Yilmaz M, et al. Marjolin's ulcer and chronic burn scarring. *J Wound Care*. March 1998;7(3):121–122.

48. Marx J. Cancer research. Inflammation and cancer: the link grows stronger. *Science*. November 2004;306(5698):966–968.

49. Jellouli-Elloumi A, Kochbati L, Dhraief S, et al. Cancers arising from burn scars: 62 cases. *Ann Dermatol Venereol*. April 2003; 130(4):413–416.

50. Love RL, Breidahl AF. Acute squamous cell carcinoma arising within a recent burn scar in a 14-year-old boy. *Plast Reconstr Surg*. October 2000;106(5):1069–1071.

51. Friedman R, Hanson S, Goldberg LH. Squamous cell carcinoma arising in a Leishmania scar. *Dermatol Surg*. November 2003;29(11):1148–1149.

52. Yu HS, Liao WT, Chai CY. Arsenic carcinogenesis in the skin. *J Biomed Sci*. Jun 2006 [Epub ahead of print].

53. Col M, Col C, Soran A, et al. Arsenic-related Bowen's disease, palmar keratosis, and skin cancer. *Environ Health Perspect*. August 1999;107(8):687–689.

54. Agency for Toxic Substances and Disease Registry (ATSDR). Toxicological Profile for creosote. 1996. Atlanta, GA: U.S. Department of Health and Human Services, Public Health Service.

55. Ding J, Li, J, Chen J, et al. Effects of polycyclic aromatic hydrocarbons (PAHs) on vascular endothelial growth factor induction through phosphatidylinositol 3-kinase/AP-1-dependent, HIF-1alpha-independent pathway. *J Biol Chem* [serial online]. April 2006;281(14):9093–9100. Accessed February 6, 2006.

56. WHO. "PAHs." Air Quality Guidelines, 2nd ed. Denmark: WHO Regional Office for Europe;2000;1–24.

57. Freiman A, Bird G, Metelitsa AI, et al. Cutaneous effects of smoking. *J Cutan Med Surg*. November/December 2004; 8(6):415–423.

58. Smith JB, Fenske NA. Cutaneous manifestations and consequences of smoking. *J Am Acad Dermatol*. May 1996;34(5 pt 1):717–732.

59. Nagomi-Obradovic L. Effects of cigarette smoke constituents on the immune system with special consideration of patients with tuberculosis. *Med Pregl*. 2004;57(suppl 1):33–35.

60. Stern RS, Members of the Photochemotherapy Follow-up Study. Genital tumours among men with psoriasis exposed to psoralens and ultraviolet A radiation (PUVA) and ultraviolet B radiation. *N Engl J Med*. 1990;322:1093–1097.

61. Stern RS, Lange R. Nonmelanoma skin cancer occurring in patients treated with PUVA five to ten years after first treatment. *J Invest Dermatol*. 1988;91:120–124.

62. Forman AB, Roenigk HH Jr, Caro WA, et al. Long term follow up of skin cancer in the PUVA-48 Co-operative Study. *Arch Dermatol*. 1989;125:515–519.

63. Lindelof B, Sigurgeirsson B, Tegner E, et al. PUVA and cancer: a large-scale epidemiological study. *Lancet*. 1991;338: 91–93.

64. Brynzeel I, Bergmann W, Hartevelt HM, et al. 'High single-dose' European PUVA regimen also causes an excess of nonmelanoma skin cancer. *Br J Dermatol*. 1991;124:49–55.

65. Stern RS, Khanh TN, Vakeva LH. Malignant melanoma in patients treated for psoriasis with methoxsalen (psoralen) and ultraviolet radiation (PUVA). *N Engl J Med*. 1997;336:1041–1045.

66. Stern RS, PUVA follow up study. The risk of melanoma in association with long-term exposure to PUVA. *J Am Acad Dermatol*. 2001;44:755–761.

67. Durant ST, Paffett KS, Shrivastav M, et al. UV radiation induces delayed hyper-recombination associated with hypermutation in human cells. *Mol Cell Biol*. August 2006;26(16):6047–6055.

68. Clapp RW, Howe GK, Jacobs M. Environmental and occupational causes of cancer re-visited. *J Public Health Policy*. 2006;27(1):61–76.

69. Peate WE. Occupational skin disease. *Am Fam Physician.* September 2002;66(6): 1025–1032.
70. Lucas RM and Ponsonby AL. Ultraviolet radiation and health: friend and foe. *Med J Aust.* December 2002;177(11–12):594–598.
71. Bickers DR.Sun-induced disorders. *Emerg Med Clin North Am.* November 1985;3(4): 659–676.
72. Cavallo J, DeLeo VA. Sunburn. *Dermatol Clin.* April 1986;4(2):181–187.
73. Van Laethem A, Claerhout S, Garmyn M: The sunburn cell: regulation of death and survival of the keratinocyte. *Int J Biochem Cell Biol.* August 2005;37(8):1547–1553.
74. Claerhout S, Van Laethem A, et al. Pathways involved in sunburn cell formation: deregulation in skin cancer. *Photochem Photobiol Sci.* February 2006; 5(2):199–207 [Epub 2005 Sep 5].
75. Rivers JK. Melanoma. *Lancet.* March 1996;347(9004):803–806.
76. Kennedy C, Bajdik CD, et al. The influence of painful sunburns and lifetime sun exposure on the risk of actinic keratoses, seborrheic warts, melanocytic nevi, atypical nevi, and skin cancer. *J Invest Dermatol.* June 2003;120(6):1087–1093.
77. Abdulla FR, Feldman SR, Williford PM, Krowchuk D, Kaur M. Tanning and skin cancer. *Ped. Dermatol.* 2005;22(6):501–512.

CHAPTER 5

The Genetic Basis of Common Forms of Skin Cancer

Sena Lee, M.D., Ph.D.
Steven S. Fakharzadeh, M.D., Ph.D.

BOX 5-1   Overview

- A number of specific genes have been implicated in the pathogenesis of each major form of skin cancer through genetic studies involving familial and/or sporadic skin cancer. Their role in cutaneous tumorigenesis is confirmed by functional analysis in animal model systems.
- *CDKN2A* and *CDK4* defects are associated with both familial and sporadic cutaneous malignant melanoma. Deregulation of *RAS* signaling, through either *RAS* mutation (*N-RAS*) or activation of MAP kinase (*BRAF*) and PI3′ kinase (*PTEN*, *PKB/AKT*) *RAS* effector pathways, contributes to melanoma tumorigenesis.
- Mutations in the *TP53* gene are common in squamous cell carcinoma and precursor lesions, suggesting that p53 inactivation represents an early step in development of this form of skin cancer. *CDKN2A* defects may occur in squamous cell carcinoma as well. *RAS* activation may cooperate with other genetic aberrations in causing cutaneous squamous cell carcinoma tumorigenesis.
- Aberrations involving the *PTCH* gene have been implicated in both hereditary and sporadic forms of basal cell carcinoma. In addition, mutations in genes encoding other mediators of *SHH* signaling have been associated with sporadic tumors. Defects in the *TP53* tumor suppressor gene are frequently observed in basal cell carcinoma as well.
- Although significant progress has been made in identifying gene defects that promote skin cancer development, additional genes likely play a role in the pathogenesis of each major form of skin cancer.

INTRODUCTION

Tumorigenesis is a multistep process that derives from various acquired, and in some cases inherited, genetic aberrations.[1] Together, these alterations lead to imbalances between critical cellular processes including proliferation, differentiation, and cell death. Consequently, such imbalances allow for clonal cell expansion and ultimately tumor development. Significant advances in delineating the genetic basis of skin cancers have been made. Specific gene[†] defects implicated in the pathogenesis of cutaneous neoplasia have been identified through studies of both hereditary and/or sporadic skin cancer. In turn, functional studies in animal model systems confirm the role of many of these gene defects in skin cancer development. Here we review and summarize the current understanding of the genetic basis of the three most common types of skin cancer: melanoma, squamous cell carcinoma, and basal cell carcinoma.

CUTANEOUS MALIGNANT MELANOMA (CMM)

BOX 5-2   Summary

- *CDKN2A* and *CDK4* represent the only known familial melanoma genes, yet they account for a minority of hereditary cases of melanoma. Mouse models recapitulate melanoma susceptibility conferred by defects in these genes. *CDKN2A* and *CDK4* defects are associated with sporadic melanoma as well.
- Deregulation of *RAS* signaling, through either *RAS* mutation (*N-RAS*) or activation of MAP kinase (*BRAF*) and PI3′ kinase (*PTEN*, *PKB/AKT*) *RAS* effector pathways, contributes to melanoma tumorigenesis. *BRAF* mutations are the most commonly observed in human melanoma.
- *MC1R* represents a low-penetrance melanoma susceptibility gene and variants may confer risk for melanoma independently of skin pigmentation phenotype.
- *MITF* and *NEDD9* are melanoma-associated genes recently identified through genome-wide searches.

Familial Melanoma

CDKN2A (*INK4A* AND *ARF*) GENE DEFECTS

Although most melanomas are thought to arise in a sporadic fashion, it has been

---

[†]*Nomenclature note:* Genes are designated by italicized letters. Proteins are designated by nonitalicized letters. Human genes and proteins are capitalized; mouse genes and proteins have the first letter capitalized and are followed by lower case letters, e.g., *SHH*: human gene; SHH: human protein; *Shh*: mouse gene; Shh: mouse protein.

---

estimated that familial melanomas comprise up to 10% of all cases.[2] Genetic studies of such families predisposed to developing CMM led to the identification of the first melanoma susceptibility gene. Early studies provided initial clues for a melanoma locus by demonstrating cytogenetic aberrations and deletions involving the short arm of chromosome 9 in both primary CMMs and melanoma cell lines.[3] Linkage analysis confirmed these findings and localized a putative melanoma tumor suppressor gene to the 9p21 region.[4] Subsequently, germline mutations were detected within the *CDKN2A* locus, which maps to 9p21, in several affected members of CMM families showing linkage to this region.[5,6] The frequency of *CDKN2A* mutation in familial CMM varies depending on the population; overall, mutations have been detected in 20 to 40% of the families with three or more affected members and in 10% of the families with at least two cases of CMM. Of those individuals that inherit *CDKN2A* mutations, 55 to 100% ultimately develop CMM. Thus, the CMM susceptibility phenotype associated with *CDKN2A* mutations is highly penetrant.[7]

The *CDKN2A* locus encodes two proteins, p16^{INK4A} and p14^{ARF} (reviewed in [8,9]). The two genes share overlapping sequences; however, they give rise to two completely distinct proteins. Independent promoters are used to initiate transcription of these genes, and different first exons are incorporated into each transcript (Fig. 5-1). Alternative mRNA splicing joins each first exon with the same second and third exons. However, different translational reading frames (hence designation of p14 as *ARF* for alternative reading frame) are used for the shared exons, thus yielding proteins with distinct amino acid sequences that lack homology.

The p16^{INK4A} protein negatively regulates cell proliferation by arresting cells at the G1 phase of the cell cycle (Fig. 5-2).[8,9] Progression through G1 is dependent on a protein complex formed by cyclin D1 and CDK4 (cyclin-dependent kinase 4). The CDK4 portion of this complex phosphorylates the retinoblastoma tumor suppressor protein (RB), which then releases E2F family transcription factors. After they are released, E2F transcription factors induce genes required for progressing through G1 and entering the S phase of the cell cycle. Binding of p16^{INK4A} to CDK4 inhibits its kinase activity, leading to inhibition of cell

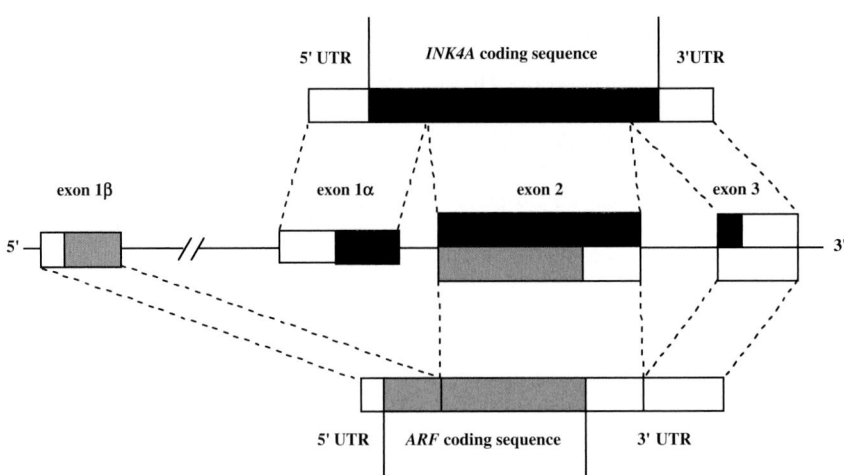

▲ **FIGURE 5-1** *INK4A* and *ARF* transcripts expressed from the *CDKN2A* locus. Both *INK4A* and *ARF* share overlapping sequences within the *CDKN2A* locus. Use of different promoters allows for transcription of distinct first exons, 1α (*INK4A*) and 1β (*ARF*). Alternative mRNA splicing permits joining of each first exon with the same second and third exons. However, the p16[INK4A] and p14[ARF] proteins are derived from different translational reading frames in exons 2 and 3 (*INK4A* black; *ARF* gray). Thus each protein has a distinct amino acid sequence that shares no homology with the other.

tumorigenesis independent of p16[INK4A]. However, mutations that affect only the p14[ARF] protein have been found in some CMM families, indicating that it represents a bonafide melanoma susceptibility gene in its own right. Deletions within a region of *ARF* exon 1β that do not disrupt *INK4A* coding sequences have been identified in melanoma families.[12,13] A germline insertion into exon 1β sequences that introduces a translational frame shift and premature termination codon exclusively disrupting *ARF* expression was observed in a subject with multiple CMMs.[14] Similarly, germline mutations altering the splice donor site of exon 1β, thus compromising expression of p14[ARF] from this allele, have been detected in a number of melanoma families.[15,16] An example of a germline missense mutation specifically involving *ARF* exon 1β, has been described in an additional melanoma family.[13] Together these findings demon-

cycle progression. In turn, phosphorylation of RB protein is hindered, and release of E2F transcription factors by RB becomes impaired. Consequently, the cell cycle stalls in the G1 phase. Therefore, loss of p16[INK4A] activity through either *CDKN2A* mutation or deletion would eliminate a critical suppressor of cell cycle progression and tumor development. Most germline *CDKN2A* mutations that confer CMM susceptibility interfere with p16[INK4A] binding to CDK4.[10,11] This, in essence, would render p16[INK4A] functionally inactive. However, mutations in noncoding regions of *CDKN2A* have also been identified.

The p14[ARF] protein is also involved in cell cycle regulation, but it exerts its influence via stabilization of p53, an important tumor suppressor that regulates cell cycle arrest and programmed cell death (p53 is discussed in detail in the section on cutaneous squamous cell carcinoma, (Fig. 5-4). The p14[ARF] gene product binds to the human homolog of murine Mdm2 (HDM2); this blocks HDM2-mediated ubiquitination of p53, which in turn prevents p53 degradation. Consequently, stabilization of p53 promotes cell cycle arrest. Thus, both products of the *CDKN2A* locus, p16[INK4A] and p14[ARF], block progression of the cell cycle through distinct, yet critical, alternative pathways.

Because the two proteins are encoded within the same locus, it has been difficult to discern the role of p14[ARF] in CMM

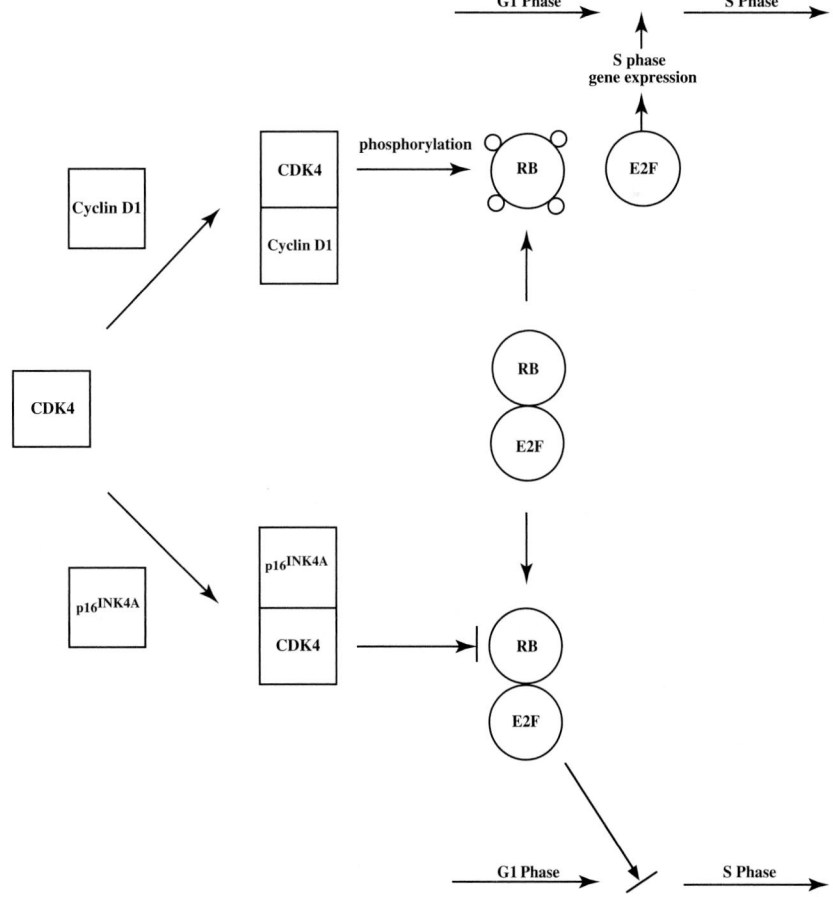

▲ **FIGURE 5-2** CDK4 and p16[INK4A] regulation of the cell cycle. (upper panel) CDK4 and cyclin D1 bind each other to form a complex that phosphorylates RB through the kinase activity of CDK4. After it becomes phosphorylated, RB releases E2F transcription factors, which induce expression of various genes needed for progressing from G1 to S phase of the cell cycle. (lower panel) p16[INK4A] binds CDK4 and inhibits its kinase activity. This leads to hypophosphorylation of RB, which prevents release of E2F transcription factors and inhibits progression to S phase.

strate that germline defects specific to *ARF* may raise increased susceptibility to CMM in a manner independent of *INK4A*.

A variety of mouse models developed for functional analysis of the *CDKN2A* locus corroborate findings derived from mutation analysis in familial CMM, and directly implicate *CDKN2A* defects in melanoma tumorigenesis. Mice carrying a targeted deletion that disrupts the expression of both p16^{INK4A} and p19^{ARF} (the murine homolog of human p14^{ARF}) show normal development. Nonetheless, these mice are predisposed to developing spontaneous tumors early in life and are highly susceptible to tumorigenesis induced by carcinogenic agents.[17] However, directing expression of an activated *H-RAS* or *N-RAS* gene to melanocytes in p16^{INK4A}/p19^{ARF}-deficient mice specifically leads to development of melanoma.[18,19] Similarly, melanocyte-directed expression of activated *H-RAS* in mice with targeted deletion of the genes encoding either p16^{INK4A} or p19^{ARF} alone develop melanoma as well. However, these mice generate tumors with a greater latency period compared to mice deficient for both genes.[9] These studies provide direct evidence for a causal relationship between *CDKN2A* aberrations and development of CMM. Furthermore, they demonstrate that cooperation between defects in *CDKN2A* and *RAS* pathway genes may be important in the pathogenesis of melanoma (*RAS* involvement in melanoma tumorigenesis is discussed below).

***CDK4* GENE DEFECTS** Given that most *CDKN2A* mutations inhibit p16^{INK4A} binding to CDK4, it would be predicted that defects in CDK4 that inhibit its interaction with p16^{INK4A} would similarly lead to unregulated CDK4 activity. Therefore, it is not surprising that CMM families harboring germline *CDK4* mutations have been identified.[11] Notably, all *CDK4* mutations detected to date are missense mutations for the arginine at residue 24, which is normally important for facilitating binding between the CDK4 and p16^{INK4A} proteins. Similar to *CDKN2A* mutations, carriers of *CDK4* mutations show high penetrance of the CMM susceptibility phenotype. Although *CDK4* mutations have been found in only a handful of CMM families to date, detection of *CDK4* mutations in familial melanoma further indicates that disruption of p16^{INK4A} interaction with CDK4 contributes to CMM tumorigenesis.

Studies using a mouse model that recapitulates the germline *CDK4* mutation identified in some CMM families

provide functional evidence implicating it in melanoma tumorigenesis. Mice expressing a "knock in" variant of *CDK4* with an arg24cys mutation that abrogates binding to p16^{INK4A} are susceptible to developing melanocytic tumors and invasive melanomas induced by treatment with topical carcinogens.[20] In addition, mice expressing both the arg24cys variant of *CDK4* and an activated *H-RAS* gene develop spontaneous melanomas and show increased susceptibility to melanoma tumorigenesis in response to UV irradiation.[21]

Thus, mouse models carrying each type of germline mutation detected in familial melanoma have been generated. Each faithfully reproduces the human susceptibility to CMM and provides functional evidence implicating the defects in these genes in melanoma tumorigenesis.

ALTERNATIVE GENE DEFECTS In addition to the *CDKN2A* locus and the *CDK4* gene, substantial evidence suggests that other gene defects may underlie cases of familial melanoma. Approximately 25 to 40% of melanoma families have been shown to harbor defects involving the *CDKN2A* locus.[2] Of those kindreds that do not carry *CDKN2A* aberrations, several show, nonetheless, genetic linkage to chromosome 9p. The *CDKN2B* gene, which encodes p15, another protein that inhibits cell cycle progression similar to p16^{INK4A}, represents an obvious CMM candidate gene. The *CDKN2B* gene and the *CDKN2A* locus lie in close proximity to each other, and both are frequently deleted in CMM. However, mutation screening did not reveal any germline *CDKN2B* aberrations in subjects from over 200 melanoma families.[13,22] Further evidence supporting the presence of an alternative CMM locus at 9p derives from studies showing loss of chromosomal markers in regions distinct from the *CDKN2A* locus in sporadic melanoma.[23] However, no alternative CMM tumor suppressor gene has yet been identified in this region.

Similarly, genetic linkage studies performed on additional CMM families have identified alternative loci that potentially may carry genes conferring melanoma susceptibility. It is worth noting that a locus at 1p36 was the first to be defined by genetic linkage analysis of families predisposed to CMM.[24] However, the presence of dysplastic nevi was included as a clinical feature of affected individuals in this study. This may have obscured the findings in this report, and no subsequent studies have demonstrated genetic link-

age to 1p36 in familial melanoma.[8] Nonetheless, deletion of chromosomal markers from 1p36 has been seen in sporadic melanomas, suggesting that a putative melanoma tumor suppressor gene may indeed reside in this region.[25] In addition, genetic linkage analysis of 49 Australian melanoma families lacking *CDKN2A* or *CDK4* defects defined a new melanoma susceptibility locus at chromosomal region 1p22. Linkage to this region was associated with the development of CMM at an early age.[26] However, no specific familial melanoma gene has yet been identified within this region.[27]

Sporadic Melanoma

***CDKN2A* GENE DEFECTS** Studies discussed above have established a clear association between *CDKN2A* aberrations and familial melanoma. Evidence of involvement of *CDKN2A* defects in sporadic CMM derives from studies of both cultured and uncultured melanoma cells. Inactivation of the *CDKN2A* locus through deletion, mutation, or promoter methylation has been detected in nearly all melanoma cell lines.[28] In contrast, *CDKN2A* defects have been observed less frequently in uncultured melanomas. Data derived from a number of reports revealed that about half of uncultured melanomas (54%) show evidence for loss of DNA markers flanking the *CDKN2A* locus. Intragenic *CDKN2A* mutations (8%) and *CDKN2A* inactivation through promoter methylation (6%) were seen in still fewer samples.[22]

There may be several reasons for these discrepancies between melanoma cell lines and uncultured melanomas. Admixture of otherwise normal cells, such as stromal cells, in samples of tumor tissue may obscure identification of gene defects specific to melanoma cells. Detection of homozygous deletions would be particularly difficult in this context. Furthermore, establishing tumor cells in culture may select for cells with a growth advantage derived from acquired *CDKN2A* mutations. Nonetheless, these studies provide further evidence supporting that *CDKN2A* defects contribute to the pathogenesis of sporadic CMM. Notably, however, mutations localizing specifically to *ARF* exon 1β leading to its inactivation in a manner independent of *INK4A* have not been detected in sporadic CMM.[29]

***CDK4* GENE DEFECTS** Given that *CDK4* mutations have been identified in some cases of familial melanoma, it follows that similar defects have been observed in sporadic CMM as well. Specifically, the arg24cys mutation that prevents p16[INK4A] from binding to and inhibiting CDK4 has been observed in samples of sporadic CMM.[30] However, as is the case with germline *CDK4* mutations in familial CMM, *CDK4* defects in sporadic melanoma are exceptionally rare.[31] In addition, a recent study detected amplification and overexpression of *CDK4* in 5 to 6% of sporadic CMMs examined.[32] It is worth noting that the amplification and overexpression of *HDM2* was observed in these tumors as well. Thus, genomic co-amplification of *CDK4* and *HDM2* presumably represents an alternative mechanism for inactivating the RB and p53 pathways, respectively, in sporadic melanoma.

RAS GENE DEFECTS The *RAS* family of genes (*N-RAS*, *K-RAS*, and *H-RAS*) encodes membrane-associated GTPases that control intracellular signaling through the MAP (mitogen-activated protein) kinase pathway and the PI3′ kinase pathway to regulate cell proliferation and survival (Fig. 5-3) (reviewed in [33]). Activation of *RAS* genes through mutation is commonly observed in human cancers, and may play a role in the pathogenesis of CMM development.[34] As discussed previously, *RAS* activation in conjunction with inactivation of p16[INK4A]/p19[ARF] promotes tumor progression in murine models for melanoma.[18,19,21] Similarly, melanocyte-targeted expression of an activated *RAS* gene combined with hTERT expression and inhibition of either the p53 or RB pathways gives rise to melanocytic neoplasia in reconstituted human skin equivalents after transplantation onto immunodeficient mice.[35]

These experimental studies correlate with the observation that activating *RAS* mutations are common in familial CMMs. Activating *N-RAS* mutations were detected in 95% (20 of 21) of primary melanomas from patients harboring germline mutations in the *CDKN2A* gene.[36] In contrast, *RAS* mutations are much less frequent (4 to 31%) in uncultured sporadic melanomas and melanoma cell lines.[37-39] Nearly all were activating mutations at codon 61 of the *N-RAS* gene, while *H-RAS* mutations were rarely detected.[37]

BRAF GENE DEFECTS The discrepancy between the high frequency of *RAS* mutations in familial CMMs and the relative lack of *RAS* mutations seen in sporadic melanomas may relate, in part, to the high rate of *BRAF* mutations in the latter.[40] Members of the RAF family of proteins are serine/threonine kinases that function downstream of RAS proteins in the MAP kinase signaling pathway (Fig. 5-3).[33] RAF family proteins localize to the plasma membrane by virtue of their interaction with RAS proteins, and become activated through dimerization and phosphorylation. Activated RAF proteins affect signal transduction by phosphorylating MEK1/2, which in turn phosphorylates ERK1/2. Various transcription factors are targeted for phosphorylation by ERK1/2, thus permitting them to regulate expression of a series of target genes. Given that RAF proteins function immediately downstream of RAS proteins, activating *RAF* mutations could influence MAP kinase pathway activation in a manner similar to *RAS* mutations.

Activating mutations in the *BRAF* gene represent the most frequently observed genetic aberration in human CMM (reviewed in [41]), and have been detected in up to 70% of sporadic tumors.[40-43] Mutations in *BRAF* commonly localize to sequences encoding the kinase domain, and the vast majority of these consist of the identical valine to glutamic acid substitution at residue 599 (V599E). These mutations lead to constitutive BRAF kinase activity, permitting BRAF to drive downstream signaling through the MAP kinase pathway in an unregulated manner. It is worth noting that *BRAF* and *N-RAS* mutations tend to be mutually exclusive in CMM; tumors harboring *BRAF* mutations typically lack *N-RAS* defects and vice versa. This suggests functional overlap between *BRAF* and *N-RAS* mutations in stimulating MAP kinase activity and CMM tumorigenesis. However, activated *BRAF*, in contrast to activated *N-RAS*, failed to induce formation of invasive melanoma in an experimental model for human CMM.[35] Thus, further investigation is required to fully elucidate the role of B-RAF mutation in the pathogenesis of sporadic melanoma.

Nonetheless, given that *BRAF* mutations are common in sporadic CMMs, members of families with increased susceptibility to melanoma were screened for germline *BRAF* mutations. Many of the families tested showed no evidence for defects involving the *CDKN2A* locus or the *CDK4* gene. However, no *BRAF* mutations were identified in 168 cases of familial CMM, indicating that *BRAF* does not represent a familial melanoma susceptibility gene.[44-46] In contrast, *BRAF* mutations are very common in benign melanocytic lesions. The same V599E mutation has been identified in over 80% of melanocytic nevi examined in some studies.[47,48] This observation suggests that *BRAF* mutation leading to activation of MAP kinase pathway signaling may represent a common, early step in melanocytic neoplasia, and that acquisition of additional aberrations would be

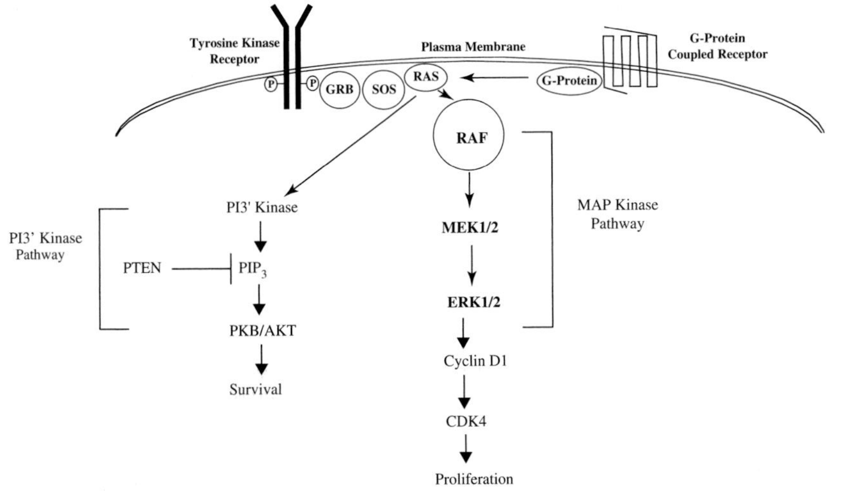

▲ **FIGURE 5-3** RAS signaling pathway. RAS-mediated signaling may be activated by tyrosine kinase or G-protein-coupled cell surface receptors. RAS activates the MAP kinase and PI3′ kinase effector pathways. RAF serine/threonine kinases function immediately downstream of RAS and activate signaling through the MAP kinase pathway, resulting in cell proliferation. PI3′ kinase activity produces PIP$_3$, leading to phosphorylation of PKB/AKT and promoting survival. The PI3′ kinase pathway may be inhibited by PTEN, which dephosphorylates PIP$_3$.

required for development of invasive melanoma.

PTEN GENE DEFECTS

Genomic markers mapping to chromosome 10q are often deleted in CMM, and specifically defects in the *PTEN* gene at 10q23 have been identified. *PTEN* is a tumor suppressor gene that may undergo deletion or mutation in a wide range of cancers. In addition, germline *PTEN* mutations cause Cowden syndrome, a hereditary disorder that predisposes affected individuals to developing hamartomatous lesions and malignancies in a variety of tissues, including skin, breast, thyroid and colon. However, CMM is not typically associated with Cowden syndrome.

The protein encoded by the *PTEN* gene functions is both a lipid and protein phosphatase, and may influence a number of cellular processes.[49] In particular, the PTEN phosphatase may serve as a tumor suppressor by attenuating signal transduction within the PI3′ kinase effector arm of the *RAS* pathway (Fig. 5-3).[33] PTEN dephosphorylates phosphoinositide-3,4,5-trisphosphate (PIP_3), which is normally produced through activity of PI3′ kinase. Activation of the PI3′ kinase pathway promotes intracellular accumulation of PIP_3, resulting in phosphorylation and subsequent activation of protein kinase B (PKB or AKT). Phosphorylation of PKB/AKT, in turn, leads to inactivation of proteins that suppress cell cycle progression or induce apoptosis. Normally, PTEN maintains low cellular levels of PIP_3. However, when PTEN is deficient, PIP_3 levels increase and PKB/AKT becomes hyperphosphorylated. Consequently, these events promote cell proliferation and survival.

Several studies have examined sporadic CMM for aberrations involving the *PTEN* gene. Although variable results have been reported, *PTEN* defects have been observed in approximately 30 to 60% of melanoma cell lines and approximately 5 to 20% of uncultured melanomas.[49–53] Conversely, selective activation of the AKT3 isoform was detected in up to 60% of sporadic melanomas.[54] Putative mechanisms accounting for this observation may include loss of the *PTEN* gene or gains in copy number of the *AKT3* gene leading to increased levels of its expression. Taken together, these findings indicate that genomic aberrations resulting in diminished PTEN function and AKT3 activation may contribute to the pathogenesis of sporadic CMMs.

Functional evidence supporting this derives from studies in which *PTEN*

expression was reconstituted in melanoma cells lacking PTEN.[55,56] *PTEN* expression suppressed cell growth and attenuated the ability of melanoma cells to form tumors when introduced into mice. In addition, inhibition of AKT3 activity also reduced the survival and proliferation of human melanoma cells upon transplantation in immunodeficient mice.[54] These experimental models suggest that *PTEN* may be important in maintaining a check on cellular proliferation via the activated PKB/AKT pathway and thus suppress melanoma formation and progression.

Notably, *N-RAS* mutations and *PTEN* defects are mutually exclusive in melanoma.[33] Similarly, as discussed above, *N-RAS* mutations are not observed in the context of *BRAF* mutations in melanoma. Given these observations, it appears that inactivation of both major arms of *RAS*-mediated signaling, the MAP kinase and PI3′ kinase pathways, may be achieved through either mutation in *N-RAS* alone or acquisition of defects in both *PTEN* and *BRAF*.

MC1R VARIATION

Variation within the gene encoding the melanocortin 1 receptor (MC1R) represents a major determinant of skin pigmentation (reviewed in [57]). The *MC1R* gene encodes a G-protein coupled receptor for alpha-MSH (or alpha-melanocyte stimulating hormone). Binding of alpha-MSH to MC1R results in activation of adenylate cyclase in melanocytes and increased cAMP production. Elevated levels of cAMP induce a switch in melanin production from red/yellow pheomelanin to brown/black eumelanin.

Several studies provide evidence supporting that variants of the *MC1R* gene are associated with an increased risk of CMM (reviewed in [57]). In general, most studies indicate that variation within the *MC1R* gene confers an approximately two- to four-fold increased risk of melanoma, although certain specific variants may be associated with an even greater risk for CMM.[59-64] Individuals with two allelic variants of the *MC1R* gene display a still higher risk compared to those carrying just one variant. Notably, in studies where risk analysis was stratified according to hair color or skin type, the increased risk for developing CMM appeared to be independent of pigmentation phenotype.

In addition, *MC1R* variants may influence development of melanoma in patients from families with high susceptibility to CMM. Patients harboring both *MC1R* variants and a germline *CDKN2A*

mutation tend to develop melanoma at an earlier age compared to patients carrying a *CDKN2A* mutation alone[65–67] Taken together, these studies indicate that the *MC1R* gene represents a low penetrance melanoma susceptibility gene, given the modest, yet significant association between variants of this gene and CMM. However, it may also represent a modifier gene when risk variants are inherited in the context of germline *CDKN2A* mutations.[68]

MITF DEFECTS

Recent studies have implicated the gene encoding Microphthalmia-associated transcription factor (MITF) in melanoma. Normally, MITF serves as a "master regulator" of differentiation, function and survival of melanocytes (reviewed in [69]). Waardenburg syndrome type IIA, which has features of white forelock, as well as ocular and auditory defects due to deficient melanocytes, is caused by mutations in the *MITF* gene. In addition, mice lacking a functional *Mitf* gene lack pigment, whereas mice with partial *Mitf* function may show white belly spotting or premature graying due to impaired survival of melanocytes. Expression of *MITF* is induced as a consequence of alpha-MSH binding to MC1R; *MITF* expression may also be induced by PAX3 and β-catenin through WNT pathway signaling. MITF, in turn, increases transcription of various genes that regulate melanin synthesis, as well as genes that control cell cycle progression. It is worth noting that in otherwise normal melanocytes, MITF may cause cell cycle arrest by inducing expression of p16[INK4A].

A recent genome-wide search for melanoma susceptibility genes led to the discovery of increased copy number at chromosome 3p14-3p13, the region that includes the *MITF* gene, in several melanoma cell lines.[70] Increased expression of *MITF* was found to correlate with chromosomal amplification in these cell lines. Subsequently, melanoma samples were screened for similar changes, and *MITF* amplification was observed in 10% of CMM, and 15 to 20% of metastatic melanomas. In addition, functional studies have provided further evidence that amplification and overexpression of *MITF* may contribute to melanoma tumorigenesis. Coexpression of *MITF* with activated *BRAF* in TERT-expressing, p53- and RB-deficient melanocytes was found to promote colony growth in soft agar. Although *MITF* expression can be quite variable among melanoma samples,[71,72] these findings suggest that increased levels of MITF may contribute to tumorigenesis in some proportion of human melanomas, perhaps through promoting cell survival.

ALTERNATIVE GENE DEFECTS Despite identification of several genes that contribute to melanoma tumorigenesis, considerable evidence indicates that additional gene defects likely play a role in the pathogenesis of CMM. Loss of heterozygosity, cytogenetic, and comparative genomic hybridization (CGH) studies of sporadic melanomas have defined a number of genomic regions that may harbor other, novel melanoma genes. Among these, loci at chromosomes 1p, 3p, 6q, 6p, 10q, 11q, and 17p demonstrate nonrandom, recurrent aberrations indicative of activation or inactivation of specific genes.[73–75]

The advent of array-based technologies has facilitated more refined, high resolution, and global analysis of gene expression profiles and genomic aberrations in melanomas. Transcription profiling studies have defined different molecular subtypes of melanoma and have identified distinct patterns of gene expression for different stages of melanoma tumor progression.[76,77] Similarly, distinct patterns of genomic gains and losses of have been observed using array-based CGH, which may allow for further classification of melanomas at a molecular level.[78]

In addition, use of these approaches may facilitate identification of novel genes that contribute to melanoma tumorigenesis. Recent studies used array-based CGH to compare patterns of genomic changes in metastatic and nonmetastatic tumors derived from a murine model for melanoma.[79] Nonrandom, recurrent amplification of a region syntenic to human chromosome 6p24-25 was identified in metastatic lesions. Expression analysis of candidate genes in the region revealed upregulation of *NEDD9* in a pattern showing correlation with human melanoma progression, thus implicating it as a putative melanoma gene. Further studies using similar approaches should permit identification of still additional melanoma-associated genes.

■ **CUTANEOUS SQUAMOUS CELL CARCINOMA (SCC)**

BOX 5-3 Summary

- Mutations in the *TP53* gene are prevalent in SCC and SCC precursor lesions, suggesting that p53 inactivation may represent an early step in development of this form of skin cancer.

- Activating *RAS* mutations are common in SCC. Experimental models demonstrate that *RAS* activation may cooperate with other genetic aberrations, such as *TP53* inactivation or *CDK4* activation, in squamous cell carcinoma neoplasia.
- Chromosomal deletions and mutations at the *CDKN2A* locus occur in SCC, and may contribute to their pathogenesis.
- Perturbation of TGFβ pathway signaling and SMAD4 activity may lead to SCC tumorigenesis in experimental models.

Evidence supports that cutaneous SCC arises as the end result of a multistep mutagenic process in which cumulative ultraviolet (UV) exposure plays a large role. Accordingly, disruption of mechanisms that function to repair UV-induced damage to DNA facilitates this process and predisposes to SCC tumorigenesis. Such is the case in xeroderma pigmentosum (XP), a recessive hereditary disorder characterized largely by defects in nucleotide excision repair (NER). Eight XP complementation groups and the gene defects underlying each have been identified (reviewed in [87]). Defects involving various steps in NER, including error recognition by repair proteins, open complex formation through helicase unwinding of DNA, and dual repair incision to remove the damaged region have been characterized in XP patients. Consequently, failure to repair UV-induced DNA damage leads to extreme susceptibility to a variety of skin cancers, including SCC, BCC, and CMM.

Despite these insights, no hereditary disorder that specifically increases the risk of SCC has been identified. Thus genetic analysis has been somewhat more complicated for SCC compared to CMM and BCC. Consequently, most studies have focused on screening sporadic SCCs for mutations in oncogenes and tumor suppressor genes that are known to influence tumorigenesis in other forms of cancers and functional analysis of molecular pathways that may be altered by such gene defects. We discuss here studies focusing on the role of several genes in development of cutaneous SCC.

TP53 Gene Defects

The *TP53* tumor suppressor gene is perhaps the most commonly altered gene in human cancers, and it has been implicated in cutaneous SCC tumorigenesis. The protein encoded by the *TP53* gene functions to regulate progression of the cell cycle and apoptosis in response to DNA damage induced by insults such as UV irradiation.[81] Breakage of DNA strands leads directly to induction of p53 expression (Fig. 5-4). Consequently, p53

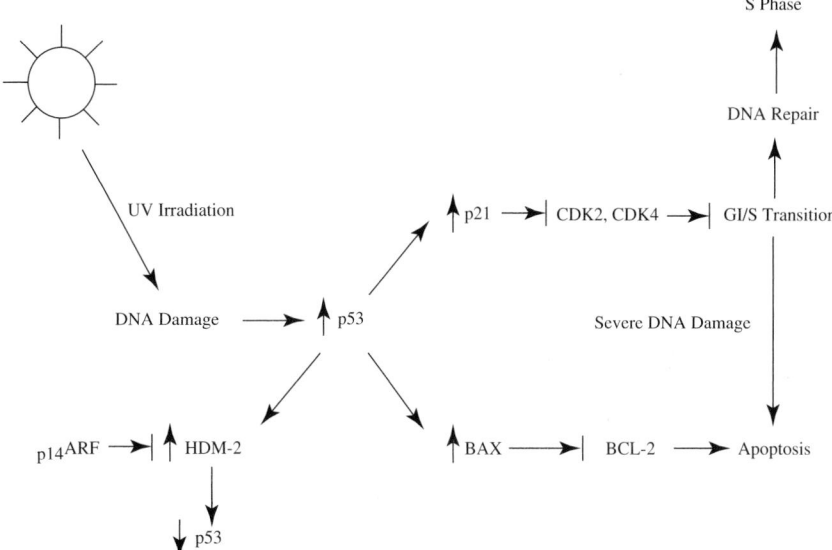

▲ **FIGURE 5-4** *TP53* tumor suppressor gene function. DNA damage resulting from insults such as UV irradiation induces p53 expression. In turn, p53 induces expression of p21^Cip1, which prevents progression of the cell cycle from G1 to S phase by inhibiting CDK2 and CDK4. Cell cycle blockade permits repair of DNA before replication in S phase to prevent retention of acquired mutations. If DNA damage is severe, cells undergo programmed cell death mediated by p53-induced BAX. In addition, p53 induces expression of HDM-2, which, in turn, down regulates p53 to permit cell cycle progression when appropriate. p14ARF inhibits HDM-2 to promote stabilization of p53. Inactivation of the *TP53* gene would eliminate p53-induced cell cycle blockade and the cell death response to severe DNA damage, thus preventing mutations from being repaired and allowing them to accumulate.

triggers expression of p21^{Cip1}, which blocks cell cycle progression in the G1 phase by binding to and inhibiting cyclin-dependent kinases (CDKs) 2 and 4. Blockade of the cell cycle permits DNA repair prior to replication in the S phase, and consequently eliminates mutations that may have been acquired. When extreme damage to DNA is incurred, however, p53 induces expression of BAX. This, in turn, leads to programmed cell death as BAX binds to BCL-2 and inhibits its anti-apoptotic activity.

However, when p53 is inactivated, blockade of cell cycle progression would not occur in response to DNA damage. This would prevent repair of mutations prior to DNA replication and facilitate their retention in genomic DNA. Moreover, inactivation of p53 would prevent induction of programmed cell death in response to severe DNA damage. Therefore, damaged cells that have acquired mutations would persist. Any given cell gaining a mutation that provides some form of growth or survival advantage could subsequently undergo clonal proliferation and ultimately give rise to tumorigenesis. Thus, the TP53 gene, in essence, functions as a "guardian of the genome" and represents a critical tumor suppressor.

There is considerable evidence implicating defects in the TP53 gene specifically in SCC tumorigenesis. Several studies have determined that TP53 gene defects are common in SCC, although the frequency of TP53 mutations varies among different reports. Three different studies detected TP53 mutations in 41, 58, and 69% of SCC tumor samples.[82–84] These findings suggest that functional defects in p53 may play a critical role in SCC tumor development. Furthermore, TP53 mutations have been identified in actinic keratoses (AKs) and early SCC lesions as well. Roughly 50 to 60% of AKs[83,84] and 35% of in situ SCCs studied[85] were shown to harbor TP53 mutations in separate reports. A high proportion of the TP53 mutations displayed the characteristic UV signature CC → TT or C → T tandem transitions at dipyrimidine sequences.[83] Moreover, clonal expansions of keratinocytes in otherwise normal sun-exposed skin have been shown to carry TP53 mutations,[86,87] although one study failed to identify a definitive genetic association between such TP53 clones, AKs and SCCs.[88] Nonetheless, together these findings provide further evidence to support the fact that UV-induced DNA damage is critical in the pathogenesis of SCC and that alterations in the TP53

gene likely occur in the early stages of squamous cell neoplasia.

Surprisingly, however, patients with Li-Fraumeni syndrome, which is caused by germline mutation of the TP53 gene, do not display increased susceptibility to cutaneous SCC.[89] The molecular basis underlying this discrepancy between acquired and inherited TP53 gene defects in relationship to SCC development is unclear.

Nonetheless, animal studies further support a role for p53 in SCC tumorigenesis. Patches of keratinocytes that express mutant p53 protein develop in the skin of UV-irradiated SKH1 hairless mice; furthermore, their density correlates with tumor risk in these mice.[90,91] Mutations in the p53 gene were detected in nearly 2/3 of patches immunostaining for mutant p53 protein in one study.[92] Moreover, p53 "hotspot" mutations previously observed in SCC tumors in similar tumorigenesis studies in hairless mice[93,94] were detected in these p53 patches. Together, these findings further suggest that p53 defects occur early in the process of SCC neoplasia and that patches of mutant p53 expressing keratinocytes represent lesions that may progress to SCC.

Similarly, premalignant lesions resembling AKs and frank SCCs developed in response to UV irradiation in p53 null mice.[95,96] Furthermore, histologic examination of UV-treated skin from normal and p53 null mice revealed more clues into early events involved in development of these lesions.[97] The epidermis of normal mice harbored so-called "sunburn cells" (apoptotic keratinocytes); however, similar sunburn cells were not seen in the epidermis of p53 null mice. This finding indicates that p53-deficient keratinocytes were unable to initiate programmed cell death in response to UV irradiation. Consequently, cells that accumulated DNA damage would have persisted in the epidermis of p53 null mice. In turn, acquired mutations activating proto-oncogenes and/or inactivating of tumor suppressor genes would have facilitated clonal cell proliferation and ultimately tumorigenesis. These studies convincingly establish that p53 may play an important role in guarding against early events that lead to squamous neoplasia.

RAS Gene Defects

Similar to TP53 gene defects, RAS mutations are among the most frequently observed genetic aberrations in human cancers. Specifically, activating mutations

constitutively drive molecular signaling pathways downstream of RAS, such as the MAP kinase pathway discussed above, which in turn may influence certain cell functions, such as proliferation (Fig. 5-3).[33] Given that RAS mutations are common in other types of cancer, several studies were performed to determine whether sporadic SCCs harbor activating RAS mutations. Although reports of the frequency of RAS mutations in SCC range widely, it appears that RAS mutations are relatively common in cutaneous SCC. In one study, 46% of SCCs carried activating mutations converting the valine at amino acid 12 of the H-RAS gene to glycine. In contrast, mutations in the K-RAS gene and amplification of the N-RAS gene were less frequently detected.[98] Similarly, mutations altering the valine at amino acid 12 of the H-RAS gene were identified in 35% of SCCs examined in another study.[99] Further still, mutations leading to activation of either the H-RAS or K-RAS genes were seen in 12% of SCCs and in 16% of actinic keratoses (AKs) in another report.[100] Given that SCCs may develop from precursor AK lesions, RAS mutation may play a role early in the pathogenesis of SCC. Taken together, these findings support that RAS activation may be involved in the development of cutaneous SCCs.

Studies using murine keratinocytes have also shown that early ras (ras for mouse, RAS for human) activation is important in SCC tumorigenesis (reviewed in [101]). Primary mouse keratinocytes engineered to express the oncogenic v-ras^{Ha} variant have been shown to give rise to benign squamous papillomas when grafted onto immunodeficient mice. Expression of oncogenic ras may lead to downstream events that are regulated by altered patterns of protein kinase C (PKC) activity, and depend on activation of the epidermal growth factor receptor (EGFR). However, activation of ras in the absence of other cellular events is not sufficient to give rise to SCC tumorigenesis and instead may induce growth arrest. Further genetic alterations and modifications in expression of other genes are required for premalignant cells to progress and undergo malignant transformation.

Circumvention of ras-induced growth arrest may be achieved through loss of inhibition of cell cycle progression mediated by p53. Primary mouse keratinocytes that both express the oncogenic v-ras^{Ha} variant and lack p53, proliferate and develop into frank carcinomas when grafted onto immunodeficient mice.[102] Similarly, primary murine keratinocytes deficient for p19^{ARF} (the mouse equivalent of p14^{ARF}) bypass *ras*-induced growth arrest, proliferate and form tumors as well.[103] Given that p19^{ARF} plays a role in stabilizing p53 protein, lack of p19^{ARF} would have a similar effect and lead to impairment of p53 function. Thus, either direct (through a p53 defect) or indirect (through a p19^{ARF} defect) mechanisms for circumventing p53-mediated blockade of the cell cycle would bypass *ras*-induced growth arrest and lead to cell proliferation. Taken together, these results provide experimental support for cooperation between defects in ras and p53 pathways in promoting SCC tumorigenesis.

Models for SCC tumorigenesis using human keratinocytes have provided additional insights into the consequences of *RAS* activation. Similar to other cell types, studies have shown that activated *H-RAS* expression alone in primary human keratinocyte cultures induces growth arrest.[104,105] Furthermore, *RAS*-induction of CDK inhibitors and restriction of *CDK4* expression, leading to blockade of cell cycle progression at G1, appears to regulate growth arrest. However, when primary keratinocytes are manipulated to express an activated form of *RAS* with *CDK4* and are then engrafted onto immunodeficient mice, they give rise to tumors resembling invasive SCCs.[104] Similar findings were observed in studies in which IκBα was coexpressed with activated *RAS* in human keratinocytes. IκBα inhibits NF-κB, a transcription factor that stimulates cell proliferation and guards against apoptosis in many cell types, yet paradoxically suppresses primary keratinocyte proliferation.[106] Notably, these studies showed that *CDK4* expression was induced by IκBα in keratinocytes.[105] Consequently, either direct or IκBα-induced expression of *CDK4* may serve to bypass *RAS*-mediated growth arrest, resulting in unregulated cell proliferation.

In addition, these studies demonstrated that activated *RAS* signaling may inhibit apoptosis.[107,108] Although IκBα favors cell proliferation through activation of CDK4, increased susceptibility to apoptosis by suppressing NF-κB function could represent a potential consequence of IκBα expression. However, Dajee et al[105] showed that coexpression of *RAS* with IκBα opposes susceptibility to apoptosis in primary human keratinocytes. Taken together, these studies indicate that cooperation between *CDK4* and *RAS* pathways may (1) circumvent growth arrest to promote cell proliferation, and (2) block apoptosis, leading to primary human keratinocyte transformation and SCC tumorigenesis.

CDKN2A Gene Defects

Deletions of portions of chromosomes are frequently observed in SCC (see below). In particular, deletions involving the short arm of chromosome 9 are common. Approximately 30 to 50% of SCCs show evidence for loss of 9p genomic markers,[109,110] suggesting frequent LOH for a tumor suppressor gene in this region. The *CDKN2A* locus maps to 9p21; consequently, studies were undertaken to examine sporadic SCCs for mutations that inactivate p16^{INK4a}/p14^{ARF}. Mutations at the *CDKN2A* locus were detected in 9 to 42% of cutaneous SCCs, indicating that disruption of p16^{INK4a}/p14^{ARF} may contribute to SCC development.[110,111] Furthermore, one study[112] reported deletion of DNA markers surrounding the *CDKN2A* locus in both AKs and SCCs. Loss of the *CDKN2A* locus was seen in 21% of AKs and 46% of SCCs, respectively. Given that deletions in this region were more commonly observed in SCCs, inactivation of the *CDKN2A* locus might represent a late event involved in the progression of premalignant AK to malignant SCC in some cases.

The TGFβ Pathway and SMAD4

The TGFβ pathway is involved in many biological processes, including epidermal development and neoplasia. Specifically, several studies have demonstrated that disruption of TGFβ pathway signaling may contribute to SCC tumorigenesis. Targeted disruption of TGFβ1 in keratinocytes expressing the v-ras^{Ha} oncogene resulted in tumor formation when these cells were grafted onto nude mice.[113] Another study showed that transgenic mice expressing a dominant negative type II TGFβ receptor developed epidermal hyperplasia and had increased susceptibility to chemically induced SCCs.[114] Intracellular signaling through the TGFβ pathway is mediated by the family of SMAD proteins.[115] SMAD2 and 3 are associated with TGFβ and activin signaling, whereas SMAD1, 5, and 8 are associated with BMP signaling. SMAD4 is a common mediator for both pathways.

Given the central role SMAD4 plays in TGFβ signaling, a number of studies have investigated the consequences of manipulating SMAD4 on cutaneous tumorigenesis. Although *Smad4*-deficient mice die during embryogenesis, mice heterozygous for a *Smad4* null allele develop cutaneous SCCs, in addition to gastric polyps and cancer.[116] These findings indicate that Smad4 plays an essential role not only in embryonic development but in tumor suppression as well. Accordingly, targeted disruption of *Smad4* specifically in mouse skin resulted in epidermal hyperplasia, and all mutant mice developed spontaneous malignant skin tumors, most of which were SCCs.[117] Infrequently, these mice also developed basal cell carcinomas, trichoepitheliomas, and sebaceous adenomas, indicating that disruption of *Smad4* and TGFβ signaling may influence development of other cutaneous tumors as well.

Interestingly, inactivation of the Pten tumor suppressor gene and activation of Akt, were observed in *Smad4*-deficient tumors. However, neither change was detected in otherwise normal *Smad4*-deficient mouse skin. These findings suggest that alteration of other genes is required for SCC tumorigenesis in the context of *Smad4* inactivation, and that TGFβ and BMP signaling likely interact with the Pten and PI3′ kinase pathways in this process. Despite these findings, PTEN coding region mutations were not detected in a set of 21 cutaneous SCCs in one study.[118] Similarly, activating AKT mutations were not observed in epithelial tumors, including SCC, in another study.[119] Whether human cutaneous SCC tumors harbor mutations in the *SMAD4* gene remains to be determined.

Alternative Gene Defects

Despite advances in identifying genes that contribute to the pathogenesis of SCC, it is likely that additional genes contribute to this process as well. Evidence for this derives from identification of recurrent chromosomal aberrations through genome-wide analysis of SCC tumors. Quinn, et al found that loss of microsatellite markers mapping to several chromosomes was common in SCCs. In addition to loss of heterozygosity at 9p (41%), as discussed previously, frequent losses at 3p (23%), 13q (46%), 17p (33%), and 17q (33%) were observed.[120] Similarly, AKs showed a high frequency of loss of chromosomal markers in the same regions.[121,122] This finding suggests that loss of potential tumor suppressor genes mapping to these loci may contribute to the pathogenesis of both AKs and SCCs, and provides further support for AKs representing precursor lesions to SCCs. However, SCCs often demonstrated multiple karyotypic aberrations and genetic heterogeneity within the same tumor, suggesting that further genetic abnormalities are required for progression to SCC.[119]

Additional studies using comparative genomic hybridization have further substantiated results from microsatellite marker studies discussed above. Ashton et al observed chromosomal losses at 9p in 67% of 15 SCCs studied.[123] Less frequent losses were detected at 3p (53%), 18q (47%), 17p (33%), 4q (27%), 11p, 13q, and still other loci (20%). In addition, losses were seen at 9p and 13q in 58% of 12 AK samples, while losses at 3p, 4q, 11p, and 17p were identified in 25% of AKs. Similarly, chromosomal gains were prevalent at 3q, 4p, 17q, and several other regions in both SCCs and AKs. These studies demonstrated considerable overlap in the spectrum of chromosomal losses and gains detected in SCCs and AKs, thus providing still further evidence for SCCs being derived from AKs. Nonetheless, SCCs generally showed more frequent and more numerous chromosomal aberrations indicating that additional genetic changes are necessary for transformation of AKs to SCCs.

While the *CDKN2A* locus (9p) and *TP53* gene (17p) may represent targets for deletion in some AKs and SCCs, potential novel tumor suppressor genes or oncogenes that contribute to SCC development may localize to other areas of chromosomal loss or gain, respectively. In particular, losses at 18q appear to be somewhat specific for SCC as this finding was seen in 47% of SCCs, yet in just 8% of AKs.[123] Further studies using more focused approaches to evaluate larger numbers of tumors may permit fine mapping and identification of a putative 18q tumor suppressor gene, and possibly other genes involved in squamous neoplasia.

In addition, investigators have performed gene expression profiling using high-density oligonucleotide arrays as an alternative approach for global gene analysis of SCCs.[124] Gene expression in SCCs was compared to site-matched control skin and hyperplastic psoriatic lesions. Notably *TP53* and *CDK4* expression showed no difference in SCC compared to matched normal skin, while *CDKN2A* showed increased, yet statistically insignificant, expression in some SCCs. Nonetheless,

several genes involved in epidermal differentiation or regulation of proliferation were upregulated in both psoriatic skin and SCCs. Other genes, including WNT receptor frizzled homolog 6 (*FZD6*), the prostaglandin-metabolizing enzyme hydroxyprostaglandin dehydrogenase (*HGPD*), various matrix metalloproteinases, and *STAT3*, showed increased expression specifically in SCC. However, how and to what extent various differentially expressed genes contribute to SCC tumorigenesis are yet to be elucidated.

■ BASAL CELL CARCINOMA (BCC)

> **BOX 5-4 Summary**
>
> - Mutations in the *PTCH* tumor suppressor gene causes Gorlin syndrome, a hereditary BCC susceptibility disorder. Inactivation of *PTCH* is a frequent occurrence in sporadic BCC as well.
> - *PTCH* regulates activity of the *SHH* signaling pathway. Mutations in genes encoding other components of the *SHH* pathway, particularly *SMO*, may also contribute to sporadic BCC tumorigenesis.
> - Mutations in the *TP53* tumor suppressor gene are common in sporadic BCC as well. Mutations in *TP53* may be seen in association with *PTCH* gene defects suggesting that inactivation of both genes may promote BCC tumorigenesis in a cooperative manner.

Hereditary Basal Cell Carcinoma

PTCH GENE DEFECTS: GORLIN SYNDROME

Initial clues regarding the molecular basis of basal cell carcinoma (BCC) came from genetic analysis of families with Gorlin syndrome (basal cell nevus syndrome, nevoid basal cell carcinoma syndrome).[125,126] Although affected subjects have normal-appearing skin early in life, they may develop hundreds of BCCs in a generalized distribution over the course of their lifetime. Additional cutaneous findings in this disorder may include palmoplantar pitting and epidermal inclusion cysts. Patients with Gorlin syndrome are susceptible to developing other forms of malignant and benign internal tumors, such as medulloblastoma, meningioma, rhabdomyosarcoma, and ovarian tumors. Other common features include odontogenic jaw cysts, skeletal anomalies, such as bifid ribs and tall stature, intracranial calcification, and various craniofacial defects, such as cleft palate and coarse facies.

Gorlin syndrome follows an autosomal dominant pattern of inheritance. Linkage analysis of families with Gorlin syndrome mapped the chromosomal locus for the disorder to 9q22.3.[127] In addition, deletion of this region has been frequently detected in both BCC from Gorlin syndrome patients and sporadic BCC.[127] Taken together, these findings indicated that a tumor suppressor gene associated with BCC susceptibility localized to this locus. Subsequently, inactivating mutations in the human homolog of the Drosophila *patched* gene, were detected in Gorlin syndrome patients and implicated in BCC tumorigenesis.[128,129]

In vertebrate models, the *Ptc* gene has been shown to influence development of a variety of structures and tissues, including neural tube, skeleton, limbs, craniofacial structures, skin, and hair follicles. At the molecular level, *Ptc* regulates the *Hedgehog* (*Hh*) signaling pathway.[130] Vertebrates harbor three *Hh* homologs; *Sonic* (*Shh*), *Desert* (*Dhh*), and *Indian* (*Ihh*). Of these, *Shh* has been most extensively characterized in normal development and tumorigenesis. The *Ptc* gene encodes a membrane-bound protein that normally suppresses activity of Smoothened (Smo), a G-protein-coupled transmembrane receptor protein (Fig. 5-5). Shh is a secreted factor that binds to and inhibits Ptc. Consequently, Ptc-mediated suppression of Smo is relieved, permitting Smo to convey a signal influencing expression of a variety of downstream target genes through *Gli* effector genes.

The *Gli* genes (*Gli1*, *Gli2*, and *Gli3*) give rise to a family of DNA-binding, zinc-finger transcription factors.[131] An activation domain at its C-terminal end allows Gli1 to induce expression of target genes upon activation of Shh signaling. In contrast, both Gli2 and Gli3 carry N-terminal repressor and C-terminal activator domains. Thus Gli2 and Gli3 may function as transcriptional activators or repressors. However, Gli3 may be more proficient as a transcriptional repressor of Shh-responsive genes, whereas Gli2 may play more of a role in activating gene expression.

Shh signaling induces cell proliferation, which may lead to tumorigenesis if normal regulation of pathway activity is compromised. Evidence suggests that both Shh and Ptc may directly influence progression of the cell cycle.[130] Shh may block activity of p21[Cip1], a CDK inhibitor that restricts transition through the cell cycle. In addition, Shh induces expression of D and E cyclins, which

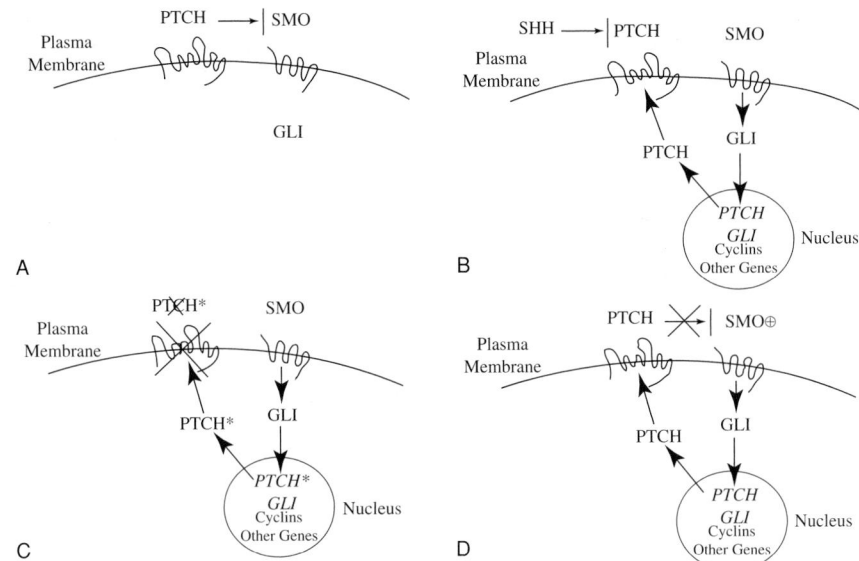

▲ **FIGURE 5-5** *SHH* signaling pathway. **A.** *PTCH* encodes a membrane-bound protein that normally inhibits SMO activity. **B.** Binding of SHH inactivates PTCH, permitting SMO to transmit its signal to induce transcription of target genes including *SHH* mediators, such as the *PTCH* and *GLI* genes, and genes that stimulate cell proliferation. Induction of *PTCH* expression re-establishes suppression of SMO and prevent uncontrolled pathway activity. **C.** When *PTCH* is inactivated (designated by *), SMO functions without restraint and the *SHH* pathway becomes constitutively activated. PTCH protein derived from a mutant allele is nonfunctional and incapable of suppressing *SHH* pathway signaling. **D.** Activating *SMO* mutations (designated by ⊕), cause it to become unresponsive to PTCH repression, allowing *SHH* pathway signaling to proceed without inhibition.

promote progression through G1 into S phase.[132] Ptc is known to bind phosphorylated cyclin B1 and alter its distribution within cells, thus blocking transition from G2 to M.[133] Conversely, loss of Ptc results in increased translocation of cyclin B1 into the nucleus and promotes cell cycle progression.[134] Ptc inactivation also leads to nuclear accumulation of cyclin D1. Therefore, inactivation of the *Ptc* gene may promote cell proliferation through compromise of checkpoints regulating transition through the G1-S and G2-M stages of the cell cycle.[134]

An understanding of the molecular components that mediate *SHH* signaling further clarifies the role of *PTCH* as a tumor suppressor gene in Gorlin syndrome (reviewed in [135]). Affected individuals harbor a germline mutation involving one *PTCH* allele. Inactivation of the other, normal *PTCH* allele in a given cell would lead to complete absence of PTCH function. This would lead to constitutive *SHH* pathway signaling as a result of unrestrained SMO activity (Fig. 5-5). Consequently, cell proliferation would be unregulated and ultimately give rise to tumor formation. Experimental evidence confirming that *PTCH* defects indeed play a causative role in Gorlin syndrome derives from studies using mouse models

for this disorder. Mice heterozygous for a *Ptc* knockout allele represent genetic murine equivalents of humans with Gorlin syndrome. These mice display findings analogous to those seen in patients, such as skeletal limb defects and susceptibility to developing medulloblastoma. In addition, these mice spontaneously develop primordial hair follicle lesions resembling trichoblastoma.[136] Moreover, they develop tumors with features similar to BCC in response to UV or ionizing radiation.[136,137] Results from these functional studies, therefore, corroborate findings from genetic analysis of Gorlin syndrome and directly implicate loss of *PTCH* function in BCC tumorigenesis.

ALTERNATIVE GENE DEFECTS: NON-GORLIN SYNDROME BCC SUSCEPTIBILITY DISORDERS In addition to Gorlin syndrome, other genetic disorders predispose to BCC tumorigenesis. However, these disorders may not be attributable to mutations in *PTCH*. Linear unilateral basal cell nevus (LUBCN) is a rare disorder manifesting increased susceptibility to BCCs and basaloid follicular hamartomas (BFH) in a limited, unilateral distribution.[138] An underlying mutation in *PTCH* has been ruled out in at least one patient with this disorder (our unpub-

lished observations). Bazex–Dupré–Christol syndrome has features of follicular atrophoderma, hypotrichosis and predisposition to BCC tumorigenesis at an early age. This syndrome follows an X-linked pattern of inheritance and linkage analysis has mapped a genetic locus for this disorder to Xq24-q27.[139] Similarly, subjects with Rombo syndrome develop findings such as multiple BCCs, trichoepitheliomas, vermiculate atrophoderma, milia, hypotrichosis, and peripheral vasodilation with cyanosis.[140] Neither a specific gene nor a genetic locus for this disorder has been identified. Given phenotypic differences compared to Gorlin syndrome, it may be that this syndrome is not caused by *PTCH* mutation. Characterization of the gene defect underlying each of these disorders may identify novel BCC genes and provide further insight into mechanisms that contribute to BCC tumorigenesis.

Sporadic Basal Cell Carcinoma and Other Forms of Basaloid Neoplasia

***SHH* PATHWAY GENE DEFECTS** Evidence for *PTCH* inactivation in Gorlin syndrome raised speculation that *PTCH* gene defects may contribute to the pathogenesis of sporadic BCCs as well. Subsequent studies detected mutations in *PTCH* in 12 to 67% of sporadic BCCs examined.[141–143] In addition, deletion of DNA markers flanking the *PTCH* locus has been observed in 40 to 67% of sporadic BCCs.[127,142,144] These findings indicate that *PTCH* defects are common in sporadic BCC, and suggest that both hereditary and sporadic BCCs may develop through common mechanisms.

Further still, mutations in genes encoding other components of the *SHH* pathway were speculated to play a role in BCC tumorigenesis. Activating mutations in *SMO* were seen in 6 to 20% of sporadic BCCs[143,145,146] and rarely *SHH* mutation has been reported in BCC as well.[147] Additionally, mutation of the *PTCH2* gene, which shows strong homology to *PTCH*, and the *SUFUH* gene, both of which participate in *SHH* signaling, have been described.[143,148] Thus, mutations in different pathway mediators may be involved in deregulating *SHH* signaling and consequently contribute to BCC tumorigenesis.

In addition, evidence supports that altered *SHH* signaling may play a role in the pathogenesis of other, more benign types of cutaneous basaloid tumors. Precedence for this derives from studies implicating *PTCH* defects in sporadic trichoepitheliomas. Deletions involving the *PTCH* locus at 9q22.3 were detected in approximately 50% of trichoepithelioma samples studied in one report,[149] whereas mutations in *PTCH* were identified in sporadic trichoepitheliomas in another study.[150] Sebaceous nevi are congenital cutaneous lesions that may develop foci of basal cell carcinoma over time. Up to 40% of sebaceous nevi in one study showed evidence for loss of heterozygosity for at least one genomic marker at 9q22.3, suggesting a role for *PTCH* inactivation in development of these lesions.[151] Lastly, increased expression of mRNA for *PTCH* and other pathway target genes provides evidence for deregulation of *SHH* signaling in BFH.[152,153] However, BFH showed lower levels and an altered distribution of transcripts for these genes compared to BCC, suggesting that the magnitude and/or pattern of *SHH* signaling may influence tumor phenotype.

Studies using experimental mouse models corroborate these observations. Aberrant expression of various mediators of *SHH* signaling to induce or mimic *Ptc* inactivation gives rise to basaloid tumorigenesis in transgenic mice. Overexpression of *SHH* to bypass Ptc suppression of Smo in skin gives rise to growths comparable to BCC.[147] Similarly, primary human keratinocytes engineered to overexpress *SHH* develop into lesions resembling BCC upon transplantation onto immunodeficient mice.[154] Further still, transgenic mice expressing an activated, mutant variant of human *SMO* generate basaloid lesions resembling BFH.[145,153]

Similar findings have been observed in functional studies of downstream effectors of *SHH* signaling. Transgenic mice that direct expression of *GLI*1 to basal epidermis produce both BCCs and trichoepitheliomas,[155] whereas transgenic mice that express *GLI*2 in the skin develop BCCs as well.[156] Taken together, these studies provide considerable experimental evidence supporting that deregulation of *SHH* signaling, through inactivation of *Ptc* or activation of either upstream or downstream pathway components, plays a central role in mediating development of BCC and other related forms of basaloid neoplasia.

***TP53* GENE DEFECTS** Given that the *TP53* tumor suppressor gene is a commonly altered gene in many forms of human cancer, a number of studies examined BCCs for *TP53* mutations. Approximately half of sporadic BCCs studied were found to carry *TP53* mutations.[82,157,158,143] As is the case for cutaneous SCC, inactivating *TP53* mutations typically display UV signature

(C → T or CC → TT) features in BCC, implicating mutagenesis through solar irradiation.[158] Deletion of the *TP53* locus, however, appears to be an infrequent event in BCC.[159]

Once defects specifically involving the *PTCH* region were identified in BCCs, studies were performed to determine whether both *TP53* and 9q/*PTCH* aberrations frequently occur in the same tumors. Of 18 tumors evaluated in one study, 11 (61%) BCCs displayed loss of 9q DNA markers and 11 (61%) had *TP53* mutations; 7 (39%) maintained alterations of both genes.[159] Similarly, in another report, 38% of early onset BCCs examined showed mutations in both *PTCH* and *TP53* genes, although this study likely underestimated *PTCH* defects as allelic loss at 9q was not assessed.[160] Yet another study observed both allelic loss of *PTCH* and *TP53* mutations in six of eight (75%) sporadic BCCs.[161] Taken together, these findings indicate that defects in both *PTCH* and *TP53* genes may be frequently associated in BCC and suggest that inactivation of both genes may promote BCC tumorigenesis in a cooperative manner.

ALTERNATIVE GENE DEFECTS Despite substantial evidence implicating mutations in mediators of *SHH* signaling in BCC, it is possible that defects in other genes may contribute to BCC tumorigenesis. Although mutations in *PTCH* or *SMO* have been detected in a majority of sporadic BCCs as discussed above, mutations in neither gene have been identified in a significant proportion of these tumors. Although this, in part, may reflect limitations of the approaches used for mutation screening, a plausible alternative explanation for this observation is that mutations in other genes may be involved in the pathogenesis of these BCCs. Mutations in alternative genes commonly associated with other forms of skin cancer, such as *RAS* family and *CDKN2A* genes, are rare in sporadic BCC,[143,162-164] suggesting that other, unknown genes may play some role.

Additional evidence supporting that alternative genes may contribute to BCC neoplasia derives from genome-wide screenings for chromosomal aberrations in tumor-derived DNA. In addition to recurrent losses at 9q encompassing the *PTCH* region, recurrent chromosomal gains were observed at five loci by comparative genomic hybridization (CGH) in a panel of BCC.[165] In particular, regional gains at 6p were detected in 47% of tumors studied. This finding suggests that an oncogene localizing to

6p may become activated by virtue of its amplification and overexpression in a significant proportion of sporadic BCCs. Similarly, high resolution SNP genotyping identified genomic losses at 6q23 to q27 in 5 of 14 (36%) BCCs, suggesting the presence of a putative tumor suppressor gene in this region.[166]

Lastly, experimental mouse models may provide still further evidence for alternative BCC genes. The *Notch*1 gene regulates normal development in various tissues, and altered Notch1 signaling has been associated with tumorigenesis. Mice designed to selectively inactivate *Notch*1 in keratinocytes develop epidermal hyperplasia and skin tumors resembling BCC.[167] Moreover, tumors derived from these mice show elevated and constitutive expression of *Gli*2, a *SHH* pathway effector gene. Although involvement of *NOTCH*1 in human BCC has not been reported, it is conceivable that defects in the *NOTCH*1 gene or other genes associated with *NOTCH*1 signaling may play a role in the pathogenesis of some BCCs.

■ FINAL THOUGHTS

Significant advances have been made in defining oncogenes and tumor suppressor genes, which when activated or inactivated, respectively, lead to CMM, SCC, and BCC. Identification of such genes has allowed investigation of molecular pathways involved in tumor development and how mutations in different genes may interact or cooperate with each other to sway the balance between cell proliferation, differentiation, and death in favor of tumorigenesis. However, our understanding of the genetic and molecular mechanisms underlying these cancers is far from complete.

There is considerable evidence indicating that additional genes may be involved in the pathogenesis of CMM, SCC, and BCC. The various mutation screening studies discussed in this chapter have identified defects in specific genes in only a portion of tumors examined. Although this, in part, may reflect limitations of techniques used to identify mutations or use of alternative mechanisms to effect gene activation or inactivation, it is plausible that aberrations in different genes may provide significant contributions to tumorigenesis. In addition, many tumor types harbor recurrent, nonrandom genomic aberrations that may activate proto-oncogenes (through gains in copy number) or inactivate tumor suppressor genes (through deletion). Such aberrations frequently occur in chromosomal regions distinct from sites of known cancer genes, indicating that they may contain novel genes that promote tumorigenesis. Lastly, defects in alternative genes are likely to be responsible for causing various hereditary skin cancer syndromes. Specific germline gene defects have not been identified in the majority of melanoma families, and a number of genetic disorders that increase susceptibility to BCC appear to be unrelated to the *PTCH* gene.

In the course of future investigation, and with advances in technology, novel skin cancer genes will certainly be discovered. Further study will elucidate the normal function of these genes, the consequences of perturbing their activities, and how they interact with other known cancer genes to promote tumorigenesis. As novel skin cancer genes are discovered and studied, a more complete understanding of the genetic and molecular basis of skin cancer will be achieved. Ultimately, this may permit development of novel therapies that target specific gene defects and the molecular pathways gone awry to treat skin cancer.

REFERENCES

1. Hanahan D, Weinberg RA. The hallmarks of cancer. *Cell*. 2000;100:57–70.
2. Hayward NK. Genetics of melanoma predisposition. *Oncogene*. 2003;22:3053–3062.
3. Fountain JW, Karayiorgou M, Ernstoff MS, et al. Homozygous deletions within human chromosome band 9p21 in melanoma. *Proc Natl Acad Sci*. 1992;89:10557–10561.
4. Cannon-Albright LA, Goldgar DE, Meyer LJ, et al. Assignment of a locus for familial melanoma, MLM, to chromosome 9p13–p22. *Science*. 1992;258:1148–1152.
5. Hussussian CJ, Struewing JP, Goldstein AM, et al. Germline p16 mutations in familial melanoma. *Nat Genet*. 1994;8:15–21.
6. Kamb A, Shattuck-Eidens D, Eeles R, et al. Analysis of the p16 gene (CDKN2) as a candidate for the chromosome 9p melanoma susceptibility locus. *Nat Genet*. 1994;8:23–26.
7. Walker GJ, Hussussian CJ, Flores JF, et al. Mutations of the CDKN2/p16INK4 gene in Australian melanoma kindreds. *Hum Mol Genet*. 1995;4:1845–1852.
8. Piepkorn M. Melanoma genetics: an update with focus on the CDKN2A(p16)/ARF tumor suppressors. *J Am Acad Dermatol*. 2000;42:705–722.
9. Sharpless E, Chin L. The INK4a/ARF locus and melanoma. *Oncogene*. 2003;22:3092–3098.
10. Ranade K, Hussussian CJ, Sikorski RS, et al. Mutations associated with familial melanoma impair p16INK4 function. *Nat Genet*. 1995;10:114–116.
11. Zuo L, Weger J, Yang Q, et al. Germline mutations in the p16INK4a binding domain of CDK4 in familial melanoma. *Nat Genet*. 1996;12:97–99.
12. Randerson-Moor JA, Harland M, Williams S, et al. A germline deletion of p14(ARF) but not CDKN2A in a melanoma-neural system tumour syndrome family. *Hum Mol Genet*. 2001;10:55–62.
13. Laud K, Marian C, Avril MF, et al. Comprehensive analysis of CDKN2A (p16INK4A/p14ARF) and CDKN2B genes in 53 melanoma index cases considered to be at heightened risk of melanoma. *J Med Genet*. 2006:43:39–47.
14. Rizos H, Puig S, Badenas C, Malvehy J, Darmanian AP, Jimenez L, Mila M, Kefford RF. A melanoma-associated germline mutation in exon 1beta inactivates p14ARF. *Oncogene*. 2001;20:5543–5547.
15. Hewitt C, Lee Wu C, Evans G, et al. Germline mutation of ARF in a melanoma kindred. *Hum Mol Genet*. 2002;11:1273–1279.
16. Harland M, Taylor CF, Chambers PA, et al. A mutation hotspot at the p14ARF splice site. *Oncogene*. 2005;24:4604–4608.
17. Serrano M, Lee H, Chin L, et al. Role of the INK4a locus in tumor suppression and cell mortality. *Cell*. 1996;85:27–37.
18. Chin L, Pomerantz J, Polsky D, et al. Cooperative effects of INK4a and ras in melanoma susceptibility in vivo. *Genes Dev*. 1997;11:2822–2834.
19. Ackermann J, Frutschi M, Kaloulis K, et al. Metastasizing melanoma formation caused by expression of activated N-RasQ61K on an INK4a-deficient background. *Cancer Res*. 2005;65:4005–40011.
20. Sotillo R, Garcia JF, Ortega S, et al. Invasive melanoma in Cdk4-targeted mice. *Proc Natl Acad Sci*. 2001;98:13312–13317.
21. Hacker E, Muller HK, Irwin N, et al. Spontaneous and UV radiation-induced multiple metastatic melanomas in Cdk4R24C/R24C/TPras mice. *Cancer Res*. 2006;66:2946–2952.
22. Pollock PM, Trent JM. The genetics of cutaneous melanoma. *Clin Lab Med*. 2000;20:667–690.
23. Holland EA, Beaton SC, Edwards BG, et al. Loss of heterozygosity and homozygous deletions on 9p21–22 in melanoma. *Oncogene*. 1994;9:1361–1365.
24. Bale SJ, Dracopoli NC, Tucker MA, et al. Mapping the gene for hereditary cutaneous malignant melanoma-dysplastic nevus to chromosome 1p. *N Engl J Med*. 1989;320:1367–1372.
25. Poetsch M, Woenckhaus C, Dittberner T, et al. An increased frequency of numerical chromosomal abnormalities and 1p36 deletions in isolated cells from paraffin sections of malignant melanomas by means of interphase cytogenetics. *Cancer Genet Cytogenet*. 1998;104:146–152.
26. Gillanders E, Hank Juo SH, Holland EA et al. Localization of a novel melanoma susceptibility locus to 1p22. *Am J Hum Genet*. 2003;73:301–313.
27. Walker GJ, Indsto JO, Sood R, et al. Deletion mapping suggests that the 1p22 melanoma susceptibility gene is a tumor suppressor localized to a 9-Mb interval. *Genes Chromosomes Cancer*. 2004:41:56–64.
28. Castellano M, Pollock PM, Walters MK, et al. CDKN2A/p16 is inactivated in most melanoma cell lines. *Cancer Res*. 1997;57:4868–4875.
29. Peris K, Chimenti S, Fargnoli MC, et al. UV fingerprint CDKN2a but no p14ARF mutations in sporadic melanomas. *J Invest Dermatol*. 1999;112:825–826.
30. Wolfel T, Hauer M, Schneider J, et al. A p16INK4a-insensitive CDK4 mutant targeted by cytolytic T lymphocytes in a human melanoma. *Science*. 1995;269:1281–1284.
31. Guldberg P, Kirkin AF, Gronbaek K, et al. Complete scanning of the CDK4 gene by denaturing gradient gel electrophoresis: a novel missense mutation but low overall frequency of mutations in sporadic metastatic malignant melanoma. *Int J Cancer*. 1997;72:780–783.
32. Muthusamy V, Hobbs C, Nogueira C, et al. Amplification of CDK4 and MDM2 in malignant melanoma. *Genes Chromosomes Cancer*. May 2006;45(5):447–454.
33. Rodriguez-Viciana P, Tetsu O, Oda K, Okada J, Rauen K, McCormick F. Cancer targets in the Ras pathway. *Cold Spring Harb Symp Quant Biol*. 2005;70:461–467.
34. Herlyn M, Satyamoorthy K. Activated ras. Yet another player in melanoma. *Am J Pathol*. 1996;149:739–744.
35. Chudnovsky Y, Adams AE, Robbins PB, Lin Q, Khavari PA. Use of human tissue to assess the oncogenic activity of melanoma-associated mutations. *Nat Genet*. 2005;37:745–749.
36. Eskandarpour M, Hashemi J, Kanter L, et al. Frequency of UV-inducible NRAS mutations in melanomas of patients with germline CDKN2A mutations. *J Natl Cancer*. Inst 2003;95:790–798.
37. Albino AP. Nanus DM. Mentle IR. et al. Analysis of ras oncogenes in malignant melanoma and precursor lesions: correlation of point mutations with differentiation phenotype. *Oncogene*. 1989;4:1363–1374.
38. Demunter A, Stas M, Degreef H, et al. Analysis of N- and K-ras mutations in the distinctive tumor progression phases of melanoma. *J Invest Dermatol*. 2001;117:1483–1489.
39. Omholt K, Karsberg S, Platz A, et al. Screening of N-ras codon 61 mutations in paired primary and metastatic cutaneous melanomas: mutations occur early and persist throughout tumor progression. *Clin Cancer Res*. 2002;8:3468–3474.
40. Davies H, Bignell GR, Cox C, et al. Mutations of the BRAF gene in human cancer. *Nature*. 2002;417:949–954.
41. Thomas NE. BRAF somatic mutations in malignant melanoma and melanocytic naevi. *Melanoma Res*. 2006;16:97–103.
42. Uribe P, Wistuba II, Gonzalez S. BRAF mutation: a frequent event in benign, atypical, and malignant melanocytic lesions of the skin. *Am J Dermatopathol*. 2003;25:365–70.
43. Daniotti M, Oggionni M, Ranzani T, et al. BRAF alterations are associated with complex mutational profiles in malignant melanoma. *Oncogene*. 2004;23:5968–5977.
44. Lang J, Boxer M, MacKie R. Absence of exon 15 BRAF germline mutations in

familial melanoma. *Hum Mutat.* 2003;21: 327–330.

45. Meyer P, Klaes R, Schmitt C, et al. Exclusion of BRAFV599E as a melanoma susceptibility mutation. *Int J Cancer.* 2003;106:78–80.

46. Laud K, Kannengiesser C, Avril MF, BRAF as a melanoma susceptibility candidate gene. *Cancer Res.* 2003;63: 3061–3065.

47. Pollock PM, Harper UL, Hansen KS, High frequency of BRAF mutations in nevi. *Nat Genet.* 2003;33:19–20.

48. Kumar R, Angelini S, Snellman E, Hemminki K. BRAF mutations are common somatic events in melanocytic nevi. *J Invest Dermatol.* 2004;122:342–348.

49. Wu H, Goel V, Haluska FG. PTEN signaling pathways in melanoma. *Oncogene.* 2003;22:3113–3122.

50. Pollock PM, Walker GJ, Glendening JM, et al. PTEN inactivation is rare in melanoma tumours but occurs frequently in melanoma cell lines. *Melanoma Res.* 2002;12:565–575.

51. Celebi JT, Shendrik I, Silvers DN, Peacocke M. Identification of PTEN mutations in metastatic melanoma specimens. *J Med Genet.* 2000;37:653–657.

52. Reifenberger J, Wolter M, Bostrom J, et al. Allelic losses on chromosome arm 10q and mutation of the PTEN (MMAC1) tumour suppressor gene in primary and metastatic malignant melanomas. *Virchows Arch.* 2000;436:487–493.

53. Tsao H, Zhang X, Fowlkes K, Haluska FG. Relative reciprocity of NRAS and PTEN/MMAC1 alterations in cutaneous melanoma cell lines. *Cancer Res.* 2000;60:1800–1804.

54. Stahl JM, Sharma A, Cheung M, et al.. Deregulated Akt3 activity promotes development of malignant melanoma. *Cancer Res.* 2004;64:7002–70010.

55. Robertson GP, Furnari FB, Miele ME, et al. In vitro loss of heterozygosity targets the PTEN/MMAC1 gene in melanoma. *Proc Natl Acad Sci.* 1998;95:9418–9423.

56. Stahl JM, Cheung M, Sharma A, et al. Loss of PTEN promotes tumor development in malignant melanoma. *Cancer Res.* 2003;63:2881–2890.

57. Rees JL. The genetics of sun sensitivity in humans. *Am J Hum Genet.* 2004;75: 739–751.

58. Sturm RA. Skin colour and skin cancer - MC1R, the genetic link. *Melanoma Res.* 2002;12:405–416.

59. Valverde P, Healy E, Sikkink S, et al. The Asp84Glu variant of the melanocortin 1 receptor (MC1R) is associated with melanoma. *Hum Mol Genet.* 1996;5: 1663–1666.

60. Palmer JS, Duffy DL, Box NF, et al. Melanocortin-1 receptor polymorphisms and risk of melanoma: is the association explained solely by pigmentation phenotype. *Am J Hum Genet.* 2000;66:176–186.

61. Kennedy C, ter Huurne J, Berkhout M, et al. Melanocortin 1 receptor (MC1R) gene variants are associated with an increased risk for cutaneous melanoma which is largely independent of skin type and hair color. *J Invest Dermatol.* 2001;117:294–300.

62. Matichard E, Verpillat P, Meziani R, et al. Melanocortin 1 receptor (MC1R) gene variants may increase the risk of melanoma in France independently of clinical risk factors and UV exposure. *J Med Genet.* 2004;41:e13.

63. Landi MT, Kanetsky PA, Tsang S, et al. MC1R, ASIP, and DNA repair in sporadic and familial melanoma in a Mediterranean population. *J Natl Cancer Inst.* 2005;97:998–1007.

64. Stratigos AJ, Dimisianos G, Nikolaou V, et al. Melanocortin receptor-1 gene polymorphisms and the risk of cutaneous melanoma in a low-risk southern European population. *J Invest Dermatol.* 2006;126:1842–1849.

65. Box NF, Duffy DL, Chen W, et al. MC1R genotype modifies risk of melanoma in families segregating CDKN2A mutations. *Am J Hum Genet.* 2001;69:765–773.

66. van der Velden PA, Sandkuijl LA, Bergman W, et al. Melanocortin-1 receptor variant R151C modifies melanoma risk in Dutch families with melanoma. *Am J Hum Genet.* 2001;69:774–779.

67. Chaudru V, Laud K, Avril MF, et al. Melanocortin-1 receptor (MC1R) gene variants and dysplastic nevi modify penetrance of CDKN2A mutations in French melanoma-prone pedigrees. *Cancer Epidemiol Biomarkers Prev.* 2005;14: 2384–2390.

68. Pho L, Grossman D, Leachman SA. Melanoma genetics: a review of genetic factors and clinical phenotypes in familial melanoma. *Curr Opin Oncol.* 2006; 18:173–179.

69. Levy C, Khaled M, Fisher DE. MITF: master regulator of melanocyte development and melanoma oncogene. *Trends Mol Med.* 2006;12:406–414.

70. Garraway LA, Widlund HR, Rubin MA, et al. Integrative genomic analyses identify MITF as a lineage survival oncogene amplified in malignant melanoma. *Nature.* 2005;436:117–122.

71. Steingrimsson E, Copeland NG, Jenkins NA. Melanocytes and the microphthalmia transcription factor network. *Annu Rev Genet.* 2004;38:365–411.

72. Miller AJ, Du J, Rowan S, et al. Transcriptional regulation of the melanoma prognostic marker melastatin (TRPM1) by MITF in melanocytes and melanoma. *Cancer Res.* 2004;64:509–516.

73. Healy E, Rehman I, Angus B, et al. Loss of heterozygosity in sporadic primary cutaneous melanoma. *Genes Chromosomes Cancer.* 1995;12:152–156.

74. Thompson FH, Emerson J, Olson S, et al. Cytogenetics of 158 patients with regional or disseminated melanoma. Subset analysis of near-diploid and simple karyotypes. *Cancer Genet Cytogenet.* 1995;83:93–104.

75. Bastian BC, LeBoit PE, Hamm H, et al. Chromosomal gains and losses in primary cutaneous melanomas detected by comparative genomic hybridization. *Cancer Res.* 1998;58:2170–2175.

76. Bittner M, Meltzer P, Chen Y et al. Molecular classification of cutaneous malignant melanoma by gene expression profiling. *Nature.* August 3, 2000;406(6795):536–540.

77. Haqq C, Nosrati M, Sudilovsky D, et al. The gene expression signatures of melanoma progression. *Proc Natl Acad Sci.* 2005;102:6092–6097.

78. Curtin JA, Fridlyand J, Kageshita T, et al. Distinct sets of genetic alterations in melanoma. *N Engl J Med.* 2005;353: 2135–2147.

79. Kim M, Gans JD, Nogueira C, et al. Comparative oncogenomics identifies NEDD9 as a melanoma metastasis gene. *Cell.* 2006;125:1269–1281.

80. Stary A, Sarasin A. The genetics of the hereditary xeroderma pigmentosum syndrome. *Biochimie.* 2002;84:49–60.

81. Nataraj AJ, Trent JC, Ananthaswamy HN. p53 gene mutations and photocarcinogenesis. *Photochem Photobiol.* 1995;62: 218–230.

82. Bolshakov S, Walker CM, Strom SS, et al. p53 mutations in human aggressive and nonaggressive basal and squamous cell carcinomas. *Clin Cancer Res.* 2003;9: 228–234.

83. Brash DE, Rudolph JA, Simon JA, et al. A role for sunlight in skin cancer: UV-induced p53 mutations in squamous cell carcinoma. *Proc Natl Acad Sci.* 1991;88:10124–10128.

84. Nelson MA, Einspahr JG, Alberts DS, et al. Analysis of the p53 gene in human precancerous actinic keratosis lesions and squamous cell cancers. *Cancer Lett.* 1994;85:23–29.

85. Campbell C, Quinn AG, Ro YS, et al. p53 mutations are common and early events that precede tumor invasion in squamous cell neoplasia of the skin. *J Invest Dermatol.* 1993;100:746–748.

86. Nakazawa H, English D, Randell PL, et al. UV and skin cancer: specific p53 gene mutation in normal skin as a biologically relevant exposure measurement. *Proc Natl Acad Sci.* 1994;91:360–364.

87. Jonason AS, Kunala S, Price GJ, et al. Frequent clones of p53-mutated keratinocytes in normal human skin. *Proc Natl Acad Sci.* 1996;93:14025–14029.

88. Ren ZP, Ahmadian A, Ponten F, et al. Benign clonal keratinocyte patches with p53 mutations show no genetic link to synchronous squamous cell precancer or cancer in human skin. *Am J Pathol.* 1997;150:1791–1803.

89. Malkin D. The Li-Fraumeni syndrome. In: The Genetic Basis of Human Cancer, Vogelstein B, Kinzler K, eds. 1998; 393–407. New York: McGraw-Hill.

90. Berg RJ, van Kranen HJ, Rebel HG, et al. Early p53 alterations in mouse skin carcinogenesis by UVB radiation: immunohistochemical detection of mutant p53 protein in clusters of preneoplastic epidermal cells. *Proc Natl Acad Sci.* 1996: 93:274–278.

91. Rebel H, Mosnier LO, Berg RJ, et al. Early p53-positive foci as indicators of tumor risk in ultraviolet-exposed hairless mice: kinetics of induction, effects of DNA repair deficiency, and p53 heterozygosity. *Cancer Res.* 2001;61:977–983.

92. Kramata P, Lu YP, Lou YR, et al. Patches of mutant p53-immunoreactive epidermal cells induced by chronic UVB Irradiation harbor the same p53 mutations as squamous cell carcinomas in the skin of hairless SKH-1 mice. *Cancer Res.* 2005;65:3577–3585.

93. Van Kranen HJ, De Gruijl FR, De Vries A, et al. Frequent p53 alterations but low incidence of ras mutations in UV-B-induced skin tumors of hairless mice. *Carcinogenesis.* 1995:16:1141–1147.

94. Dumaz N, van Kranen HJ, de Vries A, et al. The role of UV-B light in skin

carcinogenesis through the analysis of p53 mutations in squamous cell carcinomas of hairless mice. *Carcinogenesis*. 1997:18:897–904.

95. Li G, Tron V, Ho V. Induction of squamous cell carcinoma in p53-deficient mice after ultraviolet irradiation. *J Invest Dermatol*. 1998;110:72–75.

96. Jiang W, Ananthaswamy HN, Muller HK, et al. p53 protects against skin cancer induction by UV-B radiation. *Oncogene*. 1999;18:4247–4253.

97. Ziegler A, Jonason AS, Leffell DJ, Sunburn and p53 in the onset of skin cancer. *Nature*. 1994;372:773–776.

98. Pierceall WE, Goldberg LH, Tainsky MA, et al. Ras gene mutation and amplification in human nonmelanoma skin cancers. *Mol Carcinog*. 1991;4:196–202.

99. Kreimer-Erlacher H, Seidl H, Back B, et al. High mutation frequency at Ha-ras exons 1–4 in squamous cell carcinomas from PUVA-treated psoriasis patients. *Photochem Photobiol*. 2001;74:323–330.

100. Spencer JM, Kahn SM, Jiang W, et al. Activated ras genes occur in human actinic keratoses, premalignant precursors to squamous cell carcinomas. *Arch Dermatol*. 1995;131:796–800.

101. Yuspa SH. The pathogenesis of squamous cell cancer: lessons learned from studies of skin carcinogenesis. *J Dermatol Sci*. 1998;17:1–7.

102. Weinberg WC, Azzoli CG, Kadiwar N, et al. p53 gene dosage modifies growth and malignant progression of keratinocytes expressing the v-rasHa oncogene. *Cancer Res*. 1994;54:5584–5592.

103. Lin AW, Lowe SW. Oncogenic ras activates the ARF-p53 pathway to suppress epithelial cell transformation. *Proc Natl Acad Sci*. 2001;98:5025–5030.

104. Lazarov M, Kubo Y, Cai T, et al. CDK4 coexpression with Ras generates malignant human epidermal tumorigenesis. *Nat Med*. 2002;8:1105–1114.

105. Dajee M, Lazarov M, Zhang JY, et al. NF-kappaB blockade and oncogenic Ras trigger invasive human epidermal neoplasia. *Nature*. 2003;421:639–643.

106. Seitz CS, Lin Q, Deng H, et al. Alterations in NF-kappaB function in transgenic epithelial tissue demonstrate a growth inhibitory role for NF-kappaB. *Proc Natl Acad Sci*. 1998;95:2307–2312.

107. Bonni A, Brunet A, West AE, et al. Cell survival promoted by the Ras-MAPK signaling pathway by transcription-dependent and -independent mechanisms. *Science*. 1999;286:1358–1362.

108. Stambolic V, Mak TW, Woodgett JR. Modulation of cellular apoptotic potential: contributions to oncogenesis. *Oncogene*. 1999;18:6094–6103.

109. Quinn AG, Sikkink S, Rees JL. Delineation of two distinct deleted regions on chromosome 9 in human non-melanoma skin cancers. *Genes Chromosomes Cancer*. 1994;11:222–225.

110. Saridaki Z, Liloglou T, Zafiropoulos A, et al. Mutational analysis of CDKN2A genes in patients with squamous cell carcinoma of the skin. *Br J Dermatol*. 2003;148:638–648.

111. Kreimer-Erlacher H, Seidl H, Back B, et al. High frequency of ultraviolet mutations at the INK4a-ARF locus in squamous cell carcinomas from psoralen-plus-ultraviolet-A-treated psoriasis

patients. *J Invest Dermatol*. 2003;120: 676–682.

112. Mortier L, Marchetti P, Delaporte E, et al. Progression of actinic keratosis to squamous cell carcinoma of the skin correlates with deletion of the 9p21 region encoding the p16(INK4a) tumor suppressor. *Cancer Lett*. 2002;176:205–214.

113. Tremain R, Marko M, Kinnimulki V, et al. Defects in TGF-beta signaling overcome senescence of mouse keratinocytes expressing v-Ha-ras. *Oncogene*. 2000;19:1698–1709.

114. Amendt C, Schirmacher P, Weber H, Blessing M. Expression of a dominant negative type II TGF-beta receptor in mouse skin results in an increase in carcinoma incidence and an acceleration of carcinoma development. *Oncogene*. 1998;17:25–34.

115. Grady WM. Transforming growth factor-beta, Smads, and cancer. *Clin Cancer Res*. 2005;11:3151–3154.

116. Redman RS, Katuri V, Tang Y, Dillner A, Mishra B, Mishra L. Orofacial and gastrointestinal hyperplasia and neoplasia in smad4+/− and elf+/−/smad4+/− mutant mice. *J Oral Pathol Med*. 2005;34: 23–29.

117. Qiao W, Li AG, Owens P, et al. Hair follicle defects and squamous cell carcinoma formation in Smad4 conditional knockout mouse skin. *Oncogene*. 2006; 25:207–217.

118. Kubo Y, Urano Y, Hida Y, Arase S. Lack of somatic mutation in the PTEN gene in squamous cell carcinomas of human skin. *J Dermatol Sci*. 1999;19:199–201.

119. Waldmann V, Wacker J. Mutations of the PH domain of protein kinase B (PKB/AKT) are absent in human epidermal skin tumors. *Dermatology*. 2001;203:284–288.

120. Quinn AG, Sikkink S, Rees JL. Delineation of two distinct deleted regions on chromosome 9 in human non-melanoma skin cancers. *Genes Chromosomes Cancer*. 1994;11:222–225.

121. Rehman I, Quinn AG, Healy E, et al. High frequency of loss of heterozygosity in actinic keratoses, a usually benign disease. *Lancet*. 1994;344:788–789.

122. Rehman I, Takata M, Wu YY, Rees JL. Genetic change in actinic keratoses. *Oncogene*. 1996;12:2483–2490.

123. Ashton KJ, Weinstein SR, Maguire DJ, et al. Chromosomal aberrations in squamous cell carcinoma and solar keratoses revealed by comparative genomic hybridization. *Arch Dermatol*. 2003;139:876–882.

124. Haider AS, Peters SB, Kaporis H, et al. Genomic analysis defines a cancer-specific gene expression signature for human squamous cell carcinoma and distinguishes malignant hyperproliferation from benign hyperplasia. *J Invest Dermatol*. 2006:126:869–881.

125. Gorlin RJ. Nevoid basal cell carcinoma syndrome. *Dermatol Clin*. 1995;13:113–125.

126. Kimonis VE, Goldstein AM, Pastakia B, et al. Clinical manifestations in 105 persons with nevoid basal cell carcinoma syndrome. *Am J Med Genet*. 1997;69:299–308.

127. Gailani MR, Bale SJ, Leffell DJ, et al. Developmental defects in Gorlin syndrome related to a putative tumor suppressor gene on chromosome 9. *Cell*. 1992;69:111–117.

128. Hahn H, Wicking C, Zaphiropoulous PG, et al. Mutations of the human homolog of Drosophila patched in the nevoid basal cell carcinoma syndrome. *Cell*. 1996;85:841–851.

129. Johnson RL, Rothman AL, Xie J, et al. Human homolog of patched, a candidate gene for the basal cell nevus syndrome. *Science*. 1996;272:1668–1671.

130. Wetmore C. Sonic hedgehog in normal and neoplastic proliferation: insight gained from human tumors and animal models. *Curr Opin Genet Dev*. 2003;13: 34–42.

131. Ruiz i Altaba A, Sanchez P, Dahmane N. Gli and hedgehog in cancer: tumours, embryos and stem cells. *Nat Rev Cancer*. 2002;2:361–372.

132. Duman-Scheel M, Weng L, Xin S, et al. Hedgehog regulates cell growth and proliferation by inducing Cyclin D and Cyclin E. *Nature*. 2002;417:299–304.

133. Barnes EA, Kong M, Ollendorff V, et al. Patched1 interacts with cyclin B1 to regulate cell cycle progression. *EMBO J*. 2001;20:2214–2223.

134. Adolphe C, Hetherington R, Ellis T, Wainwright B. Patched1 functions as a gatekeeper by promoting cell cycle progression. *Cancer Res*. 2006;66:2081–2088.

135. High A, Zedan W. Basal cell nevus syndrome. *Curr Opin Oncol*. 2005;17:160–166.

136. Aszterbaum M, Epstein J, Oro A, et al. Ultraviolet and ionizing radiation enhance the growth of BCCs and trichoblastomas in patched heterozygous knockout mice. *Nature Med*. 1999;5: 1285–1291.

137. Mancuso M, Pazzaglia S, Tanori M, et al. Basal cell carcinoma and its development: insights from radiation-induced tumors in Ptch1-deficient mice. *Cancer Res*. 2004;64:934–941.

138. Bleiberg J, Brodkin RH. Linear unilateral basal cell nevus with comedones. *Arch Dermatol*. 1969;100:187–190.

139. Vabres P, Lacombe D, Rabinowitz LG, et al. The gene for Bazex-Dupre-Christol syndrome maps to chromosome Xq. *J Invest Dermatol*. 1995;105:87–91.

140. Michaelsson G, Olsson E, Westermark P. The Rombo syndrome: a familial disorder with vermiculate atrophoderma, milia, hypotrichosis, trichoepitheliomas, basal cell carcinomas and peripheral vasodilation with cyanosis. *Acta Derm Venereol*. 1981;61:497–503.

141. Gailani MR, Stahle-Backdahl M, Leffell DJ, et al. The role of the human homologue of Drosophila patched in sporadic basal cell carcinomas. *Nature Genet*. 1996;14:78–81.

142. Aszterbaum M, Rothman A, Johnson RL. et al. Identification of mutations in the human PATCHED gene in sporadic basal cell carcinomas and in patients with the basal cell nevus syndrome. *J Invest Dermatol*. 1998;110:885–888.

143. Reifenberger J, Wolter M, Knobbe CB, et al. Somatic mutations in the PTCH, SMOH, SUFUH and TP53 genes in sporadic basal cell carcinomas. *Br J Dermatol*. 2005;152:43–51.

144. Holmberg E, Rozell BL, Toftgard R. Differential allele loss on chromosome 9q22.3 in human non-melanoma skin cancer, *Br J Cancer*. 1996;74:246–250.

145. Xie J, Murone M, Luoh SM, et al. Activating Smoothened mutations in sporadic basal-cell carcinoma. *Nature.* 1998;391:90–92.

146. Lam CW, Xie J, To KF, et al. A frequent activated smoothened mutation in sporadic basal cell carcinomas. *Oncogene.* 1999;18:833–836.

147. Oro AE, Higgins KM, Hu Z, et al. Basal cell carcinomas in mice overexpressing sonic hedgehog. *Science.* 1997;276:817–821.

148. Smyth I, Narang MA, Evans T, et al. Isolation and characterization of human patched 2 (PTCH2), a putative tumour suppressor gene in basal cell carcinoma and medulloblastoma on chromosome 1p32. *Hum Mol Genet.* 1999;8:291–297.

149. Matt D, Xin H, Vortmeyer AO, et al. Sporadic trichoepithelioma demonstrates deletions at 9q22.3. *Arch Dermatol.* 2000;136:657–660.

150. Vorechovsky I, Unden AB, Sandstedt B, et al. Trichoepitheliomas contain somatic mutations in the overexpressed PTCH gene: support for a gatekeeper mechanism in skin tumorigenesis. *Cancer Res.* 1997;57:4677–4681.

151. Xin H, Matt D, Qin, JZ, et al. The sebaceous nevus: a nevus with deletions of the PTCH gene. *Cancer Res.* 1999;59: 1834–1836.

152. Jih, DM, Shapiro M, James WD, et al. Familial basaloid follicular hamartoma: lesional characterization and review of the literature. *Am J Dermpathol.* 2003;25: 130–137.

153. Grachtchouk V, Grachtchouk M, Lowe L, et al. The magnitude of hedgehog signaling activity defines skin tumor phenotype. *EMBO J.* 2003;22:2741–2751.

154. Fan H, Oro AE, Scott MP, et al. Induction of basal cell carcinoma features in transgenic human skin expressing Sonic Hedgehog. *Nat Med.* 1997;3:788–792.

155. Nilsson M, Unden AB, Krause D, et al. Induction of basal cell carcinomas and trichoepitheliomas in mice overexpressing GLI-1. *Proc Nat Acad Sci.* 2000; 97:3438–3443.

156. Grachtchouk M, Mo R, Yu S, et al. Basal cell carcinomas in mice overexpressing Gli2 in skin. *Nature Genet.* 2000;24:216–217.

157. Rady P, Scinicariello F, Wagner RF Jr, et al. p53 mutations in basal cell carcinomas. *Cancer Res.* 1992;52:3804–3806.

158. Ziegler A, Leffell DJ, Kunala S, et al. Mutation hotspots due to sunlight in the p53 gene of nonmelanoma skin cancers. *Proc Natl Acad Sci.* 1993;90: 4216–4220.

159. Gailani MR, Leffell DJ, Ziegler A, et al. Relationship between sunlight exposure and a key genetic alteration in basal cell carcinoma. *J Natl Cancer Inst.* 1996;88:349–354.

160. Zhang H, Ping XL, Lee PK, et al. Role of PTCH and p53 genes in early-onset basal cell carcinoma. *Am J Pathol.* 2001;158:381–385.

161. Ling G, Ahmadian A, Persson A, et al. PATCHED and p53 gene alterations in sporadic and hereditary basal cell cancer. *Oncogene.* 2001;20:7770–7778.

162. Wilke WW, Robinson RA, Kennard CD. H-ras-1 gene mutations in basal cell carcinoma: automated direct sequencing of clinical specimens. *Mod Pathol.* 1993;6:15–19.

163. Kubo Y, Urano Y, Fukuhara K, et al. Lack of mutation in the INK4a locus in basal cell carcinomas. *Br J Dermatol.* 1998;139:340–341.

164. Saridaki Z, Koumantaki E, Liloglou T, et al. High frequency of loss of heterozygosity on chromosome region 9p21–p22 but lack of p16INK4a/p19ARF mutations in greek patients with basal cell carcinoma of the skin. *J Invest Dermatol.* 2000;115:719–725.

165. Ashton KJ, Weinstein SR, Maguire DJ, et al. Molecular cytogenetic analysis of basal cell carcinoma DNA using comparative genomic hybridization. *J invest Dermatol.* 2001;117:683–686.

166. Teh MT, Blaydon D, Chaplin T, et al. Genomewide single nucleotide polymorphism microarray mapping in basal cell carcinomas unveils uniparental disomy as a key somatic event. *Cancer Res.* 2005;65:8597–8603.

167. Nicolas M, Wolfer A, Raj K, et al. Notch1 functions as a tumor suppressor in mouse skin. *Nat Genet.* 2003;33: 416–421.

CHAPTER 6

Basal Cell Carcinoma

Keyvan Nouri, M.D.
Christopher J. Ballard, B.S.
Asha R. Patel, B.S.
Rana Anadolu Brasie, M.D.

BOX 6-1   Overview

- Basal cell carcinoma (BCC) is a non-melanoma skin cancer and is the most common type of cancer in humans worldwide.
- A combination of environmental factors, phenotype, and genetic predisposition account for the main etiologic causes of BCC.
- The majority of BCC cases are triggered by DNA mutations produced by UV radiation. The most common mutations are seen in the *patched* (*PTCH1*) gene and in the *p53* gene.
- UV-induced inflammation may also play some role.
- Genodermatoses, such as Gorlin's syndrome (basal cell nevus syndrome) and xeroderma pigmentosum (XP), have BCCs appear prominently in their clinical presentations.
- BCCs have many subtypes that include the following: nodular/noduloulcerative, pigmented, superficial, morpheaform (sclerosing or fibrosing), basosquamous/metatypical, infiltrative, micronodular, field-fire, and giant.
- Treatment via surgical means are standard for BCC removal; however, examples of the variety of treatment modalities used today are simple surgical excision, curettage and electrodesiccation, cryosurgery, radiation therapy, Mohs' micrographic surgery, laser surgery, photodynamic therapy, imiquimod, and 5-fluorouracil.
- Taking preventative measures is absolute key in decreasing the incidence of skin cancer around the world. Abstinence from sun exposure is highly recommended but nearly impossible to comply with. Therefore, appropriate application of sunscreen and protective clothing must be enforced.

INTRODUCTION

The incidence of skin cancer has markedly increased over the past few decades. At this time, between 2 and 3 million nonmelanoma skin cancers (NMSCs) and approximately 132,000 melanoma skin cancers occur globally each year. Alarmingly, one in every three cancers diagnosed is a skin cancer. The Skin Cancer Foundation currently estimates that one in every five Americans will develop skin cancer in their lifetime due to the ever-decreasing ozone layer, increased recreational exposure to the sun, and more histories of blistering sunburns.[1] Basal cell carcinoma (BCC), squamous cell carcinoma (SCC), and malignant melanoma are commonly grouped together under the term "skin cancer." BCC and SCC are the two most common cancers that are distinctly labeled as NMSC.[2] NMSCs are the most common forms of cancer in the United States[3] and account for nearly 90% of all skin cancers diagnosed in the world.[4] They are not only common in the Caucasian population of the United States,[3] but also in Australia.[5] NMSCs are rising at a disturbing rate in most European nations as well;[6,7] NMSCs have the highest prevalence at regions and countries nearest to the equator.[4] Out of the NMSCs, BCC is the most frequently occurring cancer.[1,4,5,8] BCC is described as an abnormal growth of epidermal keratinocytes immediately above the basement membrane[9] in the form of indolent malignant neoplasm of the hair follicle.[10] This chapter will primarily focus on the epidemiology, pathogenesis, diagnosis, treatment, and prevention of BCC.

EPIDEMIOLOGY

BOX 6-2   Summary

- BCC is the most frequent type of cancer found in humans; an estimated 75% of all diagnosed skin cancers in the United States are BCCs.
- A definite correlation exists between NMSC's incidence and sun exposure, specifically UV radiation.
- The face, head, neck, arms, and back of the hands are most commonly affected by BCCs. The structures of the head that are most susceptible to BCCs include the nose, scalp, eyelids, ears, and lips.
- Patients with light hair, light eyes, freckles, a fair complexion, Celtic ancestry (Scottish, Irish, Welsh), and Fitzpatrick skin types I and II have an increased incidence of NMSCs.
- Besides sun exposure, other known factors also increase the risk of NMSC such as genetic susceptibility, exposure to chemical carcinogens such as arsenic, tobacco, coal-tar, ionized radiation, asphalt, soot, crude paraffin, anthracene, pitch, organic and inorganic solvents, organophosphatic compounds, burns, scars, and chronic ulcerations.

More than 1 million cases of NMSC occur in the United States every year. Approximately 75% of all diagnosed skin cancers in the United States are BCCs.[8] The incidence of BCC in the United States, Canada, Australia, and Europe increases roughly by 3 to 6% per year.[11] Various epidemiological studies demonstrate that there is a definite correlation between NMSC incidence and sun exposure, specifically UV radiation.[1,2,5,8,11,12] The incidence of skin cancer has been linked to latitude. The regions closer to the equator have a greater prevalence of NMSC.[4,13] The state of Hawaii reports an annual incidence of BCC four times more than the incidence of mainland United States.[13] Nearly 80% of all cases of this cancer arise on areas exposed by the sun, such as the face, head, neck, arms, and back of the hands.[12] The structures of the head that are most susceptible to BCC include the scalp, eyelids, ears, nose, and lips.[11] In most cases, sun exposure plays a role in the pathogenesis of the carcinoma, but areas on the body not regularly exposed to UV rays may also be affected by BCC.[13] These startling incidence rates have started to impose an extreme financial burden in many countries,[14] including the United States. Presently in the United States, NMSCs are the fifth most costly cancer for patients.[15]

The patient's race and ethnicity are important factors in determining the incidence of skin cancer.[4] Patients with light hair, light eyes, freckles, a fair complexion, Celtic ancestry (Scottish, Irish, Welsh), and Fitzpatrick skin types I and II have an increased incidence of NMSCs.[4,16–18] The phenotypes with red[7] or blonde hair, blue or green eyes, and Fitzpatrick skin type I (patients who burn the fastest and never tan) have the highest incidence of NMSCs.[19,20] In a large multicenter southern European study, "Helios," a tendency to sunburn, an inability to tan, and a history of sunburn at youth were warning flags for an increased incidence of BCC.[21] Individuals with a darker skin tone or African, Asian, and Mediterranean ethnic groups have a lower incidence of skin cancer.[4] Therefore, melanin, the pigment responsible for darker skin coloring, could possibly protect the skin from these types of cancers.[4,22] Reports of albinism in Africans show that they have an incidence of BCC comparable with white Caucasians, further supporting the role of melanin as a protective agent against skin cancer.[4]

The incidence of NMSC is on the rise, but fortunately the death rates are declining. The mortality estimate from NMSC is extremely low, with a total 5-year survival rate of greater than 95%.[18] The American Cancer Society believes that approximately 1000 to 2000 people die each year from NMSC. Most of these mortalities are in the elderly, immunosuppressed, and untreated people.[8] In 1991, it was estimated that a 10% reduction in the ozone layer would cause 12 million extra cases of skin cancer along with 200,000 more deaths in the United States by the year 2050.[18] The rule of thumb is that a 10% reduction in the ozone layer thickness will cause an approximate 20% increase in UV radiation and an overwhelming 40% increase in skin cancers. More specifically, for every 1% decrease in total column atmospheric ozone, an increase of 2.7% in NMSCs should be expected. Only a small change in the thickness of ozone layer makes a big impact on the incidence of skin cancer.[23]

People with occupational or recreational outdoor sun exposure and those living at latitudes close to the equator have an increased risk of NMSC. The influence of today's society, culture, and fashion has made a deep impact upon incidence rates of skin cancer. For example, the obsession to obtain deep and dark suntans and its association with higher socioeconomic status has driven skin cancer to epidemic proportions.[23] BCC is no longer exclusively associated with the middle-aged or elderly population. Unfortunately, it has now encroached upon younger age groups because of the dangerous and unprotected levels of sun exposure.[8]

For decades, radiation from the sun and elsewhere has been proposed to have damaging effects. Ultraviolet B (UVB) light, which has wavelengths ranging from 290 to 320 nm, creates carcinogenic mutations in the skin that manifest as cancer at an older age. The UVB light impairs and damages the DNA, as well as leads to suppression of the immune system response. This inhibits the body from detecting the damaged genetic material. The altered DNA goes unchecked and eventually leads to cancer.[4] BCC incidence is highly related to sun exposure. Other known factors also increase the risk of NMSC such as genetic susceptibility, diet, exposure to chemical carcinogens, tobacco, coal-tar, ionized radiation, asphalt, soot, crude paraffin, anthracene, pitch, organic and inorganic solvents, mineral oils, organophosphatic compounds, burns, scars,

and chronic ulcerations.[4,6,24] Inorganic arsenic has been proven to induce superficial BCC lesions on areas of the body protected from the sun, such as the trunk.[4,25] Contact with fiberglass dust and dry cleaning agents also increase the chance of BCC.[26] The human papillomavirus (HPV) is currently being researched for having a possible role in triggering superficial BCC.[11] Lowered immunity states, such as patients with xeroderma pigmentosum (XP), organ transplantation, and HIV, increase the possibility of developing NMSC.[4] The immunosuppressive state is conducive to an increased cancer rate for two main reasons.[27] First, medications and agents used in transplant and seriously ill patients have a certain degree of toxicity, and perhaps may also be mutagenic.[28,29] Secondly, the immune system is not optimally functioning because of the patient's health status; therefore, the body's natural defenses are inhibited.[4,30,31]

Primary (previously untreated) BCCs also have a tendency to recur. Nearly two-thirds of BCCs will recur in the following 3 years after treatment. Between the 5th and 10th year after treatment, about 18% of BCCs will return.[32] The American Cancer Society has reported that patients with a single basal cell lesion will develop a new skin tumor within the next 5 years.[8]

■ PATHOGENESIS

BOX 6-3   Summary

- BCC is the indolent malignant neoplasm of the hair follicle and emerges from keratinocyte stem cells in hair follicles, sebaceous glands, or interfollicular basal cells.
- The radiation from the UV rays induces DNA mutations in certain genes within cells, such as the *p53* gene for BCC and SCC and the *patched* (*PTCH1*) gene for BCC.
- The most frequent UVB-induced alteration seen is the C → T, CC → TT base substitutions at dipyrimidine sites; these dimers have been named UV signatures.
- UV-induced inflammation via COX-2 plays a role in BCC pathogenesis as well as SCC in the skin.
- The most frequent mutation is associated with the *p53* tumor-suppressor gene; UVB irradiation causes direct alteration to the *p53*, which eventually inhibits apoptosis and the development of skin cancer.
- Alterations of *p53* have been found in nearly 56% of human BCC cases.
- Alterations of *PTCH1* have been found in 30 to 40% of sporadic BCCs.

- Two hereditary disorders, Gorlin's syndrome (autosomal dominant) and xeroderma pigmentosum (autosomal recessive), have indications of *PTCH1* gene mutations. The mutation of the *PTCH1* gene inactivates the suppressor function, leading to uncontrolled cell proliferation and tumor formation.

BCC is the most frequent type of cancer found in humans.[1,5,8,33,34] Usually, BCCs emerge from keratinocyte stem cells, in hair follicles, sebaceous glands, or interfollicular basal cells.[33,35] Generally, most BCC cases are sporadic, but BCCs may also appear in genetic disorders such as Gorlin's syndrome (basal cell nevus syndrome) and XP.[33] The majority of sporadic cases are induced by sunlight, specifically UVB rays.[4,34] The radiation from the UV rays induces DNA mutations in certain genes within cells. The genes that undergo the most substantial mutations are the *p53* gene for BCC and SCC and the *patched* (*PTCH1*) gene for BCC.[33] UV-induced inflammation in the skin contributes to the pathogenesis of BCC as well as SCC. UV-induced inflammation is mediated by increased prostaglandin synthesis mainly through cyclooxygenase-2 (COX)-2. Erythema and inflammation associated with COX-2 can be inhibited by systemic administration of COX-2 inhibitors. Animal studies have shown that these agents have a chemopreventive effect on already ongoing photocarcinogenesis, and reduce the number of BCC and SCCs in mice.[36–38]

The *p53* and *PTCH1* genes are tumor-suppressor genes.[33] The *p53* gene is responsible for encoding a protein that controls the cell cycle and apoptosis.[39] The *PTCH1* gene encodes for a receptor in an inhibitory pathway.[35] An alteration to these tumor-suppressor genes leads to their inactivation, triggering mutated cell proliferation.[33]

The most frequent UVB-induced alteration seen is the C → T, CC → TT base substitutions at dipyrimidine sites. These unique dimers have been titled as the "UV signature" because of their frequency in photodamaged skin.[33] These signatures are commonly seen in lighter skin compared to darker skin because the greater amount of melanin in darker skin leads to better filtering of radiation, which is more protective.[34]

The mutation associated with the *p53* gene is more frequent in SCC than in BCC in the skin. UVB irradiation causes direct alteration to the *p53* tumor-suppressor gene, which eventually inhibits apoptosis and the development of skin cancer. There are *p53* mutations in various BCC lesions including the earliest and smallest ones. Alterations of *p53* have been found in nearly 56% of human BCC cases and the "UV signature" is in approximately 65% of these.[33,40]

The *PTCH1* gene is a human tumor-suppressor gene that was initially discovered as the gene accountable for the onset of Gorlin's syndrome. Alterations of *PTCH1* have been found in 30 to 40% of sporadic BCCs and the "UV signature" has been found in 41% of these *PTCH1* altered lesions.[33,35] This gene is located on chromosome 9q22.3 and is responsible for the repression of genes that direct embryonic cell development, growth, and differentiation, such as the *hedgehog* gene. If this gene and its pathway are abnormally activated, it can lead to various types of tumorigenesis, one type being BCC.[33,34] The *PTCH1* gene encodes for a large transmembrane glycoprotein that is part of a receptor complex with another transmembrane glycoprotein. The latter transmembrane glycoprotein is the product of the *smoothened* gene (SMO),[33,40] which is a seven-transmembrane-domain protein that has a significant role in the *hedgehog* pathway.[41] The glycoprotein receptor complex is actually the main receptor for *hedgehog*'s extracellular signaling molecule. When this complex binds with specific ligands, it initiates a conformational change within the *PTCH1* gene. This change then activates the *smoothened* gene.[33,40]

PTCH1 inhibits the *smoothened* repressor function.[41] Abnormal activation of *smoothened* results in an unrestrained, continuous transmission of signals into the nucleus. This activates gene transcription regulated by the GLI transcription factor family.[35,41]

Two hereditary disorders, Gorlin's syndrome and XP, have indications of *PTCH1* gene mutations. The mutation of the *PTCH1* gene inactivates the suppressor function, leading to cell proliferation and tumor formation. Gorlin's syndrome is an autosomal dominant disorder characterized by keratocysts, skeletal defects, and numerous BCCs. These patients have a germline mutation of *PTCH1*.[33] XP is an autosomal recessive disorder where the person cannot repair UV-mutated DNA due to the genetic absence of that mechanism. These patients have a higher incidence of skin cancer because of the lack of a repairing mechanism. In XP BCCs, a higher amount of UV-induced alterations of the *PTCH1* gene are found compared to that in non-XP patients. There are also many more "UV signatures." In half of the

XP BCCs, the *PTCH1* gene and the *p53* gene reveal UV-induced alterations. Since only half of the *PTCH1* genes show UV-induced changes, there is a high probability that another cause unrelated to UV radiation may cause *PTCH1* damage and tumorigenesis.[33,40,42]

Not only is damage inflicted upon the *PTCH1* gene and the *hedgehog* pathway, but downstream targets such as the *Wnt* gene are abnormally activated as well.[43,44] Once binding of Wnt to its receptor (frizzled) occurs, a signaling intermediate (β-catenin) is dephosphorylated.[43,45] β-Catenin's dephosphorylation is significant because it allows this newly altered β-catenin to travel to the nucleus and perform as part of a transcription activation complex so other genes can activate.[43,46] β-Catenin has been under scrutiny for a correlation with BCC because it is actually a molecule that aids in the bonding of actin bundles, structures necessary for epithelial cell-to-cell adhesion.[43,47] One immunohistochemical study investigated the distribution of β-catenin in the cells of sporadic BCCs via antibodies directed against β-catenin. The study resulted in surprising confirmation that nuclear β-catenin distribution is a feature of BCC. In this study, atopic dermatitis, psoriasis, and SCC did not have nuclear β-catenin localization, further supporting the theory that nuclear β-catenin distribution is unique to BCC pathogenesis.[43]

Other genes, besides the ones mentioned earlier, are also speculated to have a part in BCC development. *PTCH2*, on chromosome 1p32.1–32.3, is currently under analysis since alterations of this gene have been found in a case of BCC.[33,48] The biological role of *PTCH2* is still not understood, but it has been hypothesized to take part in the *hedgehog* pathway at a certain level.[35] Another target for research are transcription factors, the Gli 1 and Gli 2 zinc finger proteins, which are the activators of the *hedgehog* pathway in mammalian cells. These transcription factors' genetic material are greatly expressed in BCC lesions. Researchers predict that mutations that lead to a high expression of Gli 1 zinc finger protein in basal cells are more likely to induce BCC.[33,49] The transcription factor Gli1 has an activating function specifically for a platelet-derived growth factor receptor, PDGFRα. Scientists have found an elevated PDGFRα level expressed in BCCs of mice and humans. A theory has been developed that this growth factor and its receptor play an essential role in the mutation mechanism of the *hedgehog* pathway, thus instigating tumorigenesis.[41]

Certain gene polymorphisms have been shown to be associated with certain phenotypic features in BCC patients such as young age, multiple lesions, and lesions on the trunk. Glutathione *S*-transferase and cytochrome P450 genotypes are associated with multiple BCCs.[50,51] Other known associations include vitamin D receptor (VDR) genes and tumor necrosis factor alpha (TNF-α) microsatellite polymorphisms.[52,53]

BCC is classified as a nonendocrine tumor of the skin; however, endocrine cell differentiation within BCC tumors has been discovered. Furthermore, BCC is the first classified nonendocrine tumor to present with endocrine cells.[54,55] The peculiar endocrine cells in BCCs resemble Merkel cells, the only epidermal endocrine cells. Since true Merkel cells are not present in BCC, these non-Merkel endocrine cells in BCC may contribute to its pathogenesis.[54]

■ DIAGNOSIS

BOX 6-4   Summary

- Nodular/noduloulcerative BCCs are the most common. Look for pearly, waxy papules or nodules with raised or rolled borders and central small ulcers covered with crust in the latter.
- Superficial BCCs occur more on the trunk and extremities than on the head and neck, and affect younger patients more than do nodular BCCs.
- Morpheaform BCCs may appear similar to a scar. They may grow quite extensively. They have high risk of recurrence and microscopic extension.
- Basosquamous/metatypical carcinoma is more aggressive than is typical BCCs. It shows features of both basal and squamous cell carcinomas.
- Pigmented BCCs mimic pigmented nevi, pigmented seborrheic keratosis, and even melanoma.
- Infiltrative BCCs have an opaque whitish yellow color that may blend with the surrounding skin; this clinical presentation is challenging for clinical diagnoses. These, as well as micronodular BCCs, tend to have high recurrence rates.
- Giant BCCs are at least 5 cm in diameter, and can result from recurrent tumors and neglect.
- Nevoid basal cell carcinoma syndrome is an autosomal dominant disorder that has a mutation of the *Patched1* gene on chromosome 9q22.3. They have numerous BCCs, jaw cysts, skeletal abnormalities, ectopic calcification, and palmar and plantar pits.

As with many dermatologic entities, BCCs can be recognized clinically. A discerning eye is necessary when examining a patient's skin. Although these lesions have typical characteristics, the clinical presentations can vary. A definitive diagnosis cannot be established until a biopsy is taken and proven to be a BCC. A shave biopsy is usually adequate for most BCC lesions, such as the nodular and superficial types. However, if an infiltrative or morpheaphorm-type is suspected, a punch or excisional biopsy should be taken to verify the diagnosis. Unlike SCCs, BCCs do not have a known precursor lesion; instead, they arise *de novo*. Numerous subtypes of BCCs exist and are usually found on hair-bearing skin; they almost never occur on mucous membranes. They are generally seen in adults, although there are reports of BCCs in children. BCCs, in general, metastasize very rarely. Reports have described a metastasis rate between 0.0028[56] and 0.1%.[57] Clinically and histologically, numerous forms can be differentiated, and the most common types are described below.

NODULAR/NODULOULCERATIVE BASAL CELL CARCINOMA

BOX 6-5 Summary

- This form is the most common type of BCC and is commonly found on the head and neck regions. Lesions clinically manifest as pink or red papules, have a pearly or waxy appearance, and have telangiectasias.
- Under microscopic examination, nodular/noduloulcerative BCCs are composed of well-defined, smooth-bordered basophilic staining islands of neoplastic cells. Under higher power, the cells have large homogenous, oval, elongated nuclei with scant cytoplasm. The BCC cells have a high nuclear-to-cytoplasmic ratio and lack well-formed intercellular bridges.
- This subtype of BCC is indolent in growth; however, if left untreated for enough time, this tumor can invade critical structures of the head and neck and increase morbidity.

The most common form of BCC is the nodular/noduloulcerative type. These are most frequently found on the head and neck, and account for 62 to 70% of all BCCs.[58]

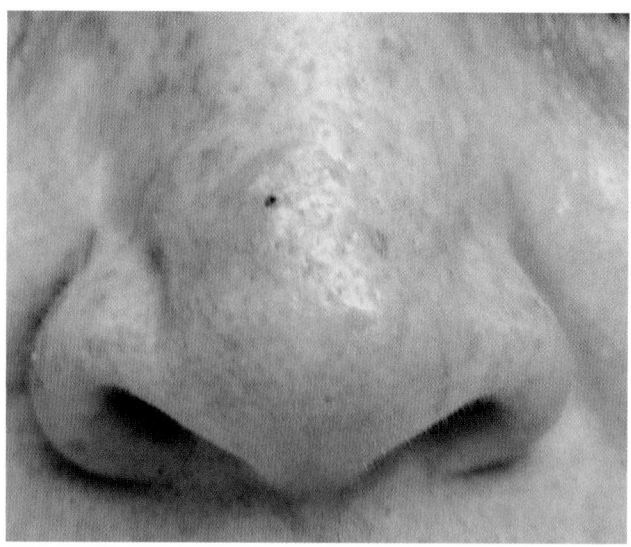
▲ **FIGURE 6-1** Early BCC papule on the nose.

Clinical Presentation

They usually appear as red or pink papules with raised, rolled borders that slowly enlarge (Fig. 6-1). Typically, they are described as having a *pearly, waxy,* or translucent appearance. Telangiectasias are prominent features on the surface of the tumor that can sometimes present with bleeding (Fig. 6-2). Noduloulcerative BCCs have indurated edges and central painless ulcerations that are covered with crust: "rodent ulcers."

Dermatopathology

Under the microscope with scanning magnification, nodular/noduloulcerative BCC is composed of well-defined, smooth-bordered basophilic staining islands of neoplastic cells. BCC islands classically stain much more basophilic than do overlying normal epidermis and normal hair follicle epithelium in H&E-stained sections. These neoplastic islands are made of basaloid cells that show pronounced peripheral palisading of nuclei. Retraction artifacts due to stromal shrinkage in the form of clefts around the tumor islands is a frequent finding[59,60] (Fig. 6-3). BCCs may arise from normal epidermis, pilosebaceous units, or in conjunction with them (Fig. 6-4). BCC is usually characterized by surrounding stroma with a high content of mucin (Fig. 6-5). Inflammatory response in varying degree usually presents in the surrounding stroma too.

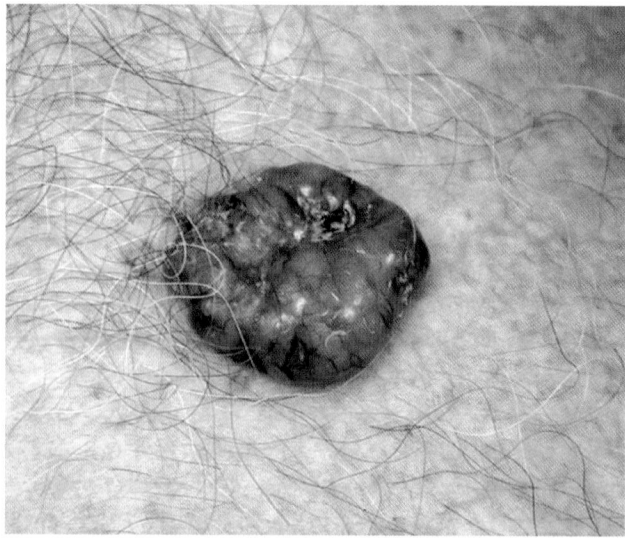
▲ **FIGURE 6-2** Typical nodular BCC with rolled borders decorated with prominent telangiectasia.

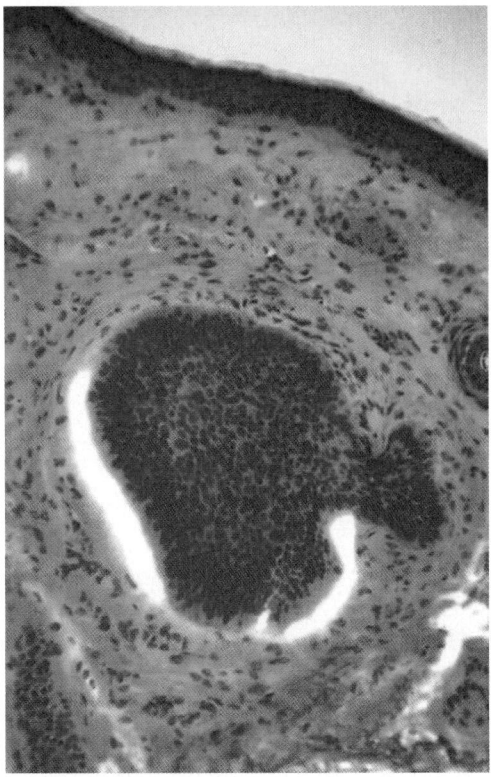

▲ **FIGURE 6-3** Early nodular BCC H&E basophilic nodular BCC tumor island with prominent clefting.

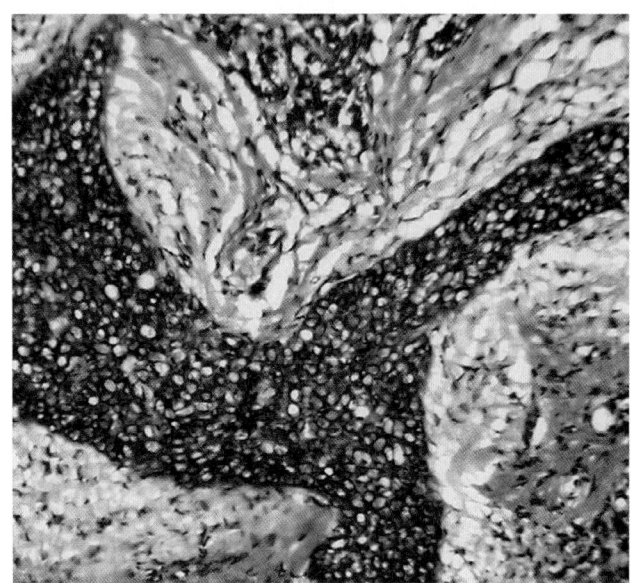

▲ **FIGURE 6-5** BCC with peri tumoral mucinous fibrosis.

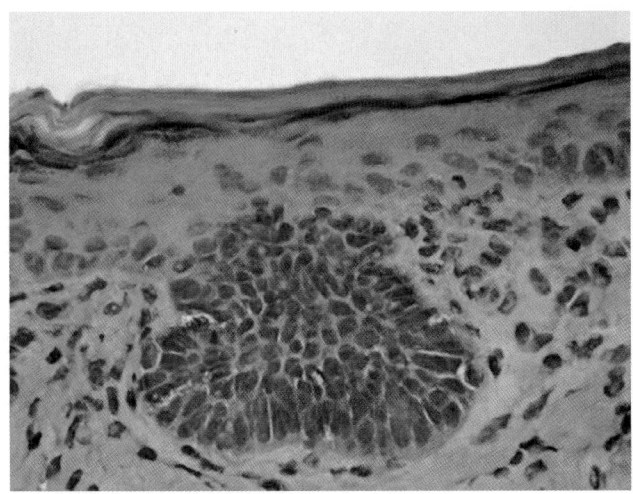

▲ **FIGURE 6-4** BCC arising from surface epidermis H&E.

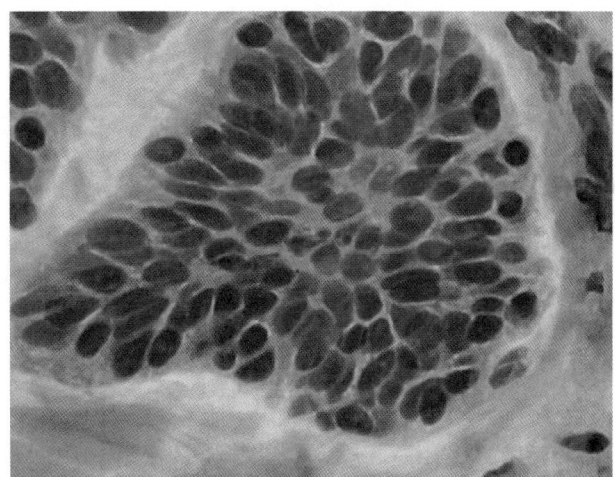

▲ **FIGURE 6-6** BCC with peripheral palisading of the nuclei, basophilic staining neoplastic cells have a high nuclear ratio and show pleomorphism.

In higher magnification, BCC cells have large homogenous, oval, elongated nuclei with scant cytoplasm. These cells have a high nuclear-to-cytoplasmic ratio and are devoid of well-formed intercellular bridges (Fig. 6-6). Even though they are malignant, it is rare for BCC cells to demonstrate atypical mitoses.[61] Necrotic cells and necrosis *en masse* are frequent findings in BCC islands, which the latter reflects itself as ulceration clinically (Fig. 6-7). BCC may show sebaceous, eccrine, apocrine, ductal, glandular, matrical, tricholemmal, squamous, myoepithelial, neuroendocrine, and combined mixed (folliculosebaceous, apocrine/eccrine) differentiations[62] (Figs. 6-8 to 6-11).

Prognosis

Most nodular BCCs grow at a slow rate and have only limited growth; however, they can invade local structures and cause significant damage. The longer they are allowed to grow, the greater the potential for morbidity and destruction. For example, on the face, nodular BCCs can invade the nose or eyes to an extent that these structures need to be removed to eradicate the tumor.

PIGMENTED BASAL CELL CARCINOMA

BOX 6-6   Summary

- This form of BCC consists of a brown, black, or gray blue color that can present on the head, neck, trunk, and/or extremities.

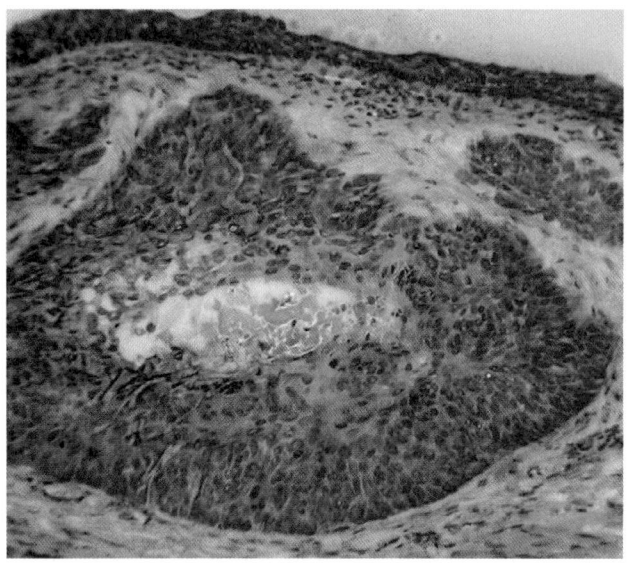

▲ **FIGURE 6-7** BCC on the eyelid with necrosis *en mass*.

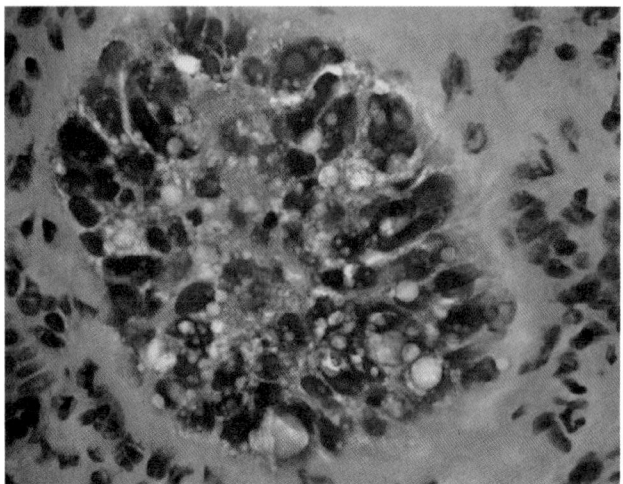

▲ **FIGURE 6-8** BCC with prominent sebaceous differentiation.

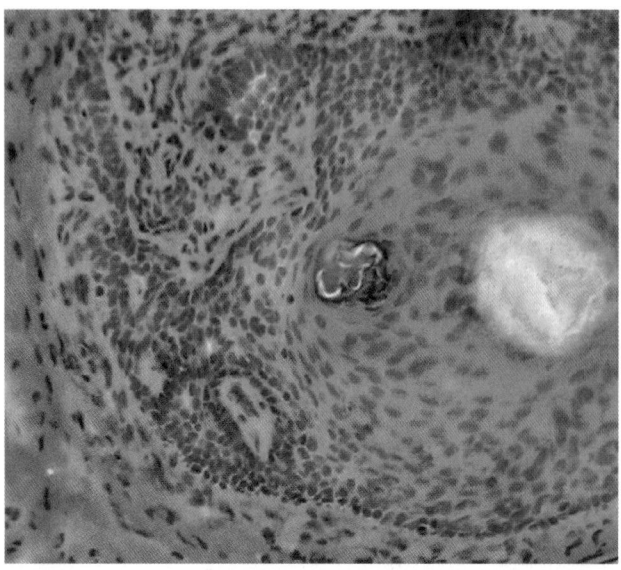

▲ **FIGURE 6-9** BCC with squamous differentiation.

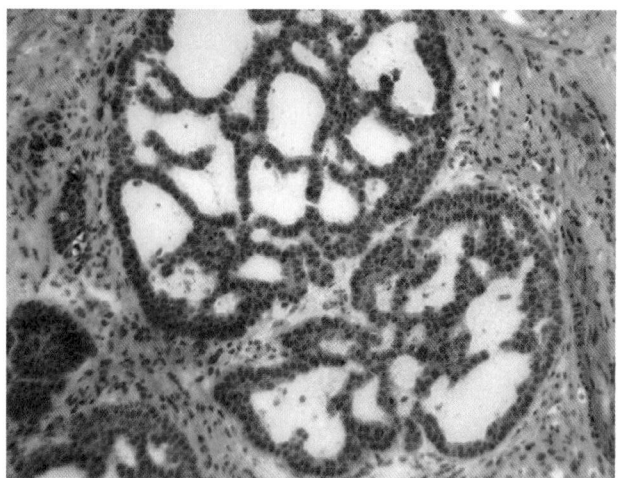

▲ **FIGURE 6-10** BCC with glandular differentiation.

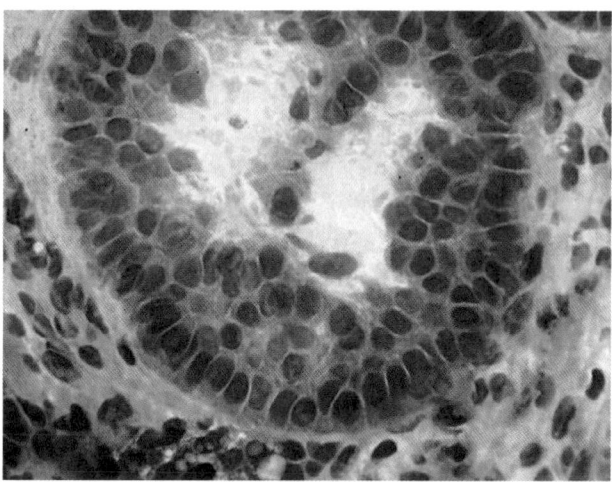

▲ **FIGURE 6-11** BCC with apocrine glandular differentiation.

- Pigmented BCCs can belong to either the nodular/noduloulcerative/micronodular subtype or the superficial multicentric subtype.
- Keep in mind the important differential diagnoses for this type of BCC: pigmented nevi, melanoma, pigmented seborrheic keratosis, and pigmented Bowen's disease.

These BCCs are characterized with brown, black, or grayish blue pigmentation and constitute approximately 6% of all BCCs.

Clinical Presentation

Pigmented BCCs can occur in either nodular/noduloulcerative/micronodular or superficial multicentric clinical types with additional prominent pigmented components (Figs. 6-12 and 6-13). Nodular/noduloulcerative forms frequently are located in the head and neck, whereas the superficial multicentric type can occur often on the trunk and extremities as well. Depending upon the amount and location of melanin present in these lesions, clinical presentation

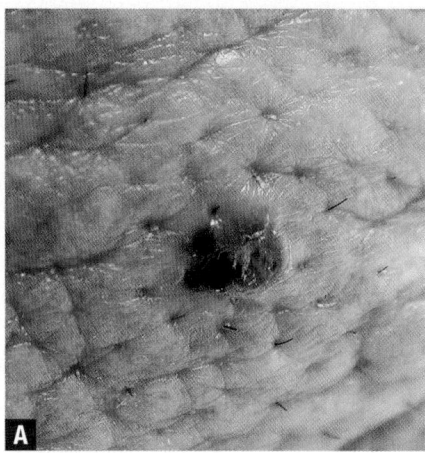
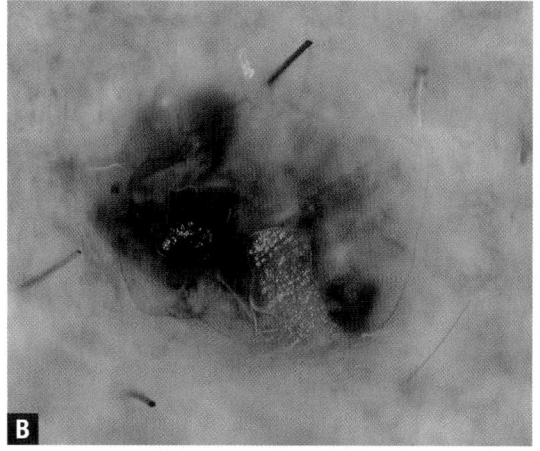

▲ FIGURE 6-12 **A.** Nodular BCC with prominent melanin pigmentation. **B.** Dermoscopic view of the pigmented nodular BCC.

vary but mostly manifest itself as a pigmented lesion of the skin. Pigmented nevi, melanoma, pigmented seborrheic keratosis, and pigmented Bowen's disease are the most frequent clinical differential diagnoses for such lesions.

Dermoscopy is very helpful in clinical assessment of pigmented BCCs. These lesions are reported to be more often adequately excised with tumor-free margins possibly due to more prominent clinically visible margins secondary to the pigmentation.[63]

SUPERFICIAL MULTIFOCAL BASAL CELL CARCINOMA

BOX 6-7   Summary

- This subtype of BCC is the second most common and presents more often on the trunk and extremities. Clinically, lesions present as flat, red to pink, scaly patches with ulcerations and/or crusting.
- Under microscopic examination, these BCCs have a single or multiple basophilic staining tumor sheets or buds extending

from the lower part of the epidermis into the papillary dermis.
- These tumors tend to grow laterally and can cause significant damage to local tissue and structures, if not treated.

The second most common form, occurring with a frequency of 9 to 17.5% of all BCCs, is the superficial type.[58] These lesions are found more on the trunk and extremities compared to nodular BCCs, which are found more often on the face. And patients with superficial BCCs usually present at a younger age than those with nodular types (average age 57.5 vs. 65.5 years, respectively).[11]

Clinical Presentation

Superficial multifocal BCCs can appear as flat or slightly raised red to pink, scaly,

eczematous patches that can have superficial ulcerations or crusting (Fig. 6-14). The borders can be slightly elevated or rolled. Superficial BCCs can be mistaken for nummular eczema, psoriasis, or Bowen's disease (SCC *in situ*).[64] This subtype can also present as a pigmented variant with a central brown to black pigmentation from the presence of melanin within the lesion. They initially grow laterally, and can reach substantial sizes. Horizontal growth allows these tumors to extend significantly beyond the clinical borders. As with all BCCs, these lesions are likely to invade local tissues and structures the longer they remain untreated.

Dermatopathology

Superficial multifocal BCCs have a single or multiple basophilic staining tumor sheets or buds extending from the lower

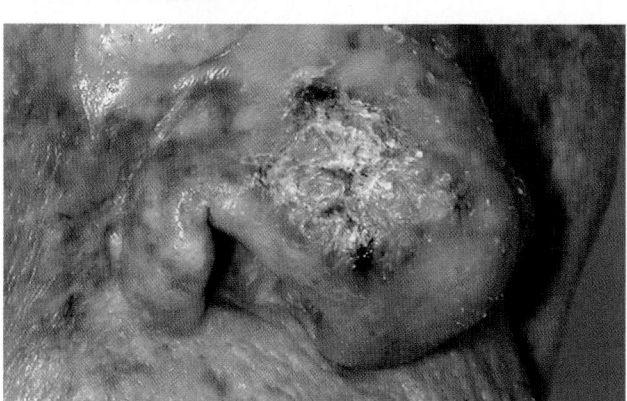

▲ FIGURE 6-13 Pigmented, recurrent infiltrative BCC on the nose.

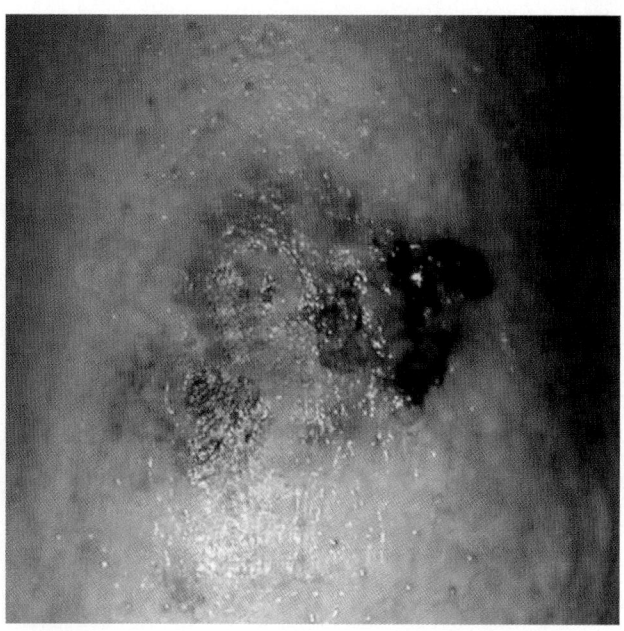

▲ FIGURE 6-14 Pigmented superficial multicentric BCC.

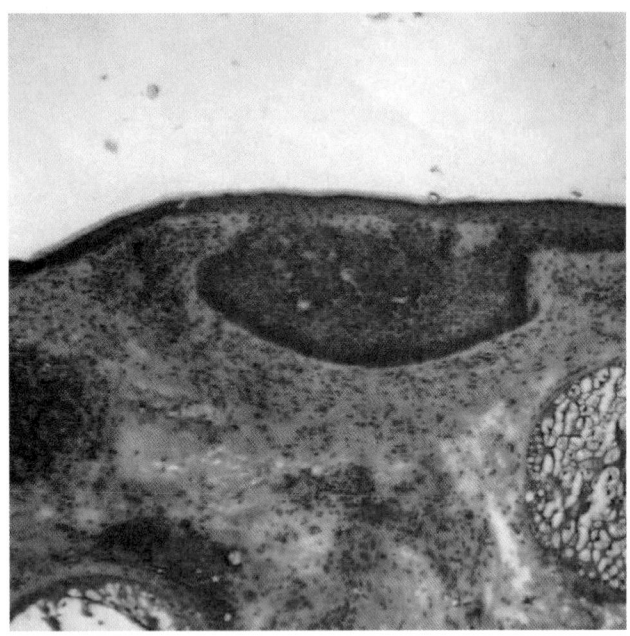

▲ **FIGURE 6-15** Superficial multifocal BCC H&E.

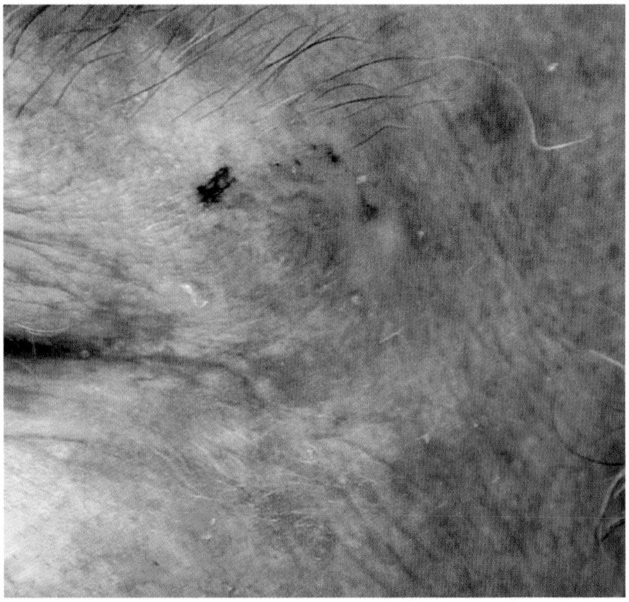

▲ **FIGURE 6-16** Morpheaform BCC.

part of the epidermis into the papillary (superficial) dermis with pronounced peripheral palisading and spaces of stromal retraction around the neoplastic islands (Fig. 6-15). Superficial BCCs usually do not extend into the deep dermis, and a nonspecific inflammatory infiltrate may be seen in the papillary dermis.[59–61] Although superficially located, this particular type of BCC needs special attention in diagnosis and treatment, as most of the time the neoplastic islands are discohesive and can be separated by large pieces of normal tissue.

MORPHEAFORM (SCLEROSING OR FIBROSING) BASAL CELL CARCINOMA

BOX 6-8   Summary

- This subtype is not as common and is found on the head and neck region. Morpheaform is also known to be an aggressive type of BCC that is more likely to recur, approximately 60%.
- Morpheaform BCCs present as skin-colored, pink, or white plaques, and may appear as a smooth shiny scar.
- Under the microscope, there is a fibrotic dermis that contains small, linear, and branching collections of tumor cells. It has BCC islands that are not well circumscribed and do not have prominent peripheral palisading of nuclei. Histopathologically, morpheaform BCC cells can reach deep into the dermis.
- Mohs' micrographic surgery is the treatment of choice.

This subtype occurs much less often than do the previous forms, with a frequency of about 2 to 3% of all BCCs diagnosed. They occur mainly on the head and neck.[58,65] Morpheaform BCCs represent a more aggressive tumor that has a greater tendency to recur. Aggressive behavior in skin cancers has been highly associated with *p53* expression, whereas Bcl-2 was associated with nonaggressive behavior.[66]

Clinical Presentation

Morpheaform BCC presents clinically as a skin-colored, pink, or white indurated plaque with poorly defined borders. The overall appearance is somewhat shiny and looks like a smooth, firm scar (Fig. 6-16). These lesions are reported to be more frequent on the face in women and may be associated with smoking.[67] The

underlying tumor may grow quite extensively before the overlying skin begins to ulcerate. Unfortunately, these lesions are often misdiagnosed, leading to greater tumor growth and delayed treatment. The tumor's extension is often underestimated, leading to incomplete excision.

Dermatopathology

Morpheaform BCCs are composed of numerous small cords or clusters of basaloid cells embedded in a dense fibrotic stroma.[58] The characteristic fibrotic dermis contains small, linear, and branching collections of tumor cells. Unlike the nodular type, morpheaform BCC islands typically are not well circumscribed and do not demonstrate prominent peripheral palisading of nuclei. Morpheaform BCC cells can reach far deeper into the dermis (Fig. 6-17). The lesions can be

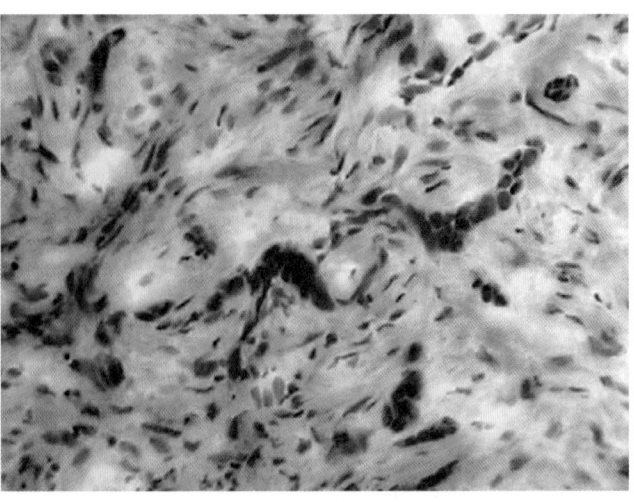

▲ **FIGURE 6-17** Morpheaform BCC H&E high.

mistaken for other desmoplastic neoplasms such as microcystic adnexal carcinoma and metastatic carcinoma, especially from the breast.[60,61]

Prognosis

Even though the overall risk is still low, morpheaform BCCs have a greater tendency to be more aggressive and invade into deep layers of the skin more often than do the former subtypes. Recurrence has been reported up to 60% due to frequent microscopic extension beyond the clinical borders.[59] Since morpheaform BCCs have a higher rate of recurrence and metastasis, Mohs' micrographic surgery (MMS) is the treatment of choice. In general, the larger the tumor size, the greater the subclinical extension and the greater the chance of recurrence.

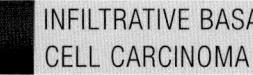
INFILTRATIVE BASAL CELL CARCINOMA

BOX 6-9   Summary

- Infiltrative BCCs present with an opaque whitish yellow color and blend in with surrounding normal skin.
- BCCs found on embryonic fusion lines are more likely to be the infiltrative subtype.
- Histopathologically, infiltrative BCCs present itself with basophilic staining, and elongated islands and strands of basaloid neoplastic cells with jagged or spiky borders. Usually, the deep or peripheral portions of these neoplasms exhibit more of an infiltrative pattern with no prominent fibrosis in the stroma.
- Mohs' micrographic surgery (MMS) is indicated for these types of tumors and long-term follow-up must be instituted for these patients.

The infiltrative form of BCC is a more aggressive subtype than are some others, and is more likely to recur. The infiltrative subtype can occur solely or more frequently be a component of a mixed-type BCC.

Clinical Presentation

Solely infiltrative BCCs have an opaque whitish yellow color. They do not have a sharp or rolled border; and blend with the normal surrounding skin.[68] When present as a component of a mixed-type BCC such as nodular, the clinical picture carries both characteristic findings. BCCs on the embryonic fusion lines are reported to be more infiltrative type.

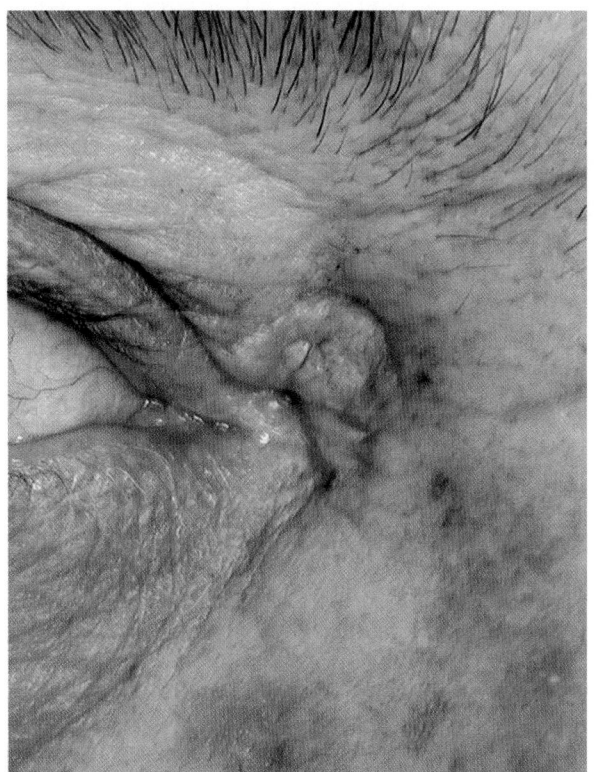
▲ **FIGURE 6-18** Infiltrative BCC on inner canthus.

Overall, this type of BCC clinically has less well-defined borders than do nodular types (Fig. 6-18).

Dermatopathology

In scanning magnification, histopathologically infiltrative BCCs present itself with basophilic staining and elongated islands and strands of basaloid neoplastic cells with jagged or spiky borders. As the neoplastic islands are no longer round or oval, peripheral palisading is also no longer an impressive finding (Fig. 6-19). The neoplastic islands may vary in size and shape, and are also frequently associated with more nodular, micronodular, or other histological patterns. Generally, the deep or peripheral portions of such neoplasms exhibit more of an infiltrative pattern with no prominent fibrosis in the stroma. This latter finding differentiates infiltrative BCC from morpheaform BCC in which fibrosis in the stroma is an important finding. The surrounding stroma may contain increased acid mucopolysaccharides.[68] The tumor cells show little cellular differentiation.[69] Predominant or not, infiltrative growth pattern have to be mentioned in the histopathology report when observed, as implies the high recurrent rate.

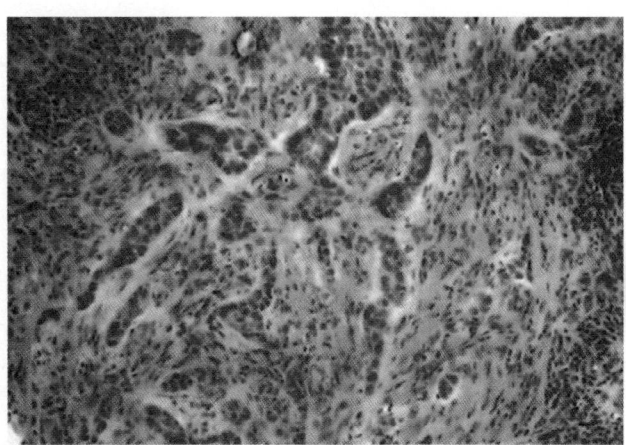
▲ **FIGURE 6-19** Infiltrative BCC among lymphocytes and coarse collagen bundles.

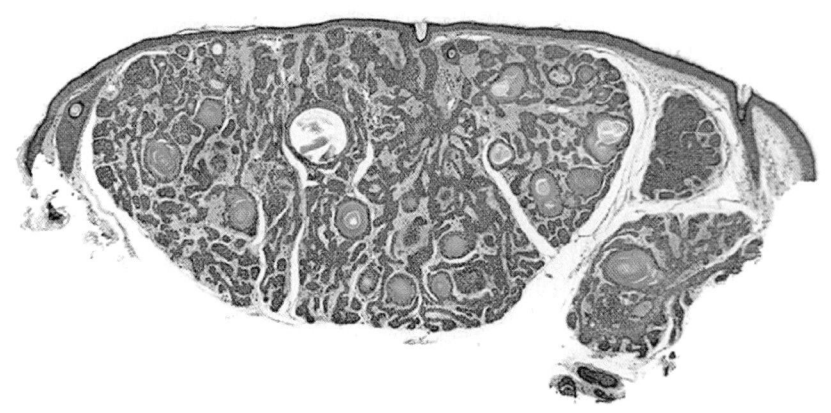

▲ **FIGURE 6-20** Infundibulocystic BCC H&E.

Prognosis

Infiltrative subtypes tend to show more aggressive behavior than do most of the BCC forms. Also, these tumors have a greater propensity to recur. Following surgical excision, infiltrative BCCs are more likely to have positive margins compared to nodular BCCs. In addition to their infiltrative nature, these neoplasms are usually much larger than they appear clinically. Mohs' micrographic surgery (MMS) is indicated for infiltrative BCCs. Patients should be followed for long-term to gauge any recurrence.[68,69]

INFUNDIBULOCYSTIC BASAL CELL CARCINOMA

BOX 6-10   Summary

- This subtype was recently categorized as a genuine subtype of BCC and presents as a small, shiny, flesh-colored papule on the head, neck, trunk, and/or extremities. Clinically, this tumor can resemble skin tags.
- Histopathologically, infundibulocystic BCCs have a distinctive combination of follicular differentiation that includes follicular germs and infundibula. With H&E staining, cords and strands of palisading basaloid cells can be demonstrated with scattered infundibular cysts.
- Indolent growth is characteristic of this subtype of BCC; either Mohs' micrographic surgery or nonsurgical treatments are options for therapy.

Infundibulocystic BCC was justified as a true variant of BCC in 1990.[70] Since then, it has been quite recognized as its own distinct entity and correct identification of this lesion can lead to appropriate treatment and management.

Clinical Presentation

Infundibulocystic BCCs present as small to minute shiny flesh-colored papules on the head, neck, trunk, and extremities of individuals. Ages can vary from adolescents to elderly individuals. In addition, these neoplasms are very slow-growing and may resemble "skin tags."[71]

Dermatopathology

It has been reported in the literature that infundibulocystic BCCs have a unique combination of follicular differentiation that includes follicular germs and infundibula.[70] Under scanning magnification with H&E staining, infundibulocystic BCC demonstrates cords and strands of palisading basaloid cells with few scattered infundibular cysts. Hyperchromasia and rare mitoses may also exist[71] (Fig. 6-20).

Prognosis

Infundibulocystic BCCs grow at a slow pace and are recognized to be a less ag-

gressive subtype.[70] Treatments such as MMS and nonsurgical management may be successfully used for such neoplasms.[71]

GIANT BASAL CELL CARCINOMA

BOX 6-11   Summary

- This subtype of BCC is characterized by its clinical size, diameter of at least 5 cm.
- Tumors appear on the trunk and also have a more aggressive nature.
- Preferred treatment is surgical; however, because of the sheer size, postoperative morbidity needs to be discussed with the patient.

Giant BCCs are defined as tumors of at least 5 cm as their greatest diameter[72] (Fig. 6-21) and they only make up about 1% of all BCCs.[73] These tumors typically appear on the trunk, and display an aggressive behavior, resulting in an increased risk of local recurrence and metastasis.[74,75] Some of these large tumors are merely the result of neglect,[76] but others can represent recurrent skin cancers.[73] Nonsurgical modalities are relatively ineffective for giant BCCs. However, the surgical operation for an aggressive giant skin cancer may leave the patient with functional loss, major deformity, and serious postoperative complications.[72]

CONTROVERSIAL ENTITIES

Basosquamous (Metatypical) Carcinoma

BOX 6-12   Summary

- This type of carcinoma has both histopathological features of BCC and

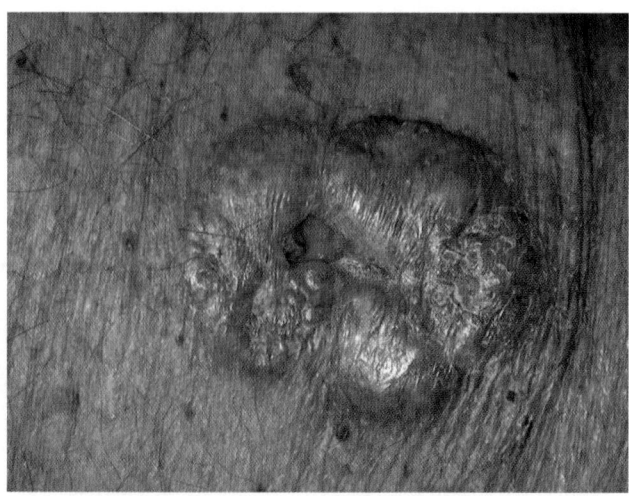

▲ **FIGURE 6-21** Giant BCC on the back, lesion size 5.5 × 4 cm.

SCC; however, it must be noted that this is a controversial category.

- BSC may be even more aggressive than SCC, leading to a higher prevalence of metastasis.
- Clinical presentation can vary from papules to ulcerating tumors and can be found on the head and neck regions.
- Histopathologically, BSC has three components: (1) basaloid components exhibit the features of BCC; (2) cribriform or adenoid growth pattern may be present in this part of the neoplasm as well as Ber EP4 positivity; (3) squamous components show SCC-like features, this part of the neoplasm is expected to be EMA-positive.
- BSCs are likely to recur, have lymph node metastasis, and distant metastasis.
- Mohs' micrographic surgery is indicated for these types of tumors and long-term follow-up must be instituted for these patients to assess for recurrence.

Basosquamous carcinoma (BSC) is reported to constitute approximately 0.4 to 12% of all BCCs.[77,78] It has also been called basaloid squamous carcinoma, basaloid SCC, and metatypical BCC. Controversy exists as to whether or not this is a unique entity and a form of SCC, or if it is merely a collision of two cancers (BCC and SCC).[79] The term BSC should be used only to define lesions that bear both typical histopathological features of BCC and SCC in conjunction with a transitional zone. BCC with keratinization or the cases of simultaneous BCC and SCC on the same site but as two separate neoplasms should not be included into this already not well-defined category.

BSC is reported to have a higher prevalence of metastasis,[80] even higher than SCCs. In this regard, biological behavior of BSC is much more similar if not more aggressive to SCC rather than to BCC.

True basosquamous/metatypical features in skin neoplasms should be seen as an alarming finding and these lesions are best treated and followed up as carefully as SCCs, in terms of the risk of deep invasion, recurrence, and metastasis.

CLINICAL PRESENTATION These rare tumors occur mostly on the face, neck, and ears.[78,80] The clinical presentation vary in between flat to slightly raised lesions red papules to large ulcerated tumors[80] (Fig. 6-22).

DERMATOPATHOLOGY True BSC has three major components: basaloid components exhibit the features of BCC with basaloid, dark staining, well-circumscribed tumor blends that show peripheral palisading and peritumoral clefting. Cribriform or adenoid growth pattern may be present in this part of the neoplasm, as well as Ber EP4 positivity. Squamous components show SCC-like features with larger, lighter stained cells with a tendency to keratinize consistently with epidermal involvement. This part of the neoplasm is expected to be EMA positive. The intermediate component is the transition zone in between two polar differentiation attempts where the neoplastic cells have neither typical features of BCC nor of SCC but rather in between. Typical strong Ber EP4 or EMA immunostainings diminish in this area. There are cases also associated with undifferentiated spindle cell tumor components that have been reported in the literature[61,77,81–86] (Fig. 6-23).

PROGNOSIS These tumors have a markedly higher risk for metastases than do BCCs or SCCs alone. BSCs have a propensity for recurrence, lymph node, and distant metastasis,[78,87] with a metastasis rate reported at 7.4%.[80] Sentinel lymph node biopsies should be considered for high-risk BSCs that are larger than 2 cm and those with perineural and lymphatic invasion. Predictors of tumor recurrence include male sex, positive surgical margins, lymphatic invasion, and perineural invasion. MMS is appropriate for these tumors and it is important to maintain long-term follow-up to assess for neoplastic recurrence or metastasis.

Micronodular Basal Cell Carcinoma

BOX 6-13   Summary

- Micronodular BCCs have a deeper and more subclinical presentation, and therefore, are much larger than they clinically present as.
- Histopathologically, these BCCs have a pattern that consists of round tumor islands less than 0.15 mm in diameter nodules. Also neoplastic islands are present that tend to be round and well circumscribed with peripheral palisading. Retraction spaces may not be as prominent.
- Mohs' micrographic surgery is the treatment modality of choice.

In 1996, the micronodular subtype was reported as a histopathological BCC form that was more difficult to cure than were nodular BCCs, since it was more likely to have positive surgical margins following excision. Micronodular BCC is a histopathological description rather than a distinctive clinical form. Micronodular BCCs may comprise 15% of all BCCs,[88,89] yet micronodular pattern can also be a component of mixed-type BCC. Micronodular BCCs may have deeper and more subclinical extension

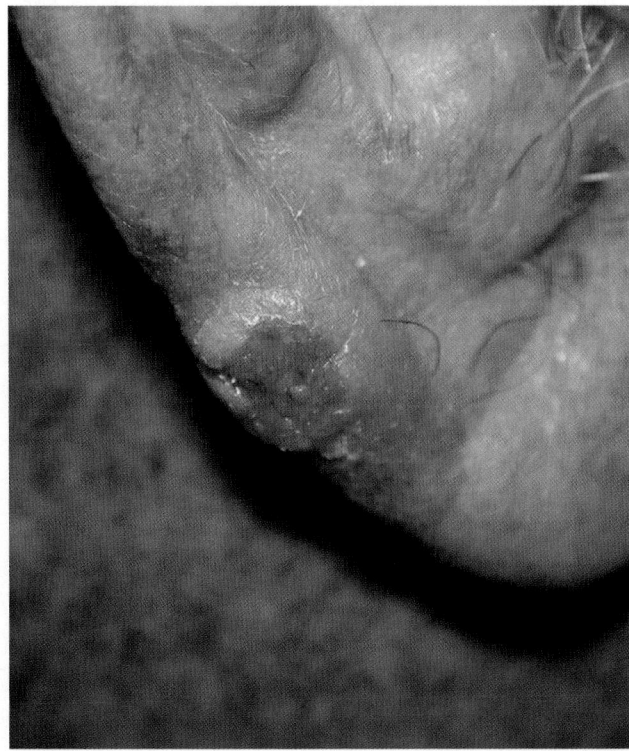

▲ **FIGURE 6-22** Basosquamous carcinoma on the ear helix.

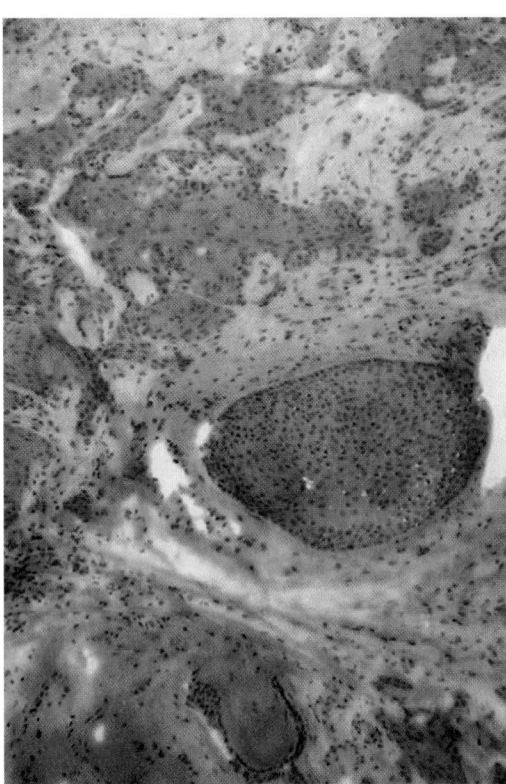

▲ **FIGURE 6-23** Basosquamous Carcinoma H&E.

than do nodular BCCs; therefore, micronodular BCCs are much larger than they appear. Some authors believe that this subtype should deserve the same consideration as the morpheaform and infiltrative forms of BCC.[89]

DERMATOPATHOLOGY Micronodular histopathologic pattern is consistent with round tumor islands less than 0.15 mm in diameter nodules similar to, but smaller than, those in nodular BCC. The neoplastic islands tends to be round, well-circumscribed with peripheral palisading. Retraction spaces may not be as prominent as in nodular BCC. It is not rare to observe two or more types of BCC within one lesion.

PROGNOSIS This type of BCC is reported to be a more difficult form to treat and more prone to recurrence because it tends to stretch beyond its visible clinical borders. The treatment of choice is MMS, because of its ill-defined borders and widespread subclinical extension.[89]

Field Fire Basal Cell Carcinoma

BOX 6-14 Summary

- This type of BCC is a variant of the noduloulcerative subtype and presents as multiple, scarred, crusting, and ulcerating tumors in a single area.

- Lesions extend laterally and can grow to large sizes.
- Incomplete treatment after electrodessication and curettage can lead to scarring and recurrence.

Considered a variant of the nodulo-ulcerative type, the "field-fire" BCC presents with multiple tumors in a single area. They appear as a combination of scarring, crusting, and ulceration. These lesions tend to spread laterally and can grow to significant sizes.[90] This clinical presentation can also be associated with previous and uncompleted treatments of BCCs with modalities such as electrodessication and curettage, which lead both to scarring and discohesive recurrence.

Fibroepithelioma of Pinkus (FEP)

BOX 6-15 Summary

- These tumors are described as skin-colored, red to pink, smooth, pedunculated nodules on the trunk or extremities.
- Histopathologically, fibroepitheliomas have strands of basophilic tumor cells joining together in a fibrous, edematous stroma reaching from the epidermis into the deep dermis.
- Fibroepithelioma of Pinkus has also been categorized as a fenestrated trichoblastoma rather than as a type of BCC.

CLINICAL PRESENTATION Described by Pinkus in 1953,[91] these lesions are commonly located on the trunk and extremities; fibroepitheliomas can be mistaken for fibromas clinically. They appear as skin-colored red to pink, smooth, pedunculated nodules that are somewhat firm on palpation. FEP is reported to be more common in females and not frequently associated with sun damage.

DERMATOPATHOLOGY Fibroepitheliomas have strands of basophilic tumor cells joining together in a fibrous, edematous stroma reaching from the epidermis into the deep dermis. Hints of follicular bulb and dermal papilla formations can be observed. Bowen et al redefined FEP as a fenestrated trichoblastoma rather than a type of BCC.[60,92,93]

 GENODERMATOSES ASSOCIATED WITH BCC

Nevoid Basal Cell Carcinoma Syndrome (NBCCS)

BOX 6-16 Summary

- NBCCS is an autosomal dominant disorder and is characterized by (1) numerous BCCs at an early age, (2) odontogenic cysts, (3) skeletal abnormalities, (4) ectopic calcification, and (5) palmar/planta pits.
- NBCCS is caused by a mutated *Patched* gene on chromosome 9.
- The most frequent locations for BCCs are on the face, back, and chest. On the face, the BCCs appear around the eyes, on the eyelids, nose, and upper lip.

The nevoid basal cell carcinoma syndrome (NBCCS), also known as basal cell nevus syndrome, Gorlin–Goltz syndrome, and Gorlin's syndrome, is an autosomal dominant disorder with complete penetrance and variable expression characterized by numerous BCCs. The mutated *Patched* gene is a tumor-suppressor gene found on chromosome 9q22.3. Most are rearrangements that result in the truncation of the *Patched1* (*PTCH1*) protein. Approximately 30% of NBCCS also have mutations in *p53*.[94]

Five features are characteristic of NBCCS[95]:

1. numerous, usually aggressive, BCCs that appear at an early age,
2. jaw (odontogenic) cysts,
3. skeletal abnormalities including the ribs, spine, and skull,
4. ectopic calcification,
5. palmar and plantar pits.

About 0.4% of all BCCs are NBCCS[96] and 2% of patients under 45 years with BCCs have this syndrome.[97] NBCCS is estimated to affect nearly 1 in 60,000 people.[98,99] This condition affects mostly whites, with an equal number of males and females. African Americans typically have many fewer tumors than do Caucasians.[100] The BCCs present in patients between puberty and 35 years, but may occur as early as 2 years of age. The most frequent locations for BCC development are on the face, back, and chest. On the face, the BCCs appear around the eyes, on the eyelids, nose, and upper lip. Milia may be seen among the tumors. The number of tumors may range from only a few to thousands, with sizes from 1 to 10 mm in diameter. Tumor invasion should be suspected when a BCC enlarges or begins to bleed or crust.[94] Only a few cases of NBCCS have been associated with metastasis; however, it can be associated with other tumors. For example, up to 5% of NBCCS may be associated with medulloblastoma. Patients most affected by medulloblastomas with NBCCS are under 5 years of age. Following radiation treatment, BCCs can become activated and turn progressively invasive within the next 10 years.[94]

Histologically, the carcinomas of NBCCS cannot be distinguished from those of BCCs from patients without the syndrome. Pitting can occur on the hands, feet, or both; it occurs in nearly two-thirds of patients with NBCCS. The pits are from an incomplete lack or total lack of a stratum corneum. These pits can measure 1 to 3 mm deep by 2 to 3 mm in diameter, with some confluent pits even greater in size. Under the microscope, one can see basal cell epitheliomas forming in the epidermis under the pit. These pits are asymptomatic and permanent.[95]

Bazex–Dupré–Christol Syndrome

> **BOX 6-17   Summary**
>
> - This disorder has a dominant inheritance and is linked to Xq24–q27.
> - Characteristics of this syndrome are (1) congenital diffuse hypotrichosis, (2) follicular atrophoderma, and (3) basocellular neoformations, including BCCs and basal cell nevi.

Bazex–Dupré–Christol (BDC) syndrome was described by Bazex et al in 1966.[101] This disorder is presumed to have dominant inheritance linked to Xq24–q27.[87]

BDC is characterized by congenital hypotrichosis, follicular atrophoderma, and basocellular neoformations, including BCCs and basal cell nevi.[102] Follicular atrophoderma is usually limited to the face, dorsa of the hands and feet, and extensor surfaces of the knees and elbows.[102] Bazex et al originally described the hypotrichosis as diffuse, involving all body parts with hair but without any specific hair shaft abnormality.[101] However, patients have been described without hypotrichosis.[102] Microscopically, some hairs demonstrate twisting and trichorrhexis nodosa.[103]

Rombo Syndrome

> **BOX 6-18   Summary**
>
> - Rombo syndrome is hypothesized to be autosomal dominant and is characterized by peripheral vasodilation with cyanosis and follicular atrophy in sun-exposed areas. Manifestations tend to appear between the ages of 7 and 10 years.
> - Atrophic skin has a "worm-eaten" appearance termed atrophoderma vermiculatum.
> - Histopathologically, irregular elastin patterns with a lymphocytic infiltrate and vascular proliferation is visualized.
> - Patients with Rombo syndrome have a greater susceptibility to BCCs, which may develop at about 35 years of age.

Having similarities to the BDC syndrome is the Rombo syndrome. Manifestations of this rare syndrome begin at ages around 7 to 10, with redness in a cyanotic distribution as well as follicular atrophy in sun-exposed areas. Telangiectasias and milia-like papules appear later, and atrophic skin becomes more prominent (some have likened this to a "worm-eaten" appearance called atrophoderma vermiculatum). Patients may also present with vellus hair cysts. Under the microscope, the upper dermis of Rombo syndrome skin demonstrates irregular elastin patterns with a lymphocytic infiltrate and vascular proliferation.[104] These patients have a greater susceptibility to BCCs, which may develop at about 35 years of age. The gene for Rombo syndrome has not been mapped yet, but it may have autosomal dominant inheritance.[87,104]

■ TREATMENT

> **BOX 6-19   Summary**
>
> - Surgical excision is one of the most common treatments.

- Excision has a high cure rate for primary BCCs, but has the potential complications of infection and scarring. Excision may require multiple sessions to clear the tumor.
- Curettage and electrodesiccation is another common technique for small (<1 cm), well-demarcated tumors. The C&E cycle is usually performed two to six times; it should not be used for recurrent tumors.
- Cryosurgery lowers the skins temperature to −50 to −60°C; crystals form within the cell and disrupt the cell membrane. It can be used for single or multiple tumors. Cryosurgery is not advised for aggressive BCCs subtypes.
- Radiation therapy is good for medium-sized tumors in patients of age over 60 years. It is also a good option for patients who are not good surgical candidates or do not want a surgical procedure. Remember the risks of chronic radiodermatitis and the potential for more aggressive cancers to arise at the site of previous irradiation.
- Mohs' micrographic surgery has the advantages of microscopic examination of the clinical borders, as well as being a tissue-sparing technique. It can achieve very high cure rates.
- Mohs' micrographic surgery is the treatment of choice for large tumors (>2 cm), aggressive subtypes (such as morpheaform, basosquamous, micronodular, and infiltrative BCCs), and high-risk anatomic locations.
- Laser surgery and photodynamic therapy have not yet been accepted as primary therapies, but they show promising results in the treatment of BCCs.
- Interferon is a costly method that is a viable nonsurgical alternative, but long-term cure rates are still needed. Interferon can have systemic side effects such as flu-like symptoms, which may decrease patient's compliance.
- Imiquimod recently gained Food and Drug Administration's (FDA) approval for the treatment of superficial BCCs. It is an immune response modifier that promotes a cell-mediated response, and induces the production of numerous cytokines.
- 5-Fluorouracil is a topical chemotherapeutic agent used in low-risk BCCs, especially superficial BCCs. Application-site inflammation, irritation, crusting, and swelling may decrease patient's compliance. It can be used both topically and intralesionally.
- Nonsurgical modalities do not allow for histologic tissue examination.
- Chemoprevention, such as with retinoids and cyclooxygenase inhibitors, is still controversial. More research is needed before this becomes an accepted option.

Once a BCC has been diagnosed, it is time to decide among the various therapeutic options available. Since BCCs can grow to large sizes, invade local tissues and structures, and even metastasize, they almost always need to be treated.[105] When choosing among the numerous modalities, several factors should be considered. Tumor size, location, histologic subtype, morphology, and whether the tumor has invaded any local structures influence the method chosen.[106] Physicians also need to consider a patient's age, health condition, and cosmetic expectations before beginning a procedure. Ideally, a treatment should be cost-effective, convenient, and acceptable to the patient.

Surgical Excision

BOX 6-20 Summary

- Surgical excision is a primary treatment option for NMSC.
- Margins are generally 3 to 6 mm for small and well-delineated BCCs; however, large tumors, clinical extension, rate of growth, and local structures involved need to be considered to merit larger excision margins.
- Surgical defects are repaired with primary closure, flaps, grafts, or are left to heal by secondary intention.
- Surgical excision cure rates range from 90 to 98%.

Surgical excision is one of the primary treatment modalities for NMSC. This option is most appropriate for well-delineated tumors located in less cosmetically sensitive areas such as the extremities. Conventional excision is the method of choice for most physicians when the lesion is less than 2 cm in diameter, is located in a lower risk area such as the trunk or extremities, and is a low-risk subtype such as a nodular or superficial form. The margins required for surgical removal are on the order of 3 to 6 mm for small, well-demarcated BCCs.[64,107–109] However, this is not a universal rule, as larger tumors, degree of clinical spread, rate of growth, and amount of adjacent skin penetrated may warrant wider margins. Recurrent tumors and those with more aggressive subtypes (i.e., morpheaform, infiltrative, basosquamous, and micronodular) may extend beyond the clinical margins, and therefore, may also require greater surgical margins. Some suggest taking 5 to 10 mm margins for recurrent BCCs.[109]

The overall goal of conventional excision is to resect the entire tumor until histologic margins show no residual neo-plastic cells at the surgical borders. Surgical defects are repaired with primary closure, flaps, or grafts, or are left to heal by secondary intention. Excision can produce good cosmetic results. Excisional wounds tend to heal more quickly than do those after curettage and electrodesiccation or cryosurgery.[64,110] A further benefit of surgery is the ability to evaluate a lesion histologically (either by frozen or embedded sections) to determine the tumor's subtype and if further treatment is necessary.[111] Potential drawbacks to conventional surgery include possible infection, scarring, longer procedural time than those of some nonsurgical methods, and more normal tissue removed than with MMS. If margins are still positive after the first surgery, treatment may require multiple sessions.[107]

A recent study showed that clinicians might leave positive margins in nearly 16% of patients. Of those still positive, half did not receive any further treatment, which only led to a 3.2% recurrence over 3.6 years. This gives further support to those who believe in a "wait and see" policy.[112]

Studies have shown surgical excision to have a very respectable cure rate, typically from 90 to 98%.[113–115] Overall, in the short term (<5 years), only about 2.8% of primary BCCs recurred after surgical removal. This gives a clearance rate of 97.2%. For the patient, long-term cure rates are most important. At 5 years, clearance rates between 89.9 and 95.2% have been achieved for primary lesions.[32,116] Proper curettage to better define the BCC's borders prior to excision may increase the cure rate for primary lesions.[109]

Previously treated tumors tend to be more difficult to treat. Therefore, there was a higher rate of recurrence found in this group with 11.6% at 5-year follow-up.[116] The same study also found that there was a trend toward greater recurrence in men and in aged people. Recurrences at various anatomic sites were compared. BCCs occurring on the head (including the scalp, eyes, periocular area, nose, perinasal area, etc.) had a much higher predilection to recur (6.6%) compared to all other bodily areas such as the neck, trunk, and extremities (0.7%). An evaluation of BCCs on the head revealed a trend toward increasing recurrence rates with increasing BCC diameter.[116]

A prospective study compared surgical excision with radiotherapy. After 4 years, the surgical group had only 0.7% recurrence, compared to 7.5% with radiotherapy. This is a high cure rate for excision, and is closer to those reported for MMS. Four years after completing therapy, patients who underwent conventional excision rated their cosmetic outcome higher than those who had radiation.[111]

Curettage and Electrodessication

BOX 6-21 Summary

- Curettage and electrodesiccation (C&E) is one of the most commonly used treatment modalities for the removal of BCCs.
- It is appropriate to use this treatment option for small well-demarcated cutaneous tumors. However, this modality is not usually recommended for large-diameter BCCs, aggressive subtypes, or BCC involving high-risk anatomic areas because of the high recurrence rates in these types of situations.
- A C&E wound does not usually require sutures; wounds generally have a satisfactory cosmetic result.

Compared to normal skin, there are significantly fewer desmosomes present in BCC cells. These components are important in mediating cell–cell attachment.[117,118] In addition, BCCs have fewer connections to the basement membrane. Hemidesmosomes occupy nearly 45% of the normal basal cell layer, but in BCCs they account only for 7%.[119] Therefore, these features allow a curet to separate cancerous cells from the normal surrounding cells in the skin.

Curettage refers to the use of a curet, which has both a blunt and a sharp side for separating and cutting the tumor from the skin. *Electrodesiccation* refers to the use of electrocautery, in which a high-frequency electrical current is directly applied to the tissue. The current obtains hemostasis and may destroy some tumor cells. This modality should be used with caution in patients with pacemakers or implantable cardioverter defibrillators.[120]

The tissue is locally infiltrated with anesthetic prior to the procedure. A sharp curet is essential to properly cut and debulk the tumor. Smaller curets may be used during the initial debulking. The patient's skin should be held taut, to stabilize and hold the operating field firm. During the curetting, the physician should feel a difference between tumor and normal skin. BCCs typically feel soft and easily breakable, but the dermis will feel coarse and more difficult to scrape. The curet begins in the center of the tumor and is scraped in several directions, continuing throughout the field until the entire area has a gritty feel. Electrocautery is then applied to the entire curetted area. This cycle is typically repeated two to six times in a single visit.[120]

Curettage and electrodesiccation (C&E) is one of the most commonly used treatments for BCCs.[121] It is typically utilized for small (<1 cm), well-delineated cutaneous tumors. This modality may not be appropriate for BCCs with large diameters, aggressive subtypes, or in high-risk anatomic areas such as the mid-face, because of the increased rate of residual tumor and high recurrence rates in these locations.[122] Also, delicate locations such as the eyelid may not be as amenable to C&E.[120] C&E does not provide adequate tissue for a histologic examination to ensure that margins are tumor-free.[110] Recurrent tumors are not very amenable to C&E, because they are trapped in fibrous tissue. Without the contrast in texture between normal and cancerous cells, curettage of recurrent tumors is difficult.[123]

C&E is an easy technique to learn; it is cost-effective and convenient.[122] It can be done rapidly in an outpatient setting and requires only minimal equipment. Also, the C&E wound does not usually disrupt the structure of the underlying dermis or require sutures. Only an experienced physician should perform C&E, as clearance and recurrence rates can vary greatly based on ability.[124] Recurrence rates also depend on the BCC subtype, anatomic location, and tumor diameter. Subtypes most appropriate for this technique are the superficial and nodular forms.[120] This procedure usually has a favorable cosmetic result, with minimal scarring and a majority of sites considered to have good or acceptable cosmetic outcomes.[106,122] However, the wound from this technique may take 4 to 6 weeks to heal—longer than surgical excision. It can also leave a hypopigmented or hypertrophic scar.[110,125]

C&E achieved a 5-year recurrence rate of 5.7 to 13.2% for primary BCCs; for previously treated (recurrent) BCCs, 18.1% recurred.[115,122,126] Also, the lesion's diameter is correlated with the chance of recurrence. Generally, the larger the BCC, the greater the recurrence rate. For example, BCCs 0 to 5 mm in diameter had a 5-year 8.5% recurrence rate compared to BCCs with a diameter of 20 mm or more, which had a recurrence rate of 26.1%. In high-risk areas (such as the perinasal, perioral, periocular, and mandibular areas), there was at least a 16.3% recurrence. Fewer BCCs recurred at medium-risk sites (such as the scalp, forehead, and pre- and postauricular areas) at a rate between 10.7 and 13.4%. Low-risk sites (including the neck, trunk, and extremities) achieved recurrence rates of 9.5% or less with this modality.[122] Studies have shown that residual BCC may be found histologically in more than one-third of all sites after C&E.[127,128] The inflammation and proliferative phase of wound healing were not found to have any effect on tumor clearance following C&E, so the exact mechanism of eradication after C&E remains unclear.[121] It is not recommended that C&E be used to treat recurrent BCCs, as this can result in a high recurrence rate of up to 41 to 60%.[120]

There is some controversy over whether C&E may be used to treat BCCs along embryonal fusion lines and in higher risk areas such as the mid-facial region. Some have advocated that this modality is not appropriate for high-risk locations. However, other data supports the possible use of C&E for tumors that are 5 mm in diameter or less. They only had a 4.5% 5-year recurrence rate, compared to those 6 mm and larger, which had a recurrence of 17.6%.[122]

It seems that all tumors with diameters less than 10 mm in low-risk sites may be treated with C&E. In medium-risk locations, tumors greater than 10 mm should not be cleared with this modality. However, smaller BCCs in these areas can be managed appropriately with this treatment.[122]

Cryosurgery

BOX 6-22   Summary

- Cryosurgery uses various mechanisms to treat carcinoma by rapidly forming crystals, demonstrating recrystallization patterns as the cells thaw, exposing cells to high electrolyte concentrations in adjacent thawing and nonfrozen fluids, and causing ischemic damage from vascular stasis and destruction.
- Cryosurgery has high cure rates and the overall recurrence rate for primary BCCs is approximately 4.3%.
- Use caution when treating patients with a darker skin tone. This mode of treatment may cause a hyperpigmentation, postinflammatory hypopigmentation, or even a white depigmentation.
- Cryosurgery is a quick, low-cost, and safe treatment option that remains a viable nonsurgical option to treat BCCs.

Cryosurgery employs the use of a cryogen to form an ice ball. Different cryogens are available, including ethyl chloride, freon, carbon dioxide, and nitrous oxide, but most procedures use liquid nitrogen. This inexpensive cryogen has a boiling point of −196°C and can be readily stored in an insulated container. In an office setting, liquid nitrogen is sprayed from a handheld unit or applied with a cotton-tipped applicator. Numerous nozzles may be used on the handheld unit to change the stream size delivered. Changing the operator's pressure on the applicator controls the freeze depth. Longer durations are associated with a deeper freeze. An ice ball will appear and grow deeper with greater pressure and freezing applied.[120]

Most superficial tumors can be treated with a 10-second freeze, while keeping the BCC frozen and white. The lesion should thaw for approximately 20 to 45 seconds. Cryosurgery should also include a 4 to 6 mm border of normal skin to treat the tumor margins and decrease recurrence.[120,129] With this quick procedure, typically only two freeze–thaw cycles are required for treatment. As a rule, it is better to freeze quickly and thaw slowly.

Cryosurgery effects tumor clearance through different mechanisms: rapidly forming crystals, recrystallization patterns as the cells thaw, cell exposure to high electrolyte concentrations in adjacent thawing and nonfrozen fluids, and ischemic damage from vascular stasis and destruction. As the skin's temperature is lowered to −50 to −60°C, crystals form within the cell and disrupt the cell membrane.[120,130]

Cryosurgery is a widely used technique for single or multiple BCCs, but the tumors must be judiciously chosen. Very high-risk BCCs, with aggressive histology or located in critical facial sites, are not appropriate for cryosurgery.[109] Most dermatologists only use cryosurgery for superficial and small nodular BCCs.[120] High cure rates can be achieved with cryosurgery. The overall recurrence rate for primary BCCs is approximately 4.3%.[131] And on average, recurrent tumors return at a rate 13% after treatment.[115] Kuflik[132] found a cure rate of 94% for primary tumors, and 70% in recurrent BCCs. Another report gave a recurrence rate of 7.6%; notably, this study included morpheaform BCCs.[133] Another study of 22 patients with eyelid BCCs saw no recurrences after 5 years, but the authors caution that patient selection was a crucial part of treatment success.[134] One of the largest studies published the results of 4228 skin cancers (about 92% were BCCs) treated with cryosurgery. With 5-year follow-up, about 97% of the cancers were cured. Interestingly, most of the recurrences appeared within the first 3 years after therapy.[135]

Cryosurgery can be combined with curettage to achieve a high cure rate on the nose. In one study, a total of 61 BCCs on the nose of at least 10 mm in diameter were first curetted and then treated with cryosurgery. After at least 5 years follow-up, only one tumor recurred. Cryosurgery is typically inadequate to treat lesions on the nose, because this is a high-risk location for recurrence. However, the curettage delineates the tumor's margins and removes the majority of the BCC; the deep freezing eradicates the rest. This technique is not recommended for morpheaform BCCs.[136]

Complications associated with cryosurgery include immediate pain, redness, and edema at the treated site. Throbbing may be felt up to 30 min after the procedure. Within the first day after cryosurgery, the patient may develop a blister, which can be hemorrhagic and scab. Small wounds usually heal within 6 weeks, but it may take 14 weeks or longer for larger wound areas and those found on the trunk or extremities.[129,130] Caution is required when treating patients with darker colored skin. Cryosurgery may produce a hyperpigmentation, postinflammatory hypopigmentation, or even a white depigmentation, which can be permanent. Infrequently, patients may develop a hypertrophic scar.[129,137] When using cryosurgery, one must be careful when treating BCCs of the lip, nasal ala, or eyelid because contraction can lead to unfavorable cosmetic results, asymmetry, and free margin retraction.[129] Nearby structures may be permanently damaged with deep-freezing, such as nerves or the cornea.[120] Unlike surgical excision, histologic margins are not examined with this method. Overall, cryosurgery is a quick, low-cost, and safe procedure that remains a viable nonsurgical option to clear BCCs.

Radiation Therapy (Radiotherapy)

BOX 6-23 Summary

- Radiation is an appropriate treatment option for patients that are not candidates for surgical procedures or if their skin carcinoma is considered unresectable.
- Recommended locations include facial structures and usually patients are greater than 60 years of age and have medium- to large-sized tumors.
- The most common types of radiation used in dermatologic practices include superficial X-rays, Grenz rays, contact therapy, supervoltage therapy, electron beam therapy, and radiation from implanted radioactive isotopes.
- Chronic treatment can cause radiodermatitis and cutaneous atrophy.
- Radiation postoperatively should be used in patients with advanced lesions, positive surgical margins, lymph node metastasis, and perineural invasion.

Most BCCs are sensitive to doses of radiation therapy that can be endured by normal surrounding skin.[138] This modality is indicated for patients who are not candidates for surgery or who have skin cancers deemed unresectable.[137] Radiotherapy may be appropriate for primary BCCs of the head and neck[139] as well as for recurrent ones. Most high-risk tumors can be managed with MMS, but this option is not desirable or available to all patients.[140] It has also been recommended for medium-sized tumors in older patients (>60 years of age).[141] Suitable locations to consider X-ray radiation include the eyelids, ears, nose, and lips, where surgery could be disfiguring. These areas retain excellent functional and cosmetic results after treatment.[138,140] Cosmetic outcomes may not be as favorable for tumors of the trunk and extremities.[138] With higher doses used, there is a greater risk of damaging normal skin and having worse cosmetic results.[139] The most common types of radiation used in dermatology include superficial X-rays, Grenz rays, contact therapy, supervoltage therapy, electron beam therapy, and radiation from implanted radioactive isotopes.[138] During irradiation, protect sensitive structures nearby, such as the eye or lacrimal gland. Protective materials used include lead, gold, or tungsten.[139]

When conventional surgery was compared to radiation, surgical excision was preferred for its better cosmetic results and lower recurrence rates.[111] Radiotherapy is a good option for patients with physical or psychological impairments and can be used concomitantly with most medications. Patients also benefit from this procedure being painless and performed on an outpatient basis without anesthesia. Radiotherapy can be useful for incompletely excised tumors and those inadequately removed by C&E. Some disadvantages of the technique are the inability to histologically examine the treated tissue, potential threat of a radiation-induced malignancy in the future, and possibly increased surgical complica-

tion and difficulties if the radiotherapy is not successful.[139] Tumors that recur following radiation tend to be more aggressive, invasive, and difficult to treat than are the primary lesions. Side effects include cutaneous atrophy, telangiectasia, and dyspigmentation of the treatment area. Redness, skin necrosis, and hair loss can also be seen.[129]

Contraindications include tumors arising from burns, scars of chronic ulcers, or osteomyelitis scars. Additional radiation treatments should not be performed on skin cancers in the location of chronic radiodermatitis. For patients who are especially prone to developing multiple cancers (i.e., basal cell nevus syndrome, XP, etc.), irradiating the tumors may actually induce new cancer formations.[138] However, recent evidence suggests that select basal cell nevus syndrome patients may benefit from superficial radiotherapy.[142]

It is important not to forget the danger of chronic radiodermatitis with X-ray therapy. After total therapeutic doses of 40 to 60 Gy, the associated skin can become intensely erythematous while sloughing and oozing. This acute radiodermatitis is generally not painful, and slowly heals in 3 to 6 weeks but can remain noticeable for many years. Radiation therapy can also induce a slow cutaneous atrophy after 3 to 24 months.[138] This treatment may not be as appropriate for younger patients with the potential decline in cosmetic appearance following treatment.[139]

Radiotherapy should be spread over 2 to 6 weeks for better results. Overall cure rates are usually greater than 90% for primary BCCs.[138,139,143] Previously treated tumors recur at a rate of approximately 82%.[139,143] Up to 89% of eyelid, nose, and ear skin cancers can be locally cured.[144-146] The cure rates are comparable with conventional surgery. Radiation can even be used for larger (>2 cm), more clinically advanced tumors with a reported 13% recurrence.[147] Caution is required when treating larger lesions, as the amount of radiation required approaches levels that can harm nearby tissue.[109] But more aggressive forms, like morpheaform BCCs, may still have high recurrences.[66]

Postoperative radiation should be used in patients with advanced lesions, positive surgical margins, lymph node metastasis, and perineural invasion.[139] Radiation therapy is appropriate for patients who are in poor health, elderly, or have large facial tumors.[66] X-ray irradiation, when performed properly and with appropriate precautions, can be a safe and efficacious BCC therapy.[138]

Mohs' Micrographic Surgery

BOX 6-24   Summary

- Mohs' micrographic surgery is the treatment modality that has the highest cure rates along with the best tissue conservation and patient's satisfaction record.
- Dr. Frederic E. Mohs developed this surgical technique that currently consists of a fresh-tissue technique with precise microscope-guided excision.
- Mohs' micrographic surgery is indicated for NMSCs and a variety of other rare and aggressive skin lesions.
- Overall Mohs' micrographic surgery 5-year cure rates are greater than 99% and 96% with primary BCC and recurrent BCC, respectively.

Currently, Mohs' micrographic surgery (MMS) is the technique that offers patients the lowest cancer recurrence rates. In addition to its high cure rate, MMS has the highest tissue conservation rate, has a higher patient satisfaction rate, and is a safe procedure that is primarily performed in an outpatient setting.[3] Dr. Frederic E. Mohs, who developed the MMS, stumbled upon his technique as a medical student in 1932. Mohs discovered that zinc chloride paste was an ideal way to chemically fix a tumor's architecture *in situ*. The idea of fixation *in situ* combined with microscope-aided excision was the basis of all future improvements in this surgical practice.[148–150]

Presently, the majority of MMS is a fresh-tissue technique, which incorporates the use of a local anesthetic (preferably 1% lidocaine solution combined with epinephrine 1:100,000), as opposed to the old fixed-tissue technique that used zinc chloride paste. Mohs also incorporated the use of horizontal tissue sections as opposed to vertical layers or "bread-loafing." This method of cutting the tumor lets the surgeon visualize tumor margins more effectively.[151,152] The tumor must be contiguous for MMS to be completely successful.[152]

MMS is principally used for the treatment of aggressive BCCs and SCCs, but it has successfully treated a variety of other aggressive and rare cutaneous cancers.[153] Since BCCs are the most common type of skin malignancy in the United States,[154,155] the majority of MMS cases are for BCC (Table 6-1).[152,156]

Overall MMS 5-year cure rates of greater than 99 and 96% are achieved with primary BCC and recurrent BCC, respectively.[152,157–159] In contrast, 5-year

Table 6-1

BCC Histologic Subtypes Most Amenable to Mohs' Micrographic Surgery

Morpheaform/sclerosing/fibrosing
Infiltrative
Micronodular
Metatypical/basosquamous

cure rates achieved with other treatment modalities are not as successful.[152,160,161]

Cure rates rely upon BCC subtype, location, size, and whether the lesion is primary or recurrent (Table 6-2).[152] MMS is indicated for the more aggressive histologic subtypes of BCC, which include morpheaform, infiltrative, micronodular, and basosquamous.[152,156,162]

Morpheaform BCCs are more likely to have elongations of tumor cells leading to subclinical, silent spread; therefore, MMS is indicated.[152,156] In a series of 51 morpheaform BCCs, the average length of tumor extension from the clinically apparent cancer was 7.2 mm.[163] The infiltrative BCCs are capable of deep tumor infiltration, upon rare occasions even leading to perineural invasion. Thus, MMS is indicated for such an aggressive tumor that has the potential to destroy such delicate and essential structures.[152,156] Micronodular BCCs are found to have significant tumor extensions as opposed to its counterpart, the nodular BCC.[89] Although superficial BCCs can be successfully treated with traditional surgical excision, these lesions may exhibit extensive subclinical spread[152,156] with follicular involvement. MMS is indicated in these complicated cases because of its precision with tumor margins and unprecedented tissue conservation.[156]

MMS is strongly recommended for the above BCC variants. These aggressive histologic subtypes of BCC are dangerous because they are more likely to have significant silent spread, high recurrence rates, and a potential to metastasize.

Table 6-2

Locations Most Amenable to Mohs' Micrographic Surgery

Nose
Medial and lateral canthi
Preauricular and postauricular areas
Philtrum
Lip
Eyelids
Digits
Anogenital region
Other areas that require ultimate tissue
 conservation

Laser Surgery

BOX 6-25   Summary

- Laser therapy is a fairly novel option for the treatment of BCC and has not been widely studied.
- Lasers that have been tested are the 585-nm pulsed-dye laser (PDL), the Nd:YAG laser, and the CO_2 laser with inconclusive results.
- Lasers may prove to be effective in the future; however, more clinical studies are warranted to test the efficacy of lasers alone and in combination with other therapies.
- Presently, lasers are still not a well-accepted primary treatment for basal cell carcinomas.

Lasers are used to treat a variety of conditions, such as port-wine stains, hemangiomas, and telangiectasias. They are relatively new options for NMSCs, and have not been widely used in the treatment of BCCs. But they offer the potential benefits of being less invasive than are surgical alternatives, and more selective, affecting only the laser-treated area and sparing surrounding tissues. A 585-nm pulsed-dye laser (PDL) has been attempted, but the recurrence and cure rates were unacceptable in comparison to other more commonly used treatments such as Mohs' or excisional surgery.[164] Operating at 585 nm, this laser selectively targets hemoglobin in vessels. The PDL is a nonablative laser that operates on the theory of selective photothermolysis; this leads to a microvascular thrombosis within the targeted vessel.[165]

A small number of patients have been treated with a neodynium:yttrium, aluminum, garnet (Nd:YAG) laser. The Nd:YAG heats the skin to cytotoxic levels above 41 C to kill the cancerous cells. With a 3- to 5-year follow-up, 97.3% of BCCs were cleared; only 1 of the 37 lesions recurred (2.7%).[166]

Another laser used is the carbon dioxide (CO_2) laser, which emits infrared light at a wavelength of 10,600 nm. This is an ablative laser that targets water in the skin to create a localized thermal injury. Laser ablation can have significant side effects such as hypertrophic scarring, crusting, bleeding, and dyspigmentation. Another potential drawback is that there is no histologic tissue evaluation after the procedure to assess therapeutic efficacy.[129] It has been tried in large BCCs and in basal cell nevus syndrome in which surgery was either contraindicated or undesirable.[167] Some suggest treating superficial BCCs along with a 4-mm border of normal skin. The resulting wound is allowed to heal by second intention.[168]

Controversy exists over the efficacy of this modality. A study of 370 superficial BCCs showed that the CO_2 laser combined with curettage achieved complete eradication with no recurrence after an average follow-up period of about 20 months.[169] Another study of 61 BCCs used the CO_2 laser and found a 97% cure rate, with a mean follow-up of 41.7 months.[170] In contrast, when 24 lesions were treated, 50% recurred by the end of the first year.[171] Compared to conventional surgery, the CO_2 laser was faster and more cost-efficient.[172] Good candidates for laser surgery include patients with multiple or large BCCs on the trunk or extremities. Basal cell nevus syndrome and immunosuppressed patients may not be candidates for conventional surgery, where removal of every lesion may not be possible. Finally, lasers are a noninvasive method that may appeal to elderly patients with many medications and concomitant afflictions.[170] Lasers may prove to be efficacious in the future, most likely in combination with other therapies. But they are still not well-accepted primary treatments of BCCs.

Photodynamic Therapy (PDT)

BOX 6-26   Summary

- Photodynamic therapy is a treatment option for select patients with BCCs in areas where tissue loss or scarring might be functionally or cosmetically unfavorable.
- Superficial BCCs have the highest cure rate with this treatment modality, approximately reaching 79 to 100%.
- The most successful treatments have been seen in superficial BCCs less than 2-mm thick.

Photodynamic therapy (PDT) utilizes a photosensitizer like 5-aminolevulinic acid (5-ALA) to make the tumor more susceptible when treated with a light source. 5-ALA may be used alone or with a substance such as dimethylsulfoxide to enhance tissue penetration. The methyl ester of 5-ALA, methyl aminolevulinate (MAL), may offer greater permeation into a lesion due to its increased lipophilic nature and its enhanced predilection for neoplastic cells.[173]

5-ALA is a precursor to the photosensitizer protoporphyrin IX (PpIX) in the heme biosynthetic pathway. When 5-ALA absorbs light, it is converted into PpIX. This generates oxygen singlet species and radicals to induce cell death.[174] Numerous light sources and lasers have been attempted, including UV, blue, and red lights.[173,175] PpIX has absorptions near 410 and 635 nm. Blue lights do not penetrate deeply enough to be effective, but red light irradiation targets the second peak and effects greater tissue penetration.[176] PDT works because the photoactive derivative, PpIX, accumulates more in the mitochondria of rapidly dividing tumor cells than in the surrounding normal skin cells.[174] The process results in localized tissue destruction, while preserving adjacent tissues. This may be a good option for BCCs in areas where tissue loss or scarring might be functionally or cosmetically unfavorable. Compared to cryotherapy, PDT had a shorter healing time, less scarring, and a superior cosmetic outcome.[177] Elderly patients and others who may not be good surgical candidates or do not desire surgery may consider this noninvasive option. Large areas and multiple tumors, such as in basal cell nevus syndrome, have been treated successfully with ALA-PDT.[178] Side effects include a localized burning or stinging sensation, pain, redness, crusting, and photosensitivity in the days or weeks following treatment. MAL-PDT may be less painful than ALA-PDT.[179]

Even though it is convenient and leaves an excellent cosmetic result, the recurrence rates after a single PDT session can be unacceptably high. PDT appears to be more effective in superficial BCCs than in the nodular subtype.[180] Clearance rates typically range from 79 to 100% for superficial BCCs.[176,181–184] Nodular BCCs, which tend to be thicker and deeper, may not allow the photosensitizer to penetrate as well or reach as deep into the tumor. The response rate is between 10 and 75%, but may improve to 100% after multiple treatments.[184–187] Recurrence rates range from 2 to 43%, with many of the higher recurrences in studies that include nodular and morpheaform BCCs.[176]

When MAL-PDT was compared to surgery in nodular BCC eradication, the two methods did not differ significantly. However, the MAL-PDT had better cosmetic outcomes, but did trend toward having a higher recurrence rate.[188] When treating recurrent lesions, PDT cured 82% of previously treated BCCs, although most required multiple treatments.[189]

Long-term cure rates for PDT have been disappointing, and treatment may require multiple sessions to increase the clearance rate. This modality may still prove to be a good option for select patients. Since the photosensitizers may have limited penetration and diffusion, BCCs should be of the superficial subtype and less than 2-mm thick to increase the chances of successful tumor treatment. Consider this treatment when patients have large and numerous superficial tumors. PDT is not recommended for the treatment of more aggressive subtypes (i.e., morpheaform, etc.). More studies are needed before PDT becomes a primary treatment. Until then, it will remain an adjunctive addition to the current treatment armamentarium for BCCs.

Interferon

BOX 6-27   Summary

- Treatment with interferon is an adjuvant therapy that can be recommended in certain situations.
- Intralesional treatment is most effective with superficial and nodular BCCs, and clinical improvement may take up to 16 weeks to visualize.
- Interferon treatment may induce side effects such as flu-like symptoms that may lead to decreased patient's compliance.
- This treatment modality is expensive and requires a major time commitment from the patient. As of now, cure rates are not comparable to other established treatment modalities; however, long-term clinical studies are warranted to justify its use as a primary treatment.

Interferons (IFNs) are additional therapies for BCCs. These natural glycoproteins are secreted in response to different inducers, including viral infections. IFN-α induces BCC cells to express FasR. Since FasL is also still expressed, the neoplastic cells are subjected to the FasR/FasL-mediated apoptotic pathway.[190,191] Intralesional IFN-α generally achieves cure rates between 70 and 100%,[192–195] and is effective for both nodular and superficial BCCs. Clinical improvement can be seen after about 8 weeks, with the greatest difference at 16 weeks. When the tumor appears cured clinically, this usually correlates with histologic clearance as well.[196] But the cure rate becomes dismal with more aggressive, unresponsive forms such as morpheaform and recurrent tumors. With these tumors, the clearance rate falls to only 27%.[197] A study combining INF-α2a and IFN-α2b found the combination to be no more effective than each IFN by itself.[198] IFN-β1a had a similar cure rate at 67%.[199]

Side effects of systemic IFN are flu-like symptoms (i.e., fever, headache, fatigue, chills, anorexia, and arthralgias), which may cause decreased patient's compliance.[174,195] Giving IFN is not only expensive, but also time-consuming since frequent visits are needed for multiple injections. Cure rates are not equivalent to other treatments.

IFN is minimally invasive and does not leave a large scar. If positive margins exist after surgery, IFN has been used successfully to control the remaining neoplasm. It is still an investigational treatment with long-term cure rates lacking. This may be another nonsurgical alternative to contemplate in patients not suitable for surgery.[109,195]

Imiquimod

BOX 6-28 Summary

- Imiquimod is a recently approved topical immune response modifier for superficial BCCs.
- Patients who are appropriate candidates for this treatment include the elderly, non-surgical candidates, those with lesions on areas prone to scarring if surgically treated, and patients who do not favor a surgical option.
- This topical medication is approved by Food and Drug Administration (FDA) only for superficial BCCs as large as 2 cm in diameter located on the neck, trunk, or extremities.
- Local side effects of this medication include erythema, hardened skin, edema, vesiculation, erosion, ulceration, scabbing, and flaking. Systemic effects of this medication include headaches, gastrointestinal disturbances, nausea, and vomiting.
- Cure rates for nonaggressive subtypes of BCC have ranged from 60 to 100%.

Previously indicated only for genital and anal warts, in 2004, imiquimod cream gained Food and Drug Administration's approval as a treatment for superficial BCCs. Indications include elderly patients who may not be surgical candidates, superficial BCCs in areas where scarring may be problematic, and for patients who simply do not favor surgery. After using the cream, patients typically experience very little to no scarring. This cream is only approved for biopsy-proven superficial BCCs up to 2 cm in diameter located on the neck, trunk, or extremities.

Imiquimod is a type of immune response modifier, which promotes a cell-mediated response. Binding to Toll-like receptor-7 on macrophages and dendritic cells induces the production of interferon (IFN)-α, tumor necrosis factor-α, and interleukins 1, 5, 6, 8, 10, and 12. Imiquimod upregulates the body's IFN to remove tumors.[200,201] The neoplastic cells also become more apoptotic, as imiquimod decreases the expression of Bcl-2.[201]

Even though only approved for superficial BCCs, studies show imiquimod also to be effective for nodular subtypes.[200] Cure rates for these nonaggressive subtypes range from 60 to 100%, depending on the dosing schedule and tumor size treated.[201–206] It has been used even in some aggressive forms such as infiltrative BCCs.[201] Transplant recipients[207] as well as patients with basal cell nevus syndrome[208] and XP[205] have also benefited from this noninvasive therapy.

This medication is not always a benign treatment. It can have systemic effects such as headache, gastrointestinal disturbances, nausea, and vomiting. Local side effects include erythema, hardened skin, edema, vesiculation, erosion, ulceration, scabbing, and flaking. These are generally well tolerated by patients, and do not cause patients to stop therapy.[210] Even though this modality's cure rates are not as good as destructive methods, this may still be a desirable nonsurgical alternative for some patients. Also, it is generally prescribed for at least 6 weeks, and compliance might be a concern. The local irritation, erythema, other possible side effects, and weeks of therapy must be weighted against a single surgical intervention.

5-Fluorouracil

BOX 6-29 Summary

- 5-Fluorouracil is a topical agent that is used to treat low-risk superficial BCCs, particularly on the face.
- Cure rates have been reported to be 95% with superficial BCCs.
- Application site irritation, inflammation, crusting, and swelling may occur during treatment sessions.

Treatment of BCCs with 5-fluorouracil (5-FU), a topical chemotherapeutic agent, is usually used in cases of low-risk BCCs (e.g., those not on the nose, ears, and central zone of the face), especially superficial BCCs.[109] However, this compound is not strong enough to eliminate tumors with extensive invasion or involving a patient's follicles. Since this treatment can be easily applied by the patient and spread on relatively large areas, 5-FU can be used for multiple BCCs on the trunk and extremities,[109] but it is not indicated for nodular BCCs.[211] 5-FU is an analog of thymine and inhibits thymidylate synthetase, which disturbs DNA synthesis and leads to cell death. It can cure up to 95% of superficial BCCs.[129] Results can be improved if the lesion is curetted before starting topical therapy.[212] The final cosmetic outcome is very good. However, during treatment, patients may experience considerable tenderness as well as application-site irritation, inflammation, crusting, and swelling, which may decrease patients' compliance.[129]

5-FU can also be injected directly into the lesion. This procedure is safe and effective in superficial and nodular BCCs. This may clear 80 to 90% of lesions, which makes it a viable, noninvasive alternative for treatment.[213]

Chemoprevention (Retinoids and COX-2 Inhibitors)

BOX 6-30 Summary

- Oral retinoids is suggested to be an appropriate chemopreventative agent for patients that are predisposed to multiple NMSCs.
- Studies have shown that retinoids supplementation is connected to reduced and delayed skin carcinoma formation. However, this outcome diminishes over a few months span once supplementation is terminated.
- Topical retinoids, such as tazarotene, may have beneficial effects in treating BCC; however, preliminary results are inconclusive.
- Known side effects of excessive retinoids are osteoporosis, ligament and tendon calcification, and liver abnormalities. Retinoids are also teratogenic during pregnancy, and isotretinoin has a possible link to depression.

Many of the studies performed in chemoprevention of NMSCs have focused on actinic keratoses and SCCs. However, studies are emerging to determine the effects of these compounds on BCCs.

RETINOIDS

Retinoids are derivatives of vitamin A, and are essential to maintaining cellular differentiation. They also play a role in cell growth and apoptosis. When present in physiologic to supra-physiological levels, retinoids can impede the progression of epithelial carcinogenesis. The chemopreventative effect may be exerted at the retinoic acid receptor (RAR) level. Mice models of cancerous skin cells had decreased RAR expression during tumor malignancy progression. Retinoids, at supra-physiological levels, may be able to increase the expression of RARs, and offset the negative tumor-promoting effects.[214]

Oral retinoids (such as acitretin and isotretinoin) may be indicated for those with predilections for multiple NMSCs, such as XP and basal cell nevus syndrome.[110,215,216] Others include organ-transplant recipients and patients with greatly sun-damaged skin.[110,215] These supplements have been associated with reduced and delayed tumor formation while taking the drugs, but the favorable effects diminish within months of completing therapy.[215] However, some studies have found isotretinoin to have no significant effect in the prevention of BCCs when compared to placebo or retinol.[217,218] In addition, dietary retinoids in 73,000 female nurses and 43,000 male health care professionals failed to show any association between dietary intake and BCC development risk.[219,220]

Topical retinoids, such as tazarotene, may have beneficial effects in treating BCCs.[221] After 24 weeks, 76.7% of superficial and nodular BCCs had regressed by more than half. Of these, 46.7% were completely cleared with no recurrence for 2 years. The antitumor effect was likely from increased apoptosis and increased RAR expression, similar to oral retinoids.[222]

The current evidence does not support the use of retinoids, either natural or synthetic, in the treatment of NMSC. There may be some indications where these substances may be useful, such as in patients with high susceptibility to skin cancer development. But patients should be warned and monitored for signs of adverse events similar to excessive vitamin A intake such as osteoporosis, ligament and tendon calcification, and liver abnormalities.[223,224] Other potential complications include the known teratogenic risks of retinoids during pregnancy and isotretinoin's possible link to depression.[224]

CYCLOOXYGENASE INHIBITORS

BOX 6-31   Summary

- Drugs that are considered to be in this group are aspirin, piroxicam, and indomethacin. These drugs are known as nonsteroidal anti-inflammatory drugs (NSAIDS).
- Selective COX-2 inhibitors, such as celecoxib, have been shown to prevent UV-induced skin cancers in animal models.
- A growing need for an effective and safe chemopreventive agent warrants more long-term clinical trials to justify this agent to be used for chemoprevention.

Cyclooxygenase (COX)-1 and -2 are enzymes involved in the conversion of arachidonic acid to prostaglandins. COX-2 gene expression is increased and even overexpressed in some cancers of the esophagus, stomach, colon, breast, and lung. Drugs such as aspirin, piroxicam, and indomethacin nonselectively inhibit both COX-1 and COX-2 enzymes. Collectively, these medications are known as nonsteroidal anti-inflammatory drugs (NSAIDs).[36] Several studies have even shown that regular NSAID usage decreases the risk of death and incidence of breast and colorectal cancers.[225–229] Selective COX-2 inhibitors like celecoxib are thought to avoid the unwanted gastrointestinal side effects associated with nonselective agents.

Interestingly, COX-2 upregulation may contribute to the promotion and progression of skin cancers.[230] A number of animal models show that use of both selective and nonselective cyclooxygenase inhibitors may be able to prevent UV-induced skin cancers.[36,231–234] However, it remains to be seen if these results will translate into a treatment and preventative measure for human skin cancer. Also, when using these drugs, remember the possible link between selective COX-2 inhibitors and increased heart disease risk.[235]

◼ PREVENTION

BOX 6-32   Summary

- Prevention is the most critical measure one can take to decrease the risk of developing skin cancer.
- Avoid sun exposure between the hours of 10 a.m. and 4 p.m.
- Sunscreen that protects against UVA and UVB rays should be applied liberally everyday.
- Wearing sunscreen, with a protective factor index of at least 30 or higher, may decrease the risk of NMSCs.
- Protective clothing is essential such as long-sleeved shirts, long pants, and wide-brimmed hats.
- Preventative education must be implemented to encourage patients to be proactive against skin cancer.

Prevention is the most critical measure one can take to decrease the risk of developing skin cancer. Avoiding extreme and unnecessary sun exposure is imperative, especially between the hours of 10 a.m. and 4 p.m. when the sun is brightest. Wearing sunscreen, with a protective factor index of at least 30 or higher during the first 18 years of life, may decrease the chance of NMSCs by 78%. Consumers should take care when choosing a sunscreen. Most sunscreens in the past protected only against UVB rays, and UVA protection was rarely included. Presently, sunscreen manufacturers are including protection against both types of rays.[3,236] UVB is mostly associated with skin cancer. UVA rays are emitted year-round, and cause lines and wrinkles by destroying collagen and elastin in the dermis. UVB rays are most intense during the summer and are the main cause of sunburn.[3] Sunscreen and protective clothing are essential. Whenever possible, one should wear long sleeves and long pants while outdoors.[3,4] Wide-brimmed hats are also advised because they can provide complete coverage of the head, neck, and face.[4] Even sunscreen incorporated into special clothing has been manufactured for maximum protection. SPF 30 or higher is available in various clothing and accessories.[237] Tanning beds are extremely hazardous and should be avoided at all costs.

Because NMSC is so common, and various treatments can be expensive, it is predicted that the cost to manage BCC is on the rise. Although mortality is not high in NMSC, the frequency of the cancer is a burden upon insurance companies. To reduce financial problems, the public must be educated about skin cancer because it is, for the most part, preventable.[15] Physicians must implement preventative education measures along with routine physical exams. Patients should know how to distinguish skin cancers and be more prudent toward the subject of skin cancer.[3] Physicians must insist on a follow-up every 3 to 6 months for the first year after treatment.

Subsequently, 6 months is an adequate interval for a routine checkup. Physicians and patients should note scars that thicken or alter in color or texture. These observations could justify further examination and possibly may prevent a recurrence of the cancer.[4] With public awareness, liberal use of sunscreens, and protective clothing, the BCC epidemic can be reduced and controlled.

◼ FINAL THOUGHTS

BCC is by far the most common cancer in the world and is the main cause of the skin cancer epidemic we are now facing. Fortunately, the majority of BCC cases are also preventable due to the chief etiologic factor, UV radiation. An ever-increasing amount of evidence, linking the dangers of UV radiation to cancer, is discovered and imposed upon the health care field and the general public. With this evidence in hand, it is the job of physicians to reinforce and educate patients until the message is understood. Many treatment modalities are also becoming available, including topical regimens. It is necessary to explore these newer agents with large clinical trials to prove their efficacy to have them available in the near future for our patients. With new treatment options and preventative measures in hand, the BCC crisis may be finally under control.

◼ REFERENCES

1. Available at: www.who.int.
2. Armstrong BK, Kricker A. The epidemiology of UV induced skin cancer. *J Photochem Photobiol B*. 2001;63:8–18.
3. Anthony ML. Surgical treatment of non-melanoma skin cancer. *AORN J*. 2000;71 (3):552–564.
4. Garner KL, Rodney WM. Basal and squamous cell carcinoma. *Prim Care*. 2000; 27(2):447–458.
5. Available at: www.cancer.org.au.
6. Gallagher RP, Hill GB, Bajdik CD, et al. Sunlight exposure, pigmentary factors, and risk of nonmelanocytic skin cancer. I. Basal cell carcinoma. *Arch Dermatol*. 1995;131(2):157–163.
7. Davies TW, Treasure FP, Welch AA, et al. Diet and basal cell skin cancer: results from the EPIC–Norfolk cohort. *Br J Dermatol*. 2002;146(6):1017–1022.
8. Available at: www.cancer.org.
9. Salasche SJ. Epidemiology of actinic keratoses and squamous cell carcinoma. *J Am Acad Dermatol*. 2000;42(1, pt 2):4–7.
10. Kruger K, Blume-Peytavi U, Orfanos CE. Basal cell carcinoma possibly originates from the outer root sheath and/or the bulge region of the vellus hair follicle. *Arch Dermatol Res*. 1999;291(5): 253–259.
11. Bastiaens MT, Hoefnagel JJ, Bruijn JA, et al. Differences in age, site distribution, and sex between nodular and superficial basal cell carcinoma indicate different types of tumors. *J Invest Dermatol*. 1998; 110(6):880–884.
12. Scotto J, Fears TR, Fraumeni JF. *Incidence of Nonmelanocytic Skin Cancer in the United States*. Bethesda, MD: National Institutes of Health; 1983 (publication #83-2433).
13. Stone JL, Reizer G, Scotto J. Incidence of nonmelanoma skin cancer in Kauai during 1983. *Hawaii Med J*. 1986;45:281–286.
14. Stockfleth E, Sterry W. New treatment modalities for basal cell carcinoma. *Recent Results Cancer Res*. 2002;160: 259–268.
15. Housman TS, Feldman SR, Williford PM, et al. Skin cancer is among the most costly of all cancers to treat for the medicare population. *J Am Acad Dermatol*. 2003;48(3):425–429.
16. Pennello G, Devesa S, Gail M. Association of surface ultraviolet B radiation levels with melanoma and nonmelanoma skin cancer in United States blacks. *Cancer Epidemiol Biomarkers Prev*. 2000; 9(3):291–297.
17. Leong GK, Stone JL, Farmer ER, et al. Nonmelanoma skin cancer in Japanese residents of Kauai, Hawaii. *J Am Acad Dermatol*. 1987;17(2, pt 1):233–238.
18. Gloster HM, Jr, Brodland DG. The epidemiology of skin cancer. *Dermatol Surg*. 1996;22(3):217–226.
19. Lear JT, Tan BB, Smith AG, et al. Risk factors for basal cell carcinoma in the UK: case–control study in 806 patients. *J R Soc Med*. 1997;90(7):371–374.
20. Marks R. Epidemiology of non-melanoma skin cancer and solar keratoses in Australia: a tale of self-immolation in Elysian fields. *Australas J Dermatol*. 1997;38(suppl 1):S26–S29.
21. Zanetti R, Rosso S, Martinez C, et al. The multicentre south European study 'Helios'. I. Skin characteristics and sunburns in basal cell and squamous cell carcinomas of the skin. *Br J Cancer*. 1996; 73(11):1440–1446.
22. Kaidbey KH, Agin PP, Sayre RM, et al. Photoprotection by melanin—a comparison of black and Caucasian skin. *J Am Acad Dermatol*. 1979;1(3):249–260.
23. Diepgen TL, Mahler V. The epidemiology of skin cancer. *Br J Dermatol*. 2002;146 (suppl 61):1–6.
24. Zak-Prelich M, Narbutt J, Sysa-Jedrzejowska A. Environmental risk factors predisposing to the development of basal cell carcinoma. *Dermatol Surg*. 2004; 30(2, pt 2):248–252.
25. Mowad CM, Jaworsky C, Werth VP. Numerous erythematous truncal plaques. Multiple basal cell carcinomas associated with arsenic ingestion. *Arch Dermatol*. 1996;132(9):1105–1106,1108–1109.
26. Gallagher RP, Bajdik CD, Fincham S, et al. Chemical exposures, medical history, and risk of squamous and basal cell carcinoma of the skin. *Cancer Epidemiol Biomarkers Prev*. 1996;5(6):419–424.
27. Berg D, Otley CC. Skin cancer in organ transplant recipients: epidemiology, pathogenesis, and management. *J Am Acad Dermatol*. 2002;47(1):1–17.
28. Hojo M, Morimoto T, Maluccio M, et al. Cyclosporine induces cancer progression by a cell-autonomous mechanism. *Nature*. 1999;397(6719):530–534.
29. Kelly GE, Meikle W, Sheil AG. Effects of immunosuppressive therapy on the induction of skin tumors by ultraviolet irradiation in hairless mice. *Transplantation*. 1987;44(3):429–434.
30. Servilla KS, Burnham DK, Daynes RA. Ability of cyclosporine to promote the growth of transplanted ultraviolet radiation-induced tumors in mice. *Transplantation*. 1987;44(2):291–295.
31. Boyle J, MacKie RM, Briggs JD, et al. Cancer, warts, and sunshine in renal transplant patients. A case–control study. *Lancet*. 1984;1(8379):702–705.
32. Rowe DE, Carroll RJ, Day CL, Jr. Long-term recurrence rates in previously untreated (primary) basal cell carcinoma: implications for patient follow-up. *J Dermatol Surg Oncol*. 1989;15(3):315–328.
33. Lacour JP. Carcinogenesis of basal cell carcinomas: genetics and molecular mechanisms. *Br J Dermatol*. 2002;146(suppl 61): 17–19.
34. Kim M, Park HJ, Baek S, et al. Mutations of the p53 and PTCH gene in basal cell carcinomas: UV mutation signature and strand bias. *J Dermatol Sci*. 2002;29(1):1–9.
35. Kogerman P, Krause D, Rahnama F, et al. Alternative first exons of PTCH1 are differentially regulated *in vivo* and may confer different functions to the PTCH1 protein. *Oncogene*. 2002;21(39):6007–6016.
36. Orengo IF, Gerguis J, Phillips R, et al. Celecoxib, a cyclooxygenase 2 inhibitor as a potential chemopreventive to UV-induced skin cancer: a study in the hairless mouse model. *Arch Dermatol*. 2002; 138(6):751–755.
37. Pentland AP, Schoggins JW, Scott GA, Khan KN, Han R. Reduction of UV-induced skin tumors in hairless mice by selective COX-2 inhibition. *Carcinogenesis*. 1999;20(10):1939–1944.
38. Fischer SM, Lo HH, Gordon GB, et al. Chemopreventive activity of celecoxib, a specific cyclooxygenase-2 inhibitor, and indomethacin against ultraviolet light-induced skin carcinogenesis. *Mol Carcinogen*. 1999;25(4):231–240.
39. Gaspari AA, Sauder DN. Immunotherapy of basal cell carcinoma: evolving approaches. *Dermatol Surg*. 2003;29(10): 1027–1034.
40. Soehnge H, Ouhtit A, Ananthaswamy ON. Mechanisms of induction of skin cancer by UV radiation. *Front Biosci*. 1997; 2:d538–d551.
41. Xie J, Aszterbaum M, Zhang X, et al. A role of PDGF alpha in basal cell carcinoma proliferation. *Proc Natl Acad Sci USA*. 2001;98(16):9255–9259.
42. Bodak N, Queille S, Avril MF, et al. High levels of patched gene mutations in basal-cell carcinomas from patients with xeroderma pigmentosum. *Proc Natl Acad Sci USA*. 1999;96(9):5117–5122.
43. Yamazaki F, Aragane Y, Kawada A, et al. Immunohistochemical detection for nuclear beta-catenin in sporadic basal cell carcinoma. *Br J Dermatol*. 2001;145(5): 771–777.
44. Hammerschmidt M, Brook A, McMahon AP. The world according to hedgehog. *Trends Genet*. 1997;13(1):14–21.
45. Ikeda S, Kishida S, Yamamoto H, et al. Axin, a negative regulator of the wnt signaling pathway, directly interacts with adenomatous polyposis coli and regulates the stabilization of beta-catenin. *J Biol Chem*. 1998;273(18): 10823–10826.

46. Morin PJ, Sparks AB, Korinek V, et al. Activation of beta-catenin-Tcf signaling in colon cancer by mutations in beta-catenin or APC. *Science*. 1997;275(5307): 1787–1790.

47. Wijnhoven BP, Dinjens WN, Pignatelli M. E-cadherin–catenin cell–cell adhesion complex and human cancer. *Br J Surg*. 2000;87(8):992–1005.

48. Smyth I, Narang MA, Evans T, et al. Isolation and characterization of human patched 2 (PTCH2), a putative tumour suppressor gene in basal cell carcinoma and medulloblastoma on chromosome 1p32. *Hum Mol Genet*. 1999;8(2):291–297.

49. Ghali L, Wong ST, Green J, et al. Gli1 protein is expressed in basal cell carcinomas, outer root sheath keratinocytes and a subpopulation of mesenchymal cells in normal human skin. *J Invest Dermatol*. 1999;113(4):595–599.

50. Ramachandran S, Lear JT, Ramsay H, et al. Presentation with multiple cutaneous basal cell carcinomas: association of glutathione S-transferase and cytochrome P450 genotypes with clinical phenotype. *Cancer Epidemiol Biomarkers Prev*. 1999;8(1):61–67.

51. Yengi L, Inskip A, Gilford J, et al. Polymorphism at the glutathione S-transferase locus GSTM3: interactions with cytochrome P450 and glutathione S-transferase genotypes as risk factors for multiple cutaneous basal cell carcinoma. *Cancer Res*. 1996;56(9):1974–1977.

52. Hajeer AH, Lear JT, Ollier WE, et al. Preliminary evidence of an association of tumor necrosis factor microsatellites with increased risk of multiple basal cell carcinomas. *Br J Dermatol*. 2000, 142(3): 441–445.

53. Ramachandran S, Fryer AA, Lovatt TJ, et al. Combined effects of gender, skin type, and polymorphic genes on clinical phenotype: use of rate of increase in numbers of basal cell carcinomas as a model system. *Cancer Lett*. 2003;189(2):175–181.

54. Foschini MP, Eusebi V. Divergent differentiation in endocrine and nonendocrine tumors of the skin. *Semin Diagn Pathol*. 2000;17(2):162–168.

55. Eusebi V, Mambelli V, Tison V, et al. Endocrine differentiation in basal cell carcinoma. *Tumori*. 1979;65(2):191–199.

56. Paver K, Poyzer K. The incidence of basal cell carcinoma and their metastases in Australia and New Zealand. *Australas J Dermatol*. 1973;14:53.

57. Von Domarus H, Stevens PJ. Metastatic basal cell carcinoma. *J Am Acad Dermatol*. 1984;10:1043–1060.

58. Scrivener Y, Grosshans E, Cribier B. Variations of basal cell carcinomas according to gender, age, location and histopathological subtype. *Br J Dermatol*. 2002;147:41–47.

59. Goldberg LH, Leis P, Pham HN. Basal cell carcinoma on the neck. *Dermatol Surg*. 1996;22:349–353.

60. Hood AF, Kwan TH, Mihm MC, et al. Neoplastic patterns of the epidermis. In: *Primer of Dermatopathology*. 3rd ed. Philadelphia, PA: Lippincott Williams and Wilkins; 2002:101–130.

61. Kirkham N. Tumors and cysts of the epidermis. In: Elder D, Elenitsas R, Jaworsky C, Johnson B, eds. *Lever's Histopathology of the Skin*. 8th ed. Philadelphia, PA: Lippincott-Raven; 1997:719–747.

62. Hutcheson ACS, Fisher AH, Lang PG. Basal cell carcinomas with unusual histologic patterns. *JAAD*. 2005;53(5):833–837.

63. Maloney ME, Jones DB, Sexton FM. Pigmented basal cell carcinoma: investigation of 70 cases. *JAAD*. 1992;27(1):74–78.

64. Sachs DL, Marghoob AA, Halpern A. Geriatric dermatology. *Clin Geriatr Med*. 2001;17(4, pt 1):715–738.

65. Lesher JL, d'Aubermont PC, Brown V. Morpheaform basal cell carcinoma in a young black woman. *J Dermatol Surg Oncol*. 1988;14:200–203.

66. Zagrodnik B, Kempf W, Seifert B, et al. Superficial radiotherapy for patients with basal cell carcinoma. Recurrence rates, histologic types, and expression of p53 and bcl-2. *Cancer*. 2003;98(12):2708–2714.

67. Erbagci Z, Erkilic S. Can smoking and/or occupational UV exposure have any role in the development of the morpheaform basal cell carcinoma? A critical role for peritumoral mast cells. *Int J Dermatol*. 2002;41(5):275–278.

68. Seigle RJ, MacMillan J, Pollack SV. Infiltrative basal cell carcinoma:a nonsclerosing type. *J Dermatol Surg Oncol*. 1986;12(8):830–836.

69. Hendrix JD, Jr, Parlette HL. Duplicitous growth of infiltrative basal cell carcinoma: analysis of clinically undetected tumor extent in a paired case–control study. *Dermatol Surg*. 1996;22(6):535–539.

70. Walsh N, Ackerman AB. Infundibulocystic basal cell carcinoma: a newly described variant. *Mod Pathol*. 1990;3(5): 599–608.

71. Kelly SC, Ermolovich T, Purcell SM. Non-syndromic segmental multiple infundibulocystic basal cell carcinomas in an adolescent female. *Dermatol Surg*. 2006;32 (9):1202–1208.

72. Takemoto S, Fukamizu H, Yamanaka K, et al. Giant basal cell carcinoma: improvement in the quality of life after extensive resection. *Scand J Plast Reconstr Surg Hand Surg*. 2003;37:181–185.

73. Randle HW. Basal cell carcinoma. Identification and treatment of the high-risk patient. *Dermatol Surg*. 1996;22:255–261.

74. Copcu E, Aktas A. Simultaneous two organ metastases of the giant basal cell carcinoma of the skin. *Int Semin Surg Oncol*. 2005;2(1):1.

75. Scanlon EF, Volkmer DD, Oviedo MA, Khandekar JD, Victor TA. Metastatic basal cell carcinoma. *J Surg Oncol*. 1980; 15:171–180.

76. Kokavec R, Fedeles J. Giant basal cell carcinomas: a result of neglect? *Acta Chir Plast*. 2004;46(3):67–69.

77. Cherpelis BS, Marcusen C, Lang PG. Prognostic factors for metastasis in squamous cell carcinoma of the skin. *Dermatol Surg*. 2002;28:268–273.

78. Martin RC, Edwards MJ, Cawte MJ, et al. Basosquamous carcinoma. Analysis of prognostic factors influencing recurrence. *Cancer*. 2000;88(6):1365–1369.

79. Maloney ML. What is basosquamous carcinoma? *Dermatol Surg*. 2000;26:505–506.

80. Bowman PH, Ratz JL, Knoepp TG, et al. Basosquamous carcinoma. *Dermatol Surg*. 2003;29:830–833.

81. Sendur N, Karaman G, Dikicioglu E, et al. Cutaneous basosquamous carcinoma infiltrating cerebral tissue. *JEADV*. 2004;18:334–336.

82. Beer TW, Shepard P, Theaker JM. Ber EP4 and epithelial membrane antigen aid distinction of basal cell, squamous cell and basosquamous carcinomas of the skin. *Histopathology*. 2000;37:218–223.

83. Mitsuhashi T, Itoh T, Shimizu Y, et al. Squamous cell carcinoma of the skin: dual differentiations to rare basosquamous and spindle cell variants. *J Cutan Pathol*. 2006;33:246–252.

84. de Faria JL, Navarrete MA. The histopathology of the skin basal cell carcinoma with areas of intermediate differentiation. A metatypical carcinoma? *Pathol Res Pract*. 1991;187(8):978–985.

85. Barnes L, Ferlito A, Altavilla G, Mac-Millan C, Rinaldo A, Doglioni C. Basaloid squamous cell carcinoma of the head and neck: clinicopathological features and differential diagnosis. *Ann Otol Rhinol Laryngol*. 996;105:75–82.

86. Coletta RD, Almeida OP, Vargas PA. Cytokeratins 1, 7 and 14 immunoexpression are helpful in the diagnosis of basaloid squamous carcinoma. *Histopathology*. 2006;48:773–774.

87. Saldanha G, Fletcher A, Slater DN. Basal cell carcinoma: a dermatopathological and molecular biological update. *Br J Dermatol*. 2003;148:195–202.

88. Sexton M, Jones GB, Maloney M. Histologic pattern analysis of basal cell carcinoma. *J Am Acad Dermatol*. 1990;23: 1118–1126.

89. Hendrix JD, Jr, Parlette HL. Micronodular basal cell carcinoma. A deceptive histologic subtype with frequent clinically undetected tumor extension. *Arch Dermatol*. 1996;132:295–298.

90. Kuflik EG. The "field-fire" basal-cell carcinoma: treatment by cryosurgery. *J Dermatol Surg Oncol*. 1980;6(4):247–249.

91. Pinkus H. Premalignant fibroepithelial tumors of skin. *Arch Derm Syph*. 1953; 67:598.

92. Pinkus H. Epithelial and fibroepithelial tumors. *Arch Dermatol*. 1965;91:24–37.

93. Bowen AR, LeBoit PE. Fibroepithelioma of Pinkus is a fenestrated trichoblastoma. *Am J Dermatopathol*. 2005;27(2):149–154.

94. Gorlin RJ. Nevoid basal cell carcinoma (Gorlin) syndrome. *Genet Med*. 2004;6(6): 530–539.

95. Howell JB, Mehregan AH. Pursuit of the pits in the nevoid basal cell carcinoma syndrome. *Arch Dermatol*. 1970;102: 586–597.

96. Maddox WD, Winkleman RK, Harrison EG, et al. Multiple nevoid basal cell epitheliomas, jaw cysts and skeletal defects. *JAMA*. 1964;188:106–111.

97. Rahbari H, Mehregan AH. Basal cell nevus epithelioma [cancer in children and teenagers]. *Cancer*. 1982;49:350–353.

98. Manfredi M, Vescovi P, Bonanini, et al. Nevoid basal cell carcinoma syndrome: a review of the literature. *Int J Oral Maxillofac Surg*. 2004;33:117–124.

99. Evans DG, Birch JM, Orton CI. Brain tumours and the occurrence of severe invasive basal cell carcinoma in first degree relatives with Gorlin syndrome. *Br J Neurosurg*. 1991;5(6):643–646.

100. Goldstein AM, Pastakia B, DiGiovanna JJ, et al. Clinical findings in two African-American families with the nevoid basal cell syndrome (NBCC). *Am J Med Genet*. 1994;50:272–281.

101. Bazex A, Dupré A, Christol B. Follicular atrophoderma, baso-cellular proliferations and hypotrichosis. *Ann Dermatol Syphiligr (Paris)*. 1966;93(3):241–254.

102. Goeteyn M, Geerts ML, Kint A, et al. The Bazex–Dupré–Christol syndrome. *Arch Dermatol*. 1994;130(3):337–342.

103. Colomb D, Ducros B, Boussuge N. Le syndrome de Bazex, Dupré et Christolia propos d' un cas aveclcuemie prolymphocytaire. *Ann Dermatol Venereol*. 1989; 116:381–387.

104. Van Steensel MA, Jaspers NG, Steijlen PM. A case of Rombo syndrome. *Br J Dermatol*. 2001;144:1215–1218.

105. Lear JT, Smith AG. Basal cell carcinoma. *Postgrad Med J*. 1997;73(863):538–542.

106. Stulberg DL, Crandell B, Fawcett RS. Diagnosis and treatment of basal cell and squamous cell carcinomas. *Am Fam Phys*. 2004;70:1481–1488.

107. Reynolds PL, Strayer SM. Treatment of skin malignancies. *J Fam Pract*. 2003;52(6): 456–464.

108. Wolf DJ, Zitelli JA. Surgical margins for basal cell carcinoma. *Arch Dermatol*. 1987;123:340–344.

109. Telfer NR, Colver GB, Bowers PW. Guidelines for the management of basal cell carcinoma. *Br J Dermatol*. 1999; 141(3):415–23.

110. Wong CSM, Strange RC, Lear JT. Basal cell carcinoma. *BMJ*. 2003;327:794–798.

111. Avril MF, Auperin A, Margulis A, et al. Basal cell carcinoma of the face: surgery or radiotherapy? Results of a randomized study. *Br J Cancer*. 1997;76(1): 100–106.

112. Hallock GG, Lutz DA. A prospective study of the accuracy of the surgeon's diagnosis and significance of the positive margins in nonmelanoma skin cancers. *Plast Reconstr Surg*. 2001;107(4): 942–947.

113. Dubin N, Kopf AW. Multivariate risk score for recurrence of cutaneous basal cell carcinomas. *Arch Dermatol*. 1983;119 (5):373–377.

114. Roenigk RK, Ratz JL, et al. Trends in the presentation and treatment of basal cell carcinomas. *J Dermatol Surg Oncol*. 1986; 12(8):860–865.

115. Rowe DE, Carroll RJ, Day CL, Jr. Mohs surgery is the treatment of choice for recurrent (previously treated) basal cell carcinoma. *J Dermatol Surg Oncol*. 1989; 15:424–431.

116. Silverman MK, Kopf AW, Bart RS, et al. Recurrence rates of treated basal cell carcinomas. Part 3: Surgical excision. *J Dermatol Surg Oncol*. 1992;18:471–476.

117. Kumakiri M, Hashimoto K. Ultrastructural resemblance of basal cell epithelioma to primary epithelial germ. *J Cutan Pathol*. 1978;5:53–67.

118. Luzi P, Miracco C, Del Vecchio MT, et al. Stereological study of desmosomes in basal cell carcinoma and seborrheic keratosis. *J Submicrosc Cytol*. 1987;19: 337–343.

119. McNutt NS. Ultrastructural comparison of the interface between epithelium and stroma in basal cell carcinoma and control human skin. *Lab Invest*. 1976;35: 132–142.

120. Orengo I, Katta R, Rosen T. Techniques in the removal of skin lesions. *Otolaryngol Clin North Am*. 2002;35(1): 153–170.

121. Nouri K, Spencer J, Taylor J, et al. Does wound healing contribute to the eradication of basal cell carcinoma following curettage and electrodessication? *Dermatol Surg*. 1999;25:183.

122. Silverman MK, Kopf AW, Grin CM, et al. Recurrence rates of treated basal cell carcinomas. Part 2: Curettage-electrodessication. *J Dermatol Surg Oncol*. 1991; 17:720–726.

123. Rowe DE. Comparison of treatment modalities for basal cell carcinoma. *Clin Dermatol*. 1995;13(6):617–620.

124. Alexiades-Armenakas M, Ramsay D, Kopf AW. The appropriateness of curettage and electrodessication for the treatment of basal cell carcinomas. *Arch Dermatol*. 2000;136(6):800.

125. Spencer JM, Tannenbaum A, Sloan L, et al. Dose inflammation contribute to the eradication of basal cell carcinoma following curettage and electrodessication? *Dermatol Surg*. 1997;23:625–631.

126. Kopf AW, Bart RS, Schrager D, et al. Curettage-electrodessication treatment of basal cell carcinoma. *Arch Dermatol*. 1977;113:439–443.

127. Edens BL, Bartlow GA, Haghighi P, Astarita RW, Davidson TM. Effectiveness of curettage and electrodessication in the removal of basal cell carcinoma. *J Am Acad Dermatol*. 1983;9(3): 383–388.

128. Swetter SM. Malignant melanoma from the dermatologic perspective. *Surg Clin North Am*. Dec. 1996;76(6):1287–1298.

129. Padgett JK, Hendrix JD. Cutaneous malignancies and their management. *Otolaryngol Clin North Am*. 2001;34(3): 523–553.

130. Kuflik EG. Cryosurgery updated. *J Am Acad Dermatol*. 1994;31:925–944.

131. Thissen M, Neumann M, Schouten LJ. A systematic review of treatment modalities for primary basal cell carcinomas. *Arch Dermatol*. 1999;135:1177–1183.

132. Kuflik EG. Cryosurgery for carcinoma of the eyelids: a 12-year experience. *J Dermatol Surg Oncol*. 1985;11:243–246.

133. Tuppurainen K. Cryotherapy for eyelid and periocular basal cell carcinomas: outcome in 166 cases over an 8-year period. *Graefes Arch Clin Exp Opthalmol*. 1995;233:205–208.

134. Lindgren G, Larko O. Long-term follow-up of cryosurgery of basal cell carcinoma of the eyelid. *J Am Acad Dermatol*. 1997;36:742–746.

135. Zacarian SA. Cryosurgery of cutaneous carcinomas. 1983;9:947–956.

136. Nordin P, Larko O, Stenquist B. Five-year results of curettage-cryosurgery of selected large primary basal cell carcinomas on the nose: an alternative treatment in a geographical area underserved by Mohs' surgery. *Br J Dermatol*. 1997; 136:180–183.

137. Kibarian MA, Hurza GJ. Nonmelanoma skin cancer. *Postgrad Med*. 1995;98(6): 39–58.

138. Panizzon RG. Radiotherapy of skin tumors. *Recent Results Cancer Res*. 2002; 160:234–239.

139. Vora SA, Garner SL. Role of radiation therapy for facial skin cancers. *Clin Plast Surg*. 2004;31(1):33–38.

140. Thom GA, Heywood JM, Cassidy B, et al. Three-year retrospective review of superficial radiotherapy for skin conditions in a Perth radiotherapy unit. *Australas J Dermatol*. 2003;44:174–179.

141. Mitusuhashi N, Hawakawa K, Yamakawa M, et al. Cancer in patients aged 90 years or older: radiation therapy. *Radiology*. 1999;211:829–833.

142. Caccialanza M, Percivalle S, Piccinno R. Possibility of treating basal cell carcinomas of nevoid basal cell carcinoma syndrome with superficial X-ray therapy. *Dermatology*. 2004;208(1):60–63.

143. Lovett RD, Perez CA, Shapiro SJ, et al. External irradiation of epithelial skin cancer. *Int J Radiat Oncol Biol Phys*. 1990; 19:235–242.

144. Fitzpatrick PJ, Thompson GA, Easterbrook WM, et al. Basal and squamous cell carcinoma of the eyelids and their treatment by radiotherapy. *Int J Radiat Oncol Biol Phys*. 1984;10:449–454.

145. Morrison W, Garden AS, Ang KK. Radiation therapy for nonmelanoma skin carcinomas. *Clin Plast Surg*. 1997;24(4): 719–729.

146. Mazeron JJ, Chassagne D, Crook J, et al. Radiation therapy of carcinomas of the skin of nose and nasal vestibule: a report of 1676 cases by the Groupe Europeen de Curietherapie. *Radiother Oncol*. 1988; 13(3):165–173.

147. Kwan W, Wilson D, Moravan V. Radiotherapy for locally advanced basal cell and squamous cell carcinomas of the skin. *Int J Radiat Oncol Biol Phys*. 2004; 60(2):406–411.

148. Mohs FE. Chemosurgery. In: *Cancer, Gangrene and Infections*. Springfield, IL: Charles C Thomas Publishing; 1956:3–6.

149. Mohs FE. Mohs micrographic surgery. A historical perspective. *Dermatol Clin*. 1989;7(4):609–611.

150. Mohs FE. Contemporaries: Frederick E. Mohs, M.D. *J Am Acad Dermatol*. 1983;9 (5):806–814.

151. Lang PG, Jr. Mohs micrographic surgery fresh-tissue technique. *Dermatol Clin*. 1989;7(4):613–626.

152. Shriner DL, McCoy DK, Goldberg DJ, et al. Mohs micrographic surgery. *J Am Acad Dermatol*. 1998;39(1):79–97.

153. Rapini RP. Mohs surgery for unusual tumors. In: Gross KG, Steinman HK, Rapini RP, eds. *Mohs Surgery: Fundamentals and Techniques*. St. Louis, MO: Mosby;1999:193–208.

154. Gloster HM, Broadland DG. The epidemiology of skin cancer. *Dermatol Surg*. 1996;22:217–226.

155. Silverberg E, Lubera JA. Cancer statistics, 1988. *CA Cancer J Clin*. 1988;38(1):5–22.

156. Lang PG, Jr, Osguthorpe JD. Indications and limitations of Mohs micrographic surgery. *Dermatol Clin*. 1989;7:627–644.

157. Tulli A. Mohs' micrographic surgery. In: Chu AC, Edelson RL, eds. *Malignant Tumors of the Skin*. London, UK: Arnold; 1999:381–395.

158. Martinez JC, Otley CC. The management of melanoma and non-melanoma skin cancer: a review for the primary care physician. *Mayo Clin Proc*. 2001;76: 1253–1265.

159. Lawrence CM. Mohs micrographic surgery for basal cell carcinoma. *Clin Exp Dermatol*. 1999;24:130–133.

160. Mohs FE. Chemosurgical techniques. In: *Chemosurgery. Microscopically Controlled Surgery for Skin Cancer*. Springfield, IL: Charles C Thomas; 1978:1–29,153–164.

161. Leslie DF, Greenway HT. Mohs micrographic surgery for skin cancer. *Australas J Dermatol.* 1991;32:159–164.

162. Lang PG, Maize JC. Histologic evolution of recurrent basal cell carcinoma and treatment implications. *J Am Acad Dermatol.* 1986;14:186–196.

163. Salasche SJ, Ammonette RA. Morpheaform basal cell epitheliomas. A study of subclinical extensions in a series of 51 cases. *J Dermatol Surg Oncol.* 1981;7: 387–393.

164. Allison KP, Kiernan MN, Waters RA, et al. Pulsed dye laser treatment of superficial basal cell carcinoma: realistic or not? *Lasers Med Sci.* 2003;18(2):125–126.

165. Tanzi EL, Lupton JR, Alster TS. Lasers in dermatology: four decades of progress. *J Am Acad Dermatol.* 2003;49(1):1–31.

166. El-Tonsy MH, El-Domyati MM, El-Saxy AE, et al. Continuous-wave Nd:Yag laser hyperthermia: a successful modality in treatment of basal cell carcinoma. *Dermatol Online J.* 2004;10(2):3.

167. Nouri K, Chang A, Trent JT, et al. Ultrapulse CO₂ used for the successful treatment of basal cell carcinomas found in patients with basal cell nevus syndrome. *Dermatol Surg.* 2002;28: 287–290.

168. Humphreys TR, Malhotra R, Scharf MJ, et al. Treatment of superficial basal cell carcinoma and squamous cell carcinoma *in situ* with a high-energy pulsed carbon dioxide laser. *Arch Dermatol.* 1998;134: 1247–1252.

169. Wheeland RG, Bailin PL, Ratz JL, et al. Carbon dioxide laser vaporization and curettage in the treatment of large or multiple superficial basal cell carcinomas. *J Dermatol Surg Oncol.* 1987;13:119–125.

170. Iyer S, Bowes L, Kricorian G, et al. Treatment of basal cell carcinoma with the pulsed carbon dioxide laser: a retrospective analysis. *Dermatol Surg.* 2004;30 (9):1214–1218.

171. Adams EL, Price NM. Treatment of basal-cell carcinomas with a carbon-dioxide laser. *J Dermatol Surg Oncol.* 1979; 5(10):803–806.

172. Horlock N, Grobbelaar AO, Gault DT. Can the carbon dioxide laser completely ablate basal cell carcinomas? A histological study. *Br J Plast Surg.* 2000;53:286–293.

173. Siddiqui MA, Perry CM, Scott LJ. Topical methyl aminolevulinate. *Am J Clin Dermatol.* 2004;5(2):127–137.

174. Miller SJ. Biology of basal cell carcinoma (part II). *J Am Acad Dermatol.* 1991;24: 161–175.

175. Ahmadi S, McCarron PA, Donnelly RF, et al. Evaluation of the penetration of 5-aminolevulinic acid through basal cell carcinoma: a pilot study. *Exp Dermatol.* 2004;13(7):445–451.

176. Clark C, Bryden A, Dawe R, et al. Topical 5-aminolaevulinic acid photodynamic therapy for cutaneous lesions: outcome and comparison of light sources. *Photodermatol Photoimmunol Photomed.* 2003;19: 134–141.

177. Wang I, Bendsoe N, Klinteberg CA, et al. Photodynamic therapy vs. cryosurgery of basal cell carcinomas: results of a phase III clinical trial. *Br J Dermatol.* 2001;144(4):832–840.

178. Oseroff AR, Shieh S, Frawlet NP, et al. Treatment of diffuse basal cell carcinomas and basaloid follicular hamartomas

179. in nevoid basal cell carcinoma syndrome by wide-area 5-aminolevulinc acid photodynamic therapy. *Arch Dermatol.* 2005;141:60–67.

179. Wiegell SR, Stender IM, Na R, et al. Pain associated with photodynamic therapy using 5-aminolevulinic acid or 5-aminolevulinic acid methylester on tape-stripped normal skin. *Arch Dermatol.* 2003;139(9):1173–1177.

180. Naidenov N, Dencheva R, Tsankov N. Recurrence rate of basal cell carcinoma after topical aminolevulinic acid-based photodynamic therapy. *Acta Dermatovenereol Croat.* 2004;12(3):157–161.

181. Soler AM, Warloe T, Berner A, et al. A follow-up study of recurrence and cosmesis in completely responding superficial and nodular basal cell carcinomas treated with methyl 5-aminolaevulinate-based photodynamic therapy alone and with prior curettage. *Br J Dermatol.* 2001;145(3):467–471.

182. Soler AM, Warloe T, Tausjo J, et al. Photodynamic therapy by topical aminolevulinic acid, dimethylsulphoxide and curettage in nodular basal cell carcinoma: a one-year follow-up study. *Acta Derm Venereol.* 1999;79(3):204–206.

183. Kennedy JC, Pottier RH, Pross DC. Photodynamic therapy with endogenous protoporphyrin IX: basic principles and present clinical experience. *J Photochem Photobiol B.* 1990;6(1/2):143–148.

184. Svanberg K, Andersson T, Killander D, et al. Photodynamic therapy of non-melanoma malignant tumours of the skin using topical delta-amino levulinic acid sensitization and laser irradiation. *Br J Dermatol.* 1994;130(6):743–751.

185. Dijkstra AT, Majoie IM, van Dongen JW, et al. Photodynamic therapy with violet light and topical 6-aminolaevulinic acid in the treatment of actinic keratosis, Bowen's disease and basal cell carcinoma. *J Eur Acad Dermatol Venereol.* 2001;15(6):550–554.

186. Kalka K, Merk H, Mukhtar H. Photodynamic therapy in dermatology. *J Am Acad Dermatol.* 2000;42(3):389–413.

187. Stockfleth E, Sterry W. New treatment modalities for basal cell carcinoma. *Recent Results Cancer Res.* 2002;160: 259–268.

188. Rhodes LE, de Rie M, Enstrom Y, et al. Photodynamic therapy using topical methyl aminolevulinate vs. surgery for nodular basal cell carcinoma: results of a multicenter randomized prospective trial. *Arch Dermatol.* 2004;140(1):17–23.

189. Soler AM, Angell-Petersen E, Warloe T, et al. Photodynamic therapy of superficial basal cell carcinoma with 5-aminolevulinic acid with dimethylsulfoxide and ethylendiaminetetraacetic acid:a comparison of two light sources. *Photochem Photobiol.* 2000;71(6):724–729.

190. Buechner S. Regression of basal cell carcinoma by intralesional interferon-alpha treatment is mediated by CD95 (Apo1/Fas)-CD95 ligand induced suicide. *J Clin Invest.* 1997;100:2691–2696.

191. Villa AM, Berman B. Immunomodulators for skin cancer. *J Drugs Dermatol.* 2004;3(5):533–539.

192. Buechner S. Intralesional interferon-alpha 2b in the treatment of basal cell carcinoma. *J Am Acad Dermatol.* 1991;24: 731–734.

193. Dogan B, Harmanyeri Y, Baloglu H, et al. Intralesional alfa-2a interferon therapy for basal cell carcinoma. *Cancer Lett.* 1995;91(2):215–219.

194. Greenway HT, Cornell RC, Tanner DJ, et al. Treatment of basal cell carcinoma with intralesional interferon. *J Am Acad Dermatol.* 1986;15(3):437–443.

195. Kim KH, Yavel RM, Gross VL, et al. Intralesional interferon alpha-2b in the treatment of basal cell carcinoma and squamous cell carcinoma: revisited. *Dermatol Surg.* 2004;30(1):116–120.

196. Cornell RC, Greenway HT, Tucker SB, et al. Intralesional interferon therapy for basal cell carcinoma. *J Am Acad Dermatol.* 1990;23(4, pt 1):694–700.

197. Stenquist B, Wennberg AM, Gisslen H, et al. Treatment of aggressive basal cell carcinoma with intralesional interferon: evaluation of efficacy by Mohs surgery. *J Am Acad Dermatol.* 1992;27(1):65–69.

198. Alpsoy E, Yilmaz E, Basaran E, et al. Comparison of the effects of intralesional interferon alfa-2a, 2b and the combination of 2a and 2b in the treatment of basal cell carcinoma. *J Dermatol.* 1996;23(6):394–396.

199. Kowalzick L, Rogozinski T, Wimheuer R, et al. Intralesional recombinant interferon beta-1a in the treatment of basal cell carcinoma: results of an open-label multicentre study. *Eur J Dermatol.* 2002; 12(6):558–561.

200. Huber A, Huber JD, Skinner RB, Jr, et al. Topical imiquimod treatment for nodular basal cell carcinomas: an open-label series. *Dermatol Surg.* 2004;30(3):429–430.

201. Vidal D, Matias-Guiu X, Alomar A. Open study of the efficacy and mechanism of action of topical imiquimod in basal cell carcinoma. *Clin Exp Dermatol.* 2004;29(5):518–525.

202. Beutner KR, Geisse JK, Helman D, et al. Therapeutic response of basal cell carcinoma to the immune response modifier imiquimod 5% cream. *J Am Acad Dermatol.* 1999;41(6):1002–1007.

203. Marks R, Gebauer K, Shumack S, et al. Imiquimod 5% cream in the treatment of superficial basal cell carcinoma: results of a multicenter 6-week dose-response trial. *J Am Acad Dermatol.* 2001; 44(5):807–813.

204. Geisse JK, Rich P, Pandya A, et al. Imiquimod 5% cream for the treatment of superficial basal cell carcinoma: a double-blind, randomized, vehicle-controlled study. *J Am Acad Dermatol.* 2002; 47(3):390–398.

205. Shumack S, Robinson J, Kossard S, et al. Efficacy of topical 5% imiquimod cream for the treatment of nodular basal cell carcinoma: comparison of dosing regimens. *Arch Dermatol.* 2002;138(9):1165–1171.

206. Sterry W, Ruzicka T, Herrera E, et al. Imiquimod 5% cream for the treatment of superficial and nodular basal cell carcinoma: randomized studies comparing low-frequency dosing with and without occlusion. *Br J Dermatol.* 2002;147(6): 1227–1236.

207. Vidal D, Alomar A. Efficacy of imiquimod 5% cream for basal cell carcinoma in transplant patients. *Clin Exp Dermatol.* 2004;29(3):237–239.

208. Kagy MK, Amonette R. The use of imiquimod 5% cream for the treatment of superficial basal cell carcinomas in a

basal cell nevus patient. *Dermatol Surg.* 2000;26:577–578.

209. Weisberg NK, Varghese M. Therapeutic response of a brother and sister with xeroderma pigmentosum to imiquimod 5% cream. *Dermatol Surg.* 2002;28: 518–523.

210. Bath-Hextall F, Bong J, Perkins W, et al. Interventions for basal cell carcinoma of the skin: systematic review. *BMJ.* 2004; 329(7468):705.

211. Reymann F. Treatment of basal cell carcinoma of the skin with 5-fluorouracil ointment. *Dermatologica.* 1979;158(5): 368–372.

212. Epstein E. Fluorouracil paste treatment of thin basal cell carcinomas. *Arch Dermatol.* 1985;121(2):207–213.

213. Miller BH, Shavin JS, Cognetta A, et al. Nonsurgical treatment of basal cell carcinomas with intralesional 5-fluorouracil/epinephrine injectable gel. *J Am Acad Dermatol.* 1997;36:72–77.

214. Hansen LA, Sigman CC, Andreola F, et al. Retinoids in chemoprevention and differentiation therapy. *Carcinogenesis.* 2000;21(7):1271–1279.

215. Marks R, Motley RJ. Skin cancer recognition and treatment. *Drugs.* 1995;50(1): 48–61.

216. Hodak E, Ginzburg A, David M, et al. Etretinate treatment of nevoid basal cell carcinoma syndrome. Therapeutic and chemopreventive effect. *Int J Dermatol.* 1987;26:606–609.

217. Tangrea JA, Edwards BK, Taylor PR, et al. Long-term therapy with low-dose isotretinoin for prevention of basal cell carcinoma: a multicenter clinical trial. *J Natl Cancer Inst.* 1992;84: 328–332.

218. Levine N, Moon T, Cartmel B, et al. Trial of retinol and isotretinoin in skin cancer prevention: a randomized, double-blind, controlled trial. *Cancer Epidemiol Biomarkers Prev.* 1997;6:957–961.

219. Van Dam RM, Zhiping H, Giovannucci E, et al. Diet and basal cell carcinoma of the skin in a prospective cohort of men. *Am J Clin Nutr.* 2000;7:135–141.

220. Hunter DJ, Colditz GA, Stampfer MJ, et al. Diet and risk of basal cell carcinoma of the skin in a prospective cohort of women. *Ann Epidemiol.* 1992;2: 231–239.

221. Peris K, Fargnoli MC, Chimenti S. Preliminary observations on the use of topical tazarotene to treat basal-cell carcinoma. *N Engl J Med.* 1999;341: 1767–1768.

222. Orlandi A, Bianchi L, Costanzo A, et al. Evidence of increased apoptosis and reduced proliferation in basal cell carcinomas treated with tazarotene. *J Invest Dermatol.* 2004;122:1037–1041.

223. Bialy TL, Rothe MJ, Grant-Kels JM. Dietary factors in the prevention and treatment of nonmelanoma skin cancer and melanoma. *Dermatol Surg.* 2002;28: 1143–1152.

224. De Graaf YG, Euvrard S, Bouwes Bavinck JN. Systemic and topical retinoids in the management of skin cancer in organ transplant recipients. *Dermatol Surg.* 2004;30(4, pt 2):656–661.

225. Smalley W, Ray WA, Daugherty J, et al. Use of nonsteroidal anti-inflammatory drugs and incidence of colorectal cancer: a population-based study. *Arch Intern Med.* 1999;159(2):161–166.

226. Neugut AI, Rosenberg DJ, Ahsan H, et al. Association between coronary heart disease and cancers of the breast, prostate, and colon. *Cancer Epidemiol Biomarkers Prev.* 1998;7(10):869–873.

227. Langman MJ, Cheng KK, Gilman EA, et al. Effect of anti-inflammatory drugs on overall risk of common cancer: case–control study in general practice research database. *BMJ.* 2000;320(7250):1642–1646.

228. Gann PH, Manson JE, Glynn RJ, et al. Low-dose aspirin and incidence of colorectal tumors in a randomized trial. *J Natl Cancer Inst.* 1993;85(15):1220–1224.

229. Harris RE, Namboodiri KK, Farrar WB. Nonsteroidal antiinflammatory drugs and breast cancer. *Epidemiology.* 1996;7 (2):203–205.

230. Muller-Decker K, Scholz K, Marks F, et al. Differential expression of prostaglandin H synthase isozymes during multistage carcinogenesis in mouse epidermis. *Mol Carcinogen.* 1995;12(1):31–41.

231. Bissett DL, Chatterjee R, Hannon DP. Photoprotective effect of topical anti-inflammatory agents against ultraviolet radiation-induced chronic skin damage in the hairless mouse. *Photodermatol Photoimmunol Photomed.* 1990;7(4):153–158.

232. Lowe NJ, Connor MJ, Breeding J, et al. Inhibition of ultraviolet-B epidermal ornithine decarboxylase induction and skin carcinogenesis in hairless mice by topical indomethacin and triamcinolone acetonide. *Cancer Res.* 1982;42(10): 3941–3943.

233. Reeve VE, Matheson MJ, Bosnic M, et al. The protective effect of indomethacin on photocarcinogenesis in hairless mice. *Cancer Lett.* 1995;95(1/2):213–219.

234. Haedersdal M, Poulsen T, Wulf HC. Effects of systemic indomethacin on photocarcinogenesis in hairless mice. *J Cancer Res Clin Oncol.* 1995;121(5):257–261.

235. Mamdani M, Juurlink DN, Lee DS, et al. Cyclo-oxygenase-2 inhibitors versus non-selective non-steroidal anti-inflammatory drugs and congestive heart failure outcomes in elderly patients:a population-based cohort study. *Lancet.* 2004; 363(9423):1751–1756.

236. Roth J, Granick M. Squamous cell and adnexal carcinomas of the skin. *Clin Plast Surg.* 1997;24:695.

237. Available at: www.aad.org.

CHAPTER 7

Squamous Cell Carcinoma of the Skin

Rana Anadolu-Brasie, M.D.
Asha R. Patel, B.S.
Shalu S. Patel, B.S.
Anita Singh, M.S.
Keyvan Nouri, M.D.

BOX 7-1 Overview

- Squamous cell carcinoma (SCC) is a non-melanoma skin cancer. It is the second most common type of cancer in humans worldwide.
- SCC pathogenesis is a multistep process that involves both extrinsic and intrinsic factors that ultimately lead to carcinogenesis.
- The main etiologic factors that lead to SCC are natural, occupational, or artificial cumulative UV exposure. Others include HPV infection, chronic immunosuppression, ionizing radiation, scarring, and exposure to certain carcinogens.
- UV-induced DNA mutations in the p53 tumor suppressor gene are reported to be associated with 90% of SCCs.
- Genodermatoses such as XP, epidermodysplasia verruciformis (EV), and oculocutaneous albinism (OCA) are associated with high incidence of early onset and multiple SCC.
- SCCs, both *in situ* and invasive forms, present in many clinical forms with different biological behavior. These include AK, AC, BD, EQ, common invasive SCC, BSC, verrucous carcinoma, KA, spindle cell SCC, lymphoepithelial carcinoma, acantholytic SCC, DSCC, as well as others.
- The diagnosis of SCC is based on patient history, clinical manifestations, and most importantly histopathologic examination of the lesion.
- The gold standard for the treatment of SCC is to remove or destroy the neoplastic tissue by means of simple surgical excision, Mohs surgery, cryotherapy, and laser ablation. Topically applied antimetabolites can also be used and these include 5-flourouracil (5-FU), immunomodulators, anti-inflammatory agents, or PDT.
- Chemoprevention of SCC is achievable, both by using topical or systemic UV protectors, and possibly by topical and systemic anti-inflammatory and immunomodulator agents.
- Acknowledging and learning appropriate prevention techniques is an essential component to decrease the risk of SCC.

INTRODUCTION

Squamous cell carcinoma (SCC) is the malignant neoplasm of keratinocytes that constitutes the epidermis, mucosal epithelium, and the epithelium of adnexal structures. SCC is the second most common malignant skin neoplasm, and can arise *de novo* in the skin, as well as preceded by natural or artificial ultraviolet (UV) damage, human papillomavirus (HPV) infection, human immunodeficiency virus (HIV) infection, immunosuppression, radiation, scarring, adjacent chronic ulcer, sinus or fistula formation, and exposure to carcinogens.

SCC has many clinical and histopathologic variants that show different biological behavior. The term SCC *in situ* defines the malignant neoplasm that is only confined to the epidermis or the epithelium. When the neoplasm extends through or presents beneath the basement membrane zone in the dermis or even deeper in the skin, then it is called invasive SCC. There are a significant number of invasive SCCs shown to develop from a preceding *in situ* SCC at the same site.

Actinic keratosis (AK) is a form of SCC *in situ* that may evolve into invasive carcinoma; however, it rarely metastasizes to the regional lymph nodes. On the other hand, certain types of SCCs such as the ones arising on radiation or burn scars, or in immunocompromised patients, usually behave more aggressively and frequently metastasize to the regional lymph nodes and even distantly to other sites. SCCs of the skin that carry the potential of being locally destructive, and being able to metastasize locally, and rarely systemically, require early diagnosis and adequate treatment as well as preventive measures.

EPIDEMIOLOGY

BOX 7-2 Summary

- Skin cancers constitute about half the cases of all cancers combined.
- Most cases of skin cancers are BCCs and SCCs.
- Death is an uncommon outcome of non-melanoma skin cancers.

- Many cancer registries still do not have the exact numbers of nonmelanoma skin cancers, but BCC is calculated to be four times more frequent than SCC.
- The overall increase in the number of SCC and BCC during the last decade is attributed mostly to increased UVR exposure due to both lifestyle changes and the depleted stratospheric ozone layer.
- Another factor that may be important in determining the increase in the numbers of SCCs and BCCs is increased public awareness.
- Among all skin cancers, SCC seems to be the one, which is the most positively correlated with total and occupational UVR exposure.
- SCCs are mostly located on body sites that have the highest cumulative UVR exposure such as the head and neck region.
- UVB radiation is more associated with SCCs and the amount of UVB radiation is also dependent on the latitude.
- SCCs in general are expected to be more frequent in individuals older than 45 to 50 and more common in males than females, with the highest incidence among skin type I and II Caucasians.
- SCCs in other ethic groups are usually non-UV related and associated with other risk factors.
- SCC incidence is increased in transplant patients associated with HPV

Among all cancers, skin cancer (both melanoma and nonmelanoma) constitutes about half of the cancer cases.[1] An estimated number of 1 million new cases per year is diagnosed as nonmelanoma skin cancer in the United States and 2 to 3 million throughout the world. These cases are mostly comprised of basal cell carcinomas (BCCs) and SCCs.[2,3] Despite the high frequency, death is an uncommon outcome of nonmelanoma skin cancers, excluding the very aggressive or advanced types or in the elderly and immunocompromised patients. Although mortality is not the main concern, morbidity of these skin cancers can be very high. However, many cancer registries still do not have the exact numbers for nonmelanoma skin cancers including SCC.[1,4]

A population-based study revealed a 1% incidence rate for SCC in Australia.[4] The estimated incidence of SCC in the United States is 100,000 to 200,000 cases per year, and BCC is four times more frequent than SCC according to the cancer statistics in 1990.[5] Miller et al. estimated the lifetime risk of developing SCC as

7 to 10% for a child born in 1994.[6] The age-adjusted incidence rates for SCC were given as 81 to 136 for males and 26 to 59 for females per 100,000 individuals in a 1-year period among the U.S. Caucasian population.[6] Holme et al. reported a significant rise in the incidence of nonmelanoma skin cancer over a 10-year period between 1988 and 1998 in South Wales, and indicated a 16% increase in SCC crude rate alone from 35.8 to 41.2 per 100,000 population.[7]

The overall increase in the number of SCCs and BCCs over the last decade is attributed mostly to increased UV radiation (UVR) exposure due to both lifestyle changes and the depleted stratospheric ozone layer. It is predicted that for every 10% decrease in ozone layer, a 40% increase in skin cancer has to be expected.[8] Another factor that may be important in determining the increase in the numbers of SCCs and BCCs is increased public awareness. This may have an impact on the number of patients that seek medical examination and diagnosed as having an SCC or BCC.

Among all skin cancers, SCC seems to be the one which is the most positively correlated with total and occupational UVR exposure.[9] SCCs are mostly located on body sites that have the highest cumulative UVR exposure, such as the head and neck region. On the other hand, BCC and melanoma seem to be more related to nonoccupational UVR exposure and an early-age sunburn history. Experimental studies have shown that the peak values of the UVR spectrum are 293 to 380 nm in inducing SCC in the animal models. These peak values are mostly within the UVB waveband range.[9] The amount of UVB radiation is also dependent on the latitude. The incidence of SCC has been shown to increase at latitudes closer to the equator. In fact, there is a two-fold increase in SCC incidence for every 10° decline toward the equator.[10]

Cumulative UVR exposure is closely related to the age of the individual, as well as, the skin type. SCCs in general are expected to be more frequent in individuals older than 45 to 50 and more common in males than females, with the highest incidence among skin type I and II Caucasians.[1,4,11–13] The incidence of nonmelanoma skin cancer in general and SCC in particular increases with age.[1,11,14] Recently, the increase is reported to be even more significant in younger age groups. Males between the ages of 36 and 39 are found to have two times more SCCs than the females in the same age group.[14] SCC is not common among other ethnic groups (e.g.,

Black, Asian, or Hispanics). SCCs that occur in these individuals are usually non-UV related and associated with other risk factors.

PATHOGENESIS

BOX 7-3 Summary

- SCC pathogenesis is a multistep process that involves both extrinsic and intrinsic factors that ultimately lead to carcinogenesis.
- Mutations in protooncogenes and tumor suppressor genes are important to the pathogenesis of SCC.
- The most important extrinsic risk factor for the development of SCC is UV radiation. UVA causes indirect damage through the production of ROS, while UVB is responsible for more direct and destructive biological mutation.
- UV exposure is known to induce an inflammatory response within the skin. Specific inflammatory factors include prostaglandins, TNF, and interleukin-1 alpha.
- Another important extrinsic factor is infectious diseases, most importantly the DNA virus and human papillomavirus (HPV). HPV E7 and E6 oncoproteins have been found to functionally inactivate tumor suppressor genes RB and p53.
- Other extrinsic factors include chemical carcinogens, arsenic, polycyclic aromatic hydrocarbons, tobacco, and ionizing radiation. These agents are dose-dependent and the time period between exposure and carcinoma may be decades.
- Important intrinsic risk factors include immune status and genetics of the host. Organ transplant recipients, xeroderma pigmentosum (XP) patients, and oculocutaneous albinism (OCA) patients are more prone to SCC development.
- Immunosuppressants, such as azathioprine and cyclosporine A are potentially mutagenic.

The multistage model of skin carcinogenesis is the basic foundation of understanding SCC pathogenesis. The multiple cellular events that result in SCC development are believed to include both extrinsic and intrinsic factors. Extrinsic risk factors comprise various environmental exposures and infectious disease. SCC incidence is increased in transplant patients associated with HPV. Intrinsic risk factors include genetic predispositions including certain phenotypes and specific pathogenic mutations. These factors are believed to work synergistically, thereby using a multistep process resulting in carcinogenesis.[15,16]

The combination of risk factors affects normal keratinocytes ultimately by causing a series of mutations within certain genes. These genes are regulators of cell growth and development and are known as protooncogenes and tumor suppressor genes. Protooncogenes are responsible for growth signaling and, if mutated, they result in oncogenes. Oncogenes trigger constitutive activation of growth, thereby allowing tumor cells to grow out of proportion compared to surrounding normal cells. Tumor suppressor genes allow cells to restrict their growth by promoting apoptosis and limiting growth factors primarily. If these genes are mutated, the cells are not restricted or regulated and may result in carcinogenesis. In general, protooncogenes need only one mutation of a single copy ("single hit") to result in a carcinogenic manifestation whereas tumor suppressor genes need both copies of the gene to be inactivated ("double hit").[16,17]

The most infamous extrinsic risk factor is known to be UV radiation,[18,19] which is subdivided into two wavebands, UVA (315 to 400 nm) and UVB (280 to 315 nm).[19] UVA is known to cause indirect damage by producing reactive oxygen species (ROS) that results in oxidative damage to DNA, proteins, and lipids. Certain ROS that have been identified in the epidermis are superoxides and hydrogen peroxide. UVB has been known to be responsible for more of the direct and destructive biological mutations.[18]

The epidermal lining of the skin is naturally equipped with antioxidant enzymes such as superoxide dismutase, glutathione peroxidase, and catalase, which dispose off harmful ROS produced by UV radiation.[20] However, it has been reported that the amplified ROS production after UV contact can diminish these natural defenses thus resulting in a higher susceptibility to biological damage.[21] ROS also induce gene point mutations, specifically affecting guanine bases mutating them to either thymine, cytosine, or adenine.[18] Another mechanism of indirect damage secondary to UV radiation is the production of reactive nitrogen species that are known to cause nitrosylation of tyrosine, lipid peroxidation, and general disruption of cellular function. These changes occur because UVA and UVB activate nitric oxide synthase in the epidermis, which increases nitric oxide (NO) concentration. The excess NO then combines with UV-induced superoxide to form peroxynitrite, the free radical known to damage DNA.[18,22,23] Another consequence of peroxynitrite production is the activation of poly(ADP-ribose) polymerase (PARP) that reduces ATP formation which may lead to energy loss and cell death in severe cases.[18,24]

UV exposure is known to induce an inflammatory response within the skin. An increase in blood flow to the exposed site transports macrophages, neutrophils, and other innate inflammatory factors to the area. Inflammatory factors and cells produce ROS that add to the cycle of biological damage. Specific inflammatory factors that have been reported to produce ROS are prostaglandins (PGE2), tumor necrosis factor (TNF), and interleukin 1α (IL-1α). Therefore, UV exposure induces inflammation that further instigates DNA defects via production of ROS.[18]

As mentioned earlier, UVB causes more direct DNA damage. This direct damage is actually a trademark of UVB and consists of actual mutations from Guanine-Cytosine (GC) → Adenine-Thymine (AT) when occurring at tandem dipyrimidine (Py-Py) sites or pyrimidine (Py) sets. This specific mutation is known as a UVB fingerprint mutation.[25]

It has also been suggested that UV radiation affects the immune system via various methods of suppression. Different theories are focusing on the reduction of enzymes, immune cells, and signaling cascades in the areas exposed to UV radiation. More interestingly, recent studies have shown a stronger connection with UVA radiation as opposed to formerly thought UVB radiation. However, more discussion and research are needed to investigate these newfound theories.[18]

Another extrinsic factor that has had a great impact on the pathogenesis of SCC is infectious disease, most importantly the DNA virus, HPV. The virus is a member of the *Papovaviridae* family and is part of the *Papillomavirus* genus.[26] There are certain types that have been found to be more oncogenic than others. Types 16, 18, 31, 33, 35, and 58 are believed to contribute to cervical cancer.[15] Types 36, 38, and 8 have been identified in cutaneous carcinomas, indicating that these specific strains may be involved in skin neoplastic changes.[15,26] Oncoproteins such as HPV E7 and E6 have been identified to functionally inactivate tumor suppressor genes RB and p53; thereby behaving like direct mutations caused by UV radiation.[16] It is important to note that these findings are still controversial and that HPV is also found in skin without any evidence of neoplastic changes.[15,26] Other infectious diseases such as human herpesvirus (HHV) type 6 and type 1 are also under study, detecting yet another possible association between viral etiology

and nonmelanoma skin cancer.[27] Further research is warranted to garner more evidence regarding the correlation between HPV and skin carcinoma.[26,28,29]

It should also be mentioned that extrinsic factors such as chemical carcinogens have undoubtedly been associated with SCC development. Compounds such as arsenic, polycyclic aromatic hydrocarbons, and tobacco are sources of carcinogenic agents that progressively lead to the neoplastic changes characteristic of SCC. These agents are dose-dependent and the time period between exposure and carcinoma may be decades.[30–32] However, current knowledge has steadily decreased SCC incidence secondary to these preventable factors. Ionizing radiation has also been indicated in the formation of skin cancer. This risk factor strongly existed in the era when radiotherapy was used as treatment for benign processes such as acne, hypertrichosis, and hemangiomas. In those times, protection from X-rays was nonexistent due to the lack of knowledge regarding its carcinogenic potential. Occupational risk still may exist today as physicians, technicians, and engineers among others are exposed to varying amounts of radiation.[33]

Intrinsic risk factors of SCC mostly depend upon the immune status and genetics of the host. It is a known fact that both the degree and chronicity of immunosuppression play a role in developing carcinoma. There have been many research analyses regarding the strong association between organ transplant recipients receiving various immunosuppressants and the incidence of nonmelanoma skin carcinoma.[34] SCC is the most common post-transplantation malignancy.[35] Studies by Glover, Jensen, and most recently Kasiske showed statistically significant associations between certain regimens of medication and SCC.[36–38] Iatrogenic immunosuppression along with slight histoincompatibilities between host and donor antigens may allow for a subclinical chronic immune response that may facilitate tumor growth. Immunosuppressants such as azathioprine and cyclosporine A are also potentially mutagenic, compounding the issue further.[39] It should also be mentioned that genodermatoses such as xeroderma pigmentosum (XP) and oculocutaneous albinism (OCA) are more prone to SCC development. Both conditions are autosomal recessive and patients tend to acquire skin carcinomas at a younger age due to their inability to naturally protect themselves from UV radiation. XP patients have a deficit in the excision repair mechanism for

UV-induced signature mutations. OCA is characterized by the congenital absence of melanin, a pigment that naturally protects against UV radiation.[40,41]

CLINICAL MANIFESTATIONS AND DIAGNOSES OF SQUAMOUS CELL CARCINOMA

BOX 7-4 Summary

- Cutaneous SCC has two main forms: SCC *in situ* and invasive SCC. These two variants carry different clinical and prognostic features.
- *In situ* SCCs include: AK, AC, BD, erythroplasia of Queyrat, and leukoplakia.
- Invasive SCCs include: common invasive SCC, *de novo* invasive SCC, solitary KA, Bowen type of invasive SCC, verrucous carcinoma, epithelioma cuniculatum, verrucous carcinoma of the oral mucosa, acantholytic SCC, spindle cell SCC, papillary SCC, signet ring SCC, pigmented SCC, DSCC, clear cell SCC, adenosquamous carcinoma, BSC, malignant proliferating pilar tumor/cyst, SCC arising in adnexal cysts, FSCC, squamoid eccrine ductal carcinoma, lymphoepithelioma-like carcinoma, and tricholemmal carcinoma.
- Prognostically, SCC variants can be divided into four categories: (1) low-risk SCCs (metastatic rate < 2%), (2) intermediate-risk SCCs (metastatic rate 3 to 10%), (3) high-risk SCCs (metastatic rate ≥ 10%), and (4) SCCs with indeterminate risk.
- SCC uses the Broders grading system, which correlates biologic behavior of the tumor with the degree of histologic differentiation.
- The diagnosis of SCC is based on history, clinical manifestations, and histopathologic examination of the lesion.

Cutaneous SCC arises from malignant proliferation of the keratinocytes in the epidermis and adnexa. This neoplasm develops predominantly on sun-exposed areas of the skin and is considered the second most common skin cancer.

Cutaneous SCC manifests itself in two main forms: (1) SCC *in situ*, where the neoplasm is confined to the epidermis, and (2) Invasive SCC, where the neoplasm extends beyond the epidermis. These two forms have many clinical and histopathologic variants that carry different clinical and prognostic features. For SCC *in situ* and even locally invasive SCC, appropriate therapy is usually curative. Nonetheless, SCC may metastasize to lymph nodes and organs, can cause significant morbidity and even death.[42] In the case of invasive SCC, the degree of histopathologic differentiation of the tumor is of extreme importance. Well-differentiated SCC has a cure rate of 99.4% following Mohs surgery, whereas in poorly differentiated SCC, this rate decreases down to 42.1%.[43]

The major factors that have a great impact on treatment choice, follow-up regimen, and prognosis include: the clinical size of the neoplasm; location of the neoplasm; history of previous treatment followed by recurrence; anatomical depth of the tumor, in regard to, cutaneous layers and structures; the vertical histopathologic tumor thickness in millimeters; presence of perineural, muscle, subcutaneous fat, and cartilage invasion; and local and/or distant metastases.[44–48]

Prognostically, SCC variants can be divided into four categories: (1) low-risk SCCs (metastatic rate < 2%), (2) intermediate-risk SCCs (metastatic rate 3 to 10%), (3) high-risk SCCs (metastatic rate ≥ 10%), and (4) SCCs with indeterminate risk. Low-risk SCCs include: *in situ* SCCs, invasive SCCs derived from AK, invasive SCC solitary keratoacanthoma (KA) type, HPV-associated invasive SCC, tricholemmal carcinoma, and spindle cell SCC that is not associated with radiation. Intermediate-risk SCCs include: acantholytic invasive SCC and lymphoepithelioma-like carcinoma of the skin. High-risk subtypes include: *de novo* invasive SCCs; SCC arising in association with predisposing factors such as, radiation, burns, scars, and immunosuppression; invasive Bowen disease (BD); adenosquamous carcinoma; basosquamous carcinoma (BSC); desmoplastic SCC (DSCC); and invasive SCC arising from proliferating pilar tumor/cyst (malignant proliferating pilar tumor). The indeterminate category includes signet ring cell invasive SCC, follicular SCC, papillary SCC, SCC arising in eccrine and apocrine sweat gland cysts, squamoid eccrine ductal carcinoma, and clear-cell SCC.[45,49–59]

SCC uses the Broders grading system, which correlates biologic behavior of the tumor with the degree of histologic differentiation. Broders grade 1 represents well-differentiated to moderately well-differentiated cells that microscopically show abundant keratinization, little nuclear anaplasia, and less than 25% undifferentiated cells. Broders grade 2 represents moderately differentiated cells that are 50% keratinizing. In addition, in grade 2, there is nuclear anaplasia present and less than 50% undifferentiated cells. Broders grade 3 represents moderately to poorly differentiated

cells. These cells are less than 25% keratinizing, extensive nuclear anaplasia, and less than 75% undifferentiated cells. Finally, Broders grade 4 represents poorly differentiated cells. Grade 4 has extensive nuclear anaplasia, little or no keratinization, includes spindle cell and undifferentiated carcinomas, and greater than 75% undifferentiated cells.[60]

In situ Squamous Cell Carcinomas

SCC *IN SITU*—ACTINIC KERATOSIS/ACTINIC CHELITIS TYPE

BOX 7-5   Summary

- AKs are the most common type of *in situ* SCC of the skin among light-skinned individuals.
- AK is the initial manifestation of a continuum of clinical and histopathologic abnormalities that progress into invasive SCC.
- Clinical manifestations of AK are usually very subtle and asymptomatic. In the most common form, AK appears as an ill-defined, subtle, erythematous macule with a slightly hyperkeratotic surface on sun-exposed areas.
- The key to clinical diagnosis on physical examination is the sandpaper-like sensation felt on touching the surface of these persistent skin lesions on sun-damaged skin.
- AC is the mucosal analog of AK and is located primarily on the lip. This lesion mostly occurs on the lower lip as slight scaling on an erythematous base.
- The gold standard in diagnosing AK/AC type of SCC *in situ* is histopathologic examination of the affected skin/mucosa biopsy specimen.

Actinic Keratosis (AK), also known as solar keratoses (SK), are the most common type of *in situ* SCC of the skin among light-skinned individuals. These lesions are confined to the epidermis and develop solely on sun-damaged skin. Up to 25% of the adult population in the Northern hemisphere has at least one AK. In addition, the incidence is strikingly increased with latitudes close to the equator.[61]

Dubreuilh was the first author to describe AK as a separate entity in 1896 and emphasized its relation to skin aging and skin cancer. From then on, AK/SK has been recognized and eventually classified as a "precancerous" skin lesion that is common in the elderly.[62,63] Ackerman suggested AK/AC is not a "precancerous" skin lesion, but, in fact, SCC *in situ*.[64–67] Although the subject is still a matter of discussion for some authors, especially due to the unknown

natural course of untreated AK, as well as treatment and reimbursement issues, there is an increasing consensus among dermatologists that AK/AC is representative of SCC *in situ*.[68–83]

AK is the initial manifestation of a continuum of clinical and histopathologic abnormalities that progress into invasive SCC.[67,68,70–75,83,84] The risk of progression to invasive SCC has been estimated to range from 0.25 to 20% per year.[85] One study actually showed that AK was contiguous with SCC in 72% of the cases.[86]

Clinical manifestations of AK are usually very subtle and asymptomatic. In the most common form, AK appears as an ill-defined, subtle, erythematous macule with a slightly hyperkeratotic surface on sun-exposed areas of the head and neck, forearms, hands, and upper back. Lesions can be multiple, usually less than 1 cm in diameter. Multiple adjacent lesions can merge and become confluent patches with time or become slightly elevated in the form of subtle flat plaques. AKs may appear pigmented with a tan-brown color, as well as red or skin color with no well-defined borders. In addition, the surface of AKs has a dry, firmly adherent scale with a rough, sandpaper-like consistency. The key to clinical diagnosis on physical examination is the sandpaper-like sensation felt on touching the surface of these persistent skin lesions on sun-damaged skin (Figs. 7-1 and 7-2).

AKs may manifest themselves in many different clinical forms other than

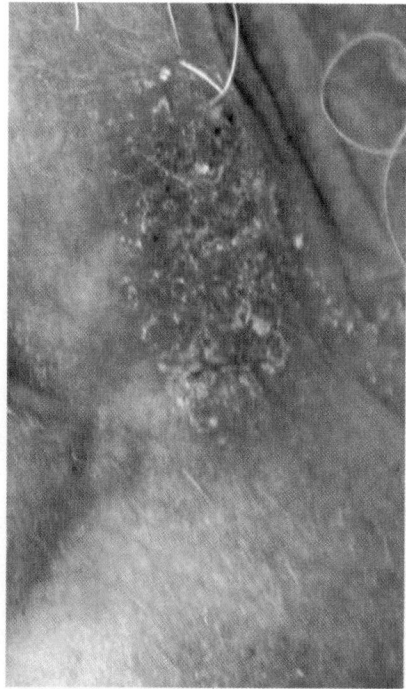

▲ **FIGURE 7-1** Solitary AK on the face of an elderly male.

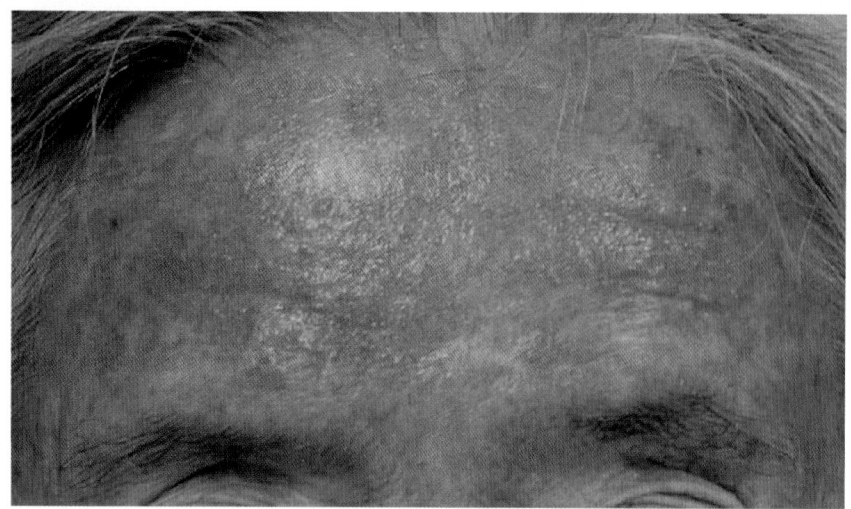

▲ **FIGURE 7-2** Confluent AK on the forehead of an elderly female.

the earlier-mentioned classical clinical descriptions. These other clinical forms include: atrophic, keratotic papular, verrucous/papillomatous, hyperplastic, pigmented, and cutaneous horn. The cutaneous horn type displays marked visible hyperkeratosis, leading to a horn-like mass.[67,69,70,72,87] Clinical differential diagnoses of AK include inflammatory conditions like: seborrheic dermatitis, psoriasis vulgaris, contact dermatitis, pitriasis rosea, lichen planus, lichen planus-like keratosis, invasive SCC, lentigines, seborheic keratosis, Bowen disease (BD), melanoma in situ, superficial multicentric BCC, as well as others.

Actinic chelitis (AC) is the mucosal analog of AK, and is located primarily on the lip. This lesion mostly occurs on the lower lip as slight scaling on an erythematous base (Fig. 7-3). Small wrinkles may also appear on the lip. Commonly, the entire lower lip can be involved. In one study done in 2004,[88] the mean age at the time of diagnosis of AC was 53.1 ± 11.4 years and it was found that 60% used tobacco, while 66.2% had an outdoor occupation. This study revealed three clinical forms of AC, which are: white nonulcerated lesions, erosions or ulcers of the lip, and mixed white and erosive. The clinical picture is almost indistinguishable from chelitis simplex or contact dermatitis of the lip in many cases. Surrounding skin and mucosa generally show other signs of sun damage, which include atrophy, solar lentigines, telengiectasias, etc.[70,89–91]

When AC progress into invasive SCC of the lip, usually the lesion becomes more circumscribed, which is associated with slight infiltration, and the vermilion border of the lip loses its usual plasticity. Eventually, ulceration follows as a definitive sign of invasive SCC. One study showed that intense inflammatory infiltrate in the corium may also be a warning sign for the possibility of microinvasive SCC in the nearby tissue.[92] This study also showed that 85% of ACs were immunoreactive to the p53 protein, but the conclusion was that it would not be helpful to add the p53 protein immunohistochemical study to histopathologic criteria because no statistically significant correlation was found between the p53 expression and any other histopathologic criterion.

The gold standard in diagnosing AK/AC type of SCC in situ is histopathologic examination of the affected skin/mucosa biopsy specimen. Histopathologically, AK/AC specimens show the very early findings of SCC in situ most prominently and characteristically at the basal layer of the epidermis. The typical findings in the basal layer are: proliferation of atypical keratinocytes that exhibit nuclear hyperchromasia, pleomorphism, atypical and increased mitosis, high nuclear/cytoplasmic ratio, and loss of polarity of the nuclei.[67,69,72] The increased number of atypical cells in the basal layer results in a crowded appearance, and eventually leads to slight budding extensions toward the superficial papillary dermis.[67,69] Thickening of the upper layers of the epidermis can be found in the form of acanthosis, where keratinocytes with ample eosinophilic cytoplasms reach the upper layers of the epidermis, exhibiting hyperparakeratosis and occasional dyskeratosis. Typically, in early AK, follicular and acrosyringeal epithelium are spared or less affected by the neoplastic process, and alternating columns of hyperparakeratosis and hyperorthokeratosis are observed.[65,93]

Histopathologic characteristics of AC include: alterations of the thickness of the spinous cell layer, increased thickness of the keratin layer, epithelial dysplasia, connective tissue changes, perivascular inflammation, and basophilic changes of the connective tissue.[88,94] In the dermis, varying degrees of solar elastosis accompany the typical overlying epidermal changes. Slight to moderately dense inflammatory cell infiltration may also be observed, composed of mainly mononuclear cells with occasional eosinophils and plasma cells.[67,69] Parallel to the clinical expressions and variations, additional findings such as epidermal atrophy, prominent or verrucous epidermal hyperplasia, increased melanin pigmentation, lichenoid or band-like inflammatory infiltrate, cutaneous horn formation, neoplastic intraepidermal acantholysis, as well as others may be present.[71,95,96]

The histopathologic distinction between a superficial SCC and a thick or hyperplastic AK/AC is often very difficult. Remembering the description of in situ carcinoma can be helpful. However, it is not always possible to decide whether or not the neoplastic process is still confined to and within the boundaries of an intact epidermal basement membrane (Figs. 7-4 to 7-9).

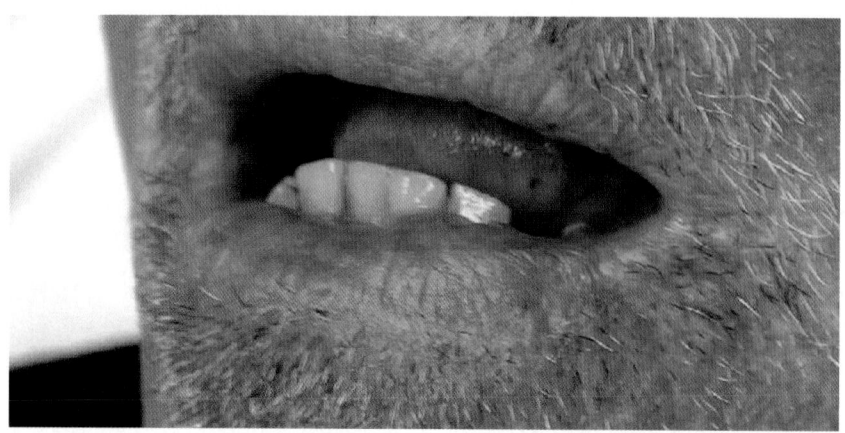

▲ **FIGURE 7-3** AC on the lower lip.

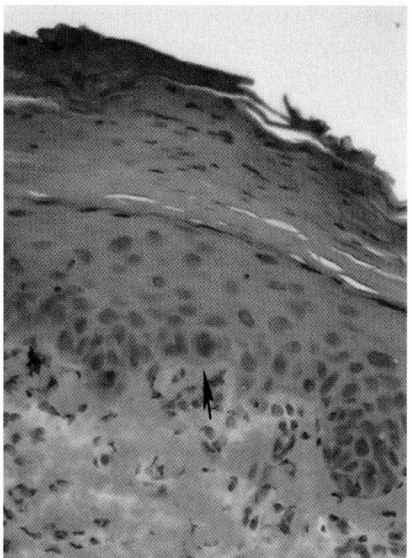

▲ **FIGURE 7-4** AK—early H&E, atypical keratinocyte at the basal layer (*arrow*).

SCC *IN SITU* BOWEN TYPE: BOWEN DISEASE (BD)

BOX 7-6 Summary

- BD is a type of SCC *in situ* with dysplasia at all levels of the epidermis.
- BD occurs both on the skin and mucosal surfaces, which further augments clinical manifestations and complicates nomenclature with various clinical entities.
- BD occurs mainly in the elderly and, in general, affects both sexes with a slight female predominance.
- The lesions mostly occur both on sun-exposed skin and mucosa, with the head and neck the most commonly affected anatomic locations, followed by the limbs.
- Clinically, BD appears as an erythematous, scaly, and/or crusty macule, patch, papule, or plaque with sharply defined borders.
- BD can be found on the oral, anal, as well as both male and female genital mucosa.
- Histopathologically, the lesions of BD on the skin and mucosa share many similar features of SCC *in situ* throughout all levels of the epidermis.

BD is a type of SCC *in situ* with dysplasia at all levels of the epidermis. Bowen described this entity in 1912 in two patients and defined it as a precancerous dermatosis.[97] The relationship between BD and the increased incidence of internal malignancy in these patients has been widely discussed by several authors.[98–100] It is possible that some common neoplastic initiator or promoter factors, e.g., ingested carcinogens or oncogenic virus infections, such as

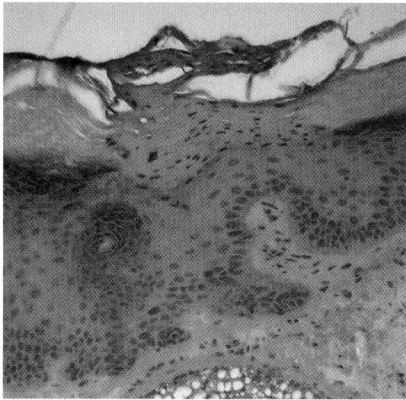

▲ **FIGURE 7-5** AK—hyperparakeratosis, acanthosis, crowding of the keratinocyte nuclei in the basal layer, prominent solar elastosis in the upper dermis (H&E high magnification).

HPV, may play a role in these cases rather than BD being the only paraneoplastic manifestation.[101–103]

This type of SCC *in situ* occurs both on the skin and mucosal surfaces, which further augments clinical manifestations, and complicates nomenclature with various clinical entities, such as erythroplasia of Queyrat, malignant erythroplakia, malignant leukoplakia, bowenoid papulosis, vulvar intraepidermal neoplasia (VIN), kraurosis vulva, and anal intraepidermal neoplasia, of which all possibly belong to the category of SCC *in situ*.[102–111] Without proper treatment, BD may develop into an invasive SCC.

BD occurs mainly in the elderly, and, in general, affects both sexes with a slight female predominance.[102,103,112] The lesions mostly occur both on sun-exposed skin and mucosa, with the head and neck being the most commonly affected anatomic locations, followed by the limbs. Eighty percent of the cases present with a single lesion, and patients with multiple lesions may be due to HPV infection, arsenic, and other carcinogen ingestion.[103]

Clinically, BD appears as an erythematous, scaly, and/or crusty macule, patch, papule, or plaque with sharply defined borders. The lesions can vary in size and tend to enlarge very slowly. Plaques may be composed of reddish lenticular papules, tending to extend gradually in an annular or polycyclic pattern. Occasionally, the lesions may be fissured, verrucous, or pigmented. On the nail bed, it may present as a periungual scaling or an erosion with crusting and nail discoloration.[70,103,112]

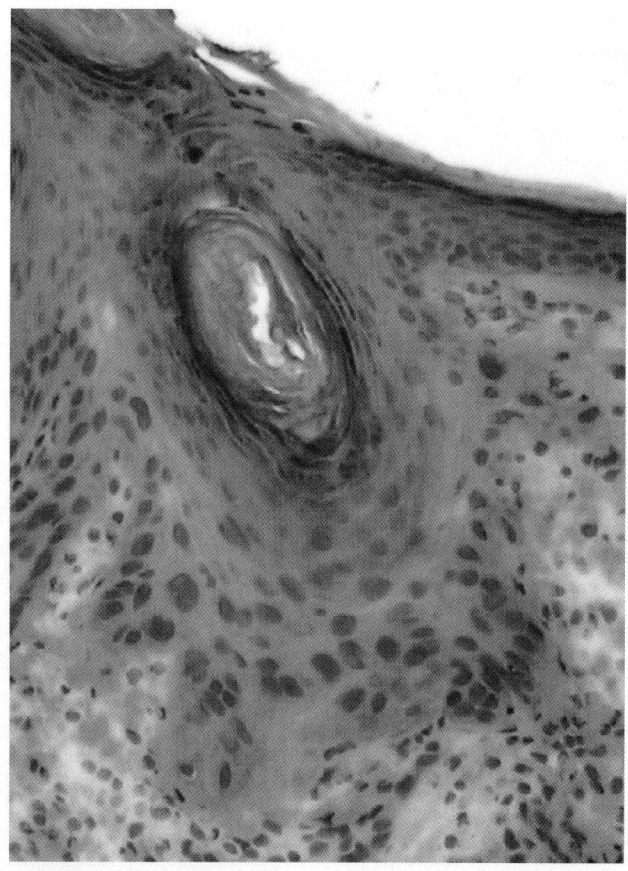

▲ **FIGURE 7-6** Superficial SCC developing from AK type SCC *in situ*, (H&E) multiple atypical keratinocytes showing nuclear pleomorphism at the basal layer.

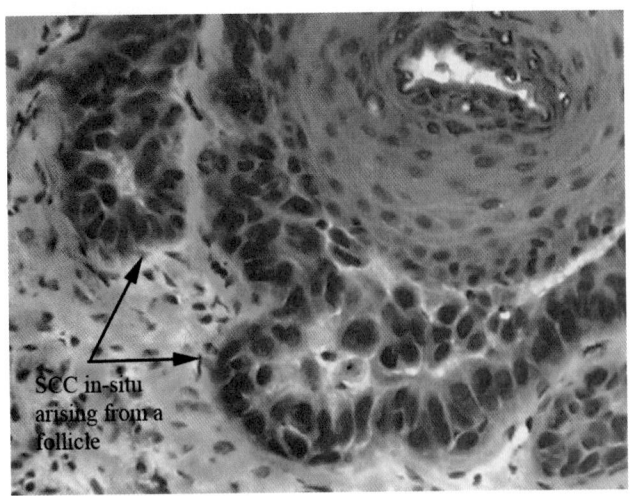

▲ **FIGURE 7-7** Superficial SCC arising from the follicle.

SCC in-situ arising from a follicle

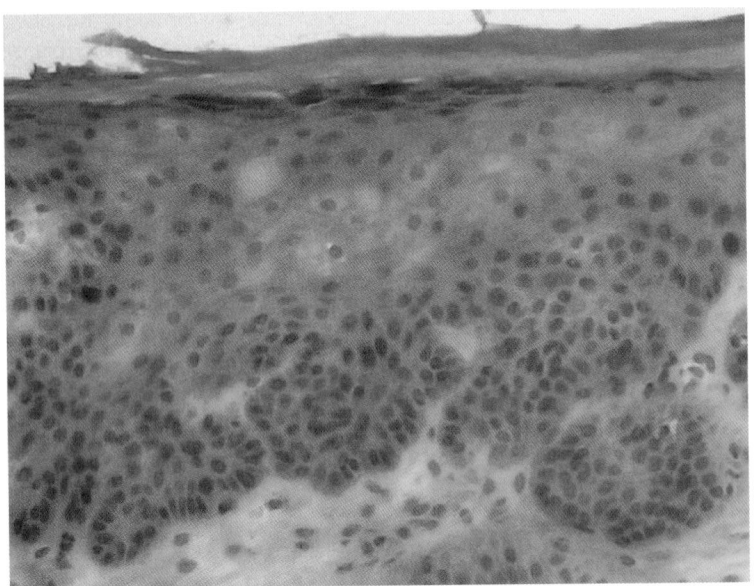

▲ **FIGURE 7-8** Superficial SCC arising from AC on the lower lip (H&E).

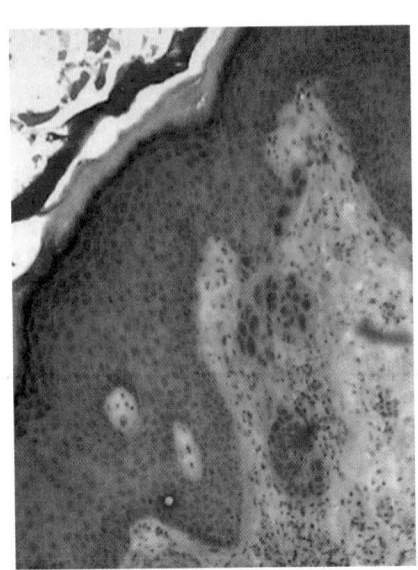

▲ **FIGURE 7-9** Early superficially invasive SCC arising from overlying SCC *in situ*, (H&E).

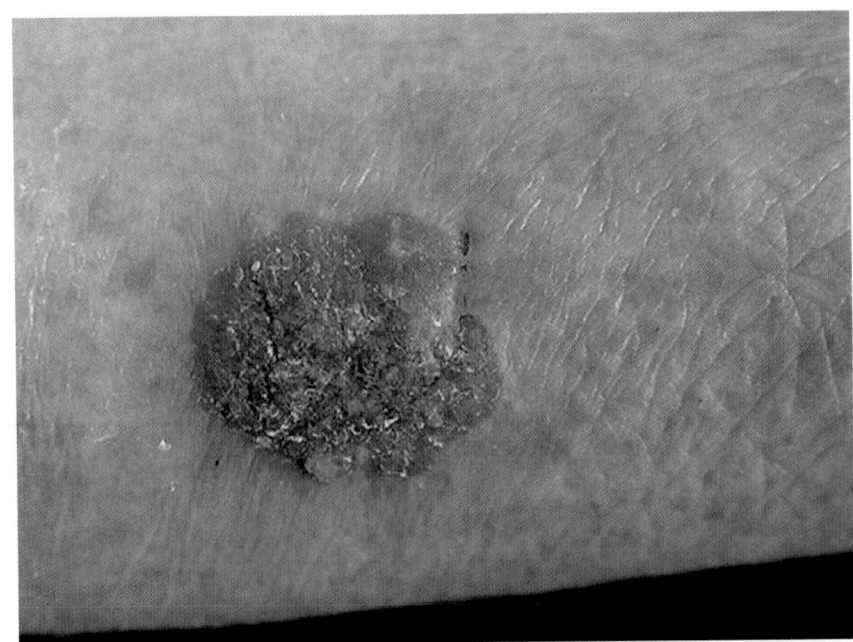

▲ **FIGURE 7-10** SCC *in situ* Bowen type, clinical.

Usually, BD lesions are either symptomatically silent or slightly pruritic or tender (Fig. 7-10). The differential diagnoses of BD on the skin include: contact dermatitis, psoriasis, tinea corporis, AK/AC, mammary and extramammary Paget's disease, and superficial multicentric and pigmented types of BCC, and melanoma *in situ* must be taken into account.

BD of the mucosa is not uncommon. It can be found on the oral, anal, as well as both male and female genital mucosa. The most favorable mucosal sites are the oral mucosa, vulva, vagina, penis, conjunctiva, larynx, and nasal mucosa. On mucous membranes, BD may appear as a verrucous, polypoid, erythroplakic patch, or as a velvety erythematous plaque.[50,113,114] The differential diagnoses of mucosal BD include: mucosal lichen planus; pemphigus; AC; pathogen candida infections; simple inflammatory conditions of mucosal surfaces such as stomatitis, conjunctivitis, vaginitis; sexually transmitted diseases such as syphilis, ulcus molle, herpes, and HIV and HPV infections.

Histopathologically, the lesions of BD on the skin and mucosa share many similar features of SCC *in situ* throughout all levels of the epidermis. On the skin, hyperparakeratosis is a prominent feature; the epidermis/epithelium shows acanthosis, which bears atypical keratinocytes that have large, hyperchromatic and pleomorphic nuclei. Once again, the usual orderly nuclear alignment of the epithelial cells is disrupted not only at the basal layer but throughout the epidermis; in addition, atypical

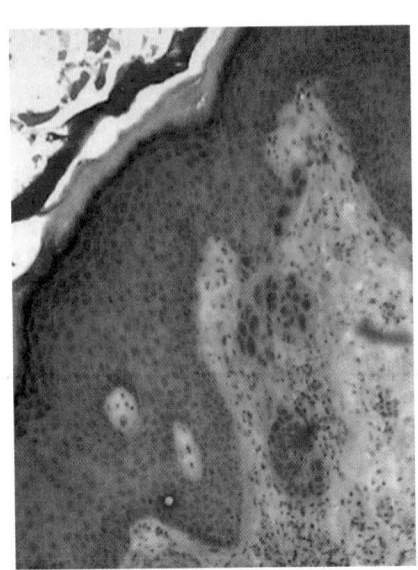

SKIN CANCER

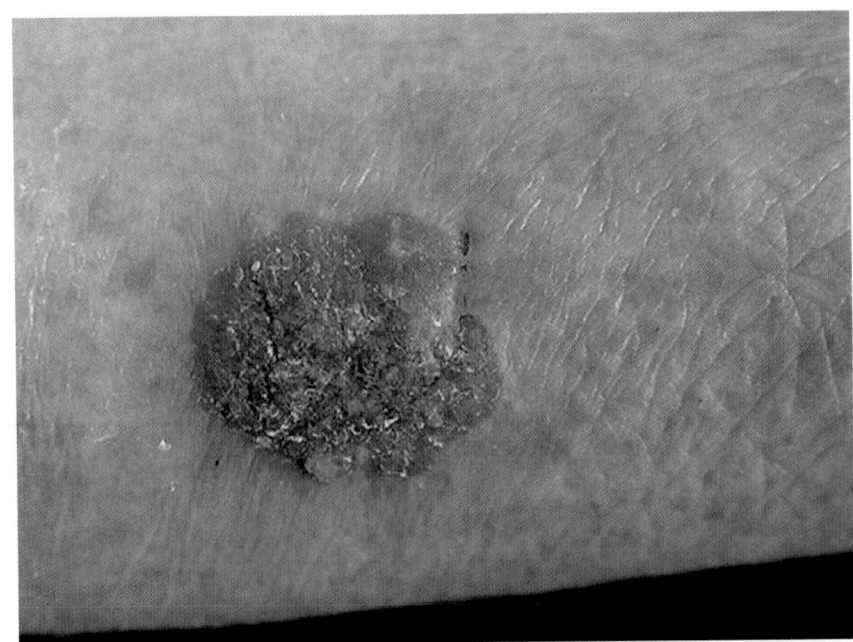

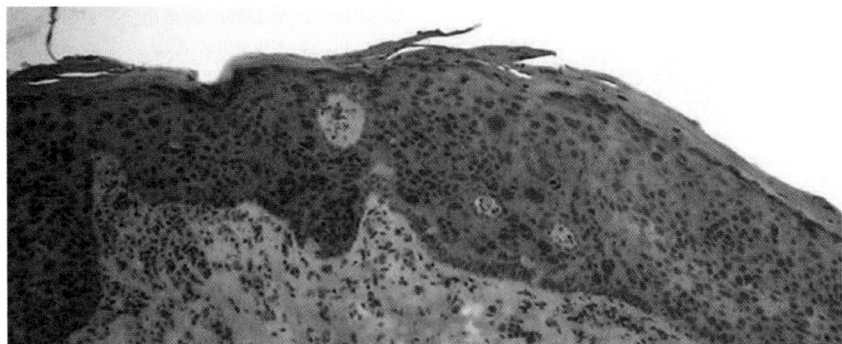

▲ **FIGURE 7-11** SCC *in situ* Bowen type proliferation, atypical keratinocytes in all layers of the epidermis. In contrast to AKs in Bowen Disease, the basal layer may be spared (H&E low magnification).

and explosive mitotic figures are not rare. Single atypical keratinocytes that show multinucleation and/or dyskeratosis may scatter within the epidermal layers in pagetoid BD specimens (Figs. 7-11 and 7-12).

The earlier-mentioned prominent epidermal changes are still confined to the epidermis, and frequently accompanied by varying degrees of mainly mononuclear inflammatory infiltrate in the upper dermis. Lesions on the sun-exposed skin are usually accompanied by prominent solar elastosis in the upper and middermis.[50,57,115] Occasionally, specimens from young patients, or even mucosal lesions may exhibit HPV-like changes in the form of coarse and large keratohyaline granules, and halo-like spaces around piknotic nuclear material in the form of coilocytes within upper reaches of the epidermis.[111,116–118] Ulceration may occur in time on any BD lesion and is usually a sign of invasive SCC. The risk of progression of BD to invasive SCC is reported to be between 3 and 20%.[103,119,120] Partial or complete spontaneous regression is also reported in the literature.[121–123]

ERYTHROPLASIA OF QUEYRAT (EQ)

BOX 7-7   Summary

- Erythroplasia of Queyrat refers to penile carcinoma *in situ*, particularly on the glans and prepuce of the penis.
- EQ usually manifests as solitary or multiple cutaneous lesions with minimally raised, erythematous plaques. It is seen almost exclusively in uncircumcised men.
- Presenting symptoms can vary and may include redness, crusting, scaling, ulceration, bleeding, pain, pruritis, dysuria, penile discharge, and difficulty retracting the foreskin.

Erythroplasia of Queyrat, which is BD of the glans penis was first reported by Tarnovsky in 1891 and later recognized as a penile disease by Fournier and Darier in 1893. EQ refers to penile carcinoma *in situ*, particularly on the glans and prepuce of the penis. EQ arises from the squamous epithelial cells of the glans penis or inner lining of the prepuce. It is seen almost exclusively in uncircumcised men. EQ usually manifests as solitary or multiple cutaneous lesions with minimally raised, erythematous plaques. An individual lesion may be 10 to 15 mm in diameter. The plaques may be smooth, velvety, scaly, crusty, or verrucous.[124,125]

With time, clinical ulceration or distinct papillomatous papules may occur and tend to correlate with histologic evidence of invasive SCC. Presenting symptoms can vary and may include redness, crusting, scaling, ulceration, bleeding, pain, pruritis, dysuria, penile discharge, and difficulty retracting the foreskin (Figs. 7-13 and 7-14). EQ is treatable if there is no underlying invasive carcinoma; however, up to 10% of patients with these lesions may already have invasive SCC in the primary lesion.[124,125]

SCC *IN SITU* OF THE ORAL MUCOSA: LEUKOPLAKIA TYPE

BOX 7-8   Summary

- Leukoplakia is a white patch or plaque that cannot be scraped off and cannot be characterized clinically or pathologically as any other disease.
- Leukoplakia manifests as a well-circumscribed white patch.
- Leukoplakia may or may not be associated with any physical, chemical, or viral causative agent such as tobacco, HPV, and EBV.
- Clinically, oral leukoplakia can appear in two different forms: homogenous leukoplakia and verrucous leukoplakia.
- The current standard for diagnosis of leukoplakia is histopathologic observation of prominent cellular atypia and "dysplasia" within the epithelium.

Leukoplakia is defined by the World Health Organization as "a white patch or plaque that cannot be scraped off and cannot be characterized clinically or pathologically as any other disease." Therefore, a process of exclusion establishes the diagnosis of the disease. Leukoplakia manifests as a well-circumscribed white patch. There may be single or multiple lesions. The surfaces of the patches are slightly raised above the surrounding mucosa. Individuals with oral leukoplakia are not

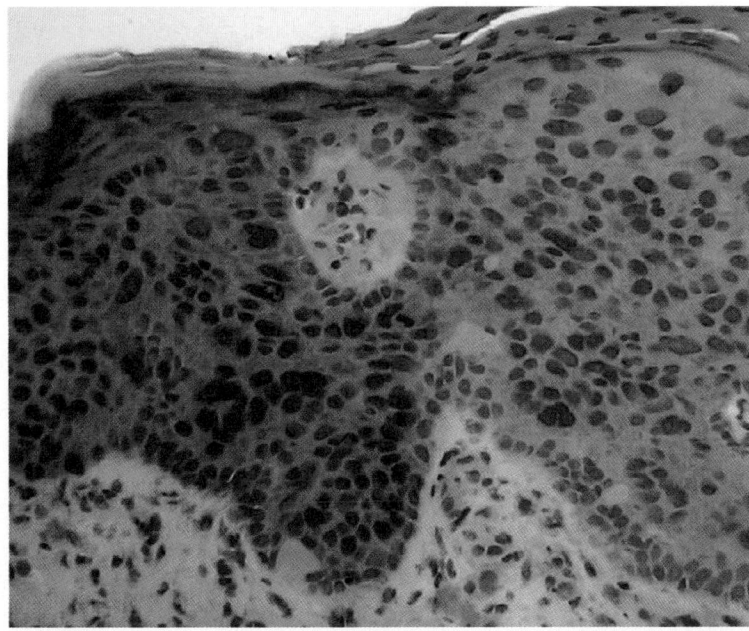

▲ **FIGURE 7-12** SCC *in situ* Bowen type—atypical keratinocytes with prominent nuclear pleomorphism in all layers of the epidermis (H&E high magnification).

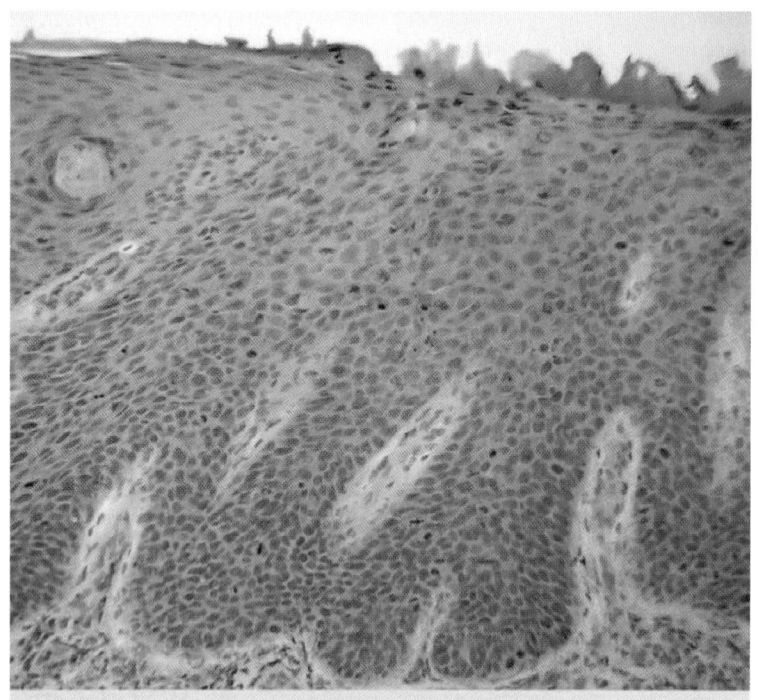

▲ **FIGURE 7-13** Erythroplasia of Queyrat—atypical keratinocytic proliferation in all layers of the epithelium of the male prepuce (H&E low magnification).

symptomatic.[126-128] Leukoplakia of the oral mucosa is not an uncommon lesion, the pooled global prevalence is estimated at 2.6%, and it is approximately three times more prevalent in males.[129]

Leukoplakia may or may not be associated with any physical, chemical, or viral causative agent such as tobacco, HPV, and EBV.[130-132] Not all leukoplakias are *in situ* carcinomas and not all types of leukoplakias are associated with increased risk of invasive SCC of the oral mucosa. The overall incidence of developing an invasive SCC from all forms of leukoplakia varies between 4.4 and 36% with an annual rate of 2.9%.[129,133-136]

Clinically, oral leukoplakia can appear in two different forms. The most common form is uniform white plaques, which are called homogenous leukoplakia. They are prevalent on the buccal mucosa, and usually have low potential to develop into SCC. The second type is speckled or verrucous leukoplakia, which has a stronger potential to develop into invasive SCC. Speckled leukoplakia consists of white flecks or fine nodules on an atrophic erythematous base. There are certain clinical criteria that when seen on a lesion indicates higher possibility of SCC *in situ*. These are nonhomogenous types including: verrucous type of leukoplakia, erosion within the lesion, and oral leukoplakia of the anterior floor of the mouth and undersurface of the tongue, which is strongly associated with high risk. Presence of a nodule or ulceration, and a lesion that is hard on its periphery is probably already associated with invasive SCC.[126,135,137-139] Up to 48% of the definitive invasive SCC lesions of the oral mucosa are reported to be associated with adjacent leukoplakia.[140]

Clinical differential diagnoses include: non-SCC *in situ* leukoplakias, oral lichen planus, candidiasis, leukoedema, morsicatio buccarum/linguarum, frictional oral hyperkeratoses, secondary syphilis, sanguinaria-associated oral white patches, and oral hairy leukoplakia.[141]

In diagnosing true leukoplakia-type SCC *in situ*, clinical criteria are not fully reliable. Histopathologic examination is usually helpful, but not for all the cases. The current standard for diagnosis is histopathologic observation of prominent cellular atypia and "dysplasia" within the epithelium. These include cells with large and hyperchromatic nuclei, increased nuclear/cytoplasmic ratio, cellular and nuclear pleomorphism, increased and atypical mitosis, presence of mitosis in the upper layers of the epithelium, individual dyskeratotic cells, and increased thickness of the epidermis due to these early cytologic changes.

Observation of the earlier-mentioned criteria in a leukoplakia is diagnostic, yet the reverse is not enough for excluding the possibility of SCC *in situ* in a persistent white oral lesion.[126,142,143] Detecting p53 protein overexpression, loss of heterozygosity (alleleic imbalance), and DNA aneuploidy in leukoplakia tissue samples can be helpful in coming to a definitive diagnosis.[126,141,143]

Invasive Squamous Cell Carcinomas

Invasive SCC of the skin is believed to occur both *de novo*, as well as preceded by any of the earlier-mentioned *in situ* forms. Approximately 60% of all invasive SCCs have been reported to be associated with SCC *in situ*. Being an epithelial cancer itself, hypothetically all invasive SCCs must have gone through an *in situ* phase, except for metastatic SCCs.

COMMON INVASIVE SCC: INVASIVE SCC ASSOCIATED WITH PREEXISTING SCC *IN SITU* AK/AC TYPE—LOW-RISK INVASIVE SCC

BOX 7-9 Summary

- Common invasive SCC that is associated with preexisting SCC *in situ* AK/AC type is the most common form of invasive SCC in the skin.
- It represents the majority of the cases and lesions are located always on the sun-exposed areas of the body, predominantly on the head and neck and distal extremities.
- Clinically, sharp circumscription, increase in size, thickness/infiltration, erosion/ulceration, prominent increase in scaling, hyperkeratosis or crusting, exophitic growth especially on a preexisting lesion on sun-damaged skin are the signs of invasive SCC.
- Histopathologically, the common invasive SCC is characterized by the malignant proliferation of keratinocytes in the form of large buds extending from or in conjunction with the surface epidermis, or islands, and/or sheets of neoplastic cells infiltrating the dermis and the deeper tissue.

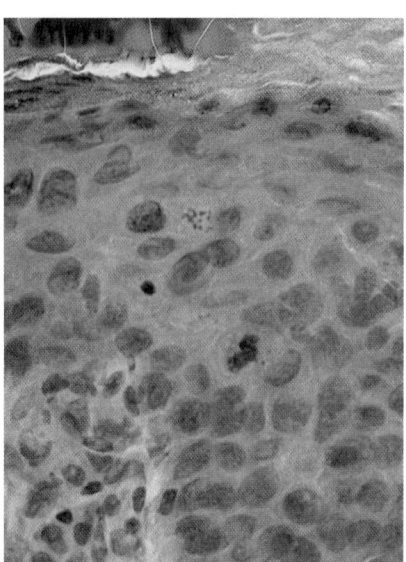

▲ **FIGURE 7-14** Erythroplasia of Queyrat—atypical mitosis, cellular and nuclear pleomorphism (H&E high magnification).

- Prognostically, the common invasive SCC of the skin is reported to be generally associated with low risk of metastases and favorable prognosis.

Common invasive SCC that is associated with preexisting SCC *in situ* AK/AC type is the most common form of invasive SCC in the skin.[65,71,84,86,144–146] It represents the majority of the cases, and lesions are located always on the sun-exposed areas of the body, predominantly on the head and neck and distal extremities. This type of SCC is more common in middle age to elderly males.[45,57,71,146,147] Fair-skinned individuals with extensive UV exposure may develop AK/AC, as well as common invasive SCC at a relatively early age. The manifestations of chronic UV damage, such as solar lentigines, fine wrinkles, telengiectasias, atrophy, AKs, AC-like lesions, history of chronic natural or artificial UV exposure, and a history of previous skin cancer are important factors in determining the high-risk individuals.

Clinically, sharp circumscription, increase in size, thickness/infiltration, erosion/ulceration, prominent increase in scaling, hyperkeratosis or crusting, and exophitic growth especially on a preexisting lesion on sun-damaged skin are the signs of invasive SCC. Depending upon the type of preexisting *in situ* lesion, duration, location, host response, neglect, and many other factors that are not fully known to us, common invasive SCC can manifest itself in many different clinical forms (Figs. 7-15 to 7-18).[45,55,148–150]

Histopathologic examination of the adequate biopsy specimen taken from the lesion usually leads to a definitive diagnosis. Histopathologically, the common invasive SCC is characterized by the malignant proliferation of keratinocytes in the form of large buds extending from or in conjunction with the surface epidermis, or islands, and/or sheets of neoplastic cells infiltrating the dermis and the deeper tissue.

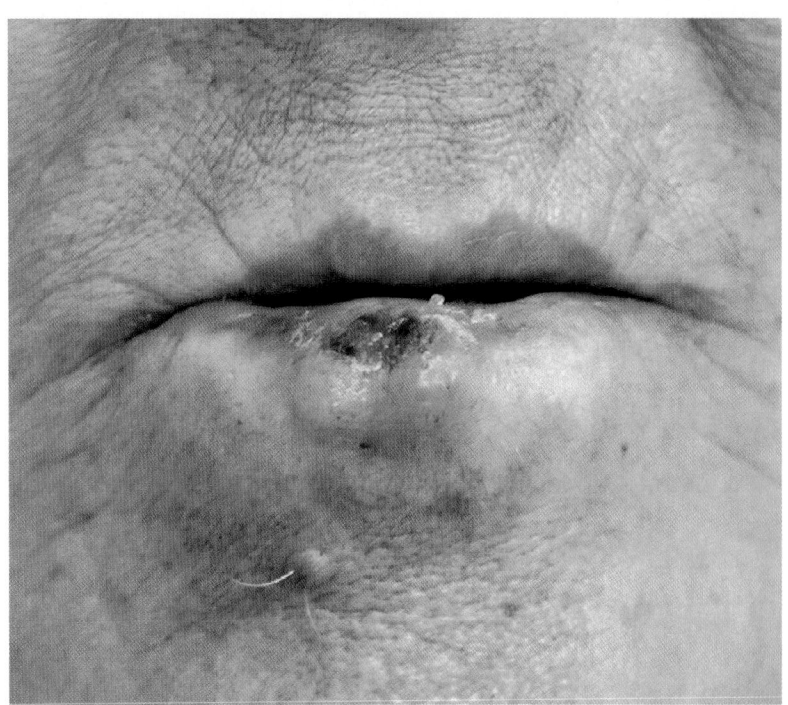
▲ **FIGURE 7-16** Common invasive SCC on the lower lip associated with AC.

The neoplasm shows different degrees of differentiation, namely well differentiated, moderately differentiated, and less differentiated. The differentiation of invasive SCC is mainly determined by the keratinization capability of the neoplastic cells. Well-differentiated SCC is characterized by clusters of highly keratinized atypical keratinocytes that are capable of complete keratinization and producing eosinophilic horn pearls in the tissue (Fig. 7-19). These neoplastic cells tend to have large eosinophilic cytoplasms, and easily recognizable intercellular bridges.

As the differentiation of the tumor decreases, the degree of complete keratinization also decreases and even diminishes. Individual cell keratinization in the form of dyskeratotic cells, increasing amount of cellular and nuclear pleomorphism, frequent mitosis and atypical mitotic figures, less prominent intercellular bridges, higher nuclear/cytoplasmic ratio, and occasional necrotic neoplastic cells are the features of moderately to less differentiated SCC (Figs. 7-20 to 7-23). Although in the case of indifferentiated invasive SCC, cells do not exhibit keratinization; however, they tend to become more spindle shaped and more pleomorphic, with almost no visible intercellular bridges, high number of atypical mitosis, and necrosis in the mass being frequent findings (Figs. 7-24 and 7-25). Depending upon the depth of the tumor and the degree of host response, an inflammatory infiltrate, mainly composed of lymphocytes, eosinophils, and plasma cells in varying density usually is found in the dermis within and surrounding the neoplasm.[151] Prognostically, the common invasive SCC of the skin is reported to be generally associated with low risk of metastases and favorable prognosis.[45,57,58,152,153]

DE NOVO INVASIVE SCC

BOX 7-10   Summary

- *De novo* invasive SCC is an invasive SCC of the skin, mucosa, and adnexal epithelium that is not associated with or preceded by an in situ component.
- *De novo* invasive SCC is reported to be a high-risk SCC.
- *De novo* malignancies, including *de novo* SCC of the skin and mucosa, are reported to be increasingly associated with organ transplant and immunosuppressed patients.

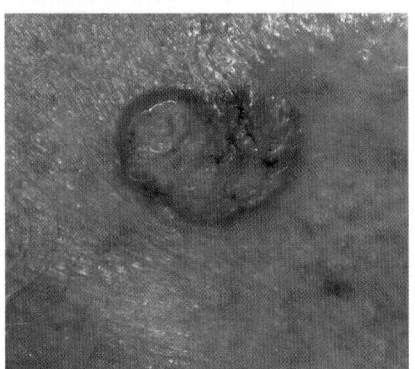
▲ **FIGURE 7-15** Common invasive SCC on sun-damaged skin.

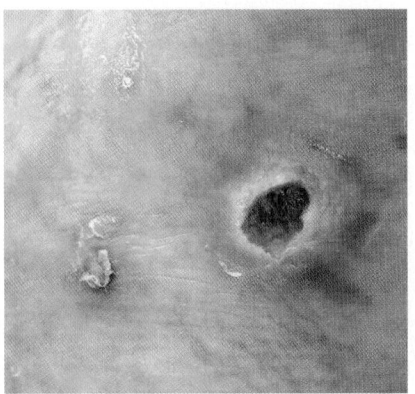
▲ **FIGURE 7-17** Invasive SCC presenting as a nonhealing small ulcer on the distal extremity—AKs on the surrounding skin.

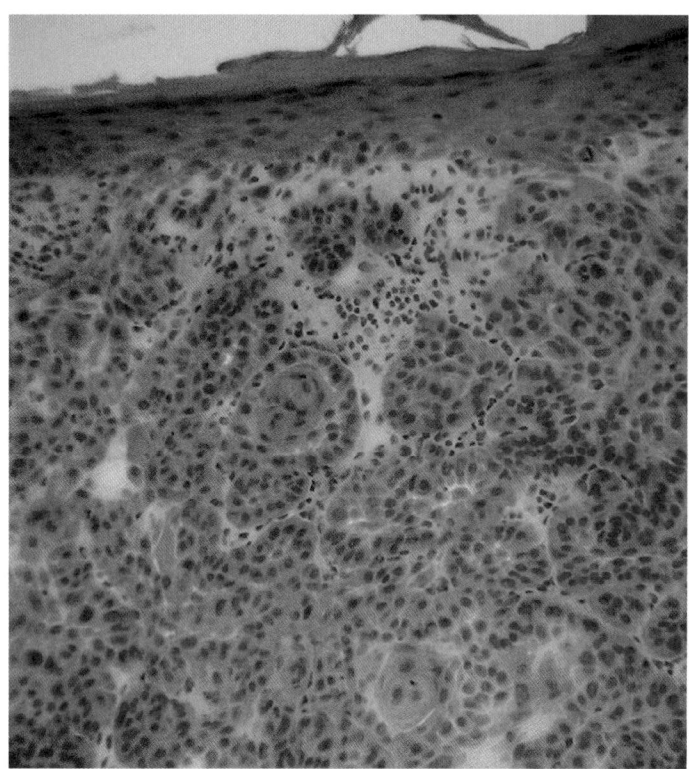

▲ **FIGURE 7-18** Well-differentiated common invasive SCC associated with SCC *in situ* on the surface of sun-damaged skin.

De novo invasive SCC is an invasive SCC of the skin, mucosa, and adnexal epithelium that is not associated with or preceded by an *in situ* component. It is reported to be a high-risk SCC.[49] It is known that chronic inflammation can lead to cancer formation in various tissues, including skin. Recent studies have shown that chronic inflammation induces *de novo* epithelial carcinogenesis in transgenic mice and this process is B-lymphocyte dependent.[154] On the other hand, again in animal model, inhibition of Notch signaling has shown to result in *de novo* spontaneous SCC formation, as well as AK-like lesions in the skin.[155]

De novo malignancies, including *de novo* SCC of the skin and mucosa, are reported to be increasingly associated with organ transplant and immuno-suppressed patients.[156–158] *De novo* invasive SCCs are considered high-risk lesions as they tend to be more aggressive and associated with poor prognosis. The incidence of local and/or distant metastases in this type of invasive SCC is approximately 8 to 14%.[49,159,160]

INVASIVE SCC—SOLITARY KERATOACAN-THOMA TYPE

> **BOX 7-11 Summary**
>
> - Solitary KA is a common type of invasive SCC that is a rapidly growing neoplasm with a central keratin plug that demonstrates a histologic pattern resembling that of a typical SCC.
> - KAs occur most commonly on sun-damaged skin in middle-aged and older individuals.
> - Clinically, KA is characterized by a rapidly growing papule/nodule over 1 to 2 months, followed by spontaneous regression over 3 to 6 months leaving a depressed scar.
> - Histopathologically, KAs are replicas of well-differentiated invasive SCCs.
> - Although spontaneous complete resolution is the frequently expected course of solitary KA, it is not always possible to differentiate solitary KA from more aggressive forms of invasive SCC, clinically and histopathologically.

Solitary KA is a common type of invasive SCC, in which the clinical course of SCC is both more rapid and results in complete spontaneous resolution, possibly due to host response and other not fully known factors in this low-risk type of SCC.[50,56,59,65,115] KA was first described as a "crateriform ulcer of the face" in 1889 by Jonathan Hutchinson. It is a rapidly growing neoplasm with a central keratin plug that demonstrates a histologic pattern resembling that of a typical SCC. KAs occur most commonly on sun-damaged skin in middle-aged and older individuals.[63]

Clinically, KA is characterized by a rapidly growing papule/nodule over 1 to 2 months, followed by spontaneous

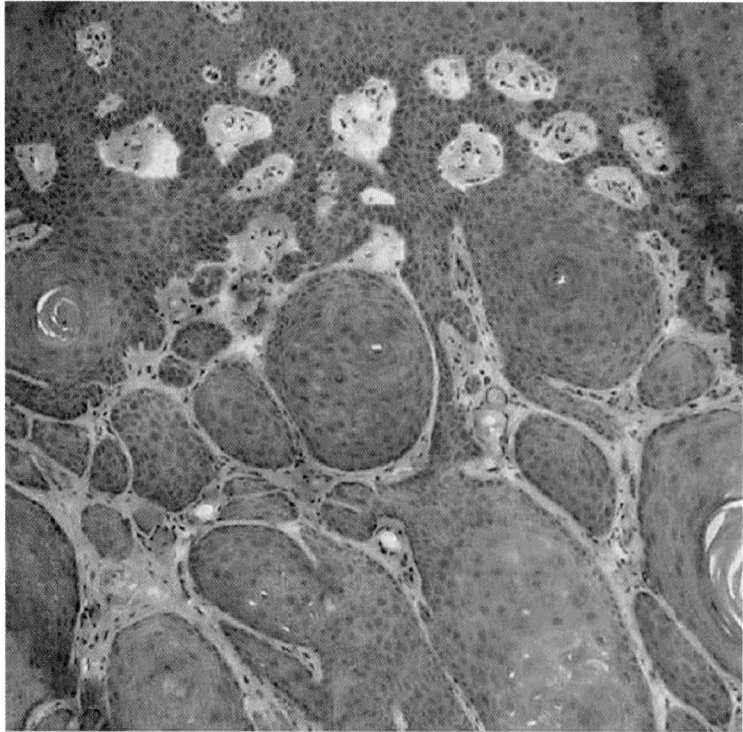

▲ **FIGURE 7-19** Well-differentiated SCC—islands of highly keratinized neoplastic keratinocytes are capable of complete keratinization in the form of eosinophilic horn pearls (H&E low magnification).

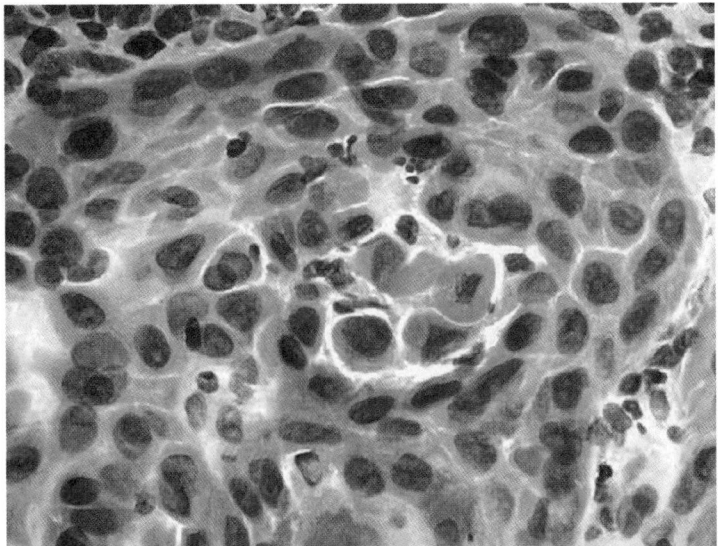

▲ **FIGURE 7-20** Moderately differentiated SCC—individual cell keratinization and pleomorphism (H&E high magnification).

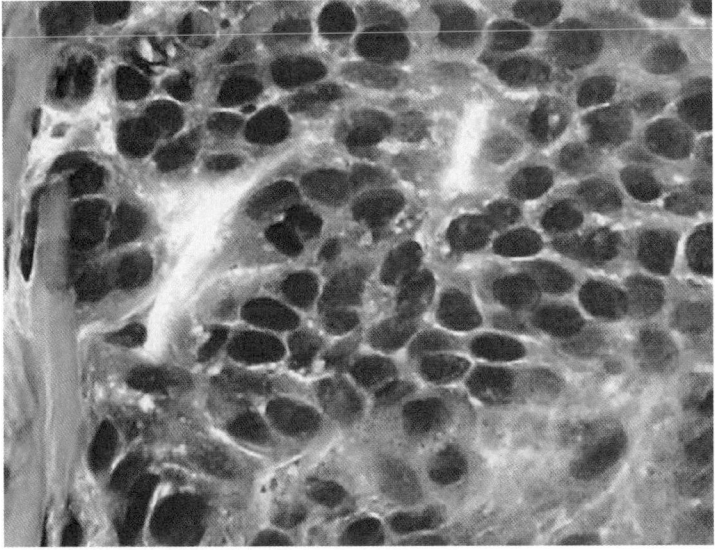

▲ **FIGURE 7-21** SCC poorly differentiated—prominent pleomorphism (*arrow*), atypical mitosis.

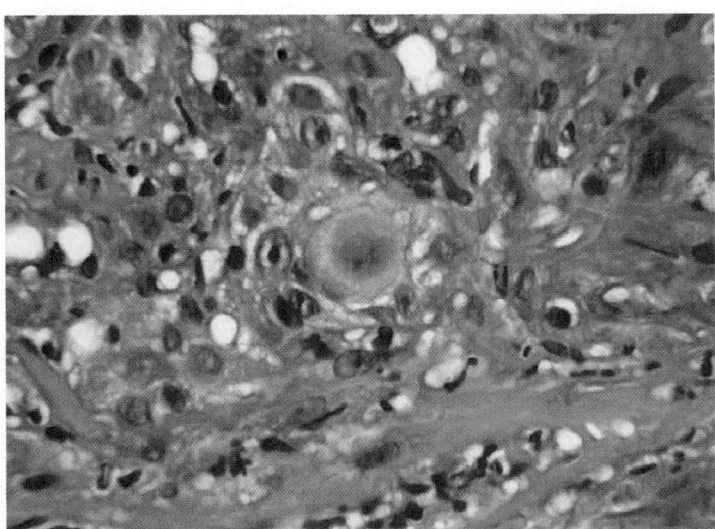

▲ **FIGURE 7-22** Poorly differentiated SCC with single-cell keratinization (H&E high magnification).

regression over 3 to 6 months leaving a depressed scar. KA usually presents as a solitary, flesh to pink-red colored dome-shaped nodule, couple of centimeters in diameter, with a central keratin plug. The most common locations are the face and extremities, although they may occur on any body site (Fig. 7-26). Three evolutionary stages—namely proliferation, maturation, and involution—that frequently lead to complete clinical regression are typical for solitary KA (Fig. 7-27).

There are several clinical variants of KA, which include: giant KAs (lesions > 3 cm in diameter); KA centrifugum marginatum, which is characterized by continuous peripheral growth and central healing without complete resolution; subungal KAs, which grow rapidly, are destructive, and fail to regress; and multiple KAs: Ferguson-Smith and Grzybowski types.[49,50]

Histopathologically, KAs are replicas of well-differentiated invasive SCC. They are neoplastic proliferation of keratinocytes extending from the overlying acanthotic epidermis into various depths of dermis in the form of large buds or sheets of cells with abundant eosinophilic cytoplasms and prominent keratinization. Typically, the dome-shaped lesion is well-circumscribed with a large, keratin-filled crater in the center and varying degrees of mixed-cell inflammatory infiltration within and surrounding the neoplasm. The peripheral deep portions of a still enlarging KA in proliferating stage may reveal less differentiated SCC features with more prominent cytological atypia and many mitoses. A mature KA is characterized by neoplastic proliferation of well-differentiated keratinocytes with glassy pale pink cytoplasm, rich in keratin. However, in a resolving involution-stage KA, a dense lichenoid mononuclear cell inflammatory infiltrate with occasional multinucleated histiocytes results in prominent fibrosis which effaces the neoplasm leading to complete spontaneous resolution with scarring (Figs. 7-28 to 7-30).[50,55,56,65,93]

Although spontaneous complete resolution is the frequently expected course of solitary KA, it is not always possible to differentiate solitary KA from more aggressive forms of invasive SCC, clinically and histopathologically. Therefore, complete surgical removal is the recommended treatment of choice for these lesions. Metastasizing solitary KA and large solitary KA associated with local tissue destruction are also reported.[50,56,63]

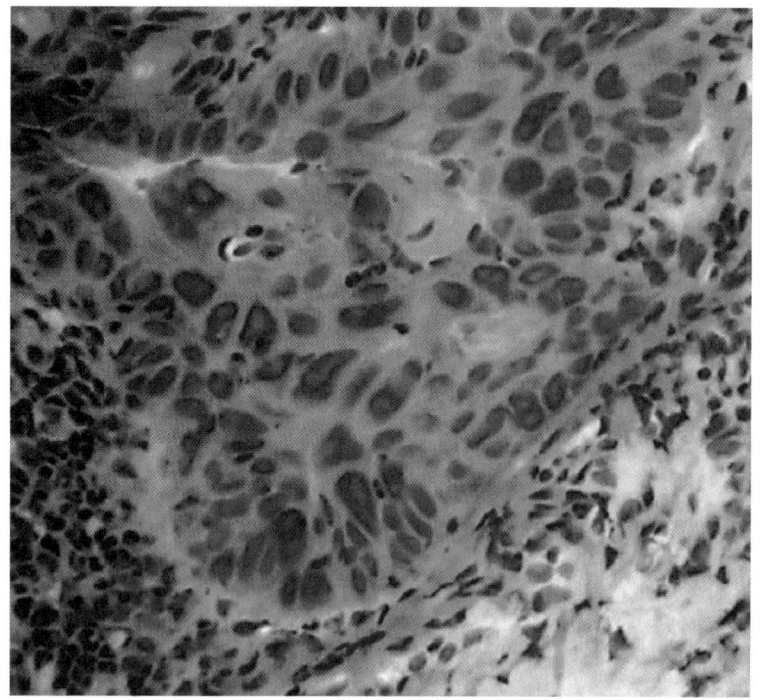

▲ FIGURE 7-23 Poorly differentiated SCC with pleomorphic nuclei (H&E high magnification).

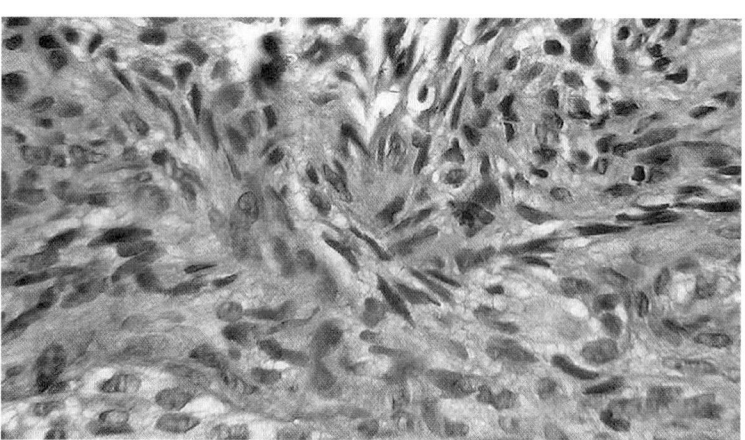

▲ FIGURE 7-24 Indifferentiated SCC—spindle-shaped cells with pleomorhic and spindle-shaped nuclei (H&E high magnification).

INVASIVE SCC—BOWEN TYPE

BOX 7-12   Summary

- Invasive BD, or Bowen carcinoma, is an invasive SCC developing in BD.
- The risk of metastasis in invasive SCC depends on histologic characteristics, as well as clinical characteristics.
- The most common presentation is a rapidly growing, ulcerated tumor occurring in a scaly or erythematous patch, which is present for months to years.
- Invasive BD occurs most often on the head and neck, followed by the extremities and trunk.

Invasive BD, or Bowen carcinoma, is an invasive SCC developing in BD. It is very rare and specific features are not well defined. It develops in 3 to 5% of untreated or recurrent BD. Metastatic disease from the invasive component may occur in up to 13% of cases with death from metastases occurring in 10% of those patients.[161] The risk of metastasis in invasive SCC depends on histologic characteristics including degree of differentiation, depth of invasion, and the presence of perineural invasion, as well as clinical characteristics such as tumor size, location, and duration, previous treatment, patient age, smoking history, and immune status.[162]

The most common presentation is a rapidly growing, ulcerated tumor occurring in a scaly or erythematous patch, which is present for months to years (Fig. 7-31). The invasive change most commonly seen is a poorly differentiated SCC with a basaloid differentiation pattern. Invasive BD occurs most often on the head and neck, followed by the extremities and trunk.[161–162]

INVASIVE SCC—VERRUCOUS CARCINOMA TYPE

BOX 7-13   Summary

- Verrucous carcinoma is a variant of differentiated SCC with low-grade malignancy, slow growth, and little metastatic potential. These lesions are mostly found in the oral mucosa.
- HPV and chemical carcinogens, such as tobacco, may play an important role in the development of verrucous SCC of the skin.
- The special feature of this tumor type is that it appears macroscopically malignant but histologically more benign.
- Early oral verrucous carcinoma can appear as white, translucent patches on an erythematous base; later, they may become white cauliflower-like papillomas.

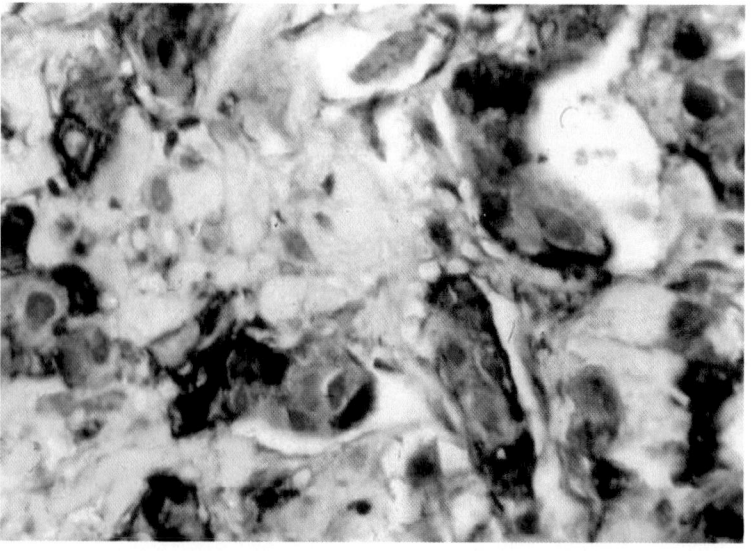

▲ FIGURE 7-25 Indifferentiated SCC—cytokeratin+, avidin-biotin peroxidase (courtesy of Ankara University School of Medicine).

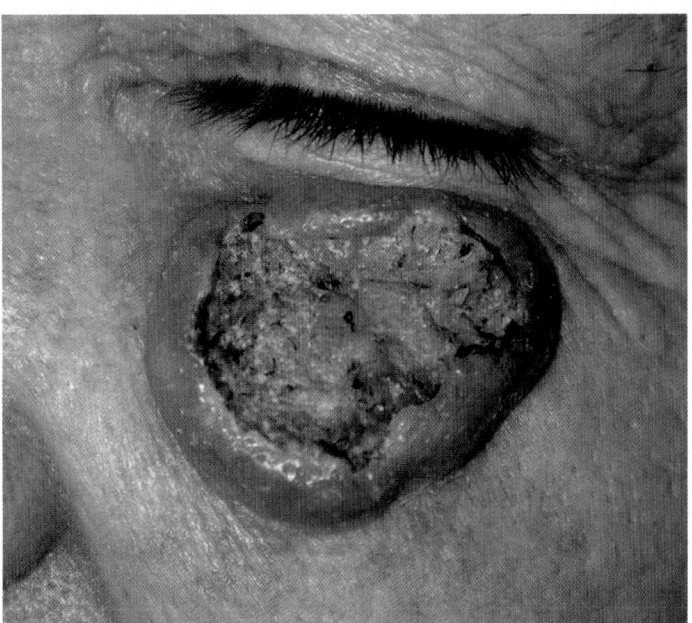

▲ **FIGURE 7-26** Invasive SCC, solitary KA type on the face.

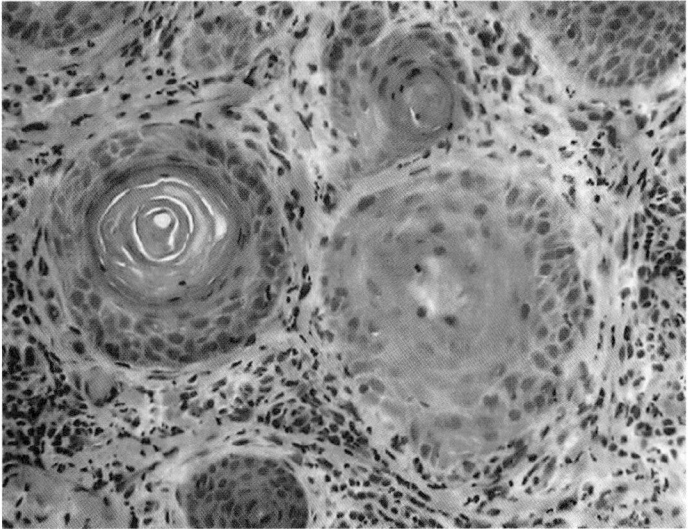

▲ **FIGURE 7-27** Well-differentiated SCC (H&E high magnification).

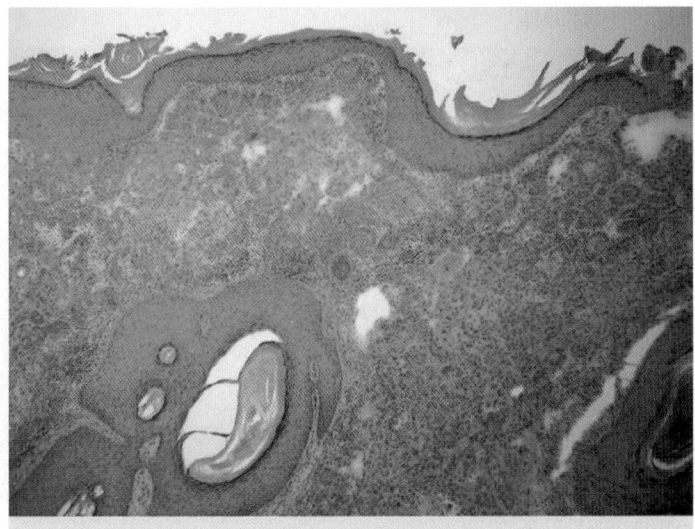

▲ **FIGURE 7-28** Invasive SCC, solitary KA type (H&E low magnification).

Verrucous carcinoma is a variant of differentiated SCC with low-grade malignancy, slow growth, and little metastatic potential. These tumors can be locally invasive and recurrent after incomplete treatment. Although it has been reported at extraoral sites like the foot and genitals, the tumor is mostly found in the oral mucosa. HPV and chemical carcinogens, such as tobacco, may play an important role in the development of verrucous SCC of the skin.[163]

The special feature of this tumor type is that it appears macroscopically malignant but histologically more benign.[163] There are many different types of verrucous carcinoma depending on the location of the lesion. There is the oral type (Ackerman tumor or oral florid papillomatosis), anogenital type (Buschke–Loewenstein tumor [Fig. 7-32]), palmoplantar type (epithelioma cuniculatum), and verrucous carcinomas of other body sites have been found.[164]

Early oral verrucous carcinoma can appear as white, translucent patches on an erythematous base. Later, they may become white cauliflower-like papillomas, ulcerate, cause lymphadenopathy, and sometimes may even grow around lymph nodes. Anogenital verrucous carcinoma most commonly occurs on the glans penis, and less commonly on the bladder and other pelvic organs. These lesions appear as large cauliflower-like tumors, and tend to infiltrate deeply (Fig. 7-23).

Palmoplantar verrucous carcinomas commonly occur on the first metatarsal head, as well as the heel, toes, dorsum, on amputated limbs, and the medioplantar region. They are usually exophytic tumors with ulceration and sinuses draining foul-smelling discharge.[164,165]

EPITHELIOMA CUNICULATUM

> **BOX 7-14   Summary**
>
> - Epithelioma cuniculatum is a type of verrucous carcinoma presenting as a bulbous mass mainly on the plantar surface of the foot.
> - Initially, the tumor may resemble a plantar wart, but it may slowly progress to form a bulky, exophytic mass with foul-smelling, toothpaste-like debris.

Epithelioma cuniculatum is most often seen in older white men. It is a type of verrucous carcinoma presenting as a bulbous mass mainly on the plantar surface of the foot. Initially, the tumor may resemble a plantar wart, but it

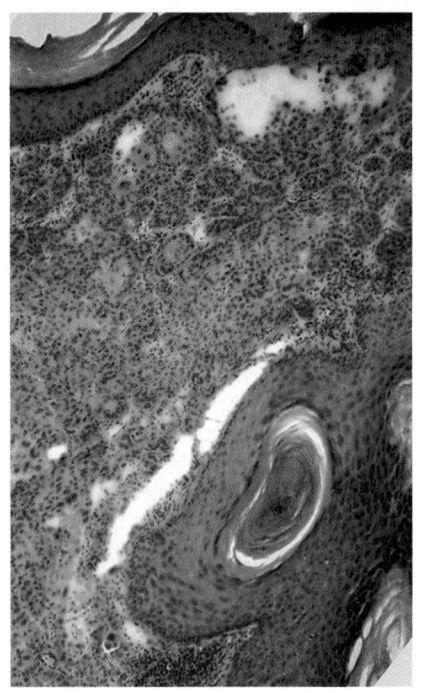

▲ **FIGURE 7-29** Invasive SCC, solitary KA type (H&E).

may slowly progress to form a bulky, exophytic mass. It may become ulcerated and develop multiple sinuses from which a foul-smelling, toothpaste-like, keratinous debris can be emitted. It has often been described as a "squashy" mass. The tumor enlarges slowly, and may penetrate into deeper tissues, but rarely causes distant metastases. It can be deforming and painful, leading to difficulty with ambulation (Fig. 7-33).[119,164]

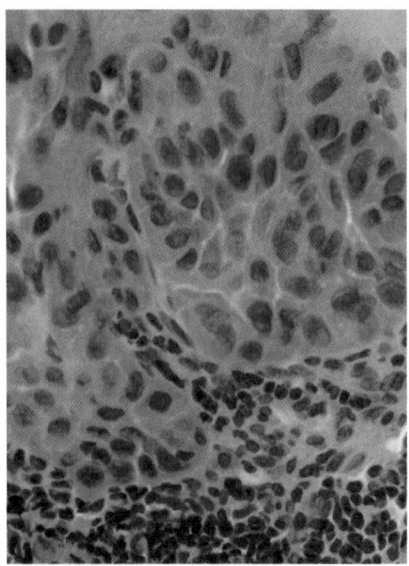

▲ **FIGURE 7-30** Invasive SCC, solitary KA type—base of the lesion with prominent nuclear pleomorphism (H&E high magnification).

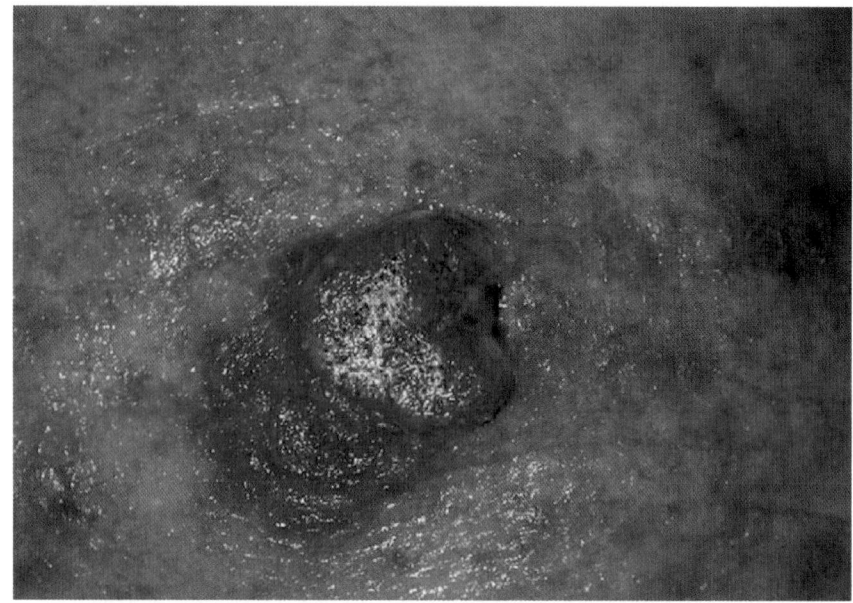

▲ **FIGURE 7-31** Invasive Bowen-type SCC on the scalp.

VERRUCOUS CARCINOMA OF THE ORAL MUCOSA

> **BOX 7-15 Summary**
>
> • Verrucous carcinoma of the oral mucosa most frequently occurs on the buccal mucosa.
> • Clinically, this tumor is initially soft and well defined. Over time, however, it becomes more indurated, firm, and more tufted.

The term "verrucous carcinoma" was first used by Ackerman in 1948 to describe a carcinoma of the oral cavity.[165] Verrucous carcinoma of the oral mucosa most frequently occurs on the buccal mucosa. However, lesions can be found on the alveolar ridge or gingival and the floor of the mouth. Clinically, this tumor is initially soft and well defined. Over time, however, it becomes more indurated, firm, and more tufted. There are numerous papillary projections that protrude from the surface. These projections are heavily keratinized and in some areas appear nodular, pebbled, or fungating, usually without ulceration. Lesions of the buccal mucosa may extend into the buccal sulcus and adjacent alveolar ridge and have the ability to destroy bone slowly after becoming fixed to the overlying periosteum, usually of the mandible. Painful nonmalignant lymphadenopathy can be seen with concurrent infection. If metastases do occur, they usually remain limited to the regional lymph nodes.[165–167]

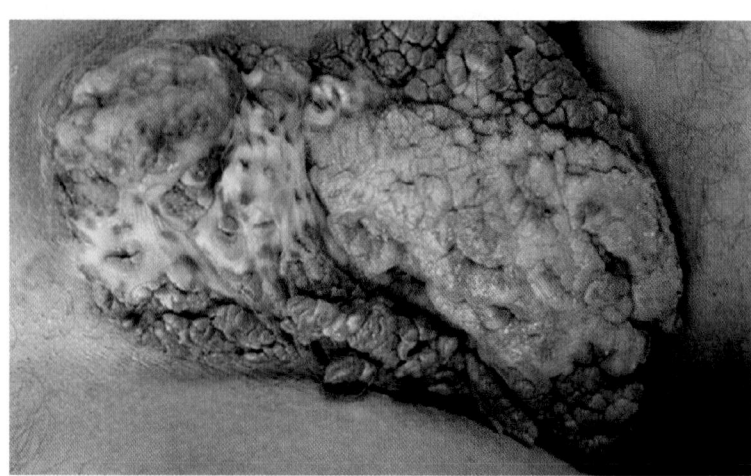

▲ **FIGURE 7-32** Verrucous carcinoma, Buschke–Loewenstein tumor (courtesy of Ankara University School of Medicine).

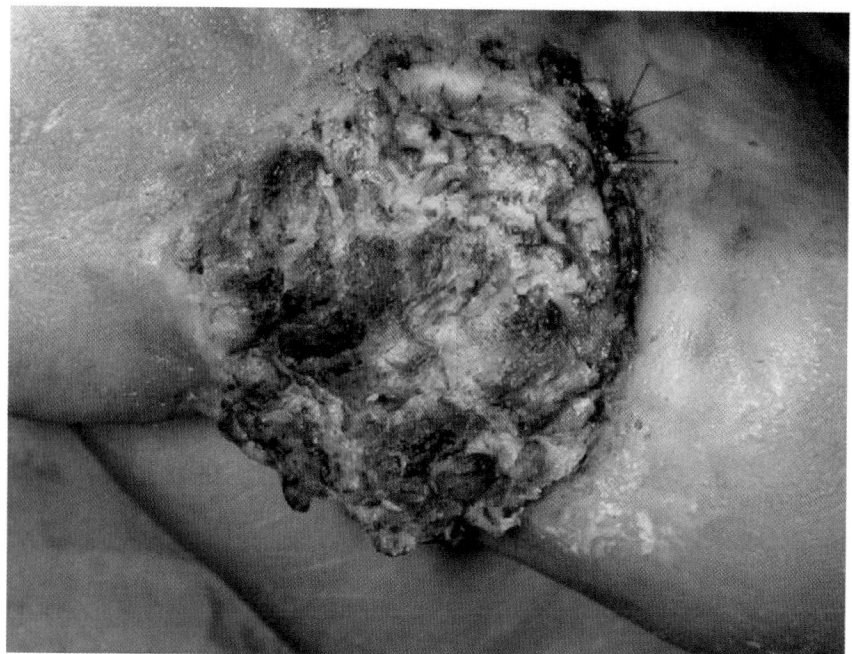

▲ **FIGURE 7-33** Epithelioma cuniculatum/verrucous carcinoma type invasive SCC on the sole (courtesy of Ankara University School of Medicine).

INVASIVE SCC—ACANTHOLYTIC TYPE

BOX 7-16   Summary

- Acantholytic invasive SCC is an uncommon and histologically distinctive variant of SCC.
- Acantholytic invasive SCC develops preferentially on the sun-exposed areas of elderly individuals, following AK with acantholysis.
- These lesions have an overwhelming male predominance.

Acantholytic invasive SCC, also known as pseudoglandular or adenoid SCC, is an uncommon and histologically distinctive variant of SCC. This tumor was initially described in 1947 as a tumor composed of both solid and gland-like epithelial proliferations extending into the dermis. It has a typical SCC pattern, but with acantholysis, gland-like formation, and dyskeratotic cells.[168]

Acantholytic invasive SCC develops preferentially on the sun-exposed areas of elderly individuals, following actinic keratosis with acantholysis. This lesion has an overwhelming male predominance. In one study, only three females were affected out of a total of 155 patients.[169] These lesions can appear as eroded nodules in sun-exposed areas, especially on the face and ears (Figs. 7-34 and 7-35). Acantholytic invasive SCC on the skin and mucosal areas of the head and neck has a worse prognosis than conventional SCC. The rate of metastasis can range from 3 to 19%, and local growth can be rapid.[170]

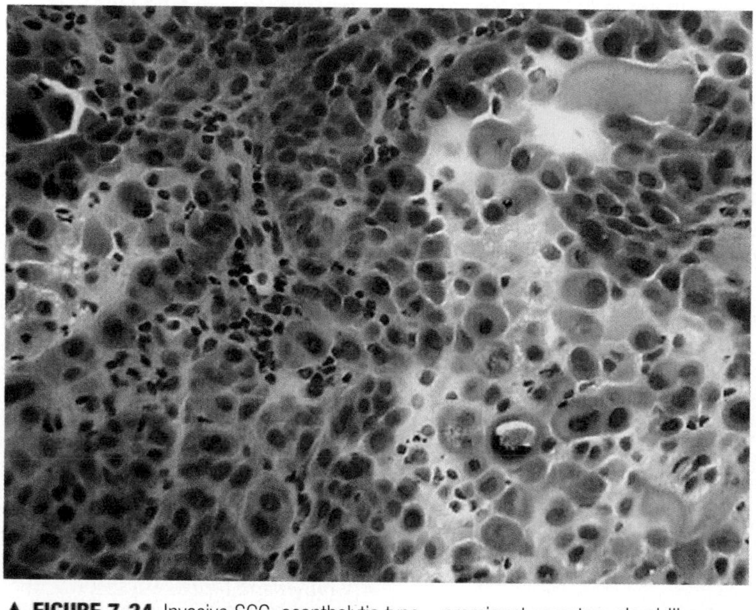

INVASIVE SCC—SPINDLE CELL TYPE

BOX 7-17   Summary

- Spindle cell SCC is a rare high-risk type of invasive SCC.
- It has been proposed that often, spindle cell SCC arise from areas of previous radiation exposure.
- Clinically, this tumor appears as an ulcerated, polypoid, exophytic, or fungating mass that occurs in the head-and-neck area.

Spindle cell SCC is a rare high-risk type of invasive SCC. This variant of SCC was initially reported by Martin and Stewart in 1935.[171] It has been proposed that often, spindle cell SCCs arise from the area of previous radiation exposure. These lesions tend to have a more aggressive course than those that are not related to radiation. Spindle cell SCCs have also been reported to arise in renal transplant patients, where up to 1:4 of these patients developed metastatic disease. There have not been any large studies conducted to determine the prognosis of this variant of SCC, especially comparing *de novo* tumors with radiation-associated tumors.

Clinically, these tumors appear as ulcerated, polypoid, exophytic, or fungating mass that occur in the head-and-neck area (Fig. 7-36).[171,172] Surface ulceration is common in these tumors. The ulcerated lesion has a tendency to become infected and, therefore, may be associated with abscess or pus exudation. These lesions are quite aggressive, with metastasis occurring in up-to 25% of patients. The rate of local recurrence may also be high, as these lesions are commonly associated with perineural invasion (Figs. 7-37 and 7-38).[163,171,172]

▲ **FIGURE 7-34** Invasive SCC, acantholytic type—prominent secretory gland-like areas in the neoplasm with malignant acantholysis and individual cell keratinization (H&E).

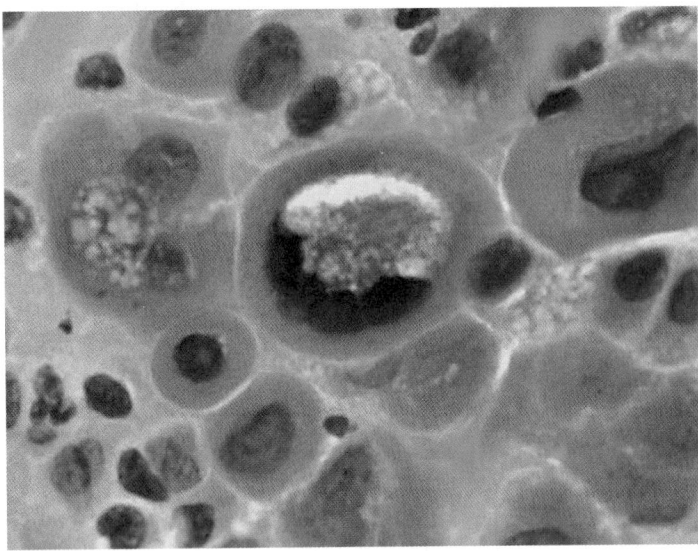

▲ **FIGURE 7-35** Invasive SCC, acantholytic type—pleomorphic nuclei and individual cell keratinization (H&E high magnification).

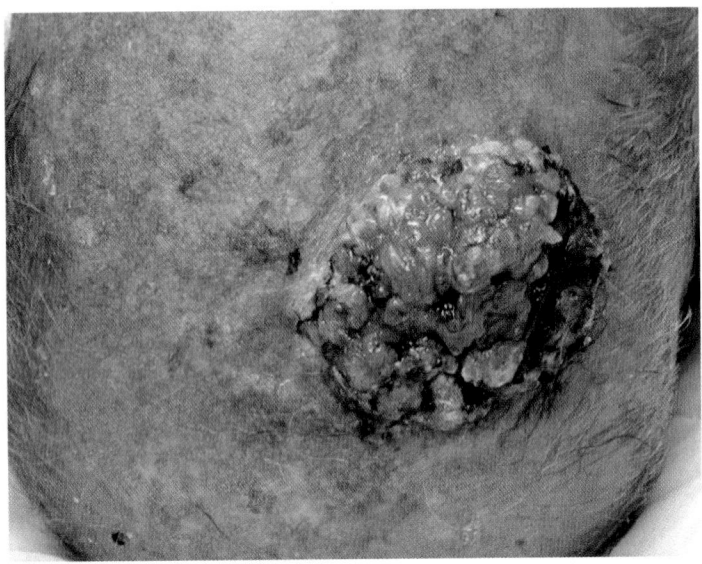

▲ **FIGURE 7-36** Invasive SCC, spindle cell type—verrucous exophitic mass on the scalp, AK on the surrounding skin.

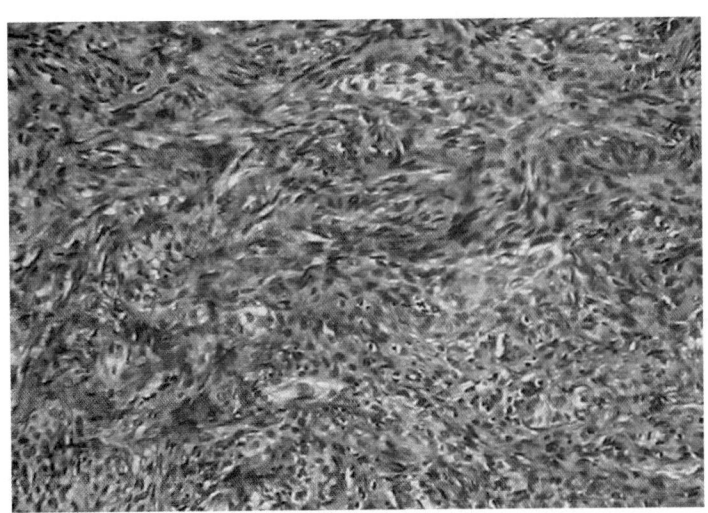

▲ **FIGURE 7-37** Invasive SCC, spindle cell type, poorly differentiated—both neoplastic cells and their nuclei are spindle shaped (H&E low magnification).

INVASIVE SCC—PAPILLARY TYPE

BOX 7-18 Summary

- Papillary SCC has been reported at many locations in the body. These include the skin, uterine, cervix, eye, larynx, oropharynx, nasal septum, and nasopharynx.
- Most patients present with an exophytic, red-tan, enlarging lesion on sun-exposed skin. The size of these lesions ranges from less than 1 to greater than 5.0 cm and the location determines the symptoms.

Landman and his colleagues first described papillary SCC in 1990. They reported two elderly women with lesions that had an exophytic papillary growth pattern which was histologically distinct from verrucous carcinoma. These lesions occurred on the face of these patients and appeared as red nodules or tumors that looked like SCC or pyogenic granuloma. Both of these cases were treated by electrodesiccation and curettage, and no recurrence was found.[173]

Papillary SCC has been reported at many locations in the body. These include the skin, uterine, cervix, eye, larynx, oropharynx, nasal septum, and nasopharynx. These lesions are usually exophytic, fungiform masses. Most patients present with an exophytic, red-tan, enlarging lesion on sun-exposed skin. The size of these lesions range from less than 1 cm to greater than 5.0 cm and the location determines the symptoms. These lesions occur in both male and females, with men being more affected. The mean age of presentation is in the 60s, but can range from 30 to 80 years.[173,174]

INVASIVE SCC—SIGNET RING TYPE

BOX 7-19 Summary

- Signet ring SCC is very rare. This tumor contains signet ring cells, which typically have nuclear displacement and compression by cytoplasmic contents.
- Clinically, these lesions appear as ulcerated erythematous, scaly plaques or nodules.

Signet ring SCC is very rare. This tumor contains signet ring cells, which typically have nuclear displacement and compression by cytoplasmic contents. Clinically, these lesions appear as ulcerated erythematous, scaly plaques or nodules. This variant of SCC was first described by Cramer and Heggeness in 1989, and a second case was reported by McKinley and his colleagues in 1998. Since there has

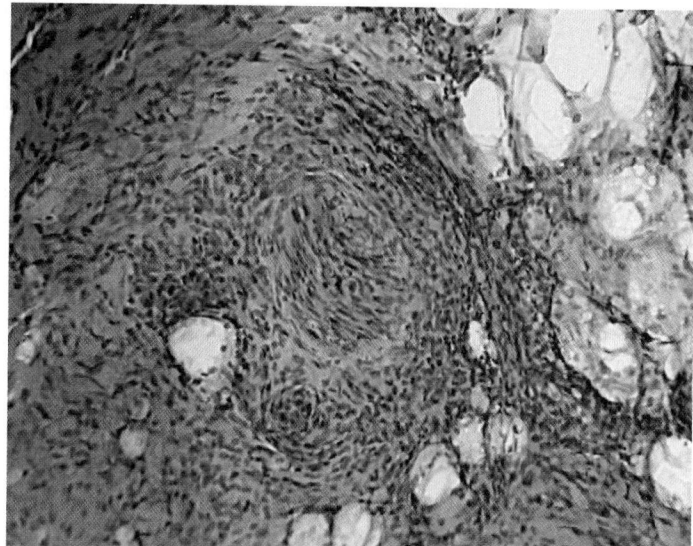

▲ **FIGURE 7-38** Invasive SCC, spindle cell type with perineural invasion (H&E low magnification).

only been two cases reported, it is almost impossible to determine its biologic behavior. In Cramer and Heggeness' case, the lesion behaved very aggressively, with local invasion, lymph-node metastasis, and eventually leading to death. Further cases need to be reported to determine this tumor's true biologic behavior.[175,176]

INVASIVE SCC—PIGMENTED TYPE

> **BOX 7-20   Summary**
>
> - Pigmented SCC is a very rare. Clinically, it can be confused with pigmented BCC and melanoma.
> - These lesions are rapidly growing, crusted, pigmented papules on actinically damaged skin of elderly individuals.
> - Most lesions occur on the face, but can also occur on the scrotum, in the oral mucosa, and on the conjunctiva and cornea.

Pigmented SCC is also a very rare clinical type. Clinically, it can be confused with pigmented BCC and melanoma, in particular, melanomas associated with pseudoepithelomatous hyperplasia. These lesions are rapidly growing, crusted, pigmented papules on actinically damaged skin of elderly individuals. Most occur on the face, but can also occur on the scrotum, in the oral mucosa, and on the conjunctiva and cornea.[177,178]

There have only been few reports of infiltrating pigmented SCC of the skin described in the literature. In one study, which evaluated five cases of pigmented SCCs, all these tumors presented as rapidly growing crusted papules on actinically damaged skin of the face. After the lesion was excised, the average follow-up of 4 years did not reveal any recurrence or metastasis. Since there have only been few reports of pigmented SCCs, it is difficult to come to a conclusion regarding the malignant potential of these lesions.[178]

INVASIVE SCC—DESMOPLASTIC TYPE

> **BOX 7-21   Summary**
>
> - DSCC is a rare, high-risk variant of SCC characterized by thin strands or groups of infiltrative spindle cells associated with a dense stromal response.
> - DSCC tends to arise more often in the head and neck region of elderly male patients.
> - Aggressive treatment is recommended, with wider excision margins, lymph-node examination, and lymph-node dissection for lesions deeper than 5 mm.

Desmoplastic SCC (DSCC) is a rare, high-risk variant of SCC characterized by thin strands or groups of infiltrative spindle cells associated with a dense stromal response, which, by definition, occupies at least 30% of the tumor volume. DSCC was first described by Haneke in 1989.[179] DSCC tends to arise more often in the head and neck region of elderly male patients. There is a high incidence of DSCC on the ears, cheeks, and nose, and a relatively low incidence on the trunk and extremities.[49]

One study reviewed 44 cases of DSCCs that were treated with Mohs and followed up to 5 years. The DSCCs were found to metastasize six times more often and have local recurrences 10 times more often than common SCCs. This study concluded that desmoplasia is a significant prognostic factor for SCC and is associated with the development of metastases or recurrence. Aggressive treatment is recommended, with wider excision margins, lymph-node examination, and lymph-node dissection for lesions deeper than 5 mm.[49,57,58,115,180]

INVASIVE SCC—CLEAR CELL TYPE

> **BOX 7-22   Summary**
>
> - Clear cell carcinoma has widespread hydropic change, with accumulation of intracellular fluid.
> - Clear cell carcinoma occurs mostly in elderly white men with an extensive history of sun exposure.
> - Clinically, it appears as a nodule or mass that may sometimes be ulcerated.

Clear cell carcinoma, also known as hydropic SCC, was first described in 1980 by Kuo. Clear cell carcinoma has widespread hydropic change, with accumulation of intracellular fluid. It occurs mostly in elderly white men with an extensive history of sun exposure. The cases that have been reported have occurred in the head and neck region, with the mandible being the most common site. Clinically, it appears as a nodule or mass that may sometimes be ulcerated. With only a few cases reported, more studies are necessary before a clear prognosis of this variant of SCC can be ascertained.[181]

ADENOSQUAMOUS CARCINOMA

> **BOX 7-23   Summary**
>
> - Primary cutaneous adenosquamous carcinoma is very rare. It is usually aggressive and has true glandular differentiation.
> - Most cases occur in elderly patients and the incidence is practically the same between males and females. The lesions tend to involve the head and neck region.
> - The lesions usually appear as elevated, indurated, keratotic plaques, measuring from 1 to 6 cm in size.

Primary cutaneous adenosquamous carcinoma is very rare. This variant was first described by Weidner and Foucar in 1985. It is usually aggressive and has true glandular differentiation. Most of the reported cases thus far have been associated with sun-damaged skin and have shown areas of typical SCC. Most cases occur in elderly patients. The incidence is practically the same between males and females, and the lesions tend to involve

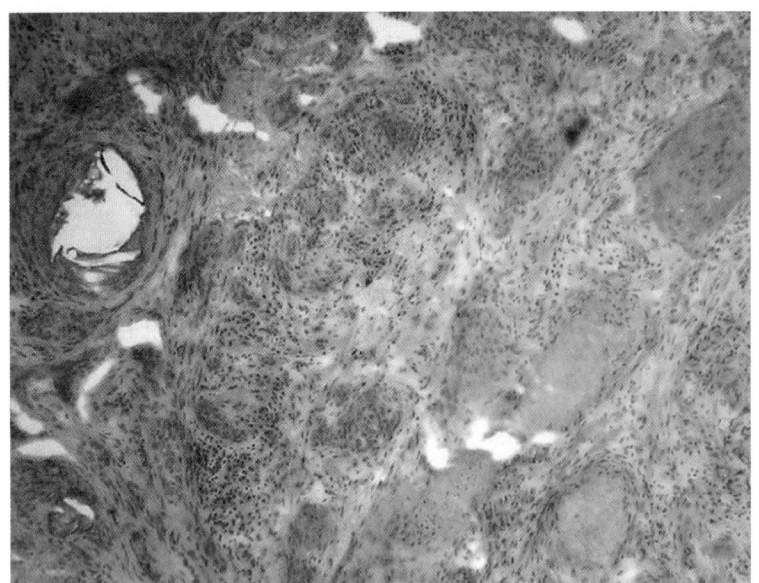

▲ **FIGURE 7-39** BSC (H&E low magnification).

the head and neck region. However, the penis is a very common site. The lesions usually appear as elevated, indurated, keratotic plaques, measuring from 1 to 6 cm in size. Adenosquamous carcinoma has been shown to be very aggressive, with a high rate of recurrence and metastasis. One study revealed that five out of 10 patients died of this carcinoma, and two were alive with extensive disease.[45,182,183]

BASOSQUAMOUS CARCINOMA

> **BOX 7-24   Summary**
>
> - BSC is an entity that has been classified under BCC for a long period; however, clinically, the lesions are more akin to SCC.
> - BSC is a malignant skin neoplasm predominantly induced by UV radiation.
> - Histopathologically, this entity comprises two distinct neoplastic components, one of which is BCC and the other is well-differentiated SCC.
> - BSCs have been reported to be associated with high recurrence rates after initial treatment regardless of treatment choice.

Basosquamous Carcinoma (BSC) is an entity that has been classified under BCC for a long period (see the Chapter 6); however, clinically the lesions are more akin to SCC. These lesions have also been called metatypical carcinoma and BCC with squamous differentiation.

BSC is a malignant skin neoplasm, predominantly induced by UV radiation, as the lesions are located mostly on sun-exposed areas of the body and commonly associated with other manifestations of sun-damaged skin. Histopathologically,

this entity is composed of two distinct neoplastic components, one of which is BCC and the other is well-differentiated SCC. In between these two polar cellular ends, a third transitional component shows neoplastic cells that are neither typical of BCC nor SCC histopathologically and immunohistochemically (Fig. 7-39).[51,63] True BSC has to be differentiated from simultaneous occurrence of SCC and BCC at the same location.

BSCs have been reported to be associated with high recurrence rates after initial treatment regardless of treatment choice. The overall rate of metastases is also

reported to be much higher than BCC and even higher than ordinary SCC types. In this sense, BSC is nosologically still controversial, yet clinically and prognostically, it can be emphasized that the biologic behavior of BSC is much more aggressive than an average BCC. The earlier-mentioned features support the approach of several authors who classify BSC as a type of SCC rather than BCC.[50,57,63]

MALIGNANT PROLIFERATING PILAR (TRICHOLEMMAL) TUMOR/CYST (INVASIVE SCC ARISING FROM PTT)

> **BOX 7-25   Summary**
>
> - PPT are rare malignant neoplasms, found more commonly in elderly women and on the scalp.
> - Clinically, the neoplasm is a multinodular cystic mass, with occasional ulceration, present on the scalp of an older patient.
> - The tumor is often slow-growing, and though local recurrences are common, metastases are rare.

Proliferating pilar (tricholemmal) tumor/cyst (PPT) was initially described by Wilson–Jones in 1966.[184] These are rare malignant neoplasms that are found more commonly in elderly women and on the scalp. The average age of presentation for these lesions is 60. Clinically, the neoplasm is a multinodular cystic mass, with occasional ulceration present on the scalp of an older patient (Fig. 7-40).

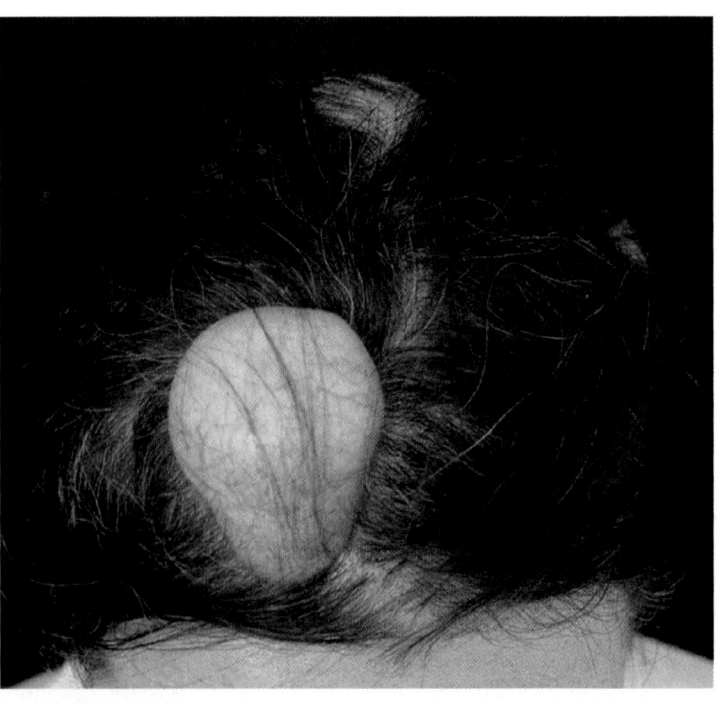

▲ **FIGURE 7-40** Proliferating pilar tumor/cyst on the scalp (courtesy of Ankara University School of Medicine).

The tumor is often slow-growing, and though local recurrences are common, metastases are rare.[49,185,186] On the other hand, one study found that 10 PPT cases out of 63 had features of infiltrating carcinoma. However, only one recurred and one metastasized after complete excision. It has been concluded that PPTs should be regarded as benign cystic squamous neoplasms with the potential for recurrence and progression to invasive SCC.[45,187]

INVASIVE SCC—ARISING IN ADNEXAL CYSTS

BOX 7-26 Summary

- Invasive SCC arising in adnexal cysts appear as nodules which are ill-defined, fixed, and do not appear to involve the overlying epidermis.
- No recurrence of these lesions has been found after complete excision.

Skelton et al. first described SCC arising in adnexal cysts. This study reported two elderly white males with SCC arising from eccrine and apocrine hidrocystomas. The SCCs in both these patients came from the cyst walls and invaded the surrounding dermis. The lesions appeared as a nodule which was ill-defined, fixed, and did not appear to involve the overlying epidermis. It was found in both cases that both the patients were positive for HPV-16. This finding could possibly suggest a pathogenic role for this virus. There was no recurrence of the lesion after complete excision in both patients. However, more cases need to be reported to confirm a nonaggressive course of this tumor.[188]

FOLLICULAR SQUAMOUS CELL CARCINOMA

BOX 7-27 Summary

- FSCC occurs most commonly on sun-damaged skin.
- These lesions are mostly located on sun-damaged skin of the head and commonly affect elderly individuals.
- Clinically, they appear as a dome-shaped, nonulcerated nodule with sharply demarcated borders.

Follicular SCC (FSCC) occurs most commonly on sun-damaged skin. Clinically, FSCC most commonly affects elderly individuals. The lesions are mostly located on sun-damaged skin of the head. The gross appearance is a dome-shaped, nonulcerated nodule with sharply demarcated borders. In a study done by Diaz-Cascajo, 16 cases occurred on the face of elderly patients. Of these, there were only two recurrences and no metastases reported. However, even though FSCC seems to display nonaggressive behavior, more studies are needed to conclude a definitive prognosis.[45,52]

SQUAMOID ECCRINE DUCTAL CARCINOMA

BOX 7-28 Summary

- Squamoid eccrine ductal carcinomas present as solitary dermal nodules found on the head and neck and extremities of elderly patients.
- More patients need to be examined to determine the malignant potential of this tumor.

Squamoid eccrine ductal carcinoma was reported in 1997 by Wong et al. These lesions had overlapping ductal and squamoid features. They presented as solitary dermal nodules found on the head and neck and extremities of elderly patients. One patient in this study suffered several recurrences after excision. It is difficult to give a prognosis for this variant of SCC because only a small number of cases have been reported. More patients need to be examined to determine the malignant potential of this tumor.[45,189]

LYMPHOEPITHELIOMA-LIKE CARCINOMA OF THE SKIN

BOX 7-29 Summary

- LELCS is a rare cutaneous neoplasm.
- LELCS typically presents as a flesh-colored or red, firm nodule or plaque. These lesions usually occur on the head and neck region, but can occur on the trunk as well.
- LELCS typically affects middle-aged to elderly patients and occurs in equal incidence in males and females.

Lymphoepithelioma-like carcinoma of the skin (LELCS) is a rare cutaneous neoplasm. Its nosologic classification as a type of invasive SCC is still subject to further discussion. LELCS typically presents as a flesh-colored or red, firm nodule or plaque. These lesions usually occur on the head and neck, but can occur on the trunk as well. LELCS typically affects middle-aged to elderly patients and occurs in equal incidence in males and females. It can be clinically and histologically confused with other benign and malignant tumors. Despite its poorly differentiated histology,

LELCS prognosis is relatively good. However, recurrences from incomplete excision, metastasis to regional lymph nodes, and one case of fatal distant metastasis have been reported.[190,191]

TRICHOLEMMAL CARCINOMA

BOX 7-30 Summary

- TLC is a cutaneous adnexal tumor with external hair sheath differentiation.
- These tumors occur in hair bearing, sun-exposed skin, and involve the scalp, face, trunk, or upper extremities.
- The lesions are usually slightly raised, pale tan or reddish, and keratotic. They are usually present for less than 1 year and can measure from 0.4 to 2.0 cm.
- TLC has an aggressive growth pattern, but it has an indolent clinical course.

Trichilemmal carcinoma (TLC) was originally described by Headington as a "histologically invasive, cytologically atypical clear cell neoplasm of adnexal keratinocytes which is in continuity with the epidermis and/or follicular epithelium." TLC is a cutaneous adnexal tumor with external hair sheath differentiation. These tumors occur in hair bearing, sun-exposed skin, and involve the scalp, face, trunk, or upper extremities. The lesions are usually slightly raised, pale tan or reddish, and keratotic. They are usually present for less than 1 year, and can measure from 0.4 to 2.0 cm. TLC can be frequently misdiagnosed clinically as BCC. Despite an aggressive growth, it has an indolent clinical course. No cases of recurrence or metastasis have been reported.[192–195]

DIAGNOSES AND TREATMENT PLANNING IN SCC

BOX 7-31 Summary

- The diagnosis of SCC is based on patient history, clinical manifestations, and most importantly histopathologic examination of the lesion.
- SCC is a common malignant neoplasm that can be cured by adequate and complete removal of the tumor.
- The clinical features that are mostly associated with high risk in SCC are: high-risk clinical types of SCC, patients with preexisting conditions, radiation or burn scars, chronic ulcer/sinus sites, other scarring skin diseases, immunosupression, organ transplantation, and HIV infection.

- The histopathologic features that are most commonly associated with high risk in SCC are: high-risk SCC subtypes such as spindle cell SCC, DSCC, adenosquamous carcinoma, malignant proliferating pilar tumor, invasive Bowen, and BSC. This is in addition to poorly differentiated neoplasms, Broders grade 3 to 4, tumors with maximal vertical thickness greater than 4 mm, Clark level IV to V, infitrative growth, growth pattern, and perineural, lymphatic, or vascular invasion.

The diagnosis of SCC is based on the earlier-mentioned features in history, clinical manifestations, and most importantly histopathologic examination of the lesion. Excisional biopsy or total excision should be preferred whenever possible in order to simplify the pathology adequately. The overall histopathologic architecture is as important, if not more important, than the clinical architecture of the lesion in coming to a definitive diagnosis and in shaping the treatment and follow-up based on prognostic assessment.

SCCs with typical histopathologic features and with some degree of differentiation usually do not require additional immunohistochemical (IHC) studies to confirm the diagnoses. However, in the case of challenging histopathologic subtypes, (e.g., indifferentiated, spindle cell, sarcomatous, pleomorphic with multinucleation, pigmented, clear cell, small cell, or signet ring cell types) epithelial marker positivity, such as cytokeratins and epithelial membrane antigen is very helpful, as well as negative staining with S-100, Vimentin, Actin, Melan-b, CEA, and LCA, in coming to the definitive diagnoses of SCC.

Cytokeratins (CK) are polypeptides that are expressed in epithelial cells of various levels of differentiation. There are 30 types of CKs in human epithelia and more than 100 monoclonal antibodies for labeling them. A panel of class I and II CK subtypes Abs: CK1, 5/8, 7, 10, 14, and 19 are usually helpful in diagnosing keratinizing and nonkeratinizing epithelial in situ and invasive SCCs, as well as their metastases.

There are certain IHC and molecular genetic markers that are reported to be associated with invasive and metastatic SCC. IHC markers such as Ki-67 (mib-1), p53, p63, bcl-2, EGFr, epithelial adhesion molecule (EpCAM), P16, matrix metalloproteinase (MMP) 2 and 9, and oncogenic nuclear transcription factor (Ets-1) show increased positivity in invasive SCCs. Genetic abnormalities like DNA aneuploidy, loss of genomic material, and loss of heterozygosity (LOH) in the lesions are in favor of malignancy in early lesions, although it is still not possible to used them routinely. Ber-EP4 is also a useful diagnostic marker in differentiating BCC with squamous differentiation from SCC.

SCC is a common malignant neoplasm that can be cured by adequate and complete removal of the tumor, especially when diagnosed and treated before any lymphatic or distant metastatic involvement. Yet, certain groups of patients are clearly at a higher risk of locally invasive-recurrent disease and/or metastases and these patients are more associated with major morbidity and poor prognostic outcome.[47,57]

It is necessary to look for the possible clinical and histopathologic signs of high-risk SCC in each patient. When present, these high-risk, poor prognostic features should lead the clinician to more meticulous search for already-existing occult regional or distant involvement or invasion. The search should include, if applicable, sentinel lymph-node excision, magnetic resonance imaging (MRI), positron emission tomography (PET) imaging, more proactive treatment planning, adding adjunctive treatment modalities, and close long-term follow-up. These options are not always possible, feasible, or necessary for thousands of common low-risk cutaneous SCCs on patients.

The clinical features that are mostly associated with high risk in SCC are: high-risk clinical types of SCC, patients with preexisting conditions such as XP and OCA, radiation or burn scars, chronic ulcer/sinus sites, other scarring skin diseases, immunosupression, organ transplantation, and HIV infection. Other features that are associated with high risk include: previous history of incomplete treatment, recurrent tumor, large tumor size (maximal clinical diameter > 2 cm), and high-risk locations (preauricular, around or on external ear, lower lip, non-sun-exposed skin sites).[47,57,61,196]

While assessing SCC of the skin, a detailed histopathologic description is necessary. This includes the maximum vertical thickness of the tumor in millimeters (measuring from the granular layer of the epidermis), histopathologic subtyping, pattern of tumor invasion and the degree of differentiation, grading, and presence of perineural, lymphatic, or vascular invasion. These are all of extreme importance and have to be mentioned in the histopathology report.

The histopathologic features that are most commonly associated with high risk in SCC are: high-risk SCC subtypes such as spindle cell SCC, DSCC, adenosquamous carcinoma, malignant proliferating pilar tumor, invasive Bowen, and BSC. This is in addition to poorly differentiated neoplasms, Broders grade 3 to 4, tumors with maximal vertical thickness > 4 mm, Clark level IV to V, infitrative growth, growth pattern, and perineural, lymphatic, or vascular invasion.[3,47,49,50,57,61,196]

■ TREATMENT OF SQUAMOUS CELL CARCINOMA

BOX 7-32 Summary

- The type of treatment should be based on the histology of the lesion and its size, location, and degree of metastasis.
- MMS offers the highest 5-year cure rate for SCC, and may be the treatment of choice for those considered high-risk tumors.
- Surgical excision is the treatment of choice for lower-risk SCC tumors and provides the second-highest cure rate.
- Cryosurgery offers good short-term cure rates for low-risk tumors; however, the treatment does not provide histologic control which may lead to recurrence.
- Laser therapy, in particular the carbon dioxide laser and diode laser, is useful in treating BD at certain locations.
- Radiation therapy can be a primary or adjuvant treatment ideal for lower-staged SCC tumors. Side effects must be taken into consideration when choosing this treatment.
- Chemotherapy with topical 5-fluorouracil, PDT, or immunomodulators such as interferon or imiquimod has been proven beneficial in the prevention and treatment of BD and superficial SCC. Potential side effects are associated with these therapies.
- Retinoids, specifically oral isotretinoin, have proven effective in the prevention of SCC. They can also be used in combination with other therapies for the treatment of advanced SCC.
- NSAIDS, specifically topical 3% diclofenac, have been effective in the prevention and treatment of AK. Side effects have been associated with this therapy.
- Follow-up evaluations are recommended after any treatment because SCC has a high metastatic potential and may recur at a local or distant site.

As with most medical treatments, a detailed history and physical examination must be taken prior to initiating any therapy. This is important to possibly avoid harmful drug interactions or other surgical complications that may arise.

A biopsy is performed to confirm whether a lesion is benign or malignant (see the Chapter 36). If the tumor is determined to be cancerous, a treatment plan including one or more therapies can be designed based on the individual patient and an assessment of four basic characteristics of the lesion: histology, size, location, and degree of metastasis. Also, long-term follow-up is very important for SCC due to its significant metastatic potential.

In the United States, more than 90% of the patients with cutaneous SCC are cured by local therapy alone (surgery and/or radiotherapy), and 10% need a new therapeutic approach.[197] Determining whether tumors are low-risk or high-risk can help determine which treatment option will be the most effective. Low-risk tumors (those that are slow-growing, small, well-differentiated) may be treated with topical therapy or excision. High-risk tumors (those that are large, fast-growing, recurrent, or in transplant or otherwise immunosuppressed patients) should be managed with Mohs micrographic surgery or standard surgical excision.[198] This section will discuss both surgical and nonsurgical treatment options for SCC.

Surgical Treatments

MOHS MICROGRAPHIC SURGERY (SEE ALSO THE CHAPTER 40) Mohs micrographic surgery (MMS) offers arguably the highest long-term cure rate of any therapies for SCC discussed in this chapter. It is most commonly indicated for high-risk tumors (those that are large or located on the head and neck). Both primary and recurrent SCC tumors can be treated using this technique. In a recent, large study evaluating the long-term outcome of MMS, a 3.9% overall recurrence rate was found at the 5-year follow-up.[199] For patients who had a primary SCC tumor, the recurrence rate was 2.6%. For those who had recurrent SCC tumors, the recurrence rate was 5.9%. In a review of a large population with primary SCC treated with surgical excision, Rowe et al.[200] found that local recurrences after 5 years are less frequent when MMS is used as opposed to surgical excision.

SURGICAL EXCISION (SEE ALSO THE CHAPTER 39) Surgical excision is considered the treatment of choice for most cutaneous SCC tumors.[201] This is because it, along with MMS, allows for histologic control of the margins during treatment. Five-year cure rates for primary SCCs have reached 92%, and those for recurrent SCCs have

touched 77%.[200] For smaller tumors (less than 2 cm), a 4-mm margin of normal skin is recommended.[201,202] For larger primary tumors, up to a 10-mm margin may be necessary.[201,202] For these higher risk tumors, MMS may be considered the treatment of choice.

CRYOSURGERY (SEE ALSO THE CHAPTER 43)
Cryosurgery can be used to treat small and well-defined tumors, considered low-risk. Good short-term recurrence rates have been reported.[201,202] This treatment is contraindicated in large or recurrent tumors considered high-risk. It is also not recommended in certain areas such as the head and neck. Common side effects include edema and hypopigmentation. More serious adverse effects include atrophy and hypertrophic scarring. Also, recurrence is possible as this treatment does not provide histologic control.

LASER THERAPY Case reports indicate that the carbon dioxide laser is considered to be useful in the management of some cases of BD. In one study of BD on the digits, four out of five cases had no recurrence within 3 years of treatment, and no patient suffered a loss of function.[203] The cosmetic outcome was also acceptable. In another study of three patient cases of BD in hair-bearing areas, a combination of the CO_2 laser and a diode laser allowed for deeper ablation.[204] In a follow-up evaluation of 4 months, no clinical recurrence was noted.

Nonsurgical Treatments

RADIATION THERAPY (SEE ALSO THE CHAPTER 47) Radiation therapy, also called radiotherapy, can be used as a primary treatment for SCC or as a form of adjuvant therapy with other methods discussed in this section. Because it is less invasive than surgical interventions, it is ideal for patients who desire good cosmetic and functional outcomes,[201] for example, on the eyelids, and for the elderly. However, these cosmetic benefits are mostly short-term, and thus younger patients tend to avoid this therapy.[202] Studies indicate that radiation therapy has yielded both short and long-term cure rates.[201] It is most effective when used on tumors of the head and neck, specifically on the lip, nasal vestibule, and ear.[201] It can be used as an adjuvant therapy when there is evidence of metastasis or if residual disease is suspected. Also, it can be combined with other modalities for large, aggressive, or recurrent tumors.

The cure rates that have been reported in studies vary with the stage

of the disease. For T1 tumors, those that are 2 cm or less, cure rates of approximately 90% have been reported.[202] However, for higher-staged tumors or recurrent tumors, cure rates decline and thereby invalidate radiation therapy as a viable treatment option. In a recent study by Kwan et al.,[205] which included patients with SCC staged at T2 or above, or patients with nodal involvement of the disease, it was concluded that locoregional failure, or recurrence of the disease at the primary site or in nearby lymph nodes, is the main cause of death for patients with recurrent SCCs. Also, the median length of time for recurrence was 5 months after radiotherapy. Interestingly, prophylactic radiation of regional lymph nodes in patients without nodal involvement proved to reduce locoregional failure by 10%. Thus, it can be inferred from the results of the study that the presence of lymph-node involvement greatly affects recurrence of the disease and patient survival, and radiotherapy may offer a means of alleviating this problem.

A disadvantage of this therapy is that there is no means for testing margins to confirm if the whole lesion has been treated. Also, it can become expensive and multiple treatment sessions are needed.

There are potential side effects and complications associated with radiation therapy. First, because radiation is being used, there is a risk of inducing other cancers and tumors in the long term. Second, some follow-up studies have noted atrophy, hypopigmentation, and telangiectasia of the treated areas, primarily in the trunk and extremities.[202] Also, some patients may develop radiation necrosis such as osteoradionecrosis if the treatment is performed over bony structures.[202]

CHEMOTHERAPY Topical chemotherapy is a treatment option for SCC and BD, also known as SCC *in situ*. Three major vehicles of chemotherapy are: topical 5-fluorouracil (5-FU), an antimetabolite, photodynamic therapy, and immunomodulators such as imiquimod.

Topical 5-Fluorouracil (see also the chapter 49) 5-FU has been used for actinic keratoses with good results. In one study comparing a treatment of 0.5% fluorouracil once a day with 5% fluorouracil twice a day, a total clearance of approximately 43% was noted for both regimens, though the former was considered more tolerable and convenient.[206] In a more recent study evaluating long-term clinical outcomes, the continuous treatment of 5% imiquimod two or three times a week proved to be clinically beneficial in most patients with limited long-term safety concerns.[207]

For BD, 5-FU is recognized as a reliable treatment option, though careful and long-term follow-up is advised. It is ideal in cases of multiple lesions, or when surgical treatment is difficult or refused.[208] A typical course of therapy calls for an application of 5% cream two times a day for 4 to 8 weeks. In some cases, a lack of penetration into the epithelium can lower the response rates. For these situations, efficacy can be strengthened by using adjuvant therapies such as topical tretinoin or interferon, or by changing drug delivery methods (using an occlusive dressing to cover the lesion while being treated or using iontophoresis to increase penetration.[208] In a recent study designed to evaluate long-term effectiveness of 5-FU by taking biopsies at the follow-ups, a treatment period of 9 weeks was used, though it was shortened for certain patients due to adverse reactions.[208] The researchers found that only two of the 26 lesions present at the start of the study recurred during the follow-up evaluations, indicating that a longer therapeutic period may enhance efficacy. As with most skin cancer treatments, there are side effects that must be considered. A common side effect of topical 5-FU is inflammation, especially when it is being used to treat BD. Other common side effects include pain, erythema, edema, scarring, ulceration, and infections.

Photodynamic Therapy (see also the chapter 46) Photodynamic therapy (PDT) is another common topical chemotherapy for superficial cutaneous SCC. When topical 5-aminolevulinic acid is administered along with PDT, better responses due to longer photosensitivity are achieved. This method of treatment lacks evidential support from long-term follow-up studies. In a recent review of studies,[209] use of PDT delivered up to 100% clearance rates for SCC *in situ*, but only 8% for more invasive SCC. Further, recurrence rates were up to 52% for SCC *in situ* and up to 82% for invasive SCC. Because SCC is known for its dangerously high metastatic potential, the use of PDT as an effective treatment is limited at this time.

Immunomodulators (see also the chapter 48) There are two main groups of immunomodulators that can be used to treat BD and SCC: interferon and imiquimod. A treatment regimen using IFNα-2b three times a day for 3 weeks proved to be effective.[210] Interferon can also be used in combination therapies. For example,

patients with transplant-associated metastatic SCC are effectively treated with retinoids (discussed later) and interferon.[210] An advantage of intralesional interferon treatment is that it is minimally invasive and scarring is rare. In a recent study, intralesional IFNα-2b was injected over a period of 9 to 12 weeks, and follow-up evaluations indicated no recurrence of SCC.[211]

Imiquimod (Aldara) is a common treatment used for BD and SCC. In a recent study of 16 patients, most of whom had lower leg BD lesions, 93% had no residual tumors after a 16-week treatment.[212] Anogenital lesions respond well to imiquimod treatment. Common side effects of the treatment include pain, erythema, and infections.[202] In another study using 5% imiquimod cream treatment for 16 weeks, 73% of the patients achieved clearance and no recurrence by the 9-month follow-up.[213] No serious side effects were reported. This cream can also be used for invasive SCC, with a regimen of five times a week for 12 weeks or up to 19 weeks, as noted by a few recent studies.[214,215] These cases also had great cosmetic outcomes.

RETINOIDS Retinoids are said to be better in the chemoprevention of SCC than in the treatment of it. Studies have shown a relationship between vitamin A deficiency and cancer. Therefore, retinoic acid, being a metabolite of vitamin A, may aid in treatment or prevention by regulating genes involved in tumor promotion.[197] Long-term systemic isotretinoin may be used as a method of chemoprevention for high-risk patients (those with XP or transplant patients).[197] Further, for post-transplant patients, it was found that cells involved in organ rejection were reduced by oral isotretinoin therapy.[197]

Various studies have been done to evaluate the efficacy of this treatment. The best responses can be seen when combination therapies are used, especially for advanced SCC. For example, many preclinical trials have suggested that a treatment of both isotretinoin and IFN-α may be more beneficial in terms of response, though adverse effects can be greater as well.[197] This combination with the addition of cisplatin was also tested and achieved a longer response, but side effects were still present.[197]

NSAIDS (SEE ALSO THE CHAPTER 50) NSAIDs, or nonsteroidal anti-inflammatory drugs, can be used for the prevention

and treatment of SCC. The mechanism involves cyclooxygenase-2 (COX-2) inhibition. The topical NSAID treatment for AKs, potential precursors of SCC, has been evaluated in many studies with varying results.[216] Out of five published trials using topical 3% diclofenac therapy in a 2.5% hylauronan base two times a day to treat AKs, four trials ranging from 1 to 6 months showed clearance rates from 33 to 81%, while the placebo groups in these trials showed 10 to 20% clearance.[216] Also, through these trials, a clear correlation between the length of treatment and clearance rates was evident. Side effects of topical diclofenac include mild to moderate skin irritation, dryness, pruritus, rash, and dermatitis.[216] However, any NSAID can have a variety of adverse effects on the body, specifically on the skin, kidneys, heart, and gastrointestinal system.

Post-treatment Considerations

Because SCC has a high potential for metastasis and some of the earlier-mentioned treatments lack histologic control, routine follow-ups are essential. Recurrence usually appears within 5 years after treatment, so frequent follow-ups, either quarterly, biannually, or annually, depending on the risk level of the initial tumor, are recommended.

■ PREVENTION

BOX 7-33 Summary

- Acknowledging and learning appropriate prevention techniques is an essential component to decrease the risk of SCC.
- Chemoprevention, a new aspect of prevention, is defined as a dietary or pharmacologic preparation, which can be applied topically or ingested orally, to reduce or reverse the development of skin cancer.
- One of the most recognized and proven chemopreventive agents are the class of retinoids.
- It was found that several retinoids are capable of inhibiting tumor growth through multiple mechanisms; however, the FDA has not currently approved retinoids for the use of chemoprevention.
- Other chemopreventive agents include COX-2 selective inhibitors and nonselective NSAIDS. These induce apoptosis and cause a reduction in cell numbers in head and neck SCCs.
- Currently, randomized phase II and phase III trials are being conducted to see the chemopreventive celecoxib benefits in humans.

- Nutritional supplements, such as green tea polyphenols, green tea with curcumin, citrus peel consumption, vitamin D, silymarin, and isoflavone genistein are also being studied as chemopreventive agents.
- There has been found some correlation between dietary fat intake and a risk of SCC. Certain fats can alter the lipid membrane of cells and these cells may become more responsive to growth factors.

Acknowledging and learning appropriate prevention techniques is an essential component to decrease the risk of SCC. It is already a known fact that skin cancer is chiefly caused by excessive exposure to UV. Education geared toward the general public has primarily focused on sun protection and avoidance (see the chapter 6).

A new aspect of prevention has emerged in recent years. Chemoprevention is defined as a dietary or pharmacologic preparation, which can be applied topically or ingested orally, to reduce or reverse the development of skin cancer.[217] This area of research has grown at an incredible rate and many realistic possibilities are on the horizon.

One of the most recognized and proven chemopreventive agents are the class of retinoids. The term retinoids encompasses vitamin A (retinol) and all of its natural derivatives.[217] It has been shown that retinoids are essential for normal skin growth, epithelial maturation, differentiation, and apoptosis.[218,219] Retinoids are mediated through retinoic acid receptors (RARs) and retinoid X receptors (RXRs). These alter gene expression via transcription factors and it was shown that suppression of these retinoid receptors is associated with growth of SCC.[219] Cancer growth is also controlled by degradation of extracellular matrix which is mediated primarily by metalloproteinase (MMP). A study found that several retinoids are capable of specifically inhibiting MMP synthesis in SCC tumor lines, thereby inhibiting tumor growth.[220] Another study showed that retinoids inhibit the growth of SCC by altering gap junctional intercellular communication; therefore, disrupting growth signals and inhibiting the growth of the tumor.[221] Essentially, retinoids interfere with tumor promotion and progression rather than tumor initiation.[222] Thus, multiple mechanisms of SCC inhibition have been discovered through retinoids alone.

With basic science investigational research supporting retinoids as a successful chemoprevention agent, many recent clinical research literature have also exhibited promising results. The Southwest Skin Cancer Prevention Study Group held a randomized, double-blind, controlled trial to evaluate the effectiveness of oral retinoids in moderate-risk subjects. Their conclusion was that daily supplements of 25,000 IU of retinol was effective in preventing SCCs, while not in the case of BCCs.[223]

Studies analyzing the chemopreventive qualities of retinoids in organ transplant recipients have also been done. One prospective study in Australia evaluated Acitretin in renal transplant patients and found that SCC incidence was significantly lower in treated time periods as opposed to drug-free periods.[224] Another retrospective study in the United Kingdom researched the long-term efficacy of systemic retinoids (0.2 to 0.4 mg/kg per day for 12 months minimum) in organ transplant recipients. They found that low-dose systemic retinoids are significant in reducing SCCs in transplant patients for the first 3 years of treatment and the medication effect may last for up to 8 years.[225]

Oral retinoids have also been found to be successful in chemoprevention for psoriasis patients treated with psoralen-UVA. It was found in a recent nested cohort study that SCC risk was significantly decreased with oral retinoids whereas BCC risk was not considerably affected.[226] Further studies are required to achieve optimal dosages for the indications mentioned earlier; however, these preliminary results are quite hopeful. To note, oral retinoids are teratogenic and, therefore, caution must be administered when advising this medication. To date, the Food and Drug Administration (FDA) has not approved retinoids for the use of chemoprevention.[217]

Another potential chemopreventive agent are NSAIDs. Their mechanism of action is to inhibit the cyclooxygenase (COX) enzyme. Both isoforms of the COX enzyme, COX-1 and COX-2, produce prostaglandins. COX-2 has been found to be highly expressed in areas of the epidermis that have been radiated with UVB.[227] It has also been demonstrated that COX-2 and subsequently the prostaglandin E2 that it produces, strongly correlate with the progression and metastasis of cancer.[228] Therefore, it is only natural that NSAIDs are studied for chemoprevention.[217] Studies have found that COX-2 selective inhibitors and nonselective NSAIDs induce apoptosis and cause a reduction in cell numbers in head and neck SCCs.[229] In a murine SCC cancer cell line study, tumor growth was assessed in surgical wounds. Specifically, Celecoxib (COX-2 selective) was found to significantly inhibit tumor progression in surgical wounds.[230] Another novel study in rats evaluated concurrent treatment of celecoxib and all-trans retinoic acid (atRA) loaded microspheres. The study found that though the celecoxib maintained the atRA concentration at a higher level in the plasma, yet it prevented inflammatory responses of the retinoid. This new combination of medication is suggested for future use in the chemoprevention of SCC cases.[231] Currently, randomized phase II and phase III trials are being conducted to see the chemopreventive celecoxib benefits in humans.[217]

Another researched area in regard to chemoprevention is nutritional supplements. Green tea polyphenols, extracts, and its chief component, (-)-epigallocatechin gallate, in topical and oral applications have shown hopeful results in mice studies and human tumor lines; however, clinical trials in humans are needed to justify these primary results.[232-234] The combinations of green tea with curcumin (yellow pigment in the spice turmeric) applied topically to hamsters actually decreased the proliferation index of SCC; tea alone increased the apoptotic index in dysplasia and SCC. This original approach also needs to be further investigated and eventually tested on humans to determine the benefits.[235] Other agents that have been suggested for chemoprevention are: citrus peel consumption,[236] vitamin D,[237] silymarin,[238] and isoflavone genistein.[239,240] Follow-up studies in humans are needed to assess risks and benefits of such a preventive treatment.

Further nutritional supplements have also been tested, yet have been found to be ineffective in chemoprevention. A randomized 12-year study with beta-carotene supplementation was found to not affect the development of both BCC and SCC.[241] Other studies have also found beta-carotene to be unsuccessful, along with supplementation of vitamins A, C, and E, folate, and α-tocopherols.[242-245]

Additionally, studies have shown some correlation with dietary fat intake and risk of SCC. One study displayed that there is a consistent decreased risk of SCC when there is an increased intake of diets with a high ratio of n-3 to n-6 fatty acids.[246] It has been studied that certain fats can alter the lipid membrane of cells and have these cells abnormally more responsive to growth factors.[245] With the general public being well aware of sun safety and awareness, chemoprevention and dietary/nutritional education may well become the future target for general skin cancer prevention.

FINAL THOUGHTS

SCC has many clinical and histopathologic variants that show different biological behavior. Most SCCs are not serious; when identified early and treated promptly, the patient can be cured. However, if overlooked, they are harder to treat and can cause disfigurement. The best way to avoid developing more SCCs is to protect the skin from further sun damage. In addition, learning the signs of skin cancer, checking the skin once a month, and promptly seeking care for any suspicious growth is the key to preventing more serious outcomes.

REFERENCES

1. American Cancer Society. Cancer facts and figures 2003. Available at: http://www.cancer.org/downloads/STT/CAFF2003PWSecured.pdf.
2. Centers for Disease Control. Facts and statistics about skin cancer. Available at: http://www.cdc.gov/cancer/skin/statistics
3. World Health Organization. How common is skin cancer? Available at: http://www.who.int/uv/faq/skincancer/en/index1.html.
4. Diepgen TL, Mahler V. The epidemiology of skin cancer. *Br J Dermatol.* April 2002;146(suppl 61):1–6.
5. Silverberg E, Boring CC, Squires TS. Cancer statistics 1990. *CA Cancer J Clin.* 1990;40:9–26.
6. Miller DL, Weinstock MA. Non-melanoma skin cancer in the United States: Incidence. *J Am Acad Dermatol.* May 1994;30:774–778.
7. Holme SA, Malinovszky K, Roberts DL. Changing trends in non-melanoma skin cancer in South Wales 1988–1998. *Br J Dermatol.* 2000;143:1224–1229.
8. Oikarinen A, Raitio A. Melanoma and other skin cancers in circumpolar areas. *Int J Circumpolar Health.* 2000;59:52–56.
9. Armstrong BK, Kricker A. The epidemiology of UV-induced skin cancer. *J Photochem Photobiol B, Biol.* October 2001;63(1–3):8–18.
10. Giles G, Marks R, Foley P. Incidence of nonmelanocytic skin cancer treated in Australia. *Br Med J.* 1988;269:13–17.
11. Gray DT, Suman VJ, Su WP, et al. Trends in the population-based incidence of squamous cell carcinoma of the skin first diagnosed between 1984 and 1992. *Arch Dermatol.* 1997;133:735–740.
12. Gallagher RP, Ma B, McLean DI, et al. Trends in basal cell carcinoma, squamous cell carcinoma, and melanoma of the skin from 1973 through 1987. *J Am Acad Dermatol.* 1990;23:413–421.
13. Ceylan C, Ozturk G, Alper S. Non-melanoma skin cancers between the years of 1990 and 1999 in Izmir, Turkey: Demographic and clinicopathological characteristics. *J Dermatol.* February 2003;30(2):123–131.
14. Christenson LJ, Borrowman TA, Vachon CM, et al. Incidence of basal cell and squamous cell carcinomas in a population younger than 40 years. *JAMA.* August 2005;294(6):681–690.
15. Boukamp P. Non-melanoma skin cancer: What drives tumor development and progression? *Carcinogenesis.* 2005;26:1657–1664.
16. Tsai KY, Tsao H. The genetics of skin cancer. *Am J Med Genet.* 2004;131C:82–88.
17. Rudin CM, Thompson CB. Apoptosis and cancer. In: Vogelstein B, Kinzler KW, eds. *The Genetic Basis of Human Cancer.* New York: McGraw-Hill; 1997:193.
18. Halliday GM. Inflammation, gene mutation, and photoimmunosuppression in response to UVR-induced oxidative damage contributes to photocarcinogenesis. *Mutat Res.* 2005;571:107–120.
19. Aziz MH, Wheeler DL, Bhamb B, Verma AK. Protein kinase C δ overexpressing transgenic mice are resistant to chemically but not to UV radiation-induced development of squamous cell carcinomas: A possible link to specific cytokines and cyclooxygenase-2. *Cancer Res.* 2006;66:713–721.
20. Moysan A, Clementlacroix P, Michel L, Dubertret L, Morliere P. Effects of ultraviolet and antioxidant defense in cultured fibroblasts and keratinocytes. *Photodermatol Photoimmunol Photomed.* 1996;11:192–197.
21. Podda M, Traber MG, Weber C, Yan LJ, Packer L. UV-radiation depletes antioxidants and causes oxidative damage in a model of human skin. *Free Radic Biol Med.* 1998;24:55–65.
22. Villiotou V, Deliconstantinos G. Nitric oxide, peroxynitrite, and nitroso-compounds formation by ultraviolet A (UVA) irradiated human squamous cell carcinoma: Potential role of nitric oxide in cancer prognosis. *Anticancer Res.* 1995;15:931–942.
23. Deliconstantinos G, Villiotou V, Stavrides JC. Increase of particulate nitric oxide synthase activity and peroxynitrite synthase in UVB-irradiated keratinocytes membranes. *Biochem J.* 1996;320:997–1003.
24. Virag L, Szabo E, Bakondi E, et al. Nitric oxide-peroxynitrite-poly(ADP ribose) polymerase pathway in the skin. *Exp Dermatol.* 2002;11:189–202.
25. Agar NS, Halliday GM, Barnetson RS, Ananthaswamy HN, Wheeler M, Jones AM. The basal layer in human squamous tumors harbors more UVA than UVB fingerprint mutations: A role for UVA in human skin carcinogenesis. *PNAS.* 2004;101:4954–4959.
26. Masini C, Fuchs PG, Gabrielli F, et al. Evidence for the association of human papillomavirus infection and cutaneous squamous cell carcinoma in immunocompetent individuals. *Arch Dermatol.* 2003;139:890–894.
27. Leite JL, Stolf HO, Reis NA, Ward LS. Human herpesvirus type 6 and type 1 infection increases susceptibility to non-melanoma skin tumors. *Cancer Lett.* 2005;224:213–219.
28. Purdie KJ, Surentheran T, Sterling JC, et al. Human papillomavirus gene expression in cutaneous squamous cell carcinomas from immunosuppressed and immunocompetent individuals. *J Invest Dermatol.* 2005;125;98–107.
29. Weissenborn SJ, Nindl I, Purdie K, et al. Human papillomavirus-DNA loads in actinic keratoses exceed those in non-melanoma skin cancers. *J Invest Dermatol.* 2005;125;93–97.
30. Everall J, Dowd P. Influence of environmental factors excluding ultraviolet radiation on the incidence of skin cancer. *Bull Cancer.* 1978;65:241–248.
31. Waterhouse J. Cutting oils and cancer. *Ann Occup Hyg.* 1971;14:161–170.
32. De Hertog, Wensveen CAH, Bastiaens MT, et al. Relation between smoking and skin cancer. *J Clin Oncol.* 2001;19:231–238.
33. Alam M, Ratner D. Cutaneous squamous-cell carcinoma. *N Engl J Med.* 2001;34:975–983.
34. Durando B, Reichel J. The relative effects of different systemic immunosuppressives on skin cancer development in organ transplant patients. *Dermatol Ther.* 2005;18:1–11.
35. Jensen P, Hansen S, Moller B, et al. Skin cancer in kidney and heart transplant recipients and different longterm immunosuppressive therapy regimens. *J Am Acad Dermatol.* 1999;40:177–186.
36. Glover MT, Deeks JJ, Raftery MJ, et al. Immunosuppression and risk of non-melanoma skin cancer in renal transplant recipients. *Lancet.* 1997;34:398.
37. Jensen P, Hansen S, Moller B, et al. Are renal transplant recipients on CsA-based immunosuppressive regimens more likely to develop skin cancer than those on azathioprine and prednisolone? *Transplant Proc.* 1999;31:1120.
38. Kasiske BL, Zinder JJ, Gilbertson DT, Wang C. Cancer after kidney transplantation in the United States. *Am J Transplant.* 2004;4:905–913.
39. Bernstein S, Lim K, Brodland D, Heidelberg K. The many faces of squamous cell carcinoma. *Dermatol Surg.* 1996;22:243–254.
40. Cleaver J. Defective repair replication of DNA in xeroderma pigmentosum. *Nature.* 1968;21:652–656.
41. Odom R, James W, Berger T. Albinism. In: *Andrew's Diseases of the Skin: Clinical Dermatology.* Philadelphia, PA: WB Saunders; 2000:1069–1071.
42. Padgett JK. Cutaneous lesions: Benign and malignant. *Facial Plast Surg Clin North Am.* May 2005;13(2):195–202.
43. Mohs FE. Chemosurgery: Microscopically controlled surgery for skin cancer. Springfield, IL: Charles C. Thomas; 1978.
44. Dinehart SM, Peterson S. Evaluation of the American Joint Committee on cancer staging system for cutaneous squamous cell carcinoma and proposal of a new staging system. *Dermatol Surg.* November 2005;31(11 pt 1):1379–1384.
45. Cassarino DS, Derienzo DP, Barr RJ. Cutaneous squamous cell carcinoma: A comprehensive clinicopathologic classification. *J Cutan Pathol.* March 2006;33(3):191–206.
46. Khanna M, Fortier-Riberdy G, Smoller B, et al. Reporting tumor thickness for cutaneous squamous cell carcinoma.

J Cutan Pathol. July 2002;29(6):321–323.

47. Veness MJ. Defining patients with high-risk cutaneous squamous cell carcinoma. *Aust J Dermatol*. February 2006;47(1):28–33.

48. Quaedvlieg PJ, Creytens DH, Epping GG, et al. Histopathological characteristics of metastasizing squamous cell carcinoma of the skin and lips. *Histopathology*. September 2006;49(3):256–264.

49. Cassarino DS, Derienzo DP, Barr RJ. Cutaneous squamous cell carcinoma: A comprehensive clinicopathologic classification—part two. *J Cutan Pathol*. April 2006;33(4):261–279.

50. Rinker MH, Fenske NA, Scalf LA, et al. Histologic variants of squamous cell carcinoma of the skin. *Cancer Control*. July–August 2001;8(4):354–363.

51. Bowman PH, Ratz JL, Knoepp TG, et al. Basosquamous carcinoma. *Dermatol Surg*. August 2003;29(8):830–832.

52. Diaz-Cascajo C, Borghi S, Weyers W, et al. Follicular squamous cell carcinoma of the skin: A poorly recognized neoplasm arising from the wall of hair follicles. *J Cutan Pathol*. January 2004;31(1):19–25.

53. Beham A, Regauer S, Soyer HP, et al. Keratoacanthoma: A clinically distinct variant of well-differentiated squamous cell carcinoma. *Adv Anat Pathol*. September 1998;5(5):269–280.

54. Tronnier M. Keratoacanthoma. A variant of highly differentiated squamous cell carcinoma and its differential diagnosis. *Pathologe*. January 2002;23(1):65–70.

55. Bernstein SC, Lim KK, Brodland DG, et al. The many faces of squamous cell carcinoma. *Dermatol Surg*. March 1996;22(3):243–254.

56. Hodak E, Jones RE, Ackerman AB. Solitary keratoacanthoma is a squamous-cell carcinoma: Three examples with metastases. *Am J Dermatopathol*. August 1993;15(4):332–342.

57. Petter G, Haustein UF. Rare and newly described histological variants of cutaneous squamous epithelial carcinoma. Classification by histopathology, cytomorphology and malignant potential. *Hautarzt*. April 2001;52(4):288–297.

58. Lohmann CM, Soloman AR. Clinicopathologic variants of cutaneous squamous cell carcinoma. *Adv Anat Pathol*. January 2001;8(1):27–36.

59. Manstein CH, Frauenhoffer CJ, Besden JE. Keratoacanthoma: Is it a real entity? *Ann Plast Surg*. May 1998;40(5):469–472.

60. Broders AC. Practical points on the microscopic grading of carcinoma. *State J Med*. 1932;32:667-671.

61. American Academy of Dermatology. Actinic keratoses and skin cancer. Available at: http://www.aad.org/public/News/Derminfo/ActKerSkCancer FAQ.htm.

62. Dubreuilh WA. Des hyperkeratoses circonscrites (1). *Ann Dermatol Venereol*. 1896;27:1158–1204.

63. Lever WF. *Histopathology of the Skin*. Philadelphia, PA: JB Lippincott; 1949:279–280.

64. Ackerman AB. Editorial. Respect at last for solar keratosis. *Dermatopathol Pract Concept*. 1997;3:101–103.

65. Ng P, Ackerman AB. The major types of squamous-cell carcinoma. *Dermatopathol Pract Concept*. 1999;5:250–252.

66. Ackerman AB. Actinic keratoses—malignant or not? *J Am Acad Dermatol*. 2001;45:466–469.

67. Ackerman AB, Mones JM. Solar (actinic) keratosis is squamous cell carcinoma. *Br J Dermatol*. July 2006;155(1):9–22.

68. Cockerell CJ. Histopathology of incipient intraepidermal squamous cell carcinoma ("actinic keratosis"). *J Am Acad Dermatol*. January 2000;42(1 pt 2):11–17.

69. Cockerell CJ, Wharton JR. New histopathological classification of actinic keratosis (incipient intraepidermal squamous cell carcinoma). *J Drugs Dermatol*. July–August 2005;4(4):462–467.

70. Butani AK, Arbesfeld DM, Schwartz RA. Premalignant and early squamous cell carcinoma. *Clin Plast Surg*. April 2005;32(2):223–235.

71. Anwar J, Wrone DA, Kimyai-Asadi A, et al. The development of actinic keratosis into invasive squamous cell carcinoma: Evidence and evolving classification schemes. *Clin Dermatol*. May–June 2004;22(3):189–196.

72. Lober BA, Lober CW. Actinic keratosis is squamous cell carcinoma. *South Med J*. July 2000;93(7):650–655.

73. Fu W, Cockerell CJ. The actinic (solar) keratosis: A 21st-century perspective. *Arch Dermatol*. January 2003;139(1):66–70.

74. Ehrig T, Cockerell C, Piacquadio D, et al. Actinic keratoses and the incidence of occult squamous cell carcinoma: A clinical-histopathologic correlation. *Dermatol Surg*. October 2006;32(10):1261–1265.

75. Babilas P, Landthaler M, Szeimies RM. Actinic keratoses. *Hautarzt*. June 2003;54(6):551–560.

76. Wheeland RG. The pitfalls of treating all actinic keratoses as squamous cell carcinomas. *Semin Cutan Med Surg*. September 2005;24(3):152–154.

77. Marks R. Who benefits from calling a solar keratosis a squamous cell carcinoma? *Br J Dermatol*. July 2006;155(1):23–26.

78. Higashi MK, Veenstra DL, Langley PC. Health economic evaluation of nonmelanoma skin cancer and actinic keratosis. *Pharmacoeconomics*. 2004;22(2):83–94.

79. Lebwohl M. Actinic keratosis: Epidemiology and progression to squamous cell carcinoma. *Br J Dermatol*. November 2003;149 (suppl 66):31–33.

80. Ortonne JP. From actinic keratosis to squamous cell carcinoma. *Br J Dermatol*. April 2002;146 (suppl 61):20–23.

81. Flaxman BA. Actinic keratoses—malignant or not? *J Am Acad Dermatol*. September 2001;45(3):466–467.

82. Moy RL. Clinical presentation of actinic keratoses and squamous cell carcinoma. *J Am Acad Dermatol*. January 2000;42(1 pt 2):8–10.

83. Salasche SJ. Epidemiology of actinic keratoses and squamous cell carcinoma. *J Am Acad Dermatol*. January 2000;42(1 pt 2):4–7.

84. Guenthner ST, Hurwitz RM, Buckel LJ, et al. Cutaneous squamous cell carcinomas consistently show histologic evidence of in situ changes: A clinicopathologic correlation. *J Am Acad Dermatol*. September 1999;41(3 pt 1):443–448.

85. Halpern AC, Hanson LJ. Awareness of, knowledge of, and attitudes to nonmelanoma skin cancer (NMSC) and actinic keratosis (AK) among physicians. *Int J Dermatol*. September 2004;43(9):638–642.

86. Czarnecki D, Meehan CJ, Bruce F, et al. The majority of cutaneous squamous cell carcinomas arise in actinic keratoses. *J Cutan Med Surg*. May–June 2002;6(3):207–209.

87. Berman B, Bienstock L, Kuritzky L, et al. Actinic keratoses: Sequelae and treatments. Recommendations from a consensus panel. *J Fam Pract*. May 2006;55(suppl 5):1–8.

88. Markopoulos A, Albanidou-Farmaki E, Kayavis I. Actinic cheilitis: Clinical and pathologic characteristics in 65 cases. *Oral Dis*. July 2004;10(4):212–216.

89. Picascia DD, Robinson JK. Actinic cheilitis: A review of the etiology, differential diagnosis, and treatment. *J Am Acad Dermatol*. August 1987;17(2 pt 1):255–264.

90. Huber MA, Terezhalmy GT. The patient with actinic cheilosis. *Gen Dent*. July–August 2006;54(4):274–282.

91. Dufresne RG Jr, Curlin MU. Actinic cheilitis. A treatment review. *Dermatol Surg*. January 1997;23(1):15–21.

92. Neto Pimentel DR, Michalany N, Alchorne M, et al. Actinic cheilitis: Histopathology and p53. *J Cutan Pathol*. August 2006;33(8):539–544.

93. Ackerman AB, Ragaz AR. In: *Lives of Lesions*. New York: Masson; 1984:210–219.

94. Kaugars GE, Pillion T, Svirsky JA, et al. Actinic cheilitis: A review of 152 cases. *Oral Surg Oral Med Oral Pathol Oral Radiol Endod*. August 1999;88(2):181–186.

95. Berhane T, Halliday GM, Cooke B, et al. Inflammation is associated with progression of actinic keratoses to squamous cell carcinomas in humans. *Br J Dermatol*. 2002;146:810–815.

96. Goldberg LH, Joseph AK, Tschen JA. Proliferative actinic keratosis. *Int J Dermatol*. 1994;33:341–345.

97. Bowen JT. Precancerous dermatoses: A study of two cases of chronic atypical epithelial proliferation. *J Cutan Dis*. 1912;30:241–255.

98. Callen JP, Headington J. Bowen's and non-Bowen's squamous intraepidermal neoplasia of the skin: Relationship to internal malignancy. *Arch Dermatol*. 1980;116:422–426.

99. Graham JH, Helwig EB. Bowen's disease and its relationship to systemic cancer. *Arch Dermatol*. 1959;80:133–159.

100. Epstein E. Association of Bowen's disease with visceral cancer. *Arch Dermatol*. 1960;82:349–351.

101. Braverman IM. Bowen's disease and internal cancer. *JAMA*. 1991;266:842–843.

102. Lee MM, Wick MM. Bowen's disease. *Clin Dermatol*. January–March 1993;11(1):43–46.

103. Cox NH, Eedy DJ, Morton CA. Guidelines for management of Bowen's disease. British Association of Dermatologists. *Br J Dermatol*. October 1999;141(4):633–641.

104. Sanders N, Bedotto C. Recurrent carcinoma in situ of the conjunctiva and cornea (Bowen's disease). *Am J Ophthalmol*. 1972;74:688–693.

105. Marchesa P, Fazio VW, Oliart S, et al. Perianal Bowen's disease: A clinico-

pathological study of 47 patients. *Dis Colon Rectum*. 1997;40:1286–1293.

106. Obalek S, Jablonska S, Beaudenon S, et al. Bowenoid papulosis of the male and female genitalia: Risk of cervical neoplasia. *J Am Acad Dermatol*. 1986;14:433–444.

107. Hart WR. Vulvar intraepithelial neoplasia: Historical aspects and current status. *Int J Gynecol Pathol*. January 2001;20(1):16–30.

108. Schwartz RA, Janniger CK. Bowenoid papulosis. *J Am Acad Dermatol*. February 1991;24(2 pt 1):261–264.

109. Pala S, Poleva I, Totino F, et al. Bowenoid papulosis: Myth or reality? *Minerva Ginecol*. December 2000;52(12 suppl 1):68–74.

110. Cleary RK, Schaldenbrand JD, Fowler JJ, et al. Perianal Bowen's disease and anal intraepithelial neoplasia: Review of the literature. *Dis Colon Rectum*. July 1999;42(7):945–951.

111. Bertagni A, Vagliasindi A, Ascari Raccagni A, et al. Perianal Bowen's disease: A case report and review of the literature. *Tumori*. July–August 2003;89(suppl 4):16–18.

112. Kossard S, Rosen R. Cutaneous Bowen's disease. An analysis of 1001 cases according to age, sex, and site. *J Am Acad Dermatol*. September 1992;27(3):406–410.

113. Canavan TP, Cohen D. Vulvar cancer. *Am Fam Physician*. October 2002;66(7):1269–1274.

114. Raju RR, Goldblum JR, Hart WR. Pagetoid squamous cell carcinoma *in situ* (pagetoid Bowen's disease) of the external genitalia. *Int J Gynecol Pathol*. April 2003;22(2):127–135.

115. Kane CL, Keehn CA, Smithberger E, et al. Histopathology of cutaneous squamous cell carcinoma and its variants. *Semin Cutan Med Surg*. March 2004;23(1):54–61.

116. Hadzic B, Djurdjevic S, Hadzic M, et al. Morphologic manifestations of human papillomavirus infection in the vulvar and anogenital region. *Med Pregl*. May–June 1998;51(5–6):265–270.

117. Stafford EM, Greenberg H, Miles PA. Cervical intraepithelial neoplasia III in an adolescent with Bowenoid papulosis. *J Adolesc Health Care*. November 1990;11(6):523–526.

118. Gross G. Clinical aspects and therapy of anogenital warts and papillomavirus-associated lesions. *Hautarzt*. January 2001;52(1):6–17.

119. Kao GF. Carcinoma arising in Bowen's disease. *Arch Dermatol*. 1986;122:1124–1126.

120. Akhdari N, Amal S, Ettalbi S. Bowen disease. *CMAJ*. September 2006;175(7):739.

121. Chisiki M, Kawada A, Akiyama M, et al. Bowen's disease showing spontaneous complete regression associated with apoptosis. *Br J Dermatol*. May 1999;140(5):939–944.

122. Nihei N, Hiruma M, Ikeda S, et al. A case of Bowen's disease showing a clinical tendency toward spontaneous regression. *J Dermatol*. July 2004;31(7):569–572.

123. Murata Y, Kumano K, Sashikata T. Partial spontaneous regression of Bowen's disease. *Arch Dermatol*. April 1996;132(4):429–432.

124. Buechner SA. Common skin disorders of the penis. *BJU Int*. September 2002;90(5):498–506.

125. Narayana AS, Olney LE, Loening SA, et al. Carcinoma of the penis: Analysis of 219 cases. *Cancer*. May 1982;49(10):2185–2191.

126. Scully C, Sudbo J, Speight PM. Progress in determining the malignant potential of oral lesions. *J Oral Pathol Med*. May 2003;32(5):251–256.

127. Ben Slama L. Precancerous lesions of the buccal mucosa. *Rev Stomatol Chir Maxillofac*. April 2001;102(2):77–108.

128. Lingen MW, Kumar V. Chapter 16—head and neck. In: Kumar V, ed. *Robbins and Cotran: Pathologic Basis of Disease*. 7th ed. Philadelphia, PA: Elsevier Saunders; 2005:778–781.

129. Petti S. Pooled estimate of world leukoplakia prevalence: A systematic review. *Oral Oncol*. December 2003;39(8):770–780.

130. Bologna-Molina RE, Castaneda-Castaneira RE, Molina-Frechero N, et al. Human papilloma virus and its association with oral cancer. *Rev Med Inst Mex Seguro Soc*. Mar–April 2006;44(2):147–153.

131. Proia NK, Paszkiewicz GM, Nasca MA, et al. Smoking and smokeless tobacco-associated human buccal cell mutations and their association with oral cancer—a review. *Cancer Epidemiol Biomarkers Prev*. June 2006;15(6):1061–1077.

132. Slots J, Saygun I, Sabeti M, et al. Epstein–Barr virus in oral diseases. *J Periodontal Res*. August 2006;41(4):235–244.

133. Lind PO. Malignant transformation in oral leukoplakia. *Scand J Dent Res*. 1987;95:449–455.

134. Lee JJ, Hong WK, Hittelman WN, et al. Predicting cancer development in oral leukoplakia: 10 years of translational research. *Clin Cancer Res*. 2000;6:1702–1710.

135. Silverman S Jr, Gorsky M, Lozada F. Oral leukoplakia and malignant transformation: A follow-up study of 257 patients. *Cancer*. 1984;53:563–568.

136. Schepman KP, van der Meij EH, Smeele LE, et al. Malignant transformation of oral leukoplakia: A follow-up study of a hospital-based population of 166 patients with oral leukoplakia from the Netherlands. *Oral Oncol*. 1998;34:270–275.

137. Cawson RA, Speight P, Binnie WH, et al. *Luca's Pathology of Tumors of the Oral Tissues*. 5th ed. New York: Churchill Livingstone; 1998.

138. Shafer WG, Hine MK, Levy BM. *A Textbook of Oral Pathology*. 4th ed. Philadelphia, PA: WB Saunders; 1983.

139. Lodi G, Sardella A, Bez C, et al. Interventions for treating oral leukoplakia. *Cochrane Database Syst Rev*. October 2006;18(4):CD001829.

140. Hogewind WF, van der Waal I, van der Kwast WA, et al. The association of white lesions with oral squamous cell carcinoma. A retrospective study of 212 patients. *Int J Oral Maxillofac Surg*. 1989;18:163–164.

141. Neville BW, Day TA. Oral cancer and precancerous lesions. *CA Cancer J Clin*. July–August 2002;52(4):195–215.

142. Kuffer R, Lombardi T. Premalignant lesions of the oral mucosa. A discussion about the place of oral intraepithelial neoplasia (OIA). *Oral Oncol*. 2002;38:125–130.

143. Reibel J. Prognosis of oral pre-malignant lesions: Significance of clinical, histopathological, and molecular biological characteristics. *Crit Rev Oral Biol Med*. 2003;14(1):47–62.

144. Mittelbronn MA, Mullins DL, Ramos-Caro FA, et al. Frequency of pre-existing actinic keratosis in cutaneous squamous cell carcinoma. *Int J Dermatol*. 1998;37:677.

145. Suchniak JM, Baer S, Goldberg LH. High rate of malignant transformation in hyperkeratotic actinic keratoses. *J Am Acad Dermatol*. 1997;37:392.

146. Haydon RC. Cutaneous squamous carcinoma and related lesions. *Otolaryngol Clin North Am*. 1993;26:57–71.

147. Johnson TM, Rowe DE, Nelson BR, et al. Squamous cell carcinoma of the skin (excluding lip and oral mucosa). *J Am Acad Dermatol*. 1992;26:467–484.

148. Wade TR, Ackerman AB. The many faces of squamous-cell carcinomas. *J Dermatol Surg Oncol*. 1978;4:291.

149. Alam M, Ratner D. Cutaneous squamous cell carcinoma. *NEJM*. 2001;344:975.

150. Sober AJ, Burstein JM. Precursors to skin cancer. *Cancer*. 1995;75:645.

151. Lever WF, Schaumburg-Lever G. In: *Histopathology of the skin*. Philadelphia, PA: JB Lippincott; 1990:542–563.

152. Lund HZ. How often does squamous cell carcinoma of the skin metastasize? *Arch Dermatol*. 1965;92:635.

153. Lund HZ. Metastasis from sun-induced squamous cell carcinoma of the skin: An uncommon event. *J Dermatol Surg Oncol*. 1984;10:169.

154. de Visser KE, Korets LV, Coussens LM. *De novo* carcinogenesis promoted by chronic inflammation is B lymphocyte dependent. *Cancer Cell*. May 2005;7(5):411–423.

155. Proweller A, Tu L, Lepore JJ, et al. Impaired notch signaling promotes *de novo* squamous cell carcinoma formation. *Cancer Res*. August 2006;66(15):7438–7444.

156. Beatty ME, Habal MB. *De novo* cutaneous neoplasm: Biologic behavior in an immunosuppressed patient. *Plast Reconstr Surg*. October 1980;66(4):623–627.

157. Baccarani U, Adani GL, Montanaro D, et al. *De novo* malignancies after kidney and liver transplantations: Experience on 582 consecutive cases. *Transplant Proc*. May 2006;38(4):1135–1137.

158. Fung JJ, Jain A, Kwak EJ, et al. *De novo* malignancies after liver transplantation: A major cause of late death. *Liver Transpl*. November 2001;7(11 suppl 1):S109–S118.

159. Baloglu H, Dogan B. An unusual presentation of primary cutaneous squamous cell carcinoma. *J Eur Acad Dermatol Venereol*. 2003;17:556.

160. Graham JH. Selected precancerous skin and mucocutaneous lesions. In: Clark RL, ed. *Proceedings of the Annual Clinical Conference on Cancer by the University of Texas M.D. Anderson Hospital and Tumor Institute; Neoplasms of the Skin and Malignant Melanoma*. Chicago: Year Book Medical; 1976:82.

161. Kao GE. Carcinoma arising in Bowen's disease. *Arch. Dermatol.* 1986;122:1124–1126.

162. Rowe DE, Carroll RJ, Day CL Jr. Prognostic factors for local recurrence, metastasis, and survival rates in SCC of the skin, ear, and lip. Implications for treatment modality selection. *J Am Acad Dermatol.* 1992;26:976–990.

163. Rudolph R, Zelac DE. Squamous cell carcinoma of the skin. *Plast Reconstr Surg.* November 2004;114(6):82e–94e.

164. Schwartz RA. Verrucous carcinoma of the skin and mucosa. *J Am Acad Dermatol.* January 1995;32(1):1–21.

165. Ackerman LV. Verrucous carcinoma of oral cavity. *Surgery.* 1948;23:670–678.

166. Goethals PL, Harrison EG, Devine K. Verrucous squamous carcinoma of the oral cavity. *Am J Surg.* 1963;106:845–851.

167. Kraus FT, Perezmesa C. Verrucous carcinoma. Clinical and pathologic study of 105 cases involving oral cavity, larynx, and genitalia. *Cancer.* January 1966;19(1):26–38.

168. Toyama K, Hashimoto-Kumasaka K, Tagami H. Acantholytic squamous cell carcinoma involving the dorsum of the foot of elderly Japanese: Clinical and light microscopic observations in five patients. *Br J Dermatol.* 1995;133:141–142.

169. Johnson WC, Helwig EB. Adenoid squamous cell carcinoma (adenoacanthoma). A clinicopathologic study of 155 patients. *Cancer.* 1966;19:1639–1650.

170. Mauriello JA, Abdelsalam A, McLean IW. Adenoid squamous carcinoma of the conjunctiva—a clinicopathological study of 14 cases. *Br J Ophthalmol.* November 1997;81(11):1001–1005.

171. Martin HE, Stewart FW. Spindle cell epidermoid carcinoma. *Am J Cancer.* 1935;24:273–297.

172. Benninger MS, Kraus D, Sebek B, et al. Head and neck spindle cell carcinoma: An evaluation of current management. *Cleve Clin J Med.* September–October 1992;59(5):479–482.

173. Landman G, Taylor RM, Friedman KJ. Cutaneous papillary squamous cell carcinoma that stimulates sebaceous carcinoma. *Am J Surg Pathol.* 1980;86:108–115.

174. Ferlito A, Devaney KO, Rinaldo A, Putzi MJ. Papillary squamous cell carcinoma versus verrucous squamous cell carcinoma of the head and neck. *Ann Otol Rhinol Laryngol.* March 1999;108(3):318–322.

175. Cramer SF, Heggeness LM. Signet-ring squamous cell carcinoma. *Am J Clin Pathol.* 1989;91:488–491.

176. McKinley E, Valles R, Bang R, et al. Signet-ring squamous cell carcinoma: A case report. *J Cutan Pathol.* 1998;25:176–181.

177. Chapman MS, Ouitadamo MJ, Perry AE. Pigmented squamous cell carcinoma. *J Cutan Pathol.* February 2000;27(2):93–95.

178. Morgan MB, Lima-Maribona J, Miller RA, et al. Pigmented squamous cell carcinoma of the skin: Morphologic and immunohistochemical study of five cases. *J Cutan Pathol.* September 2000;27(8):381–386.

179. Haneke E. Histologische barianten des plattenepithelkarzinoms der haut undihre dignitat. In: Breuninger H, Rassner G, eds. *Operationsplanung und Erfolgskontrolle.* Berlin, Germany: Springer-Verlag; 1989:79–85.

180. Breuninger H, Schaumburg-Lever G, Holzschuh J, et al. Desmoplastic squamous cell carcinoma of skin and vermilion surface: A highly malignant subtype of skin cancer. *Cancer.* 1997;79:915–919.

181. Kuo T. Clear cell carcinoma of the skin: A variant of the squamous cell carcinoma that stimulates sebaceous carcinoma. *Am J Surg Pathol.* 1980;4:573–583.

182. Weidner N, Foucar E. Adenosquamous carcinoma of the skin. An aggressive mucin-and gland-forming squamous carcinoma. *Arch Dermatol.* 1985;121:775.

183. Banks ER, Cooper PH. Adenosquamous carcinoma of the skin: A report of 10 cases. *J Cutan Pathol.* 1991;18:227.

184. Wilson-Jones E. Proliferating epidermoid cysts. *Arch Dermatol.* 1966;94:11.

185. Arico M, La Rocca E, Noto G, et al. Proliferating tricholemmal tumour with lymph node metastases. *Br J Dermatol.* December 1989;121(6):793–797.

186. Noto G, Pravata G, Arico M. Malignant proliferating trichilemmal tumor. *Am J Dermatopathol.* April 1997;19(2):202–204.

187. Sau P, Graham JH, Helwig EB. Proliferating epithelial cysts. *J Cutan Pathol.* 1995;22:394.

188. Skelton HG, Flax S, Chang L, et al. Squamous cell carcinomas arising from adnexal ductal cysts. *Arch Pathol Lab Med.* January 2002;126(1):76–78.

189. Wong TY, Suster S, Mihm MC. Squamoid eccrine ductal carcinoma. *Histopathology.* March 1997;30(3):288–293.

190. Glaich AS, Behroozan DS, Cohen JL, et al. Lymphoepithelioma-like carcinoma of the skin: A report of two cases treated with complete microscopic margin control and review of the literature. *Dermatol Surg.* February 2006;32(2):316–319.

191. Dudley CM, Snow SN, Voytovich MC, et al. Enlarging facial nodule on an elderly patient. Lymphoepithelioma-like carcinoma of the skin (LELCS). *Arch Dermatol.* December 1998;134(12):1628–1629, 1631–1632.

192. Headington JT. Tricholemmal carcinoma. *J Cutan Pathol.* April 1992;19(2):83–84.

193. Swanson PE, Marrogi AJ, Williams DJ, et al. Tricholemmal carcinoma: Clinicopathologic study of 10 cases. *J Cutan Pathol.* April 1992;19(2):100–109.

194. Wong TY, Suster S. Tricholemmal carcinoma. A clinicopathologic study of 13 cases. *Am J Dermatopathol.* October 1994;16(5):463–473.

195. Boscaino A, Terracciano LM, Donofrio V, et al. Tricholemmal carcinoma: A study of seven cases. *J Cutan Pathol.* April 1992;19(2):94–99.

196. Motley R, Kersey P, Lawrence C, et al. Multiprofessional guidelines for the management of the patient with primary cutaneous squamous cell carcinoma. *Br J Plast Surg.* March 2003;56(2):85–91.

197. Jones E, Korzenko A, Kriegel D. Oral isotretinoin in the treatment and prevention of cutaneous squamous cell carcinoma. *J Drugs Dermatol.* 2004;3(5):498–502.

198. Carruci JA. Cutaneous oncology in organ transplant recipients: Meeting the challenge of squamous cell carcinoma. *J Invest Dermatol.* 2004;123:809–816.

199. Leibovitch I, Huilgol SC, Selva D, et al. Cutaneous squamous cell carcinoma treated with Mohs micrographic surgery in Australia. I. Experience over 10 years. *J Am Acad Dermatol.* 2005;53:253–260.

200. Rowe DE, Carroll RJ, Day CL Jr. Prognostic factors for local recurrence, metastasis, and survival rates in squamous cell carcinoma of the skin, ear, and lip. Implications for treatment modality selection. *J Am Acad Dermatol.* 1992;26(6):976–990.

201. Motley R, Kersey P, Lawrence C. Multiprofessional guidelines for the management of the patient with primary cutaneous squamous cell carcinoma. *Br J Plast Surg.* 2003;56:85–91.

202. Chartier TK. Treatment of cutaneous squamous cell carcinoma. In: Up To Date, Waltham, MA, 2005.

203. Gordon KB, Garden JM, Robinson JK. Bowen's disease of the distal digit. Outcome of treatment with carbon dioxide laser vaporization. *Dermatol Surg.* 1996;22:723–728.

204. Fader DJ, Lowe L. Concomitant use of a high-energy pulsed CO_2 laser and a long-pulsed (810 nm) diode laser for squamous cell carcinoma *in situ*. *Dermatol Surg.* 2002;28:97–100.

205. Kwan W, Wilson D, Moravan V. Radiotherapy for locally advanced basal cell and squamous cell carcinomas of the skin. *Int J Radiat Biol Phys.* 2004;60(2):406–411.

206. Loven K, Stein L, Furst K, Levy S. Evaluation of the efficacy and tolerability of 0.5% fluorouracil cream and 5% fluorouracil cream applied to each side of the face in patients with actinic keratosis. *Clin Ther.* 2002;24(6):990–1000.

207. Lee PK, Hawell WB, Loven KH, et al. Long-term clinical outcomes following treatment of actinic keratosis with imiquimod 5% cream. *Dermatol Surg.* 2005;31(6):659–664.

208. Bargman H, Hochman J. Topical treatment of Bowen's disease with 5-fluorouracil. *J Cutan Med Surg.* 2003;7(1):101–105.

209. Marmur ES, Schmults CD, Goldberg DJ. A review of laser and photodynamic therapy for the treatment of nonmelanoma skin cancer. *Dermatol Surg.* 2004;30:264–271.

210. Villa AM, Berman B. Immunomodulators for skin cancer. *J Drugs Dermatol.* 2004;3(5):533–539.

211. Kim KH, Yavel RM, Gross VL, et al. Intralesional interferon α-2b in the treatment of basal cell carcinoma and squamous cell carcinoma: Revisited. *Dermatol Surg.* 2004;30:116–120.

212. Urosevic M, Dummer R. Role of imiquimod in skin cancer treatment. *Am J Clin Dermatol.* 2004;5(6):453–458.

213. Patel GK, Goodwin R, Chawla M, et al. Imiquimod 5% cream monotherapy for cutaneous squamous cell *in situ* (Bowen's disease): A randomized, double-blind, placebo-controlled trial. *J Am Acad Dermatol.* 2006;54:1025–1032.

214. Konstantopoulou M, Lord MG, Macfarlane AW. Treatment of invasive squamous cell carcinoma with 5-percent imiquimod cream. *Dermatol Online J.* 2006;12(3):10.

215. Martin-Garcia RF. Imiquimod: An effective alternative for the treatment of invasive cutaneous squamous cell carcinoma. *Dermatol Surg.* 2005;31(3):371–374.

216. Asgari M, White E, Chren M. Nonsteroidal anti-inflammatory drug use in the prevention and treatment of squamous cell carcinoma. *Dermatol Surg.* 2004; 30:1335–1342.

217. Wright TI, Spencer JM, Flowers FP. Chemoprevention of nonmelanoma skin cancer. *JAAD.* 2006;54(6):933–946.

218. Hansen LA, Sigman CC, Andreola F, Ross SA, Kelloff GJ, De Luca LM. Retionoids in chemoprevention and differentiation therapy. *Carcinogenesis.* 2000;21:1271–1279.

219. Xu XC, Wong WY, Goldberg L, et al. Progressive decreases in nuclear retinoid receptors during skin squamous carcinogenesis. *Cancer Res.* 2001; 61(11):4306–4310.

220. Schoenermark MP, Mitchell TI, Rutter JL, Reczek PR, Brinckerhoff CE. Retinoid-mediated suppression of tumor invasion and matrix metalloproteinase synthesis. *Ann N Y Acad Sci.* 1999;878:466–486.

221. Rudkin GH, Carlsen BT, Chung CY, et al. Retinoids inhibit squamous cell carcinoma growth and intercellular communication. *J Surg Res.* 2002;103(2):183–189.

222. Jones E, Korzenko A, Kriegel D. Oral isotretinoin in the treatment and prevention of cutaneous squamous cell carcinoma. *J Drugs Dermatol.* 2004;3(5): 498–502.

223. Moon TE, Levine N, Cartmel B, et al. Effect of retinol in preventing squamous cell skin cancer in moderate-risk subjects: A randomized, double-blind, controlled trial. Southwest Skin Cancer Prevention Study Group. *Cancer Epidemiol Biomarkers Prev.* 1997;6(11):949–956.

224. George R, Weightman W, Russ GR, Bannister KM, Mathew TH. Acitretin for chemoprevention of non-melanoma skin cancers in renal transplant recipients. *Aust J Dermatol.* 2002;43(4):269–273.

225. Harwood CA, Leedham-Green M, Leigh IM, Proby CM. Low-dose retinoids in the prevention of cutaneous squamous cell carcinomas in organ transplant recipients: A 16-year retrospective study. *Arch Dermatol.* 2005;141(4):456–464.

226. Nijsten TEC, Stern RS. Oral retinoid use reduces cutaneous squamous cell carcinoma risk in patients with psoriasis treated with psoralen-UVA: A nested cohort study. *JAAD.* 2003;49(4):644–650.

227. Buckman SY, Gresham A, Hale P, et al. COX-2 expression is induced by UVB exposure in human skin: Implications for the development of skin cancer. *Carcinogenesis.* 1998;19:723–729.

228. Lozano Y, Taitz A, Petruzzelli GJ, Djordjevic A, Young MR. Prostaglandin E2-protein kinase A signaling and protein phosphatases-1 and -2A regulate human head and neck squamous cell carcinoma motility, adherence, and cytoskeletal organization. *Prostaglandins.* 1996;51:35–48.

229. Pelzmann M, Thurnher D, Gedlicka C, Martinek H, Knerer B. Nimesulide and indomethacin induce apoptosis in head and neck cancer cells. *J Oral Pathol Med.* 2004;33(10):607–613.

230. Roh JL, Sung MW, Kim KH. Suppression of accelerated tumor growth in surgical wounds by celecoxib and indomethacin. *Head Neck.* 2005;27(4):326–332.

231. Park K, Yang JH, Choi Y, Lee C, Kim SY, Byun Y. Chemoprevention of 4-NQO-induced oral carcinogenesis by co-administration of all-*trans* retinoic acid loaded microspheres and celecoxib. *J Control Release.* 2005;104:167–179.

232. Wang ZY, Agarwal R, Bickers DR, Mukhtar H. Protection against ultraviolet B radiation-induced photocarcinogenesis in hairless mice by green tea polyphenols. *Carcinogenesis.* 1991;12:1527–1530.

233. Wang ZY, Huang MT, Ferraro T, et al. Inhibitory effect of green tea in the drinking water on tumorigenesis by ultraviolet light and 12-O tetradecanoyl-phorbol-13-acetate in the skin of SKH-1 mice. *Cancer Res.* 1992;52: 1162–1170.

234. Valcic S, Timmermann BN, Alberts DS, et al. Inhibitory effect of six green tea catechins and caffeine on the growth of four selected human tumor cell lines. *Anticancer Drugs.* 1996;7:461–468.

235. Li N, Chen X, Liao J, et al. Inhibition of 7,12-dimethylbenz[a]anthracene (DMBA)-induced oral carcinogenesis in hamsters by tea and curcumin. *Carcinogenesis.* 2002;23(8):1307–1313.

236. Hakim IA, Harris RB, Ritenbaugh C. Citrus peel use is associated with reduced risk of squamous cell carcinoma of the skin. *Nutr Cancer.* 2000;37(2):161–168.

237. Kamradt J, Rafi L, Mitschele T, et al. Analysis of the vitamin D system in cutaneous malignancies. *Recent Results Cancer Res.* 2003;164:259–269.

238. Katiyar SK, Korman NJ, Mukhtar H, Agarwal R. Protective effects of silymarin against photocarcinogenesis in a mouse skin model. *J Natl Cancer Inst.* 1997;89:556–566.

239. Wei H, Bowen R, Zhang X, Lebwohl M. Isoflavone genistein inhibits the initiation and promotion of two-stage skin carcinogenesis in mice. *Carcinogenesis.* 1998;19:1509–1514.

240. Wei H, Saladi R, Lu Y, Wang Y, et al. Isoflavone genistein: Photoprotection and clinical implications in dermatology. *J Nutr.* 2003;133 (suppl 1): 3811S–3819S.

241. Frieling UM, Schaumberg DA, Kupper TS, Muntwyler J, Hennekens CH. A randomized, 12-year primary-prevention trial of beta-carotene supplementation for nonmelanoma skin cancer in the physicians' health study. *Arch Dermatol.* 2000;136:179–184.

242. Wernighaus K, Meydani M, Bhawan J, Margolis R, Blumberg JB, Gilchrest BA. Evaluation of the photoprotective effect of oral vitamin E supplementation. *Arch Dermatol.* 1994;130:1257–1261.

243. Fung TT, Spiegelman D, Egan KM, Giovannucci E, Hunter DJ, Willett WC. Vitamin and carotenoid intake and risk of squamous cell carcinoma of the skin. *Int J Cancer.* 2003;103:110–115.

244. Dorgan JF, Boakye NA, Fears TR, et al. Serum carotenoids and α-tocopherol and risk of nonmelanoma skin cancer. *Cancer Epidemiol Biomarkers Prev.* 2004;13(8):1276–1282.

245. McNaughton SA, Marks GC, Green AC. Role of dietary factors in the development of basal cell cancer and squamous cell cancer of the skin. *Cancer Epidemiol Biomarkers Prev.* 2005;14(7):1596–1607.

246. Hakim IA, Harris RB, Ritenbaugh C. Fat intake and risk of squamous cell carcinoma of the skin. *Nutr Cancer.* 2000;36(2): 155–162.

CHAPTER 8

Congenital Melanocytic Nevi

Christopher J. Steen, M.D.
Jerry Rothenberg, M.D.
Robert A. Schwartz, M.D., M.P.H.

BOX 8-1   Overview

- Congenital melanocytic nevi are benign nevomelanocytic proliferations which are present at birth.
- Congenital melanocytic nevi, particularly large congenital melanocytic nevi, are at increased risk of developing malignant melanoma.
- Histological criteria may help distinguish congenital melanocytic nevi from acquired nevi.
- Congenital melanocytic nevi are a component of neurocutaneous melanocytosis, a rare congenital syndrome with melanocytic neoplasms of the skin and central nervous system.
- Management of congenital melanocytic nevi varies with the size and location of the lesion.
- Management strategies include careful monitoring, surgical excision, dermabrasion, curettage, and laser treatment.

INTRODUCTION

Congenital melanocytic nevi are defined as benign nevomelanocytic proliferations that are present at birth. Occasionally, nevi that are clinically and histologically indistinguishable from congenital melanocytic nevi develop in children during the first 2 years of life. This type is referred to as congenital nevus tardive and can be treated similar to a congenital nevus. Congenital melanocytic nevi are present in approximately 1% of newborn infants and are important for three reasons. First, they can be cosmetically disfiguring, depending on the size and location. Second, congenital melanocytic nevi, particularly large ones, are at an increased risk of developing melanoma. Third, and most importantly, melanoma that develops in large congenital melanocytic nevi most often occurs deep within the dermis where it is not easily detectable on clinical examination until at an advanced stage.

PATHOGENESIS

BOX 8-2   Summary

- Melanocytes are derived from neuroectoderm.
- Congenital melanocytic nevi may result from an external insult that alters the migration and development of melanocytes from neuroectoderm-derived precursors.
- Congenital melanocytic nevi develop between the 9th and 20th weeks of gestation.

The etiology of congenital melanocytic nevi is uncertain. The melanocytes of the skin and leptomeninges originate in the neuroectoderm, although the specific cell type from which they are derived is unknown. One theory of the origin of melanocytes in the skin considers that the pluripotential nerve sheath precursor cells migrate from the neural crest to the skin along paraspinal ganglia and peripheral nerve sheaths, and differentiate into melanocytes upon reaching the skin.[1,2] One explanation for the development of a congenital melanocytic nevus is that some type of external insult results in a mutation that disrupts the normal morphogenesis of the embryonic neuroectoderm and migration of precursor cells to the skin. Based on the observation of divided congenital melanocytic nevi found on adjacent parts of the upper and lower eyelids, it has been concluded that they develop between the 9th and 20th week of fetal development, as this is the period during which the eyelids are fused.[3]

CLASSIFICATION

BOX 8-3   Summary

- Congenital melanocytic nevi have been arbitrarily divided into three groups.
- Small congenital melanocytic nevi are less than 1.5 cm in diameter; medium congenital melanocytic nevi are between 1.5 cm and 20 cm in diameter; large congenital melanocytic nevi are 20 cm or larger in diameter.

Congenital melanocytic nevi have been arbitrarily categorized into three groups. The most common method of classification is based on the size of the lesion during infancy. Small congenital melanocytic

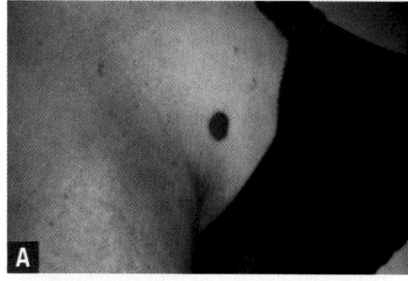
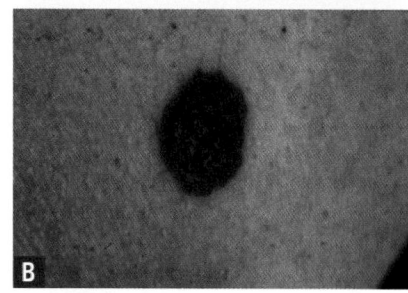

▲ FIGURE 8-1 (A and B) Small congenital melanocytic nevus on the back.

nevi (Fig. 8-1A and B) are defined as those lesions less than 1.5 cm at the greatest diameter, medium congenital melanocytic nevi as those between 1.5 and 20 cm, and large or giant congenital melanocytic nevi (Fig. 8-2) as those with a diameter of 20 cm or greater.[4] Large congenital melanocytic nevi may have smaller surrounding satellite nevi. Congenital melanocytic nevi have also been classified based on the ease of surgical removal. Small congenital melanocytic nevi can usually be removed with simple excision. Medium congenital melanocytic nevi, depending on size, may require skin grafts or flaps for closure. In cases where large congenital melanocytic nevi can be removed, they often require staged excisions using tissue expanders and skin grafts. Other classification schemes take into account the percentage of body surface area covered by a lesion based on anatomic location.

HISTOPATHOLOGY

BOX 8-4   Summary

- Histological criteria may help differentiate congenital melanocytic nevi from acquired nevi.
- Histological features of congenital melanocytic nevi include the following: presence of nevus cells within the deeper two-thirds of the dermis, involvement of nevus cells within neurovascular structures

- and deep dermal appendages, splaying of nevus cells within collagen bundles of the reticular dermis, and a perifollicular and perivascular distribution of nevus cells simulating an inflammatory reaction.
- Typical histological features are most often seen in large congenital melanocytic nevi; small and medium sized lesions may display all, some, or none of these features.

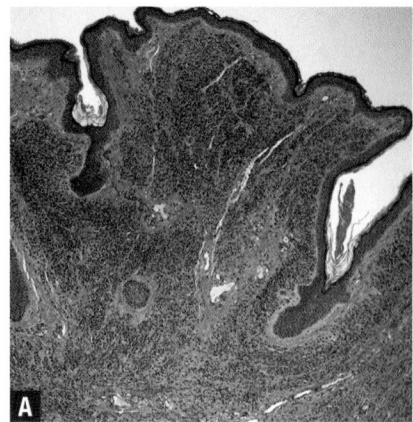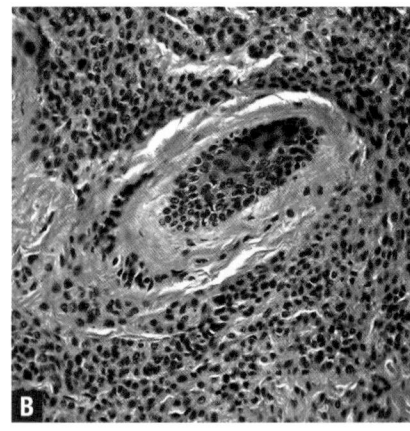

▲ **FIGURE 8-3** Congenital nevus. Sections showing a proliferation of nevus cells within the papillary and reticular dermis with permeation of the appendageal and neurovascular structures, splaying between collagen bundles, and progressive diminution in size, i.e., maturation, with depth into the dermis (hematoxylin–eosin stain).

Distinguishing congenital melanocytic nevi from acquired nevi on the basis of histology is not always possible. However, a set of distinctive histological features may help differentiate between the two. Congenital melanocytic nevi (Fig. 8-3) classically display the following elements: (1) the presence of nevus cells within the deeper two-thirds of the dermis with possible extension into the subcutaneous tissue, (2) involvement of nevus cells around and within neurovascular structures and deep dermal appendages including hair follicles, arrector pili muscles, sebaceous glands, nerves, and walls of blood vessels, (3) infiltration or splaying of nevus cells between collagen bundles of the reticular dermis either as single cells or cords of cells, and (4) a perifollicular and perivascular distribution of nevus cells simulating an inflammatory reaction.[5–8] Although these features are not pathognomonic for congenital nevi, they are most consistently observed in large congenital melanocytic nevi. Small and medium congenital melanocytic nevi may show all, some, or none of these features and

may be histologically indistinguishable from acquired nevi. In contrast to congenital melanocytic nevi, acquired nevi are usually composed of nevomelanocytes that do not involve the appendages and are limited to the papillary and upper reticular dermis. Large congenital melanocytic nevi may demonstrate a number of patterns including intradermal or compound nevus, blue nevus, neural nevus, and spindle nevus.[7,9] The nevus cells of congenital melanocytic nevi are also typically positive for the markers S-100, Melan-A, and HMB-45.[10] In the absence of a clear history, the aforementioned features can be useful in establishing the likelihood that a nevus is a congenital melanocytic nevus rather than an acquired one.

NEUROCUTANEOUS MELANOCYTOSIS

BOX 8-5 Summary

- Neurocutaneous melanocytosis is a rare congenital syndrome characterized by melanocytic neoplasms of the skin and central nervous system.
- Neurocutaneous melanocytosis may cause seizures or increased intracranial pressure due to hydrocephalus or a mass lesion.
- Symptomatic neurocutaneous melanocytosis has a poor prognosis.

Neurocutaneous melanocytosis is a rare congenital syndrome characterized by the presence of congenital melanocytic nevi and melanocytic neoplasms of the central nervous system.[11] This syndrome was first described by Rokitansky in 1861.[12] The current diagnostic criteria for neurocutaneous melanocytosis include the following: (1) one large (>20 cm) or more than three small or medium congenital nevi in association with meningeal melanosis or melanoma, (2) no evidence of meningeal melanoma except in patients with cutaneous lesions that are histologically benign, and (3) no evidence of cutaneous melanoma except in patients with meningeal lesions that are histologically benign.[13] This syndrome may result from an error in the morphogenesis of the neuroectoderm, which gives rise to the melanotic cells of both the skin and meninges. Clinically, patients with neurocutaneous melanocytosis may present with either seizures or increased intracranial pressure due to hydrocephalus or a mass lesion. A study in 2006 found that in a group of patients

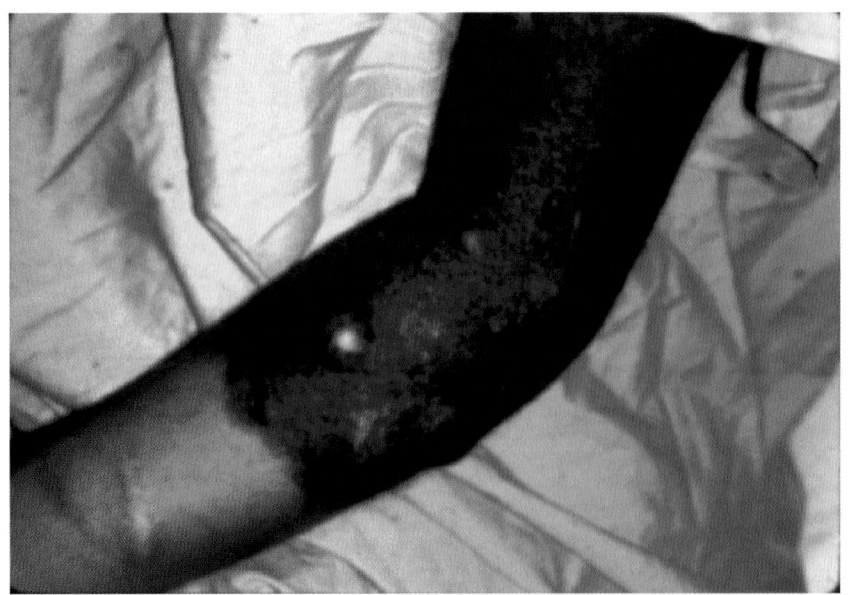

▲ **FIGURE 8-2** Large congenital melanocytic nevus covering most of an arm.

with large congenital melanocytic nevi, the percentage of patients with diagnosed or presumptive neurocutaneous melanocytosis was 7.5% in those with a large truncal congenital melanocytic nevus.[14] The prognosis for patients with symptomatic neurocutaneous melanocytosis is poor. In one review of 39 cases of symptomatic neurocutaneous melanocytosis, death occurred in >50% of the patients within 3 years of the onset of neurological symptoms. Most deaths were in patients younger than 10 years of age.[13]

CONGENITAL MELANOCYTIC NEVI AND MELANOMA

BOX 8-6   Summary

- Congenital melanocytic nevi, particularly large congenital melanocytic nevi, have an increased risk of developing malignant melanoma.
- The lifetime risk of developing melanoma in patients with large congenital melanocytic nevi has been estimated to be 5 to 20%.
- Melanoma developing within large congenital melanocytic nevi often develops during childhood and usually arises deep within the dermis where it is not easily detectable on clinical examination until it reaches an advanced stage.
- The lifetime risk of developing melanoma in patients with small and medium congenital melanocytic nevi has not been well established.
- Melanoma developing within small congenital melanocytic nevi often develops in adulthood and usually arises in the epidermis where it can be detected at an early stage by clinical examination.

Large Congenital Melanocytic Nevi

Patients with large congenital melanocytic nevi are at an increased risk of developing melanoma within the lesion, at distant cutaneous locations, and at noncutaneous sites.[15,19] A study of 1008 patients with large or multiple congenital melanocytic nevi found a 2.9% incidence of melanoma in patients with large congenital melanocytic nevi.[15] Another study found that in patients with large congenital melanocytic nevi, the 5-year cumulative risk of developing melanoma was 2.3%.[18] An analysis by Marghoob et al found a 5-year cumulative risk of developing melanoma of 4.5% in patients with large congenital melanocytic nevi.[17] Likewise, another study found a 5.7% 5-year cumulative

risk of developing melanoma.[20] An analysis of patients with large congenital melanocytic nevi demonstrated an increased risk of melanoma in patients with either higher numbers of satellite lesions or a larger diameter primary lesion.[16] Other works have suggested a lifetime risk of developing melanoma of 5 to 20% in patients with large congenital melanocytic nevi.[19,21,22] Melanomas arising within large congenital melanocytic nevi develop deep within the dermis up to two-thirds of the time, which delays clinical detection.[21,23,24] Additionally, more than half of the melanomas arising within large congenital melanocytic nevi develop during the first 10 years of life.[25] The highest rate of malignancy appears to occur during the first 5 years of life.[25]

Although patients with large congenital melanocytic nevi are undoubtedly at an increased risk of developing melanoma, the quantification of this risk has proven difficult. The variation in risk of developing melanoma cited by these different studies is further compounded by a number of factors including the fact that a significant percentage of patients with large congenital melanocytic nevi undergo treatment because of both prophylactic and cosmetic concerns, which undoubtedly influences the incidence of melanoma in this group. Many studies also focus on a younger cohort of patients, which makes it difficult to assess lifetime risk of melanoma. Additionally, in the vast majority of studies, the incidence of melanoma cited does not distinguish between melanoma developing within the large congenital melanocytic nevus, at distant cutaneous sites, or at noncutaneous sites.

Small and Medium Congenital Melanocytic Nevi

Assessing the melanoma risk in patients with small and medium congenital melanocytic nevi has proven challenging and controversial. A cohort study of 265 patients with congenital melanocytic nevi found no incidence of melanoma in its sampling of patients with nevi smaller than 5% of body surface area.[26] A study of 227 patients with medium congenital melanocytic nevi found no incidence of melanoma within the nevi during a 6.7-year follow-up period.[27] Melanomas arising within small and medium congenital melanocytic nevi develop most often in the epidermis, where they are more easily detected on clinical examination.[5,23] Reports indicate that melanoma arising within small con-

genital melanocytic nevi occurs most often in adulthood.[5,28] The melanoma risk associated with small and medium congenital melanocytic nevi, although not well defined by current studies, appears to be significantly less than the risk associated with large congenital melanocytic nevi.

MANAGEMENT OF CONGENITAL MELANOCYTIC NEVI

BOX 8-7   Summary

- Management of congenital melanocytic nevi varies depending on the size and location of the lesion.
- When possible, large congenital melanocytic nevi are excised during early childhood to reduce the risk of melanoma.
- Small congenital melanocytic nevi are often under close clinical monitoring; if prophylactic excision is desired, it can be done just prior to puberty
- Several other modalities, including dermabrasion, curettage, and laser treatment, have been used to improve cosmesis in patients with congenital melanocytic nevi, although the effects of these treatments on melanoma risk are unknown.

Management of congenital melanocytic nevi is guided by two factors: risk of malignancy and cosmetic impact. Many treatment options have been used in an attempt to reduce the rate of melanoma and/or improve the cosmetic appearance of patients with congenital melanocytic nevi. Different management strategies have included careful monitoring, serial photography, surgical excision, dermabrasion, curettage, and laser treatment. Many factors must be taken into consideration when managing these lesions, including the perceived risk of melanoma, size and location of the lesion, cosmetic impact, proximity to vital structures, psychosocial effects, risks of invasive intervention, and likely cosmetic outcome. An open discussion with patients and/or family members, including management options, realistic outcome expectations, and the relative scarcity of evidence-based data is essential.

Although the great majority of patients with congenital melanocytic nevi of any size will never develop melanoma, the presence of large congenital melanocytic nevi clearly places an individual at increased risk of malignancy. Because melanoma develops at an early age in large congenital melanocytic nevi and often originates deep to the epidermis where it cannot easily be detected on clinical examination, watchful waiting is not the recommended approach. Surgical excision of these lesions at an early age remains the mainstay of treatment for those seeking prophylactic therapy. One study, which examined the physical and psychosocial effects of large congenital melanocytic nevi and their surgical removal, suggests 6 to 9 months as an optimal age for surgical excision.[29] Unfortunately, surgical excision down to fascia does not entirely eliminate the risk of melanoma as it is not possible to ensure the removal of all nevus cells, some of which may be found deep to the fascia within muscle and nerve. Additionally, excisions of very large congenital melanocytic nevi that pose the greatest risk of melanoma, are often very difficult or impossible, and frequently produce unacceptable cosmesis. There is also a lack of published evidence to quantify the reduction of melanoma risk following prophylactic surgery.

Patients with small congenital melanocytic nevi appear to be at an increased lifetime risk of melanoma, although not to the same extent as patients with large congenital melanocytic nevi. Given the current evidence, watchful waiting with regular follow-up, dermatoscopic and photographic evaluation, and monitoring by parents is an appropriate management strategy for most of these lesions. Unlike the case of large congenital melanocytic nevi, careful clinical observation will detect malignant changes in these lesions because melanomas arising in small congenital melanocytic nevi are almost always epidermal in origin. When prophylactic removal is desired, it can generally be delayed until just prior to puberty because melanoma in these lesions develops almost exclusively during adulthood.

Management of medium congenital melanocytic nevi is the most difficult of the three classes of congenital melanocytic nevi. While they do not appear to present the same melanoma risk as large congenital melanocytic nevi, an accurate risk assessment has not been established. There is also insufficient data to suggest that one management strategy is superior. Some have suggested taking a biopsy of these lesions prior to excision.[23] If histologic patterns are similar to those of acquired nevi, then the lesions could be managed similarly to the case of small congenital melanocytic nevi. If patterns of deep dermal growth are observed, as in large congenital melanocytic nevi, the risk

of clinically undetectable melanoma presumably would be higher and warrant prophylactic excision as early as possible. Because the risk of prepubertal melanoma in these lesions is small, others have suggested excision of these lesions in the pubertal years when the risks of anesthesia are lower than during childhood.[5]

FINAL THOUGHTS

Congenital melanocytic nevi are nevomelanocytic proliferations which are at increased risk of developing melanoma. Surgical excision early in life remains the primary management strategy for large congenital melanocytic nevi that are at the greatest risk of developing melanoma at a young age. The risk of melanoma arising in small and medium congenital melanocytic nevi appears to be less than in large congenital melanocytic nevi, although the magnitude of the risk has not been clearly established. Consequently, recommended management strategies for these lesions are not well defined. Because melanoma does not typically develop in these lesions until adulthood and almost always occurs at a superficial level where it can be detected clinically, careful monitoring during childhood is a viable alternative to surgical excision in infancy. Excision of small and medium congenital melanocytic nevi, when desired, can be performed just prior to puberty.

Other strategies for treatment of congenital melanocytic nevi include the use of lasers and dermabrasion. Laser treatment of congenital melanocytic nevi has been described using several different types of laser including Q-switched ruby, Q-switched alexandrite, Erbium:YAG, and high energy pulsed carbon dioxide.[30–35] Unfortunately, laser treatment of congenital melanocytic nevi remains controversial because although this modality can significantly improve the appearance of these lesions, the long term influence of laser treatment on malignant potential is unknown. On one hand, laser treatment of congenital melanocytic nevi destroys superficial melanocytes which may result in improved cosmesis and also leaves fewer cells with the potential for malignant transformation, while on the other hand, deeper melanocytes often escape complete destruction. This complicates the clinical monitoring of these lesions because if melanoma does arise, it is more likely to develop deeper in the skin where it may be clinically undetectable until at an advanced stage. Finally, the

effects of sublethal fluences of laser irradiation on the remaining melanocytes are poorly understood. Studies of the effects of laser irradiation on various melanoma cell lines have shown that sub-lethal laser treatment may alter gene expression as well as affect the quantity and function of cell surface regulatory and adhesion molecules.[36,37] While not definitive, these findings raise the possibility that laser treatment of congenital melanocytic nevi may increase the risk of malignant transformation in the remaining melanocytes. Additionally, inadvertent laser treatment of an undiagnosed melanoma within one of these lesions may result in increased motility and greater metastatic potential.

There are also reports of neonatal dermabrasion resulting in improved cosmesis in congenital melanocytic nevi.[38,39] However, as with laser therapy, the long-term effects of dermabrasion on malignant potential are unknown. Both laser treatment and dermabrasion have their own associated risks and side effects that must be considered prior to treatment. Finally, although these modalities offer promising options for improving the cosmetic appearance of congenital melanocytic nevi, it is imperative to discuss with patients the insufficient knowledge regarding the long-term effects of these modalities on the development of malignant melanoma.

REFERENCES

1. Cramer SF. The histogenesis of acquired melanocytic nevi. Based on a new concept of melanocytic differentiation. *Am J Dermatopathol.* 1984;6(suppl):289–298.
2. Cramer SF. The melanocytic differentiation pathway in congenital melanocytic nevi: theoretical considerations. *Pediatr Pathol.* 1988;8:253–265.
3. John SM, Hamm H, Happle R. Der geteilte navus ein embryologisches experiment der natur. *Hautarzt.* 1990;41:696–698.
4. Precursors to malignant melanoma. National Institutes of Health Consensus Development Conference Statement, Oct. 24–26, 1983. *J Am Acad Dermatol.* 1984;10:683–688.
5. Tannous ZS, Mihm MC, Jr., Sober AJ, et al. Congenital melanocytic nevi: clinical and histopathologic features, risk of melanoma, and clinical management. *J Am Acad Dermatol.* 2005;52:197–203.
6. Rhodes AR, Silverman RA, Harrist TJ, et al. A histologic comparison of congenital and acquired nevomelanocytic nevi. *Arch Dermatol.* 1985;121:1266–1273.
7. Mark GJ, Mihm MC, Liteplo MG, et al. Congenital melanocytic nevi of the small and garment type. Clinical, histologic, and ultrastructural studies. *Hum Pathol.* 1973;4:395–418.

8. Everett MA. Histopathology of congenital pigmented nevi. *Am J Dermatopathol.* 1989;11:11–12.

9. Reed WB, Becker Sr SW, Becker Jr SW, et al. Giant pigmented nevi, melanoma, and leptomeningeal melanocytosis: a clinical and histopathological study. *Arch Dermatol.* 1965;91:100–119.

10. Evans MJ, Sanders DS, Grant JH, et al. Expression of Melan-A in Spitz, pigmented spindle cell nevi, and congenital nevi: comparative immunohistochemical study. *Pediatr Dev Pathol.* 2000;3:36–39.

11. Cruz MA, Cho ES, Schwartz RA, et al. Congenital neurocutaneous melanosis. *Cutis.* 1997;60:178–181.

12. Rokitansky K. Ein ausgezeichneter fall von pigment-mal mit ausgebreiteter pigmentirung der inneren hirn- und rückenmarkshäute. *Allg Wien Med Z.* 1861:6:113–116.

13. Kadonaga JN, Frieden IJ. Neurocutaneous melanosis: definition and review of the literature. *J Am Acad Dermatol.* 1991;24:747–755.

14. Bett BJ. Large or multiple congenital melanocytic nevi: occurrence of neurocutaneous melanocytosis in 1008 persons. *J Am Acad Dermatol.* 2006;54:767–777.

15. Bett BJ. Large or multiple congenital melanocytic nevi: occurrence of cutaneous melanoma in 1008 persons. *J Am Acad Dermatol.* 2005;52:793–797.

16. Hale EK, Stein J, Ben-Porat L, et al. Association of melanoma and neurocutaneous melanocytosis with large congenital melanocytic nevi—results from the NYU-LCMN registry. *Br J Dermatol.* 2005;152:512–517.

17. Marghoob AA, Schoenbach SP, Kopf AW, et al. Large congenital melanocytic nevi and the risk for the development of malignant melanoma. A prospective study. *Arch Dermatol.* 1996;132:170–175.

18. Bittencourt FV, Marghoob AA, Kopf AW, et al. Large congenital melanocytic nevi and the risk for development of malignant melanoma and neurocutaneous melanocytosis. *Pediatrics.* 2000;106:736–741.

19. Makkar HS, Frieden IJ. Congenital melanocytic nevi: an update for the pediatrician. *Curr Opin Pediatr.* 2002;14:397–403.

20. Egan CL, Oliveria SA, Elenitsas R, et al. Cutaneous melanoma risk and phenotypic changes in large congenital nevi: a follow-up study of 46 patients. *J Am Acad Dermatol.* 1998;39:923–932.

21. Rhodes AR, Wood WC, Sober AJ, et al. Nonepidermal origin of malignant melanoma associated with a giant congenital nevocellular nevus. *Plast Reconstr Surg.* 1981;67:782–790.

22. Precursors to malignant melanoma. National Institutes of Health Consensus Development Conference Statement, Oct. 24–26, 1983; *JAMA.* 1984;251:1864–1866.

23. Kanzler MH, Mraz-Gernhard S. Primary cutaneous malignant melanoma and its precursor lesions: diagnostic and therapeutic overview. *J Am Acad Dermatol.* 2001;45:260–276.

24. Marghoob AA, Agero AL, Benvenuto-Andrade C, et al. Large congenital melanocytic nevi, risk of cutaneous melanoma, and prophylactic surgery. *J Am Acad Dermatol.* 2006;54:868–870. Discussion 871–873.

25. Kaplan EN. The risk of malignancy in large congenital nevi. *Plast Reconstr Surg.* 1974;53:421–428.

26. Swerdlow AJ, English JS, Qiao Z. The risk of melanoma in patients with congenital nevi: a cohort study. *J Am Acad Dermatol.* 1995;32:595–599.

27. Sahin S, Levin L, Kopf AW, et al. Risk of melanoma in medium-sized congenital melanocytic nevi: a follow-up study. *J Am Acad Dermatol.* 1998;39:428–433.

28. Illig L, Weidner F, Hundeiker M, et al. Congenital nevi less than or equal to 10 cm as precursors to melanoma. 52 cases, a review, and a new conception. *Arch Dermatol.* 1985;121:1274–1281.

29. Backman ME, Kopf AW. Iatrogenic effects of general anesthesia in children: considerations in treating large congenital nevocytic nevi. *J Dermatol Surg Oncol.* 1986;12:363–367.

30. Kim S, Kang WH. Treatment of congenital nevi with the Q-switched Alexandrite laser. *Eur J Dermatol.* 2005;15:92–96.

31. Kono T, Ercocen AR, Nozaki M. Treatment of congenital melanocytic nevi using the combined (normal-mode plus Q-switched ruby laser in Asians: clinical response in relation to histological type. *Ann Plast Surg.* 2005;54:494–501.

32. Kono T, Nozaki M, Chan HH, et al. Combined use of normal mode and Q-switched ruby lasers in the treatment of congenital melanocytic naevi. *Br J Plast Surg.* 2001;54:640–643.

33. Michel JL. Laser therapy of giant congenital melanocytic nevi. *Eur J Dermatol.* 2003;13:57–64.

34. Michel JL, Caillet-Chomel L. Traitement par laser CO_2 superpulsé des naevus congénitaux géants. *Arch Pediatr.* 2001;8:1185–1194.

35. Reynolds N, Kenealy J, Mercer N. Carbon dioxide laser dermabrasion for giant congenital melanocytic nevi. *Plast Reconstr Surg.* 2003;111:2209–2214.

36. Chan HH, Xiang L, Leung JC, et al. In vitro study examining the effect of sublethal QS 755 nm lasers on the expression of p16INK4a on melanoma cell lines. *Lasers Surg Med.* 2003;32:88–93.

37. Zhu NW, Perks CM, Burd AR, et al. Changes in the levels of integrin and focal adhesion kinase (FAK in human melanoma cells following 532 nm laser treatment. *Int J Cancer.* 1999;82:353–358.

38. De Raeve LE, De Coninck AL, Dierickx PR, et al. Neonatal curettage of giant congenital melanocytic nevi. *Arch Dermatol.* 1996;132:20–22.

39. De Raeve LE, Roseeuw DI. Curettage of giant congenital melanocytic nevi in neonates: a decade later. *Arch Dermatol.* 2002;138:943–947.

CHAPTER 9

Spitz Tumors and Variants

Raymond L. Barnhill, M.D.

BOX 9-1 Overview

- Spitz tumors are uncommon melanocytic neoplasms defined by characteristic enlarged spindled and epithelioid melanocytes.
- A number of congenital and acquired variants have been described including agminated, plaque-type, desmoplastic, pigmented (including pigmented spindle cell variants), and finally, atypical and biologically indeterminate Spitz tumors.
- Spitz tumors most commonly develop in young individuals usually less than 20 to 30 years of age, but may occur at any age.
- Spitz tumors often present on the extremities or head and neck as nondescript pink papules or nodules frequently with smooth surface, and uncommonly as pigmented lesions.
- The most typical variants of Spitz tumor measure up to 5 to 6 mm in diameter, are symmetrical and well-defined, and exhibit maturation of the dermal component and uniform cytological features.
- Atypical variants of Spitz tumor are defined by one or more abnormal features such as diameter >1 cm, asymmetry, effacement or ulceration of the epidermis, confluent and hypercellular proliferation of melanocytes, involvement of the subcutaneous fat, diminished or absent maturation, significant mitotic rates of the dermal component, and significant cytological atypia.
- Both typical and atypical Spitz tumors are commonly confused with melanoma; however, a subset of atypical Spitz tumors is often impossible to distinguish from melanoma.
- Atypical Spitz tumors should be carefully evaluated for the abnormal features present (risk stratification) and appropriate management.
- With rare exceptions, all Spitz tumors should be completely excised for complete histopathological evaluation and to prevent recurrence.
- Spitz tumors with significant atypia (high risk) including biologically indeterminate variants should probably be excised with wider margins, e.g., about 1 cm, until more definitive data concerning appropriate therapy is available.

- At present considerable controversy surrounds the biological significance of positive sentinel lymph nodes associated with Spitz tumors and atypical Spitzoid neoplasms.

INTRODUCTION

The Spitz tumor and its closely related variants remain a relatively uncommon, yet profoundly important, and highly perplexing group of lesions among melanocytic neoplasia.[1-41] The distinct importance of the Spitz tumor is directly related to its continuing ambiguous and close relationship to conventional melanoma. Furthermore, it may represent a unique melanocytic neoplasm potentially with a continuum of risk (from negligible to high) for aggressive behavior. The characteristic histopathologic appearance that sets the Spitz tumor apart from other melancytic lesions (but not necessarily from melanoma) is the presence of large epithelioid and/or spindled melanocytes. This singular group of lesions requires much more rigorous study in order to better define their biological nature and risk to individual patients. Several variants have been described; however, a detailed discussion of all variants of Spitz tumor is not possible in this chapter.[1-9]

CLINICAL FEATURES

BOX 9-2 Summary

- *Configuration:* plaque, papule or nodule, often dome-shaped
- *Size:* small (usually <1 cm)
- *Profile:* smooth surface topography
- *Color:* pink/red; darker forms occur
- *Age:* majority in children and adolescents
- *Location:* face and extremities, most common
- *Number:* usually solitary; rare multiple forms occur
- *Symptoms:* commonly asymptomatic; rarely pruritic
- *History of growth:* months; usually less than a year

Spitz tumors are usually acquired, but rarely may be congenital. The great majority of lesions develop in children, adolescents, and young adults (<20 to 30 years of age). However, Spitz tumors are more common in adults than has been previ-

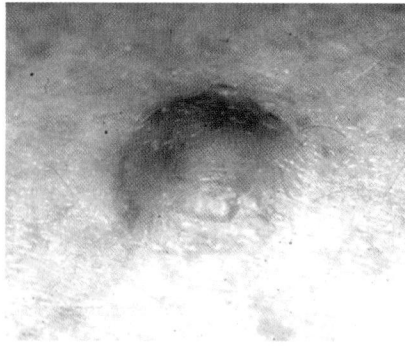

▲ **FIGURE 9-1** Spitz tumor. Shows symmetrical, reddish-pink, dome-shaped nodule with uniform smooth surface.

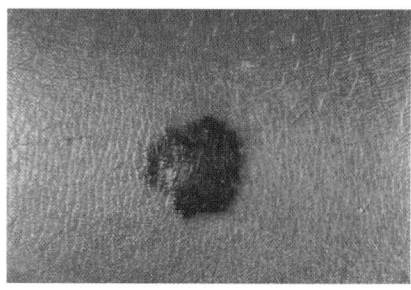

▲ **FIGURE 9-2** Pigmented Spitz tumor. The lesion has plaque-type topography, and uniform brown-black color centrally.

ously appreciated and may occur at any age. The lesions most often present as a solitary, asymptomatic, red/pink or skin-colored, hairless, dome-shaped, smooth nodule measuring less than 1 cm in diameter (Fig. 9-1). Some lesions may be tan, brown, or even black in color (Fig. 9-2). Pedunculated and polypoid forms occur. Spitz tumors may involve any site; however, there is a predilection for the face and the extremities. They may be slightly more common in females. Multiple Spitz tumors may occur in either a grouped (agminate) or disseminated pattern.[10] The disseminated type is characterized by numerous, up to hundreds of Spitz tumors, all over the body, typically sparing the palms, soles, and mucous membranes.

The vast majority of *typical* Spitz tumors are benign and present little, if any, risk to the individual. However, because of the histologic resemblance of Spitz tumors to some melanomas, the presence of atypical variants, and rare metastases from such lesions, there is some justification for the belief that uncommonly or rarely atypical variants may result in recurrence and aggressive behavior.[17,41] The exact nature and classification of these lesions is a subject of ongoing research.

BOX 9-3   Summary

- Cytologic features
  - Spindle and/or epithelioid cell type
  - Overall monomorphous population of cells
  - Occasional striking pleomorphism in a minority of cells
- Architectural features
  - Symmetry
  - Sharp lateral demarcation
  - Zonation in depth (e.g., "maturation")
  - Orderly nondisruptive infiltration of collagen by Spitz cells
- Other helpful diagnostic features
  - Absent or rare, but not atypical, mitoses in deep parts
  - Giant nevus cells
  - Irregular contours of growth at deep margin
  - Kamino bodies
  - Paucity or absence of single-cell upward spread
  - Junctional clefts
  - Loss of cohesion between cells (retraction spaces)
  - Perivascular or diffuse inflammatory infiltrate
  - Superficial distribution of pigmentation
  - Telangiectasia and edema
  - Epidermal hyperplasia

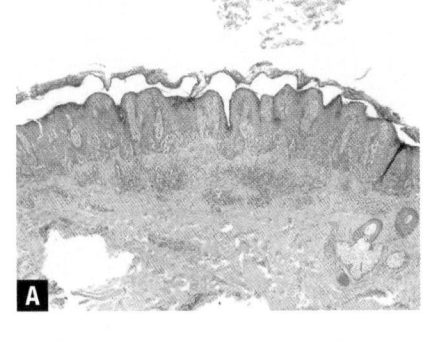
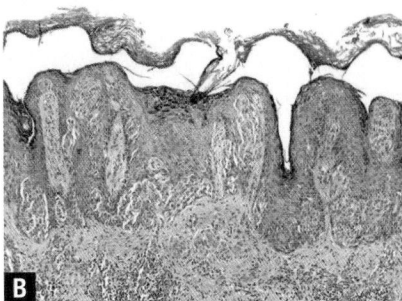
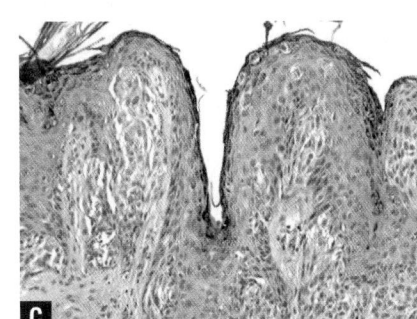
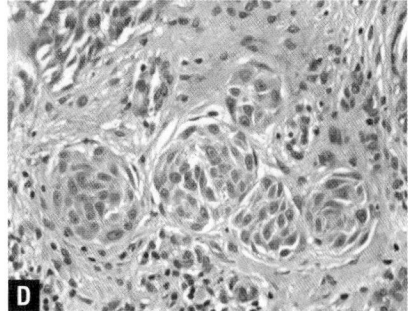

▲ **FIGURE 9-3** Compound Spitz tumor without significant atypicality. The lesion measures less than 10 mm in diameter and 0.61 mm in Breslow thickness. The tumor shows no asymmetry, sharp circumscription, no ulceration, only minimal focal pagetoid spread, and there are no mitoses in the small dermal component. This lesion requires complete excision and the patient follow-up examinations at least once a year. **A.** Scanning magnification shows a slightly raised tumor with general symmetry. **B.** The lesion demonstrates orderly appearance with regular junctional nesting and small dermal component. **C.** The lesion shows focal pagetoid spread and fairly regular junctional nesting of melanocytes. **D.** Note uniformity of the spindle and epithelioid cells in dermis.

Histopathologic Features

The majority of Spitz tumors (about two-thirds or more) are compound, 5 to 10% of the cases are junctional, and 12 to 20% are dermal.[1–9]

The most distinctive histologic features (Figs. 9-3 and 9-4) and an absolute prerequisite for diagnosis are large spindle-shaped and/or epithelioid melanocytes (Fig. 9-4C). The *spindle cells* are elongated, fusiform, often plump, and may exhibit dendrites. The cells possess centrally located nuclei, comparable in size to or even larger than the nuclei of keratinocytes. Nuclear contours are typically smooth and regular. The chromatin pattern is usually finely dispersed or slightly vesicular. Typically, a distinct, single, centrally located, and round eosinophilic or amphophilic nucleolus is present. The spindle cells are arranged in fascicles or elongated nests, characteristically in vertical orientation or concentric arrangements within nests.

The epithelioid cells are large, round, oval, polygonal, rhomboidal, or polyangular cells with distinct cellular borders (Fig. 9-4C) and have nuclei that are similar to those in the spindle cells, but also sometimes irregularly shaped or lobu-lated. Multinucleated cells are often seen when epithelioid forms constitute the predominant cell type. The cytoplasm of the spindle and epithelioid cells is usually abundant with a homogeneous eosinophilic or bluish, "ground-glass," or rarely granular appearance. Melanin is typically absent or scarce.

The two cell types may be admixed in varying proportions, but either may occur alone. Regardless of the proportion of spindle or epithelioid cells, one of the most characteristic features of Spitz tumor is the uniformity of the cells and nuclei. From side to side, in horizontal zones, the cells tend to show a strikingly uniform appearance and size. In all age groups, Spitz tumors with predominant spindle cell morphology are the most common type and are especially prevalent in adults. Spitz tumors of the epithelioid cell type are observed mainly in childhood.

While spindle and/or epithelioid cells are a prerequisite for diagnosis, they must appear in an appropriate architectural arrangement. The major architectural criteria include symmetry, sharp lateral demarcation, size (generally <1 cm), maturation (zonation), lack of deep extension, and lack of significant pagetoid spread. These and other criteria, such as few or no deeply located mitoses, and the lack of significant cytologic atypia, which are thought to reflect ordered growth, favor benignancy.[9]

MATURATION (ZONATION) Maturation (zonation) refers to the appearance of layers of differing morphology from "top to bottom." There is transition from larger nests at the dermoepidermal junction to smaller nests and single cells near the deep margin of the nevus. With this transition from top to bottom, the cellular elements exhibit a nondisruptive insinuation among collagen bundles without induction of new stroma (Fig. 9-4). The distribution of pigment may also be zonal. If melanin is present in Spitz tumors, it is largely confined to cells immediately subjacent to the epidermis. The cytologic features of the spindle and/or epithelioid cells may change from above, downwards leading to a gradient in cell size and shape, such as from large plump cells at the top to smaller or slender cells at the bottom.

MITOTIC RATE AND LOCATION OF MITOSES The mitotic rate is variable and is commonly less than two per square millimeter and rarely greater than six per square millimeter. Mitoses most commonly

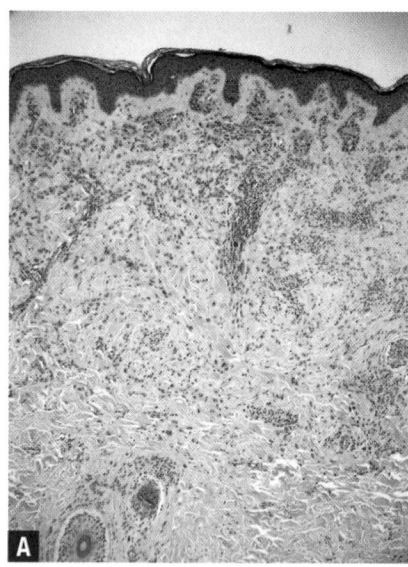 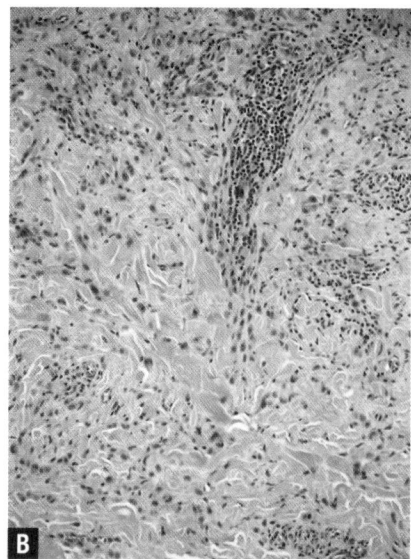 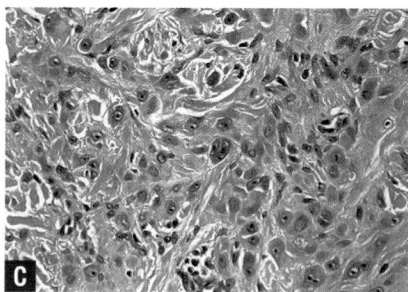

▲ **FIGURE 9-4** Dermal desmoplastic Spitz tumor. **A.** The lesion shows a general symmetry, no ulceration, maturation, and slight sclerosis of collagen. **B.** Higher magnification demonstrates maturation. **C.** The melanocytes show diminished cellularity with depth with smaller cytoplasms and nuclei. (Part C from Barnhill RL, Crowson AN, eds. *Textbook of Dermatopathology*. 2nd ed. New York: McGraw-Hill; 2004:652.)

occur in the upper portion of the lesion and are usually bipolar. Although an occasional mitosis in the deeper parts of the lesion or a rare atypical mitosis may be observed, they should nonetheless prompt careful evaluation for melanoma.

KAMINO BODIES Eosinophilic amorphous globules, either singly or in aggregates, at the dermoepidermal junction, occur frequently in Spitz tumors,[13] and are useful since they are found less frequently in melanoma. However, they are nonspecific.[14] Ultrastructurally, Kamino bodies are composed of amorphous masses and bundles of filaments. Immunohistochemically, they contain basement membrane components, including collagen types IV and VII, as well as laminin. Degenerate material derived from melanocytes and keratinocytes may also be present.[15]

PAGETOID MELANOCYTOSIS Pagetoid spread of single melanocytes occurs less commonly in the Spitz tumor than in melanoma and is often related to external insult. Upward migration of melanocytes in the Spitz tumor usually takes the form of transepidermal elimination of nests of two or more cells.

JUNCTIONAL CLEAVAGE At the dermoepidermal junction, the fascicles of spindle cells are often separated by a cleft-like retraction space from the adjacent epidermis, a result of tissue shrinkage during processing.

ADNEXAL INVOLVEMENT Spitz tumors and its variants have a propensity to involve

hair follicles and eccrine ducts. In most instances, intraepidermal fascicles of cells track along the adventitial sheaths of appendageal structures into the papillary dermis and often into the reticular dermis.

PERIVASCULAR OR DIFFUSE INFLAMMATORY INFILTRATE The distribution of the inflammatory infiltrate tends to be perivascular but may also be diffuse in some Spitz tumors.

EPIDERMAL HYPERPLASIA Epidermal hyperplasia is a common finding in Spitz tumors.

SPITZ TUMOR WITH ATYPICAL FEATURES (ATYPICAL SPITZ TUMOR)

BOX 9-4 Summary

- Organizational criteria
  - Diameter in millimeters (≥10 mm considered abnormal)
  - Depth in millimeters (involvement of subcutaneous fat considered abnormal)
  - Ulceration
  - Poor circumscription
  - Pagetoid melanocytosis over a large front
  - Prominent confluence of melanocytes
  - High cellular density
  - Lack of zonation and maturation
  - Asymmetry
  - Few or no dull pink (Kamino) bodies
- Proliferational criteria
  - Significant mitotic rate greater than 2–6/mm^2

- Deep/marginal mitoses
- Proliferation index, i.e., Ki-67 expression between 2 and 10% (Vollmer[19]) ≥10% (Kapor et al[20])
- Cytological criteria
  - Granular vs ground glass cytoplasm
  - High nuclear to cytoplasmic ratios
  - Loss of delicate or dispersed chromatin patterns
  - Thickening of nuclear membranes
  - Hyperchromatism
  - Large nucleoli

Spitz tumors with atypical features are not uncommonly encountered, yet remain controversial, as there may be difficulty in distinguishing such lesions from conventional Spitz tumors on one hand and melanoma on the other (Figs. 9-5 to 9-7). However, criteria for recognizing or categorizing such lesions have been proposed.[9,17,18,41] In general, atypical features may be subdivided into those involving primarily the epidermis and/or the dermis/subcutis (Fig. 9-6). Recently a grading protocol for evaluating Spitz tumors with atypical features in childhood and adolescence has been formulated (Table 9-1). The grading scheme attempts to estimate potential risk for metastases based on cumulative scores from quantifiable or objective parameters including diameter (greater than or less than 1 cm), presence or absence of ulceration, depth, mitotic rate per square millimeter, and age (greater than or less than 10 years).[18]

Molecular techniques have also been recently utilized in an effort to shed more light on the biological nature of Spitz

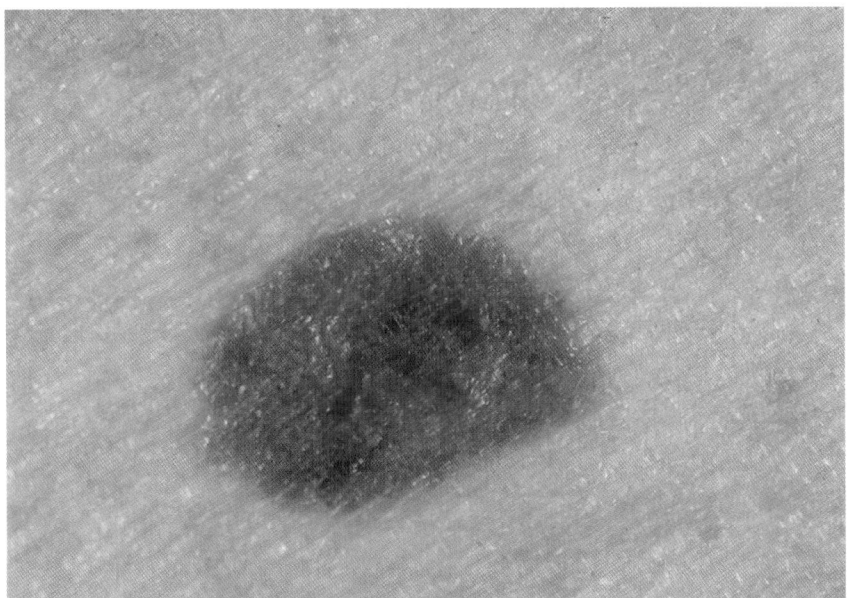

▲ **FIGURE 9-5** Spitz tumor with atypical features. The lesion is well defined, symmetrical, and has reddish-pink color centrally with brown tones at periphery.

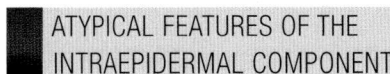

Table 9-1

Assessment of Spitz Tumors in Children and Adolescents for Risk for Metastasis[18]

PARAMETER	SCORE[a]
AGE (years)	
• 0–10	0
• 11–17	1
DIAMETER (mm)	
• 0–10	0
• >10	1
INVOLVEMENT OF SUBCUTANEOUS FAT	
• Absent	0
• Present	2
ULCERATION	
• Absent	0
• Present	2
MITOTIC ACTIVITY (mm^2)	
• 0–5	0
• 6–8	2
• >9	5

[a]Total score indicates increasing risk for metastasis. Low risk: 0–2; High risk: 5–11.

tumors. In particular, gains on chromosome 11p (by comparative genomic hybridization), mutations in the HRAS gene by fluorescence *in situ* hybridization,[21,22] and loss of heterozygosity on chromosome 9p have been described,[23,24] suggesting some evidence of tumor progression in some Spitz tumors.

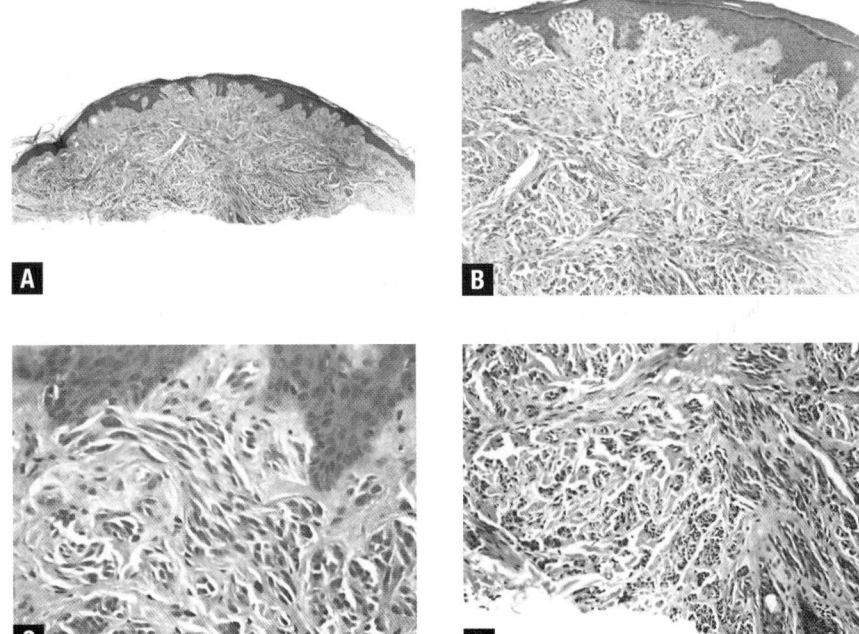

▲ **FIGURE 9-6** Compound Spitz tumor with atypical features. The tumor measures less than 10mm in diameter and at least 2.1 mm in Breslow thickness. Other attributes are: slight asymmetry, reasonable circumscription, no ulceration, no pagetoid melanocytosis, lack of maturation, high cellular density and confluence of melanocytes in dermis, mitotic rate of two per square millimeter, deep mitosis, and prominent nuclear pleomorphism. This lesion lacks sufficient atypicality for conventional melanoma. Such a lesion requires re-excision with margins of about 1 cm and careful follow-up at least every 6 months. **A.** Scanning magnification shows a raised dome-shaped tumor with the general appearance of Spitz tumor and slight asymmetry. **B.** Note lack of maturation of dermal component. **C.** The lesion exhibits junctional nesting of melanocytes but no pagetoid spread. The nests of melanocytes display prominent cellularity and confluence. **D.** There is no maturation at the base of the tumor.

ATYPICAL FEATURES OF THE INTRAEPIDERMAL COMPONENT

BOX 9-5   Summary

- Architectural disorder
  - Disordered intraepidermal melanocytic proliferation
  - Lentiginous or single-cell pattern
  - Disordered junctional nesting
    - Variation in size, shape, orientation, spacing, cellular cohesion of nests
    - Horizontal confluence and bridging of nests
    - Pagetoid spread
  - Asymmetry
  - Poorly circumscription
  - Effacement of epidermis
  - Lateral extension of intraepidermal component ("shoulder phenomenon")
- Cytologic atypia
  - Nuclear pleomorphism
  - Variation in nuclear chromatin patterns
  - Nuclear enlargement
  - Variation in nucleoli
- Host response
  - Patchy to band-like mononuclear infiltrates in papillary dermis
  - Fibroplasia

Spitz tumors (and pigmented spindle cell nevi) may show abnormal morphologic features observed in conventional atypical nevi and/or cytologic atypia. The essential criteria for diagnosis are (1) large diameter (greater than 1 cm),

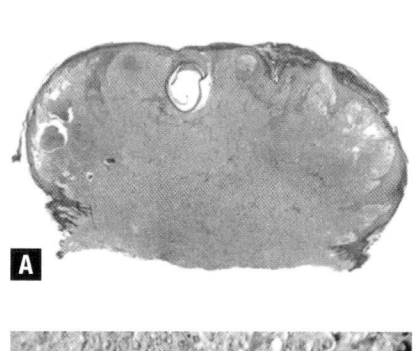
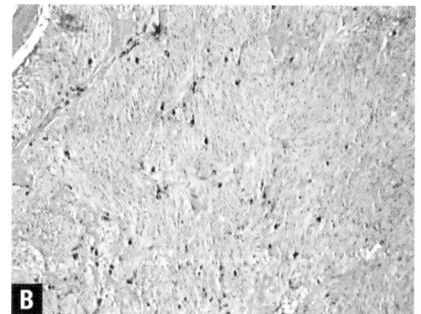
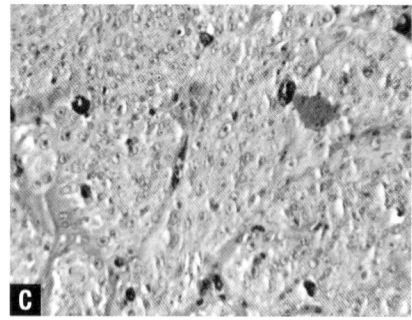
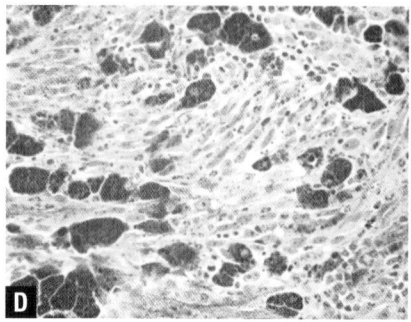

▲ **FIGURE 9-7** Metastasizing Spitz tumor (malignant Spitzoid neoplasm) in a young boy involving left back. The tumor measures 9 mm in diameter and at least 4.4 mm in Breslow thickness. Other attributes are as follows: asymmetry, reasonable circumscription, no ulceration, no pagetoid melanocytosis, no maturation, high cellular density and confluence of melanocytes throughout dermis, mitotic rate of nine per square millimeter, deep mitoses, and prominent cytological atypia. The lesion apparently grew back after the initial shave biopsy in a matter of months. At the time of complete excision, two sentinel lymph nodes contained large deposits of an atypical melanocytic tumor. Long-term follow-up will be needed to determine if there is disease progression or not. **A.** Scanning magnification shows a large raised polypoid tumor with slight asymmetry. **B.** The superficial portion of the tumor is characterized by confluent sheets of melanocytes replacing dermis. **C.** Note striking density of melanocytes at base with cytological atypia. Many nuclei contain prominent nucleoli. **D.** Sentinel lymph node containing large tumoral deposit replacing a large part of node. Note the pronounced cytological atypia of spindled melanocytes.

asymmetry, ulceration, irregular pattern of the epidermis, disordered architectural patterns of the intraepidermal component, i.e., lentiginous melanocytic proliferation and/or significant variation in junctional nesting (variation in size, shape, orientation, spacing of junctional nests; horizontal confluence and bridging of nests; diminished cellular cohesion of nests), and (2) cytologic atypia of melanocytes beyond what is considered acceptable for a Spitz tumor.[9,17,18,41]

INTRAEPIDERMAL OR MAINLY INTRAEPIDERMAL SPITZ TUMORS WITH PROMINENT PAGETOID SPREAD (PAGETOID SPITZ TUMOR)

A distinctive variant is the mainly intraepidermal subtype with a prominent pagetoid pattern.[9,25] This variant may occur anywhere in an individual, but is most commonly encountered on the lower extremities of young women.

The most important reason for recognizing this lesion is its frequent misdiagnosis as *in situ* or microinvasive melanoma. Most lesions measure less than 5 or 6 mm. Scanning magnification usually discloses a mainly intraepidermal proliferation of enlarged epithelioid cells usually devoid of melanin with an overall symmetry from side-to-side and reasonably well-defined margins. However, some lesions have ill-defined margins. Many of these lesions show a combination of both a single-cell and nested proliferation of epithelioid melanocytes. The single-cell proliferative pattern is often both basilar and pagetoid and commonly varies within the lesion. Typical junctional nests of epithelioid cells with associated clefting are also usually present and may be quite small in size. Nests of cells or single Spitz tumor cells may or may not be present in the papillary dermis. Often the degree of pagetoid spread is focal or limited; however, it may be prominent in some lesions, raising the possibility of melanoma *in situ*.

ATYPICAL FEATURES OF THE DERMAL COMPONENT

BOX 9-6 Summary

- Architectural disorder
  - Expansile nodules
  - Increased cellularity
  - Asymmetry
  - Deep extension, e.g., into subcutis
  - Lack of maturation or orderly infiltration of collagen
  - Ulceration
  - Necrosis
- Cytologic atypia (as above)
- Mitotic activity
  - Numerous mitoses (greater than six per square millimeter)
  - Mitoses at base of lesion
  - Atypical mitoses
- Host response
  - Prominent mononuclear cell infiltrates
  - Formation of tumor stroma

As already alluded to, atypicality of the dermal component includes cohesive cellular nodules, increased cellularity, asymmetry, deep extension into the lowermost dermis or subcutis, lack of maturation or orderly infiltration of collagen, cytologic atypia as mentioned above, mitotic activity especially deep, and mononuclear infiltrates (Figs. 9-6 and 9-7).[9,17] Because of the rarity of such lesions and the lack of sufficient follow-up in many instances, the significance of these various features has not been elucidated. There is little question that the presence of these various features in any given lesion is highly worrisome for melanoma and that as these features increase in number and severity, the likelihood of melanoma increases.

In evaluating such lesions, a number of factors should be weighed in the final interpretation (see above). Clinical factors such as the age of the patient, location of the tumor, clinical appearance, history of recent change in long-standing stable lesions, size greater than 1 cm, and family history of melanoma should be carefully considered. The older the patient, especially if beyond the age of 30 years, the greater is the likelihood of malignancy. As a general rule, one's threshold for diagnosing melanoma in such lesions should correlate inversely with the age of the patient, i.e., a higher threshold for very young individuals and a lower threshold for elderly individuals. The location of atypical tumors on sites less commonly involved by Spitz tumor, such as the back, is also another factor that warrants careful scrutiny of the lesion for melanoma. When, even after weighing these various factors, a clear-cut diagnosis of melanoma cannot be made, the practical approach is to communicate this situation to the clinician and patient.

DIFFERENTIAL DIAGNOSIS

BOX 9-7 Summary

- Melanocytic lesions
  - Malignant melanoma
  - Atypical nevi with features of Spitz tumor
  - Variants of tumors with spindle and/or epithelioid cells
  - Pigmented spindle cell tumor
  - Desmoplastic Spitz tumor
  - Plexiform spindle cell tumor/deep penetrating nevus
  - Cellular blue nevus
  - Various "combined" nevi
- Nonmelanocytic lesions
  - Epithelioid cell histiocytoma
  - Reticulohistiocytoma
  - Cellular neurothekeoma

The intraepidermal or junctional variants of Spitz tumors must first of all be discriminated from in situ or early invasive melanoma. These intraepidermal Spitz tumors often show relatively small size, symmetry, evidence of growth control, and sharp circumscription compared to melanoma. Of particular importance are the cytologic characteristics of the epithelioid cells; they tend to be fairly monotypic with abundant pinkish cytoplasm that has a ground glass appearance, rather than the granular cytoplasm often observed in melanoma cells. The nuclei of Spitz tumor cells are also fairly uniform with evenly dispersed chromatin versus the pleomorphism of melanoma cells.

Compound and dermal Spitz tumors and their atypical variants must also be discriminated from invasive melanoma. The features outlined above provide guidelines for this distinction. However, many Spitz lesions show atypical features. The absence or incomplete development of major diagnostic features, such as symmetry or sharply demarcated lateral borders are of concern and should prompt a careful search for features of melanoma. Even if symmetry and sharp lateral demarcation are observed, the presence of extensive pagetoid spread, the lack of maturation in depth, prominent cellularity of the dermal component, nuclear pleomor-

phism of more than a small proportion of cells, cohesive cellular nodules in the dermis, or deeply located (albeit rare) mitoses are worrisome.

Detailed knowledge of diagnostic criteria and their relative weight are critical in the histologic assessment of such atypical lesions. When an atypical lesion is present, one must attempt to determine the approximate degree of risk for recurrence (risk stratification). Depending on the severity of the atypia, one should acknowledge that melanoma cannot be completely excluded. A diagnosis of malignancy should not be made unless there is sufficient histologic evidence, so that overtreatment and undue psychological burden for the patient can be avoided.

Nonmelanocytic lesions that need to be considered in the differential diagnosis include juvenile xanthogranuloma, cellular neurothekeoma, epithelioid cell histiocytoma, and reticulohistiocytoma.

METASTASIZING SPITZ TUMOR

Melanocytic lesions classified as Spitz tumors have been reported to spread to regional and sentinel lymph nodes apparently without further neoplastic progression, i.e., the absence of visceral and distant metastases.[11,17,18,38-41] A priori all such reports must be viewed with due diligence and caution. These various "metastasizing" melanocytic neoplasms, have included a heterogenous assortment (even "waistbasket") of lesions often with attributes of ranging from those of typical Spitz tumors (commonly in children and adolescents with microscopic sentinel lymph node involvement)[38-41] to unusual Spitzoid lesions that have often been uncharacteristically large, deep, ulcerated, or commonly showing other atypical features (see above) (Fig. 9-7).[11,17,18] Definitive long-term studies are needed to clarify the nature of these various types of Spitzoid tumors, their lymph node deposits, and their biological nature. Until more information is available, many of these lesions (particularly in children) should not necessarily be considered melanoma or malignant without additional documentation of neoplastic progression. However, all such tumors must be managed on an individual basis with careful attention to adequate surgical excision, the avoidance of excessive surgery without good reason, and close long-term monitoring of patients for regional and distant tumor spread.[41]

DESMOPLASTIC SPITZ TUMOR (SCLEROSING SPITZ TUMOR, DESMOPLASTIC NEVUS)

Clinical Features

BOX 9-8 Summary

- Firm papule or nodule
- Adults (peak incidence in third decade)
- Most commonly located on extremities

Although the desmoplastic Spitz tumor is considered by many to be an unusual variant of Spitz tumor,[26] some authors maintain that this lesion is a distinct entity.[27,28] In fact, both of the latter perspectives are correct since desmoplastic or sclerosing nevi may be comprised of varying proportions of enlarged epithelioid cells, spindle cells, or smaller conventional nevus cells. Desmoplastic Spitz tumor typically presents as a firm, dome-shaped, flesh-colored papule or nodule, measuring up to 1 cm along the greatest diameter, is most often located on the extremities, and suggests a dermatofibroma. This variant of Spitz tumor primarily affects adults with a peak incidence in the third decade of life.

Histopathologic Features

BOX 9-9 Summary

- Spindle and/or epithelioid cells
- Predominantly intradermal location of melanocytes
- Sometimes junctional component
- Dermal stroma with increased collagen
- Usually circumscribed, but with ill-defined borders
- Often vaguely wedge shaped
- Usually diffuse distribution of cells with low cell density
- Typically small nests and single melanocytes
- Maturation often present
- Mitoses absent or rare
- Multinucleated giant cells not uncommon (usually superficial)
- Melanin usually sparse or absent

The desmoplastic Spitz tumor is a poorly circumscribed growth of large polygonal or elongated melanocytes in a collagen-rich stromal background (Fig 4.).[26-28] It is usually a wholly intradermal lesion. The desmoplastic changes in Spitz tumors may comprise the entire lesion or any portion of it. In the superficial dermis, melanocytes may be grouped in nests or aggregates, while in the deeper parts of the lesions, they tend to infiltrate singly between typically thickened collagen bundles (Fig. 4B and D). The latter phenomenon is maturation. Scattered multinucleated giant cells or large pleomorphic forms may be present. Cytologically, the melanocytes of desmoplastic Spitz tumors are characterized by nuclei that are often hyperchromatic with clumped or finely dispersed chromatin. Nucleoli are commonly inconspicuous, but may be prominent, especially in larger cells. The size of the nuclei tends to diminish as melanocytes approach the base of the lesion, which is usually ill defined. Mitoses are rare (usually greater than one per square millimeter).

Differential Diagnosis

BOX 9-10   Summary

- Desmoplastic melanoma
- Sclerosing blue nevus
- Dermatofibroma

The major differential diagnostic problem with desmoplastic Spitz tumor is its distinction from desmoplastic melanoma. The desmoplastic Spitz tumor may present in a fashion similar to desmoplastic melanoma, i.e., an indurated amelanotic or slightly pigmented nodule. However, in other respects, the desmoplastic Spitz tumor is different from desmoplastic melanoma. There is a predilection for the extremities of young individuals vs. the head and neck of elderly persons in desmoplastic melanoma. Histologically, desmoplastic Spitz tumors tend to be small, well circumscribed, superficial lesions whereas desmoplastic melanomas are often larger, poorly demarcated, and characterized by deep involvement of the dermis or subcutis. The desmoplastic variant of Spitz tumor also shows maturation, i.e., isolation of individually smaller cells with increasing depth versus little or no such transition in desmoplastic melanoma. The cell types in the two processes tend to be rather different. Desmoplastic Spitz tumors contain typical large epithelioid or fusiform cells whereas desmoplastic melanoma is notable for pleomorphic spindle cells often with hyperchromatic nuclei.

Although the blue nevus may have pronounced sclerosing features, it is usually a more ill-defined melanocytic lesion than desmoplastic Spitz tumor, and is composed of a more slender and more diffusely pigmented melanocytic population than the plumper cells of Spitz tumor.

Nonmelanocytic dermal spindle cell lesions that may share morphologic features of desmoplastic Spitz tumor are dermatofibroma, reticulohistiocytoma, and epithelioid cell histiocytoma (see earlier discussion).

PIGMENTED SPINDLE CELL TUMOR (PIGMENTED SPINDLE CELL NEVUS OF REED)

Clinical Features

BOX 9-11   Summary

- Peak incidence in the third decade of life
- Most often located on extremities (especially thigh)
- Women > men
- Small (usually smaller than 0.6 cm)
- Symmetric
- Pigmented (usually evenly, often heavily)
- Sharply circumscribed
- Papule or nodule
- History of recent onset

The pigmented spindle cell tumor (PSCT) is a distinctive clinicopathologic entity, important to recognize because of its frequent confusion with melanoma.[16,33–37] PSCT usually presents as a symmetric, sharply circumscribed, dark brown or black papule or nodule (Fig. 9-8). It is typically a small lesion, often measuring less than 0.6 cm in diameter. PSCT is preferentially located on the extremities. It appears to affect women slightly more than men.

Histopathology

BOX 9-12   Summary

- Junctional or compound nevus
- Predominantly spindle cells, but occasional epithelioid cells
- Spindle cells more slender and delicate than in Spitz nevi
- Uniform population of cells from side to side
- Symmetrical configuration
- Predominance of junctional nests or fascicles
- Typically ovoid nests with fusiform cells oriented vertically
- Often confluence of nests leading to irregular shapes
- Sharp lateral borders, occasional lentiginous lateral spread
- Usually abundant coarse melanin
- Uniform nuclear features
- Decrease in cell size from top to bottom ("maturation")
- Mitoses not uncommon in intraepidermal component
- Absent or rare dermal mitoses

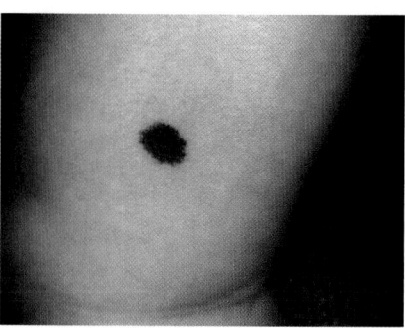

▲ **FIGURE 9-8** Pigmented spindle cell melanocytic tumor. The lesion is small with regular well-defined borders and uniform brown-black color. The tumor also demonstrates slightly elevated plaque-type topography.

These lesions are usually relatively small, strikingly well circumscribed, and remarkable for a slightly elevated, flat-topped plaque-like appearance of the epidermis (Fig. 9-9).[16,33–37] Although the PSCT may be junctional or compound, many are almost entirely intraepidermal. If papillary dermal involvement occurs, the base of PSCT is typically broad with pushing borders.

The PSCT contains uniform, delicate, spindle cells present in tightly packed fascicles. These fascicles tend to have a fairly uniform and symmetric spacing and size within the epidermis and are often vertically oriented. The fusiform cells are often slightly more slender than the spindle cells of "classic" Spitz tumor (Fig. 9-9C). Their nuclei are equal in size or smaller than the nuclei of adjacent keratinocytes. Nucleoli are usually inconspicuous. Some PSCT, particularly in children, may show florid upward migration of single melanocytes closely simulating melanoma *in situ*. Also, in contrast to ordinary Spitz tumor, melanocytes of PSCT contain variable amounts of granular melanin. Heavy pigmentation may also involve the adjacent keratinocytes, cornified layer, and papillary dermis.

There is a histologic continuum of Spitz tumor and PSCT.[16] One will encounter many nevi showing varying degrees of transition between these two poles of the spectrum. For example, some nevi may exhibit slender spindle cells, typical of PSCT, yet at the same time contain somewhat larger fusiform cells and epithelioid cells that are less heavily melaninized.

PIGMENTED SPINDLE CELL TUMOR WITH ATYPICAL FEATURES

The same discussion applies to the atypical variants of PSCT as for atypi-

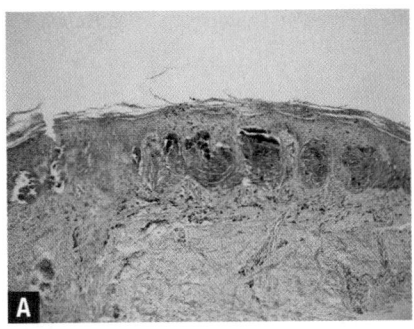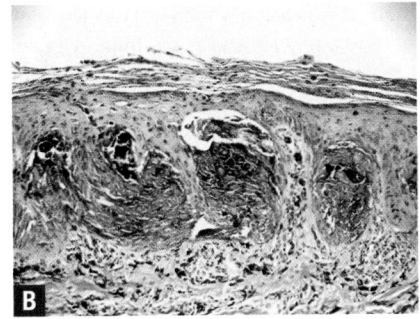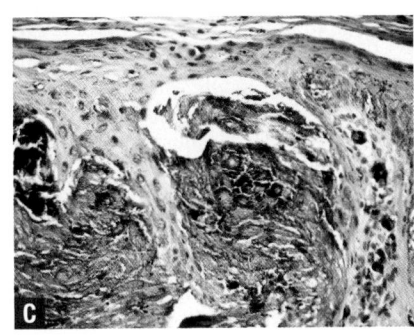

▲ **FIGURE 9-9 A.** Pigmented spindle cell melanocytic tumor. Histologically, the tumor is a uniform well-circumscribed plaque comprised of hyperplastic epidermis and the junctional aggregates of pigmented spindled melanocytes. **B.** Intraepidermal nests and vertically oriented fascicles of spindle cells are regularly and unobstrusively arrayed within the fabric of the epidermis. **C.** The spindle cells are uniform with delicate basophilic chromatin.

cal forms of Spitz tumor[16] (see earlier sections). However, most atypical variants of PSCT are primarily intraepidermal. Some overlap may occur with conventional atypical (dysplastic) nevi.

Differential Diagnosis

BOX 9-13   Summary

- Lentiginous melanoma
- Pagetoid melanoma
- Atypical (dysplastic) nevus

Pigmented spindle cell tumor and its atypical variants must be distinguished from *in situ* or microinvasive melanoma and from atypical nevus.

PSCT (particularly atypical forms of PSCT) and lentiginous melanocytic proliferations of sun-exposed skin (SMPS, lentigo maligna) may show considerable similarity on occasion.[16] Both are typically composed of pigmented spindle cells that may be arranged in junctional nests and may involve skin appendages. Discrimination of the two is based on clinical features, the usual small size, sharp circumscription, predominantly nested pattern, and uniformity of cell type in PSCT. SMPS with atypia, on the other hand, tends to be broader, poorly circumscribed, and usually typified by a mainly basilar single-cell proliferation of pleomorphic melanocytes. Rare lesions may show such overlap that distinction may not be possible. Such lesions should be completely excised with a cuff of normal tissue, and the patients carefully monitored.

PSCT and atypical variants of PSCT are often confused with pagetoid variants of melanoma because of prominent pagetoid spread.[16] One must

again rely on clinical factors, i.e., young age, anatomic site, (e.g., the extremities), as well as the overall morphologic appearance. PSCT are typically small, well demarcated, symmetric, and orderly. Even with striking pagetoid spread in some lesions, the latter features argue strongly in favor of a benign process, especially if present in a young individual and on a site such as the thigh. However, atypical forms of PSCT are extremely challenging, and all of the clinical and histologic features must be carefully weighed. In many instances, a clearcut diagnosis of melanoma cannot be made. Such lesions should be designated as pigmented spindle cell tumor (or melanocytic proliferation) with atypical features and appropriate surgery and careful follow-up of the patient arranged. Recurrence of such lesions appears to be extremely rare.

The same features characteristic of PSCT, such as cytologic uniformity and nuclear regularity, as well as its tendency to contain vertically disposed melanocytes ("raining down") to the epidermal surface, help to distinguish PSCT from atypical (dysplastic) nevus, in which the melanocytes are oriented more parallel to the epidermal surface and show more cytologic variability and atypia. Atypical (dysplastic) nevi are generally less cellular and often display a pronounced lentiginous melanocytic proliferation with elongation of the rete ridges and associated papillary dermal fibrosis, which are not typical features of PSCT. However, some atypical forms of PSCT show substantial overlap with conventional atypical nevi. Discrimination of the two lesions thus may not be reproducible. Such lesions may be designated as PSCT with atypical features or as atypical (dysplastic) nevus with features of PSCT.

■ MANAGEMENT CONSIDERATIONS

BOX 9-14   Summary

- Examination of the entire lesion
- Application of all histopathological, clinical, and other attributes for assessing abnormalities present
- Seek consultation
- Placement into risk category (Table 9-1)
- Complete excision of nonatypical and low-risk Spitz tumors
- Excision of high-risk and biologically indeterminate lesions with approximately 1 cm margins
- Individualized regular long-term follow-up examinations of patients

BOX 9-15   Summary

- Spitz tumor without atypicality
- Atypical Spitz tumor (Spitz tumor with one or more atypical features)
  - Low-risk lesions
  - High-risk lesions with indeterminate biological potential (lesions difficult to classify as unquivocally benign or malignant)
- Malignant neoplasm

One should adopt a pragmatic approach to the management of individuals with Spitzoid lesions in order to avoid overdiagnosis of malignancy and underrecognition of potentially aggressive lesions and consequently the inappropriate management of patients. As outlined above, a well-defined protocol allows for the systematic and rigorous evaluation of Spitzoid lesions utilizing all histopathologic, clinical, and ancillary information available.[41] Having collected this information, one can then assign a given lesion to one of three categories: (1) Spitz tumors without appreciable abnormality,

(2) Spitz tumors with one or more atypical features (atypical Spitz tumor) including those with indeterminate biological or malignant potential, and (3) malignant neoplasm. Admittedly this exercise remains largely subjective and is dependent on the knowledge, experience, and common sense of the pathologist and other physicians involved in the care of the patient.

The author recommends that all Spitz tumors be fully resected in order to facilitate complete histopathologic examination and also to diminish the risk of recurrence. Atypical Spitz tumors obviously require comparable excision for the same reasons but with greater clearance (up to 1cm) in order to provide even greater assurance that they are "wholly out." The reasons for recommending excision with margins free of the tumor are as follows: (1) Spitz tumors not completely excised may persist (recur) at the same site and potentially may progress to an aggressive neoplasm, and (2) some persistent/recurrent Spitz tumors may be more atypical than the original lesions and even more difficult to distinguish from melanoma.[41] Some of the latter tumors have resulted in metastases [41] (R.L. Barnhill, personal observations, 2005). It is the author's opinion that Spitz-like melanocytic tumors assigned an indeterminate biological potential require surgical margins of approximately 1 cm as this is considered to be the minimum standard of care for melanoma. Although of unproven benefit, sentinel lymph node biopsy may be considered for selected lesions (generally greater than 1 mm in thickness). Patients should be carefully monitored by regular examinations for recurrence (and metastasis in the case of atypical Spitz tumors). All patients should be managed on an individual basis and efforts made to avoid both overly aggressive and suboptimal management strategies.

FINAL THOUGHTS

Spitzoid lesions may represent a type of melanocytic neoplasm distinct from conventional melanocytic nevi and malignant melanoma perhaps with different biological properties and prognosis. Patients with Spitzoid lesions benefit from the comprehensive evaluation and classification of their lesions into three categories: (1) Spitz tumor without significant abnormality, (2) Spitz tumors with one or more atypical features (atypical Spitz tumor), including those judged to have indeterminate biological potential, and (3) malignant neoplasm, rather than classification into the two categories of "Spitz nevus" and melanoma. A priori, the author recommends that Spitzoid lesions should be completely excised for complete histopathologic study and to avoid recurrences and potential neoplastic transformation to a more aggressive tumor. Managing physicians should also refrain from overly aggressive surgical and therapeutic interventions. The rigorous characterization of sufficient numbers of Spitzoid lesions and long-term follow-up of patients should finally provide objective information about the biological nature of these lesions and their most appropriate therapy.

REFERENCES

1. Spitz S. Melanomas of childhood. *Am J Pathol.* 1948;24:591–609.
2. Allen A, Spitz S. Malignant melanoma: A clinico-pathological analysis of the criteria for diagnosis and prognosis. *Cancer.* 1953;6:1–45.
3. Kernen J, Ackerman L. Spindle cell nevi and epithelioid cell nevi (so-called juvenile melanomas) in children and adults: A clinicopathological study of 27 cases. *Cancer.* 1960;13:612–625.
4. Echevarria R, Ackerman L. Spindle and epithelioid nevi in the adult. Clinicopathologic report of 26 cases. *Cancer.* 1967;20:175–189.
5. Paniago-Pereira C, Maize J, Ackerman A. Nevus of large spindle and/or epithelioid cells (Spitz's nevus). *Arch Dermatol.* 1978;114:1811–1823.
6. Weedon D, Little J. Spindle and epithelioid cell nevi in children and adults. A review of 211 cases of the Spitz nevus. *Cancer.* 1977;40:217–225.
7. Weedon D. The Spitz nevus. *Clin Oncol.* 1984;3:493–507.
8. Binder S, Asnog C, Paul E, Cochran A. The histology and differential diagnosis of Spitz nevus. *Semin Diagn Pathol.* 1993;10:36–46.
9. Busam KJ, Barnhill RL: The spectrum of spitz tumors. In: Kirkham N, Lemoine NR eds. *Progress in Pathology.* Vol. 2. Churchill Livingstone; Edinburgh: 1995;31–46.
10. Hamm H, Happle R, Broecker E. Multiple agminate Spitz nevi: review of the literature and report of a case with distinctive immunohistological features. *Br J Dermatol.* 1987;117:511–522.
11. Smith K, Skelton H, Lupton G, Graham J. Spindle cell and epithelioid cell nevi with atypia and metastasis (malignant Spitz nevus). *Am J Surg Pathol.* 1989;13:931–939.
12. Merot Y, Frenk E. Spitz nevus (large spindle and/or epithelioid cell nevus). Age-related involvement of the suprabasal epidermis. *Virchows Arch A (Pathol Anat).* 1989;415:97–101.
13. Kamino H, Misheloff E, Ackerman A, Flotte T, Greco M. Eosinophilic globules in Spitz's nevi. New findings and a diagnostic sign. *Am J Surg Pathol.* 1979;1:319–324.
14. Arbuckle S, Weedon D. Eosinophilic globules in the Spitz nevus. *J Am Acad Dermatol.* 1982;7:324–327.
15. Havenith M, van Zandvoort E, Cleutjens J, Bosman F. Basement membrane deposition in benign and malignant nevomelanocytic lesions: An immunohistochemical study with antibodies to type IV collagen and laminin. *Histopathology.* 1989;15:137–46.
16. Barnhill RL, Barnhill MA, Berwick M, Mihm MC Jr. The histologic spectrum of pigmented spindle cell nevus: a review of 120 cases with emphasis on atypical variants. *Hum Pathol.* 1991;22:52–58.
17. Barnhill RL, Argenyi ZB, From L, et al. Atypical Spitz nevi/tumors: lack of consensus for diagnosis, discrimination from melanoma, and prediction of outcome. *Hum Pathol.* 1999;30:513–520.
18. Spatz A, Calonje E, Handfield-Jones S, Barnhill RL. Spitz Tumors in Children: A grading system for risk stratification. *Arch Dermatol.* 1999;135:282–285.
19. Vollmer RT. Use of Bayes rule and MIB-1 proliferation index to discriminate Spitz nevus from malignant melanoma. *Am J Clin Pathol.* 2004;122:499–505.
20. Kapor P, Selim MA, Roy LC, et al. Spitz nevi and atypical Spitz nevi/tumors: a histologic and immunohistochemical analysis. *Mod Pathol.* 2005;18:197–204.
21. Bastian BC, Wesselman U, Pinkel D, LeBoit PE. Molecular cytogenetic analysis of Spitz nevis shows clear differences to melanoma. *J Invest Dermatol.* 1999;113:1065–1069.
22. Bastian BC, LeBoit PE, Pinkel D. Mutations and copy number increase of HRAS in Spitz nevi with distinctive histopathologic features. *Am J Pathol.* 2000;157:967–972.
23. Healy E, Belgaid C, Takata M, Vahlquist A, Rehman I, Rigby H, Rees J. Allelotypes of primary cutaneous melanoma and benign melanocytic *nevi. Cancer Res.*1996;56:589–593.
24. Bogdan I, Burg G, Boni R. Spitz nevi display allelic deletions. *Arch Dermatol.* 2001;137:1417–1420.
25. Busam KJ, Barnhill RL. Pagetoid Spitz nevus. *Am J Surg Pathol.* 1995;19:1061–1067.
26. Barr R, Morales R, Graham J. Desmoplastic nevus. A distinct histologic variant of mixed spindle and epithelioid cell nevus. *Cancer.* 1980;46:557–564.
27. MacKie RM, Doherty VR. The desmoplastic melanocytic naevus: a distinct histological entity. *Histopathology.* 1992;20:207–211.
28. Harris GR, Shea CR, Horenstein MG, Reed JA, Burchette JL, Prieto VG. Desmoplastic (sclerotic) nevus an underrecognized entity that resembles dermatofibroma and desmoplastic melanoma. *Am J Surg Pathol.* 1999;23(7):786–794.
29. Harvell JD, Meehan SA, LeBoit PE. Spitz's nevi with halo reaction: a histopathological study of 17 cases. *J Cutan Pathol.* 1997;24:611–619.
30. Spatz A, Peterse S, Fletcher CD, Barnhill RL. Plexiform Spitz nevus: an intradermal Spitz nevus with plexiform growth pattern. *Am J Dermatopathol.* 1999;21:542–546.
31. Harvell JD, Bastian BC, LeBoit PE. Persistent (recurrent) Spitz nevi: a histopathologic, immunohistochemical, and molecular pathologic study of 22 cases. *Am Journ Surg Pathol.* 2002;26(5):654–661.
32. Burg G, Kempf W, Hochli M, et al. "Tubular" epithelioid cell nevus: a new variant of Spitz's nevus. *J Cutan Pathol.* 1998;25:475–478.
33. Reed R, Ichinose H, Clark W, Mihm MC. Common and uncommon melanocytic

nevi and borderline melanomas. *Sem Oncol.* 1975;2:119–147.

34. Gartmann H. Der pigmentierte Spindel-zellentumor. *Z Hautkrankh.* 1981;56:862–876.

35. Sagebiel R, Chinn E, Egbert B. Pigmented spindle cell nevus. Clinical and histologic review of 90 cases. *Am J Surg Pathol.* 1984; 8:645–653.

36. Smith N. The pigmented spindle cell tumor of Reed: an underdiagnosed lesion. *Sem Diagn Pathol.* 1987;4:75–87.

37. Barnhill RL, Mihm MC. Pigmented spindle cell nevus and its variants: distinction from melanoma. *Br J Dermatol.* 1989;121: 717–726.

38. Lohman CM, Coit DG, Brady MS, Berwick M, Busam KJ. Sentinel lymph node biopsy in paitents with diagnositically controversial spitzoid melanocytic tumors. *Am J Surg Pathol.* 2002;26(1):47–55.

39. Su LD, Fullen DR, Sondak VK, Johnson TM, Lowe L. Sentinel lymph node biopsy for patients with problematic spitzoid melanocytic lesions: a report on 18 patients. *Cancer.* 2003;15;97(2):499–507.

40. Roaten JB, Partrick DA, Pearlman N, Gonzalez RJ, Gonzalez R, McCarter MD. Sentinel lymph node biopsy for melanoma and other melanocytic tumors in adolescents. *J Pediatr Surg.* 2005;40(1):232–235.

41. Barnhill RL. The Spitzoid lesion: rethinking Spitz tumors, atypical variants, and risk assessment. *Mod Pathol.* 2006;19:S21–S33.

CHAPTER 10

Atypical Melanocytic Nevi

Raymond L. Barnhill, M.D.
Olivier Gaide, M.D., Ph.D.
Harold S. Rabinovitz, M.D.
Ralph Braun, M.D.

BOX 10-1   Overview

- Atypical melanocytic nevi (AMN) constitute a clinical and histological spectrum of melanocytic nevi between ordinary (banal) nevi and melanoma
- AMN are important risk markers for melanoma
- AMN are less well established as precursors to melanoma
- AMN may mimic melanoma both clinically and histologically
- Clinically atypical nevi commonly range from about 4 to 12 mm, have irregular and ill-defined margins, and irregular coloration
- Histologically atypical nevi usually exhibit architectural abnormalities and cytological atypia of melanocytes
- AMN raising significant concern for melanoma usually require histological examination
- Patients with numerous ordinary nevi and AMN may benefit from periodic examinations aided by (often total body) photography, dermoscopy, and "mole monitoring"(although the latter measures have not yet been shown to reduce mortality from melanoma)
- Much remains to be learned about the biological significance of AMN

INTRODUCTION

Since the description of atypical or "dysplastic" melanocytic nevi (AMN) in the setting of melanoma-prone families over 20 years ago and subsequently in individuals outside such kindreds, these lesions have remained highly controversial.[1–51] This has largely resulted from the failure to reach consensus about the nature of these lesions, an inability to formulate precise criteria for recognition, and finally a lack of understanding about their biological significance. Specifically, this relates to criteria for individual lesions and for the so-called "dysplastic nevus syndrome," i.e., how many clinically AMN are needed and what are the minimal essential morphological criteria needed for the diagnosis of an individual lesion. One particular problem dating back to the original studies on AMN in hereditary melanoma kindreds has been the tendency to consider that histopathologic diagnosis of AMN is the gold standard; whereas it has been shown that the histopathologic features ascribed to AMN lack specificity (see below).[24,49,50]

In order to have some appreciation of the nature of the problem, one must recognize as with any biological system, that there is considerable clinical and histopathologic heterogeneity among benign melanocytic nevi. This is present to such a degree that there is substantial disagreement among many as to how to categorize a significant proportion of nevi with atypical, aberrant, or unusual features and their role as risk markers for precursors to melanoma. Furthermore some authors consider "dysplastic" nevi to be distinctly different from other unusual nevi such as small congenital-pattern nevi and nevi occurring on particular anatomic sites such as the vulva, breast, and acral skin, despite the frequent presence of histomorphologic features ascribed to "dysplastic" nevi in these other nevi. In principle, the authors contend that all melanocytic nevi even normal-appearing ones may demonstrate atypical histologic features ranging from common nevi to melanoma. By and large, the biological significance of such abnormal features remains to be established. The goal of ongoing research, if possible, is to determine and reliably recognize at what point in the histopathologic spectrum of nevi increased melanoma risk develops.[51]

Many pathologists have been sufficiently well schooled to be able to reliably recognize a prototypic "dysplastic" nevus. However, significant problems arise when these pathologists encounter the upper and lower limits of this histopathologic spectrum, there are many variations of nevi that do not fit the textbook picture of a "dysplastic" nevus, and the reproducible assessment of architecture and cytological atypia in such nevi. Accordingly, much remains to be learned about the development and natural history of nevi, their variation with anatomic site, age, etc. and how many external or intrinsic factors induce reactive vs. neoplastic alterations in nevi, or both. As a result, there is currently no consensus about histopathologic definitions of atypical nevi.

Following from this, one cannot estimate the prevalence or melanoma risk related to them, except in the instance of specific gross morphologic features and numbers of nevi. Thus, many studies have established that irrespective of histology, melanoma risk is directly related to numbers of ordinary nevi (>50 or 100 on the total skin surface), the presence and number of atypical nevi as defined by size (e.g., >5, 6, or 8 mm), irregular or ill-defined borders, variation in color, and macular component. On the other hand, despite the seemingly logical conclusion that histopathologically atypical nevi should be associated with increased melanoma risk, this has not been convincingly demonstrated in objective studies. Furthermore, studies examining the relationship between clinically AMN and histopathologically AMN have shown a poor correlation. Therefore, the "dysplastic" nevus cannot be considered a distinct clinicopathological entity as the histopathologic features ascribed to histopathologically AMN lack specificity as already mentioned. At present, melanoma risk assessment of patients is based solely on gross morphological parameters of nevi, i.e., total numbers of nevi on the skin surface and the presence and number of clinically AMN, along with other factors such as personal or family history of melanoma.

Therefore, at present, AMN encompasses a large and heterogeneous group of nevi: (1) nevi with atypical clinical features, which have been termed "atypical nevi," (2) nevi with abnormal histopathologic features, (3) nevi with both abnormal clinical and histopathologic features, and (4) nevi with histopathologic features that are equivocal or of unknown significance. The latter group of nevi may demonstrate findings that may be reactive or proliferative in nature rather than neoplastic.[19]

The immediate significance of such lesions is whether they are markers of increased melanoma risk, whether they are precursors of melanoma, and, in practical terms, their histologic distinction from outright melanoma. Because of the controversy surrounding these nevi, an NIH Consensus Conference has recently recommended that the term dysplastic nevus be abandoned in favor of nevus with architectural disorder and/or cytologic atypia.[32]

THE SIGNIFICANCE OF THE AMN

Markers of Increased Melanoma Risk

Based on studies of hereditary melanoma kindreds,[1–5,10,11,29,36,46] the presence of AMN on individuals in these families confers a significantly increased risk for the development of melanoma. In fact, because of the presence of AMN in this setting, there is a 48.9% cumulative risk for melanoma by the age 50 years.[36] In prospective follow-up, only family members with AMN developed melanoma whereas those without AMN did not develop melanoma. Individuals in the general population have AMN,[46] which also serve as markers for increased melanoma risk, although not nearly so great as in familial melanoma.[5,11] Estimates of the relative risk for melanoma in persons with sporadic AMN may be in the range of 7 to 20%.[44,46] The prevalence of individuals with sporadic AMN has been difficult to gauge accurately but has been estimated anywhere from 0.5 to 20%.[6,29] One particular reason for the difficulty in estimating prevalence of AMN has been the lack of standardized clinical and histopathologic criteria for AMN and also what constitutes the minimum essential criteria for the AMN phenotype, e.g., 50 or 100 or more clinically atypical nevi.[25] Classifications have been devised for individuals with AMN and the extent to which they have a personal or family history of melanoma and AMN. Although much more information is needed on this subject, risk-stratification protocols have been formulated to facilitate assessment of melanoma risk and the management of patients. Melanoma risk is probably a continuum with risk directly related to family history of melanoma, especially for individuals with at least two first-degree blood relatives with melanoma, total number of nevi on the skin surface, total number of clinically atypical nevi, and personal history of melanoma.[25,33]

AMN as Precursors to Melanoma

AMN occasionally is associated with melanoma and may possibly serve as precursors to melanoma. This progression has been observed through the use of serial photographs and the histologic documentation of focal melanoma developing in an otherwise stable AMN.[10] Various authors have also reported remnants of AMN associated with melanoma with an average fre-

quency of about 33%.[18] A confounding problem in this situation is the inability in all instances to clearly distinguish the intraepidermal component of melanoma from AMN.

CLINICAL FEATURES

BOX 10-2   Summary

- Increased numbers of typical and atypical nevi (for example, >50)
- Variation in gross morphologic features among nevi
- Increased numbers of nevi on scalp, female breasts, buttocks
- Nevus characteristics
  - Increased size (4 to 12 mm, but not always)
  - Asymmetry
  - Macular component
  - Irregular border
  - Ill-defined border
  - Altered topography, pebbled or cobblestone surface
  - Haphazard, variegated or greater complexity of coloration

---

The number of clinically atypical nevi on the individual patient may vary from few to hundreds (Fig. 10-1).[1,2,10,11]

Although the majority of AMN occur on the trunk, these nevi show a peculiar propensity for the scalp, female breasts, buttocks, and dorsal surfaces of the feet. AMN tend to show considerable variation in size, shape, and coloration from nevus to nevus.

AMN[8,9,25] tend to be larger than common nevi and are usually smaller than melanoma and generally measure 3 to 12 mm. They often show asymmetry, irregular and ill-defined borders, and a relatively flat surface (at least part of the lesion is entirely flat) (Fig. 10-2). The surface may also be "pebbled" or have a cobblestone appearance (Fig. 10-3). AMN in general have a more complex color than ordinary nevi (Fig. 10-4). There are often more than two colors present, i.e., tan, brown, dark brown, and the colors have an irregular or haphazard pattern.

DERMOSCOPIC FEATURES   AMN have dermoscopic criteria of benign melanocytic lesions, but also may demonstrate some criteria shared with melanomas. In general, AMN tend to be rather uniform in color and preserve an architectural symmetry versus the usual asymmetry of melanomas. Dermoscopically one is able to recognize AMN with benign and those with uncertain patterns.

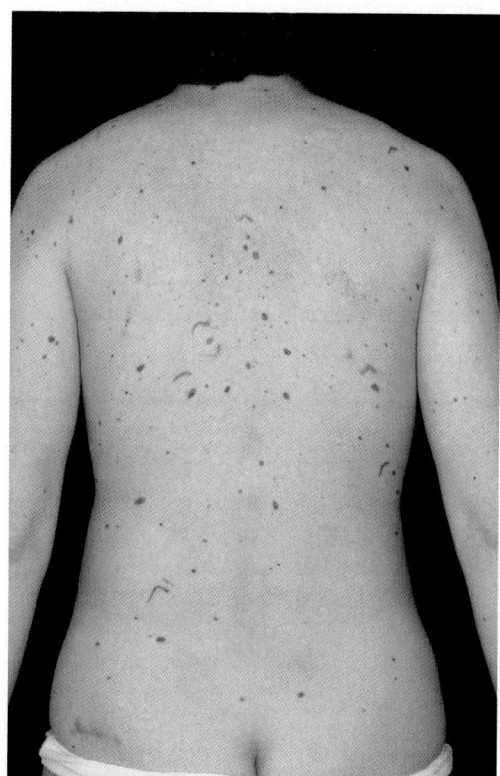

▲ **FIGURE 10-1** Back of a patient with dysplastic nevus syndrome showing a multitude of AMN.

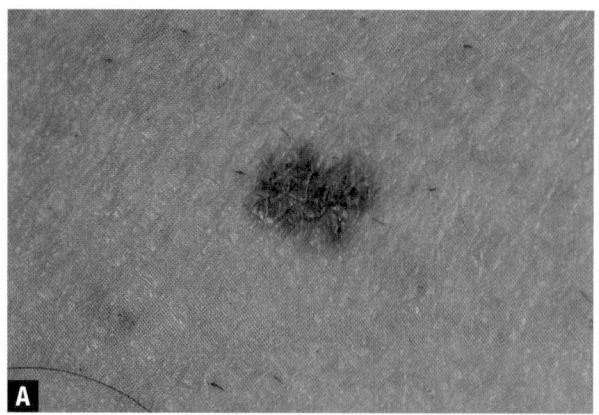

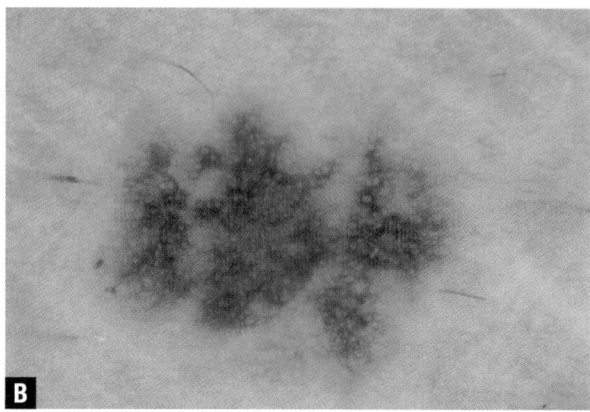

▲ **FIGURE 10-2 A.** Clinical image of AMN. **B.** Dermoscopy of (**A**) showing a patchy network.

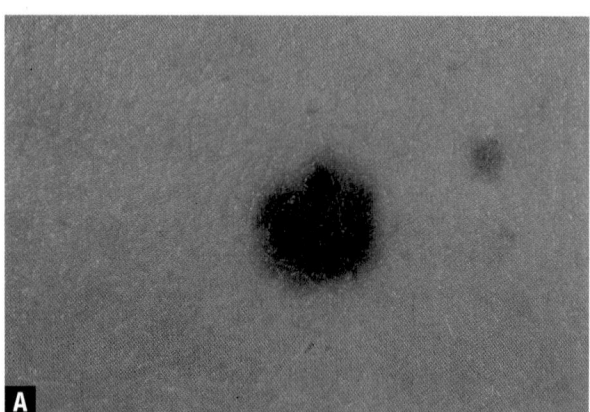

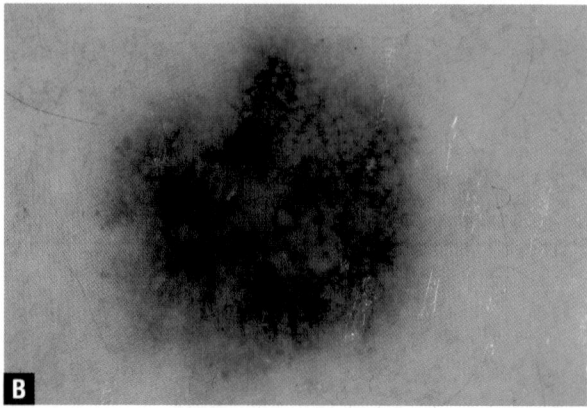

▲ **FIGURE 10-4 A.** Clinical image of a dysplastic nevus (AMN). **B.** Dermoscopy of (**A**) showing an irregular pigment network with central structureless architecture and some branched streaks as well as some peripheral globules.

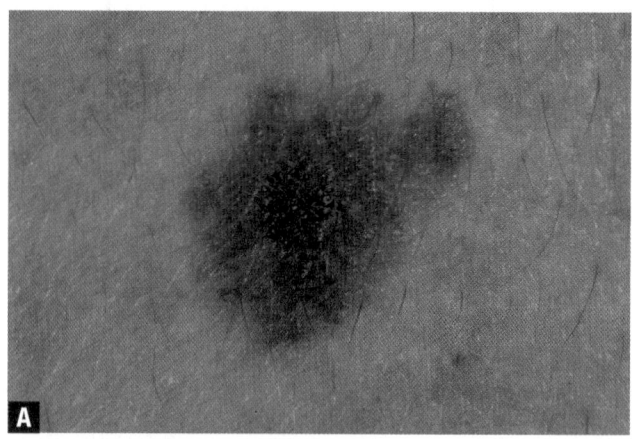

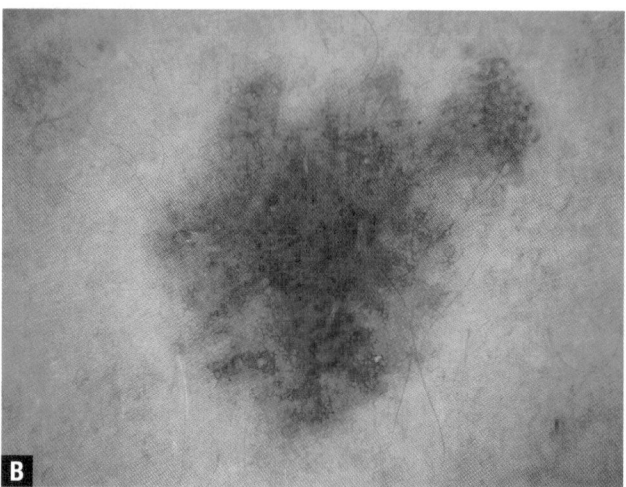

▲ **FIGURE 10-3 A.** Clinical image of a dysplastic nevus (AMN). **B.** Dermoscopy of (**A**) showing peripheral pigment network and central globules (reticular globular architecture).

"Benign Pattern" AMN

Despite some clinical overlap with melanoma, i.e., the ABCDs , most AMN on dermoscopic examination can be readily identified as having benign patterns. By dermoscopy, these lesions can have appearances seen in common melanocytic nevi. Often the patterns, colors and structures are relatively organized. Structureless (homogeneous) areas are more frequently observed than in common melanocytic nevi. Dots, globules, black blotches, network, vascular patterns, and colors can vary greatly within the lesion. Segments of the margin of AMN can be abrupt. Generally, AMN lose some or all of the architectural order (symmetry, uniformity, sparseness of colors) seen in common melanocytic nevi. Compared to common melanocytic nevi, which are usually less than 6 mm in diameter, it is not unusual for AMN to be 10 to 15 mm or more along the largest diameter.

An important diagnostic clue in the differential diagnosis of congenital melanocytic nevi and AMN is the lack of hypertrichosis and the usual lack of a

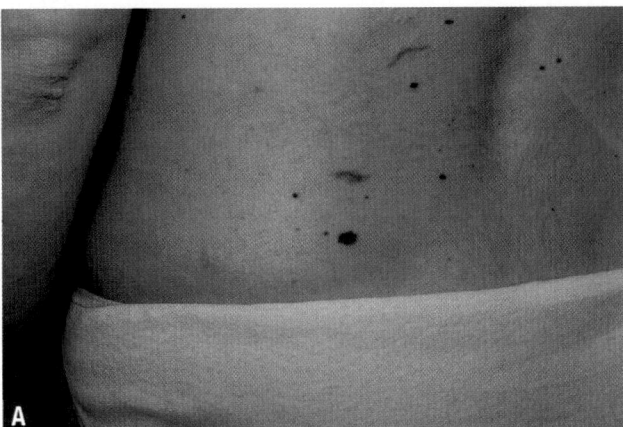

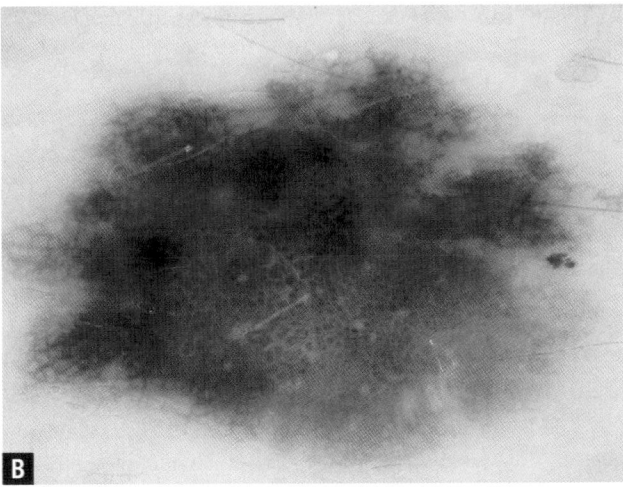

▲ **FIGURE 10-5 A.** Clinical image of a dysplastic nevus (AMN). **B.** Dermoscopy of (**A**) showing irregular pigment network at the periphery, erythema throughout the lesion as well as reversed pigment network in the center of the lesion

melanocytic proliferation or variation in junctional nesting is acceptable.)

- Lentiginous melanocytic proliferation*
- Variation in size, shape, and location of junctional nests with bridging or confluence*
- Lack of cellular cohesion of junctional nests
- Lateral extension (the "shoulder" phenomenon) of junctional component
- Cytologic features
  - Spindled cell (with prominent retraction artifact of cytoplasm) pattern
  - Epithelioid cell pattern
- Discontinuous nuclear atypia (not all nuclei atypical)*
  - Nuclear enlargement
  - Nuclear pleomorphism
  - Nuclear hyperchromatism
  - Prominent nucleoli
  - Prominent pale or "dusty" cytoplasm
  - Large melanin granules
- Host response
  - Lymphocytic infiltrates
  - Fibroplasia
  - Concentric eosinophilic pattern
  - Lamellar pattern
  - Prominent vascularity

The histological criteria include parameters of architectural disorder, cytologic atypia, and host response (Figs. 10-6 to 10-8).[2,4,7,9,14,16,19,21–23,25,28,47,48]

The majority of AMN, perhaps 80%, are compound and the remainder junctional. Most are relatively flat with only slight expansion of the papillary dermis by limited dermal components. Many (but not all) AMN are lentiginous, i.e., the epidermal rete ridges are elongated, often club-shaped, accompanied by melanocytic hyperplasia, and increased melanin content of the epidermis (Fig. 10-6). Many heavily pigmented AMN also contain melanin macroglobules in the basilar epidermis, an entirely nonspecific finding. Many (perhaps the vast majority) compound AMN have lateral extension and poor circumscription of the intraepidermal components (Fig. 10-6A). The latter features refer to the intraepidermal melanocytic component extending laterally or peripherally beyond the papillary dermal nevus elements (the "shoulder" phenomenon) and gradually diminishing in cellularity without clear-cut demarcation. Although not a fundamental component of dysplasia as outlined above, lateral extension is a useful feature in recognizing most compound AMN, particularly at scanning magnification, and does correlate with the peripheral macular annulus observed clinically in many

blue hue in AMN. There are five patterns found invariably to be benign in patients who have the classic atypical mole syndrome (i.e., patients who have the triad of 100 or more melanocytic nevi, at least one nevus 8 mm or larger in diameter and at least one dysplastic nevus). These patterns are:

- diffuse network pattern;
- patchy network pattern (Fig. 10-2);
- peripheral network pattern with central hypopigmentation pattern;
- peripheral network pattern with central hyperpigmentation;
- peripheral network pattern with central uniform globules (Fig. 10-3).

In each of these five patterns, the network must be uniform and fade at the periphery of the lesion.

"Uncertain Pattern" AMN

The implication of classifying the AMN as "uncertain" is that it is not possible to dermoscopically differentiate the lesion from melanoma (Fig. 10-5). "Uncertain" AMN patterns have a very broad spectrum of dermoscopic features.

At one end of this spectrum are AMN that have dermoscopic features that slightly deviate from the typical benign patterns. These lesions should be considered for closer follow-up or sequential dermoscopic imaging. At the other end of the spectrum, there are AMN that are dermoscopically impossible to distinguish from early melanoma. Although rare "malignant-pattern" AMN may show white scar-like depigmentation, streaks/pseudopods, blue-white veil, regression with peppering, and multiple colors (tan, dark brown, black, gray, blue, and red). These lesions should be biopsied to rule out melanoma.

HISTOPATHOLOGIC FEATURES

BOX 10-3 Summary

- Architectural features (*Essential features needed for diagnosis. Either lentiginous

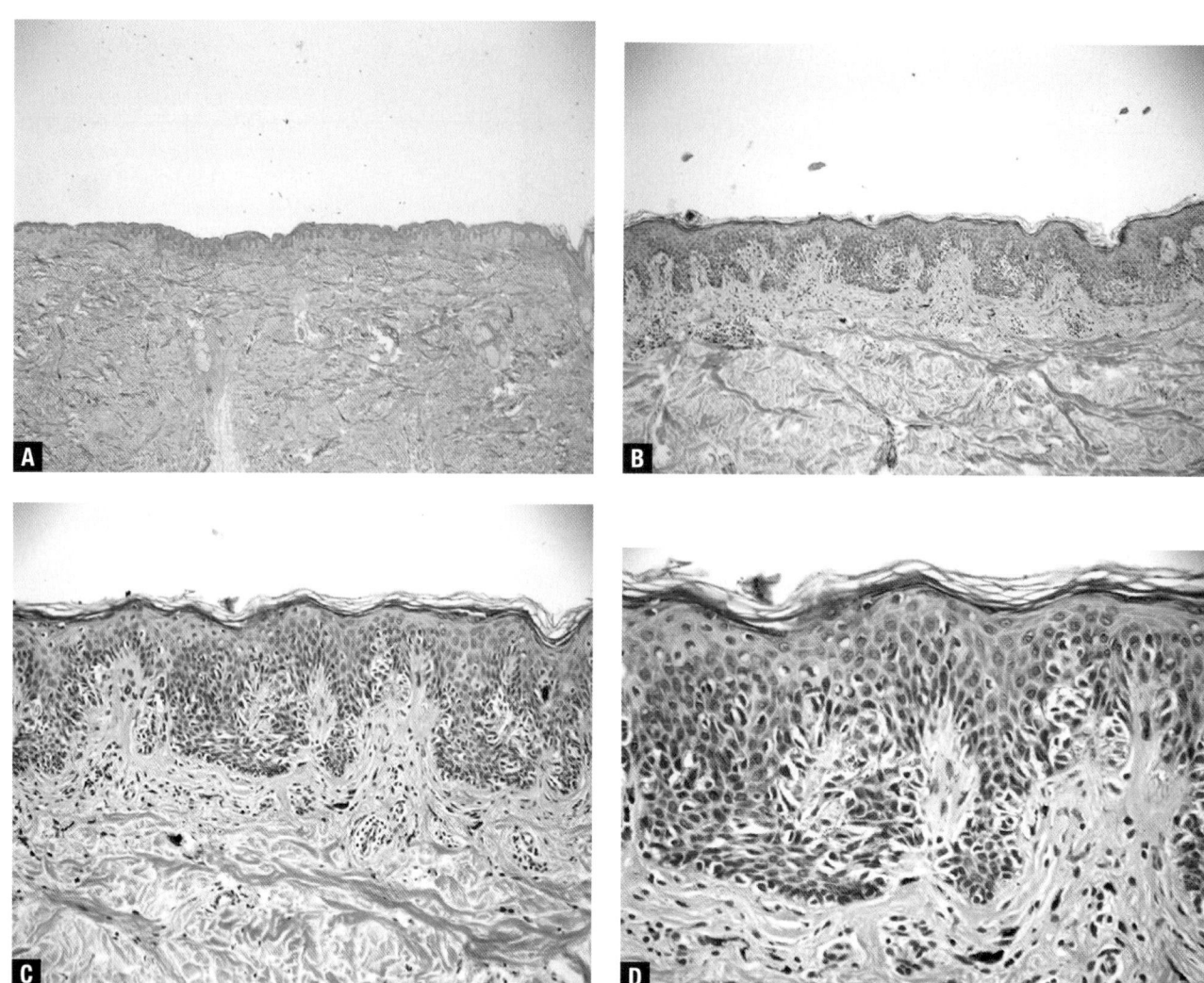

▲ **FIGURE 10-6** Atypical compound (dysplastic) nevus. **A.** This field demonstrates the poorly defined appearance of the intraepidermal component. **B** and **C.** Higher magnification discloses variation in size, shape, and staining of nuclei of basilar melanocytes. **D.** Some melanocytes have nuclei larger than those in spinous layer keratinocytes.

AMN. Junctional AMN by definition do not display lateral extension, but tend to be poorly circumscribed.

The essential architectural feature is disordered intraepidermal melanocytic proliferation[25,26] which includes two patterns: (1) disordered or irregular junctional nesting (Fig. 10-7A and B), and (2) lentiginous melanocytic proliferation (Fig. 10-7C and D). Both patterns are often present in varying degrees in many AMN, but either pattern may be present alone. The frequency of melanocytes in AMN is, as a rule greater than in a lentigo, often reaching confluence and replacing basilar keratinocytes. In its most extreme version, the proliferation of melanocytes may result in multilayered confluence of cells along the dermal–epidermal junction, often "bridging" between rete (Fig. 10-7A and B). The melanocytes present in this pattern commonly exhibit retraction of cytoplasm resulting in a vacuo-

lated appearance of the basal layer, almost suggesting basal layer vacuolopathy. The nuclei within these vacuolated cells are commonly pleomorphic with angulated contours.[23,25]

Compared to typical nevi, junctional nests in AMN tend to vary significantly in size, shape (ovoid, elongate, or confluent along the dermal–epidermal junction), and spacing (nests are not present at equidistant intervals). Junctional nests, instead of being located at the tips of rete, are irregularly distributed on the sides and between rete, often with no regular pattern ("irregularly irregular"). Bridging of nests between rete is another feature of the abnormal nesting pattern (Fig. 10-7A and B). Often paralleling the variation in nesting is the loss of cellular cohesion in junctional nests. The individual nevus cells literally appear to fall apart with clear spaces forming between individual cells and aggregates of cells.

Although upward migration of melanocytes throughout the epidermis is not a common feature of AMN, it is seen occasionally, is often limited, focal, or orderly in appearance.

CYTOLOGIC FEATURES One of the fundamental criteria for AMN is variable (or discontinuous) cytologic atypia of intraepidermal melanocytes.[9,22,23,25] The latter refers to intraepidermal melanocytes that are not uniformly atypical but tend to vary from cell to cell as to the degree of nuclear atypia (Figs. 10-6 to 10-8). In general, this nuclear atypia is a continuum and characterized by gradual nuclear enlargement, pleomorphism, variation in nuclear chromatin pattern, and the eventual development of prominent nucleoli. The beginnings of nuclear atypia may be almost imperceptible and may not be reproducible. Commonly with slight or low-grade cytologic atypia, the cells show

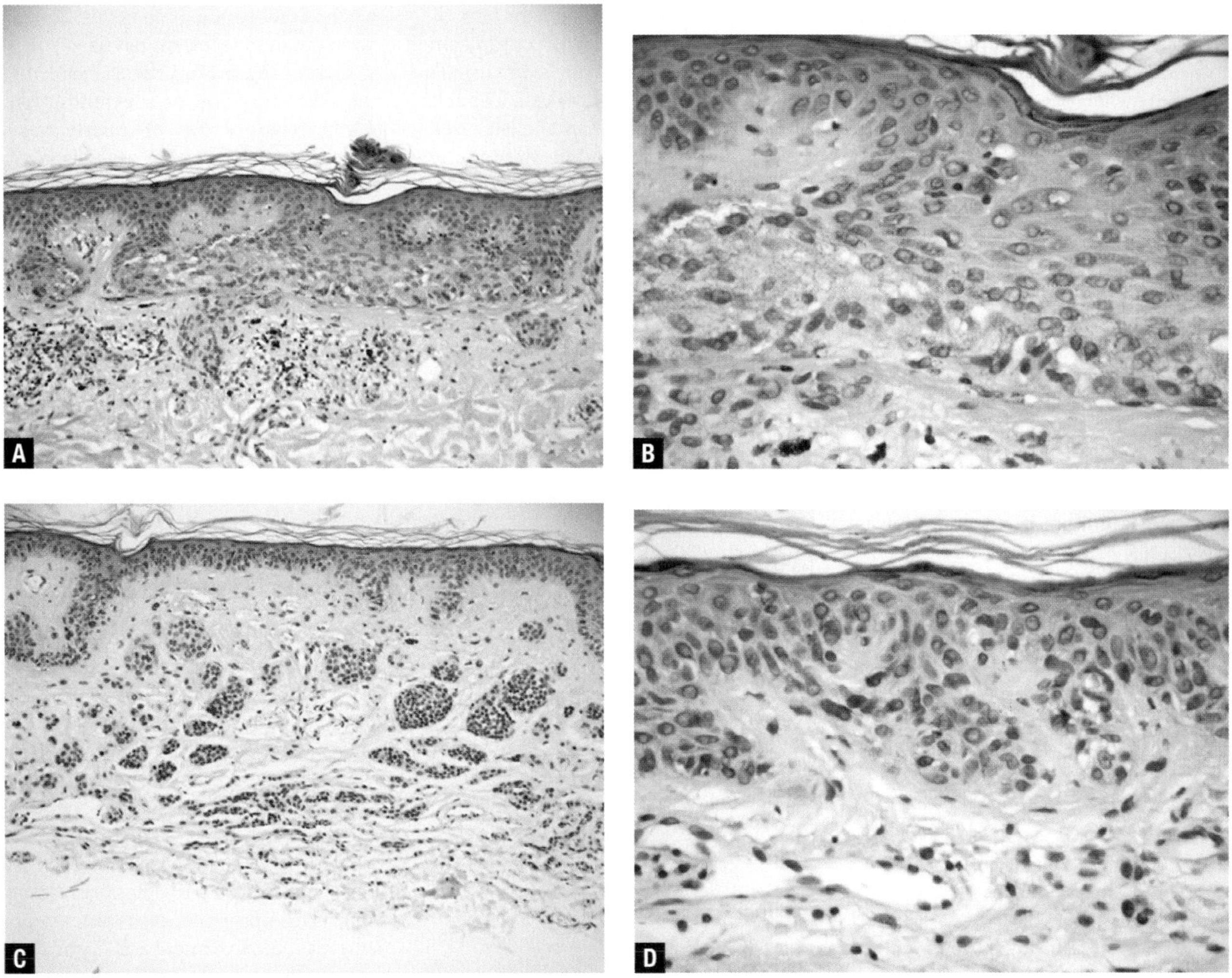

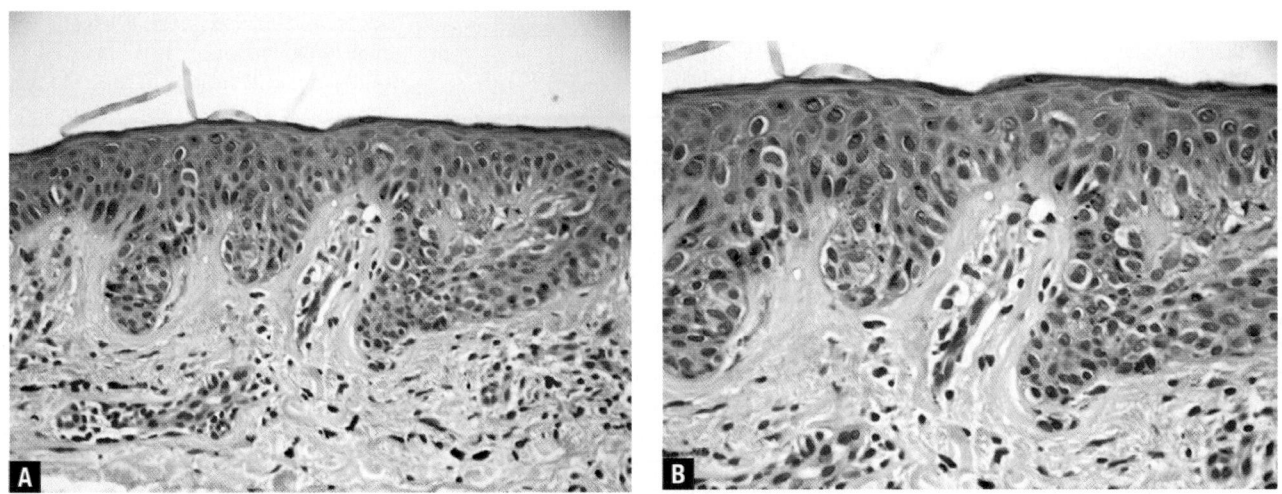

▲ **FIGURE 10-7** Atypical compound (dysplastic) nevus. **A.** Junctional nests contain epithelioid melanocytes and show bridging between epidermal rete. Perivascular lymphocytic infiltrates are present in papillary dermis. **B.** The melanocytes are enlarged and demonstrate nuclear enlargement and pleomorphism. **C.** Predominant lentiginous pattern. **D.** Higher magnification shows striking nuclear enlargement and pleomorphism.

▲ **FIGURE 10-8** Atypical compound (dysplastic) nevus. **A.** Lentiginous and junctional nested pattern. **B.** The melanocytes show significant nuclear enlargement, pleomorphism, and variation in chromatin patterns.

retraction of cytoplasm and the size of the melanocytic nuclei is increased and approximates that of or is slightly larger than the nuclei of spinous layer keratinocytes (Fig. 10-6D). With greater (moderate) atypia, the nuclei are somewhat larger than the nuclei of spinous layer keratinocytes, and nucleoli are more commonly visible (Fig. 10-7B and D). With severe cytologic atypia, the melanocytes may contain abundant cytoplasm, which often has a granular eosinophilic appearance or may contain finely-divided ("dusty") melanin. The nuclei may be enlarged to twice the size of spinous layer keratinocyte nuclei, or larger (Fig. 8A and B). Nucleoli are often enlarged and may be eosinophilic. The ultimate endpoint is a uniformly atypical population of cells, which marks the development of melanoma.

The cell types that comprise AMN include basilar melanocytes with retracted cytoplasm, small rounded nevus cells, spindle cells, sometimes pigmented, and epithelioid cells .The basilar melanocytes with retraction of cytoplasm are often observed in predominantly lentiginous forms of AMN while the epithelioid cell type is often present in a much less prevalent, predominantly nested form of AMN (so-called "epithelioid cell" dysplasia).

HOST RESPONSE Among mononuclear-cell infiltrates, fibroplasia, and prominent vascularity, the first two have received considerable attention as criteria for AMN.[9,22,23,25] Lymphocytic infiltrates are present in the overriding majority of AMN. These infiltrates vary from sparse perivascular lymphoid infiltrates (Fig. 10-7A) to dense band-like infiltrates filling the papillary dermis.

The more common form of fibroplasia is concentric eosinophilic fibrosis, which is hyalinized collagen that is compactly disposed about the epidermal rete ridges. Lamellar fibroplasia is less prevalent and notable for delicate stacking of horizontally-disposed collagen, subjacent to the epidermal rete ridges. Mesenchymal spindle cells typically line these filamentous strands of collagen. Both patterns of fibroplasia may be present in the same lesion or occur separately.

HISTOLOGIC VARIANTS OF AMN

Epithelioid Cell Variant

The "epithelioid" cells resemble the cell type in pagetoid melanoma except that they tend to be less cytologically atypical.[9] The cells are round or polygonal

and contain abundant pink or "dusty" (finely-divided melanin) cytoplasm. Relatively small round nuclei are usually present in the center of the cell. The cells tend to have an almost exclusively nested distribution often without an associated lentiginous element.

Halo Nevus Variant

These AMN display dense mononuclear cell infiltrates filling the papillary dermis and obscuring any nests of nevus cells present. These nevi are distinguished from benign halo nevi by aberrant architectural features and cytologic atypia.

SPECIFICITY OF HISTOLOGIC FEATURES OF ATYPICAL MELANOCYTIC NEVUS

Disordered arrangements of cells and cytological atypia are encountered in a number of lesions thought to be distinct from conventional AMN.[33] The latter findings are often similar to those observed in AMN and provide evidence that almost any melanocytic proliferation may progress to an "intermediate" stage and possibly have some potential for giving rise to melanoma. Because these other melanocytic lesions with atypical features, such as acral nevi, congenital nevi, Spitz nevi, and genital/flexural nevi have received considerably less attention than conventional AMN, little information is available concerning their melanoma risk. It is proposed that these various lesions may be subjected to the same guidelines as have AMN (see the following sections).

DIFFERENTIAL DIAGNOSIS

BOX 10-4 Summary

- *In situ* and invasive melanoma
- Lentiginous melanocytic nevi
- Pigmented spindle cell nevi
- Spitz tumors
- Halo nevi and nevi with halo reactions
- Melanocytic nevi with histological attributes related to anatomic site, e.g., genitalia
- Congenital nevi
- Recurrent/persistent nevi

The AMN must be distinguished from *in situ* or invasive melanoma, solar atypical lentiginous melanocytic proliferations and melanoma *in situ* of sun-damaged skin (historically termed lentigo maligna and Hutchinson's melanotic freckle), lentiginous nevi, pigmented spindle cell

nevus, Spitz tumor, halo nevus, congenital nevus, and recurrent nevus.

One of the most difficult problems is the discrimination of severely atypical AMN from *in situ* or microinvasive melanoma. In one sense, this distinction is somewhat arbitrary and subjective since no consensus has been reached regarding criteria for separating the two entities. However, in another sense, the central issue is whether a particular lesion retains some degree of growth control, an orderly nevic appearance, and variable or discontinuous nuclear atypia vs. loss of growth control, loss of an orderly nevic appearance, and continuous nuclear atypia.

AMN and lentiginous melanocytic proliferations (SIMP) and melanoma *in situ* of sun-damaged skin show histologic similarities on occasion and may be difficult to separate. SIMP is distinguished from AMN in most instances because SIMP is an atypical melanocytic proliferation secondary to cumulative sun-exposure and consequently develops on markedly sun-exposed skin of the elderly (average age of 60 years). The most common locations are the cheek and nose which are unusual sites for conventional AMN. SIMP is usually a de novo melanocytic dysplasia since dermal nevus components are uncommon, whereas approximately 80% of AMN contain dermal nevus cells.

SIMP developing on the central face most commonly shows a basilar proliferation of variably atypical melanocytes that often involve the appendageal epithelium. The epidermis is usually effaced, i.e., has no rete ridge pattern, and there is prominent solar elastosis in the dermis. In contrast, the AMN generally has elongated rete ridges with concentration of basilar melanocytes and many junctional nests along the rete ridges, and solar elastosis is usually minimal. Solar melanoma *in situ* may also have junctional nests, but they are often discohesive elongate nests composed of pigmented spindled cells. The latter nests on occasion show striking involvement of hair follicles and eccrine ducts, a finding not typically observed in AMN.

SIMP and solar melanoma *in situ* may show a rete-ridge pattern and thus present an even greater problem in differential diagnosis. Discriminating features favoring SIMP include a mainly lentiginous pattern of melanocytic proliferation, prominent involvement of appendages, presence of pigmented spindle cells, and solar elastosis. Overlap with AMN on occasion may be so great that separation may be difficult, often arbitrary, and not necessary. The various clinical and histologic features present must be assessed. If discrimination is not possible, a reasonable approach is a descriptive diagnosis, e.g., intraepidermal melanocytic proliferation with features of both SIMP and AMN and severe cytologic atypia.

Another conundrum is the distinction of AMN from lentiginous nevi, particularly those from acral skin. Here, the main problem is one of threshold, i.e., whether there is sufficient disordered architecture and cytologic atypia for the diagnosis of AMN. Such lesions should be evaluated for poor circumscription, asymmetry, substantially increased frequency of basilar melanocytes, irregularity of junctional nesting with elongated confluent nests, bridging of nests between rete ridges, and finally, cytologic atypia of intraepidermal melanocytes. Lesions having equivocal changes should not be diagnosed as AMN. It is reasonable to designate the latter lesions as showing some architectural disorder or, alternatively, as having atypical or unusual features.

As discussed below, a number of types of melanocytic nevi such as pigmented spindle cell nevus, Spitz nevus, and congenital nevus may on occasion demonstrate disordered architectural patterns and cytologic atypia. Yet, at the same time, these various nevi retain many of the histologic features that make them distinctive, e.g., fascicles of slender pigmented spindle cells in pigmented spindle cell nevus, large epithelioid cells in Spitz nevus, and extensive involvement of the reticular dermis in congenital nevus.

Recurrent melanocytic nevi may on occasion enter into the differential diagnosis of AMN (see the previous paragraphs).

GRADING OF ATYPICAL (DYSPLASTIC) NEVI

The following guidelines are suggested: (1) severely atypical or high-grade AMN should be recognized because of their overlap with melanoma in situ. Such lesions should be completely excised with margins of at least 5 mm. (2) AMN with moderate atypia (see earlier discussion) should be completely removed with clear margins. Because DNA aneuploidy has been documented in such lesions, there may possibly be a greater potential for progression to melanoma than less atypical lesions.[39] (3) AMN with slight or minimal atypia need not have re-excision if the bulk of the lesion has been removed, even if the margins

are involved. Such lesions are common, and reproducible distinction from lentiginous nevi with architectural disorder and no cytologic atypia may not be possible. In general, slightly atypical AMN do not exhibit DNA aneuploidy.[39]

HISTOPATHOLOGIC REPORTING OF ATYPICAL (DYSPLASTIC) NEVI

The pathologist should communicate clearly to the clinician the nature of the lesion and its significance, regardless of the terminology used. In one sense, the significance of the individual lesion is related to the degree of atypicality in that lesion. The immediate concern is to insure proper management of the individual lesion, i.e., degree of atypicality is properly assessed and the need for additional therapy, i.e., surgery, if any, is communicated to the clinician. In another sense, the significance of AMN must be viewed from the perspective of global melanoma risk in the patient. Thus, the significance of the individual AMN can be viewed in quantitative terms and is directly related to family history of melanoma, family history of AMN, personal history of melanoma, the patient's nevus phenotype (total number of typical and atypical nevi on the skin surface), degree of atypia of previously removed nevi, and other risk factors for melanoma.

Practical Considerations and Treatment

BOX 10-5 Summary

- In general, only clinically atypical lesions suspicious for melanoma should be removed
- Overly aggressive surgery should be avoided
- Patients with many AMN may benefit from total body photography, mole monitoring, dermoscopy, etc.

By definition AMN clinically have features of melanoma and should, in theory, be excised. In reality, patients with 50 AMN do not benefit from the excision of all AMN. Common sense should therefore prevail at all times and the physician must avoid overly aggressive procedures. The goal is to excise AMN that are or will become melanomas. This goal is virtually impossible to achieve as the AMN is difficult to distinguish from

melanoma. Considerations such as the morbidity of the excisions, especially if multiple, must be weighted against the probability of diminishing the mortality from melanoma.

The decision to surgically remove AMN depends on the number of AMN present, a personal history of melanoma, a familial history of melanoma or multiple AMN.

Individuals with AMN may present with several different scenarios. A patient may have one AMN, a few AMN, or many AMN. An isolated AMN is considered by many to be an "ugly duckling" lesion (ugly duckling nevus) and should be considered for either excision or mole monitoring. In patients with many AMN, the majority of these lesions have dermoscopic features that allow classification as benign lesions. Those lesions that have uncertain patterns should either be biopsied or monitored. Finally, lesions that have "malignant" patterns should be biopsied.

For patients with multiple AMN, total body photography and monitoring using digital dermoscopy may be helpful.

Total body photography enables the physician to monitor the pigmented lesions of a patient and to detect new lesions as well as change within existing lesions. However, it should be noted that new nevi may appear and that old nevi may enlarge or change, especially during the first three decades of life. Again, subtle alterations such as color changes occurring over a long period of time are less likely to reveal a melanoma than surface and volume changes occurring over a short period of time.

For this reason, mole monitoring using digital dermoscopy is very helpful. The criteria for digital mole monitoring have been defined. This technique allows for the detection of macroscopic changes within AMN which should be considered for removal. Some of these when biopsied are clinically and dermoscopically featureless melanomas.

Once the decision to excise a lesion has been communicated to the patient, the lesion must be excised. Excision with wide margins is not justified, and minimal margins are sufficient.

There is a strong tendency for physicians to overstate the risk of melanoma associated with AMN. This often places undue stress on the patient. This should be avoided until the biological significance of AMN is better defined.

New research tools are being developed for evaluating AMN. A confocal microscope can detect pagetoid melanocytosis in the epidermis. Since pagetoid melanocytosis suggests melanoma, visualizing AMN with the confocal microscope may prevent unnecessary excision in the future. However, the latter technique requires validation, remains costly and thus is unlikely to be utilized in the routine management of patients in the foreseeable future.

FINAL THOUGHTS

AMN have continued to be a highly controversial and polarizing subject for almost three decades. Despite the accumulation of much information on the subject, there has been a failure to reach consensus about critical aspects of the problem, as e.g., criteria for diagnosis and management of patients, research on the subject, and consequently, the biological significance of AMN. Until more definitive data are available, the authors recommend a pragmatic nomenclature of: (1) clinically atypical nevi and (2) histologically atypical nevi (or nevi with architectural disorder and cytological atypia), and also a sensible approach to the management of patients. Physicians should strive to only remove clinical lesions that are truly concerning for melanoma and to avoid raising unwarranted anxiety in patients about AMN and melanoma risk.

ACKNOWLEDGMENTS

The authors would like to thank Brandon Einstein for the review of the manuscript.

REFERENCES

1. Lynch HT, Frichot BC III, Lynch JF. Familial atypical multiple mole-melanoma syndrome. *J Med Genet.* 1978;15:352–356.
2. Clark WH Jr, Reimer RR, Greene M, Ainsworth AM, Mastrangelo MJ. Origin of familial malignant melanomas from heritable melanocytic lesions: The B-K mole syndrome. *Arch Dermatol.* 1978; 114:732–738.
3. Elder DE, Goldman LI, Goldman SC, Greene MH, Clark WH Jr. Dysplastic nevus syndrome: A phenotypic association of sporadic cutaneous melanoma. *Cancer.* 1980 1980;46:1787–1794.
4. Elder DE, Greene MH, Bondi EE, Clark WH Jr. Acquired melanocytic nevi and melanoma: The dysplastic nevus syndrome. In: Ackerman AB, ed. *Pathology of Malignant Melanoma.* New York: Masson, 1981:85–215.
5. Kraemer KH, Greene MH, Tarone R, et al. Dysplastic naevi and cutaneous melanoma risk [letter]. *Lancet.* 1983;2:1076–1077.
6. Crutcher WA, Sagebiel RW. Prevalence of dysplastic nevi in a community practice (letter). *Lancet.* 1984;1:729.
7. NIH Consensus Conference. Precursors to malignant melanoma. *JAMA.* 1984;251: 1864–1866.
8. Ackerman AB, Mihara I. Dysplasia, dysplastic melanocytes, the dysplastic nevus syndrome, and the relation between dysplastic nevi and malignant melanoma. *Hum Pathol.* 1985;16:87–91.
9. Elder DE. The dysplastic nevus. *Pathology.* 1985;17:291–297.
10. Greene MH, Clark WH Jr, Tucker MA, et al. Acquired precursors of cutaneous malignant melanoma. The familial dysplastic nevus syndrome. *N Engl J Med.* 1985;312:91–97.
11. Greene MH, Clark WH Jr, Tucker MA, Kraemer KH, Elder DE, Fraser MC. High risk of malignant melanoma in melanoma-prone families with dysplastic nevi. *Ann Intern Med.* 1985;102:458–465.
12. Nordlund JJ, Kirkwood J, Forget BM, et al. Demographic study of clinically atypical (dysplastic) nevi in patients with melanoma and comparison subjects. *Cancer Res.* 1985;45:1855–1861.
13. Kelly JW, Crutcher WA, Sagebiel RW. Clinical diagnosis of dysplastic melanocytic nevi: A clinicopathological correlation. *J Am Acad Dermatol.* 1986;14: 1044–1052.
14. Roush GC, Barnhill RL, Duray PH, Titus LJ, Ernstoff MS, Kirkwood JM. Diagnosis of the dysplastic nevus in different population. *J Am Acad Dermatol.* 1986;14: 419–425.
15. Seywright MM, Doherty VR, MacKie RM. Proposed alternative terminology and subclassification of so-called "dysplastic naevi." *J Clin Pathol.* 1986;39:189–194.
16. Bergman W, Ruiter DJ, Scheffer E, van Vloten WA. Melanocytic atypia in dysplastic nevi: Immunohistochemical and cytophotometrical analysis. *Cancer.* 1988; 61:1660–1666.
17. Steijlen PM, Bergman W, Hermans J, Scheffer E, van Vloten WA, Ruiter DJ. The efficacy of histopathological criteria required for diagnosing dysplastic naevi. *Histopathology.* 1988;12:289–300.
18. Gruber SB, Barnhill RL, Stenn KS, Roush GC. Nevomelanocytic proliferations in association with cutaneous malignant melanoma: A multivariate analysis. *J Am Acad Dermatol.* 1989;21(4 Pt 1):773–780.
19. Piepkorn M, Meyer LJ, Goldgar D. The dysplastic melanocytic nevus—a prevalent lesion that correlates poorly with clinical phenotype. *J Am Acad Dermatol.* 1989;20:407–415.
20. Rigel DS, Rivers JK, Kopf AW, et al. Dysplastic nevi markers for increased risk of melanoma. *Cancer.* 1989;63:386–389.
21. Ahmed I, Piepkorn MW, Rabkin MS, et al. Histopathologic characteristics of dysplastic nevi. Limited association of conventional histologic criteria with melanoma risk group. *J Am Acad Dermatol.* 1990; 22:727–733.
22. Barnhill RL, Roush GC. Histopathologic spectrum of clinically atypical melanocytic nevi: Studies of nonfamilial melanoma, II. *Arch Dermatol.* 1990;126(10):1315–1318.
23. Barnhill RL, Roush GC, Duray PH. Correlation of histologic and cytoplasmic features with nuclear atypia in atypical (dysplastic) nevomelanocytic nevi. *Hum Pathol.* 1990;21:51–58.
24. Klein LJ, Barr RJ. Histologic atypia in clinically benign nevi. A prospective study. *J Am Acad Dermatol.* 1990;22:275–282.
25. Barnhill RL. Current status of the dysplastic melanocytic nevus. *J Cutan Pathol.* 1991;18:147–159.
26. Barnhill RL, Roush GC. Correlation of clinical and histopathological features in clinically atypical melanocytic nevi. *Cancer.* 1991;67:3157–3164.
27. Clark WH Jr. Tumour progression and the nature of cancer. *Br J Cancer.* 1991;64: 631–644.
28. Clemente C, Cochran AJ, Elder DE, et al. Histopathologic diagnosis of dysplastic nevi: Concordance among pathologists convened by the World Health Organization Melanoma Programme. *Hum Pathol.* 1991; 22:313–319.
29. Halpern AC, Guerry D, Elder DE, et al. Dysplastic nevi as risk markers of sporadic (nonfamilial) melanoma. *Arch Dermatol.* 1991;127:995–999.
30. Roush GC, Barnhill RL. Correlation of clinical pigmentary characteristics with histopathologically-confirmed dysplastic nevi in nonfamilial melanoma patients. Studies of melanocytic nevi IX. *Br J Cancer.* 1991;64(5):943–947.
31. Duray PH, DerSimonian R, Barnhill RL, et al. An analysis of interobserver recognition of the histopathologic features of dysplastic nevi from a mixed group of nevomelanocytic lesions. *J Am Acad Dermatol.* 1992;27(5 Pt 1):741–749.
32. NIH Consensus Development Panel on Early Melanoma: Diagnosis and treatment of early melanoma. *JAMA.* 1992;268:1314–1319.
33. Barnhill RL. Melanocytic nevi and tumor progression: Perspectives concerning histomorphology, melanoma risk, and molecular genetics. *Dermatology.* 1993;187:86–90.
34. Bruijn JA, Berwick M, Mihm MC Jr, Barnhill RL. Common acquired melanocytic nevi, dysplastic melanocytic nevi, and malignant melanomas: An image analysis cytometric study. *J Cutan Pathol.* 1993;20(2):121–125.
35. Duncan LM, Berwick MA, Bruijn JA, Byers HR, Mihm MC Jr, Barnhill RL. Histopathologic recognition and grading of dysplastic melanocytic nevi: An interobserver agreement study. *J Invest Dermatol.* 1993;100(S3):318S–321S.
36. Tucker MA, Fraser MC, Goldstein AM, Elder DE, Guerry DP IV, Organic SM. Risk of melanoma and other cancers in melanoma-prone families. *J Invest Dermatol.* 1993;100:350S–355S.
37. Halpern AC, Guerry DP IV, Elder DE, Trock B, Synnestvedt M. A cohort study of melanoma in patients with dysplastic nevi. *J Invest Dermatol.* 1993;100:346S–349S.
38. Piepkorn MW, Barnhill RL, Rabkin MS, et al. Histologic diagnosis of the dysplastic nevus: An analysis of inter- and intra-observer concordance, correlation with clinical phenotype, and prevalence in population controls. *J Am Acad Dermatol.* 1994;30:707–714.
39. Schmidt B, Hollister K, Weinberg D, Barnhill RL. Analysis of dysplastic nevi by DNA image cytometry. *Cancer.* 1994;73:2971–2977.
40. Kang S, Barnhill RL, Mihm MC Jr, Fitzpatrick TB, Sober AJ. Melanoma risk in individuals with clinically atypical nevi. *Arch Dermatol.* 1994;130:999–1001.
41. Hastrup N, Clemmensen OJ, Spaun E, Sondergarrd K. Dysplastic naevus;

Histological criteria and their inter-oberver reproducibility. *Histopathology*. 1994;24: 503–509.

42. Garbe C, Buttner P, Weiss J, et al. Risk factors for developing cutaneous melanoma and criteria for identifying persons at risk: Multicenter case-control study of the central malignant melanoma registry of the German Dermatological Society. *J Invest Dermatol*. 1994;102:695–699.

43. Garbe C, Buttner P, Weiss J, et al. Associated factors in the prevalence of more than 50 common melanocytic nevi, atypical melanocytic nevi, and actinic lentigines: Multicenter case-control study of the central malignant melanoma registry of the German Dermatological Society. *J Invest Dermatol*. 1994;102: 700–705.

44. Marghoob AA, Kopf AW, Rigel DS, et al. Risk of cutaneous malignant melanoma in patients with "classic" atypical-mole syndrome: A case-control study. *Arch Dermatol*. 1994;130:993–998.

45. Slade J, Marghoob AA, Salopek TG, Riegel D, Kopf AW, Bart RS. Atypical mole syndrome: Risk factor for cutaneous malignant melanoma and implications for treatment. *J Am Acad Dermatol*. 1995;32:479–494.

46. Tucker MA, Halpern A, Holly EA, et al. Clinically recognized dysplastic nevi: A central risk factor for cutaneous melanoma. *JAMA*. 1997;277:1439–1444.

47. Blessing K. Benign atypical naevi: Diagnostic difficulties and continued controversy. *Histopathology*. 1999;34: 89–198.

48. Shea CR, Vollmer RT, Prieto VG. Correlating architectural disorder and cytological atypia in Clark (dysplastic) melanocytic nevi. *Hum Pathol*. 1999;30(5):500–505.

49. Annesi G, Cattaruzza MS, Abeni D. Correlation between clinical atypia and histologic dysplasia in acquired melanocytic nevi. *J Am Acad Dermatol*. 2001;45(1):77–85.

50. Pozo L, Naase M, Cerio R, et al. Critical analysis of histologic criteria for grading atypical (dysplastic) melanocytic nevi. *Am J Clin Pathol*. 2001;115:194–204.

51. Shors AR, Argenyi Z, Barnhill RL, et al. Nevi with moderate to severe histologic atypia: A risk factor for melanoma. *Br J Dermatol*. 2006;155(5):988–993.

CHAPTER 11

Malignant Melanoma

Raymond L. Barnhill, M.D.
Martin C. Mihm, Jr., M.D.
George Elgart, M.D.

BOX 11-1 Overview

- Cutaneous melanoma has become a major health concern among Caucasian populations worldwide over the past three or more decades.
- The principal etiologic factors responsible for the rapid increase in melanoma incidence rates appear to be most likely environmental and behavioral, due to increased recreational sun exposure.
- However, melanoma also seems to have distinct developmental pathways that are related to genetic and other host factors interacting with the environment.
- The major forms of melanoma include those developing in chronically sun-exposed skin, intermittently sun-exposed skin, and sun-protected or completely shielded sites.
- Unusual variants of melanoma meriting attention because of difficulty of diagnosis include amelanotic melanoma, desmoplastic-neurotropic melanoma, "nevoid" melanoma, small-cell melanoma, and melanoma resembling or developing in cellular blue nevus.
- The principal clinical criteria for melanoma include the ABCDEs: Asymmetry, irregular and notched orders, irregular or "variegated" or jet black Color, Diameter often >5–6 mm, Elevation from the Bskin surface, a persistently Evolving lesion, ulceration, and bleeding.
- Histopathologic diagnosis usually involves several criteria including asymmetry, diameter >5–6 mm, organizational aberrations including pagetoid melanocytosis, prominent confluence and high cellular density of melanocytes, diminished or absent maturation, effacement or ulceration of epidermis, significant cytologic atypia, and mitoses in the dermal component.
- Lesions suspicious for melanoma should be biopsied by excision, if possible, for histopathologic examination.
- The principal prognostic factors are the stages of melanoma, e.g., localized primary melanoma, regional lymph node or distant metastatic disease and Breslow thickness for localized melanomas.

- Surgery is the only effective therapy at present and may be virtually curative for many melanomas measuring less than 1 mm and without other adverse prognostic indicators.
- There is no objective evidence that any medical intervention influences the course of advanced melanoma (or perhaps melanoma at any stage).

INTRODUCTION

Malignant melanoma of the skin is increasingly an important global health problem. The reasons for this are immediately apparent: (1) The rate of incidence of cutaneous melanoma continues to rise almost inexorably in populations of European origin worldwide. (2) Diagnosis of melanoma at an early stage is almost curable. (3) There is currently no effective treatment for advanced melanoma. (4) Probably a large proportion of melanomas can be ascribed to a single (modifiable) risk factor—sun exposure. (5) It has not been established whether medical intervention of any kind influences the outcome in the case of melanoma. Major initiatives in recent years have concentrated on education about sun avoidance, the importance of skin awareness and skin examination, and the screening of populations at high risk for melanoma. However, it is unclear whether any of the latter measures have had any significant influence on mortality from melanoma.

This chapter discusses the most salient clinical and histologic features of cutaneous melanoma and their differential diagnosis.

CLASSIFICATION AND ETIOLOGIC CONSIDERATIONS

BOX 11-2 Summary

- Melanoma is thought to be one disease, but this may be an oversimplification because melanomas have distinct developmental pathways that are related to anatomic site, degree of sun exposure, genetics, and potentially other factors.

Because almost all melanomas are initially localized to squamous epithelium for some period of time, a classification of melanoma based on the presence or absence and patterns of intraepidermal involvement was described and utilized

Table 11-1
Historical Classification of Malignant Melanoma

PRESENCE OF RADIAL GROWTH PHASE

- Superficial spreading
- Lentigo maligna
- Acral lentiginous
- Unclassified

ABSENCE OF RADIAL GROWTH PHASE

- Nodular melanoma

for many years.[1–6] One idea behind such a classification was that particular intraepidermal patterns (also termed radial or horizontal growth phases) might correlate with differences in etiology and possibly prognosis. Four clinicopathologic subtypes of melanoma were thus proposed (Table 11-1).[7,8–14] Nevertheless, an objective assessment of the classification of melanoma according to intraepidermal pattern or growth phase is that such a classification is in many respects artificial.[8,15,16] The reasons for this view are: (1) the tremendous morphologic heterogeneity of melanoma, (2) morphologic patterns may correlate with anatomical site, (3) the intraepithelial components of many melanoma are not easily classified (because of overlapping features) and classification is not reproducible,[17] (4) some intraepithelial components are difficult to recognize as either clearly benign, i.e., a potential precursor such as an atypical nevus, or malignant, (5) the idea that nodular melanomas develop as de novo invasive tumors without any initial intraepithelial melanocytic proliferation[13] is theoretically possible but has not been proved, and (6) after adjustment for Breslow thickness, the pattern of the intraepidermal component has no effect on prognosis.

However, the idea that melanoma is one disease also appears oversimplified, and recent evidence supports the longstanding hypothesis that melanomas indeed seem to have distinct developmental pathways that are related to anatomic site, degree of sun exposure, genetics, and potentially other factors.[18]

MAJOR FORMS OF MELANOMA

BOX 11-3 Summary

- Melanomas of intermittently sun-exposed skin are found in young adults. It has an

- adjacent pagetoid intraepidermal component and a frequent association with BRAF mutations.
- Lentigo maligna (solar) melanoma has a strong correlation with sunlight exposure, onset in older persons, uncommon association with melanocytic nevi and a pattern of genomic aberrations.
- Acral and mucosal melanomas develop in relatively or completely sun-protected sites, have infrequent *BRAF* mutations, and show greater numbers of chromosomal aberrations.
- Nodular melanoma is a descriptive term that refers to melanomas with no adjacent intraepithelial component. This is thought to indicate simply a heterogenous group of melanoma showing rapid tumor progression.

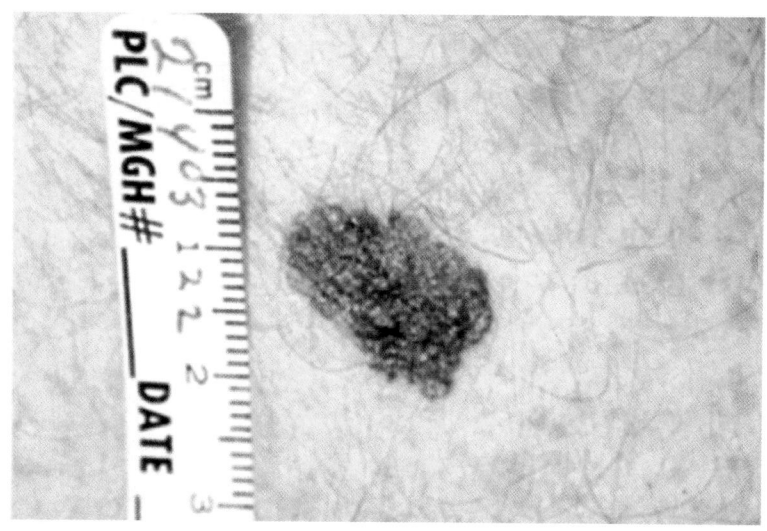

▲ **FIGURE 11-1** Melanoma of intermittently sun-exposed skin. Note the asymmetry, large diameter, irregular borders, and complex coloration.

Continued research is needed to validate differences among the latter variants and to identify clearly avenues for preventive and therapeutic intervention that have real impact on patient suffering and mortality from melanoma. Such substantiation of unique differences among melanomas that provide the basis for meaningful intervention is the only rationale for the continued use of any classification of melanoma. Otherwise, there is no real rationale for recording descriptive information in pathology reports other than information such as Breslow thickness and margins, etc. that has been validated to have a direct bearing on prognosis and patient management.

Melanoma of Intermittently Sun-Exposed Skin

This group of melanomas which account for the great majority of melanomas in Caucasians often (but not always) have an adjacent pagetoid intraepidermal component, a frequent association with *BRAF* mutations and melanocytic nevi (also with *BRAF* mutations), and development in relatively young adults.[18]

Lentigo Maligna (Solar) Melanoma

Melanomas of chronic sun-damaged skin are distinct from other forms of melanoma irrespective of intraepidermal pattern of melanocytic proliferation because of their strong correlation with cumulative sunlight exposure, onset in older persons, uncommon association with melanocytic nevi, and finally, the pattern of genomic aberrations. This group of melanomas seems to have significantly

fewer chromosomal aberrations as compared to acral and mucosal melanomas, in general an absence of *BRAF* mutations, frequent gains in *CCND1* and regions of chromosome 22, and losses from chromosome 4q.[18]

Acral (and Mucosal) Melanoma

These melanomas also appear distinctive since they develop in relatively or completely sun-protected sites, have infrequent *BRAF* mutations, and show greater numbers of chromosomal aberrations as compared to the latter melanomas.[18]

Nodular Melanoma

This descriptive term refers to melanomas with no adjacent intraepithelial component and is thought to simply indicate a heterogenous group of melanoma showing rapid tumor progression irrespective of intraepithelial pattern or location.[13,18]

GENERAL CLINICAL FEATURES OF CUTANEOUS MELANOMA

BOX 11-4   Summary

- Most commonly affects adult Caucasians, and the incidence is essentially equal between men and women.
- The most common sites that melanomas are found include the trunk (back) followed by the upper extremities and head and neck for men; and the lower extremities followed by the back, upper extremities, and head and neck for women.
- Amelanotic melanoma and those resembling keratoses are particularly difficult to

diagnose without a high index of suspicion
- Acral melanoma is the most frequent form of melanoma among Asians, Africans, and other ethnic groups of color.
- Subungual melanoma (SM) is a distinctive variant of acral melanoma that most often involves the nail bed of the great toe or thumb.

In general, cutaneous melanoma most commonly affects adult Caucasians and is rarely observed before puberty.[19,20] Men and women are equally affected although some European studies have suggested a higher incidence in females. Patients are diagnosed with melanoma most commonly in the fourth through seventh decades. The most common sites include the trunk (back) followed by the upper extremities and head and neck for men and the lower extremities followed by the back, upper extremities, and head and neck for women. Gross morphologic features of melanoma include size often >1 cm (range 2 mm to >15 cm), irregular or notched borders, asymmetry, complexity of color including a variable admixture of tan, brown, blue, black, red, pink, gray, and white, and ulceration and bleeding (Fig. 11-1).[19,20] Early melanomas especially those involving chronic sun-exposed and acral sites may be completely flat but with progression usually develop a papular or nodular component (Figs. 11-2 to 11-4). Melanomas lacking pigment (amelanotic melanoma) and those resembling keratoses are particularly difficult to diagnose without a high index of suspicion (Fig. 11-5). Acral melanoma, although accounting for 5% or less of melanomas among Caucasians, is the

141

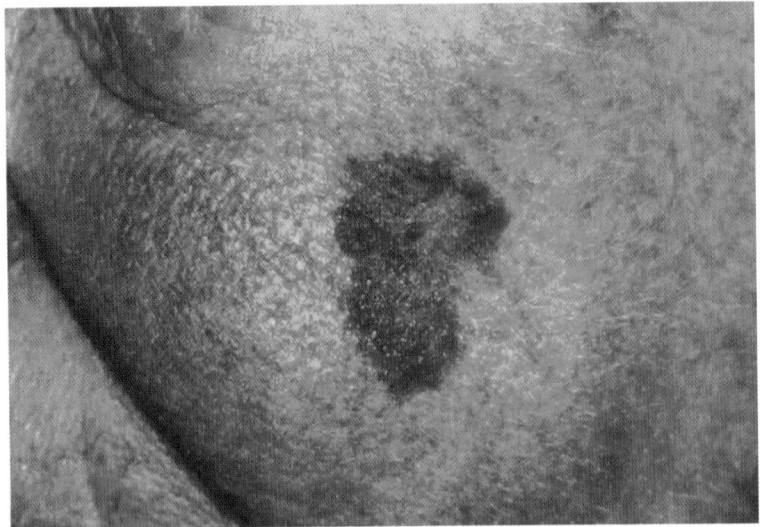

▲ **FIGURE 11-2** Solar melanoma (melanoma of chronically sun-exposed skin). This lesion involves the cheek. The lesion has macular and papular components, asymmetry, large diameter, irregular borders, and complex coloration.

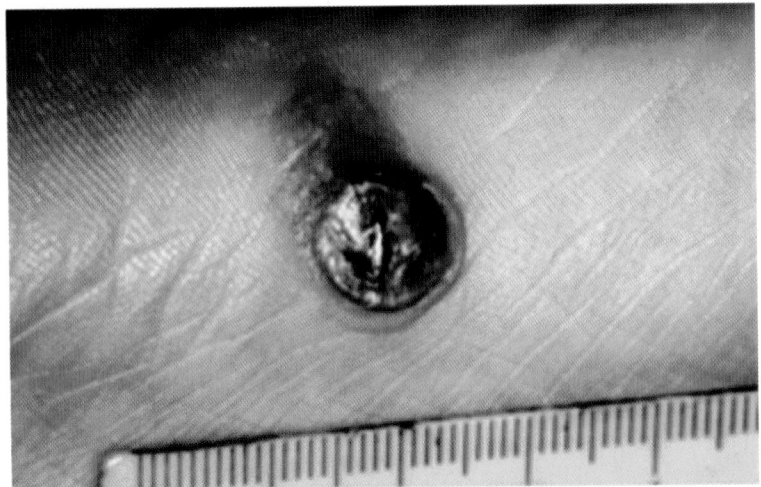

▲ **FIGURE 11-3** Acral melanoma. This lesion demonstrates macular and large nodular components.

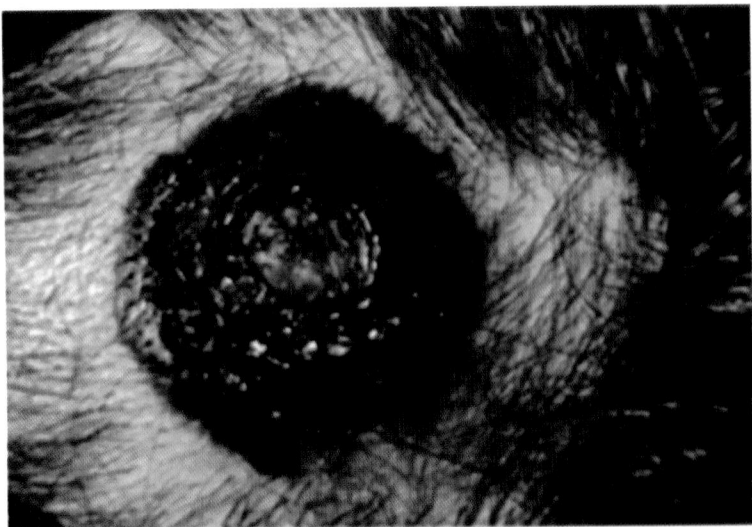

▲ **FIGURE 11-4** "Nodular" melanoma. Melanoma on the scalp, without demonstrable surrounding component. Melanomas with this configuration may develop on any anatomic site with or without a clearly identifiable adjacent intraepithelial proliferation of melanoma.

most frequent form of melanoma among Asians, Africans, and other ethnic groups of color (Fig. 11-3).[7,13,18,19] However, approximately the same incidence of acral melanoma occurs in all ethnic groups. Subungual melanoma (SM) is a distinctive variant of acral melanoma that most often involves the nail bed of the great toe or thumb[21–25] where it commonly presents as an ulcerated tumor.[22] However, the initial manifestations may include a longitudinal pigmented band of the nail plate (frequently ≈9 mm wide) or a mass under the nail plate (Fig. 11-6).[25] A useful clinical sign is pigmentation extending from the nail onto the surrounding periungual skin (Hutchinson's sign).

GENERAL HISTOPATHOLOGIC FEATURES

BOX 11-5 Summary

- Essentially all melanomas begin as a proliferation of melanocytes initially confined to the epidermis.
- Increasing cytologic atypia of melanocytes accompanies the aberrant architectural appearance of melanomas.
- After the period of intraepidermal proliferation, there is often invasion of the papillary dermis, primarily as single cells and small aggregates of cells.
- Breslow thickness (in mm) of melanoma is one of the most important factors determining prognosis and theraphy.
- Melanomas with prominent invasive components may display polypoid morphologies.

Intraepithelial Component

Almost all melanomas begin as a proliferation of melanocytes initially confined to the epidermis (Fig. 11-7).[1–16] The latter proliferation may develop with or without a detectable melanocytic nevus. Estimates of the frequency of melanomas developing in continuity with a nevus of any kind vary widely. Approximately a third of melanomas have nevus remnants. The duration of this intraepidermal phase ranges from months to many years, during which these proliferative lesions show progressive degrees of architectural and cytologic atypicality.

Increasing cytologic atypia of melanocytes accompanies the aberrant architectural appearance. The melanocytes vary in degree of atypia and the proportion of cells with nuclear atypia. However, atypical melanocytes usually have enlarged nuclei that exhibit variation in nuclear shapes and chromatin

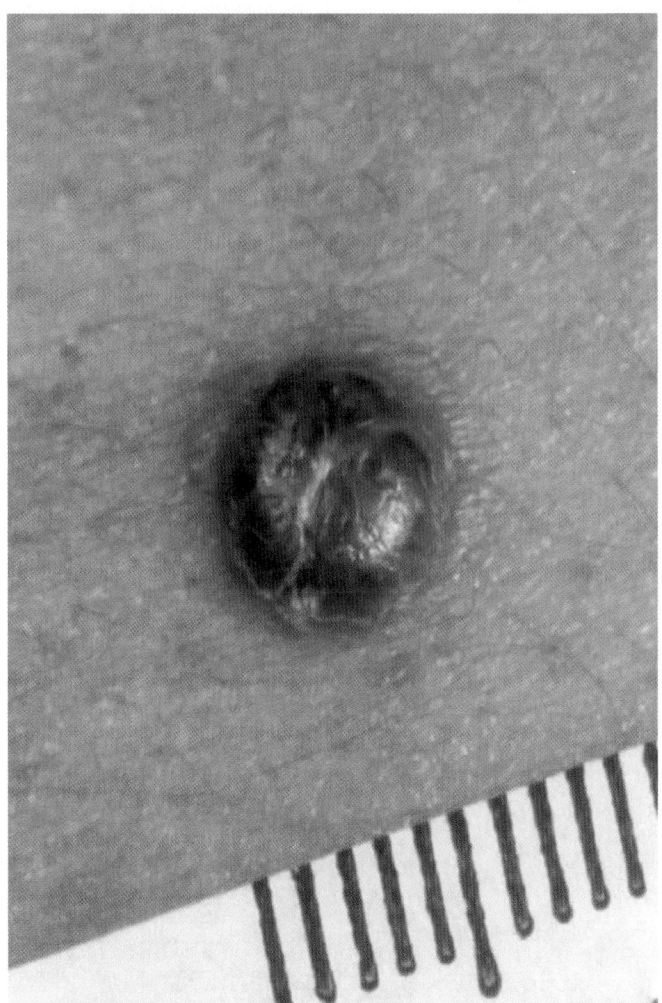

▲ **FIGURE 11-5** Amelanotic "nodular" melanoma. This type of lesion may develop at any location and is indistinguishable from metastatic melanoma.

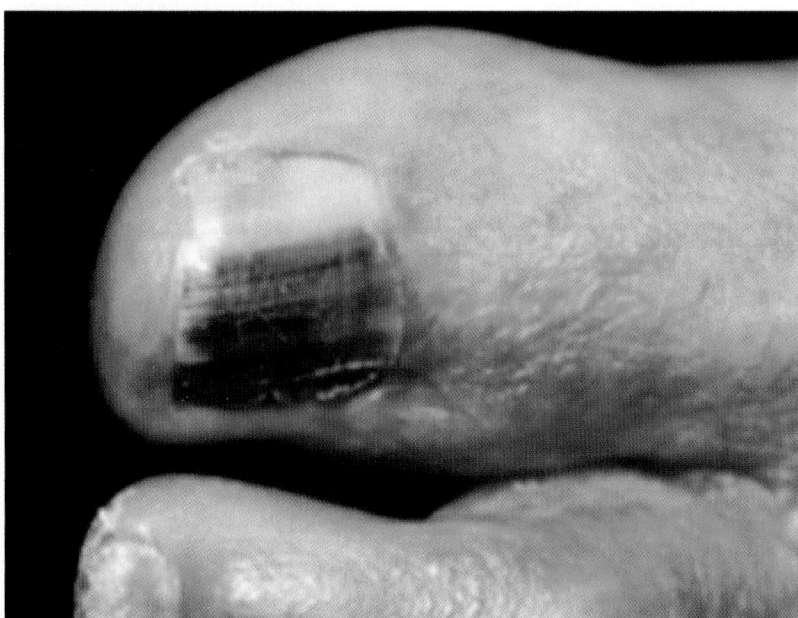

▲ **FIGURE 11-6** Subungual melanoma. Note broad irregularly pigmented band involving nail plate. Pigmentation extends onto periungual skin (Hutchinson's sign).

patterns, and may have large nucleoli. Thickening of nuclear membranes and irregular nuclear contours are also characteristic features. The cytoplasm of such melanocytes may be abundant with a pink granular quality, may contain granular or finely divided ("dusty") melanin (Figs.11-7 to 11-9), or show retraction, resulting in a clear space around the nuclei. Melanocytes with scant cytoplasm typically have high nuclear-to-cytoplasmic ratios. Such proliferations have been variously labeled atypical melanocytic hyperplasia, premalignant melanosis, melanocytic dysplasia, and "pagetoid melanocytic proliferation," as well as melanoma *in situ*.[26,27]

Invasive Melanoma

After the period of intraepidermal proliferation, there is often invasion of the papillary dermis, primarily as single cells and small aggregates of cells (Table 11-2). Microinvasive melanoma is also remarkable for a striking host response in the papillary dermis, typically a dense cellular infiltrate of lymphocytes and monocyte/macrophages. Presumably, in consequence of this host reaction, regression, often focal, is common in up to 50% of microinvasive melanomas (see the following sections).[28]

The term "vertical growth phase" ("VGP") has been used by some to describe the proliferation of invasive melanoma cells as cohesive aggregates (Fig. 11-10).[29,30] It has been postulated that the so-called VGP may signify the onset of the metastatic phenotype since it may be indistinguishable from metastatic melanoma.[30] However, melanomas lacking the morphology of the VGP have resulted in metastases.

Melanomas with prominent invasive components may display polypoid morphologies such that more than half (sessile forms) or virtually all (pedunculated forms) of the tumor is above the epidermal surface. Amelanotic variants also may develop in any type of melanoma.

Table 11-2
Anatomic Levels of Invasion

Level I	Entirely intraepidermal; melanoma *in situ*
Level II	Microinvasive into papillary dermis
Level III	Expansion of papillary dermis by cohesive cellular nodule or plaque (but confined to papillary dermis)
Level IV	Invasion of reticular dermis
Level V	Invasion of subcutaneous fat

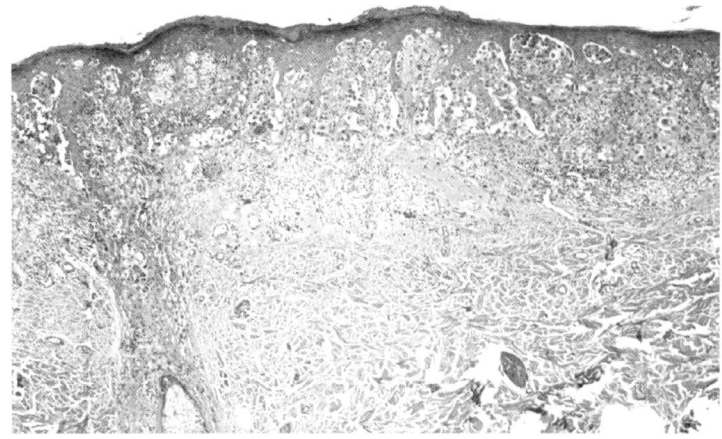

▲ **FIGURE 11-7** Melanoma of intermittently sun-exposed skin (pagetoid melanoma) Scanning magnification shows pagetoid spread of epithelioid melanoma cells.

MELANOMAS OF INTERMITTENTLY SUN EXPOSED SKIN

BOX 11-6   Summary

- *Clinical Features*
  - In general onset after puberty but all ages affected
  - Most frequent ages 30–70 years
  - Caucasians affected much greater than Africans, Asians
  - Women ≥ men
  - Most common sites are lower extremities and trunk of women and
  - Trunk (back) of men
  - Pain, pruritus
  - Size often >1 cm (range 2 mm to >15 cm)
  - Initially macular, later stages may be papular and nodular
  - Asymmetrical
  - Irregular and often notched borders
  - Complexity and variation in color often with admixtures of tan, brown, black, blue, gray, white, red
  - May be entirely skin-colored (amelanotic) or black
  - Ulceration and bleeding may be present
- *Histopathologic Criteria*
  - *Architecture*
    - ➤ Asymmetry
    - ➤ Heterogeneity of lesion
    - ➤ Large size (>6 mm) but many exceptions
    - ➤ Poor circumscription of proliferation
    - ➤ Melanin not uniformly distributed
    - ➤ Organizational abnormalities of intraepidermal component
    - ➤ Pagetoid spread
      - Upward migration of melanocytes in random pattern, single cells predominate over nests
      - Cells often reach granular and cornified layers
    - ➤ Lentiginous melanocytic proliferation
      - Melanocytes reach confluence
      - Nesting of melanocytes (sun-damaged skin)
      - Melanocytes not equidistant
      - Proliferation of melanocytes along adnexal epithelium
    - ➤ Nested pattern
      - Variation in size, shape, placement of nests
      - Nests replace large portions of squamous epithelium
      - Diminished cohesiveness of cells in nests
      - Confluence of nests
    - ➤ Loss of epidermal rete pattern (effacement)
    - ➤ Mononuclear cell infiltrates, often band-like
    - ➤ Fibroplasia of papillary dermis
    - ➤ Regression frequently present
  - *Cytology*
    - ➤ Nuclear changes
      - Majority of melanocytes uniformly atypical
      - Nuclear enlargement
      - Nuclear pleomorphism (variation in sizes and shapes)
      - Nuclear hyperchromasia with coarse chromatin
      - One or more prominent nucleoli
    - ➤ Cytoplasmic changes
      - of cytoplasm
    - ➤ Mitoses (in dermal component)
    - ➤ Atypical mitoses
    - ➤ Necrotic cells
- *Invasive Component in Dermis*
  - *Architecture*
    - ➤ Tumefactive cellular aggregates
    - ➤ Pushing, expanding pattern without regard for stroma
    - ➤ Hypercellularity
    - ➤ Less host response
  - *Cytology*
    - ➤ As above
    - ➤ Increased nuclear to cytoplasmic ratios
    - ➤ Mitoses in dermal component
    - ➤ Atypical mitoses
    - ➤ Necrotic cells

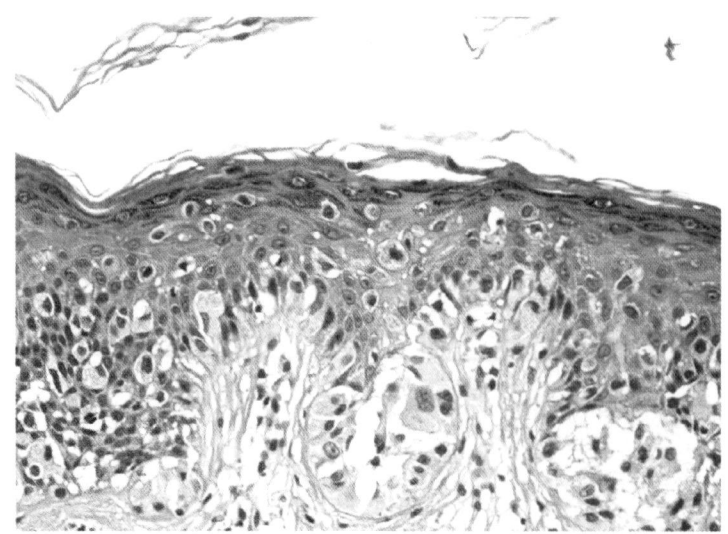

▲ **FIGURE 11-8** Melanoma of intermittently sun-exposed skin (pagetoid melanoma) Higher magnification demonstrating pagetoid pattern and the beginnings of dermal invasion by melanoma cells.

Pagetoid spread (transepidermal migration of cells in a manner analogous to Paget's disease of the breast)[1-9,31] refers to single cells and small groups of cells are randomly scattered throughout the epidermis reaching the granular layer and stratum corneum. The melanoma cells often have an epithelioid cell appearance, i.e., they resemble epithelial cells because of abundant cytoplasm that is usually granular and eosinophilic or contains

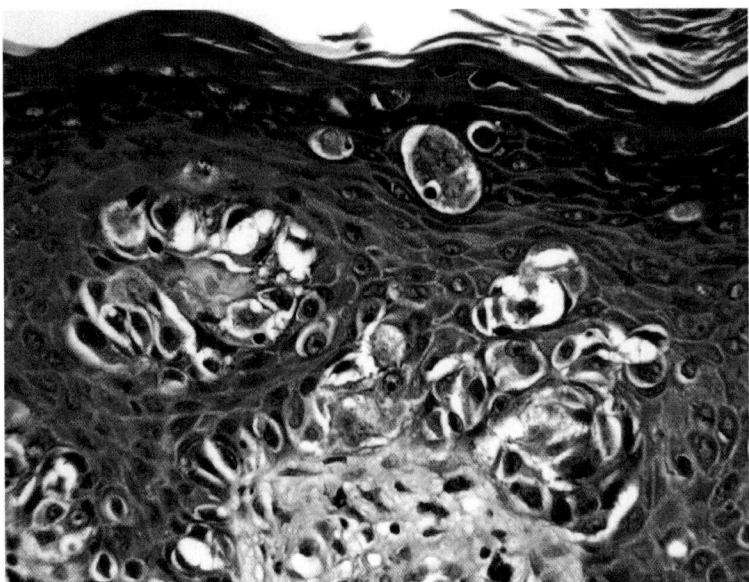

▲ **FIGURE 11-9** Melanoma of intermittently sun-exposed skin (pagetoid melanoma) Pagetoid melanocytosis with large epithelioid melanoma cells.

finely divided ("dusty") melanin (Figs. 11-7 to 11-9). The cells are usually larger than (sometimes two to three times) the surrounding keratinocytes. The epidermis may be hyperplastic, the epidermal rete pattern is often lost (effaced), and the surface of the epidermis abutting the intraepidermal tumor may exhibit a characteristically scalloped contour. Melanoma cells often proliferate as variably sized nests and horizontally disposed aggregates immediately underneath this scalloped epidermis. These aggregates have frequently large size and diminished cohe-

sion of cells. In some instances, the latter proliferative pattern may predominate with little or no pagetoid spread.

The most common cell in the invasive component is epithelioid (Fig. 11-10). Less frequently, spindle cells, small cells or large bizarre mononuclear or multinucleate cells may predominate or may be admixed with the other cell types. Many melanomas show considerable heterogeneity of cell type, such that the cells vary in nuclear size and shape and the amount of cytoplasm from one focus to another.

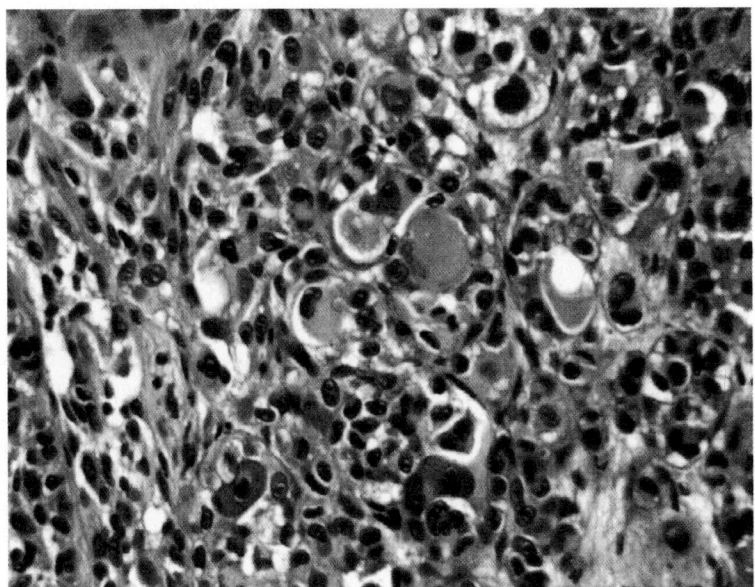

▲ **FIGURE 11-10** Melanoma of intermittently sun-exposed skin (pagetoid melanoma). Invasive component- containing epithelioid melanoma cells.

Differential Diagnosis

BOX 11-7 Summary

- Markedly atypical (dysplastic) nevi
- Halo nevi
- Spitz tumors
- Pigmented spindle cell melanocytic tumors
- Recurrent/persistent melanocytic nevi
- Congenital nevi

The differential diagnosis of melanomas with pagetoid intraepidermal components includes various melanocytic proliferations: markedly atypical (dysplastic) nevi (AMN), halo nevi, Spitz tumors, pigmented spindle cell tumors, recurrent/persistent melanocytic nevi, and congenital nevi, particularly in the first year of life. Nevi associated with prominent pagetoid spread are commonly confused with melanoma.

AMN with pronounced atypia may be misdiagnosed as melanoma because of focal or minimal pagetoid spread, confluence of cellular aggregates along the dermal/epidermal junction, prominent variation in nesting pattern, significant cytologic atypia, entrapment of nests of dermal nevus cells in the papillary dermis, and dense mononuclear cell infiltrates. On occasion, the distinction of AMN from melanoma is exceedingly difficult. Nonetheless, discrimination of melanoma from AMN is usually possible because of the larger size, greater asymmetry, disorder, cellularity, and cytologic atypia encountered in melanoma. Usually AMN will maintain an overall symmetry, a nevic appearance as exemplified by fairly organized junctional nesting, a basilar proliferation of melanocytes that is still concentrated along the epidermal rete and with greater density toward the lower poles of the rete. Thus, the intervening epidermis between rete will contain a lesser density of melanocytes compared to that on the epidermal rete. If pagetoid spread is present, this architectural pattern is often more prominent about epidermal rete and confined to the lowermost epidermis. Occasionally, AMN exhibit effacement of the epidermal rete pattern and confluence of melanocytic cells along the dermal/epidermal junction in this zone. The latter changes are commonly associated with dense mononuclear cell infiltrates and may strongly suggest melanoma. These findings must be carefully interpreted in the overall context of the lesion. AMNs are generally characterized by variable or discontinuous cytologic atypia, i.e., the degree of nuclear enlargement, pleomorphism, and hyperchromatism varies from cell to cell.[9] This cytologic feature is very helpful in discriminating AMN from the more uniform or contiguous cytologic atypia of melanoma.

A finding that raises the possibility of melanoma is entrapment of atypical nevus cells in a fibrotic papillary dermis of an AMN. Such findings may even suggest partial regression of melanoma. A distinction from melanoma should be based on an assessment of all the cytologic and architectural characteristics of the lesion. Importantly, the dermal nevus cells in question usually lack the marked and uniform cytologic atypia, especially manifested as hyperchromasia, of melanoma cells.

In general, halo nevi have dense mononuclear cell infiltrates, histologic regression in some instances, and varying degrees of architectural and cytologic atypia that may suggest melanoma. The typical halo nevus of children and adolescents is characterized by small size, overall symmetry, orderly appearance, and little or no cytologic atypia.[9] The lymphoid cells that permeate the dermal nevus have a uniform density and regular horizontal contour. The nevus cells of halo nevi may demonstrate cellular enlargement with prominent eosinophilic cytoplasm, but their nuclear details are usually little altered. In contrast, there is a variant of halo nevus that has aprominent pattern and cellular atypia, and is perhaps best categorized as an AMN. The discussion of AMN (above) is relevant to this form of (atypical) halo nevus.

The misdiagnosis of other melanocytic nevi including acral nevi, Spitz tumors (see Chapter 19), pigmented spindle cell tumors, congenital nevi, recurrent melanocytic nevi, and nevi in children as melanoma is primarily related to misinterpretation of patterns of pagetoid spread. Overall symmetry and a well-organized appearance, as well as little or no cytologic atypia, favor a benign melanocytic proliferation. Pagetoid spread in benign melanocytic nevi is generally characterized by an orderly pattern and is generally limited to the lower epidermis and aggregates of cells predominate over single cells.

LENTIGO MALIGNA (SOLAR) MELANOMA

BOX 11-8   Summary
- *Clinical Features*
  - Age 60–70 years

- Men = women
- Sun-exposed surfaces: cheek (most common), nose, forehead, ears, neck,
- Dorsal surfaces of hands
- 0.2–20 cm
- Initial tan macule suggesting a varnish-like stain
- Tan, brown, black macule or patch (black flecks characterisitic) (early lesions)
- Pink, gray, white with progression and areas of regression
- Papule or nodule, pigmented or amelanotic (advanced)
- Ulceration and bleeding
- Asymmetry
- Irregular, notched borders
- *Histopathologic Criteria*
  - Effacement and thinning of epidermis common
  - Prominent solar elastosis
- *Solar Intraepidermal Melanocytic Neoplasia (Lentigo Maligna)*
  - Solar intraepidermal melanocytic proliferation (insufficient for melanoma *in situ*)
    ➤ Lentiginous melanocytic proliferation
    ➤ Pleomorphic melanocytes (variable cytologic atypia)
    ➤ Extension of melanocytic proliferation downward along appendages
    ➤ Usual absence of nesting and pagetoid spread
- *Melanoma in situ*
    ➤ Contiguous or near contiguous lentiginous melanocytic proliferation
    ➤ Intraepidermal nesting of melanocytes
    ➤ Pagetoid spread
    ➤ Promient extension of melanocytic proliferation downward along appendages, often with nesting
    ➤ Significant cytologic atypia
    ➤ Melanocytes somewhat spindled to increasingly epithelioid
- *Pigmented spindle cell variant (often on ears)*
  - Prominent intraepidermal discohesive nesting of atypical spindle cells
  - Spindle cells often comprise invasive component but polygonal, small cells common
  - Appendage-associated nesting of atypical melanocytes suggests invasion and may be florid (not true invasion)
  - Partial regression relatively common
  - Precursor nevus present ~3% of cases
  - Desmoplasia, neurotropism, angiotropism common

Lentigo maligna (also known as melanoma with adjacent predominately lentiginous intraepidermal component of sun-exposed skin (historically lentigo maligna melanoma; Hutchinson's melanotic freckle.) is a confusing term since it has been used to describe a histologic spectrum from slightly increased numbers of basilar melanocytes with variable, low-grade cytologic atypia,[1–9,32,33] that is not clearly melanoma *in situ*, to a contiguous and often nested intraepidermal proliferation of highly pleomorphic melanocytic cells, that is, melanoma *in situ*.[32,33] Furthermore, some pathologists consider all lentigo maligna to be melanoma *in situ*[16] while others obviously do not,[9,34,35] hence the confusion. Irrespective of terminology used, the pathologist must clearly communicate to the clinician the meaning of the pathologic terms used to describe these lesions. For clarity, the author recommends the term "solar intraepidermal melanocytic proliferation" with atypia (SIMP) (atypia may be graded as slight, moderate, or severe according to guidelines proposed for atypical nevi) for lesions judged to fall short of melanoma *in situ*; otherwise, solar melanoma *in situ* should be used for lesions showing sufficiently disordered melanocytic proliferation and cellular atypia, i.e., contiguous proliferation of uniformly markedly atypical melanocytes.

In addition to a mainly basilar proliferation of melanocytes (Figs. 11-11 and 11-12), this form of melanoma is also characterized by atrophy and effacement of the epidermis, involvement of appendageal structures, and marked solar elastosis.[1–9,32,36,37] However, the presence of the latter changes may simply be related to anatomic site, i.e., the skin of the cheek in older individuals usually exhibits a flattened epidermis and prominent solar elastosis. There may be prominent involvement of appendageal epithelium with large cellular nests. Recognition of prominent appendageal involvement by melanoma is of critical importance because the lesion should not be misdiagnosed as invasive rather than simply as intraepithelial or *in situ*. The most typical cell type has retracted cytoplasm and often an elongate, stellate, or spindled configuration[1–9,36] and a high nuclear-cytoplasmic ratio. The nuclei are commonly pleomorphic and hyperchromatic. With progression, the cells become more epithelioid in appearance and exhibit nuclear enlargement and prominent nucleoli. Another characteristic feature is the presence of prominent spindle cell differentiation with formation of confluent fascicles of spindle cells along the dermal–epidermal junction and appendages. One particular variant may closely simulate pigmented spindle cell tumor.[9]

Extension of melanoma into the dermis may be difficult to recognize because of prominent cellularity of the

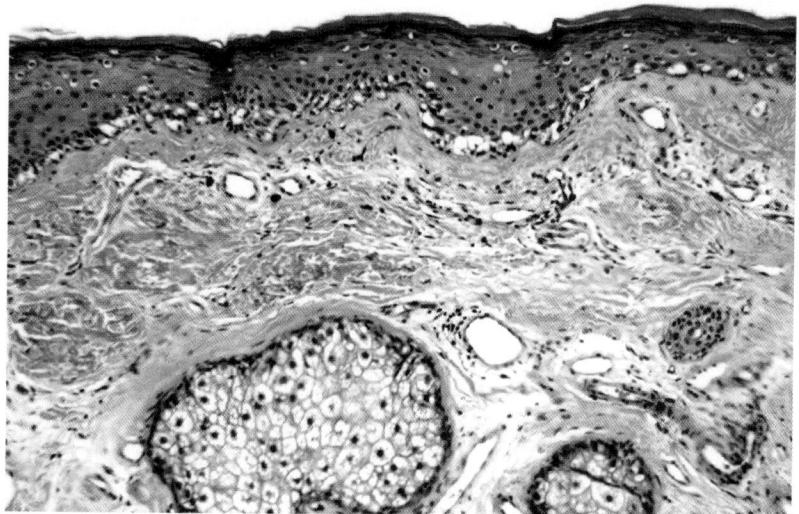

▲ **FIGURE 11-11** Solar melanoma *in situ*. There is a striking basilar proliferation of variably atypical melanocytes in the epidermis.

- Occurrence with nevi, fibrous papule, basal cell carcinoma, actinic keratosis, etc.
- Atypical intraepidermal melanocytic proliferation, not otherwise specified
- Solar lentiginous junctional or compound melanocytic nevi with or without atypia (may overlap atypical (dysplastic) nevi)
- Pigmented spindle cell tumor
- Pigmented actinic keratosis
- Squamous cell carcinoma, spindle cell type
- Atypical fibroxanthoma
- Cellular neurothekeoma
- Malignant peripheral nerve sheath tumor
- Angiosarcoma
- Kaposi's sarcoma
- Leiomyosarcoma

stroma, activation of mesenchymal cells, and the frequent adnexal involvement by melanoma. The invasive dermal component is frequently composed of spindle cells. They occur singly or in bundles with varying stromal desmoplasia and invasion of nerve twigs (see desmoplastic melanoma). However, the invasive component may contain any cell type. Invasion of the dermis may originate from appendageal-associated melanoma cells or nests. In the latter instances, depth of invasion (Breslow thickness) should not be measured from the granular layer of the epidermis since this value would overestimate tumor depth. The measurement of tumor thickness instead should ideally be taken from the granular layer of the hair follicle or sweat gland.

Differential Diagnosis

BOX 11-9   Summary

- Solar lentigo
- Solar melanocytic hyperplasia (photoactivation)
  - *de novo*

Solar melanocytic proliferations with atypia (SIMP) and lentiginous melanomas from markedly sun-damaged skin must be distinguished from solar lentigo, AMN, and pigmented spindle cell tumor (see previous discussions[32,33]). The former lesions may in fact develop from some varieties of solar lentigo. Well-differentiated forms of SIMPS and solar melanoma *in situ* with spindle cells may cause confusion with pigmented spindle cell tumor (PSCT). Typical PSCT usually involves covered skin and commonly occurs in children and young adults; whereas SIMP and solar melanoma *in situ* invariably develops in sun-exposed skin and usually in older persons. An effaced epidermis, cellular nests with diminished cohesion and a prominent basilar single cell proliferation of markedly atypical spindle cells argue in favor of SIMP and solar melanoma *in situ*. Pigmented spindle cell tumors are usually well circumscribed with well-formed, orderly, and regular fascicles of pigmented spindle cells. Epidermal hyperplasia usually encountered in PSCT contrasts with the atrophy of SIMP and solar melanoma *in situ*. Cytologically, PSCT is usually composed of monotonous fusiform cells with nuclei containing delicate chromatin.

ACRAL (AND MUCOSAL) MELANOMAS

BOX 11-10   Summary

- *Clinical Features*
  - Age 60–70 years
  - Men = women
  - Equal incidence in all racial groups

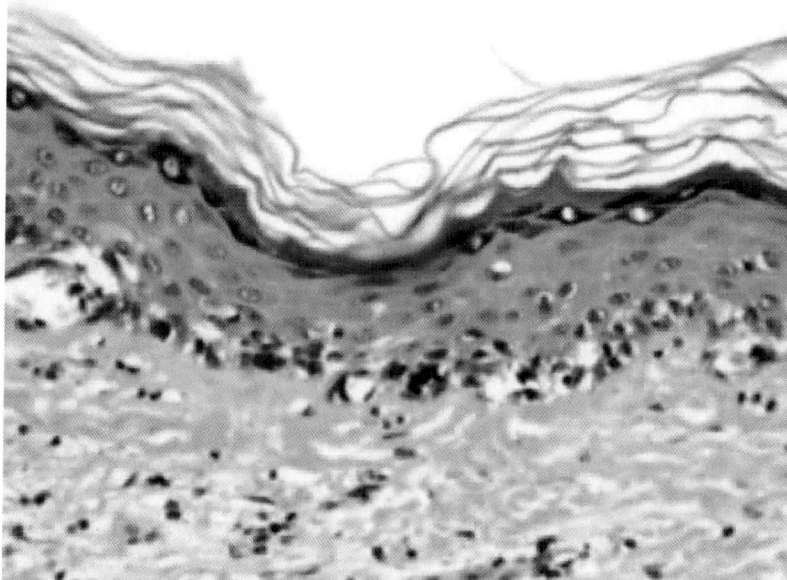

▲ **FIGURE 11-12** Solar lentiginous melanoma. Higher magnification shows atypia of basilar melanocytes.

- Most prevalent form of melanoma in Africans, Asians, Native Americans, other peoples of color
- Glabrous (volar) skin and nail unit
  ➤ Palms, soles, digits 85% of AM
  ➤ Nail unit 15%
- Feet 90% of cases
  ➤ Soles 68 to 71%
  ➤ Toes 11%
  ➤ Nail units 16 to 20%
  ➤ Palms 4 to 10%
  ➤ Fingers 2%
- 0.3–12 cm
  ➤ Often 0.7cm or larger
  ➤ <0.7 cm with irregular borders, color, or "parallel ridge" pattern on epiluminescence microscopy
- Often jet-black macule early but also tan, brown, gray, blue, pink, white
- Pigmented or amelanotic papule or nodule (advanced) with ulceration, bleeding, eschar
- Irregular borders, notching
- *Histopathologic Criteria*
  - Prominent acanthosis with elongated epidermal rete common
  - Thickened stratum corneum
  - Contiguous or near contiguous lentiginous melanocytic proliferation in almost all lesions
  - Intraepidermal melanocytes appear to lie in lacunae (clear spaces)
  - Variable cytologic atypia with minimal atypia in early lesions
  - Pagetoid spread (particularly in more advanced lesions)
  - Intraepidermal nesting (particularly in more advanced lesions)
  - Proliferation of melanocytes downward along eccrine ducts (even into deep dermis and subcutis)
  - Pronounced pagetoid spread, large intraepidermal nests, significant numbers of melanocytes in stratum corneum in advanced lesions
  - Polygonal to spindled melanocytes often with prominent dendrites
  - Nuclear enlargement, hyperchromatism, pleomorphism prominent
  - Invasive component
    ➤ Cohesive nests, sheets of cells, or loosely aggregated files of cells
    ➤ Spindle cells common but also polygonal, small, and highly pleomorphic cells are noted
    ➤ Nevoid and sarcomatoid variants occur
  - Desmoplasia, neurotropism, angiotropism common

Acral and mucosal melanomas (also known often as melanomas (but not necessarily) with adjacent predominately lentiginous intraepithelial component of acral skin, the nail apparatus, and mucosal surfaces) are usually advanced, often ulcerated, and charac-terized by a tumor nodule frequently extending deeply into the stroma.[1–12,21–25] Scanning magnification will usually reveal a hyperplastic epidermis and frequent lentiginous proliferation of atypical melanocytic cells (Figs. 11-13 to 11-15). These cells are commonly contiguous with occasional clustering, appear to lie within lacunae, and display prominent dendrites that extend through the epidermis. Pagetoid patterns are also observed frequently, either alone or associated with lentiginous proliferation. The nuclei are enlarged, hyperchromatic, and often highly pleomorphic (Fig. 11-14). With tumor progression, there is a tendency for greater pagetoid melanocytosis and dermal invasion. Variable degrees of melanization are present.

The dermal component is most often composed of spindle cells but epithelioid cells, small nevus-like cells, and highly pleomorphic cell types are occasionally noted.[1–12] A small proportion exhibit desmoplasia and neurotropism (see the next section).

Differential Diagnosis

BOX 11-11 Summary

- Melanotic macule
- Lentigo
- Atypical intraepidermal melanocytic proliferation, not otherwise specified
- Acral melanocytic nevus with or without atypia (may overlap atypical (dysplastic) nevus)

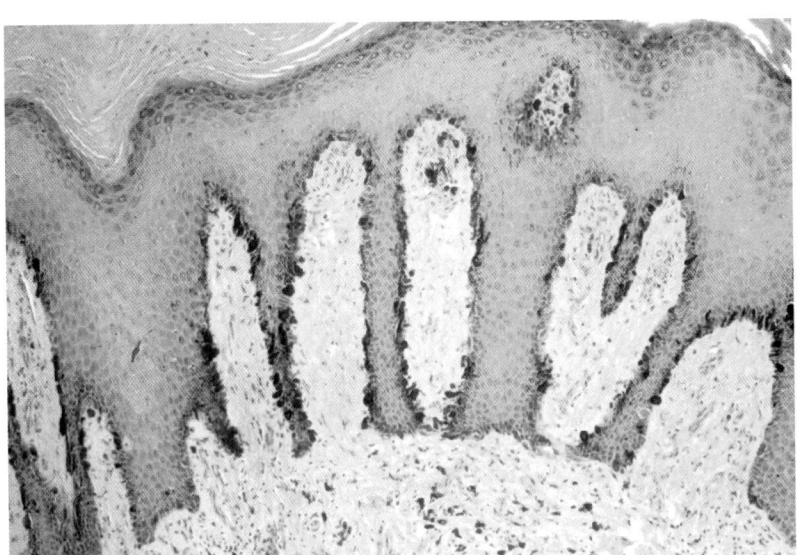

▲ **FIGURE 11-13** Acral melanoma. The epidermal is hyperplastic and exhibits characteristic lentiginous proliferation of pleomorphic melanoma cells.

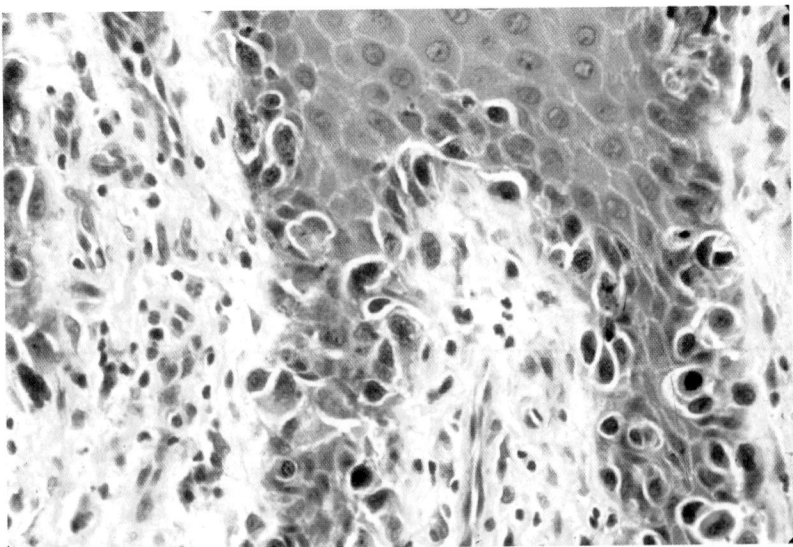

▲ **FIGURE 11-14** Acral melanoma. Higher magnification shows striking pleomorphism of melanoma cells.

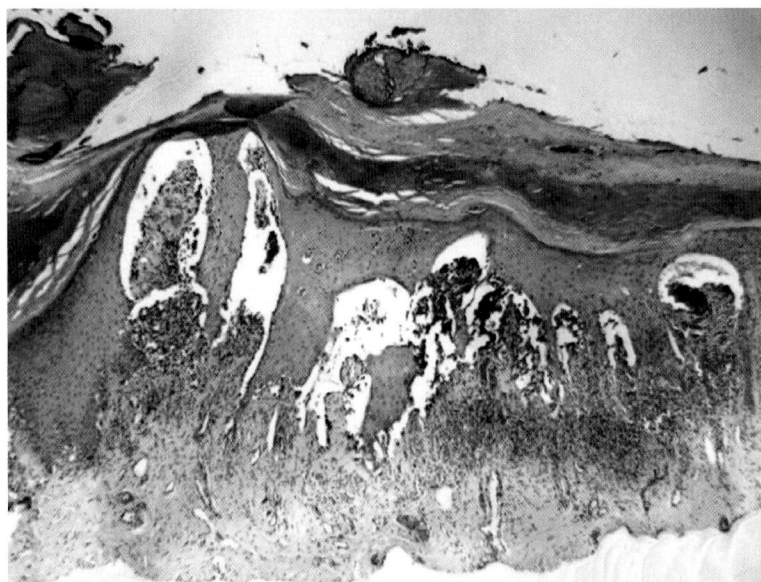

▲ **FIGURE 11-15** Acral melanoma. Hyperplastic epidermis exhibits irregular and confluent nesting of melanoma cells.

- Pigmented spindle cell tumor
- Squamous cell carcinoma, spindle cell type
- Atypical fibroxanthoma
- Cellular neurothekeoma
- Malignant peripheral nerve sheath tumor
- Angiosarcoma
- Kaposi's sarcoma
- Leiomyosarcoma

The differential diagnosis for acral melanoma primarily includes lentigines and lentiginous melanocytic nevi of acral skin. Lentigines of acral skin usually do not exhibit the frequency of melanocytic proliferation or cytologic atypia that is typical of acral melanoma.[9] Occasional acral nevi may have alarming features such as upward migration of cells throughout the epidermis, prominent lentiginous melanocytic proliferation, and some degree of cytologic atypia. Although upward migration may be noted in acral nevi, particularly in children, the constituent cells seldom reveal more than low-grade cytologic atypia and the pattern of pagetoid spread is usually orderly and confined to the lowermost epidermis. Other characteristics of acral nevi include regular size, spacing, and cohesive qualities of the junctional nesting. One particular note of caution is that well-differentiated acral melanoma may exhibit dermal components with little or no inflammatory response. In such cases, careful evaluation for cytologic atypia, necrotic cells, and mitotic activity are helpful in recognizing melanoma.

"NODULAR" MELANOMA

BOX 11-12   Summary

- *Clinical Features*
  - Age 30–70 years (often 40–50 but any age)
  - Men = women
  - Any site especially trunk dorsal surfaces of hands
  - 0.4 to 5 cm
  - Often rapid evolution, e.g., 4 month to 2 years
  - Papule or nodule, pigmented or amelanotic (advanced)
    ➤ Often protuberant, polypoid
    ➤ Black, blue-black, pink

- Ulceration, bleeding
- Asymmetry but symmetry may be present
- Often well-defined borders
- *Histopathologic Criteria*
- Dome-shaped polypoid or sessile tumor often
- May be pedunculated
- Asymmetry
- Epidermis commonly thinned, effaced, ulcerated
- Overlying intraepidermal component may or may not be present and usually does not extend peripherally beyond dermal invasive tumor
- Pagetoid spread, lentiginous melanocytic proliferation, intraepithelial nesting may be present
- Cohesive aggregate or aggregates of tumor cells fill subjacent dermis, subcutis
- Usually no maturation
- Host response at base and/or tumor-infiltrating lymphocytes common
- Epithelioid cells often comprise invasive component but spindle cells, small cuboidal cells common and often heterogeneity is present
- Partial regression relatively uncommon
- Precursor nevus present ~6% of cases

Scanning magnification discloses a raised, dome-shaped, or polypoid tumor often but not always exhibiting some asymmetry (Fig. 11-16).[1–9,13] The epidermis over the tumor is usually thin, effaced, and may be ulcerated. Variable upward migration of melanoma cells in the epidermis may be present but intraepidermal spread should not extend beyond the margins of the tumor. The dermal component is typified by a cohesive nodule or smaller nests of tumor cells having a pushing or expansile pattern of growth (Fig. 11-16). The tumor cells

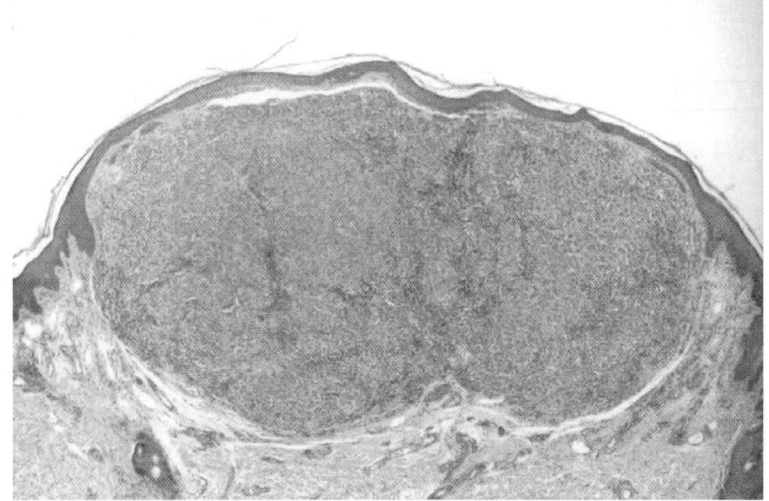

▲ **FIGURE 11-16** "Nodular" melanoma. The tumor has an asymmetrical dome-shaped configuration.

most frequently are epithelioid. However, other cell types including spindle cells and small epithelioid cells resembling nevus cells may predominate or be admixed with other cell types.[1–9]

Differential Diagnosis

"Nodular" melanoma (NM) may be confused with metastatic melanoma, Spitz tumor, and atypical varieties of cellular blue nevus, squamous cell carcinoma, atypical fibroxanthoma, fibrous histiocytoma, leiomyosarcoma, myoid fibroma, cellular capillary hemangioma, and Kaposi's sarcoma. Epidermotropic metastatic melanoma involving the papillary dermis may prove difficult to distinguish from NM.[38] Metastatic melanoma is often fairly monomorphous with little stromal response while NM are often polymorphous and exhibit greater stromal response. However, distinction may be impossible in certain cases and discrimination must rely on clinical information and clinical course.

Spitz tumors, particularly those with atypia, enter into the differential diagnosis of NM. Clinical information is pertinent to the diagnosis since melanoma is uncommon in the young, whereas atypical lesions are more suspicious for melanoma in adults.

On occasion, nonmelanocytic lesions are considered in the differential diagnosis of melanoma. The principal conditions include Paget's disease, either mammary or extramammary, squamous cell carcinoma *in situ*, sebaceous carcinoma, epidermotropic eccrine carcinoma, cutaneous T cell lymphoma, and other epidermotropic carcinomas. In most instances, the dilemma can be resolved simply by careful attention to histologic details in routinely stained sections.[39]

UNUSUAL VARIANTS OF MELANOMA

These rare variants of melanoma exhibit a continuum of histologic features corresponding to the neuroectodermal origin of the melanocyte.[7–9,40–56] The phenotype of the tumor may thus include any combination of the following:

1. *Desmoplasia*—fibroblast-like spindle cells usually in fascicles (predominant pattern);

2. *Neurotropism (perineurial invasion)*—invasion of nerve structures by tumor cells;

3. *Neural differentiation (both Schwannian and perineurial)*—formation of nerve-like structures recapitulating perineurium and endoneurium or delicate sheets of spindle cells reminiscent of neurofibroma, and less commonly myofibrocytic or neuroendocrine differentiation, as in Merkel cell carcinoma.

Desmoplastic Melanoma (DM)

DM most frequently arises in association with lentiginous melanomas,[9,46,47] however, *de novo* variants of desmoplastic melanoma also occur.[47]

The pathogenesis of desmoplasia and the true nature of the spindle cells in desmoplastic melanoma remain a subject of controversy.[41,42] Some authors maintain that the fibroplasia results from the induction of collagen synthesis by benign fibroblasts while others believe that melanoma cells function as adaptive fibroblasts to promote collagenization in these tumors. The latter conclusion is based on ultrastructural and immunohistochemical studies, and because melanocytes are capable of collagen production as well as melanin synthesis and schwannian differentiation.

CLINICAL FEATURES The usual presentation is as a raised, firm nodule that is skin-colored or associated with variable pigmentation (Fig. 11-17).[20,40,43–47] The

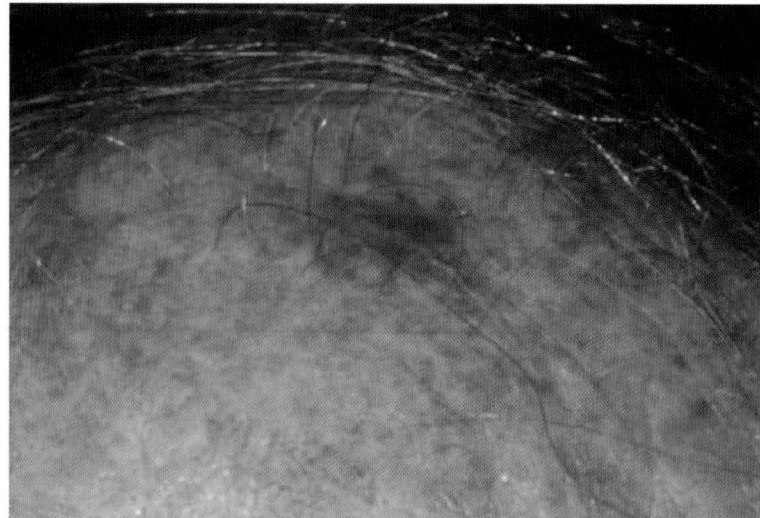

▲ **FIGURE 11-17** Desmoplastic melanoma involving vertex of scalp. The lesion is seen as a firm pink nodule.

irregular and variegated features of an associated intraepithelial component such as melanoma *in situ* may be the most visible feature of desmoplastic melanoma. Difficulty in recognizing desmoplastic melanoma, clinically and histologically, usually causes a delay in recognition and appropriate surgery.

HISTOPATHOLOGIC FEATURES Scanning magnification usually discloses a fibrous nodule displacing the normal dermal collagen or lamina propria and often extending into subcutaneous fat (Fig. 11-18).[40–47] Intraepidermal melanocytic proliferation is usually observed in the majority of cases.[47]

The most common histologic pattern of DM is a predominantly desmoplastic presentation.[47] Interspersed among dense collagenous fibers are individual spindle cells and variably sized fascicles of cells (Figs. 11-19 and 11-20). The nuclei may show minimal to pronounced pleomorphism and wavy or serpiginous nuclear morphology (Fig. 11-20), though most nuclei are enlarged with tapering contours. However, some nuclei are plump and occasional bizarre multinucleate giant cell forms are noted. Most desmoplastic melanomas lack pigment but occasional cells may contain fine melanin granules within cellular processes. The tumor stroma is usually fibrous, but myxoid alteration is occasionally encountered and uncommonly may be prominent. A finding typical of desmoplastic melanoma and useful in its recognition is variably dense perivascular lymphocytic infiltrates usually scattered throughout the tumor.[47] The tumor cells in desmoplastic melanoma are also notable for infiltrating walls of blood vessels (angiotropism). Mitotic figures are often scant, less than one or two per square millimeter, but can usually be found even in the most paucicellular forms of this tumor.[46,47]

Desmoplastic melanoma is usually diagnosed at an advanced stage, e.g., usually at least 4 or 5 mm in thickness and level IV or V.[43–48] Because of misdiagnosis, they are commonly first recognized as recurrent or metastatic tumors. Desmoplastic melanomas frequently recur (range 25 to 82%).[43–45] Based on a series of 45 cases, local recurrence was associated with the following factors: failure to diagnose the tumor correctly, inadequate surgery (resection margins less than 1 cm), location on the head and neck, anatomic level V, and thickness greater than 4 mm.[45] Failure to completely extirpate desmoplastic melanoma is related to the difficulty of assessing margins, infiltration of nerves, and the fact that they are usually amelanotic.

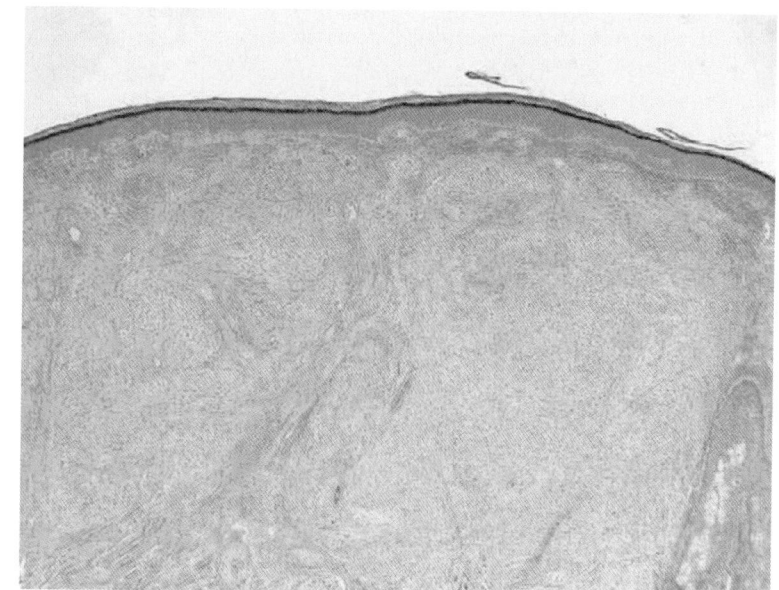

▲ **FIGURE 11-18** Desmoplastic melanoma. Fibrotic nodule occupies dermis.

Neurotropic Melanoma

BOX 11-15 Summary

- Neurotropic melanomas involve the perineurium and/or endoneurium of cutaneous nerves.
- Histologic clues to nerve involvement include the presence of hyperchromatic spindle cells in the perineurium or endoneurium and mucinous alteration of the nerve.
- Melanoma spindle cells involving cutaneous nerves usually show nuclear enlargement, hyperchromatism, and pleomorphism.

The term neurotropism refers to the involvement of perineurium and/or endoneurium of cutaneous nerves by melanoma cells (Fig. 11-21).[45,49–51] There may be considerable thickening of the perineurium and expansion of the endoneurial space by the tumor involvement. Extension of tumor along the cutaneous nerves may, however, be extensive and subtle. Histologic clues to nerve involvement include the presence of hyperchromatic spindle cells in the perineurium or endoneurium and mucinous alteration of the nerve.

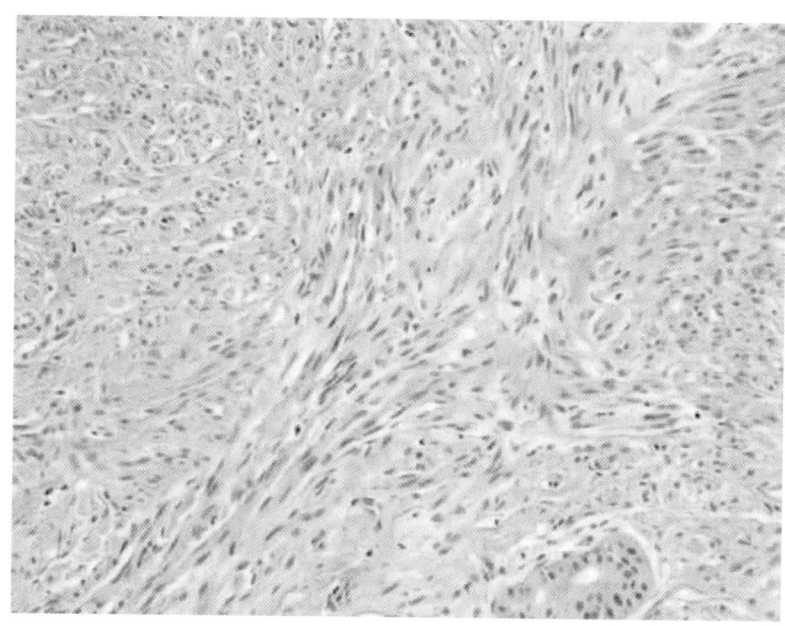

▲ **FIGURE 11-19** Desmoplastic melanoma showing intersecting fascicles of spindle cells with dense fibrous stroma.

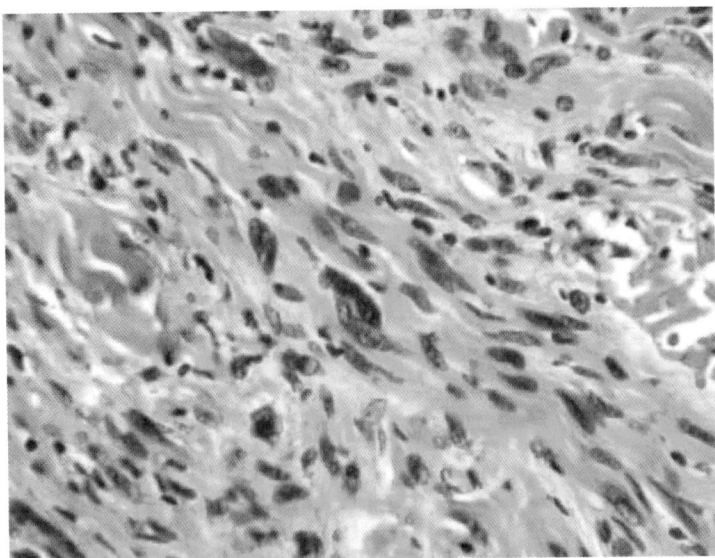

▲ **FIGURE 11-20** Desmoplastic melanoma. Spindled melanoma cells display nuclear pleomorphism and hyperchromatism.

- Desmoplastic (sclerosing) Spitz nevus
- Neurothekeoma, particularly cellular variants
- Malignant peripheral nerve sheath tumors
- Myxoma
- Dermatofibroma
- Dermatofibrosarcoma protuberans
- Atypical fibroxanthoma
- Malignant fibrous histiocytoma
- Scar
- Fibromatosis
- Spindle cell squamous cell carcinoma
- Leiomyosarcoma

Careful examination of cutaneous nerves at the surgical margins is mandatory to assess adequate excision. Melanoma spindle cells involving cutaneous nerves usually show nuclear enlargement, hyperchromatism, and pleomorphism.

The term neurotropic (or neurogenic) melanoma also describes neural or Schwannian differentiation in a pattern resembling peripheral nerve sheath tumors such as neurofibromas or neuromas and the recapitulation of perineurium and endoneurium.[45–47,49–51] The tumor cells in such areas are characterized by serpiginous or wavy nuclear configurations and filamentous cytoplasmic processes. The cells are embedded in a variably mucinous and fibrous stroma. In some instances, the stromal may be so sufficiently myxoid to suggest a myxoma. However, the tumor cells demonstrate loose fascicular arrangements, cytologic atypia, and occasional mitotic figures.

Differential Diagnosis

BOX 11-16 Summary

- Sclerosing blue nevi including variants with hypercellularity

The spectrum of tumors potentially confused with desmoplastic and neurotropic melanoma is varied and includes spindle cell proliferations and tumors with a fibrous appearance.[40,43–48] The principal lesions to be considered include sclerosing blue nevus,[46,47] desmoplastic Spitz tumor,[9] neurothekeoma,[57] malignant peripheral nerve sheath tumor, dermatofibroma, atypical fibroxanthoma, malignant fibrous histiocytoma, scar, fibromatosis, myxoma, spindle cell squamous cell carcinoma, and leiomyosarcoma.[46,47] The epidermal lentiginous melanocytic proliferation commonly found in desmoplastic melanoma is usually absent in the other conditions.

Sclerosing blue nevus and desmoplastic Spitz tumor both are characterized by an orderly infiltration of the fibrotic stroma and an overall benign cytologic appearance. Mitotic figures, usually encountered in desmoplastic melanoma, are exceedingly rare or absent in sclerosing blue nevus, but early forms of desmoplastic melanoma may be extremely difficult to distinguish from sclerosing blue nevus and it is vital to weigh all clinical and histologic features. For example, desmoplastic melanoma in a young individual on an anatomic site besides the head and neck or acral areas would be highly unusual and such circumstances would argue against a diagnosis of desmoplastic melanoma.

The desmoplastic Spitz tumor is characterized by symmetry, a wedge-shaped configuration, and infiltration of the dermis by relatively monotonous epithelioid or spindle cells, allowing its distinction from desmoplastic melanoma in most instances. Desmoplastic melanoma may also show a fascicular arrangement of cells that is generally lacking in desmoplastic Spitz tumor.

Relatively cellular variants of neurothekeoma (nerve sheath myxoma) may suggest desmoplastic melanoma.[57] Neurothekeoma commonly arises in the head and neck region, as does desmoplastic melanoma. Neurothekeoma generally

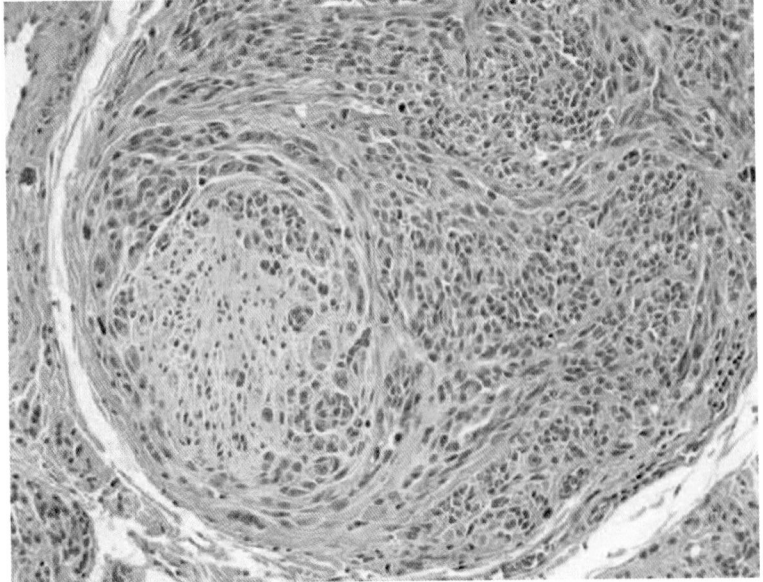

▲ **FIGURE 11-21** Desmoplastic-neurotropic melanoma. A cutaneous nerve shows pronounced nodular perineurial and endoneurial infiltration by melanoma cells (neurotropism).

occurs in young individuals (average age 20 years), does not demonstrate an intraepidermal melanocytic proliferation and is typified by a lobular architecture in the dermis. Concentric and fascicular arrangements of cells are often noted in neurothekeoma, the constituent cells may be epithelioid, or bipolar and stellate and multinucleate forms are seen. Low-grade nuclear pleomorphism and occasional mitotic figures are occasionally encountered. Distinction from desmoplastic melanoma is based on a regular, organized appearance, orderly infiltration of the dermis and a lesser degree of cytologic atypia.

Because of prominent Schwannian differentiation, discrimination of desmoplastic-neurotropic melanoma from peripheral nerve sheath tumors may be difficult or impossible. All clinical and histologic characteristics must be considered. Tumors of the head and neck of elderly patients associated with lentiginous melanomas are usually not a diagnostic problem. Tumors in other anatomic sites without an intraepidermal component will cause difficulty and immunohistochemistry may be of particular value in them.[47,52,58,59]

Lesions demonstrating fibrous or fibrohistiocytic differentiation figure prominently in the differential diagnosis of desmoplastic melanoma and include dermatofibroma (fibrous histiocytoma), juvenile xanthogranuloma, dermatofibrosarcoma protuberans and atypical fibroxanthoma, superficial forms of malignant fibrous histiocytoma, scar, and fibromatosis. These lesions generally lack intraepidermal melanocytic proliferation, melanin pigment, and neurotropism. Atypical fibroxanthoma and malignant fibrous histiocytoma enter the differential diagnosis and often require immunohistochemical evaluation, though they may contain xanthoma cells, not usually seen in desmoplastic melanoma. Fibrohistiocytic tumors as a general rule do not display neurotropism.

Desmoplastic melanomas with extensive mucin may raise problems of differential diagnosis, suggesting, e.g., a myxoma. However, myxomas generally lack the cytologic atypia and neurotropism of desmoplastic-neurotropic melanoma and the myxomatous variants of desmoplastic melanoma usually have zones of prominent cellularity.

Spindle cell squamous carcinoma and cutaneous leiomyosarcoma may be confused with desmoplastic melanoma, but neither entity usually shows intraepidermal melanocytic proliferation or melanin synthesis. Squamous cell carcinoma may show keratinization, dyskeratosis, and intercellular bridges. Leiomyosarcoma may exhibit the cytologic characteristics of smooth muscle cells, but immunohistochemistry may be essential for diagnosis (desmin and/or actin expression).

Because of the serious consequences of this tumor, immunohistochemistry is needed in most desmoplastic melanomas to confirm the diagnosis. Almost 100% of desmoplastic-neurotropic melanomas demonstrate immunoreactivity with antibodies against vimentin, S-100 protein, and p75 neurotrophin receptor[47,48,52,56,58,59] but uniquely almost all are negative for HMB-45, Mart-1, MITF, and tyrosinase. If there is positive immunostaining for HMB-45 and the latter markers in DM, it involves nondesmoplastic foci only, i.e., an intraepidermal component or superficial dermal focus of conventional melanoma cells.[47] A battery of markers must be utilized to evaluate such tumors. Other antibodies with variable reactivity with desmoplastic melanoma are neuron specific enolase and NK1/C3. Antibodies against keratin, desmin, actin, and Leu-7 (specific for peripheral nerve sheath differentiation but is negative in melanocytic tumors), in general, are negative in desmoplastic melanoma.[47]

ANGIOTROPIC MELANOMA

BOX 11-17 Summary

- *Clinical Features*
  - Age 30–70 years (often 40–50 years, but any age)
  - Men = women
  - Any site
  - 0.4–5 cm
- *Histopathologic Criteria*
  - Any type of melanoma
  - Melanoma cells cuff microvessels in pericytic location
  - Often at least level IV
  - Increased frequency of neurotropism

Angiotropic melanoma has been reported anecdotally in the literature, more as a curiosity than as an important biological entity. However, importance of angiotropism as a biological phenomenon and prognostic factor in localized melanoma and as the likely correlate of *extravascular migratory metastasis* has recently been emphasized.[60–63] Angiotropism is observed much more frequently than vascular invasion, e.g., in a series of 650 consecutive invasive melanomas, the frequency of vascular/lymphatic invasion was 1.4%.[15] In a recently published study of metastasing melanomas carefully matched with non-metastasizing melanomas for Breslow thickness, age, gender, and site, the presence of angiotropism strongly correlated with the development of metastases whereas vascular invasion was not observed in any cases.[64]

Angiotropic melanoma is defined by the cuffing of (the close opposition to) the external surfaces of either blood or lymphatic channels (in a *pericyte-like location*), or both, by aggregates of melanoma cells in at least two or more foci (Fig. 11-22).[63] By definition there is no tumor present within vascular lumina. Angiotropic foci

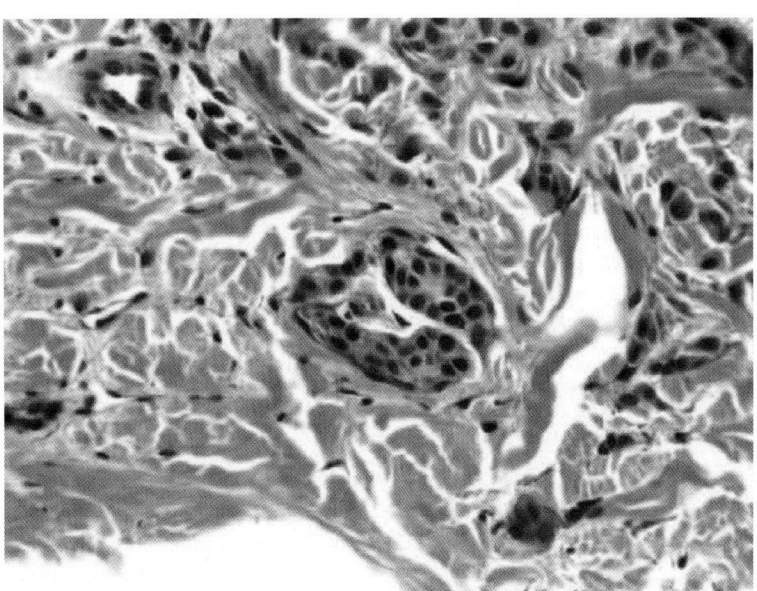

▲ **FIGURE 11-22** Angiotropic melanoma. Melanoma cells cuff microvessel in dermis without intravasation.

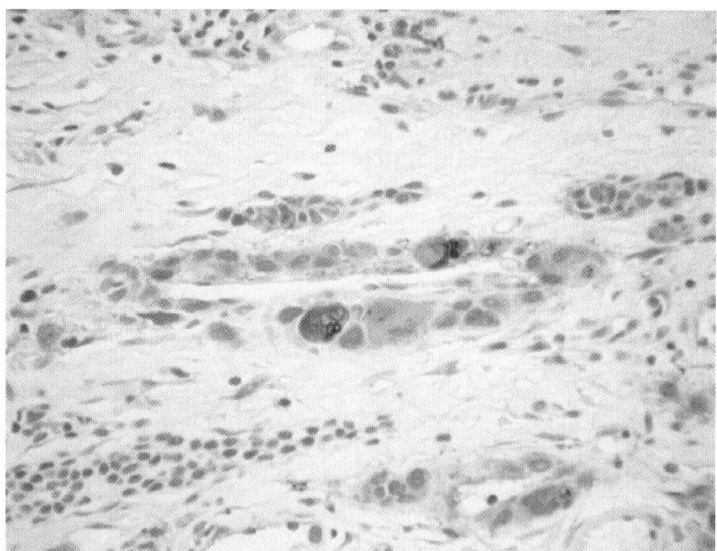

▲ **FIGURE 11-23** Angiotropic melanoma. Immunostaining of angiotropic melanoma cells with S100 protein.

must be located either at the advancing front of the tumor or some distance (usually within 1 to 2 mm) from the main tumoral mass. Although angiotropism is likely to be present within the mass of an invasive tumor, there is no specific means at present to differentiate simple entrapment of vessels by tumor from angiotropism. Immunohistochemisty with markers such as S100 protein or Mart-1 may aid in the identification or confirmation of angiotropism (Fig. 11-23). Angiotropism is observed with greater frequency in melanomas also demonstrating desmoplasia and neurotropism suggesting closely related mechanisms.

NEVOID MELANOMA

BOX 11-18 Summary

- *Clinical Features*
  - Women = men
  - All ages, commonly fifth decade
  - Occurs anywhere, but trunk and lower extremities most common
  - No distinctive features, but may have verrucous appearance
  - Any size, often relatively small diameter but up to 2 cm or more
- *Histopathologic Features*
  - Striking resemblance to banal compound or dermal nevus at scanning magnification
  - Symmetry common
  - Well-circumscribed lateral margins
  - Pagetoid spread not common
  - Often limited intraepidermal component
  - Relatively small nevus-like cells, monomorphous appearance
  - Some maturation may be present but often incomplete or absent
  - Single-cell infiltration at base
  - Cytologic atypia
    - ➤ Nuclear pleomorphism
    - ➤ Angulated nuclei
    - ➤ Hyperchromatism
    - ➤ Prominent nucleoli may be present
  - Mitoses in dermal component, particularly deep
  - Infiltration of adnexal structures
  - Little or no inflammation

In very broad terms, the term "nevoid" melanoma could connote any form of melanoma having some resemblance to or mimicking any type of melanocytic nevus.[65–68] An objection to this term is that a large number of melanomas may more or less resemble banal nevi and that the application of the term may be rather subjective. A variety of other terms have been employed to describe this general group of melanomas depending upon how stringent are the criteria for inclusion, e.g., minimal deviation melanoma, verrucous and pseudonevoid melanoma and closely related terms (see below), Spitzoid melanoma, small-diameter melanoma, and small cell melanoma. Some nevoid melanomas might also be characterized as having a small diameter or small melanoma cells, i.e., small cell melanoma. However, the term is used rather restrictively in this chapter (as have most other authors) to describe melanomas that closely resemble ordinary compound or dermal nevi; the latter lesions generally fall into four groups: (1) those with a raised, dome-shaped or poly-poid (nodular nonverrucous) configuration and resemble a predominately dermal nevus, (2) those with a distinctly papillomatous or verrucous surface, (3) those resembling a lentiginous melanocytic nevus arising in sun-exposed skin of older individuals, and (4) those with a predominately or exclusively intraepidermal nested appearance mimicking a junctional or compound nevus.

The importance of this rare group of melanomas cannot be overstated because of the profound diagnostic difficulty they pose to pathologists. The latter conclusion is simply based on the fact that many such lesions are often diagnosed only in retrospect after the development of recurrences or metastases.

The concept that melanomas may closely resemble melanocytic nevi probably dates back at least to the introduction of the term minimal deviation melanoma. Schmoeckel and his colleagues first coined the term "nevoid" melanoma in their description of 33 melanomas with histologic features suggesting a melanocytic nevus.[65] The latter authors noted that 15 patients developed metastases, and they concluded that nevoid melanoma did not seem to have any better prognosis than conventional melanoma. About 70 additional cases have subsequently been reported in the literature.[66–68]

Clinical Features

There are no distinctive clinical features compared to conventional melanomas; however, verrucous or papillomatous variants may suggest a verruca, seborrheic keratosis, or warty nevus. Most tumors reported have been in adults.

Histopathologic Features

The essential histopathologic criteria for diagnosis are as follows: (1) at scanning magnification, the lesion has a striking resemblance to an ordinary compound or dermal nevus (Figs. 11-24 and 11-25), (2) an overall symmetry (some asymmetry may be present), (3) a rather sharp circumscription at the peripheries of the lesion, (4) the absence of or often only a limited intraepidermal component, commonly with little or no pagetoid spread, (5) a monomorphous population of nevus-like cells in the dermis usually characterized by a confluent or sheet-like growth pattern in some portion of the lesion (Fig. 11-26), and (6) dermal mitotic figures.[9,65–68] Other features commonly but not invariably present that may suggest a banal nevus include diameter under 5 to 6 mm and changes suggesting maturation.

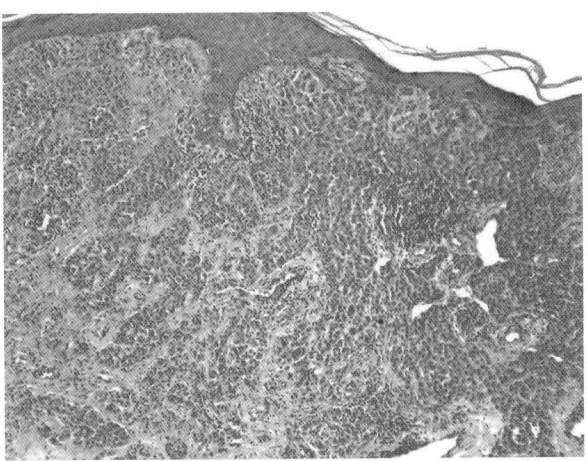

▲ **FIGURE 11-24** Nevoid melanoma. The lesion resembles a compound nevus at scanning magnification displaying striking hypercellularity.

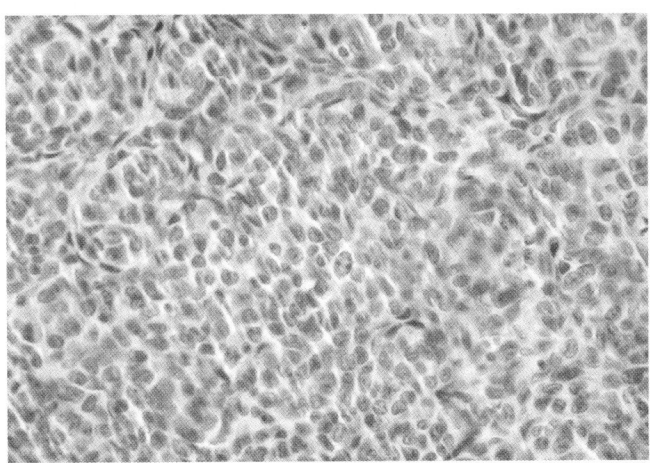

▲ **FIGURE 11-26** Verrucous small cell melanoma. The melanoma is comprised of sheets of small melanoma cells.

As mentioned above, there are four general morphologic variants: (1) the non-verrucous papular or nodular forms that present with only limited or no epidermal hyperplasia and (2) the verrucous or papillomatous variants that have the configuration suggesting a common verruca, seborrheic keratosis or papillomatous nevus (Fig. 11-25),[68–70] (3) the lentiginous variants arising in sun-exposed skin of older individuals,[71,72] and (4) the striking intraepidermal nested variants mimicking a junctional nevus (see earlier discussions).

As mentioned above, there may be no intraepidermal melanocytic component in a large proportion of cases. The intraepidermal component if present may be subtle or limited in nature. One may observe melanocytes arranged as single cells and/or in junctional nests along the dermal–epidermal junction. The latter nesting may result in conflu-

ence of nested aggregates of melanocytes replacing the basilar portion of the epidermis. The epidermis is frequently effaced, thinned, and associated with dermal–epidermal separation. Pagetoid spread may be present in a proportion of cases and is an important finding in confirming a diagnosis of melanoma; however, it is often not a conspicuous feature.

The principal finding in the dermis includes a sheet-like or confluent arrangement of relatively small cuboidal or polygonal melanocytes closely mimicking nevus cells. Often the dermale melanocytic population fills the papillary dermis and is closely opposed to the epidermis resulting in a strikingly crowded or hypercellular appreareance. In many cases, the melanocytes extend into the reticular dermis with some diminished cellular density and also some reduction in cellular and nuclear sizes suggesting some maturation. In some lesions, one

may observe fairly discreet nesting of melanocytes in some areas suggesting a nevus; however, other parts of the lesion usually demonstrate the confluence and hypercellulariy that favors melanoma. Furthermore, the heterogeneity of the lesion is another feature consonant with melanoma. Although the lateral margins are commonly well demarcated, the base of the melanoma is often poorly defined and characterized by the presence of single cells infiltrating collagen. In most instances, there is no host inflammatory response.

The melanocytes comprising NM at least in the superficial part of the lesion and perhaps throughout are generally polygonal or epithelioid cells (mimicking the so-called "type A" or epithelioid nevus cells) sufficiently small to suggest nevus cells. They, nonetheless, demonstrate definite but sometimes, subtle nuclear enlargement, pleomorphism, and often hyperchromatism; rather prominent nucleoli may be present. As mentioned above, many NM may suggest maturation, i.e., diminished cytoplasmic and nuclear diameters with depth and a transition to smaller "type B" or lymphocye-like cells and perhaps "type C" or Schwann-like cells. At the same time, the latter transition may be aocompanied by diminished cellularity with deph and loss of pigment synthesis. Nonetheless, major clues to diagnosis of NM are the presence of definite nuclear pleomorphism and in particular irregular nuclear contours, hyperchromatism, and nucleoli and continued pigment synthesis in the deepest parts of the dermal component. Generally, one observes well-defined nests of relatively small cuboidal cells in the deepest portions of NM with the latter characteristics.

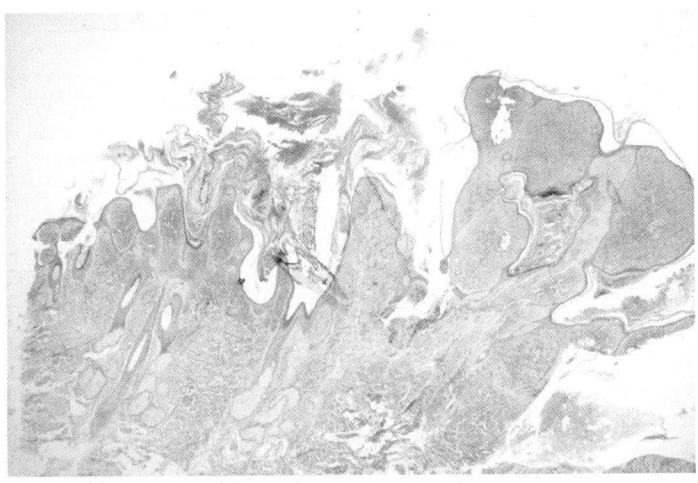

▲ **FIGURE 11-25** Verrucous small cell melanoma. The verrucoid epidermal configuration resembles a papillomatous nevus.

One of the most important and sometimes the single most important criterion for diagnosis is the presence of mitoses in the dermal component.[9,68] The latter finding is often the first clue to considering melanoma in the differential diagnosis. The presence of one or a small number of dermal mitoses does not constitute sufficient evidence for diagnosis of melanoma but it should prompt the histopathologist to search for additional criteria for melanoma and to either confirm or exclude the diagnosis (if possible). Mitoses are present in virtually all cases and their absence should provoke skepticism about melanoma. The mitotic rate is commonly relatively low, often less than six per square millimeter. Increasing mitotic rate, deeply situated mitoses, and atypical forms also provide progressively more support for NM. The author has found that the presence or absence of mitotic figures in the deepest portion of a lesion can be a decisive factor in confirming or ruling out NM.

Differential Diagnosis

BOX 11-19   Summary

- Papillomatous or cellular melanocytic nevi
- Metastatic melanoma

The principal dilemma is discrimination of such melanomas from melanocytic nevi, especially papillomatous dermal nevi, and metastatic melanoma. One's confidence in rendering a diagnosis of nevoid melanoma directly correlates with the number of abnormal features present. The following attributes are of critical importance in distinguishing NM from a nevus: (1) Dermal mitoses, usually muliple and scattered throughout the lesion are probably mandatory for the diagnosis. The higher the absolute mitotic rate and the more deeply located the mitoses, the more certain is the diagnosis. However, the presence of rare mitoses particularly in nevi in young or pregnant individuals and in nevi without atypia must be interpreted with caution and are not proof of NM. (2) Dermal aggregates or fascicles of melanocytes showing high density and confluence, having a sheet-like appearance throughout, or showing both features. The dermal population often demonstrates a monotonous appearance. (3) Cytologic atypia of melanocytes is mandatory for the diagnosis. By definition, there are lesser degrees of atypia than in conventional melanomas. Careful scrutiny at higher magnifications is necessary to establish the presence of cytologic atypia. In general, the melanocytes may be relatively small compared to the usual enlarged epithelioid melanoma cells and thus the resemblance to a nevus.

VERRUCOUS MELANOMA

BOX 11-20   Summary

- *Clinical Features*
  - Women = men
  - All ages, commonly fifth decade
  - Occurs anywhere, but trunk and lower extremities most common
  - Verrucous appearance
  - Any size, often relatively small diameter but up to 2 cm or more
- *Histopathologic Features*
  - Papillomatous epidermal hyperplasia
  - Common resemblance to banal compound or dermal nevus at scanning magnification
  - Symmetry common
  - Well-circumscribed lateral margins
  - Pagetoid spread not common
  - Often limited intraepidermal component
  - Relatively small nevus-like cells, monomorphous appearance
  - Some maturation may be present but often incomplete or absent
  - Single-cell infiltration at base
  - Cytologic atypia
    ➤ Nuclear pleomorphism
    ➤ Angulated nuclei
    ➤ Hyperchromatism
    ➤ Prominent nucleoli may be present
  - Mitoses in dermal component, particularly deep
  - Infiltration of adnexal structures
  - Little or no inflammation

Although verrucous melanoma was initially described in his classification of melanoma in 1967,[1] Clark subsequently discarded the term since he believed that its features could be present in any type of melanoma.[2] Recent reports have emphasized the prominent clinical and histologic verrucous features of such melanomas and also the difficulty in classifying many of these lesions.[69,70] Some of these melanomas might also be described as nevoid melanoma (see section titled "Nevoid Melanoma").

Clinical and Histopathologic Features

Most lesions are well circumscribed, 1 to 2 cm in diameter, and characterized by a dark-brown, black, or grayish appearance and hyperkeratotic verrucous surface and diagnosed clinically as seborrheic keratosis or papillomatous nevi.[69,70]

The most striking feature at scanning magnification is a fairly symmetrical lesion with prominent papillomatous or verrucoid epidermal hyperplasia suggesting a seborrheic keratosis, epidermal nevus, verruca, or papillomatous melanocytic nevus (Fig. 11-25). The intraepidermal melanocytic component may vary from minimal or absent or show prominent pagetoid spread. Also common is the frequent presence of a laterally extending intraepidermal component. Some of these tumors may show a contiguous basilar and suprabasilar proliferation of atypical melanocytes, often involving adnexal epithelium. In common with nevoid melanoma, the dermal component in some melanomas may show a startling resemblance to a dermal nevus.[67–70] The cell type in the latter tumors resembles a small nevus cell, but careful inspection should disclose prominent cellular pleomorphism, little or no maturation, and cells dispersed in confluent nests and sheets without orderly infiltration of stroma. The presence of mitotic figures (e.g., greater than two or three per section) and necrotic cells in the dermal component also argues against a benign process.

Differential Diagnosis

BOX 11-21   Summary

- Papillomatous or cellular melanocytic nevi

Verrucous melanoma may suggest nonmelanocytic tumors such as seborrheic keratosis, verruca, and epidermal nevus. However, the melanocytic nature of the lesion should become clear with careful inspection. Of particular concern is the potential misdiagnosis of verrucous melanoma as a benign nevus, especially a papillomatous dermal nevus.[9]

SMALL CELL MELANOMA

BOX 11-22   Summary

- *Clinical Features*
  - *High-grade small cell melanoma mimicking Merkel cell carcinoma*
    ➤ Extremely rare
    ➤ Adults (any age)
    ➤ Any site
    ➤ Often 0.4–2 cm
    ➤ Often amelanotic papule or nodule
  - *Small cell melanoma arising in predominately sun-damaged skin*
    ➤ Often >50 years of age (range 18–91)

- ➤ Men > women (2:1)
- ➤ Backs of men, legs of women
- ➤ Usually >1 cm
- ➤ Variegated color
- ➤ Often tan, brown, black, gray
- • *Histopathologic Features*
  - • *High-grade small cell melanoma mimicking Merkel cell carcinoma*
    - ➤ Melanin and intraepidermal involvement may or may not be present
    - ➤ Often cohesive nests, cords, sheets of small round cells
    - ➤ Cells with scant cytoplasm
    - ➤ Round to oval nuclei
    - ➤ Prominent mitotic rate and necrosis
  - • *Small cell melanoma arising in predominately sun-damaged skin*
    - ➤ Intraepidermal component often extensive, lentiginous and nested
    - ➤ Usually some pagetoid spread
    - ➤ Elongated epidermal rete ridges common
    - ➤ Effacement and thinning of epidermis also common
    - ➤ Small cuboidal melanocytes with scant cytoplasm
    - ➤ Melanocytes larger that those in nevi
    - ➤ Nuclear pleomorphism
    - ➤ Irregular nuclear contours
    - ➤ Dense chromatin
    - ➤ Prominent nucleoli
    - ➤ Dermal nests often large, nodular, cohesive, anatomosing
    - ➤ Often absence of maturation
    - ➤ Continued pigment synthesis with depth
    - ➤ Mitotic figures rare
    - ➤ Solar elastosis
    - ➤ Host response with fibroplasia, partial regression common

The term small cell melanoma has been introduced into the literature to describe a heterogenous assortment of melanomas from several settings perhaps related only by the common denominator of *small* melanoma cells. This term has been used to refer to (1) rare melanomas developing in children and adolescents on the scalp,[9] (2) melanomas developing in congenital melanocytic nevi of children and adolescents,[9] (3) melanomas developing in any setting but particularly adults that resemble small round cell malignancies such as Merkel cell carcinoma,[73] (4) melanomas developing in sun-damaged of older individuals in a setting of solar melanocytic neoplasia or atypical lentiginous nevi,[71,72,74] and (5) melanomas in adults that have the characteristics of nevoid melanoma, as described above. Since there is considerable overlap of small cell melanomas and

nevoid melanomas in adults (see the previous section), the following section will deal only with two entities.

1. Small cell melanoma mimicking Merkel cell (neuroendocrine carcinoma);
2. Exceptionally rare melanomas that mimic high-grade small round cell malignancies.

Small cell melanoma mimicking Merkel cell (neuroendocrine carcinoma)

These variants of melanoma are so rare that one can only make anecdotal remarks about them.[73] Perhaps they have been most commonly recognized as metastases presumably indicating progression or de-differentiation to high-grade blastlike tumors. Nonetheless, primary tumors occur in adults. The lesions are primarily defined by a small round cell population arranged in nests, cords, and sheets. Melanin and intrepidermal involvement may or may not be present. These tumors feature cells with scant cytoplasm, round to oval nuclei, high mitotic rates, and scattered nectrotic cells. Amelanotic tumors resemble neuroendocrine carcinoma, primary or metastatic; lymphoma; other small cell carcinomas; and metastatic small cell carcinoma of the lung. Immunohistochemisty is of fundamental importance for confirming a melanocytic origin versus the other entities mentioned above. In particular, neuroendocrine carcinoma, metastatic small cell carcinoma of the lung, and other small cell carcinomas may show intraepidermal involvement including nesting and pagetoid spread.

Small Cell Melanomas Arising Predominately in Sun-Damaged Skin of Elderly Individuals

Another variant of small cell melanoma, that also might be subsumed under the general category of "nevoid melanoma", occurring in sun damaged skin of individuals generally over the age of 50 years has been proposed by Kossard and Wilkinson[71,72] and Blessing et al.[74] While undoubtedly some proportion of or many these lesions may in fact be melanoma, the banal appearance of and resemblance of such lesions to lentiginous nevi, a negligible mitotic rate, and the lack of follow-up call into question the diagnosis of melanoma. Thus, the latter group of 131 cases may possibly include an admixtue of atypical nevi,

biologically indeterminate lesions, and melanomas. Although the author is confident that this entity exists, it is certain that these lesions as a group require further study.

CLINICAL FEATURES Such lesions generally develop in sun-exposed skin of older individuals with about 80% being 50 years or older (range 18 to 91 years).[72] Men outnumber women by a ratio of about 2:1. These tumors are most common on the backs of men and the lower extremities of women.

HISTOPATHOLOGIC FEATURES The lesions described by Kossard and Wilkinson suggest a lentiginous junctional or compound nevus at scanning magnification. Features favoring melanoma include large diameter, i.e., up to 1 cm or more, asymmetry, poorly defined margins, effacement and atrophy of the epidermis, host response including partial regression, large junctional and dermal nests of melanocytes that tend to confluence, some pagetoid spread often subtle, and the lack of maturation (Fig. 11-26).

Differential Diagnosis

BOX 11-23   Summary

- • *High-grade small cell melanoma mimicking Merkel cell carcinoma*
  - • Metastatic melanoma
  - • Primary and metastatic neuroendocrine carcinoma
  - • Metastatic small cell carcinoma
  - • Lymphoma
  - • Other small round cell malignancies
- • *Small cell melanoma arising in predominately sun-damaged skin*
  - • Atypical lentiginous nevi of sun-exposed skin

Distinguishing such lesions from atypical lentiginous compound nevi is the major challenge; some lesions prove so difficult that they can only be categorized as biologically indeterminate. Unfortunately, since dermal mitoses are generally rare or absent, a major aid to diagnosis is lacking. Of particular utility is the recognition of melanoma *in situ* and contiguity of the latter with the dermal component. Effacement and thinning of the epidermis, confluent nesting of melanocytes along the dermal–epidermal junction, some pagetoid spread, and sufficient atypia of the melanocytes allow for a diagnosis of intraepidermal melanoma.

SPITZOID MELANOMA

BOX 11-24 Summary

- *Clinical Features*
  - Women = men
  - Any age
  - Occurs anywhere
  - Any appearance
  - Any size, often relatively small diameter but up to 2 cm or more
- *Histopathologic Features*
  - Plaque-type, dome-shaped, or polypoid configuration
  - Epidermal hyperplasia common
  - Striking resemblance to Spitz tumor at scanning magnification
  - Asymmetry common
  - Size often >1 cm
  - Usually enlarged epithelioid to spindled melanocytes
  - Diminished or absent maturation
  - Mitotic rate >2–6 mm^2
  - Cytologic atypia
    - ➤ Nuclear pleomorphism
    - ➤ Angulated nuclei
    - ➤ Hyperchromatism
    - ➤ Prominent nucleoli may be present
  - Mitoses deep

The term Spitzoid melanoma if used at all should be reserved for melanomas that truly have a striking morphologic resemblance to Spitz tumors.[9,75] The term probably best describes a rare group of tumors often developing in young individuals that are only diagnosed as melanoma in retrospect, i.e., after the development of metastases and an aggressive course.

Differential Diagnosis

BOX 11-25 Summary

- Atypical Spitz tumor

Given the profound difficulty of distinguishing some Spitz or Spitz-like tumors from melanoma, the author discourages the use of term Spitzoid melanoma since it may result in the indiscriminate labeling of a heterogeneous group of lesions including benign Spitz tumors, lesions that are biologically indeterminant, conventional melanomas, and also a rare controversial group of tumors previously termed "metastasizing Spitz nevus/tumor." The latter group of lesions includes some that have given rise to single lymph node metastases without subsequent recurrence of melanoma on long-term follow-up.

The authors recommend such melanocytic proliferations be categorized if at all possible into one of the following groups: (1) Spitz tumor, (2) Spitz-like melanocytic tumor with atypical features (atypical Spitz tumor) and possibly indeterminate biological potential (describing the abnormal features present such as large size, deep involvement, ulceration, lack of maturation, mitotic rate, presence of deep mitoses), and (3) melanoma.

MELANOMA ARISING IN COMPOUND OR DERMAL NEVI

BOX 11-26 Summary

- *Clinical Features*
  - Women = men
  - All ages, commonly 40–60 years
  - Occurs anywhere, but head and neck most common
  - Any size, often larger that ordinary nevi
  - Often history of recent change or enlargement
- *Histopathologic Features*
  - Often eccentric and/or asymmetrical nodule in melanocytic nevus
  - Nodule shows confluence and hypercellularity
  - Often abrupt interface with surrounding nevus
  - Lack of maturation
  - Cytologic atypia
    - ➤ Nuclear pleomorphism
    - ➤ Angulated nuclei
    - ➤ Hyperchromatism
    - ➤ Prominent nucleoli may be present
  - Mitoses in dermal component >2–3/mm^2

The development of melanoma in the dermal component of an acquired nevus is an uncommon or rare event.[76–78] Some of these melanomas may originate from adnexal-associated nevus elements.

Clinical and Histopathologic Features

Most patients are approximately 40 to 60 years of age and the most common site is the head and neck area.[77] The lesions are often larger than ordinary dermal nevi, e.g., 1 to 2 cm, and there is usually a history of recent change or enlargement.

Usually within an otherwise ordinary dermal nevus, one encounters a distinct nodule of cytologically atypical melanocytes.[77] There is usually an abrupt transition from the ordinary dermal nevus component to the nodular aggregate of atypical cells. The latter cells are most commonly enlarged with abundant cytoplasm and pleomorphic nuclei. Mitotic figures are found usually within the cellular nodule.

Differential Diagnosis

BOX 11-27 Summary

- Cellular nodules (typical or atypical) present in melanocytic nevi

The most obvious dilemma is the differentiation of a focus of melanoma from dermal nevus, especially a nevus with cytologically bizarre nevus cells as in ancient schwannoma or a distinct focus of epithelioid or fusiform cells, i.e., MNPH or the so-called "combined" nevus, "inverted type A" nevus, or melanocytic nevus with focal dermal epithelioid cell component or dermal nodules.[9] The nodular area in question should demonstrate a cohesive or expansile aggregate of cells with unequivocal cytologic atypia. Although these melanocytic cells will usually have a monomorphous or clonal appearance, inspection of individual cells should disclose substantial nuclear pleomorphism and often-prominent nucleoli and hyperchromatism. Mitotic figures should also be present in this focus. A dermal nevus with bizarre or ancient cytologic features usually does not show mitoses. One should also consider clinical factors such as the age of the patient (melanoma usually in persons greater than 40 years of age), size (such lesions are often >1 cm in diameter), and history of recent change or enlargement. On the other hand, MNPH are often present in younger individuals, are characterized by a small dark nodule or papule in a relatively small symmetric nevus, and are characterized usually by low-grade or no cytologic atypia of the epithelioid/fusiform cells. Often the latter cells display prominent melaninization of melanocytes and are accompanied by melanophages.

MALIGNANT MELANOMA ORIGINATING FROM OR RESEMBLING A BLUE NEVUS (MALIGNANT BLUE NEVUS)

BOX 11-28 Summary

- *Clinical Features*
  - Two-thirds men
  - All ages, mean age about 46 years

- All ages, mean age about 46 years
- Scalp most common site
- Usually >1–2 cm
- Blue-black multinodular appearance
- *Histopathologic Features*
- Often overtly malignant component juxtaposed to benign usually cellular blue nevus
- Nodule shows confluence and hypercellularity
- Often abrupt interface with surrounding nevus
- Lack of maturation
- Cytologic atypia
  ➤ Nuclear pleomorphism
  ➤ Angulated nuclei
  ➤ Hyperchromatism
  ➤ Prominent nucleoli may be present
- Sarcoma-like presentation without distinct benign and malignant components
  ➤ Hypercellular fascicles or nodules
- Cellular blue nevus-like lesion with additional atypical features
  ➤ Mitoses in dermal component >2–3/mm^2

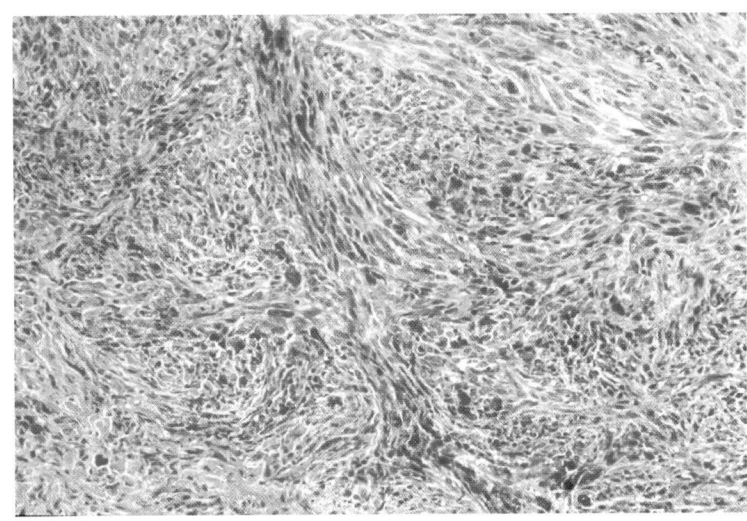

▲ **FIGURE 11-27** Malignant blue nevus (melanoma arising in association with a cellular blue nevus). Fascicular arrangements of atypical spindle cells, many of which contain melanin, can be observed in this field.

Malignant blue nevus (MBN) is an extremely rare form of melanoma originating from or associated with a preexisting blue nevus and characterized by a dense proliferation of variably pigmented spindle cells without involvement of the epidermis. Approximately 80 cases of MBN have thus far been reported.[9,79–82]

Clinical Features

The average age at diagnosis is 46 years, two-thirds of the patients are men, and the commonest site is the scalp. MBN most frequently present as blue or blue-black plaques or nodules ranging from 1 to 4 cm (mean 2.9 cm),[79–82] that are often multinodular. There is usually a history of recent enlargement or change in a previously stable blue nevus. MBN are highly aggressive with metastasis to lymph nodes and a variety of visceral sites.

Histopathologic Features

MBN usually presents in one of three patterns: (1) a lesion with an overtly malignant component (Fig. 11-27) juxtaposed to a benign blue nevus component, usually a CBN, (2) a more subtle sarcoma-like presentation (without florid benign and malignant components) initially suggesting CBN but exhibiting large densely cellular fascicles or nodules of spindle cells that on closer inspection have sufficient atypicality for malignancy and are distinctly more abnormal that the usual small fascicular

or alveolar patterns in CBN, and (3) a lesion suggesting a benign CBN with additional atypical features such as large diameter, asymmetry, prominent cellular density, nuclear pleomorphism, and some mitotic activity at least focally but not obviously malignant that subsequently results in malignant behavior (the author terms such lesions biologically indeterminate). In the most common presentation MBN are characterized by nodular or multinodular aggregations of spindle cells in tightly packed fascicles in the dermis and often the subcutis (Figs. 11-27). By definition, there is sparing of the epidermis. Occasional epithelioid cells and multinucleate giant cells are encountered. Melanin pigment and cytoplasmic vacuolization are noted in approximately two-thirds of cases.[81] Necrosis, a feature previously thought characteristic of MBN, is observed in only about one-third of cases.[82] In general, there is striking cytologic atypia, prominent nuclear pleomorphism, infrequent mitotic figures (approximately one to two mitoses per square millimeter) and uncommonly atypical mitoses. Most MBN have a component of cellular blue nevus (CBN), but elements of common blue nevus (pigmented dendritic melanocytes, fibrosis, and melanophages) and rarely nevus of Ota or Ito may be observed.

Differential Diagnosis

BOX 11-29   Summary

- Cellular blue nevus and atypical variants
- Metastatic melanoma
- Clear cell sarcoma

MBN must be distinguished from CBN and its atypical variants (see differential diagnosis for CBN)[9,81,82] and primary or metastatic melanoma, and clear cell sarcoma. Because there are no histologic features specific for MBN, a contiguous remnant of blue nevus should be identified or a history of an antecedent blue nevus documented to distinguish MBN from either nodular or metastatic melanoma.

■ BALLOON CELL MELANOMA

BOX 11-30   Summary

- No distinctive clinical features
- At least 50% of melanoma cells have abundant vacuolated cytoplasms
- Balloon cells are large round or polyhedral cells with clear or eosinophilic cytoplasms
- The nuclei are irregularly placed and exhibit only slight to moderate atypia

Balloon cell melanoma (BCM) exhibits ballooning in at least 50% of the melanoma cells.[83,84] The individual "balloon cells' have abundant vacuolated cytoplasms that impart a clear cell appearance. Knowledge of BCM is important so that it is distinguished from the much more common balloon cell nevus and from other clear cell tumors of the skin. BCM is reported to have a particular propensity for multiple skin and subcutaneous metastases.[83]

Clinical and Histopathologic Features

There were no distinctive clinical features of BCM. The balloon cells are large, round, or polygonal cells with clear or eosinophilic, slightly granular cytoplasm.[83,84] The nuclei are irregularly placed and exhibit only slight to moderate atypia. Mitotic activity is also generally low. Melanin has been noted in about a quarter of cases.[84] Metastases from BCM often show balloon cell change but maybe difficult to diagnosis because of they are amelanotic and fail to exhibit nesting. Virtually all BCM studied thus far show positive immunostaining with S-100 protein and HMB-45.[84] A small number may be positive for carcinoembryonic antigen.

Differential Diagnosis

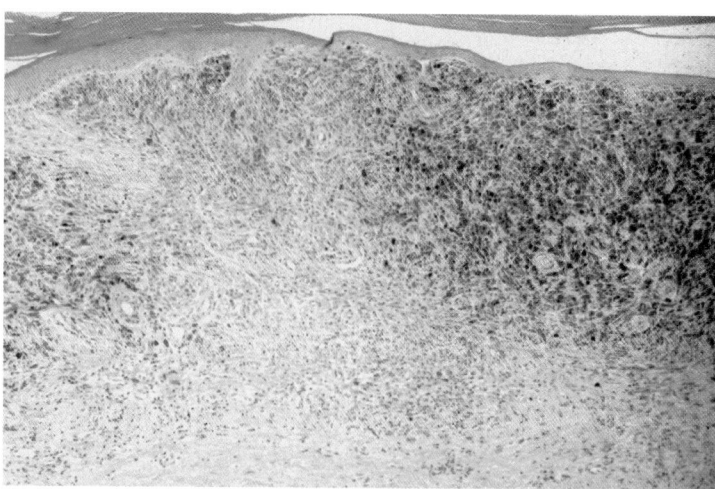

▲ **FIGURE 11-28** Tumoral melanosis. There is complete regression of melanoma with residual aggregates of melanophages.

BOX 11-31   Summary

- Balloon cell nevus
- Xanthoma
- Hibernoma
- Granular cell tumor
- Primary and metastatic clear cell carcinomas, such as renal cell carcinoma
- Liposarcoma
- Clear cell cutaneous appendageal tumors
- Metastatic melanoma

BCM may be confused with balloon cell nevus, xanthoma, hibernoma, granular cell tumor, metastatic clear cell carcinomas such as renal cell or adenocarcinoma, liposarcoma, and clear cell appendage tumors.[83,84] Perhaps, the greatest problem is distinction of BCM from balloon cell nevus. In general, balloon cell nevi occur in young individuals (under age 30 years), show "maturation" of nevus cells (decreased size of cells and nuclei with depth), the presence of multinucleate giant cells, in contrast to BCM that tends to develop in older patients, to lack "maturation" of melanoma cells, and to have cellular atypia and mitotic activity.

REGRESSION

BOX 11-32   Summary

- *Early (or active)*: Zone of papillary dermis and epidermis within a recognizable melanoma, characterized by dense infiltrates of lymphocytes disrupting/replacing nests of melanoma cells within the papillary dermis and possibly the epidermis, as compared to adjoining zones of tumor; degenerating melanoma cells should be recognizable. There is no obvious fibrosis.
- *Intermediate*: Zone of papillary dermis and epidermis within a recognizable

melanoma, characterized by reduction (loss) in the amount of tumor (a disruption in the continuity of the tumor) or absence of tumor in papillary dermis and possibly within the epidermis, compared to adjacent zones of tumor, and replaced by varying admixtures of lymphoid cells and increased fibrous tissue (as compared to normal papillary dermis) in this zone. Variable telangiectasia (and new blood vessel formation), and melanophages may also be present.
- *Late*: Zone of papillary dermis and epidermis within a recognizable melanoma, characterized by marked reduction in the amount of tumor compared to adjacent areas of tumor, or absence of tumor in this zone, and replacement and expansion of the papillary dermis in this zone by extensive fibrosis (usually dense fibrous tissue, horizontally disposed) and variable telangiectasia (and new blood vessel formation), melanophages, sparse or no lymphoid infiltrates, and effacement of the epidermis (other than fibrosis, the latter features are frequently present but not essential for recognizing regression).

Melanoma is notable for its frequency of spontaneous regression.[9,85–92] The prevalence of histologic regression varies according to the definition of regression used and the thickness range of the melanomas reported.[85–87] In a study of 563 cases of primary melanoma, histologic regression was noted in 46% of thin (<1.5 mm), 32% of intermediate (1.5–3.0 mm), and 9% of thick (>3.0 mm) melanomas.[86] McGovern has also recorded regression in 58% of melanomas ~0.70 mm in thickness.[87] Complete regression of melanoma is uncommon and has been reported to

occur with a frequency of 2.4 to 8.7% (Fig. 11-28).[88,89] Many cases of metastatic melanoma with unknown primary are thought to be explained by spontaneous regression of the primary melanoma.[89,90]

Spontaneous regression is considered to be immunologically mediated because of mononuclear cell infiltrates containing T lymphocytes, and monocyte/macrophages at the site of regression.[91] Regression is seen most often in microinvasive or thin melanoma and is present as focal, partial, and rarely complete regression of the tumor. The changes of regression form a continuum, but may be arbitrarily categorized into three stages (see earlier discusions).[92]

METASTATIC MELANOMA

BOX 11-33   Summary

- Melanoma metastasizes through lymphatic channels, vascular channels, and along the surfaces of vessels (angiotropism)
- Lymph nodes are the most common sites of metastases
- Cutaneous metastases are common and include local satellite, in transit (between primary lesion and regional lymph nodes), and epidermotropic metastases

Melanoma can spread hematogenously, through lymphatic channels, by migration along vascular channels (angiotropism) or by direct local invasion and thus may occur in any site of the body. Metastases are more frequent to lymph nodes, skin, and subcutaneous tissue (nonvisceral sites) than to visceral organs.[9,93–101] Lymph nodes are the most common site of metastases and 60 to 80% of patients with metastatic melanoma develop lymph node metastases.[96,97] The lymph node groups most commonly involved are ilioinguinal, axillary, intraparotid and cervical lymph nodes. The metastatic tumor may be clinically apparent (macroscopic metastasis) or detected only by histologic examination (microscopic metastasis).

Nearly half of the patients with metastatic melanoma develop skin metastases,[97] which may occur in the area of locoregional lymphatic drainage or at a remote location. Two subtypes of regional cutaneous metastases are arbitrarily distinguished by their distance from the primary melanoma.[97]

Cutaneous satellites are discontinuous tumor cell aggregates that are located in the dermis and/or subcutis within 5 cm of the primary tumor, whereas in-transit metastases are located more than 5 cm away from the primary melanoma. The finding of the latter metastases has poor prognostic implications, since the majority of patients with such lesions develop disseminated metastatic disease. Although virtually any organ may be involved, the most common first sites of visceral metastases reported in clinical studies are lung (14 to 20%), liver (14 to 20%), brain (12 to 20%), bone (11 to 17%), and intestine (1 to 7%), while first metastases at other sites are very rare (<1%).[97,99]

Metastatic melanoma has a tendency to grow in nests, sheets or fascicles, often with an infiltrative border, pleomorphism, mitoses and necrosis.[9,97] Cytologically, epithelioid and/or spindle cells are commonly found in metastatic melanoma.[9,97] Melanin, which greatly facilitates the recognition of metastatic melanoma, may be apparent, subtle or absent (amelanotic melanoma).

Diagnostic Problems Concerning Metastatic Melanoma

BOX 11-34 Summary

- May mimic a wide spectrum of neoplastic lesions
- Amelanotic tumors
- Primary versus metastatic melanoma
- Nodal nevus deposits versus metastatic melanoma in lymph nodes
- Metastatic melanoma with unknown primary
- Melanosis in metastatic melanoma

Several situations may arise in which the diagnosis of metastatic melanoma is not straightforward. The problem may lie in the identification of a metastatic-appearing lesion as melanocytic or in the distinction between a primary and secondary melanoma.[9]

MELANOMA SIMULATING OTHER NEOPLASMS Metastatic melanoma may assume a great variety of morphologic appearances and may mimic a number of nonmelanocytic tumors, such as lymphoma, undifferentiated carcinoma, adenocarcinoma, a variety of sarcomas and many others.[102,103] The differential diagnosis is particularly difficult in amelanotic melanoma. Often, additional studies are needed, such as melanin stains, immunohistochemistry using a panel of antibodies, and electron microscopy, to identify conclusively a metastatic tumor as melanocytic.

PRIMARY CUTANEOUS VERSUS CUTANEOUS METASTATIC MELANOMA

BOX 11-35 Summary

	Primary Melanoma	Cutaneous Metastasis
Location of tumor	Usually both dermis and epidermis	Dermis and/or subcutis
If epidermal involvement	Usually prominent; pagetoid horizontal and vertical spread commonly present; usually epidermal component extends laterally beyond dermal component	Usually dermal component extends laterally beyond epidermal component; pagetoid spread less common
Size	Nearly always >0.4 cm and usually >1.0 cm	Often small; may be <1.0 cm and occasionally <0.3 cm
Epidermal collarette	Usually less common	More likely present
Cytology	Usually pleomorphic	Usually monotonous
Reactive fibrosis	May be marked	Usually mild
Vascular invasion	Rarely seen	Angiotropism

A common problem is distinguishing an epidermotropic metastasis from a primary melanoma (or possibly a nevus in some instances) (Fig. 11-29).[98,100,101] Cutaneous metastases usually lie within the reticular dermis or subcutis and only rarely involve the overlying epidermis, while primary cutaneous melanomas typically have an intraepidermal component. In addition, metastases tend to be smaller (often <4 mm) than primary tumors (usually >4 or 5 mm). In cases of metastatic melanoma showing epidermotropism, the epidermal component is usually relatively limited compared to the dermal component (Fig. 11-29). If the dermal metastasis is superficial, the overlying epidermis may be thinned and the lateral borders may show hyperplastic elongated rete ridges turned inward forming a *collarette*. Tumor cells showing angiotropism within vascular lumina are more likely to be found in and around a metastatic lesion than near a primary tumor.

Primary tumors generally display more pleomorphism than metastatic lesions, which often appear as an atypical, but rather monomorphous population of cells. Primary tumors tend to show more variation in the overall composition of the lesion. There is often

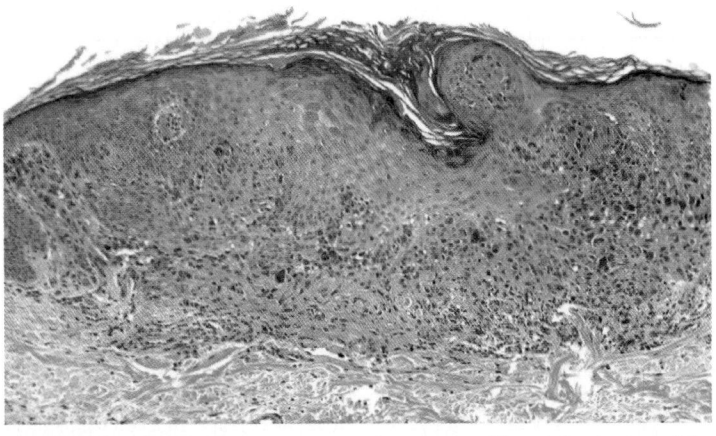

▲ **FIGURE 11-29** Epidermotropic metastatic melanoma. There is involvement of the epidermis by melanoma cells.

more fibrosis and more of an inflammatory host response. When deciding whether a melanocytic tumor is a metastasis or a primary lesion, one must weigh the histologic appearance against a detailed clinical history to arrive at the correct diagnosis. The importance of having precise clinical information is mandatory since there are exceptions to all of the guidelines for diagnosis mentioned above.[101]

MELANOCYTIC AGGREGATES VERSUS MICROMETASTASES Collections of small melanocytes are occasionally seen within lymph nodes (sentinel or other) draining the skin.[104–107] These aggregates are usually small and inconspicuous but may occupy as much as a third of a lymph node. They are usually located in the fibrous capsule or trabeculae of the node rather than the marginal sinus,[105] but rarely can be found in the lymphatic tissue proper. Their bland appearance, frequent resemblance to nevus cells, and their location in the fibrous capsule of the lymph node help to distinguish them from micrometastases. However, especially in frozen sections or in the rare situation of intranodal location, such aggregates in lymph nodes may lead to diagnostic confusion. There has been considerable debate as to whether these nodal melanocytic lesions derive from aberrant migration of melanoblasts from the neural crest during embryogenesis or represent lymphatic spread from a benign cutaneous nevus.

METASTATIC MELANOMA WITH UNKNOWN PRIMARY SITE Approximately 4 to 12% of patients with melanoma develop metastases without a clinically detectable primary tumor.[108,109] While it is possible that some melanomas may arise *de novo* within a lymph node or visceral site, it is generally believed that many of these of these cases are related to complete regression of a primary cutaneous melanoma.[110,112] Metastatic melanomas with unknown primary site are twice as common in men as in women, which is in agreement with the observation that tumor regression is more commonly observed in men as in women.[112] The most common site of presentation is in lymph nodes (64%)[1120] whereas 21% of the cases present with visceral metastases.

MELANOSIS IN METASTATIC MELANOMA Cutaneous or generalized melanosis is a rare complication of metastatic melanoma.[113–115] Hyperpigmentation may be focal or diffuse, limited to the skin or generalized, involving internal organs.

Histologic Diagnosis of Malignant Melanoma

BOX 11-36 Summary

- Size usually >5–6 mm
- Asymmetry
- Poor circumscription
- Pagetoid melanocytosis
- Diminished or absent maturation
- Confluence and high cellular density of melanocytes
- Effacement of epidermis
- Dermal mitoses
- Cytologic atypia of melanocytes

The histologic diagnosis of melanoma remains subjective and usually depends on the recognition of a constellation of histologic features, no single feature being diagnostic of melanoma.[9] Because there are so many exceptions to the conventional criteria for melanoma, one must always utilize as much information as possible and common sense at all times. On the other hand, a large percentage of melanomas are diagnosed correctly by a majority of knowledgeable observers. It is also true that a small percentage of melanocytic tumors is histologically challenging and will produce no consensus even among experts (see following sections).

In general, melanomas are characterized by an overall asymmetry and disorder, whereas benign melanocytic lesions tend to have symmetry and order. Although there is no absolute size criterion, the larger the lesion is in breadth (generally over 5 to 6 mm and especially over 10 mm), the greater is the likelihood that the lesion is melanoma. Melanomas are also often characterized by poor circumscription of the peripherally extending intraepidermal component and heterogeneity. Other architectural attributes suggesting melanoma include a contiguous proliferation of single (often basilar) melanocytes, considerable variation in the sizes and shapes of intraepidermal cellular nests, and diminished cohesiveness of the nests of cells. There may be a confluence of melanoma cells along the dermal–epidermal junction. The epidermis is frequently significantly altered, e.g., thinning, effacement, ulceration, hyperplasia, lack of uniformity from side to side, hyperkeratosis, parakeratosis, and replaced by melanoma as compared to that in benign melanocytic lesions.

One of the features most characteristic of melanoma, yet one that is not specific to melanoma, is upward migration or pagetoid melanocytosis of melanocytes with involvement of the superficial epidermis. A predominance of single cells over small aggregates or nests typifies this pattern in melanoma. Melanoma cells are usually present at all levels of the epidermis including the granular and cornified layers.

Characteristics of the dermal component suggesting melanoma include asymmetry, confluent or sheet-like patterns of melanocytes without maturation, heterogeneity, hypercellularity, mitoses particularly in significant-numbers, deeply located, and atypical, necrosis, and prominent host response.

Cytologic atypia is mandatory for a diagnosis of melanoma. There is a uniformity or monomorphous quality of the atypia in melanoma rather than the discontinuous pattern of atypia often found in atypical nevi. Melanoma is also notable for cellular and nuclear enlargement, nuclear pleomorphism, hyperchromatic nuclei, high nuclear to cytoplasmic ratios of melanoma cells, and often prominent nucleoli. Large polygonal melanoma cells often have abundant pink granular cytoplasms, finely divided ("dusty") melanin granules, or less commonly opaque cytoplasms. The melanin granules may vary considerably in size and shape.

DIAGNOSIS OF THE BORDERLINE OR CONTROVERSIAL LESION SUGGESTING MELANOMA

BOX 11-37 Summary

- Benign lesion
- Biologically indeterminate lesion
- Malignant melanoma

Not all melanocytic lesions at present can be classified as benign or malignant. One must make use all information available in order to interpret as precisely as possible a difficult melanocytic lesion and to place it into one of three categories: (1) benign, (2) biologically indeterminate, or (3) malignant, for the optimal communication to and management of the patient. A biologically indeterminate lesion is defined as one that has some potential (uncertain) risk for local recurrence and metastasis but one that cannot also be interpreted as malignant utilizing all criteria currently available. The diagnostic exercise should be comprehensive and include information such as age, gender, site, clinical characteristics, presence or absence of ulceration, diameter, thickness in mm, mitotic rate per square millimeter, possibly immunostaining for proliferative rate (e.g., with Ki 67) and other markers, etc. in order to quantify as much as possible the abnormalities present that favor or argue against melanoma. The diagnostic evaluation of such a difficult lesion should probably include obtaining the opinion of a recognized authority in the field.

PROGNOSTIC FACTORS IN MELANOMA

BOX 11-38   Summary

Prognostic factor	Effect on prognosis
Tumor thickness (mm)	Worse with increasing thickness
Levels of invasion	Worse with deeper levels
Ulceration	Worse with ulceration
Mitotic rate	Worse with increasing mitotic rate
Tumor-infiltrating lymphocytes (TILs)	Better with TILs
Regression	Unsettled; some studies have shown an adverse outcome while others no effect, or a favorable outcome
Microscopic satellites	Worse prognosis
Angiotropism	Worse prognosis
Vascular/lymphatic invasion	Worse prognosis but rare
Tumor cell type	Better prognosis with spindle cells versus other cell types
Age	Worse prognosis with increasing age
Sex	Women have better prognosis than men
Anatomic site	Extremity lesions have better prognosis than axial lesions (trunk, head and neck, palms and soles)

Over the past 20 to 30 years, there has been extensive investigation of prognostic factors in melanoma using large databases and multivariate techniques.[2,14,15,116–119] The most powerful predictors of survival from many such studies have been thickness of the primary melanoma (measured in mm from the granular layer of the epidermis vertically to the greatest depth of tumor invasion) and stage or extent of disease, i.e., localized tumor, nodal metastases, distant metastases.

Although a number of studies have described "breakpoints" for tumor thickness and prognosis, e.g., patients with melanomas <0.76 mm have almost 100% 5-year survival,[116] there is now good evidence that this inverse relationship between thickness and survival is essentially linear. While thickness is the best prognostic factor available for localized melanoma, there are occasional melanomas that defy this relationship, i.e., thin melanomas that metastasize

and thick ones that do not. A number of other factors also have been reported to influence outcome in patients with localized melanoma. However, many of these various factors largely derive their effect from a correlation with melanoma thickness and generally fail to remain significant after multivariate analysis. Five-year survival for all melanoma patients currently approaches 90%.

However, once regional lymph-node metastases have developed 5-year survival drops to the range of about 10 to 50%, which is largely related to the number and extent of lymph nodes involved. The median survival for patients with distant metastases is approximately 6 months. The only factors influencing the time to death include number of metastatic sites, surgical resectability of the metastases, duration of remission, and location of metastases, i.e., nonvisceral (skin, subcutaneous tissue, and distant lymph nodes) vs. visceral sites (lung, liver, brain, and bone).

HISTOPATHOLOGIC REPORTING OF MELANOMA

BOX 11-39   Summary

- *Essential information*
  - Diagnosis: malignant melanoma, *in situ* or invasive
  - Measured depth (in millimeters)
  - Presence of histologic ulceration
  - Presence of microscopic satellites
  - Adequacy of surgical margins
- *Other prognostic information reported to be significant in some databases*

- Mitotic rate (per square millimeter)
- Tumor-infiltrating lymphocytes
- Anatomic level, i.e, I, II, III, IV, and V
- Angiotropism
- Vascular/lymphatic invasion
- Desmoplasia-neurotropism
- Degree of regression, particularly >50% of lesion
- Radial or vertical growth phase
- Histologic subtype

The pathology report should include the following minimum information: diagnosis, i.e., malignant melanoma, *in situ* or invasive; depth of tumor invasion in mm measured vertically from the granular layer of the epidermis or from the surface of an ulcer with an ocular micrometer; and the adequacy of surgical margins.[9] The following histologic changes should also be mentioned if present: ulceration and microscopic satellites because of new staging guidelines. Other prognostic factors that may be reported are: mitotic rate per square millimeter, angiotropism, true vascular/lymphatic invasion, marked or virtually complete regression, desmoplasia, neurotropism, anatomic level, histologic type of melanoma, radial or vertical growth phase, and tumor-infiltrating lymphocytes. However, some of the latter factors are highly correlated with tumor thickness. Thus, there may be no additional significant information beyond thickness.

MANAGEMENT CONSIDERATIONS

BOX 11-40   Summary

- Optimal biopsy for examination of entire lesion if possible
  - Elliptical excision or incision for lesions suspicious for melanoma
- Complete skin and physical examination; scanning of visceral organs if specifically indicated
- Sentinel lymph node biopsy may be considered for melanomas >1.0 mm in thickness
- Surgical margins
  - Melanoma *in situ*: 0.5 cm margins
  - Melanomas ≤2 mm in thickness: 1 cm margins
  - Melanomas ≥2 mm in thickness: 2 cm margins
- Follow-up examinations related to Breslow thickness, stage, etc.
  - Every 3–6 months for first 5 years
  - Every 6–12 months for the remaining 5 to 10 years

Biopsy

The optimal method of sampling any pigmented lesion suspicious for melanoma is complete elliptical excision with narrow surgical margins of approximately 2 mm. Much has been written about the inappropriate use of shave and even punch biopsy techniques for suspected melanomas. Examination of the entire pigmented lesion allows for the greatest chance of accurate diagnosis and also for the measurement of Breslow thickness and the assessment of other prognostic factors. However, particular circumstances such as an excessively large pigmented lesion, a cosmetically or anatomically difficult site may render complete excision unfeasible and thus necessitate partial biopsy as with a punch or incisional technique.

Examination and Staging

Patients with newly diagnosed melanoma require a complete cutaneous and physical examination with particular attention to lymphadenopathy and hepatomegaly, and a baseline chest radiograph. If the latter examinations fail to detect any evidence of metastatic disease and the patient has no other symptoms or signs, no further laboratory evaluation is indicated. However, patients with melanoma exceeding 1 mm in thickness and with no other evidence of metastatic disease are candidates for sentinel lymph node biopsy. Selected patients with melanomas measuring <1 mm in thickness may be considered for SLN biopsy if the primary melanoma is ulcerated, Clark level IV, or shows extensive regression. Patients with palpable lymphadenopathy and other signs and symptoms require additional evaluation with various scanning techniques and possible lymph node biopsy, etc.

Sentinel Lymph Node Biopsy

The introduction of sentinel lymph node (SLN) biopsy has provided the means to examine regional lymph nodes for evidence of metastasis in lieu of a major surgical intervention. If one or more SLNs harbor bona fide deposits of metastatic melanoma (versus nodal nevi or indeterminate deposits), completion lymphadenectomy is performed. Although SLN biopsy is a currently accepted staging procedure, only long-term clinical trials will determine if the procedure has any significant effect on survival of melanoma patients.

Therapy for Melanoma

Surgery remains the only effective therapy for melanoma if it is diagnosed and completely excised at a localized and early stage of development, i.e., <1 to 1.5 mm in thickness. There is currently no effective treatment for advanced melanoma, and only a small percentage of patients survive long after (even limited) the documentation of regional metastatic disease.

Surgical Margins for Melanoma

The practical and theoretical benefits accruing from excising melanoma with some cuff of normal tissue are: (1) greater assurance that the primary melanoma is indeed removed with truly clear margins and (2) the potential removal of microscopic metastatic foci near the primary melanoma. Although much has been published on the subject of surgical margins for melanoma, no definitive data currently exist on this issue.[120] However, it appears that surgical margins may have no real influence on survival in melanoma, and margins probably in excess of 3 cm (and possibly even 1 cm) may provide no benefit to patients. Problems clouding the issue of margins for melanoma are the lack of sufficient knowledge about initial mechanisms of melanoma metastasis at the primary site, melanoma recurrence versus persistence of the primary melanoma and melanoma metastasis, and other considerations such as field effects. When the mechanisms of melanoma metastasis, etc. are better understood, the information needed to address finally the question of optimal margins would be available.

For the time being, the current (rather arbitrary) guidelines for the surgical management of melanoma are complete excision of the primary lesion with margins of 0.5 cm for melanomas *in situ*, 1 cm for melanomas ≤2 mm in thickness and 2 cm margins for melanomas >2 mm. It is clear that exceptions exist for these guidelines such as desmoplastic-neurotropic melanoma, e.g., wider margins of at least 3 cm are probably indicated, and anatomic sites necessitating narrower margins.

Follow-up Examinations

Follow-up of melanoma patients is related to the stage of disease, e.g., patients with documented distant or visceral metastases require the most vigilant surveillance, followed by individuals with regional lymph node, in transit or satellite metastases; and finally those with localized primary melanomas. The frequency of follow-up examinations is individualized, but usually at least every 3 months initially for regional and distant metastatic disease. Patients with localized primary melanomas of thickness >1 to 1.5 mm commonly undergo physical examination at 3-month intervals for the first 3 years (the period of highest risk for the development of metastases), every 6 months thereafter for 2 years, and once annually for an additional 5 years. Patients with low-risk melanomas (<1 mm) are generally followed at 6-month intervals for 3 years and annually thereafter.

■ FINAL THOUGHTS

The importance of malignant melanoma as a potentially fatal skin cancer among Caucasian populations worldwide has received critical attention in recent years. As compared to other life-threatening malignancies such as breast or prostate carcinoma, melanoma may be diagnosed by simple inspection of the skin surface with 80 to 90% accuracy. However, there is currently no objective evidence that medical intervention of any kind significantly alters the clinical course of melanoma, potentially other than the complete excision of localized melanoma at an early stage, e.g., generally <1 mm in thickness. Future investigations is needed to establish whether education and modification of behavior such as reduced sun exposure and various methodologies of skin examination have a significant impact in reducing mortality from melanoma. Future research must also attempt to identify useful therapeutic interventions for metastatic melanoma.

REFERENCES

1. Clark WH, Jr. A classification of malignant melanoma in man correlated with histogenesis and biologic behavior. In: Montagna W, Hu F, eds. *Advances in the Biology of the Skin.* Vol. VIII. New York, NY: Pergamon Press; 1967:621–647.
2. Clark WH, Jr, From L, Bernardino EA, Mihm MC. The histogenesis and biologic behavior of primary human malignant melanomas of the skin. *Cancer Res.* 1969;29:705–727.
3. McGovern VJ, Mihm MC, Jr, Bailly C, Booth JC, Clark WH, Jr, Cochran AJ, Hardy EG, Hicks JD, Levene A, Lewis MG, Little JH, Milton GW. The classification of malignant melanoma and its histologic reporting. *Cancer.* 1973;32:1446–1457.
4. Reed RJ. The pathology of human cutaneous melanoma. In: Costanzi JJ, ed. *Malignant Melanoma I.* The Hague, The Netherlands: Martinus Nijhoff; 1983:85–116.

5. Clark WH Jr, Elder DE, Van Horn M. The biologic forms of malignant melanoma. *Human Pathol.* 1984;17:443–450.

6. Heenan PJ, Armstrong BK, English DE, et al. Pathological and epidemiological variants of cutaneous malignant melanoma. In: Elder DE, ed. *Pathobiology of Malignant Melanoma.* Basel, Switzerland: Karger; 1987:107–146.

7. Barnhill RL, Mihm MC, Fitzpatrick TB, Sober AJ. Neoplasms: malignant melanoma. In: Fitzpatrick TB, Eisen AZ, Wolff K, Freedberg IM, Austen KF, eds. *Dermatology in General Medicine.* New York, NY: McGraw-Hill; 1993: 1078–1115.

8. Barnhill RL, Mihm MC, Jr. The histopathology of cutaneous malignant melanoma. *Semin Diagn Pathol.* 1993; 10:47–75.

9. Barnhill RL. *The Pathology of Melanocytic Nevi and Malignant Melanoma.* Boston, MA: Butterworth-Heineman; 1995.

10. Reed RJ. Acral lentiginous melanoma. In: *New Concepts in Surgical Pathology of Skin.* New York, NY: Wiley; 1976:89–90.

11. Arrington JH III, Reed RJ, Ichinose H, Krementz ET. Plantar lentiginous melanoma: A distinctive variant of human cutaneous malignant melanoma. *Am J Surg Pathol.* 1977;1:131–143.

12. Kuchelmeister C, Schaumburg-Lever G, Garbe C. Acral cutaneous melanoma in Caucasians: Clinical features, histopathology and prognosis in 112 patients. *Br J Dermatol.* 2000;143:275–280.

13. Heenan PJ, Holman CDJ. Nodular malignant melanoma: A distinct entity or a common end stage? *Am J Dermatopathol.* 1982;4:477–478.

14. Vollmer RT. Malignant melanoma: a multivariate analysis of prognostic factors. *Pathol Ann.* 1989;24:383.

15. Barnhill RL, Fine J, Roush GC, Berwick M. Predicting five-year outcome from cutaneous melanoma in a population-based study. *Cancer.* 1996;78:427–432.

16. Ackerman AB. Malignant melanoma: A unifying concept. *Human Pathol.* 1980;11: 591–595.

17. Heenan PJ, Matz LR, Blackwell JB, Kelsall GR, Singh A, Ten Seldam RE, Holman CD. Inter-observer variation between pathologists in the classification of cutaneous malignant melanoma in Western Australia. *Histopathol.* 1984;8:717–729.

18. Curtin JA, Fridlyand J, Kageshita T, Patel HN, Busam KJ, Kutzner H, Cho K-H, Aiba S, Brocker E-B, LeBoit PE, Pinkel D, Bastian BC. Distinct sets of genomic alterations in melanoma. *N Engl J Med.* 2005;535:2135–2147.

19. Mihm MC Jr, Fitzpatrick TB, Brown MM, Raker JW, Malt RA, Kaiser JS. Early detection of primary cutaneous malignant melanoma. A color atlas. *N Engl J Med.* 1973;289:989–996.

20. Barnhill RL, Fitzpatrick TB, Fandrey K, Kenet RO, Mihm MC, Jr, Sober AJ. *The Pigmented Lesion Clinic: A Color Atlas and Synopsis of Benign and Pigmented Lesions.* New York, NY: McGraw-Hill, Inc.; 1995.

21. Patterson RH, Helwig EB. Subungual malignant melanoma: A clinical-pathologic study. *Cancer.* 1980;46:2074–2087.

22. Saida T, Yoshida N, Ikegawa S, Ishihara K, Nakajima T. Clinical guidelines for the early detection of plantar malignant melanoma. *J Am Acad Dermatol.* 1990;23:37–40.

23. Blessing K, Kernohan NM, Park KGM. Subungual malignant melanoma: clinicopathological features of 100 cases. *Histopatholgy.* 1992;19:425–429.

24. Rigby HS, Briggs JC. Subungual melanoma: A clinicopathological study of 24 cases. *Br J Plast Surg.* 1992;45:275–278.

25. Saida T, Ohshima Y. Clinical and histopathologic characteristics of early lesions of subungual malignant melanoma. *Cancer.* 1989;63:556–560.

26. Ten SR, Helwig E, Sobin L, et al. Histological typing of skin tumours. In: *Histological Typing of Skin Tumours. International Histological Classification of Tumors,* no. 12. Geneve, Switzerland: World Health Organization; 1974.

27. Clark WH, Jr, Evans HL, Everett MA, et al. Early melanoma: histologic terms. *Am J Dermatopathol.* 1991;13:579–582.

28. McGovern VJ. Spontaneous regression of melanoma. *Pathology.* 1975;7:91–99.

29. Clark WH Jr, Elder DE, Guerry D IV, et al. Model predicting survival in Stage I melanoma based on tumor progression. *J Natl Cancer Inst.* 1989;81:1893–1904.

30. Herlyn M, Clark WH, Rodeck U, Mancianti ML, Jambrosic J, Koprowski H. Biology of tumor progression in human melanocytes. *Lab Invest.* 1987; 56:461–474.

31. Price NM, Rywlin AM, Ackerman AB. Histologic criteria for the diagnosis of superficial spreading malignant melanoma: formulated on the basis of proven metastatic lesions. *Cancer.* 1976; 38:2434–2441.

32. Weyers W, Bonczkowitz M, Weyers I, Bittinger A, Schill W. Melanoma in situ versus melanocytic hyperplasia in sun-damaged skin. Assessment of the significance of histopathologic criteria for differential diagnosis. *J Am Acad Dermatol.* 1996;18:560–566.

33. Acker S, Nicholson JH, Rust PF, Maize JC. Morphometric discrimination of melanoma in situ of sun-damaged skin from chronically sun-damaged skin. *J Am Acad Dermatol.* 1998;39:239–245.

34. Flotte TJ, Mihm MC. Lentigo maligna and malignant melanoma in situ, lentigo maligna type. *Hum Pathol.* 1999;30:533-536.

35. Tannous ZS, Lerner LH, Duncan LM, Mihm MC Jr, Flotte TJ. Progression to invasive melanoma from malignant melanoma, lentigo maligna type. *Hum Pathol.* 2000;31:705–708.

36. Clark WH Jr, Mihm MC, Jr. Lentigo maligna and lentigo maligna melanoma. *Am J Pathol.* 1969;55:39–67.

37. Somach SC, Taira FW, Pitha FV, Everett MA. Pigmented lesions in actinically damaged skin. Histopathologic comparison of biopsy and excisional specimens. *Arch Dermatol.* 1996;132: 1297–1302.

38. Elder DE. Metastatic melanoma. In: Elder DE, ed. *Pigment Cell;* vol. 8. Basel, Switzerland: Karger; 1987:182–204.

39. Fitzpatrick JE. The histologic diagnosis of intraepithelial pagetoid neoplasms. *Clin Dermatol.* 1991;9:255–259.

40. Conley J, Lattes R, Orr W. Desmoplastic malignant melanoma (a rare variant of spindle cell melanoma). *Cancer.* 1971;28: 914–936.

41. Valensi QJ. Desmoplastic malignant melanoma. A light and electron microscopic study of two cases. *Cancer.* 1979;43:1148–1155.

42. From L, Hanna W, Kahn HJ, Gruss J, Marks A, Baumal R. Origin of the desmoplasia in desmoplastic malignant melanoma. *Hum Pathol.* 1983;14:1072–1080.

43. Egbert B, Kempson R, Sagebiel R. Desmoplastic malignant melanoma. A clinico-histopathologic study of 25 cases. *Cancer.* 1988;62:2033–2041.

44. Jain S, Allen PW. Desmoplastic malignant melanoma and its variants. A study of 45 cases. *Am J Surg Pathol.* 1989;13:358–373.

45. Smithers BM, McLeod GR, Little JH. Desmoplastic, neural transforming and neurotropic melanoma: a review of 45 cases. *Aust N Z J Surg.* 1990;60:967–972.

46. Bruijn JA, Mihm MC Jr, Barnhill RL. Desmoplastic melanoma. *Histopathology.* 1992;20:197–205.

47. Carlson JA, Dickersin GR, Sober AJ, Barnhill RL. Desmoplastic neurotrpoic malignant melanoma: a clinicopathologic analysis of 28 cases. *Cancer.* 1994;75:478–494.

48. Skelton HG, Smith KJ, Laskin WB, McCarthy WF, et al. Desmoplastic malignant melanoma. *J Am Acad Dermatol.* 1995;32:717–725.

49. Reed RJ, Leonard DD. Neurotropic melanoma: a variant of desmoplastic melanoma. *Am J Surg Pathol.* 1979;3: 301–311.

50. Kossard S, Doherty E, Murray E. Neurotropic melanoma. A variant of desmoplastic melanoma. *Arch Dermatol.* 1987;123:907–912.

51. Barnhill RL, Bolognia JL. Neurotropic melanoma with prominent melaninization. *J Cutan Pathol.* 1995;22:450–459.

52. Anstey A, Cerio R, Ramnarain N, Orchard G, Smith NP, Jones EW. Desmoplastic malignant melanoma. An immunocytochemical study of 25 cases. *Am J Dermatopathol.* 1994;16:14–22.

53. Baer, SC, Schultz, D, Synnestvedt M, Elder, DE. Desmoplasia and Neurotopism: prognostic variables in patients with Stage I melanoma. *Cancer.* 1995; 76:2242–2247.

54. Longacre TA, Egbert BM, Rouse RV. Desmoplastic and spindle cell malignant melanoma. An immunohistochemical study. *Am J Surg Pathol.* 1996;20:1489–1500.

55. Kilpatrick SC, White WL, Browne JD. Desmoplastic malignant melanoma of the oral mucosal: an underrecognized diagnostic pitfall. *Cancer.* 1996;78:383–389.

56. Quinn MJ, Crotty KA, Thompson JF, Coates AS, O'Brien CJ, McCarthy WH. Desmoplastic and desmoplastic neurotropic melanoma: experience with 280 patients. *Cancer.* 1999;83:1128–1135.

57. Barnhill RL, Mihm MC. Cellular neurothekeoma: a distinctive variant of neurothekeoma mimicking nevomelanocytic tumors. *Am J Surg Pathol.* 1990;14:113–120.

58. Iwamoto S, Burrows RC, Agoff SN, Piepkorn M, Bothwell M, Schmidt R. The p75 neurotrophin receptor, relative to other Schwann cell and melanoma markers, is abundantly expressed in spindled melanomas. *Am J Dermatopathol.* 2001;23:288–294.

59. Xu X, Chu AY, Pasha TL, Elder DE, Zhang PJ. Immunoprofile of MITF,

165

Tyrosinase, Melan-a, and MAGE-1 in HMB45-Negative Melanomas. *Am J Surg Pathol.* 2002;26(1):82–87.

60. Lugassy C, Eyden BP, Christensen L, Escande JP. Angio-tumoral complex in human malignant melanoma characterised by free laminin: ultrastructural and immuno-histochemical observations. *J Submicrosc Cytol Pathol.* 1997;29:19–28.

61. Lugassy C, Dickersin GR, Christensen L, et al. Ultrastructural and immunohistochemical studies of the periendothelial matrix in malignant melanoma: evidence for an amorphous matrix containing laminin. *J Cutan Pathol.* 1999;26:78–83.

62. Lugassy C, Shahsafaei A, Bonitz P, Busam KJ, Barnhill RL. Tumor microvessels in melanoma express the beta-2 chain of laminin. Implications for melanoma metastasis. *J Cutan Pathol.* 1999;26:222–226.

63. Barnhill RL, Lugassy C. Angiotropic malignant melanoma and extravascular migratory metastasis: description of 36 cases with emphasis on a new mechanism of tumour spread. *Pathology.* 2004;36:485–490.

64. Barnhill R, Dy K, Lugassy C. Angiotropism in cutaneous melanoma: a prognostic factor strongly predicting risk for metastasis. *J Invest Dermatol.* 2002;119:705–706.

65. Schmoeckel C, Castro CE, Braun-Falco O. Nevoid malignant melanoma. *Arch Ermatol Res.* 1985;277:362–369.

66. Wong TY, Suster S, Duncan LM, Mihm M Jr. Nevoid melanoma: a clinicopathological study of seven cases of malignant melanoma mimicking spindle and epithelioid cell nevus and verrucous dermal nevus. *Human Pathol.* 1995;26:171–179.

67. McNutt NS, Urmacher C, Hakimian, Hoss DM, Lugo J. Nevoid malignant melanoma: morphologic patterns and immunohistochemical reactivity. *J Cutan Pathol.* 1995;22:502–517.

68. Zembowicz A, McCusker M, Chiarelli C, et al. Morphological analysis of nevoid melanoma: a Study of 20 Cases With A Review of the Literature. *Am J Dermatopathol.* 2001;23:167–175.

69. Steiner A, Konrad K, Pehamberger H, Wolff K. Verrucous malignant melanoma. *Arch Dermatol.* 1988;124:1534–1537.

70. Blessing K, Evans AT, Al-Nafussi A. Verrucous naevoid and keratotic malignant melanoma: a clinico-pathological study of 20 cases. *Histopathology.* 1993;23:453–458.

71. Kossard S, Wilkinson B. Nucleolar organizer regions and image analyis nuclear morphometry of small cell (nevoid) melanoma. *J Cutan Pathol.* 1995;22:132–136.

72. Kossard S, Wilkinson B. Small cell (naevoid) melanoma: a clinicopathologic study of 131 cases. *Australas J Dermatol.* 1997;38 (suppl):S54–S58.

73. House N, Fedok F, Maloney ME, Helm KF. Malignant melanoma with clinical and histologic features of Merkel cell carcinoma. *J Am Acad Dermatol.* 1994;31:839–842.

74. Blessing K, Grant JJH, Sanders SDA, Kennedy MM, Husain A, Coburn P. Small cell malignant melanoma: a variant of naevoid melanoma. Clinicopathological features and histological differential diagnosis. *J Clin Pathol.* 2000;53:591–595.

75. Okun MR. Melanoma resembling spindle and epithelioid cell nevus. *Arch Dermatol.* 1979;115:1416–1420.

76. Okun M, Bauman L. Malignant melanoma arising from an intradermal nevus. *Arch Dermatol.* 1965;92:69–72.

77. Okun MR, Di Mattia A, Thompson J, Pearson SH. Malignant melanoma developing from intradermal nevi. *Arch Dermatol.* 1974;110:599–601.

78. Benisch B, Peison B, Kannerstein M, Spivack J. Malignant melanoma originating from intradermal nevi. A clinicopathologic entity. *Arch Dermatol.* 1980;116:696–698.

79. Temple-Camp CRE, Saxe N, King H. Benign and malignant cellular blue nevus. A clinicopathological study of 30 cases. *Am J Dermatopathol.* 1988;10:289–296.

80. Goldenhersh MA, Savin RC, Barnhill RL, Stenn KS. Malignant blue nevus. *J Am Acad Dermatol.* 1988;19:712–722.

81. Connelly J, Smith JL, Jr. Malignant blue nevus. *Cancer.* 1991;67:2653–2657.

82. Granter SR, McKee PH, Calonje E, Mihm MC, Busan K. Melanoma associated with blue nevus and melanoma mimicking cellular blue nevus: a clinicopathologic study of 10 cases on the spectrum of so-called 'malignant blue nevus'. *Am J Surg Pathol.* 2001;25:316–323.

83. Peters MS, Su WPD. Balloon cell malignant melanoma. *J Am Acad Dermatol.* 1985;13:351–354.

84. Kao GF, Helwig EB, Graham JH. Balloon cell malignant melanoma of the skin: a clinicopathologic study of 34 cases with histochemical, immunohistochemical, and ultrastructural observations. *Cancer.* 1992;69:2942–2952.

85. McGovern VJ. Melanoma—growth patterns, multiplicity and regression. In: *Melanoma and Skin Cancer. Proceedings of the International Cancer Conferenc.* Sydney. VCN Blight: Government Printer, 1972;95–106.

86. Blessing K, McLaren KM. Histological regression in primary cutaneous melanoma: recognition, prevalence and significance. *Histopathology.* 1992;20:315–322.

87. McGovern VJ, Shaw HM, Milton GW. Prognosis in patients with thin malignant melanoma: influence of regression. *Histopathology.* 1983;7:673–680.

88. Pack GT, Miller TR. Metastatic melanomas with indeterminate primary site. *JAMA.* 1961;176:55–56.

89. Smith JL Jr, Stehlin JS, Jr. Spontaneous regression of primary malignant melanomas with regional metastases. *Cancer.* 1965;18:1399–1415.

90. Barr RJ. The many faces of completely regressed malignant melanoma. *Pathology (Phila).* 1994;2:359–370.

91. Tefany FJ, Barnetson RS, Halliday GM, McCarthy SW, McCarthy WH. Immunocytochemical analysis of the cellular infiltrate in primary regressing and non-regressing malignant melanoma. *J Invest Dermatol.* 1991;97:197–202.

92. Kang S, Barnhill RL, Mihm MC, Sober AJ. Regression in malignant melanoma: an interobserver concordance study. *J Cutan Pathol.* 1993;20:126–129.

93. Balch C, Milton G. Diagnosis of metastatic melanoma at distant sites. In: Balch, Milton, Shaw, Soong, eds. *Cutaneous Melanoma. Clinical Management and Treatment Results Worldwide.* Philadelphia, PA: J.B. Lippincott; 1985:221–250.

94. McNeer G, Das GT. Life history of melanoma. *AJR.* 1956;93:686–694.

95. Peterson N, Bodenham D, Lloyd O. Malignant melanoma of the skin: a study of the origin, development, etiology, spread, treatment, and prognosis. *Br J Plast Surg.* 1962;15:49–116.

96. Balch CM, Urist MM, Maddox WA, Milton GW, McCarthy WH. Management of regional metastatic melanoma. In: Balch CM, Milton GW, Shaw HM, Soon S-J, eds. *Cutaneous Melanoma. Clinical Management and Treatement Results Worldwide.* Philadelphia, PA: J.B. Lippincott; 1985:93–130.

97. Elder DE, Murphy G. Metastatic malignant melanoma. In: Elder DE, Murphy G, eds. *Melanocytic Tumors of the Skin.* Washington, DC: American Registry of Pathology, Armed Forces Institute of Pathology; 1991:191–205.

98. Kornberg R, Harris M, Ackerman A. Epidermotropically metastatic malignant melanoma. *Arch Dermatol.* 1978;114:67–69.

99. Elder DE, Ainsworth A, Clark W. The surgical pathology of cutaneous malignant melanoma. In: Clark W, ed. Human Malignant Melanoma. New York, NY: Grune and Stratton; 1979:55–108.

100. Bengoechea-Beeby M, Velasco-Oses A, Fernandez F, Reguilon-Rivero M, Remon-Garijo L, Casado-Perez C. Epidermotropic metastatic melanoma. *Cancer.* 1993;72:1909–1913.

101. White WL, Hitchcock MG. Dying dogma: the pathological diagnosis of epidermotropic metastatic malignant melanoma. *Semin Diag Pathol.* 1998;15:176–188.

102. Nakhleh RE, Wick MR, Rocamora A, Swanson PE, Dehner LP. Morphologic diversity in malignant melanomas. *Am J Clin Pathol.* 1990;93:731–740.

103. Banerjee SS, Harris M. Morphological and immunphenotypic variations in malignant melanoma. *Histopathology.* 2000;36:387–402.

104. McCarthy S, Palmer A, Bale P, Hist E. Nevus cells in lymph nodes. *Pathology.* 1974;6:351–358.

105. Johnson W, Helwig E. Benign nevus cells in the capsule of lymph nodes. *Cancer.* 1969;23:747–753.

106. Ridolfi R, Rosen P, Thaler H. Nevus cell aggregates associated with lymph nodes: estimated frequency and clinical significance. *Cancer.* 1977;39:164–171.

107. Andreola S, Clemente C. Nevus cells in axillary lymph nodes from radical mastectomy specimens. *Pathol Res Pract.* 1985;179:616–618.

108. Das Gupta T, Bowden L, Berg J. Malignant melanoma of unknown primary origin. *Surg Gynecol Obstetr.* 1963;117:341–345.

109. Giuliano A, Cochran AJ, Morton D. Melanoma from unknown primary site and amelanotic melanoma. *Semin Oncol.* 1982;9:442–447.

110. Pellegrini A. Regressed primary malignant melanoma with regional meta-

stases. *Arch Dermatol.* 1980;116:585–586.

111. Chang P, Knapper W. Metastatic melanoma of unknown primary. *Cancer.* 1982;49:1106–1111.

112. Reintgen D, McCarty K, Woodard B, Cox E, Seigler H. Metastatic malignant melanoma with an unknown primary. *Surg Gynecol Obstet.* 1983;156:335–340.

113. Silberberg I, Kopf A, Gumport S. Diffuse melanosis in malignant melanoma. *Arch Dermatol.* 1968;97:671–677.

114. Eide J. Pathogenesis of generalized melanosis with melanuria and melanoptysis secondary to malignant melanoma. *Histopathology.* 1981;5:285–294.

115. Rowden G, Sulicca V, Butler T, Manz H. Malignant melanoma with melanosis. Ultrastructural and histological studies. *J Cutan Pathol.* 1980;7:125–139.

116. Day Cl Jr, Lew RA, Mihm MC Jr, Harris MN, Kopf AW, Sober AJ, et al. The natural break points for primary tumor thickness in clinical stage I melanoma [letter]. *N Engl J Med.* 1981;305:1155.

117. Keefe M, MacKie RM. The relationship risk of death from clinical stage I cutaneous melanoma and thickness of primary tumour: no evidence for steps in risk. *Br J Cancer.* 1991;64:598–602.

118. Balch CM, Soong S-J, Murad TM, Ingalls AL, Maddox WA. A multifactorial analysis of melanoma: 111. Prognostic factors in melanoma patients with lymph node metastases (stage II). *Ann Surg.* 1981;193:377.

119. Balch CM, Soong S-J, Shaw HM, et al. An analysis of prognostic factors in 8500 patients with cutaneous melanoma. In: Balch CM, Houghton AN, Milton GW, et al, eds. *Cutaneous Melanoma.* 2nd ed. Philadelphia, PA: J.B. Lippincott; 1992:165–187.

120. Thomas JM, Newton-Bishop J, A'Hern R, et al. Excision margins in high-risk malignant melanoma. *N Engl J Med.* 2004;350:757–766.

CHAPTER 12

Cutaneous Lymphomas and Leukemias

Roger H. Weenig, M.D.
Lawrence E. Gibson, M.D.

BOX 12-1   Overview

- Cutaneous lymphomas and leukemias represent a broad group of hematologic malignancies that involve the skin as the primary disease presentation or with secondary skin involvement of systemic disease.
- The diagnosis of hematologic malignancies in the skin requires knowledge of the clinical, histologic, immunphenotypic, and molecular features of the malignancy in question as well as conditions that mimic skin lymphoma.
- Primary cutaneous T-cell lymphoma (CTCL) is the most common hematologic malignancy involving the skin. B-cell lymphomas affect the skin more commonly than previously recognized.
- CTCL represents a diverse group of T-cell lymphomas with varied clinical and histologic presentations, prognoses, and treatments.
- MF is the most common form of CTCL, but several clinical and histologic variants are recognized.
- As treatment of MF rarely influences survival, therapy is based on clinical stage and symptomatology.
- Cutaneous involvement by leukemia (leukemia cutis) has a varied clinical presentation and must be distinguished from reactive dermatoses (leukemids) that frequently accompany leukemia.
- During the initial presentation or relapse of leukemia, skin may be the only involved organ (aleukemic leukemia cutis).

INTRODUCTION

Cutaneous lymphomas include lymphoid malignancies that initially present in the skin (primary cutaneous lymphomas) or spread to the skin (secondary cutaneous lymphomas) from nodal or extranodal sites. Leukemia is a malignancy of bone marrow-derived cells that may involve the skin secondarily (leukemia cutis), or primarily (aleukemic leukemia cutis). Previous designations for cutaneous lymphomas were named eponymically, by the clinical presentation, or by histopathologic findings. Recent advances in immunohistochemistry and molecular biology has fostered classification schemes based on cellular lineage. These advances have led to greater precision in diagnosis and identification of distinct disease entities and disease subgroups. In this chapter, we strive to incorporate the 2004 EORTC/WHO combined classification for cutaneous lymphomas, but also discuss historical designations where relevant.

While the precise etiology for most lymphoproliferative disorders is largely unknown, specific genetic aberrations have recently been determined for several entities, but are not discussed in this chapter. An infectious cause has been associated with several lymphomas that present in the skin (Table 12-1).

PRIMARY CUTANEOUS T-CELL LYMPHOMA (CTCL)

CTCL represents a diverse group of T-cell malignancies with distinct clinical presentations, prognoses, and treatments. Therefore, we avoid the common practice of using the term "CTCL" unqualified or as interchangeable with mycosis fungoides (MF). Additionally, the current TNMB staging scheme for CTCL should be restricted to mycosis fungoides and Sézary syndrome, as the criteria do not apply to other forms of CTCL (Table 12-2). Moreover, the term "CTCL" should not be used to describe systemic T-cell lymphomas with secondary cutaneous involvement. Table 12-3 lists the relative frequency and subtypes of CTCL

Table 12-1
Selected Lymphoid Neoplasms and Associated Infections

DIAGNOSIS	ASSOCIATED INFECTIOUS AGENT
Extranodal NK/T-cell lymphoma	Epstein-Barr virus infection of NK cells
Angioimmunoblastic T-cell lymphoma	Epstein-Barr virus infection of B-cells
Some diffuse large B-cell lymphomas	Epstein-Barr virus infection of B-cells
Lymphomatoid granulomatosis	Epstein-Barr virus infection of B-cells
Immuosuppression-related lymphoproliferative disorders	
• Posttransplant lymphoproliferative disorder	Epstein–Barr virus infection of B-cells (usually), T-cells (occasionally), or NK cells (rarely)
• Methotrexate associated lymphoproliferative disorder	
Adult T-cell leukemia—lymphoma	Human lymphotrophic virus I
Oral plasmablastic lymphoma	Human herpes virus 8

In patients that present early in the course of their disease, a definitive diagnosis of CTCL may not be rendered. In these situations, "pre-mycosis fungoides," "pre-Sézary," "parapsoriasis," "CTCL Stage T0," and other historical or descriptive terms are evoked. With close clinical follow-up, repeat biopsies, immunophenotyping, and molecular genetic studies, most cases of CTCL are diagnosable over time. Yet, considerable expertise in clinicopathologic correlation in these early or "borderline" cases is required for diagnosis.

MYCOSIS FUNGOIDES (MF)

BOX 12-2   Summary

- Most common cutaneous lymphoma.
- Presents with solitary or multiple erythematous patches, plaques, or tumors.
- Diagnostic histopathologic findings include a cutaneous proliferation of medium-large, clonal T-cells that infiltrate the epidermis (epidermotropism).
- Clinical course is frequently characterized by a protracted course over many years, but progression usually occurs.
- Treatment of early stage MF consists of topical therapies and phototherapy.
- Treatment of advanced disease includes radiation therapy, chemotherapy, and bone marrow transplantation.

MF the most common form of primary cutaneous T-cell lymphoma, was described by Alibert 200 years ago.[5] The incidence of MF varies ethnically and regionally, with rates ranging from two cases per million person-years among white Americans to eight cases per million person-years for African Americans.[6]

Table 12-2
TNMB Staging for MF and Sézary Syndrome[1-3]

TUMOR STAGE	OBSERVATION
T_0	Lesions clinically or histologically equivalent to MF or SS
T_1	Patches or plaques involving <10% BSA
T_2	Patches or plaques involving >10% BSA
T_3	Tumors
T_4	Erythroderma
NODAL STAGE	
N_0	No palpable nodes; negative nodal histology
N_1	Palpable nodes; negative nodal histology
N_2	No palpable nodes; positive nodal histology
N_3	Palpable nodes; positive nodal histology
METASTATIC (VISCERAL) STAGE	
M_0	No visceral involvement by CTCL
M_1	Visceral involvement by CTCL
BLOOD STAGE	
B_0	No peripheral blood involvement
B_1	Sézary cell count >20% of peripheral blood lymphocytes or Sézary cell count >5% and a positive T-cell clone in peripheral blood
CLINICAL STAGE	
Ia	$T_1N_0M_0$
Ib	$T_2N_0M_0$
IIa	$T_{1-2}N_1M_0$
IIb	$T_3N_{0-1}M_0$
III	$T_4N_{0-1}M_0$
IVa	$T_{1-4}N_{2-3}M_0$
IVb	$T_{1-4}N_{0-3}M_1$

BSA—body surface area, MF—mycosis fungoides, SS—Sézary syndrome.

TABLE 12-4
MF Subtypes

Adnexotropic mycosis fungoides
- Pilotropic (folliculotropic) mycosis fungoides
- Syringotropic mycosis fungoides
Angiotropic mycosis fungoides
Bullous mycosis fungoides
Dyshidrotic mycosis fungoides
Erythrodermic mycosis fungoides
Purpuric dermatotis-like mycosis fungoides
Granulomatous mycosis fungoides
Hyperpigmented (melanoerythroderma) mycosis fungoides
Hypopigmented mycosis fungoides
Ichthyosiform mycosis fungoides
Interstitial mycosis fungoides
Invisible mycosis fungoides
Pagetoid reticulosis
- Unilesional/solitary (Woringer–Kolopp)
- Generalized (Goodman–Ketron)
Palmar/plantar mycosis fungoides
Parapsoriasis
- Large plaque (most cases = MF)
- Small plaque (some cases = MF)
Poikiloderma vasculare atrophicans
Pustular mycosis fungoides
Verrucous mycosis fungoides

The disease typically afflicts middle-aged adults, but may present at any age.

Myriad clinical and pathologic presentations of MF have been described, yielding many designations and disease subgroups (Table 12-4). The consistent theme of MF is that the neoplastic T-lymphocytes are prone to infiltrate epithelium (epitheliotropic), which is most common in the epidermis (epidermotropic), but also occurs in the follicular epithelium (pilotropic) or sweat gland epithelium (syringotropic).

MF presents as solitary, focal, or multifocal patches, plaques, nodules, or tumors on any cutaneous site (Fig. 12-1). Lesions of MF impart a variety of colors, most commonly as a shade of red, but also as hyperpigmented, hypopigmented, or yellow patches; the latter carries the designation *xanthoerythroderma perstans*. Mucous membrane involvement is rare in MF. Ulceration is uncommon in patches or plaques of MF, but frequent in tumor stage disease. Rarely, pustules or marked dermal neutrophilia may occur on or

Table 12-3
Primary Cutaneous T-cell Lymphomas (CTCL): Subtypes, Frequency, and Survival

LYMPHOMA TYPE	FREQUENCY (%)[a]	5-YEAR SURVIVAL (%)[a]
PRIMARY CUTANEOUS T-CELL LYMPHOMA (CTCL)		
MF and variants	44	80–88
Sézary syndrome	3	24
Subcutaneous panniculitis-like T-cell lymphoma	1	82
Anaplastic large T-cell lymphoma	8	95
Lymphomatoid Papulosis	12	100
Aggressive epidermotropic CD8+ cutaneous T-cell lymphoma	<1	18
Cutaneous gamma-delta T-cell lymphoma	<1	0
Granulomatous slack skin	<1	100
Pagetoid reticulosis	<1	100
Peripheral T-cell lymphoma, unspecified	2	16

[a]Based on Dutch and Austrian cutaneous lymphoma registries.[4]

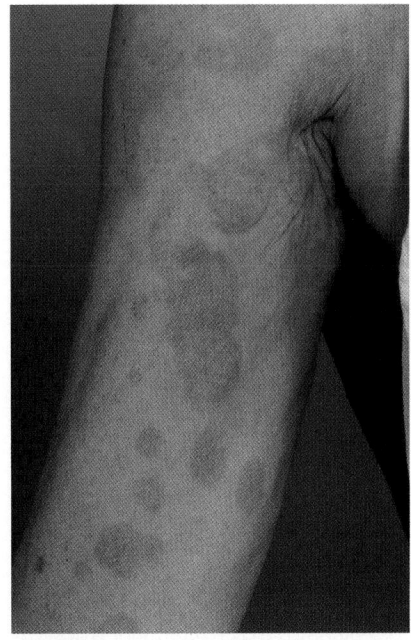

▲ **FIGURE 12-1** Annular erythematous patches of MF on the arm.

distant from MF lesions. These cases have been labeled as pustular MF or neutrophilic dermatosis associated MF. An aggressive and fatal clinical course was reported in three patients in whom MF and a neutrophilic dermatosis were implicated to be simultaneously active in the same clinical lesions.[7] Aside from a secondary infection accompanying an MF lesion; it is tenuous to assign a second inflammatory disease to MF lesions. Terms such as pustular MF or granulomatous MF may aid in the clinical recognition or management of such cases, but designating the same skin lesion as "neutrophilic dermatosis and MF" or "sarcoidosis and MF" is unlikely to aid clinicians or patients. Most cutaneous lymphoma experts recognize that other inflammatory cells (neutrophils, eosinophils, plasma cells, and histocytes) may accompany, and perhaps be recruited by the neoplastic T-lymphocytes of MF.

Although many patients show a gradual progression from patches or plaques to tumors, some patients with MF have tumors on initial presentation. Patients with erythrodermic MF may present with Sézary cells in the peripheral blood and an overall clinical picture indistinguishable from Sézary syndrome (SS). Erythrodermic MF is separated from SS by a proceeding history of typical MF (e.g. patches or plaques). Without such history patients should be diagnosed as SS. In addition, patients in whom MF progress to erythroderma should not be designated as "Sézary syndrome." However, erythrodermic MF and Sézary syndrome are placed in the same stage (T4) with the current, but antiquated TMNB staging scheme (Table 12-2). Most studies on survival have used the TNMB staging scheme and therefore, do not distinguish between erythrodermic MF and SS. Extracutaneous involvement by MF is usually a late-stage event.

The histopathology of a patch or plaque of MF demonstrates a superficial dermal lymphoid infiltrate with invasion of the overlying epidermis (epidermotropism). Invasion of hair follicles and sweat glands or ducts by neoplastic lymphocytes may be observed in addition to epidermal involvement or as an isolated finding (pilotropic MF and syringotropic MF respectively). The pattern of epidermal lymphoid infiltration is variable and may be subtle, but is usually accompanied by minimal, if any, spongiosus. Identification of singular (often haloed) lymphoid cells along the basal layer of the epidermis (basilar lymphocytosis), or in clusters within the epidermis (Pautrier collections) is highly suggestive of MF.

Table 12-5
MF Staging (WHO)[9]

CLINICAL/PATHOLOGIC FINDINGS	STAGE	TREATMENT OPTIONS
Disease confined to the skin	I	Phototherapy, Interferon, topical or
Limited patches or plaques	Ia	systemic retinoids alone or in combination, nitrogen mustard, topical steroids
Disseminated patches or plaques	Ib	Above therapies +/−
Tumors	Ic	photopheresis, radiation, total body electron beam radiation
Enlarged lymph nodes (negative histology)	II	
Enlarged lymph nodes (positive histology)	III	Systemic chemotherapy, bone
Visceral involvement	IV	marrow transplantation

The lymphoid cells in MF are usually enlarged, but not markedly so. Irregular, convoluted nuclear contours (cerebriform nuclei) of the lymphoid cells is a common but less specific finding. In chronic lesions, epidermal hyperplasia and dermal fibrosis may be appreciated. A biopsy obtained from a tumor of MF shows diffuse dermal and even subcutaneous lymphoid infiltration. However, epidermotropism is frequently less or absent in tumors compared with patches or plaques of MF. Large cell transformation in MF is diagnosed when aggregates or sheets of large cells are observed within the lymphoid infiltrate, a finding that often portends a worse prognosis. Large cell transformation in MF must be distinguished from lymphomatoid papulosis and anaplastic large cell lymphoma. Clinicopathologic correlation is required to differentiate these entities.

The immunohistochemical profile of MF is usually positive for pan-T-cell antigens (CD2, CD3, CD5, and CD7). Loss of CD2, CD3, or CD5 expression is unusual in the early stages of MF, but indicates T-cell neoplasia. As lack of CD7 expression may be observed in neoplastic or non-neoplastic skin-homing T-cells, this finding is not diagnostic of T-cell neoplasia or MF. Most cases of MF are CD4-positive and CD8-negative. Rare cases of otherwise typical MF may exhibit a CD4-negative/CD8-positive immunophenotype. The large cells in large cell transformation of MF are usually (but not always) CD30-positive.

The course of MF is usually protracted for years or even decades and no standardized therapy providing a consistent survival advantage exists. Therefore, the primary consideration for the treatment of MF should focus on the patient's quality of life. Moreover, as there is no evidence that therapeutic intervention in the earlier stages of the disease modifies disease progression or lengthens survival of MF, therapy must be tailored to each patient.[8]

Some patients experience severe pruritus and/or emotional distress with clinically mild disease. Others may have extensive cutaneous involvement for years without significant symptoms or a demonstrable reduction in their quality of life. For minimally symptomatic disease, the adverse effects or the burden of the frequent clinic visits inherent with some therapies may not be justifiable. Additionally, patients with mild disease may be subjected to various chemotherapeutic trials and experience significant adverse drug-related events or progression of lymphoma. Thus, patients with MF must be carefully selected for clinical trials, fully informed regarding the risks and benefits of a specific therapy, and potent chemotherapeutic agents should be reserved for advanced or rapidly progressive disease. Staging and treatment options for MF are summarized in Table 12-5.

Extensive skin colonization or infection by Staphylococcus aureus, herpes viruses, and other infectious agents may be associated with exacerbation of MF in the sites of skin infection. Additionally, skin barrier compromise and local immune dysregulation from MF leads to higher bacterial colonization and risk for infection. Thus, in addition to good skin care, early diagnosis and treatment of skin infection is paramount in managing patients with MF.

SÉZARY SYNDROME (SS)

BOX 12-3 Summary

- Leukemic variant of MF
- Triad of erythroderma, lymphadenopathy, and Sézaremia
- Distinguished from erythrodermic MF by preceeding clinical history of typical MF
- Disease may be prolonged in some patients, but eventual progression is expected

- Treatment includes extracorporeal photophoresis, systemic retinoids, low-dose chlorambucil/prednisone, interferon, controlling pruritus, paying close attention to infection.

The classic triad of Sézary syndrome (SS) includes: erythroderma, lymphadenopathy, and a peripheral blood lymphocytosis with an increased number of large (>11 μm) convoluted CD4+ T-cells (Sézaremia). Winkelman and Peters suggested an absolute Sézary count of 1×10^9 cells/L as diagnostic for SS.[10] Although Sézaremia may be observed erythrodermic MF, SS is differentiated from the former by an absence of a proceeding history of the typical patches and plaques observed in MF.

The clinical findings of SS include generalized erythroderma (Fig. 12-2), secondary excoriations, ectropion, alopecia, poikiloderma, varying degrees of palmar/plantar keratoderma (Fig. 12-3), and lymphadenopathy.

Although the absolute number of circulating CD4+ cells is increased in SS, these cells are dysfunctional and result in defective immune function. Consequently, infection is a significant cause of morbidity and mortality in Sézary patients. The impaired immune function coupled with the skin barrier compromise resulting from erythroderma and accompanied excoriations, Staphalococcal aureus bacteremia is a frequent and serious complication in SS.

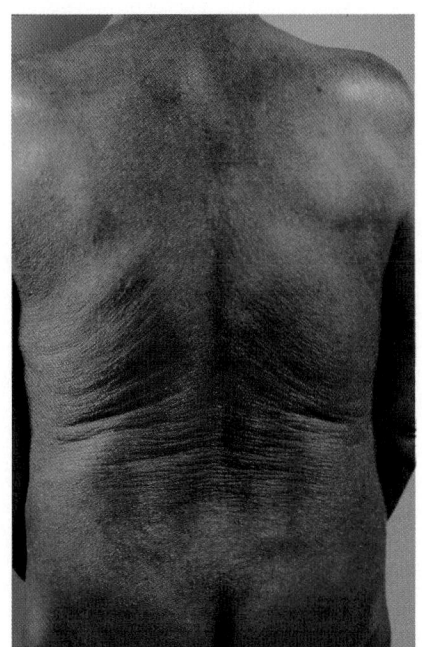

▲ **FIGURE 12-2** Generalized erythroderma of Sézary syndrome.

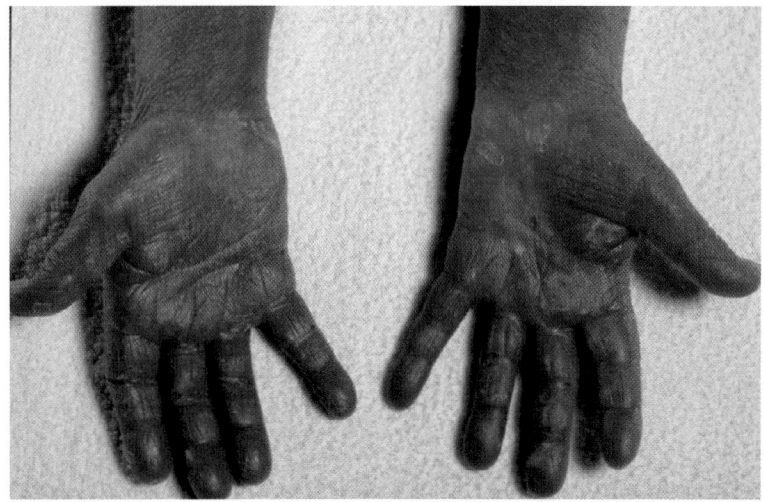

▲ **FIGURE 12-3** Diffuse palmar erythema with foci of keratoderma in Sézary syndrome.

Biopsies obtained from skin affected by SS demonstrate a superficial to mid-dermal infiltrate composed of medium-to-large lymphoid cells with cerebriform nuclei. Epidermotropism may be identified, but is usually less than is observed in MF. Features of poikiloderma (epidermal atrophy, vascular ectasia, and dermal pigment deposition) may be seen as well. The majority of the atypical lymphoid cells are CD4-positive/CD8-negative T-cells.

The prognosis of SS is poor, but varies considerably among published series of patients. Factors adversely affecting prognosis include a positive T-cell clone in the peripheral blood, tumor burden in the peripheral blood, age greater than 65 years at diagnosis, Epstein–Barr virus genome in epidermal keratinocyes, an elevated lactate dehydrogenase level >10% above normal, and 10 candidate genes identified by cDNA microarray technology.[11–14]

OTHER PRIMARY CUTANEOUS T-CELL LYMPHOMAS

CD30-Positive Lymphoproliferative Disorders (CD30+LPD)

BOX 12-4   Summary

- Includes: lymphomatoid papulosis and variants, primary cutaneous anaplastic large cell lymphoma, systemic anaplastic large cell lymphoma.
- Clinical presentation ranges from scattered red papules to large plaques and tumors, but ulceration is common in all types.
- Histologic findings vary depending on the disorder and chronicity, but the hallmark of the disease is the identification of CD30-positive cells.
- Disease spectrum ranges from indolent (LyP) to aggressive (systemic ALCL).
- Treatment includes observation, topical therapy, phototherapy, and methotrexate for LyP and localized primary cutaneous ALCL. Chemotherapy and/or radiation are usually employed for extensive primary cutaneous or systemic ALCL.

The CD30-positive lymphoproliferative disorders represent a spectrum of diseases that includes lymphomatoid papulosis and variants, primary cutaneous anaplastic large cell lymphoma, and secondary cutaneous involvement by systemic anaplastic large cell lymphoma. While the diagnosis rests on identifying CD30-positive cells, many conditions may be associated with an increased number of activated, CD30-positive cells, including: infections, infestations, inflammatory dermatoses, and other neoplastic conditions.[15] Therefore, clinical data is crucial to correctly diagnosing CD30-positive lymphoproliferative disorders.

LYMPHOMATOID PAPULOSIS Lymphomatoid papulosis (LyP) is a T-cell lymphoproliferative disorder characterized by relapsing and recurring, few to numerous crops of red papules that generally progress to necrotic, punctuate ulcers (Fig. 12-4) that over days to weeks resolve with hyperpigmented, atrophic scars.

Three histopathologic presentations are observed for LyP, including: (1) classic, Type A lesions displaying a dense perivascular, wedge-shaped, lymphoid infiltrate with its apex in the reticular dermis, admixed with eosinophils, dermal hemorrhage, and clusters of large

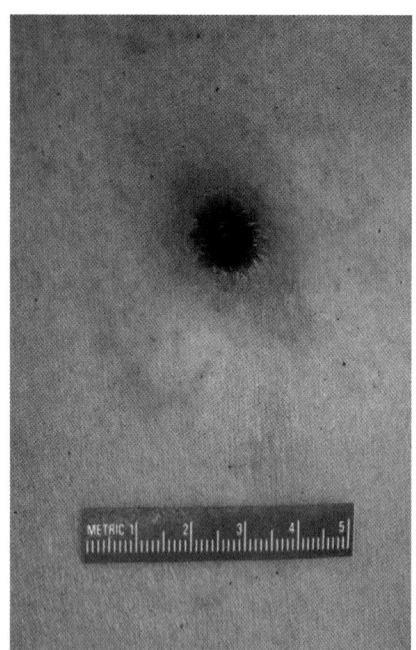

▲ **FIGURE 12-4** Punctate necrotic papule of lymphomatoid papulosis.

CD30-positive lymphoid cells, (2) MF-like, Type B lesions exhibiting a band-like lymphoid infiltrate in the superficial dermis, epidermotropism, and scattered (but not many) CD30-positive lymphoid cells, and (3) ALCL-like, Type C lesions indistinguishable from ALCL with diffuse dermal infiltration by sheets of large CD30-positive lymphoid cells. Established lesions for all types LyP tend to result in vascular injury and destruction with associated dermal hemorrhage, epidermal necrosis, and ulceration. Most cases of LyP exhibit a T-helper (CD4-positive) phenotype, however CD8-positive cases do occur. Cytotoxic markers (TIA-1 and granzyme B) are positive in CD30-positive lymphoproliferative disorders, including LyP. The rate of T-cell clonality detected in LyP is variable, but depends on the type of tissue (formalin-fixed or fresh frozen) and the method employed (polymerase chain reaction or Southern blot analyses).

The prognosis of LyP is excellent, with an estimated 5-year survival of 100%.[4] However, an associated lymphoma may be observed in 20% of patients.[16] Lymphomas associated with LyP include Hodgkin lymphoma, mycosis fungoides, and anaplastic large cell lymphoma, with the latter being the most frequently associated lymphoma. The temporal relationship of LyP with an associated lymphoma varies and is unpredictable. Therefore, evaluation to identify a second lymphoma should be entertained on initial presentation of LyP and follow-up.

Treatment of LyP should be based on the severity of symptoms, as well as the number and frequency of eruptions, and include observation, phototherapy, methotrexate, interferon, systemic corticosteroids, or retinoids.

PRIMARY CUTANEOUS ANAPLASTIC LARGE CELL LYMPHOMA (cALCL)

cALCL presents as solitary or multiple, persistent or recurrent, plaques, nodules, or tumors.

Unlike the spontaneously resolving and relapsing papulonecrotic lesions characteristic of lymphomatoid papulosis, cALCL lesions are often more persistent and tumofactive. However, spontaneous regression has been reported to occur in up to 42% of cases.[17] A preceeding history of the typical patches and plaques of MF and supportive histopathology is needed to distinguish MF with large-cell transformation from cALCL. Moreover, systemic ALCL cannot be distinguished from cALCL histologically, so a thorough staging evaluation at presentation and longitudinal follow-up is necessary to precisely diagnose and correctly manage these patients.

The histopathology of cALCL consists of a pan-dermal to subcutaneous lymphoid infiltrate comprised of mostly (>75% of the lymphoid cells) large, Reed–Sternberg-like, CD30-positive T-cells. In opposition to systemic ALCL, anaplastic lymphoma kinase-1 (ALK-1) is negative in cALCL. However, the exception would be ALK-1-negative systemic ALCL with secondary cutaneous involvement.

As cALCL is histologically indistinguishable from type-C lymphomatoid papulosis (LyP) and may resemble MF with large cell transformation, clinical information is critical to a correct diagnosis.

Treatment of cALCL may include excision or X-ray irradiation of limited disease and chemotherapy for extracutaneous disease.

CYTOTOXIC LYMPHOMAS (CL)

BOX 12-5   Summary

- Includes aggressive epidermotropic CD8-Postive CTCL, subcutaneous panniculitis-like T-cell lymphoma, cutaneous gamma/delta T-cell lymphoma, and extranodal NK/T-cell lymphoma.

- Clinically varied group of disorders, but subcutaneous nodules, skin necrosis, and ulceration are common.
- Histologic presentation is also varied, but subcutaneous infiltration, tissue necrosis, vascular invasion/destruction, and a lichenoid tissue reaction may be observed.
- Cytotoxic protein (TIA-1, Granzyme B, and Perforin) expression is observed in each disorder.
- An aggressive clinical course is observed in most of the cytotoxic lymphomas and systemic chemotherapy and/or bone marrow transplantation is usually required.

AGGRESSIVE, EPIDERMOTROPIC CD8-POSITIVE CUTANEOUS T-CELL LYMPHOMA

In opposition to the indolent development of patches and plaques typical of MF, aggressive epidermotropic CD8-positive CTCL presents relatively acutely with large plaques or tumors, frequent ulceration, and a tendency for extracutaneous involvement.[18,19]

Aggressive epidermotropic CD8-positive CTCL must be distinguished from pagetoid reticulosis and MF, both of which may express the CD8 antigen. Other diagnoses to consider include cutaneous gamma/delta T-cell lymphoma, pityriasis lichoides, and other causes of lichenoid tissue reactions. Skin biopsy reveals a dense, predominantly CD8-positive, pleomorphic T-cell infiltrate forming nodules or an infiltration of the dermis and/or subcutaneous tissue.

Fortunately, this is a rare lymphoma, as the estimated 5-year survival is less than 20%.[4] Treatment is systemic chemotherapy, and bone marrow transplantation may be considered.

SUBCUTANEOUS PANNICULITIS–LIKE T-CELL LYMPHOMA (SPTCL)

Subcutaneous panniculitis-like T-cell lymphoma (SPTCL) is malignancy of cytotoxic, CD8+ T-lymphocytes that presents and usually remains confined to the subcutaneous tissue. SPTCL represents approximately 1% of all CTCL and commonly affects women in the third to fifth decade of life.

Patients usually present with relapsing and recurring, variably tender flesh-colored to red subcutaneous nodules.

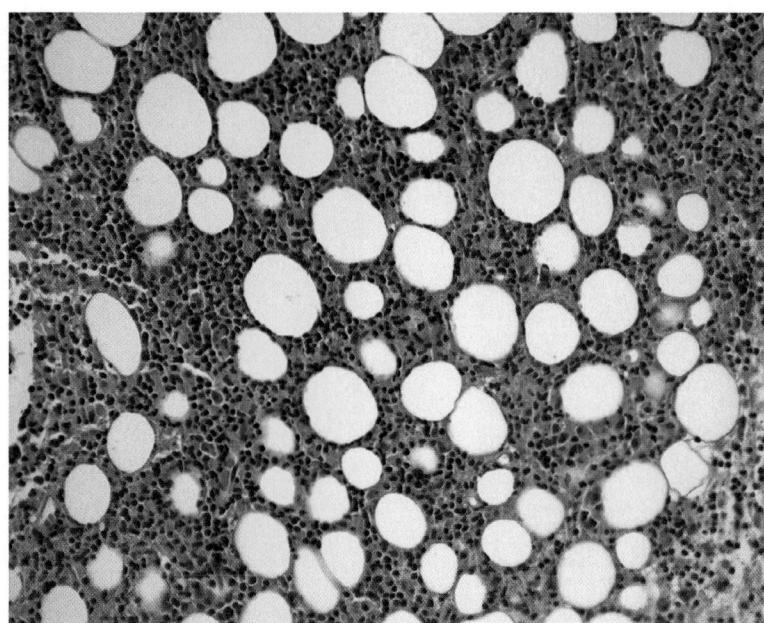

▲ **FIGURE 12-5** Lobular pannicular lymphohistiocytic infiltrate in subcutaneous panniculitis-like T-cell lymphoma (H&E stain at 50× original magnification).

B-symptoms are observed in approximately 50% of patients. Hemophagocytic syndrome may complicate SPTCL and is associated with a high mortality rate.[20]

Histopathologic findings of SPTCL include a dense lobular lymphohistiocytic infiltrate composed of small, medium, or large lymphocytes that characteristically rim individual adipocytes (Fig. 12-5). Fragmentation of lymphocyte nuclei (karryorhexis) and cytophagocytosis of lymphocytes by activated macrophages is frequently encountered. The neoplastic T-lymphocytes in SPTCL express T-cell antigens (CD2, CD3, CD5, and CD7), CD8, and cytotoxic markers (TIA-1, granzyme B, and perforin). Molecular genetic studies identify a clonal population of T-cells.

The new combined WHO/EORTC classification of cutaneous lymphomas recommends restriction of SPTCL to cases that demonstrate surface expression of the alpha/beta T-cell receptor. Another cytotoxic T-cell lymphoma, cutaneous gamma/delta T-cell lymphoma (CGDTL), shares clinical and histologic features with SPTCL. However, reproducible clinical, histologic, and prognostic differences lead most experts to conclude that distinction of these two entities is warranted. The most compelling argument for separating these entities is an estimated 5-year survival of SPTCL of 80% compared with 0% for CGDTL.[4,21]

Treatment of SPTCL is usually combination chemotherapy, but some patients have responded well to less potent immunosuppression, such as systemic corticosteroids. Other patients experienced complete remission and long-term disease-free intervals after bone marrow transplantation.[22] However, most prior series on therapy and outcome of SPTCL included alpha/beta and gamma/delta cases (CGDTL), as well as patients with and without hemophagocytic syndrome. Therefore, larger studies of pure alpha/beta SPTCL are needed to determine the best therapeutic options. Patients with an associated hemophagocytic syndrome should receive chemotherapy or other intensive therapies.

CUTANEOUS GAMMA/DELTA T-CELL LYMPHOMA (CGDTL)

Cutaneous gamma/delta T-cell lymphoma (CGDTL) is designated as a provisional entity under the new combined WHO/EORTC classification of cutaneous lymphomas. Due to the propensity for involvement of the subcutaneous tissue and given the composition of cytotoxic neoplastic T-cells, previously reported cases of CGDTL were designated as subcutaneous panniculitis-like T-cell lymphoma (SPTCL). However, clinical, histologic, immunhistochemical, and prognostic differences are evident. Patients with CGDTL may present with subcutaneous nodules, but in opposition to SPTCL, indurated plaques and ulceration are more common in CGDTL and rarely occur in SPTCL. Spontaneous resolution is reported in most patients with SPTCL, but is rare in CGDTL. The neoplastic cells in CGDTL tend to infiltrate the dermis and occasionally the epidermis, whereas this is not observed in SPCTL. CGDTL runs an aggressive clinical course and the disease responds poorly to treatment. The 5-year survival of SPTCL and CGDTL is estimated at approximately 80 and 0%, respectively.[4]

The histopathologic findings of CGDTL consists of variably sized lymphoid cells that infiltrate various components of the skin, including the epidermis, dermis, and subcutis. As in SPTCL, karyorrhexis, adipocyte rimming, and lymphocyte cytophagocytosis by macrophages is variably observed. Diffuse dermal infiltration and epidermotropism are common findings, the latter of which may be accompanied by a marked lichenoid tissue reaction (Fig. 12-6). T-cell antigens (CD2, CD3, CD5, and CD7) are expressed by CGDTL, but loss of expression of one or more of these is frequent. CGDTL does not usually stain for CD4 and CD8 antigens (double negative), but stains for cytotoxic proteins (TIA-1, Granzyme B, and perforin) are positive.

By definition, surface expression of the gamma/delta T-cell receptor is present on the neoplastic lymphoid cells in CGDTL and, by mutual exclusion, these cells do not express the alpha/beta T-cell receptor. An important distinction should be made between T-cell receptor gene rearrangements and cellular surface expression of the T-cell receptor (TCR). T-cells that express the alpha/beta TCR are designated "alpha/beta T-cells," while those that express the gamma/delta TCR are "gamma/delta T-cells." As the gamma chain gene is the first of the T-cell receptor genes to undergo rearrangement, all normal or neoplastic peripheral T-cells (alpha/beta or gamma/delta T-cells) will contain a gamma rearrangement. In other words, identification of a gamma gene rearrangement in a T-cell lymphoma does *not* establish a gamma/delta T-cell lymphoma. Many labs are able to identify surface expression of the alpha/beta TCR to identify alpha/beta T-cells on paraffin-embedded tissue. Identification of gamma/delta TCR expression is currently available only for use on frozen tissue. Therefore, if frozen tissue is unavailable, a gamma/delta T-cell is usually inferred by establishing a T-cell clone and negative alpha/beta surface expression. Identification of a T-cell clone is necessary because natural killer cells also lack alpha/beta expression but do not undergo TCR gene rearrangements. Of future interest, a gamma/

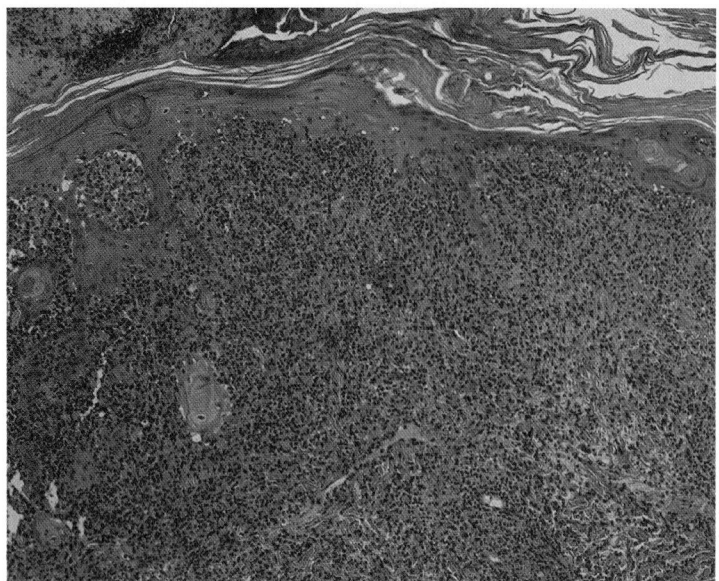

▲ **FIGURE 12-6** Dense dermal lymphoid infiltrate with lichenoid interface pattern in cutaneous gamma/delta T-cell lymphoma (H&E stain at 100× original magnification).

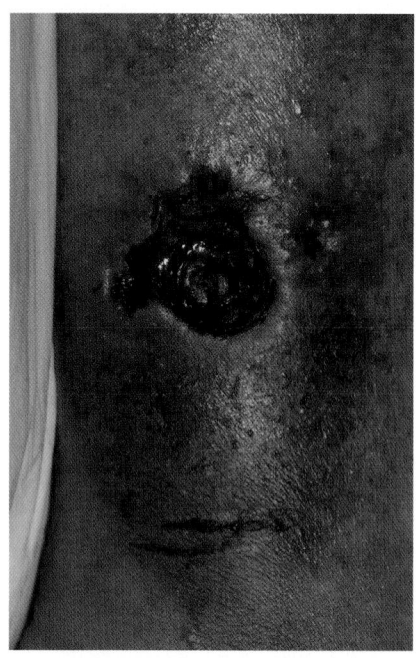

▲ **FIGURE 12-7** Necrotic ulceration with surrounding indurated erythema of the lower leg in NK/T-cell lymphoma.

delta T-cell may be confirmed by the identification of a rearrangement of the delta TCR gene as the delta TCR gene is in the open reading frame of the alpha TCR gene. Thus, a delta positive TCR gene rearrangement would preclude an alpha TCR gene rearrangement and consequently alpha/beta TCR expression.

Treatment for CGDTL includes systemic chemotherapy with early consideration of bone marrow transplantation.

EXTRANODAL NK/T-CELL LYMPHOMA, NASAL TYPE (NK/TL)

Due to the frequency of involvement of the nasal cavity, "nasal type" has been added to the designation of extranodal NK/T-cell Lymphoma (NK/TL). Many cases of so-called midline lethal granuloma were NK/TL. Although the shared immunophenotypic features between NK-cells and cytotoxic T-cells provide for the NK/T-cell designation, NK/TL is likely of natural killer cell lineage.

Following the nasal cavity, skin is the second most frequent site of involvement by NK/TL. Skin is often the initial organ involved by NK/TL, usually presenting as indurated plaques or tumors with a frequent necrosis and ulceration (Fig. 12-7). The tendency for necrosis is due to the propensity for NK/TL to invade and destroy blood vessels ("angioinvasion" and "angiodestruction"), affording the previous designation of NK/TL, angiocentric T-cell lymphoma (Fig. 12-8). However, as other T-cell and B-cell lymphomas may also produce an angiocentric and angiodestructive pattern, this

presentation should not be considered diagnostic of NK/TL without further immunophenotypic and molecular investigation.

The histopathologic findings in NK/TL include a diffuse or nodular dermal or dermal and subcutaneous lymphohistiocytic infiltrate that tends to invade and destroy blood vessels. Cutaneous hemorrhage and necrosis are often marked. Small punch biopsies adjacent to cutaneous ulceration can provide a suboptimal histologic presentation and misinterpretation of the findings as nonneoplastic inflammatory changes. The immunophe-

notype of NK/TL usually shows reactivity for CD2, CD7, CD56, and cytotoxic proteins (TIA-1, granzyme B, and perforin) and no reactivity for CD4, CD5, CD8, and T-cell receptor surface expression (alpha/beta or gamma/delta TCR). NK-cells express the cytoplasmic portion of CD3 but not the surface portion. However, the anti-CD3 antibody used by most laboratories will react with both surface and cytoplasmic CD3. Consequently, true NK-cells are CD3-

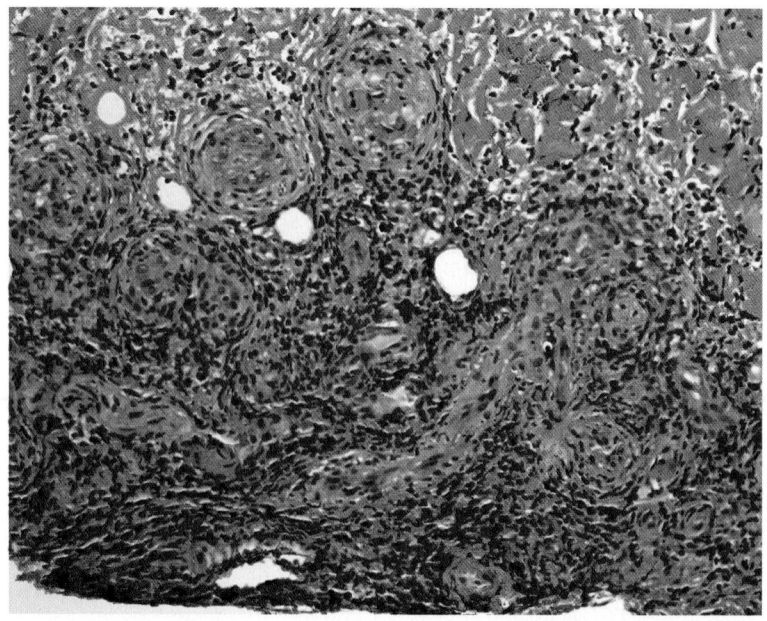

▲ **FIGURE 12-8** Deep dermal, nodular lymphoid infiltrate with angioinvasion and angiodestruction in NT/T-cell lymphoma (H&E stain at 200× original magnification).

Table 12-6
Immunophenotype of Selected Cytotoxic Lymphoproliferative Disorders

	SUBCUTANEOUS PANNICULITIS-LIKE T-CELL LYMPHOMA	EXTRANODAL, NK/T-CELL LYMPHOMA	CUTANEOUS GAMMA/DELTA LYMPHOMA	ALCL/LYMPHOMATOID PAPULOSIS
CD2	+	+	+	+
CD3[a]	+	+	+	+
CD4	−	−	−	+ (most)
CD5	+/−	−	+/−	+/−
CD7	+/−	+	+/−	+/−
CD8	+	−	−	− (most)
CD30	−	−	−	+
CD56	−	+	+/weak/−	−
α/β TCR surface expression	+	−	−	+
γ/δ TCR surface expression	−	−	+	−
TIA-1	+	+	+	+
Granzyme B	+	+	+	+
Clonal TCR rearrangement	+	−	+	+ (most)
Epstein–Barr virus	−	+	−	−

[a]The cytoplasmic (but not surface) portion of the CD3 receptor is expressed on NK cells. Many laboratories use a polyclonal anti-CD3 antibody that reacts with both surface and cytoplasmic CD3, and therefore will stain NK and T-cells.

positive with this technique and cannot be distinguished from T-cells without an extended battery of immunoperoxidase stains. As NK-cells do not undergo rearrangement of the T-cell receptor gene, identification of a TCR gene rearrangement excludes an NK-cell lymphoma. Differentiation of NK/TL from other cytotoxic lymphoproliferative disorders often requires expanded immunophenotyping, studies for Epstein–Barr virus infection, and molecular genetic studies (Table 12-6).

The prognosis of NK/TL is poor with an estimated 5-year survival of 0%.[23] Treatment of NK/TL includes systemic chemotherapy. Bone marrow transplantation has shown promise in improving survival in a recent series of patients.[24]

PERIPHERAL T-CELL LYMPHOMA, UNSPECIFIED (PTLU)

BOX 12-6 Summary
- PTLU are T-cell lymphomas that cannot be designated according to current classification schemes.
- Represents 50% of lymphomas diagnosed in the United States
- Nodal disease is usually identified at presentation.
- Aggressive course is typical and chemotherapy is usually administered.

Peripheral T-cell lymphoma, unspecified (PTLU) represents approximately 50% of all T-cell lymphomas diagnosed in the United States. PTLU most commonly present with nodal disease, but cutaneous involvement is a frequent site of involvement. Some cases of PTLU that primarily affect the skin likely belong to known subsets of CTCL described above, but clinical, histologic, or immunophenotypic features permitting assignment to a specific entity under current lymphoma classification schemes is lacking. Other cases may represent unique T-cell lymphomas yet to be described.

Skin lesions of PTLU are variable, with red to violaceous plaques or nodules localized or widely distributed. Patches and plaques typical of MF are not usual for PTLU. When skin biopsy identifies PTLU, a clinical staging to identify extracutaneous involvement is required. Patients with extracutaneous involvement by PTLU experience an aggressive clinical course and are ill with B-symptoms at presentation. In contrast, the clinical course in patients with primary cutaneous PTLU is usually more indolent and spontaneous remission has been observed.[21] Peripheral blood involvement by PTLU is common, as is the bone marrow, liver and spleen.

The histologic presentation of PTLU in the skin is variable. A diffuse or nodular dermal to subcutaneous lymphoid or lymphohistiocytic infiltrate with small atypical lymphoid cells is identified. Isolated subcutaneous involvement has also been reported.[25] Immunohistochemical study identifies a neoplastic T-cell phenotype, with most tumor cells expressing CD4 but not CD8. Epstein–Barr virus is usually negative in neoplastic T-lymphocytes. Some cases express cytotoxic granules. A clonal T-cell population is identified in most cases.

Treatment options for PTLU include systemic chemotherapy. Bone marrow transplantation should also be considered for advanced disease.[26]

SECONDARY CUTANEOUS INVOLVEMENT BY T-CELL LYMPHOMA

In general, cutaneous involvement is uncommon in systemic T-cell lymphomas, but varies widely in frequency from one entity to another. Some systemic T-cell lymphomas clinically and histologically resemble primary cutaneous T-cell lymphomas (CTCL), including MF. Therefore, combined clinical, pathologic, and staging information is essential for accurate diagnosis and appropriate management. Here it is re-emphasized that systemic T-cell lymphomas with secondary cutaneous involvement should not be designated as CTCL, an error that may lead to considerable confusion and inappropriate or delayed therapy.

ANGIOIMMUNOBLASTIC T-CELL LYMPHOMA (AITL)

BOX 12-7 Summary
- Rare peripheral T-cell lymphoma that presents in elderly.
- The cutaneous findings are often subtle, mimicking a drug eruption or viral infection, but many patients present with B-symptoms.
- Histologic findings are also subtle, with a perivascular mixed-cell infiltrate with prominent endothelial cells.
- Prognosis is poor.

Angioimmunoblastic T-cell Lymphoma (AITL) is a rare peripheral T-cell lymphoma affecting the skin in approximately 10 to 50% of cases. The onset of disease is usually in the sixth or seventh decade of life.

Cutaneous findings in AITL are nonspecific, variable and usually subtle, including scattered erythematous papules on the trunk and extremities resembling viral or drug exanthema. Erythroderma and purpura have also been reported manifestations of disease. Most patients have systemic involvement at presentation. Close to half of patients present with B-symptoms.

Biopsies obtained from skin involved by AITL reveals a mildly dense, perivascular, dermal infiltrate composed of small-to-medium-sized lymphoid cells with a various admixture of other reactive inflammatory cells (lymphocytes, eosinophils, plasma cells, and histocytes) and a proliferation of venules or capillaries containing a prominent endothelium. The neoplastic T-lymphocytes exhibit a T-helper cell phenotype (CD4-positive) and express CD10. Admixed, benign CD8-positive cells may be observed. B-cells with latent Epstein–Barr virus infection are usually absent or present in small numbers in the skin and have an uncertain relationship to the T-cell lymphoma.[27] A recent case showed more extensive infiltration of EBV-positive cells in the skin.[28]

The prognosis is generally poor, but data on large series of patients are lacking.

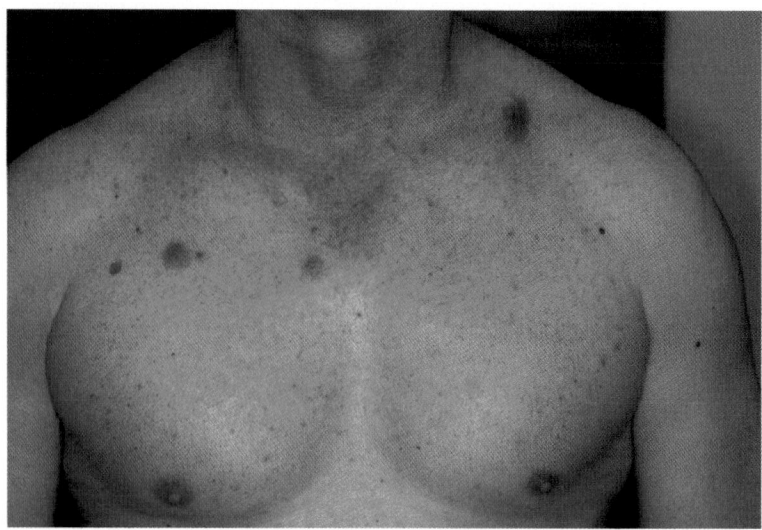

▲ **FIGURE 12-9** Red indurated papules and plaques on the upper chest in follicle center cell lymphoma.

PRIMARY CUTANEOUS B-CELL LYMPHOMA (cBCL)

BOX 12-8   Summary

- Clinical presentation varies by lymphoma type, but red to purple dermal nodules or plaques are common.
- The histologic and immunophenotypic presentation of primary cutaneous B-cell lymphomas often varies from its lymph node counterpart.
- An extensive immunohistochemical battery is frequently needed to precisely diagnose cutaneous B-cell lymphomas.

- The clinical course ranges from indolent to aggressive depending on the B-cell lymphoma type and extent of disease.
- Treatment varies for the type B-cell lymphoma and the extent of disease.
- Radiation is frequently effective for limited disease.
- Rituximab is being found effective for treating several types of cutaneous B-cell lymphomas.

Primary cutaneous B-cell lymphomas represent approximately 20% of all cutaneous lymphomas, which is much more common than previously recognized. Clinical presentation, immunohistochemical profiling, and molecular genetic studies are often required to distinguish reactive B-cell cutaneous infiltrates (B-cell pseudolymphomas) from cutaneous B-cell lymphomas.[29] Table 12-7 presents the immunophenotypic profiles of some B-cell lymphomas that present in the skin. It is important to recognize that

B-cell lymphomas may loose CD20 expression after treatment with rituximab (anti-CD20) and additional B-cell immunoperoxidase stains (such as CD79a) may be required for diagnosis.

CUTANEOUS FOLLICULE CENTER CELL LYMPHOMA (FCCL)

Cutaneous Follicle center cell lymphoma (FCCL) is the most common B-cell lymphoma occurring in the skin which resembles nodal follicular lymphomas (FCCL, follicular pattern) or diffuse large B-cell lymphoma (FCCL, diffuse pattern) on histopathology examination.

The skin lesions of FCCL consist of solitary or multiple indurated red papules, plaques, or tumors most frequently located on the head and neck or trunk (Fig. 12-9).

As mentioned above, two histologic patterns are observed in follicle center cell lymphoma, a follicular pattern and a diffuse pattern. The follicular pattern poses

Table 12-7
Immunophenotypic Profile of Selected B-cell Lymphomas

LYMPHOMA TYPE	CD5	CD10	CD19, CD79[a]	CD20[a]	CD23	BCL-2	BCL-6	CYCLIN D-1	MUM-1
Follicle center cell lymphoma	−	+	+	+	NA	−/+	+	−	NA
Diffuse large B-cell lymphoma	−/+	−/+	+	+	NA	+/−	+/−	−	−
Large B-cell lymphoma, leg type	−/+	−/+	+	+	NA	+/−	+	−	+
Intravascular large B-cell lymphoma	−/+	NA	+	+	NA	+/−	+	−	NA
Extranodal marginal zone lymphoma (MALT)	−	−	+	+	NA	+/−	−	−	NA
Mantel cell lymphoma	+	−	+	+	−	+	−	+	NA
B-cell chronic lymphocytic leukemia/small lymphocytic lymphoma	+	−	+	+	+	+/−	−	−	NA

NA—not applicable
[a]May be negative in patients treated with rituximab

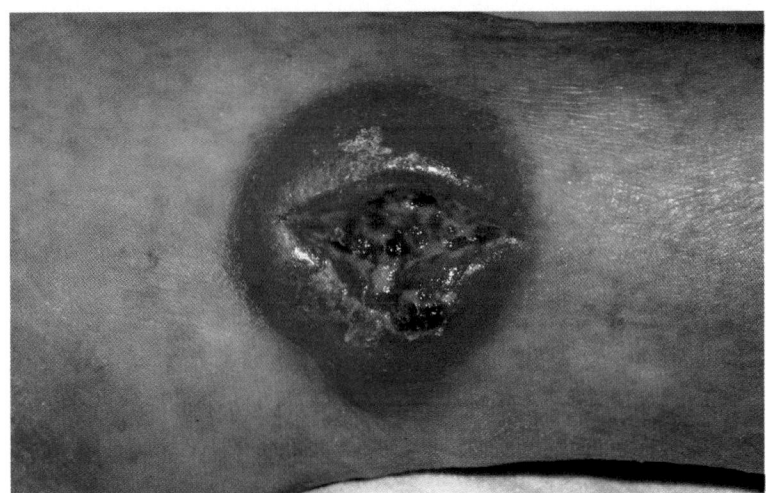

▲ **FIGURE 12-10** Deep-red ulcerated tumor on the leg in large B-cell lymphoma, leg type.

less diagnostic challenge, with nodular aggregates of variably sized cleaved cells with a diminished mantle region, admixed centroblasts, and surrounding T-cells. Conversely, the diffuse pattern lacks well-formed follicles and resembles diffuse large B-cell lymphoma (DLBCL), but the centroblasts remain scattered in FCCL in opposition to the diffuse sheets of centroblasts observed in DLBCL. The neoplastic B-lymphocytes express CD20, CD10, and BCL-6. Unlike nodal follicular lymphoma, most cases of FCCL lack BCL-2 expression. This distinction is important in terms of prognosis and therapy, as DLBCL follows a more aggressive course and is usually treated with systemic chemotherapy.

Treatment of FCCL is usually radiation and/or excision for localized disease. Rituximab alone or incombination with systemic chemotherapy may be considered for multifocal or advanced disease.[30,31]

LARGE B-CELL LYMPHOMA, LEG TYPE (LBLLT)

Although, large B-cell lymphoma, leg type may occur at any cutaneous site, the high predilection for involvement of the leg has afforded "leg type" to the designation. This is analogous to the appellation of "nasal type" to extranodal NK/T-cell lymphoma.

Large B-cell lymphoma, leg type (LBLLT) most commonly afflicts elderly females. Patients usually present with solitary or a few red tumors or plaques on one or occasionally both legs and lesions have a tendency to ulcerate (Fig. 12-10).

The histopathology of large B-cell lymphoma, leg type reveals a diffuse dermal and often pannicular infiltrate composed of sheets of large centrob-

lasts. The immunophenotype of LBLLT shows expression of B-cell antigens (CD20, CD79a), BCL-2, BCL-6, and MUM-1). A clonal rearrangement of the immunoglobulin heavy chain gene is identified in most cases.

The prognosis of LBLLT shows an intermediate behavior with a 5-year survival estimated at 58%.[32]

Treatment approaches for LBLLT include surgery and radiation for localized disease and systemic chemotherapy for widespread disease.

EXTRANODAL MARGINAL ZONE LYMPHOMA OF MUCOSAL ASSOCIATED LYMPHOID TISSUE (cMALT)

Cutaneous involvement by extranodal marginal zone lymphoma of mucosal associated lymphoid tissue (cMALT lymphoma), behind follicle center cell lymphoma, is the second most common B-cell lymphoma to present primarily in the skin. Differentiation of cMALT from low-grade follicle center cell lymphomas and reactive lymphoid hyperplasia may be challenging.

Patients with cMALT lymphoma usually present with solitary to multiple, red to violaceous indurated papules or nodules.

The histopathology of cMALT lymphoma is characterized by a nodular or diffuse dermal lymphoid infiltrate composed of small lymphoid cells and numerous plasma cells. A common observation is remnant follicular germinal centers of various size infiltrated by small lymphoid cells with so-called "boomerang nuclei" and numerous plasma cells located on the periphery of the lymphoid nodules. A clonal popula-

tion of B-cells and plasma cells is usually evident with kappa/lamda immunoperoxidase staining or may be confirmed by molecular genetic techniques.

Treatment of cMALT includes excision of solitary lesions, and radiation therapy or interferon for localized disease. Rutiximab has shown to be effective for cMALT as well.[33] Systemic chemotherapy is reserved for extracutaneous spread.

SECONDARY CUTANEOUS B-CELL LYMPHOMA (2⁰cBCL)

> **BOX 12-9 Summary**
>
> - May occur in any systemic B-cell lymphoma.
> - Common in intravascular larger B-cell lymphoma and lymphomatoid granulomatosis, but rare in mantel cell lymphoma and Hodgkin lymphoma.
> - Frequently portends a poor prognosis.
> - Treatment includes combination chemotherapy, rituximab, and/or bone marrow transplantation
> - Secondary cutaneous B-cell lymphomas may occur in any type of systemic B-cell.

Secondary cutaneous involvement by B-cell lymphoma is uncommon, but occurs with greater frequency in some types (intravascular large B-cell lymphoma, lymphomatoid granulomatosis) than in others (Mantel cell lymphoma, Hodgkin lymphoma). Treatment of the cutaneous disease is typically the same as treating systemic counterpart.

INTRAVASCULAR LARGE B-CELL LYMPHOMA (IVLBL)

Intravascular Large B-cell lymphoma (IVLBL) is a variant of diffuse large, B-cell lymphoma characterized by an absence of nodal or marrow disease at presentation and the trapping of large neoplastic B-lymphocytes within vascular lumina. Luminal occlusion results in ischemic tissue injury, which may be localized or widespread.

Skin and central nervous system signs and symptoms are most common, but nonspecific, including livedo reticularis, subcutaneous nodules, erythema nodosum-like lesions, stroke-like symptoms, dementia, or focal neurologic deficits. Other clinical manifestations of IVLBL include testicular ischemia, vasculo-occlusive lung disease, fever of

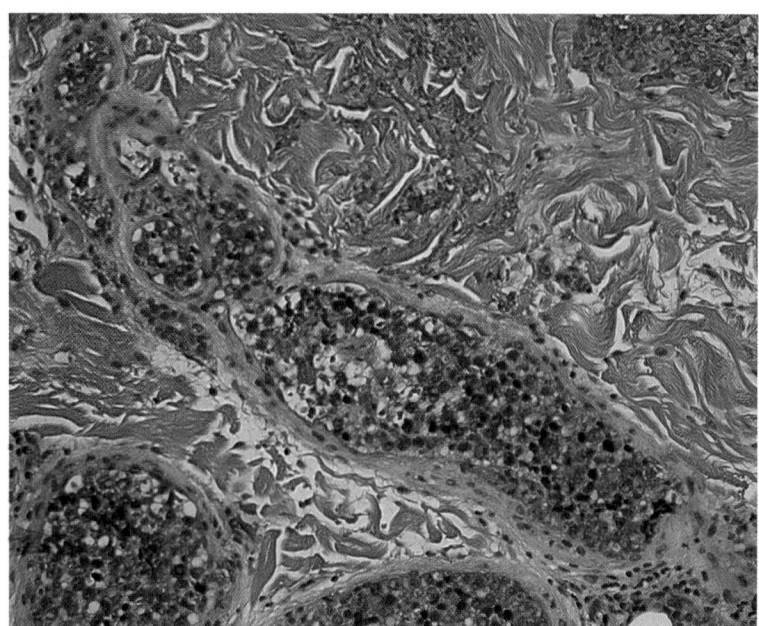

▲ **FIGURE 12-11** Deep dermal blood vessels, dilated and congested by large neoplastic B-cells in intravascular large B-cell lymphoma (H&E stain at 400× original magnification).

unknown origin, cytopenias and other hematologic complications.

Skin biopsy of IVLBL reveals clusters of large atypical lymphoid cells within dilated vascular channels (Fig. 12-11). Fibrin thrombi may also be identified. The lymphoid cells are decorated with B-cell antigens (CD19, CD20, CD79a). Intravascular localization or identification of lymphoma is not restricted to IVLBL, as cases with a T-cell or NK-cell phenotype have been reported.

The prognosis of IVLBL is extremely poor, as many cases are diagnosed postmortem. Early diagnosis, systemic chemotherapy and bone marrow transplantation may prove to provide the best outcome for this aggressive lymphoma.

LYMPHOMATOID GRANULOMATOSIS (LyG)

Lymphomatoid granulomatosis (LyG) is an angioinvasive and angiodestructive T-cell rich, Epstein–Barr virus associated, B-cell lymphoproliferative disorder. The clinicopathologic spectrum of LyG ranges from a self-limited course to fulminant progression to large B-cell lymphoma. Followed by the lung, the skin is the second most common organ involved by LyG. Pulmonary involvement is close to universal during the course of LyG, but may be preceded by skin involvement. Therefore, a high degree of clinical suspicion is usually necessary to establish a diagnosis of cutaneous involvement by LyG.

Skin lesions of LyG are characterized by red nodules or plaques that are frequently ulcerated. Skin biopsies of LyG show a nodular dermal to subcutaneous lymphohistiocytic infiltrate composed of small-to-medium-sized lymphocytes which frequently infiltrate and destroy cutaneous blood vessels.

The histologic appearance of LyG in the skin is often interpreted as an infection, "reactive" lymphohystiocytic process, or T-cell malignancy. Moreover, skin lesions of LyG often contain small numbers of neoplastic B-cells and studies for Epstein–Barr virus may be negative. If neoplastic B-cells are present, they are usually enlarged, overtly atypical, and clonal. The infiltrate tends to surround, infiltrate, and destroy dermal blood vessels with consequential skin necrosis.

Treatment of LyG depends on the extent and grade of extracutaneous disease. Systemic chemotherapy is usually employed. Rituximab has shown mixed results as monotherapy.[34–36] Bone marrow transplantation was associated with a prolonged remission in a recently published case of LyG.[37]

MANTLE CELL LYMPHOMA (MCL)

Mantle cell lymphoma (MCL) only occasionally involves the skin, and usually as a secondary event. Most patients have advanced disease at presentation.

The skin lesions of mantle cell lymphoma are nonspecific, but include red to purple papules or nodules. Biopsy from skin lesions involved by MCL demonstrate a nodular or diffuse dermal infiltrate composed of monomorphous, small, blue lymphoid cells with irregular nuclear contours. The blastoid variant appears to occur in the skin with greater frequency than other sites. The neoplastic cells of mantle cell lymphoma express CD20, CD5, and cyclin D-1. CD5-negative MCL is rare, but appears to be less aggressive.[38] The prognosis of MCL is poor, with most patient succumbing to progressive disease within 3 to 5 years.

Combination chemotherapy combined with rituximab and bone marrow transplantation has been recently advocated as first-line therapy of MCL.[39]

LEUKEMIA CUTIS (LC)

BOX 12-10   Summary

- Defined by the presence of leukemic cells in the skin.
- Leukemia may present in skin without blood or bone marrow involvement (aleukemic leukemia cutis).
- Histologic findings vary, but commonly reveal an interstitial pattern of leukemic cell infiltration in the dermis.
- Treatment of leukemia cutis is the same as treatment of its bone marrow counterpart.

Cutaneous infiltration in leukemia (leukemia cutis) varies in frequency according to leukemia subtype, with the acute myeloid leukemia (monocytic variants) being the most common. Cutaneous involvement by acute lymphoblastic leukemia (ALL) is rare. Correspondingly, the propensity for AML to affect adults and ALL to affect children accounts for the relative high rate of leukemia cutis in adulthood and its rarity in childhood.

Three points should be considered by clinicians and pathologists with regard to skin eruptions in leukemia patients, namely leukemids, leukemic cells that may accompany "reactive" dermatoses, and the atypical appearance of leukocytes following chemotherapy. Several inflammatory dermatoses occur with an increased frequency in the setting of leukemia, and are designated as leukemids. Leukemids are not specific for leukemia, but likely represent a state of "hyperreactivity" secondary to a dysregulated immune system. Examples of leukemids include some cases of drug eruption, persistent arthropod bite reaction, Sweet's syndrome, pyoderma gangrenosum, neutrophilic eccrine hidradenitis, and other neutrophilic dermatoses. Although leukemids by definition do not contain leukemic cells, identification of leukemic cells in skin biopsies of an otherwise typical reactive dermatosis in patients with leukemia should *not* always be interpreted as "leukemia cutis." In some cases, the composition of the cutaneous infiltrate includes leukemic cells because of their presence in high numbers in the peripheral blood and does not represent progression of the leukemia per se. Although the leukemic cells in the skin are identical morphologically and immunohistochemically to those in the peripheral blood and bone marrow, admixed lymphocytes, neutrophils, or eosinophils usually accompany the infiltrate. Clinical findings are also essential for a definitive diagnosis. Lastly, the leukocytes in skin biopsies of skin eruptions from patients that have recently completed chemotherapy may have an "immature" or "blast-like" appearance and should not be mistaken for leukemia cutis.

The skin lesions of leukemia cutis vary substantially in clinical appearance, but include red to purple papules, nodules, or plaques (Fig. 12-12).

Skin biopsies of leukemia cutis most often show a dermal mononuclear cell infiltrate that tends to infiltrate between collagen bundles in an "interstitial pattern." In AML, immunohistochemical stains identify a CD3-negative, CD20-negative, CD43-positive infiltrate, with myeloid markers (myeloperoxidase) or

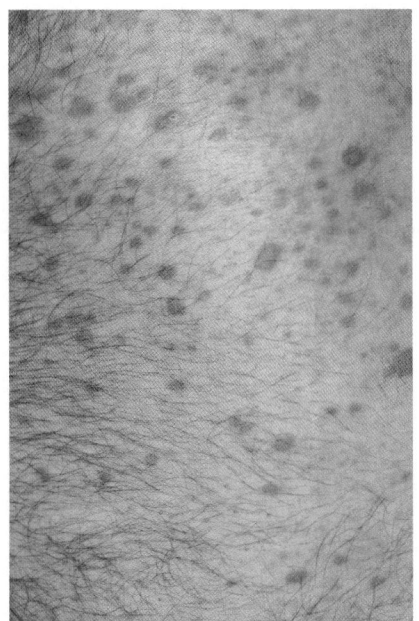

▲ **FIGURE 12-12** Scattered red papules on the chest in acute myeloid leukemia.

monocytic markers (CD4, CD68, lysozyme) showing variable expression depending on cellular differentiation. Terminal deoxynucleotidyl transferase (TdT) is usually positive in ALL and in some cases of AML. Specific cutaneous involvement by chronic lymphocytic leukemia (CLL) is not common, but does occur. The cells in CLL coexpress CD20 and CD5.

Treatment of leukemia cutis is the same as treatment of the specific type of leukemia if identified in the peripheral blood or bone marrow.

PRECURSOR HEMATODERMIC NEOPLASM (BLASTIC NK-CELL LYMPHOMA)

Precursor hematodermic neoplasm (also known as *CD4+/CD56+* hematodermic neoplasm and previously as blastic NK-cell lymphoma) is a rare, usually fatal neoplasm, the understanding of which is in evolution. Precursor hematodermic neoplasm (PHDN) was previously believed to be a natural killer lymphoma due to CD56-positivity, but an increasing body of data implicates a plasmacytoid dendritic cell origin rather than an NK-cell lineage. Given the clinical and histologic presentation, the high propensity to develop a leukemic phase, as well as a treatment approach similar to acute myeloid leukemia, we place PHDN under the rubric of leukemia cutis.

Comprising less than 1% of all primary cutaneous lymphomas in the French Study Group on Cutaneous Lymphomas, PHDN is rare. Males are affected with PHDN twice as frequently as females. The median survival of PHDN is 14 months overall, 38 months for patients less than 40 years of age and 10 months for patients over 40 years of age.

Cutaneous involvement in PHDN is nearly universal at initial presentation and at relapse. Extracutaneous involvement is present in approximately 40% of patients at first presentation, but most patients ultimately develop a leukemic phase during the disease course. Skin lesions are typically characterized by deep red to purple papules or nodules that may be few and scattered or innumerable and confluent (Fig. 12-13).

Histopathologic examination of skin biopsies in PHDN may resembles cutaneous involvement by acute myeloid leukemia, with a diffuse dermal and frequently subcutaneous infiltrate composed of medium-sized, monomorphous blast-like cells with scant cytoplasm. These cells do not stain for B-cell,

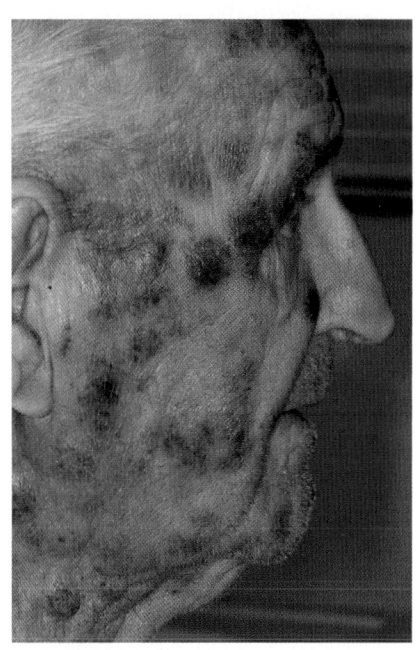

▲ **FIGURE 12-13** Deep red and purple nodules on the face in precursor hematodermic neoplasm.

T-cell, or myeloid cell markers, but do stain for CD4 and CD56. No clone is identified with T-cell receptor and immunoglobulin heavy chain gene rearrangement studies.

Treatment of PHDH is usually similar to that of acute myeloid leukemia, but early treatment with bone marrow transplantation may improve survival.[40]

FINAL THOUGHTS

In conclusion, cutaneous lymphomas and leukemias represent a diverse group of diseases that are vastly different in terms of clinical presentation, histologic findings, molecular genetic alterations, infectious disease associations, prognoses, and treatments. Recent advances in molecular techniques and collaborations between the researchers around the globe have led to a dramatic increase in the understanding of this complex area of cutaneous neoplasia. However, until we precisely understand the causes and find more effective treatments for these vexing diseases, we will always have much to learn.

REFERENCES

1. Bunn P, Lamberg S. Report of the committee on staging and classification of cutaneous T-cell lymphoma. *Cancer Treat Rep.* 1979;63:725–728.
2. Sausville EA, Eddy JL, Makuch RW, et al. Histopathologic staging at initial diagnosis of mycosis fungoides and Sézary syndrome: definition of three distinctive prognostic groups. *Ann Int Med.* 1988; 109:372–382.

3. Russell-Jones R, Whittaker S. TCR gene analysis in the diagnosis of Sézary syndrome. *J Am Acad Dermatol*. 1999;41:254–259.

4. Willemze R, Jaffe ES, Burg G, Cerroni L, et al. WHO-EORTC classification for cutaneous lymphoma. *Blood*. 2005;105:3768–3785.

5. Alibert JLM. Tableau de plan fongoides: description des maladies de la peau observee a l'hospital St. Louis, et exposition des meilleures methods suivies pour leur traitement. Paris, France, Barrior l'Anine et Files, 1806.

6. Weinstock MA, Gardstein B. Twenty-year trends in the reported incidence of myocosis fungoides and associated mortality. *Am J Public Health*. 1999;89:1240–1244.

7. Franck N, Carlotti A, Gorin I, et al. Mycosis Fungoides-type cutaneous T-cell lymphoma and Neutrophilic Dermatosis. *Arch Dermatol*. 2005;141:353–356.

8. Kaye FJ, Bunn PA Jr, Steinberg SM, et al. A randomized trail comparing combination electron-beam radiation and chemotherapy with topical therapy in the initial treatment of mycosis fungoides. *N Engl J Med*. 1989;321:1784–1790.

9. Ralfkiaer E, Jaffe ES. Mycosis fungoides and Sézary syndrome. In: Jaffe ES, Harris NL, Stein H, Vardiman JW, eds. *World Health Organization Classification of Tumours: Tumours of Haematopoietic and Lymphoid Tissues*. Lyon: IARC Press; 2001;216–220.

10. Winkelmann RK, Peters MS. Absolute number of circulating Sézary cells. *Arch Dermatol*. 1981;117:382.

11. Fraser-Andrews E, Woolford AJ, Russell-Jones R, et al. Detection of a peripheral blood T cell clone is an independent prognostic marker in Sézary syndrome. *J Inv Dermatol*. 2000;114:117–121.

12. Scarisbrick JJ, Whittaker S, Evans AV, et al. Prognostic significance of tumor burden in the blood of patients with erythrodermic primary cutaneous T-cell lymphoma. *Blood*. 2001;97:624–630.

13. Foulc, P. N'Guyen, J M. Dreno, B. Prognostic factors in Sézary syndrome: a study of 28 patients. *Br J Dermatol*. 2003;149:1152–1158.

14. Kari L, Loboda A, Nebozhyn M, et al. Classificaiton and prediction of survival in patients with the leukemic phase of cutaneous T-cell lymphoma. *J Exp Med*. 2003;197:1477–1488.

15. Kempf W. CD30+ lymphoproliferative disorders: histopathology, differential diagnosis, new variants, and simulators. *J Cutaneous Pathol*. 2006;33(suppl 1):58–70.

16. El-Azhary RA, Gibson LE, Kurtin PJ, et al. Lymphomatoid papulosis: a clinical and histopathologic review of 53 cases with leukocyte immunophenotyping, DNA flow cytometry, and T-cell receptor gene rearrangement studies. *J Am Acad Dermatol*. 1994;30:210–218.

17. Bekkenk MW, Geelen FA, van Voorst Vader PC, et al. Primary and secondary cutaneous CD30+ lymphoproliferative disorders: a report from the Dutch Cutaneous Lymphoma Group on long-term follow-up data of 219 patients and guidelines for diagnosis and treatment. *Blood*. 2000;95:3653–3661.

18. Berti E, Tomasini D, Vermeer MH, et al. Primary cutaneous CD8-positive epidermotropic cytotoxic T cell lymphomas. A distinct clinicopathological entity with an aggressive clinical behavior. *Am J Pathol*. 1999;155:483–492.

19. Marzano AV, Ghislanzoni M, Gianelli U, et al. Fatal CD8+ epidermotropic cytotoxic primary cutaneous T-cell lymphoma with multiorgan involvement. *Dermatology*. 2005;211:281–285.

20. Weenig RH, Ng CS, Perniciaro C. Subcutaneous panniculitis-like T-cell lymphoma: an elusive case presenting as lipomembranous panniculitis and a review of 72 cases in the literature. *Am J Dermatopathol*. 2001;23:206–215.

21. Santucci M, Pimpinelli N, Massi D, et al. Cytotoxic/natural killer cell cutaneous lymphomas. Report of EORTC Cutaneous Lymphoma Task Force Workshop. *Cancer*. 2003;97:610–627.

22. Ghobrial IM, Weenig RH, Pittlekow MR, et al. Clinical outcome of patients with subcutaneous panniculitis-like T-cell lymphoma. *Leuk Lymphoma*. 2005;46:703–708.

23. Massone C, Chott A, Metz D. Subcutaneous, blastic natural killer (NK), NK/T-cell, and other cytotoxic lymphomas of the skin. *Am J Surg Pathol*. 2004;28:719–735.

24. Murashige N, Kami M, Kishi Y, et al. Allogeneic haematopoietic stem cell transplantation as a promising treatment for natural killer-cell neoplasms. *Br J Haematol*. 2005;130:561–567.

25. Futagami A, Aoki M, Kawana S. A case of peripheral T-cell lymphoma unspecified involving subcutaneous tissue. *Leuk Lymphoma*. 2005;46:785–788.

26. Zaja F, Russo D, Silvestri F, Fanin R, et al. Retrospective analysis of 23 cases with peripheral T-cell lymphoma, unspecified: clinical characteristics and outcome. *Haematologica*. 1997;82:171–177.

27. Dogan A, AttyGalle AD, Kyriakou C. Angioimmunoblastic T-cell lymphoma. *Br J Haematol*. 2003;121:681–691.

28. Brown H, Macon WR, Kurtin PJ, Gibson LE. Cutaneous involvement by angioimmunoblastic T-cell lymphoma with remarkable heterogeneous Epstein–Barr virus expression. *J Cutaneous Pathol*. 2001; 28:432–438.

29. Kazakov DV, Burg G, Kempf W. Primary cutaneous B-cell lymphomas and pseudolymphomas: review of histopathological features. *Cesk Patol*. 2002;38:147–154.

30. Fierro MT, Savoia P, Quaglino P, et al. Systemic therapy with cyclophosphamide and anti-CD30 antibody (rituximab) in relapsed primary cutaneous B-cell lymphoma: a report of 7 cases. *J Am Acad Dermatol*. 2003;49:281–287.

31. Gellrich S, Muche JM, Pelzer K, et al. Anti-CD20 antibodies in primary cutaneous B-cell lymphoma. Initial results in dermatologic patients. *Hautarzt*. 2001;52:205–210.

32. Fink-Puches R, Zenahilik P, Bäck B, et al. Primary cutaneous lymphomas: applicability of current classification schemes (European Organization for Research and Treatment of Cancer, World Health Organization) based on clinicopathologic features observed in a large group of patients. *Blood*. 2002;99:800–805.

33. Soda R, Costanzo A, Cantonetti M, et al. Systemic therapy of primary cutaneous B-cell lymphoma, marginal zone type, with rituximab, a chimeric anti-CD20 monoclonal antibody. *Acta Derm Venereol*. 2001;81:207–208.

34. Jordan K, Grothey A, Grothe W, et al. Successful treatment of mediastinal lymphomatoid granulomatosis with rituximab monotherapy. *Eur J Haematol*. 2005; 74:263–266.

35. Polizzotto MN, Dawson MA, Opat SS. Failure of rituximab monotherapy in lymphomatoid granulomatosis. *Eur J Haematol*. 2005;75:172–173.

36. Moudir-Thomas C, Foulet-Roge A, Plat M, et al. Efficacy of rituximab in lymphomatoid granulomatosis. *Rev Mal Respir*. 2004;21:1157–1161.

37. Johnston A, Coyle L, Nevell D. Prolonged remission of refractory lymphomatoid granulomatosisafter autologous hemopoietic stem cell transplantation with post-transplantation maintenance interferon. *Leuk Lymphoma*. 2006;47:323–328.

38. Kaptain S, Zukerberg LR, Ferry JA, et al. BCL-1 cyclin-D1+ CD5− mantle cell lymphoma. *Modern Pathol*. 1998;11:133.

39. de Guibert S, Jaccard A, Bernard M, et al. Rituximab and DHAP followed by intensive therapy with autologous stem-cell transplantation as first-line therapy for mantle cell lymphoma. *Haematologica*. March 2006;91(3):425–426.

40. Yamaguchi M, Maekawa M, Nakamura Y, et al. Long-term remission of blastic natural killer-cell lymphoma after autologous peripheral blood stem-cell transplantation. *Am J Hematol*. 2005;80:124–127.

CHAPTER 13

Merkel Cell Carcinoma

Jerry D. Brewer, M.D.
David L. Appert, M.D.
Randall K. Roenigk, M.D.

BOX 13-1 Overview

- Merkel cell carcinoma (MCC) is a rare cutaneous neoplasm occurring on the head and neck of elderly Caucasian patients.
- MCC is one of the more deadly carcinomas, comparing with small cell lung cancer and melanoma in mortality.
- MCC has a high local recurrence rate and spreads to regional lymph nodes often, making curative treatment difficult in spite of the primary tumor usually being small in size (<2 cm).
- MCC is usually treated with wide local excision of at least 2 cm of clinically free margins with adjuvant radiation to the tumor site and draining lymph nodes.
- Combination chemotherapy plays an important role in metastatic disease and as adjuvant treatment for high-risk patients.
- Combination chemotherapy is sometimes used as a radiosensitizing agent.
- In spite of aggressive treatment, MCC remains an aggressive tumor with a high mortality rate.

INTRODUCTION

Friedrich Sigmund Merkel first described a unique nonkeratinocyte, nondendritic epidermal cell, which he labeled as a tactile cell, or "tastzelle," in 1875. This cell eventually bore his name and was viewed as a primary touch receptor, providing information about touch and hair movement.[1] Merkel cells have been described as being primary neural cells, derived from neural crest cells, and found as either single cells within the basal layer of the epidermis or in groups as a component of the tactile hair disc of Pinkus, functioning as slowly adapting type I mechanoreceptors.[2,3] Although Merkel cells have been widely believed to be derived from neural crest cells, they have been found to express a number of both neuronal and epithelial markers. This has led

some authors to conclude that Merkel cells are actually keratinocyte-derived and epidermal in origin. This conclusion is being more recently accepted.[4–6]

In 1972, Toker documented five cases of a trabecular cell carcinoma of the skin, originally thought to be derived from sweat glands.[7] However, 6 years later, Tang and Toker reported the presence of dense-core granules in these cells, characteristic of Merkel cells and other neuroendocrine cells.[8] In 1980, De Wolf-Peeters suggested the name Merkel cell carcinoma (MCC) for this trabecular-looking tumor, and it has been hypothesized that MCC is derived from Merkel cells.[9] To date, there have been over 2000 cases of MCC reported in the literature, with approximately 470 new cases diagnosed yearly in the United States.[10] Other names which have been used to describe this tumor include trabecular carcinoma of the skin, primary small cell carcinoma of the skin, and cutaneous apudoma; but the most common alternative name is primary neuroendocrine carcinoma of the skin.

Current management guidelines for MCC are based mostly on well documented phase I and phase II trials. Due to the rarity of MCC, no phase III randomized controlled trials have been performed, and patients are often rendered treatment based on clinic experience rather than evidence-based medicine.[11]

EPIDEMIOLOGY

BOX 13-2 Summary

- MCC is a rare cutaneous malignancy of the elderly.
- MCC occurs more often in males with a male-to-female ratio of 2:1 to 3:1.
- The average age of patients who are diagnosed with MCC is 67 to 69 years.
- MCC has been found in patients from 7 to 104 years of age.
- MCC can occur anywhere on the body, but has a predilection for sun-exposed skin, especially the head and neck (especially periorbitally), extremities, and trunk.

MCC is a rare cutaneous malignancy of the elderly with an incidence of 0.23 per 100,000 in Caucasians and 0.01 per 100,000 in African Americans per the US Surveillance, Epidemiology, and End Results (SEER) Program as well as a defined patient population at the Mayo

Clinic.[12–16] Men seem to be more commonly affected with a male-to-female ratio of 2:1 to 3:1, according to SEER data[16]; however, there have been a few case series reporting a higher incidence in women.[17,18] Medina-Franco et al reviewed 1024 cases reported in 20 series and determined the male-to-female ratio to be 1.4:1.[19] Most cases of MCC occur in the elderly population with the average age at diagnosis of 67 to 69 years, and only 5% of cases occurring before the age of 50.[10,16–18,20–22] The reported age range in patients diagnosed with MCC is 7 to 104.[13,23–26] The sites of the body most often harboring a primary MCC are usually the sun-exposed areas. These include the head and neck area (periorbital in particular), extremities, and trunk.

PATHOGENESIS

BOX 13-3 Summary

- MCC has been linked to photo exposure.
- MCC occurs more frequently in areas close to the equator and has a correlation with the UVB index.
- Methoxsalen and UVA therapy increases the incidence of MCC 100 fold.
- MCC has also been associated with arsenic and infrared light.
- Immunosuppression is associated with a higher incidence of MCC, a younger age at onset, and a more aggressive course.
- The frequency of secondary malignancies in the setting of MCC is as high as 25%.
- Conditions seen in conjunction with MCC include congenital ectodermal dysplasia, Cowden's disease, and Hodgkin's disease.

Little is known about the etiology of MCC; however, it has been linked to photo exposure, as it occurs more frequently in areas of proximity to the equator geographically as well as on parts of the body which are more exposed to sunlight anatomically. In addition, the frequency of MCC correlates with the UVB index, much like melanoma.[16] One study was able to demonstrate a typical p53 mutation in MCC, which commonly occurs in UVB-induced carcinomas.[27] Methoxsalen and UVA used for the treatment of psoriasis has also been correlated with MCC.[10] In fact, it has been suggested that methoxsalen and UVA therapy for psoriasis increase the incidence of MCC 100 fold.[28] Other correlations include arsenic[29] and infrared light.[30]

An interesting association is immuno-suppression, with cases of MCC being linked to organ transplantation,[31,32] HIV infection (with a relative risk in acquired immunodeficiency of 13.4), and chronic lymphocytic leukemia.[33–36] In transplant patients, the incidence of MCC is 0.9% of all *de novo* malignancies, and MCC tends to occur at an earlier age (mean of 46 years) and has a worse prognosis in these patients.[37] MCC has also been seen with synchronous or metachronous squamous cell carcinoma (SCC) as well as basal cell carcinoma (BCC).[38–43] The frequency of secondary malignancy in MCC is as high as 25% (only 5.8% in melanoma), an association which also pretends an immunologic basis for the development of MCC.[43] Other conditions seen in conjunction with MCC include congenital ectodermal dysplasia, Cowden's disease, and Hodgkin's disease.[44]

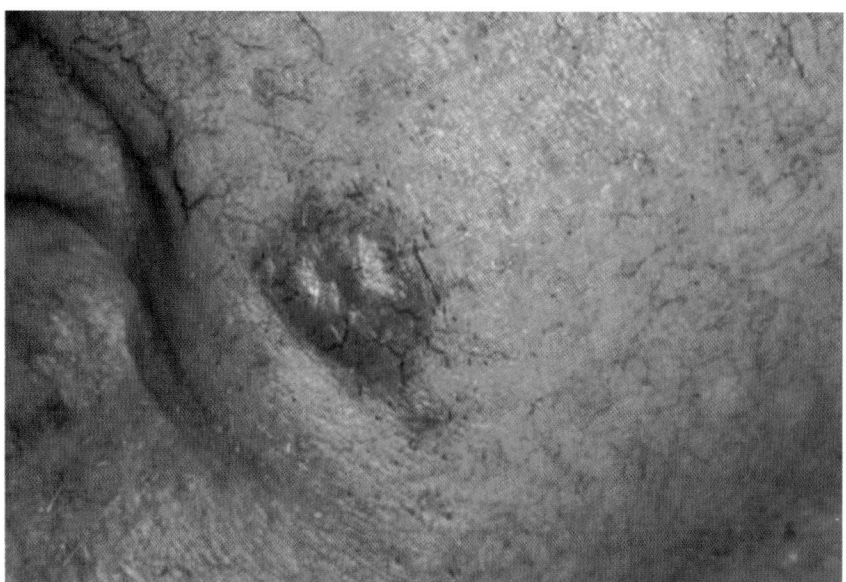

▲ **FIGURE 13-1** Merkel cell carcinoma presenting as an erythematous painless, raised, cutaneous nodule with overlying telangiectasia on the cheek of an elderly patient.

CLINICAL PRESENTATION

BOX 13-4   Summary

- MCC presents as a painless, firm, red, pink, blue, or violaceous appearing intracutaneous mass with overlying telangiectasia.
- Most MCCs are less than 2 cm in diameter at diagnosis.
- The diagnosis of MCC is rarely made clinically as it is often confused with BCC, SCC, amelanotic melanoma, cutaneous lymphoma, and lipomas.
- The number of patients presenting with localized disease is 70 to 80%.
- There is a greater than 50% likelihood of lymphatic metastasis or hematogenous spread at some time during the course of the illness.
- Secondary malignancies include SCC, hematologic malignancies, and adenocarcinomas of the breast and ovary.
- No universally accepted staging system exists for MCC.
- A simple staging system has been proposed. Stage I for local disease, Stage II for locoregional disease, and Stage III for distant metastasis.

MCC typically presents as a painless, firm, raised intracutaneous mass (most often nodular but can also be plaque-like) with a shiny surface and frequent overlying telangiectasia. This lesion is usually red, pink, blue, or violaceous in appearance (Figs. 13-1 and 13-2).[23] Tumor sizes range from 0.2 to 20 cm in diameter, with the majority measuring less than 2 cm (81%) at diagnosis. There is often a history of rapid growth of the lesion during the weeks prior to biopsy, and the lesion may even be ulcerated.[45,46] Occasionally a patient may present with metastatic disease to the lymph nodes without evidence of a primary tumor, and 10 to 20% of these cases will present with no obvious primary site. Interestingly, patients with an occult primary tumor have been found to have a more favorable prognosis when compared to patients with metastatic disease and a known primary tumor.[47] As mentioned previously, MCC tends to occur on sun-exposed areas, with 50% being located on the head and neck, and frequently involving the eyelids.[48–50] MCC also occurs on the extremities and trunk, roughly 40 and 10% of the time respectively (both sites being more common in younger patients).[13,19,23,44,51–59] Rare reports have documented MCC in areas such as the oral mucosa,[60] vulva,[61] and penis,[10,26,62] which are not exposed to the sun.

Patients usually have local symptoms only, related to tumor growth and/or lymph node involvement. There are, however, reported cases of superior vena cava syndrome due to an obstructing tumor mass[63] and paraneoplastic syndromes[64] associated with MCC.

Because MCC is a rare tumor, the diagnosis is rarely made clinically, and the presentation can be confused with BCC, SCC, amelanotic melanoma, cutaneous lymphoma, and even a lipoma. Any vio-

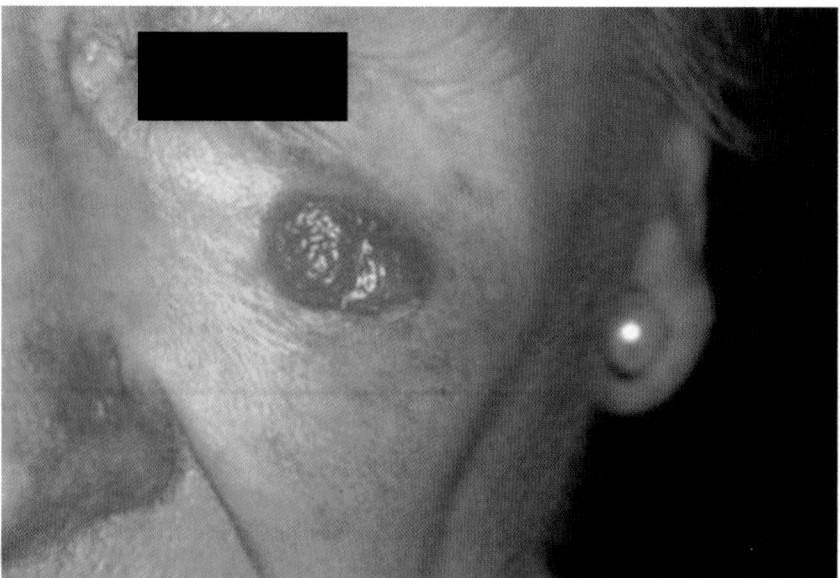

▲ **FIGURE 13-2** Patient with Merkel cell carcinoma presenting as a painless, raised, red to violaceous cutaneous nodule on the cheek.

laceous dermal nodule occurring on sun-exposed skin should be evaluated carefully. Dermal spread via the lymphatics is a common occurrence, and multiple satellite lesions may be seen clinically.

About 70 to 80% of patients with MCC will present with localized disease, and a small percentage with in-transit metastases. It has been estimated that between 20 and 33% of patients have clinically involved regional lymph nodes at presentation, and less than 5% are found to have distant metastases when diagnosed.[10,13,54] Although the tumor is usually small at presentation and the majority of patients appear to have localized disease only, there is still a very high risk of tumor spread. In fact, it has been suggested that the overall risk of lymphatic metastasis and/or hematogenous spread is greater than 50% at some point during the course of the illness, reflecting the aggressive nature of this carcinoma (Figs. 13-3 to 13-5).[23,51] Nodal status at presentation is the strongest predictor of distant spread. The most likely sites of distant metastasis include the skin (28%), lymph nodes (27%), liver (13%), lung (10%), bone (10%), and central nervous system (6%).[15,19]

There have been a few cases of spontaneous regression of MCC with no signs of recurrence after long periods of follow-up. The incidence of this occurrence has been estimated to be 1.7%.[65]

As mentioned previously, there is a high incidence of secondary malignancy (25%) in patients with MCC. SCC makes

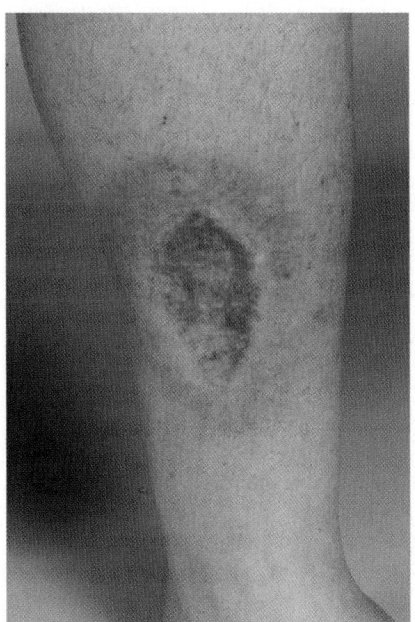

▲ FIGURE 13-3 Recurrent Merkel cell carcinoma on the lower extremity status post wide local excision.

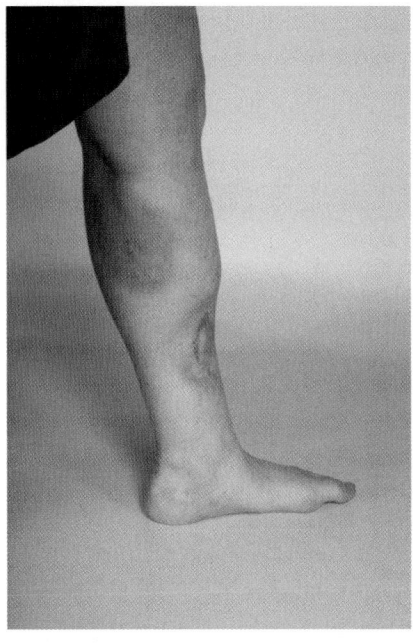

▲ FIGURES 13-4 View from the side of recurrent Merkel cell carcinoma of the lower extremity in the same patient as in Fig. 13-3. Note the multiple wide local excisions due to multiple in-transit metastases.

up roughly half of these secondary cancers, the remainder being mostly hematologic malignancies, and adenocarcinomas of the breast and ovary. After appropriate therapy for MCC, patients still have a 2.1% risk of manifesting a second malignancy each year, and patients with secondary malignancies tend to

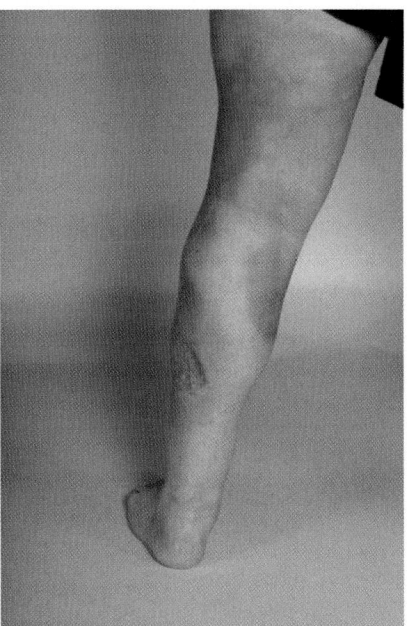

▲ FIGURES 13-5 View from the back of recurrent Merkel cell carcinoma of the lower extremity in the same patient as in Fig. 13-3. Note the multiple wide local excisions due to multiple in-transit metastases.

Table 13-1
Staging for Merkel Cell Carcinoma

STAGE		DESCRIPTION
I		Local disease
	• IA	Tumor size ≤2.0 cm in diameter
	• IB	Tumor size >2.0 cm in diameter
II		Locoregional disease with regional lymph node involvement
III		Metastatic disease

have a worse prognosis and a greater chance of dying from MCC.[43]

Staging

No universally accepted staging system for MCC exists, but there are a few commonly used systems. The most commonly adopted staging system, which was proposed by Yiengpruksawan et al, separates patients into three stages: stage I for patients with local disease only, stage II for patients with locoregional disease, and stage III for patients with distant metastasis (Table 13-1).[46]

Another system used less often is the American Joint Committee on Cancer (AJCC) staging system for skin cancer in general (Table 13-2).

When looking at the staging system in Table 13-1, 70 to 80% of patients will present with stage I disease, 10 to 30% with stage II, and 1 to 4% with stage III.[10,17,45,46,52] It has been proposed that the use of the simpler staging system outlined by Yiengpruksawan et al can effectively categorize patients into different treatment regimens. Patients with stage I and stage II disease should be treated with a curative intent and stage III patients palliatively.

■ HISTOLOGY

BOX 13-5   Summary

- There are three histologic types of MCC, namely intermediate, small cell, and trabecular.
- MCC is composed of small blue cells and can be confused with small cell lung cancer, lymphoma, neuroblastoma, Ewing's sarcoma, melanoma, or BCC
- Immunohistochemical staining with CK 20, TTF 1, and CK 7, as well as CAM 5.2 can help distinguish MCC from other entities, especially small cell lung cancer.
- The c-kit receptor tyrosine kinase (CD 117) is expressed in 95% of MCC, but does not seem to impact prognosis.

Table 13-2
The American Joint Committee on Cancer Staging System for Skin Cancer

STAGE	DESCRIPTION		
PRIMARY TUMOR (T)			
• TX	Primary tumor cannot be assessed		
• T0	No evidence of primary tumor		
• Tis	Carcinoma *in situ*		
• T1	Tumor ≤2 cm in greatest dimension		
• T2	Tumor >2 cm, but <5 cm in greatest dimension		
• T3	Tumor >5 cm in greatest dimension		
• T4	Tumor invades deep extradermal structures (i.e., cartilage, muscles, or bone)		
REGIONAL LYMPH NODES (N)			
• NX	Regional lymph nodes cannot be assessed		
• N0	No regional lymph node metastasis		
• N1	Regional lymph node metastasis		
DISTANT METASTASIS (M)			
• MX	Distant metastasis cannot be assessed		
• M0	No distant metastasis		
• M1	Distant metastasis		
STAGE GROUPING			
• Stage 0	Tis	N0	M0
• Stage I	T1	N0	M0
• Stage II	T2	N0	M0
	T3	N0	M0
• Stage III	T4T	N0	M0
	Any	N1	M0
• tage IV	Any T	Any N	M1

MCC is composed of small blue cells with hyperchromatic nuclei, small nucleoli, and scant cytoplasm (reversal of the nucleus to cytoplasm ratio). Mitoses are common and apoptosis is frequently extensive (Fig. 13-6).[44] In addition, lymphovascular invasion is often present.[58] Three different subtypes of MCC have been described histologically, namely, intermediate (most common), small cell, and trabecular (least common).[66] There does not seem to be any differences in prognosis among these different histologic types of MCC, and a combination of the three is commonly seen.

The intermediate variant of MCC is characterized by diffuse sheets of basophilic cells, a scant amount of cytoplasm, and round to oval vesicular nuclei with dispersed chromatin giving the pathognomonic "watery appearance." The small cell variant appears identical to other small cell carcinomas, having irregular, hyperchromatic cells, often with crush artifact and frequent nuclear molding. It is difficult to distinguish this variant from metastatic pulmonary small cell carcinoma, and immunohistochemical staining is indicated. In the trabecular variant, ribbons of small basophilic cells are

seen which typically display nuclear molding. In addition to these three common variants, spindle-cell forms

have been described, and keratinization and ductal differentiation may also be seen.

MCC usually arises in the dermis, can extend to the subcutaneous tissue, and is considered one of the "small blue cell tumors". The overlying epidermis is commonly intact; however, ulceration or rarely, squamous cell carcinoma *in situ* (SCCIS) may be seen.[67] In a small number of other patients, the epidermis may have tumor involvement, either as neuroendocrine carcinoma *in situ* or as single cells randomly scattered throughout the epithelium.[58,68]

With hematoxylin and eosin (H&E)-stained sections, MCC may be confused with small cell lung cancer, lymphoma, neuroblastoma, Ewing's sarcoma, melanoma, or BCC. Another histologic differential diagnosis is peripheral primitive neuroectodermal tumor. Paranuclear whorls of intermediate filaments can be seen histologically, which helps differentiate MCC from the most often contended diagnosis of oat cell carcinoma metastatic to the skin.

Immunohistochemical staining helps to differentiate MCC from other small cell blue tumors (Table 13-3). MCC characteristically expresses both neuroendocrine and cytokeratin markers. The neuroendocrine markers expressed in MCC include neurone specific enolase, synaptophysin, and chromogranin. Expressed cytokeratins include cytokeratin (CK) 20 (Fig. 13-7) and CAM 5.2

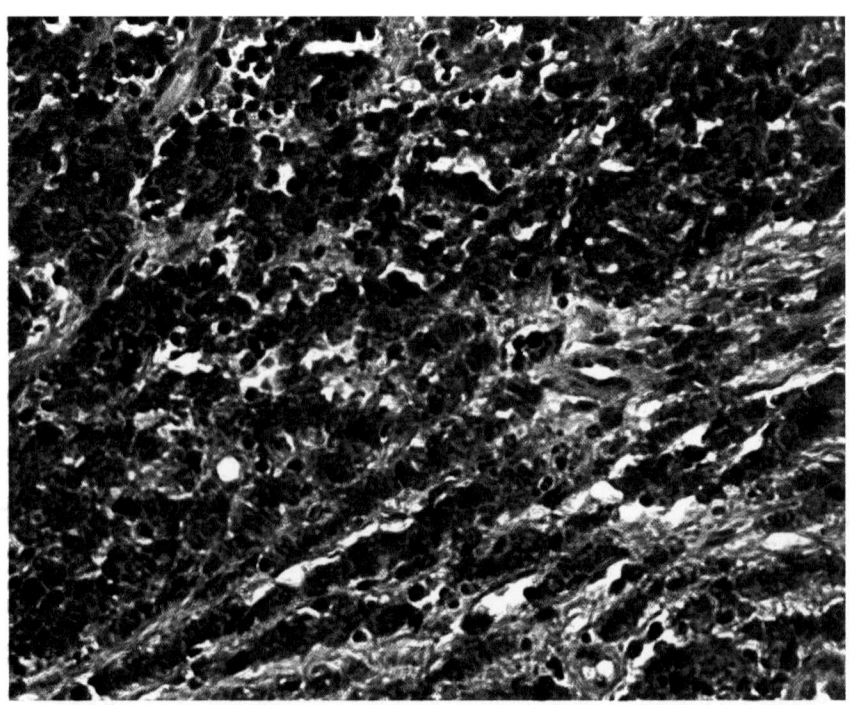

▲ **FIGURE 13-6** Sheets and clusters of small blue cells within the dermis. Cells contain vesicular nuclei with several nucleoli (H&E at 400× original magnification).

Table 13-3
Immunocytochemic Differential Diagnosis of Merkel Cell Carcinoma

TUMOR	CK20	S100	TTF 1	CK7	LCA	NFP	CD99	NSE
Merkel cell carcinoma	+	−	−	−	−	+	Rarely + (cytoplasmic)	+
Small cell lung carcinoma	−	−	+	+	−	+/−	Rarely + (cytoplasmic)	+
Lymphoma	−	−	−	−	+	−	−	−
Peripheral primitive neuroectodermal tumor	−	−	−	−	−	Rarely +	+ (membranous)	+
Small cell melanoma	−	−	−	−	−	−	−	+

CD99—cluster of differentiation antigen 99, CK7—cytokeratin 7, CK20—cytokeratin 20, LCA—leucocyte common antigen, NFP—neurofilament protein, NSE—neurone specific enolase, S100—S100 protein, TTF1—thyroid transcription factor 1, + (positive stain), − (negative stain).

seen as a paranuclear dot.[69–76] Epithelial membrane antigen and BER-EP4 may also be expressed.[77,78] MCC is usually negative for S100, leukocyte common antigen, and thyroid transcription factor (TTF) 1 (commonly expressed in pulmonary small cell tumors).[79–82] In addition, MCC is usually negative for CK 7 (also commonly expressed in pulmonary small cell tumors). Thus, combining CK 20, TTF 1, and CK 7, as well as CAM 5.2, one can differentiate fairly well between pulmonary small cell tumors and MCC.[83,84] Additionally, neurofilament protein, which is commonly positive in MCC, is absent in small cell carcinomas of the lung.[85–88] These markers can also be used to detect micrometastatic disease present in lymph nodes after sen-

tinel lymph node surgery has been performed. This technique identifies tumor cells in 22% of nodes that were previously pronounced negative on hematoxylin-eosin (H&E) stained sections.[89] The c-kit receptor tyrosine kinase (CD 117) is expressed in 95% of MCC, but does not seem to impact prognosis. The presence of CD 117 in most patients with MCC has been the catalyst to recent discussion as to the possible role of imatinib mesylate (Gleevec), a tyrosine kinase inhibitor, in the treatment of this difficult to manage tumor.[90,91]

Electron microscopy examination of MCC reveals electron dense granules (80 to 200 nm) and paranuclear aggregates of keratin and neurofilament protein.

DIAGNOSIS

BOX 13-6   Summary

- A biopsy is essential to the diagnosis of MCC.
- CT, MRI, and PET scans are helpful in evaluating extent of disease and for staging purposes.
- Sentinel lymph node biopsy is also helpful for staging, and will show positive lymphatic spread in 24% of cases.

Due to the rarity of MCC, the diagnosis is most commonly made after histopathologic evaluation. After the histologic diagnosis of MCC has been made, particular attention should be given to the primary site and to the regional lymph nodes (Table 13-4). The primary tumor should be assessed for satellite lesions as well as dermal seeding. The regional lymph nodes should be carefully examined for clinical signs of regional spread.

The patient with MCC should undergo further imaging studies for staging purposes as well as to exclude other sites as possible primary sources of small cell carcinoma. Computed tomography (CT) of the chest will evaluate for any lung masses (to rule out small cell carcinoma of the lung) as well as provide information regarding metastatic disease. In addition, abdominal and pelvic CT scans should be obtained to assess for metastases (especially in the liver).[92] Additional imaging studies such as bone scans and magnetic resonance imaging (MRI) of the brain are not indicated without supporting symptoms.

The presence of lymphatic spread is a negative predictor for overall survival in MCC but can be treated with excision, external radiation, and chemotherapy. Thus, it is important to know whether lymphatic spread has occurred. Elective lymph node dissection could be considered, but has potential complications

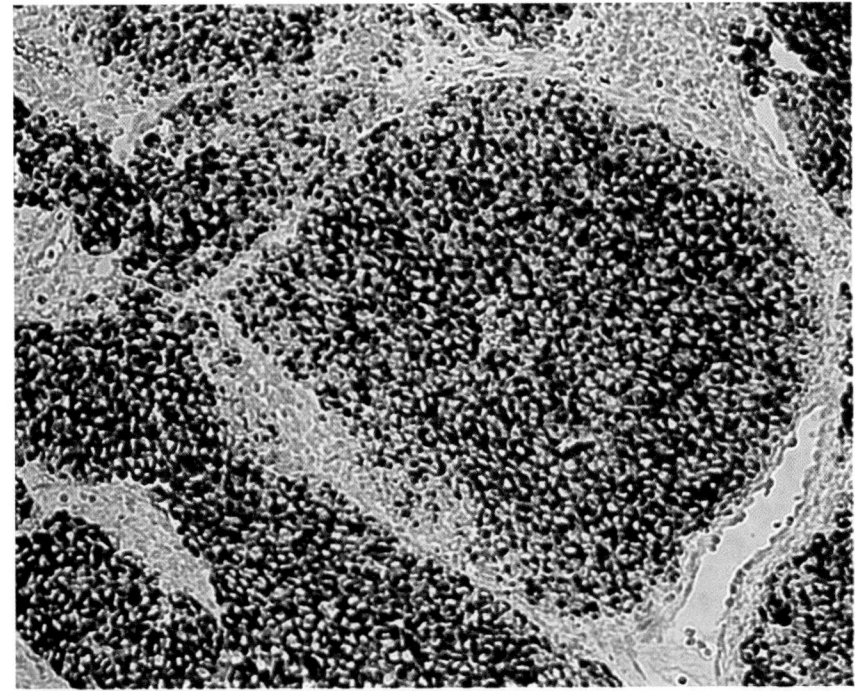

▲ **FIGURE 13-7** Photomicrograph of tumor specimen stained with cytokeratin (CK) 20 showing characteristic perinuclear dot staining, typical for Merkel cell carcinoma (immunoperoxidase stain with cytokeratin 20 at 200× original magnification).

Table 13-4

Approach to the Patient With Merkel Cell Carcinoma

STEP OF INVESTIGATION	DESCRIPTION
COMPLETE HISTORY AND PHYSICAL	
• Focus on the primary site	Look for satellite lesions and dermal seeding
• Focus on the regional lymph nodes	Look for signs of lymphatic spread
ADDITIONAL IMAGING	
• CT Chest	Rule out small cell cancer of the lung
• CT Abdomen	Look for metastases (especially of the liver)
• CT Pelvis	Look for metastases
• Nuclear[a]	Can be supplementary
CONSIDER SENTINAL LYMPH NODE MAPPING AND BIOPSY OR ELECTIVE DISSECTION	Evaluate for regional spread in high risk patients

[a]Octreotide, PET, and sentinal node scintigraphy.

including misidentification of the draining basin, chronic lymphedema, and nerve damage. Sentinal lymph node biopsy via mapping with radioactive colloid and blue dye has been used instead of elective lymph node dissection in many cases of MCC.[93,94] As mentioned previously, some sentinel lymph nodes may be evaluated as negative via H&E, but found to be positive for micrometastases when immunohistochemical stains are applied.[89,95] Pan et al evaluated 95 patients with MCC who underwent sentinal lymph node mapping and biopsy, and found lymphatic spread to be present in 24%.[26] Little, however, is known regarding the negative predictive value of this test in MCC, and further research is needed.

Nuclear medicine evaluation including sentinel-node scintigraphy, somatostatin-receptor scintigraphy, and positron emission tomography (PET), can be used to supplement cross-sectional scans for greater diagnostic accuracy.[96,97] Octreotide (or somatostatin) analogue scans have been used for detection of various neuroendocrine carcinomas, especially of the gastrointestinal tract, since the early 1990s,[98] and several authors feel that this modality may be more sensitive for MCC evaluation than CT scans.[99–105] However, Durani et al demonstrated false positives or false negatives in 5 of 11 patients with an overall sensitivity and specificity of 78 and 96%, respectively.[106,107] The regular use of octreotide scans for staging purposes in MCC cannot be recommended fully until further evaluation has been done. PET scans using 18-fluorodeoxyglucose [18F] have also been used with success in staging and evaluating MCC, as well as carcinoid, pheochromocytoma, and neuroblastoma; however, further experience is needed here as well before formal recommendations can be made.[108–110]

■ MOLECULAR ASPECTS

BOX 13-7   Summary

- Mutations in *p53* and loss of heterozygosity on chromosome 1 are commonly seen in MCC.
- Loss of heterozygosity in chromosome 3p21 has also been seen in MCC, the same region affected in more than 90% of small cell lung cancer patients.

MCC has been characterized by a wide range of chromosomal anomalies. Chromosomes most frequently affected include chromosome 1, 3, 5, 6, 11, and 13, with the short arm of chromosome 1, long arm of chromosome 3, and a gain of 5p material being common.[111] A deletion of 1p36 (short arm of chromosome 1) has been seen in MCC as well as neuroblastoma and melanoma, leading some to believe a tumor suppressor gene may be located here that contributes to the development of these tumors.[112–117] Interestingly, *p73* is found at chromosome 1p36.33, however, a recent investigation found mutations of *p73* in only 1 out of 10 patients with MCC (also an infrequent finding in melanoma).[27,118] *P53* is a tumor suppressor which is thought to be transiently expressed in MCC. Recently, evidence that chronic sun exposure may be a contributing factor in MCC has surfaced, and UVB induced mutations in *p53* and HRAS genes have been found in some MCC cell lines.[27] In a small series, mutant *p53* was found in six of nine patients. These 6 patients had worse clinical outcomes when compared to a group of 10 patients with MCC that did not have mutant *p53*.[119]

Another interesting abnormality is loss of heterozygosity in chromosome 3p21. This is the same region affected in more than 90% of patients with small cell lung cancer. The ras association domain family 1 gene (RASSF1A) is the proposed tumor suppressor gene of this region which may be implicated in the development of MCC and/or small cell lung carcinoma.[120–122] Loss of heterozygosity has also been seen in chromosome 10q[123] and chromosome 13, associated with frequent deletions of the retinoblastoma gene in one report.[124–126] In addition, multiple numbers of chromosome X have been seen in MCC, while only one copy is demonstrated in normal Merkel cells.[127]

A new DNA-binding protein has recently been identified in MCC, called the Merkel nuclear factor. This factor has been identified as POU4F3, a member of the POU domain family of transcription factors. This factor has also been found in normal human Merkel cells and in animal models has been shown to play a crucial role in neuroendocrine differentiation as well as normal Merkel cell function.[128]

Other specific mutations that have been seen in MCC include trisomy 1,[124,129,130] trisomy 6,[129,131,132] trisomy 11,[124,131] trisomy 18,[127] and deletion of chromosome 7.[131]

Leonard et al looked at the number of chromosomal aberrations present, particularly on chromosome 1 in patients with MCC. Seventy-three percent of tumors were found to have a loss of heterozygosity in one locus and 58% had a loss of heterozygosity in more than one locus. This has led some authors to believe that multiple tumor suppressor genes play a role in the development of MCC.[116]

While many tumor suppressor and oncogenes have been studied as to their relationship in the pathogenesis of MCC, no clear gene has been implicated conclusively. Much remains speculative in regard to the molecular genetics of MCC, and little is known regarding the prognostic implications of specific chromosomal aberrations.

■ PROGNOSIS

BOX 13-8   Summary

- The major determinant of survival is stage of disease at diagnosis.
- In spite of aggressive treatment, MCC remains difficult to control.
- Patients with nodal involvement have a median survival of 13 months.
- MCC has a high recurrence rate, especially when located on the lower extremities.
- Future prognostication may focus on the identification of transcription factors.

The major determinant of survival is the stage of the disease at diagnosis.[19] The 5-year survival for stage I and stage II disease has been documented as 64 and 47%, respectively.[10] Stage III disease carries a grave prognosis with a median survival of only 9 months, and a 5-year survival of practically 0%.[10,15]

Despite advances in treatment options, MCC remains an aggressive tumor that can prove difficult to control. When appropriate combinations of surgery and radiation are utilized, however, locoregional control can be obtained in 85 to 90% of cases.[133]

There are several characteristics which portend to a poor prognosis. Nodal disease is a powerful predictor of future metastatic disease, and ultimately of survival.[54,134] In one study, patients with involved nodes had a median survival of 13 months, compared to 40 months in patients without nodal disease.[13] In the Trans-Tasman Radiation Oncology Group (TROG) Study 96:07 trial in which high-risk MCC patients were treated with a standard chemotherapy/radiation protocol, the markers of local control and survival were tumor site and nodal disease.[47] The presence of either of these factors, however, did not influence locoregional control of the carcinoma, which demonstrates the effectiveness of radiation in securing local control of the tumor, even when nodal disease is present.

MCC is commonly undertreated and has a high likelihood of recurrence when located on the lower extremity (Table 13-5). One reason is that lower extremities have a poor blood supply, especially in the elderly. Because of this reason, and concerns regarding wound healing, adequate wide local excision on the lower extremities of patients with MCC is difficult to obtain. Additionally, the lower limbs do not tolerate high-dose radiation well. Due to these factors, MCC on the lower extremities has been associated with a worse outcome.[11] Other poor prognostic indicators include male sex,[54] primary size greater than 2 cm,[135] older than 60 years of age at diagnosis,[21] and lack of radiotherapy for management.[136] A negative surgical margin has been reported as a good prognostic indicator; however this did not influence the course of disease when radiation was given postoperatively.[137]

Future prognostication may focus on the identification of transcription factors, (i.e., HATH-1, Brn-3c and the previously mentioned Merkel nuclear factor), which have been identified in MCC as well as normal Merkel cells, and are essential for normal function and neuroendocrine differentiation.[128] These transcription factors are only expressed in the classic variant of MCC, where neurosecretory granules are present. A variant form of MCC exists which does not have neurosecretory granules, nor does it express these transcription factors.[128] Whether or not these transcription factors prove to be of prognostic significance remains to be seen.

TREATMENT

BOX 13-9 Overview

- General considerations
  - The primary goal to treating MCC is to control the primary site and the locoregional lymph nodes.
  - Treatment modalities include surgery, radiotherapy, and chemotherapy.
- Surgical treatment
  - Surgery plays a major role in the treatment of MCC.
  - Controversy exists regarding optimal margins, however, most authors suggest WLE with 2 to 3 cm margins.
  - Conflicting reports exist regarding the use of Mohs micrographic surgery in the setting of MCC.
  - Better outcomes are seen when radiotherapy is added postoperatively.
- Treatment of lymph nodes
  - Pathologic involvement of lymph nodes is seen in 10 to 30% of patients.
  - Prophylactic lymph node dissection is not recommended.
  - Lymphoscintigraphy and sentinel lymph node biopsy have been proposed as alternatives to lymph node dissection.
  - Patients with known lymph node disease should undergo surgical removal supplemented with postoperative radiotherapy.
- Radiation therapy
  - MCC is a radiosensitive tumor.
  - Strong evidence suggests the use of radiotherapy to the primary site in addition to the draining lymph node basin after surgical excision of the primary tumor.
  - Radiotherapy is usually employed 4 weeks postoperatively at a dose between 45 to 70 Gy.
  - Radiation can be used palliatively for patients experiencing pain, bleeding, infection, ulceration, and metastatic disease to the bone or brain.
- Chemotherapy
  - Chemotherapy is mostly used palliatively in patients with hematogenous spread, or stage III disease.
  - Chemotherapy can be used as an adjuvant in high risk stage II patients and as a radiosensitizing agent.
  - Common combination chemotherapy regimens used include cyclophosphamide, doxorubicine (or epirubicin), and vincristine (CAV), as well as etoposide and cisplatin (or carboplatin).
  - Isolated limb perfusion with chemotherapy, mostly melphalan, can be used to gain better locoregional control, especially of the lower extremities.
- Other therapeutic options
  - Biologics such as interferon (IFN) and tumor necrosis factor (TNF) have been used to treat MCC.
  - Rare reports exist documenting the treatment of MCC with other therapeutics such as octreotide, *bcl-2* antisense oligonucleotides, imatinab mesylate (Gleevec), topical dinitrochlorbenzol, and Imiquimod (Aldara).

Due to the rare nature of MCC, no prospective studies have been performed to assess the efficacy of surgery, radiation, or chemotherapy. A general treatment approach according to stage is presented in Table 13-6.[46]

The primary goal of treating patients with MCC is to control the primary site as well as the locoregional lymph nodes. Because uncontrolled locoregional disease has a tremendous impact on the quality of life, on the risk of local recurrence, risk of lymphatic and hematologic spread, as well as on survival, it is very important to control the tumor at the primary site as well as at the lymph nodes. In addition, once there is a recurrence, it is much more difficult to gain control of the tumor, which tends to be more aggressive. For this reason, it is

Table 13-5
Prognostic Factors of Merkel Cell Carinoma

PROGNOSIS	INDICATORS
WORSE PROGNOSIS	Lymph node disease
	Immunosuppression
	Male sex
	Tumor size >2 cm
	Age >60 years
	Lack of radiotherapy
	Location of tumor on the lower extremities
BETTER PROGNOSIS	Tumor size <2 cm
	Surgic margins free of tumor[a]
	Absence of nodal disease

[a]Does not hold for patients receiving postoperative radiation therapy.

Table 13-6
Staging, Overall Survival, and Recommended Treatment for Merkel Cell Carcinoma

STAGE	MEDIAN SURVIVAL (month)	5-YEAR SURVIVAL (%)	TREATMENT RECOMMENDATIONS
I Localized disease		64	*Surgery:* loc excision with >2 cm margins[a] *XRT:* adjuvant treatment to tumor site and draining LNs *Chemotherapy:* Could consider as adjuvant or radiosensitizing agent
IA ≤2.0 cm	30		
IB >2.0 cm	26		
II Lymph node involvement	18	47	*Surgery:* Same as for stage I [a] *XRT:* Same as for stage I *Chemotherapy:* Same as for stage I
II Distant metastases	5	0	*Surgery:* No real role for surgery *XRT:* For palliation of pain, ulceration, bone or brain mets *Chemotherapy:* CAV or EP are most commonly used

Key: LN—lymph nodes, XRT—Radiotherapy, CAV—cyclophosphamide, doxorubicin, vincristine, EP—etoposide, cisplatin (or carboplatin).
[a]Could consider sentinel lymph node dissection in these patients depending on whether radiotherapy is to be delivered to the draining LN basin.

important to be aggressive in the primary treatment of MCC. The secondary goals when treating MCC include reducing the risk of metastasis, minimizing the toxicity of treatment, maintaining function, and preserving cosmesis.

Treatment of MCC proves to be difficult because many patients are elderly and have a low tolerance to extensive surgery, radiation, and chemotherapy. In addition, the location of MCC often presents a challenge for adequate surgical margins as MCC has a predilection for the head and neck, especially the periorbital area. Poor blood supply in the lower extremities of elderly patients can cause poor wound healing following wide local excision, which in turn compromises further treatment options and leads to adverse outcomes.

The treatment plan should consider all of the factors previously mentioned, and be tailored to the individual patient's needs. It is often beneficial to formulate a treatment plan in a multidisciplinary fashion, taking into account information from the pathologist, oncologist, and surgeon.

Surgic Treatment

Surgery plays an important role in patients with stage I and II disease. Controversy exists regarding the optimal margins for wide loc excision (WLE) due to the lack of randomized controlled trials; however, due to MCC's propensity for dermal seeding and spread to the

lymphatics, most authors recommend WLE with 2 to 3 cm margins.[44,46,52,53,138,139] Most MCC tumors are less than 2 cm in diameter at presentation, and WLE with these margins is not problematic, however, many times margins of only 5 mm are possible, especially in the head and neck region, particularly in the periorbital areas. If radiation is to be used as an adjuvant to surgical removal, then surgical margins become less relevant.

There have been several studies demonstrating high rates of recurrence after WLE with large margins when surgery is used as the only method of treatment, some studies reporting recurrence rates of 89, 81, and even 100%.[13,54,134] In contrast, many retrospective comparisons have demonstrated a favorable outcome when radiation is added postoperatively.[19,23,51,53,54,140–144] When radiotherapy is provided to the primary site postoperatively (usually 4 weeks after surgery to give the wound adequate time to heal) as well as to the regional lymph nodes, the relapse rate is significantly reduced, even when only 2 cm surgical margins are used. It is important to treat the draining lymph nodes as well as the primary site with radiation, as patients who do not have draining lymph nodes treated will experience recurrence rates of 46 to 76%.[145] It is thought that the high failure rate seen with surgery alone is most likely due to positive margins and dermal lymphatic spread,[66,146] suggesting that radiotherapy is capable of treating tumor at

wound margins as well as lymphatic disease.[18]

Mohs micrographic surgery may be an alternative to WLE for the treatment of MCC. A study at the Mayo clinic demonstrated a decrease in local recurrence and distant metastasis in patients who were treated with Mohs, compared to standard surgical excision.[147] However, Brissett et al compared Mohs to WLE alone or WLE with additional nodal dissection, and found the 2-year survival to be 33, 68, and 100% respectively, suggesting Mohs to be an inadequate therapeutic option for MCC.[148] Like in WLE, it has been shown that patients do better when radiotherapy is combined as an adjunct even after Mohs surgery.[147,149] While Mohs has been proposed to be a good method of obtaining clear margins, especially on areas not conducive to wide loc excision, conflicting reports exist, and additional clinical studies are needed.

Treatment of Lymph Nodes

Pathologic involvement of regional lymph nodes is present in 10 to 30% of patients presenting with MCC.[45,46] However, prophylactic lymph node dissection is generally not recommended as a routine therapeutic measure.[53,66] Some surgeons recommend a prophylactic lymph node dissection for patients who are considered highrisk for recurrence (i.e., tumor >2 cm, mitotic figures >10 per high power field, histologic evidence of lymphatic permeation, and small cell histologic pattern), or in younger patients with larger lesions or tumors located on the head and neck.[46,52,53,150] However, elective lymph node dissection would still not be indicated if the patient were to receive radiotherapy, especially if a lymph node dissection would delay the delivery of radiation, considering that MCC is a radiosensitive tumor. It has been argued that prophylactic nodal resection may reduce the chance of recurrence.[151] To date, however, there does not appear to be any survival advantage associated with prophylactic lymph node dissection.[152]

Lymphoscintigraphy and sentinel lymph node biopsy has been proposed as an alternative to lymph node dissection in patients with MCC.[94,153–160] Though it is true that sentinel lymph node biopsies may decrease unnecessary lymphadenectomies,[161] if postoperative radiotherapy becomes a routine practice, this argument becomes a little more questionable.

Nodal recurrence can occur in up to 76% of patients with MCC,[21,44,46,53,140,151,161] and patients found to have nodal disease have a significantly increased risk of developing distant metastasis.[47] If nodal disease is discovered, then surgical removal should be supplemented with postoperative radiotherapy.

Radiation Therapy

It is known that MCC is a radiosensitive tumor, having been shown to be radiosensitive *in vitro*[162] (in contrast to melanoma which has unpredictable responses to radiotherapy). Sixty-six percent of patients who experience locoregional recurrences will ultimately die of disease.[52] Because of this, locoregional control of the tumor is of utmost importance. Owing to the recurrent and aggressive nature of MCC, as well as the documented high failure rates after surgery alone, radiation therapy is used as an adjuvant therapy after primary resection as well as after resection of local recurrences. In spite of the evidence that adjuvant radiation decreases recurrences when used with surgery, there have only been two studies suggesting an overall survival advantage associated with the use of adjuvant radiation,[18,54] and other authors report no benefit from adjuvant radiation.[46,56] In spite of these conflicting reports, it is now common practice to use radiation therapy in addition to surgical treatment of MCC, with studies supporting this practice from the United States,[18,142,163–165] Australia,[54,161] Israel,[139] France,[166] Germany,[167] and the United Kingdom.[146] In addition to being an adjunct therapy, radiotherapy has also been used alone as definitive treatment with fairly good local control, demonstrating MCC's radiosensitivity.[13,146,161,168] This would be a consideration when surgery is not possible, or in bulky stage II disease.[169] In addition to radiotherapy, the concomitant use of hyperthermia has been shown to be of benefit in the case of a few patients.[170,171]

Due to the aggressive nature of MCC, radiotherapy should be employed as soon as possible after local resection. This is usually done around 4 weeks postoperatively, giving the incision site adequate time to heal. Radiotherapy is commonly delivered to the primary site with 3 to 5 cm margins, ensuring the dermal lymphatics adjacent to the incision site are adequately treated. In addition, radiotherapy should be employed to the regional lymph nodes as well. It has been shown that when the draining lymph nodes are not treated with radiotherapy, recurrence rates become 46 to 76%.[145] Doses of radiation vary between 45 to 70 Gy. Higher doses are used in bulky stage II lymphatic disease, and lower doses are employed in areas of the body with lower tolerances like the lower extremities, or when blood supply is compromised in elderly patients.

Finally, radiotherapy can be used for palliative measures. Indications for palliative radiotherapy in patients with MCC include pain, bleeding, infection, ulceration, and metastatic disease to the bone or brain. Multiple sessions can be employed, but patients often begin to feel relief, especially from bony metastatic pain, after the first dose of radiotherapy.

Chemotherapy

Chemotherapy is mostly used in MCC patients who have hematogenous spread, or stage III disease.[15,172] In these patients, treatment is mostly palliative. Distant metastatic disease is common in MCC occurring between 28 and 70% of the time. Response to chemotherapy is usually short lived, and these patients usually die of their disease.[173,174] It was initially thought that MCC was for the most part resistant to chemotherapy, however, regimens similar to those used in small cell lung cancer and neuroendocrine tumors have been reported to result in increased response rates.[175,176]

Additional evidence has been reported which supports chemotherapy as an adjuvant in high risk, stage II patients.[47,177–179] The use of adjuvant chemotherapy in these patients may be employed as a curative measure.[47] In addition to targeting metastatic disease, chemotherapy can also be used as a radiosensitizing agent.[47] Because MCC is morphologically similar to and demonstrates a propensity to recur and spread much like small cell lung cancer, combination chemotherapy regimens already known to be beneficial in small cell lung cancer are usually chosen for the treatment of MCC.[172] Chemotherapeutic agents most frequently used include doxorubicin (or epirubicin), anthracyclines, cisplatin, carboplatin, etoposide, cyclophosphamide, irinotecan, and vincristine.[172] Response rates to first line chemotherapy have been reported to be 57 to 59% in patients with distant metastasis, and 68 to 69% in patients with locally advanced disease.[15,172] Common combination chemotherapy regimens used include cyclophosphamide, doxorubicine (or epirubicin), and vincristine (CAV), as well as etoposide and cisplatin (or carboplatin) with complete response rates of 35.1 and 36%, respectively. No randomized controlled trials have been performed with chemotherapeutic regimens in MCC, and thus the exact impact chemotherapy has on survival and quality of life still remains speculative. In addition, chemotherapy is not without risks, with toxic deaths occurring in 3.4 and 7.7% of patients in two separate series.[15,172] Myelosuppression and neutropenia are other common side effects seen in MCC patients treated with these chemotherapeutic agents.[15,172]

CAV and etoposide/platinum combinations are reasonable choices in MCC patients with few comorbidities. Patients with cardiac disease will not be suitable for administering doxorubicin, or the CAV combination. When using etoposide/carboplatin or cisplatin, it should be remembered that carboplatin is not as toxic, has less side effects when compared to cisplatin, and may be a better choice when used in the elderly. In addition, many of the elderly population have renal, cardiac, or hearing impairment, which would also be an indication to use carboplatin instead of cisplatin.

Adjuvant chemotherapy is used in efforts to decrease the occurrence of regional and distant spread in patients with MCC.[177] TROG study demonstrated that patients with MCC who received a therapeutic regimen consisting of carboplatin, etoposide, and radiotherapy had a 3-year survival, locoregional control, and distant control of 76, 75, and 76%, respectively, even though 62% of patients had lymphatic disease (stage II) at presentation. There was however, a 40% incidence of neutropenic fever.[47]

Isolated limb perfusion with chemotherapy, most often using melphalan, has also been used as a way to gain better locoregional control of MCC, especially in uncontrolled disease of the lower extremities. Additionally, isolated hyperthermic limb perfusion has been used for the same reason. It is thought that heat may act as a cytotoxic agent supporting the rationale behind this option.[180]

Other Therapeutic Options

Several biologic agents, including interferon (IFN)[180–183] and tumor necrosis factor (TNF)[180,184–186] have been used to treat MCC. Two reports from Japan have documented complete remission of MCC after direct intratumoral injection of TNF.[184,185]

In addition, complete remission has been reported in a patient with metastatic somatostatin receptor positive MCC treated with octreotide.[103] However, other reports using this treatment modality in neuroendocrine tumors have been disappointing.[187]

Due to the frequent overexpression of *bcl-2* in MCC cells compared to that in normal Merkel cells,[188–190] a recent trial using *bcl-2* antisense oligonucleotides was reported in SCID mice with MCC, where inhibition of human MCC growth was observed.[191]

Also, MCC cells express the c-kit receptor tyrosine kinase 95% of the time. This has lead to recent speculation regarding the use of imatinab mesylate, or Gleevec. Gleevec was first developed as an ATP-competitive inhibitor of *bcr-abl*,[192] but was found to bind to and specifically inhibit other tyrosine kinases. The use of Gleevec as a treatment modality in MCC, however, remains purely speculative at this point, and no reports exist as to its use in treating this tumor.

Finally, there is a report documenting complete remission of MCC of the scalp with local and regional metastases after the topic use of dinitrochlorbenzol.[193]

Some authors are also considering immunotherapy in the treatment of MCC. A colleague at this institution is currently treating a patient with Imiquimod (Aldara), after having a history of five local recurrences of MCC on the lower extremity over the course of 5 years. After using Imiquimod (Aldara), the most recent recurrence has disappeared clinically. Additional follow-up and experience with more patients will be needed to assess the effectiveness of this treatment.

If surgery is used as the only treatment modality in patients with MCC, surgical margins should be at least 2 to 3 cm when possible. Postoperative radiotherapy is an important adjuvant to any surgical treatment (even Mohs) and should be delivered to the primary site postoperatively as well as to the draining lymph nodes. This practice is widely accepted and felt to be important in patients with stage I and stage II disease. Combination chemotherapy can be used for metastatic disease, as an adjuvant in high-risk patients, as well as a radiosensitizing agent. At present, the effectiveness of chemotherapy in any of these situations is still being determined.

■ PREVENTION

BOX 13-10 Summary

- MCC is a rare cutaneous malignancy and little is know regarding preventative measures.
- Because MCC has been linked to sun exposure, it is reasonable to assume sun protective measures to be somewhat preventative.

Due to the rare nature of MCC, little is known regarding its pathogenesis, risk factors, and effective preventative measures. Because MCC has been linked to photoexposure, it is reasonable to assume effective sun-protective habits to be somewhat preventative, as in all carcinomas involving the skin.

■ FINAL THOUGHTS

MCC has proven to be one of the most aggressive forms of cutaneous malignancy. Treatment of MCC should be focused on the primary site as well as the draining lymph nodes. Therapy is best when developed in a multidisciplinary approach, utilizing the pathologist, surgeon, and oncologist. When excising a primary focus of MCC, margins should be at least 2 to 3 cm when possible, and radiation should be administered promptly to the primary site as well as to the draining lymph nodes, especially in stage I and stage II patients. The role of adjuvant chemotherapy is still being developed, as are multiple other treatment options, including immunotherapy. Despite the small size of most MCCs at presentation, aggressive treatment is needed initially as recurrence occurs often and is a marker for worse outcomes.

REFERENCES

1. Merkel F. Tastzellen und Tastkörperchen bei den Haustieren und beim Menschen. *Archiv für Mikroskopische Anatomie und Entwicklungsmechanik.* 1875;11:636–652.
2. Pinkus F. Über einen bisher unbekannten Nebenapparat am Haarsystem des Menschen. Haarscheiben. *Dermatologische Zeitschrift.* 1902;9:465–469.
3. Winkelmann RK, Breathnach AS. The Merkel cell. *J Invest Dermatol.* 1973;60:2–15.
4. Frigerio B, Capella C, Eusebi V, et al. Merkel cell carcinoma of the skin: The structure and origin of normal Merkel cells. *Histopathology.* 1983;7:229–249.
5. Moll I, Zieger W, Schmelz M. Proliferative Merkel cells were not detected in human skin. *Arch Dermatol Res.* 1996;288:184–187.
6. Szeder V, Grim M, Halata Z, Sieber-Blum M. Neural crest origin of mammalian Merkel cells. *Dev Biol.* 2003;253:258–263.
7. Toker C. Trabecular carcinoma of the skin. *Arch Dermatol.* 1972;105:107–110.
8. Tang C, Toker C. Trabecular carcinoma of the skin: an ultrastructural study. *Cancer.* 1978;42:2311–2321.
9. De Wolf-Peeters C, Marien K, Mebis J, et al. A cutaneous APUDoma or Merkel cell tumor? A morphologically recognizable tumor with a biologic and histologic malignant aspect in contrast with its clinic behavior. *Cancer.* 1980;46:1810–1816.
10. Goessling W, McKee PH, Mayer R. Merkel cell carcinoma. *J Clin Oncol.* 2002;20:588–598.
11. Poulsen M. Merkel-cell carcinoma of the skin. *Lancet Oncol.* 2004;5(10):593–599.
12. Chuang TY, Su WP, Muller SA. Incidence of cutaneous T cell lymphoma and other rare skin cancers in a defined population. *J Am Acad Dermatol.* 1990;23:254–256.
13. Morrison WH, Peters LJ, Silva EG, et al. The essential role of radiation therapy in securing locoregional control of Merkel cell carcinoma. *Int J Radiat Oncol Biol Phys.* 1990;19:583–591.
14. Anderson LL, Phipps TJ, McCollough ML. Neuroendocrine carcinoma of the skin (Merkel cell carcinoma) in a black. *J Dermatol Surg Oncol.* 1992;18:375–380.
15. Voog E, Biron P, Martin JP, et al. Chemotherapy for patients with locally advanced or metastatic Merkel cell carcinoma. *Cancer.* 1999;85:2589–2595.
16. Miller RW, Rabkin CS. Merkel cell carcinoma and melanoma: etiologic similarities and differences. *Cancer Epidemiol Biomarkers Prev.* 1999;8:153–158.
17. Meyer-Pannwitt U, Kummerfeldt K, Boubaris P, et al. Merkel cell tumor or neuroendocrine skin carcinoma. *Langenbecks Arch Chir.* 1997;382:349–358.
18. Ott MJ, Tanabe KK, Gadd MA, et al. Multimodality management of Merkel cell carcinoma. *Arch Surg.* 1999;134:388–393.
19. Medina-Franco H, Urist MM, Fiveash J, et al. Multimodality treatment of Merkel cell carcinoma: case series and literature review of 1024 cases. *Ann Surg Oncol.* 2001;8:204–208.
20. Kroll MH, Toker C. Trabecular carcinoma of the skin: further clinicopathologic and morphologic study. *Arch Pathol Lab Med.* 1982;106:404–408.
21. Boyle F, Pendlebury S, Bell D. Further insights into the natural history and management of primary cutaneous neuroendocrine (Merkel cell) carcinoma. *Int J Radiat Oncol Biol Phys.* 1995;31:315–323.
22. Smith DF, Messina JL, Perrott R, et al. Clinic approach to neuroendocrine carcinoma of the skin (Merkel cell carcinoma). *Cancer Control.* 2000;7:72–83.
23. Goepfert H, Remmler D, Silva E, et al. Merkel cell carcinoma (endocrine carcinoma of the skin) of the head and neck. *Arch Otolaryngol.* 1984;110:707–712.
24. Schmid C, Beham A, Feichtinger J, et al. Recurrent and subsequently metastasizing Merkel cell carcinoma in a 7-year-old girl. *Histopathology.* 1992;20:437–439.
25. Sonak RA, Trede K, Gerharz CD. Merkel cell tumor of the hand in a 104-year-old patient: case report with review of the literature. *Handchir Mikrochir Plast Chir.* 1996;28:43–45.
26. Pan D, Narayan D, Ariyan S. Merkel cell carcinoma; 5 reports using sentinel node biopsy and review of 110 cases. *Plast Reconstr Surg.* 2002;110(5):1259–1265.
27. Van Gele M, Kaghad M, Leonard JH, et al. Mutation analysis of P73 and TP53 in Merkel cell carcinoma. *Br J Cancer.* 2000;82:823–826.
28. Lunder EJ, Stern RS. Merkel-cell carcinomas in patients treated with methoxsalen and ultraviolet A radiation. *N Engl J Med.* 1998;339:1247–1248.

29. Tsuruta D, Hamada T, Mochida K, et al. Merkel cell carcinoma: Bowen's disease and chronic occupational arsenic poisoning. *Br J Dermatol.* 1998;139:291–294.

30. Hewitt JB, Sherif A, Kerr KM, et al. Merkel cell and squamous cell carcinomas arising in erythema ab igne. *Br J Dermatol.* 1993;128:591–592.

31. Buell JF, Trofe J, Hanaway MJ, et al. Immunosuppression and Merkel cell cancer. *Transplant Proc.* 2002;34:1780–1781.

32. Bordea C, Wonjnarowska F, Millard PR, et al. Skin cancers in renal-transplant recipients occur more commonly than previously recognized in a temperate climate. *Transplantation.* 2004;77:574–579.

33. Safadi R, Pappo O, Okon E, et al. Merkel cell tumor in a woman with chronic lymphocytic leukemia. *Leuk Lymphoma.* 1996;20:509–511.

34. Quaglino D, Di Leonardo G, Lalli G, et al. Association between chronic lymphocytic leukaemia and secondary tumours: Unusual occurrence of a neuroendocrine (Merkel cell) carcinoma. *Eur Rev Med Pharmacol Sci.* 1997;1:11–16.

35. Ziprin P, Smith S, Salerno G, et al. Two cases of Merkel cell tumour arising in patients with chronic lymphocytic leukaemia. *Br J Dermatol.* 2000;142:525–528.

36. Engels E, Frisch M, Goedart J, et al. Merkel cell carcinoma and HIV infection. *Lancet.* 2002;359:497–498.

37. Penn I, First MR. Merkel's cell carcinoma in organ recipients: report of 41 cases. *Transplantation.* 1999;68:1717–1721.

38. Gomez LG, DiMaio S, Silva EG, et al. Association between neuroendocrine (Merkel cell) carcinoma and squamous carcinoma of the skin. *Am J Surg Pathol.* 1983;7:171–177.

39. Silva EG, Mackay B, Goepfert H, et al. Endocrine carcinoma of the skin (Merkel cell carcinoma). *Pathol Annu.* 1984;19(pt 2):1–30.

40. Jones CS, Tyring SK, Lee PC, et al. Development of neuroendocrine (Merkel cell) carcinoma mixed with squamous cell carcinoma in erythema ab igne. *Arch Dermatol.* 1988;124:110–113.

41. Cerroni L, Kerl H. Primary cutaneous neuroendocrine (Merkel cell) carcinoma in association with squamous and basal-cell carcinoma. *Am J Dermatopathol.* 1997;19:610–613.

42. Iacocca MV, Abernethy JL, Stefanato CM, et al. Mixed Merkel cell carcinoma and squamous cell carcinoma of the skin. *J Am Acad Dermatol.* 1998;39:882–887.

43. Brenner B, Sulkes A, Rakowsky E, et al. Second neoplasms in patients with Merkel cell carcinoma. *Cancer.* 2001;91:1358–1362.

44. Haag ML, Glass LF, Fenske NA. Merkel cell carcinoma: diagnosis and treatment. *Dermatol Surg.* 1995;21:669–683.

45. Hitchcock CL, Bland KI, Laney RG III, et al. Neuroendocrine (Merkel cell) carcinoma of the skin: Its natural history, diagnosis, and treatment. *Ann Surg.* 1988;207:201–207.

46. Yiengpruksawan A, Coit DG, Thaler HT, et al. Merkel cell carcinoma: prognosis and management. *Arch Surg.* 1991;126:1514–1519.

47. Poulsen M, Rischen D, Walpole E, et al. High risk Merkel cell carcinoma of the skin treated with synchronous carbo-platin/etoposide and radiation: a Trans-Tasman Radiation Oncology Group Study—TROG 96:07. *J Clin Oncol.* 2003;21(23):4371–4376.

48. Soltau JB, Smith ME, Custer PL. Merkel cell carcinoma of the eyelid. *Am J Ophthalmol.* 1996;121:331–332.

49. Metz KA, Jacob M, Schmidt U, et al. Merkel cell carcinoma of the eyelid: histologic and immunohistochemical features with special respect to differential diagnosis. *Graefes Arch Clin Exp Ophthalmol.* 1998;236:561–566.

50. Gackle HC, Spraul CW, Wagner P, et al. Merkel cell tumor of the eyelids: review of the literature and report of 2 patients. *Klin Monatsbl Augenheilkd.* 2000;216:10–16.

51. Raaf JH, Urmacher C, Knapper WK, et al. Trabecular (Merkel cell) carcinoma of the skin: treatment of primary, recurrent, and metastatic disease. *Cancer.* 1986;57:178–182.

52. Shaw JH, Rumball E. Merkel cell tumour: clinic behaviour and treatment. *Br J Surg.* 1991;78:138–142.

53. Ratner D, Nelson BR, Brown MD, et al. Merkel cell carcinoma. *J Am Acad Dermatol.* 1993;29:143–156.

54. Meeuwissen J, Bourne R, Kearsley J. The importance of postoperative radiotherapy in the treatment of merkel cell carcinoma. *Int J Radiation Oncol Biol Phys.* 1995;31:325–331.

55. Meyer-Pannwitt U, Kummerfeldt K, Boubaris P, et al. Merkel cell tumor or neuroendocrine skin carcinoma. *Langenbecks Arch Chir.* 1997;382:349–358.

56. Savage P, Constenla D, Fisher C, et al. The natural history and management of Merkel cell carcinoma of the skin: a review of 22 patients treated at the Royal Marsden Hospital. *Clin Oncol (R Coll Radiol).* 1997;9:164–167.

57. Skelton HG, Smith KJ, Hitchcock CL, et al. Merkel cell carcinoma: analysis of clinical, histologic, and immunohistologic features of 132 cases with relation to survival. *J Am Acad Dermatol.* 1997;37:734–739.

58. Gollard R, Weber R, Kosty MP, et al. Merkel cell carcinoma: review of 22 cases with surgical, pathologic, and therapeutic considerations. *Cancer.* 2000;88:1842–1851.

59. Angelli M, Clegg LX. Epidemiology of primary Merkel cell carcinoma in the United States. *J Am Acad Dermatol.* 2003;49:832–841.

60. Hauschild A, Rademacher D, Rowert J, et al. Merkel cell carcinoma: follow-up of 10 patients—current diagnosis and therapy. *Langenbecks Arch Chir.* 1997;382:185–191.

61. Chen KT. Merkel's cell (neuroendocrine) carcinoma of the vulva. *Cancer.* 1994;73:2186–2191.

62. Tomic S, Warner TF, Messing E, et al. Penile Merkel cell carcinoma. *Urology.* 1995;45:1062–1065.

63. Routh A, Hickman BT, Johnson WW. Superior vena cava obstruction from Merkel cell carcinoma. *Arch Dermatol.* 1987;123:714–716.

64. Eggers SD, Salomao DR, Dinapoli RP, et al. Paraneoplastic and metastatic neurologic complications of Merkel cell carcinoma. *Mayo Clin Proc.* 2001;76:327–330.

65. Connelly TJ, Cribier B, Brown TJ, Yanguas I. Complete spontaneous regression of Merkel cell carcinoma: a review of the 10 reported cases. *Dermatol Surg.* 2000;26:853–856.

66. Pilotti S, Rilke F, Bartoli C, et al. Clinicopathologic correlations of cutaneous neuroendocrine Merkel cell carcinoma. *J Clin Oncol.* 1988;6:1863–1873.

67. Iacocca MV, Abernethy JL, Stefanato CM, et al. Mixed Merkel cell carcinoma and squamous cell carcinoma of the skin. *J Am Acad Dermatol.* 1998;39:882–887.

68. LeBoit PE, Crutcher WA, Shapiro PE. Pagetoid intraepidermal spread in Merkel cell (primary neuroendocrine) carcinoma of the skin. *Am J Surg Pathol.* 1992;16:584–592.

69. Domagala W, Lubinski J, Lasota J, et al. Neuroendocrine (Merkel-cell) carcinoma of the skin: cytology, intermediate filament typing and ultrastructure of tumor cells in fine needle aspirates. *Acta Cytol.* 1987;31:267–275.

70. Pettinato G, De Chiara A, Insabato L. Diagnostic significance of intermediate filament buttons in fine needle aspirates of neuroendocrine (Merkel cell) carcinoma of the skin. *Acta Cytol.* 1989;33:420–421.

71. Skoog L, Schmitt FC, Tani E. Neuroendocrine (Merkel-cell) carcinoma of the skin: immunocytochemic and cytomorphologic analysis on fine-needle aspirates. *Diagn Cytopathol.* 1990;6:53–57.

72. Layfield LJ, Glasgow BJ. Aspiration biopsy cytology of primary cutaneous tumors. *Acta Cytol.* 1993;37:679–688.

73. Gottschalk-Sabag S, Ne'eman Z, Glick T. Merkel cell carcinoma diagnosed by fine-needle aspiration. *Am J Dermatopathol.* 1996;18:269–272.

74. Alvarez-Gago T, Bullon MM, Rivera F, et al. Intermediate filament aggregates in mitoses of primary cutaneous neuroendocrine (Merkel cell) carcinoma. *Histopathology.* 1996;28:349–355.

75. Shin HJ, Caraway NP. Fine-needle aspiration biopsy of metastatic small cell carcinoma from extrapulmonary sites. *Diagn Cytopathol.* 1998;19:177–181.

76. Collins BT, Elmberger PG, Tani EM, et al. Fine-needle aspiration of Merkel cell carcinoma of the skin with cytomorphology and immunocytochemic correlation. *Diagn Cytopathol.* 1998;18:251–257.

77. Jimenez FJ, Burchette JL Jr, Grichnik JM, et al. Ber-EP4 immunoreactivity in normal skin and cutaneous neoplasms. *Mod Pathol.* 1995;8:854–858.

78. Kontochristopoulos GJ, Stavropoulos PG, Krasagakis K, et al. Differentiation between Merkel cell carcinoma and malignant melanoma: an immunohistochemic study. *Dermatology.* 2000;201:123–126.

79. Collaco L, Silva JP, Goncalves M, et al. Merkel cell carcinoma of the eyelid: a case report. *Eur J Ophthalmol.* 2000;10:173–176.

80. Leland JY, Shah RP, Adelman HM. A skin lesion found by serendipity. *Hosp Pract.* 2000;35:32–33.

81. Agoff SN, Lamps LW, Philip AT, et al. Thyroid transcription factor-1 is expressed in extrapulmonary small cell carcinomas but not in other extrapulmonary neuroendocrine tumors. *Mod Pathol.* 2000;13:238–242.

82. Cheuk W, Kwan MY, Suster S, et al. Immunostaining for thyroid transcription factor 1 and Cytokeratin 20 aids the distinction of small cell carcinoma from Merkel cell carcinoma, but not pulmonary from extrapulmonary small cell carcinomas. *Arch Pathol Lab Med.* 2001; 125:228–231.

83. Moll R, Lowe A, Laufer J, et al. Cytokeratin 20 in human carcinomas: a new histodiagnostic marker detected in monoclonal antibodies. *Am J Pathol.* 1992;140(2):427–447.

84. Byrd-Gloster Al, Khoor A, Glass LF, et al. Differential expression of thyroid transcription factor-1 (TTF-1) in small cell carcinoma and Merkel cell carcinoma. *Hum Pathol.* 2000;31(1):58–62.

85. Shah IA, Netto D, Schlageter MO, et al. Neurofilament immunoreactivity in Merkel-cell tumors: a differentiating feature from small-cell carcinoma. *Mod Pathol.* 1993;6:3–9.

86. Narisawa Y, Hashimoto K, Kohda H. Immunohistochemic demonstration of the expression of neurofilament proteins in Merkel cells. *Acta Derm Venereol.* 1994;74:441–443.

87. Alvarez-Gago T, Bullon MM, Rivera F, et al. Intermediate filament aggregates in mitoses of primary cutaneous neuroendocrine (Merkel cell) carcinoma. *Histopathology.* 1996;28:349–355.

88. Schmidt U, Muller U, Metz KA, et al. Cytokeratin and neuro- filament protein staining in Merkel cell carcinoma of the small cell type and small cell carcinoma of the lung. *Am J Dermatopathol.* 1998;20:346–351.

89. Su LD, Lowe L, Bradford CR, et al. Immunostaining for cytokeratin 20 improves the detection of micometastatic Merkle cell carcinoma in sentinel lymph nodes. *J Am Acad Dermatol.* 2002;46: 661–666.

90. Su LD, Fullen DR, Lowe L, et al. CD 117 (KIT receptor) expression in Merkel cell carcinoma. *Am J Dermatopathol.* 2002; 4:289–293.

91. Feinmesser M, Halpern M, Kaganovsky E, et al. C-kit expression in primary and metastatic merkel cell carcinoma. *Am J Dermatopathol.* 2004;26(6): 458–62.

92. Gollub MJ, Gruen DR, Dershaw DD. Merkel cell carcinoma: CT findings in 12 patients. *Am J Roentgenol.* 1996;167: 617–620.

93. Wasserberg N, Schachter J, Fenig E, et al. Applicability of the sentinel node technique to Merkel cell carcinoma. *Dermatol Surg.* 2000;26:138–141.

94. Rodrigues LK, Leong SP, Kashini-Sabet M, Wong JH. Early experience with sentinel lymph node mapping for Merkel cell carcinoma. *J Am Acad Dermatol.* 2001;45:303–308.

95. Allen PJ, Busam K, Hill AD, et al. Immunohistochemic analysis of sentinel lymph nodes from patients with Merkel cell carcinoma. *Cancer.* 2001;92: 1650–1655.

96. Nguyen B, McCullough A. Imaging of Merkel cell carcinoma. *Radiographics.* 2002;22:367–376.

97. Nguyen BD. Positron emission tomographic imaging of Merkel cell carcinoma. *Clin Nucl Med.* 2002;27: 922–923.

98. Carnaille B, Nocaudie M, Pattou F, et al. Scintiscans and carcinoid tumors. *Surgery.* 1994;116:1118–1121.

99. Kwekkeboom DJ, Hoff AM, Lamberts SW, et al. Somatostatin analogue scintigraphy: a simple and sensitive method for the *in vivo* visualization of Merkel cell tumors and their metastases. *Arch Dermatol.* 1992;128:818–821.

100. Kau RJ, Wagner-Manslau C, Saumweber DM, et al. Detection of somatostatin receptors in tumors in the area of the head and neck and their clinic importance. *Laryngorhinootologie.* 1994;73:21–26.

101. Lastoria S, Maurea S, Vergara E, et al. Comparison of labeled MIBG and somatostatin analogs in imaging neuroendocrine tumors. *Q J Nucl Med.* 1995; 39:145–149.

102. Kau R, Arnold W. Somatostatin receptor scintigraphy and therapy of neuroendocrine (APUD) tumors of the head and neck. *Acta Otolaryngol.* 1996; 116:345–349.

103. Cirillo F, Filippini L, Lima GF, et al: Merkel cell tumor: report of case and treatment with octreotide. *Minerva Chir.* 1997;52:1359–1365.

104. Lobrano MB, McCarthy K, Adams L, et al. Metastatic carcinoid tumor imaged with CT and a radiolabeled somatostatin analog: a case report. *Am J Gastroenterol.* 1997;92:513–515.

105. Straka JA, Straka MB. A review of Merkel cell carcinoma with emphasis on lymph node disease in the absence of a primary site. *Am J Otolaryngol.* 1997;18: 55–61.

106. Durani B, Klein A, Henze M, et al. Somatostatin analogue scintigraphy in Merkel tumours. *Br J Dermatol.* 2003;148: 1135–1140.

107. Guitera-Rovel P, Lumbroso J, Gautier-Gougis M, et al. Indium-111 octreotide scintigraphy of Merkel cell carcinoma and their metastases. *Ann Oncol.* 2001; 12:807–811.

108. Lampreave JL, Benard F, Alavi A, et al. PET evaluation of therapeutic limb perfusion in Merkel's cell carcinoma. *J Nucl Med.* 1998;39:2087–2090.

109. Wong CO, Pham AN, Dworkin HJ. F-18 FDG Accumulation in an octreotide negative Merkel cell tumor. *Clin Positron Imag.* 2001;3:71–73.

110. Scanga D, Martin W, Delbeke D. Value of FDG PET imaging in the management of patients with thyroid, neuroendocrine and neural crest tumours. *Clin Nucl Med.* 2004;29:86–89.

111. Van Gele M, Leonard JH, Van Roy N, et al. Combined karyotyping, CGH and M-FISH analysis allows detailed characterization of unidentified chromosomal arrangements in Merkel cell carcinoma. *Int J Cancer.* 2002;101(2): 137–145.

112. Harnett PR, Kearsley JH, Hayward NK, et al. Loss of allelic heterozygosity on distal chromosome 1p in Merkel cell carcinoma: a marker of neural crest origins? *Cancer Genet Cytogenet.* 1991;54:109–113.

113. Van Gele M, Van Roy N, Ronan SG, et al. Molecular analysis of 1p36 breakpoints in two Merkel cell carcinomas. *Genes Chromosomes Cancer.* 1998;23:67–71.

114. Maris JM, Matthay KK. Molecular biology of neuroblastoma. *J Clin Oncol.* 1999;17:2264–2279.

115. Judson H, van Roy N, Strain L, et al. Structure and mutation analysis of the gene encoding DNA fragmentation factor 40 (caspaseactivated nuclease), a candidate neuroblastoma tumour suppressor gene. *Hum Genet.* 2000;106: 406–413.

116. Leonard JH, Cook AL, Nancarrow D, et al. Deletion mapping on the short arm of chromosome 1 in Merkel cell carcinoma. *Cancer Detect Prev.* 2000;24:620–627.

117. Smedley D, Sidhar S, Birdsall S, et al. Characterization of chromosome 1 abnormalities in malignant melanomas. *Genes Chromosomes Cancer.* 2000;28: 121–125.

118. Tsao H, Zhang X, Majewski P, et al. Mutational and expression analysis of the p73 gene in melanoma cell lines. *Cancer Res.* 1999;59:172–174.

119. Carson HJ, Lueck NE, Horten BC. Comparison of mutant and wild-type p53 proteins in Merkel cell carcinoma. *Clin Diagn Lab Immunol.* 2000;7:326 (Letter).

120. Leonard JH, Williams G, Walters MK, et al. Deletion mapping of the short arm of chromosome 3 in Merkel cell carcinoma. *Genes Chromosomes Cancer.* 1996;15: 102–107.

121. Dammann R, Li C, Yoon JH, et al. Epigenetic inactivation of a RAS association domain family protein from the lung tumour suppressor locus 3p21.3. *Nat Genet.* 2000;25:315–319.

122. Burbee DG, Forgacs E, Zochbauer-Muller S, et al. Epigenetic inactivation of RASSF1A in lung and breast cancers and malignant phenotype suppression. *J Natl Cancer Inst.* 2001;93:691–699.

123. Van Gele M, Leonard JH, Van Roy N, et al. Frequent allelic loss at 10q23 but low incidence of PTEN mutations in Merkel cell carcinoma. *Int J Cancer.* 2001;92: 409–413.

124. Leonard JH, Leonard P, Kearsley JH. Chromosomes 1, 11, and 13 are frequently involved in karyotypic abnormalities in metastatic Merkel cell carcinoma. *Cancer Genet Cytogenet.* 1993;67: 65–70.

125. Leonard JH, Hayard N. Loss of heterozygosity of chromosome 13 in Merkel cell carcinoma. *Genes Chromosomes Cancer.* 1997;20:93–97.

126. Van Gele M, Speleman F, Vandesompele J, et al. Characteristic pattern of chromosomal gains and losses in Merkel cell carcinoma detected by comparative genomic hybridization. *Cancer Res.* 1998;58:1503–1508.

127. Amo-Takyi BK, Tietze L, Tory K, et al. Diagnostic relevance of chromosomal in-situ hybridization in Merkel cell carcinoma: targeted interphase cytogenetic tumour analyses. *Histopathology.* 1999;34(2):163–169.

128. Leonard JH, Cook AL, Van Gele M, et al. Proneural and proneuroendocrine transcription factor expression in cutaneous mechanoreceptor (Merkel) cells and Merkel cell carcinoma. *Int J Cancer.* 2002;101:103–110.

129. Harle M, Arens N, Moll I, et al. Comparative genomic hybridization (CGH) discloses chromosomal and subchromosomal copy number changes in Merkel cell carcinomas. *J Cutan Pathol.* 1996;23:391–397.

130. Vortmeyer AO, Merino MJ, Boni R, et al. Genetic changes associated with primary Merkel cell carcinoma. *Am J Clin Pathol.* 1998;109(5):565–570.

131. Sandbrink F, Muller L, Fiebig HH, et al. Short communication: deletion 7q, trisomy 6 and 11 in a case of Merkel-cell carcinoma. *Cancer Genet Cytogenet.* 1988; 33:305–309.

132. Larsimont D, Verhest A. Chromosome 6 trisomy as sole anomaly in a primary Merkel cell carcinoma. *Virchows Arch.* 1996;428:305–309.

133. Poulsen M, Harvey J. Is there a diminishing role for surgery in Merkel cell carcinoma of the skin? A review of the current management. *ANZ J Surg.* 2002;72(2):142–146.

134. Fenig E, Brenner B, Katz A, et al. The role of radiation therapy and chemotherapy in the treatment of Merkel cell carcinoma. *Cancer.* 1997;80: 881–885.

135. Koljonen V, Bohling T, Granhroth G, Tukianinen E. Merkel cell carcinoma: a clinicopathologic study of 34 patients. *Eur J Surg Oncol.* 2003;29:697–710.

136. Eich HT, Eich D, Staar S, Mauch C. Role of post-operative radiotherapy in the management of Merkel cell. *Am J Clin Oncol.* 2002;25:50–56.

137. Coit DG. Merkel cell carcinoma. *Ann Surg Oncol.* 2001;8(suppl):S99–S102.

138. O'Connor WJ, Brodland DG. Merkel cell carcinoma. *Dermatol Surg.* 1996;22: 262–267.

139. Al Ghazal SK, Arora DS, Simpson RH, et al. Merkel cell carcinoma of the skin. *Br J Plast Surg.* 1996;49(7):491–496.

140. Bourne RG, O'Rourke MG. Management of Merkel cell tumour. *Aust N Z J Surg.* 1988;58:971–974.

141. Tennvall J, Bjorklund A, Johansson L, et al. Merkel cell carcinoma: management of primary, recurrent and metastatic disease: a clinicopathologic study of 17 patients. *Eur J Surg Oncol.* 1989;15:1–9.

142. Marks ME, Kim RY, Salter MM. Radiotherapy as an adjunct in management of Merkel cell carcinoma. *Cancer.* 1990;65:60–64.

143. Kokoska ER, Kokoska MS, Collins BT, et al. Early aggressive treatment for Merkel cell carcinoma improves outcome. *Am J Surg.* 1997;174:688–693.

144. Herbst A, Haynes HA, Nghiem P. The standard of care for Merkel cell carcinoma should include adjuvant radiation and lymph node surgery. *J Am Acad Derm.* 2002;46(4):640–642.

145. Suntharalingam M, Rudoltz MS, Mendenhall WM, et al. Radiotherapy for Merkel cell carcinoma of the skin of the head and neck. *Head Neck.* 1995;17: 96–101.

146. Ashby M, Jones DH, Tasker AD, et al. Primary cutaneous neuroendocrine (Merkel cell or trabecular carcinoma) tumour of the skin: a radiosensitive tumour. *Clin Radiol.* 1989;40:85–87.

147. O'Connor WJ, Roenigk RK, Brodland DG. Merkel cell carcinoma: comparison of Mohs micrographic surgery and wide excision in eighty-six patients. *Dermatol Surg.* 1997;23:929–933.

148. Brissett AE, Olsen KD, Kasperbauer JL, et al. Merkel cell carcinoma of the head and neck: a retrospective case series. *Head Neck.* 2002;24(11):982–988.

149. Boyer JD, Ziltelli JA, Brodland DG, et al. Loc control of primary Merkel cell carcinoma: review of 45 cases treated. *J Am Acad Derm.* 2002;47(6):885–892.

150. Smith DE, Bielamowicz S, Kagan AR, et al. Cutaneous neuroendocrine (Merkel cell) carcinoma: A report of 35 cases. *Am J Clin Oncol.* 1995;18:199–203.

151. Victor NS, Morton B, Smith JW. Merkel cell carcinoma: is prophylactic lymph node dissection indicated? *Am Surg.* 1996; 62:879–882.

152. Allen PJ, Zhang ZF, Coit DG. Surgic management of Merkel cell carcinoma. *Ann Surg.* 1999;229(1):97–105.

153. Pfeifer T, Weinberg H, Brady MS. Lymphatic mapping for Merkel cell carcinoma. *J Am Acad Dermatol.* 1997;37: 650–651.

154. Messina JL, Reintgen DS, Cruse CW, et al. Selective lymphadenectomy in patients with Merkel cell (cutaneous neuroendocrine) carcinoma. *Ann Surg Oncol.* 1997;4:389–395.

155. Bilchik AJ, Giuliano A, Essner R, et al. Universal application of intraoperative lymphatic mapping and sentinel lymphadenectomy in solid neoplasms. *Cancer J Sci Am.* 1998;4:351–358.

156. Ames SE, Krag DN, Brady MS. Radiolocalization of the sentinel lymph node in Merkel cell carcinoma: a clinic analysis of seven cases. *J Surg Oncol.* 1998;67:251–254.

157. Hill AD, Brady MS, Coit DG. Intraoperative lymphatic mapping and sentinel lymph node biopsy for Merkel cell carcinoma. *Br J Surg.* 1999;86: 518–521.

158. Wasserberg N, Feinmesser M, Schachter J, et al. Sentinel-node guided lymph-node dissection for Merkel cell carcinoma. *Eur J Surg Cancer.* 1999;25: 444–446.

159. Wasserberg N, Schachter J, Fenig E, et al. Applicability of the sentinel node technique to Merkel cell carcinoma. *Dermatol Surg.* 2000;26:138–141.

160. Zeitouni NC, Cheney RT, Delacure MD. Lymphoscintigraphy, sentinel lymph node biopsy, and Mohs micrographic surgery in the treatment of Merkel cell carcinoma. *Dermatol Surg.* 2000;26:12–18.

161. Pacella J, Ashby M, Ainslie J, et al. The role of radiotherapy in the management of primary cutaneous neuroendocrine tumors (Merkel cell or trabecular carcinoma): experience at the Peter MacCallum Cancer Institute (Melbourne, Australia). *Int J Radiat Oncol Biol Phys.* 1988;14:1077–1084.

162. Leonard JH, Ramsay JR, Kearsley JH, et al. Radiation sensitivity of Merkel cell carcinoma cell lines. *Int J Radiat Oncol Biol Phys.* 1995;32:1401–1407.

163. Wilder RB, Harari PM, Graham AR, et al. Merkel cell carcinoma: improved locoregional control with postoperative radiation therapy. *Cancer.* 1991;68:1004–1008.

164. Nathu RM, Mendenhall WM, Parsons JT. Merkel cell carcinoma of the skin. *Radiat Oncol Investig.* 1998;6:233–239.

165. Gillenwater Am, Hessel AC, Morrison WH, et al. Merkel cell carcinoma of the head and neck: effect of surgic excision and radiation on recurrence and survival. *Arch Otolaryngol Head Neck Surg.* 2001;127(2):149–154.

166. Bedane C, Clavere P, Lavignac C, et al. Neuroendocrine primary cutaneous carcinoma: therapeutic aspects in 13 patients. *Ann Dermatol Venereol.* 1996; 123:443–446.

167. Bischof M, van Kampen M, Huber P, et al. Merkel cell carcinoma: the role of radiation therapy in general management. *Strahlenther Onkol.* 1999;175:611–615.

168. Mortier L, Mirabel X, Fournier C, et al. Radiotherapy alone for primary Merkel cell carcinoma. *Arch Dermatol.* 2003; 139(12):1587–1590.

169. Poulsen M. Merkel cell carcinoma of skin: diagnosis and management strategies. *Drugs Aging.* 2005;22(3):219–29.

170. Knox SJ, Kapp DS. Hyperthermia and radiation therapy in the treatment of recurrent Merkel cell tumors. *Cancer.* 1988;62:1479–1486.

171. Muggianu M, Rainero ML, Panarese P, et al. Radiotherapy and hyperthermia in the treatment of primary Merkel cell carcinoma of the skin: a case report. *Bull Cancer Radiother.* 1994;81:237–240.

172. Tai PT, Yu E, Winquist E, et al. Chemotherapy in neuroendocrine/Merkel cell carcinoma of the skin: case series and review of 204 cases. *J Clin Oncol.* 2000;18:2493–2499.

173. Feun LG, Savaraj N, Legha SS, et al. Chemotherapy for metastatic Merkel cell carcinoma, Review of the M.D. Anderson Hospital's experience. *Cancer.* 1988;62:683–685.

174. Sharma D, Flora G, Grunsberg S. Chemotherapy of metastatic Merkel cell carcinoma: case report and review of the literature. *Am J Clin Oncol.* 1991;14:166–169.

175. George TK, di Sant'agnese PA, Bennett JM. Chemotherapy for metastatic Merkel cell carcinoma. *Cancer.* 1985;56: 1034–1038.

176. Wynne CJ, Kearsley JH. Merkel cell tumor: a chemosensitive skin cancer. *Cancer.* 1988;62:28–31.

177. Davis M, Miller E, Rau R, et al. The use of VP16 and cisplatin in the treatment of Merkel cell carcinoma. *J Dermatol Surg Oncol.* 1990;16:276–278.

178. Fenig E, Lurie H, Klein B, Sulkes A. The treatment of advanced Merkel cell carcinoma: a multimodality chemotherapy and radiation treatment approach. *J Dermatol Surg Oncol.* 1993;19:860–864.

179. Fenig E, Lurie H, Sulkes A. The use of cyclophosphamide, methotrexate, and 5-fluorouracil in the treatment of Merkel cell carcinoma. *Am J Clin Oncol.* 1993;16:54–57.

180. Olieman AF, Lienard D, Eggermont AM, et al. Hyperthermic isolated limb perfusion with tumor necrosis factor alpha, interferon gamma, and melphalan for locally advanced nonmelanoma skin tumors of the extremities: A multicenter study. *Arch Surg.* 1999;134:303–307.

181. Durand JM, Weiller C, Richard MA, et al. Treatment of Merkel cell tumor with interferon-alpha-2b. *Br J Dermatol.* 1991; 124:509.

182. Bajetta E, Zilembo N, Di Bartolomeo M, et al. Treatment of metastatic carcinoids and other neuroendocrine tumors with recombinant interferon-alpha-2a: a study by the Italian trials in

Medic Oncology Group. *Cancer.* 1993; 72:3099–3105.

183. Zilembo N, Buzzoni R, Bajetta E, et al. Salvage treatment after r-interferon alpha-2a in advanced neuroendocrine tumors. *Acta Oncol.* 1993;32:245–250.

184. Ito Y, Kawamura K, Miura T, et al. Merkel cell carcinoma: a successful treatment with tumor necrosis factor. *Arch Dermatol.* 1989;125:1093–1095.

185. Hata Y, Matsuka K, Ito O, et al. Two cases of Merkel cell carcinoma cured by intratumor injection of natural human tumor necrosis factor. *Plast Reconstr Surg.* 1997;99:547–553.

186. Lampreave JL, Benard F, Alavi A, et al. PET evaluation of therapeutic limb perfusion in Merkel's cell carcinoma. *J Nucl Med.* 1998;39:2087–2090.

187. di Bartolomeo M, Bajetta E, Buzzoni R, et al. Clinic efficacy of octreotide in the treatment of metastatic neuroendocrine tumors: a study by the Italian trials in Medic Oncology Group. *Cancer.* 1996; 77:402–408.

188. Moll I, Gillardon F, Waltering S, et al. Differences of bcl-2 protein expression between Merkel cells and Merkel cell carcinomas. *J Cutan Pathol.* 1996;23:109–117.

189. Kennedy MM, Blessing K, King G, et al. Expression of bcl-2 and p53 in Merkel cell carcinoma: an immunohistochemic study. *Am J Dermatopathol.* 1996;18: 273–277.

190. Feinmesser M, Halpern M, Fenig E, et al. Expression of the apoptosis-related oncogenes bcl-2, bax, and p53 in Merkel cell carcinoma: can they predict treatment response and clinic outcome? *Hum Pathol.* 1999;30:1367–1372.

191. Schlagbauer-Wadl H, Klosner G, Heere-Ress E, et al. Bcl-2 antisense oligonucleotides (G3139) inhibit Merkel cell carcinoma growth in SCID mice. *J Invest Dermatol.* 2000;114:725–730.

192. Buchdunger E, Zimmermann J, Mett H, et al. Inhibition of the Abl protein-tyrosine kinase *in vitro* and *in vivo* by a 2-phenylaminopyrimidine derivative. *Cancer Res.* 1996;56(1):100–104.

193. Herrmann G, Groth W, Krieg T, Mauch C. Complete remission of Merkel cell carcinoma of the scalp with loc and regional metastases after topic treatment with dinitrochlorbenzol. *J Am Acad Dermatol.* 2004;50(6): 965–969.

CHAPTER 14

Fibrohistiocytic Tumors

Bernhard Zelger, M.D., M.Sc.
Walter HC Burgdorf, M.D.

BOX 14-1   Overview

- Dermatofibromas
  - Synonyms and stereotypical presentation
  - Clinicopathologic variants with architectural and/or cytologic peculiarities
  - Relatives of dermatofibromas
- Xanthogranulomas
  - Synonyms and stereotypical presentation
  - Clinicopathologic variants including a unifying concept
  - Immunohistochemistry and differential diagnoses including myths
- Malignant fibrous histiocytomas (MFH)
  - Undifferentiated pleomorphic sarcoma (pleomorphic MFH)
  - Undifferentiated pleomorphic sarcoma with giant cells (giant cell MFH)
  - Undifferentiated pleomorphic sarcoma with prominent inflammation (inflammatory MFH)
- Myxofibrosarcoma (myxoid MFH)
- Angiomatoid fibrous histiocytoma (angiomatoid MFH)
- Atypical fibroxanthoma

■ INTRODUCTION

"Fibrohistiocytic tumors" is a satisfying phrase which unfortunately does not stand up well on close inspection. "Fibro" refers to a proliferation of fibroblasts, which can easily be appreciated in the common dermatofibroma (DF), which is generally accepted to be a reactive inflammatory process. The term "histiocytic" is more problematic because histiocytes have never been defined unequivocally. Though histiocytes are mostly equated with macrophages, monocytes which have escaped from circulation and transformed into tissue phagocytes, many entities designated as histiocytic are of different histogenesis or so only with a reactive admixture of macrophages. Therefore, histiocytosis X and atypical regressive histiocytosis are today well accepted as Langerhans cell disease and

CD30-positive lymphoma, respectively. Many accept the concept that malignant fibrous histiocytoma is a reaction pattern of a variety of dedifferentiated malignancies, while the nature of the dermal counterpart, atypical fibroxanthoma (AFX), is still controversial (in our experience most cases are dedifferentiated squamous cell carcinomas). Finally, other fibrohistiocytic lesions such as dermatofibrosarcoma protuberans and its juvenile variant giant cell fibroblastoma are low-grade fibrosarcomas which will be discussed in the chapter on sarcomas.

The classification of fibrohistiocytic tumors is currently undergoing dramatic changes and is soon be replaced by a more sophisticated histogenetic approach, rather than that of the mysterious concept of a fibrohistiocyte. This evolution was prophesied by Terry Headington over 20 years ago in an editorial for the *Archives of Dermatology* entitled *"The Histiocyte: in memoriam"*.[1] He nicely concluded his article in 1986 with the final sentence *"Histiocyte, requiescat in pace"*. We completely agree with Headington and would like to include the "fibrohistiocyte" in the same final resting place.

■ DERMATOFIBROMAS

BOX 14-2   Summary

- Fibrosing dermatitis with paracrine melanocytic hyperplasia
- Characteristic clinical miscue as melanocytic nevus
- Dimpling (or Montgomery) sign helpful for diagnosis
- There are many clinicopathologic variants
- May be misinterpreted and thus mismanaged as malignancies
- Optional therapy is simple excision

DF is a fibrosing dermatitis characterized by an increased number of fibrocytes in the dermis and occasionally in the subcutis, a variable admixture of macrophages, and other inflammatory cells frequently including lymphocytes, and more rarely eosinophils, neutrophils, and/or plasma cells. Coarse collagen bundles in haphazard array, often with peripheral entrapment, and hyperplasia of adjacent structures (epidermis, hair follicles) or cells (melanocytes) are also seen.

Synonyms

The most common synonym for DF in Europe is *histiocytoma* and it is the least

helpful. The concept of histiocytes (from Greek "to histion" for "tissue") is flawed. What could be less specific than a "tissue cell"? Most modern classifications today identify two types of bone-marrow derived cells capable of antigen presentation and phagocytosis. Dendritic cells, including the Langerhans cells of the skin, are professional antigen-presenting cells, while macrophages are primarily phagocytic cells. Early lesions of DF may be rich in macrophages and these cellular variants are often called histiocytomas. In *fibrous xanthoma,* prominent xanthomatized macrophages (lipophages) are due to lipids from the lipid membranes of extravasated erythrocytes or from involvement of the subcutaneous fat. Later, as both cellular and fibrous elements are seen, the term *fibrous histiocytoma* is used.

Many other cells may be present including neutrophils, lymphocytes, dendritic cells including Langerhans cells, and occasionally eosinophils and mast cells. Variable presence of these inflammatory cells leads to pseudolymphomatous DF or DF with diffuse eosinophilic infiltrate.

Later lesions of DFs have few cells, and consist mostly of fibrocytes and collagen. In addition, endothelial cells, nerves, and smooth muscle fibers may be involved. Such lesions have been termed *fibroma durum, subepidermal nodular fibrosis* or *sclerosis*, and even *sclerotic* or *sclerosing fibroma* (synonym: storiform collagenoma) or *keloidal dermatofibroma*. Sometimes the endothelial cells are very prominent and this may explain the now extinct name of *sclerosing hemangioma*. In our opinion, DF is the most appropriate term, both clinically as well as pathologically.

Etiology

Our concept is that DFs are a local response to some type of inflammation or trauma—be it an arthropod bite reaction, a ruptured hair follicle (these are the two most common), a ruptured follicular or mucous cyst, a viral wart, or the presence of foreign bodies such as a wood splinter or suture material. Initially, there is an inflammatory response with granulation tissue, neutrophils, macrophages, dendritic cells, lymphocytes, and fibroblasts, while later, the reparative fibrous response dominates. Fibroblasts are activated fibrocytes which present as epithelioid cells with round-to-oval, hypochromatic nuclei and ill-defined cytoplasm in a loose stroma of mucin, but without or only minor amounts of thin collagen bundles. In haematoxylin and eosin (H&E) stain test, such cells are frequently difficult or impossible to differentiate from macrophages, Langerhans cells, activated endothelial cells, or other epithelioid cells. Immunohistochemically, they are positive for vimentin, while markers for other lines of differentiation are negative. The only exception is myofibroblasts which immunohistochemically are positive for smooth muscle-specific actin; histologically, they are half-way between fibroblasts and fibrocytes, i.e., spindly cells with long cytoplasmic extensions and slender elongated nuclei. In contrast to fibrocytes, their cytoplasm is more prominent and brightly eosinophilic, which is due to the presence of the contractile components. On the other hand, fibrocytes are slender, spindly to wavy cells with hyperchromatic nuclei and moderate amounts of cytoplasm, embedded into a stroma with more or less prominent/thick collagen bundles which may become wiry, storiform, and/or sclerotic. A single process, fibrosing dermatitis, is seen and described at different moments of its life history.[2]

Epidemiology

DFs are an extremely common form of fibrosing dermatitis. It appears to be more common in females with predilection for the lower extremities. The peak incidence occurs in the third to fourth decade of life, but rare cases are found in children and on the face.

Stereotypical Presentation

DF is the most common fibrocytic lesion, except for scars.[3] It may develop at any age; nearly every adult has at least one. The most characteristic setting is on the shins or calves of young adult females. Usually, a DF is a single, round, oval to targetoid slightly elevated, asymptomatic papule to nodule. Early lesions are red or red-brown; older ones, brown to skin-colored, frequently with a darker peripheral rim (Fig. 14-1A). Lesions are moderately well circumscribed and firm. The "dimpling" or Fitzpatrick sign, when lesions are squeezed between the thumb and index finger, is characteristic. Thereby smooth pressure forces the DF down into the subcutis; this phenomenon is caused by the altered arrangement of collagen in the reticular dermis. After years, these lesions may completely involve or leave slightly atrophic macules with some faint brown discoloration.

Histology shows a dense infiltrate of fibrocytes and/or macrophages in the reticular dermis, and, sometimes, the

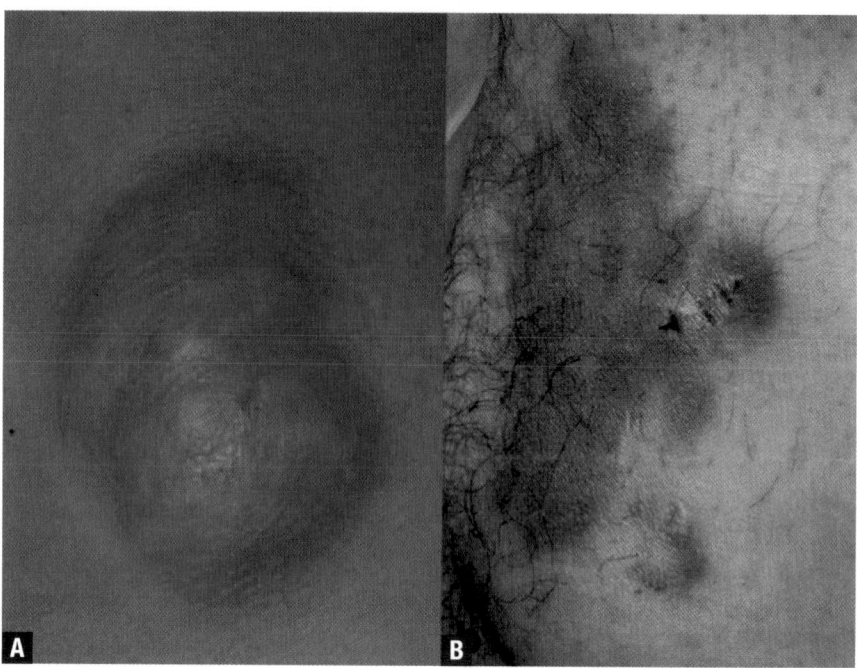

▲ **FIGURE 14-1** **A.** Ill-defined, reddish dermatofibroma with brown peripheral rim. **B.** Plaque-like variant of giant dermatofibroma; note satellite lesions [Courtesy Dr. M. Hagedorn, M.D. (Darmstadt)].

upper part of the subcutis. Early lesions are rich in macrophages, some of which may be siderophages, and/or lipophages, others multinucleate, e.g., Touton or foreign body giant cells. At times foam cells may be prominent in deeper areas adjacent to subcutaneous fat. Late lesions (Fig. 14-2) show prominent fibrocytes and coarse bundles of collagen in a haphazard fashion, frequently arranged in short fascicles that interweave ("storiform"), sometimes with a sclerotic center. Lesions are ill defined because of splaying of both fibrocytes and macrophages between thickened collagen bundles at the periphery of the lesion (often called "entrapment of collagen"). Epidermal, melanocytic, and folliculosebaceous hyperplasia is characteristically found above the lesions, while rarely smooth muscle or neural proliferation is observed. The epidermal hyperplasia is most common and can be so prominent that buds of hair follicles mimic superficial basal cell carcinoma. It may be minimal or absent in late or deep-seated lesions. Lymphocytes

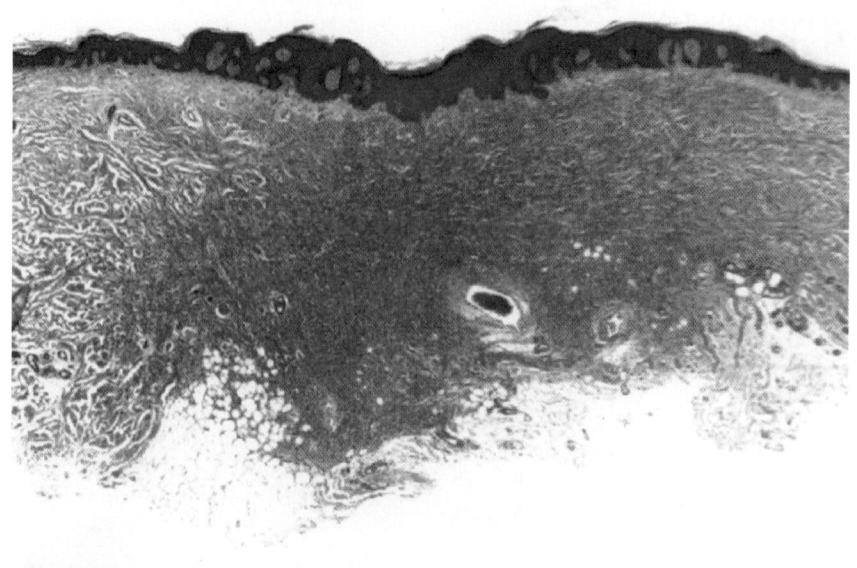

▲ **FIGURE 14-2** Characteristic silhouette of dermatofibroma.

Table 14-1
Clinicopathologic Characteristics of DF Variants

DF Variant	Predilection Sex, Age (Year), Site	Clinical Pitfalls	Histopathologic Pitfalls
Variants With Mostly Architectural (Usually Low Power) Peculiarities			
Atrophic DF	F, 20–40, shoulder	Basal cell carcinoma	
Aneurysmal FH	F, 20–40, lower legs	Hemangioma, melanoma	Kaposi sarcoma
Haemangiopericytoma-like FH	F, 20–40, lower legs	Hemangioma, melanoma	Infantile myofibroma(tosis)
Plaque-like and deep penetrating DF (giant DF)	F, 20–40 upper and lower limbs, trunk	DFSP	DFSP
Multinucleate cell angiohistiocytoma	F, 40–70, trunk, proximal extremities	Sarcoidosis, Kaposi sarcoma, tufted angioma	Kaposi sarcoma
Sclerotic DF	F, 20–40, acral	Indicator of Cowden syndrome	
Keloidal DF	F, 20–40, upper and lower extremities		Keloid
Myxoid DF	F, 20–40, hands and feet		Myxoma, mucous cyst
Cholesterotic/lipidized FH (ankle-type DF)	F, 20–40, ankle	Cyst, xanthoma	Gout
Palisading cutaneous FH	F, 20–40, hands and feet		Schwannoma
Ossifying DF	F, 20–40, lower legs		Extraskeletal osteosarcoma
Variants With Mostly Cytologic (Usually High Power) Peculiarities			
Pseudolymphomatous DF	F, 20–40, lower legs		Pseudolymphoma
DF with diffuse eosinophilic infiltrate	F, 20–40, lower legs		Langerhans cell disease
Hemosiderrhotic DF	F, 20–40, lower legs	Melanocytic nevus, melanoma	Melanoma
Clear cell DF	F, 20–40, lower legs		Renal cell carcinoma metastasis, myomelanocytic tumor ("PEComa")
Granular cell DF	M, 20–40, shoulder		Granular cell tumor
Epithelioid cell histiocytoma	M, 10-30, upper limbs	Spitz melanocytic nevus	Spitz melanocytic nevus
Cellular benign FH	M, 10-30, limbs, head, neck		Leiomyosarcoma, rarely fibro- or angiosarcoma
Myofibroblastic DF	F, 20–40, lower legs		Myofibroblastoma
Atypical/pseudosarcomatous FH, DF with monster cells	F, 20–40, lower legs		Atypical fibroxanthoma

DFSP: Dermatofibrosarcoma protuberans; F: female, FH: fibrous histiocytoma; M: male

are often spread throughout the lesion with frequent prominence at the periphery, but may be lacking in later stages.

Clinicopathological Variants

A wide variety of clinicopathologic variants (Table 14-1) may, in a minor proportion of cases (2 to 3%), cause difficulties in correct interpretation and subsequently lead to clinical mismanagement, such as further or even wide excisions, superfluous internal investigations, long-term follow-up, stigmatization of patients with a malignancy, and unnecessary costs.[4]

Atrophic DF reveals a skin-colored plaque on the shoulder, frequently supposed to be a basal cell carcinoma, a characteristic clinical miscue. Histology reveals a DF which by shrinkage of fibroplasia is substantially thinner than the surrounding dermis.

In *aneurysmal fibrous histiocytoma* spontaneous or traumatic hemorrhage may rapidly enlarge a previously asymptomatic lesion and frequently is painful. *Angiomatoid fibrous histiocytoma* is a confusing synonym which should not be used for this DF variant. The term should be restricted for a lesion which previously was known as *angiomatoid malignant fibrous histiocytoma,*[5] nowadays best regarded as a low-grade malignancy of uncertain differentiation (see below).

Plaque-like variants of DF (Fig. 14-1B) up to more than 20 cm in diameter and deep penetrating DFs with tumors of several centimeters diameter have been grouped together as *giant DFs.*[6] Both may be confused with dermatofibrosarcoma protuberans.

Occasionally, there may be a few, up to several dozen, sometimes grouped ("agminated") papules.[2] The latter variant occurs on the trunk or proximal extremities of young adults with clusters of blue-brown papules. Clinically, sarcoidosis or Kaposi sarcoma is most frequently sus-

pected. Besides typical features of DF, these lesions reveal ectatic vessels and multinucleate giant cells. One could view these multinucleate cell angiohistiocytomas as combined DFs[4] consisting of grouped papules with features of sclerosing hemangioma and bizarre giant cells of DF with monster cells. Similar papules are sometimes seen close to plaque-like variants of DF (Fig. 14-1B).

Multiple widespread DFs are regarded as a marker of immune suppression; they have been observed most often in black females with systemic lupus erythematosus, as well as in patients with other autoimmune diseases (Sjögren syndrome, pemphigus vulgaris, myasthenia gravis, and ulcerative colitis), and in those with inborn, acquired, or iatrogenic immunosuppression such as Cowden syndrome, HIV/AIDS, or transplant recipients, respectively. In Cowden syndrome, multiple, often acral sclerotic DFs most likely represent regressing or fibrotic HPV

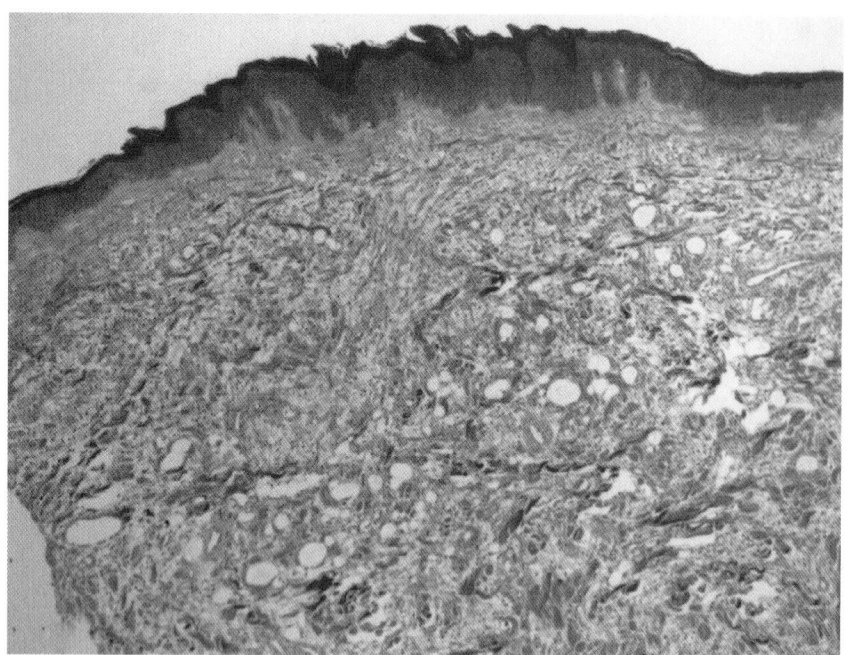

▲ **FIGURE 14-3** Clear cell dermatofibroma with epidermal hyperplasia, prominent collagen bundles, and characteristic cytology.

infections, as Cowden syndrome patients have other warty lesions, such as trichilemmomas.[7]

Apart from unusual architecture, DFs may present with stromal and cellular peculiarities such as myxoid DFs with mucin between dendritic fibrocytes or rare cases of ossifying DF, which reveal bone formation with osteoclast-like giant cells. Very unusual cytologic features of DFs are seen in clear (Fig. 14-3) and granular cell DFs, which may mimic renal cell carcinoma metastasis and granular cell tumor, respectively.

More commonly seen is epithelioid cell histiocytoma (Fig. 14-4) with scalloped eosinophilic cells, a mimicry of Spitz melanocytic nevi. It has been suggested that the location in the papillary dermis with a moderate amount of loose collagen fibers allows cells more easily to develop epithelioid features than in the reticular dermis where the much more restricted tissue constrictions favor a spindle-cell appearance. Alternatively, the age of a lesion may play a role, so that the early phases show epithelioid fibroblasts, whereas the later ones show spindle cells. While most epithelioid cell histiocytomas are confined to the papillary dermis with a prominent collarette of epidermis and adnexal epithelium lateral to the exophytic papule, some lesions can extend deeply into the reticular dermis and even subcutis, either diffusely or with fascicles or nests. In our experience such deep penetrating epithelioid cell histiocytomas are part of the spectrum which in the literature is known as *cellular or atypical benign fibrous histiocytoma* (Fig. 14-5),[8] most commonly located on the trunk, back, and upper arm, and which is frequently misinterpreted as leiomyosarcoma, fibrosarcoma, or even angiosarcoma, the latter in particular when additional hemorrhage is prominent.

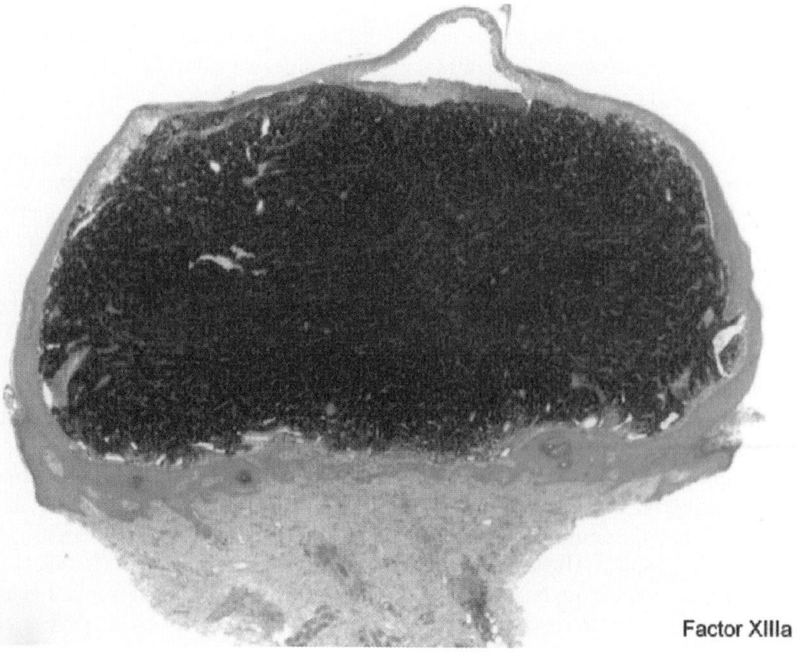

Relatives of Dermatofibromas

In our experience, subungual osteochondroma (synonyms: *subungual exostosis* and *fibroosseous pseudotumor of the digit*) overlaps with or is intimately connected with subungual or acral counterparts of DF. Peripheral ossifying fibroma in the oral cavity is a DF-like lesion which invariably contains bone. The special anatomy with bone and cartilage close to the skin or mucosa and the susceptibility to trauma are responsible for the involvement of these components in otherwise typical fibrosing inflammation.

The various types of superficial fibromatoses[3] such as palmar Dupuytren contracture, plantar Ledderhose disease, or penile Peyronie contracture all share features with DF. They can be interpreted as late-stage variants of such a fibrosing process complicated by the sequels of shrinkage. Similarly, giant cell fibroma and fibroma of tendon sheath, which by most are regarded as benign neoplasms,[5] share fibrocytic features with or without sheets of lipo- and siderophages, which from an alternative point of view can be interpreted as early-stage variants of a reactive tissue response. In contrast, in the subcutis or deeper tissues the more loose tissue conditions give rise to other presentations: "connective tissue culture"-like appearance in nodular fasciitis; a biphasic mixture of fibrocytes and collagen with osteoclast-like giant cells within fatty tissue in plexiform fibrohistiocytic tumor (Fig. 14-6); with epithelioid, sometimes giant cells with homogenous cytoplasm ("ganglion"-like cells) in proliferative fasciitis; or with analogous

Factor XIIIa

▲ **FIGURE 14-4** Reactivity for factor XIIIa in epithelioid cell histiocytoma.

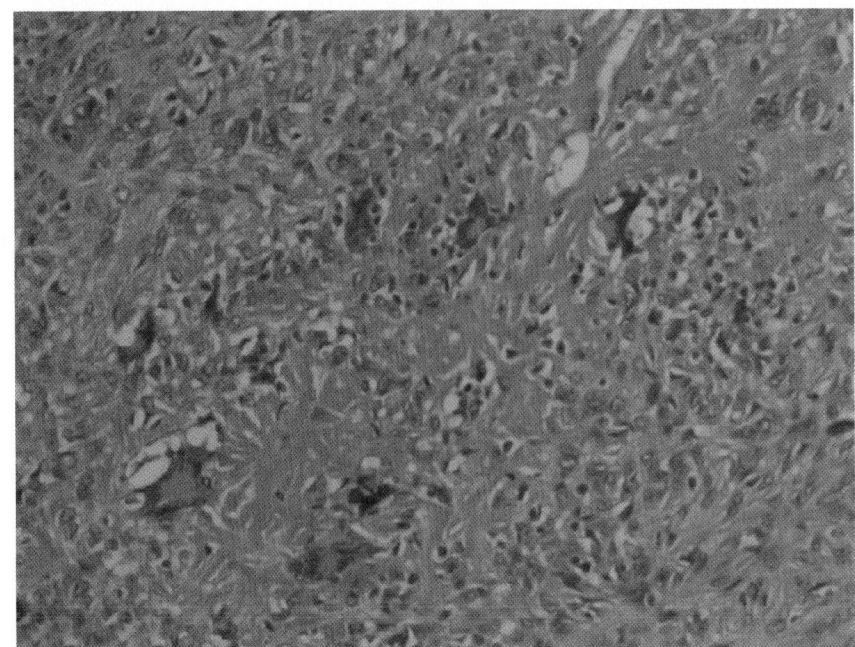

▲ **FIGURE 14-5** Atypical/pseudosarcomatous fibrous histiocytoma with prominent atypia, including monster cells.

features in deep muscle tissue as proliferative, sometimes ossifying myositis.[9]

Immunohistochemistry

DFs reveal a variable immunohistochemical profile which reflects the stage of the inflammatory response. Early lesions are rich in reactivity for macrophage markers such as Ki-M1p, PGM1, or KP1 (CD68). Frequent labeling for factor XIIIa is seen in early phases (Fig. 14-4) and indicates activity of a protease involved in tissue linkage mechanisms, e.g., covalently connecting the numerous monomer structures of fibrin and collagen. This reactivity is mostly seen at the periphery and continuously diminishes with the aging of the lesion to be completely absent in atrophic variants.

Predominance of factor XIIIa positive dendritic cells have given rise to the concept of dermal dendrocytomas.[10] In our experience, dermal dendrocytomas are just another variation on the theme of an early fibrosing dermatitis which consists of a variably mixed population of fibrocytes and dendritic macrophages positive for factor XIIIa. Langerhans cells are not a predominate cell type of these lesions, but frequently may be scattered through the lesion, as shown by cells positive for CD1a dispersed in a starry sky pattern.

A time cycle in the profile of an immunohistochemical marker is also observed with proliferation markers such as proliferating cell nuclear antigen and Ki-67 (Mib1). Rapidly evolving lesions such as early DFs show prominent mitoses, while sclerotic variants have none.

Other variably expressed markers include smooth muscle specific actin, NKIC3 (CD56), and neuron specific enolase. Labeling for smooth muscle specific actin is most prominently seen in *myofibroblastic dermatofibroma*, which shows slim, spindle-shaped nuclei with slender cytoplasmic cell extensions. NKIC3 (CD56) is encountered in 10 to 20% of all DFs, at least focally, and in particular is frequently very prominent in those with myofibroblastic, granular, and clear cell differentiation. Our experience is similar with neuron specific enolase. Exceptional cases with characteristic histologic features of DF show diffuse reactivity for CD34[11]; other rare cases express S100 protein.

Differential Diagnoses

The most important histologic differential diagnoses are dermatofibrosarcoma protuberans and Kaposi sarcoma. Dermatofibrosarcoma protuberans is poorly circumscribed, usually much broader and deeper with irregular dissection of subcutis, and shows cells with wavy nuclei in association with delicate fibrillary bundles of collagen frequently arranged in a storiform pattern. In contrast to DF, it is regularly positive for CD34. Kaposi sarcoma in the nodular and tumor stage is characterized by erythrocytes extravasated into slits between interweaving fascicles of spindle-shaped cells; often, tiny pink hyaline globules that represent degenerated erythrocytes are found in these spindle-shaped endothelial cells. Lesions are positive for CD34 and vascular markers such as CD31. In times prior to immunohistochemistry and modern techniques such as PCR which can detect HHV8 in Kaposi sarcoma lesions, differentiation of nodular Kaposi sarcoma from aneurysmal fibrous histiocytoma was occasionally a difficult task.

Prognosis

We view DF as an entirely *benign* reactive process. Yet, we are aware of well-differ-

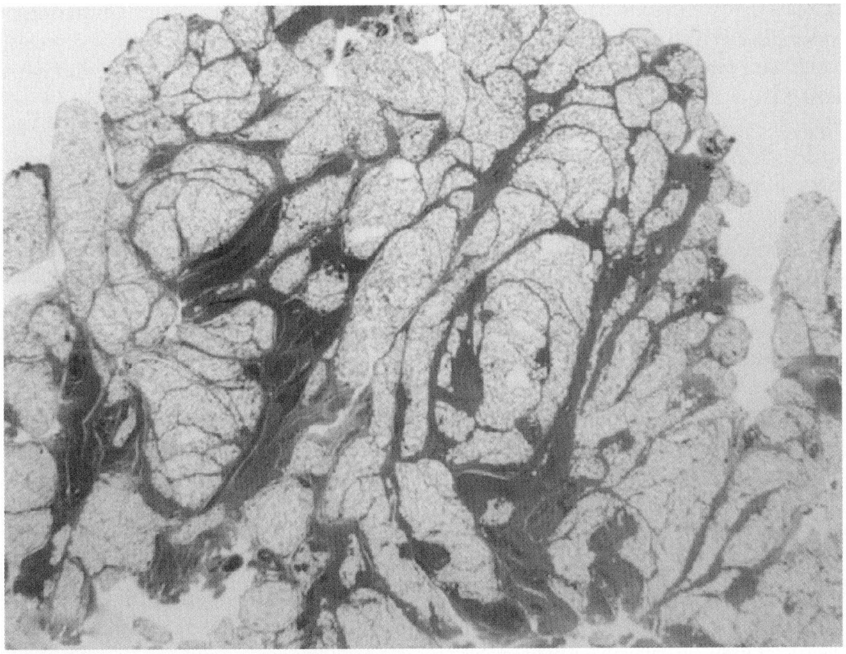

▲ **FIGURE 14-6** Plexiform fibrohistiocytic tumor with characteristic biphasic pattern of fibrosis and nodules of macrophages within fatty tissue.

entiated fibrosarcomas (negative for CD34), which histologically closely mimic DFs. They show predilection for the face and acral sites, invariably recur when incompletely excised, and may metastasize ("metastasizing DF") and potentially kill the patient.[12] These exceptionally rare cases have raised the claim that DFs are a neoplasia. This interpretation is supposed to be substantiated by recent cytogenetic FISH and RT-PCR[13] and molecular studies by the HUMARA technique,[14] which has documented clonality in a minority of lesions.[15] Clonality alone is by no means a proof of a neoplastic disease as, for example, it is seen in a variety of inflammatory disorders including atopic dermatitis, lichen sclerosus atrophicans, or psoriasis.

Both recurrences and rare metastases have been described in "atypical benign fibrous histiocytomas"[9] and some forms of "facial DFs".[16] None of the publications which we are aware of unequivocally document the "progression" of a DF into a malignant process. Authors may show medium or high power views with bland features and say that these lesions were clonal, recurred, or even metastasized; or they show atypical areas with high cellularity, atypia, mitoses, and even necroses taken from lesions which behaved in a benign fashion. Consistently missing is a scanning magnification (or a clinical photograph) which would allow us to use architectural as well as clinical criteria such as asymmetry, irregular demarcation, nonhomogenous appearance, or destruction of preexisting structures for differentiation of a benign fibrosing dermatitis from a malignant neoplasia.

These features must not be confused with DFs with monster cells or atypical/pseudosarcomatous fibrous histiocytomas (Fig. 14-5). In our experience, these are ancient/degenerative features in long-standing lesions; they always behave in a benign fashion, and do not histologically show high cellularity, necroses, or atypical mitoses. These lesions must also be differentiated from AFXs; but here growth pattern, cytologic atypia, numerous mitoses, and a greater prominence of xanthomatized macrophages allow easier separation.

XANTHOGRANULOMAS

BOX 14-3   Summary

- Nodular to diffuse dermatitis by macrophages ("granulomatous dermatitis")
- Originally opposed to Langerhans cell disease ("histiocytosis X")

- Frequently (multiple) papules to nodules; less commonly plaques and tumors.
- Macrophages are vacuolated, xanthomatized, spindly, dendritic to scalloped, and oncocytic
- Immunohistochemically positive with Ki-M1p, negative for CD1a
- Ultrastructurally, various (phago-)lysosomal structures, but without Birbeck granules
- Varying presentation according to age, location, number and cellular composition of lesions, and concomitating disorders (autoimmune and neoplastic disorders)
- Spontaneous regression in kids; apart from excision there is no effective therapy in adults

Xanthogranuloma (XG) is one type of a granulomatous dermatitis[2] characterized by a nodular-to-diffuse infiltrate of macrophages in the dermis, occasionally subcutis and other organs, clinically presenting mostly as solitary, localized, generalized, or systemic papules or nodules, but rarely patches or plaques. Macrophages may present in variable number and composition as mononuclear (vacuolated, xanthomatized, spindle-shaped, dendritic-scalloped, or oncocytic) and multinucleate cells (Touton and ground glass type) with a variable admixture of fibrocytes and other inflammatory cells frequently including lymphocytes, but rarely eosinophils, neutrophils, and/or plasma cells.

Synonyms

XG is the prototype of *non-Langerhans cell histiocytoses*,[17] which includes *generalized eruptive histiocytoma, multicentric reticulohistiocytosis,* and *progressive nodular histiocytosis* to mention a few examples (Table 14-2). Originally, they were known as *non-X histiocytoses*[18] as opposed to *histiocytosis X*. This term had been proposed by Lichtenstein[19] in the 1950s to unify several previously identified disorders (Abt-Letterer-Siwe disease, Hand-Schüller-Christian disease, eosinophilic granuloma of the bone, and later self-healing reticulohistiocytosis Hashimoto–Pritzker) after he astutely observed similar histological features. In due course, Langerhans cell differentiation was recognized and the Histiocyte Society replaced the "X" with *Langerhans cell histiocytosis*[20] (and non-Langerhans cell histiocytoses, respectively), but this classification is not much better than the older eponyms. Other classifications such as *Langerhans cell granulomatosis* (and *non-Langerhans cell granulomatosis*) are even worse. Dendritic cells cannot form granulomas, which by defin-

ition are an aggregation of macrophages (without further need for non-Langerhans cell disclosure). Not surprisingly, we prefer to speak of Langerhans cell disease, XGs, and their variants.

Etiology

The schematic drawing (Fig. 14-7) shows our classification of the many variants of XGs.[17] While we favor a unifying approach to these disorders, for purposes of communication we have retained the traditional unwieldy terminology. The etiology of all these disorders is unknown. Moreover, the literature is inconclusive about the exact nature of disease, be it neoplastic or inflammatory.[21] In our experience, there are hints indicating that infectious stimuli in association with a deregulated cytokine concert have pathogenetic importance.[22] Adults with chronic persistent, widespread lesions may have immunologic disorders such as lupus erythematosus, dermatomyositis, or Hashimoto thyroiditis as well as a wide variety of neoplastic diseases; while in juvenile variants, similar immunologic defects could be associated with transient intrauterine or postpartum infections.[23] In some cases, the disease may represent a paraneoplastic phenomenon, waxing and waning with the underlying disorder, e.g., mycosis fungoides.[24]

All of these diseases show differentiation towards monocytes/macrophages. Macrophages derive from stem cells in the bone marrow, circulate as monocytes via blood through the organism, and then leave the blood system into the various tissues. There is marked trafficking with recruitment to sites of inflammation.[25] Macrophages are capable of phagocytosis, which has led to a variety of synonyms such as siderophages or lipophages.

XG, including all variants, must be separated from other granulomatous dermatitides (macrophage disorders) such as palisading (granuloma annulare, necrobiosis lipoidica, necrobiotic xanthogranuloma, rheumatoid nodule, and gout), sarcoidal (sarcoidosis, silica, and beryllium reactions), tuberculoid (tuberculosis, acne agminata, some forms of leprosy, leishmaniasis, and syphilis), suppurative (deep fungal infections, atypical mycobacteriosis, halogenoderma, and follicular occlusion disease), suppurative tuberculoid (geographical necrosis with palisading macrophages and admixture of neutrophils or eosinophils as seen in cat scratch disease, yersiniosis, *Campylobacter jejuni* infections, and Wegener and Churg-Strauss granulomas), and foreign body granulomas to

Table 14-2
Clinicopathologic Characteristics of Xanthogranuloma (XG) Variants

XG VARIANT	PREDILECTION SEX, AGE (YEAR), SITE	PREDOMINANT MACROPHAGE TYPE	PECULARITIES
Benign cephalic histiocytosis	F = M, small children, cheek and forehead	Vacuolated	Early manifestation of XG, may precede to classic XG
Mononuclear variant (Shapiro)	F = M; children, trunk	Vacuolated	Solitary (or a few) lesion(s)
Generalized eruptive histiocytoma	F = M, adults, generalized	Vacuolated	May precede XG or other variants; sometimes paraneoplastic (mycosis fungoides)
Xanthoma disseminatum (Montgomery disease) or disseminated xanthosiderohistiocytosis	F < M, childhood, young adults, eyelids, flexures, (oral) mucosa (50%), diabetes insipidus (40%)	Dendritic to scalloped in early, xanthomatized in late stages	Cave conjunctival (blindness) or respiratory involvement (may need tracheotomy); many other internal organs; mostly persistent to progressive, only rarely regressive
Scalloped cell xanthogranuloma	F = M, adults, trunk	Dendritic to scalloped	Rare solitary variant similar to adult XG
Papular xanthoma	F = M, children or adults, solitary or localized to head, neck, genitalia	Xanthomatized with extensive Touton giant cells	No associated hyperlipidemia
Xanthelasma	F = M, adults, upper more than lower eyelids	Xanthomatized without extracellular lipids	No associated hyperlipidemia (usually)
Verruciform xanthoma (histiocytosis Y; Shafer disease)	F = M, adults, gingival and alveolar mucosa, anogenital	Xanthomatized within papillary dermis	Verrucous plaques, associated with viral warts, CHILD nevus, lupus erythematosus, psoriasis a.o.m.
Normolipemic plane xanthomas (with paraproteinemia)	F = M, adults, trunk and extremities	Xanthomatized	Widespread macular version of papular xanthoma; also seen in atopic dermatitis, chronic actinic dermatitis and mycosis fungoides
Reticulohistiocytoma	F = M, adults, trunk	Oncocytic cells and giant cells with ground glass appearance	"Overlap" to classic XG
Multicentric reticulohistiocytosis	F > M, 40–60, hands (coral bead sign), ears, lips, nares (leonine face)	Oncocytic cells and giant cells with ground glass appearance	Destructive arthritis (telescoping fingers) before (50%), simultaneously with (30%) or following skin lesions;
Progressive nodular histiocytosis	F < M, 40–60, trunk, extremities and face (leonine facies)	Spindle-shaped in nodules beside classic dermal XG	Rare combination of classic dermal papules of XG with subcutaneous nodules of spindle cell XG, sometimes hemorrhagic and then painful
Spindle cell xanthogranuloma	F = M, adults, trunk	Spindle shaped	Rare solitary variant similar to adult XG
Dermal dendrocytomas	F = M, 40–60, trunk	Spindle shaped	Variant of spindle cell XG with multiple lesions; overlap to generalized DFs
Progressive mucinous histiocytosis	F > M, 40–60, trunk, extremities, face	Spindle shaped with prominent mucin	Variant of spindle cell XG

various exogenous and endogenous subjects (splinters, metal, glass fragments; keratin). In addition to granulomatous reactions, congenital and acquired metabolic diseases and deposit disorders, such as eruptive, tuberous, and plane xanthomas in hyperlipidemias, or sitosterolemia, cerebrotendinous xanthomas, and sea blue histiocytic syndrome show prominent macrophage participation.

Epidemiology

The incidence of XG is two to three cases per 100,000 people per year and is most common on the scalp, face, and neck. It occurs mostly in children, is multiple in this group and occurs without sexual predilection. XG is less frequent in adults, is mostly single in this group, and occurs on the trunk or limbs.

Stereotypical Presentation

XG most commonly occurs in children, justifying the alternative name of *juvenile xanthogranuloma*. Yet, every experienced dermatologist has seen a few in adults (*adult xanthogranuloma*). The lesions are typically red-brown papules or nodules (Fig. 14-8), usually with a yellowish hue and sometimes with telangiectases. Most common sites in children include

UNIFYING CONCEPT OF XANTHOGRANULOMA FAMILY

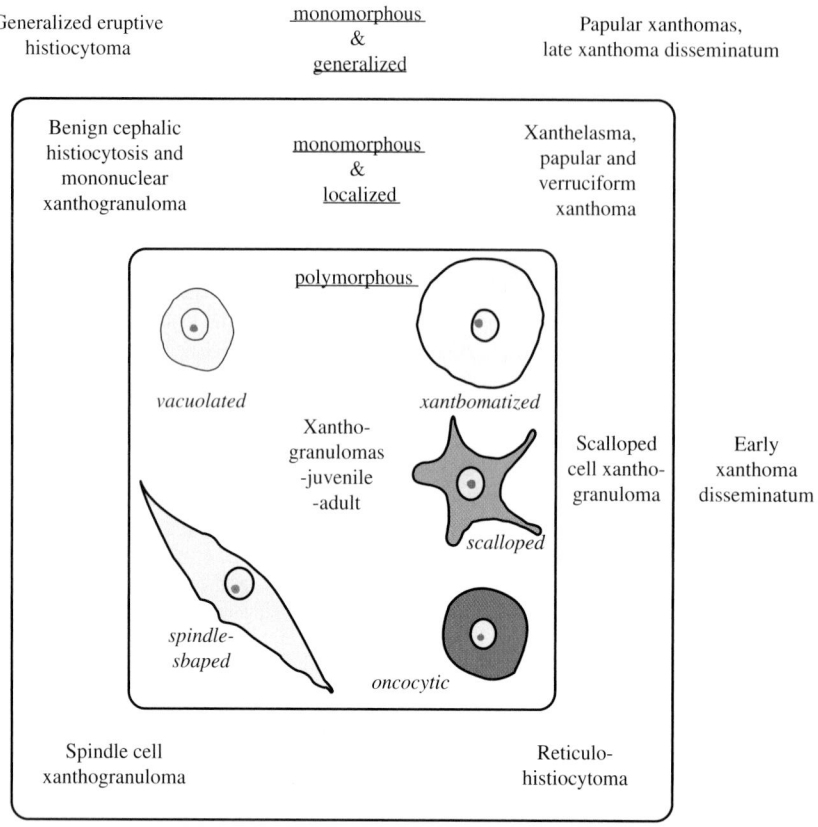

▲ **FIGURE 14-7** Schematic drawing of a unifying concept of xanthogranuloma family. This figure is a slightly modified version of a schematic drawing originally published as Fig. 14-12 in the review article by Zelger et al.[17] (Reproduced with permission of the publisher, Lippincott Williams & Wilkins, Inc.)

tion, giant XG has been defined as a lesion >2 cm in diameter.

Apart from cutaneous lesions, XG may also affect subcutaneous fat and soft tissue. Ocular changes involve the iris or ciliary body leading to glaucoma or bleeding into the anterior chamber (hyphema). Conjunctival, bulbar, or retinal lesions are extremely uncommon. Other internal involvement is less clear; CNS changes are the most life threatening, while pulmonary and bony changes may also be seen. Internal manifestations may be much more common than generally believed as subtle lesions may not cause any clinical problems or serologic changes, except in problematic regions such as the sella turcica where they can produce diabetes insipidus. Moreover, papules similar to those in the skin might easily be overlooked or even be too small for all our modern imaging techniques. Yet, there are rare cases with clearly documented internal manifestations.[26]

Erdheim—Chester disease has been defined as the association of subcutaneous XG with bony defects. Radiographically, symmetrical sclerosis involving the diametaphyseal aspects of long bones and, pathologically, characteristic xanthogranulomatous changes are diagnostic. Nonosseous disease includes hypothalamus/pituitary involvement with diabetes insipidus, renal and retroperitoneal infiltration, and lung lesions.[27] In the skin xanthomas, the most frequent finding is particularly around the eyes. The clinical course of Erdheim–Chester disease varies

the flexural areas and scalp. Children typically have several lesions, which usually tend to regress within several months to years. In contrast, most adults have only a single lesion and are often permanent.

Many clinical variations on juvenile XG have been described. There may be patches, papules, plaques, and subcutaneous tumors. The Cyrano form refers to disfiguring nasal involvement. In children, lesions usually regress leaving an atrophic scar. Lesions in adults are more likely to be solitary and are often permanent. A distinction has been made between micronodular disease with many small lesions and an increased likelihood of ocular involvement, as compared to macronodular disease with fewer lesions, but a greater risk of internal organ involvement. While the terms micro- and macronodular well describe the cutaneous patterns, they do not accurately predict internal involvement. In addi-

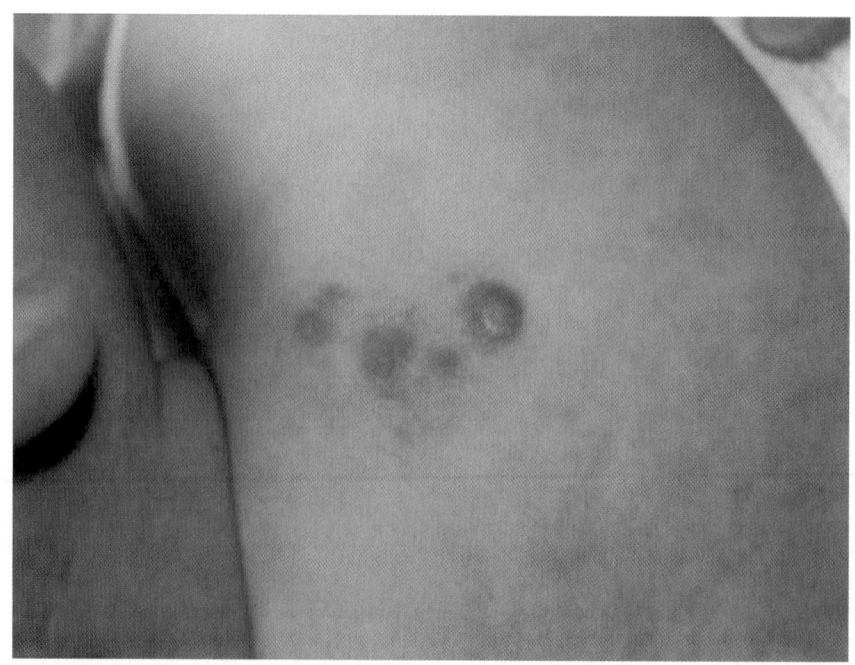

▲ **FIGURE 14-8** Juvenile xanthogranuloma with a cluster of yellow papules (Courtesy Dr. L Hefel, M.D., Dornbirn, Austria).

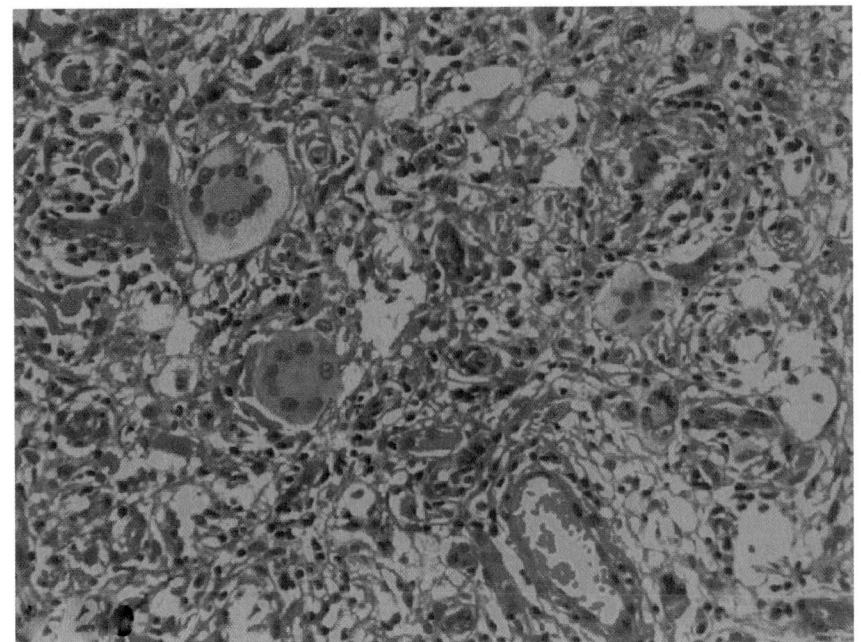

▲ **FIGURE 14-9** Xanthomatized macrophages and Touton giant cells of xanthogranuloma.

and is dependent on the extent and distribution of extraosseous involvement. From our point of view, Erdheim–Chester disease is a variant of XGs with mostly osseous and internal involvement.

Histology reveals a diffuse infiltrate of macrophages with prominent Touton giant cells, in which a wreath of nuclei enclose a paler central area (Fig. 14-9). The macrophages of XGs may be vacuolated with a finely stippled cytoplasm; they may be xanthomatized with prominent lipid vacuoles within greatly enlarged cells; some cells may become spindly, others dendritic to scalloped with long extending spider-like cytoplasmic extensions (Fig. 14-10A); and still other cells may show a finely granular, prominently eosinophilic cytoplasm in epithelioid to polygonal cells—the so-called "oncocytic cells" from Greek "onkein", to swell (Fig. 14-10B). A variable number of lymphocytes, sometimes also eosinophils, and rarely neutrophils, are found in between or surrounding the macrophages.

Clinicopathological Variants

The concept of xanthogranulomas is best understood when one knows the multiple aspects of cytological presentation of macrophages as shown in the schematic drawing (Fig. 14-7). Generally, XGs show a mixture of all the cell types discussed above, but are dominated by the eye-catching Touton giant cells which are regularly mixed up with xanthomatized mononuclear macrophages. When the infiltrate becomes less polymorphous and one cell type dominates, then characteristic clinicopathologic entities may be described. These lesions may be solitary (Fig. 14-11A), localized (Fig. 14-11B), generalized, or systemic (Fig. 14-12) (Table 14-2). Accordingly, there is plentiful variation, and once again, "overlaps" are the rule. If one is a fanatical pigeon holer, these disorders are guaranteed to increase anxiety.

The association of generalized and systemic variants with immunologic disorders and malignancies is assured. This is particularly regarding multicentric reticulohistiocytosis, but in a minor percentage also involves multiple adult xanthogranulomas, progressive nodular histiocytosis, and rarely generalized eruptive histiocytoma and xanthoma disseminatum. Diseases which may be found include lupus erythematosus, dermatomyositis, Sjögren syndrome, vasculitis, primary biliary cirrhosis, and many others, while malignant neoplasms have been identified in a range of organs.[28] Of special importance, the multicentric reticulohistiocytosis is diagnosed first in 75% of cases; the malignant neoplasm or associated disease in 25%. Histology reveals mononuclear and multinucleate oncocytic cells; the latter are also known as giant cells with ground glass appearance.

Immunohistochemistry

XG are positive for macrophage markers such as Ki-M1p, PGM1, and KP1 (CD68) or HAM56 (Fig. 14-13). Other markers are variably expressed such as labeling for factor XIIIa, which is seen in "early" lesions histologically characterized by vacuolated or dendritic to scalloped macrophages (benign cephalic histiocytosis, generalized eruptive histiocytoma, or early xanthoma disseminatum). Later on, when xanthomatized, macrophages may show adherence for the lectin peanut agglutinin, or, when spindle-shaped, for smooth muscle actin. Ultrastucturally, a variety of (phago-)lysosomal structures is loosely associated with certain variants such as dense bodies in generalized eruptive histiocytoma, pleomorphic cytoplas-

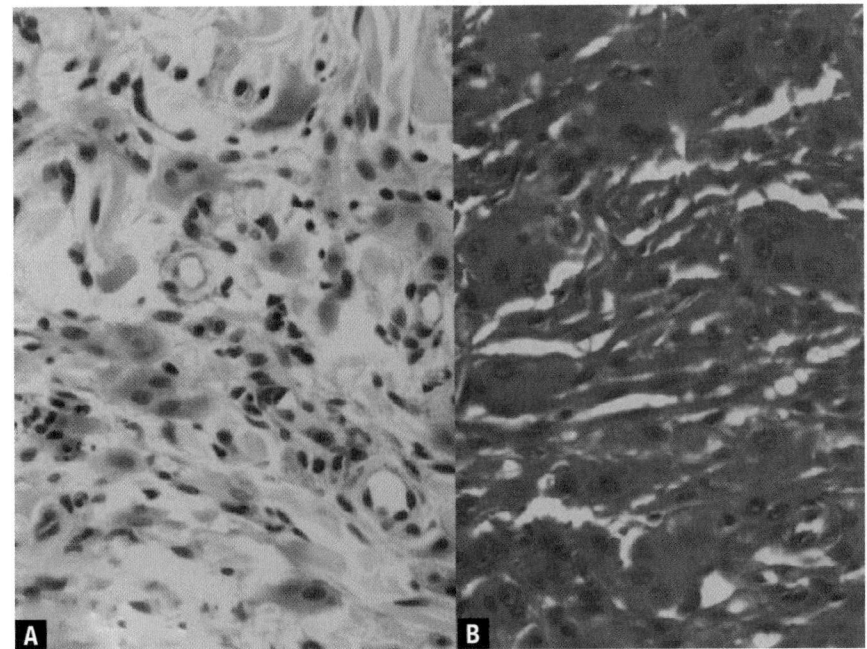

▲ **FIGURE 14-10 A.** Dendritic to scalloped macrophages of a scalloped cell xanthogranuloma. **B.** Oncocytic macrophages and giant cells with ground glass appearance of multicentric reticulohistiocytosis.

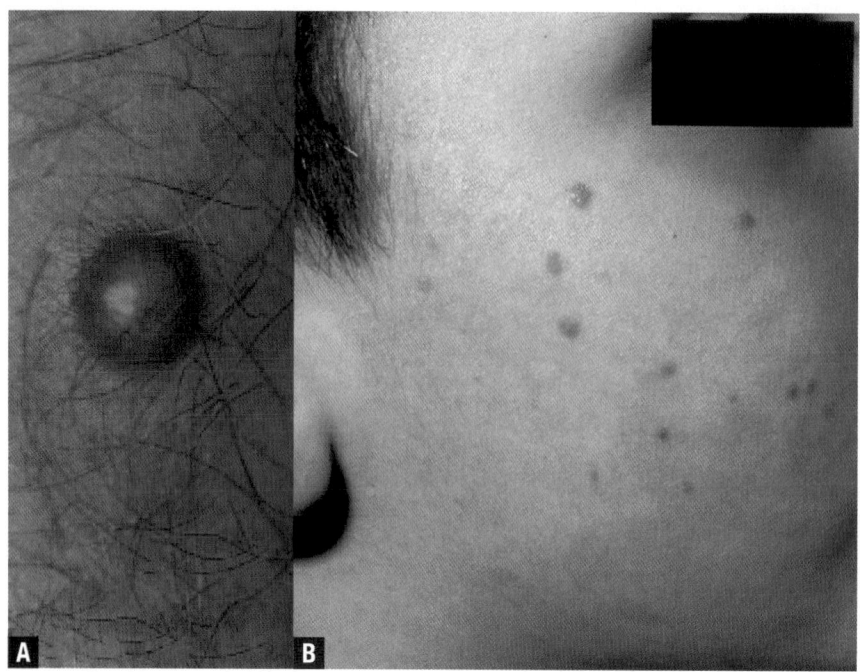

▲ **FIGURE 14-11 A.** Yellow papule of solitary papular xanthoma. **B.** Red-brown papules of benign cephalic histiocytosis.

mic inclusions in reticulohistiocytoma and multicentric reticulohistiocytosis, or myeloid bodies in papular xanthoma and late xanthoma disseminatum to mention but a few examples. Again, overlap is the rule and not the exception. Thus, electron microscopy in multicentric reticulohistiocytosis identifies a variety of lipids within the giant cells, leading to the old name of *lipoid dermatoarthritis*.

In our experience, XG and its variants may, in a minor proportion of cases (<5%, show diffuse reactivity for S100

protein. Such labeling usually is less prominent than positive internal controls of Langerhans cells and nerves, but it is reproducible, restricted to macrophages, and thus allows no smear artefact, which sometimes can be seen with various markers in inflammatory disorders. In the past, such entities have been filed as *indeterminate cell histiocytosis*, defined as a disease with both Langerhans cell and macrophage characteristics. The concept derives from immunohistochemical observations which were thought to

prove such lineage infidelity. While in the original definition, these lesions were said to also label for CD1a, but without ultra-structural detection of Birbeck granules;[29] in later case reports and series reactivity for CD1a was reported as focal and probably outlined a background reaction. Moreover, basic science research has neither provided a clear definition nor a likely function of this indeterminate cell. We are thus skeptical of the utility of this diagnosis and have expressed this previously in a review on non-Langerhans cell histiocytoses in childhood: *"The indeterminate cell-in indeterminate cell histiocytosis-is really as vague as its name suggests."*[24] We do not think that it is really justified to separate entities according to differences in one immunohistochemical marker only.[30] Having seen more than 25 cases of what is thought to be indeterminate cell histiocytosis in consultation, we think that this phenomenon describes a mixture of entities, on one hand when positive for CD1a a Langerhans cell disease, which failed to reveal Birbeck granules ultrastructurally, on the other a macrophage disorder positive for S100 protein, but consistently negative for CD1a and without Birbeck granules.[31]

The latter seems to be related to sinus histiocytosis with massive lymphadenopathy (Rosai-Dorfman disease). It typically involves children and young adults who present with extreme cervical lymphadenopathy. Again, the etiology is unknown; HHV-6 was just a scare, yet an infectious process is likely. In most instances the disease resolves spontaneously. A small percentage of patients die from their disease while others have persistent problems. About 10% of these patients with full-blown disease have cutaneous findings, usually red-brown papules or nodules, which also may occur as the only manifestation of disease. Histology reveals sheets of pale to eosinophilic S100 positive (CD1a negative) macrophages some of which have taken up many lymphocytes. This phenomenon is nothing else than phagocytosis, yet the literature euphemistically speaks of "emperipolesis", and the affected cells have been called "bean bag cells".

Differential Diagnoses

The classic historical mimicry is Langerhans cell disease. Their coffee-bean or kidney-shaped nuclei, immunohistochemistry for CD1a and lag antigen, and electron microscopy with trilamellar Birbeck granules usually allow easy diagnosis. Yet, one has to be cautious as late

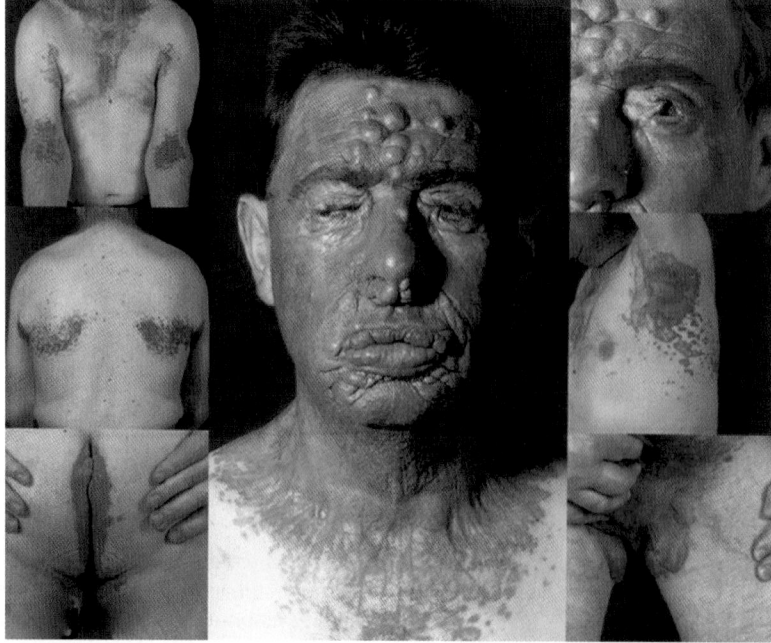

▲ **FIGURE 14-12** Xanthoma disseminatum.

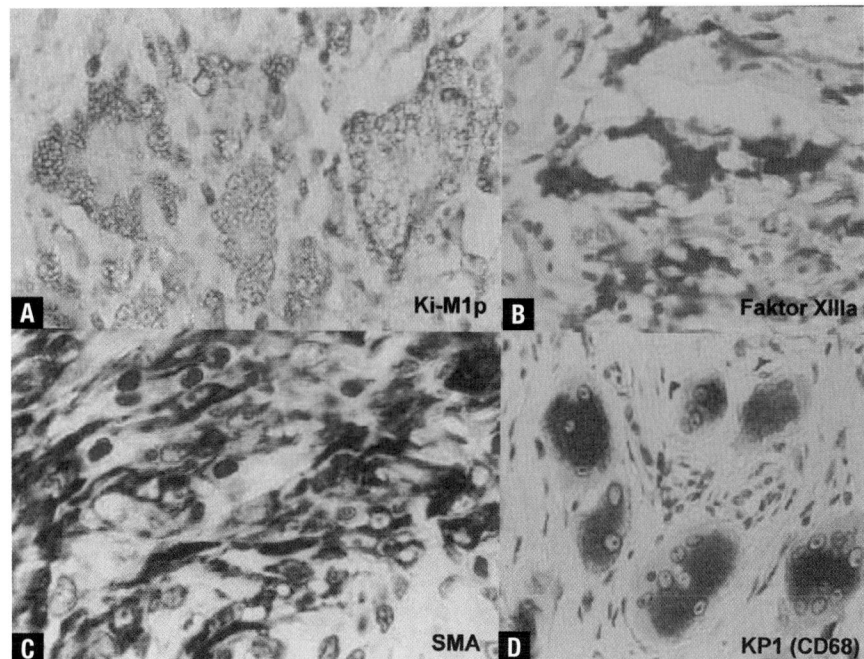

▲ **FIGURE 14-13** **A.** Xanthomatized macrophages positive with Ki-M1p. **B.** Dendritic to scalloped macrophages positive for factor XIIIa. **C.** Spindle-shaped macrophages positive for smooth muscle actin. **D.** Giant cells with ground glass appearance positive with KP1 (CD68).

stages sometimes are poor in Langerhans cells, but instead show numerous xanthomatized macrophages. Other classic differential diagnostic considerations in children are Spitz melanocytic nevus and mast cell tumor.

Further difficulties arise regarding sharp demarcation from DFs. Basically, the latter are dominated by fibrocytes (or fibroblasts), show prominent fibroplasia (entrapment of collagen bundles), and a concomitating hyperplasia of nearby or surrounding tissue components, in particular a hyperplastic epidermis. Yet, sometimes a borderline between variants of either type is a challenge to draw, outlining their overall relation as an inflammatory response. Therefore, delineation may be difficult between (juvenile) XG and histiocytoma, scalloped cell XG and epithelioid cell histiocytoma, spindle cell XG and DF, or papular xanthoma and fibrous xanthoma.

Prognosis

Prognosis depends on two factors. In solitary lesions, excision is diagnostic as well as curative. When generalized in children, watchful waiting is also fine as spontaneous resolution usually occurs within months to years. Rarely, ocular involvement with glaucoma may require surgery in juvenile XG. In contrast, there is no satisfactory therapy in generalized adult variants. The vast majority progress or at least persist; only a minority spontaneously regress. This partially correlates with the

waxing and waning of underlying disorders which must be carefully looked for. All forms of treatment have been disappointing including corticosteroids, chemotherapeutic regimens, interferon gamma, and various lipid antimetabolites. Diabetes insipidus can usually be managed with standard measures. Excision of single lesions, or in case of multiple lesions those most disfiguring, is the therapy of choice. Alternatively, destruction by laser treatment (tunable dye, carbon dioxide) is an elegant modern method.

■ MALIGNANT FIBROUS HISTIOCYTOMA

BOX 14-4 Summary

- Encloses undifferentiated pleomorphic sarcoma, undifferentiated pleomorphic sarcoma with giant cells, and undifferentiated pleomorphic sarcoma with prominent inflammation
- No definitive disease, but reaction patterns of a variety of dedifferentiated malignancies exist; thus, MFH has become a diagnosis of exclusion
- Electron microscopy, immunohistochemistry, and molecular techniques (FISH, PCR, RT-PCR, microarray) have been helpful tools
- Usually grave prognosis with <50% 5-year survival
- Therapy includes wide excision frequently combined with radiochemotherapy

The term malignant fibrous histiocytoma (MFH) was first introduced by Ozello, Stout, and Murray in 1963 and became more popular by Enzinger`s seminal paper in 1977.[32] He subdivided this entity into five categories: (storiform-)pleomorphic, myxoid, giant cell, inflammatory, and angiomatoid variants. Over the years, the whole concept of MFH, previously the most frequent sarcoma in adults, has become questionable. In most cases of the so-called pleomorphic MFH, a line of differentiation can be established (fibro-, myofibro-, leio- and rhabdomyo-, liposarcoma; carcinoma, melanoma) and the few remaining cases are best regarded as pleomorphic sarcomas not otherwise specified. This diagnosis has become a diagnosis of exclusion accounting for <5% of adult sarcomas. Similarly, the morphological features of the so-called giant cell and inflammatory MFH are shared by a number of specific tumor types. Finally, myxofibrosarcoma (formerly known as myxoid MFH) and the so-called angiomatoid MFH represent distinct entities. In 2002, the latter had been downgraded from a high- to a low-grade malignancy in the latest WHO classification on soft tissue tumors and accordingly been termed angiomatoid fibrous histiocytoma.[5]

Undifferentiated Pleomorphic Sarcoma (Pleomorphic MFH)

The term pleomorphic MFH is nowadays reserved for a small group of undifferentiated pleomorphic sarcomas; both terms are used interchangeably.[33] Current techniques do not reveal a definable line of differentiation.

For many years, pleomorphic MFH was the prototypic form of MFH and thereby the most common soft tissue sarcoma in adults.[34] Based on morphology and tissue culture techniques, it was originally thought to represent a pleomorphic spindle cell malignant neoplasm with fibrocytic and facultative "histiocytic" (macrophage) differentiation. Today, it is well established that this pattern may be seen in a wide variety of poorly differentiated neoplasms (Fig. 14-14) including carcinomas, melanoma, and lymphoma. Moreover, it is also now agreed that these lesions show no evidence of true macrophage differentiation. Consequently, the incidence of pleomorphic MFH has fallen dramatically over the past decade.

EPIDEMIOLOGY MFH was previously the most common type of sarcoma in adults over the age of 40 years. There are one to two cases per 100,000 people, but the

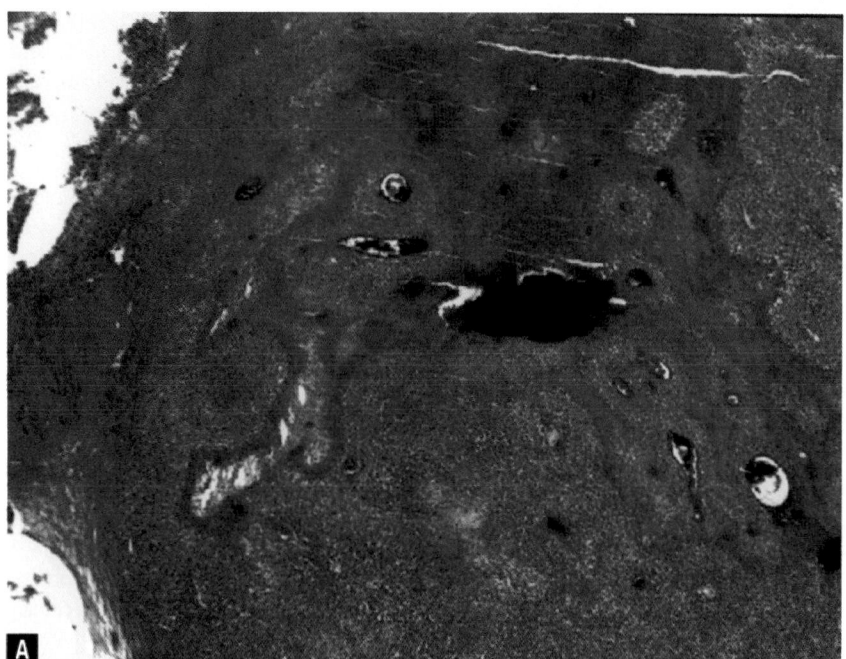

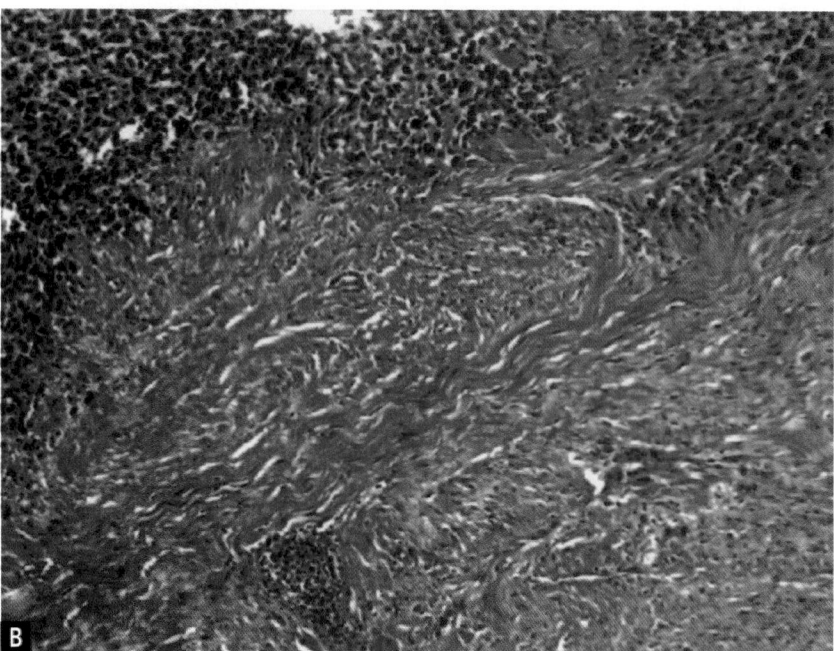

▲ **FIGURE 14-14 A.** Anaplastic growth pattern of pleomorphic MFH; note geographical necroses. **B.** Higher magnification focally reveals fascicles with neuroid differentiation (wavy nuclei) positive for S100 protein indicating malignant peripheral nerve sheath tumor.

often grow rapidly and then may be painful. Imaging methods and macroscopy reveal well-circumscribed masses with heterogeneous composition. Pale fibrous and fleshy areas are admixed with zones of (cystic) necroses, hemorrhage, or myxoid features.

Undifferentiated pleomorphic sarcomas are a diagnosis of exclusion following thorough sampling and critical use of ancillary diagnostic techniques (including immunohistochemistry, electron microscopy, cytogenetics with FISH, PCR and RT-PCR, microarrays, etc).[35] Lesions are very heterogeneous in appearance and cellularity, since some have extensive fibrous stroma. Characteristically, lesions reveal prominent pleomorphism with marked atypia, numerous atypical mitoses, and bizarre giant cells, frequently with xanthomatized to oncocytic or rhabdoid cytoplasmic appearance. A storiform growth pattern and variable chronic inflammatory cells are common. Undifferentiated pleomorphic sarcomas have an overall 5-year survival of roughly 50%. Yet over the years, it became clear that there are prognostic subgroups among lesions previously summarized as pleomorphic MFH. Therefore, dedifferentiated liposarcoma has a metastatic rate of only 15 to 20%, high-grade myxofibrosarcoma of 30 to 35%, while pleomorphic leio- and rhabdomyosarcoma are much more aggressive with higher rates of metastases and shorter disease free and overall survival times.[36] The clinical and therapeutic benefits of this sub-classification are just beginning to be appreciated.

Undifferentiated Pleomorphic Sarcoma with Giant Cells (Giant Cell MFH).

Similar to undifferentiated pleomorphic sarcoma, this MFH pattern may be shared by a variety of malignancies, in particular, extraskeletal osteosarcoma (Fig. 14-15), giant cell tumor of soft tissue, leiomyosarcoma, and osteoclast-rich carcinoma.[37] Organs in which giant cell-rich or osteoclastoma-like carcinomas are most common include pancreas, thyroid, breast, and kidney. The term "giant cell MFH" is reserved for undifferentiated pleomorphic sarcomas with prominent osteoclastic giant cells (synonyms: malignant giant cell tumor of soft parts, malignant osteoclastoma, giant cell sarcoma)[38]; again, this diagnosis is gradually disappearing from common usage in soft tissue pathology.[39] Most of these lesions occur in the deep soft tissue of the extremities and trunk of older adults without sex predilection. Most lesions are large (>5cm), painless masses with prominent hemorrhage and

prevalence increases with age. The peak incidence occurs during the sixth and seventh decade of life, but rare cases occur in adolescents and young adults. MFH also has a slight male predominance.

PATHOGENESIS The etiology of MFH is unknown. A minority (<2 to 3% occur at a site of previous radiation with rare cases at a site of chronic ulceration and scarring. Genomic imbalances frequently occur with a loss of 2p24-pter, 2q32-qter, and chromosomes 11, 13, and 16, with a gain of 7p15-pter, 7q32, and

1p31. Proto-oncogenes are frequently involved mapping to 12q13-15: *SAS, MDM2, CDK4, DDIT3,* or *HMGIC.* Other mutations and/or deletions regard *TP53, RB1,* and *CDKN2*A.

CLINICOPATHOLOGICAL EVALUATION Most undifferentiated pleomorphic sarcomas occur in the deep subfascial soft tissue of the lower limb and less often the trunk; roughly 10% are primarily subcutaneous. At presentation, lesions are frequently tumors between 5 and 15 cm of diameter; less than 5cm in subcutis,

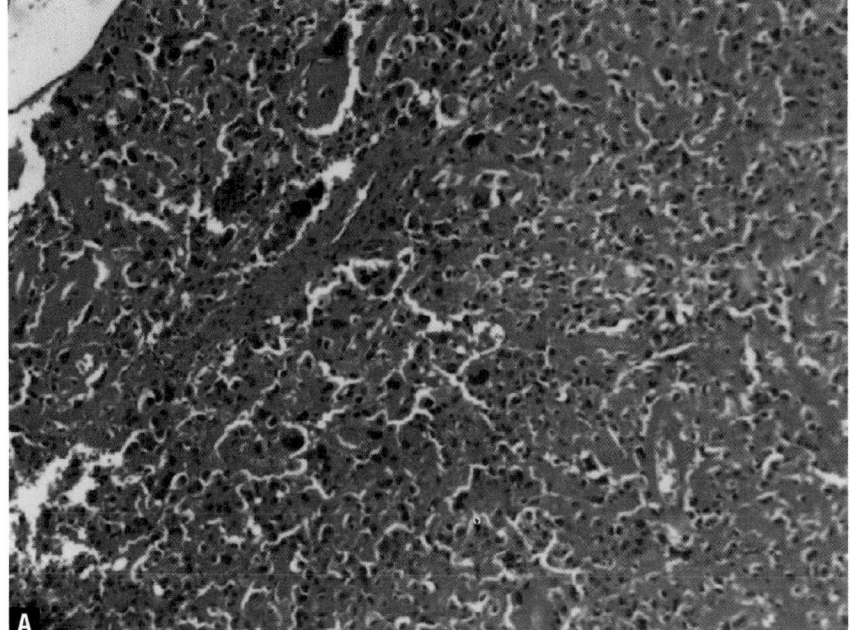

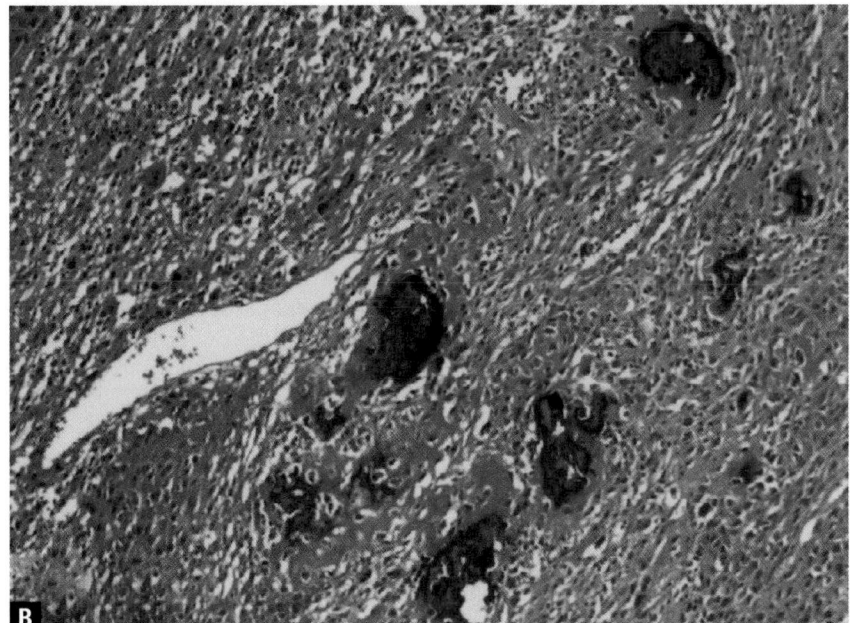

▲ **FIGURE 14-15** **A.** Growth pattern of giant cell MFH; note bizarre giant cells (left site) beside osteoid formation (right site). **B.** Other tumor parts revealed neoplastic bone formation characteristic of extraskeletal osteosarcoma.

Undifferentiated Pleomorphic Sarcoma with Prominent Inflammation (Inflammatory MFH)

This MFH variant is characterized by numerous xanthomatous cells (synonyms: xanthomatous MFH, malignant fibrous xanthoma, xanthosarcoma), morphologically both benign and malignant, admixed with atypical ovoid to spindle-shaped cells and acute and chronic inflammatory cells (Fig. 14-16A). Such a pattern is seen in mesenchymal as well as epithelial neoplasms. Inflammatory MFH is rare[40]; it mostly occurs in patients older than 40 years of age, without sexual predilection in deep location (retroperitoneum, deep soft tissue of extremities, and trunk).[41] Apart from local symptoms and respective imaging features, patients frequently suffer from fever, weight loss, leukocytosis, and eosinophilia due to cytokines.[42] Like undifferentiated pleomorphic sarcomas with or without giant cells, undifferentiated pleomorphic sarcoma with prominent inflammation is a diagnosis of exclusion and could represent an inflammatory dedifferentiated component shared by different neoplasms such as carcinomas, lymphomas, leiomyosarcomas, inflammatory myofibroblastic tumors, and liposarcomas (Fig. 14-16B). In the retroperitoneum, dedifferentiated liposarcoma is the most common simulant. Another option is large cell anaplastic lymphoma. Immunohistochemistry for CD30 (BerH2) and/or cytogenetics for CD12; 16 translocation may be helpful to recognize these entities. Two-thirds of the retroperitoneal cases die from persistence of the malignancy and local problems; one-third from metastases.[37,40]

 MYXOFIBROSARCOMA (MYXOID MFH)

BOX 14-5 **Summary**

- Sarcoma with fibroblastic differentiation
- Frequently affects subcutis (or deeper tissues) of lower limbs
- Multinodular growth pattern with ill-defined margins and discohesive growth
- Variable cellularity (according to grade I-III) beside mucin and curvilinear vessels
- Wide excisions of 3 to 5 cm essential to avoid recurrences
- Prognosis varies from nearly 100% (grade I) to 30% 5-year survival (grade III)

Nowadays, most experts regard myxofibrosarcoma, formerly known as myxoid MFH,[43] as a distinct sarcoma with fibroblastic differentiation.[44]

necroses. Histology reveals variably pleomorphic oval to spindle-shaped cells with prominent osteoclastic giant cells. Aside from these features common to all undifferentiated pleomorphic sarcoma with giant cells, morphology is largely influenced by the specific tumor type. Therefore, a giant-cell rich extraskeletal osteosarcoma shows variably prominent osteoid between atypical cells (Fig. 14-15A), a giant cell tumor of soft tissue usually has a multinodular growth pattern and cytologically resembles its analogue in bone, and, finally, a giant cell-rich leiomyosarcoma shows at least small areas with characteristic smooth muscle cytology and a fascicular growth pattern. In addition, immunohistochemistry is helpful as it shows reactivity for desmin or caldesmon or as it helps to confirm the keratogenous differentiation of osteoclast-rich carcinoma. Prognosis of undifferentiated pleomorphic sarcomas with prominent ostoclastic giant cells is similar to other pleomorphic sarcomas. In particular, the prognosis is very bad in extraskeletal osteosarcoma and leiomyosarcoma.

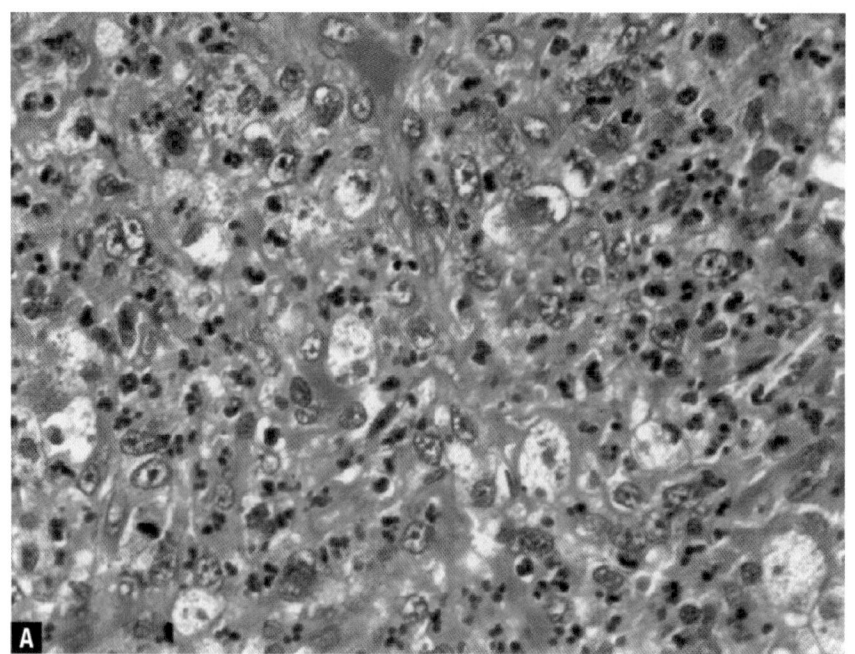

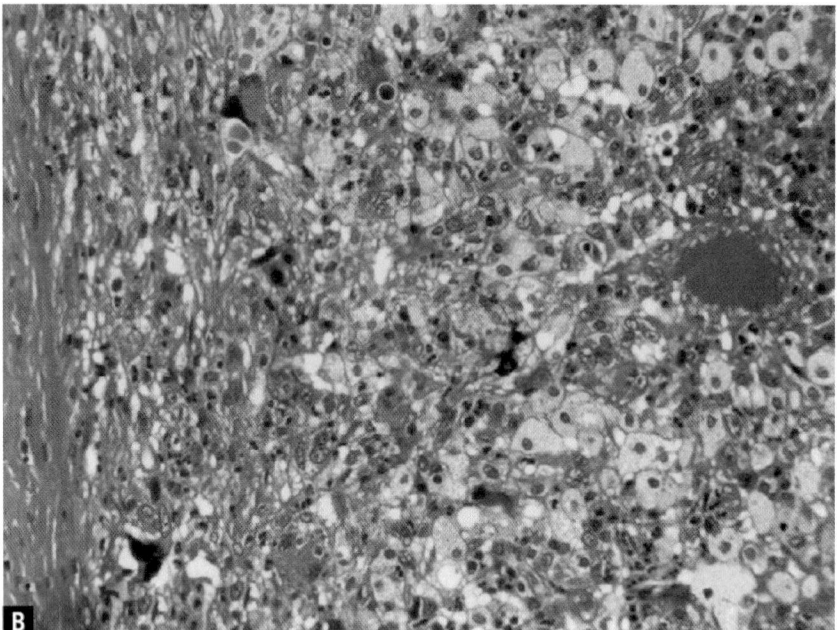

▲ **FIGURE 14-16** **A.** Inflammatory MFH reveals plentiful neutrophils beside siderophages. **B.** Other tumor parts revealed hyperchromatic giant cells and xanthomatized macrophages beside focal lipoblasts characteristic of dedifferentiated liposarcoma, inflammatory type.

Epidemiology

Myxofibrosarcoma is one of the most common sarcomas in elderly patients with a peak incidence occurring in the sixth to eighth decade of life. Very rare cases occur in adolescents and young adults (below 20 years). In addition, there is a slight male predominance.

Pathogenesis

The etiology of myxofibrosarcoma is unknown. Complex karyotypes with great intratumoral heterogeneity and chromosome numbers in triploid and tetraploid range in the majority of cases; some with ring chromosome (Chr20q). Genomic imbalances frequently occur with loss of 6p, and a gain of 9q and 12q.

Clinicopathological Evaluation

Most cases occur in the limbs including the limb girdles (lower > upper extremities); trunk, head, and neck are rarely involved while the retroperitoneum is exceptionally involved. Two-thirds of these lesions arise in dermal/subcutaneous tissue, the rest in the underlying fascia and skeletal muscle. Most patients present with slowly enlarging and painless masses in a multinodular pattern (Fig. 14-17). According to the variable composition lesions appear soft to gelatinous (mucin), firm (fibrosis), or fleshy (cellular). Inadequately, narrow excisions result in often-repeated recurrences in 50 to 60% of lesions unrelated to tumor grade. In contrast, metastases and disease-related mortality are closely related to tumor grade, almost none in grade I, 20 to 35% in grade II, and 60 to 70% in grade III. Metastases affect the lung and bone as well as, in a small but significant number, the locoregionary lymph nodes. The longer the lesions exist and (following inadequate excision) persist, the higher the tumor grade they transform into, and thus the more problematic. Histology reveals a broad spectrum of cellularity, atypia, and mitoses. Characteristically, lesions show a multinodular pattern with incomplete fibrous septa, a myxoid stroma of hyaluronic acid (Fig. 14-18A), and a distinctive curvilinear vascular pattern. Low-grade variants are hypocellular with only few, noncohesive, moderately hyperchromatic and pleomorphic nuclei within a plump, spindle-shaped to stellate, ill-defined, slightly eosinophilic cytoplasm (Fig. 14-18B). Frequently, the cytoplasm of fibroblasts is vacuolated due to acid mucin (pseudolipoblasts). At this stage mitoses are rare. Accentuation of neoplastic cells together with lymphocytes and plasma cells is prominent around curvilinear vessels. In contrast, high-grade neoplasms show large areas of a storiform-pleomorphic neoplasm with numerous atypical mitoses, areas of hemorrhage, and necroses. Bizarre multinucleate giant cells with abundant eosinophilic cytoplasm (resembling myoid cells) and irregular nuclei are frequently prominent. High-grade lesions focally show features of a lower grade neoplasm with more diagnostic features as described above. Subcutaneous myxofibrosarcoma commonly is ill defined, frequently extending beyond clinically suspected extensions. Lesions are immunohistochemically positive for vimentin and sometimes for actin (the latter suggesting myofibroblastic differentiation), while desmin and macrophage markers are negative. Electron microscopy also shows evidence of fibroblastic differentiation, i.e., fusiform or oval neoplastic cells with elongated, occasionally clefted nuclei with a prominent, often dilated endoplasmic reticulum within a myxoid matrix.[45]

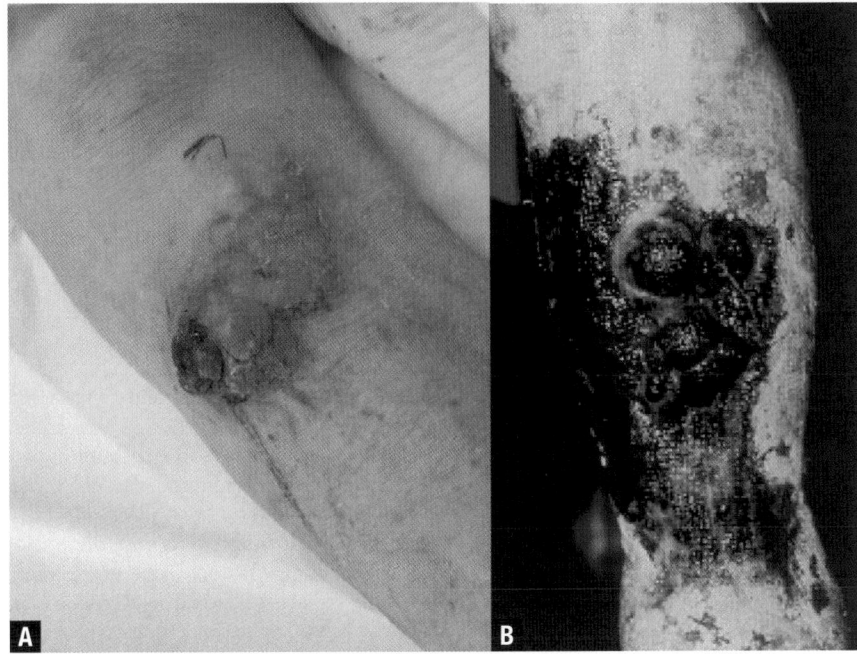

▲ **FIGURE 14-17 A.** Irregular multinodular growth pattern of myxofibrosarcoma. (Courtesy Dr. P Petzlbauer, M.D., Vienna, Austria.) **B.** Dedifferentiated myxofibrosarcoma (myxoid MFH).

ANGIOMATOID FIBROUS HISTIOCYTOMA (ANGIOMATOID MFH)

BOX 14-6 Summary

- Low-grade malignancy of uncertain differentiation
- Dermal to subcutaneous location in lymph node regions
- Frequently imitates hematoma
- Histology shows a multinodular growth of epithelioid to spindly cells within pseudoangiomatoid spaces and a "lymph node" character
- Wide excisions of 2 to 3 cm are essential to avoid recurrences
- Less than 1% metastases to lymph nodes; rare deaths due to distant metastases

Originally described by Enzinger in 1979 as an angiomatoid variant of MFH,[46] this lesion is nowadays considered to be a distinct entity of uncertain differentiation. As angiomatoid MFH shows a comparatively benign course with only low metastatic potential. The last[5] WHO classification on soft tissue tumors in 2002 changed the term to angiomatoid fibrous histiocytoma and listed this entity under the group of low-grade lesions. As mentioned before, it should not be confused with aneurysmal fibrous histiocytoma, a DF variant.

Epidemiology

Angiomatoid fibrous histiocytoma makes up approximately 5% of all MFH and 0.3% of all soft tissue tumors. It occurs in a wide range of ages (from infants to the elderly), yet is most common in children and young adults. There is a slight female predominance and a predilection for the lower limbs, less commonly the trunk and face.

Pathogenesis

The etiology for angiomatoid fibrous histiocytoma is unknown and there is an uncertain/disputed line of differentiation. Complex rearrangements of chromosomes 2, 12, 16, and 17 exist, along with a translocation of the FUS gene (16p11) fused with ATF1 gene (12q13); the chimeric FUS/ATF1 protein is similar to the EWS/ATF1 chimeric protein seen in clear cell sarcomas with a t(12;22) (q13;q12).

Clinicopathologic Evaluation

The extremities are most commonly involved, followed by the trunk, head, and neck. The majority occurs in regions where lymph nodes may be found such as the antecubital fossa, popliteal fossa, axilla, inguinal area, supraclavicular fossa, and anterior and posterior neck.[47] Clinically, lesions grow slowly, preferentially involve the subcutis and dermis, and often simulate a hematoma. Sometimes patients report a trauma, but pain is generally missing. Interestingly, occasional

cases show systemic symptoms such as fever, anemia, and weight loss, probably due to cytokine production and release by the lesion, similar to hematopoietic tumors or follicular dendritic cell tumors. Palpation frequently reveals a spongy consistency, which correlates with fluid-filled levels, indicating hemorrhage (by MRI scanning), similar to that seen in an aneurysmal bone cyst. Histology (Fig. 14-19) reveals characteristic features: a multinodular proliferation of eosinophilic spindle-shaped to epitheliod (myoid) cells, pseudoangiomatoid spaces, a thick fibrous capsule, and a pericapsular infiltrate of lymphocytes and plasma cells. The neoplastic cells are monomorphous with ovoid vesicular nuclei and a remarkable immunoprofile: 50% of cases are positive for desmin,[48] 40% for EMA, and many with macrophage markers (KP1/CD68, Ki-M1p); also, 50% with MIC1 (CD99), while markers for follicular dendritic cell tumor (CD21, CD35), S100 protein, HMB45, keratins, CD34, and vascular markers (CD31 and factor VIII related antigen) are negative.[49] The infiltrate of lymphocytes and plasma cells frequently forms germinal centers which together with the thick fibrous capsule imitate lymph nodes; yet, this infiltrate frequently lies outside the capsule and shows no marginal and hilar sinus. Some lesions show myxoid change, or cellular pleomorphism and increased mitotic activity, particularly in spindle-shaped lesions. This does not correlate with the outcome. In general, a small number of cases (2 to 11%) show persistence (lesions with infiltrating margins and location on the head and neck, or in deep muscle) and less than 1% metastases, generally nonfatal to regional lymph nodes[47] and rare deaths due to late distant metastases.[49] Wide local excision is the adequate treatment of primary lesions.

ATYPICAL FIBROXANTHOMA

BOX 14-7 Summary

- No definitive disease, but reaction pattern of a variety of dedifferentiated malignancies
- This encloses most frequently squamous cell carcinoma, rarely melanoma, basal cell carcinoma, and leiomyosarcoma
- Undifferentiated AFX (5%) is rare; a diagnosis of exclusion
- Electron microscopy, immunohistochemistry, and molecular techniques have been helpful tools
- Usually complete excision is curative

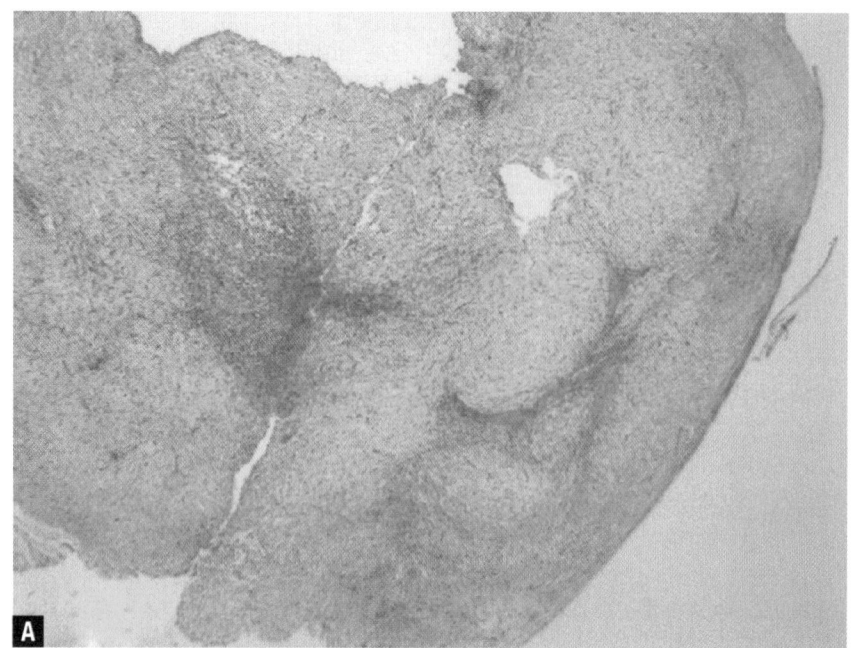

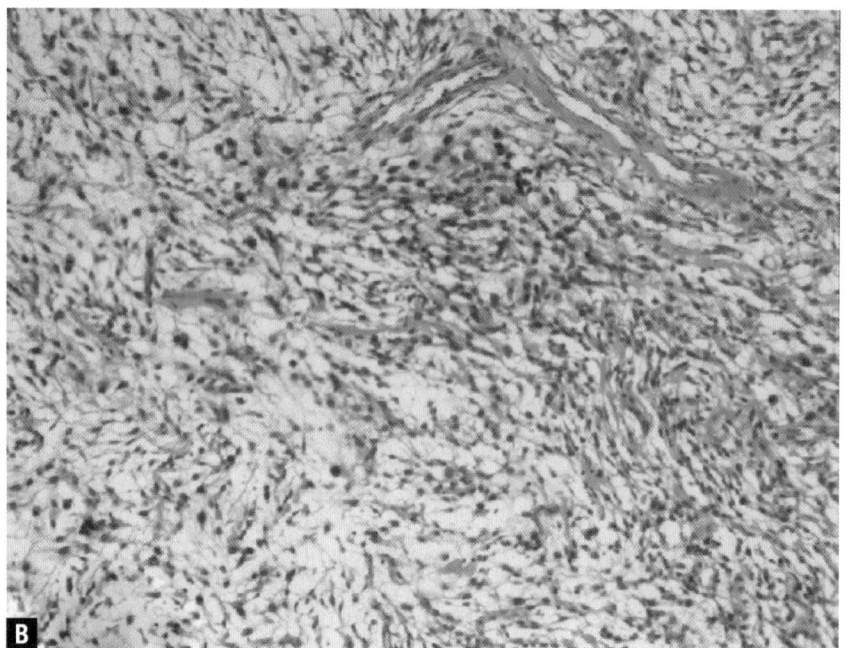

▲ **FIGURE 14-18** **A.** Myxofibrosarcoma, grade II, reveals a multinodular growth pattern of myxoid and more cellular areas. **B.** Higher magnification reveals hyperchromatic pleomorphic cells in a myxoid stroma beside characteristic curvilinear vessels.

Epidemiology

The incidence of AFX is 10 cases per 100,000 people per year. The peak incidence occurs during the sixth to eighth decade of life, is rare in adolescents and young adults, and has a male predominance. The sun-exposed areas of face (forehead, temple, ear, nose, bald scalp) or dorsal hands are the most common places for AFX.

Pathogenesis

Most cases occur in areas of massive solar damage (UV-carcinogenesis), but some cases occur in radiation exposure areas. There is an increased frequency and more serious course of disease in immunocompromized patients. Frequently, there is a long-standing history of preexisting actinic keratoses (squamous cell carcinoma *in situ* and various types of invasive squamous cell carcinomas) or subsequent development following excision of invasive squamous cell carcinomas. Genomic changes are similar to or identical to those of other *in situ* and invasive squamous cell carcinomas (pyrimidine mutations in p53 gene).

Clinicopathologic Evaluation

AFX characteristically occurs in the sun-exposed skin of elderly patients and is more common in males than in females.[52] While there is frequently a long-standing history of preexisting actinic keratoses, lesions usually grow within several weeks as exophytic, eroded, fleshy nodules to tumors (Fig. 14-20). Patients themselves, or in case of mental disability, guided by their relatives, usually rapidly seek medical advice. Clinical diagnosis frequently is squamous cell carcinoma.

Histology (Fig. 14-21) reveals an exophytic dermal nodule, frequently eroded or covered by a serohemorrhagic crust; the surrounding skin often shows severe solar damage. Lesions are usually confined to the dermis, but they may invade subcutis (or deeper structures). Characteristically, AFX shows sheaths of epithelioid to spindly cells; rare variants exhibit prominent clear cells, granular cells, pigmentation, or osteoclastic giant cells.[54] All types are characterized by prominent atypia, numerous, frequently atypical mitoses, single and mass necroses, and variable xanthomatization. These latter cells may be atypical or bland. In the latter instance, immunohistochemistry reveals those cells as macrophages while neoplastic cells are negative for all markers including Ki-M1p and CD68 (KP1 or PGM1), except vimentin. Obviously, macrophages are

AFX was originally described by Helwig in 1963 for a lesion he considered was a reactive process.[50] About the same time, Bourne described similar lesions of what he considered to be paradoxical fibrosarcomas (pseudosarcomas).[51] Since then, the concept that AFX is a neoplasm has been confirmed, and the distinctive clinicopathologic features have been established.[52] Most authors in the past considered this lesion as proliferation of fibrocytes and macrophages ("histiocytes").

Analogous to Fletcher who recognized pleomorphic MFH as a reaction pattern of a variety of dedifferentiated neoplasms,[33] we consider AFX as a reaction pattern of a predominantly dermal (superficial) dedifferentiated neoplasm including squamous cell carcinomas, basal carcinomas, melanomas, leiomyosarcomas, and rarely other dedifferentiated malignancies. In our experience the vast majority are dedifferentiated squamous cell carcinomas.[53]

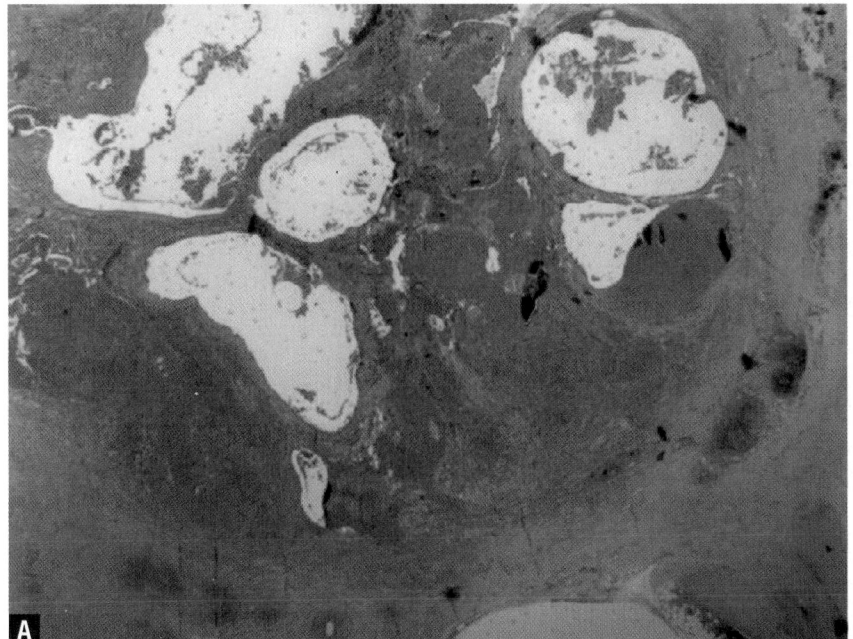

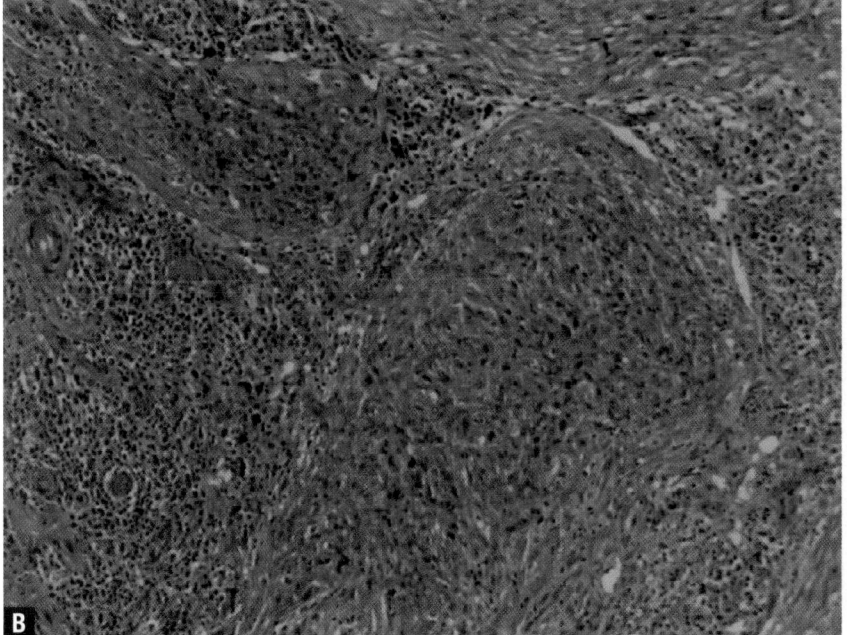

▲ **FIGURE 14-19** **A.** Angiomatoid fibrous histiocytoma (previously angiomatoid MFH) with nodules to sheaths of epithelioid cells and prominent hemorrhage surrounded by a thick fibrous capsule and inflammatory response with lymph follicle formation. **B.** Higher magnification reveals epitheliod nodule demarcated by lymphoctes, plasma cells, and prominent siderophages.

keratin markers, AFX usually is negative. Yet, when performing serial sections, often a reactivity of clusters of cells is detected. Moreover, even complete negativity does not exclude keratogenous differentiation. In contrast to better differentiated squamous cell carcinomas that often are keratin positive/vimentin negative, dedifferentiated variants, including those thought to be AFX, are keratin negative/vimentin positive. The latter immunoprofile is also often observed in the basal layer of solar keratoses. A switch from keratin positive/vimentin negative to an inverse profile is also known to occur in a variety of carcinomas such as thyroid, stomach, colon, and kidney.[52] Finally, while ultrastructural studies mostly fail to detect keratin filaments, rare lesions show tonofilaments and desmosome-like structures.

Differential diagnoses include other dedifferentiated malignancies with AFX pattern such as melanoma, basal cell carcinoma, and leiomyosarcoma. In these instances, at least parts of the lesion usually reveal more characteristic histopathologic features such as epidermal (pagetoid) spread of melanocytes, remnants of basal cell carcinoma with basophilic basaloid cells in peripheral palisading, and with retraction artifacts or less dedifferentiated areas with fascicles of elongated cells with cigar-shaped nuclei and perinuclear vacuolization in leiomyosarcoma. Moreover, nowadays there is a broad panel of markers for melanocytic and myogenic lesions including S100 protein, Melan-A, HMB45, or MITF and desmin, caldesmon, or calponin, respectively. Other differential diagnoses include pseudosarcomatous fibrous histiocytoma and reticulohistiocytoma, which were discussed earlier.

In short, a detailed examination of lesions supposed to be AFX can pro-

reactive and result from the destruction of existing epidermal and folliculosebaceous epithelium, tumor cell necroses, or hemorrhage. In those few lesions in which reactivity of neoplastic cells is prominent, there seems to be correlation with phagocytosis of neoplastic cells.[55]

Another clue for the keratogenous differentiation of these lesions derives from dyskeratotic cells and hints of intercellular bridges. Moreover, a solar keratosis is often contiguous or continuous; serial sec-

tions often revealing a merging of the solar keratosis and the purported AFX. Occasionally, another morphologic expression of squamous cell carcinoma (morbus Bowen, verrucous carcinoma, or squamous cell carcinoma with keratoacanthomatous features) may blend imperceptibly into what is thought to be an AFX.[53]

While immunohistochemistry of some lesions that are histomorphologically indistinguishable from AFX, reveal prominent reactivity for AE1/3 or other

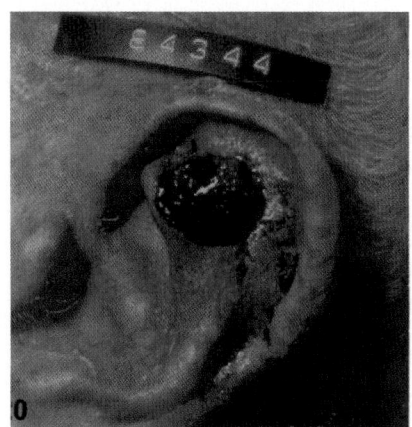

▲ **FIGURE 14-20** Fleshy nodule of AFX. Note hyperkeratosis of nearby helix characteristic of actinic keratosis (squamous cell carcinoma *in situ*).

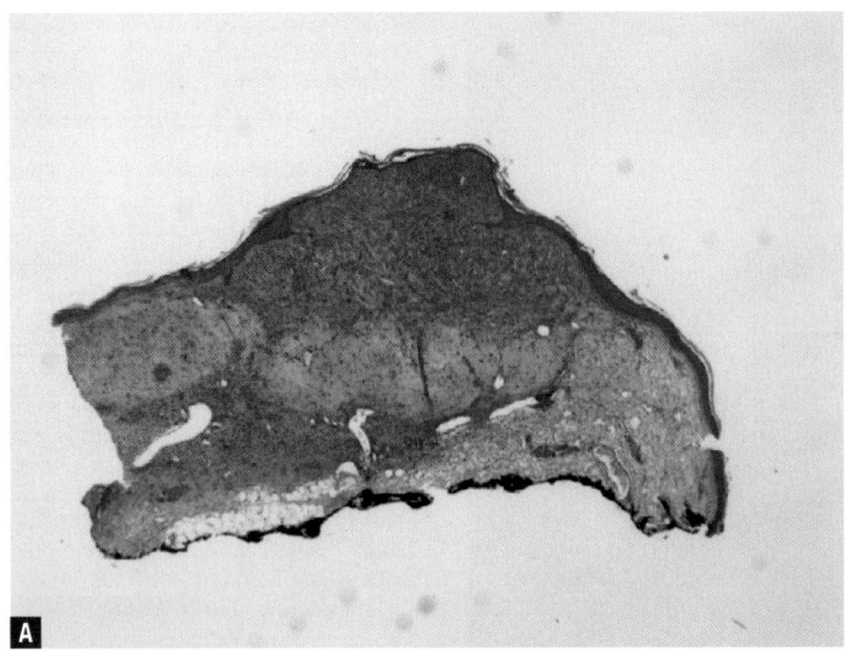

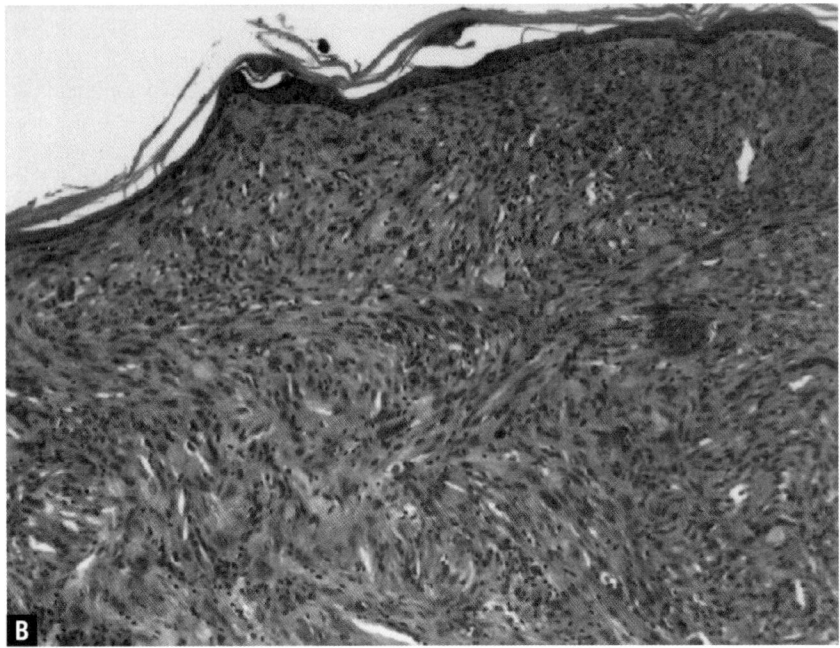

▲ **FIGURE 14-21 A.** Irregular exoendophytic nodule of AFX. Note the thick band of basophilic solar elastosis. **B.** Higher magnification reveals storiform-pleomorphic growth pattern with focal xanthomatization. The majority of these lesions (>95%) are dedifferentiated squamous cell carcinomas.

vide a definitive diagnosis for a vast majority of cases (95%), chief among those being squamous cell carcinoma. For a minority of cases (5%), AFX becomes a diagnosis of exclusion, defying definitive diagnosis by current techniques analogous to the phenomenon of MFH.

Complete excision with free margins of 0.5 cm usually cures AFX. Recurrences may occur in up to 10% of cases, in particular when inadequately excised or with deep subcutaneous extension. Only rare cases have metastasized to regional lymph nodes or into the lung, exceptionally leading to tumor-related death.

FINAL THOUGHTS

The concept of the fibrohistiocyte and the classification of fibrohistiocytic tumors do not stand up well to close inspection including results from modern techniques. A more sophisticated histogenetic approach is currently causing dramatic changes of classification, which hopefully, will contribute to a better general understanding of these previously often enigmatic entities.

ACKNOWLEDGEMENT

The authors are grateful to following colleagues for providing clinical photographs: Hagedorn M, MD (Darmstadt; Fig. 14-1B), Hefel L, MD (Dornbirn, Austria; Fig. 14-8), and Petzlbauer P, MD (Vienna, Austria; Fig. 14-17A). We thank Dr. Parwaresch, Department of Pathology, University of Kiel, Germany, for kindly providing us with the macrophage marker Ki-M1p.

REFERENCES

1. Headington JT. The histiocyte: In memoriam. *Arch Dermatol.* 1986;122:532.
2. Ackerman AB, Chongchitnant N, Sanchez J, Guo Y, Bennin B, Reichel M, Randall MB, eds. *Histologic Diagnosis of Inflammatory Skin Disorders. An Algorithmic Method Based on Pattern Analysis.* 2nd ed. Baltimore, MD: Williams & Wilkins; 1997.
3. LeBoit PE, Burg G, Weedon D, Sarasin A. Pathology and genetics of skin tumours. In: Kleihues P, Sobin L, eds. *World Health Organization (WHO) Classification of Tumours.* Lyon: IARC Press; 2006.
4. Zelger BG, Sidoroff A, Zelger B. Combined dermatofibroma: co-existence of two or more variant patterns in a single lesion. *Histopathology.* 2000;36:529.
5. Fletcher CDM, Unni KK, Mertens F. Pathology and genetics of tumours of soft tissue and bone. In: Kleihues P, Sobin L, eds. *World Health Organization (WHO) Classification of Tumours.* Lyon: IARC Press; 2002.
6. Weedon D, ed. *Skin Pathology.* Edinburgh: Churchill Livingstone; 1997:930.
7. Schaller J, Rohwedder A, Burgdorf WH, et al. Identification of human papilloma virus DNA in cutaneous lesions of Cowden syndrome. *Dermatology.* 2003;207:134.
8. Calonje E, Mentzel Th, Fletcher CDM. Cellular benign fibrous histiocytoma. Clinicopathologic analysis of 74 cases of a distinctive variant of cutaneous fibrous histiocytoma with frequent recurrence. *Am J Surg Pathol.* 1994;18:668.
9. Weiss SW, Goldblum JR, eds. *Enzinger's Soft Tissue tumors.* 4th ed. St. Louis: Mosby; 2001.
10. Nestle FO, Nickoloff BJ, Burg G. Dermatofibroma: an abortive immunoreactive process mediated by dermal dendritic cells? *Dermatology.* 1995;190:265.
11. Zelger B. It's a dermatofibroma, CD34 is irrelevant! *Am J Dermatopathol.* 2002;24:453.
12. Guillou L, Gebhard S, Salmeron M, et al. Metastasizing fibrous histiocytoma of the skin: a clinicopathologic and immunohistochemical analysis of three cases. *Mod Pathol.* 2000;13:654.
13. Vanni R, Fletcher CDM, Sciot R, et al. Cytogenetic evidence of clonality in cutaneous benign fibrous histiocytomas: a report of the CHAMP study group. *Histopathology.* 2000;37:212.
14. Chen TC, Kuo TT, Chan HL. Dermatofibroma is a clonal proliferative disease. *J Cutan Pathol.* 2000;27:36.
15. Hui P, Glusac EJ, Sinard JH, et al. Clonal analysis of cutaneous fibrous histiocytoma (dermatofibroma). *J Cutan Pathol.* 2002;29:385.
16. Mentzel T, Kutzner H, Rütten A, et al. Benign fibrous histiocytoma (dermatofi-

broma) of the face: clinicopathologic and immunohistochemical study of 34 cases associated with an aggressive clinical course. *Am J Dermatopathol.* 2001;23:419.

17. Zelger B, Sidoroff A, Orchard G, et al. Non-Langerhans cell histiocytoses-a new unifying concept. *Am J Dermatopathol.* 1996;18:490.

18. Winkelmann RK. Cutaneous syndromes of Non-X Histiocytosis-a review of the macrophage-histiocyte diseases of the skin. *Arch Dermatol.* 1981;117:667.

19. Lichtenstein L. Histiocytosis X. Integration of eosinophilic granuloma of bone, "Letterer-Siwe Disease", and "Schüller-Christian Disease" as related manifestations of a single nosologic entity. *Arch Pathol.* 1953;56:84.

20. Writing Group of the Histiocyte Society. Histiocytosis syndromes in Children. *Lancet.* 1987;i:208.

21. Arceci RJ, Brenner MK, Pritchard J. Controversies and new approaches to treatment of Langerhans cell histiocytosis. *Hematol Oncol Clin North Am.* 1998;12:339.

22. Tokura Y, Yagi J, O'Malley M, et al. Superantigenic staphylococcal exotoxins induce T-cell proliferation in the presence of Langerhans cells or class II-bearing keratinocytes and stimulate keratinocytes to produce T-cell-activating cytokines. *J Invest Dermatol.* 1994;202:31.

23. Rodriguez-Jurado R, Duran-McKinster C, Ruiz-Maldonado R. Benign cephalic histiocytosis progressing into juvenile xanthogranuloma. A non-Langerhans cell histiocytosis transforming under the influence of a virus? *Am J Dermatopathol.* 2000;22:70.

24. Zelger B, Burgdorf WH. The cutaneous "histiocytoses". *Adv Dermatol.* 2001;17:77.

25. Cline MJ. Histiocytes and histiocytoses. *Blood.* 1994;84:2840.

26. Freyer DR, Kennedy R, Bostrom BC, et al. Juvenile xanthogranuloma. Forms of systemic disease and their clinical implications. *J Pediatr.* 1996;129:227.

27. Rush WL, Andriko JAW, Galateau-Salle F, et al. Pulmonary pathology of Erdheim-Chester disease. *Mod Pathol.* 2000;13:747.

28. Valencia IC, Colsky A, Berman B. Multicentric reticulohistiocytosis associated with breast carcinoma. *J Am Acad Dermatol.* 1998;39:864.

29. Wood GS, Hu C-H, Beckstead JH, et al. The indeterminate cell proliferative disorder: report of a case manifesting as an unusual cutaneous histiocytosis. *J Dermatol Surg Oncol.* 1985;11:1111.

30. Tomaszewski MM, Lupton GP. Unusual expression of S-100 protein in histiocytic neoplasms. *J Cutan Pathol.* 1998;25:129.

31. Ratzinger G, Burgdorf W, Zelger BG, et al. Indeterminate cell histiocytosis: fact or fiction? *J Cutan Pathol.* 2005;32:552.

32. Enzinger FM. Recent developments in the classification of soft tissue sarcomas, in management of primary bone and soft tissue sarcomas. Chicago, IL: Year Book Medical Publishers Inc.; 1977.

33. Fletcher CD. Pleomorphic malignant fibrous histiocytoma: fact or fiction? A critical reappraisal based on 159 tumors diagnosed as pleomorphic sarcoma. *Am J Surg Pathol.* 1992;16:213.

34. Weiss SW. Malignant fibrous histiocytoma. A reaffirmation. *Am J Surg Pathol.* 1982;6:773.

35. Mertens F, Fletcher CD, Dal Cin P, et al. Cytogenetic analysis of 46 pleomorphic soft tissue sarcomas and correlation with morphologic and clinical features: a report of the CHAMP study group. *Genes Chromosomes Cancer.* 1998;22:16.

36. Fletcher CD, Gustafson P, Rydholm A, et al. Clinicopathologic reevaluation of 100 malignant fibrous histiocytomas: prognostic relevance of subclassification. *J Clin Oncol.* 2001;19:3045.

37. Hollowood K, Fletcher CD. Malignant fibrous histiocytoma: morphologic pattern or pathologic entity? *Semin Diagn Pathol.* 1995;12:210.

38. O'Connell JX, Wehrli BM, Nielsen GP, et al. Giant cell tumors of soft tissue: a clinicopathologic study of 18 benign and malignant tumors. *Am J Surg Pathol.* 2000;24:386.

39. Oliveira AM, Dei Tos AP, Fletcher CD, et al. Primary giant cell tumor of soft tissues: a study of 22 cases. *Am J Surg Pathol.* 2000;24:248.

40. Kyriakos M, Kempson RL. Inflammatory fibrous histiocytoma. An aggressive and lethal lesion. *Cancer.* 1976;37:1584.

41. Khalidi HS, Singleton TP, Weiss SW. Inflammatory malignant fibrous histiocytoma: distinction from Hodgkin's disease and non-Hodgkin's lymphoma by a panel of leukocyte markers. *Mod Pathol.* 1997;10:438.

42. Melhem MF, Meisler AI, Saito R, et al. Cytokines in inflammatory malignant fibrous histiocytoma presenting with leukemoid reaction. *Blood.* 1993;82:2038.

43. Weiss SW, Enzinger FM. Myxoid variant of malignant fibrous histiocytoma. *Cancer.* 1977;39:1672.

44. Mentzel T, Calonje E, Wadden C, et al. Myxofibrosarcoma. Clinicopathologic analysis of 75 cases with emphasis on the low-grade variant. *Am J Surg Pathol.* 1996;20:391.

45. Kindblom LG, Merck C, Angervall L. The ultrastructure of myxofibrosarcoma. A study of 11 cases. *Virchows Arch A Pathol Anat Histol.* 1979;381:121.

46. Enzinger FM. Angiomatoid malignant fibrous histiocytoma: a distinct fibrohistiocytic tumor of children and young adults simulating a vascular neoplasm. *Cancer.* 1979;44:2147.

47. Fanburg-Smith JC, Miettinen M. Angiomatoid (malignant) fibrous histiocytoma: a clinicopathologic study of 158 cases and further exploration of the myoid phenotype. *Hum Pathol.* 1999;30:1336.

48. Costa MJ, McGlothlen L, Pierce M, et al. Angiomatoid features in fibrohistiocytic sarcomas. Immunohistochemical, ultrastructural, and clinical distinction from vascular neoplasms. *Arch Pathol Lab Med.* 1995;119:1065.

49. Hasegawa T, Seki K, Ono K, et al. Angiomatoid (malignant) fibrous histiocytoma: a peculiar low-grade tumor showing immunophenotypic heterogeneity and ultrastructural variations. *Pathol Int.* 2000; 50:731.

50. Helwig EB. Atypical fibroxanthoma. Proceedings of the 18th Annual Tumor Seminar of San Antonio Society of Pathologists, *Tex State J Med.* 1963;59:664.

51. Bourne RG. Paradoxical fibrosarcoma of skin (pseudosarcoma): a review of 13 cases. *Med J Aust.* 1963;1:504.

52. Fretzin DF, Helwig EB. Atypical fibroxanthoma of the skin: a clinicopathologic study of 140 cases. *Cancer.* 1973;31:1541.

53. Zelger B, Soyer HP. Between scylla and charybdis: mythology in dermatopathology. *Dermatopath: Pract Concept.* 2000;6: 348.

54. Murali R, Palfreeman S. Clear cell atypical fibroxanthoma—report of a case with review of the literature. *J Cutan Pathol.* 2006;33:343.

55. Smith KJ, Skelton III HG, Morgan AM, et al. Spindle-cell neoplasms coexpression cytokeratin and vimentin (metaplastic squamous cell carcinoma). *J Cutan Pathol.* 1992;19:286.

CHAPTER 15

Sarcomas

Matthew Halpern, M.D.
Elbert Chen, M.D.
Desiree Ratner, M.D.

BOX 15-1 Overview

- Sarcomas are malignant tumors of the soft tissues of the body.
- Liposarcomas appear as nodules or masses arising in the deep soft tissues of the extremities, the retroperitoneum, and the intra-abdominal cavity.
- Subcutaneous liposarcomas generally do not cause distant metastases while tumors of the deep soft tissues are associated with an overall 5-year survival of less than 50%.
- Treatment of liposarcomas is wide local excision.
- Leiomyosarcomas of the skin present as frequently painful, umbilicated or pedunculated nodules on the lower extremities.
- Cutaneous leiomyosarcomas rarely produce distant metastases, while subcutaneous leiomyosarcomas metastasize in 30 to 40% of cases.
- Cutaneous and subcutaneous leiomyosarcomas are treated with wide local excision.
- Dermatofibrosarcoma protuberans is a low-grade, locally aggressive malignant fibrohistiocytic tumor that presents as a slow-growing, asymptomatic plaque on the trunk or proximal extremities.
- Dermatofibrosarcoma protuberans is associated with 11 to 53% local recurrence after conventional wide excision while treatment with Mohs micrographic surgery results in a significantly lower recurrence rate of 2 to 6.6%.
- Epithelioid sarcoma is a rare aggressive tumor that commonly presents as a painless nodule on the distal extremities of young adults.
- Local recurrence of epithelioid sarcoma is common as are distant metastases to scalp and lung.
- Wide local excision combined with radiotherapy is considered standard of care for treatment of epithelioid sarcomas.
- Fibrosarcoma is an uncommon soft tissue tumor of the deep soft tissues or bone that most commonly presents as a slow-growing deep-seated painful nodule in young to middle-aged adults.

Table 15-1

The Five Histologic Subtypes of Liposarcoma According to the World Health Organization are Each Associated with a Given Peak Incidence, Characteristic Cytogenetic Alterations, and Histopathologic Changes

SUBTYPE	PEAK INCIDENCE (YEAR)	CYTOGENETICS	HISTOLOGY
Well differentiated	50–70	12q13–15 ring	Mature adipocytes
Dedifferentiated	50–70	12q13–15 ring	Nonlipogenic areas
Myxoid	30–50	T(12q13;16p11)	Myxoid matrix
Round cell	30–50	T(12q13;16p11)	Uniform round cells
Pleomorphic	50–70	Not characterized	Pleomorphic spindle cells

- The 5-year survival rate for patients with fibrosarcoma is reported to be 39 to 41%, and wide excision is the first line of treatment.

INTRODUCTION

Sarcomas are a group of malignant tumors arising from or differentiating towards the cells that constitute the soft tissues of the body. This includes fibroblasts, adipocytes, myocytes, chondrocytes, osteoblasts, and endothelial cells, which can give rise to a diverse group of neoplasms. This chapter will focus on liposarcoma, leiomyosarcoma, dermatofibrosarcoma protuberans, epithelioid sarcoma and fibrosarcoma, all of which have the potential to involve the skin or subcutaneous tissue. Other sarcomas commonly involving the skin are discussed elsewhere in this text such as malignant fibrous histiocytoma, atypical fibroxanthoma (see Chapter 14), Kaposi's sarcoma and angiosarcoma (see Chapter 20).

LIPOSARCOMA

BOX 15-2 Summary

- Most common soft tissue sarcoma in adults.
- Occur as nodules or masses in the deep soft tissues of the extremities, the retroperitoneum and the intra-abdominal cavity.
- Five distinct histologic subtypes: well differentiated, dedifferentiated, myxoid, round cell and pleomorphic.
- Tumors occurring in the dermis or subcutis may recur locally but generally do not cause distant metastasis or patient mortality.
- Liposarcomas of the deep soft tissue are extremely malignant.
- Wide excision is the first line of treatment for liposarcomas.

Liposarcoma is the most common soft tissue sarcoma in adults, representing approximately 20% of all cases.[1] This heterogeneous group of malignant neoplasms is characterized by a variable degree of adipocytic differentiation, and according to the most recent World Health Organization classification, there are five distinct histologic subtypes: well-differentiated, dedifferentiated, myxoid, round cell and pleomorphic (Table 15-1).[2] An additional spindle cell variant has also been described.[3] Because of the high degree of variability within this category of soft tissue sarcomas, there is significant divergence in the clinical behavior and metastatic potential among the different subtypes.

Pathogenesis

Liposarcomas are thought to arise *de novo* and do not represent dedifferentiation of preexisting lipomas. Unlike other soft tissue sarcomas, ultraviolet radiation does not appear to be involved in the genesis of these tumors.[4] Cytogenetic analysis has been used to further evaluate the morphologic subtypes of liposarcomas. Both well-differentiated and dedifferentiated liposarcomas exhibit ring or free-floating marker chromosomes composed of chromosome 12q13-15 that result in gene amplification.[5–8] Myxoid and round cell liposarcomas feature a reciprocal chromosome translocation at (12q13;16p11) in 75% of cases and it is generally accepted that round cell liposarcomas represent a high-grade variant of the myxoid subtype.[7,8]

Clinical Presentation

Liposarcomas most commonly occur as nodules or masses in the deep soft tissues of the extremities, the retroperitoneum, and the intra-abdominal cavity.

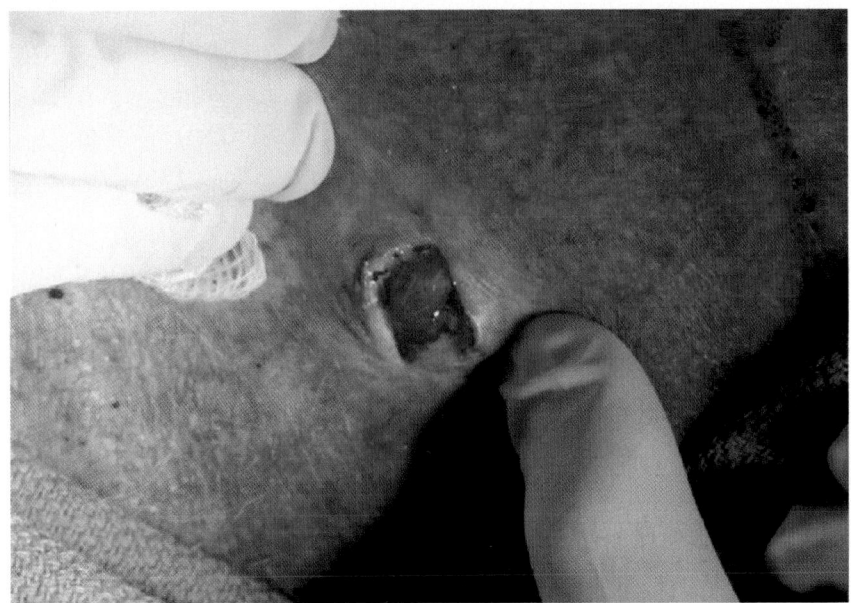

▲ **FIGURE 15-1** The large nodule of the left upper back had been slowly growing for 1 year and was thought clinically to be a lipoma. After the initial incision was made, mucinous yellow-brown adipose tissue was noted, which did not have the usual lobular configuration of normal adipose tissue, and a tentative clinical diagnosis of liposarcoma was made. Histopathologic evaluation of a tissue sample taken from the center of the lesion confirmed the presence of low-grade liposarcoma. The patient was ultimately referred to surgical oncology for evaluation and management.

Less frequent locations include the head and neck, paratesticular regions and the mediastinum.[8] The myxoid and round cell variants have a peak incidence between the third and fifth decades, whereas well-differentiated, dedifferentiated and pleomorphic liposarcomas occur between the fifth and seventh decades.[8] Rare cases occur in children 10 years or older, but are not reported in younger children.[9]

Liposarcoma predominantly arises in the deep soft tissue and its occurrence in the skin and subcutis is extremely rare (Figs. 15-1 and 15-2). A recently reported series suggests that primary cutaneous lesions represent approximately 1% of all cases.[10] In this series, seven cases of purely dermal liposarcoma were identified and described. These tumors all grew in an exophytic manner and presented as small dome-shaped or polypoid lesions. Moreover, although this case series demonstrated an increased incidence of the high-grade pleomorphic subtype of liposarcomas, there were no associated metastases or deaths and only two patients developed local recurrences.[10] Tumors occurring in the dermis or subcutis may demonstrate local recurrence; however, they generally do not cause distant metastasis or patient mortality.[4] Liposarcomas of the deep soft tissues, in contrast, exhibit extremely malignant behavior, and are associated with an overall 5-year survival of less than 50%.[11]

Histopathology

All subtypes of liposarcoma feature the presence of immature fat cells known as lipoblasts which contain well-demarcated cytoplasmic lipid accumulation and hyperchromatic, scalloped nuclei. In well-differentiated liposarcomas there is a variable number of lipoblasts intermixed with mature adipocytes. Myxoid liposarcomas are characterized by the presence of lipoblasts, plexiform capillaries, a myxoid matrix and mucopolysaccharide lakes. Round cell liposarcoma features a proliferation of uniform round cells with atypical, hyperchromatic nuclei intermixed with lipoblasts. Pleomorphic liposarcomas demonstrate pleomorphic spindle cells and variable numbers of lipoblasts. Dedifferentiated liposarcoma consists of areas of well-differentiated liposarcoma mixed with areas of nonlipogenic sarcoma. No specific immunohistochemical marker exists to identify liposarcomas, and the main utility in performing these marker studies is to exclude other malignant spindle cell tumors.[2,12]

Treatment

Wide excision is considered to be first line treatment for liposarcomas in order to prevent recurrence and dedifferentiation. As the majority of lesions will involve deep soft tissues, preoperative CT and MRI scanning may be helpful in defining the underlying extent of tumor. For tumors limited to the skin and subcutis, surgical therapy is considered to be adequate.[4,10] Adjuvant radiation therapy and systemic chemotherapy may be helpful for deeper lesions; however, these modalities remain experimental at this time.[13]

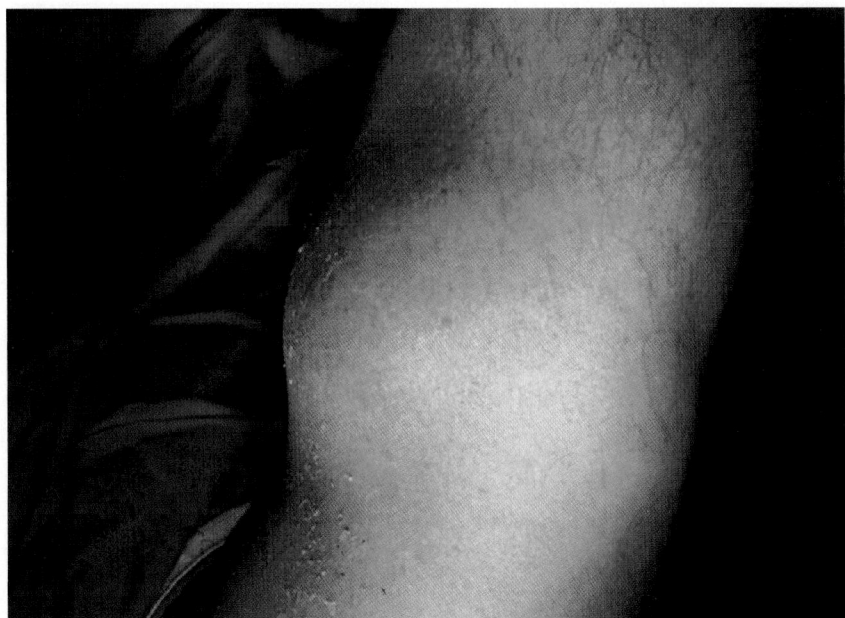

▲ **FIGURE 15-2** High-grade liposarcoma of the right upper arm. This subcutaneous nodule grew rapidly over a period of 3 months.

BOX 15-3   Summary

- Cutaneous and subcutaneous leiomyosarcomas account for 2 to 3% of total superficial sarcomas.
- Predilection for the lower extremities of middle-aged white patients.
- 32% of cutaneous leiomyosarcomas locally recur following excision, but distant metastases are rare.
- Subcutaneous leiomyosarcomas metastasize in 30 to 40% of cases.
- Treatment with wide local excision with 3 to 5 cm margins and deep extension to fascia has the highest reported cure rates.

SKIN CANCER

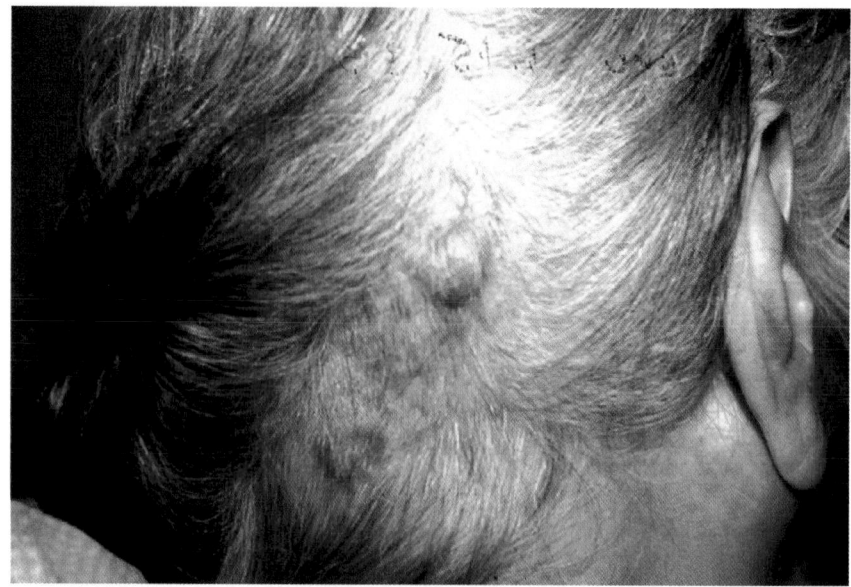

▲ **FIGURE 15-3** Cutaneous metastases of the scalp in a patient with known retroperitoneal leiomyosarcoma. The patient shown here underwent excision of a number of these exquisitely tender lesions from her scalp, trunk, and extremities over a period of 6 months.

Introduction

Leiomyosarcoma accounts for 7 to 10% of all adult soft tissue sarcomas.[11] This malignant tumor is typically divided into three categories based on clinical location. Retroperitoneal and intra-abdominal tumors include uterine and gastrointestinal leiomyosarcomas and are the most common type. Leiomyosarcomas of deep vascular origin represent a separate tumor subtype that is less common. Finally, the superficial variant of leiomyosarcomas accounts for only 2 to 3% of total superficial sarcomas. Superficial leiomyosarcomas are further subdivided into either cutaneous or subcutaneous groups. Although the classification of a given lesion is not always clinically evident because of tumor progression, it has been shown to have significant prognostic implications and thus remains a useful framework (Table 15-2).[14,15]

Pathogenesis

Cutaneous leiomyosarcoma derives from the arrector pili muscles of hair and sweat glands. Subcutaneous leiomyosarcoma is thought to arise from the muscular layer of blood vessels.[16] Case reports and anecdotes suggest a number of potential predisposing factors including trauma, preexisting leiomyomas and exposure to radiation.[17]

Clinical Presentation

Leiomyosarcomas are most common in white patients and the majority of cases occur between the ages of 40 and 60 years. Superficial leiomyosarcomas have a predilection for the lower extremities, with the cutaneous variant occurring most commonly in areas of increased hair follicle density.[14] Pain is usually a prominent symptom although it is not invariably present.[16] Classically, the lesion presents as a solitary, well-circumscribed nodule that may be pedunculated or umbilicated. Cutaneous tumors tend to have a red color and are adherent to the overlying epidermis, while subcutaneous tumors are skin-colored and freely mobile. Cutaneous tumors also tend to be smaller (<2 cm) and slow-growing compared to the subcutaneous variants.[15]

Cutaneous leiomyosarcomas have an excellent prognosis. Although 32% may have local recurrence following excision, distant metastases are rare.[14] Subcutaneous leiomyosarcomas metastasize in 30 to 40% of cases (Figure 15-3).[14,18] The risk of metastasis for both types of superficial leiomyosarcomas appears to be directly related to the size and depth of the primary tumor.[14,15] Metastasis frequently involves the lungs via hematogenous spread followed by invasion of local lymph nodes.[16]

Histopathology

Cutaneous leiomyosarcomas are moderate to well-differentiated spindle cell neoplasms arising in the dermis. In some areas the nuclei are elongated and plump while in other less differentiated regions, nuclei are anaplastic and bizarre with visible mitoses. A fascicular, infiltrative growth pattern reflects the fact that this tumor originates in the arrector pili muscle.[12]

Subcutaneous leiomyosarcomas are usually well-circumscribed, irregular aggregates of atypical smooth muscle cells arising in the subcutaneous fat. A rim of compressed collagen bundles often surrounds the tumor and the fascicular pattern of the cutaneous variant is not seen.[12] Mitoses are easily seen but there seems to be no correlation between the degree of histologic atypia and the occurrence of metastases.[19]

Immunohistochemical staining demonstrates expression of desmin and muscle

Table 15-2

Superficial Leiomyosarcomas are Subdivided into Cutaneous and Subcutaneous Groups which Reflects Their Distinct Cells of Origin, Histology, and Prognosis

SUBTYPE	TISSUE ORIGIN	HISTOLOGY	PROGNOSIS
Cutaneous	Arrector pili	Well-differentiated, dermal spindle cells	32% local recurrence; rare distant metastasis
Subcutaneous	Vascular muscularis	Atypical smooth muscle cells in fat	30–40% distant metastases

specific actin in the large majority of cutaneous leiomyosarcomas and in approximately 50% of subcutaneous leiomyosarcomas.[12,19] Cytokeratin staining may be positive as well.[12,20]

Treatment

The treatment of superficial leiomyosarcoma is wide local excision. Although standardized guidelines do not exist, the most effective results reported excision with 3 to 5 cm margins and deep extension to fascia.[14,15] Inadequate excision appears to be a significant concern, as recurrent tumors tend to be larger and deeper and thus present a higher risk of metastasis and death.[15] Mohs micrographic surgery has been used to treat 15 documented cases of leiomyosarcoma and demonstrates a favorable recurrence rate of 13% compared to that of wide excision (30 to 45%).[21] Radiation therapy and chemotherapy have also been sporadically reported, but appear to be less effective in the treatment of this tumor.[14]

DERMATOFIBROSARCOMA PROTUBERANS

BOX 15-4 Summary

- Low-grade, locally aggressive malignant fibrohistiocytic tumor.
- Commonly presents as a slow-growing, asymptomatic plaque on the trunk or proximal extremities.
- Recurrence after conventional wide excision is estimated at 11 to 53%.
- Small risk of distant metastasis, most commonly to lung, followed by regional lymph nodes, brain, bone and heart.
- Treatment with Mohs micrographic surgery is associated with significantly lower rates of recurrence compared to wide excision.

Introduction

Dermatofibrosarcoma protuberans (DFSP) is a rare, low-grade malignant fibrohistiocytic tumor. It was first described in 1924 by Darier and Ferrand as a progressive and recurring dermatofibroma.[22] This tumor represents approximately 1% of all soft tissue sarcomas and is estimated to occur in 5 to 8 patients per one million persons per year.[23,24]

Pathogenesis

The etiology of DFSP is uncertain and it may be classified as a histiocytic, fibroblastic or neural tumor. Current evidence suggests that the tumor originates from either a fibroblastic or mesenchymal stem cell precursor.[25] Antecedent trauma, thermal burns and surgical scars have all been reported in association with DFSP, although no causal relationship has been established.[26] Greater than 90% of DFSPs have been shown to involve a translocation of chromosomes 17 and 22 that places transcriptional control of the platelet derived growth factor β gene (17q22) under the promoter of the collagen 1α1 gene (22q13).[27] This results in increased production of a COL1A1-PDGFβ fusion protein that is processed to form mature platelet derived growth factor β. This protein exerts its effects through both autocrine and paracrine stimulation of the PDGFβ receptor expressed on the cell surface of DFSP.[28]

Clinical Presentation

DFSPs most commonly occur between the ages of 20 and 50 years, affecting all races equally, and displaying a slight male predominance. The tumors present most frequently on the trunk and proximal extremities and less often on the head and neck and distal extremities. The lesions begin as skin-colored, slow-growing, asymptomatic plaques.[26,29] As they progress they become indurated and develop a brown to violaceous color. With time, DFSPs often become nodular, and generally overlie an ill-defined firm or atrophic plaque (Fig. 15-4A and B).[26]

DFSP tend to be locally aggressive, invading deeper adjacent structures including fat, muscle and bone. Recurrence after conventional wide excision is quite high and estimated at 11 to 53% depending on the extent of the excisional margin taken.[29–31] Local recurrences tend to occur early, with 40% seen within 1 year of excision and 75% within 3 years.[29] The high recurrence rate is likely due to the asymmetric and unpredictable growth pattern of this tumor, which often results in a poor correlation between preoperative tumor size and the extent of final defect after clearance by Mohs micrographic surgery.[32] DFSP carries a small risk of distant metastasis, most commonly to lung, followed by regional lymph nodes, brain, bone and heart.[33–35]

Histopathology

On biopsy, DFSP demonstrates a dermal and often subcutaneous tumor composed of individual spindle cells dispersed between collagen bundles. Minimal nuclear atypia and rare mitotic figures may be seen. As the tumor progresses, the spindle cells assume a characteristic storiform appearance and frequently infiltrate into the underlying subcutaneous tissue in a honeycomb pattern. Involvement of the deeper fascia and muscle may occur in advanced tumors.[12]

There are several histologic variants of DFSP. Myxoid tumors contain a vascular proliferation of characteristic thin-walled vessels. Pigmented DFSP is composed of small numbers of melanin-containing cells and is also referred to as a Bednar tumor. Fibrosarcomatous areas are recognized as having a fascicular pattern of spindle cells and are thought of as a more aggressive variant.[36] Finally, some tumors may demonstrate the presence of giant cells.[12]

Immunohistochemistry can be helpful in confirming the diagnosis of DFSP. Spindle-shaped cells stain positively for anti-CD34 antibody but are negative for anti-Factor XIIIA antibodies. This immunostaining pattern is particularly useful in distinguishing DFSP from cellular dermatofibromas, which are Factor XIIIA positive/CD34 negative.[12]

Treatment

The treatment paradigm for DFSP has shifted in the last several years. Treatment by wide excision down to fascia with 1 to 3 cm margins was once considered to be the treatment of choice. Retrospective studies suggest recurrence rates that range from 11 to 53% depending on the extent of the excisional margin.[33,34] The use of standardized margins assumes a concentric tumor growth pattern. However, it has been demonstrated that DFSP often exhibits a deeply infiltrative and asymmetric growth pattern rendering such standardized excisions potentially inadequate and accounting for the high rates of local recurrence with this technique.[32] Mohs micrographic surgery, which permits histopathologic examination of all peripheral and deep margins of the excisional specimen, is associated with significantly lower recurrence rates ranging from 2 to 6.6%.[32,37] This may be of particular clinical importance given the fact that recurrent lesions appear to have the highest likelihood of dedifferentiation into higher grade sarcomas and subsequent metastatic disease.[33,38–41] Some authors have noted the potential difficulty in distinguishing DFSP from residual scar tissue using frozen sections and advocate the use of an additional stage for permanent sections or rapid immunohistochemical stains, such as

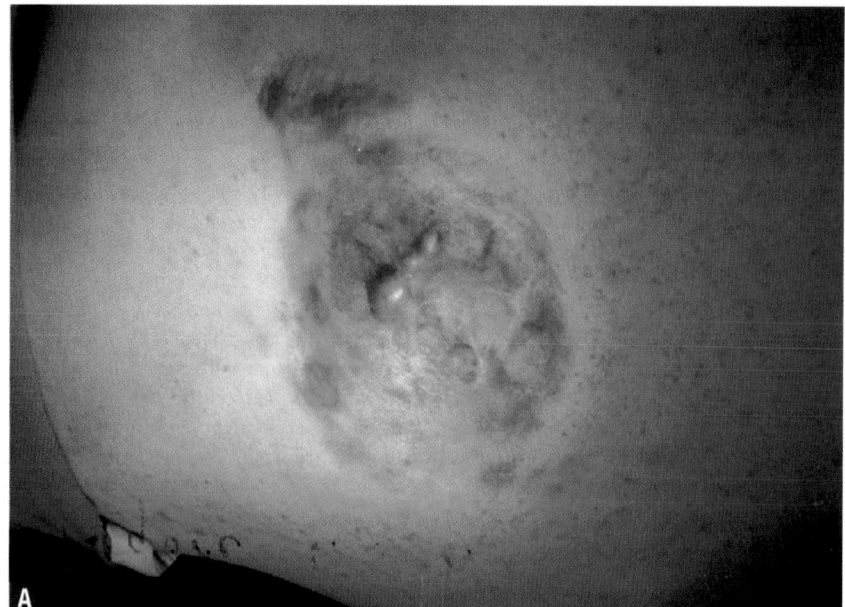

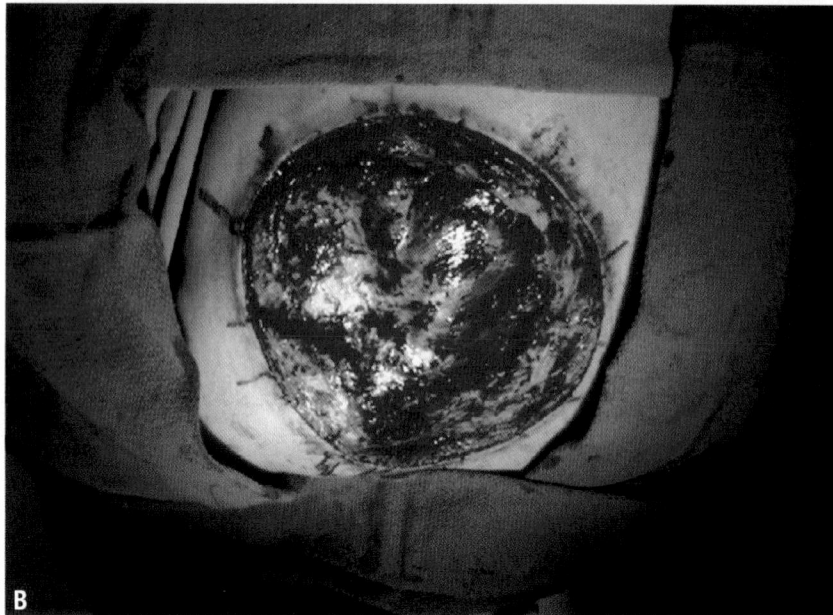

▲ **FIGURE 15-4** **A.** Preoperative view of a 16-year-old boy with a congenital atrophic DFSP of the right upper back, which had been previously diagnosed as a congenital vascular malformation. While the lesion had appeared to grow with him over time, it had become nodular over the preceding several years. Incisional biopsy revealed the true diagnosis. **B.** Post Mohs micrographic surgical defect. The final wound dimensions measured 15.0 cm × 20.8 cm and extended to the level of the muscularis. The patient was subsequently repaired by plastic surgery with a split thickness skin graft and has been free of disease for 18 months.

CD34, in conjunction with traditional Mohs surgery.[42,43] Sondak et al have developed a hybrid procedure that combines standard excision with complete peripheral margin examination and report no instances of recurrence in 45 consecutive DFSP cases treated over 10 years.[44] Several studies have demonstrated that pre or post-operative radiation therapy in conjunction with wide excision is also effective in decreasing the rate of local recurrence relative to treatment with wide excision alone.[45-47] There are also several reports of successful treatment of DFSP using radiation as primary therapy, but this method has not been systematically evaluated in a controlled study.[46,48]

The identification of deregulated expression of the tyrosine kinase receptor agonist PDGF in a high number of tumors (>70%) has generated interest in the potential use of imatinib mesylate (Gleevec) a PDGF tyrosine kinase inhibitor. In the largest case series to date, eight patients with locally advanced DFSP underwent treatment with imatinib mesylate and clinical improvement was observed in 50% of patients. DFSP with fibrosarcomatous histologic differentiation did not appear to be responsive to the treatment.[49] The role that this and other chemotherapies will play in the treatment of DFSP remains to be seen pending the outcome of future investigations.

■ EPITHELIOID SARCOMA

BOX 15-5   Summary

- Rare aggressive soft tissue sarcoma
- Commonly presents as a painless nodule on the distal extremities of young adults
- Local recurrence is common as well as distant metastases to scalp and lung.
- Wide local excision combined with radiotherapy is considered standard of care.

Introduction

Epithelioid sarcoma is a rare tumor first described in 1961 by Laskowski, who originally named this neoplasm sarcoma aponeuroticum to reflect its tendency to grow along fascial planes, tendon sheaths and aponeuroses.[50] It was characterized further by Enziger as a sarcoma which mimics a granuloma or carcinoma.[51]

Pathogenesis

Cytogenetic studies indicate that the most frequent alterations associated with epithelioid sarcoma affect chromosomes 22 and 11.45% of tumors have been shown to contain a mutation in the 150-kb region of chromosome 22q11 containing the SMARCB1/INI1 gene, a tumor suppressor gene frequently inactivated in infantile malignant rhabdoid tumors. Most commonly, this mutation seems to occur in the "proximal" subtype of epithelioid sarcomas that have a more aggressive course. Overall, these results point to *SMARCB1/INI1* gene involvement in the genesis and/or progression of epithelioid sarcomas.[52] Other studies have identified overexpression of the Cyclin D1 gene located on chromosome 11q13 in 96% of epithelioid sarcomas. This positive cell cycle regulator has also been shown to be upregulated in mantle cell lymphomas and breast carcinomas.[53]

Clinical Presentation

Epithelioid sarcomas most commonly occur in young adults with the majority of tumors found between the ages of 20 and 40 years and in males twice as frequently as in females. It typically presents on the distal extremities as a painless tan or white nodule or several grouped nodules that enlarge slowly.[54] The tumor also rarely occurs on the pelvis, perineum and vulva.[55] The recently reported large-cell "proximal-type" variant is characterized by increased aggressiveness, deep location, preferential occurrence in proximal/axial regions of older patients, and rhabdoid features.[56] Superficial lesions tend to be smaller (0.5 to 5 cm) and are frequently ulcerated, while deeper lesions are larger (3 to 6 cm) and are attached to the underlying tendons and fascia. Tumors with nerve involvement may present with pain, paresthesias and muscle atrophy. The tumor is described as having a high propensity for spreading along fascial and neurovascular structures as well as by lymphatics. Local recurrences of epithelioid sarcomas are common as are distant metastases to scalp and lungs.[54]

Histopathology

Biopsy of epithelioid sarcoma reveals a nodular proliferation of spindle-shaped, round, or polygonal cells containing small nuclei with minimal pleomorphism and abundant eosinophilic cytoplasm.[54] The tumor is frequently associated with fascia, periosteum, tendons and nerves.[57] Mitotic figures may be scattered throughout the lesion. A lymphohistiocytic inflammatory infiltrate often surrounds the tumor nodule.[54] Central necrosis of the tumor is seen more frequently in larger tumors. Growth along neurovascular bundles is a common finding. The proximal subtype is characterized by the presence of sheets of large epithelioid cells with rhabdoid inclusions. Central necrosis is not typically seen in this variant.[58]

Immunochemistry is necessary to definitively identify epithelioid sarcomas. Tumor cells stain positively for cytokeratins, EMA, vimentin, CD34, and muscle-specific actin. Staining for S-100, HMB-45, and CD31 is not present.[59]

Prognosis and Treatment

Rates of local recurrence range from 35 to 77%, while rates of distant metastasis range from 40 to 47% respectively.[60–64] A recent retrospective analysis of 37 patients with epitheliod sarcoma reported a median survival of 8 months following the development of distant metastases.[60]

Because of the high rates of local recurrence and distant metastasis seen with this high-grade malignant sarcoma, aggressive therapy is warranted. Wide local excision combined with radiotherapy is considered the standard of care, and recurrence rates following this treatment regimen compare favorably with those achieved by radical surgery including amputation.[61]

FIBROSARCOMA

BOX 15-6   Summary

- Uncommon soft tissue sarcoma originating from the deep soft tissues or bone.
- Most commonly presents as a slow-growing deep-seated painful nodule in young to middle-aged adults.
- 5-year survival rate reported to be 39 to 41%.
- Wide excision is the first line of treatment.

Introduction

Fibrosarcoma is a neoplasm most likely derived from a multipotential primitive mesenchymal cell, which differentiates into a fibroblastic cell.[65] It occurs as either a tumor of the deep soft tissues or bone. There is considerable debate about the exact nature of this sarcoma variant and its relationship to other malignant neoplasms of bone and soft tissue, such as malignant fibrous histiocytoma and monophasic synovial sarcoma, dating back to the original description of fibrosarcoma in the 1940s.[66,67]

Pathogenesis

Fibrosarcoma has been reported in association with previous radiation therapy as well as in scars from thermal burns.[68] Patients with neurofibromatosis are believed to have a 10% lifetime risk of developing either fibrosarcoma or neurosarcoma.[69] Fibrosarcoma has also been reported in patients following metallic implants used for fracture fixation as well as in patients with preexisting bone disease such as Paget's disease, chronic osteomyelitis and fibrous dysplasia.[70,71]

Clinical Presentation

Fibrosarcoma most commonly presents as a slow-growing deep-seated painful nodule in young to middle-aged adults. Congenital or infantile fibrosarcomas have been reported but appear to be extremely rare and follow a less aggressive course. The lower extremities, upper extremities, trunk, head and neck are the most frequent sites of the tumor.[72,73] Fibrosarcoma originates in the deep soft tissue or bone and involvement of the overlying subcutis and skin is secondary to tumor extension. Patients with soft tissue tumors may present for treatment later than patients with tumors of bone because pain is a relatively late symptom. High-grade variants can metastasize to the lungs and less commonly to bone via hematogenous spread.[73]

HISTOPATHOLOGY Fibrosarcoma consists of a proliferation of relatively uniform spindle cells intermixed with collagen fibers in a herringbone pattern. Mitoses are usually easily identifiable and focal myxomatous change may be present. More aggressive tumors may demonstrate a higher degree of nuclear atypia, increased mitoses, necrosis, and loss of the typical herringbone pattern.[73] Several variants have been identified including sclerosing epithelioid fibrosarcoma, low-grade myxofibrosarcomas and fibromyxoid sarcomas.[72,74] Immunohistochemistry shows positive staining for vimentin and muscle specific actin.[4]

Prognosis and Treatment

The 5-year survival rate for patients with fibrosarcoma is reported to be 39 to 41%.[72,75] Local recurrence occurs in 23% of patients at 1 year, 37% at 2 years and 42% at 5 years. Distant metastases occur in 34% of patients at 1 year, 52% at 2 years and 63% at 5 years.[73]

Wide excision is the first line of treatment for fibrosarcoma. Inadequate surgical margins are associated with a significantly increased rate of local recurrence (79% at 5 years) as well as decreased 5-year survival rate (29%).[73] Several studies have reported that increased survival may be possible when surgical resection is combined with adjuvant radiation or systemic chemotherapy.[76,77]

FINAL THOUGHTS

In conclusion, sarcomas are a diverse group of malignant neoplasms. Clinical presentation, treatment and prognosis vary greatly among the various subtypes. A multidisciplinary approach involving dermatology, oncology, surgical oncology and radiation oncology is ideal for evaluating the patient who presents with a soft tissue sarcoma and for devising the appropriate treatment course.

REFERENCES

1. Mack, TM. Sarcomas and other malignancies of the soft tissue, retroperitoneum, peritoneum, pleura, heart, mediastinum, and spleen. *Cancer.* 1995; 75(suppl):211–244.

2. Weiss, SW. *WHO Histological Typing of Soft Tissue Tumors.* 2nd ed. Berlin: Springer-Verlag; 1994.

3. Dei Tos AP, Mentzel T, Newman PL Fletcher CDM. Spindle cell liposarcoma: a hitherto unrecognized variant of well-differentiated liposarcoma. Analysis of six cases. *Am J Surg Pathol.* 1994;18:913–921.

4. Bolognia JL, Jorizzo JL, Rapini RP. *Dermatology.* New York: Mosby; 2003: 1863–1897.

5. Fletcher CD, Akerman M, Dal Cin P et al. Correlation between clinicopathological features and karyotype in lipomatous tumors. A report of 178 cases from the CHAMP Collaborative Study Group. *Am J Pathol.* 1996;148:623–630.

6. Dal Cin P, Kools P, Sciot R, et al. Cytogenetic and fluorescence *in situ* hybridization investigation of ring chromosomes characterizing a specific pathologic subgroup of adipose tissue tumors. *Cancer Genet Cytogenet.* 1993;68:85–90.

7. Sreekantaiah C, Karakousis CP, Leonig SP, et al. Cytogenetic findings in liposarcoma correlate with histopathologic subtypes. *Cancer.* 1992;69:2484–2495.

8. Mentzel T. Cutaneous lipomatous neoplasms. *Sem Diag Path.* 2001;18(4): 250–257.

9. Shmookler BM, Enzinger FM. Liposarcoma occurring in children: an analysis of 17 cases and review of the literature. *Cancer.* 1983;52:567.

10. Dei Tos AP, Primary liposarcoma of the skin: a rare neoplasm with unusual high grade features. *Am J Dermatopath.* 1998; 20(4):332–338.

11. Weiss SW, Goldblum JR. *Enzinger and Weiss's Soft Tissue Tumors.* 4th ed. Philadelphia: Mosby-Harcourt; 2001.

12. Elder D, Elenitsas R, Jaworsky C, Johnson B Jr. *Lever's Histopathology of the Skin.* New York: Lippincott, Williams & Wilkins; 1997.

13. Jones RL, Fisher C, Al-Muderis O, Judson IR. *Eur J Cancer.* November 2005.

14. Fields JP, Helwig EB. Leiomyosarcoma of the skin and subcutaneous tissue. *Cancer.* 1981;47:156–169.

15. Bernstein SC, Roenigk RK. Leiomyosarcoma of the skin. *Dermatol Surg.* 1996;22: 631–635.

16. Spencer JM, Amonette RA. Tumors with smooth muscle differentiation. *Derm Surg.* 1996;22:761–768.

17. Davidson LL, Frost ML, Hanke CW, Epinette WW. Primary leiomyosarcoma of the skin. Case report and review of the literature. *J Am Acad Dermatol.* 1989;21: 1156–1160.

18. Dahl I, Angervall L. Cutaneous and subcutaneous leiomyosarcoma. A clinicopathologic study of 47 patients. *Pathol Eur.* 1974;9:307–315.

19. Hashimoto, H, Daimaru Y, Tsuneyoshi M, Enjoji M. Leiomyosarcoma of the external soft tissue. *Cancer.* 1986;57: 2077.

20. Lundgren L, Kindblom LG, Seidal T, Angervall L. Intermediate and fine cytofilaments in cutaneous and subcutaneous leiomyosarcomas. *APMIS.* 1991; 99:820.

21. Humphreys TR, Finkelstein MD, Lee JB. Superficial leiomyosarcoma treated with mohs micrographic surgery. *Dermatol Surg.* 2004;30:108–112.

22. Darier J, Ferrand M. Dermatofibromas progressifs et recidivants ou fibrosarcomes de la peau. *Ann Dermatol Syph.* 1924;5:545.

23. Bendix-Hansen K, Myhre-Jensen O, Kaae S. Dermatofibrosarcoma protuberans. A clinico-pathological study of nineteen cases and review of world literature. *Scand J Plast Reconstr Surg.* 1983;17:247–252.

24. Chuang TY, Su WP, Muller SA. Incidence of cutaneous T cell lymphoma and other rare skin cancers in a defined population. *J Am Acad Dermatol.* 1990;23:254–256.

25. Fletcher CD, Evan BJ, MacArtney JC, et al. Dermatofibrosarcoma protuberans: a clinicopathological and immunohistochemical study with a review of the literature. *Histopathology.* 1985;9:921–938.

26. Fish FS. Soft tissue sarcomas in dermatology. *Dermatol Surg.* 1996;22:268–273.

27. Sandberg AA, Bridge JA. Updates on the cytogenetics and molecular genetics of bone and soft tissue tumor: Dermatofibrosarcoma protuberans and giant cell fibroblastoma. *Cancer Genet Cytogenet.* 2003;140:1–12.

28. Maki RG, Awan RA, Dixon RH, Jhanwar S, Antonescu CR. Differential sensitivity to imatinib of 2 patients with metastatic sarcoma arising from dermatofibrosarcoma protuberans. *Int J Cancer.* 2002; 100(6):623–626.

29. Taylor HB, Helwig EB. Dermatofibrosarcoma protuberans: a study of 115 cases. *Cancer.* 1962;15:717.

30. Hajdu SI. *Pathology of Soft Tissue Tumors.* Philadelphia: Lea and Febiger; 1979; 60–83.

31. Roses DF, Valensi Q, LaTrenta G, et al. Surgical treatment of dermatofibrosarcoma protuberans. *Surg Gynecol Obstet.* 1986;162:449–452.

32. Ratner D, Thomas CO, Johnson TM, et al. Mohs micrographis surgery for the treatment of dermatofibrosarcoma protuberans, results of a multiinstitutional series with an analysis of the extent of microscopic spread. *J Am Acad Dermatol.* 1997;37:600–613.

33. McPeak CJ, Cruz T, Nicastri AD. Dermatofibrosarcoma protuberans: an analysis of 86 cases—five with metastasis. *Ann Surg.* 1967;166:803–816.

34. Pack GT, Tabah EF. Dermatofibrosarcoma protuberans: a report of thirty-nine cases. *Arch Surg.* 1951;62:391–411.

35. Rutgers EJ, Kroon BBR, Albus-Lutter CE, Gortzak E. Dermatofibrosarcoma protuberans: treatment and prognosis. *Eur J Surg Oncol.* 1992;18:241–248.

36. Bowne WB, Antonescu CR, Leung DH, et al. Dermatofibrosarcoma protuberans. A clinicopathologic analysis of patients treated and followed at a single institution. *Cancer.* 2000;88:2711–2720.

37. Gloster HM, Harris KR, Roenigk RK. A comparison between Mohs micrographic surgery and wide surgical excision for the treatment of dermatofibrosarcoma protuberans. *J Am Acad Dermatol.* 1996; 35:82–87.

38. Adams JT, Saltzstein SL. Metastasizing dermatofibrosarcoma protuberans. *Ann Surg.* 1963;29:878–886.

39. Bonnabeau RC Jr, Soughton WB, Armanious AW, Cuono CV, Mossburg WL, Lancaster JR. Dermatofibrosarcoma protuberans: report of a case with pulmonary metastasis and multiple intrathoracic recurrences. *Oncology.* 1974;29:1–12.

40. Kahn LB, Saxe N, Gordon W. Dermatofibrosarcoma protuberans with lymph node and pulmonary metastases. *Arch Dermatol.* 1978;114:599–601.

41. Barnes L, Coleman JA Jr, Johnson JT. Dermatofibrosarcoma protuberans of the head and neck. *Arch Otolaryngol.* 1984; 110;398–404.

42. Rowsell AR, Poole MD, Godfrey AM. Dermatofibrosarcoma protuberans: the problems of surgical management. *Br J Plast Surg.* 1986;39:262–264.

43. Jiminez FN, Frichnikik JM, Buchana MD, Clark RE. Immunohistochemical margin control applied to Mohs micrographic surgical excision of dermatofibrosarcoma protuberans. *J Dermatol Surg Oncol.* 1994;20:687–689.

44. Sondak VK, Cimmino VM, Lowe LM, Dubay DA, Johnson TM. Dermatofibrosarcoma protuberans: what is the best surgical approach? *Surg Oncol.* 1999;8:183–189.

45. Dagan R, Morris CG, Zlotecki RA, Scarborough MT, Mendenhall WM. Radiotherapy in the treatment of dermatofibrosarcoma protuberans. *Am J Clin Oncol.* 2005;28(6):537–539.

46. Suit H, Spiro I, Mankin HJ, et al. Radiation in management of patients with dermatofibrosarcoma protuberans. *J Clin Oncol.* 1996;14:2365–2369.

47. Sun LM, Wang CJ, Huang CC, et al. Dermatofibrosarcoma protuberans: treatment results of 35 cases. *Radiother Oncol.* 2000;57:175–181.

48. Marks LB, Suit HD, Rosenberg AE, Wood WC. Dermatofibrosarcoma protuberans treated with radiation therapy. *Int J Radiat Oncol Biol Phys.* August 1989;17(2): 379–384.

49. McArthur GA, Demetri GD, van Oosterom A, et al. Molecular and clinical analysis of locally advanced dermatofibrosarcoma protuberans treated with imatinib: imatinib target exploration consortium study B2225. *J Clin Oncol.* 2005;23:866–873.

50. Laskowski J. Sarcoma aponeuroticum. *Nowotory.* 1961;11:61–67.

51. Enziger FM. Epithelioid sarcoma: a sarcoma simulating a granuloma or carcinoma. *Cancer.* 1970;26:1029–1041.

52. Modena P, Lualdi E, Facchinetti F, et al. SMARCB1/INI1 tumor suppressor gene is frequently inactivated in epithelioid sarcomas. *Cancer Res.* 2005;65:4012–4019.

53. Lin L, Hicks D, Xu B, et al. Expression profile and molecular genetic regulation of cyclin D1 expression in epithelioid sarcoma. *Mod. Pathol.* 1005;18:705–709.

54. Chase DR, Enzinger FM. Epithelioid sarcoma. Diagnosis, prognostic indicators, and treatment. *Am J Surg Pathol.* 1985;9: 241–263.

55. Zevallos-Giampietri EA, Abarrionuevo C. Proximal-type epithelioid sarcoma: report of two cases in the perineum: differential diagnosis and review of soft tissue tumor with epithelioid and/or rhabdoid features. *Appl. Immunohistochem. Mol. Morphol.* September 2005;13(3): 221–230.

56. Guillou L, Wadden C, Coindre JM, Krausz T, Fletcher CD. "Proximal-type" epithelioid sarcoma, a distinctive aggressive neoplasm showing rhabdoid features. Clinicopathologic, immunohistochemical, and ultrastructural study of a series. *Am. J. Surg. Pathol.* February 1997; 21(2):130–146.

57. Evans HL, Baer SC. Epithelioid Sarcoma: a clinicopathologic and prognostic study of 26 cases. *Sem Diag Pathol.* 1993;10(4): 286–291.

58. Hasegawa T, Matsuno Y, Shimoda T, Umeda T, Yokoyama R, Hirohashi S. Proximal-type epithelioid sarcoma: a clinicopathologic study of 20 cases. *Mod Pathol.* July 2001;14(7):655–663.

59. Humble SD, Prieto VG, Horenstein MG. Cytokeratin 7 and 20 expression in epithelioid sarcoma. *J Cutan Pathol.* April 2003;30(4):242–246.

60. Spillane AJ, Thomas JM, Fisher C. Epithelioid sarcoma: the clinicopathological complexities of this rare soft tissue sarcoma. *Ann. Surg. Oncol.* April 2000;7(3): 218–225.

61. Callister MD, Ballo MT, Pisters PWT, et al. Epithelioid sarcoma: results of conservative surgery and radiotherapy. *Int J of Rad Onc Biol Phys.* 2001;51(2):384–391.

62. Halling AC, Wollan PC, Pritchard DJ. Epithelioid sarcoma: a clinicopathologic review of 55 cases. *Mayo Clin Proc.* 1996; 71:636–642.

63. Ross HM, Lewis JJ, Woodruff JM. Epithelioid sarcoma: clinical behavior and prognostic factors of survival. *Ann Surg Oncol.* 1997;4:491–495.

64. Steinberg BD, Gelberman RH, Mankin HJ. Epithelioid sarcoma in the upper extremity. *J Bone Joint Surg.* 1992;74:28–35.

65. Antonescu CR, Erlandson RA, Huvos AG. Primary fibrosarcoma and malignant fibrous histiocytoma of bone—a comparative ultrastructural study: evidence of a spectrum of fibroblastic differentiation. *Ultrastruct Pathol.* 2000;24:83–91.

66. Hajdu SI. Fibrosarcoma. A historic commentary. *Cancer.* 1998;82:2081–2089.

67. Scott SM, Reiman HM, Pritchard DJ, Ilstrup DM. Soft tissue fibrosarcoma. A clinicopathologic study of 132 cases. *Cancer.* 1989;64:925–931.

68. Wilkund TA, Blomquist CP, Raty J. Postirradiation sarcoma. Analysis of a nationwide cancer registry material. *Cancer.* 1991;68:524–531.

69. Menon AG, Anderson KM, Riccardi VM, et al. Chromosome 17p deletions and p53 gene mutations associated with the formation of malignant neurofibrosarcomas in von Recklinghausen neurofibromatosis. *Proc Natl Acad Sci USA.* July 1990;87(14):5435–5439.

70. Hadjipavlou A, Zucker J. *Sarcoma in Paget's Disease of Bone. Current Concepts of Diagnosis and Treatment of Bone and Soft Tissue Tumors.* Berlin: Springer-Verlag; 1984:383–394.

71. Hinarejos P, Escuder MC, Monllau JC, et al. Fibrosarcoma at the site of a metallic fixation of the tibia—a case report and literature review. *Acta Orthop Scand.* June 2000; 71(3):329–332.

72. Meis-Kindblom JM, Kindblom LG, Enzinger FM. Sclerosing epithelioid fibrosarcoma. A variant of fibrosarcoma simulating carcinoma. *Am J Surg Pathol,* 1995;19(9):979–993.

73. Scott SM, Reiman HM, Pritchard DJ, Ilstrup DM. Soft tissue fibrosarcoma: a clinicopathologic study of 132 cases. *Cancer.* 1989;64:925–931.

74. Antonescu CR, Baren A. Spectrum of low-grade fibrosarcomas: a comparative ultrastructural analysis of low-grade myxofibrosarcoma and fibromyxoid sarcoma. *Ultrastruct Pathol.* 2004;28:321–332.

75. Pritchard DJ, Soule EH, Taylor WF, Ivins JC. Fibrosarcoma: a clinicopathologic and statistical study of 199 tumors of the soft tissue of the extremities and trunk. *Cancer.* 1974;33:888–897.

76. Eilber FN, Morton DL, Eckhardt J, Grant T, Weisenburger T. Limb salvage for skeletal and soft tissue sarcomas: multidisciplinary preoperative therapy. *Cancer.* 1984;53:2579–2584.

77. Karakousis CP, Emrich LG, Rao U, Krishnamsetty RM. Feasibility of limb salvage and survival in soft tissue sarcomas. *Cancer.* 1986;57:484–491.

CHAPTER 16

Sweat Gland Tumors

Darius Mehregan, M.D.
David Mehregan, M.D.
Viktor Goncharuk, M.D.

BOX 16-1   Overview

- **BENIGN NEOPLASM (TREATMENT WITH EXCISIONAL BIOPSY)**
  - Hidrocystoma
  - Syringocystadenoma Papilliferum
  - Hidradenoma Papilliferum
  - Erosive adenomatosis of the nipple
  - Tubular Apocrine Adenoma
  - Cylindroma
  - Eccrine Spiradenoma
  - Eccrine Poroma
  - Eccrine Syringofibroadenoma
  - Hidroacanthoma Simplex
  - Papillary Eccrine Adenoma
  - Syringoma
  - Chondroid Syringoma
  - Clear Cell Hidradenoma
  - Aggressive Digital Papillary Adenoma
- **MALIGNANT NEOPLASM (TREATMENT WITH COMPLETE EXCISION OR Mohs)**
  - Syringocystadenocarcinoma
  - Cylindrocarcinoma
  - Malignant Spiradenoma
  - Eccrine Porocarcinoma
  - Malignant Hidroacanthoma
  - Malignant Hidradenoma
  - Digital Papillary Adenocarcinoma
  - Syringoid Eccrine Carcinoma
  - Microcystic Adnexal Carcinoma
  - Mucinous Carcinoma
  - Adenocystic Carcinoma
  - Apocrine Carcinoma
  - Adnexal Carcinoma

INTRODUCTION

Sweat gland tumors have been historically divided into those with eccrine and apocrine features. Most of these tumors are named based on their degree of resemblance to normal constituents of the eccrine and apocrine glands and ducts. It is helpful to organize these tumors by degree of differentiation toward eccrine or apocrine sweat glands rather than stating categorically that a tumor arose from a specific part of the sweat gland.[1] The morphologic similarities between the intradermal portions of the eccrine and apocrine duct lead to difficulties in segregating tumors with ductal differentiation into definite categories of "apocrine" and "eccrine" tumors. Markers of apocrine differentiation include histologic identification of columnar cells with decapitation secretion, and identification of lysozymal enzymes including acid phosphatase and B-glucuronidase.[2] A definite immunohistochemical marker of eccrine or apocrine differentiation does not currently exist.

The eccrine and apocrine neoplasms are primarily intradermal neoplasms. For this reason, punch biopsy or excisional biopsy is recommended. The differential diagnosis may include a primary adnexal carcinoma or metastatic adenocarcinoma. In these cases, architectural features are of paramount importance and may only be observed in an adequate biopsy specimen. In cases of benign adnexal neoplasms with an adequate biopsy that samples the entire lesion, further surgery or therapy may not be necessary.

EPIDEMIOLOGY

Tumors with eccrine and apocrine sweat gland differentiation are relatively unusual. Benign tumors of the sweat glands, although uncommon, may be seen in clinical practice. In a review of over 100,000 cases from a private dermatopathology laboratory, eccrine poroma, syringoma, and hidrocystoma represented three of the more common glandular tumors representing approximately 0.04% of all specimens received. Eccrine spiradenoma, syringocystadenoma papilliferum, hidradenoma, and cylindroma represent less common benign sweat gland tumors, making up less than 0.1% of all specimens received. Malignant neoplasms with eccrine and apocrine differentiation are relatively rare and represent approximately two to three specimens per 100,000 received. Although relatively rare, it is important to recognize the benign sweat gland tumors to avoid confusion with basal cell carcinoma and squamous cell carcinoma and subsequent aggressive surgical therapy. In addition, many of the malignant sweat gland tumors may show more aggressive clinical behavior including metastases and death. For this reason, it is important to differentiate these from basal cell carcinoma and squamous cell carcinoma to allow for appropriate treatment and follow-up.

MALIGNANT TRANSFORMATION OF BENIGN SWEAT GLAND TUMORS

Malignant transformation of benign eccrine, apocrine, and follicular neoplasms although rare has been described.[3,4] These lesions typically show histologic transition from typical benign adnexal tumors to areas of malignant degeneration. The malignant portions show some loss of the characteristic histologic pattern of the underlying primary lesion.[4] In these areas, an invasive growth pattern and/or areas of squamous differentiation may be seen.[5,6] Benign adnexal neoplasms are marked by lack of cellular pleomorphism and mitotic activity and in these areas of malignant degeneration, irregularly shaped and hyperchromatic nuclei with increased numbers of mitotic figures may be observed.[6]

HIDROCYSTOMA

BOX 16-2   Summary

- Flesh-colored to bluish papule on the head and neck
- Cystic space lined by apocrine or eccrine epithelium
- Cyst wall made up of two layers of cells

The hidrocystoma may present as a flesh-colored, translucent or bluish papule primarily on the head and neck (Fig. 16-1). Lesions are common around the eyes, primarily found in adult patients and found equally in men and women. Clinically, the lesions may be mistaken for a pigmented basal cell carcinoma or melanocytic neoplasm.[7] Hidrocystomas may show either apocrine or eccrine differentiation. Histologically, single or multiple cystic spaces are present within the dermis. The cystic spaces are lined by either apocrine-type or eccrine-type epithelium (Fig. 16-2). In the eccrine hidrocystoma, the cyst lining consists of a cuboidal layer of glandular cells and a peripheral flattened layer of myoepithelial cells surrounded by a thin fibrous stroma. Squamous metaplasia may occur. The cytokeratin pattern in these tumors is similar to the dermal eccrine duct.[8] In the apocrine hidrocystoma, an inner layer of high columnar cells may be seen with an outer layer of elongated myoepithelial

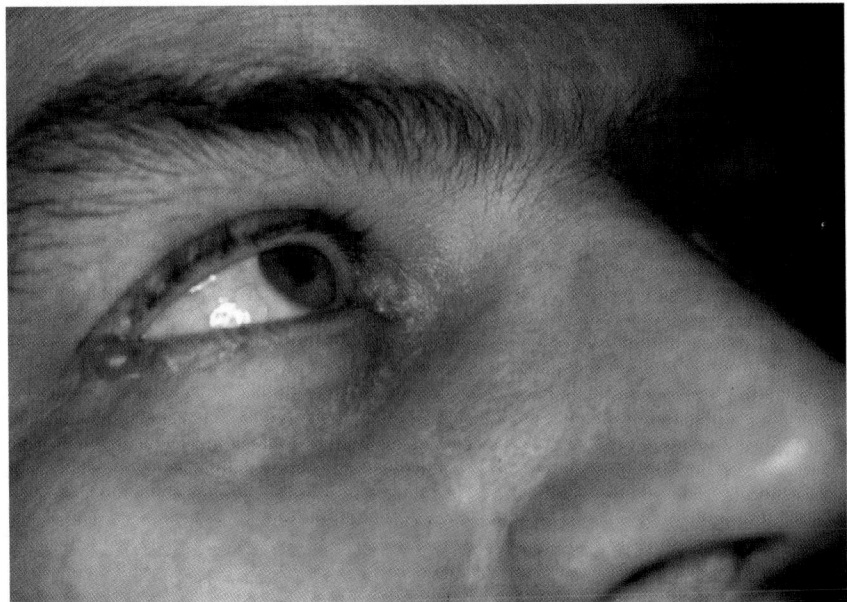

▲ **FIGURE 16-1** Hidrocystoma presenting as a clear to bluish papule on the face, commonly around the eyes. (Courtesy of Dr. James Ulery.)

cells. The columnar cells may show areas of decapitation secretion into the central cystic space. The cystic space contains amorphous secretory material. Papilliferous projections of columnar epithelial cyst lining into the central cyst cavity may be observed.[9] In pigmented variants, melanin may be seen in the epithelial lining cells.[10]

Surgical excision is curative. However, some patients may present with multiple lesions in which surgical excision may be either disfiguring or impractical. Other treatment modalities which have been described include ablation with trichloracetic acid and inhibition of secretion by either injection of botulinum toxin or application of topical atropine.[11–13] Ablation by CO_2, pulsed dye, 1450 nm diode and argon lasers have also been described.[14–17]

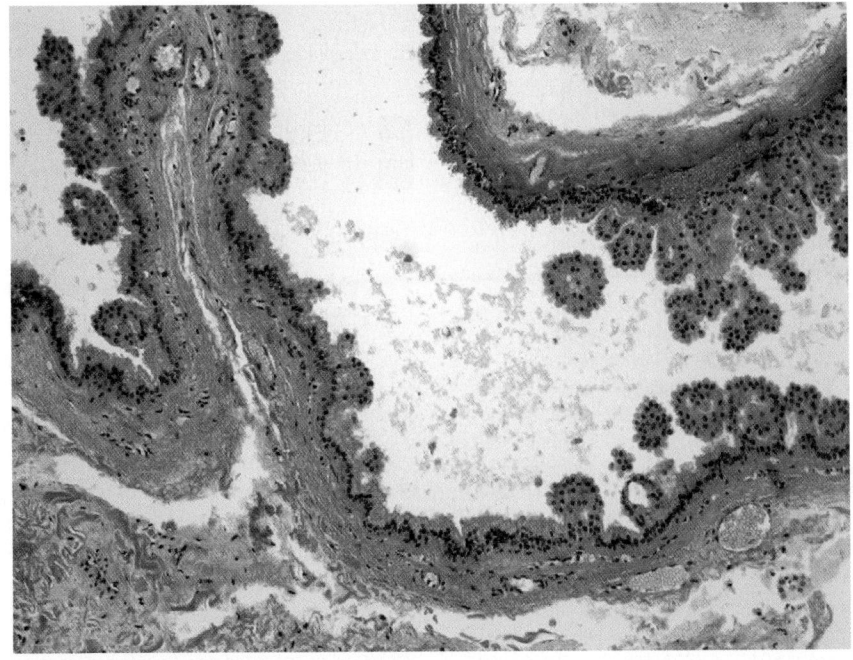

▲ **FIGURE 16-2** Hidrocystoma showing a large cystic space lined by two layers of glandular epithelium.

SYRINGOCYSTADENOMA PAPILLIFERUM

BOX 16-3   Summary

- Verrucous or papillomatous nodule or plaque, most commonly on the head and neck
- Often associated with nevus sebaceus of Jadassohn (organioid nevus)
- Multiple cystic invaginations and papillary projections in the dermis lined by columnar epithelium with decapitation secretion
- Plasma cells in the stroma
- Treatment is by surgical excision

The syringocystadenoma papilliferum may occur as a primary neoplasm or on the background of a preexisting nevus sebaceus of Jadassohn (organoid nevus) (Fig. 16-3).[18] Lesions are found most commonly on the scalp, but may be found elsewhere on the head and neck and less commonly on the trunk.[19] They may present clinically as a verrucous or papillomatous nodule or plaque, often with a central discharge. The lesions form a well-circumscribed tumor extending from the epidermis into the mid-to-deep dermis. There are one or multiple cystic invaginations from the epidermis into the dermis. At the point of invagination, the epithelial lining consists of stratified keratinizing epithelium, which shows transformation into high columnar epithelium with an inner layer of luminal cells resting on a basal layer of flattened myoepithelial cells. The luminal cells may show focal decapitation secretion. These papillary projections extend into the dermis and are surrounded by a fibrovascular stroma containing a large number of plasma cells. The well-circumscribed nature of the neoplasm, lack of nuclear pleomorphism, lack of mitotic activity and connection to the overlying epidermis helps differentiate this from a metastatic carcinoma. The presence of a plasma cell rich stroma differentiates this tumor from other glandular tumors with apocrine differentiation, including hidradenoma papilliferum and erosive adenomatosis of the nipple. Tumors with evidence of apocrine and eccrine differentiation have been described.[20]

Surgical excision is curative. Ablation by CO_2 laser has also been described for lesions not amenable to excision.[21]

Syringocystadenocarcinoma has been described as a rare malignant variant.[22] These may arise *de novo* or in

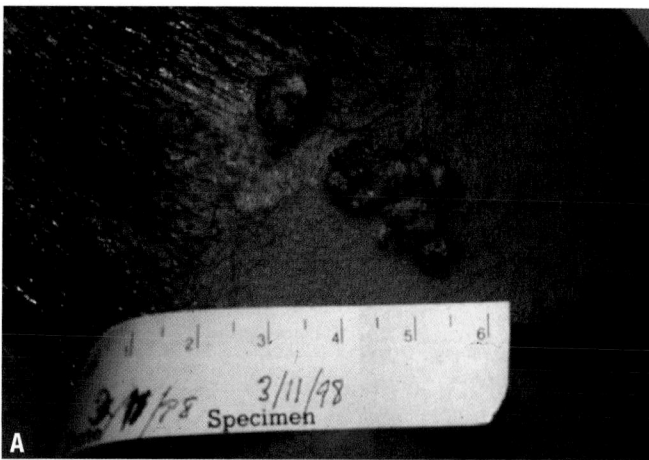

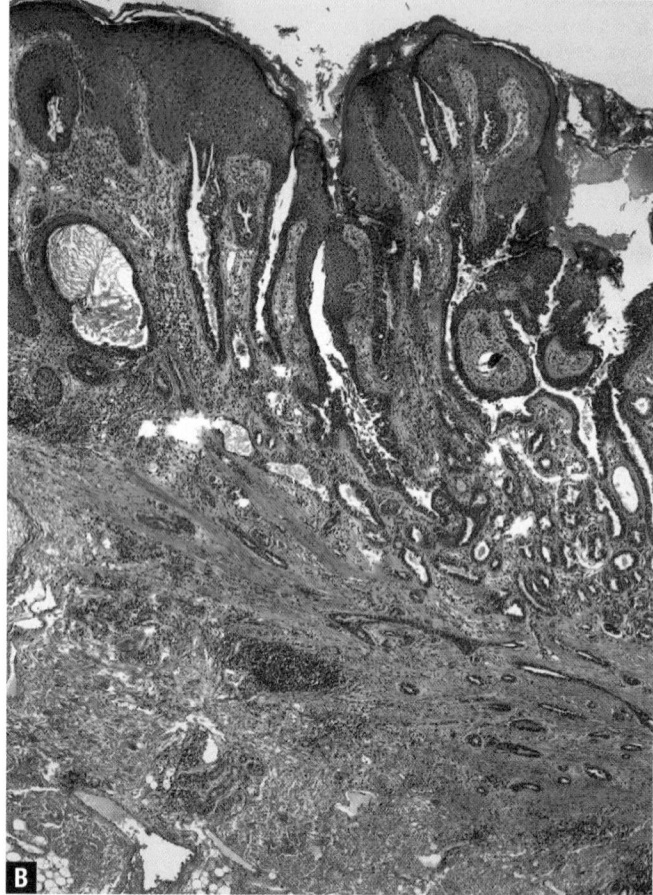

▲ **FIGURE 16-3** Syringocystadenoma presenting as multiple invaginations arising from the epidermis and extending down into the dermis. The upper portions of the invaginations are keratinized with a granular cell layer whereas deeper portions show evidence of glandular differentiation. The surrounding stroma contains numerous plasma cells. This lesion is arising on the background of a nevus sebaceus of Jadassohn. (Courtesy of Dr. Robert Schoenfeld.)

association with a previous syringocystadenoma papilliferum or nevus sebaceus.[22] The histologic pattern is similar to syringocystadenoma papilliferum with an invasive ductal component extending into the deep dermis and subcutaneous fat.[22] Treatment is by surgical excision or Mohs micrographic surgery.[23]

■ HIDRADENOMA PAPILLIFERUM

BOX 16-4   Summary

- Subcutaneous flesh-colored cystic nodule in the vulva or perineum of elderly women
- Relatively circumscribed cystic cavity with numerous papillary projections

- Secretory cells with decapitation secretory and flattened myoepithelial cells
- Rare plasma cells in the stroma
- Treatment is by surgical excision

Clinically, the hidradenoma papilliferum presents as an asymptomatic subcutaneous flesh-colored cystic nodule primarily in the vulva or perineum of middle-aged to elderly women.[24] A central opening or erosion may be present. Histologically, the lesions are relatively circumscribed and composed of a central cystic cavity filled with numerous papillary projections lined by high columnar apocrine-type secretory epithelium (Fig. 16-4). The luminal layer of secretory cells shows evidence of decapitation secretion. There is a flattened basal layer of myoepithelial cells. Plasma cells are rarely found within the stroma. In addition, the overall architecture is cystic as opposed to the multiple invaginations seen in syringocystadenoma papilliferum. Nuclear pleomorphism and mitotic figures are not prominent features. This, along with the well-circumscribed nature of the neoplasm, helps differentiate this from a primary adnexal carcinoma or metastatic adenocarcinoma.

Surgical excision is curative. Consultation with a gynecologic or colorectal surgeon may be of benefit for large lesions involving the vagina or anal sphincter.

A rare case of malignant adenocarcinoma arising in a hidradenoma papilliferum has been described.[25] This case showed cellular atypia and infiltrating growth pattern and was marked by metastasis and fatal outcome.[25]

■ EROSIVE ADENOMATOSIS OF THE NIPPLE

BOX 16-5   Summary

- Nodular enlargement of the nipple with superficial erosions and serous discharge in elderly females.
- Well-defined lesion with numerous branching ductal structures extending from the epidermis to the deep dermis.
- Usually is not connected with underlying glandular breast tissue.
- The epithelial lining shows squamous epithelium in the upper portions and columnar cells in the intradermal portions with outer layer of myoepithelial cells.
- No nuclear pleomorphism or mitotic figures.
- Treatment is by surgical excision or Mohs surgery as a nipple sparing technique.

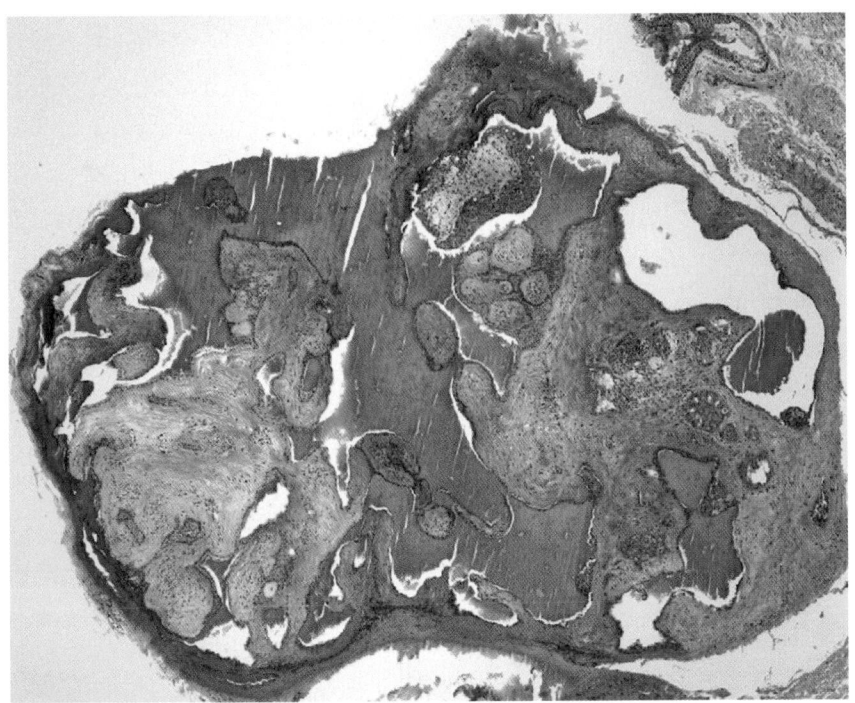

▲ **FIGURE 16-4** Hidradenoma papilliferum representing a well-circumscribed nodular proliferation of cystic spaces with glandular differentiation.

This lesion presents clinically as a nodular enlargement of the nipple with superficial erosions and serous discharge, which may be bloody. The tumor may be confused with Paget's disease of the nipple or an eczematous plaque. The majority of patients are middle aged or elderly females with fewer than 5% of cases occurring in males.[26] Histologically, the lesion is well defined and shows numerous branching ductal structures extending from the surface of the epidermis deep into the dermis (Fig. 16-5). Superficial portions of the cystic invaginations may be lined by squamous epithelium. The intradermal portions of the branching ductal structures are lined by an inner layer of tall columnar cells and an outer layer of flattened cuboidal cells. Decapitation secretion may be seen in the luminal layer of columnar cells. Histologic features may resemble syringocystadenoma papilliferum; however, there is no evidence of increased numbers of plasma cells within the surrounding fibrovascular stroma. The primary differential diagnosis includes a primary adenocarcinoma of the breast.[26] Erosive adenomatosis of the nipple is a relatively circumscribed lesion. Connection to underlying glandular breast tissue is not observed. The nuclei are relatively uniform in size and shape with no evidence of pleomorphism or increased numbers of mitotic figures.

Complete excision of the lesion is recommended. This may require removal

of the nipple.[27] For this reason Mohs micrographic surgery has been proposed as a nipple sparing technique.[28]

TUBULAR APOCRINE ADENOMA

BOX 16-6   Summary

- Slow-growing flesh-colored dermal nodule in adults, most commonly on the scalp and may be associated with nevus sebaceous.
- Well-circumscribed cystic and tubular structures surrounded by a fibrovascular stroma.
- The intracystic papillary projections lined by columnar cells resting on the outer layer of cuboidal cells.
- No nuclear pleomorphism or mitosis.
- Treatment is by surgical excision.

The tubular apocrine adenoma presents clinically as a slow-growing, flesh-colored dermal nodule, most commonly in adults. The lesions may occur in any anatomic site, but are more common on the scalp,

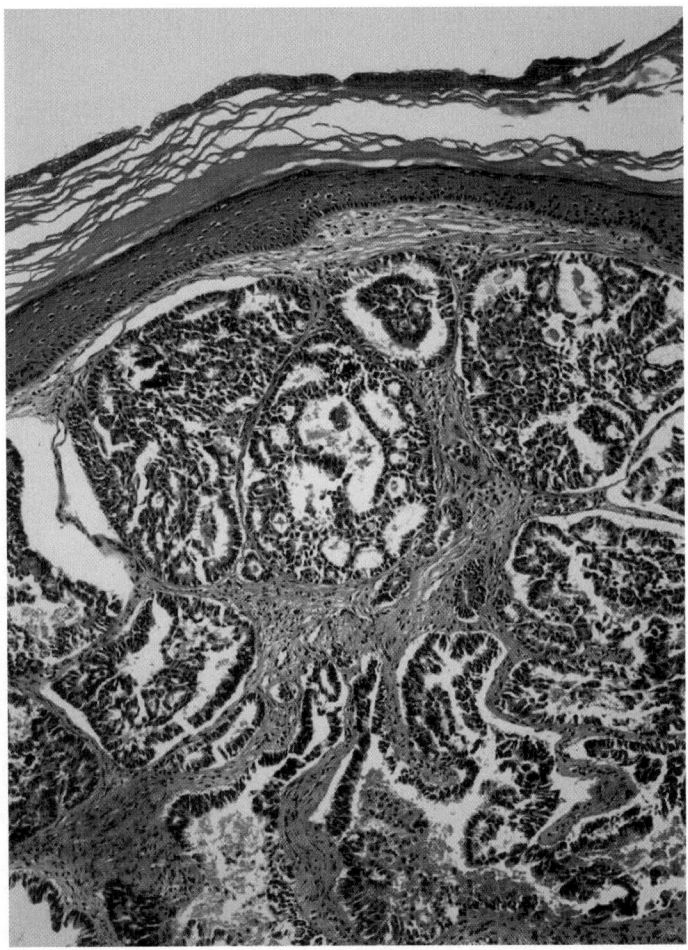

▲ **FIGURE 16-5** The erosive adenomatosis of the nipple showing invaginations of glandular epithelium from the epidermis into the dermis. Areas of nuclear pleomorphism or increased mitotic activity are not observed.

face, axillae, and genital skin. Lesions occurring on the scalp may be associated with nevus sebaceus of Jadassohn.[29] Histologically, the lesion shows evidence of multiple dilated cystic and branching tubular structures surrounded by a fibrovascular stroma.[30] The lesion is well circumscribed. The lining of the tubular structures is composed of an inner layer of columnar cells showing focal decapitation secretion resting over an outer layer of flattened or cuboidal cells. Papillary projections of glandular epithelium into cystic spaces may be observed. The lesions are histologically similar to the papillary eccrine adenoma.[31] The differential diagnosis includes a metastatic adenocarcinoma. The absence of nuclear pleomorphism and mitotic activity helps to differentiate the tubular apocrine adenoma from metastatic adenocarcinoma. Surgical excision is curative.

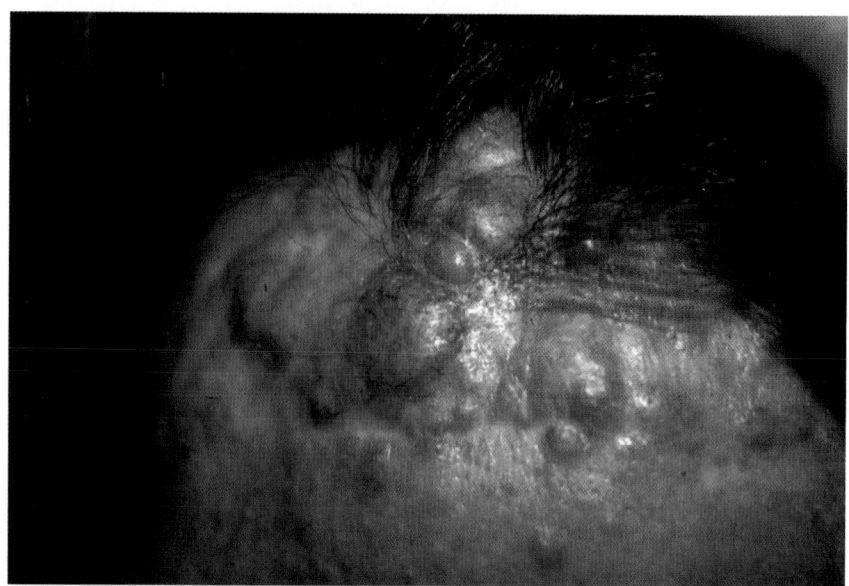

▲ **FIGURE 16-6** The cylindroma often presents as a red to flesh-colored nodule in the scalp. (Courtesy of Dr. James Ulery.)

CYLINDROMA

BOX 16-7 Summary

- Slow-growing subcutaneous or intradermal nodule on the face and scalp
- Associated with Brooke-Spiegler syndrome and is linked to mutations of the CYLD gene
- Well-circumscribed dermal proliferation of basaloid cells arranged in "jigsaw puzzle"
- Basaloid islands are surrounded by eosinophilic hyaline bands of PAS positive material
- Treatment is by surgical excision or YAG or CO_2 laser debulking

A cylindroma often presents as a slow growing smooth surfaced subcutaneous or intradermal nodule primarily on the face and scalp (Fig. 16-6).[32] Lesions may be tender or painful. Tumors may be sporadic or multiple with an autosomal dominant inherited pattern. Multiple lesions may be observed involving the forehead and scalp in a so-called "turban" distribution, becoming confluent throughout the scalp. Inherited patterns may also present with multiple trichoepitheliomas, eccrine spiradenomas, and milia in the Brooke-Spiegler syndrome.[33] This syndrome is linked to mutations in the CYLD gene, a tumor suppressor gene found on chromosome 16q 12-13.[34] Mutations in this gene have also been described in familial cylindromatosis and multiple familial trichoepitheliomas.[33,34] Histologically, the cylindroma is marked by a well-circumscribed dermal proliferation of nests of basaloid

cells. The small nests of basaloid cells are irregularly shaped and closely juxtaposed within the dermis like pieces of a jigsaw puzzle (Fig. 16-7). Basaloid islands are surrounded by a layer of PAS positive hyaline sheath and show small

hyaline globules within the basaloid nests that represent invagination of stroma into tumor lobules. Glandular lumina may be found within the basaloid islands, some of which may show decapitation secretion. The tumors

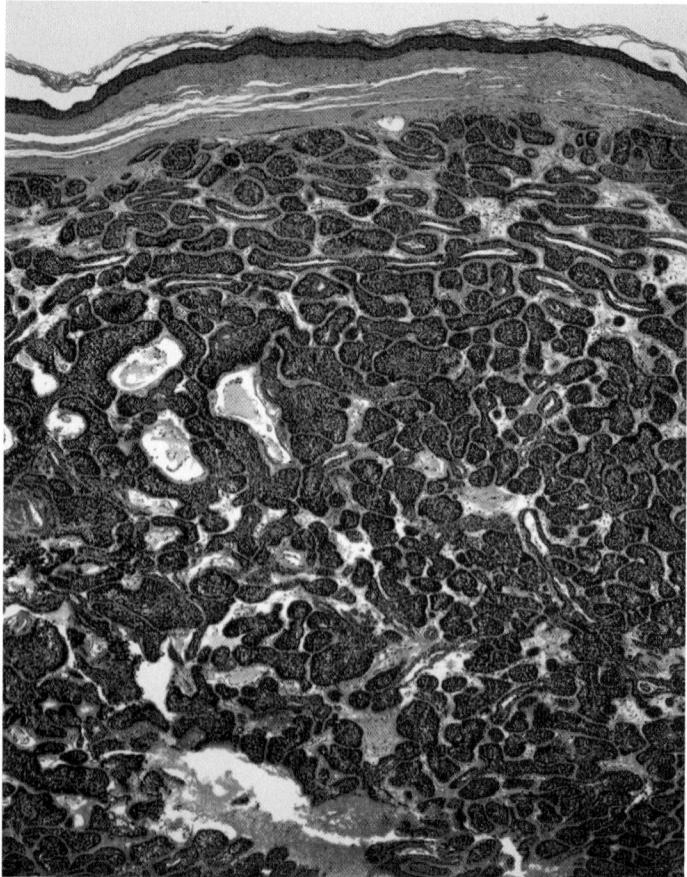

▲ **FIGURE 16-7** Cylindroma showing areas of basaloid cells surrounded by a thick eosinophilic cuticle which fit together in a jigsaw puzzle-like pattern within the dermis.

should be considered poorly differentiated glandular neoplasms. The cylindroma may express focal S-100 positivity suggestive of eccrine differentiation and human milk fat globulin consistent with apocrine differentiation as well as keratins 7, 8, and 18 consistent with secretory coil differentiation.[35,36] Similar staining patterns are also seen in the spiradenoma.[37]

The differential diagnosis may include a basal cell carcinoma. The presence of a thick PAS positive hyaline membrane and the absence of clefting between the basaloid islands and the surrounding stroma help in differentiation. The cutaneous cylindroma shows no evidence of nuclear pleomorphism or mitotic figures. Lesions of cylindroma are typically well circumscribed within the dermis, although they may rarely show extension into the subcutaneous fat.

Treatment of isolated lesions is by surgical excision. Removal of all lesions in patients with multiple cylindromas is not always practical. In these cases treatment with laser ablation using Nd:YAG or CO_2 laser debulking may provide cosmetically acceptable results.[38,39]

Malignant change in a cylindroma may be heralded clinically by rapid growth or ulceration.[40] Cylindrocarcinoma is most common in elderly patients arising in scalp lesions.[40] Metastasis to lymph nodes and internal viscera have both been reported. Areas of malignant change show an infiltrating growth pattern adjacent to areas of typical cylindroma.[41] Malignant changes include loss of the peripheral palisading of tumor cells and loss of the hyaline membrane surrounding tumor lobules as well as nuclear pleomorphism and increased mitotic activity. Complete surgical excision with tumor free margins is indicated.

ECCRINE SPIRADENOMA

BOX 16-8 Summary

- Painful solitary intradermal nodule with bluish discoloration
- Multiple lesions associated with Brooke-Spiegler syndrome
- Intradermal lobules of basaloid cells with no connection to the overlying epidermis
- A hyaline mantle of basement membrane material or intralobular droplets of hyaline material may be seen
- Cytologic atypia should not be seen and mitoses are exceedingly rare
- Complete excision

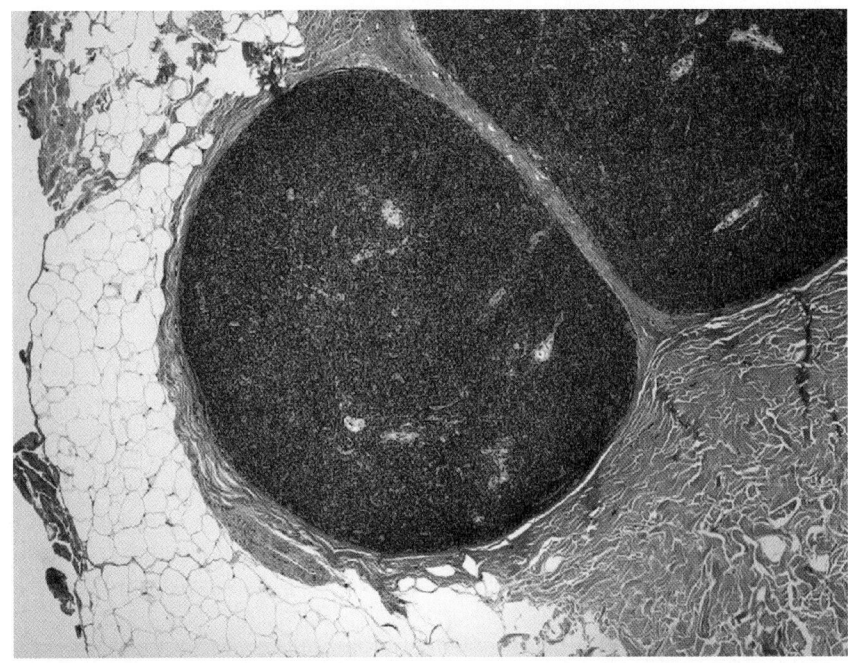

▲ **FIGURE 16-8** Eccrine spiradenoma showing a proliferation of basaloid cells in the deep dermis and subcutaneous fat. The lesions are well circumscribed and composed of one or few well demarcated lobules surrounded by an eosinophilic cuticle.

The eccrine spiradenoma presents as an intradermal nodule on the head or trunk.[42] Lesions are typically solitary and may be painful.[42] Multiple eccrine spiradenomas and cylindromas may occur in patients with autosomal dominantly inherited trichoepitheliomas in the Brooke-Spiegler syndrome.[43] The tumors are composed of deep dermal or subcutaneous, well-circumscribed proliferations of basaloid cells (Fig. 16-8). The tumors are typically formed by one or few large lobules of basaloid cells surrounded by a thick eosinophilic cuticle that is PAS positive and diastase resistant. The tumor is surrounded by a richly vascular stroma. Within the tumor lobules are thin anastomosing cords of two types of cells. The outer cells are small with compact nuclei and appear darker staining. The inner cells are large with more cytoplasm and appearing lighter staining. Central lumina may be seen. Areas of eosinophilic hyaline deposition may be found between the thin anastomosing cords. The cytokeratin expression pattern is consistent with differentiation towards the transitional portion between the secretory and coiled duct of the eccrine gland.[44] Surgical excision is curative.

Rare malignant variants have been reported which histologically show transition from benign to malignant areas (Fig. 16-9). The malignant variants tend to be large and may be found on the head, trunk and extremities.[45] Disorganization, nuclear pleomorphism, increased mitoses and squamous metaplasia may be seen.[46]

Malignant areas show loss of the two cell types typically seen in eccrine spiradenoma.[47] Metastases and death have been reported.[47,48] Because of the aggressive nature complete excision either with wide margins or by Mohs micrographic technique is recommended. Sentinal lymph node biopsy has been used; however, its role remains undetermined at this time.[49]

ECCRINE POROMA

BOX 16-9 Summary

- Pink to red asymptomatic verrucous nodule on the acral areas of the body
- Proliferation of elongated strands of pale cuboidal cells arising from the undersurface of the epidermis and extending into the dermis

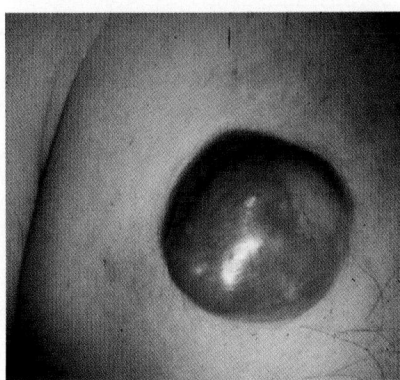

▲ **FIGURE 16-9** Fast-growing nodule representing a spiradenocarcinoma arising in a previous eccrine spiradenoma.

- Small ductal structures within the tumor lobules
- Variably hyalinized and fibrotic stroma, frequently hemorrhagic
- Surgical excision is curative

The eccrine poroma represents a benign tumor showing differentiation toward the intraepidermal portion of the eccrine duct.[50] Clinically, these are most common on the acral areas of the body, particularly the hands and feet, where eccrine glands are abundant (Fig. 16-10). However, they may also present on the face and trunk. Multiple lesions have been described as eccrine poromatosis. Lesions typically present as a pink to red verrucous nodule or plaque. They may bleed easily. Histologically, the lesions show a proliferation of pale staining cuboidal cells arising from the undersurface of the epidermis and extending into the dermis.[50] Multiple connections to the overlying epidermis are typically seen (Fig. 16-11). The tumor cells have round to slightly oval nuclei and pale staining cytoplasm, which contains glycogen on staining with PAS technique.[50] The pale staining cells show a sharp line of demarcation between tumor epithelium and the overlying epidermis. Within the tumor lobules, small ductal structures may be found. Intercellular desmosomal attachments are inconspicuous.[50] Keratinization is not observed. Within the dermis is a highly vascular stroma. Dendritic melanocytes may be found within the tumor lobules leading to a pigmented variant of eccrine poroma. Tumor cells stain for cytokeratin 5/6 and EMA consistent with acrosyringeal differentiation.[51]

A primarily intradermal variant without obvious epidermal connection has been reported as dermal duct tumor.[52] These lesions present as smooth dermal nodules (Fig. 16-12). Histologic features are similar to eccrine poroma although the lesions lack an epidermal connection.[52]

Surgical excision is curative. Treatment of an isolated case with topical imiquimod has been reported.[53]

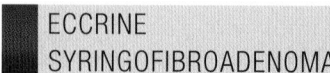

ECCRINE SYRINGOFIBROADENOMA

BOX 16-10   Summary

- Solitary or multiple papules and nodules on the acral surfaces of the hands and feet in adults
- Multiple lesions associated with ectodermal dysplasia and Schopf syndrome
- Thin anastomozing strands of uniform small epithelial cells with focal ductal differentiation
- The epithelial strands enclose fibrovascular stroma
- Surgical excision in symptomatic lesions

Eccrine syringofibroadenoma presents primarily on the acral surfaces of the hands and feet of adults.[54] Lesions are typically pink to red with smooth to verrucous surface that may show a linear distribution. Histologically, the epithelial islands form a sponge like proliferation of thin strands and septae of acrosyringeal-type cells (Fig. 16-13). The acrosyringeal cells show evidence of pale staining cytoplasm containing PAS positive glycogen. Small ducts may be seen within the anastomosing strands. Keratinization is not present which may help to differentiate this tumor from the fibroepithelioma of Pinkus. The thin strands are surrounded by an extensive fibrovascular stroma. The luminal cells stain for CEA and cytokeratins 6, 8, 18, and 19 consistent with acrosyringeal and dermal duct differentiation.[54] Similar changes can be seen as reactive changes in the setting of a chronic dermatosis.[55] A case of malignant change has been described by Katane with an invasive dermal growth pattern.[56] Symptomatic lesions may be treated by surgical excision.

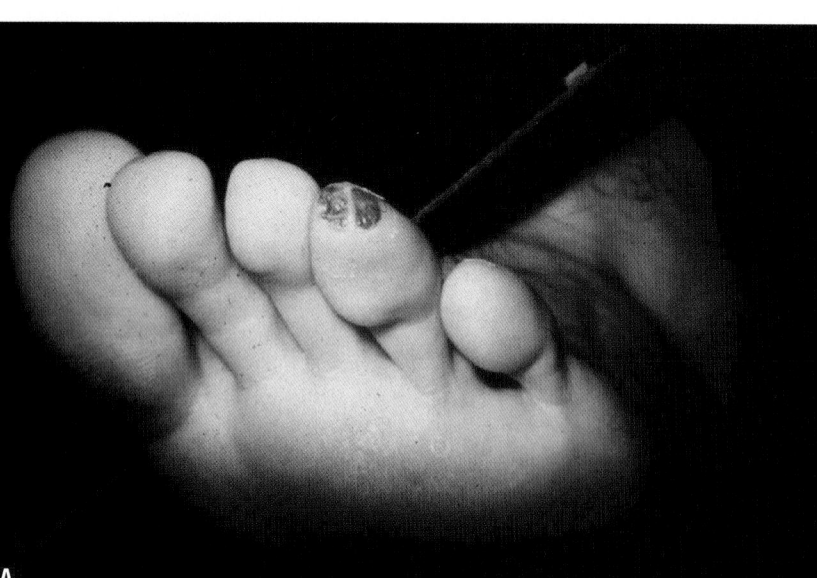

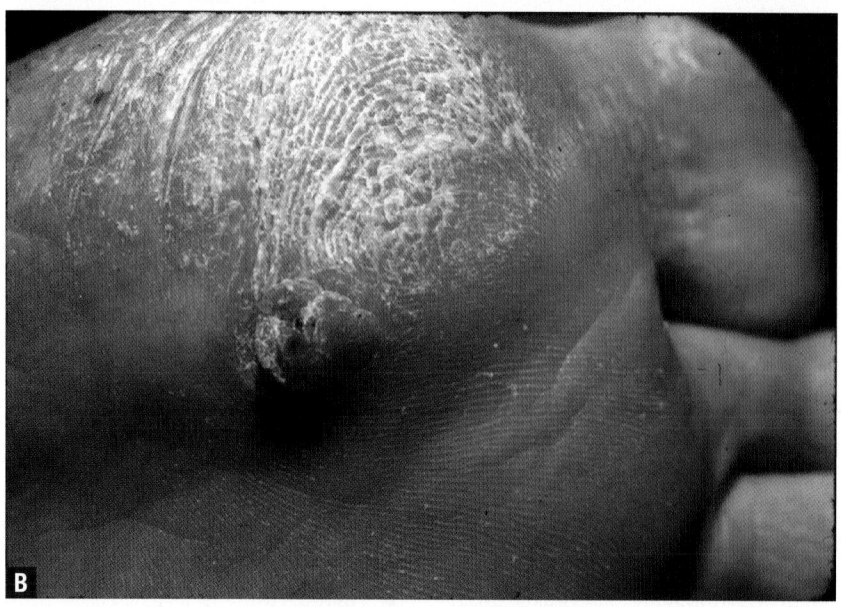

▲ **FIGURE 16-10** Eccrine poroma presenting as a flesh-colored to red papule most commonly on the acral surfaces. (Courtesy of Dr. James Ulery and Dr. Robert Schoenfeld.)

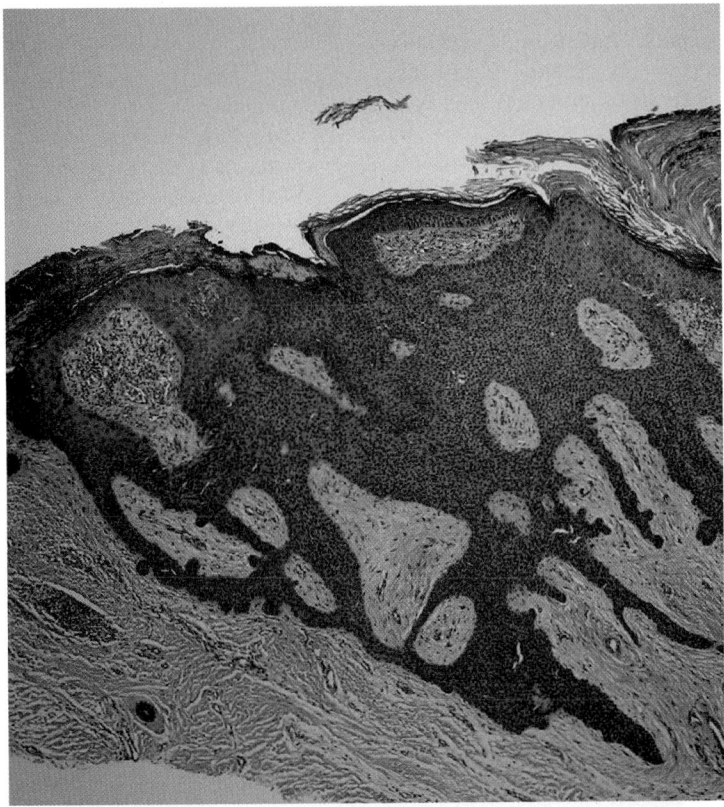

▲ **FIGURE 16-11** Eccrine poroma showing a proliferation of pale staining cuboidal cells arising from the undersurface of the epidermis extending into the dermis. This is surrounded by a vascular stroma.

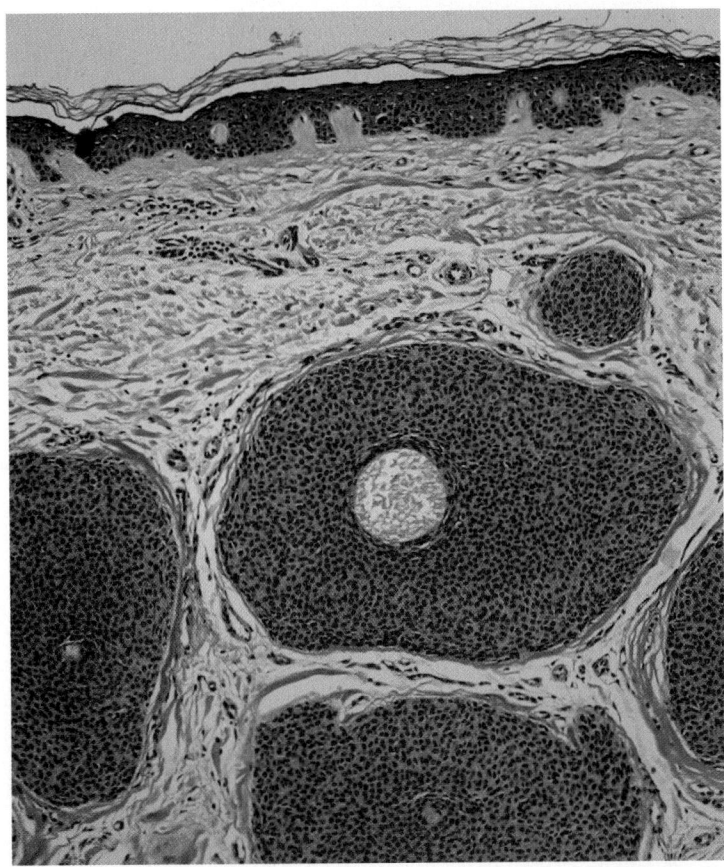

▲ **FIGURE 16-12** Dermal duct tumor showing similar histologic features without an obvious epidermal connection.

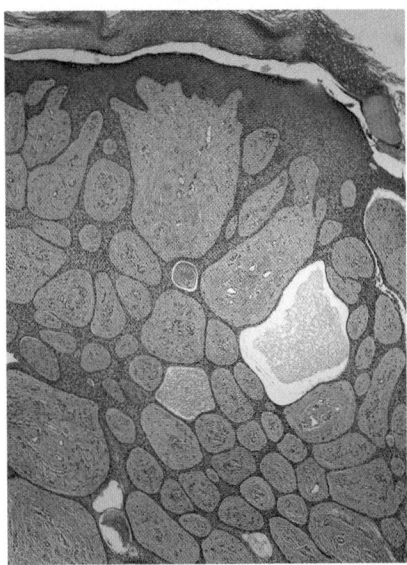

▲ **FIGURE 16-13** Eccrine syringofibroadenoma showing anastomosing strands of cuboidal to pale-staining cells in a highly vascular stroma.

HIDROACANTHOMA SIMPLEX

> **BOX 16-11 Summary**
>
> - Well-demarcated pink to tan, flat scaly plaque
> - Well-circumscribed islands of pale uniform cuboidal cells in an intraepidermal distribution
> - Small eccrine ductal structures may be found within the tumor lobules
> - Complete surgical excision is recommended

The hidroacanthoma simplex represents a superficial intraepidermal eccrine neoplasm clinically appearing as a well-demarcated pink to tan, flat, slightly scaly plaque.[57] Clinically, these may be misinterpreted as a flat seborrheic keratosis or Bowen's disease.[57] Histologically, the lesions show circumscribed islands of uniform-appearing cuboidal cells resembling those of an eccrine poroma, and may be considered an intra-epidermal variant of poroma. The tumor islands are present in an intra-epidermal distribution. The surrounding epidermis may be acanthotic. The tumor cells appear as lighter staining and contain glycogen, which helps to differentiate them from the surrounding acanthotic epidermis. Special stains may highlight a decreased number of Langerhans cells and melanin in hidroacanthoma simplex in contrast to a clonal seborrheic keratosis.[57] Small eccrine ductal structures may be found both entering into the tumor lobules from the dermis and within the tumor lobules. The syringoacanthoma represents a benign variant occurring in an acanthotic and

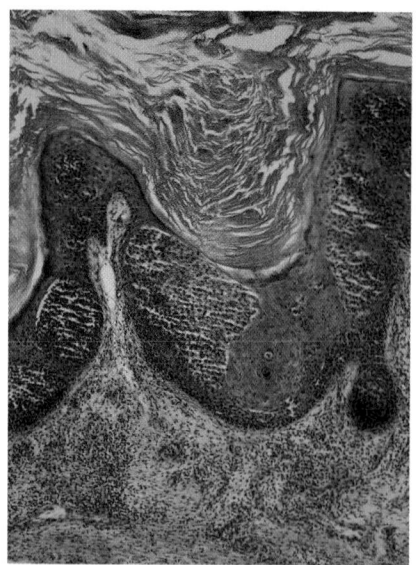

▲ **FIGURE 16-14** Syringoacanthoma showing a proliferation of pale staining cells with areas of ductal differentiation within an acanthotic and hyperkeratotic epidermis.

hyperkeratotic epidermis (Fig. 16-14). Lesions may be locally destructive.[59] A rare malignant variant has been reported in which the tumor cells show extensive nuclear pleomorphism with mitotic figures.[60] These malignant variants may be considered as porocarcinoma arising in a pre-existing hidroacanthoma simplex or malignant hidroacanthoma.[61] This rare association of hidroacanthoma and porocarcinoma has prompted some authors to recommend complete excision of lesions of hidroacanthoma simplex.[62]

PAPILLARY ECCRINE ADENOMA

BOX 16-12   Summary

- Intradermal papule or nodule on the distal extremities
- Well-circumscribed proliferation of dilated and branching ductal structures
- Papillary projections with a double layer of uniform cuboidal cells; no decapitation secretion, nuclear atypia, or mitoses
- Dense fibrosis and hyalinization of stroma
- Surgical excision is curative

The papillary eccrine adenoma presents as an intradermal papule or nodule. People of all ages may be affected. The lesions are slow growing and asymptomatic. Histologically, the lesion is characterized by a well-circumscribed proliferation of dilated and branching ductal structures.[63] The ductal structures are lined by an inner layer of columnar cells with an outer layer of flattened myoepithelial cells. The inner cells show evi-

dence of papillary projections into the cystic lumina. Amorphous secretory material may be found within the lumina. The ductal structures stain with immunohistochemical stains to S-100 protein, CEA, and EMA and cytokeratin 8, consistent with differentiation towards the transitional portion of the eccrine duct and secretory coil of the eccrine gland.[63,64]

The relative circumscribed architecture, lack of nuclear pleomorphism, and lack of mitotic figures help to differentiate this from metastatic adenocarcinoma. The presence of papillary projections and absence of decapitation secretion helps to differentiate this from the tubular apocrine adenoma, which has otherwise similar architectural features. Surgical excision is curative.

SYRINGOMA

BOX 16-13   Summary

- Flesh-colored to yellowish papules on the face
- In eruptive variant, the disseminated lesions involve the trunk of young adults and patients with Down syndrome
- Relatively well-circumscribed interconnecting eccrine strands and ducts within a fibrous stroma
- The strands have a tadpole or comma shape
- Surgical excision in solitary lesions or electrodessication in multiple variant

The syringoma presents as flesh-colored to yellowish papules, primarily on the face. Lesions are most commonly found in a periorbital distribution (Fig. 16-15). However, widespread eruptive lesions

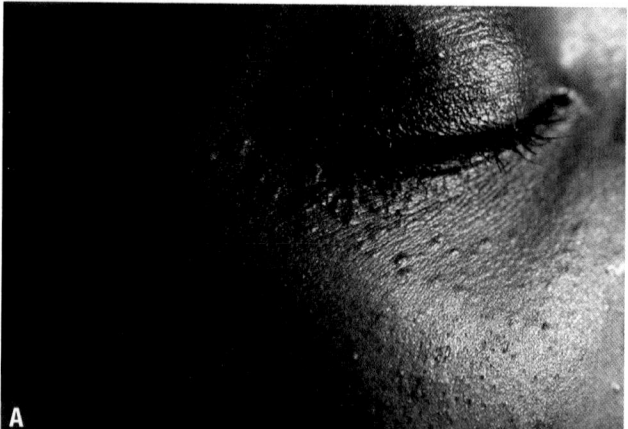

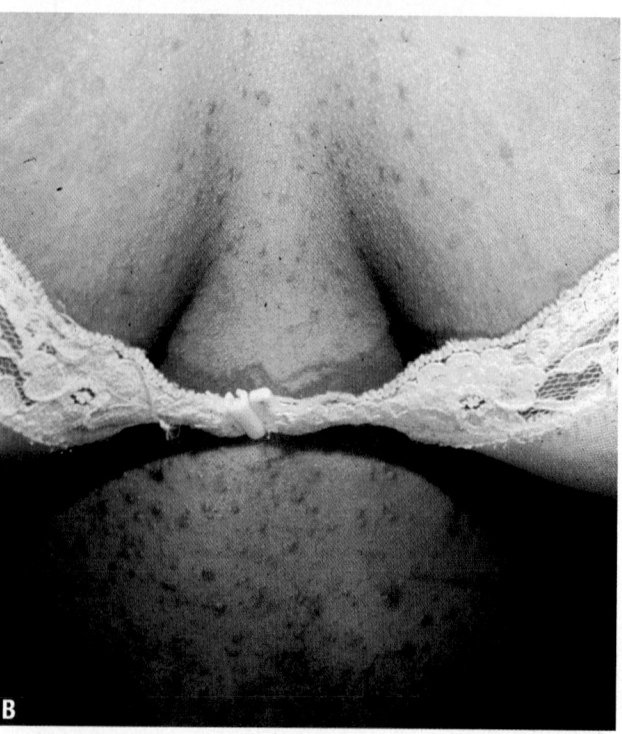

▲ **FIGURE 16-15** Syringoma may present as a single or multiple flesh-colored to yellowish papules around the periorbital area. Widespread lesions may be found on the trunk, axilla, and genital skin. (Courtesy of Dr. James Ulery.)

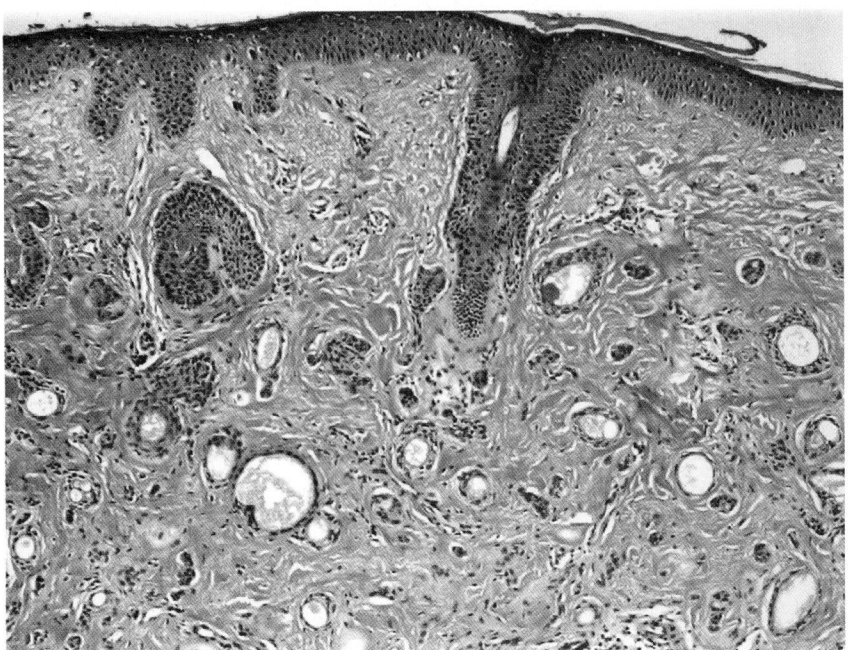

▲ **FIGURE 16-16** Syringoma showing areas of small epithelial islands, some of which show ductal differentiation in a fibrotic stroma where the tumor is well-circumscribed and located primarily in the upper to mid dermis.

may be found on the trunk, axillae, anterior arms, and genital skin.[65] Facial lesions are more common in young adults and the elderly while the widespread eruptive variety often begins in childhood.[65] Eruptive syringomas are more common in young girls with disseminated lesions involving the trunk. A familial autosomal dominant presentation has been described. Lesions may also be associated with Down syndrome.[66] Histologically, the lesions are marked by a proliferation of small epithelial tumor lobules in the dermis surrounded by a fibrotic stroma (Fig. 16-16). The epithelial lobules may show evidence of duct formation, containing PAS positive diastase resistant material. Some of the epithelial structures have "comma-like" tails, which may also have a resemblance to "tadpoles". Nuclear pleomorphism and mitotic activity are not observed. A clear cell variant marked by epithelial islands with abundant pale staining cytoplasm containing glycogen is present (Fig. 16-17). The clear cell variant may be associated with diabetes.[67] Syringomas express luminal CEA and cytokeratins 1, 5, 10, 11, and 19, similar to the upper dermal sweat duct.[68,69] The superficial nature of the tumor, well-circumscribed architecture, and lack of nuclear pleomorphism help to differentiate the syringoma from microcystic adnexal carcinoma.

The syringoma is a benign neoplasm that is easily removed by excision or punch biopsy technique. In cases of multiple syringomas, destruction by intralesional electrodessication or electrodessication with curettage may provide a cosmetically acceptable alternative.[70,71] Destruction with CO_2 laser, with or without pretreatment by TCA peel has also been described.[72,73] Treatment with erbium YAG laser has also been reported with good cosmetic results.[74]

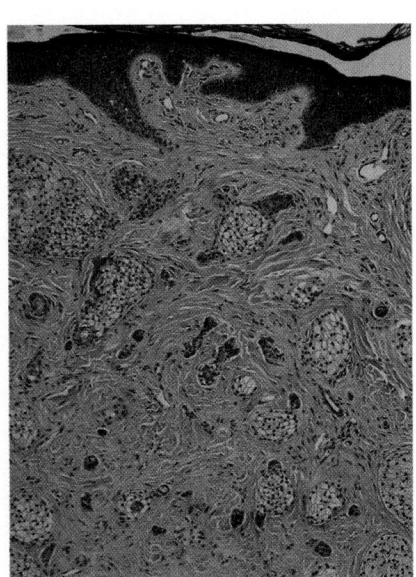

▲ **FIGURE 16-17** Clear cell syringoma showing similar histologic features as the syringoma; however, the epithelial islands contain abundant glycogen forming clear cells.

■ CHONDROID SYRINGOMA

BOX 16-14 Summary

- Intradermal or subcutaneous flesh-colored nodule on the head and neck of elderly patients
- Well-circumscribed intradermal nodule
- Composed of epithelial and stromal component
- Small ductal structures and larger anastomosing branching epithelial islands surrounded by a distinctive myxomatous or "chondroid" stroma
- Surgical excision with a narrow margin of normal tissue

The chondroid syringoma (mixed tumor of the skin) presents clinically as an intradermal or subcutaneous flesh-colored nodule. Lesions are noted in adults and elderly patients, particularly on the head and neck.[75] Histologically, the chondroid syringoma is composed of prominent epithelial and stromal components, hence the name mixed tumor of the skin. The lesions resemble the mixed tumor of the salivary gland. The epithelial component may consist of small ductal structures to larger anastomosing and branching epithelial islands with central lumina (Fig 16-18). These are surrounded by a loose pale staining stroma containing fibroblasts and alcian blue positive mucin with a distinctive myxomatous or "chondroid" appearance. True chondroid metaplasia may be seen. Areas of follicular and sebaceous differentiation may be observed in the epithelial component. The lesions are typically well circumscribed within the dermis and may extend down to the superficial subcutaneous fat. Luminal cells stain for CEA while the cytokeratin expression pattern suggests both apocrine ductal and follicular differentiation.[76] Lack of nuclear pleomorphism and mitotic activity helps differentiate this from metastatic carcinomas to the skin. Treatment is by surgical excision with a narrow margin of normal tissue.[75]

A malignant variant with greater cellularity containing mitotic figures and nuclear pleomorphism has been described.[77] Tumor cells stain positive for S-100, cytokeratin AE1/AE3, neuron specific enolase, and glial fibrillary acidic protein.[78] Metastasis from malignant chondroid syringoma is reported in up to 39% of cases.[78,79] Wide excision with tumor-free margins is recommended.

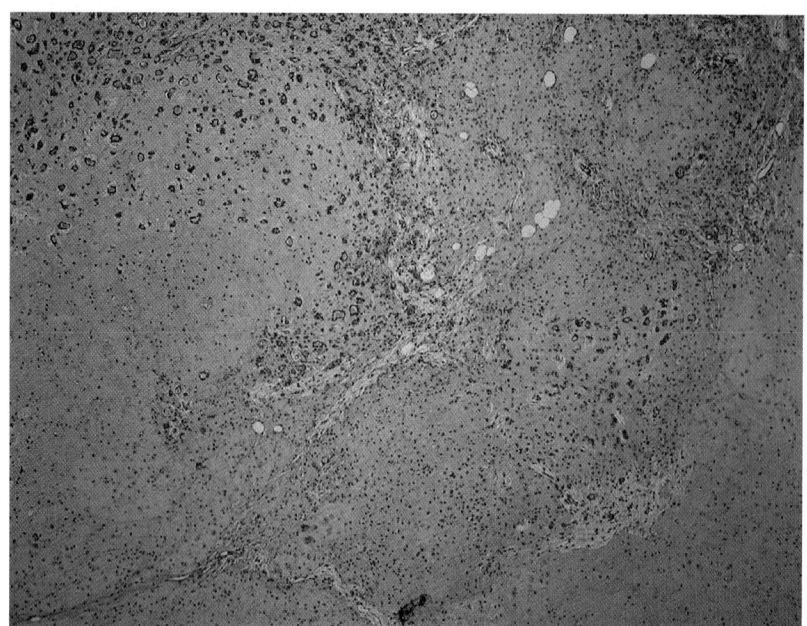

▲ **FIGURE 16-18** The chondroid syringoma shows areas of ductal differentiation surrounded by an abundant mucin-containing stroma resembling cartilage.

CLEAR CELL HIDRADENOMA

BOX 16-15 Summary

- Slow-growing flesh-colored to red-blue smooth deep dermal or subcutaneous nodules
- Well-circumscribed, dermal-based lesion with occasional epidermal connection or extension into the subcutaneous fat
- Uniform cells with small round to oval nuclei and pale "clear" cytoplasm
- The stroma may be variably fascicular, collogenous, or hyalinized
- Surgical excision is curative

The clear cell hidradenoma (eccrine acrospiroma) represents a poorly differentiated tumor thought to show eccrine differentiation (Fig. 16-19).[80] Clinically the lesions present as slow growing flesh colored to red-blue smooth deep dermal or subcutaneous nodules. Histologically, the lesions are well-circumscribed solid masses. The tumor cells are typically uniform in size and shape with small round oval nuclei and pale staining cytoplasm.[80] The cytoplasm contains abundant glycogen which is PAS positive and diastase sensitive. These variants may be termed "clear cell hidradenoma." Small lumina or large cystic spaces may both be seen. Neoplasms marked by cystic spaces may be termed "solid, cystic hidradenoma." Their surrounding stroma is less prominent, but may be highly vascular. The clear cells stain for cytokeratins 7, 8, 19 and EMA consistent with eccrine secretory coil differentiation.[51]

The histologic differential diagnosis may include metastatic renal cell carcinoma, metastatic adenocarcinoma, sebaceous carcinoma, and squamous cell carcinoma.[81] The lack of nuclear pleomorphism and mitotic figures helps to differentiate this from these various forms of primary and metastatic carcinoma. In addition, the lesions are typically well circumscribed and limited to the dermis and subcutaneous fat. Treatment is by complete surgical excision.

A malignant variant composed of clear polygonal cells has been described (Fig. 16-20). Cellular atypia including increased mitotic figures and nuclear pleomorphism is subtle. The lesions are poorly circumscribed with an invasive growth pattern.[82] Widespread metastases with fatal outcome have been reported.[82] Treatment is by wide surgical excision. Mohs micrographic surgery may also be considered.[83]

AGGRESSIVE DIGITAL PAPILLARY ADENOMA

BOX 16-16 Summary

- Painless nodule on the hands or feet of middle-aged adults
- The term of aggressive digital papillary adenocarcinoma had been applied in cases with lymph node and pulmonary metastasis
- Poorly circumscribed growth of multiple cystic lobules with both glandular and papillary architecture
- The glandular spaces are lined by one or two layers of cuboidal cells
- Invasive growth pattern, nuclear pleomorphism, necrosis, and mitotic figures in adenocarcinoma variant
- Wide surgical excision or digital amputation is the treatment of choice

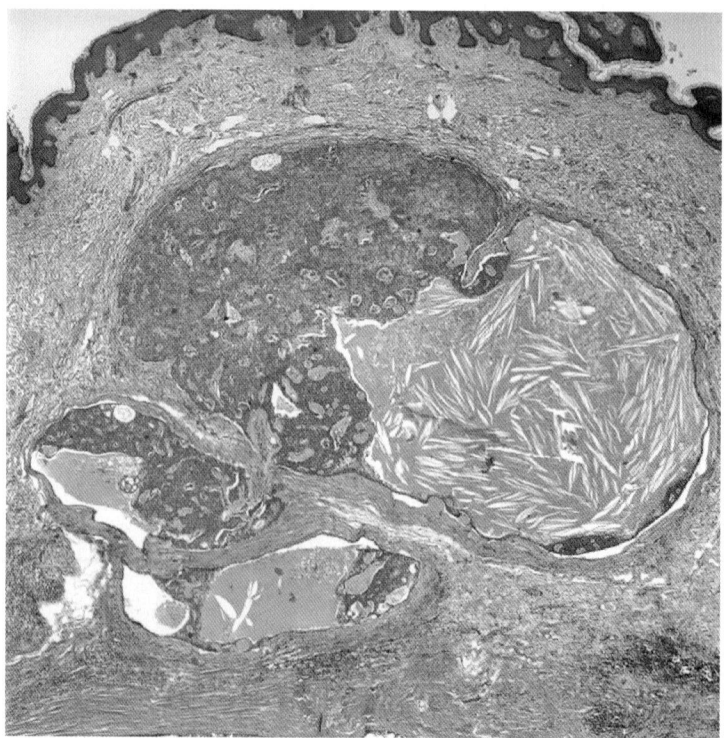

▲ **FIGURE 16-19** Solid cystic hidradenoma is composed of a nodular proliferation of pale staining cells in the dermis. There are clear cell changes made predominantly in the clear cell hidradenoma whereas cystic changes may predominate in the solid and cystic hidradenoma.

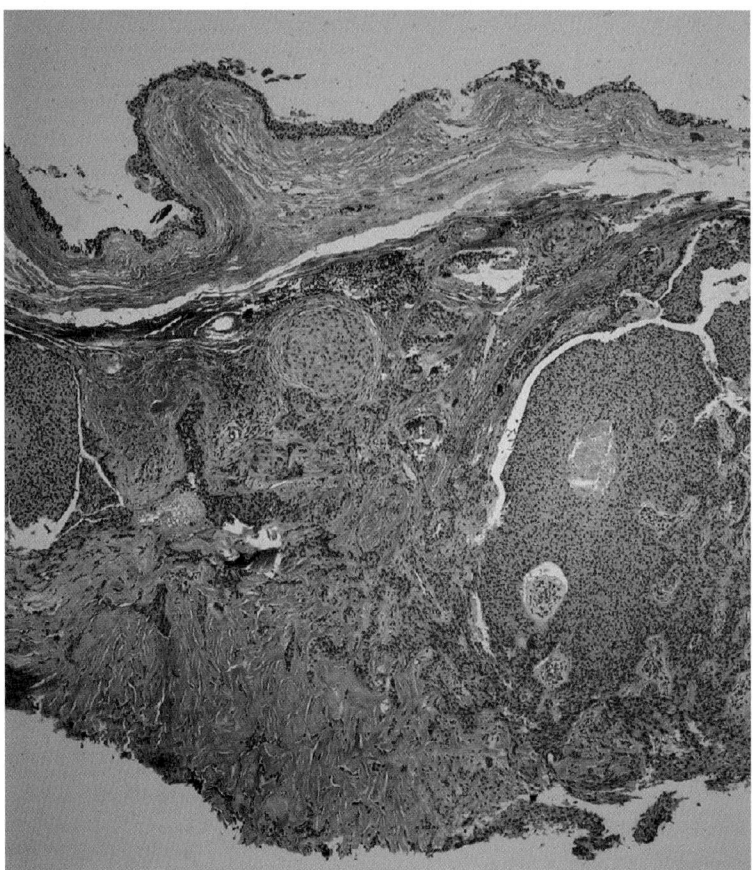

▲ **FIGURE 16-20** Malignant hidradenoma showing areas typical of hidradenoma with a proliferation of pale staining epithelium and ductal spaces; however, there are areas of an infiltrative growth pattern and squamous metaplasia.

The aggressive digital papillary adenoma presents as a painless nodule on the hands or feet of middle aged adults.[84] Lesions may be ulcerated or bleed. Regional lymph node and pulmonary metastasis have been described, and termed aggressive digital papillary adenocarcinoma.[84] Histologically, the tumor is situated in the dermis forming branching tubular and ductal structures, shows a poorly circumscribed growth pattern and often extends into the subcutaneous tissue. Within the dilated ductal structures are papillary projections. Nuclear pleomorphism, mitotic figures, poor glandular differentiation, tumor necrosis and an invasive growth pattern may be seen in the adenocarcinoma variant.[84] The lesions may show an infiltrating growth pattern into the surrounding soft tissues. Immunoperoxidase stains are positive for S-100 protein and CEA along the luminal borders and show diffuse cytokeratin staining especially in areas of squamous differentiation.[84] These tumors may also show immunohistochemical staining for antibodies to ferritin.[85] Both the adenoma and the adenocarcinoma variants show a propensity for recurrence.[84] In a large

series by Kao et al, 41% of aggressive digital papillary adenocarcinomas developed metastases, with three of seven of

these patients dying of metastatic disease 5 to 20 years after initial resection.[84] Wide surgical excision or digital amputation is the treatment of choice.[86]

ECCRINE POROCARCINOMA

BOX 16-17 Summary

- Red crusted nodules or plaque on acral surfaces of the elderly
- Infiltrating growth of well-defined islands of neoplastic cells both within the epidermis and dermis
- Tumor cells have abundant glycogen and sweat duct lumina formation
- Extensive nuclear pleomorphism and an increased number of mitotic figures
- Surgical excision with tumor-free margins

The eccrine porocarcinoma is a relatively rare neoplasm that may present clinically as a red crusted nodule or plaque.[87] Lesions are most common on acral surfaces of the elderly (Fig. 16-21). The lesion is characterized by the presence of well-defined islands of neoplastic cells, both within the epidermis and dermis. The tumor islands show an infiltrating growth pattern extending throughout the dermis down to the level of the subcutaneous fat. Intralymphatic tumor islands may be seen. The neoplastic epithelium may show sharp demarcation with the adjacent epidermis in a manner similar to that seen with eccrine poroma. Tumor cells have pale staining cytoplasm containing

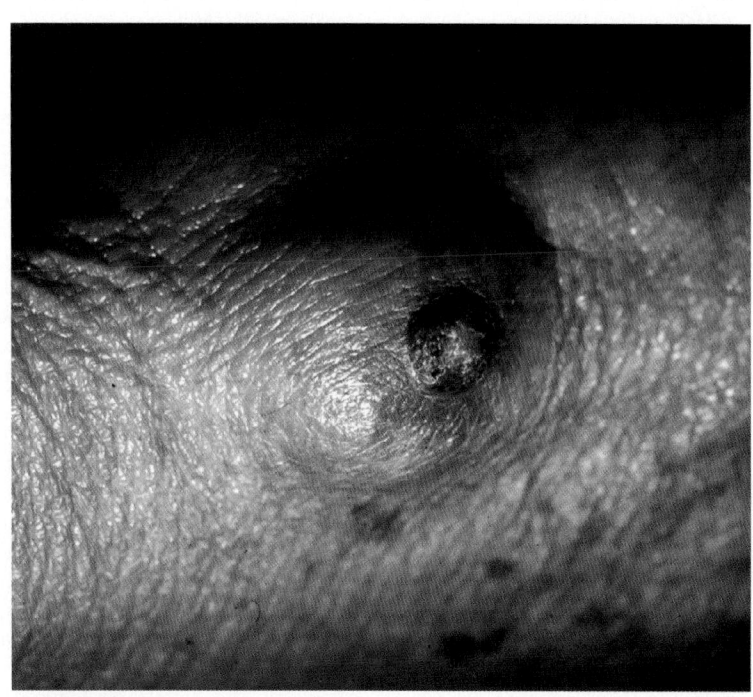

▲ **FIGURE 16-21** Eccrine porocarcinoma presenting as an ulcerated or verrucous nodule on the extremities.

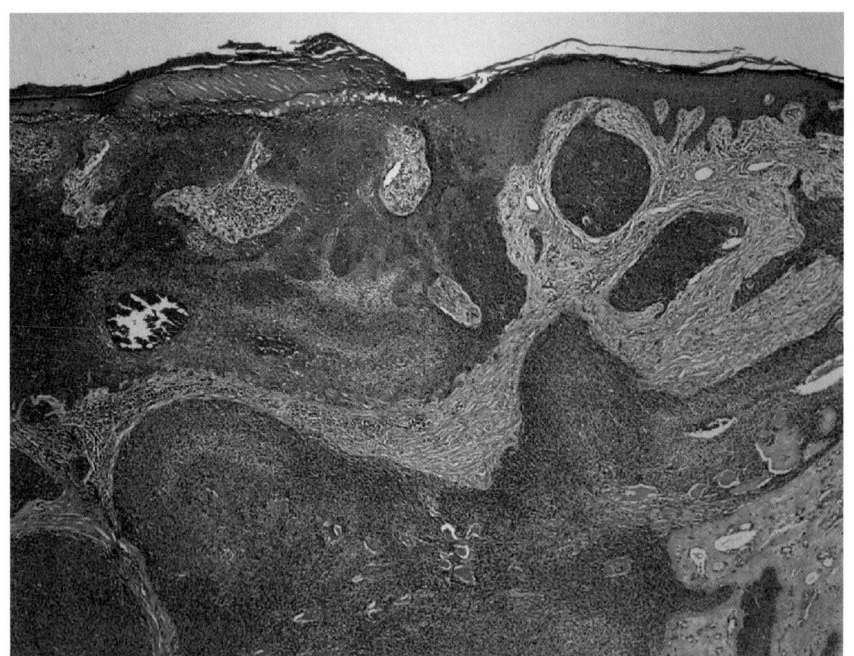

▲ **FIGURE 16-22** Porocarcinoma histologically showing areas of connection to the undersurface of the epidermis. The tumor is composed of pale staining to eosinophilic cuboidal cells resembling a poroma; however, there is extensive nuclear pleomorphism, mitotic activity, and an invasive growth pattern.

PAS positive diastase sensitive glycogen and show areas of small lumina formation.[87] There is extensive nuclear pleomorphism and an increased number of mitotic figures (Fig. 16-22). This along with the invasive growth pattern helps to differentiate this from the eccrine poroma. The presence of abundant glycogen and sweat duct lumina formation helps in differentiating the eccrine porocarcinoma from a squamous cell carcinoma.

Treatment is by surgical excision with tumor free margins. Excision by Mohs micrographic technique has been described.[88] Regional and distant metastases have been observed. Evaluation for nodal disease may be of benefit in identifying early nodal spread. Treatment of metastatic disease is difficult as the tumor responds poorly to chemotherapy.[89] Isolated response to alpha interferon and isotretinoin alone or in combination has been reported.[90,91] Intra-arterial docetaxel has also been reported to slow tumor progression.[89,92]

SYRINGOID ECCRINE CARCINOMA

BOX 16-18   Summary

- Rare solitary tumor on the head and extremities of elderly patients
- Duct and cords of atypical basaloid cells infiltrate from upper to the deep dermis and subcutaneous tissue

- Nuclear atypia and mitotic figures in the cells surrounding the ducts
- Perineural and arrector pili muscle invasion
- Surgical excision with tumor-free margins or Mohs technique

The syringoid eccrine carcinoma presents as a rare solitary lesion on the head and extremities of elderly patients, but has no characteristic clinical appearance. Tubular structures and cords of atypical basaloid cells infiltrate from the upper to the deep dermis and subcutaneous tissue.[93] A number of mitotic figures may be seen in the cells surrounding the ducts, which are lined by a single layer of cuboidal cells. Keratin-filled cysts and follicular differentiation are usually not evident. Connection to the overlying epidermis may be seen. The stroma may be vascular or fibrotic. Perineural and arrector pili muscle invasion are often seen. These tumors show an aggressive growth pattern with local recurrence and rare metastases.[94]

The histologic differential diagnosis may include a syringocystadenoma papilliferum and syringoma. However, the infiltrating growth pattern, nuclear pleomorphism and mitotic activity help to differentiate this from benign glandular neoplasms. Syringoid eccrine carcinoma may be difficult to differentiate from basal cell carcinoma (BCC), microcystic adnexal carcinoma and metastatic adenocarcinomas such as colorectal and infiltrative ductal breast carcinoma. Histologically,

they may appear similar, but CEA is expressed in benign and malignant eccrine neoplasms and is lacking in BCC.[95] The absence of expression of CK20 may exclude metastatic colorectal cancers. Expression of HMFG (human milk fat globulin) in breast carcinoma may help to differentiate syringoid eccrine carcinoma (SEC) from metastatic breast carcinoma.[96] SEC and MAC have similar immunohistochemical profiles, but SEC does not usually form keratin-filled cysts and lacks follicular differentiation. Surgical excision with tumor free margins or excision by Mohs micrographic technique is recommended.[97]

MICROCYSTIC ADNEXAL CARCINOMA

BOX 16-19   Summary

- Slow-growing plaque or nodule on the head of older patients
- The tumor demonstrates both follicular and glandular differentitation
- The islands of basaloid cells with focal squamous differentiation, keratin cyst formation, and focal sweat duct-like lumina formation
- Tendancy for a perivascular and perineural invasion, local recurrence, but rare metastasis
- Mohs micrographic surgery may be considered the treatment of choice

The microcystic adnexal carcinoma typically presents as a slow growing plaque or a nodule on the upper lip, cheeks, or forehead of middle aged to older patients.[98] Ultraviolet radiation and previous radiation therapy may be risk factors.[98,99] There is a tendency for local recurrence but metastases are rare.[100] Histologically, there is evidence of both follicular and glandular differentiation. Small basaloid islands infiltrate the full thickness of the dermis, and may extend down into the subcutaneous fat. The tumor islands are formed by small basaloid cells which may show focal squamous differentiation and keratin cyst formation. Areas of sweat duct-like lumina formation may be seen in the tumor. Tumor lobules may extend into the subcutaneous fat in a perivascular and perineural distribution. The microcystic adnexal carcinoma shows immunoreactivity for cytokeratin, EMA, and CEA. Both follicular and glandular differentiation may be exhibited.[101] The differential diagnosis includes the morpheaform basal cell carcinoma. The microcystic adnexal carcinoma lacks the thickened fibrotic stroma of morpheaform basal cell carcinoma. In addition, the morpheaform basal cell carcinoma typically shows superficial basaloid islands surrounded by clefting and a fibrovascular stroma that is more typical of basal cell carcinoma. The desmoplastic trichoepithelioma may also show small epithelial islands with areas of keratin cyst formation. However, the desmoplastic trichoepithelioma lacks the presence of sweat duct-like structures. Desmoplastic trichoepitheliomas fail to stain with CEA.[101] A superficial biopsy of microcystic adnexal carcinoma may be mistaken for syringoma.

Treatment is by surgical excision or Mohs micrographic surgery.[102] Mohs micrographic surgery may be considered the treatment of choice for microcystic adnexal carcinoma. Garcia reviewed the treatment of MAC with Mohs and found a cure rate of 89% with follow up of at least 2 years as compared to a cure rate of 47% of patients treated with other surgical techniques.[103]

MUCINOUS CARCINOMA

BOX 16-20   Summary

- Slow-growing flesh-colored intradermal nodule on the face of elderly patients
- Small nests and strands of basaloid cells with duct-like lumina surrounded by extensive depositions of acid mucopolysaccharides
- Mild nuclear pleomorphism and scattered mitotic figures
- High local recurrence, but rare metastasis
- Excision with tumor-free margins

The mucinous carcinoma presents as a slow-growing-flesh colored, red or bluish intradermal nodule most commonly on the face of elderly patients. Lesions may occur on the trunk, scalp and axillae. It has a high local recurrence rate; however, metastases are rare.[104] Small nests and strands of basaloid cells are present surrounded by extensive depositions of acid mucopolysaccharides.[104] The tumor islands may appear to be floating within pools of this Alcian blue positive mucin (Fig. 16-23). The pools of mucin are separated by thin septae of fibrocollagenous stroma. The basaloid epithelial islands may show central duct-like lumina. There is a small degree of nuclear pleomorphism with scattered mitotic figures. The histologic findings may resemble those of mucinous carcinoma of the breast. Epithelial nests stain positive for

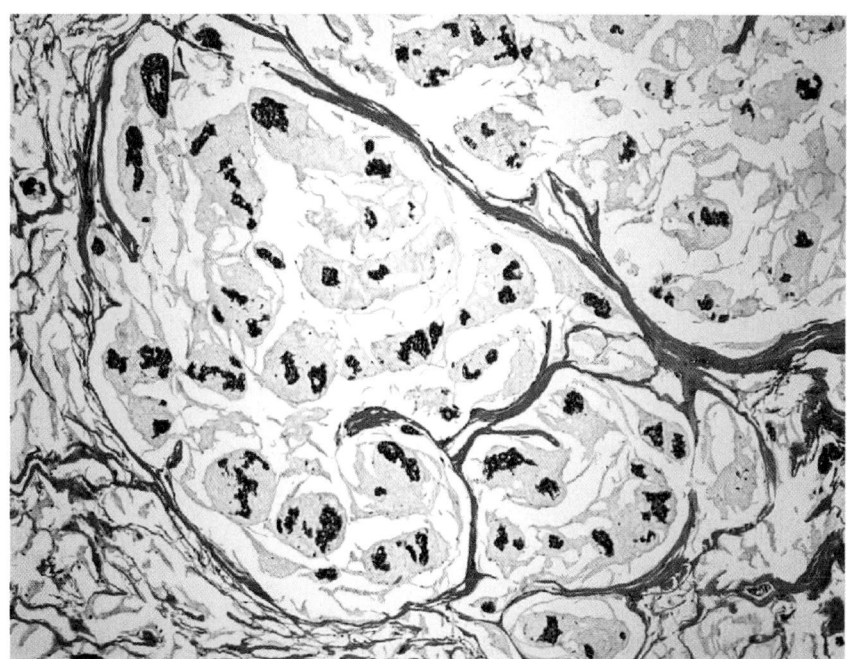

▲ **FIGURE 16-23** Mucinous carcinoma of the skin presenting with an infiltrating neoplasm of small basaloid cells surrounded by abundant mucin.

CEA and cytokeratin 7, 8, 18 and 19 suggestive of eccrine secretory coil differentiation.[105] Focal human milk fat globulin 1 expression is also suggestive of apocrine differentiation.[106] The tumor fails to stain with CK 20 which helps to differentiate it from metastatic gastrointestinal carcinoma.[105] Positive staining to estrogen and progesterone receptor antibodies has been described.[107]

Treatment is by excision with tumor free margins. Excision by Mohs micrographic surgery has been described.[108] Mohs surgery utilizing immunohistochemistry for cytokeratin has also been utilized to enhance sensitivity.[109] Metastases are rare.

ADENOCYSTIC CARCINOMA

BOX 16-21   Summary

- Slow-growing asymptomatic nodule in middle-aged patients on the head and scalp
- Invasive growth of tubular structures into the dermis and subcutis
- Branching dilated tubules lined by a single layer of luminal cells
- Nuclear pleomorphism and mitotic figures
- Surgical excision with free margins

Adenocystic carcinoma is most commonly found in middle aged to elderly patients as a slowly growing asymptomatic papule or nodule.[110] Lesions are most common on the head and scalp

but may be found elsewhere. The adenocystic eccrine carcinoma is a rare variant marked by a histologic pattern of numerous cystic dilated and branching tubular structures.[110] The tubular structures are lined by a single layer of luminal cells. These tubular structures extend into the dermis and subcutaneous fat with an invasive growth pattern. Nuclear pleomorphism and scattered mitotic figures are present. The lumina may contain PAS positive diastase resistant mucin. Immunohistochemical staining reveals the tumor islands to stain for cytokeratin, EMA, and CEA. The differential diagnosis includes the adenocystic basal cell carcinoma.

Treatment is by surgical excision with free margins. Metastases are rare. Mohs micrographic surgery may be useful to decrease the risk of recurrence.[83]

APOCRINE CARCINOMA

BOX 16-22   Summary

- Reddish painless dermal nodule in axilla and genital skin
- Rare association with nevus sebaceus
- Poorly circumscribed, invasive growth of glandular tubular structures
- Nuclear pleomorphism and increased mitotic activity
- Common lymph node metastasis
- Surgical excision and consideration of lymph node dissection

Apocrine carcinomas are rare neoplasms arising in the skin and presenting as reddish to flesh colored painless dermal nodules. These may occur in any anatomic site but are more common in areas rich in apocrine glands such as the axillae and genital skin. Apocrine carcinoma associated with nevus sebaceous has been described.[111] The tumors are more common in elderly and middle aged patients. Histologically the lesions tend to be poorly circumscribed with an invasive growth pattern. Glandular tubular structures ranging from well differentiated to poorly differentiated may be observed. Decapitation secretion is present. The infiltrating growth pattern, nuclear pleomorphism and increased mitotic activity help to differentiate this lesion from benign glandular tumors.

Surgical excision is the treatment of choice. Lymph node metastases are common and therefore therapeutic lymph node dissection may be indicated for confirmed lymph node metastases.[112] Adjuvant radiotherapy has also been described for local disease.[112] A case of recurrent disease has been reported as responding to chemotherapy with bleomycin and methotrexate.[113]

ADNEXAL CARCINOMA

BOX 16-23   Summary

- Poorly differentiated carcinoma showing divergent differentiation
- Islands of basaloid cells taking typical features of basal cell carcinoma
- Squamous metaplasia, follicular differentiation, and sweat duct-like lumina formation
- Deep dermal and subcutaneous involvement
- Common lymph node and distant metastasis
- Surgical excision and consideration of lymph node dissection

Adnexal (pilary complex) carcinomas are poorly differentiated carcinomas showing divergent differentiation.[114] In such cases, islands of basaloid cells lacking typical features of basal cell carcinoma such as palisading of nuclei and retraction spaces may be seen.[114] The basaloid islands extend into the dermis and deep subcutaneous fat. Areas of squamous metaplasia, follicular differentiation, sebaceous differentiation, and sweat duct-like lumina formation suggest a relation to the folliculosebacous apparatus.[114] Similar lesions have been rarely reported in the literature. Extension to local lymph nodes and distant metastasis has been described in these lesions.[114]

DIFFERENTIATION OF ADNEXAL TUMORS FROM METASTASES

A variety of immunohistochemical stains is available to help identify benign and malignant sweat gland tumors. However, as many of these tumors share features with metastatic adenocarcinomas, some caution must be applied. These stains need to be put into clinical and histologic context and the reader should keep in mind that this is an evolving field. p63 is a homologue of p53 which has been identified in the basal cell layer of the epidermis and adnexal structures and plays a role in epithelial development.[115] Six isoforms have been identified which have either transactivating or dominant negative effects on p53 reporter genes.[116] p63 expression has been reported in basal cell carcinoma; however, squamous cell carcinoma shows variable staining. p63 has also been identified in a majority of benign and malignant primary adnexal neoplasms; however, it is rarely present in adenocarcinomas metastatic to the skin.[117] Cytokeratin 5/6 is also more commonly expressed in primary cutaneous neoplasms, including glandular neoplasms, basal cell carcinoma and trichoepithelioma; however, it may also be expressed in a minority of metastatic carcinomas.[118,119] Staining with p63 and CK 5/6 has been reported in metastatic squamous cell carcinoma.[120] Staining of cutaneous metastases of breast carcinoma for estrogen receptors and progesterone receptors can be helpful if the primary lesion is also ER or PR positive.[121] As always, the results of immunohistochemical stains must be interpreted in the context of the histologic features. In difficult cases, a clinical evaluation followed by directed studies to rule out a source for metastases is recommended.

FINAL THOUGHTS

Sweat gland tumors are relatively uncommon neoplasms found in the skin. However, the clinician may encounter these neoplasms in routine practice of dermatology and dermatologic surgery. It is important to recognize the benign sweat gland tumors in order to prevent over-aggressive surgical therapy. An adequate biopsy specimen is crucial for the diagnosis of sweat gland tumors. An adequately biopsied benign sweat gland tumor may not require additional surgical treatment. In contrast, an inadequately biopsied specimen may require re-exicsion to ensure its complete removal and for further histologic review.

Malignant transformation of a benign sweat gland tumor may be observed, although rare. In these cases, rapid growth, ulceration, or bleeding may be observed clinically. Again, adequate biopsy is crucial for diagnosis. Excisional biopsy is recommended. Malignant sweat gland tumors require more aggressive surgical treatment including consideration of wide local excision, Mohs surgery, and possible evaluation for metastasis.

In some cases, differentiation of adnexal neoplasms from metastatic disease may be required. In this case, immunohistochemical staining may be of further utility. These must be interpreted with caution as this represents a continuously evolving field.

REFERENCES

1. Pinkus H. Premalignant Fibroepithelial Tumors of Skin. *Arch Dermat Syph.* June 1953;67:598–615.
2. Hashimoto K, Mehregan AH, Kumakiri M. Tumors of Skin Appendages. *Arch Dermat Syph.* 1987;146.
3. Wong TY, Suster S, Nogita T, Duncan LM, Dickersin RG, Mihm MC Jr. Clear cell eccrine carcinomas of the skin. A Clinicopathologic study of nine patients. *Cancer.* March 1994;73(6):1631–1643.
4. Argenyi ZB, Nguyen AV, Balogh K, Sears JK, Whitaker DC. Malignant eccrine spiradenoma. A Clinicopathologic study. *Am J Dermatopathol.* October 1992;14(5):381–390.
5. Iyer PV, Leong AS. Malignant dermal cylindromas. Do they exist? A morphological and immunohistochemical study and review of the literature. *Pathology.* October 1989;21(4):269–274.
6. Lee HH, Lee KG. Malignant eccrine spiradenoma with florid squamous differentiation. *J Korean Med Sci.* April 1998;13(2):191–195.
7. Veraldi S, Gianotti R, Pabisch S, Gasparini G. Pigmented apocrine hidrocystoma: a report of two cases and review of the literature. *Clin Exp Dermatol.* January 1991;16(1):18–21.
8. Ohnishi T, Watanabe S. Immunohistochemical analysis of cytokeratin expression in multiple eccrine hidrocystoma. *J Cutan Pathol.* February 1999;26(2):91–94.
9. Ohnishi T, Watanabe S. Immunohistochemical analysis of cytokeratin expression in apocrine cystadenoma or hidrocystoma. *J Cutan Pathol.* July 1999;26(6):295–300.
10. Kamishima T, Igarashi S, Takeuchi Y, Ito M, Fukuda T. Pigmented hidrocystoma of the eccrine secretory coil in the vulva: clinicopathologic, immunohistochemical, and Ultrastructural studies. *J Cutan Pathol.* March 1999;26(3):145–149.
11. Dailey RA, Saulny SM, Tower RN. Treatment of multiple apocrine hidrocystomas with trichloroacetic acid. *Ophthal Plast Reconstr Surg.* March 2005;21(2):148–150.
12. Blugerman G, Schavelzon D, D'Angelo S. Multiple eccrine hidrocystomas: a

new therapeutic option with botulinum toxin. *Dermatol Surg.* May 2003;29(5): 557–559.

13. Armstrong DK, Walsh MY, Corbett JR. Multiple facial eccrine hidrocystomas: effective topical therapy with atropine. *Br J Dermatol.* September 1998;139(3): 558–559.

14. Del Pozo J, Garcia-Silva J, Pena-Penabad C, Fonseca E. Multiple apocrine hidrocystomas: treatment with carbon dioxide laser vaporization. *J Dermatolog Treat.* June 2001;12(2):97–100.

15. Tanzi E, Alster TS. Pulsed dye laser treatment of multiple eccrine hidrocystomas: a novel approach. *Dermatol Surg.* October 2001;27(10):898–900

16. Echague AV, Astner S, Chen AA, Anderson RR. Multiple apocrine hidrocystoma of the face treated with a 1450-nm diode laser. *Arch Dermatol.* November 2005;141(11):1365–1367.

17. Baum U, Konigsdorffer E, Bocker T, Strobel J, Wollina U. Argon laser therapy of multiple eccrine cysts of sweat gland efferent ducts (eccrine hidrocystomas). *Klin Monatsbl Augenheilkd.* October 1996;209(4):249–251.

18. Chun K, Vazquez M, Sanchez JL. Nevus sebaceus: clinical outcome and considerations for prophylactic excision. *Int J Dermatol.* August 1995;34(8):538–541.

19. Lee HJ, Chun EY, Kim YC, Lee MG. Nevus comedonicus with hidradenoma papilliferum and syringocystadenoma papilliferum in the female genital area. *Int J Dermatol.* December 2002;41(12):933–936.

20. Ishihara M, Mehregan DR, Hashimoto K, Yotsumoto S, Toi Y, Pietruk T, Mehregan AH, Mehregan DA: staining of eccrine and apocrine neoplasms and metastatic adenocarcinoma with IKH-4, a monoclonal antibody specific for the eccrine gland. *J Cutan Pathol.* February 1998;25(2):100–105.

21. Jordan JA, Brown OE, Biavati MJ, Manning SC. Congenital syringocystadenoma papilliferum of the ear and neck treated with the CO₂ laser. *Int J Pediatr Otorhinolaryngol.* December 5 1996;38(1):81–87.

22. Hügel H, Requena L. Ductal Carcinoma Arising from a Syringocystadenoma Papilliferum in a Nevus Sebaceus of Jadassohn. *Am J Dermatopathol.* December 2003;25:490–493.

23. Chi CC, Tsai RY, Wang SH. Syringocystadenocarcinoma papilliferum: successfully treated with Mohs micrographic surgery. *Dermatol Surg.* March 2004;30(3):468–471.

24. Handa Y, Yamanaka N, Inagaki H, Tomita Y. Large ulcerated perianal hidradenoma papilliferum in a young female. *Dermatol Surg.* July 2003;29(7):790–792.

25. Bannatyne P, Elliott P, Russell P. Vulvar adenosquamous carvcinoma arising in a hidradenoma papilliferum, with rapidly fatal outcome: case report. *Gynecol Oncol.* December 1989;35(3): 395–398.

26. Rosen PP, Caicco JA. Florid papillomatosis of the nipple: a study of 51 patients, including nine with mammary carcinoma. *Am J Surg Pathol.* February 1986;10(2):87–101.

27. Rosen PP. *Rosen's Breast Pathology.* 2nd ed. Philadelphia PA: Lippincott, Williams & Wilkins; 2001:101–110.

28. Lee HJ, Chung KY. Erosive adenomatosis of the nipple: conservation of nipple by Moh's micrographic surgery. *J Am Acad Dermatol.* October 2002;47(4): 578–80.

29. Ahn BK, Park YK, Kim YC. A case of tubular apocrine adenoma with syringocystadenoma papilliferum arising in nevus sebaceus. *J Dermatol.* June 2004;31(6):508–10.

30. Tellechea O, Reis JP, Marques C, Baptista AP. Tubular apocrine adenoma with eccrine and apocrine immunophenotypes or papillary tubular adenoma? *Am J Dermatopathol.* October 1995;17(5): 499–505.

31. Ishiko A, Shimizu H, Inamoto N, Nakmura K. Is tubular apocrine adenoma a distinct clinical entity? *Am J Dermatopathol.* October 1993;15(5): 482–487.

32. Guzzo C, Johnson B. Unusual abdominal location of a dermal cylindroma. *Cutis.* October 1995;56(4):239–240.

33. Bowen S, Gill M, Lee DA, Fisher G, Geronemus RG, Espinel-Vazquez ML, Tok-Celebi J. Mutations in the CYLD gene in Brooke–Spiegler syndrome, familial cylindromatosis, and multiple familial trichoepithelioma: lack of genotype–phenotype Correlation. *J Invest Dermatol.* 2005;124:919–920.

34. Salhi A, Bornholdt D, Oeffner F, Malik S, Heid E, Happle R, Grzeschik KH: Multiple familial trichoepithelioma caused by mutations in the cylindromatosis tumor suppressor gene. *Cancer Res.* August 2004;64(15):5113–5117.

35. Tellechea O, Reis JP, Ilheu O, Baptista AP. Dermal cylindroma. An immunohistochemical study of thirteen cases. *Am J Dermatopathol.* June 1995;17(3): 260–265.

36. Wiley EL, Milchgrub S, Freeman RG, Kim ES. Sweat gland adenomas: immunohistochemical study with emphasis on myoepithelial differentiation. *J Cutan Pathol.* August 1993;20(4):337–343.

37. Meybehm M, Fischer HP. Spiradenoma and dermal cylindroma: comparative immunohistochemical analysis and histogenetic considerations. *Am J Dermatopathol.* April 1997;19(2):154–161.

38. Martins C, Bartolo E. Brooke–Spiegler syndrome: treatment of cylindromas with CO₂ laser. *Dermatol Surg.* September 2000;26(9):877–880.

39. Tarstedt M, Molin L. Nd:YAG laser for effective treatment of multiple cylindroma of the scalp. *J Cosmet Laser Ther.* May 2004;6(1):41–43.

40. Hammond DC, Grant KF, Simpson WD. Malignant degeneration of dermal cylindroma, *Ann Plast Surg.* February 1990;24(2):176–178.

41. Durani BK, Kurzen H, Jaeckel A, Kuner N, Naeher H, Hartschuh W. Malignant transformation of multiple dermal cylindromas. *Br J Dermatol.* October 2001;145(4):653–656.

42. Yoshida A, Sato T, Sugawara Y, Matsuta M, Akasaka T. Two cases of multiple eccrine spiradenoma with linear or localized formation. *J Dermatol.* July 2004; 31(7):564–568.

43. Kazakov DV, Soukup R, Mukensnabl P, Boudova L, Michal M: Brooke–Spiegler syndrome: report of a case with combined lesions containing cylindroma-

tous, spiradenomatous, trichoblastomatous, and sebaceous differentiation. *Am J Dermatopathol.* February 2005;27(1): 27–33.

44. Watanabe S, Hirose M, Sato S, Takahashi H. Immunohistochemical analysis of cytokeratin expression in eccrine spiradenoma: similarities to the transitional portions between secretory segments and coiled ducts of eccrine glands. *Br J Dermatol.* December 1994;131(6): 799–807.

45. Granter SR, Seeger K, Calonje E, Busam K, McKee PH. Malignant eccrine spiradenoma (spiradenocarcinoma): a clinicopathologic study of 12 cases. *Am J Dermatopathol.* April 2000;22(2):97–103.

46. Ishikawa M, Nakanishi Y, Yamazaki N, Yamamoto A. Malignant eccrine spiradenoma: a case report and review of the literature. *Dermatol Surg.* January 2001;27(1):67–70.

47. Herzberg AJ, Elenitsas R, Strohmeyer CR. An unusual case of early malignant transformation in a spiradenoma. *Dermatol Surg.* August 1995;21(8):731–734.

48. Leonard N, Smith D, McNamara P. Low-grade malignant eccrine spiradenoma with systemic metastases. *Am J Dermatopathol.* June 2003;25(3): 253–255.

49. Russ BW, Meffert J, Bernert R. Spiradenocarcinoma of the scalp. *Cutis.* June 2002;69(6):455–458.

50. Pinkus H, Rogin JR, Goldman P. Eccrine Poroma: tumors exhibiting features of the epidermal sweat duct unit. *Am Med Assoc.* 1956;74:511–521.

51. Demirkesen C, Hoede N, Moll R: Epithelial markers and differentiation in adnexal neoplasms of the skin: an immunohistochemical study including individual cytokeratins. *J Cutan Pathol.* December 1995;22(6):518–535.

52. Winkelmann RK, McLeod WA. The Dermal Duct Tumor. *Arch Derm.* July 1966;94:50–55.

53. Jo JH, Chin HW, Kim MB, Oh CK, Jang HS, Kwon KS. A case of eccrine poroma treated with 5% imiquimod cream. *J Dermatol.* August 2005: 32(8):691–693.

54. Komine M, Hattori N, Tamaki K. Eccrine syringofibroadenoma (Mascaro): an immunohistochemical study. *Am J Dermatopathol.* April 2000;22(2):171–175.

55. Ohnishi T, Watanabe S, Nomura K. Immunohistochemical analysis of cytokeratin expression in reactive eccrine syringofibroadenoma-like lesion: a comparative study with eccrine syringofibroadenoma. *J Cutan Pathol.* April 2000; 27(4):164–168.

56. Katane M, Akiyama M, Ohnishi T, Watanabe S, Matsuo I. Carcinomatous transformation of eccrine syringofibroadenoma. *J Cutan Pathol.* Mar 2003; 30(3):211–214.

57. Liu HN, Chang YT, Chen CC. Differentiation of hidroacanthoma simplex from clonal seborrheic keratosis — an immunohistochemical study. *Am J Dermatopathol.* June 2004;26(3):188–193.

58. Rahbari H. Syringoacanthoma. Acanthotic lesion of the acrosyringium. *Arch Dermatol.* June 1984;120(6):751–756.

59. Cribier B, Halna JM, Grosshans E. Mutilating syringoacanthoma. *Dermatology.* 1994;188(2):145–147.

60. Lee WJ, Seo YJ, Yoon JS, et al. Malignant hidroacanthoma simplex: a case report. *J Dermatol.* January 2000;27(1):52–55.

61. Rutten A, Requena L, Requena C. Clear-cell porocarcinoma *in situ*: a cytologic variant of porocarcinoma *in situ*. *Am J Dermatopathol.* February 2002;24(1):67–71.

62. Lee JB, Oh CK, Jang HS, Kim MB, Jang BS, Kwon KS. A case of porocarcinoma from pre-existing hidroacanthoma simplex: need of early excision for hidroacanthoma simplex? *Dermatol Surg.* July 2003;29(7):772–774.

63. Mizuoka H, Senzaki H, Shikata N, Uemura Y, Tsubura A. Papillary eccrine adenoma: immunohistochemical study and literature review. *J Cutan Pathol.* January 1998;25(1):59–64.

64. Ichikawa E, Okabe S, Umebayashi Y, Iijima S, Otsuka F, Watanabe S. Papillary eccrine adenoma: immunohistochemical studies of keratin expression. *J Cutan Pathol.* October 1997;24(9):564–570.

65. Tsunemi Y, Ihn H, Saeki H, Tamaki K. Generalized eruptive syringoma. *Pediatr Dermatol.* September/October 2005;22(5):492–493.

66. Jacobs S, Grussendorf-Conen EI. Disseminated eruptive syringomas in Down syndrome, *Hautarzt.* January 2004;55(1):70–72.

67. Timpanidis PC, Lakhani SR, Groves RW. Progesterone receptor-positive eruptive syringoma associated with diabetes. *J Am Acad Dermatol.* May 2003;48(5 suppl):S103–S104.

68. Ohnishi T, Watanabe S. Immunohistochemical analysis of keratin expression in clear cell syringoma. A comparative study with conventional syringoma. *J Cutan Pathol.* July 1997;24(6):370–376.

69. Eckert F, Nilles M, Schmid U, Altmannsberger M. Distribution of cytokeratin polypeptides in syringomas. An immunohistochemical study on paraffin-embedded material. *Am J Dermatopathol.* April 1992;14(2):115–121.

70. Karam P, Benedetto AV. Intralesional electrodesiccation of syringomas. *Dermatol Surg.* October 1997;23(10):921–924.

71. Stevenson TR, Swanson NA. Syringoma: removal by electrodesiccation and curettage. *Ann Plast Surg.* August 1985;15(2):151–154.

72. Frazier CC, Camacho AP, Cockerell CJ. The treatment of eruptive syringomas in an African American patient with a combination of trichloroacetic acid and CO_2 laser destruction. *Dermatol Surg.* May 2001;27(5):489–492.

73. Wang JI, Roenigk HH Jr. Treatment of multiple facial syringomas with the carbon dioxide (CO_2) laser. *Dermatol Surg.* February 1999;25(2):136–139.

74. Riedel F, Windberger J, Stein E, Hormann K. Treatment of peri-ocular skin lesions with the erbium: YAG laser. *Ophthalmologe.* November 1998;95(11):771–775.

75. Chen AH, Moreano EH, Houston B, Funk GF. Chondroid syringoma of the head and neck: clinical management and literature review. *Ear Nose Throat J.* February 1996;75(2):104–108.

76. Ohnishi T, Watanabe S. Histogenesis of mixed tumor of the skin, apocrine type: immunohistochemical study of keratin expression. *Am J Dermatopathol.* October 1997;19(5):456–461.

77. Matz LR, McCully DJ, Stokes BA. Metastasizing chondroid syringoma: case report. *Pathology.* January 1969;1(1):77–81.

78. Takahashi H, Ishiko A, Kobayashi M, Tanikawa A, Takasu H, Md MT. Malignant chondroid syringoma with bone invasion: a case report and review of the literature. *Am J Dermatopathol.* October 2004;26(5):403–406.

79. Steinmetz JC, Russo BA, Ginsburg RE. Malignant chondroid syringoma with widespread metastasis. *J Am Acad Dermatol.* May 1990;22(5 pt 1):845–847.

80. Ohnishi T, Watanabe S. Histogenesis of clear cell hidradenoma: immunohistochemical study of keratin expression. *J Cutan Pathol.* January 1997;24(1):30–36.

81. Volmar KE, Cummings TJ, Wang WH, Creager AJ, Tyler DS, Xie HB. Clear cell hidradenoma: a mimic of metastatic clear cell tumors. *Arch Pathol Lab Med.* May 2005;129(5):e113–e116.

82. Engel A, Bar-Dayan Y, Engelberg S, Levi Y. Malignant nodular hidradenoma—sweat gland tumor. *Harefuah.* May 1999;136(9):683–686, 755.

83. Wildemore JK, Lee JB, Humphreys TR. Mohs' surgery for malignant eccrine neoplasms. *Dermatol Surg.* 2004;30:1574–1579.

84. Kao GF, Helwig EB, Graham JH. Aggressive digital papillary adenoma and adenocarcinoma. A clinicopathological study of 57 patients, with histochemical, immunopathological, and ultrastructural observations. *J Cutan Pathol.* 1987;14:129–146.

85. Altman CE, Hamill RL, Elston DM. Metastatic aggressive digital papillary adenocarcinoma. *Cutis.* August 2003;72(2):145–147.

86. Inaloz HS, Patel GK, Knight AG. An aggressive treatment for aggressive digital papillary adenocarcinoma. *Cutis.* March 2002;69(3):179–182 (Quiz 210).

87. Pinkus H, Mehregan AH. Epidermotropic Eccrine Carcinoma: a case combining features of eccrine poroma and Paget's dermatosis. *Arch Dermatol.* Nov 1963;88:597–606.

88. Johr R, Saghari S, Nouri K. Eccrine porocarcinoma arising in a seborrheic keratosis evaluated with dermoscopy and treated with Mohs' technique. *Int J Dermatol.* August 2003;42(8):653–657.

89. de Bree E, Volalakis E, Tsetis D, Varthalitis Y, Panagiotidis J, Romanos J, Tsiftsis DD. Treatment of advanced malignant eccrine poroma with locoregional chemotherapy. *Br J Dermatol.* May 2005;152(5):1051–1055.

90. Barzi AS, Ruggeri S, Recchia F, Bertoldi I. Malignant metastatic eccrine poroma. Proposal for a new therapeutic protocol. *Dermatol Surg.* April 1997;23(4):267–272.

91. Huet P, Dandurand M, Pignodel C, Guillot B. Metastasizing eccrine porocarcinoma: report of a case and review of the literature. *J Am Acad Dermatol.* November 1996;35(5 pt 2):860–864.

92. Plunkett TA, Hanby AM, Miles DW, Rubens RD. Metastatic eccrine porocarcinoma: response to docetaxel (Taxotere) chemotherapy. *Ann Oncol.* Mar 2001;12(3):411–414.

93. Ohnishi T, Kaneko S, Egi M, Takizawa H, Watanabe S. Syringoid eccrine carcinoma: report of a case with immunohistochemical analysis of cytokeratin expression. *Am J Dermatopathol.* 2002;24(5):409–413.

94. Weber PJ, Gretzula JC, Garland LD, Hevia O, Menn H. Syringoid eccrine carcinoma. *J Dermatol Surg Oncol.* January 1987;13(1):64–67.

95. Swanson PE, Cherwitz DL, Neumann MP, Wick MR. Eccrine sweat gland carcinoma: an histologic and immunohistochemical study of 32 cases. *J Cutan Pathol.* April 1987;14(2):65–86.

96. Rye PD, Walker RA. Prognostic value of a breast cancer-associated glycoprotein detected by monoclonal antibody LU-BCRU-G7. *Eur J Cancer.* 1994;30A(7):1007–1012.

97. Moy RL, Rivkin JE, Lee H, Brooks WS, Zitelli JA. Syringoid eccrine carcinoma. *J Am Acad Dermatol.* 1991;24:857–859.

98. Abbate M, Zeitouni NC, Seyler M, Hicks W, Loree T, Cheney RT. Clinical course, risk factors, and treatment of microcystic adnexal carcinoma: a short series report. *Dermatol Surg.* October 2003;29(10):1035–1038.

99. Stein JM, Ormsby A, Esclamado R, Bailin P. The effect of radiation therapy on microcystic adnexal carcinoma: a case report. *Head Neck.* March 2003;25(3):251–254.

100. Ban M, Sugie S, Kamiya H, Kitajima Y. Microcystic adnexal carcinoma with lymph node metastasis. *Dermatology.* 2003;207:395–397.

101. Wick MR, Cooper PH, Swanson PE, Kaye VN, Sun TT: Microcystic adnexal carcinoma. An immunohistochemical comparison with other cutaneous appendage tumors. *Arch Dermatol.* February 1990;126(2):189–194.

102. Khachemoune A, Olbricht SM, Johnson DS. Microcystic adnexal carcinoma: report of four cases treated with Mohs' micrographic surgical technique. *Int J Dermatol.* June 2005;44(6):507–512.

103. Garcia C, Holman J, Poletti E. Mohs' surgery: commentaries and controversies, *Int J Dermatol.* 2005;44:893–905.

104. Weber PJ, Hevia O, Gretzula JC, Rabinovitz HC. Primary mucinous carcinoma. *J Dermatol Surg Oncol.* February 1988;14(2):170–172.

105. Eckert F, Schmid U, Hardmeier T, Altmannsberger M. Cytokeratin expression in mucinous sweat gland carcinomas: an immunohistochemical analysis of four cases. *Histopathology.* August 1992;21(2):161–165.

106. Ohnishi T, Takizawa H, Watanabe S. Immunohistochemical analysis of cytokeratin and human milk fat globulin expression in mucinous carcinoma of the skin. *J Cutan Pathol.* January 2002;29(1):38–43.

107. Bellezza G, Sidoni A, Bucciarelli E. Primary mucinous carcinoma of the skin. *Am J Dermatopathol.* April 2000;22(2):166–170.

108. Bindra M, Keegan DJ, Guenther T, Lee V. Primary cutaneous mucinous carcinoma of the eyelid in a young male. *Orbit.* September 2005;24(3):211–214.

109. Marra DE, Schanbacher CF, Torres A. Mohs' micrographic surgery of primary cutaneous mucinous carcinoma using immunohistochemistry for margin

control. *Dermatol Surg.* May 2004;30(5): 799–802.

110. Adamski H, Le Lan J, Chevrier S, Cribier B, Watier E, Chevrant-Breton J. Primary cutaneous cribriform carcinoma: a rare apocrine tumour. *J Cutan Pathol.* September 2005;32(8):577–580.

111. Dalle S, Skowron F, Balme B, Perrot H. Apocrine carcinoma developed in nevus sebaceus of Jadassohn. *Eur J Dermatol.* September/October 2003;13(5):487–489.

112. Chamberlain RS, Huber K, White JC, Travaglino-Parda R. Apocrine gland carcinoma of the axilla: review of the literature and recommendations for treatment. *Am J Clin Oncol.* April 1999; 22(2):131–135.

113. Morabito A, Bevilacqua P, Vitale S, Fanelli M, Gattuso D, Gasparini G. Clinical management of a case of recurrent apocrine gland carcinoma of the scalp: efficacy of a chemotherapy schedule with methotrexate and bleomycin.

Tumori. November/December 2000; 86(6):472–474.

114. Rahbari H, Mehregan AH. Pilary complex carcinoma: an adnexal carcinoma of the skin with differentiation towards the components of the pilary complex. *J Dermatol.* October 1993;20(10):630–637.

115. Dellavalle RP, Walsh P, Marchbank A, et al. CUSP/p63 expression in basal cell carcinoma. *Exp Dermatol.* June 2002; 11(3):203–208.

116. Reis-Filho JS, Torio B, Albergaria A, Schmitt FC. p63 expression in normal skin and usual cutaneous carcinomas. *J Cutan Pathol.* October 2002;29(9):517–523.

117. Ivan D, Hafeez Diwan A, Prieto VG. Expression of p63 in primary cutaneous adnexal neoplasms and adenocarcinoma metastatic to the skin. *Mod Pathol.* January 2005;18(1):137–42.

118. Qureshi HS, Ormsby AH, Lee MW, Zarbo RJ, Ma CK. The diagnostic utility of p63, CK5/6, CK7, and CK20 in dis-

tinguishing primary cutaneous adnexal neoplasms from metastatic carcinomas. *J Cutan Pathol.* February 2004;31(2): 145–152.

119. Plumb SJ, Argenyi ZB, Stone MS, DeYoung BR. Cytokeratin 5/6 immunostaining in cutaneous adnexal neoplasms and metastatic adenocarcinoma. *Am J Dermatopathol.* December 2004;26(6):447–451.

120. Kaufmann O, Fietze E, Mengs J, Dietel M. Value of p63 and cytokeratin 5/6 as immunohistochemical markers for the differential diagnosis of poorly differentiated and undifferentiated carcinomas. *Am J Clin Pathol.* December 2001;116(6): 823–830.

121. O'Connell FP, Wang HH, Odze RD. Utility of immunohistochemistry in distinguishing primary adenocarcinomas from metastatic breast carcinomas in the gastrointestinal tract. *Arch Pathol Lab Med.* Mar 2005;129(3):338–347.

CHAPTER 17

Sebaceous Carcinoma

Paul T. Martinelli, M.D.
Philip R. Cohen, M.D.
Keith E. Schulze, M.D.
Jaime A. Tschen, M.D.
Bruce R. Nelson, M.D.

BOX 17-1 Overview

- Sebaceous gland carcinoma is a rare aggressive skin cancer derived from the adnexal epithelium of sebaceous glands.
- Sebaceous carcinomas are generally divided into those occurring in ocular or extraocular locations.
- Ocular sebaceous carcinomas occur most commonly in the elderly with a predilection for females and Asian populations; they often resemble a chalazion or other chronic inflammatory conditions clinically, leading to a delay in diagnosis.
- Extraocular sebaceous carcinomas can arise on any area of the body with sebaceous glands, but present most frequently on the head and neck; they also occur most commonly in the elderly but without a racial or gender preference.
- Histologically, sebaceous carcinomas may exhibit basaloid or squamous differentiation, necessitating the use of special stains, immunohistochemical, or ultrastructural studies; clinicopathologic correlation is essential.
- Pagetoid intraepithelial spread is also common with sebaceous carcinomas.
- At the genetic level, loss of cell cycle control may contribute to the pathogenesis of sebaceous carcinomas.
- Sebaceous carcinomas have a significant risk of local recurrence, as well as regional or distant metastases.
- Current accepted treatment modalities include Mohs micrographic surgery or standard excision with frozen section control, with or without conjunctival map biopsies.
- Sebaceous gland neoplasms, including sebaceous carcinomas, may be associated with the Muir-Torre syndrome, an autosomal dominantly inherited genodermatosis with malignant potential.

INTRODUCTION

BOX 17-2 Summary

- Sebaceous carcinoma is a rare aggressive cutaneous malignancy.
- The ocular region, particularly the upper eyelid, is the most common location for sebaceous carcinomas to develop.
- The tumor frequently exhibits diverse clinical presentations and histologic patterns, often resulting in a delay in an accurate diagnosis.
- Noncontiguous multicentric histologic patterns and pagetoid spread of tumor cells are common and may contribute to the high recurrence rate of sebaceous carcinoma.
- Mohs micrographic surgery or standard excision with frozen section control represents the current mainstays of therapy.

Sebaceous gland carcinoma, also called meibomian gland carcinoma, is a rare aggressive malignant tumor derived from the adnexal epithelium of sebaceous glands. Sebaceous carcinoma may occur in either ocular or extraocular locations; the ocular region, particularly the upper eyelid, is the most common site of occurrence. This malignancy most frequently arises from the meibomian glands of the tarsi, but can also arise from the sebaceous glands of Zeis, the sebaceous glands within the caruncle and brow, and from the pilosebaceous apparatus associated with fine hair follicles located on the cutaneous surface of the eyelids and the lacrimal gland. The tumor may exhibit a myriad of clinical presentations and diverse histologic patterns, accounting for an initial misdiagnosis in approximately 50% of cases.[1] Although most cases of sebaceous carcinoma represent sporadic occurrences, the tumor may also present in the setting of the Muir-Torre syndrome,[2] and the diagnosis of a sebaceous carcinoma should prompt consideration of this genodermatosis, especially in the context of other sebaceous neoplasms or internal malignancies.

Although individual cases of sebaceous carcinoma were reported in the late 1800s, Straatsma's detailed clinical and histologic evaluation of 16 patients with sebaceous carcinoma in 1956 helped initiate a very concise and comprehensive study of this entity.[3] Since then, multiple large series and critical reviews[1,4–12] have furthered the understanding of sebaceous carcinoma and have led to its acceptance as a unique clinical and pathologic entity. Sebaceous carcinoma of the eyelid is rare in the United States and comprises 0.2 to 4.7% of malignant eyelid neoplasms[1,6,13]; however, there is a notably higher incidence of this tumor in Asian series.[14] Adequate treatment of sebaceous carcinoma is often difficult, and recurrence is common, perhaps due to a delay in initial diagnosis or a possible noncontiguous multicentric histologic pattern. Mohs micrographic surgery or standard excision with frozen section control, with or without conjunctival map biopsies, appear to represent the current standard of care.[15]

STRUCTURE AND FUNCTION OF NORMAL SEBACEOUS GLANDS

BOX 17-3 Summary

- Sebaceous glands are most numerous on the head and neck, but may be located in any hair-bearing region of the body.
- The ocular adnexae contain six types of sebaceous glands: meibomian glands in the tarsal plate, glands of Zeis associated with eyelash follicles, and sebaceous glands of the eyebrow, caruncle, lacrimal gland, and those associated with the fine hair follicles on the skin.
- The greater number of meibomian glands in the upper eyelid explains the predilection of sebaceous carcinoma for this site.

Sebaceous glands are most numerous on the skin of the head and neck, but may be found on any hair-bearing region of the body. They are associated with hair follicles and comprise a portion of the pilosebaceous unit. Each sebaceous gland possesses one to several sebaceous lobules leading to a common excretory duct composed of stratified squamous epithelium. Each lobule possesses a peripheral layer of deeply basophilic cells with no lipid droplets, and the more centrally located cells contain lipid droplets which can be detected with fat stains on frozen sections.[16]

Sebaceous glands are derived from the embryonal stratum germanitivum and are well-developed at birth. Ectopic sebaceous glands not associated with hair follicles may be found on the vermillion border of the lips and buccal mucosa (Fordyce's condition), the nipple and areola (Montgomery's areolar tubercles), as well as on the labia minora and inner aspect of the prepuce (Tyson's glands).[16] Furthermore, sebaceous differentiation in the parotid gland is also a well-described phenomenon which explains the possible presence of sebaceous tumors in this location.[17] The ocular adnexa contains six types of sebaceous glands: meibomian glands within the tarsal plate, Zeis glands associated with eyelash follicles, sebaceous glands of the eyebrow, sebaceous glands of the caruncle, and sebaceous glands associated with the fine hair follicles on the skin of the eyelids and lacrimal gland.[18,19]

The meibomian glands are modified sebaceous glands not associated with hair follicles that are located in the tarsal plates of the upper and lower eyelids. The upper eyelid contains a greater number of meibomian glands than does the lower eyelid, helping to explain the preferential involvement of the upper eyelid by sebaceous carcinoma. The glands are embedded in a single row along the length of the tarsal plates and may be visible through the conjunctiva by eversion of the lids. As they are not associated with a hair follicle, meibomian glands secrete sebum in a holocrine manner directly into a central meibomian duct that emerges onto the lid margin. This duct is lined by a stratified squamous epithelium that keratinizes in a trichilemmal fashion, helping to explain the squamous features sometimes noted histologically within sebaceous carcinomas. The secreted sebum forms the outermost layer of the precorneal tear film which helps stabilize the tear film and prevent evaporation of the underlying aqueous layer.[20]

EPIDEMIOLOGY

BOX 17-4   Summary

- Sebaceous carcinoma is the fourth most common eyelid malignancy, representing 0.2 to 5.5% of all eyelid cancers.
- The incidence of ocular sebaceous carcinoma is greater in Asian populations.
- Ocular sebaceous carcinoma typically affects adults in their sixth to eighth decades of life, and is more common in women.
- Extraocular sebaceous carcinoma most commonly arises in the head and neck region, occurs with greatest frequency in older adults, and does not exhibit a predilection for men or women.

Ocular sebaceous carcinoma is uncommon in the Western world, comprising only approximately 0.2 to 5.5% of all malignant eyelid neoplasms.[1,6,13,21] Sebaceous carcinoma is, however, the fourth most common eyelid malignancy, with basal cell carcinoma representing the most frequent malignant eyelid tumor, followed then by squamous cell carcinoma, and malignant melanoma.[8,22] Interestingly, the incidence of sebaceous carcinoma in the Asian population seems to be significantly higher. Three large series from Shanghai and Singapore reported that sebaceous carcinoma comprised approximately 10 to 34% of all eyelid malignancies and was second only to basal cell carcinoma in frequency.[9,14,23] A retrospective study of 207 eyelid tumors at a center in India also reported sebaceous carcinoma as the second most common eyelid malignancy, comprising 27% of malignant eyelid tumors in their series.[24] The reason for this apparent regional predilection has not been explained.

Ocular sebaceous carcinoma tends to occur in older adults 60 to 80 years of age; summarization of the data of several large series shows that the mean age of onset ranges between 57 and 75 years.[8,9,12–14,22] There are also reports of ocular sebaceous carcinoma developing in children after radiation therapy for retinoblastoma.[12,25] The incidence of sebaceous carcinoma appears to be somewhat greater in women and ranges between 57 and 77%.[4]

Extraocular sebaceous carcinoma also occurs most frequently in older individuals, usually in the sixth to seventh decades of life. However, as opposed to the female predilection seen in the ocular variant, extraocular sebaceous carcinoma is seen almost equally in men and women. The most common extraorbital site is the face and neck where sebaceous glands are the most numerous.

CLINICAL PRESENTATION

BOX 17-5   Summary

- Ocular sebaceous carcinoma typically presents as a small erythematous or yellowish, firm, deep-seated, slowly enlarging papule on the upper eyelid.
- Ocular sebaceous carcinoma may be indistinguishable from a chalazion, and when intraepidermal spread onto the conjunctiva is present, can be confused with keratoconjunctivitis or blepharoconjunctivitis.
- Given the varied clinical presentations of ocular sebaceous carcinoma, the mean delay from disease onset to diagnosis ranges from approximately 1 to 3 years.

- Approximately 25% of sebaceous carcinomas arise in extraocular sites, most commonly on the head and neck.
- The clinical appearance of extraocular sebaceous carcinomas is nondiagnostic, and usually presents as a pink to red-yellow nodule.
- Although generally believed to be less aggressive than their ocular counterparts, extraocular sebaceous carcinomas have the potential for local or distant metastases.

Ocular Sebaceous Carcinoma

Although sebaceous carcinoma has the potential to develop from any sebaceous gland in the body, it most commonly arises from the meibomian glands. Several large series confirmed that ocular sebaceous carcinoma arose from the meibomian glands in 51 to 70% of cases examined; 12 to 24% were found to be multicentric in origin; and 4 to 10% arose from the glands of Zeiss; the remainder originated from the caruncle or orbit.[8,9]

The clinical presentations of ocular sebaceous carcinoma are diverse and may delay an accurate diagnosis for months to years. The mean delay from onset of disease to diagnosis has been reported to be 1 to 2.9 years.[4] Upper eyelid lesions are two to three times more common than lower eyelid lesions, probably reflecting the greater number of meibomian glands in the tarsal plate of the upper eyelid.[1,6–8,12] The most common clinical presentation is a small, erythematous or possibly yellowish, slowly enlarging, firm, deep-seated papule or nodule on the upper eyelid that may be indistinguishable from that of a chalazion (Figs. 17-1 and 17-2). Chalazions, caused by inflammation of the meibomian glands or glands of Zeiss, are the most common cause of painless granulomatous inflammation of the eyelids and represent the most common clinical misdiagnosis of sebaceous carcinoma. Eventual distortion and ulceration of the eyelid may occur as the initial lesion extends beyond the tarsus.

If pagetoid or intraepithelial spread onto the conjunctiva occurs, the presentation is consistent with keratoconjunctivits or blepharoconjunctivitis, which is typically unilateral but may also occasionally be bilateral. Advanced cases with extensive pagetoid spread may result in the loss of lid lashes, eyelid eversion, erosion and ulceration, or gross ocular distortion.[6,9] Pagetoid spread may be very extensive and

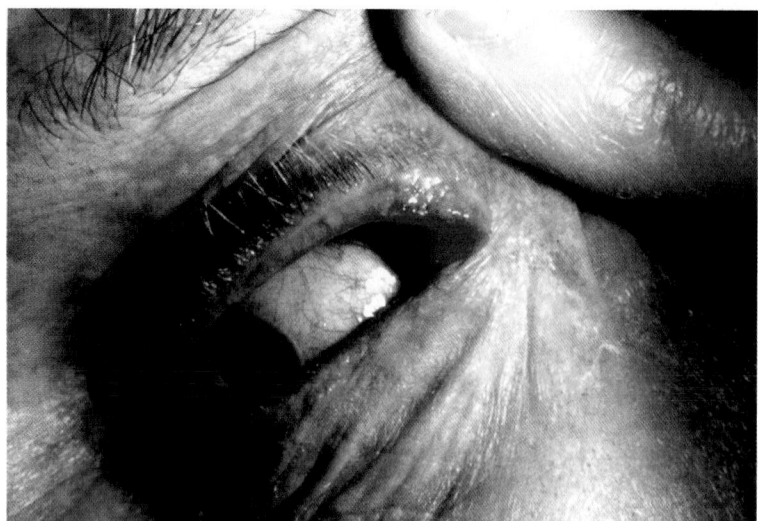

▲ **FIGURE 17-1** Sebaceous carcinoma of the left upper eyelid. The upper eyelid is the most common location for sebaceous carcinoma to develop. Note the clinical resemblance to a chalazion. (*Source:* Nelson BR, Hamlet KR, Gillard M, Railan D, Johnson TM. Sebaceous carcinoma. J Am Acad Dermatol 1995;33:1–15; reprinted with permission.)

extend well beyond clinically apparent tumor. A recent report documents the pagetoid spread of a lesion initially misdiagnosed as chronic blepharoconjunctivitis along the nasolacrimal duct, eventually producing a tumor involving the entire right nasal cavity.[26]

Numerous other inflammatory conditions, autoimmune diseases, infectious processes, and neoplasms may clinically mimic sebaceous carcinoma of the eyelid (Table 17-1). Given the myriad and diverse clinical presentations of ocular sebaceous carcinoma, a high degree of suspicion and ultimate biopsy of nonhealing lesions is critical in making the correct diagnosis. Indeed, in some unfortunate cases, a diagnosis was made only after metastases to the regional lymph node basin or parotid gland were detected.[26–28]

Extraocular Sebaceous Carcinoma

Approximately 25% of all reported cases of sebaceous carcinoma are extraocular in origin.[29] The clinical appearance of these tumors is nondiagnostic; they typically present as a pink to red-yellow nodule, 6 mm to 20 cm in diameter. Since the head and neck region contains the highest density of sebaceous glands in the body, extraocular carcinomas occur most commonly in this location (Figs. 17-3 to 17-5). Other reported locations of extraocular sebaceous carcinoma include the external genitalia, the parotid and submandibular glands, the external auditory canal, the trunk, the extremities, the laryngeal and pharyngeal cavities, the uterine cervix and ovaries, the nasal vestibule, the oral mucosa, and within an existing nevus sebaceus[4,30–38] There is also a report of a sebaceous carcinoma presenting as an endobronchial neoplasm within the left lower lobe of the lung[39]; metastatic disease was ruled out after an exhaustive search for another primary tumor. Interestingly, sebaceous tissue is not normally found in the distal trachea or bronchus, and although unlikely, the authors acknowledge that the neoplasm may represent metaplasia of salivary gland-like tissue. Although extraocular sebaceous carcinomas are generally viewed as less locally aggressive with a reduced tendency to metastasize than are the ocular tumors, there have been reports of local and regional as well as distant visceral metastases with this malignancy.[40–42]

Table 17-1

Clinical Differential Diagnosis of Sebaceous Carcinoma

Chalazion
Hordeolum
Keratoconjunctivitis
Blepharoconjunctivitis
Papillary conjunctivitis
Pyogenic granuloma
Ocular pemphigoid
Sarcoidosis
Granulomatous inflammation from syphilis or tuberculosis
Central retinal artery occlusion and proptosis
Exophthalmos
Other neoplasms
- Squamous cell carcinoma (*in situ* or invasive)
- Basal cell carcinoma
- Cutaneous horn
- Conjunctival carcinoma *in situ*
- Merkel cell carcinoma
- Benign adnexal neoplasms
- Metastatic tumors

HISTOPATHOLOGY

BOX 17-6   Summary

- Routine H&E-stained sections reveal a poorly circumscribed dermal-based tumor with variable sebaceous differentiation.
- Vacuolated cells demonstrate abundant lipid when frozen sections are stained with oil red O or Sudan black.

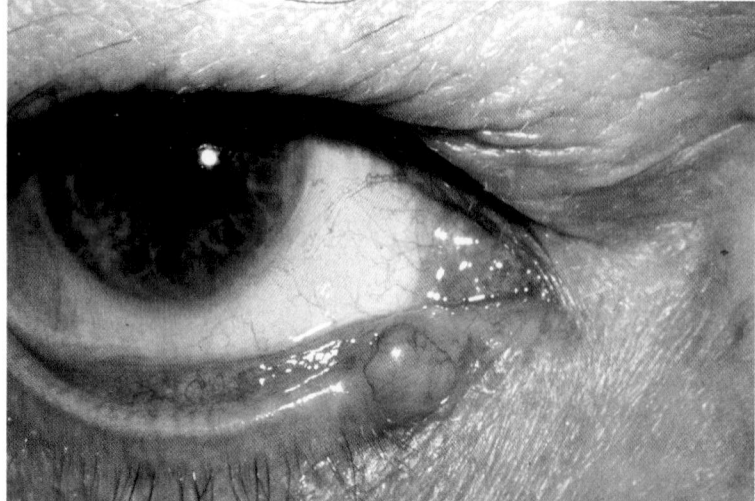

▲ **FIGURE 17-2** Sebaceous carcinoma presenting as a pink telangiectatic papule on the right medial lower eyelid. (*Source:* Nelson BR, Hamlet KR, Gillard M, Railan D, Johnson TM. Sebaceous carcinoma. J Am Acad Dermatol 1995;33:1–15; reprinted with permission.)

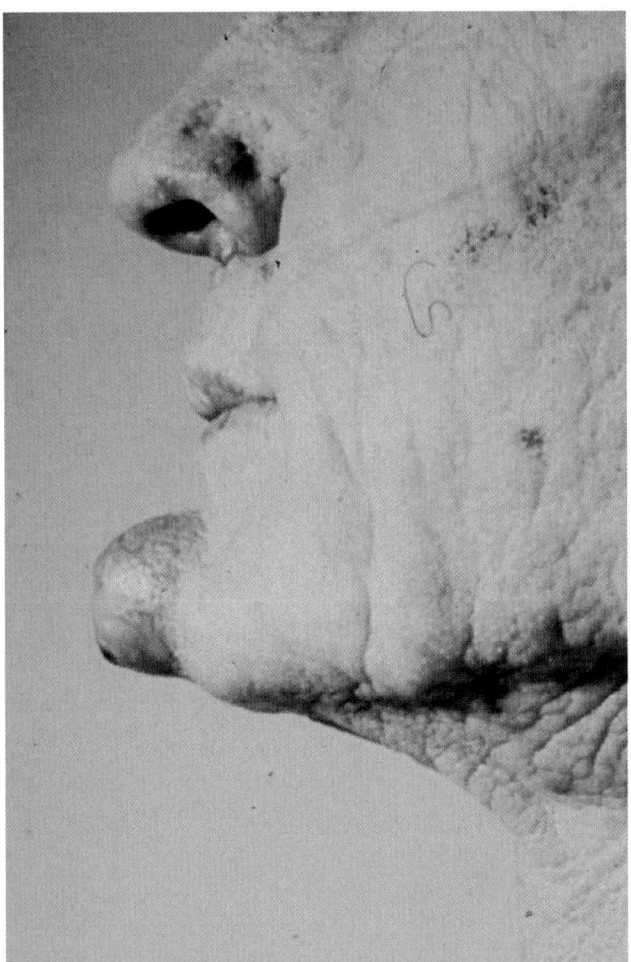

▲ **FIGURE 17-3** Extraocular sebaceous carcinoma presenting as a large tumor on this patient's chin. (*Source:* Nelson BR, Hamlet KR, Gillard M, Railan D, Johnson TM. Sebaceous carcinoma. J Am Acad Dermatol 1995;33:1–15; reprinted with permission).

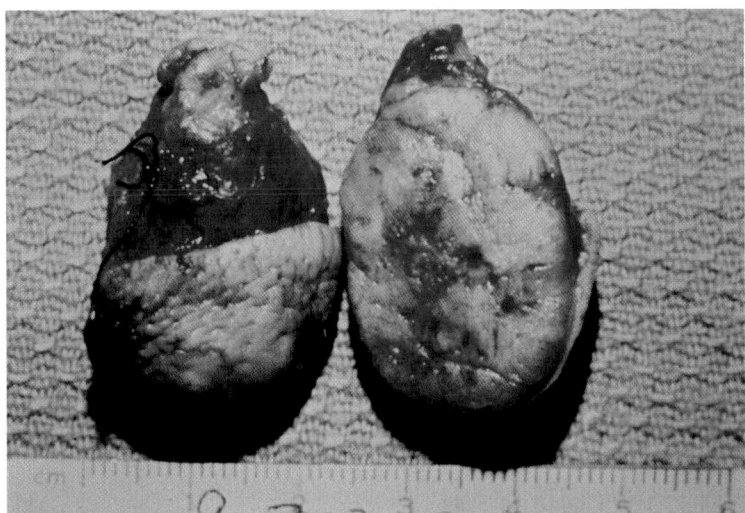

▲ **FIGURE 17-4** Gross appearance of biopsy specimen of extraocular sebaceous carcinoma from the chin. Note the yellowish hue of the tumor nodule. (*Source:* Nelson BR, Hamlet KR, Gillard M, Railan D, Johnson TM. Sebaceous carcinoma. J Am Acad Dermatol 1995;33:1–15; reprinted with permission.)

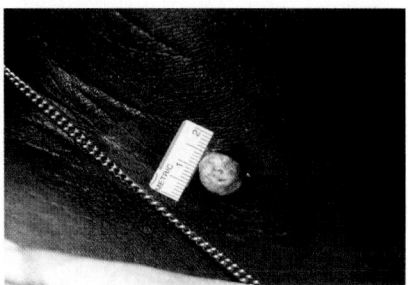

▲ **FIGURE 17-5** Extraocular sebaceous carcinoma presenting as an erythematous nodule on the right lateral neck.

- Approximately 50% of ocular sebaceous carcinomas demonstrate pagetoid spread of malignant cells.
- Tumor cells stain positively for EMA and androgen receptors, but negatively for CEA and S100 protein.
- Poor histologic prognostic factors include vascular and lymphatic invasion, poor differentiation, an infiltrative growth pattern, and large tumor size.
- Sebaceous carcinomas may exhibit basaloid or squamous differentiation, making histologic diagnosis more difficult; clinicopathologic correlation is essential.

Routine hematoxylin and eosin (H&E)-stained permanent sections demonstrate a poorly circumscribed dermal-based tumor with variably sized lobules or sheets of cells separated by a fibrovascular stroma. The cells show variable sebaceous differentiation, characterized by finely vacuolated or foamy cytoplasm (Fig. 17-6). There is typically more differentiation in the center of the nests. The vacuolated cells demonstrate abundant lipid if a frozen section is stained with oil red O or Sudan black. The nuclei are large with large nucleoli and scattered mitoses. Focal necrosis may be seen within tumor lobules resulting in a comedo-carcinoma pattern (Fig. 17-7).[7] The tumor may extend deeply and often involves the subcutaneous tissue or possibly even the underlying muscle. Adverse prognostic factors include vascular and lymphatic invasion, orbital extension, poor differentiation, an infiltrative growth pattern, and large tumor size.[16,43]

Approximately 50% of ocular sebaceous carcinomas demonstrate pagetoid spread of malignant cells in the conjunctival epithelium, the epidermis of the eyelid skin, or both[8] (Figs. 17-8 and 17-9). The pagetoid cells stain positively for fat with oil red O. It is thought that tumor cells may reach the epidermis from the

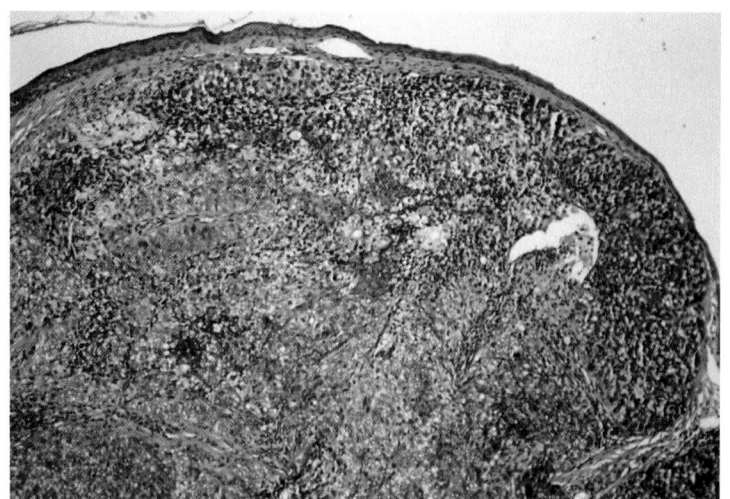

▲ **FIGURE 17-6** Microscopic examination of sebaceous carcinoma shows a dermal nodule with lobules and sheets of basaloid cells with foamy cytoplasm (H&E, 4×).

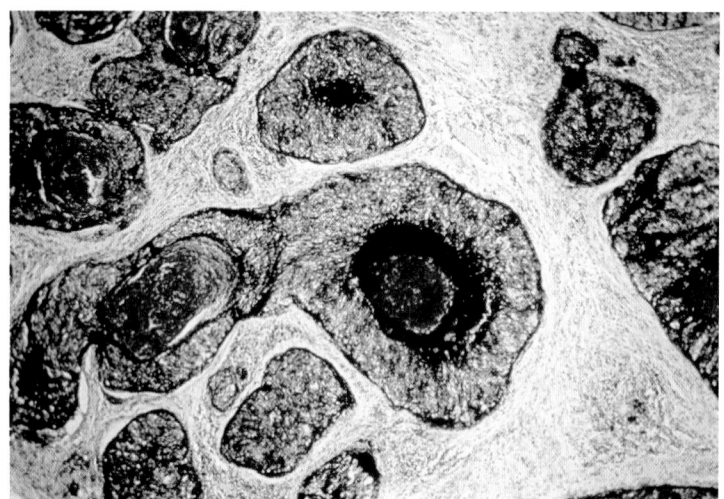

▲ **FIGURE 17-7** Comedo-carcinoma growth pattern with central necrosis and oil red O-positive staining (20×). (*Source:* Nelson BR, Johnson TM. Sebaceous carcinoma. In: Maloney M, Hoffman T, Torres A, eds. Surgical Dermatopathology. Cambridge, UK: Blackwell Scientific Publications, Inc. 1999; reprinted with permission.)

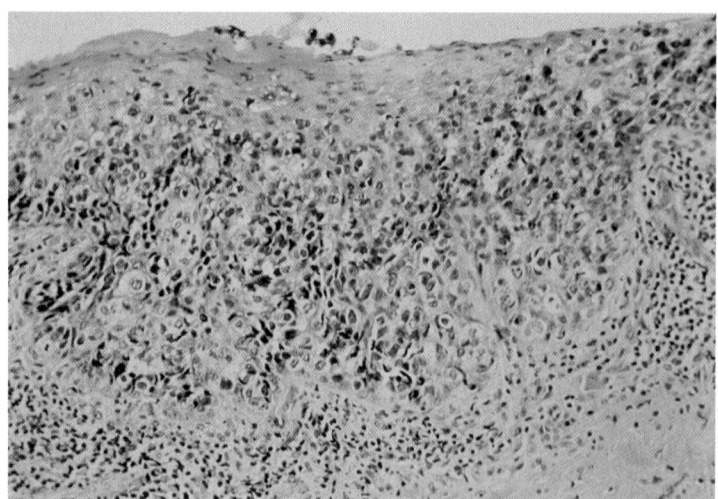

▲ **FIGURE 17-8** Sebaceous carcinoma with intraepidermal pagetoid features. (H&E, 10×). (*Source:* Nelson BR, Hamlet KR, Gillard M, Railan D, Johnson TM. Sebaceous carcinoma. J Am Acad Dermatol 1995;33:1–15; reprinted with permission.)

Table 17-2
Histologic Differential Diagnosis of Intraepidermal Pagetoid Cells[66]

Sebaceous carcinoma
Paget's disease (mammary and extramammary variants)
Squamous cell carcinoma *in situ*
Superficial spreading malignant melanoma
Pagetoid Spitz nevus
Merkel cell carcinoma with pagetoid spread
Pagetoid dyskeratosis
Cutaneous T cell lymphoma
Langerhans' cell histiocytosis
Clear cell papulosis
Eccrine porocarcinoma
Epidermotropic metastasis

underlying sebaceous glands via migration through the ductal epithelial lining to ascend the infundibulum. Alternatively, a proliferative intradermal focus of sebaceous carcinoma may breach the basement membrane from below.[11] Other entities that demonstrate pagetoid spread are listed in Table 17-2. In contrast, these changes are only rarely seen in extraocular sebaceous carcinomas.[29]

The histologic diagnosis of sebaceous carcinoma is not straightforward and other entities need to be considered in the pathologic differential diagnosis. Some tumors contain smaller basaloid cells and resemble basal cell carcinoma histologically (Fig. 17-10). The nuclei, however, are more vesicular and the cytoplasm is more foamy than that seen in basal cell carcinoma. In addition, lipid-laden histiocytes interspersed between tumor nests and positive lipid stains help distinguish between the two entities.

Also, since the central sebaceous ducts normally exhibit trichilemmal keratinization with lack of a true granular layer, it is not unusual to observe focal areas of keratinization within sebaceous carcinomas (Fig. 17-11). This observation, in addition to the perineural invasion sometimes exhibited by sebaceous carcinoma, makes it difficult to exclude squamous cell carcinoma histologically. Indeed, in a recent histopathologic review of 44 cases of sebaceous carcinoma of the eyelid, 84% were classified as poorly differentiated and 75% of these had features similar to squamous cell carcinoma, including dyskeratosis which was found in 30% of the tumors.[44]

The histologic differentiation of sebaceous carcinoma from sebaceous adenoma, sebaceous epithelioma, or normal mature sebaceous glands is based on the amount of cellular atypia, size, symmetry,

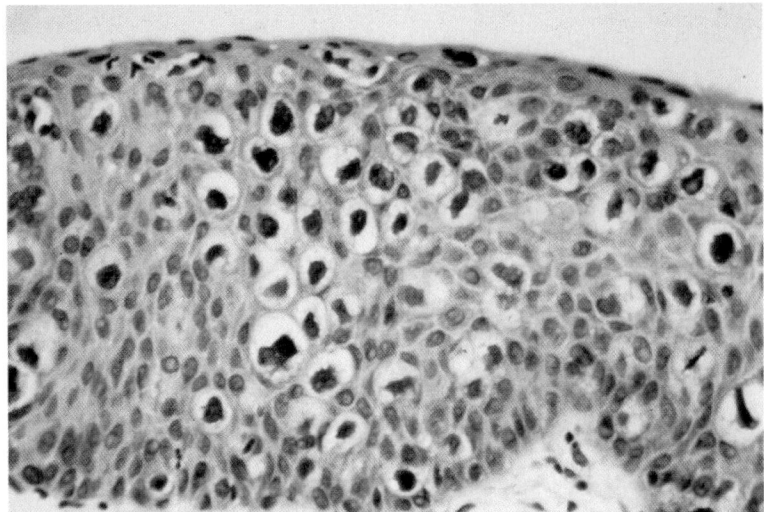

▲ **FIGURE 17-9** Higher magnification view of sebaceous carcinoma demonstrates pagetoid spread of malignant cells. (H&E, 20×).

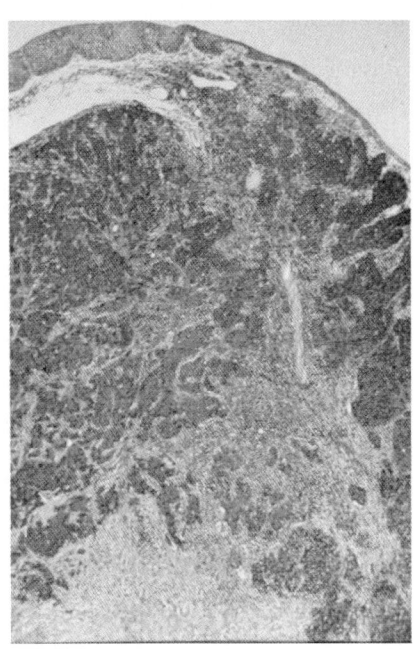

▲ **FIGURE 17-10** Sebaceous carcinoma with basaloid features. Note the resemblance to basal cell carcinoma. (H&E, 4×). (*Source:* Nelson BR, Hamlet KR, Gillard M, Railan D, Johnson TM. Sebaceous carcinoma. J Am Acad Dermatol 1995;33:1–15; reprinted with permission.)

degree of circumscription, and degree of differentiation. Furthermore, an apocrine variant with glandular structures and decapitation secretion has also been described.[45] Indeed, it is possible that pluripotent stem cells in the folliculosebaceous-apocrine unit may give rise to both sebaceous as well as apocrine stem cells.[45]

Additional histologic studies may be necessary for equivocal cases. Immunohistochemical studies may then be employed. The tumor cells stain positive for epithelial membrane antigen (EMA) and androgen receptors, but not for carcinoembryonic antigen (CEA) or S100 protein.[42] EMA staining, however, is often lost in poorly differentiated lesions, but nuclear staining for human androgen receptors is present, making it a more reliable marker.[46] It should be noted, however, that approximately 50% of basal cell carcinomas will also show focal positivity for androgen receptors.[46] Electron microscopy of tumor cells reveal cytoplasmic lipid droplets and tonofilaments inserting into well-formed desmosomes.

There are two histologic classification schemes for sebaceous carcinoma: one based on the degree of cellular differentiation and the other based on the architectural growth pattern of the tumor. These classification systems are not routinely discussed in modern texts of dermatopathology, and their interest is primarily historical. Classification schema based on the degree of differentiation are listed in Table 17-3. Well-differentiated tumors in Font's system[47] correspond to Grade I lesions in Wolfe's[10] classification;

tumors in this category contain many readily apparent sebaceous cells with abundant foamy cytoplasm (Fig. 17-12). At the other end of the spectrum, poorly differentiated to undifferentiated or Grade IV lesions display small hyperchromatic nuclei with increased mitotic activity (Fig. 17-13); additional studies are often required for correct diagnosis of these tumors. Classification systems based on tumor growth patterns are outlined in Table 17-4.

With the inherent clinical and histologic difficulties in diagnosing sebaceous carcinoma, clinicopathologic correlation is of primary importance. The diagnosis may depend on the combined knowledge and efforts of the pathologist, ophthalmologist, and dermatologist.

Table 17-3

Classification of Sebaceous Carcinoma Based on Degree of Differentiation

Classification by Font[47]

WELL DIFFERENTIATED	Contains many neoplastic cells exhibiting sebaceous differentiation with abundant finely vacuolated cytoplasm. Areas of sebaceous differentiation are often toward the center of tumor lobules.
MODERATELY DIFFERENTIATED	Only a few areas of highly differentiated sebaceous cells are seen. The majority of the tumor is composed of neoplastic cells with hyperchromatic nuclei and prominent nucleoli and abundant basophilic cytoplasm
POORLY DIFFERENTIATED	The majority of cells exhibit pleomorphic nuclei with prominent nucleoli and scant cytoplasm. A moderate increase in mitotic activity is present.

CLASSIFICATION BY WOLFE ET AL.[10]

Grade I	Well differentiated; foamy cytoplasm present in all cells.
Grade II	Large vacuolated nuclei and foamy cytoplasm seen in most cells.
Grade III	Small hyperchromatic nuclei and little cytoplasm present in most cells.
Grade IV	Undifferentiated; small hyperchromatic nuclei and little cytoplasm; diagnosis requires positive fat stain, ultrastuctural study, or areas of better differentiation.

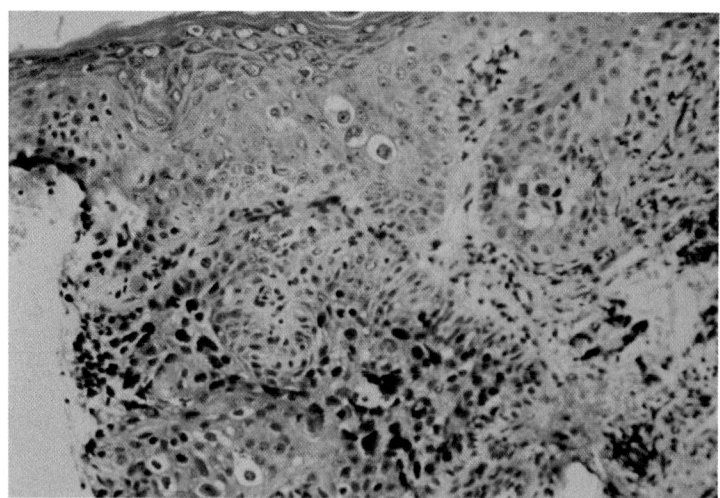

▲ **FIGURE 17-11** Sebaceous carcinoma of the eyelid demonstrating squamous features. (H&E, 2×). (*Source:* Nelson BR, Hamlet KR, Gillard M, Railan D, Johnson TM. Sebaceous carcinoma. J Am Acad Dermatol 1995;33:1–15; reprinted with permission.)

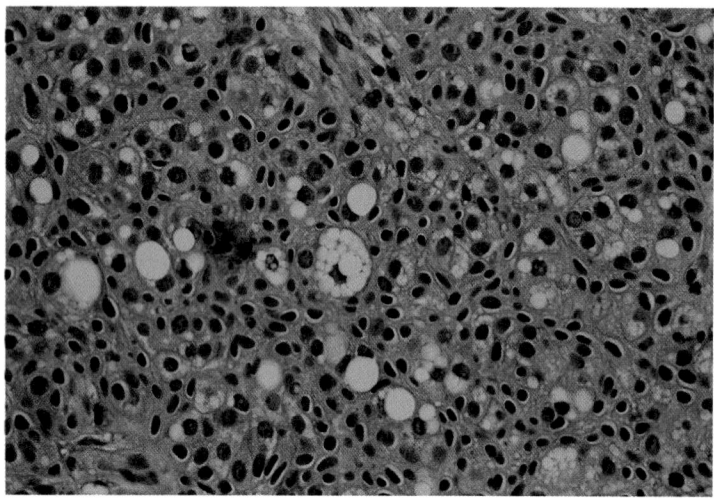

▲ **FIGURE 17-12** Well-differentiated sebaceous carcinoma. The neoplastic cells have vacuolated cytoplasm and resemble mature sebocytes. (H&E, 40×).

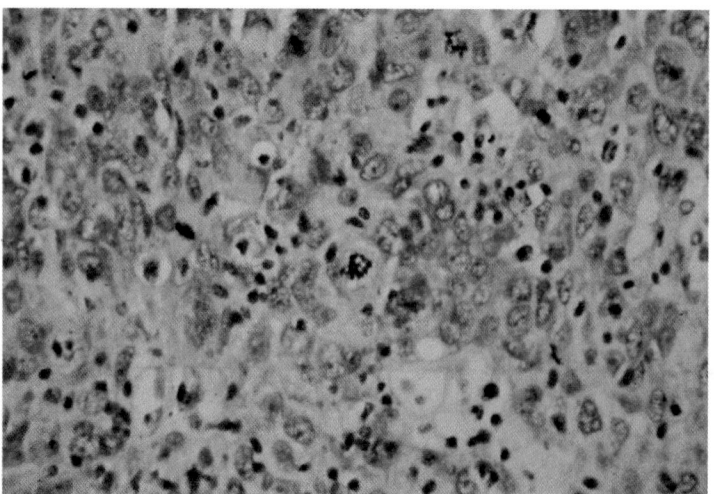

▲ **FIGURE 17-13** Poorly differentiated sebaceous carcinoma with pleomorphism, mitotic figures, and less prominent sebaceous features. (Hematoxylin-eosin, 40×). (*Source:* Nelson BR, Hamlet KR, Gillard M, Railan D, Johnson TM. Sebaceous carcinoma. J Am Acad Dermatol. 1995;33:1–15; reprinted with permission.)

Table 17-4
Classification of Sebaceous Carcinoma Based on Growth Pattern

CLASSIFICATION BY NI ET AL.[9]	CLASSIFICATION BY RAO ET AL.[7]
Squamoid	Lobular
Basaloid	Comedo-carcinoma
Adenoid	Papillary
Spindle cell	Mixed
Differentiated	

PATHOGENESIS

BOX 17-7   Summary

- Radiation is a well-documented risk factor for the development of sporadic sebaceous carcinomas (i.e., those not associated with the Muir-Torre syndrome).
- Inactivation of the tumor suppressor gene p53 or loss of the cell cycle mediator p21^{WAF1} may play a role in the pathogenesis of sebaceous carcinomas.

The cause of sporadic sebaceous carcinomas, comprising the vast majority of reported tumors, is still being elucidated. Previous radiation to the area is a well-documented risk factor especially in children being treated for retinoblastoma.[12,25] For example, there is a report of multiple eyelid sebaceous carcinomas developing in a 74-year-old woman approximately 50 years after receiving radiation therapy for facial eczema.[48]

There are also reports of sebaceous carcinoma associated with oral diuretic use[49]; thiazide diuretic-induced production of carcinogenic nitrosamines was hypothesized to play a role in the tumorigenesis of the sebaceous carcinomas in these patients. However, although interesting, no firm etiologic link exists between diuretic use and the development of sebaceous carcinoma.

The molecular mechanisms for tumor development and progression are currently being evaluated. One group of investigators,[50] in their small series of seven biopsy-proven cases of ocular sebaceous carcinoma, noted that mutational inactivation of the tumor suppressor gene p53 was present in all cases of invasive disease but was absent in patients with only *in situ* involvement. They postulated that the loss of p53 and the consequent disruption of genomic integrity might play a critical role in the progression of sebaceous carcinoma. Furthermore, their work may provide a model to explain the tendency for sebaceous carcinoma to present as a multifocal disease. Over time, the dysplastic epithelium may acquire a p53 mutation, reducing its ability to guard against further genetic damage. This process may occur at separate sites, resulting in discrete and separate foci of invasive disease.

Another group of researchers[51] have focused on the p21^{WAF1} gene product, which also plays a critical role in the cell cycle by mediating G1 cell cycle arrest and preventing progression through the cycle. They noted that there was a loss of topological control of this marker in the cases of sebaceous carcinoma evaluated, but was unaffected in normal sebaceous glands, sebaceous adenomas, and sebaceous epitheliomas. Therefore, dysregulation of cell cycle progression may be an important process in the development of sebaceous carcinomas.

ASSOCIATION WITH THE MUIR-TORRE SYNDROME

BOX 17-8 Summary

- Muir-Torre syndrome is an autosomal dominantly inherited genodermatosis defined by the presence of: (1) at least a single sebaceous gland neoplasm (adenoma, epithelioma, or carcinoma) and (2) a minimum of one internal malignancy.
- The diagnosis of Muir-Torre syndrome should be considered in patients with sebaceous neoplasms, including sebaceous carcinoma.
- The most common internal malignancies include colorectal carcinoma and genitourinary tumors.
- Germline mutations of the genes hMSH2 and hMLH1, which encode the mismatch repair proteins, MSH2 and MLH1, respectively, are well documented in patients with Muir-Torre syndrome.

The Muir-Torre syndrome is considered a genodermatosis with malignant potential.[52] It is inherited in an autosomal dominant fashion with variable penetrance and is defined by the presence of: (1) at least a single sebaceous gland tumor (adenoma, epithelioma, or carcinoma) and (2) a minimum of one internal malignancy. This syndrome has been the subject of recent comprehensive literature reviews.[2,53–55] In his review of 292 malignancies in 147 patients with Muir-Torre syndrome, Cohen et al[2] documented a median age of diagnosis of 54 years (range: 31 to 89 years) and a male-to-female ratio of nearly 2:1. Colorectal carcinoma was the most common associated visceral malignancy, occurring in 53% of

cases evaluated. Importantly, in contrast to colorectal tumors in the general population, approximately 58% of Muir-Torre syndrome patients occurred proximal to or at the splenic flexure, necessitating a complete colonoscopy for adequate evaluation. Genitourinary malignancies followed in incidence and accounted for 25% of the cancers recorded. Additional associated malignant neoplasms included carcinoma of the breast, hematologic malignancies, carcinomas of the head and neck, and cancer of the lung, stomach, pancreas, and biliary tree. Nearly half of the patients had greater than one primary malignancy.

Sebaceous gland neoplasms and keratoacanthomas represent the cutaneous stigmata in Muir-Torre syndrome patients. Sebaceous carcinoma comprised approximately 30% of sebaceous neoplasms in a large study with approximately equal distribution between ocular and extraocular sites.[53] Almost 20% of the ocular sebaceous carcinomas metastasized, resulting in the death of 1 patient with progressive pulmonary metastatic disease. Cutaneous lesions occurred prior to or concurrent with the diagnosis of an internal malignancy in 41% of the patients in this review.

Recent genetic studies have shed light on the pathogenesis of the Muir-Torre syndrome. It is currently thought that a subset of patients with Muir-Torre syndrome have a variant of the hereditary nonpolyposis colorectal cancer syndrome, another autosomal dominantly inherited disorder. Mutations in mismatch repair genes, which lead to subsequent microsatellite instability, are common to both syndromes. Specifically, germline mutations of the genes hMSH2 (human mutS homolog 2) and hMLH1 (human mutL homolog 1) on chromosomes 2p and 3p, respectively, which encode two mismatch repair proteins (MSH2 and MLH1) have been recently well documented in patients with the Muir-Torre syndrome.[56–58]

Interestingly, loss of DNA mismatch repair proteins has also been noted in the skin tumors of patients with Muir-Torre syndrome, and 1 group of researchers has suggested that immunohistochemical analysis of skin biopsies is a fast and effective method of diagnosing Muir-Torre syndrome.[59] In their series of eight Muir-Torre patients with known germline MSH2 mutations, 88% showed loss of MSH2 expression in their cutaneous neoplasms. However, loss of mismatch repair proteins in skin lesions is much less common in patients who do not have the Muir-Torre syndrome.[60]

PROGNOSIS

BOX 17-9 Summary

- Regardless of location, sebaceous carcinoma is an aggressive malignancy, with local recurrence rates after Mohs surgery reported to be 9 to 36%.
- Ocular sebaceous carcinomas may metastasize in 8 to 25% of patients, and the 5-year mortality rate for metastatic disease is approximately 50 to 67%.
- Poor prognostic factors for ocular sebaceous carcinomas include a delay in diagnosis of greater than 6 months, tumor diameter greater than 1 cm, and involvement of both upper and lower eyelids.
- Extraocular sebaceous carcinoma, though historically considered to portend a more favorable prognosis, is also capable of local recurrence, as well as regional and distant metastases.

Regardless of location, sebaceous carcinoma is an aggressive malignancy with a tendency to recur locally after surgical excision. The multicentric nature of the tumor, as well as its frequent pagetoid spread, make recognition and interpretation of frozen sections difficult, contributing to its local recurrence rate. According to one large review,[4] local recurrence after surgical excision with frozen section control tends to occur in 5 years in 9 to 36% of patients and as early as 3 to 35 months after Mohs micrographic surgery. In another recent series of 60 cases of sebaceous carcinoma followed for an average of 41 months, Shields et al[12] noted local tumor recurrence in 18% of patients at a median of 18 months. Their series, however, included several nonsurgical, as well as surgical, modes of treatment: six patients received topical chemotherapy (mitomycin C) and two patients were irradiated. The majority of patients in this study (68%) underwent excisional biopsy and chemotherapy as the initial definitive treatment.

Ocular sebaceous carcinoma may metastasize via the lymphatics, the blood vessels, by the lacrimal secretory system, and the lacrimal excretory system. Metastases occur in approximately 8 to 25% of patients, and involve regional lymph nodes, followed by spread to the liver, lungs, brain, and bones.[1,6–8,11,12] Lymphatic metastases from ocular sebaceous carcinoma often present as preauricular, submandibular, or cervical lymphadenopathy, with or without secondary parotid masses.[8,49]

The 5-year mortality rate for metastatic disease is approximately 50 to 67%.[8]

The reported metastatic rate, however, is typically higher in older series, indicating that the prognosis may be gradually improving. This may be secondary to a better understanding of the pathogenesis of this tumor. In addition, improved surveillance, early detection, definitive therapy, and close clinical follow-up may also contribute to the more recent lower rate of metastases.

Similarly, the mortality rate of sebaceous carcinoma has also improved over the last several decades. Doxanas and Green,[1] in their review of 40 cases of sebaceous carcinoma, reported a mortality rate before 1970 as 24%. In comparison, Zürcher and colleagues reported that the mortality rate for 43 patients treated from 1976–1992 was 9.3%.[13]

Several histologic features of sebaceous carcinoma may portend a more aggressive clinical course. Rao et al,[8] in his review of 104 cases of sebaceous carcinoma with a minimum of 5 years of follow-up, cited four features commonly observed in patients with fatal outcomes: multicentric origination, poor sebaceous differentiation, pagetoid spread with distortion of the overlying epithelium, and an infiltrative growth pattern. Clinical features that may predict a poor prognosis include delay of diagnosis of more than 6 months, tumor diameter exceeding 1 cm, and involvement of both upper and lower eyelids.[8]

Extraocular sebaceous carcinoma has historically been associated with a more favorable prognosis than its ocular counterpart. However, as the number of reported cases of extraocular sebaceous carcinoma has increased, several authors have disputed that notion.[41–43] In a review of 91 cases of extraocular carcinoma, metastasis was reported in 21% of the patients.[61] Ten percent of these patients had distant metastases. The recurrence rate was 29%. Therefore, although extraocular sebaceous carcinoma is generally considered to be less aggressive than the ocular variant, the significant morbidity and mortality associated with this tumor still warrant careful evaluation and management.

EVALUATION AND MANAGEMENT OF A PATIENT WITH SEBACEOUS CARCINOMA

BOX 17-10   Summary

- Physical examination should focus on a complete dermatologic and ophthalmo-

logic evaluation, as well as a thorough lymph node examination.
- An adequate biopsy specimen should be obtained for routine sectioning, special stains, and possible immunohistochemical and ultrastructural studies.
- The clinician should inquire into a personal or family history of Muir-Torre syndrome.
- Baseline studies for Muir-Torre include a chest x-ray, complete blood count, complete metabolic panel, urinalysis with cytology, rectal examination, mammogram, and colonoscopy; additional investigations should be based on specific signs or symptoms.
- Mohs micrographic surgery or standard excision with frozen section control are well-accepted therapeutic modalities for sebaceous carcinoma.
- Patients with residual conjunctival intraepithelial disease may be treated with adjunctive cryotherapy or topical mitomycin C.
- Radiation therapy should be reserved for patients unable or unwilling to undergo surgery.

Once a diagnosis of sebaceous carcinoma is considered, a detailed history and physical examination should be performed, with an emphasis on a thorough ophthalmologic and complete dermatologic evaluation. In addition, palpation of the lymph nodes and adjacent structures should be performed to help delineate the extent of disease. An adequate biopsy specimen for frozen sectioning, hematoxylin and eosin, special stains, and possible immunohistochemical or ultrastructural studies, is mandatory. The clinician should also inquire about a personal and family history suggestive of the Muir-Torre syndrome. Baseline studies should include a chest X-ray, complete metabolic panel, and complete blood count. Further screening for internal malignancies associated with the Muir-Torre syndrome should include a rectal examination, full colonoscopy, and barium enema. Additional studies may include urinalysis with cytology and a mammogram. More detailed evaluations should be based on specific signs or symptoms. A complete list of the recommended studies, in addition to those listed above, to evaluate for internal malignancy associated with Muir-Torre syndrome is provided by Cohen et al.[53]

The primary treatment of sebaceous carcinoma is complete surgical excision, when possible. There is no consensus in the literature, however, regarding the optimal size of the surgical margins and the treatment of intraepithelial neoplasia

or pagetoid involvement. Mohs micrographic surgery is a generally accepted therapeutic modality for sebaceous carcinoma, and it received strong evidence-based support in a recent review.[15]

Although no extensive prospective studies with protracted follow-up periods have been performed to assess the efficacy of Mohs surgery in treating sebaceous carcinoma, some recent reports are encouraging.[11,62,63] In his review of 49 patients with sebaceous carcinoma treated with the Mohs technique from 1987–2001 at the University of Wisconsin, Snow and colleagues[11] reported an overall cure rate of approximately 88% with a mean follow-up of 3.1 years. Six patients developed local recurrence and four of these six developed regional metastases; no deaths due to sebaceous carcinoma were reported. Intraepithelial spread was noted in 50% of the patients, but histologically discontinuous and multifocal disease was seen in only 6% of cases. The authors of the study also recommended taking an additional Mohs layer, if feasible, in patients having long-standing lesions, individuals with a history of previous treatment or trauma to the site (which may aggravate epithelial discontinuity), and/or tumors with evidence of pagetoid spread.

Standard excision with frozen section control is also a well-accepted therapeutic option. Conjunctival map biopsies may also be done at the time of surgery to assess for potential pagetoid spread and to better delineate the extent of tumor involvement. Adjunctive cryotherapy has been employed to treat patients with residual conjunctival intraepithelial disease. However, cryotherapy can be potentially associated with many damaging side effects including dry eye, symblepharon, corneal erosions, and neovascularization. Therefore, the use of cryotherapy should perhaps be limited to those patients unable to undergo definitive surgical excision. Topical mitomycin C, a non-cell cycle specific alkylating agent, has also been used as an adjunctive therapy in patients with intraepithelial involvement.[64]

Sebaceous carcinoma is relatively radioresistant. Radiotherapy and electron beam therapy have not been shown to be effective primary treatment modalities. Recurrences have been reported after periocular radiation doses exceeding 5000 rads.[15] Therefore, this form of therapy should be considered palliative and reserved for those patients unable or unwilling to undergo surgery.

Finally, metastatic disease may be treated with a combination of excision, radiation, and chemotherapy. A regimen of intralesional 5-flurouracil in conjunction with intravenous 5-fluorouracil, doxorubicin, cisplatin, and vinblastine has been employed. There are reports of long-term survival after resection of metastatic disease.[65]

◼ FINAL THOUGHTS

Sebaceous carcinoma is a rare and aggressive cutaneous malignancy with varied clinical and histologic appearances. The tumor most commonly presents on the eyelids of older adults, but may also occur in extraocular locations as well. Histologically, pagetoid or intraepithelial spread is not uncommon, especially with sebaceous carcinomas arising from the ocular adnexae, contributing to the difficulties in definitive clinical management and potential subsequent recurrences or metastases. Sebaceous gland neoplasms, including sebaceous carcinomas, may also represent the cutaneous stigmata of the Muir-Torre syndrome, and their presence should prompt consideration of this autosomal dominantly inherited genodermatosis with malignant potential. Definitive treatment is currently surgical, and a coordinated approach with ophthalmologic surgeons may be helpful when managing periocular lesions. Mohs micrographic surgery or standard excision with frozen section control, with or without conjunctival map biopsies, appear to offer the highest cure rates at this time.

REFERENCES

1. Doxanas MT, Green WR. Sebaceous gland carcinoma: review of 40 cases. *Arch Ophthalmol*. 1984;102:245–249.
2. Cohen PR, Kohn SR, Davis DA, et al. Muir-Torre syndrome. *Dermatol Clin*. 1995;13:79–89.
3. Straatsma BP: Meibomian gland tumors. *Arch Ophthalmol*. 1956;56:71–93.
4. Nelson BR, Hamlet KR, Gillard M, et al: Sebaceous carcinoma. *J Am Acad Dermatol*. 1995;33:1–15.
5. Nelson BR, Johnson TM: Sebaceous carcinoma. In: Maloney ME, Torres A, Hoffmann TJ, Helm KF. Malden MA, eds. *Surgical Dermatopathology*. Malden, MA: Blackwell Science, Inc.;1999:297.
6. Boniuk M, Zimmerman LE. Sebaceous carcinoma of the eyelid, eyebrow, caruncle, and orbit. *Trans Am Acad Ophthalmol Otol*. 1968;72:619–640.
7. Rao NA, McLean JW, Zimmerman LE. Sebaceous carcinoma of the eyelid and caruncle: correlation of clinicopathologic features with prognosis. In: Jakobiec FA, ed. *Ocular and Adnexal Tumors*. Aesculapis: Birmingham;1978:461.
8. Rao NA, Hidayat AA, McLean IW, et al. Sebaceous carcinomas of the ocular adnexa: a clinicopathologic study of 104 cases, with five-year follow-up data. *Hum Pathol*. 1982;13:113–122.
9. Ni C, Searl SS, Kuo PK, et al. Sebaceous cell carcinomas of the ocular adnexa. *Int Ophthalmol Clin*. 1982;22:23–61.
10. Wolfe JT, Yeatts RP, Wick MR, et al: Sebaceous carcinoma of the eyelid: errors in clinical and pathologic diagnosis. *Am J Surg Pathol*. 1984;8:597–606.
11. Snow SN, Larson PO, Lucarelli MJ, et al. Sebaceous carcinoma of the eyelids treated by Mohs micrographic surgery: report of nine cases with review of the literature. *Dermatol Surg*. 2002;28:623–631.
12. Shields JA, Demirci H, Marr BP, et al. Sebaceous carcinoma of the eyelids. Personal experience with 60 cases. *Ophthalmology*. 2004;111:2151–2157.
13. Zürcher M, Hintschich CR, Garner A, et al. Sebaceous carcinoma of the eyelid: a clinicopathological study. *Br J Ophthalmol*. 1998;82:1049–1055.
14. Ni C, Kuo PK. Meibomian gland carcinoma: a clinicopathological study of 156 cases with long-period follow-up of 100 cases. *Jpn J Ophthalmol*. 1979;23:388–401.
15. Cook Jr. BE, Bartley GB. Treatment options and future prospects for the management of eyelid malignancies. An evidence-based approach. *Ophthalmology*. 2001;108:2088–2100.
16. Elder D, Elenitsas R, Ragsdale BD. Tumors of the epidermal appendages. In: Elder D, Elenitsas R, Jaworsky C, Johnson B Jr, eds. *Lever's Histopathology of the Skin*. 8th ed. Philadelphia: Lippincott-Raven;1997:768.
17. Silver H, Goldstein MA. Sebaceous cell carcinoma of the parotid region. A review of the literature and a case report. *Cancer*. 1966;19:1773–1779.
18. Harvey PA, Parsons MA, Rennie IG. Primary sebaceous carcinoma of lacrimal gland: a previously unreported primary neoplasm. *Eye*. 1994;8:592–595.
19. Briscoe D, Mahmood S, Bonshek R, et al. Primary sebaceous carcinoma of the lacrimal gland. *Br J Ophthalmol*. 2001;85: 625–626.
20. Zide BM, Jelks GW, eds. *Surgical Anatomy of the Orbit*. New York: Raven Press;1985: 35.
21. Kass LG, Hornblass A. Sebaceous carcinoma of the ocular adnexa. *Surv Ophthalmol*. 1989;33:477–490.
22. Margo CE, Mulla ZD. Malignant tumors of the eyelid. A population-based study of non-basal cell and non-squamous cell malignant neoplasms. *Arch Ophthalmol*. 1998;116:195–198.
23. Lee SB, Saw SM, Eong KGA, et al. Incidence of eyelid cancers in Singapore from 1968 to 1995. *Br J Ophthalmol*. 1999;83:595–597.
24. Abdi U, Tyagi N, Maheshwari V, et al. Tumours of eyelid: a clinicopathologic study. *J Indian Med Assoc*. 1996;94:405–409.
25. Kivela T, Asko-Seljavaara S, Pihkala U, et al. Sebaceous carcinoma of the eyelid associated with retinoblastoma. *Ophthalmology*. 2001;108:1124–1128.
26. Shet T, Kelkar G, Juvekar S, et al. Masquerade syndrome: sebaceous carcinoma presenting as an unknown primary with pagetoid spread to the nasal cavity. *J Laryngol Otol*. 2004;118:307–309.
27. Seenu V, Misra MC, Khazanchi RK, et al. An eyelid swelling with a parotid mass. *Postgrad Med J*. 1997;73:123–125.
28. Mandreker S, Pinto RW, Usgaonkar U, et al. Sebaceous carcinoma of the eyelid with metastasis to the parotid region: diagnosis by fine needle aspiration cytology. *Acta Cytologica*. 1997;41:1636–1637.
29. Wick MR, Goellner JR, Wolfe JT, et al. Adnexal carcinomas of the skin II. Extraocular sebaceous carcinomas. *Cancer*. 1985;56:1163–1172.
30. Yamazawa K, Ishikura H, Matsui H, et al. Sebaceous carcinoma of the uterine cervix: a case report. *Int J Gynecol Pathol*. 2003;22:92–94.
31. Vartanian RK, McRae B, Hessler RB. Sebaceous carcinoma arising in a mature cystic teratoma of the ovary. *Int J Gynecol Pathol*. 2002;21:418–421.
32. Alawi F, Siddiqui A. Sebaceous carcinoma of the oral mucosa: case report and review of the literature. *Oral Surg Oral Med Oral Pathol Oral Radiol Endod*. 2005;99:79–84.
33. Li TJ, Kitano M, Mukai H, et al. Oral sebaceous carcinoma: report of a case. *J Oral Maxillofac Surg*. 1997;55:751–754.
34. Dasgupta S, Scott A, Skinner DW, et al. Sebaceous carcinoma of the nasal vestibule. *J Laryngol Otol*. 2001;115:1010–1011.
35. Abuzeid M, Gangopadhyay K, Rayappa CS, et al. Intraoral sebaceous carcinoma. *J Laryngol Otol*. 1996;110:500–502.
36. Miller CJ, Ioffreda MD, Billingsley EM. Sebaceous carcinoma, basal cell carcinoma, trichoadenoma, and syringocystadenoma papilliferum arising within a nevus sebaceus. *Dermatol Surg*. 2004;30: 1546–1549.
37. deGiorgi V, Massi D, Brunasso G, et al. Sebaceous carcinoma arising from nevus sebaceus: a case report. *Dermatol Surg*. 2003;29:105–107.
38. Misago N, Kodera H, Narisawa Y. Sebaceous carcinoma, trichoblastoma, and sebaceoma with features of trichoblastoma in nevus sebaceus. *Am J Dermatopathol*. 2001;23:456–462.
39. Borczuk AC, Sha KK, Hisler SE, et al. Sebaceous carcinoma of the lung: histologic and immunohistochemical characterization of an unusual pulmonary neoplasm: report of a case and review of the literature. *Am J Surg Pathol*. 2002;26: 795–798.
40. Bassetto F, Baraziol R, Sottosanti MV, et al. Biological behavior of the sebaceous carcinoma of the head. *Dermatol Surg*. 2004;30:472–476.
41. Duman DZ, Ceyhan BB, Çelikel T, et al. Extraorbital sebaceous carcinoma with rapidly developing visceral metastases. *Dermatol Surg*. 2003;29:987–989.
42. Moreno C, Jacyk WK, Judd MJ, et al. Highly aggressive extraocular sebaceous carcinoma. *Am J Dermatopathol*. 2001;23: 450–455.
43. Weedon D, ed. *Skin Pathology*. 2nd ed. London: Churchill Livingstone; 2002: 876.
44. Pereira PR, Odashiro AN, Rodrigues-Reyes AA, et al. Histopathological review of sebaceous carcinoma of the eyelid. *J Cutan Pathol*. 2005;32:496–501.
45. Misago N, Narisawa Y. Sebaceous carcinoma with apocrine differentiation. *Am J Dermatopathol*. 2001;23:50–57.
46. Bayer-Garner IB, Givens V, Smoller B. Immunohistochemical staining for

androgen receptors. A sensitive marker of sebaceous differentiation. *Am J Dermatopathol.* 1999;21:426–431.

47. Font RL. Eyelids and lacrimal drainage system. In: Spencer HW, ed. *Ophthalmic Pathology: An Atlas and Textbook.* 3rd ed. Philadelphia: WB Saunders; 1986:2169–2214.

48. Rumelt S, Hogan NR, Rubin PAD, et al. Four-eyelid sebaceous carcinoma following irradiation. *Arch Ophthalmol.* 1998; 116:1670–1672.

49. Khan JA, Grove AS Jr, Joseph MP, et al. Sebaceous carcinoma. Diuretic use, lacrimal spread, and surgical margins. *Ophthal Plast Reconstr Surg.* 1989;5:227–234.

50. Gonzalez-Fernandez F, Kaltreider SA, Patnaik BD, et al. Sebaceous carcinoma. Tumor progression through mutational inactivation of p53. *Ophthalmology.* 1998; 105:497–506.

51. McBride SR, Leonard N, Reynolds NJ. Loss of p21^{WAF1} compartmentalisation in sebaceous carcinoma compared with sebaceous hyperplasia and sebaceous adenoma. *J Clin Pathol.* 2002;55:763–766.

52. Cohen PR. Genodermatoses with malignant potential. *Am Fam Physician.* 1992; 46:1479–1486.

53. Cohen PR, Kohn SR, Kurzrock R. Association of sebaceous gland tumors and internal malignancy: the Muir-Torre syndrome. *Am J Med.* 1991;90:606–613.

54. Davis DA, Cohen PR. Genitourinary tumors in men with the Muir-Torre syndrome. *J Am Acad Dermatol.* 1995;33:909–912.

55. Cohen PR. Muir-Torre syndrome in patients with hematologic malignancies. *Am J Hematol.* 1992;40:64–65.

56. Kolodner RD, Hall NR, Lipford J, et al. Structure of the Human MSH2 locus and analysis of two Muir-Torre kindreds for msh2 mutations. *Genomics.* 1994;24:516–526.

57. Nyström-Lahti M, Parsons R, Sistonen P, et al. Mismatch repair genes on chromosomes 2p and 3p account for a major share of hereditary nonpolyposis colorectal cancer families evaluable by linkage. *Am J Hum Genet.* 1994;55:659–665.

58. Bapat B, Xia L, Madlensky L, et al. The genetic basis of Muir-Torre syndrome includes the hMLH1 locus. *Am J Hum Genet.* 1996;59:739–740.

59. Mathiak M, Rütten A, Mangold E, et al. Loss of DNA mismatch repair proteins in skin tumors from patients with Muir-Torre syndrome and MSH2 or MLH1 germline mutations. Establishment of immunohistochemical analysis as a screening test. *Am J Surg Pathol.* 2002;26:338–343.

60. Popnikolov NK, Gatalica Z, Colome-Grimmer MI, et al. Loss of mismatch repair proteins in sebaceous gland tumors. *J Cutan Pathol.* 2003;30:178–184.

61. Bailet JW, Zimmerman MC, Arnstein DP, et al. Sebaceous carcinoma of the head and neck: case report and literature review. *Arch Otolaryngol Head Neck Surg.* 1992;118:1245–1249.

62. Callahan EF, Appert DL, Roenigk RK, et al. Sebaceous carcinoma of the eyelid: a review of 14 cases. *Dermatol Surg.* 2004;30:1164–1168.

63. Dzubow LM. Sebaceous carcinoma of the eyelid: treatment with Mohs surgery. *J Dermatol Surg Oncol.* 1985;11:40–44.

64. Tumuluri K, Kourt G, Martin P. Mitomycin C in sebaceous gland carcinoma with pagetoid spread. *Br J Ophthalmol.* 2004;88:718–719.

65. Tenzel RR, Stewart WB, Boynton JR, et al. Sebaceous adenocarcinoma of the eyelid. *Arch Ophthalmol.* 1977;95:2203–2204.

66. Kohler S, Rouse RV, Smoller BR. The differential diagnosis of pagetoid cells in the epidermis. *Mod Pathol.* 1998;11:79–92.

CHAPTER 18

Hair Follicle Tumors

Darius R. Mehregan, M.D.
David A. Mehregan, M.D.
Eric Hanson, M.D.

BOX 18-1   Overview

BENIGN NEOPLASM (TREATMENT WITH EXCISIONAL BIOPSY)

- Basaloid follicular hamartoma (treatment by observation)
- Dilated pore of winer
- Fibrofolliculoma
- Inverted follicular keratosis
- Perifollicular fibroma
- Pilar sheath acanthoma
- Pilomatricoma
- Proliferating trichilemmal cyst
- Trichilemmoma
- Trichoadenoma
- Trichodiscoma
- Trichoepithelioma
- Trichofolliculoma
- Trichogerminoma
- Tumor of the follicular Infundibulum

MALIGNANT NEOPLASM (TREATMENT WITH WIDE EXCISION OR MOHS)

- Trichilemmal carcinoma
- Pilomatrical carcinoma
- Malignant proliferating trichilemmal cyst

INTRODUCTION

Hair follicle tumors can be classified by both their level of maturation (the degree to which they resemble mature hair follicles) and by the specific portion of the hair follicle to which the tumor resembles. The majority of the hair follicle tumors discussed in this chapter are benign. Their diagnostic significance often lies in their differentiation from malignant epithelial tumors. A representative biopsy specimen is necessary for the differentiation of benign follicular neoplasms from malignant epithelial tumors such as basal cell carcinoma and squamous cell carcinoma. The majority of follicular tumors form well-circumscribed symmetric neoplasms located in the upper to mid-dermis. In a smaller, superficial biopsy specimen, circumscription, symmetry, and maturation with depth cannot be adequately addressed. For this

reason, a punch biopsy or excisional biopsy specimen is recommended for diagnosis. Malignant transformation in follicular neoplasms presenting with rapid growth, pain, ulceration or bleeding has been described.[1] Excision of these lesions is recommended for diagnostic purposes and to ensure completeness of removal.

EPIDEMIOLOGY

Benign follicular tumors are uncommon, but not rare in clinical practice. Their recognition is important to prevent an inappropriate diagnosis of basal cell carcinoma or squamous cell carcinoma, which would result in inappropriately aggressive surgical techniques. The most common follicular tumors include the trichilemmoma and inverted follicular keratosis. In a review of over 100,000 specimens received in a private dermatopathology laboratory in 2005; each of these tumors accounted for 0.1% of all specimens received. Pilomatricomas and trichoepitheliomas were slightly less common, representing 0.07 and 0.03% of all specimens received. Other follicular tumors including trichoadenoma and trichofolliculoma are much less common. In contrast, malignant follicular tumors are quite rare. In a similar review of over 100,000 surgical specimens received in a private dermatopathology laboratory in 2005, malignant follicular tumors represented one specimen per 100,000.

TRICHOFOLLICULOMA

BOX 18-2   Summary

- Flesh-colored papule with central white vellus hairs
- Central dilated follicular infundibulum
- Primary hair follicles radiate from dilated infundibulum
- Secondary primitive hair follicles radiating from primary hair follicles

---

The trichofolliculoma represents a well-differentiated follicular neoplasm. Clinically, the lesion presents as a flesh-colored papule or nodule with a central depression or comedonal opening containing fine white vellus hairs (Fig. 18-1).[2] Histologically, the lesion consists of one or several dilated structures which keratinize with a thin granular cell layer, and contain delicately laminated keratin similar to that seen in the follicular

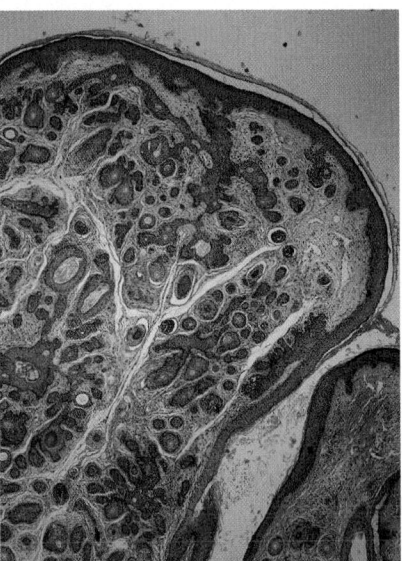
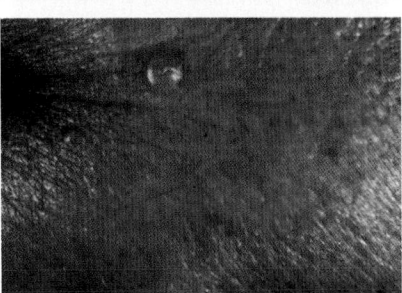

▲ **FIGURE 18-1** Trichofolliculoma shows a central comedonal opening with vellus hair follicles radiating from the central space. There are more primitive basaloid follicular germ structures radiating from the vellus hair follicles. Clinically these vellus hairs appear as a white tuft emanating from the center of the tumor. (Clinical photo courtesy of Dr. James Ulery.)

infundibulum. Radiating from this primary follicle are numerous hair follicle structures surrounded by a fibrotic stroma. Some of these hair follicle structures form small vellus hairs that empty into the central cystic space. Branching from these vellus hair-like structures are more primitive follicular germ structures. The overall architecture is relatively circumscribed, may be multinodular and tends to fill the reticular dermis. A variant of the trichofolliculoma is seen with large hyperplastic sebaceous lobules and is referred to as a sebaceous trichofolliculoma.[3]

Trichofolliculoma is a benign follicular neoplasm, which in most cases is adequately treated with re-excision if it remains beyond the initial biopsy. Local recurrence in the periocular area has been reported, and complete surgical excision was curative.[4,5]

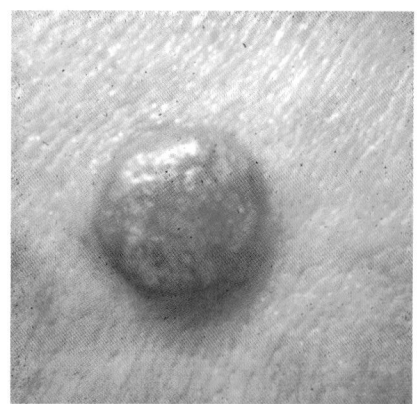

▲ **FIGURE 18-2** Trichoadenoma presents as a flesh-colored papule or nodule primarily on the face or trunk.

TRICHOADENOMA

BOX 18-3 Summary

- Flesh-colored papule
- Multiple dermal cystic structures with outer root sheath differentiation
- Pale-staining epithelial strands may interconnect cystic structures
- Fibrotic stroma surrounds cystic structures

A trichoadenoma is most commonly found as a flesh-colored papule or nodule on the face and/or trunk (Fig. 18-2).[6,7] The trichoadenoma is a moderately well-differentiated tumor consisting of numerous small cystic structures (Fig. 18-3) The cystic structures keratinize both with and without a thin granular cell layer, and contain a small amount of delicate keratin. The cystic spaces are surrounded by pale-staining follicular epithelium, which resembles the outer root sheath of the hair follicle. This pale-staining epithelium forms epithelial strands that may interconnect the cystic spaces. Follicular germ structures are not formed and no hair shafts are seen. The trichoadenoma tends to be a relatively circumscribed tumor present in the upper to mid-dermis and is surrounded by a fibrotic stroma. Rupture of the small keratin-filled cysts may produce a focal granulomatous inflammatory response.

The trichoadenoma is a benign follicular neoplasm and its treatment beyond the initial biopsy is generally not needed.

DILATED PORE OF WINER

BOX 18-4 Summary

- Flesh-colored papule with central comedonal opening
- Large dermal cystic cavity lined by epithelium with trichilemmal differentiation
- Finger-like projections extend from cyst wall into adjacent dermis

The dilated pore of Winer presents clinically as a dome-shaped or slightly raised flesh-colored papule with a central opening resembling a large open comedone.[8] Though usually solitary, multiple dilated pores have been reported in the same patient.[9] Histologically, the lesion may be considered as a follicular tumor with trichilemmal differentiation (Fig. 18-4). The large central cystic opening keratinizes with a granular cell layer, and contains delicate keratin. The acanthotic follicular epithelium shows finger-like projections into the surrounding dermis.

The dilated pore of Winer is a benign follicular neoplasm and its treatment beyond biopsy is generally not needed.

PILAR SHEATH ACANTHOMA

BOX 18-5 Summary

- Papule with central comedonal opening
- Central dermal cystic space
- Massive proliferation of epithelium with outer root sheath differentiation

The pilar sheath acanthoma presents as a slightly raised papule with a central comedonal opening similar to the dilated pore of Winer (Fig. 18-5).[10] The lesions are most commonly found on

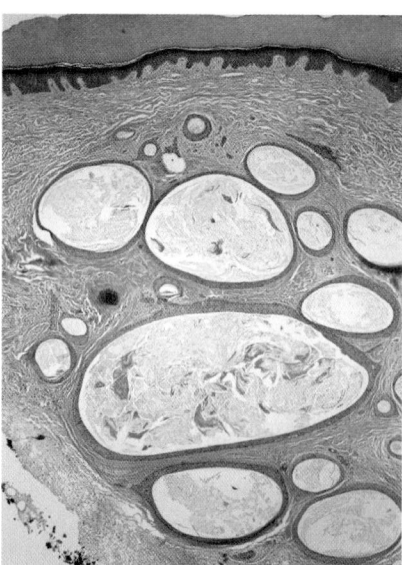

▲ **FIGURE 18-3** Histology of trichoadenoma is composed of cystic spaces which keratinize with a thin or inconspicuous granular cell layer, and contain delicate keratin. The cystic spaces are lined by pale-staining epithelium.

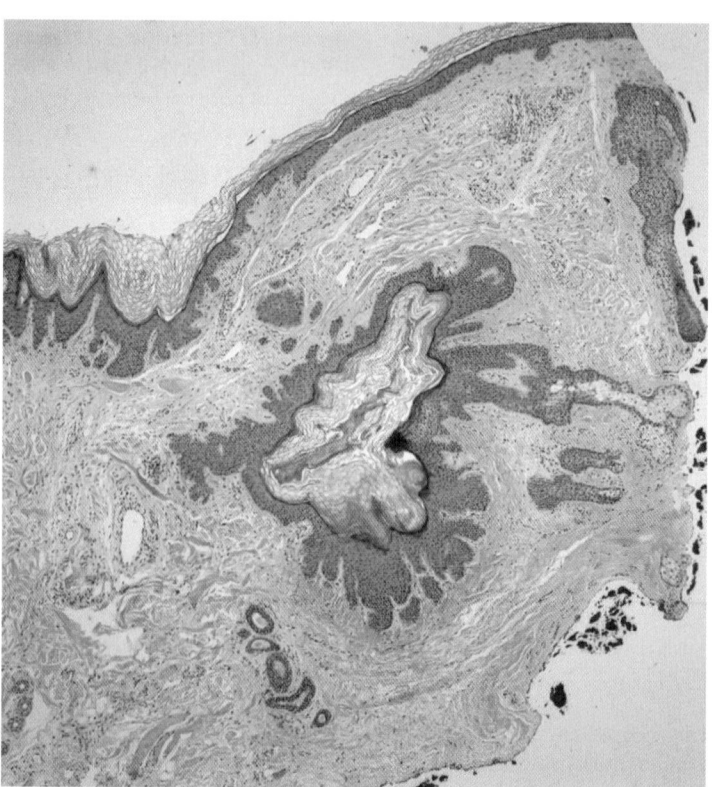

▲ **FIGURE 18-4** Histology of the dilated pore of Winer consists of a central cystic space surrounded by hypertrophic and pale-staining outer root sheath-type epithelium.

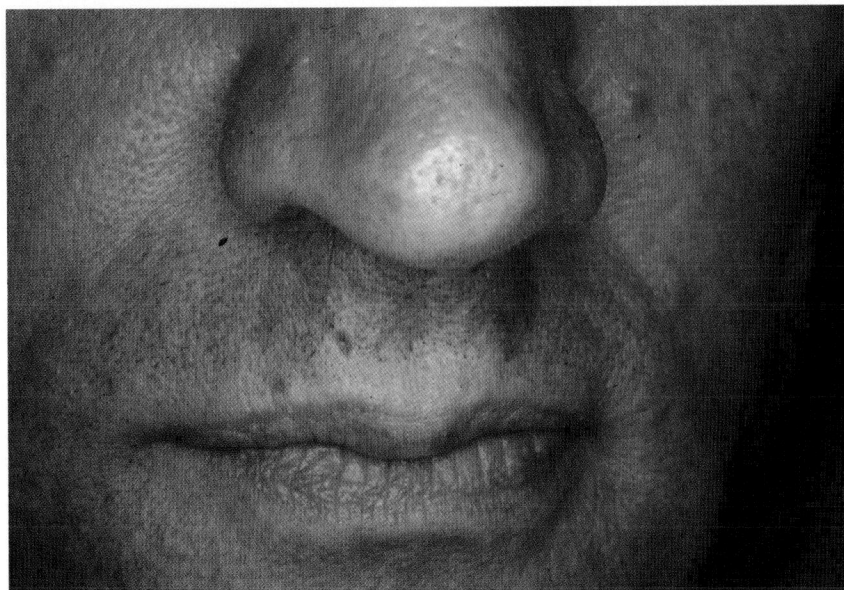

▲ **FIGURE 18-5** Pilar sheath acanthoma presents as a comedonal-like opening, most commonly on the upper lip.

the upper lip. Histologically, there is a large central cystic space that extends into the reticular dermis. The cystic space shows keratinization with a granular cell layer and delicately laminated keratin (Fig. 18-6). Rising from the central cystic space is a massive proliferation of outer root sheath epithelium that extends from the cyst cavity into the surrounding dermis in all directions and down into the deep reticular dermis.

Pilar sheath acanthoma is a benign follicular tumor that generally does not require treatment beyond the initial biopsy.

TUMOR OF THE FOLLICULAR INFUNDIBULUM

BOX 18-6 Summary

- Hypopigmented to flesh-colored slightly raised papules
- Superficial dermal cords of pale-staining cells forming a fenestrated pattern
- Multiple connections with overlying epidermis
- Hair follicles may be seen entering tumor from deeper dermis
- Association with Cowden syndrome reported

The tumor of the follicular infundibulum presents as single or multiple macular to slightly raised hypopigmented to flesh-colored 2 to 10 mm papules and macules on the face, neck, and upper chest (Fig. 18-7).[11–16] Association with Cowden syndrome has been described (see also section "Trichilemmoma").[17] Histologically, these lesions show outer root sheath differentiation. The growth pattern can resemble a superficial basal cell carcinoma. Cords and masses of pale-staining cells containing PAS positive glycogen resembling the outer root sheath of the hair follicle form a shelf or fenestrated plate beneath the epidermis (Fig. 18-8). There are multiple connections to the overlying epidermis. Hair follicles may be seen entering the tumor from the underlying dermis. The stroma is fibrotic. Lack of peripheral palisading, clefting around tumor lobules, and fibrovascular stroma containing mucin help to differentiate this lesion from superficial basal cell carcinoma.

The tumor of the follicular infundibulum is a benign follicular neoplasm and complete excision is generally curative. However, superficial laser ablation is a treatment option when multiple lesions are present.[18]

TRICHILEMMOMA

BOX 18-7 Summary

- Solitary or multiple flesh-colored papules especially on face
- Lobules of pale-staining cells extending from undersurface of epidermis

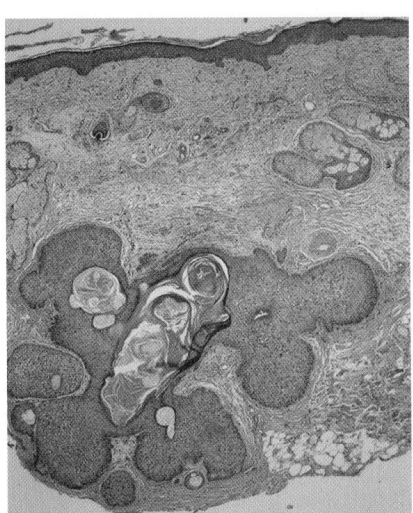

▲ **FIGURE 18-6** Pilar sheath acanthoma shows a central cystic space surrounded by hypertrophic lobules of eosinophilic pale-staining outer root sheath-type epithelium which extends into the surrounding dermis.

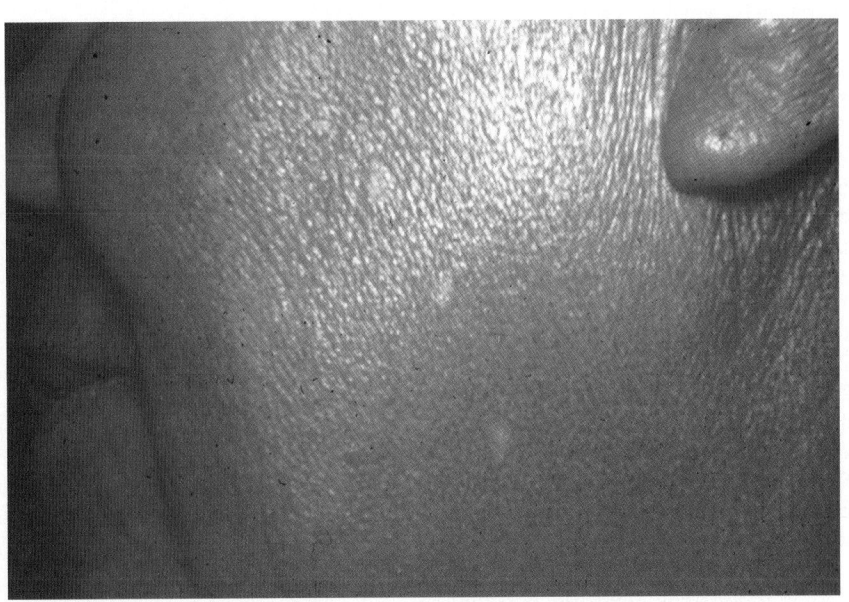

▲ **FIGURE 18-7** Tumor of the follicular infundibulum presents as a single or multiple flesh-colored papule(s) on the face, neck, and upper chest.

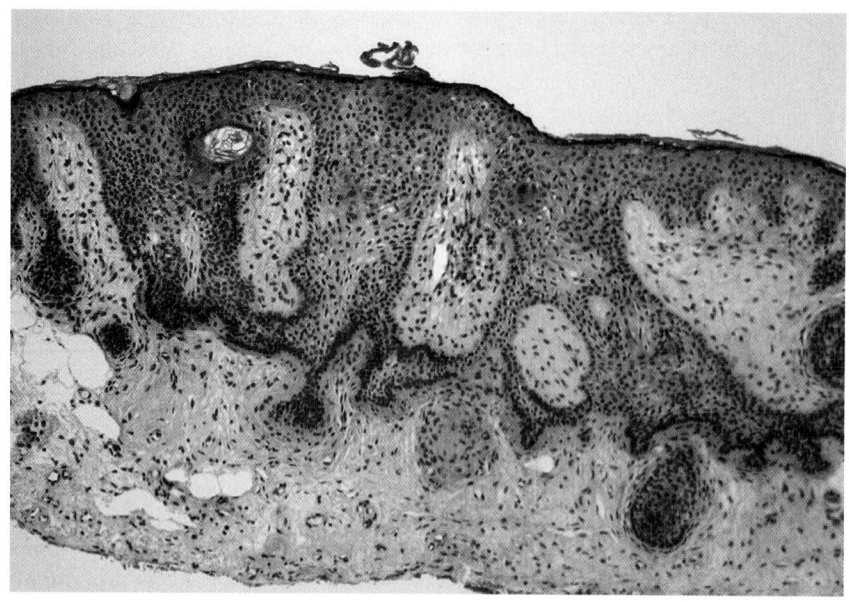

▲ **FIGURE 18-8** Histology of the tumor of follicular infundibulum shows a plate-like growth of pale-staining outer root sheath-type epithelium which connects to the undersurface of the epidermis. Primitive hair follicle structures may enter the tumor from below.

- Darker-staining cells with palisading at periphery of tumor lobules
- Desmoplastic variant has thin strands of basaloid cells in a hyalinized fibrous stroma
- Multiple trichilemmomas associated with Cowden syndrome

The trichilemmoma presents clinically as a flesh-colored to tan papule. The lesions may show evidence of hyperkeratosis or crust formation. The lesions are more common in middle-aged to elderly patients and may be mistaken clinically as a basal cell carcinoma or verruca. Trichilemmomas, especially when multiple and on the face, are commonly found in Cowden syndrome.[19,20] Other cutaneous findings in Cowden syndrome include sclerotic fibromas,[21] oral fibromas, and benign acral keratosis.[20] Cowden syndrome is an autosomal dominant genodermatosis characterized by the formation of hamartomas, colonic polyps, and rare involvement of the central nervous system with an increased susceptibility to malignancy of the breast, thyroid, and genito-urinary tract.[22–25] Germline mutations of the PTEN tumor suppressor gene in Cowden syndrome and the finding of PTEN mutations in breast and thyroid cancers further supports the association of Cowden syndrome and these malignancies. The detection of PTEN mutations opens the possibility of genetic counseling for Cowden syndrome patients and their family members for ensuring appropriate clinical screening and follow up for thyroid and breast cancers.[26,27]

Histologically, trichilemmomas represent a proliferation of follicular sheath epithelium (Fig. 18-9). There is a proliferation of pale-staining cells resembling the outer root sheath of the hair follicle seen in connection with the lower surface of the epidermis. The light staining cells contain abundant glycogen. The overlying epidermis may show focal hypergranulosis with parakeratosis and inflammatory cell crust. There is peripheral palisading of darker staining cells around the periphery of the tumor lobules. The lesion maintains a rel-atively well-circumscribed and symmetric architecture. Surrounding the proliferation of pale-staining cells is a relatively fibrotic stroma. Traumatized lesions may show increased number of mitotic figures; however, lack of nuclear pleomorphism and well-circumscribed architecture of the lesion help to differentiate the lesion from squamous cell carcinoma. There is some controversy in the literature regarding the etiology of these lesions. Some authors believe that these may represent a variant of verruca vulgaris with trichilemmal differentiation. The presence of human papilloma virus (HPV) type 23 has been identified within these lesions by some authors; however, many other investigators have failed to identify human papilloma virus in these lesions.[28–30]

Desmoplastic trichilemmoma represents a histologic variation in which thin strands of basaloid cells extend from the surface of the trichilemmoma into the surrounding dermis embedded in a dense hyalinized fibrous stroma (Fig. 18-10). In a superficial biopsy, this may give the false impression of morpheaform basal cell carcinoma. However, if the biopsy is of adequate size, it will be noted that the lesion maintains a well-circumscribed architecture with a defined lower margin. The tumor cells stain with antibodies to cytokeratins while the stromal cells stain for vimentin. Staining for human papilloma virus has failed to confirm the presence of HPV in the desmoplastic variant.[31]

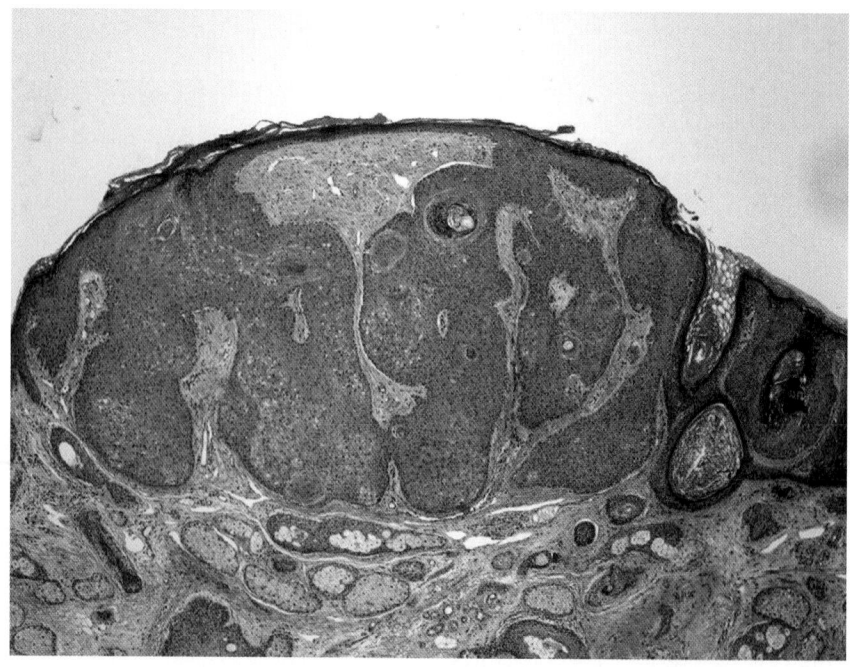

▲ **FIGURE 18-9** Trichilemmoma is a well-circumscribed exo-endophytic growth of pale-staining outer root sheath-type epithelium.

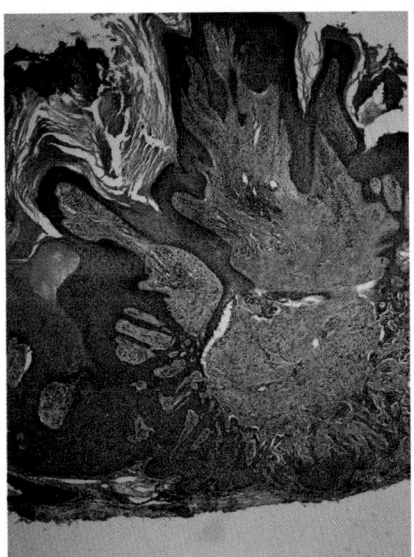

▲ **FIGURE 18-10** Desmoplastic trichilemmoma shows areas of dense hyalinized stroma within the lobules of pale-staining outer root sheath-type epithelium. However, the lesion remains well circumscribed and has a well-defined lower margin.

Solitary trichilemmomas do not require further treatment beyond diagnostic biopsy. Treatment of patients with multiple trichilemmomas with topical 5-fluorouracil, isotretinoin, curettage and laser ablation has been described.[32] One group reports successful treatment of desmoplastic trichilemmoma with Mohs micrographic surgery.[33]

TRICHILEMMAL CARCINOMA

> **BOX 18-8 Summary**
>
> - Papules or nodules on sun-exposed sites and burn scars
> - Lobular epithelium with abundant clear cytoplasm and trichilemmal keratinization
> - Palisading of nuclei and hyaline mantles at periphery of tumor lobules
> - Mitotic figures may be prominent and atypical
> - Pushing borders or invasive pattern

Trichilemmal carcinoma is a rare tumor, most often affecting the elderly at sites of sun exposure, especially the face, head and neck, but also the eyelid, extremities, and trunk.[34–37] Trichilemmal carcinoma has also been reported in burn scars.[38]

Histologically, trichilemmal carcinoma most commonly presents as an invasive lobular epithelial proliferation extending from the epidermis to the deep dermis and subcutaneous fat.

There is usually a pushing lower border but an infiltrative pattern may be seen. The tumor aggregates undergo trichilemmal keratinization with individual cells containing abundant, clear, PAS positive, diastase sensitive cytoplasm. Palisading of nuclei and a hyaline mantle may be seen at the periphery of tumor lobules. Prominent mitotic figures, some of which may be atypical, and nuclear pleomorphism are found.

Trichilemmal carcinoma has been successfully treated with wide local excision[34,36] and more recently with Mohs micrographic surgery.[39,40] Mohs surgery has also been useful for patients with multiple recurrent trichilemmal carcinomas with perineural invasion.[41] Metastasis has been reported but is rare.[42]

INVERTED FOLLICULAR KERATOSIS

> **BOX 18-9 Summary**
>
> - Flesh-colored papule
> - Endophytic lobules of basaloid cells with peripheral palisading of nuclei
> - Numerous squamous eddies within tumor lobules

The inverted follicular keratosis presents as a flesh-colored papule, most commonly on the face, especially the cheek and upper lip, and also around the eyes (Fig. 18-11). Those affected are usually the middle-aged to elderly.[43–48] Inverted follicular keratoses may crust or bleed, and are often mistaken clinically for basal cell carcinoma, squamous cell carcinoma or verruca vulgaris. Histologically, the inverted follicular keratosis shows evidence of outer root sheath differentiation, and shares some histologic features with trichilemmoma. There is a proliferation of pale-staining outer root sheath-type epithelium that is well circumscribed and surrounded by a fibrotic stroma (Fig. 18-12). Both lesions show peripheral palisading of basaloid cells at the periphery of the tumor lobules. However, in the inverted follicular keratosis, there are concentric layers of squamous cells with evidence of keratinization forming squamous eddies. As with trichilemmoma, some authors have postulated that these may represent variations of a trichilemmal verruca vulgaris. However, true koilocytic change is not present and studies searching for human papilloma virus have shown conflicting evidence.[49–52]

Inverted follicular keratosis is a benign follicular neoplasm and complete excision is generally curative.

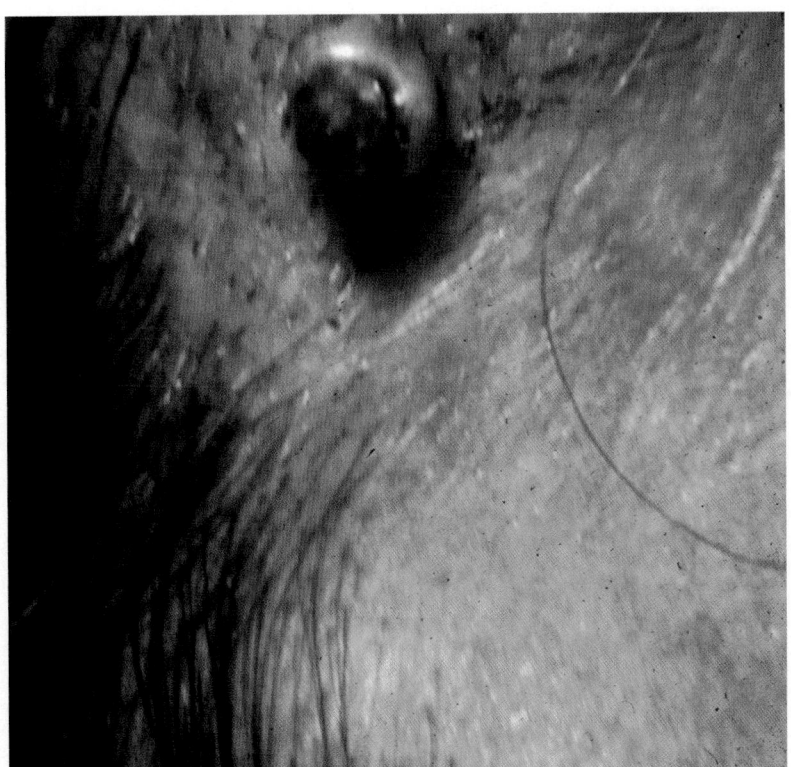

▲ **FIGURE 18-11** Inverted follicular keratosis often presents as a verrucous papule most commonly on the face.

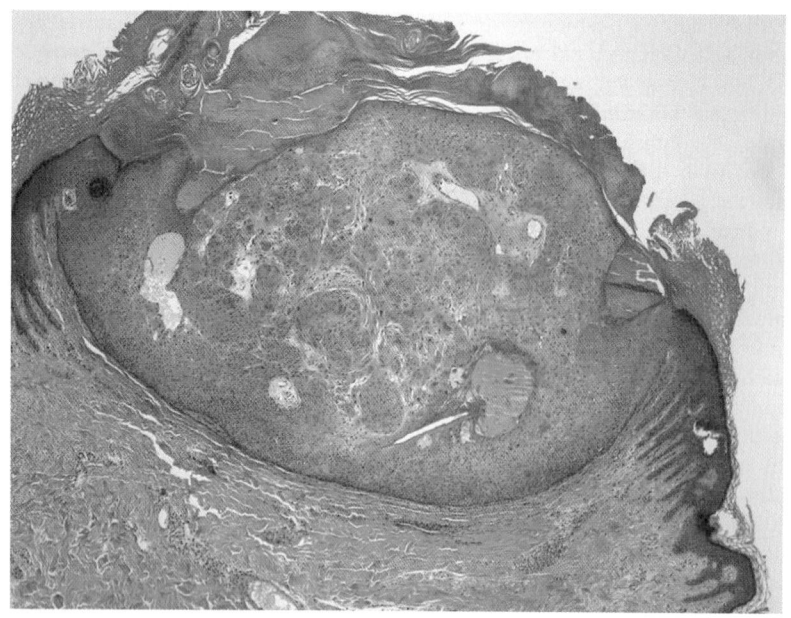

▲ **FIGURE 18-12** Histology of the inverted follicular keratosis shows a well-circumscribed neoplasm of pale-staining outer root sheath-type epithelium containing areas of squamous eddies.

PILOMATRICOMA (CALCIFYING EPITHELIOMA OF MALHERBE)

BOX 18-10   Summary

- Deep dermal nodule
- Small dark-staining cells with matrical differentiation
- Pale-staining "shadow cells" with loss of nuclei and preservation of cell contours
- Foci of calcification with possible ossification
- Multiple pilomatricomas reported in myotonic dystrophy
- Pilomatricoma-like changes reported in epidermoid cysts of Gardner syndrome

The calcifying epithelioma of Malherbe presents as a slow-growing, deep-seated dermal nodule (Fig. 18-13). These may often present clinically as inflamed nodules. Lesions are common in children, but may also be seen in adults.[53–55] Multiple pilomatricomas in the same patient have been reported in association with myotonic dystrophy.[55] Pilomatricoma-like changes have also been found in the epidermoid cysts of Gardner syndrome.[56] Histologically, the lesion begins with small dark staining cells resembling the matrical cells of the hair follicle. The basaloid matrix-type cells show transformation into fully keratinized shadow

cells (Fig. 18-14). Both trichilemmal and infundibular keratinization may be seen in the transition to shadow cells. Shadow cells consist of large masses of pale-staining eosinophilic keratin that maintain the outline of the cell surface and loss of nuclei. Calcification may occur within the areas of shadow cells and may be followed by osteoma formation. The lesions may begin with a cystic architecture, however most commonly the lesions are seen as ruptured masses within the deep dermis. Free keratin may be surrounded by areas of foreign body granuloma formation and dermal fibrosis.

Pilomatricomas are benign adnexal neoplasms that rarely recur or metastasize.[57] Complete excision with clear margins is the treatment of choice.[57–60]

PILOMATRICAL CARCINOMA

BOX 18-11   Summary

- Malignant change in a pilomatricoma
- Nuclear pleomorphism, mitotic frequency, necrosis, and squamous metaplasia
- Local invasion and metastasis may occur

Cases of malignant pilomatricoma have been reported in the literature. These show histologic features typical of pilomatricoma with additional changes of nuclear pleomorphism, increased mitotic activity, necrosis, and focal squamous metaplasia.[61] The lesions typically show areas of infiltrating growth pattern within the dermis and subcutaneous fat (Fig. 18-15).

Pilomatrical carcinoma tends to recur with a recurrence rate of 59% reported by one group.[62] Metastasis and death from local invasion have also been reported.[62–64] Complete surgical excision with clear margins is the recommended treatment for pilomatrical carcinoma.[65] Mohs micrographic surgery has also been successfully used to treat pilomatrical carcinoma.[66]

TRICHOEPITHELIOMA

BOX 18-12   Summary

- Single or multiple flesh-colored papules especially on face
- Solid epithelial aggregates of basaloid cells in dermis
- Keratinizing cysts often present within tumor aggregates
- Rudimentary hair papillae and germ structures common

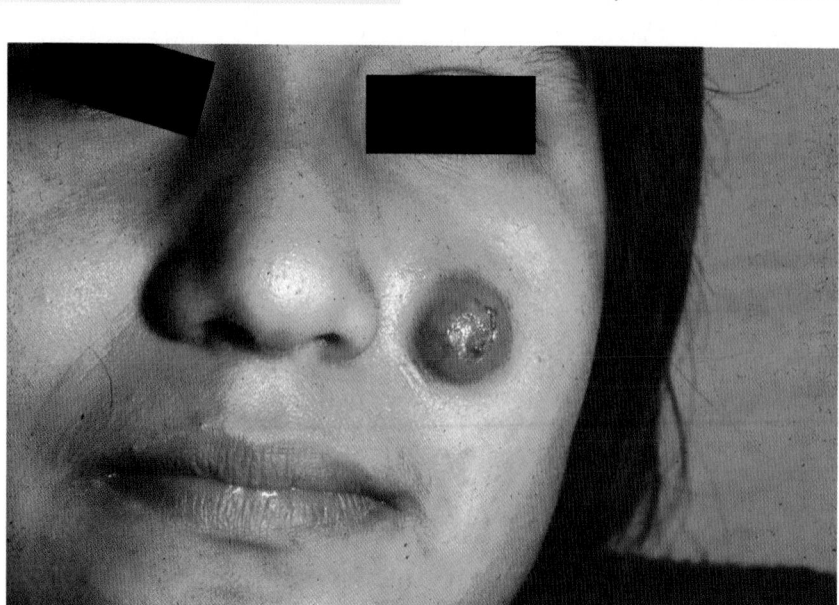

▲ **FIGURE 18-13** Calcifying epithelioma of Malherbe (pilomatricoma) often presents with an intradermal or subcutaneous nodule. The lesions are very common in children and may often be inflamed.

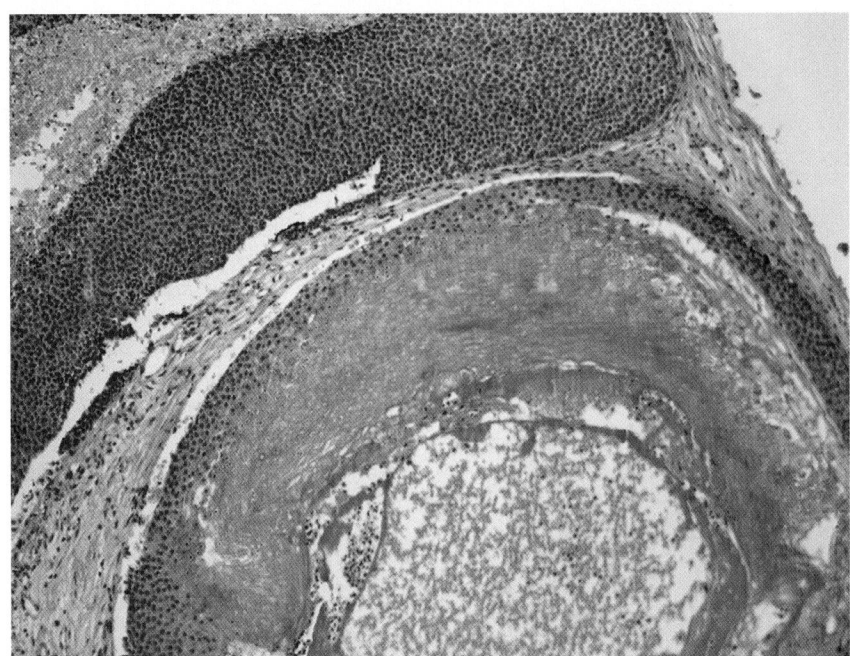

▲ **FIGURE 18-14** Pilomatricoma shows areas of matrical cells, which show both abrupt and gradual transition into eosinophilic shadow cells. Areas of ruptured keratinous debris may be surrounded by granulomatous inflammation.

- Fibrotic stroma surrounds tumor aggregates
- Multiple trichoepitheliomas may be seen in autosomal dominant inheritance pattern
- Brooke-Spiegler syndrome has multiple trichoepitheliomas, cylindromas, spiradenomas

The trichoepithelioma represents a less mature hair follicle tumor. Clinically, the lesions present as a solitary flesh-colored papule, most commonly on the faces of young patients and adults (Fig. 18-16).

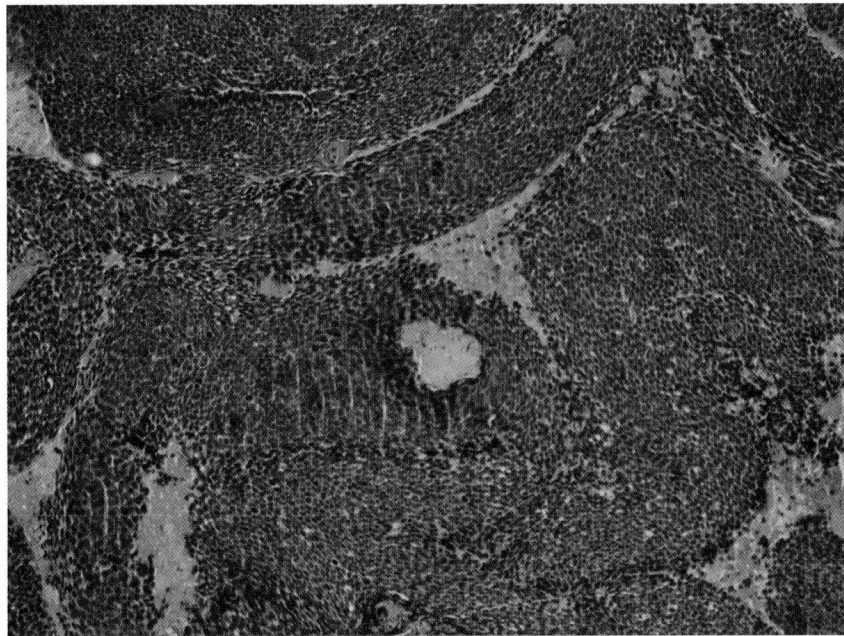

▲ **FIGURE 18-15** Pilomatrical carcinoma shows areas typical of pilomatricoma with additional changes of nuclear pleomorphism, increased mitotic activity, and focal squamous metaplasia.

However, multiple lesions may be seen (Fig. 18-17). Familial multiple trichoepitheliomas may present with an autosomal dominant-type inheritance pattern, and has been mapped to chromosome 9p21, a locus that may code for tumor suppressor genes p16 and p15.[67] Multiple trichoepitheliomas may also be seen in association with cylindromas and spiradenomas in Brooke-Spiegler syndrome. This is a genodermatosis associated with mutations in the CYLD gene on chromosome 16q21-13 and is

also discussed under "Cylindroma."[68,69] Histologically, the lesions are marked by relatively symmetric and circumscribed proliferation of basaloid cells within the dermis. There are solid epithelial and basaloid nests that often contain tiny keratinizing cysts resembling milia (Fig. 18-18). Rudimentary hair papillae and germ structures are common and are quite characteristic of trichoepithelioma. The stroma is typically fibrotic. Retraction spaces and mucin deposition are not common in trichoepitheliomas. Separation may occur within the layers of the fibrous stroma and the surrounding dermis. CD34 positive spindle cells have been identified in the stroma of trichoepithelioma, but are less common within the stroma of basal cell epithelioma. Staining with bcl-2, a marker of cellular apoptosis, shows increased staining within the tumor lobules of basal cell carcinoma. However, with trichoepithelioma, the staining tends to be limited to the periphery of the tumor lobules with a lack of staining in the center of the tumor lobules.

Histologic variations of the trichoepithelioma include the adamantinoid trichoepithelioma, trichoblastoma, and desmoplastic trichoepithelioma.

The trichoblastoma represents a poorly differentiated follicular neoplasm with hair germ differentiation.[70] Basaloid islands of hair germ like cells form a well-circumscribed neoplasm in the dermis. The stroma is fibrotic. Peripheral palisading of nuclei and clefting between tumor lobules and stroma are not present. Horn cysts and calcification are less common than in the trichoepithelioma.

Desmoplastic trichoepithelioma typically presents as a solitary firm nodule or plaque with a central depressed area most commonly on the face.[71] Lesions are more common in women and are seen in all age groups. Histologically, these show small islands of basaloid cells surrounded by fibrotic stroma, and may resemble morpheaform basal cell carcinoma and microcystic adnexal carcinoma.[71] The basaloid cells show small foci of keratin cyst formation, areas of calcification, and focal areas of foreign body-type granuloma (Fig. 18-19). Areas of follicular germ and papillae formation may be seen, which help to differentiate this from the morpheaform basal cell carcinoma and microcystic adnexal carcinoma. In addition, the microcystic adnexal carcinoma shows areas of ductal differentiation and invasion of the deep dermis and subcutaneous fat. Differentiation of the desmoplastic trichoepithelioma from morpheaform

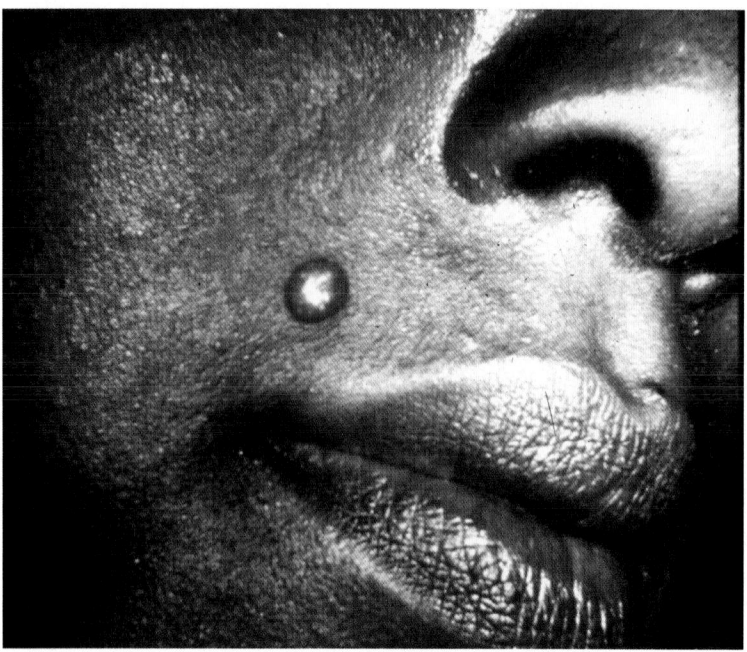

▲ **FIGURE 18-16** Trichoepithelioma presents as a solitary flesh-colored papule most commonly on the face. However, multiple lesions may be seen.

basal cell carcinoma and microcystic adnexal carcinoma is crucial to avoid overly-aggressive or disfiguring surgery. Conservative surgical excision may be sufficient for diagnosis and therapy.[72]

The cytokeratin pattern resembles the basal cells of the follicular outer root sheath.[73] The basaloid cells stain with antibodies to CK1, 5, 10, 14 and 15, ductal structures with CK7, CK8/18, and

CK 19, while cystic structures stain with CK5/8, CK6, CK10/11 and CK14.[74]

Trichoepitheliomas are benign, and if the biopsy is diagnostic, does not require further surgery. However some patients may desire removal for cosmesis. Trichoepitheliomas have been treated with many modalities including excision, electrosurgery,[75] cryosurgery,[76] dermabrasion, chemical peel,[77] and radiation.[78] Patients with multiple trichoepitheliomas have also been treated with CO_2, erbium:YAG, and argon lasers with good cosmetic results and low recurrence rates.[79–82]

■ TRICHOGERMINOMA

BOX 18-13 Summary

- Asymptomatic dermal or subcutaneous nodules
- Islands of dermal basaloid cells resemble hair bulbs
- Differentiation toward various portions of hair follicle may be present

The trichogerminoma is a rare tumor with differentiation toward the follicular germ. The lesions present as slow growing asymptomatic dermal or subcutaneous nodules on the head, trunk, and extremities.[83] Histologically, the tumors are well demarcated in the dermis and are composed of islands of basaloid cells resembling hair bulbs. Peripheral palisading of nuclei, keratinization, and differentiation toward various portions of the hair follicle may be present.[83] Retraction spaces between the tumor lobules and stroma are not present. The differential diagnosis includes basal cell carcinoma, trichoepithelioma, and trichoblastoma. Immunohistochemically, the tumor cells contain a wide range of cytokeratins including AE1/AE3, CK5/6, and Cam 5.2 but fail to stain with CK7 or CK20.[84]

Trichogerminoma is a benign neoplasm. Excision with clear margins is the treatment of choice.[83]

■ BASALOID FOLLICULAR HAMARTOMA

BOX 18-14 Summary

- Large plaque, typically unilateral
- Small dermal basaloid nests with peripheral palisading and fibrotic stroma
- May see keratin cyst formation and follicular differentiation
- Generalized forms reported in association with myasthenia gravis and alopecia

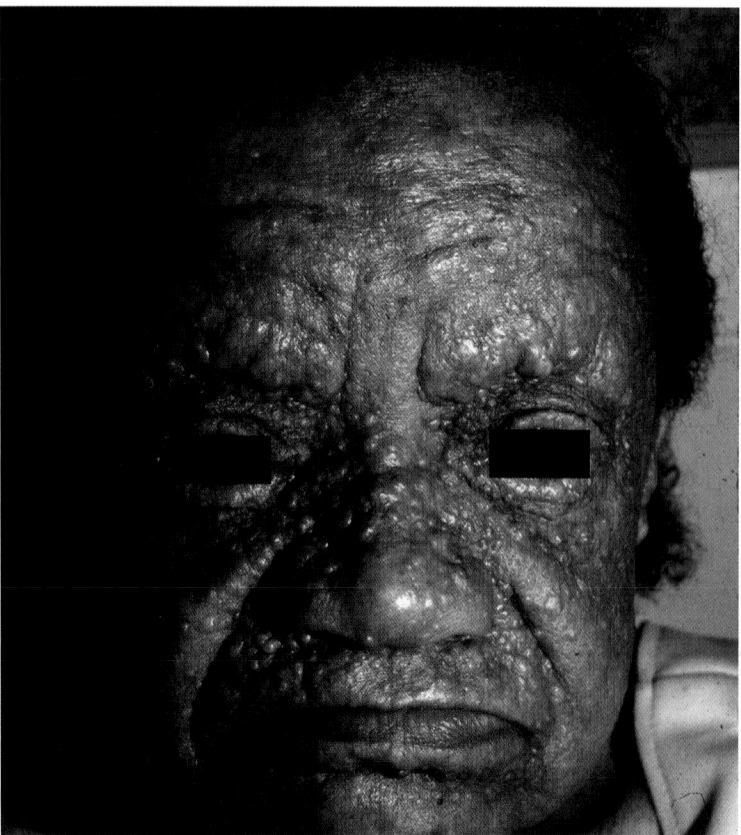

▲ **FIGURE 18-17** Patient presenting with multiple familial trichoepitheliomas and cylindromas in the Brooke-Spiegler syndrome.

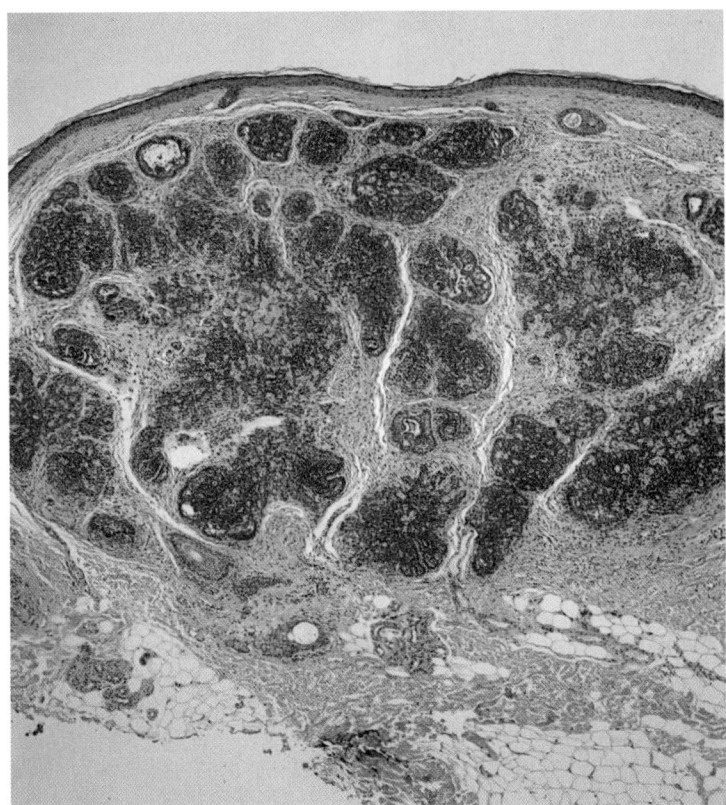

▲ **FIGURE 18-18** Trichoepithelioma presents as a well-circumscribed proliferation of basaloid cells. The basaloid cells show areas of keratin cyst formation and areas of follicular differentiation including follicular germ formation.

The basaloid follicular hamartoma presents as a large plaque, typically in a unilateral distribution resembling an epidermal nevus (Fig. 18-20). Lesions may be solitary, multiple or linear. Generalized forms that are reported have been associated with alopecia and myasthenia gravis.[85] Histologically, the basaloid follicular hamartoma shows proliferation of small basaloid nests and masses within the dermis. The level of differentiation may vary. Basaloid islands may show peripheral palisading surrounded by a fibrovascular stroma resembling a basal cell carcinoma. Other areas of the tumor may show areas of keratin cyst formation, fibrotic stroma, and follicular differentiation resembling trichoepithelioma. The unilateral or systematized presentation of a large plaque present at birth or in early childhood helps to differentiate this clinically from basal cell carcinoma or trichoepithelioma.

Small lesions may be treated with surgical excision if desired. Larger lesions do not require excision. Photodynamic therapy with 5-aminolevulenic acid was successful and well tolerated for the treatment of multiple basaloid follicular hamartomas and basal cell carcinomas in children with nevoid basal cell carcinoma syndrome.[86]

■ PERIFOLLICULAR FIBROMA

BOX 18-15 Summary

- Flesh-colored papule
- Central vellus hair follicle with concentric fibrous connective tissue
- May be seen in Birt-Hogg-Dubé syndrome

The perifollicular fibroma presents as a small, firm, flesh-colored papule primarily on the head and neck.[87] Histologically, this is marked by a central vellus hair follicle surrounded by concentric proliferation of fibrous connective tissue.

The perifollicular fibroma may occur sporadically or in association with Birt-Hogg-Dubé syndrome.[88,89] It has been suggested that perifollicular fibroma fits within the histologic spectrum of fibrofolliculoma and trichodiscoma, and may not be a distinct entity.[90] Like fibrofolliculoma and trichodiscoma, the perifolliculoma is benign and excision is curative. Destructive techniques such as CO_2 laser ablation, cryosurgery, and dermabrasion have been used when lesions are multiple.

■ FIBROFOLLICULOMA

BOX 18-16 Summary

- Single or multiple firm papules
- Central dilated follicular infundibulum
- Anastamosing strands of infundibular epithelium
- Fibrotic connective tissue stroma
- May be seen in Birt-Hogg-Dubé syndrome

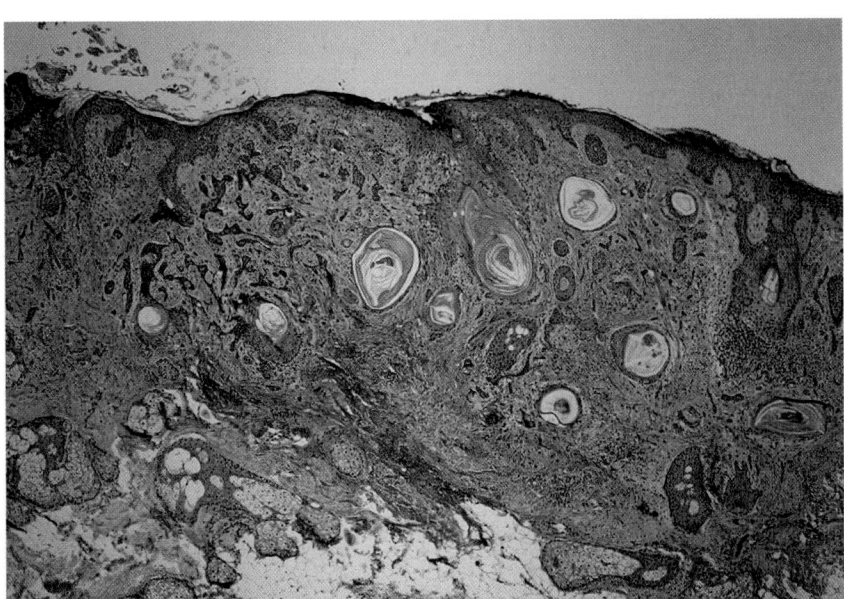

▲ **FIGURE 18-19** Desmoplastic trichoepithelioma shows small basaloid islands in the upper to mid-dermis surrounded by a fibrotic stroma. Areas of keratin cyst formation and follicular germ structures are present.

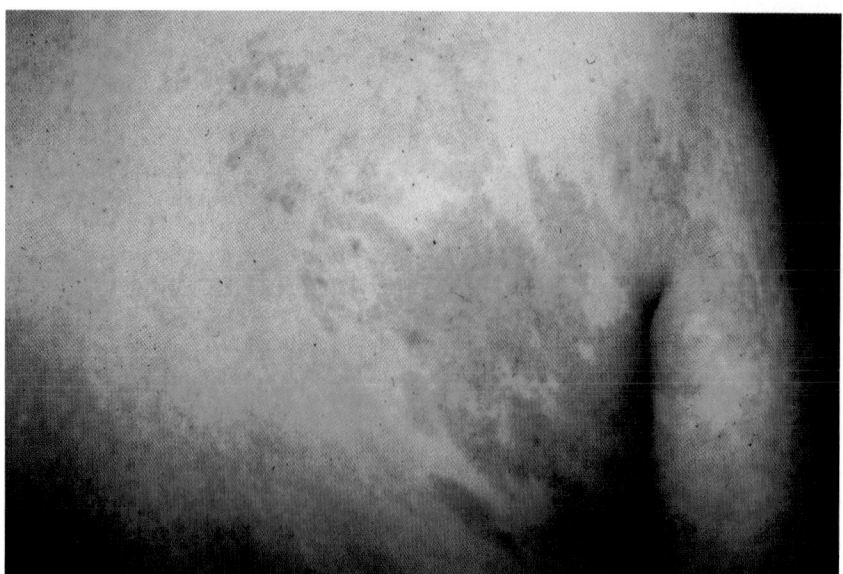

▲ **FIGURE 18-20** Basaloid follicular hamartoma presents at birth or shortly thereafter, with a large unilateral patch resembling an epidermal nevus.

The fibrofolliculoma may present as a single or multiple firm papules, primarily on the head, and neck of middle-aged patients. Histologically, the lesion shows a central dilated follicular infundibulum surrounded by proliferation of pale-staining infundibular epithelium (Fig. 18-21). The pale-staining infundibular epithelium forms interconnecting and anatomizing strands surrounded by a fibrotic connective tissue stroma. Patients with multiple fibrofolliculomas, trichodiscomas, and acrochordons may present in cancer-prone families as Birt-Hogg-Dubé syndrome.

Birt-Hogg-Dubé syndrome is an autosomal dominant genodermatosis characterized by mutation in the BHD protein folliculin, located on chromosome 17p11.2.[88,91] These patients have an increased incidence of pulmonary cysts, pneumothorax, and renal carcinoma.[88,92] It has been suggested that fibrofolliculoma fits within the histologic spectrum of trichodiscoma and perifollicular fibroma, and may not be a distinct entity.[90,93,94]

Like trichodiscoma and perifollicular fibroma, the fibrofolliculoma is benign and excision is curative. Destructive techniques such as CO_2

laser ablation,[95] cryosurgery, and dermabrasion have been used when lesions are multiple.

■ TRICHODISCOMA

BOX 18-17 Summary

- Small flesh-colored papule
- Tumor of vascular connective tissue of perifollicular sheath
- Fibroblasts embedded in loose mucinous stroma
- May be seen in Birt-Hogg-Dubé syndrome

Felix Pinkus described the hair disk (haarscheibe) as a touch receptor associated with adjacent hair follicles in the skin.[96,97] The trichodiscoma, which represents a tumor of this hair disk, presents clinically as a small flesh-colored papule (Fig. 18-22). Histologically, the lesion represents a tumor of the vascular connective tissue of the perifollicular sheath with fibroblasts embedded in a loose stroma containing abundant Alcian blue reactive mucin (Fig. 18-23). The lesions are located adjacent to a hair follicle.

The trichodiscoma may occur sporadically or in association with Birt-Hogg-Dubé syndrome.[88] It has been suggested that tricodiscoma fits within the histologic spectrum of fibrofolliculoma and perifollicular fibroma, and may not be a distinct entity.[90,93,94] Like fibrofolliculoma and perifollicular fibroma, the

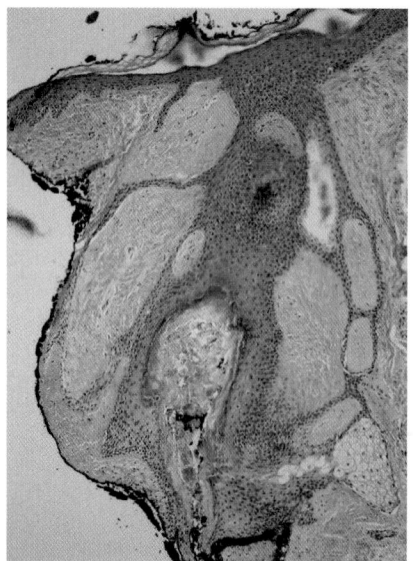

▲ **FIGURE 18-21** Fibrofolliculoma shows a central dilated follicular infundibulum surrounded by a proliferation of infundibular epithelium and a fibrotic connective tissue stroma.

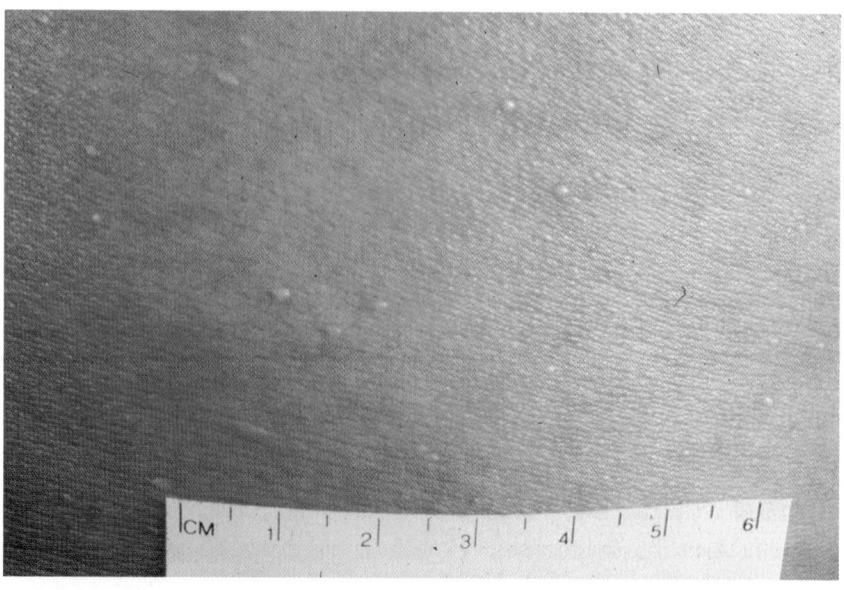

▲ **FIGURE 18-22** Trichodiscoma presents as a small flesh-colored papule.

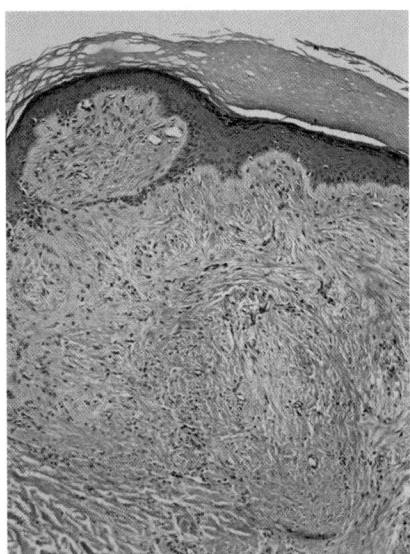

▲ **FIGURE 18-23** Trichodiscoma represents a tumor of follicular stroma.

trichodiscoma is benign and excision is curative. Destructive techniques such as CO_2 laser ablation,[95] cryosurgery, and dermabrasion have been used when lesions are multiple.

PROLIFERATING TRICHILEMMAL CYST

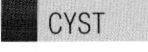

BOX 18-18 Summary

- Deep dermal nodules
- Multiple lobules of outer root sheath epithelium
- Nuclear pleomorphism and numerous mitotic figures are not common
- Associated malignant change may occur

The proliferating trichilemmal cyst or trichilemmal tumor is a multinodular neoplasm most often located on the head and scalp of elderly patients, particularly women (Fig. 18-24).[98] Histologically, the lesions are multilobular and are located in the dermis and subcutaneous fat. The lesion is composed of pale-staining outer root sheath-type epithelium with extensive trichilemmal keratinization, forming densely packed keratin without a granular cell layer (Fig. 18-25). Dermal fibrosis and chronic inflammation are common. Nuclear pleomorphism and numerous mitotic figures are not common in these tumors, and if present, should prompt consideration of squamous cell carcinoma formation.

The proliferating trichilemmal cyst is prone to local recurrence and surgical

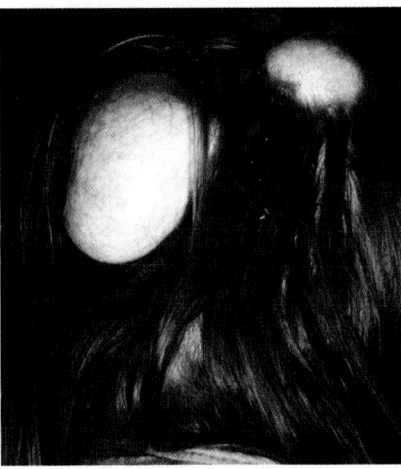

▲ **FIGURE 18-24** Proliferating trichilemmal cyst presents with a rapidly growing dermal or subcutaneous nodule primarily on the scalp of elderly patients.

excision is recommended for complete removal.

Cases of proliferating trichilemmal tumor with metastasis have been described.[99,100] For this reason, some authors believe the proliferating trichilemmal tumor to represent a well-differentiated squamous cell carcinoma. The presence of marked nuclear atypia and mitotic figures may indicate malignant change.[101] Increased proliferation may be confirmed with staining for proliferating cell nuclear antigen (PCNA).[102] In contrast, benign trichilemmal cysts show staining limited to the basal cell layer.[103] The presence of a spindle cell component may also signal malignancy.[98] These lesions should be completely excised.[104,105] Removal of these lesions with Mohs micrographic surgery has also been recommended.[99]

FINAL THOUGHTS

Benign hair follicle tumors are relatively uncommon, but may be seen in a routine dermatologic practice. These must be recognized in order to prevent confusion with basal cell carcinoma or squamous cell carcinoma with subsequent excessively aggressive surgical removal. Some follicular tumors such as the fibrofolliculoma and trichodiscoma may also be important as markers of cancer-prone families.

The management of follicular tumors begins with an adequate biopsy sample. Punch or excisional biopsy is recommended for suspicious lesions. This is important in order to differentiate follicular tumors from other neoplasms of the skin. Re-excision of a benign follicular tumor that has been adequately sampled is not always required. Malignant follicular tumors are rare and may be aggressive. Recognition of these lesions is important to ensure adequate surgical therapy including either wide local excision or removal by Mohs surgical technique.

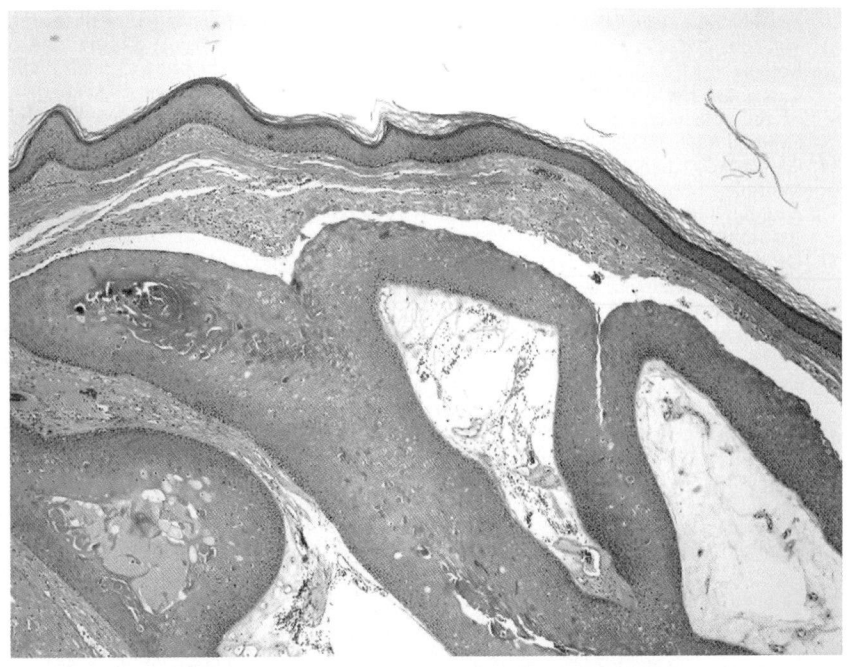

▲ **FIGURE 18-25** Proliferating trichilemmal cyst shows areas of cyst formation without a granular cell layer surrounded by a somewhat circumscribed proliferation of the pale-staining squamous epithelium.

1. Liegl B, Leibl S, Okcu M, et al. Malignant transformation within benign adnexal skin tumours. *Histopathology.* 2004;45: 162–170.

2. Pinkus H, Sutton RL Jr. Trichofolliculoma. *Arch Dermatol.* 1965;91:46–49.

3. Plewig G. Sebaceous trichofolliculoma. *J Cutan Pathol.* 1980;7:394-403.

4. Simpson W, Garner A, Collin JR. Benign hair-follicle derived tumours in the differential diagnosis of basal-cell carcinoma of the eyelids: a clinicopathological comparison. *Br J Ophthalmol.* 1989; 73:347–353.

5. Morton AD, Nelson CC, Headington JT, et al. Recurrent trichofolliculoma of the upper eyelid margin. *Ophthal Plast Reconstr Surg.* 1997;13:287–288.

6. Rahbari H, Mehregan A, Pinkus H. Trichoadenoma of Nikolowski. *J Cutan Pathol.* 1977;4:90–98.

7. Yamaguchi J, Takino C. A case of trichoadenoma arising in the buttock. *J Dermatol.* 1992;19:503–506.

8. Winer LH. The dilated pore, a trichoepithelioma. *J Invest Dermatol.* 1954;23: 181–188.

9. Konohana A, Kobayashi T. Aggregated dilated pores. *J Dermatol.* 1999;26:332–333.

10. Mehregan AH, Brownstein MH. Pilar sheath acanthoma. *Arch Dermatol.* 1978; 114:1495–1497.

11. Mehregan AH, Butler JD. A tumor of follicular infundibulum. Report of a case. *Arch Dermatol.* 1961;83:924–927.

12. Mehregan AH. Tumor of follicular infundibulum. *Dermatologica.* 1971;142: 177–183.

13. Cribier B, Grosshans E. Tumor of the follicular infundibulum: a clinicopathologic study. *J Am Acad Dermatol.* 1995;33: 979–984.

14. Hutchinson KW, Boulton JE, Sulivan TJ, et al. Clinicopathological report Periocular tumour of the follicular infundibulum. *Clin Experiment Ophthalmol.* 2001;29:100–101.

15. Kolenik SA, 3rd, Bolognia JL, Castiglione FM Jr, et al. Multiple tumors of the follicular infundibulum. *Int J Dermatol.* 1996;35:282–284.

16. Cheng AC, Chang YL, Wu YY, et al. Multiple tumors of the follicular infundibulum. *Dermatol Surg.* 2004;30: 1246–1248.

17. Cribier B, Waskievicz W, Heid E. Multiple infundibuloma. *Ann Dermatol Venereol.* 1991;118:281–285.

18. Vin-Christian K, Grekin R, McCalmont T. Hypopigmented papules of the cheeks, neck, and shoulders. *Arch Dermatol.* 1999;135:463–464, 6–7.

19. Starink TM, Hausman R. The cutaneous pathology of facial lesions in Cowden's disease. *J Cutan Pathol.* 1984;11: 331–337.

20. Brownstein MH, Mehregan AH, Bikowski JB, et al. The dermatopathology of Cowden's syndrome. *Br J Dermatol.* 1979;100:667–673.

21. Requena L, Gutierrez J, Sanchez Yus E. Multiple sclerotic fibromas of the skin. A cutaneous marker of Cowden's disease. *J Cutan Pathol.* 1992;19:346–351.

22. Blanco V, Keochgerian V. Cowden's syndrome. Case report, with reference to an affected family. *Med Oral Patol Oral Cir Bucal.* 2006;11:E12–E16.

23. Boonpipattanapong T, Phuenpathom N, Mitarnun W. Cowden's syndrome with Lhermitte-Duclos disease. *Br J Neurosurg.* 2005;19:361–365.

24. Leao JC, Batista V, Guimaraes PB, et al. Cowden's syndrome affecting the mouth, gastrointestinal, and central nervous system: a case report and review of the literature. *Oral Surg Oral Med Oral Pathol Oral Radiol Endod.* 2005;99: 569–572.

25. Reifenberger J. Hereditary tumor syndromes. Cutaneous manifestations and molecular pathogenesis of Gorlin and Cowden syndromes. *Hautarzt.* 2004;55: 942–951.

26. Bau MG, Arisio R, Cristini G, et al. Screening-detected breast carcinoma in a patient with Cowden syndrome. *Breast.* 2004;13:239–241.

27. Fistarol SK, Anliker MD, Itin PH. Cowden disease or multiple hamartoma syndrome—cutaneous clue to internal malignancy. *Eur J Dermatol.* 2002;12:411–421.

28. Rohwedder A, Keminer O, Hendricks C, et al. Detection of HPV DNA in trichilemmomas by polymerase chain reaction. *J Med Virol.* 1997;51:119–125.

29. Leonardi CL, Zhu WY, Kinsey WH, et al. Trichilemmomas are not associated with human papillomavirus DNA. *J Cutan Pathol.* 1991;18:193–197.

30. Starink TM, Hausman R. The cutaneous pathology of extrafacial lesions in Cowden's disease. *J Cutan Pathol.* 1984; 11:338–344.

31. Tellechea O, Reis JP, Baptista AP. Desmoplastic trichilemmoma. *Am J Dermatopathol.* 1992;14:107–114.

32. Kovich O, Cohen D. Cowden's syndrome. *Dermatol Online J.* 2004;10:3.

33. Schweiger E, Spann CT, Weinberg JM, et al. A case of desmoplastic trichilemmoma of the lip treated with Mohs surgery. *Dermatol Surg.* 2004;30:1062–1064.

34. Swanson PE, Marrogi AJ, Williams DJ, et al. Tricholemmal carcinoma: clinicopathologic study of 10 cases. *J Cutan Pathol.* 1992;19:100–109.

35. Boscaino A, Terracciano LM, Donofrio V, et al. Tricholemmal carcinoma: a study of seven cases. *J Cutan Pathol.* 1992;19:94–99.

36. Wong TY, Suster S. Tricholemmal carcinoma. A clinicopathologic study of 13 cases. *Am J Dermatopathol.* 1994;16: 463–473.

37. Dekio S, Funaki M, Jidoi J, et al. Trichilemmal carcinoma on the thigh: report of a case. *J Dermatol.* 1994;21: 494–496.

38. Ko T, Tada H, Hatoko M, et al. Trichilemmal carcinoma developing in a burn scar: a report of two cases. *J Dermatol.* 1996; 23:463–468.

39. Lai TF, Huilgol SC, James CL, et al. Trichilemmal carcinoma of the upper eyelid. *Acta Ophthalmol Scand.* 2003;81: 536–538.

40. Garrett AB, Azmi FH, Ogburia KS. Trichilemmal carcinoma: a rare cutaneous malignancy: a report of two cases. *Dermatol Surg.* 2004;30:113–115.

41. Allee JE, Cotsarelis G, Solky B, et al. Multiply recurrent trichilemmal carcinoma with perineural invasion and cytokeratin 17 positivity. *Dermatol Surg.* 2003;29:886–889.

42. Knoeller SM, Haag M, Adler CP, et al. Skeletal metastasis in tricholemmal carcinoma. *Clin Orthop Relat Res.* 2004: 213–216.

43. Mehregan AH. Inverted follicular keratosis. *Arch Dermatol.* 1964;89:229–235.

44. Boniuk M, Zimmerman LE. Eyelid tumors with reference to lesions confused with squamous cell carcinoma. II. Inverted follicular keratosis. *Arch Ophthalmol.* 1963;69:698–707.

45. Azzopardi JG, Laurini R. Inverted follicular keratosis. *J Clin Pathol.* 1975;28: 465–471.

46. Sassani JW, Yanoff M. Inverted follicular keratosis. *Am J Ophthalmol.* 1979;87: 810–813.

47. Mehregan AH. Inverted follicular keratosis is a distinct follicular tumor. *Am J Dermatopathol.* 1983;5:467–470.

48. Adrian JC. Inverted follicular keratosis of the lip. *Oral Surg Oral Med Oral Pathol.* 1984;57:625–630.

49. Reed RJ, Pulitzer DR. Inverted follicular keratosis and human papillomaviruses. *Am J Dermatopathol.* 1983;5:453–465.

50. Mehregan AH, Nadji M. Inverted follicular keratosis and verruca vulgaris. An investigation for the papillomavirus common antigen. *J Cutan Pathol.* 1984; 11:99–102.

51. Shih CC, Yu HS, Tung YC et al. Inverted follicular keratosis. *Kaohsiung J Med Sci.* 2001;17:50–54.

52. Ruhoy SM, Thomas D, Nuovo GJ. Multiple inverted follicular keratoses as a presenting sign of Cowden's syndrome: case report with human papillomavirus studies. *J Am Acad Dermatol.* 2004;51:411–415.

53. Marrogi AJ, Wick MR, Dehner LP. Pilomatrical neoplasms in children and young adults. *Am J Dermatopathol.* 1992;14:87–94.

54. Kaddu S, Soyer HP, Cerroni L, et al. Clinical and histopathologic spectrum of pilomatricomas in adults. *Int J Dermatol.* 1994;33:705–708.

55. Julian CG, Bowers PW. A clinical review of 209 pilomatricomas. *J Am Acad Dermatol.* 1998;39:191–195.

56. Cooper PH, Fechner RE. Pilomatricoma-like changes in the epidermal cysts of Gardner's syndrome. *J Am Acad Dermatol.* 1983;8:639–644.

57. Cigliano B, Baltogiannis N, De Marco M, et al. Pilomatricoma in childhood: a retrospective study from three European paediatric centres. *Eur J Pediatr.* 2005; 164:673–677.

58. Danielson-Cohen A, Lin SJ, Hughes CA, et al. Head and neck pilomatrixoma in children. *Arch Otolaryngol Head Neck Surg.* 2001;127:1481–1483.

59. Agarwal RP, Handler SD, Matthews MR, et al. Pilomatrixoma of the head and neck in children. *Otolaryngol Head Neck Surg.* 2001;125:510–515.

60. Lan MY, Lan MC, Ho CY, et al. Pilomatricoma of the head and neck: a retrospective review of 179 cases. *Arch Otolaryngol Head Neck Surg.* 2003;129: 1327–1330.

61. Haferkamp B, Bastian BC, Brocker EB, et al. Pilomatrix carcinoma in an unusual location. Case report and review of the literature. *Hautarzt.* 1999;50:355–359.

62. Sau P, Lupton GP, Graham JH. Pilomatrix carcinoma. *Cancer.* 1993;71:2491–2498.

63. Niedermeyer HP, Peris K, Hofler H. Pilomatrix carcinoma with multiple visceral metastases. Report of a case. *Cancer.* 1996;77:1311–1314.

64. De Galvez-Aranda MV, Herrera-Ceballos E, Sanchez-Sanchez P, et al. Pilomatrix carcinoma with lymph node and pulmonary metastasis: report of a case arising on the knee. *Am J Dermatopathol.* 2002;24:139–143.

65. Hardisson D, Linares MD, Cuevas-Santos J, et al. Pilomatrix carcinoma: a clinicopathologic study of six cases and review of the literature. *Am J Dermatopathol.* 2001;23:394–401.

66. Sable D, Snow SN. Pilomatrix carcinoma of the back treated by Mohs micrographic surgery. *Dermatol Surg.* 2004;30:1174–1176.

67. Harada H, Hashimoto K, Ko MS. The gene for multiple familial trichoepithelioma maps to chromosome 9p21. *J Invest Dermatol.* 1996;107:41–43.

68. Bowen S, Gill M, Lee DA, et al. Mutations in the CYLD gene in Brooke-Spiegler syndrome, familial cylindromatosis, and multiple familial trichoepithelioma: lack of genotype-phenotype correlation. *J Invest Dermatol.* 2005;124:919–920.

69. Zheng G, Hu L, Huang W, et al. CYLD mutation causes multiple familial trichoepithelioma in three Chinese families. *Hum Mutat.* 2004;23:400.

70. Yu DK, Joo YH, Cho KH. Trichoblastoma with apocrine and sebaceous differentiation. *Am J Dermatopathol.* 2005; 27:6–8.

71. Brownstein MH, Shapiro L. Desmoplastic trichoepithelioma. *Cancer.* 1977;40:2979–2986.

72. Koay JL, Ledbetter LS, Page RN, et al. Asymptomatic annular plaque of the chin: desmoplastic trichoepithelioma. *Arch Dermatol.* 2002;138:1091–1096.

73. Ohnishi T, Watanabe S. Immunohistochemical analysis of cytokeratin expression in various trichogenic tumors. *Am J Dermatopathol.* 1999;21:337–343.

74. Yamamoto O, Hamada T, Doi Y, et al. Immunohistochemical and ultrastructural observations of desmoplastic trichoepithelioma with a special reference to a morphological comparison with normal apocrine acrosyringeum. *J Cutan Pathol.* 2002;29:15–26.

75. Shaffelburg M, Miller R. Treatment of multiple trichoepithelioma with electrosurgery. *Dermatol Surg.* 1998;24:1154–1156.

76. Duhra P, Paul JC. Cryotherapy for multiple trichoepithelioma. *J Dermatol Surg Oncol.* 1988;14:1413–1415.

77. Bari AU, Rahman SB. Multiple familial trichoepithelioma: a rare cutaneous tumour. *J Coll Physicians Surg Pak.* 2004;14:560–561.

78. Aygun C, Blum JE. Trichoepithelioma 100 years later: a case report supporting the use of radiotherapy. *Dermatology.* 1993;187:209–212.

79. Rallan D, Harland CC. Brooke-Spiegler syndrome: treatment with laser ablation. *Clin Exp Dermatol.* 2005;30:355–357.

80. Sajben FP, Ross EV. The use of the 1.0 mm handpiece in high energy, pulsed CO_2 laser destruction of facial adnexal tumors. *Dermatol Surg.* 1999;25:41–44.

81. Rosenbach A, Alster TS. Multiple trichoepitheliomas successfully treated with a high-energy, pulsed carbon dioxide laser. *Dermatol Surg.* 1997;23:708–710.

82. Flores JT, Apfelberg DB, Maser MR, et al. Trichoepithelioma: successful treatment with the argon laser. *Plast Reconstr Surg.* 1984;74:694–698.

83. Sau P, Lupton GP, Graham JH. Trichogerminoma. Report of 14 cases. *J Cutan Pathol.* 1992;19:357–365.

84. Kazakov DV, Kutzner H, Rutten A, et al. Trichogerminoma: a rare cutaneous adnexal tumor with differentiation toward the hair germ epithelium. *Dermatology.* 2002;205:405–408.

85. Starink TM, Lane EB, Meijer CJ. Generalized trichoepitheliomas with alopecia and myasthenia gravis: clinicopathologic and immunohistochemical study and comparison with classic and desmoplastic trichoepithelioma. *J Am Acad Dermatol.* 1986;15:1104–1112.

86. Oseroff AR, Shieh S, Frawley NP, et al. Treatment of diffuse basal cell carcinomas and basaloid follicular hamartomas in nevoid basal cell carcinoma syndrome by wide-area 5-aminolevulinic acid photodynamic therapy. *Arch Dermatol.* 2005;141:60–67.

87. Zackheim HS, Pinkus H. Perifollicular fibromas. *Arch Dermatol.* 1960;82:913–917.

88. Welsch MJ, Krunic A, Medenica MM. Birt-Hogg-Dube Syndrome. *Int J Dermatol.* 2005;44:668–673.

89. Junkins-Hopkins JM, Cooper PH. Multiple perifollicular fibromas: report of a case and analysis of the literature. *J Cutan Pathol.* 1994;21:467–471.

90. Schulz T, Hartschuh W. Birt-Hogg-Dube syndrome and Hornstein-Knickenberg syndrome are the same. Different sectioning technique as the cause of different histology. *J Cutan Pathol.* 1999;26:55–61.

91. Schmidt LS, Nickerson ML, Warren MB, et al. Germline BHD-mutation spectrum and phenotype analysis of a large cohort of families with Birt-Hogg-Dube syndrome. *Am J Hum Genet.* 2005;76:1023–1033.

92. Vocke CD, Yang Y, Pavlovich CP, et al. High frequency of somatic frameshift BHD gene mutations in Birt-Hogg-Dube-associated renal tumors. *J Natl Cancer Inst.* 2005;97:931–935.

93. Vincent A, Farley M, Chan E, et al. Birt-Hogg-Dube syndrome: a review of the literature and the differential diagnosis of firm facial papules. *J Am Acad Dermatol.* 2003;49:698–705.

94. Collins GL, Somach S, Morgan MB. Histomorphologic and immunophenotypic analysis of fibrofolliculomas and trichodiscomas in Birt-Hogg-Dube syndrome and sporadic disease. J Cutan Pathol. 2002;29:529–533.

95. Kahle B, Hellwig S, Schulz T. Multiple mantleomas in Birt-Hogg-Dube syndrome: successful therapy with CO2 laser. *Hautarzt.* 2001;52:43–46.

96. Pinkus H, Coskey R, Burgess GH. Trichodiscoma. A benign tumor related to haarscheibe (hair disk). *J Invest Dermatol.* 1974;63:212-218.

97. Coskey RJ, Pinkus H. Trichodiscoma. *Int J Dermatol.* 1976;15:600–601.

98. Plumb SJ, Stone MS. Proliferating trichilemmal tumor with a malignant spindle cell component. *J Cutan Pathol.* 2002;29:506–509.

99. Tierney E, Ochoa MT, Rudkin G, et al. Mohs micrographic surgery of a proliferating trichilemmal tumor in a young black man. *Dermatol Surg.* 2005;31:359–363.

100. Weiss J, Heine M, Grimmel M, et al. Malignant proliferating trichilemmal cyst. *J Am Acad Dermatol.* 1995;32:870–873.

101. Lee SJ, Choi KH, Han JH, et al. Malignant proliferating trichilemmal tumor of the lower eyelid. *Ophthal Plast Reconstr Surg.* 2005;21:349–352.

102. Herrero J, Monteagudo C, Ruiz A, et al. Malignant proliferating trichilemmal tumours: an histopathological and immunohistochemical study of three cases with DNA ploidy and morphometric evaluation. *Histopathology.* 1998;33:542–546.

103. Rutty GN, Richman PI, Laing JH. Malignant change in trichilemmal cysts: a study of cell proliferation and DNA content. *Histopathology.* 1992;21:465–468.

104. Mathis ED, Honningford JB, Rodriguez HE, et al. Malignant proliferating trichilemmal tumor. *Am J Clin Oncol.* 2001;24:351–353.

105. Mehregan AH, Lee KC. Malignant proliferating trichilemmal tumors—report of three cases. *J Dermatol Surg Oncol.* 1987;13:1339–1342.

CHAPTER 19

Tumors of the Nail Unit

Olympia I. Kovich, M.D.
Richard K. Scher, M.D., F.A.C.P.

BOX 19-1   Overview

- This chapter will cover verrucae of the nail unit and the most common malignant neoplasms, including Bowen's disease, invasive SCC, keratoacanthoma, verrucous carcinoma, basal cell carcinoma, metastases, and malignant melanoma.
- Any benign or malignant tumor that affects the skin can also occur in the nail unit.
- As the nail unit has a limited number of responses to injury, it is often difficult to differentiate between inflammatory, infectious and neoplastic processes.
- Due to the potential clinical overlap between benign and malignant lesions, it is important to biopsy any lesion that is persistent, suspicious, or recalcitrant to treatment.

■ INTRODUCTION

Tumors of the nail unit encompass many of the same benign and malignant entities that affect the remainder of the skin. However, diagnosis and treatment are often delayed due to altered morphology of nail tumors and reluctance to biopsy the nail unit because of the risk of permanent nail dystrophy. Recognition of how nail tumors commonly present and indications to biopsy are crucial to provide appropriate treatment.

This chapter will cover malignant tumors of the nail unit. While SCC is the most common malignant tumor of the nail unit, many other malignancies have been reported, albeit rarely. It is prudent, however, to note that several benign nail tumors, including verruca vulgaris, eccrine poroma and onycholemmal cysts, may undergo malignant degeneration. As the most common benign tumor of the nail unit, verruca vulgaris will be covered in detail as well.

Since the nail unit has a limited number of responses to injury, infection, and neoplasms, there is often significant overlap in the clinical presentation of

benign and malignant entities. While certain key features may aid in their differentiation, SCC *in situ* may masquerade as melanonychia while verruca of the proximal nail fold may be mistaken for paronychia.[1-3] An overarching principle is that any lesion of the nail unit that does not respond appropriately to treatment, or is suspicious or persistent, warrants a biopsy for histopathologic confirmation of the diagnosis.

■ VERRUCA VULGARIS

Epidemiology and Clinical Presentation

BOX 19-2   Summary

- Verruca vulgaris is the most frequently encountered tumor of the nail unit.
- Verrucae of the nail unit occur most frequently in children and young adults, but may present at any age, especially in association with certain risk factors.
- While verrucae typically present as hyperkeratotic papules, unusual presentations have been reported.
- Periungual verrucae, if left untreated, may progress to involve the subungual location.

Verruca vulgaris is the most common tumor to occur in the nail unit and may present in any age group. However, children and teenagers are the patients most likely to develop warts in the periungual location, especially those who engage in the habits of nail biting or finger sucking. While the incidence of periungual verrucae is greatest between the ages of 12 and 16, they also occur more frequently in patients with occupational risk factors (including prolonged contact with water and handling of meat, fish and poultry) and those who are immunocompromised.[4] In the latter group, verrucae may be particularly recalcitrant to treatment.

Common warts have a classic presentation as hyperkeratotic papules or nodules with punctuate black dots, corresponding to thrombosed capillaries histologically, which lead to pinpoint bleeding if the lesion is pared (Fig. 19-1). Warts typically arise in the proximal and lateral nail folds and the hyponychium. Subsequent extension into the nail bed may occur, complicating treatment. Underlying bone destruction has been reported rarely.[5]

While they usually have a classic appearance, verrucae of the proximal

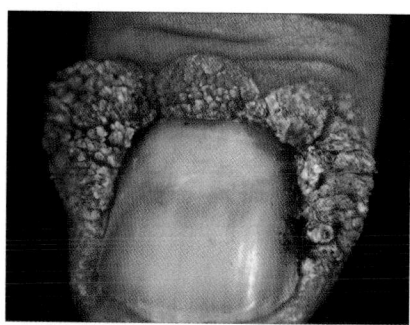

▲ **FIGURE 19-1** Verrucous papules of the proximal and lateral nail folds consistent with verrucae vulgaris.

nail fold may present as tender erythematous nodules, resembling a foreign body reaction, digital mucous cyst or paronychia.[6,7] In these atypical presentations, the smooth surface of the wart correlates histologically to tightly packed, parakeratotic mounds, rather than papillomatosis.[6] Thus, these lesions are best classified as myrmecia. Another uncommon presentation of periungual verruca is the giant wart. This requires a biopsy to rule out a wide differential diagnosis, including that of verrucous and SCCs, in addition to tuberculosis verrucosa cutis, deep mycosis and blastomycosis-like pyoderma.[8]

In addition to the differential diagnoses listed above, it is always prudent to consider the possibility of either malignant transformation of a verruca or the concomitant presence of an SCC. While the oncogenic potential of the human papilloma virus, the etiologic agents of warts, is well described in patients with epidermodysplasia verruciformis, common verrucae rarely undergo malignant change. Despite the relative rarity of malignant degeneration, there may be clinical similarities between warts and SCCs. Several case reports of SCC either mistakenly treated as verrucae or left untreated for extended periods of time emphasize the importance of an adequate biopsy for unusual, large or recalcitrant lesions.[9,10] In addition, many authors support the biopsy of any verrucous lesion of the nail unit in patients who carry a diagnosis of cervical dysplasia, cervical carcinoma, or condyloma acuminate.[11] One cannot be reassured by the presence of several verrucous lesions or a concomitant verruca; the risk of malignancy still exists.[11] In addition, patients with epidermodysplasia verruciformis are at a known increased risk for developing

Bowen disease within lesions that resemble verrucae planae.

Pathogenesis and Histology

> **BOX 19-3   Summary**
> - Periungual verrucae are most commonly caused by human papillomavirus types 1, 2 and 4.
> - Characteristic histopathologic findings are present, including "koilocytic" change.
> - Rare cases of Bowen disease and SCC arising in verrucae have been described, emphasizing the importance of careful histopathologic examination.

Of the more than 130 genotypes of the human papillomavirus (HPV), periungual verrucae are most often caused by HPV types 1, 2, and 4.[4,12] Human papillomavirus, a double-stranded DNA virus, must infect the basal cell layer of squamous epidermis or epithelium to produce clinical sequelae.[12] This mechanism explains why risk factors that generally disrupt the normal barrier of the skin predispose to infection.

Once infection has occurred, typical histopathologic changes ensue, namely hyperkeratosis, acanthosis and papillomatosis. Tiers of parakeratosis, often with hemorrhage, alternate with valleys of hypergranulosis. Cells above the basal layer often develop a characteristic appearance of a pyknotic nucleus with a surrounding clear halo; these cells are termed "koilocytes". Though rare, bowenoid change or SCC may arise in a wart; therefore, a verruca must be examined carefully for atypia.[13]

Prognosis and Treatment

> **BOX 19-4   Summary**
> - Most verrucae will regress spontaneously over time. Therefore, the potential sequelae of treatment must be weighed carefully.
> - Treatment options for periungual verrucae vary from benign neglect to topical agents, intralesional therapy, destructive methods, oral agents and surgery.
> - Treatment is dependent on patient factors and presentation, including age, immune status and extent of involvement.
> - Biopsy is indicated for lesions that are recalcitrant to treatment, long-standing or have an unusual presentation.
> - Malignant transformation, though rare, should be considered.

In general, warts exhibit a tendency toward spontaneous regression within a year or two after their appearance.[12] A review of treatment trials for verrucae demonstrated an average spontaneous rate of regression of 30% within the placebo arms.[14] While many patients elect to pursue treatment, it behoves physicians to remember the natural history of verrucae when considering more aggressive intervention. In the periungual location, this is particularly important, given the risk of permanent nail dystrophy and other potential complications of treatment.

A complete overview of the treatment of verrucae is beyond the scope of this chapter and the reader is referred to a recent review of surgical and nonsurgical approaches to the treatments of warts of the nail unit by Tosti and Piraccini.[4] In brief, treatment of verruca can be divided into several categories (Table 19-1). In immunocompetent adults, the preferred treatment for periungual verrucae that do not extend below the nail plate is often cryotherapy.[15] Invasive treatments include intralesional injection of antigens and the use of laser and related treatments, including the CO_2 laser, pulsed dye laser, potassium-titanyl-phosphate laser and photodynamic therapy. These have been used with variable success but are generally not first-line treatment. More destructive treatment modalities should be limited to recalcitrant lesions, as there are increased risks. For example, treatment with the CO_2 laser carries a risk of temporary or permanent nail dystrophy, prolonged pain, scarring and altered function.[4]

Table 19-1
Treatment Options for Cutaneous Warts

MEDICAL	
Keratolytics	Salicylic acid
Cytotoxic	Cantharidin
	5-fluorouracil
Intralesional	Bleomycin sulphate
	Interferon
	Candida Antigen
Immunotherapy	Squaric acid dibutylether (SADBE)
	Diphenylcyclopropenone (DFC)
	Imiquimod
Systemic	Cimetidine
	Retinoids
SURGICAL	
Cryotherapy	Cotton tip
Surgical excision	Cryospray

TREATMENT IN IMMUNOSUPPRESSED PATIENTS Specific consideration must be given to patients who are immunosuppressed, including HIV-infected patients and organ transplant recipients. These patients are more likely to be infected with the human papillomavirus and often have multiple HPV types within their cutaneous lesions (Fig. 19-2).[12] In addition, while malignant transformation of a common wart is rare, it has been reported more often in patients with immune suppression.[16] Finally, clinicians should have a lower threshold to biopsy suspicious lesions, as the clinical appearance of these lesions does not always mirror the histologic changes.[17]

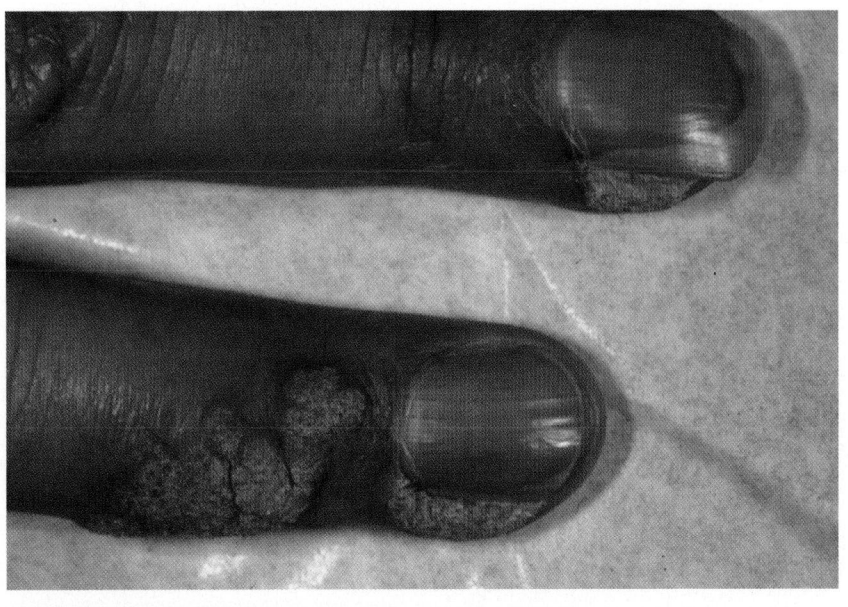

▲ **FIGURE 19-2** Multiple warts in an immunocompromised patient.

TREATMENT IN PEDIATRIC PATIENTS It is helpful to approach the treatment of verrucae with a ladder of therapy, that may differ for pediatric patients. Though benign neglect is often not acceptable to patients or their parents, other harmless therapies may be utilized, including occlusion with duct tape. A prospective, randomized controlled trial in children showed greater clearance of verruca with duct tape occlusion (85%) versus cryotherapy (60%).[18] Keratolytics, including salicylic acid, are often used in children, given their low-risk profile. Other topical treatments include topical immunotherapy with contact sensitizers. An in-depth review is beyond the scope of this chapter.

BOWEN DISEASE

Introduction

The nomenclature of malignancies arising from the epidermis of the nail unit has used numerous terms for the same entities. Some authors lump Bowen disease and SCC under the broader category of 'epidermoid carcinoma'.[19] For the purposes of this discussion, only the terms Bowen disease (namely SCC *in situ*) and invasive SCC will be used. It is worth noting that these are the two most common malignancies of the nail unit.[19,20] Three additional distinct entities, keratoacanthoma, verrucous carcinoma and basal cell carcinoma will also be discussed in the category of malignant epidermal neoplasms.

Epidemiology and Clinical Presentation

BOX 19-5   Summary

- Bowen disease is an uncommon tumor of the nail unit that usually occurs in patients
  - over the age of 60 years and has a male predominance.
- The thumb, index and middle fingers are the most common sites of Bowen disease.
- Bowen disease may be mistaken for a variety of inflammatory, infectious and neoplastic processes, due to it protean presentations.
- The occurrence of polydactylous lesions warrants a careful physical examination and close follow-up.

Bowen disease, or SCC *in situ*, though uncommon, has been reported in both the periungual and subungual location. It appears likely that it primarily affects the nail folds, with potential extension

into the remainder of the nail unit; primary involvement of the nail bed is rare.[2] It occurs predominantly in males after the fifth decade; however, patients as young as 39 years have been affected.[2,3] There is a predilection for involvement of the first three fingers. While the thumb has generally been reported as the most common site, one series found that 57% (4/7) of cases occurred on the middle finger.[3] Some authors report that Bowen disease more commonly involves fingers of the left hand.[21]

The clinical presentation of Bowen disease may be protean. In a series of seven patients with Bowen disease, Sau et al reported that three lesions resembled verruca vulgaris, two presented with nail dystrophy and onycholysis, one mimicked paronychia and one resembled acral melanoma.[3] The authors suggest that scaling and onycholysis out of proportion to the verrucous change were helpful indicators in suggesting Bowen disease.[3] Other unusual presentations have mimicked subungual hematoma, onychomatricoma, and a fibrokeratoma, both with or without melanocytic pigmentation; an erythematous band (simulating onychopapilloma) and longitudinal melanonychia have also been reported.[1,19,22–25]

The occurrence of polydactylous lesions, involving either both hands or the hands and feet, provides a rationale for avoiding overly aggressive treatment measures.[2,20] Initial close examination of all 20 nails and follow-up of the patient is warranted.

Pathogenesis and Histology

BOX 19-6   Summary

- Human papillomavirus is associated with approximately 50-60% of cases of Bowen disease of the nail unit. The occurrence of "high-risk" HPV types makes a causal relationship likely.
- Environmental factors, including repeated trauma, exposure to radiation and chemicals, and arsenic ingestion, have also been implicated as potential etiologic factors.
- Patients with certain genodermatoses, such as dyskeratosis congenita and epidermodysplasia verruciformis are at increased risk.
- Histologic examination reveals full-thickness keratinocytic atypia, loss of maturation of keratinocytes with hyperchromatic nuclei, and numerous mitoses.

Investigation into the pathogenesis of Bowen disease of the nail unit has examined the potential role of the human papillomavirus. In one series, 57% (4/7) of the cases were found to contain HPV-16 DNA by *in situ* hybridization.[3] In that series, a review of the literature to date revealed that 62% (28/45) of cases of periungual Bowen disease and SCC were associated with HPV.[3] HPV types found in Bowen disease of the nail include types 11, 16, 34, and 35; one case was found to harbor both HPV-11 and 16.[3,26] While this association does not confirm causality, it is likely that HPV plays a role in the etiology of many cases of Bowen disease.

Additional factors hypothesized to play a role in the development of Bowen disease include exposure to radiation or chemicals, repeated trauma and arsenic ingestion.[19] Therefore, query regarding these potential exposures should be included in the patient's history. While UV exposure is known to play a role in cutaneous Bowen disease, the nail plate serves as a protective barrier to most UV radiation, limiting its role at this site. Patients with epidermodysplasia verruciformis and dyskeratosis congenita are at increased risk of developing Bowen disease.[3]

A biopsy of Bowen disease reveals full-thickness atypia of a thickened epidermis/epithelium. There is a loss of maturation of keratinocytes, many of that have hyperchromatic nuclei. Numerous typical and atypical mitoses may be seen at all levels of the epidermis. It is important to note that an initial biopsy demonstrating the characteristic features of Bowen disease may, upon examination of excision specimen, reveal invasion.

Prognosis and Treatment

BOX 19-7   Summary

- Bowen disease of the nail unit is a low-grade malignancy with a moderate potential for recurrence but a low metastatic potential.
- Surgical excision, particularly with Mohs micrographic surgery, is the standard of care.
- Other avenues of treatment are either less effective or have not been adequately studied.
- Follow-up of patients should include a complete cutaneous examination, including all 20 nails, and a lymph node examination.

Bowen disease of the nail unit is generally considered to represent a low-grade malignancy and is a slow-growing tumor. It is difficult to provide specific prognostic details for Bowen disease, since it is usually grouped together with invasive SCC in the literature. While it has been reported that Bowen disease of the nail unit, when compared to its cutaneous counterpart, is more likely to become invasive, this may be due to a delay in diagnosis rather than an inherent difference in aggressiveness. In general, though recurrences have been reported, metastases are rare. Prognosis will be discussed in further depth in the section on invasive SCC.

Surgical excision is the standard of care for the treatment of Bowen disease. Prior to surgery, an X-ray to assess for the presence of underlying osseous involvement is required. Additionally, examination of lymph nodes is warranted. Many authors advocate the technique of Mohs micrographic surgery as a tissue-sparing technique in this special site. Rate of recurrence in one series treated with Mohs was 33% (2/6); the authors suggest that an additional surgical margin after the final stage may be warranted.[3] Although the benefit of complete margin control cannot be overstated, at the minimum, an adequate margin of normal surrounding tissue is requisite in treatment.

Another therapeutic approach that has been employed more recently is photodynamic therapy after application of aminolevulinic acid; two cases of subungual Bowen disease have been successfully treated with this modality.[21,27] Other treatments that have been utilized in the treatment of Bowen disease, but are not routinely recommended, include curettage with electrocautery, topical application of 5-fluorouracil or imiquimod, Grenz rays and CO_2 laser ablation.[27]

Follow-up should include regular examination of the affected site to monitor for recurrence, examination of all other digits and the entire integument, and palpation for lymphadenopathy. The likelihood of genital–digital autoinoculation is supported by the finding of an uncommon HPV type in penile and anal intraepithelial neoplasia and periungual SCC in the same patient.[28] Due to the frequent association with HPV-16, some authors recommend an examination of the anogenital area and close monitoring of female patients for cervical cancer.[29]

■ SQUAMOUS CELL CARCINOMA

Epidemiology and Clinical Presentation

BOX 19-8 Summary

- SCC is the most common malignant tumor of the nail unit.
- It usually affects men after the fifth decade.
- As with Bowen disease, its myriad presentations mimic benign inflammatory and infectious conditions.
- The differential diagnosis includes keratoacanthoma, verrucous carcinoma, and metastatic SCC.

SCC is the most common malignant tumor of the nail unit. As the prior section covered SCC *in situ* (Bowen disease), reference to SCC in this section implies invasive SCC, unless otherwise stated. SCC occurs most commonly in men after the fifth decade on the thumb and index finger, with rare occurrence on the toes.[30] Though rare in children, there are vanishingly rare reports in patients as young as 13 years.[31]

SCC may arise in any portion of the nail unit, including the lateral nail fold.[32] Due to its relatively slow growth and often subtle clinical findings, it has been misdiagnosed as onychomycosis, onycholysis, warts, nail deformity, ingrown nail, subungual exostosis, chronic osteomyelitis, traumatic dyschromia, pyogenic granuloma, paronychia, onychogryphosis, and has mimicked a fibrokeratoma with melanonychia (Figs. 19-3 to 19-5).[30,31,33] When loss of the nail plate occurs, secondary infections are common, which may mislead the clinician.[34] Features should raise suspicion for SCC include nodularity, bleeding, ulceration and an unresponsiveness to treatment.[34] Perhaps attributable to its myriad presentations, the average delay to diagnosis of a subungual SCC is 4 years.[30]

SCC has also been reported to arise in the setting a variety of primary dermatologic conditions. These include a case of SCC which developed in the nail matrix and bed of a patient with lichen planus that solely affected the nails and a well-differentiated SCC with features of a verrucous carcinoma that developed within a psoriatic nail bed.[35,36] In immunocompromised patients, SCC of the nail unit may grow more rapidly and may harbor HPV types not typically associated with malignancy.[11]

Radiographically, subungual SCC usually exhibits periosteal thickening and reactive sclerosis.[37,38] An erosive lesion in the distal phalanx has a broad differential diagnosis and, in addition to a subungual SCC, includes an implantation cyst, subungual fibroma, glomus tumor, giant cell tumor of the tendon sheath, mucous cyst, and subungual keratoacanthoma.[37] At times, it may not be possible to distinguish SCC from a keratoacanthoma radiologically.[37,38]

When a biopsy demonstrates SCC, the differential diagnosis should include metastatic SCC, which has been rarely described as secondary to primary lung and esophageal carcinomas.[39,40]

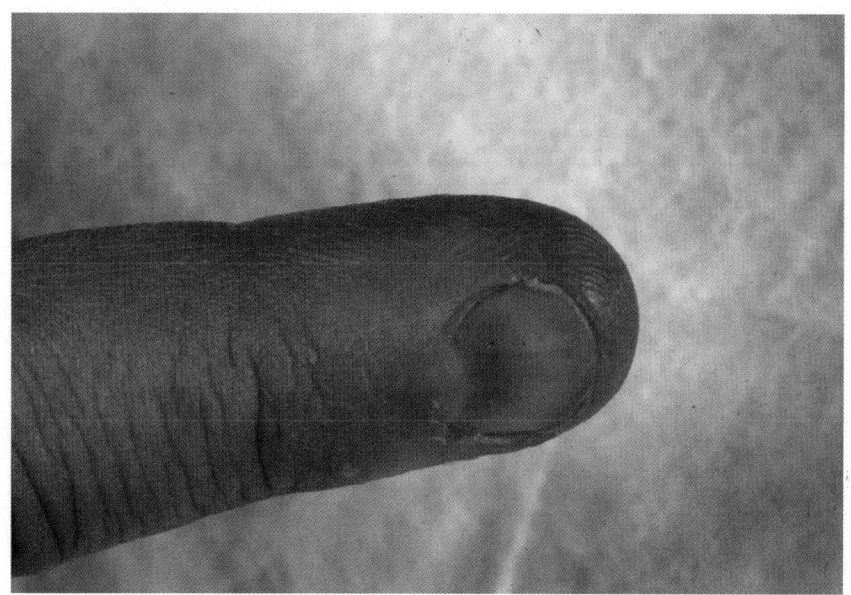

▲ **FIGURE 19-3** Erythema distal to the lunula secondary to an SCC.

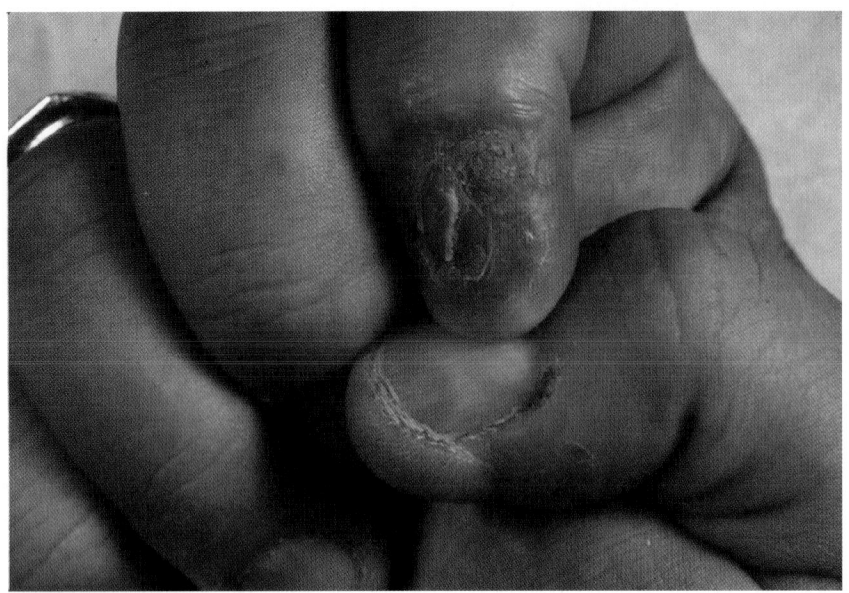

▲ **FIGURE 19-4** SCC presenting as a verrucous papule with partial loss of the nail plate and nail dystrophy.

Pathogenesis and Histology

BOX 19-9   Summary

- SCC is associated with a variety of genetic, infectious and environmental risk factors.
- Histologic examination reveals atypical keratinocytes that extend into the underlying dermis.
- Keratinocytes typically have large, hyperchromatic nuclei and mitotic figures are numerous.

Risk factors for the development of SCC are identical to those for Bowen disease, namely chronic paronychia, repeated trauma, exposure to radiation, arsenic, chemicals, and infection with human papillomavirus; there is also a higher incidence in patients with certain genodermatoses. In one series, five of seven cases (71%) of periungual SCC (two invasive SCC, three SCCIS) contained HPV-16, detected by polymerase chain reaction, in patients with no other known risk factors.[41] Another series found 80% of cases (8/10) with HPV, six of which had HPV-

16.[42] It is worth noting that HPV-16 is the most common subtype associated with cervical and genital intraepithelial neoplasia.[42] In three cases of subungual SCC arising on the toes, however, one of which was metastatic to the inguinal lymph nodes, PCR for HPV DNA was negative.[43]

The histopathologic features of invasive SCC include full-thickness atypia of the epithelium with invasion of islands of squamous cells into the dermis. SCC at this site may either be poorly or well differentiated. Typically cells are pleomorphic, with hyperchromatic nuclei and numerous mitoses. The biopsy and excision must be examined for invasion of the underlying bone and for the presence of vascular invasion.

Prognosis and Treatment

BOX 19-10   Summary

- SCC of the nail unit may invade the underlying phalanx but rarely metastasizes.
- Mohs micrographic surgery is the treatment of choice for invasive SCC.
- Extension into underlying bone necessitates amputation.
- Long-term follow-up is warranted in all cases.

Subungual SCC has been reported to invade the bone in 18 to 60% of cases.[1,37] Therefore, pre-operative evaluation should include an X-ray. Metastases have been reported in 1.7% of cases; spread to the lymph nodes has been reported in less than 2% of patients.[37,44] Post-surgical follow-up with an X-ray is often considered judicious.

It is important to consider that what appears to be bone involvement of an SCC on an X-ray obtained prior to surgery may in fact represent a reversible pressure effect due to the rapid growth of a subungual keratoacanthoma.[45] Therefore, it is often most prudent to avoid amputation as the primary treatment, except in cases of definitive histological osseous involvement.[45]

While it is mandatory to obtain an initial X-ray, it is unclear whether further investigation to evaluate for a primary tumor or for potential metastases at the time of presentation is required. In those cases reported in the literature, initial investigations have included chest, abdomen and pelvic CT scans (to rule out a primary tumor that has metastasized to the digit), lymphoscintigraphy, and whole body technetium or bone scans.[34,43,46] Other authors advocate a simple physical examination and X-ray.[11]

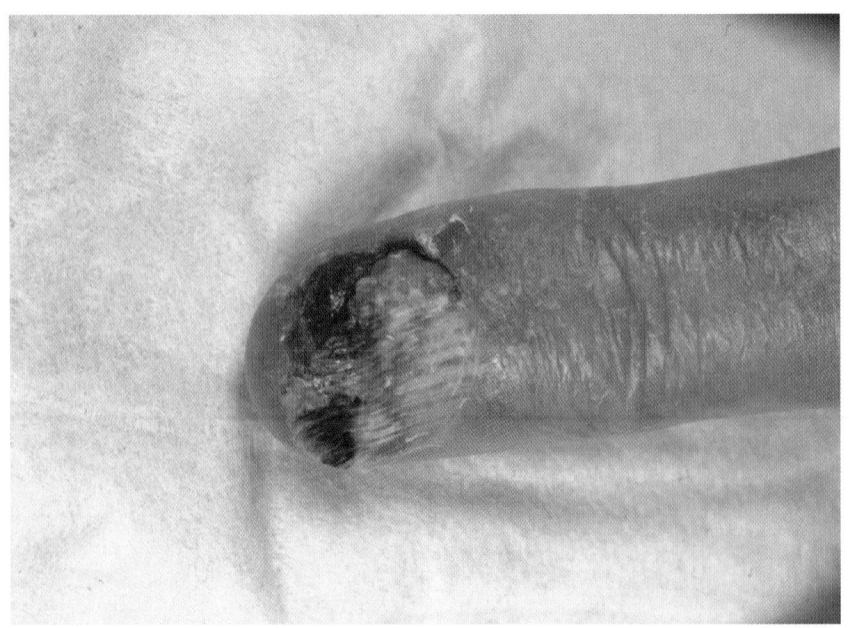

▲ **FIGURE 19-5** SCC presenting as an erythematous papule with distal onycholysis, dystrophy and discoloration of the nail plate.

Mohs micrographic surgery boasts cure rates as high as 92 to 96% and is the treatment of choice for SCC of the nail unit that does not have osseous involvement.[31,44] One series that did not have any cases of recurrence attributed their success to a modified Mohs technique in which they fixed their sections with 10% formalin and wax embedding, with examination by both the pathologist and surgeon.[47] Some authors favor wide local excision with a 5 mm margin and report that, for SCC arising in the lateral nail fold, reconstruction is more cosmetically acceptable with local flaps rather than skin grafts.[32] Sampling the periosteum of the underlying phalanx should be considered.

For SCC with bony involvement, amputation at the interphalangeal joint proximal to bone invasion has been advocated.[48] An interesting modification to simple amputation involves initial tumor resection with Mohs micrographic surgery prior to amputation, with subsequent flap repair utilizing the preserved intact sensate tissue.[48] It is worth noting that though no recurrences were reported with this modified procedure, the patients did not have histologic evidence of bony involvement despite radiographic changes that initially prompted amputation.

A reported alternative to amputation is external beam radiation, which may be considered in unresectable subungual SCC.[49]

Follow-up should extend at least 10 years, due to the risk of late metastasis.[30] In one of the few cases of periungual SCC that metastasized to an axillary lymph node 3.3 years after surgery, HPV type 35 was identified in both the primary tumor and metastasis.[50] There is also a report of a well-differentiated subungual SCC without bony involvement that metastasized despite treatment with a radical amputation.[51]

KERATOACANTHOMA

Epidemiology and Clinical Presentation

BOX 19-11   Summary

- Keratoacanthoma occurs most commonly in middle-aged Caucasian men.
- It has a distinct clinical presentation, with rapid growth within a few weeks to months, associated with pain.
- The characteristic radiographic finding of a cup-shaped lytic defect is a distinctive diagnostic clue and must be differentiated from periosteal changes seen in invasive SCC.

Two controversies arise in the discussion of keratoacanthoma (KA) of the nail unit. The first, applicable to both cutaneous and ungual keratoacanthomas involves the classification of this tumor, namely whether to consider it a distinct entity or as a subtype of SCC. It seems reasonable to consider KA as a "clinically distinct variant of well differentiated SCC capable of immunologically mediated spontaneous regression."[38] The fact that a portion of cutaneous keratoacanthomas may undergo spontaneous regression should be considered in the treatment rationale.

The second controversy regarding a subungual keratoacanthoma (SUKA) is whether it can arise in a non hair-bearing area, such as the nail unit. Keratoacanthomas are considered to originate from hair follicle epithelium; as the nail unit is devoid of hair follicles, some argue that the diagnosis of keratoacanthoma cannot be made in this location. However, histologic criteria for the diagnosis of keratoacanthoma in the nail unit appear sufficient to permit this diagnosis.

Subungual keratoacanthomas differ from typical SCCs of the nail unit. In general, patients with keratoacanthoma tend to be younger (peak incidence in the fifth decade) than those with subungual SCC (peak in the seventh decade).[37] Even patients in the second and third decades have been affected.[52] There is a male preponderance (male:female ratio of 3.5:1) and a predilection for the thumb and index finger.[53] Keratoacanthomas have solely been reported in Caucasian patients and may be solitary, multiple, eruptive or familial.[54]

The rapid evolution of keratoacanthomas, usually within several weeks to months, as well as the presence of associated pain, are the most helpful distinguishing features. Due to their rapid growth, a SUKA usually has a shorter time to presentation compared to an SCC.[53] SUKA may be associated with drainage from the nail bed that may be a firm, keratinaceous plug or a cheesy to purulent exudates.[55]

Periungual keratoacanthomas have been clinically mistaken for a verruca, epidermoid implantation cyst, SCC, melanoma, paronychia, cellulitis, osteomyelitis, deep mycosis, enchondroma, glomus tumor, metastatic carcinoma, onychomycosis and a giant cell tumor.[52,54–56]

The typical radiographic appearance of a subungual KA is a crescent- or cup-shaped lytic defect without sclerosis or periosteal reaction.[37] When compared to an SCC, it often exhibits more prominent bone erosion, possibly due to its rapid growth in a confined space.[36] These changes in the bone, however, may be reversible after removal of the keratoacanthoma; it is critical to differentiate this potentially temporary resorption in the phalanx from true invasion, as may be seen in SCC.[45]

Pathogenesis and Histology

BOX 19-12   Summary

- There are numerous risk factors for the development of a keratoacanthoma that are similar to those for SCC.
- The characteristic histology of a keratoacanthoma is a crateriform nodule of squamous epithelium with glassy cytoplasm, neutrophilic microabscesses and an infiltrate with lymphocytes and eosinophils. There are several important histologic differences between a subungual and cutaneous keratoacanthoma.

Purported predisposing factors for keratoacanthoma include trauma, exposure to coal tars and chemical carcinogens, eczema, psoriasis, atopic dermatitis, and xeroderma pigmentosum.[37] Whether ultraviolet radiation, a culprit in the etiology of cutaneous keratoacanthoma, plays a role in subungual keratoacanthoma is unclear. The question of whether HPV is involved in the development of periungual keratoacanthomas in a manner analogous to periungual SCCs was raised in a case report by Baran et al[57] In this case report, two oncogenic strains, HPV types 31 and 35, were isolated from a periungual keratoacanthoma; HPV was not identified, however, in the verruca that occurred in this same location prior to the development of a keratoacanthoma.[57] The authors suggest that inoculation with HPV was related to the transformation of the verruca.[57]

Keratoacanthomas in the nail unit have a similar histology to cutaneous lesions, with a crateriform nodule of squamous epithelium with glassy cytoplasm. Compared to a cutaneous keratoacanthoma, a SUKA has more depth than breadth, has an increased number of dyskeratotic cells, often lacks a collarette and has a less prominent inflammatory infiltrate.[52,54]

Prognosis and Treatment

BOX 19-13 Summary

- Only rare reports of spontaneous regression of subungual keratoacanthomas exist.
- Surgical treatment is the standard of care for SUKA. Curettage is an option in cases with definitive histology.
- Bone changes seen on X-ray may be reversible and a follow-up X-ray after treatment should be obtained.
- Most recurrences occur in the first several months but have been reported as late as 2 years after treatment. Long-term follow-up is therefore warranted.

The natural history of SUKA with regard to potential spontaneous resolution is not well delineated. There is one report of a lesion, clinically and radiologically consonant with a subungual keratoacanthoma, which regressed spontaneously without treatment.[38] In this case, only a mild residual deformity of the phalanx remained.[38] In a case series of 12 SUKAs, one resolved spontaneously.[56]

Most authors agree that, due to the potential overlap in histology between a keratoacanthoma and a well-differentiated SCC, a subungual keratoacanthoma should be treated surgically. However, some authors feel that curettage is also an acceptable treatment, given the relatively high cure rate of this modality, a tendency for potential recurrence within a shorter time frame, and lack of cases of metastatic keratoacanthoma.[53] Amputation is generally not warranted except for multiple recurrences or when there is histologic overlap with SCC.[54]

There are numerous reports of resolution of the bony defects associated with keratoacanthomas after treatment. Follow-up of treated lesions should therefore include an X-ray to assess for reossification.[54] Recurrences have been reported most commonly in the first 5 months, but as late as 28 months after treatment.[54] Therefore, follow-up for at least several years is indicated.

■ VERRUCOUS CARCINOMA

Epidemiology and Clinical Presentation

BOX 19-14 Summary

- Verrucous carcinoma is a rare subtype of SCC that may mimic a verruca both clinically and histologically.

- Involvement of the nail unit, either primarily or secondarily, is rare, with less than 20 reported cases in the literature.
- It is crucial to distinguish this entity, as certain modalities of treatment are contraindicated.

Verrucous carcinoma is an uncommon, well-differentiated type of SCC that typically occurs in the oral cavity, anogenital region and foot, where it is also called carcinoma cuniculatum.[58] There are fewer than 20 reported cases in the literature of verrucous carcinoma involving the nail unit. The nail unit may be the primary origin or may be secondarily involved from a tumor of the adjacent volar skin. It has been reported in approximately equal frequency on the fingers and toes, more commonly involving the thumb, great toe and fourth and fifth toes.[59]

Verrucous carcinoma may be confused both clinically and histologically with verruca vulgaris.

Dobson et al (2002) raise the potential importance of distinguishing this variant of SCC, as cases of verrucous carcinoma treated with radiation have been reported to transform to high-grade SCC.[36] In addition, they are more likely to cause local destruction and have a potential for metastasis.[36]

Pathogenesis and Histology

BOX 19-15 Summary

- Infection with human papillomavirus may play a role in the development of verrucous carcinoma.
- Due to its often-bland cytologic features, the architecture and growth pattern must be relied on to make this diagnosis and to differentiate verrucous carcinoma from benign tumors, such as verruca.

The pathogenesis of verrucous carcinoma has not been completely elucidated, though some studies point to a role for the human papillomavirus.[60]

Histologic confirmation of verrucous carcinoma may be difficult, as there is usually minimal keratinocytic atypia and rare mitoses.[60] Features that aid in the diagnosis include the presence of both an exophytic and endophytic tumor, with epithelial aggregates that extend into the dermis and form keratin-filled cysts.[58] Thus the overall architecture and growth pattern, rather than cytology, are used to differentiate verrucous carcinoma from a common verruca.

Prognosis and Treatment

BOX 19-16 Summary

- Verrucous carcinoma can be locally aggressive and the presence of osseous involvement must be evaluated prior to selecting treatment.
- While many cases have been treated by disarticulation/amputation, primary surgical excision or the use of Mohs micrographic surgery is a reasonable alternative in the absence of bony invasion.
- Radiation is contraindicated in the treatment of verrucous carcinoma as it may lead to transformation to a high-grade SCC.

While verrucous carcinoma is low-grade tumor, it is locally aggressive and involves the bone in over 10% of cases.[60] Most reported cases (8/12; 66%) have been treated with disarticulation or amputation.[59] However, excision or Mohs micrographic surgery are reasonable alternatives when there is no osseous involvement. There is a single report of the successful treatment of a verrucous carcinoma with an intra-arterial infusion of methotrexate.[59] Radiation is contraindicated as transformation of verrucous carcinoma to a high-grade SCC has been reported with use of this modality.[36]

■ BASAL CELL CARCINOMA

Epidemiology and Clinical Presentation

BOX 19-17 Summary

- Basal cell carcinoma (BCC) rarely occurs in the nail unit, but is more commonly found on the fingers and in male patients.
- Unlike its cutaneous counterpart, BCC of the nail unit does not exhibit a classic presentation. Therefore, it may mimic many infectious, inflammatory and neoplastic entities.

Basal cell carcinoma is the most common malignant cutaneous tumor and arises most often on sun-exposed skin.[61] There are 19 reported cases of basal cell carcinoma (BCC) of the nail unit.[61,62] A recent review by Martinelli et al highlighted the salient features regarding BCC of the nail unit.[62] Of the 18 cases described, BCC affected the fingers almost three times more often than the toes and exhibited a slight male predominance.[62] BCC of the nail unit rarely presented with the typical cutaneous presentation of a pearly papule with rolled borders. Instead, nail unit BCCs had a wide variety of presentations, including longitudinal melanonychia, nail plate destruction, onycholysis with subungual debris, and nail bed ulceration.[62] Due to its atypical presentations, it is not surprising that basal cell carcinomas at this site are mistaken for a wide variety of infectious, inflammatory and neoplastic entities. Ulceration may be a helpful distinguishing feature, as it occurred in 56% (10/18) of cases.[62]

Pathogenesis and Histology

> **BOX 19-18   Summary**
>
> - While sun exposure is a major causative factor in the development of cutaneous BCC, its role in BCC of the nail unit is less clear.
> - BCC of the nail unit shows identical histologic features to its cutaneous counterpart.

Basal cell carcinoma occurs more frequently on sun-exposed skin. It is unclear why BCC does not commonly involve the nail unit, though the nail plate may act as shield, limiting direct exposure of the nail epithelium to UV damage. Other purported pathogenic factors include HPV infection, trauma and chronic injury.[61] As the nail unit is an uncommon site for BCC, the history and physical examination should include investigation into genetic syndromes with a predisposition for developing basal cell carcinomas, including basal cell nevus syndrome. Additional historical factors that should be elucidated include exposure to arsenic or other chemicals, radiation exposure and history of trauma.

The histological appearance of basal cell carcinoma of the nail unit mirrors its cutaneous correlate; namely, there are aggregates of basaloid cells that exhibit peripheral palisading, clefting between tumor and stroma, numerous mitoses and individual cell necrosis.

Prognosis and Treatment

> **BOX 19-19   Summary**
>
> - There are no reported cases of nail unit BCC that have metastasized.
> - Surgical excision is the most common treatment for BCC of the nail unit.

Although there are no reported cases of metastatic BCC arising from the nail unit, BCCs that have arisen in other sun-protected areas have rarely metastasized.[63] Therefore, it is theoretically possible that a metastasis from a primary BCC of the nail unit could occur. Palpation for local lymphadenopathy should be a routine part of the physical examination when the diagnosis of BCC of the nail unit is made.

In a series of 18 cases, surgical excision was employed in the treatment of 66% (12/18) of tumors, seven of which utilized Mohs micrographic surgery.[62] While amputation was performed in several cases, this is likely not the initial treatment of choice for a localized lesion. Surgical repair may be achieved by flaps, grafts or healing by secondary intention, yielding acceptable cosmetic and functional results.[62]

■ METASTATIC CARCINOMA

Epidemiology and Clinical Presentation

> **BOX 19-20   Summary**
>
> - Subungual metastases, though uncommon, may herald the diagnosis of an unsuspected primary malignancy.
> - Subungual metastases most often eventuate from extension of an underlying bony metastasis.
> - Subungual metastases are most often mistaken for an infection and are associated with pain.
> - Oncology patients may have concomitant infections, such as paronychia or osteomyelitis.

Subungual metastases, though uncommon, have been reported in 133 patients.[64] They most often occur as a result of extension from a bony metastasis.[64] Subungual metastases are most frequently associated with a primary tumor of the lung (41%), genitourinary system (17%) and breast (9%).[64] They have also been reported to arise from tumors of the head and neck, bone, skin (melanoma), gastrointestinal tract, liver and other sites.[64] It is worth noting that in 44% of cases, a subungual metastasis was the presenting sign of an undiscovered primary malignancy.[64] This is in contrast to cutaneous metastases, which are the initial sign of a primary malignancy in only 1% of cases.[64]

Metastatic tumors typically induce pain due to their rapid growth, a feature helpful in distinguishing them from SCC.[65] They may be mistaken for an acute infection, as they often present with erythema, tenderness and edema.[64] In an oncology patient, the presentation of polydactylic onycholysis secondary to metastases may be misinterpreted as photo-onycholysis secondary to chemotherapy.[66] Subungual metastases may be limited to a single digit of the hand or foot or affect multiple fingers and/or toes. It is most common for subungual metastases to involve a single or multiple digits of the hands; bilateral symmetric involvement may occur.[64,66] As radiologic changes in the underlying phalanx are usually present, an X-ray is helpful in establishing the diagnosis and evaluating for concomitant osteomyelitis. In an oncology patient, secondary infection may occur. Thus, it is important both to evaluate for and treat any infection that is present and to consider the diagnosis of a metastasis in a lesion that is not responding appropriately to treatment.

Pathogenesis and Histology

> **BOX 19-21   Summary**
>
> - It is not known why the distal phalanges are rare sites for metastasis.
> - The histology of a subungual metastasis reflects the histology of the underlying primary tumor.

It is unclear why tumors only rarely metastasize to the fingers and toes; the factors that promote metastasis to these sites are not well understood.[64]

The histology of a subungual metastasis reflects the origin of the primary tumor. Though the potential histologic findings of a subungual metastasis encompasses the breadth of possible primary tumors, the two most common histologic types seen are renal cell carcinoma and SCC.[64]

Prognosis and Treatment

> **BOX 19-22   Summary**
>
> - Discovery of a subungual metastasis is a very poor prognostic sign.
> - Treatment is determined by the extent of disease and may involve systemic or local measures.

The presence of a subungual metastasis is associated with an extremely poor prognosis and often heralds death following a few months. In a patient with a known malignancy, a subungual metastasis reflects either progression of their disease or recurrence, necessitating evaluation by their oncologist.[64]

Treatment is determined by the treating oncologist after the full extent of disease is determined. It may consist of systemic therapy that will treat the subungual metastasis or solely localized therapies, such as radiotherapy.[64]

■ MALIGNANT MELANOMA

Epidemiology and Clinical Presentation

BOX 19-23   Summary

- Melanoma of the nail unit is more common in non-Caucasian patients, with a mean incidence in the fifth through seventh decades.
- It affects the thumb and great toe most commonly, where it usually presents as longitudinal melanonychia, which may be accompanied by Hutchinson's sign.
- While there are many caveats to consider in the differential diagnosis of longitudinal melanonychia, its occurrence on a single nail is suspicious for melanoma and necessitates a biopsy.

Melanoma of the nail unit has a predilection for non-Caucasians, in whom it accounts for 17 to 25% of all cutaneous melanomas.[67] In contrast, in Caucasians, it accounts for only 2 to 3% of cutaneous melanomas.[68] Melanoma of the nail unit differs from cutaneous melanomas by presenting somewhat later in life, with a mean incidence in the fifth through seventh decades.[67,69] In one large study of 93 patients with melanoma of the nail unit, the mean age at presentation was 55.4 years.[69] It most commonly occurs on the thumb and great toe.[67]

Pigmentation of the nail plate is the presenting sign of melanoma in 76% of cases.[67] Unfortunately, there is often a delay of several years between the appearance of pigment in the nail plate and a definitive diagnosis. A biopsy must be considered if a previously thin-pigmented streak becomes wider or exhibits color variegation. The same races that have a higher relative incidence of melanoma of the nail unit also have a higher incidence of melanonychia striata, making diagnosis more difficult. However, unless one band differs from the rest, melanoma is not usually associated with multiple digits that exhibit melanonychia striata.

Despite the frequent presence of pigmentation, melanoma of the nail unit

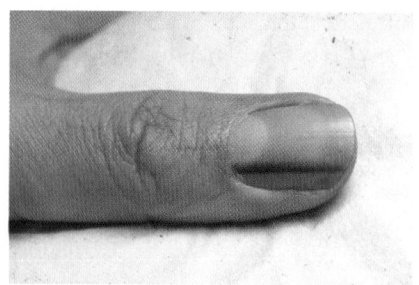

▲ **FIGURE 19-6** Longitudinal melanonychia affecting a single nail in a Caucasian patient.

can have a variety of clinical presentations and has been mistaken for onychomycosis.[70] There are numerous causes to consider in the differential diagnosis of a pigmented streak of a single nail. (Fig. 19-6) These include trauma and benign and malignant melanocytic and nonmelanocytic neoplasms.[67]

An estimated 20 to 33% of nail unit melanomas are amelanotic, a much higher proportion compared to 7% of cutaneous melanomas.[67,70] It is unclear whether amelanotic melanomas of the nail unit have an inherently worse prognosis or whether the poor outcomes associated with this subtype of melanoma are due to a delay in diagnosis.

A mnemonic that aids in the diagnosis of melanoma of the nail unit uses the letters ABCDEF.[70] In this system, *A* stands for *age* (highest incidence in the fifth to seventh decades) and *A*frican *A*mericans, *A*sians and native *A*mericans (groups with a higher incidence of melanoma of the nail unit). *B* stands for brown-black *b*and with a diameter ≥3 mm or variegated borders. *C* stands for

either a *c*hange in an existing nail band OR lack of change despite appropriate treatment. *D* stands for the *d*igit most commonly involved (thumb most often, followed by the great toe or index finger). *E* stands for *e*xtension of the pigment onto the nail fold, either proximal or lateral (namely, Hutchinson's sign) or onto the free edge of the nail plate. Finally, *F* stands for *f*amily or personal history of dysplastic nevi or melanoma.

One sign that is helpful, but not pathognomonic for melanoma of the nail unit, is Hutchinson's sign, namely the extension of pigment onto the cuticle and proximal nail fold. (Fig. 19-7) Other potential causes of pigmentation of the nail folds, which include Laugier-Hunziker syndrome and certain medications, must be excluded. The presence of Hutchinson's sign along with melanonychia striata is suspicious for melanoma. If a true Hutchinson's sign is present, an excisional biopsy is warranted; in such cases, the patient should also be examined for lymphadenopathy. However, one cannot necessarily be reassured by the absence of Hutchinson's sign. In a series of seven cases of malignant melanoma *in situ* of the nail unit in Caucasians, longitudinal melanonychia without Hutchinson's sign was the clinical presentation in 57% (4/7) of patients.[71]

Pigmentation extending onto the hyponychium, on the other hand, may be seen in both melanoma and melanocytic nevi.[72] While the dermatoscopic features of the nail plate may be identical in nevi and melanomas, hyponychial pigmentation in nevi had a

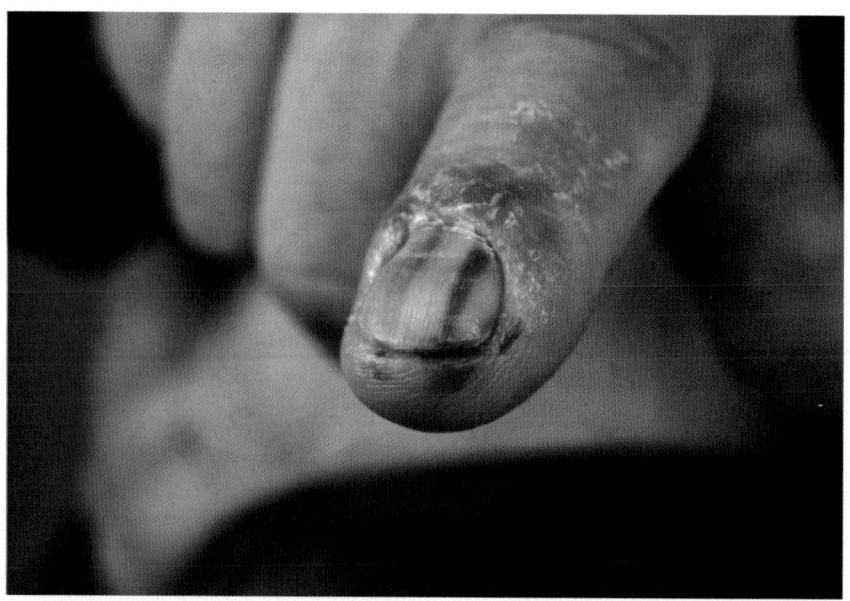

▲ **FIGURE 19-7** Malignant melanoma of the nail unit with Hutchinson's sign.

brushy linear structure across skin markings while haphazard pigmentation was seen in melanomas.[72] These findings follow the pattern of pigmentation in plantar nevi and acral lentiginous melanoma *in situ*, respectively.[72]

Dermoscopy is a tool that may aid in the evaluation of longitudinal melanonychia in several ways. A recent article describes the utility of dermoscopy of the free edge of the nail plate to determine whether pigmentation arises from the proximal or distal nail matrix.[73] This technique may provide critical information in guiding selection of the biopsy site. Biopsy site selection may also be guided by use of dermoscopy directly on the nail bed and matrix after removal of the nail plate, since dermoscopic findings of the nail plate may be nonspecific.[74] While dermoscopy of the nail plate has proven helpful in selecting cases that require biopsy, it does not replace histopathologic examination, especially in cases of uncertainty.[75]

A new pigmented streak in a Caucasian is always suspicious, and therefore, a general rule of thumb is that any such lesion, whether pigmented of not, should be biopsied if it persists after 6 to 12 weeks.[67] Features that should prompt concern for melanoma and biopsy of a pigmented streak include a width greater than 3 mm, color variegation and proximal widening.[70,76] In a study of 100 Caucasian patients with longitudinal melanonychia, the authors found no reliable criteria to differentiate melanoma from benign melanocytic

lesions.[77] In this group of patients, melanoma accounted for the longitudinal melanonychia in 5% (5/100) of patients.[77] The only reliable clue that suggested the diagnosis of a nail matrix nevus was the age at onset of the pigmented streak.[77]

Since melanonychia striata is common in non-Caucasians, monitoring these lesions requires patient involvement. During an initial evaluation, patients should be educated regarding the signs of change that would necessitate re-evaluation. Indications for biopsy of existing pigmented streaks includes a change in appearance, associated nail dystrophy, ulceration or development of Hutchinson's sign (Fig. 19-8).[67]

Melanoma, both cutaneous and of the nail unit, occurs in 0.8 to 6.3 cases per million in patients younger than 20 years of age.[70] There are only a few cases of melanoma arising in the nail unit of children reported in the literature.[78] Whether the risk of malignant transformation of a melanocytic nevus of the nail present since birth is similar to the risk of cutaneous congenital melanocytic nevi has not been studied.[78] In children, close follow-up is recommended for any new streak. Melanoma as the cause of longitudinal melanonychia is extremely rare in children and therefore every case does not need to be biopsied, but should be considered on an individual basis. Biopsy should be considered for those with a change in a pre-existing streak, especially in the setting of continued or rapid growth of a

streak that may progress to involve the entire nail.[67,70]

In summary, though patient race and age must be taken into consideration, Banfield and Dawber[76] succinctly explained the bottom line: "All patients of any race and any age with clinically suspicious LM (longitudinal melanonychia) affecting a single digit should have a diagnostic nail biopsy that must include the nail matrix."

Pathogenesis and Histology

> **BOX 19-24   Summary**
>
> - The normal distribution of melanocytes in the nail unit may mimic melanoma. Therefore, a complete understanding of the anatomy of the nail unit is essential to histologic examination of a suspicious lesion.
> - While acral lentiginous and nodular melanomas predominate, all subtypes may occur in the nail unit.
> - The pathogenesis of melanoma of the nail unit is not clear; UV radiation and trauma may play a role.

It is important to understand the normal characteristics of melanocytes in the nail unit, that differ for Caucasian and non-Caucasian patients. In Caucasian patients, melanocytes in the proximal matrix are dormant and do not produce melanin.[76] However, melanocytes of the distal matrix may be active and produce melanin, explaining the occurrence of melanonychia striata in Caucasian patients.[76] In one series of Caucasian patients with normal nails, melanocytes in the nail matrix were found both in the basal layer and above it, mimicking melanoma *in situ*; this finding may complicate the diagnosis of melanoma at this site.[79] In non-Caucasians, melanocytes in the nail unit are functionally active, producing melanin.[76] The most common histologic diagnoses of a pigmented streak in the nail plate are a benign melanotic macule (lentigo) and junctional nevus, in adults and children, respectively.[70]

Melanoma of the nail unit usually arises in the matrix, but can rarely originate in the hyponychium and nail bed[80]; therefore, the matrix should always be included in a biopsy performed to rule out melanoma. In general, an increase in the width of a pigmented streak due to melanoma correlates with the radial growth phase. Signs associated with the vertical growth phase cause deformity of the nail, either by thickening, ulceration or destruction.[70]

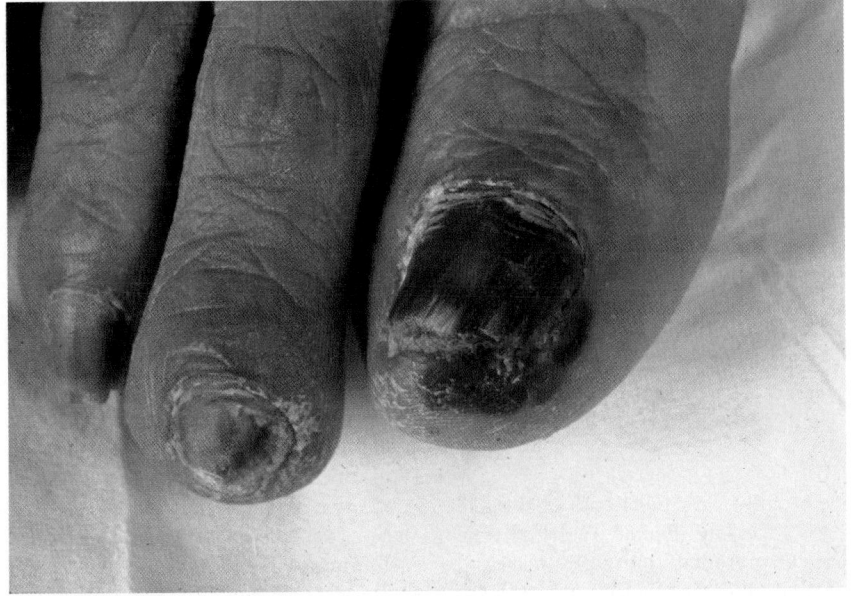

▲ **FIGURE 19-8** Malignant melanoma of the nail unit with discoloration of the entire nail plate and extension onto the hyponychium.

All four subtypes of melanoma, namely superficial spreading melanoma, lentigo maligna melanoma, nodular melanoma and acral lentiginous melanoma, can occur in the nail unit. Acral lentiginous melanoma (ALM) accounts for 38 to 62% of melanomas of the nail unit.[67] ALM, along with nodular melanoma, are the two most common subtypes to occur in the nail unit.[76] Survival does not appear to be related to the histologic subtype of melanoma.[67]

Histologic findings reflect the subtype of melanoma. In general, there is an asymmetric proliferation of enlarged melanocytes arranged as single units and irregular nests at the dermo-epithelial junction. Melanocytes are often present within the upper levels of the epithelium. Melanocytes usually have large, hyperchromatic nuclei with prominent nucleoli. Melanocytes are present in the dermis in cases of invasive melanoma. When immunohistochemistry is used to confirm the diagnosis, atypical melanocytes generally demonstrate strong positive staining with HMB-45, while weak or negative staining with S-100 has been reported in some cases.[76,81]

As almost a third of melanomas of the nail are amelanotic, it is wise to submit any lesion removed from the nail, such as a presumed pyogenic granuloma, for histologic examination.[68] When one considers that two-thirds of patients with melanoma of the nail unit have an inappropriate surgical procedure prior to a definitive diagnosis, it becomes evident that the practice of routine histologic examination of lesions would eliminate these procedures and more importantly, render the correct diagnosis.[68]

It is not uncommon for a melanoma of the nail unit to undergo partial regression and therefore care must be taken not to misdiagnose a regressed melanoma as a benign blue nevus.[82] Sometimes sentinel lymph node biopsy is warranted in these cases, which, if positive, can establish the diagnosis with certainty.[82]

An important caveat in the histopathologic examination of a pigmented lesion of the nail unit is that any malignancy of the nail unit can result in secondary hemorrhage. If only the nail plate is sampled, one cannot necessarily be reassured by the finding of hemorrhage. In one series of 33 patients with melanoma of the nail unit, 85% (28/33) of patients reported spontaneous bleeding, ulceration or suppuration.[83] Therefore, the finding of blood does not rule out an underlying malignancy.

The pathogenesis of melanoma of the nail unit has not been well delineated. It is known that the nail plate is effective in preventing transmission of UVB irradiation, while permitting UVA rays to reach the underlying nail matrix and bed. It seems that UV radiation plays less of a direct role in the pathogenesis of nail unit melanoma, compared to cutaneous melanoma.

It has been hypothesized that trauma may be involved in the etiology of melanoma of the nail unit, as between 23 to 44% of patients recall trauma that is temporally related to the appearance of the melanoma.[84] However, there are several potential explanations for this association, which include the potential proclivity of a melanoma of the nail unit to bleed with slight trauma, increased vigilance of that site due to a pre-existent abnormality or trauma-induced atypia of regenerating melanocytes.[84] In a series of 33 patients with melanoma of the nail unit, 9% (3/33) patients had a history of antecedent trauma, ranging from 6 to 50 years prior to diagnosis.[83] More prevalent than antecedent trauma in this series was injury to a clinically apparent tumor or a prior surgical procedure in 64% (21/33) of patients.[83] Those patients who experienced trauma of a clinically apparent tumor had a higher 5-year cumulative probability of recurrence and a markedly lower 5-year probability of survival.[83] The authors hypothesize that the release of cytokines during wound repair may play a role in tumor progression.[83]

Prognosis and Treatment

BOX 19-25 Summary

- Prognosis of melanoma of the nail unit is adversely affected by the long lag time between both clinical appearance of an abnormality in the nail and presentation to a physician and the subsequent delay in diagnosis.
- Increasing tumor thickness (Breslow measurement) and ulceration are associated with a worse prognosis.
- Treatment has generally been amputation at the closest joint, though there is some evidence for the use of more conservative techniques, at least for thinner lesions.
- Adjuvant therapies may be warranted in thicker lesions or for those with evidence of metastasis.

The prognosis of melanoma of the nail unit is adversely affected by the lag time between presentation to a physician and a definitive diagnosis that ranges from between 3 and 48 months.[67] The necessity of an adequate biopsy to enable a diagnosis cannot be overstated. It should include the nail matrix, bed and plate, down to the periosteum. It is worth noting that biopsies of lesions within the lateral third of the nail plate are less likely to result in permanent nail dystrophy.[67] If the clinical suspicion for melanoma is low, a 3-mm punch biopsy may be sufficient.

As for cutaneous melanoma, increasing Breslow thickness and ulceration are associated with a worse prognosis. The anatomy of the nail unit may make a precise measurement of thickness more difficult. The mean Breslow thickness at diagnosis for melanoma of the nail unit of 3.05 mm at the Sydney Melanoma Unit is comparable with other studies.[67] The presence of lymphadenopathy at diagnosis is an additional independent sign of poor prognosis.[67] Data on the validity of the mitotic rate as an indicator of prognosis is not definitive. It appears that, at the same stage of disease, melanoma of the nail unit has a poorer prognosis compared to cutaneous melanoma, with a 5-year survival of 16 to 87%.[67,70] With regard to tumor thickness, the 5-year survival for melanoma of the nail <2.5 mm compared to ≥2.5 mm, is 88 and 40%, respectively.[76] Even when controlling for advanced stage and Clark's level, African-Americans have a mortality rate that is 2.6 times greater than Caucasians.[69]

Treatment is usually amputation of the finger at the nearest uninvolved interphalangeal joint, at the neck of the proximal phalanx or interphalangeal joint of the thumb and the metatarsophalangeal joint of toes.[67,69] Some authors advocate excision with a 0.5 to 1 cm margin for early thin melanomas of the nail unit.[67] The decision of whether to perform sentinel lymph node biopsy or elective lymph node dissection is unclear as its effect on survival is unknown.[67] In a study of 93 patients with melanoma of the nail unit, there was no survival benefit of elective lymph node dissection in patients with intermediate thickness lesions (0.76 to 4 mm) in the absence of detectable nodal involvement.[69]

Some authors advocate the use of Mohs micrographic surgery, with or without the use of immunohistochemistry, particularly for cases of melanoma *in situ*.[71] In a series of 14 patients with nail unit melanomas that were 0 to 3.3 mm in depth, the author excised the lesions using the Mohs technique with a minimum of a 6-mm margin of normal skin and removal of the entire nail unit.[85] This technique resulted in a 79% disease-free survival with an average follow-up period of 7.7 years and a local recurrence rate of 21% (3/14 patients).[85]

Another technique that demonstrated results comparable with amputation was reported by Moehrle et al[86] The authors performed "functional" surgery, which consisted of excision of the tumor with a 5-mm safety margin, removal of the entire nail unit and the distal part of the distal phalanx and subsequent examination of three-dimensional histology.[86] When comparing this technique with amputation, patients treated with "functional" surgery did not have a higher probability for progression of disease due to local recurrence or metastasis.[86] These authors recommend amputation only in those cases with bony or joint space involvement.[86]

In patients with advanced stages of melanoma of the nail unit, chemotherapy, either systemic or delivered with isolated limb perfusion, immunotherapy or other modalities of treatment may be indicated.[67,69]

■ FINAL THOUGHTS

In summary, the nail unit may be affected by any benign or malignant cutaneous neoplasm. In contrast to the remainder of the integument, however, the nail matrix and bed are obscured by the nail plate. In addition, the confined space of the nail unit may alter the appearance of tumors. Therefore, tumors that occur in the nail unit may mimic inflammatory and infectious processes and unrelated neoplasms. For this reason, a biopsy at the purported site of origin of a potential tumor must be considered in every case of an altered nail that is not responding appropriately to treatment or is suspicious for a tumor.

REFERENCES

1. Sass U, et al. Longitudinal melanonychia revealing an intraepidermal carcinoma of the nail apparatus: detection of integrated HPV-16 DNA. *J Am Acad Dermatol.* 1998;39:490–493.
2. Mirza B, Muir JB. Bowen's disease of the nail bed. *Australas J Dermatol.* 2004;45: 232–233.
3. Sau P, et al. Bowen's disease of the nail bed and periungual area. *Arch Dermatol.* 1994;130:204–209.
4. Tosti A and Piraccini, BM. Warts of the nail unit: surgical and nonsurgical approaches. *Dermatol Surg.* 2001;27:235–239.
5. Gardner LW and Acker DW. Bone destruction of the distal phalanx caused by periungual warts. *Arch Dermatol.* 1973;107:275–276.
6. Holland TT, et al. Tender Periungual Nodules. *Arch Dermatol.* 1992;128:105–110.
7. Läuchli S, et al. Swelling of the proximal nail fold caused by underlying warts. *Dermatology.* 2001;202:328–329.
8. Ergun SS, et al. Giant verruca vulgaris. *Dermatol Surg.* 2004;30:459–462.
9. Robinette JW, et al. Subungual squamous cell carcinoma mistaken for a verruca. *J Am Podiatr Med Assoc.* 1999;89:435–437.
10. Fleckman P, et al. Squamous cell carcinoma of the nail bed treated as chronic paronychia and wart for fourteen years. *Cutis.* 1985;36:189–191.
11. High WA, et al. Rapidly enlarging growth of the proximal nail fold. *Dermatol Surg.* 2003;29:984–986.
12. Kirnbauer R, et al. *Human Papillomavirus in Dermatology.* Bolognia JL, Jorizzo JL, Rapini RP, eds. London:Mosby;2003: 1218, 1219, 1221.
13. Goette DK. Carcinoma *in situ* in verruca vulgaris. *Int J Dermatol.* 1980;19:98–101.
14. Bacelieri R and Johnson S. Cutaneous warts: an evidence-based approach to therapy. *Am Fam Physician.* 2005;72: 647–652.
15. Kuflik EG. Specific indications for cryosurgery of the nail unit. *J Dermatol Surg Oncol.* 1992;18:702–706.
16. Shelley WB, Wood MG. Transformation of the common wart into squamous cell carcinoma in a patient with primary lymphedema. *Cancer.* 1981;48:820–824.
17. Sterling JC, et al. Guidelines for the management of cutaneous warts. *Br J Dermatol.* 2001;144:4–11.
18. Focht DR, et al. The efficacy of duct tape vs cryotherapy in the treatment of verruca vulgaris (the common wart). *Arch Pediatr Adolesc Med.* 20022;156:971–974.
19. Ongenae K, et al. Bowen's disease of the nail. *Dermatology.* 2002;204:348–350.
20. Koch A, et al. Polydactylous Bowen's disease. *J Eur Acad Dermatol Venereol.* 2003; 17:213–215.
21. Usmani N, et al. Subungual Bowen's disease treated by topical aminolevulinic acid-photodynamic therapy. *J Am Acad Dermatol.* 2005;53:S273–S276.
22. Baran R, Perrin C. Bowen's disease clinically simulating an onychomatricoma. *J Am Acad Dermatol.* 2002;47:947–949.
23. Baran R, Perrin C. Longitudinal erythronychia with distal subungual keratosis: onychopapilloma of the nail bed and Bowen's disease. *Br J Dermatol.* 2000;143: 132–135.
24. Baran R and Perrin CH. Pseudo-fibrokeratoma of the nail apparatus with melanocytic pigmentation: a clue for diagnosing Bowen's disease. *Acta Derm Venereol.* 1994;74:449–450.
25. Baran R and Simon Cl. Longitudinal melanonychia: a symptom of Bowen's disease. *J Am Acad Dermatol.* 1988;18: 1359–1360.
26. Sato T, et al. Human papillomavirus associated with Bowen's disease of the finger. *J Dermatol.* 2004;31:927–930.
27. Tan B, et al. Photodynamic therapy for subungual Bowen's disease. *Australas J Dermatol.* 2004;45:172–174.
28. Kreuter A, et al. Human papillomavirus type 26–associated periungual squamous cell carcinoma *in situ* in a HIV-infected patient with concomitant penile and anal intraepithelial neoplasia. *J Am Acad Dermatol.* 2005;53:737–739.
29. Kaiser JF, Proctor-Shipman L. Squamous cell carcinoma *in situ* (Bowen's disease) mimicking subungual verruca vulgaris. *J Fam Pract.* 1994;39:384–387.
30. Virgili A, et al. Squamous cell carcinoma of the nail bed: a rare disease or only misdiagnosed? *Acta Derm Venereol.* 2001;81: 306–307.
31. Dominguez-Cherit J, et al. Pseudo-fibrokeratoma: an unusual presentation of subungual squamous cell carcinoma in a young girl. *Dermatol Surg.* 2003;29: 788–789.
32. Figus A, et al. Squamous cell carcinoma of the lateral nail fold. *J Hand Surg.* 2006;31B:216–220.
33. Obiamiwe PE, Gaze NR. Subungual squamous cell carcinoma. *Br J Plast Surg.* 2001;54:631–632.
34. Yip K-M, et al. Subunugal squamous cell carcinoma: report of 2 cases. *J Formos Med Assoc.* 2000;99:646–649.
35. Okiyama N, et al. Squamous cell carcinoma arising from lichen planus of nail matrix and nail bed. *J Am Acad Dermatol.* 2005;53:908–909.
36. Dobson CM, et al. Squamous cell carcinoma arising in a psoriatic nail bed: case report with discussion of diagnostic difficulties and therapeutic options. *Br J Dermatol.* 2002;147:144–149.
37. Bui-Mansfield L, et al. Subungual squamous cell carcinoma of the finger. *Am J Roentgenol.* 2005;185:174–175.
38. Sinha A, et al. Spontaneous regression of subungual keratoacanthoma with reossification of underlying distal lytic phalynx. *Clin Exp Dermatol.* 2005;30:20–22.
39. Chang SE, et al. Metastatic squamous cell carcinoma of the nail bed: a presenting sign of lung cancer. *Br J Dermatol.* 1999;141:939–940.
40. Yasaka N, et al. An acral 'inflammatory' cutaneous metastasis of oesophageal carcinoma. *Br J Dermatol.* 1999;141:938–939.
41. Ashinoff R, et al. Detection of human papillomavirus DNA in squamous cell carcinoma of the nail bed and finger detected by polymerase chain reaction. *Arch Dermatol.* 1991;127:1813–1818.
42. Moy RL, et al. Human papillomavirus type 16 DNA in periungual squamous cell carcinomas. *JAMA.* 1989;261:2669–2673.
43. Nasca MR, et al. Subungual squamous cell carcinoma of the toe: report on three cases. *Dermatol Surg.* 2004;30:345–348.
44. Zaiac MN, Weiss E. Mohs micrographic surgery of the nail unit and squamous cell carcinoma. *Dermatol Surg.* 2001;27: 246–251.
45. De Berker D. Hold on the amputation. *Br J Dermatol.* 2003;148:1077–1078.
46. Wong TC, et al. Squamous cell carcinoma of the nail bed: three case reports. *J Orthop Surg.* 2004;12:248–252.
47. de Berker DAR, et al. Micrographic surgery for subungual squamous cell carcinoma. *Br J Plast Surg.* 1996;49:414–419.
48. Peterson SR, et al. Squamous cell carcinoma of the nail unit with evidence of bony involvement: a multidisciplinary approach to resection and reconstruction. *Dermatol Surg.* 2004;30:218–221.
49. Yaparpalvi R, et al. Radiation therapy for the salvage of unresectable subungual squamous cell carcinoma. *Dermatol Surg.* 2003;29:294–296.
50. McHugh RW, et al. Metastatic periungual squamous cell carcinoma: detection of human papillomavirus type 35 RNA in the digital tumor and axillary lymph

node metastases. *J Am Acad Dermatol.* 1996;34:1080–1082.

51. Huang K-C, et al. Late inguinal metastasis of a well-differentiated subungual squamous cell carcinoma after radical toe amputation. *Dermatol Surg.* 2005;31:784–786.

52. Stoll DM, Ackerman AB. Subungual keratoacanthoma. *Am J Dermatopathol.* 1980;2:265–271.

53. Pellegrini VD, Tompkins A. Management of subungual keratoacanthoma. *J Hand Surg.* 1986;11:718–724.

54. Baran R, et al. Distal digital keratoacanthoma: two cases with a review of the literature. *Dermatol Surg.* 2001;27:575–579.

55. Lovett JE, et al. Subungual keratoacanthoma masquerading as a chronic paronychia. *Ann Plast Surg.* 1995;34:84–87.

56. Baran R, Goettman S. Distal digital keratoacanthoma: a report of 12 cases and a review of the literature. *Br J Dermatol.* 1998;139:512–515.

57. Baran R, Tosti A, DeBerker D. Periungual keratoacanthoma preceded by a wart and followed by a verrucous carcinoma at the same site. *Acta Derm Venerol.* 2003;83:232–233.

58. Vandeweyer E, et al. Cutaneous verrucous carcinoma. *Br J Plast Surg.* 2001;54:168–170.

59. Sheen M-C, et al. Subungual verrucous carcinoma of the thumb treated by intra-arterial infusion with methotrexate. *Dermatol Surg.* 2005;31:787–789.

60. Tosti A, et al. Carcinoma cuniculatum of the nail apparatus: report of three cases. *Dermatology.* 1993;186:217–221.

61. de Giorgi V, et al. Ungual basal cell carcinoma on the fifth toe mimicking chronic dermatitis: case study. *Dermatol Surg.* 2005;31:723–725.

62. Martinelli PT, et al. Periungual basal cell carcinoma: case report and literature review. *Dermatol Surg.* 2006;32:320–323.

63. Ting PT, et al. Metastatic basal cell carcinoma: report of two cases and literature review. *J Cutan Med Surg.* 2005;9:10–15.

64. Cohen PR. Metastatic tumors to the nail unit: subungual metastases. *Dermatol Surg.* 2001;27:280–293.

65. Kouskoukis CE, Scher RK, Kopf AW. Squamous cell carcinoma of the nail bed. *J Dermatol Surg Oncol.* 1982;8:853–855.

66. Lambert D, et al. Distal phalangeal metastasis of a chondrosarcoma initially presenting as bilateral onycholysis. *Clin Exp Dermatol.* 1992;17:463–465.

67. Thai K, et al. Nail apparatus melanoma. *Australas J Dermatol.* 2001;42:71–83.

68. de Georgi V, et al. Subungual melanoma: an insidious erythematous nodule on the nail bed. *Arch Dermatol.* 2005;141:398–399.

69. O'Leary, et al. Subungual melanoma: a review of 93 cases with identification of prognostic variables. *Clin Orthop Relat Res.* 2000;378:206–212.

70. Levit KE, et al. The ABC rule for clinical detection of subungual melanoma. *J Am Acad Dermatol.* 2000;42:269–274.

71. High WA, et al. Presentation, histopathologic findings and clinical outcomes in 7 cases of melanoma *in situ* of the nail unit. *Arch Dermatol.* 2004;140:1102–1106.

72. Kawabata Y, et al. Two kinds of Hutchinson's sign, benign and malignant. *J Am Acad Dermatol.* 2001;44:305–307.

73. Braun RP, Baran R, Saurat JH, Thomas L. Surgical pearl: dermoscopy of the free edge of the nail to determine the level of nail plate pigmentation and the location of its probable origin in the proximal or distal nail matrix. *J Am Acad Dermatol.* 2006;55:512–513.

74. Hirata SH, Yamada S, Almeida FA, et al. Dermoscopy of the nail bed and matrix to assess melanonychia striata. *J Am Acad Dermatol.* 2005;53:884–886.

75. Ronger S, Touzet S, Ligeron C, et al. Dermoscopic examination of nail pigmentation. *Arch Dermatol.* 2002;138:1327–1333.

76. Banfield CC, Dawber RPR. Nail melanoma: a review of the literature with recommendations to improve patient management. *Br J Dermatol.* 1999;141:628–632.

77. Tosti A, et al. Nail matrix nevi: a clinical and histopathologic study of twenty-two patients. *J Am Acad Dermatol.* 1996;34:765–771.

78. Antonovich DD, et al. Childhood subungual melanoma *in situ* in diffuse nail melanosis beginning as expanding longitudinal melanonychia. *Pediatr Dermatol.* 2005;22:210–212.

79. Perrin C, et al. Anatomic distribution of melanocytes in normal nail unit: an immunohistochemical investigation. *Am J Dermpathol.* 1997;19:462–467.

80. Daniel CR. Longitudinal melanonychia and melanoma: an unusual case presentation. *Dermatol Surg.* 2001;27:294–295.

81. Kwon IH, et al. Acral lentiginous melanoma *in situ*: a study of nine cases. *Am J Dermatopathol.* 2004;26:285–289.

82. Yang C, et al. Regressed subungual melanoma simulating cellular blue nevus: managed with sentinel lymph node biopsy. *Dermatol Surg.* 2006;32:577–581.

83. Bormann G, et al. Concomitant traumas influence prognosis in melanomas of the nail apparatus. *Br J Dermatol.* 2006;155:76–80.

84. Mohrle M, Hafner HM. Is subungual melanoma related to trauma? *Dermatology.* 2002;204:259–261.

85. Brodland DG. The treatment of nail apparatus melanoma with Mohs micrographic surgery. *Dermatol Surg.* 2001;27:269–273.

86. Moehrle, et al. "Functional" surgery in subungual melanoma. *Dermatol Surg.* 2003;29:366–374.

CHAPTER 20

Vascular Tumors of the Skin

Daniel J. Santa Cruz, M.D.
Anita Singh, M.S.

BOX 20-1   Overview

- Although well-defined clinicopathologic vascular tumors can be recognized, there is frequent morphologic overlap that defies a specific classification of an individual lesion.
- Venous lake is an acquired venular ectasia found in elderly individuals.
- Capillary aneurysms usually present as a solitary bluish papule on the face or trunk, occasionally with itching or tenderness. The principal finding is a single ectatic vascular structure (usually a vein), often containing a thrombus.
- Spider angioma is a common cutaneous vascular lesion that is often seen as an incidental finding in healthy children.
- Nevus flammeus is a congenital vascular anomaly that often involves the head and neck region.
- Angioma serpiginosum is an unusual benign vascular lesion. It typically occurs during the first two decades of life, is more common in women, and occurs at any site.
- Angiokeratomas occur as variably hyperkeratotic lesions that may be pink-red to purple, brown, or occasionally blue to black.
- Verrucous hemangioma (VH) is an uncommon vascular malformation that tends to arise near birth or in childhood.
- Cavernous hemangiomas usually presents as soft, red to purple nodules or plaques that have a compressible quality, which usually presents at birth or in childhood, but may develop in older individuals.
- Cherry angioma is one of the most common vascular tumors encountered in the skin. It often develops in adults beginning in adolescence and are especially common in older adults.
- Capillary hypercellular hemangioma is a common tumor of infancy that usually presents within the first few weeks of life as a solitary localized tumor.
- Lobular capillary hemangioma (LCH) is a commonly acquired vascular lesion that was once considered to be secondary to pyogenic infection or arising as exuberant granulation tissue in response to trauma, but now thought to be an acquired hemangioma.
- Acquired tufted angioma (ATA) arises as slowly enlarging erythematous macules and plaques that often have a deep component and typically occur on the neck and upper trunk of children and young adults.
- The glomeruloid hemangioma is considered to be a reactive endothelial proliferation, and the result of circulating angiogenic factors from activated lymphocytes.
- Angiolymphoid hyperplasia with eosinophilia presents as single or multiple, pink to red brown papules or plaques in the head and neck region of young to middle-aged adults. It occurs particularly in women, although some reports have noted a male predominance.
- Microvenular hemangioma is believed to be a type of acquired venous hemangioma. It typically occurs as a solitary asymptomatic, small, enlarging, purple-to-red plaque or nodule that favor the extremities of young to middle-aged adults of either sex.
- Targetoid hemosiderotic hemangioma typically presents as a solitary, annular, violaceous to purple papule 2 to 3 mm in diameter, with both a surrounding pale rim and a more peripheral ecchymotic ring giving a target-like appearance.
- Acro-angiodermatitis consists of reactive vascular proliferation, dermal fibrosis, and hemosiderin deposition in the setting of arteriovenous malformations and venous insufficiency.
- Intravascular papillary endothelial hyperplasia typically presents as a slowly enlarging, often tender, blue-to-red, deep dermal to subcutaneous swelling or mass. It occurs at diverse sites, the most frequent of which are the head and the extremities, particularly the fingers.
- Angiomatosis is a rare condition that usually presents in childhood as symptoms of persistent swelling of a large contiguous area of soft tissue and dermis.
- Bacillary angiomatosis typically occurs in patients with the acquired immunodeficiency syndrome (AIDS). It is a zoonotic infection linked to domestic cats.
- Malignant angioendotheliomatosis has an insidious onset and by the time it presents it has neurologic and cutaneous manifestations. It has a rapid, fatal course.
- Reactive angioendotheliomatosis (RAE) is a benign process often associated with an underlying chronic infection and various other stimuli, including hypoxia or ischemia with diffuse dermal angiomatosis.
- Arteriovenous hemangioma primarily is a tumor of middle-aged to elderly adults with a peak incidence in the fourth and fifth decades of life. It is a relatively common lesion and has a male predominance.
- Glomus tumors can be classified into solitary and multiple types. The typical solitary glomus tumor occurs in an adult as a small, blue red nodule, less than 1 cm in diameter, in the deep dermis or subcutis of the extremities. Multiple glomus tumors are uncommon, often present in childhood, are generally asymptomatic, arise in more proximal sites, only rarely occur subungually, and can be subdivided anatomically into whether they are regional or disseminated.
- Spindle cell hemangioma is a nonneoplastic, reactive vascular proliferation, associated with malformed blood vessels and repeated cycles of recanalization after thrombosis.
- Lymphangiomas are proliferations of variably dilated lymphatic vessels, usually present either at birth or within the first few years of life, and generally considered to be hamartomatous in nature.
- Benign lymphangioendothelioma is a rare entity that can offer diagnostic difficulty with low-grade angiosarcoma and the lymphangioma-like form of Kaposi sarcoma.
- "Hemangioendothelioma" was used in the past to refer to benign conditions, often present in childhood, and also to malignant vascular neoplasms.
- Epithelioid hemangioendothelioma is a rare entity that has been reported in systemic organs and in the skin as a biologically "borderline" neoplasm because of an occasional association with local recurrence or metastasis.
- Kaposi sarcoma has been primarily known as a relatively rare tumor of the elderly until the advent of the acquired immunodeficiency syndrome (AIDS) and organ transplantation. It has become endemic in Central Africa.
- Hemangiopericytoma is a relatively rare soft-tissue neoplasm that is thought to derive from the pericyte.
- Endovascular papillary angioendothelioma presents with enlarging cutaneous lesions, 4 to 9 cm in diameter, occurring as either a diffuse swelling or an intradermal tumor on the head, neck, and extremities.
- Retiform hemangioendothelioma is a recently described vascular tumor that is considered a well-differentiated and low-grade form of angiosarcoma.

- Kaposiform hemangioendothelioma is an exceedingly rare vascular tumor occurring almost exclusively in childhood and involving the deep soft tissues and skin.
- Composite hemangioendothelioma is a recently described vascular tumor considered to be a low-grade malignancy mimicking conventional angiosarcoma, but with a better prognosis.
- Angiosarcoma is a rare, malignant endothelial tumor that arises in skin, soft tissue, breast, bones, liver, and other viscera. Cutaneous AS is the most common form of angiosarcoma.
- Cutaneous angiosarcomas are aggressive angiosarcomas appearing in the setting of mammary carcinoma, radical mastectomy, and adjuvant therapy, as well as radiation therapy or chemotherapy.

INTRODUCTION

The nomenclature of vascular lesions is sometimes confusing, since the pathogenesis of many lesions is poorly understood.[1-4] Many classification schemes have been proposed, but none is entirely satisfactory at present. For example, vascular lesions may be classified based on the type and/or caliber of the vascular channel present, e.g., capillary, venule, vein, arteriole, artery, lymphatic, and glomus vessel; proliferative versus nonproliferative lesions; congenital versus acquired lesions; malformations versus reactive, proliferative, or neoplastic lesions; and other features such as distribution and multicentricity. This review discusses the various entities in general terms as (1) benign vascular lesions that will include ectasias/telangiectasias, proliferative lesions such as capillary hemangioma, and various malformations; (2) lesions with indeterminate or borderline status, e.g., the so-called hemangioendotheliomas; and (3) malignant vascular lesions such as angiosarcoma. We attempt to maintain a balanced perspective in discussing each entity without trying to resolve the often controversial issues of nomenclature and pathogenesis.

Although the capillary differentiation of hemangiomas is frequently mentioned in the literature, the vast majority of the benign vascular neoplasms have, in addition to the inner endothelial lining, a peripheral coat of smooth muscle cells. Therefore, most of the so-called capillary hemangiomas are, in fact, venular lesions. This bias is reflected in the literature by the widespread reference to endothelial cell markers as vascular markers. Furthermore, many vascular proliferations contain a specialized stroma, in addition to the vascular channels. Strictly speaking, only telangiectasias and perhaps lymphangiomas are characterized by an endothelial lining alone. Paradoxically, the so-called venous lakes do not seem to have a substantial smooth muscle component, thus better qualifying as a telangiectatic condition.

There is undoubtedly considerable heterogeneity of endothelial and smooth muscle cell phenotypes and functions in normal blood vessels that are today poorly understood. It is likely that there are specialized functions in endothelial cells, including antigen presentation and secretion of cytokines among others, beyond the simple and obvious blood-containing function.

The peripheral vascular cells pose an interesting dilemma. Anatomically, cells immediately peripheral to the endothelium are either pericytes or smooth muscle cells. Simplistically and hypothetically, pericytes would give origin to pericytomas and smooth muscle cells to leiomyomas (angioleiomyomas). While vascular smooth muscle cells have a well-defined phenotype, pericytes share with smooth muscle cells many of their morphological and phenotypic qualities. Additionally, glomus cells are epithelioid smooth muscle cells that give origin to glomus tumors. Although more or less pure forms of smooth muscle vascular neoplasms exist, overlaps are common. Thus, conditions such as glomangiomyoma and myopericytoma are recognized as distinct tumors.

Although well-defined clinicopathologic vascular tumors can be recognized, there is frequent morphologic overlap that defies a specific classification of an individual lesion.

BENIGN VASCULAR LESIONS

Secondary Telangiectases

Secondary causes of telangiectasia are manifold and include conditions such as acne rosacea, varicose veins, trauma, lupus erythematosus, dermatomyositis, scleroderma and sclerodactyly (CREST syndrome), radiation dermatitis, poikiloderma, xeroderma pigmentosum, chronic sun exposure, and mastocytosis. These are not true vascular tumors *per se*, but can at times present differential diagnosis issues with them.

VENOUS LAKE

> **BOX 20-2 Summary**
>
> - An acquired venular ectasia found in elderly individuals.
> - Lesions are usually solitary dark bluish papules, 3 to 10 mm in diameter.
> - They are ectatic, erythrocyte-filled vascular spaces localized to the superficial or middle dermis.

The venous lake is an acquired venular ectasia developing on exposed skin of the head and neck in elderly patients probably due to lack of support from the surrounding tissue.

Clinical features: The lesions are often solitary dark bluish papules, 3 to 10 mm in diameter, and commonly involve the ears, lips, face, and neck. Pyogenic granuloma arising after cryosurgery to a venous lake has been reported.[5]

Histopathological features: Venous lakes are ectatic, erythrocyte-filled vascular spaces localized to the superficial or middle dermis (Fig. 20-1). In spite of its name, most venous lakes are usually lined by a single layer of endothelium; however, smooth muscular elements

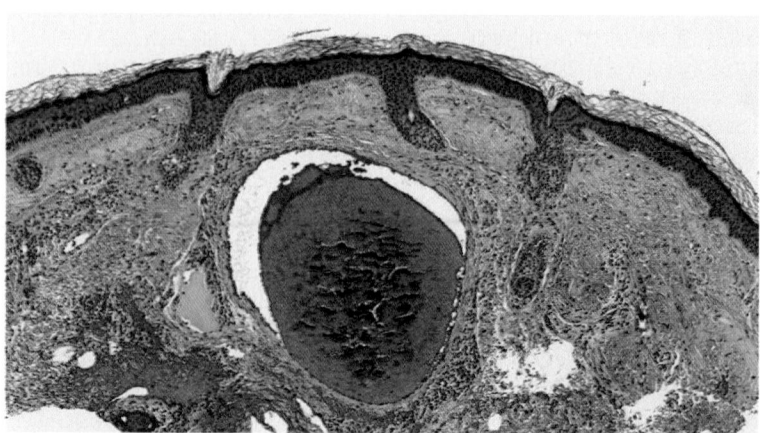

▲ **FIGURE 20-1** Venous lake. Note the thin-walled vascular structure and pronounced actinic damage.

may occasionally be associated with the wall of the vessel.[6] The surrounding dermis usually shows actinic elastosis and diminished collagen.

Differential diagnosis: The lesion is distinctive; however, other vascular ectasias might be considered in the differential diagnosis. This is particularly so if the lesion was thrombosed.

CAPILLARY ANEURYSM (OR THROMBOSED CAPILLARY ANEURYSM)

BOX 20-3   Summary

- Capillary aneurysms usually present as a solitary bluish papule on the face or trunk, occasionally with itching or tenderness.
- The principal finding is a single ectatic vascular structure (usually a vein), often containing a thrombus.
- The differential diagnosis includes venous lake, enlarged and torturous arterial and lymphatic channels, and angiokeratoma.

Clinical features: The lesion usually presents as a solitary bluish papule on the face or trunk occasionally with itching or tenderness.[7] The lesion may have developed slowly or abruptly. The sudden development of such a lesion is attributed to occlusion of the vessel by a thrombus. The primary clinical concern in many instances is to rule out melanoma. The lesion is likely produced by trauma to a preexisting vein or artery and likely does not represent a true vascular proliferation or neoplasm.

Histopathological features: The principal finding is a single ectatic vascular structure (usually a vein), often containing a thrombus.[7] The vascular channel is characterized by an unremarkable endothelial lining that is surrounded by a concentric layering of fibrous tissue without smooth muscle or elastic lumina. The thrombus may display different degrees of organization. This phenomenon may substantially alter the histologic appearance and the structure of the original vessel.

Differential diagnosis: The differential diagnosis includes other ectatic vascular channels with or without thrombosis, such as a venous lake, enlarged and torturous arterial and lymphatic channels, and angiokeratoma.

SPIDER ANGIOMA

BOX 20-4   Summary

- Spider angioma is a common cutaneous vascular lesion that is often seen as an incidental finding in healthy children.
- Spider angiomas are commonly found on the face, particularly the upper infraorbital

cheeks, the neck, trunk, and hands.
- Histologically, you can see a central artery rising into the dermis and branching into smaller vessels that supply blood to the radiating array of fine capillaries.
- The clinical appearance of spider angiomas, with its pulsatile nature, is very distinct and narrows the differential diagnosis.

Also known as nevus araneus, spider nevus, arterial spider, or spider telangiectasis. The spider angioma is a common cutaneous vascular lesion that is often seen as an incidental finding in healthy children.[8,9] Some of these lesions persist into adulthood, and other spider angiomas occur as acquired manifestations of pregnancy, hepatic cirrhosis, and thyrotoxicosis.

Clinical features: The most common sites of involvement are the face, particularly the upper infraorbital cheeks, the neck, trunk, and hands. An erythematous central punctum, which may be slightly elevated and may be seen to be pulsatile on diascopy, gives forth an array of peripherally radiating fine vessels. A spider angioma typically blanches with pressure, and upon release refills rapidly by blood flow originating from its center. Often solitary, multiple spider angiomas may occur occasionally, and particularly in the setting of chronic liver disease that may be numerous.

Histopathological features: A central artery rises in the dermis and branches into smaller vessels that supply blood to the radiating array of fine capillaries.[8] Rarely, the wall of the artery may contain glomus cells.[8]

Differential diagnosis: The clinical appearance of the spider angioma with its pulsatile nature is distinct and allows distinction from simple telangiectases. In contrast to spider angiomas, the lesions of hereditary hemorrhagic telangiectasia, an inherited mucocutaneous disorder that is described further in this chapter, are numerous and consist of nonpulsatile, punctate, or linear telangiectases.

NEVUS FLAMMEUS

BOX 20-5   Summary

- Nevus flammeus is a congenital vascular anomaly that often involves the head and neck region.
- The initial lesions present at birth are pink to reddish macules that are often irregular in configuration.
- Commonly associated with Cobb syndrome, Sturge–Weber syndrome, and Klippel–Trenaunay–Weber syndrome.

- Histologically, you can see widely dilated, thin-walled venules scattered throughout the upper dermis or throughout the entire reticular dermis.

Also known as salmon patch or port-wine stain, this congenital vascular anomaly often involves the head and neck with a unilateral distribution but may occur anywhere.[2–4,8,9] Some variants, e.g., the so-called salmon patch, may regress in the postnatal period, whereas other variants are persistent, e.g., the port-wine stain. There may be an association with syndromes involving other organs.

Clinical features: The initial lesions present at birth are pink to reddish macules that are often irregular in configuration and involve the nape of the neck (so-called stork bite), the eyelids and glabella (the salmon patch), other areas of the face, or any anatomic site. Persistent lesions may become papular and keratotic, and may be associated with particular syndromes, termed congenital dysplastic angiopathies that are highly variable in their clinical findings.[8] The following syndromes are commonly associated with port-wine stains:

- *Cobb syndrome:* Individuals with this syndrome have a vascular malformation involving the spinal cord and usually a port-wine stain in the distribution of the corresponding dermatome of the skin.[10]

- *Sturge–Weber syndrome (encephalotrigeminal angiomatosis):* This syndrome is characterized by a unilateral port-wine stain often in the distribution of the ophthalmic branch of the fifth (trigeminal) cranial nerve, seizures and hemiplegia or hemiparesis related to a vascular malformation involving the contralateral leptomeninges, possible choroidal vascular malformations, mental retardation, and glaucoma.[8,11]

- *Klippel–Trenaunay–Weber syndrome (hemihemangiectatic hypertrophy, congenital dysplastic angiopathies, angioosteohypertrophy):* In addition to a port-wine stain (usually involving the affected limb), the primary defining feature is the unilateral hypertrophy of a limb, most commonly the lower extremity, often with associated varicosities.[8,12,13] There is an overgrowth of both bone and soft tissue in most instances. Commonly, there is an underlying arteriovenous malformation, but other vascular anomalies may be present including angiokeratomas and venous (cavernous) and lymphatic malformations.

Histopathological features: The essential findings are widely dilated, thin-walled venules scattered throughout the upper dermis or throughout the entire reticular dermis.[2,3,8] Papular lesions developing in nevus flammeus are composed of a proliferation of thin-walled vascular channels with lumina that vary in size.

Differential diagnosis: Other vascular ectasias such as generalized essential telangiectasia, hereditary benign telangiectasia, hereditary hemorrhagic telangiectasia, unilateral nevoid telangiectasia, and spider angioma enter into the differential diagnosis. Nevus flammeus differs from the other conditions because of the onset of lesions at birth, rather distinctive macular to papular clinical lesions, and fairly discrete dilated venules in the upper reticular dermis.

ANGIOMA SERPIGINOSUM

BOX 20-6   Summary

- Angioma serpiginosum is an unusual benign vascular lesion.
- Angioma serpiginosum typically occurs during the first two decades of life, is more common in women, and occurs at any site.
- Clinically, there are minute violaceous red puncta, which occur in gyrate or serpiginous configurations.
- Angioma serpiginosum is characterized by increased numbers of dilated, capillaries in the upper dermis.

Angioma serpiginosum is an unusual benign vascular lesion that was first described by Hutchinson in 1889 as a peculiar form of serpiginous and infective nevoid disease. It was named by Crocker in 1894 and additional reports over time have clarified its clinicopathologic features.

Clinical features: Angioma serpiginosum typically occurs during the first two decades of life, is more common in women, and occurs at any site.[14,15] Although the lower extremities are the most common sites, the palms and soles are typically spared. Extensive involvement of the trunk and extremities occurs infrequently.[16] Minute violaceous red puncta, at times requiring magnification for adequate visualization, occur in gyrate or serpiginous configurations. Groups of puncta may coalesce into patches. Peripheral extension occurs through the formation of satellite puncta. Angioma serpiginosum usually occurs sporadically in individuals, but familial transmission has been reported. Autosomal dominant inheritance with variable penetrance

favoring women was suggested, but the possibility of recessive inheritance could not be excluded. Angioma serpiginosum may spontaneously regress but is usually slowly progressive. There may, however, be periods of relative quiescence or prolonged stability.

Histopathological features: Angioma serpiginosum is characterized by increased numbers of dilated capillaries in the upper dermis.[14,15] The overlying epidermis is normal and there is no significant inflammation. Red cell extravasation and hemosiderin are absent. The dilated capillaries are relatively thick-walled.

Differential diagnosis: The absence of red cell extravasation and hemosiderin differentiate angioma serpiginosum from pigmented purpuric dermatoses and Henoch–Schönlein purpura. Clinical similarities to angiokeratoma circumscriptum exist, but the latter condition differs from angioma serpiginosum by developing a verrucous, hyperkeratotic surface.

ANGIOKERATOMA

BOX 20-7   Summary

- There are five clinical types of angiokeratoma: Mibelli type, Fordyce type, angiokeratoma corporis diffusum, solitary or multiple type, and angiokeratoma circumsciptum.
- Angiokeratomas occur as variably hyperkeratotic lesions that may be pink red to purple, brown, or occasionally blue to black.
- Histologically, you can see ectatic, thin-walled vascular spaces in the papillary dermis intimately associated with an acanthotic epidermis with elongated rete ridges and hyperkeratosis.

Angiokeratomas traditionally occur as five clinical types:[17–20]

1. *Mibelli type,* with hyperkeratotic lesions on the dorsal fingers and toes

2. *Fordyce type,* with involvement of the scrotum and vulva

3. *Angiokeratoma corporis diffusum* (ACD), a lysosomal storage disease inherited as an X-linked recessive disorder in Fabry's disease (α-galactosidase A deficiency) but also seen with the autosomal recessive disorder, fucosidosis (α-L-fucosidase deficiency), and rarely with β galactosidase deficiency, alone or in combination with neuraminidase deficiency

4. *The solitary or multiple type* that may occur anywhere but favors the lower extremities

5. *Angiokeratoma circumscriptum,* with lesions in groups or bands usually on an extremity

However, this last type of angiokeratoma has deep angiomatous involvement in contrast to the telangiectatic nature of angiokeratomas, in general, and may be better classified with verrucous hemangiomas (VHs). The existence of a sixth type of angiokeratoma, angiokeratoma serpiginosum, clinically simulating angioma serpiginosum, has been suggested.

Clinical features: Most forms of angiokeratoma present during the first two decades of life. Angiokeratoma circumscriptum may be visible at birth. In contrast, angiokeratomas of ACD typically present in late childhood; and angiokeratoma scroti and the solitary or multiple types of angiokeratoma generally arise during the second to fourth decades or later. Vulvar angiokeratomas usually occur in the third and fourth decades and have been regarded as analogous to angiokeratoma scroti, particularly in regards to their anatomic location and a pathogenesis related to conditions of increased venous pressure. ACD is a manifestation of a systemic disorder, the clinicopathological features of which are beyond the scope of this discussion.[21]

Angiokeratomas occur as variably hyperkeratotic lesions that may be pink red to purple, brown, or occasionally blue to black. Clinically, the differential diagnosis includes hemangioma, verruca, nevus, and when thrombosed and deeply pigmented, malignant melanoma. The latter occurrence has been emphasized in individual case reports. Angiokeratomas usually offer no symptoms, but with local trauma they may become irritated and can bleed, given their highly vascular nature.

Histopathological features: All angiokeratomas are histologically similar, except for the addition of certain features for angiokeratoma corporis diffusum.[19,20] Ectatic, thin-walled vascular spaces occur in the papillary dermis intimately associated with, and variably encased by, acanthotic epidermis with elongated rete ridges and hyperkeratosis that is often slight but is accentuated on acral sites (Fig. 20-2). Partial or virtually complete occlusion of these dilated vessels by intravascular fibrin thrombi, in various degrees of organization, is common. Dilated veins often drain the vascular lacunae of angiokeratoma scroti and vulvar angiokeratoma.

Careful examination of angiokeratomas of ACD may show subtle

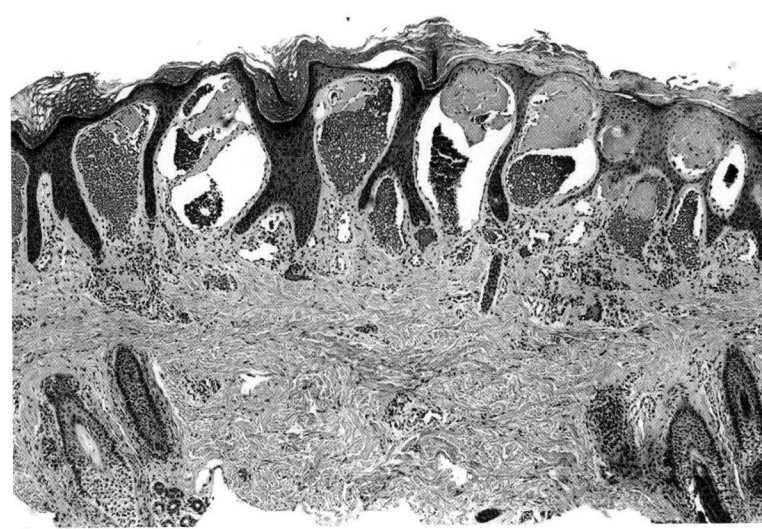

▲ **FIGURE 20-2** Angiokeratoma. The vascular lumina impinge upon the epidermis.

vacuolization of the endothelium, arrector pili muscle, and vascular smooth muscle cells, but these vacuoles are better seen by lipid stains, such as Sudan black B, or by periodic acid–Schiff stain (PAS) of the glycolipid. The lipid is doubly refractile and can be visualized in frozen tissue sections examined by polarized light. Ultrastructural examination will reveal characteristic electron-dense, lamellar inclusion bodies. Abnormal collagen was noted in the multiple angiokeratomas of a child with juvenile dermatomyositis.[22]

Differential diagnosis: The diagnosis of angiokeratoma is seldom difficult, and the clinical setting allows appropriate subclassification. It is important of course to distinguish angiokeratomas with enzyme deficiencies, due to the obvious systemic implications. Verrucous hemangiomas because of their superficial component may mimic angiokeratomas and when small may enter into the differential diagnosis. However, because angiokeratomas are telangiectasias, they lack the deep hemangiomatous component so characteristic of both verrucous hemangioma and the even more deeply extensive condition, including muscle or bone, recently reported as angiomatosis with angiokeratoma-like features in children.[23] Finally, it has been suggested that larger variants of solitary angiokeratoma, when traumatized, may eventuate into targetoid hemosiderotic hemangiomas, lesions known for involvement of both the upper and lower dermis.

VERRUCOUS HEMANGIOMA (VH)

BOX 20-8 Summary

- Verrucous hemangioma (VH) is an uncommon vascular malformation that tends to arise near birth or in childhood.
- VH typically occurs as unilateral, grouped, sometimes linear or serpiginous, discrete to confluent, hyperkeratotic angiomatous papules.
- VH is a variant of capillary or cavernous malformation that may have mixed features of both.

Verrucous hemangioma (VH) is also known as keratotic hemangioma, unilateral VH, angiokeratoma circumscriptum naeviforme, nevus keratoangiomatosus, and naevus vascularis unius lateralis. VH is an uncommon vascular malformation that tends to arise near birth or in childhood.[24–26] In 1967, Imperial and Helwig at the Armed Forces Institute of Pathology defined the clinicopathologic features of 21 VHs identified during a retrospective review of 1175 cases that previously had been classified as angiokeratoma or various types of hemangiomas.[24]

Clinical features: In Imperial and Helwig's series, approximately half of VH developed in the perinatal period whereas six others presented by the age of 17 years.[24] The most common site is the lower extremity, particularly distally. VH typically occurs as unilateral, grouped, sometimes linear or serpiginous, discrete to confluent, hyperkeratotic angioma-

tous papules. Early lesions are bluish red, well-demarcated, soft, and compressible. Over time, VHs gradually enlarge, satellite nodules may arise, and ultimately a verrucous hyperkeratotic appearance develops. The linearity of VH has been theorized to reflect genetic mosaicism.[27] VHs enlarge with body growth and tend to recur after surgical excision. Accordingly, they are best removed earlier in life when still small. In contrast to angiokeratomas, which respond to various superficial means of therapy, removal of VH requires a deep and relatively wide surgical excision. Otherwise, the lesions are apt to recur.

Histolopathological features: VH is a variant of capillary or cavernous malformation (venous malformation, cavernous hemangioma) that may have mixed features of both and is associated with secondary, reactive epidermal changes, such as acanthosis, papillomatosis, and hyperkeratosis (Fig. 20-3).[24–26] Although the superficial portion of VH may bear resemblance to an angiokeratoma, the VH is distinct in that a deep angiomatous component extends deeply into the reticular dermis and underlying subcutaneous tissue. Often, the vascularity extends laterally into adjacent skin that clinically appears normal. The upper dermis can show fibrosis, hemosiderin, and inflammation. The surface may hold inflammatory and hemorrhagic crusts, and may show occasional ulceration.

Differential diagnosis: Clinically, the differential diagnosis includes angiokeratoma, Cobb syndrome, angioma serpiginosum, lymphangioma circumscriptum, verrucae, and perhaps, pigmented tumors. Angiokeratoma corporis diffusum, scrotal angiokeratomas, and angiokeratoma of Mibelli on the fingers and toes are clinically distinct.

CAVERNOUS HEMANGIOMA

BOX 20-9 Summary

- Cavernous hemangiomas may be associated with a number of syndromes such as blue rubber bleb nevus syndrome and Mafucci's syndrome.
- The individual vascular lesion usually presents as soft, red to purple nodules or plaques that have a compressible quality, which usually presents at birth or in childhood, but may develop in older individuals.
- Cavernous hemangioma lesions are usually situated in the deep dermis or subcutis and are often well-circumscribed, but may be diffuse.

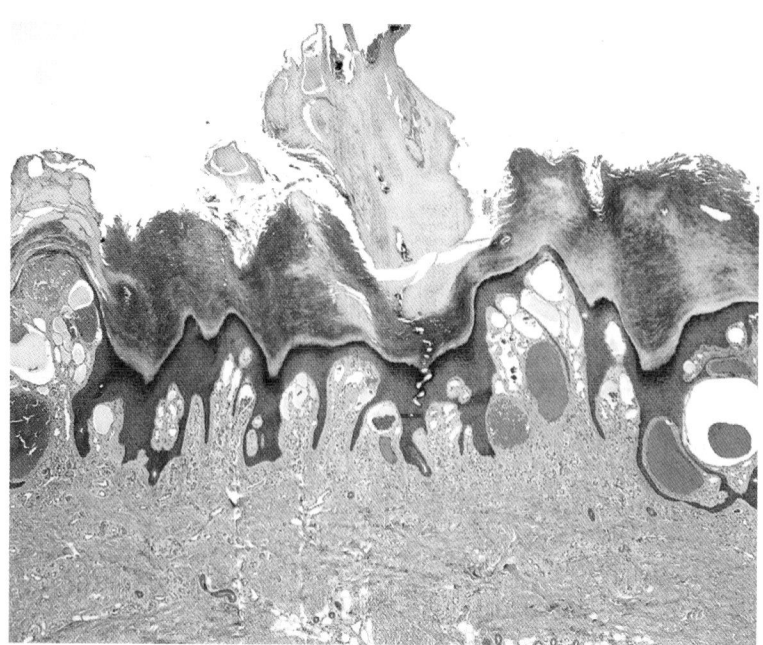

▲ **FIGURE 20-3** Verrucous hemangioma. Abundant verrucous hyperplasia of the epidermis.

Also known as a venous malformation, this rather characteristic type of vascular proliferation usually presents at birth or in childhood, but may develop in older individuals. Cavernous hemangiomas may be associated with a number of syndromes such as blue rubber bleb nevus syndrome (BRBNS) and Mafucci's syndrome.[2,3,8,28–30] The term cavernous refers to widely dilated vascular channels that resemble those in corpus cavernosum.

Clinical features: The individual vascular lesion usually presents as soft, red to purple nodules or plaques that have a compressible quality. The most common sites include the head and neck, but lesions may occur anywhere. Onset may be at birth, in the first few weeks of life, or later, and may be familial.[31,32]

Individuals with BRBNS, an autosomal dominant condition, present at birth with numerous cavernous vascular malformations involving the skin, gastrointestinal tract, central nervous system, liver, and spleen.[8,28,29] Patients may exhibit pain and hyperhidrosis from the cutaneous lesions, as well as melena and anemia from those situated in the GI tract. The principal findings with Maffucci's syndrome include three varieties of vascular lesions: cavernous malformations, lymphatic malformations, and phlebectasias; multiple enchondromas and bony deformities resulting from nonossifying cartilage in the metaphyses of growing bones; frequent fractures of bone from the latter defects; and the frequent development of chondrosarcoma and angiosarcoma in up to 50% of affected individuals.[8,30]

Histopathological features: The lesions are usually situated in the deep dermis or subcutis and are often well-circumscribed, but may be diffuse.[2,7,8] The vascular channels are often encased in fairly dense fibrous tissue that has a lobular configuration. The vessels exhibit a single layer of endothelium surrounded by fibrous tissue. Smooth muscle elements may be observed in the fibrous lining of the vessels. A subset of cavernous hemangioma, sinusoidal hemangioma, has dilated, interconnecting, thin-walled vascular channels with pseudopapillary features, a generally lobular architecture, and in areas, an ill-defined infiltrative pattern.[33]

It must be emphasized that cavernous proliferations may occur as a component of almost any complex or combined vascular malformation or as part of any of the syndromes described above. Thus, for example, one may have capillary-lymphatic, capillary-cavernous (venous), lymphaticocavernous (venous), and arteriocavernous (venous) malformations, or even more complex combinations of channels.

Differential diagnosis: Cavernous (venous) malformation must be distinguished from cavernous lymphatic malformation, glomangioma, port-wine stain, arteriovenous and other malformations, and juvenile capillary hemangioma (involuting stage).

CHERRY ANGIOMA

BOX 20-10   Summary

- Cherry angioma is one of the most common vascular tumors encountered in the skin.
- They often develop in adults beginning in adolescence and are especially common in older adults.
- They present as uniform bright to dull red papules ranging in size from 2—3 to 10 mm.
- Histologically, they are composed of fairly well-defined lobules composed of thin-walled dilated vascular channels that are largely confined to the papillary dermis.

Also known as senile angioma or Campbell de Morgan spot, the cherry angioma is one of the most common vascular tumors encountered in the skin. These lesions develop in adults and increase in number with age.[8]

Clinical features: Cherry angiomas often develop in adults beginning in adolescence and are especially common in older adults.[8] These angiomas occur at all sites, but especially involve the trunk. They present as uniform bright to dull red papules ranging in size from 2–3 to 10 mm or so.

Histopathological features: Cherry angiomas are usually raised dome-shaped lesions that exhibit an epidermal collarette. They are composed of fairly well-defined lobules comprising thin-walled dilated vascular channels that are largely confined to the papillary dermis. In one sense, they are a variant of lobular capillary hemangioma (LCH). The vascular lobules are separated by fibrous septa that vary in thickness depending on the age of the lesion. The vascular channels comprising the proliferation are venular.

Differential diagnosis: The entities to be considered include LCH and bacillary angiomatosis because of the lobular architecture and epidermal collarettes. Cherry angioma does not show the endothelial proliferation noted in pyogenic granuloma or the inflammation, granular debris, and epithelioid endothelium observed in bacillary angiomatosis.

CAPILLARY HYPERCELLULAR HEMANGIOMA (CHH)

BOX 20-11   Summary

- Common tumor of infancy that usually presents within the first few weeks of life as a solitary localized tumor.
- CHH often presents as a pink macule, involving the head and neck, and varying greatly in size. With growth these lesions become red to purplish papules or nodules that often have a rubbery texture.

- CHH is usually characterized by lobules of compact uniform endothelial cells with an admixture of pericytes and mast cells occupying the dermis and frequently the subcutaneous fat.

Also known as juvenile capillary hemangioma and strawberry hemangioma, capillary hypercellular hemangioma (CHH) is a relatively common tumor of infancy.[2–4,34,35] The majority of these lesions present in the first few weeks of life as a solitary localized tumor in the skin. However, lesions involving multiple sites may occur. The incidence at birth is 1 to 2% and rises to 12% by age of 1 year. Caucasians are most commonly affected relative to other racial groups, and females outnumber males by a ratio of 3:1. CHH is typified by a fairly predictable natural history in the great majority of cases: (1) rapid proliferation and enlargement in the first 8 to 12 months of life (the proliferating phase) and (2) regression over a period of 1 to 5 years (the involuting phase). Over 50% of patients have complete regression of the CHH by age 5 years, 70 to 90% by age 7 years, and there is a continued involution in the remainder of patients to an age of 10 to 12 years. About 90% of CHHs are associated with no adverse effects in children and do not necessitate any treatment. The remaining 10% require intervention, often because of local destructive effects or impingement on a vital structure such as an airway or the eye. In addition, large CHH may result in shunting of blood and high-output cardiac failure or entrapment of platelets and a thrombocytopenic coagulopathy and a potentially life-threatening hemorrhage (the Kasabach–Merritt syndrome or phenomenon).[36] The pathogenesis of CHH is poorly understood. There is an association with prematurity.

Clinical features: CHH often presents in the 1st month to 1st year of life as a pink macule often involving the head and neck and varying greatly in size. With growth, these lesions become red to purplish papules or nodules that often have a rubbery texture. Some may occupy large areas, greatly distorting the normal anatomy and threatening vital structures. Some may exhibit ulceration usually from rapid growth. Involuting lesions develop whitish streaks that correspond to fibrosis.

Histopathological features: In the initial proliferative phase, CHH is usually characterized by lobules of compact uniform endothelial cells with an admixture of pericytes and mast cells occupying the dermis and frequently the subcutaneous fat.[2–4,34,35] Vascular lumina may be difficult to discern but are usually present within the hypercellular lobules (Fig. 20-4). The mitotic rate is usually significant at this stage. With time, the lobular character of the tumor becomes more evident, the degree of cellularity diminishes, and the vascular lumina are more readily identified. With involution, the vascular lobules are gradually replaced by fibrous tissue.

Differential diagnosis: The clinical presentation of CHH in children is usually distinctive. However, the differential diagnosis includes vascular malformations, kaposiform hemangioendothelioma, tufted angioma, and cellular nonvascular tumors of infancy.

LOBULAR CAPILLARY HEMANGIOMA (PYOGENIC GRANULOMA)

BOX 20-12 Summary

- Commonly acquired vascular lesion that was once considered to be secondary to pyogenic infection or arising as exuberant granulation tissue in response to trauma, but now thought to be an acquired hemangioma.
- Lobular capillary hemangioma (LCH) typically appears as a solitary, rapidly growing, dark red, exophytic, raised to polypoid, vascular lesion that frequently has superficial ulceration.
- Histologically, LCHs evolve through three distinct phases.

Also known in the past as granuloma pyogenicum, granuloma gravidarum, botryomycosis humaine, and botryomycoma, this commonly acquired vascular lesion was once considered to be secondary to pyogenic infection or arising as exuberant granulation tissue in response to trauma. At present, it is best understood as an acquired hemangioma, designated lobular capillary hemangioma (LCH) because of its lobular architecture on low-power magnification.[37–40]

Clinical features: LCH typically appears as a solitary, rapidly growing, dark red, exophytic, raised to polypoid, vascular lesion that frequently has superficial ulceration. Many LCHs arise spontaneously without a known cause, and others are associated with trauma, cast immobilization,[41] pregnancy,[42] and antiretroviral therapy.[43] The most common sites for LCHs are the fingers, face, and oral cavity. In the latter location, lesions may be seen on the gingiva, lips, and tongue. The name, granuloma gravidarum or pregnancy tumor, applies to a pyogenic granuloma arising on the gingival surface during pregnancy. Oral mucosal LCHs favor female patients (2:1) while cutaneous lesions affect both sexes equally.[44] Retinoid therapy has also been associated with pyogenic granuloma-like lesions. The ones composed of granulation tissue have been described in cystic acne, treated with oral isotretinoin or secondarily infected with *Escherichia coli*.[45] Etretinate, a retinoid akin to isotretinoin, has similarly been linked with the development

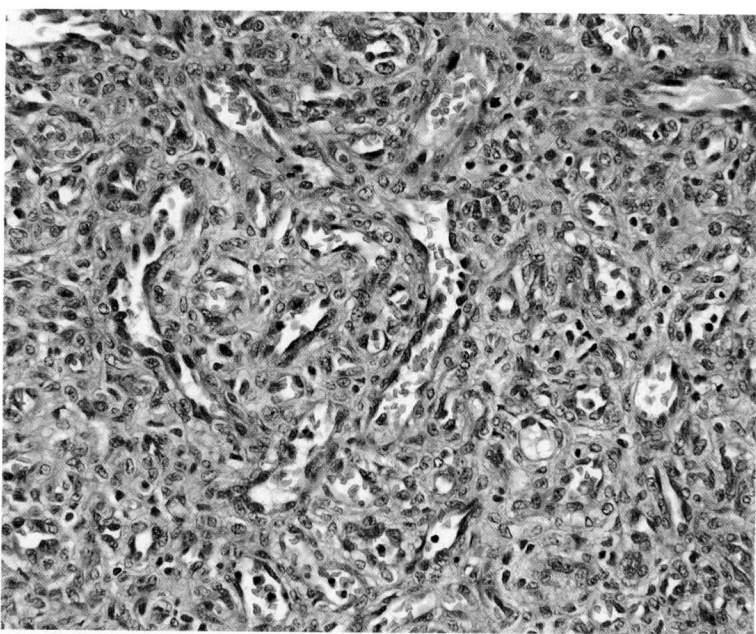

▲ **FIGURE 20-4** Capillary hypercellular hemangioma. The narrow vascular lumina are difficult to appreciate due to the compactness of the vascular proliferation.

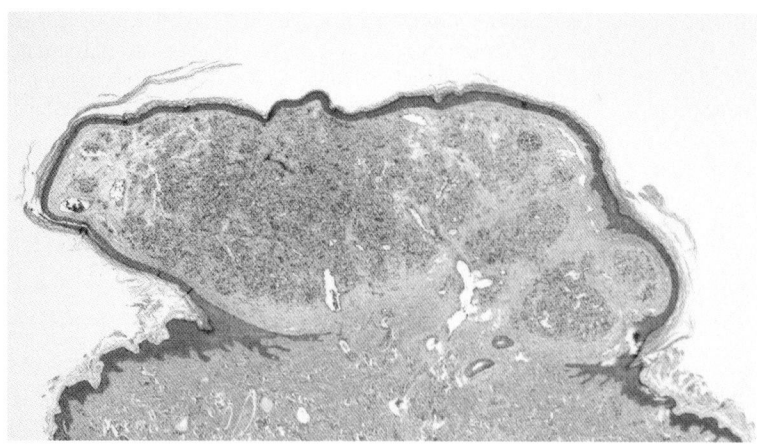

▲ **FIGURE 20-5** Lobular capillary hemangioma. Typical polypoid lesion with lobulated vascular proliferation.

BOX 20-13 Summary

- Acquired tufted angioma (ATA) arises as slowly enlarging erythematous macules and plaques that often have a deep component and typically occur on the neck and upper trunk of children and young adults.
- More than half of the cases have occurred during the first 5 years of life, and a few cases have presented at birth. Lesions have been associated with hyperhidrosis and Kasabach–Merritt syndrome.
- The hallmark of this hemangioma is the presence of small cellular, capillary tufts dispersed as "cannonballs" throughout the dermis.

of pyogenic granuloma-like lesions in patients with psoriasis.[46] Topical use of tretinoin, tazarotene, and a combination of retinoic acid and minoxidil has also been implicated.[47]

The rare phenomenon of satellite lesions arising after surgical removal, laser excision, or trauma to a pyogenic granuloma is well known. Satellite lesions usually occur on the trunk, particularly on the upper back of individuals less than 25 years of age. A rare, eruptive, disseminated, self-limited form with lesions that may number in the hundreds has been described. In most cases, they have appeared spontaneously, although they have also arisen after a second-degree burn and after the removal of an ocular neoplasm. Underlying malignancy has been documented in some patients with disseminated pyogenic granulomas, but causation has not been established. The notion of a circulating angiogenic factor being involved in the pathogenesis is certainly intriguing but is still entirely speculative. The rapid growth of LCHs may result from decreased apoptosis associated with increased expression of the Bcl-2 family of apoptotic-regulatory proteins.[48]

Histopathological features: LCHs evolve through three, more or less, distinct phases. In the early phase, there is a compact vascular proliferation of solid, largely unopened vascular structures. The histology is atypical with endothelial cells arranged seemingly in solid sheets with prominent nuclei and numerous mitotic figures. Later, there is a frank evolution into vascular structures with a multilobular arrangement and regular appearing lumina. In the final stage, there is a progressive development of pericytic cells, transformation

into spindled smooth muscle, and evolution into veins. At the beginning, one or two veins dominate each lobule, but later, there is an extensive venulization of the whole lesion. Intra- and interlobular fibrosis ensues, and the lesion becomes progressively avascular and fibrotic. Rare examples may show a cavernous hemangioma appearance, but the typical lobular arrangement can be seen elsewhere.

The typical LCH contains variably cellular but cytologically bland, lobular capillary proliferations with variable mitotic activity (Fig. 20-5). The overlying epidermis is flattened, forms a peripheral collarette, and frequently shows erosion. As a result, LCHs often show secondary changes such as edema, hemorrhage, fibrin, necrosis, and acute inflammation. One case of extramedullary hematopoiesis has been reported recently.[49] LCHs have also occurred intravenously and in subcutaneous tissue. Intravenous LCHs extend into vascular lumina as polypoid lesions that connect with the wall of the vein by a fibrovascular stalk. Immunohistochemically, the endothelial cells of the well-formed capillaries are positive for factor VIII-related antigen, Ulex europaeus lectin, CD31, and CD34.

Differential diagnosis: The differential diagnosis of LCH is as varied as its clinical presentations and evolutionary stages. It may be confused clinically with amelanotic melanoma and eccrine poroma. Histologically, LCH has features that link it with tufted hemangioma. On occasion, the endothelial cells can be prominent and epithelioid, and a differential diagnosis with ALHE (epithelioid hemangioma) is required. The dermal form is sometimes confused with a glomus tumor.

Also known as angioblastoma (Nakagawa), progressive capillary hemangioma, or tufted hemangioma, this condition was described by Wilson Jones in 1976, and additional cases have better defined its clinicopathologic features.[50–52] Progressive capillary hemangioma (MacMillan) and angioblastoma (Nakagawa), an entity better known in the Japanese literature, have been regarded by many as being similar or identical.[52] Acquired tufted angioma (ATA) is considered to be a distinct clinicopathologic entity, related to the pyogenic granuloma (LCH), and peripheral satellite nodules resembling pyogenic granulomas have been observed. Furthermore, lesions reported as dermal pyogenic granulomas have been purported to be ATA.

Clinical features: Classically, ATA arises as slowly enlarging erythematous macules and plaques that often have a deep component and typically occur on the neck and upper trunk of children and young adults.[50,51] More than half of the cases have occurred during the first 5 years of life, and a few cases have presented at birth. Lesions have been associated with hyperhidrosis[52] and with Kasabach–Merritt syndrome.[53] ATA may present in adults; however, some of these cases have arisen within a preexisting, fixed vascular blemish or port-wine stain. ATAs are usually dull red in color, but occasionally the superficial component may appear more brightly red. ATAs are benign lesions that slowly enlarge over years and may attain considerable size.

ATA generally occurs sporadically. However, there has been one report of familial lesions with an autosomal dominant inheritance. One case of eruptive ATA of the right axilla and arm appearing in an older man soon after liver transplantation is documented. Surprisingly, the lesions were self-limited, involuting spontaneously over several months. ATA of the oral mucosa has also been reported recently.[54]

Histopathological features: The hallmark of this hemangioma is the presence of small cellular, capillary tufts dispersed as "cannonballs" throughout the dermis.[50–52] The tufts tend to be larger in the middle and lower dermis. The subcutaneous tissue is spared. Dilated lymphatic-like vessels may be present in the dermis and often appear as cleft-like lumina at the periphery of capillary tufts. Protrusion of the tuft into the lumen may impart a glomerular-like appearance. The degree of cellularity within tufts may be so dense that capillary lumina may not be readily evident. Reticulin stains will reveal a rich network that ensheathes individual endothelial cells. Mitotic figures may be seen, but cellular atypia is absent.

Differential diagnosis: Although the progressive nature of ATA may invoke consideration of a low-grade angiosarcoma or Kaposi sarcoma (KS), the clinicopathologic features and particularly the early onset of most cases allow distinction. The most likely differential diagnosis is with LCH, a condition with which ATA may be related. Although the vascular lobules are very similar, the scattered nature of ATA is fairly characteristic. Glomeruloid hemangioma can also be very similar, but the systemic manifestations and the characteristic intralobular PAS-positive eosinophilic bodies are sufficient to allow the distinction. Similar thoughts are true for reactive angioendotheliomatosis. The heterogeneous appearance of the vascular lobules and different clinical presentations allow for a precise diagnosis. Dabska tumor also may have a superficial resemblance to ATA. The endotheliotropic lymphocytes are, however, characteristic.

GLOMERULOID HEMANGIOMA (GH)

BOX 20-14 Summary

- Rare hemangioma that occurs in patients with POEMS syndrome.
- The glomeruloid hemangioma is considered to be a reactive endothelial proliferation, and the result of circulating angiogenic factors from activated lymphocytes.
- The lesions are multiple, punctate-to-several-millimeter-sized, red or violaceous papules favoring the trunk and proximal limbs.

- Typical GH shows ectatic vascular spaces in the dermis and these spaces contain glomerulus-like structures formed by conglomerates of blood-filled capillaries lined generally by flat endothelial cells.

This rare hemangioma derives its name from its distinctive histologic resemblance to renal glomeruli and occurs in the setting of POEMS syndrome, a multisystem disorder consisting of polyneuropathy, organomegaly, endocrinopathy, M-protein, and skin changes.[55,56] The cutaneous manifestations include hyperpigmentation, hypertrichosis, hyperhidrosis, scleroderma-like skin thickening, and hemangiomas. Many patients with POEMS syndrome show overlapping features with multicentric Castleman disease and its characteristic angiofollicular lymphoid hyperplasia of lymph nodes.

The glomeruloid hemangioma is considered to be a reactive endothelial proliferation, perhaps akin to reactive angioendotheliomatosis, and the result of circulating angiogenic factors from activated lymphocytes. A very similar etiopathogenic situation, but with very different clinical and histologic presentation, is seen in patients with reactive angioendotheliomatosis with luminal cryoprecipitates. These patients have circulating cryoproteins that when captured by endothelial cells of peripheral vessels produce their proliferation with widespread inspissated cryoproteins in vascular lumina.

Clinical features: Glomeruloid hemangiomas appear to be more common in the Japanese than in other ethnic groups. Only a few cases have been reported in the Caucasian population, affecting the fifth to sixth decades of life with no preponderance of sex. Patients with POEMS syndrome and hemangiomas have multiple, punctate-to-several-millimeter-sized, red or violaceous papules favoring the trunk and proximal limbs. Most of the hemangiomas are actually cherry-like capillary hemangiomas, with the glomeruloid hemangiomas being fairly rare. We have seen a case associated with multiple myeloma.

Histopathological features: A precursor stage of immature vascular tissue has been suggested.[57] Typical GH shows ectatic vascular spaces in the dermis and these spaces contain glomerulus-like structures formed by conglomerates of blood-filled capillaries lined generally by flat endothelial cells (Fig. 20-6).[55,56,58] An occasional endothelial cell may be plump with pale cytoplasm, clear vacuoles, or eosinophilic globules. Similar cells that may be immature endothelial cells are interspersed as stromal cells between the capillary loops. The eosinophilic globules, PAS-positive and diastase-resistant, show polytypic immunoglobulin staining and presumably represent circulatory-derived immunoglobulin and other proteinaceous material. Mitoses are inconspicuous, numbering less than one per 10 high-power field. There is little, if any, inflammation. Irregular lumina associated with capillaries and sinusoid-like

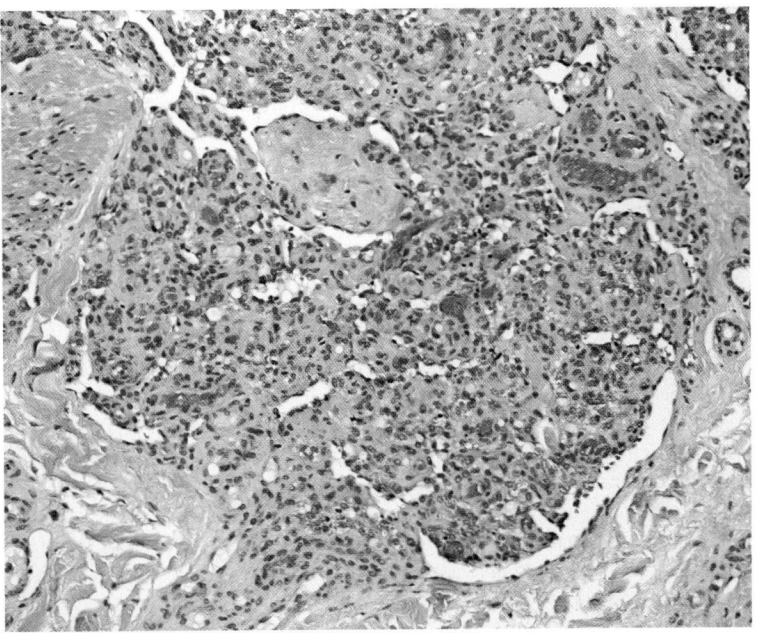

▲ **FIGURE 20-6** Glomeruloid hemangioma. Lobulated vascular proliferation resembling a renal glomerulus.

spaces have been described within the glomeruloid structures in GH.

Differential diagnosis: Acquired tufted hemangioma is frequently associated with peripheral vascular clefts, but there is no actual intravascular angiomatous growth and are devoid of eosinophilic globules. Others that need to be considered include LCH (pyogenic granuloma), intravascular papillary endothelial hyperplasia, reactive angioendotheliomatosis, and endovascular papillary angioendothelioma (Dabska tumor).

ANGIOLYMPHOID HYPERPLASIA WITH EOSINOPHILIA (ALHE)

BOX 20-15   Summary

- ALHE presents as single or multiple, pink to red brown papules or plaques in the head and neck region of young to middle-aged adults. It occurs particularly in women, although some reports have noted a male predominance.

- Most lesions of ALHE are intradermal, but deeper extension into the subcutaneous tissue may occur, and occasionally the condition may arise as primary subcutaneous nodules.

- ALHE shows blood vessel proliferation and inflammation. The vessels vary in diameter and are lined by prominent endothelial cells, a feature that is characteristic of ALHE and defines the entity.

Angiolymphoid hyperplasia with eosinophilia (ALHE) has many synonyms: epithelioid hemangioma, subcutaneous lymphoid hyperplasia with eosinophilia, subcutaneous ALHE, atypical pyogenic granuloma, inflammatory angiomatous nodules with abnormal blood vessels, pseudopyogenic granuloma, papular angioplasia, atypical vascular proliferation with inflammation, intravenous atypical vascular proliferation, nodular angioblastic hyperplasia with eosinophilia and lymphofolliculosis, and histiocytoid hemangioma. ALHE is an entity that has conceptually evolved since the 1960s and has carried various names since that time.[59–64] Moreover, ALHE had been confused with Kimura's disease, a condition that differs clinicopathologically from ALHE and is now viewed as a separate entity.[61] Opinions regarding the pathogenesis of ALHE seem to favor a reactive vascular proliferation; however, origination as a primary vascular neoplasm or hemangioma must be considered. A role for human herpesvirus 8 in the pathogenesis of ALHE has been suggested, but also refuted.[65]

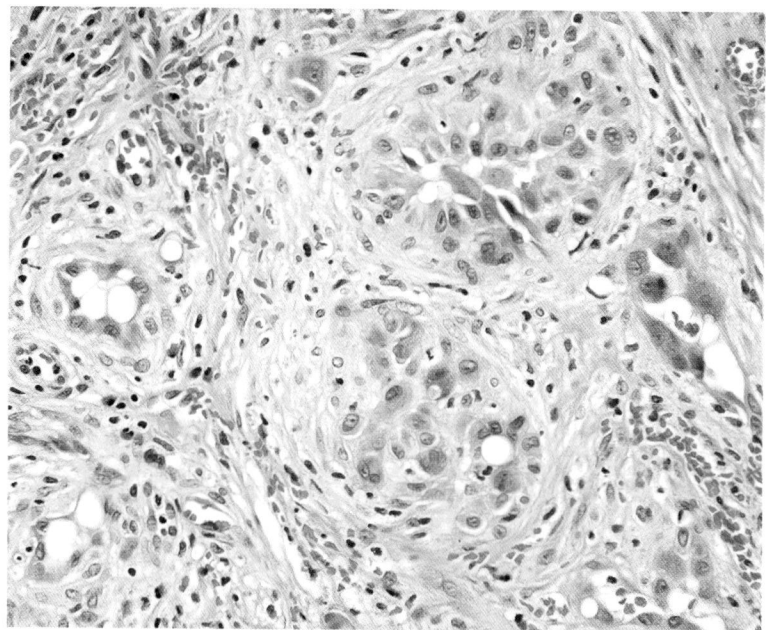

▲ **FIGURE 20-7** Angiolymphoid hyperplasia with eosinophilia. Note the epithelioid appearance of the endothelial cells and numerous intracellular lumina.

Clinical features: ALHE presents as single or multiple, pink to red brown papules or plaques in the head and neck region of young to middle-aged adults, particularly women, although some reports have noted a male predominance.[59–64] The most common sites are the ear and forehead. Uncommonly, the trunk, extremities, and hands may be involved. Disseminated lesions have been reported.[66] Most lesions of ALHE are intradermal, but deeper extension into the subcutaneous tissue may occur, and occasionally the condition may arise as primary subcutaneous nodules. Peripheral blood eosinophilia is present in a minority of cases. Lesions of ALHE are usually asymptomatic but on occasion there may be tenderness, pulsation, pruritus, or bleeding, either spontaneously or after minor trauma. Involvement of the oral mucosa was recently reported.[67]

Histopathological features: ALHE shows blood vessel proliferation and inflammation.[59–64] The vessels vary in diameter and are lined by prominent endothelial cells, a feature that is characteristic of ALHE and defines the entity. These "histiocytic" endothelial cells led to the grouping of ALHE under the name histiocytoid hemangioma, a term used to encompass lesions of other organ systems that by light microscopy had cells with a similar appearance. However, the latter term (histiocytoid hemangioma) is eschewed by many, since such a category may encompass a diverse group of specific entities that may not necessarily be related. The endothelial cells are enlarged, cuboidal to "hobnail"

in shape, with abundant eosinophilic to amphophilic cytoplasm and large vesicular nuclei. Cytoplasmic vacuoles may be present and, when large, may distort the nucleus or coalesce into small lumina by merging with the vacuoles of other cells (Fig. 20-7). There is an accompanying diffuse to nodular lymphocytic infiltrate, possibly with lymphoid follicles and germinal center formation. Variable numbers of eosinophils are present (Fig. 20-8). There is zonation of the inflammatory infiltrate toward the periphery of the lesion. Occasional thrombi may be seen, and mitotic activity is generally inconspicuous to absent. Multinucleated cells, perivascular and interstitial, were noted in one case.[68]

Subcutaneous lesions, particularly those associated with arteriovenous malformations, tend to show prominent endothelial cell proliferation, sometimes forming solid intraluminal masses. Such solid proliferations of endothelial cells may obscure the true vascular nature of the lesion and occasionally lead to confusion in diagnosis. Subcutaneous masses, developing after trauma, showing thickened small to medium-sized arteries, myxoid degeneration, and capillary vascular proliferation have been designated traumatic pseudoaneurysm and theorized to be a precursor of ALHE.[69] Some lesions of ALHE may contain a minority of epithelioid endothelial cells, while the majority resemble those of LCHs.

Differential diagnosis: Clinicopathologic differences serve to differentiate ALHE from Kimura's disease. Kimura's

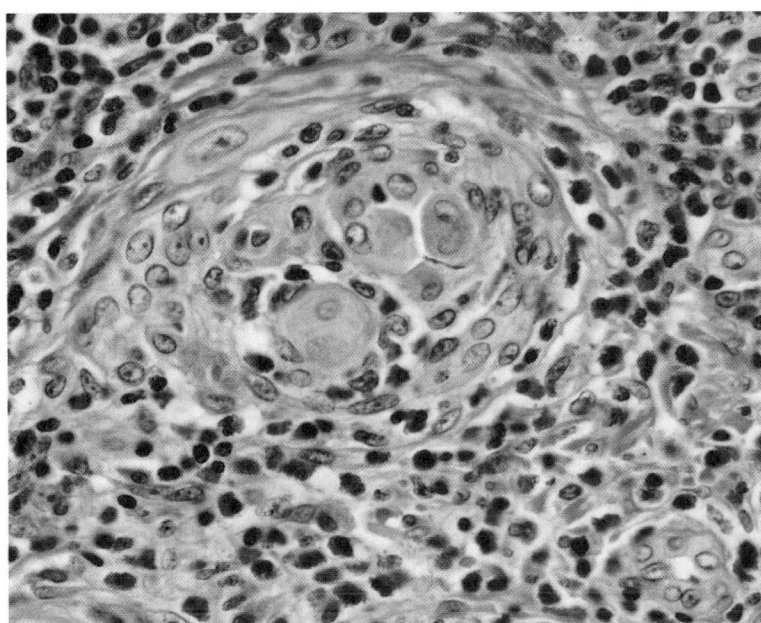

▲ **FIGURE 20-8** Angiolymphoid hyperplasia with eosinophilia. Epitheliod endothelial cells with numerous interstitial eosinophils.

disease is considered to be the result of an immunologic reaction of allergic or autoimmune nature. Mast cells are increased in lesions of less than 1 year duration.[70] Juvenile temporal arteritis recently has been speculated to be an accessory lesion of Kimura's disease.[71] In comparison to ALHE, angiosarcoma generally has conspicuous cytologic atypia, frequent mitotic figures, piling up of cells, and lack the inflammatory infiltrate of ALHE, although rare angiosarcomas can display substantial infiltrates. Solid areas of ALHE have an appearance similar to that of epithelioid angiosarcoma and even more so as of epithelioid hemangioendothelioma. However, epithelioid angiosarcoma is generally a highly malignant appearing tumor that is more apt to be mistaken for poorly differentiated carcinoma than is a lesion of ALHE.

MICROVENULAR HEMANGIOMA (MV)

BOX 20-16 Summary

- Microvenular hemangioma is believed to be a type of acquired venous hemangioma.
- Microvenular hemangiomas (MVs) typically occur as solitary asymptomatic, small, enlarging, purple to red plaques or nodules that favor the extremities of young to middle-aged adults of either sex.
- The microvenular hemangioma comprises irregularly branching, small blood vessels, often with the appearance of collapsed venules.

This hemangioma, also known as "microcapillary angioma," with its characteristic histologic appearance of small dermal blood vessels was first described by Hunt et al in 1991.[72] The clinicopathologic features of 10 cases were presented, and 2 years later, five additional cases were added to the literature by Aloi et al.[73] Microvenular hemangioma is believed to be a type of acquired venous hemangioma. A very similar if not identical appearing angioma arising in young females under the hormonal influence of pregnancy or hormonal contraceptives has been referred to as microcapillary angioma.

Clinical features: Microvenular hemangiomas (MVs) typically occur as solitary asymptomatic, small, enlarging, purple to red, plaques or nodules that favor the extremities of young to middle-aged adults of either sex. In the original series, the patients (six males and four females) ranged in age from 9 to 39 years (mean 28 years) and presented with lesions as large as 1 cm.[72] The later report showed similar demographics; however, the age range was extended to a 64-year-old woman who uniquely had two lesions, including the first described on the face.[73] Lesions in that series were slightly larger, between 1 and 2 cm. The duration of MV at presentation is usually brief, weeks to several months, but has been as long as 4 years. Clinically, MVs are generally viewed as a benign hemangioma, but the differential diagnosis has also included dermatofibroma and Kaposi Sarcoma (KS). MV in a case of Wiskott–Aldrich syndrome has been reported.[74]

Histopathological features: The microvenular hemangioma comprises irregularly branching, small blood vessels, often with the appearance of collapsed venules (Fig. 20-9).[72,73] Lumina are generally inconspicuous, narrow to absent. Endothelial cells may, at times, be a little plump, but there is no cellular atypia. Some examples of MV have prominent epithelioid cells resembling those of epithelioid (histiocytoid) hemangioma. Tufted aggregates of vessels can be seen in the deep dermis.

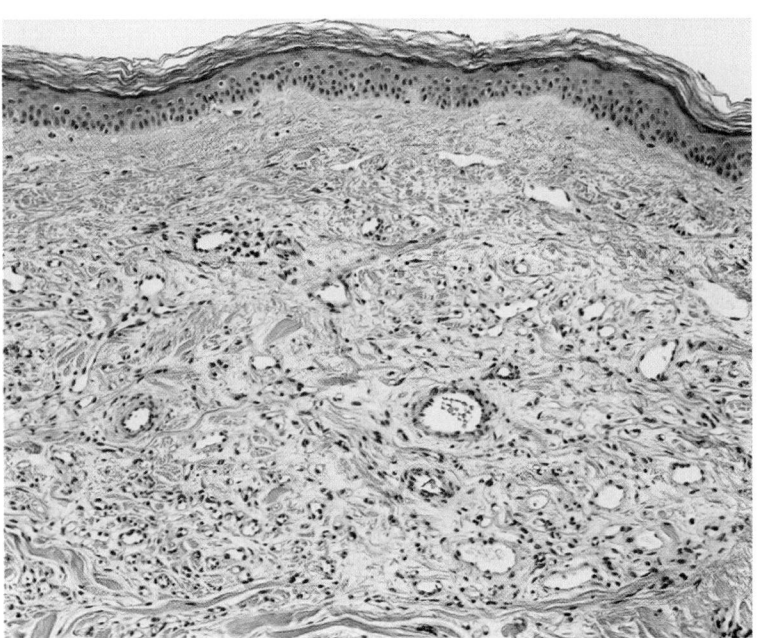

▲ **FIGURE 20-9** Microvenular hemangioma. Note the pseudoinfiltrative pattern and mature nature of the small veins.

These structures closely resemble those of LCHs and tufted hemangiomas. Examples of pyogenic granuloma merging with microvenular hemangioma have also been observed. There is a background of dermal desmoplasia with variably thickened dermal collagen. Inflammation and hemosiderin are generally scant or absent. Plasma cells and eosinophils are usually not observed.

Differential diagnosis: Microvenular hemangioma has a distinctive histologic appearance allowing little difficulty in diagnosis, although there may be some resemblance to stasis change, reactive angiogenesis of scars, early KS, and the vascular proliferations in some lesions previously included under the name, sclerosing hemangioma. The venular differentiation is also similar to that which may sometimes be seen in late stages of acquired tufted angioma and targetoid hemosiderotic hemangioma.

(TARGETOID) HEMOSIDEROTIC HEMANGIOMA (THH)

BOX 20-17   Summary

- THH typically presents as a solitary, annular, violaceous to purple papule 2 to 3 mm in diameter, with both a surrounding pale rim and a more peripheral ecchymotic ring giving a target-like appearance.
- THH does not affect one sex over the other, the age range is 5 to 72 years, and the median age is in the early fourth decade of life.
- The histology of THH varies according to the duration or age of the individual lesion.

Also known as hobnail hemangioma, targetoid hemosiderotic hemangioma (THH) is a benign vascular lesion first described in 1988.[75] More than a hundred cases have now been reported. THH is one of the histologic simulants of KS, and knowledge of its clinicopathologic features is crucial to the avoidance of misdiagnosis. The name hobnail hemangioma[76,77] has been connected with THH. This new name intends to emphasize the frequent morphology of the endothelial cell protruding into the lumen. In fact none of the lesions were clinically targetoid, nor did they contain hemosiderin.[77] Furthermore, the hobnail appearance is not a constant feature of THH, but many other vascular lesions contain similar hobnail endothelial cells.

Clinical features: THH typically presents as a solitary, annular, violaceous to purple papule 2 to 3 mm in diameter, with both a surrounding pale rim and a more peripheral ecchymotic ring giving a target-like appearance (Fig. 20-10).[75] This ring expands peripherally and then eventually disappears. Late lesions may show only a purple brown, slightly elevated papule. This event appears to be secondary to trauma or thrombosis and may not be a constant feature. This raises the question as to how many of the clinical (and histologic) features are primary and how many are secondary changes. Neither sex appears to be favored, the age range is 5 to 72 years, and the median age is in the early fourth decade of life.[75–79] THH occurs in diverse sites, favoring the proximal upper and lower extremities (particularly the thigh) and the trunk. One case of THH was reported

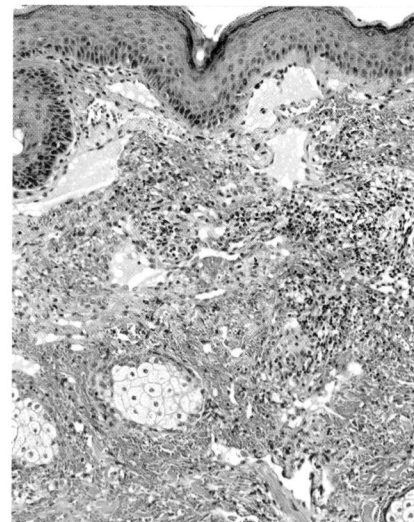

▲ **FIGURE 20-11** Targetoid hemosiderotic hemangioma. Jagged vascular lumina with both lymph and erythrocytes content.

as an acquired process developing in a congenital lesion of 17-year duration, and another involved the trunk in the belt line, both cases suggesting a role for trauma in their development. A role for trauma in the pathogenesis of THH has been further supported,[79] perhaps to a preexisting lymphangioma or hemangioma, such as a solitary angiokeratoma[78] THH is benign, may be removed by local excision, and typically does not recur.

Histopathological features: The histology of THH varies according to the duration or age of the individual lesion. The earliest finding is a proliferation of widely dilated and irregular, thin-walled vascular lumina in the superficial dermis.[75] The endothelial cells are flat or conspicuously epithelioid. Intraluminal papillary projections lined by a single layer of epithelioid, endothelial cells in "hobnail" fashion are often seen protruding into vascular lumina (Fig. 20-11). These plump endothelial cells may occasionally pileup and even obliterate vascular lumina (Fig. 20-12). Intraluminal fibrin thrombi may be present.

Vessels deeper in the reticular dermis have an inconspicuous endothelial cell lining and become angulated and irregular, appearing to be dissected collagen bundles. The vessels tend to be oriented around adnexal structures, such as eccrine coils. Other features of THH are dermal edema; variable, often intense red blood cell extravasation; hemosiderin deposition (Fig. 20-13); and an inconspicuous to mild, predominantly lymphocytic, inflammatory infiltrate. Overall on low-power magnification, THH gives a stratified or biphasic appearance with ectatic vessels containing

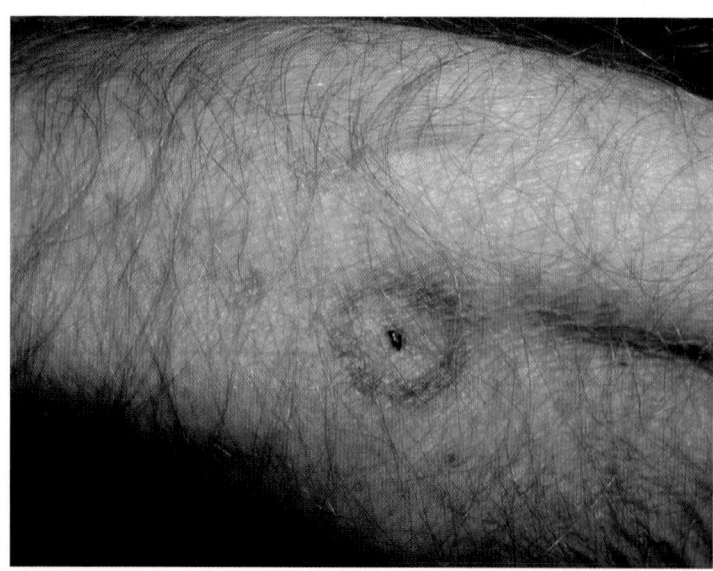

▲ **FIGURE 20-10** Targetoid hemosiderotic hemangioma. Clinical appearance of the lesion.

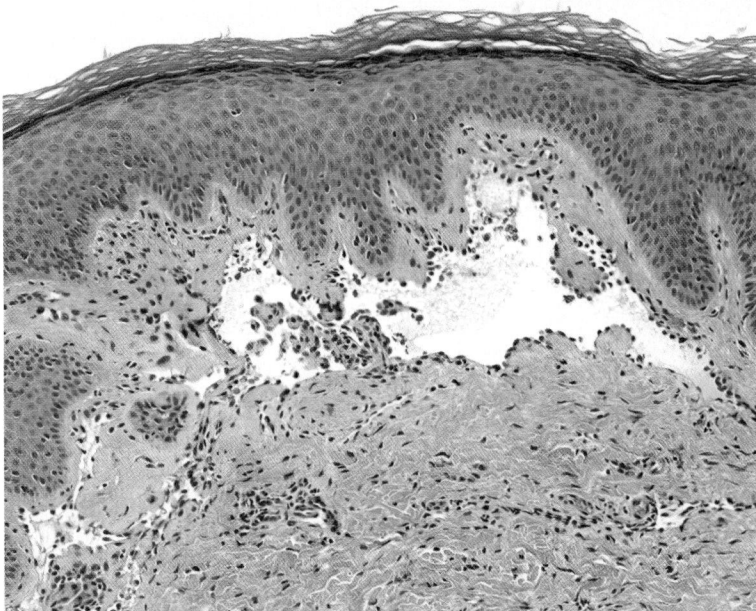

▲ **FIGURE 20-12** Targetoid hemosiderotic hemangioma. Stag horn vascular lumina with papillary projections of epithelioid appearing endothelial cells.

epithelioid endothelial cells at the top and angulated, inconspicuous vessels at the bottom. Mature lesions show most vascular lumina to be collapsed and increased cellularity of extravascular tissue. Spindle cells appear in close approximation to the vascular proliferation. Late lesions demonstrate collapsed, anastomosing, thin-walled vessels crisscrossing the dermis. Foci of elongated arborizing vessels within THH have been said to resemble benign lymphangioendothelioma and retiform hemangioendothelioma.[76,77]

Differential diagnosis: Targetoid hemosiderotic hemangioma appears histologically as an atypical vascular lesion with similarity to KS of the patch stage and lymphangiosarcoma-like types, and to benign lymphangioendothelioma. The clinical setting is helpful in differentiating these lesions because THH occurs as a solitary small lesion in healthy individuals. Lesions of KS are typically multiple and of variable size. Benign lymphangioendothelioma is clinically distinct from THH and occurs as well-demarcated dermal plaques that are larger in size than

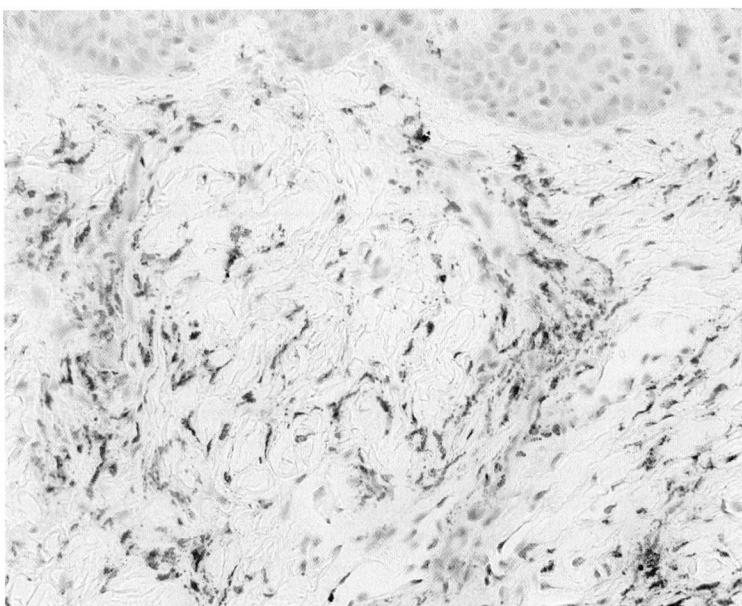

▲ **FIGURE 20-13** Targetoid hemosiderotic hemangioma. Abundant deposits of hemosiderin as demonstrated by the Perl's reaction.

those of THH, and often reach considerable proportions.

ACRO-ANGIODERMATITIS (AA)

BOX 20-18 Summary

- The name, acro-angiodermatitis is a misnomer, as the spectrum of changes is reactive in nature and does not reflect an inflammatory dermatosis.
- AA consists of reactive vascular proliferation, dermal fibrosis, and hemosiderin deposition in the setting of arteriovenous malformations and venous insufficiency.
- The clinical lesions of acro-angiodermatitis are scaly, violaceous plaques, papules, and nodules.
- Reactive epidermal acanthosis and compact hyperkeratosis are frequent features of AA. The most striking histologic changes involve the papillary and superficial to mid-reticular dermis.

Also known as stasis dermatitis, angiodermatitis, or pseudo-KS, acro-angiodermatitis (AA) is a reactive vasoproliferative condition first described in 1965 by Mali and colleagues.[80–83] Eighteen patients, with chronic venous insufficiency of the lower extremities, presented with violaceous plaques on the extensor surface of the foot and toes. In several patients, the diagnosis of KS was a clinical consideration. Since this initial report, the characteristic constellation of reactive vascular proliferation, dermal fibrosis, and hemosiderin deposition has also been reported in the setting of arteriovenous malformations and venous insufficiency. The name, acro-angiodermatitis is a misnomer, as the spectrum of changes is reactive in nature and does not reflect an inflammatory dermatosis. This name, however, is preferable to the proposed alternative of pseudo-KS.

Clinical features: In a given population, the incidence of mild forms of stasis dermatitis parallels the incidence of chronic venous insufficiency. In comparison to the incidence of chronic venous insufficiency, however, the florid clinical lesions described by Mali, and later by Strutton, are relatively uncommon and are an exaggerated vasoproliferative response to venous stasis. Most affected patients are middle-aged or older. The original paper, showed that males predominated, though the incidence of chronic venous insufficiency is higher in women.[64] Later reports, by a number of authors, have emphasized the occurrence of acro-angiodermatitis in younger patients with relative chronic venous

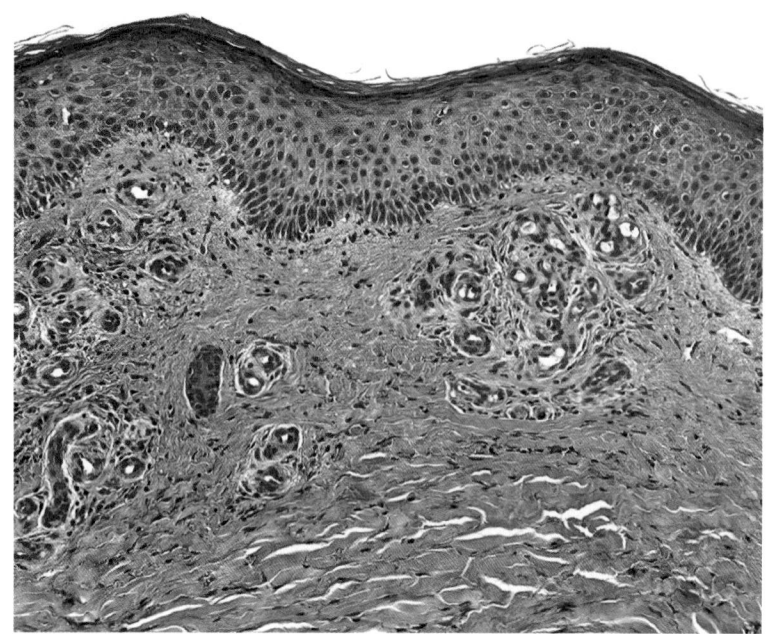

▲ **FIGURE 20-14** Acroangiodermatitis. Tufted subepidermal vascular proliferation with an overlying reactive epidermis.

insufficiency associated with arteriovenous malformations whether they be congenital or acquired.[84] In particular, AA has been reported as an acquired, iatrogenic complication of arteriovenous shunts for hemodialysis. AA has been seen in venous stasis associated with paralytic feet, in the hypertrophied leg of a patient with the Klippel–Trénaunay syndrome, and in the setting of an above-the-knee amputation stump, attributed to chronic circulatory disturbance from a poorly fitting suction-type prosthesis.

The clinical lesions of acro-angiodermatitis are scaly, violaceous plaques, papules, and nodules. In chronic venous insufficiency of the lower extremities, the lesions are most numerous over the extensor surfaces of the toes and foot. They tend to spare areas of the foot where direct pressure, either extrinsic or intrinsic, is applied. Areas of sparing include points where adjacent digits contact each other or a shoe.[64] Lesions may also occur on the lateral aspect of the ankle and anterior lower leg.[81] Surrounding tissues are edematous and show changes of stasis dermatitis. Acroangiodermatitis arising in the setting of arteriovenous malformation presents a similar clinical picture, limited to the extremity involved by the arteriovenous malformation. An unusual case of AA extending from the leg to involve the thigh and penis correlated with the presence of multiple fine arteriovenous shunts by femoral angiography.[85] Because AA is a reactive, vasoproliferative response, it is not generally amenable to direct surgical approaches, and therapy to limit progression of lesions is directed at the underlying cause.

Histopathological features: Reactive epidermal acanthosis and compact hyperkeratosis are frequent features of AA. The most striking histologic changes involve the papillary and superficial to mid-reticular dermis (Fig. 20-14). A proliferation of small blood vessels with dilated, round lumina are distributed throughout the dermis in a loose, vaguely lobular arrangement.[80–83] The vessels tend to be relatively uniform in size and regular in contour. The endothelial cells are plump and one cell layer in thickness. The cytologic features are bland. The neovascular proliferation is superimposed on a background of dermal edema and fibrosis. The contribution of each component varies from lesion to lesion and varies in individual lesions over time. The dermal edema may be quite pronounced, particularly in the papillary dermis. Fibrosis is more variable and ranges from inconspicuous, represented by a relatively sparse number of fibroblasts, to quite pronounced, with dense dermal fibrosis. Similar vascular proliferation is seen around sweat gland coils.

Extravasated erythrocytes are distributed in perivascular sites. The extent of erythrocyte extravasation is variable and often prominently associated with more superficial dermal vessels. Dermal deposition of hemosiderin may be quite exuberant and reflects chronic, ongoing erythrocyte extravasation and degradation. Hemosiderin deposition is most prominent in a perivascular pattern and may be extracellular or contained within dermal macrophages. An inconspicuous, mononuclear inflammatory infiltrate is an inconstant feature. Plasma cells are an infrequent component of the inflammatory infiltrate and never a prominent finding.

Differential diagnosis: The clinical lesions of AA may closely resemble the lesions of classic KS. A clinical history of chronic venous insufficiency and a background of stasis changes should raise the consideration of AA. Certainly, the presence of a local AV malformation or fistula should prompt consideration of AA, but the possibility of an unsuspected AV malformation should not be overlooked when a diagnosis of AA or KS is entertained in a young individual. The microscopic features of AA are distinctly different from those of KS.

Chronic lesions of atrophie blanche (hyalinizing segmental vasculitis) may have similar vasoproliferative changes, usually associated with vascular fibrin deposits. Also, the lobular pattern of vascular proliferation may be quite pronounced and may vaguely mimic the vascular proliferation of dermal pyogenic granuloma, a point emphasized by Le Boit considering the lobular proliferation of capillaries as the underlying process in a number of benign vascular tumors and reactive conditions.[82]

INTRAVASCULAR PAPILLARY ENDOTHELIAL HYPERPLASIA (IPEH)

BOX 20-19   Summary

- IPEH typically presents as a slowly enlarging, often tender, blue to red, deep dermal to subcutaneous swelling or mass. It occurs at diverse sites, the most frequent of which are the head and the extremities, particularly the fingers.

- IPEH has arisen within vascular malformations, hemangiomas of the blue rubber bleb nevus syndrome, and cervical cystic hygromas. It has also been identified in unusual sites, such as the paranasal sinus, oral mucosa, tongue, and eyelid.

- Histologically, IPEH shows conspicuous intravascular papillary structures that are formed by cores of fibrous tissue that are lined by endothelial cells that are generally flattened in appearance.

In 1923, Masson first described intravascular papillary endothelial hyperplasia (IPEH) as *vegetant intravascular hemangioendothelioma*, an unusual angiosarcoma-like proliferation in organizing thrombi of hemorrhoidal veins.[86–89]

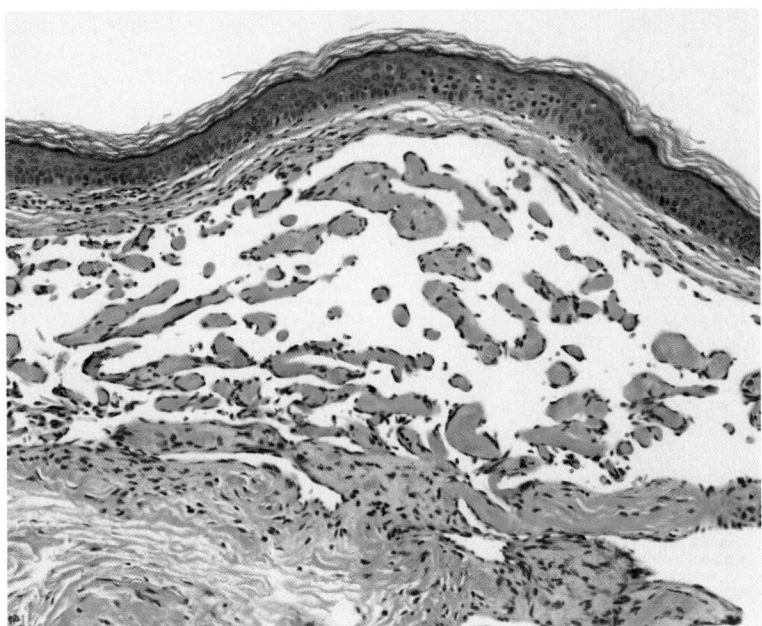

▲ **FIGURE 20-15** Papillary endothelial hyperplasia. Numerous papillary fronds fill the vascular lumina.

conglomerates of blood-filled capillaries lined by endothelial cells that may display clear vacuoles and eosinophilic globules. In addition, IPEH has papillations with fibrous cores and is largely a process resulting from the organization of thrombotic matrix.

ANGIOMATOSIS

> **BOX 20-20   Summary**
>
> - Angiomatosis is a rare condition that usually presents in childhood as symptoms of persistent swelling of a large contiguous area of soft tissue and dermis.
> - Angiomatosis is characterized by infiltration of dermis and soft tissue by a mixture of veins, cavernous vascular spaces, and capillary-sized vessels.

Clinical features: The term angiomatosis was used in several contexts. Not only as a diffuse, yet benign vascular proliferation with multiorgan involvement, usually in childhood, but also as a diffuse reactive vascular proliferation, largely involving the skin. It has been considered synonymous with reactive angioendotheliomatosis. Angiomatosis is a rare condition that usually presents in childhood as symptoms of persistent swelling of a large contiguous area of soft tissue and dermis.[92] Occasional lesions extend into bone. This condition is sometimes painful. Cases associated with visceral and central nervous system hemangiomas have been described. Angiomatosis has a very high recurrence rate, up to 90% in one series. The term angiomatosis is also sometimes used to define localized yet ill-defined vascular proliferations.

Histopathological features: Angiomatosis is characterized by infiltration of dermis and soft tissue by a mixture of veins, cavernous vascular spaces, and capillary-sized vessels.[92] A characteristic feature is the presence of large amounts of adipose tissue. This feature may cause confusion with adipose tumors. A distinctive subtype of angiomatosis is composed of capillary-sized vessels with occasional larger "feeder" vessels.

Differential diagnosis: Distinction between intramuscular hemangioma and angiomatosis essentially depends on the extent of the lesion. Intramuscular hemangioma tends to be limited to a group of muscles compared to the more extensive involvement by angiomatosis. The small size and discrete nature of angiolipoma preclude confusion with angiomatosis.

However, the phenomenon received little attention until the last two decades, when the clinicopathologic features of IPEH became better defined.

Clinical features: IPEH, also known as Masson tumor, intravascular angiomatosis, or vegetant intravascular hemangioendothelioma, occurs in patients of all ages.[86–89] The typical presentation is that of a slowly enlarging, often tender, blue to red, deep dermal to subcutaneous swelling or mass. IPEH occurs at diverse sites, the most frequent of which are the head and the extremities, particularly the fingers. The duration at presentation is often more than 1 year, and has been as long as 21 years. Multiple lesions appearing as violaceous papules and nodules on the lower extremities of an elderly woman have clinically mimicked KS. In native blood vessels, IPEH occurs within arterial thromboemboli and venous thrombi, particularly those of hemorrhoids. In the skin, IPEH occurs as a pure form without any apparent prior lesion or, more commonly, as a focal change within a preexisting pyogenic granuloma or other hemangioma. IPEH has arisen within vascular malformations, hemangiomas of the BRBNS, and cervical cystic hygromas. IPEH has also been identified in unusual sites, such as the paranasal sinus,[90] oral mucosa, tongue, and eyelid. IPEH arising in the palm in the setting of lymphedema after surgery and radiation therapy for breast cancer, thereby mimicking Stewart–Treves syndrome, has been reported.[91] Extravascular papillary

endothelial hyperplasia has occurred in an organizing hematoma of the thyroid gland. Surgical excision of IPEH is usually curative, although recurrence after excision has been reported.

Histopathological features: IPEH shows conspicuous intravascular papillary structures that are formed by cores of fibrous tissue that are lined by endothelial cells that are generally flattened in appearance (Fig. 20-15). Endothelial cells at times, however, may be plump with mildly enlarged nuclei, and there may be some piling up. Mitotic figures are generally absent or rare. IPEH may virtually fill the lumina of some blood vessels. A characteristic feature in most cases is the presence of an underlying thrombotic matrix that appears to be undergoing the process of organization. The papillary projections result from the endothelialization of fragmented thrombotic material and the ingrowth of anastomosing capillaries. Immunohistochemically, IPEH shows a pattern of reactivity similar to that of organizing thrombi. Factor VIII-related antigen is only seen in advanced lesions.

Differential diagnosis: The juxtaposition or fusion of adjacent papillae results in an irregular, vascular network reminiscent of the pattern seen in angiosarcoma. However, key histologic features in identifying IPEH are the thrombotic matrix, the intraluminal location, and the relative absence of both cytologic atypia and mitotic activity. Necrosis and solid cellular areas are rare. Glomeruloid hemangiomas differ from IPEH by showing

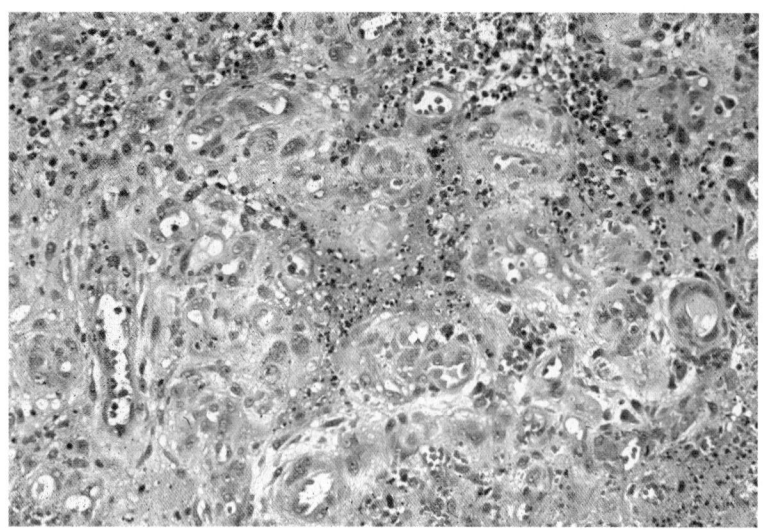

▲ **FIGURE 20-16** Bacillary angiomatosis. Proliferation of blood vessels with epithelioid features. Note the basophilic granular interstitium.

BACILLARY ANGIOMATOSIS (BA)

BOX 20-21 Summary

- BA typically occurs in patients with acquired immunodeficiency syndrome (AIDS). It is a zoonotic infection linked to domestic cats.
- It is associated with a gram-negative bacillus identified as *Bartonella henselae* or rarely *Bartonella quintana*.
- The most helpful histologic features for the recognition of BA are the presence of neutrophils and the interstitial, finely granular aggregates.

This characteristic disorder, also known as epithelioid angiomatosis, typically occurs in patients with acquired immunodeficiency syndrome (AIDS).[93–95] Bacillary angiomatosis (BA) is a zoonotic infection linked to domestic cats. It is associated with a gram-negative bacillus identified as *Bartonella* (formerly *Rochalimaea*) *henselae* or rarely *Bartonella quintana*,[94] and on low power, the lobulated vascularity may mimic a pyogenic granuloma. Older lesions fibrose, and the resemblance to KS may be striking. The clinicopathologic features allow distinction from vascular tumors such as LCH/pyogenic granuloma, ALHE (epithelioid hemangioma), KS, and angiosarcoma.

The most helpful histologic features for the recognition of BA are the presence of neutrophils and the interstitial, finely granular aggregates (Fig. 20-16). Silver stains and, if needed, electron microscopy may be used to detect the bacilli and confirm the diagnosis (Fig. 20-17). Although there may be vague lobular aggregates of blood vessels, BA lacks the well-organized lobular architecture that typifies pyogenic granulomas. In contrast to KS, BA lacks spindled cells, hyaline globules, and thin-walled vessels in "dissection" of dermal collagen. Moreover, the inflammatory cell infiltrate of KS is predominantly lymphoplasmacytic.

ANGIOENDOTHELIOMATOSIS

BOX 20-22 Summary

- Angioendotheliomatosis is a rare vascular disorder first described in 1959.
- Malignant angioendotheliomatosis has an insidious onset and by the time it presents it has neurologic and cutaneous manifestations. It has a rapid, fatal course.

In 1959, Pfleger and Tappeiner described a rare vascular disorder that they subsequently named angioendotheliomatosis proliferans systemisata.[96,97] Over subsequent years, additional cases of angioendotheliomatosis were reported, and their disparate clinical courses illustrated that there were actually two distinct categories: reactive and malignant. Reactive angioendotheliomatosis (RAE) is a benign process often associated with an underlying chronic infection, such as subacute bacterial endocarditis, and various other stimuli, including hypoxia or ischemia with diffuse dermal angiomatosis, a purported variant of RAE.

The historical term, "malignant angioendotheliomatosis," also known as neoplastic angioendotheliosis, intravascular lymphomatosis, malignant intravascular lymphomatosis,[98] intravascular malignant lymphoma, angiotropic (intravascular) large-cell lymphoma, or cerebral angioendotheliomatosis, in contrast to reactive angioendotheliomatosis, is an aggressive disease that is associated with progressive clinical manifestations leading to death.[98–100] The onset is insidious and by the time the malignancy presents itself as neurologic and cutaneous manifestations, the course is rapidly fatal. This is not a vascular neoplasm but a lymphoma. Two cases of intravascular disseminated angiosarcoma have been reported and were considered by the authors to be true malignant angioendotheliomatosis.[101]

REACTIVE ANGIOENDOTHELIOMATOSIS (RAE)

BOX 20-23 Summary

- Reactive angioendotheliomatosis (RAE) is a benign process often associated with an

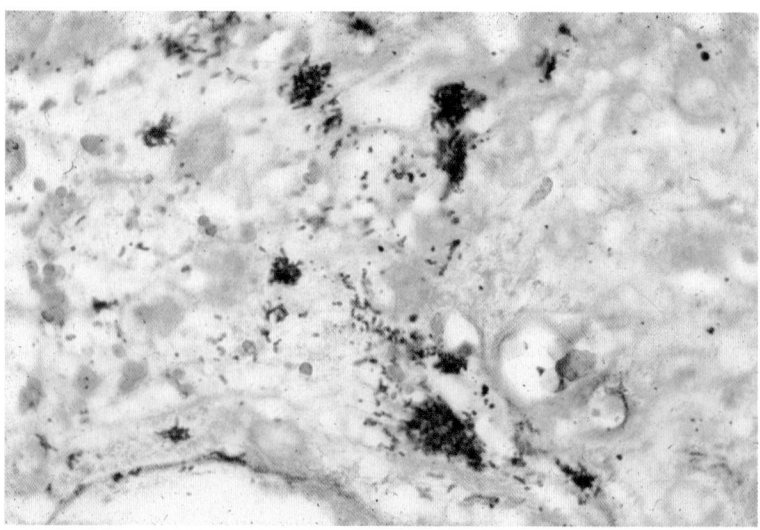

▲ **FIGURE 20-17** Bacillary angiomatosis. Warthin-Starry silver stain shows numerous bacteria.

underlying chronic infection and various other stimuli, including hypoxia or ischemia with diffuse dermal angiomatosis.

- RAE shows no sex predilection and is usually seen in adults, although patients range from infancy to the eighth decade of life. Lesions of RAE are multiple and may occur as red brown patches or plaques and purple red nodules.
- Reactive angioendotheliomatosis shows dilated dermal and subcutaneous vessels that contain proliferations of small to enlarged endothelial cells that variably fill and often occlude vascular lumina.

Also known as angioendotheliomatosis proliferans systemisata, Tappeiner–Pfleger disease, or reactive forms of proliferating or systemic angioendotheliomatosis, reactive angioendotheliomatosis is extremely rare and includes the case described by Pfleger and Tappeiner, a patient reported by Gottron and Nikolowski one year earlier, and a number of others.[102–105] The earliest case was possibly reported by Merklen and Wolf in 1928 as "arterio-capillary endotheliitis." The etiology is unknown, but inflammatory or immunologic reactions and a pathogenesis involving a circulating angiogenic factor have been suggested. An endothelial proliferative response to bacterial antigens and to cryoproteins has been proposed. RAE has been associated with chronic infections, cryoproteins, cold agglutinins,[106] immunoglobulin of a monoclonal gammopathy,[107] antiphospholipid syndrome,[108] rheumatoid arthritis,[109] iatro-genic hemodialysis-related arteriovenous fistulas,[110] dermal amyloid angiopathy,[111] and underlying hepatopathy and hypertensive portal gastropathy.[112]

Clinical features: RAE shows no sex predilection and is usually seen in adults, although patients range from infancy to the eighth decade of life. Lesions of RAE are multiple and may occur as red-brown patches or plaques and purple-red nodules.[102–105] Sites of involvement have included the face, earlobes, trunk, and limbs. Diffuse dermal angiomatosis, a reported variant of RAE, occurs on the lower extremities associated with severe atherosclerosis[113,114] but more recently has been reported on the distal upper extremities in the setting of iatrogenic, hemodialysis-related arteriovenous fistula[110] and on the breast.[115] Necrosis and ulceration can occur with RAE. An associated infection may be present, the most common of which is subacute bacterial endocarditis but individual associations with pulmonary tuberculosis, Chagas' disease, and acute otitis media have been documented. Many cases have constitutional symptoms, such as fever, malaise, and weight loss.

Histopathological features: Reactive angioendotheliomatosis shows dilated dermal and subcutaneous vessels that contain proliferations of small to enlarged endothelial cells that variably fill and often occlude vascular lumina (Fig. 20-18). Focal glomeruloid features may occur.[106] Nuclei of RAE may appear vesicular. Fibrin thrombi may be present. Being endothelial in nature, the intraluminal cells of RAE react with endothelial markers. Most of the cells stain with CD31, CD34, factor VIII-related antigen and, to a lesser degree, Ulex europaeus lectin 1.

Differential diagnosis: The reactive form of angioendotheliomatosis must be distinguished from intravascular malignant lymphoma (angiotropic lymphoma). The intravascular lymphoma displays cytologically malignant cells that mark as lymphoid cells by immunohistochemistry. Glomeruloid hemangioma (GH), associated with POEMS syndrome, in contrast to RAE, has more distinctively glomeruloid features and the presence of eosinophilic globules but perhaps GH can be viewed as a clinicopathologic variant of RAE. Diffuse dermal angiomatosis bears similarity to acro-angiodermatitis but typically is more extensive, being present throughout the dermis, and lacks the abundant hemosiderin, the extravasated red blood cells, and the vaguely lobular arrangement of acro-angiodermatitis.

ARTERIOVENOUS HEMANGIOMA (AH)

BOX 20-24 Summary

- AH primarily is a tumor of middle-aged to elderly adults with a peak incidence in the fourth and fifth decades of life. It is a relatively common lesion and has a male predominance.
- Lesions most commonly present as single, red, or violaceous papules on the head or neck.
- AH lesions are well-circumscribed but unencapsulated. They are composed of an intimate admixture of thick-walled and thin-walled blood vessels distributed within the superficial and middle dermis.

Synonyms for arteriovenous hemangioma and related terms include venous hemangioma, acral arteriovenous tumor, arteriovenous shunt, cirsoid aneurysm, and arteriovenous malformation. Biberstein and Jessner reported the first case of arteriovenous hemangioma (AH) in 1956 as "cirsoid aneurysm."[116] The entity then lay relatively dormant in the literature until 1974 when Girard et al characterized the salient clinical and histologic features of this benign entity in a report of 69 patients with histologically similar lesions that they termed arteriovenous hemangioma.[117] Subsequent reports have confirmed the benign nature of these vascular tumors and have emphasized the acral pattern of distribution by the assignment of the name acral arteriovenous tumor.[118,119]

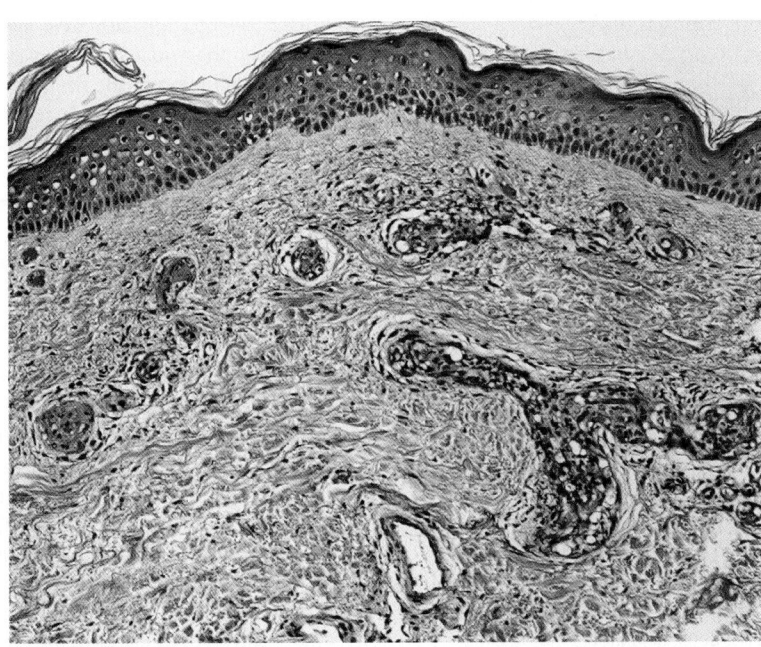

▲ **FIGURE 20-18** Angiomatosis. Vascular proliferation with hypercellularity and thrombi.

Clinical features: The exact incidence of AH is unknown. The large number of cases included in most reports suggests that AH is a relatively common lesion. Our personal case files support this observation. AH primarily is a tumor of middle-aged to elderly adults with a peak incidence in the fourth and fifth decades of life.[116–119] Rare cases have occurred in childhood, the youngest patient being 6 weeks of age.

In most series, except that of Girard et al,[117] males predominate. The lesions most commonly present as single, red, or violaceous papules on the head or neck. Fingertips may be affected.[120] AH may be cutaneous or mucosal. Tumors have ranged in size from 1 mm to 3 cm, with an average of 4 to 6 mm. All are contained within the dermis in cutaneous sites and the submucosa in mucosal sites. Most are asymptomatic, but a minority of patients complain of enlargement, pain, or pruritus. Local excision is curative. Rarely, AH has occurred in association with ALHE, verruciform xanthoma, and basal cell carcinoma.[121–123]

Histopathological features: AH lesions are well-circumscribed but unencapsulated.[116–119] They are composed of an intimate admixture of thick-walled and thin-walled blood vessels distributed within the superficial and middle dermis (Fig. 20-19). The proportion of thick-walled to thin-walled vessels is variable, although the former typically predominates. The vessels may be closely approximated to and dispersed between the cutaneous and mucosal adnexae.

The lining endothelium is a single layer in thickness and typically bland. Occasionally, the endothelial cells are prominent and protrude into the vessel lumen in a "hobnail" fashion. Thrombi, often showing organization and recanalization, are an occasional finding. The tumor stroma is characteristically collagenous. Girard and colleagues described direct communication between arteries and veins in a subset of their cases, whereas other authors have emphasized apparent "hybrid" fibromuscular channels reminiscent of the Sucquet–Hoyer canal of the glomus. Inflammation is an infrequent feature; when present it is described as a mixed, chronic inflammatory cell infiltrate associated with accentuation of fibrous changes within vessel walls.

Differential diagnosis: The morphology of AH is characteristic, and a limited number of entities enter into the differential diagnosis. Clinically, venous lakes and cherry angiomas are a consideration due to their occurrence in a distribution and age group similar to AHs. The histology of each is distinct and easily distinguished from AH. Histologically, vascular leiomyomas are a consideration. The abundance of smooth muscle associated with these lesions is distinct from AH, as is the clinical setting.

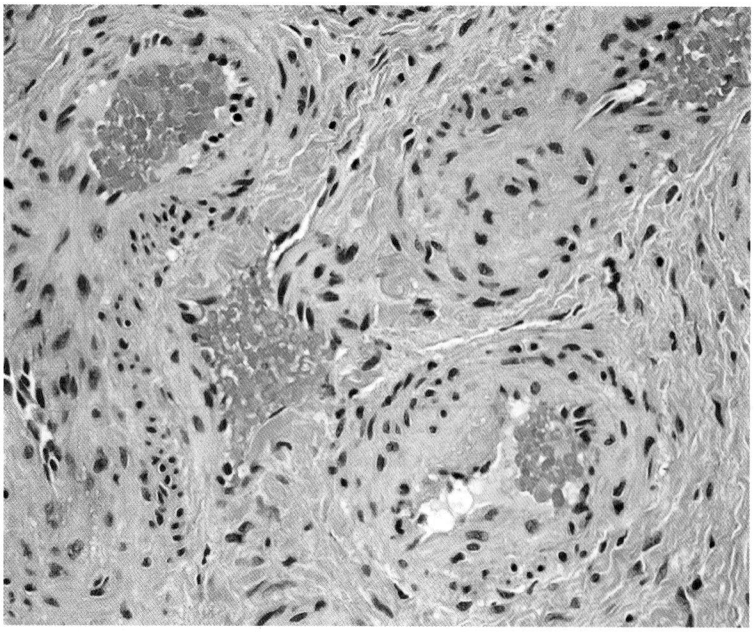

GLOMUS TUMOR

BOX 20-25 Summary

- Glomus tumors can be classified into solitary and multiple types.

- The typical solitary glomus tumor occurs in an adult as a small, blue red nodule, less than 1 cm in diameter, in the deep dermis or subcutis of the extremities.
- Multiple glomus tumors are uncommon, often present in childhood, are generally asymptomatic, arise in more proximal sites, only rarely occur subungually, and can be subdivided anatomically into whether they are regional or disseminated.
- The typical glomus cell is round or cuboidal, with a round nucleus, in an amphophilic to eosinophilic cytoplasm. It occurs in monotonous nests and sheets that are interrupted by many blood vessels, around which the glomus cells form collars.

In 1924, Masson described the glomus tumor as a distinct neoplasm with morphological similarities to the normal neuromyoarterial glomus, an arteriovenous shunt concerned with temperature regulation, located in the reticular dermis of the skin of the nailbeds, the pads of the fingers and toes, the volar side of the hands and feet, the ears, and the center of the face.[124–130] This arteriovenous anastomosis consists of a vessel with a thick, cellular wall (Suquet–Hoyer canal) connecting the two circulations prior to the ramification of the capillary bed. A neural network surrounds this thick-walled canal and peripherally there is a capsule of connective tissue.

Clinical features: Glomus tumors can be classified into solitary and multiple types.[124–130] The typical solitary glomus tumor occurs in an adult as a small, blue-red nodule, less than 1 cm in diameter, in the deep dermis or subcutis of the extremities. The most common site is the subungual region of the finger where glomus tumors typically produce a triad of symptoms: pain, which may be paroxysmal; tenderness; and temperature sensitivity. Unusual sites of glomus tumors have included the stomach, rectum, cervix, vagina, mesentery, chest wall, bone, eyelid, and nose. Intravascular or intravenous glomus tumors have been reported.[125,131] In contrast to solitary glomus tumors, multiple glomus tumors are uncommon, often present in childhood, are generally asymptomatic, arise in more proximal sites, only rarely occur subungually, and can be subdivided anatomically into whether they are regional or disseminated. Compared to the regional type, the disseminated form is often familial, with inheritance as an autosomal dominant trait. Congenital multiple patch- or plaque-like

▲ **FIGURE 20-19** Arteriovenous hemangioma. Proliferation of mature, intertwining muscular vessels.

glomus tumors (glomangioma and glomangiomyoma) have been reported, and usually are nonfamilial.[132,133] In general, multiple glomus tumors tend to be larger than solitary tumors and may reach several centimeters in size. Widespread glomangiomas presenting in infancy may mimic the BRBNS and facial glomangiomas with their blue hue may mimic venous malformations.

Glomangiosarcoma or malignant glomus tumor is rare.[134,135] These tumors typically have sarcoma accompanying a glomus tumor. Initial cases lacked metastasis and the prognosis was considered good, perhaps because early presentation secondary to pain led to excision while the tumor was still small. However, cases with widespread metastasis have now been reported[136,137] and one of these cases occurred despite the primary tumor having been excised from the hip 2 years earlier while still small, measuring only 1 cm.[138] This case was considered to be a *de novo* glomangiosarcoma; such a tumor is exceedingly rare and must be distinguished from other round cell sarcomas. In general, though, superficially situated glomus tumors with malignant-appearing histologic features behave better than similar-appearing tumors in deep locations.

Histopathological features: The histology of the glomus tumor is very distinctive.[124-130] The typical glomus cell is round or cuboidal, with a round nucleus, in an amphophilic to eosinophilic cytoplasm. It occurs in monotonous nests and sheets that are interrupted by many blood vessels, around which the glomus cells form collars (Fig. 20-20). Depending upon the relative proportions of smooth muscle and blood vessels, glomus tumors have been subclassified as glomangioma and glomangiomyoma. Solitary glomus tumors are usually encapsulated, contain numerous small blood vessels, and are associated with ample nerve fibers.

Multiple glomus tumors generally appear as glomangiomas, tumors with large, irregularly shaped vascular spaces that may resemble those of a cavernous malformation (usually termed hemangioma). These spaces may be filled with blood or contain organized thrombi. Typically, only a few layers of glomus cells surround these large spaces, and some vessels may focally lack glomus cells (Fig. 20-21). In contrast to the solitary painful tumors, nerve fibers about multiple glomus tumors are few. Glomangiomyomas are an uncommon variant of glomus tumor and show glomus cells blending with a population of smooth muscle cells (Fig. 20-22). These

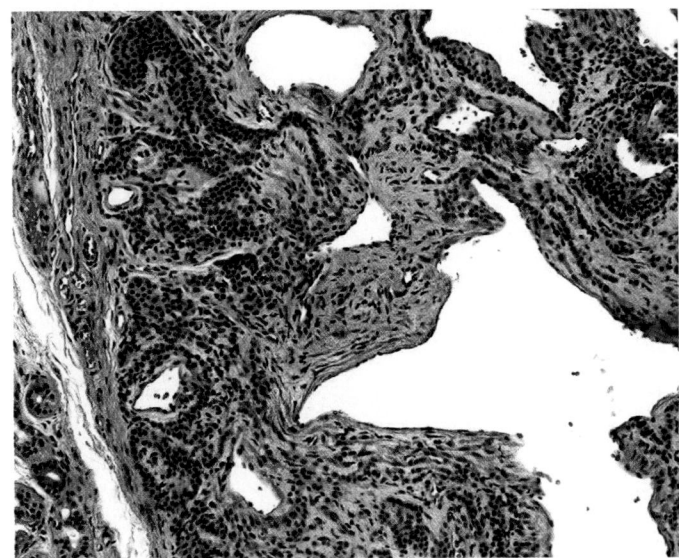

▲ **FIGURE 20-20** Glomus tumor. Cavernous lumina with numerous adventitial epithelioid glomus cells.

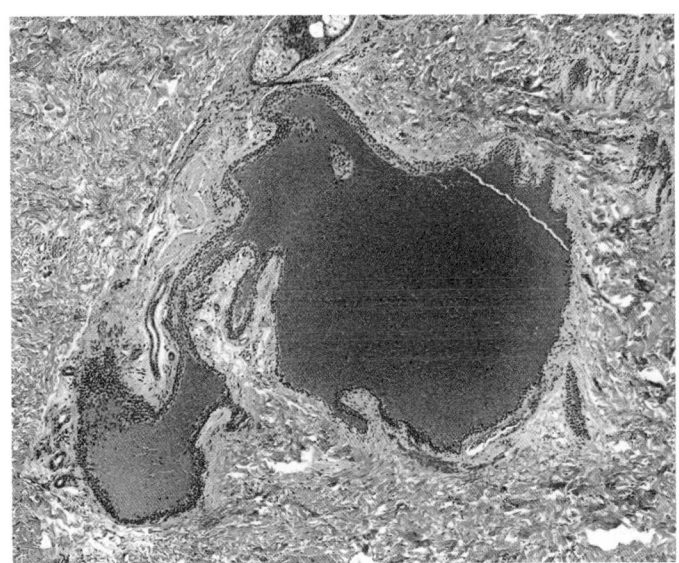

▲ **FIGURE 20-21** Glomangioma. Wide lumina filled with red blood cells and a thin peripheral rim of glomus cells.

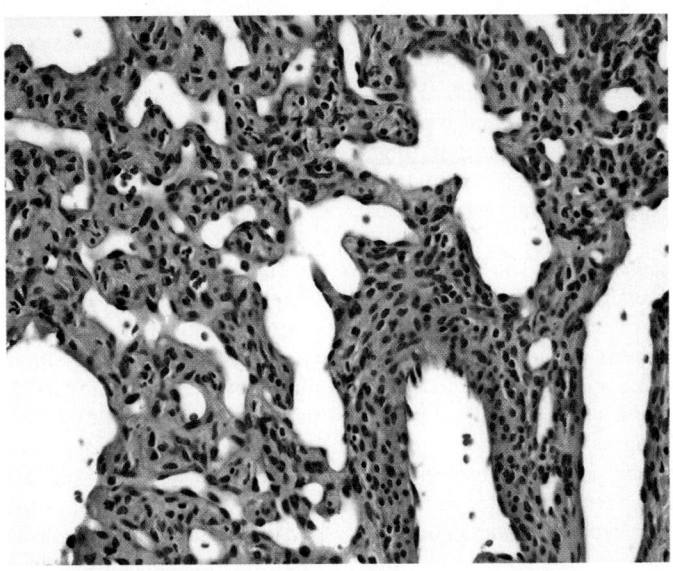

▲ **FIGURE 20-22** Glomangiomyoma. The cells have shared features of smooth muscle and glomus cells.

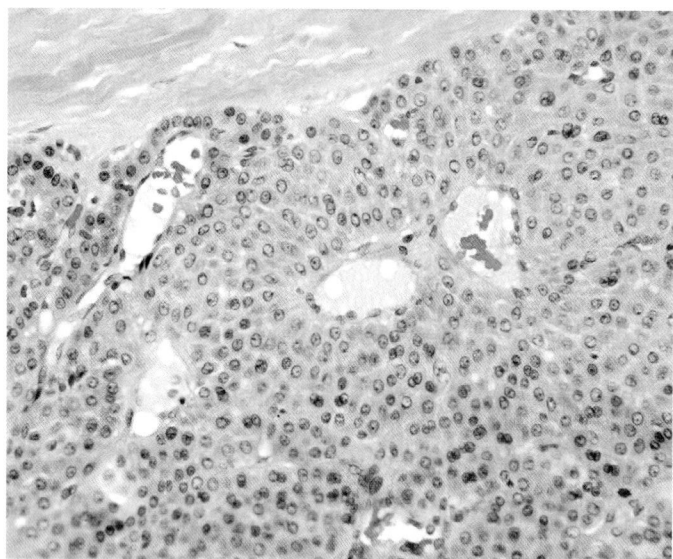

▲ **FIGURE 20-23** Glomus tumor, solid type. The absence of substantial vascular lumina makes this lesion appear more like an epithelial neoplasm.

features are best seen at the periphery of large blood vessels. Solid forms are also seen with a remarkable epithelioid appearance of solid lobules of glomus cells with scant lumen formation (Fig. 20-23).

Glomangiosarcomas are characterized by numerous mitoses, short spindle cells, disordered arrangement of cells, moderate pleomorphism, and single large nucleoli. Recently, criteria for malignant glomus tumor (reserved for lesions with marked risk of metastasis) were proposed: (1) greater than 2 cm size and a deep location, or (2) atypical mitotic figures, or (3) moderate to high nuclear grade and greater than or equal to five mitotic figures per 50 high-power field. Unusual or atypical glomus tumors failing to meet these criteria did not metastasize and were classified as glomus tumor of uncertain malignant potential (high mitotic activity and superficial location, or large size, or deep location) and as the two benign groupings: symplastic glomus tumor (high nuclear grade) and glomangiomatosis (diffuse angiomatosis and excess glomus cells).[137]

Differential diagnosis: The histology of benign glomus tumors is so characteristic that it is not easily confused with that of other tumors. An exception might be the occasional glomangioma that exhibits only a subtle, multifocal population of glomus cells. Others include mastocytomas, solid glomus tumors, pseudoangiomatous melanocytic nevi, hemangiopericytomas, glomangiopericytoma, glomangiosarcomas, and the normal anatomic structure—glomus coccygeum.

SPINDLE CELL HEMANGIOMA (SCH)

BOX 20-26 Summary

- SCH is a nonneoplastic, reactive vascular proliferation, associated with malformed blood vessels and repeated cycles of recanalization after thrombosis.
- SCH presents as either solitary or multiple, asymptomatic nodules that over a period of months or years gradually increase in size or number and often eventuate in extensive disease.
- SCH is characterized histologically by two distinctive components: (1) thin-walled, cavernous blood vessels that sometimes are filled with organizing thrombi and phleboliths and (2) more solid, cellular areas composed predominantly of spindled cells.

In 1986, Weiss and Enzinger delineated the features of this unique vascular lesion and coined the name spindle cell hemangioendothelioma.[139] It was first considered to be a low-grade angiosarcoma, with features of both a cavernous malformation and KS, to be categorized biologically with the epithelioid hemangioendothelioma and the endovascular papillary angioendothelioma (Dabska tumor) because of the favorable prognosis and limited capability for metastasis. However, additional cases were reported by Scott and Rosai in 1988, and despite the tendency toward slow progression and local recurrence, it was believed that there was insufficient evidence to view SCH as a low-grade angiosarcoma.[140] With further study, it now appears that

spindle cell hemangioma (SCH) is a nonneoplastic, reactive vascular proliferation, associated with malformed blood vessels and repeated cycles of recanalization after thrombosis.[141,142]

Clinical features: SCH occurs in individuals at any age and in both sexes.[143] Lesions have arisen as early as the perinatal period, and nearly half of the cases have presented during the third and fourth decades of life. SCH has a predilection for the extremities, particularly distally, often involving the hands and feet. Typically arising in the dermis or subcutaneous tissue, SCH presents as either solitary or multiple, asymptomatic nodules that over a period of months or years gradually increase in size or number and often eventuate in extensive disease. When lesions are multiple, they usually occur in the same general area; however, bilateral lesions of the hands have been described and rare patients may have multiple lesions on diverse sites, including the trunk, oral cavity, and genitalia.[140,143,144]

Grossly, the tumors may be several centimeters in diameter and generally appear as small, circumscribed red to red brown nodules that on sectioning show variably sized, cystic, hemorrhagic spaces. On occasion, a phlebolith may be present and "pop out" from these cavities. More than half of cases of SCH are entirely or partially intravascular, being associated with large vessels and often residing within thick-walled veins.[143] Local recurrence frequently occurs after simple excision and multiple recurrences may occur in individual patients. Although several patients have developed extensive local disease, none have developed visceral metastasis and none have died, despite having received only conservative surgical therapy.

Histopathological features: SCH is characterized histologically by two distinctive components: (1) thin-walled, cavernous blood vessels that sometimes are filled with organizing thrombi and phleboliths and (2) more solid, cellular areas composed predominantly of spindled cells (Fig. 20-24). The proportion of cavernous spaces to areas of spindled cells is variable.[139–142] The spindled cells may form a network of slit-like spaces and short fascicles. Small aggregates of plump, epithelioid cells are commonly interspersed among the spindled cells. Intracytoplasmic lumen formation is often present, usually in association with these epithelioid or "histiocytoid" areas. On occasion, these vacuolated cells may line vascular spaces. Cytologic atypia and mitotic activity are inconspicuous.

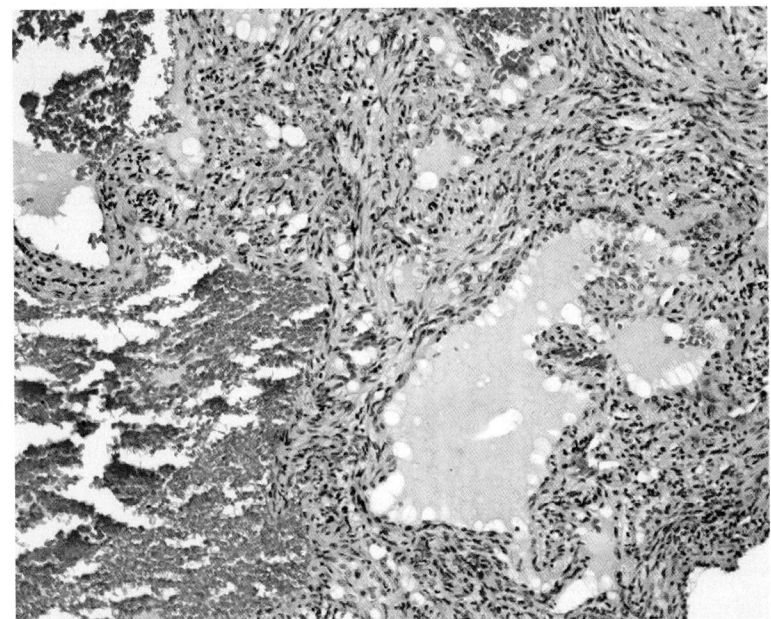

▲ **FIGURE 20-24** Spindle cell hemangioma. The lesion combines areas of cavernous lumina with solid spindle cell areas resembling Kaposi sarcoma.

The large, thick-walled veins containing SCH have abnormalities of muscular wall and intima, apparent on multiple sectioning.[143]

Differential diagnosis: The most problematic entity in differential diagnosis is KS. In particular, the solid, cellular areas of spindled cells in SCH bear a resemblance to KS but differ by containing an admixture of plump endothelial cells with clear to vacuolated cytoplasm. Ectatic, irregular vascular spaces are a component of plaque-stage KS, but frankly cavernous spaces containing thrombi and phleboliths are not. KS-associated herpesvirus (human herpesvirus 8) is not found in SCH.[145]

LYMPHANGIOMA

BOX 20-27 Summary

- Lymphangiomas are proliferations of variably dilated lymphatic vessels, usually present either at birth or within the first few years of life, and generally considered to be hamartomatous in nature.
- Various clinical types of lymphangioma have been reported: lymphangioma simplex (capillary lymphatic malformation), lymphangioma circumscriptum (localized and classic forms), cavernous lymphangioma (cavernous lymphatic malformation), and cystic hygroma. These types have different clinical presentations.
- Histologically, various lymphangiomas generally differ in the size of the lymphatic vessels.

Lymphangiomas are proliferations of variably dilated lymphatic vessels, usually present either at birth or within the first few years of life, and generally considered to be hamartomatous (malformations) in nature.[1–3,8,35,146,147] Various clinical types of lymphangioma have been reported: lymphangioma simplex (capillary lymphatic malformation), lymphangioma circumscriptum (localized and classic forms), cavernous lymphangioma (cavernous lymphatic malformation), and cystic hygroma. Cystic hygoma is an extremely dilated form of cavernous hemangioma occurring on typical clinical sites. Many lymphangiomas have a deep component, and in general, the features of the above types of lymphangioma form a continuum and may overlap, thus making the exact classification of individual cases difficult at times. Generalized lymphangiomatosis is exceedingly rare; one case report described a neonate with chylothorax and cutaneous lymphangiomas.[148]

Clinical features: Lymphangioma simplex appears in infancy as a solitary, rather well-defined, skin-colored dermal, mucosal, or subcutaneous lesion, often less than a few centimeters in size. The contour is usually smooth and slightly elevated.

Lymphangioma circumscriptum is the most common type of lymphangioma and clinically is characterized by cutaneous vesicles. Typically, the localized form is single and of small size. It may occur at any age and is the one form of lymphangioma that is most apt to arise beyond infancy. In contrast, the classic form of lymphangioma circumscriptum usually appears at birth or in early childhood, is generally of larger size, and comprises solitary or multiple patches. Common sites are the proximal extremities, limb girdle, neck, tongue, and buccal mucosa. The degree of involvement may at times be quite extensive. Both clinical forms of lymphangioma circumscriptum may include vesicles with a variably sanguinous or violaceous appearance due to presence of admixed red blood cells. Features similar to lymphangioma circumscriptum have developed as an acquired lymphangiectasias in the setting of lymphedema subsequent to mastectomy or lumpectomy and radiotherapy. Also, among such lesions are acquired vulvar lymphangiomas, which can be idiopathic but commonly arise secondary to impaired lymphatic drainage from various causes, including congenital lymphedema, infections, Crohn's disease, and surgery and/or radiotherapy of cervical carcinoma. These genital lymphangiomas may present as verrucous papules mimicking condyloma acuminatum.[149]

Cavernous lymphangioma (cavernous lymphatic malformation) is usually present at birth or by infancy. This large, ill-defined lesion may occur at many sites but favors the head, neck, mouth, and extremities. A particular subtype of cavernous lymphangioma, the cystic hygroma, has extensive, often deforming, cystic dilatations that generally occur on the neck but may involve the axilla, groin, popliteal fossa, mediastinum, and retroperitoneum. An axillary lesion with a concurrent Becker's nevus has been reported.[150]

Histopathological features: Various lymphangiomas generally differ in the size of the lymphatic vessels.[1–3,8,35,146,147] Lymphangioma simplex is composed of small capillary-sized lymphatic vessels. Lymphangioma circumscriptum has dilated lymphatic channels occupying the superficial dermis (Fig. 20-25). The overlying epidermis is often elevated and is variably thin to acanthotic. There may be papillomatosis and hyperkeratosis, particularly in the classic type of lymphangioma circumscriptum. Also, in contrast to the localized type, this classic type has deeper extension of the lymphatic vessels into the lower dermis and subcutis (Fig. 20-26). Cavernous lymphangiomas have widely dilated lymphatic channels occupying and expanding the dermis and subcutis. The intervening stroma may be inapparent or variably fibrotic. Cystic hygromas show large unilocular or multilocular thin-walled cysts. Lymphangiomas gen-

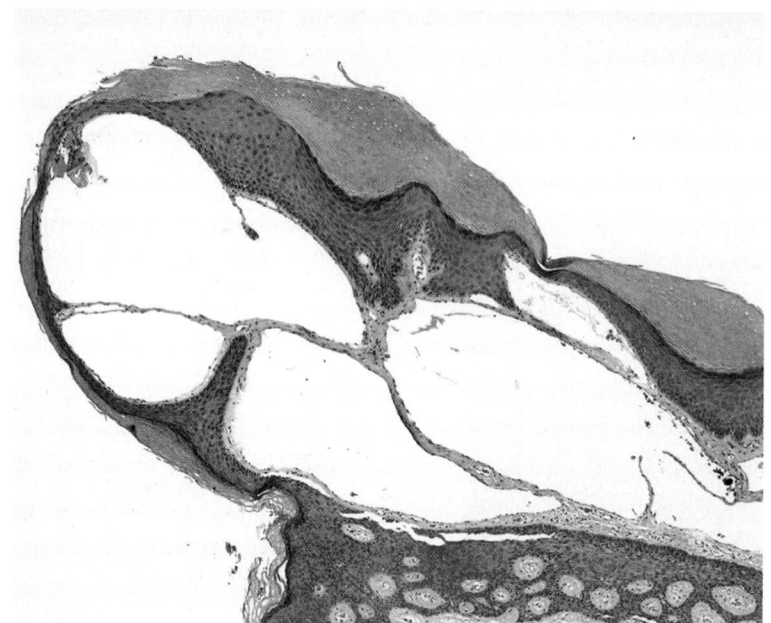

▲ **FIGURE 20-25** Lymphangioma. The lesion contains widely dilated lumina devoid of erythrocytes abutting the epidermis.

erally show homogenous, lightly stained lymph fluid within their lymphatic spaces and may have a variable number of stromal lymphocytes. Red blood cells may at times be present within lymphatic lumina. A deeper cavernous lymphangioma may occasionally underlie the classic type of lymphangioma circumscriptum. Smooth muscle bundles may be seen within the walls of some dilated lymphatic vessels in cavernous and cystic lymphangiomas.

Differential diagnosis: The diagnosis of lymphangioma (or lymphatic malformation) may have to suffice when clinical correlation is lacking and when vessels of mixed size are present. Moreover, the presence of admixed erythrocytes within a particular lymphangioma may generate consideration of a hemangioma or mixed lesion (hemolymphangioma or hemolymphatic malformation). The papillary dermal component of lymphangioma circumscriptum bears similarity to that of an angiokeratoma, and the presence of intralumenal red blood cells, whether they be present *de novo* or secondary to

trauma from a biopsy procedure, may contribute to misdiagnosis. Recognition of the deeper lymphatic component in the classic form of lymphangioma circumscriptum is useful in such situations. The diagnosis of cavernous and cystic lymphangiomas is seldom difficult, and the clinicopathologic features for the cystic hygroma, in particular, are quite unique.

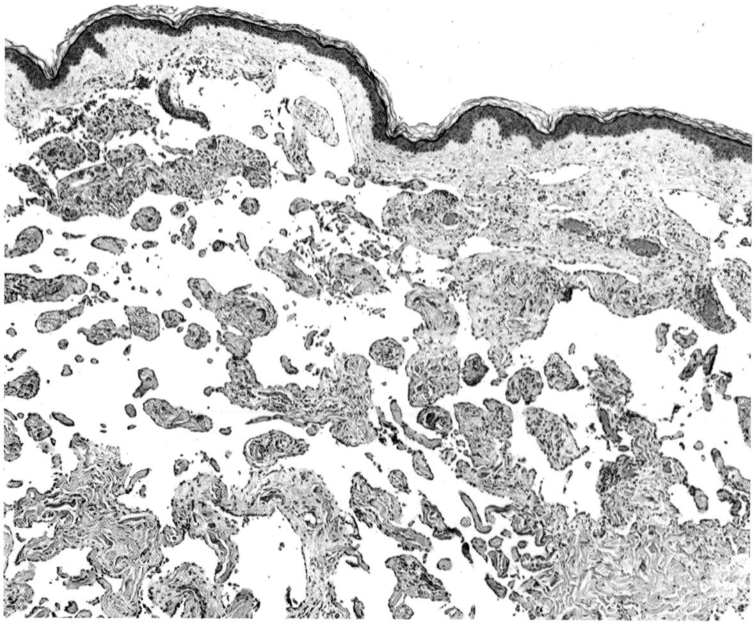

BENIGN LYMPHANGIOENDOTHELIOMA (BL)

BOX 20-28 Summary

- BL is a rare entity that can offer diagnostic difficulty with low-grade angiosarcoma and the lymphangioma-like form of Kaposi sarcoma.
- Clinical lesions are well-demarcated dermal plaques that range in color from dull pink, to dusky, to violaceous. Characteristically, the dermal plaques are painless and nontender.
- The incidence of BL is relatively similar in males and females. Patients range in age from 5 to 90 years.
- Histologically, the epidermis is unremarkable. The lesions are dermal with a tendency to involve the midpapillary dermis and superficial to midreticular dermis.

Also known as angioendothelioma (lymphatic type), or acquired progressive lymphangioma, benign lymphangioendothelioma is an entity that has undergone a nosological evolution over the three decades prior to Jones and colleagues' proposal of the name benign lymphangioendothelioma (BL) in 1990.[151,152] BL was earlier described by Gold and Jones in the late 1960s under the name angioendothelioma (lymphatic type). In the interim, a few cases were also reported as acquired progressive lymphangioma. BL is a rare entity that can offer diagnostic difficulty with a low-grade angiosarcoma and the lymphangioma-like form of KS.

Clinical features: The incidence of BL is relatively similar in males and females. Patients range in age from 5 to 90 years. The duration of clinical lesions before presentation has ranged from 2 months to 20 years.[153,154] Sites of involvement are diverse and include the head, neck, oral mucosa, trunk, breast, buttock, shoulder, forearm, thigh, and foot. Multiple sites of involvement, both synchronous and asynchronous, are documented. Cases may follow trauma to the affected area, including a report of BL arising in a traumatized birthmark,[155] as well as at the site of a tick bite.[156]

▲ **FIGURE 20-26** Deep lymphangioma. The lymphatic lumina crisscross the whole thickness of the dermis.

Clinical lesions are well-demarcated dermal plaques that range in color from dull pink, to dusky, to violaceous. The lesional borders are usually clearly delineated from the surrounding, uninvolved skin.[151,152] Characteristically, the dermal plaques are painless and nontender. The plaques tend to slowly enlarge over a period of time. In reported cases, the lesions have ranged in size from 3 to 30 cm. Presentation as a subcutaneous nodule has been reported.

Excision of BL with attainment of clear margins is curative, and clinical recurrence after excision has not been reported. Regression of two asynchronous lesions after oral prednisolone therapy and spontaneous regression of a case of BL have been documented. The significance of lesional regression after steroid therapy is uncertain and requires further investigation. Most lesions tend to pursue a relatively static clinical course, slowly increasing in size over a period of years. There are no reports of malignant transformation.

Histopathological features: The epidermis is unremarkable. The lesions are dermal with a tendency to involve the midpapillary dermis and superficial to midreticular dermis. Occasional lesions show full-thickness dermal involvement and may extend to involve superficial subcutaneous tissue.[151,152] The unifying histologic features, identified in all cases, are jagged, irregularly shaped vascular channels distributed between dermal collagen bundles. The lumina of these thin-walled vascular spaces may be dilated or collapsed and inconspicuous. The vessels are intimately associated with the dermal collagen, appearing to dissect between the collagen bundles. The thin-walled vessels tend to be arranged in a horizontal array, although they may be quite haphazard in distribution. The endothelial lining is one cell layer in thickness. The cytologic features tend to be bland, although occasional plump or hyperchromatic endothelial cells are an acceptable finding. Pronounced cytologic atypia is not a feature of BL. Exceptionally, a single case report described occasional multinucleated endothelial cells. More recent is a case with aggregated endothelial cells, resembling multinucleate giant cells.[153] Occasional, intraluminal papillary projections may be seen. Rarely, endothelial cells may detach from the vascular wall and appear to float freely within the vessel lumen. Mitotic activity is absent. The vascular spaces are typically empty but may contain a faintly eosinophilic, proteinaceous material. A scant, mononuclear, inflammatory infiltrate is a variable feature. Plasma cells, extravasated erythrocytes, spindle cell proliferation, and hemosiderin are not reported features of BL.

Differential diagnosis: Benign lymphangioendothelioma is a histologic mimic of both low-grade or well-differentiated angiosarcoma and patch-stage KS. The clinical setting for each of these entities is distinct, and an important caveat is that a diagnosis of BL should not be established on a small biopsy, in the absence of clinical history.

Cutaneous angiosarcomas, excluding the Stewart–Treves syndrome and postradiation angiosarcomas, are malignant tumors essentially confined to the head and neck of elderly individuals. If an adequate biopsy of AS is obtained, the degree of cytologic atypia far exceeds that acceptable for BL. In addition, extravasated erythrocytes, hemosiderin deposition, and an inflammatory tumor response are distinct from BL. Lymphangioma circumscriptum has one or more patches of vesicles favoring the limb girdles; contains large, dilated lymphatic vessels raising the epidermis; and lacks the dissection of collagen pattern seen in BL. Hobnail endothelial morphology, when present in BL, is only focal and not as prominent a feature as that of the typically smaller lesion known for hobnail features, the targetoid hemosiderotic hemangioma. Giant-cell fibroblastoma may in some rare settings be confused with BL. The presence of the giant cells and the endothelial marker-negative pseudolumina should allow the correct diagnosis.

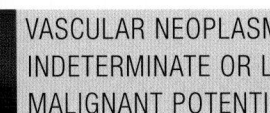

VASCULAR NEOPLASMS WITH INDETERMINATE OR LOW MALIGNANT POTENTIAL

Hemangioendotheliomas Definition

> **BOX 20-29   Summary**
>
> - "Hemangioendothelioma" was used in the past to refer to benign conditions, often present in childhood, and also to malignant vascular neoplasms.
> - Recently, the term has been reborn to define vascular neoplasms with relatively low malignant potential behavior.

The name hemangioendothelioma was used in the past to refer to benign conditions, often present in childhood, and also to malignant vascular neoplasms. Recently, the term has been reborn to define vascular neoplasms with relatively low malignant potential behavior. This is not without peril, since as more is known about these neoplasms, it may be necessary to reclassify them as either benign or definitively malignant. Such was the case of spindle cell hemangioendothelioma. Described as a low-grade angiosarcoma, it is now considered a benign or even reactive vasoproliferative condition and, thus, renamed as spindle cell hemangioma.

The nature of KS continues to baffle the "experts" in the field and its nosologic place is yet to be determined. While it is of relative indolent behavior in some patients, AIDS patients have a more disseminated form. The discovery of herpesvirus as part of this process casts additional questions about its nature.

Epithelioid Hemangioendothelioma (EH)

> **BOX 20-30   Summary**
>
> - EH is a rare entity that has been reported in systemic organs and in the skin as a biologically "borderline" neoplasm because of an occasional association with local recurrence or metastasis.
> - EH presentation on the skin is rare and occurs on the upper and lower limbs of adults of both sexes, favoring the third and fourth decades of life.
> - Cutaneous EH has varied from being asymptomatic dermal nodules to being associated with the severe burning pain, hyperesthesia, swelling, and hyperhidrosis of reflex sympathetic dystrophy.
> - EH displays "histiocytoid" or epithelioid-appearing endothelial cells that may be angiocentric and, in at least half of soft-tissue cases, arise from and expand the wall of a medium to large-size vein.

Also known as histiocytoid hemangioma, intravascular bronchioloalveolar tumor (IVBAT), sclerosing endothelial tumor, sclerosing angiogenic tumor, sclerosing interstitial vascular sarcoma, or sclerosing epithelioid angiosarcoma, epithelioid hemangioendothelioma (EH) is a rare entity that has been reported in systemic organs and in the skin as a biologically "borderline" neoplasm because of an occasional association with local recurrence or metastasis.[157–160] This condition is different, but very closely related to ALHE (epithelioid or histiocytoid hemangioma)

Clinical features: EH is an angiocentric neoplasm that may be multifocal and

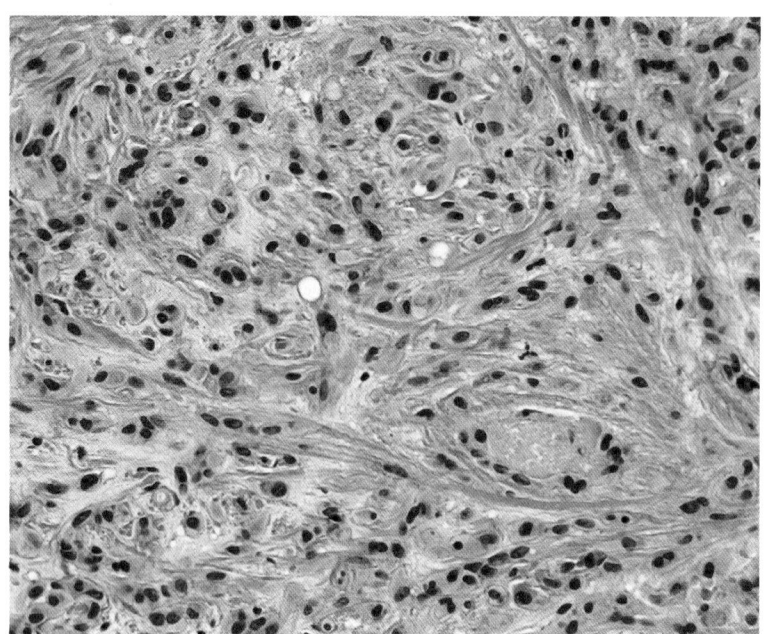

▲ **FIGURE 20-27** Epithelioid hemangioendothelioma. Note the close mimicry of an epithelial neoplasm. The small intracellular lumina are the diagnostic clue.

has been described in soft tissue and in various organs such as the lung, liver, and bones.[157–160] EH presentation on the skin is rare and occurs on the upper and lower limbs of adults of both sexes, favoring the third and fourth decades of life. Cutaneous EH is usually associated with involvement of underlying bone, although cases of EH limited to the skin have been reported. The most common site is the palm (four cases), while other sites have included the scalp, upper lip, nose, neck, thorax, knee, leg, anus, and penis.[161–164]

Cutaneous lesions of EH may be solitary or multiple. EH of soft tissue usually presents as a solitary, slightly painful mass. Cutaneous EH has varied from being asymptomatic dermal nodules to being associated with the severe burning pain, hyperesthesia, swelling, and hyperhidrosis of reflex sympathetic dystrophy. One case of ossifying EH presenting intramuscularly in the cheek as a 1-cm encapsulated nodule with a shell of mature lamellar bone has been reported.[165]

The prognosis of EH is variable. Patients with EH of the lung and liver have a higher mortality than those with EH of soft tissue. Mortality rates of 65, 35, and 13%, respectively, have been reported. Local recurrence and metastatic disease to regional lymph nodes or to lung may occur, yet less than one half of the patients with metastases succumb to their disease. Histologically benign appearing forms of EH generally have a better prognosis than those that appear malignant; however, histologically bland

appearing lesions have occasionally been associated with metastasis and death. Whether the relatively indolent tumors previously described as cutaneous epithelioid angiosarcoma belong to the spectrum of EH is unclear. Some of these patients experienced slow, protracted disease associated with numerous local recurrences and regional lymph node metastases.[160] The prognosis of primary cutaneous EH without underlying bone involvement, treated by local excision, appears good; however, the length of follow-up for reported cases is quite limited.

Histological features: EH displays "histiocytoid" or epithelioid-appearing endothelial cells that may be angiocentric and, in at least half of soft-tissue cases, arise from and expand the wall of a medium to large-size vein.[157–160] A hyaline to myxoid or myxochondroid-appearing stroma is common. The endothelial cells appear as cords or solid nests of rounded or slightly spindled epithelioid cells (Fig. 20-27). Small intracytoplasmic lumina appear as vacuoles, and on occasion, these vacuoles are large and may distort the cell, mimicking the mucin-containing cells of an adenocarcinoma. Red blood cells may be present within the intracytoplasmic lumina. In contrast to the angiocentric pattern that may be seen with EH in soft tissue, the vascularity in cutaneous EH is relatively inconspicuous and, when present, generally consists of small vascular channels that may be lined by cuboidal endothelial cells. Cutaneous EH is often associ-

ated with acanthotic epidermis, which may be accompanied by marked acrosyringeal proliferation, reminiscent of eccrine syrigofibroadenoma.[163]

"Benign"-appearing EH is cytologically bland without appreciable mitotic activity. In contrast, the features of "malignant"-appearing, clinically more aggressive cases of EH in the past have included significant cytologic atypia, more than one mitotic figure per 10 high-power fields (HPF), necrosis, and focal spindling of cells. However, a more recent review found it difficult to correlate histologic features with prognosis; only a high mitotic rate of greater than 6 per 10 HPF clearly correlated with a bad prognosis.[162]

A reticulin stain will reveal a network of reticulin fibers outlining individual cells and groups of cells. Immunohistochemically, EH usually marks with CD31, CD34, and factor VIII-related antigen and less consistently with Ulex europaeus lectin. The staining for factor VIII-related antigen is accentuated about intracytoplasmic lumina, and varies in distribution and with the degree of tissue preservation. EH is typically negative for both epithelial membrane antigen and cytokeratin; however, staining for keratin was observed in one case when frozen sections were utilized and more recently in several cases of formalin-fixed paraffin-embedded tissue.[162] By electron microscopy, EH shows features of endothelial cells such as Weibel–Palade bodies, pinocytotic vacuoles, and well-developed basal lamina. Abundant cytoplasmic intermediate filaments are present. By cytogenetic study, an identical chromosomal translocation t(1;3)(p36.3;q25) was recently detected in two cases of EH.[166]

Differential diagnosis: EH shares similarities to a variety of tumors that exhibit epithelioid histologic patterns. Among these are metastatic carcinoma, adenocarcinoma, malignant melanoma, ALHE (epithelioid hemangioma), epithelioid sarcoma, and epithelioid angiosarcoma. Carcinomas, malignant melanoma, and epithelioid angiosarcoma generally show significant cytologic atypia and mitotic activity that will distinguish them from most cases of EH. ALHE may show intracytoplasmic vacuoles; however, ALHE characteristically shows well-developed vascularity lined by hobnail endothelial cells and has a prominent inflammatory infiltrate of lymphoid follicles and eosinophils. Epithelioid sarcoma perhaps has the closest similarity to EH, but epithelioid sarcoma will generally display a nodular arrangement of cells with central cores of necrotic debris and collagen. Cutaneous mixed tumor may also enter the differential diagnosis but can be distinguished by its broader epithelial differentiation, including apocrine differentiation, squamous metaplasia, and ducts.

Kaposi Sarcoma (KS)

BOX 20-31   Summary

- KS has been primarily known as a relatively rare tumor of the elderly until the advent of the acquired immunodeficiency syndrome (AIDS) and organ transplantation. It has become endemic in Central Africa.
- Characteristically, KS lesions evolve through stages as patches, plaque, and nodules. Clinical lesions of varying stages are often present in single patient. Lesions may gradually coalesce, and nodules may eventually ulcerate.
- The isolation of herpesvirus-like DNA sequences designated KS-associated herpesvirus or human herpesvirus 8 (HHV-8) in KS from AIDS-related KS, African endemic KS, and the Mediterranean form of KS, strongly suggests a role for this agent in the pathogenesis of KS.
- The histology of cutaneous lesions associated with the various clinical forms of KS is essentially identical.

This vascular neoplasm was first described by Kaposi in 1872 under the name of "idiopathic multiple pigmented sarcoma of the skin."[167–189] The skin is the most common site, but several other organ systems may be affected. Although Kaposi sarcoma (KS) has been endemic in Central Africa for some time, KS has been primarily known as a relatively rare tumor of the elderly until the advent of the AIDS and organ transplantation. With the increase in the number of cases of KS, as well as the occurrence of the disorder in a younger population that is apt to have other, generally benign, vascular lesions, intimate knowledge of the disease spectrum of KS has become essential to make the correct diagnosis. This is particularly true for the diagnosis of early lesions of KS.

The isolation of herpesvirus-like DNA sequences designated KS-associated herpesvirus or human herpesvirus 8 (HHV-8) in KS from AIDS-related KS, African endemic KS, and the Mediterranean form of KS strongly suggests a role for this agent in the pathogenesis of KS.[190–192] This gamma herpesvirus is partially homologous to Epstein–Barr virus (EBV) and herpesvirus saimiri. HHV-8 appears to be an important infective cofactor, prone to a long period of latency before disease, with the development of KS possibly accelerated or triggered by the additional effects of EBV, HIV, other infections, immunosuppresive drugs, or age. Debate remains whether KS is a true neoplasm or a reactive hyperplasia.

Clinical features: The classic, chronic, or "European" form of KS is an uncommon disease that generally affects individuals greater than 50 years of age and shows a strong predilection for men.[167–170] There is an increased incidence of KS in Ashkenazic Jews and individuals of Mediterranean descent. KS typically begins on the distal lower extremities, either uni- or bilaterally. Over time, lesions may increase in number and arise more proximally. The upper extremities may become affected, and occasionally this may be the initial site of presentation. Characteristically, KS lesions evolve through stages as patches, plaque, and nodules, and clinical lesions of varying stages are often present in a single patient. Lesions may gradually coalesce, and nodules may eventually ulcerate. The clinical course of the classic form of KS is relatively indolent. Occasional lesions may regress while others progress. However, one should be aware that up to one-third of patients with the classic form of KS subsequently develop a second primary neoplasm, often of hematopoietic origin.

In equatorial Africa, KS is a common neoplasm. Males again predominate, but this endemic African form of KS affects a younger population than does the classic European variant, with the difference averaging a decade in most reports, and children are also affected. The disease can be subclassified into four clinical groups: nodular, florid, infiltrative, and lymphadenopathic. The nodular group presents with a limited number of circumscribed cutaneous nodules and pursues an indolent clinical course. The florid and infiltrative groups have more aggressive disease with extensive cutaneous lesions on one or more extremities, generally associated with involvement of bone. The lymphadenopathic type occurs mainly in children in whom lymph node involvement is usually the sole manifestation, and in young adults who may have concomitant skin involvement.

AIDS-associated, or epidemic KS, occurs in a population of individuals with unique demographics. This group of patients, at risk for an aggressive, often disseminated form of KS, is composed predominantly of homosexual men who comprise 95% of all cases. The remainder comprises intravenous drug users and other populations at risk for AIDS. All but very rare cases have serologic antibody titers to the human immunodeficiency virus type 1. Indirect evidence for cofactors being involved in the pathogenesis of KS is the drop in the incidence of KS in the AIDS-affected homosexual population since the early 1980s. Upon initial medical presentation, lesions of KS are often small and few in number. They may be light purple or pink rather than deeply violaceous as with more established lesions of KS (Fig. 20-28). The upper half of the body is frequently affected without the tendency

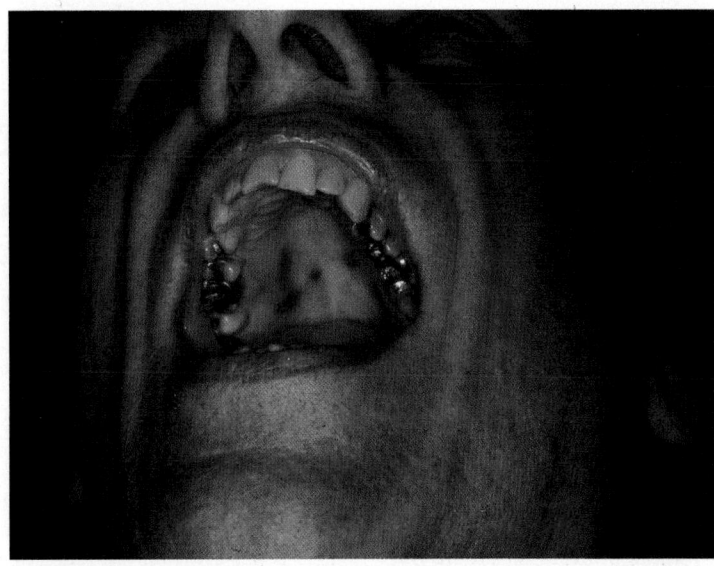

▲ **FIGURE 20-28** Kaposi sarcoma. Typical location of early lesions in a patient with AIDS.

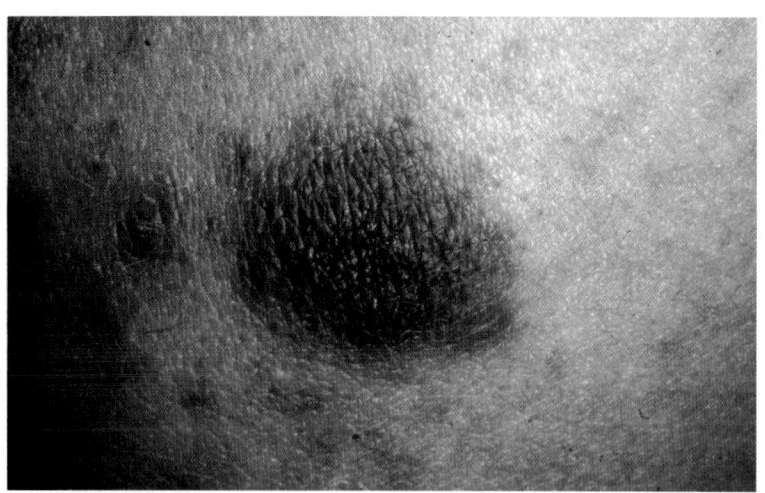

▲ **FIGURE 20-29** Kaposi sarcoma. Infiltrated brown reddish plaque.

of classic KS to first involve the distal lower extremities (Fig. 20-29). Moreover, clinically normal skin of patients with well-developed AIDS show endothelial ultrastructural abnormalities similar to those of early KS, suggesting that they too are potential sites of involvement.

Another more recent group of patients at risk for the development of KS are patients receiving immunosuppressive agents, particularly organ transplant recipients.[193] The incidence is low and after renal transplantation is estimated at about half of 1%. As with classic KS, there is a propensity toward individuals of Jewish or Mediterranean descent. However, women are more frequently affected in this group than in the other clinical forms of KS. Cutaneous and visceral involvement occur, but no particular pattern of distribution has been emphasized. The clinical course is more aggressive than is classic KS, with a significant percentage of patients perishing with disseminated disease. Lesions may regress with the reduction or withdrawal of immunosuppressive therapy.

Rarely, a Stewart–Treves-like syndrome is associated with KS, rather than angiosarcoma, developing in the setting of a chronically lymphedematous upper extremity years after an ipsilateral radical mastectomy.[194,195] Also rare is the lymphangioma-like variant of KS, the clinical hallmark of which is a bulla-like appearance that occurs in many but not all cases.[196,197]

Histopathologic features: The histology of cutaneous lesions associated with the various clinical forms of KS is essentially identical and will be described together according to their stage at presentation. Although some authors feel there are subtle differences between classic and AIDS-associated KS, others have not

confirmed this impression. The observed differences and diagnostic difficulty in AIDS-associated KS seem related to the subtle changes inherent in early lesions rather than differences unique to this form of KS. For patch-stage KS, the earliest features are inconspicuous and on initial review may be mistaken as nondiagnostic or inflammatory (Fig. 20-30). The alterations are mainly confined to the reticular dermis (involving the upper half or all of it). A variable, predominantly lymphocytic perivascular infiltrate is present, and contains a variable number of plasma cells. Subtle vascular changes can be appreciated. The earliest of these is a proliferation of miniature or irregular, jagged blood vessels around normal or ectatic dermal blood vessels

and about adnexal structures. The newly formed vessels may protrude into a vascular lumen or surround and partially isolate normal dermal structures; a feature referred to as the promontory sign. In some lesions, the vessels aggregate into clusters that resemble small hemangiomas. The endothelium may be inconspicuous or plump with a single layer in thickness and shows little atypia or mitotic activity. Irregular, branching, thin-walled bland vessels may be seen dissecting between collagen bundles. These neovascular channels tend to be contiguous with preexisting dermal blood vessels. In well-developed patch-stage lesions, KS involves the entire dermis.

A highly suggestive but subtle finding that may be seen only with careful examination of multiple levels of sections is the presence of small numbers of bland spindle cells in close association with the newly formed vessels (Fig. 20-31). Other features that are relatively inconspicuous in patch-stage KS but may be seen are apoptotic endothelial cells, extravasated erythrocytes, hemosiderin, and hyaline globules. In contrast to patch-stage KS, these features are best seen in well-developed plaques and nodules. Hyaline globules are small, faintly eosinophilic, PAS-positive, and diastase-resistant spheres that may be deposited extracellularly or may be seen intracellularly within macrophages. The globules most likely represent phagocytized red blood cells and their degenerative forms. They are a useful diagnostic criterion but are neither necessary nor sufficient

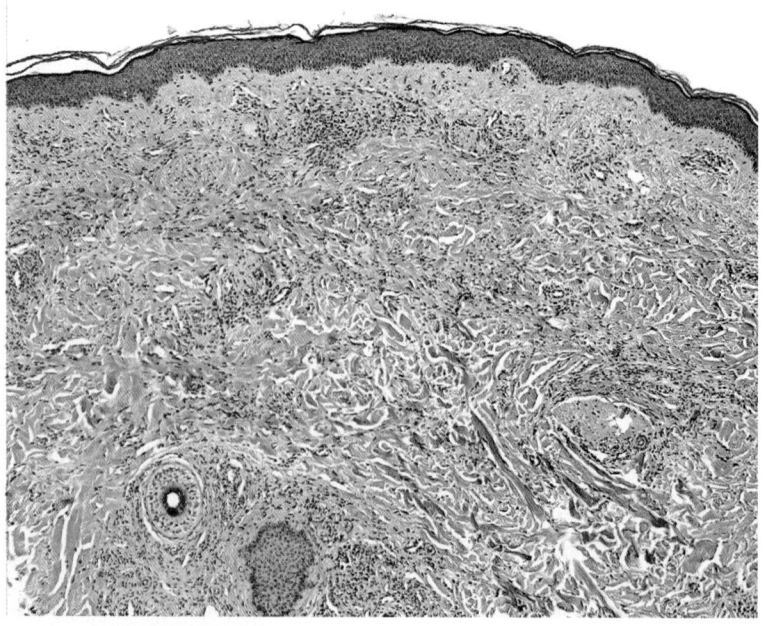

▲ **FIGURE 20-30** Kaposi sarcoma. Early patch lesion. The lesion is subtle and resembles an inflammatory process.

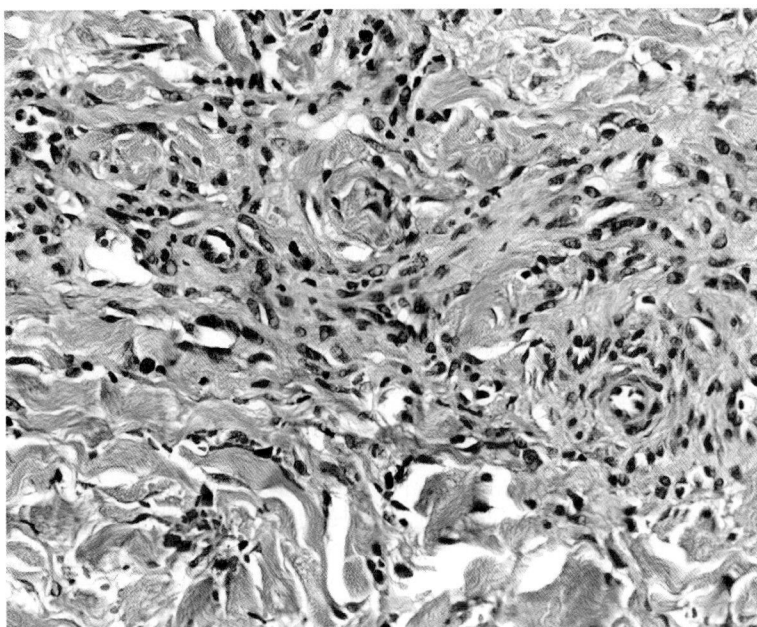

▲ **FIGURE 20-31** Kaposi sarcoma. At higher magnification, the presence of plasma cells and short fascicles of spindled cell are characteristic.

for the diagnosis of KS. These globules may be seen in other neoplastic and inflammatory processes with abundant erythrocyte extravasation, such as angiosarcomas, pyogenic granulomas, and inflammatory granulation tissue.

Plaque-stage lesions of KS show further progression of the neoplastic process, filling the entire dermis and involving the superficial subcutaneous tissue. The most characteristic feature of this stage is the presence of a significant spindle cell component. These relatively bland cells are dispersed between dermal collagen bundles and around preexisting dermal vessels. Between these spindle cells, irregular, cleft, or slit-like spaces are formed, creating new, angulated vascular channels that contain small numbers of erythrocytes (Fig. 20-32).

Hemosiderin deposits and hyaline globules are more prominent than in patch-stage KS. The vasoproliferative changes of the patch stage persist at the periphery of plaques. The predominantly lymphocytic, perivascular inflammatory infiltrate persists along with its component of plasma cells.

Nodular lesions of KS show a further proliferation of spindle cells into intersecting fascicles and sheets. Amidst these spindle cells are slit-like vascular spaces containing variable numbers of erythrocytes. The spindle cells show a degree of cytologic atypia that generally ranges from mild to moderate. Frank anaplasia of the spindle cell component is distinctly uncommon and is more frequently described in the endemic African

form of KS. Apoptotic cells, hyaline globules, and hemosiderin deposition are all readily visible. Mitotic figures vary in number but may be frequent. The dermal lymphoplasmacytic inflammatory infiltrate persists, and at the periphery of the nodules, ectatic blood vessels and lymphatics are generally noted.

Lymphangiomatous or lymphangioma-like lesions of KS have been reported as both a focal and predominant clinicopathologic pattern in otherwise typical KS.[188] The process usually

involves the entire dermis and often extends into the superficial subcutaneous tissue.[198] Angulated, irregular, narrow to ectatic, thin-walled vascular channels lined by a single layer of flattened, bland endothelium interconnect, and dissect collagen bundles. The majority of the vascular spaces lack red blood cells. Features typical of KS, such as a significant inflammatory infiltrate, extravasated erythrocytes, hemosiderin, and hyaline globules, have not been reported. Occasional cases show sparse numbers of spindle cells in close association with the vascular elements, but these cells are never a prominent feature.

The histogenesis of KS is a subject open to some debate. KS may be a lesion that arises from pluripotential stem cells variably differentiating toward blood vessel endothelium. However, an alternative theory involves multicentric hyperplasia that combines lymphatic venular anastomoses with elements of both lymphatic and blood vessel endothelium.

Despite their erythematous clinical appearance, early lesions of KS typically have thin-walled vessels with a lymphatic-like histologic appearance. Enzyme histochemistry shows these vessels to have a staining profile of lymphatic endothelium. In contrast, ultrastructural examinations of the endothelial cells in a minority of cases show Weibel–Pelade bodies and, in general, display features of poorly differentiated blood vessels. Variable immunohistochemical results have been obtained, but endothelial cells of early KS are usually negative for fac-

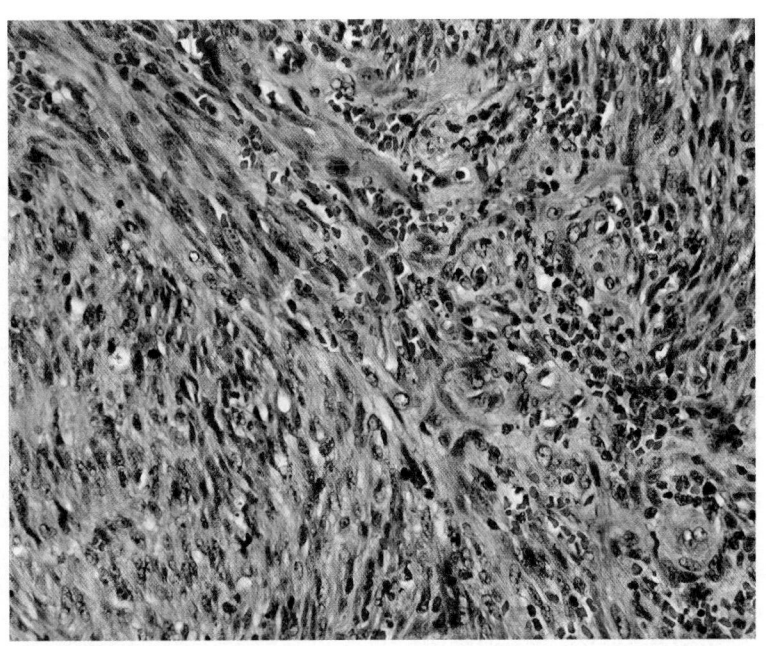

▲ **FIGURE 20-32** Kaposi sarcoma. At tumor stage, the lesion shows confluent fascicles of spindle cell with interstitial red blood cells.

tor VIII-related antigen and weakly positive for Ulex europaeus lectin 1. The spindle cells of nodular lesions of KS display only patchy reactivity for factor VIII-related antigen and show diminished reactivity for Ulex europaeus lectin 1. Moreover, it is doubtful that these two markers can reliably distinguish between blood vessel and lymphatic endothelium.

Newer markers that can react with KS are CD31, CD34, and CD40. Antibody to vascular endothelial growth factor receptor 3 (VEGFR-3), a receptor found almost exclusively in lymphatic endothelium in the adult, marked nearly all cases of KS but did not discriminate KS from borderline and malignant vascular neoplasms. All of the tested samples of both kaposiform hemangiondothelioma and endovascular papillary angioendothelioma (Dabska tumor) and half of the samples of angiosarcoma also reacted.[199]

Differential diagnosis: Difficulty in diagnosis usually occurs with early lesions of KS rather than the well-developed lesions of nodular-stage KS. Among the entities to be considered in the differential diagnosis of KS are acro-angiodermatitis, benign lymphangioendothelioma, targetoid hemosiderotic hemangioma, early scar, bacillary angiomatosis, and angiosarcoma. More cellular lesions of KS must be differentiated from aneurysmal fibrous histiocytoma and from spindle cell hemangioma. The reader is referred to sections on the above topics for discussions of the differential features. In particular, histologic findings that are often important to the diagnosis of early KS include the promontory sign, plasma cells, and newly formed thin-walled vessels that dissect dermal collagen. Important criteria of more evolved lesions include spindle cells, slit-like spaces containing erythrocytes, hyaline globules, apoptotic cells, and hemosiderin deposition. It should be recognized, however, that there is a continuum of these features from patch to nodular stage. Finally, the detection of HHV-8 by polymerase chain reaction (PCR) and the localization of the virus to specific cells by the more recent technique of reverse transcription *in situ* PCR may assist in discriminating KS from its mimics.[200,201]

Hemangiopericytoma

BOX 20-32 Summary

- Hemangiopericytoma is a relatively rare soft-tissue neoplasm that is thought to derive from the pericyte.
- Hemangiopericytomas generally occur as deep-seated soft-tissue tumors in adults, with a median age of 45 years in one large series. Typically, the tumor arises as a painless mass that is often several centimeters in size by the time of clinical presentation.
- Histologically, tumor cells are rounded or spindle-shaped and are present outside the numerous, admixed blood vessels.

The hemangiopericytoma is a relatively rare soft-tissue neoplasm that is thought to derive from the pericyte.[202–206] The diagnosis is often difficult, since other soft-tissue tumors may be highly vascular and show hemangiopericytoma-like patterns. Its occurrence in the skin proper is debatable, with some denying its existence. An example of this is the unique case report of a polypoid dermal hemangiopericytoma that has been alternatively viewed by another author as an epithelioid cell histiocytoma with prominent hemangiopericytoma-like vascularity.[207,208]

Clinical features: Hemangiopericytomas generally occur as deep-seated soft-tissue tumors in adults, with a median age of 45 years in one large series. The most common sites are the lower extremities and the pelvic retroperitoneum, but the tumor has a wide distribution. Typically, the tumor arises as a painless mass that is often several centimeters in size by the time of clinical presentation. Hypoglycemia may be associated with large retroperitoneal lesions. Hemangiopericytomas are well-vascularized tumors, and excision is often complicated by hemorrhage.

Benign and malignant forms of hemangiopericytomas have been recognized. However, there are also intermediate or borderline cases of hemangiopericytoma that resist classification and make prognostication difficult. A median survival of 19 months was reported for malignant hemangiopericytomas. Malignant tumors frequently recur and metastasize.

Histopathological features: Tumor cells are rounded or spindle-shaped and are present outside the numerous, admixed blood vessels.[202–206] A reticulin stain will demonstrate that the endothelial cells of the vessels lie inside a delicate reticulin sheath and are thus separated from the peripheral population of tumor cells. The rich network of blood vessels has a varied morphology ranging from capillaries to large sinusoidal-like spaces (Fig. 20-33). The latter spaces often appear to divide in antler-like or "staghorn" configurations. Lipomatous hemangiopericytoma of deep soft tissue has been reported and is characterized by mature adipose tissue in benign hemangiopericytoma.[209] It has been suggested that lipomatous hemangiopericytoma represents a fat-containing variant of solitary fibrous tumor.[210]

Malignant hemangiopericytomas are characterized by hemorrhage, necrosis, and increases in both cellularity and mitotic activity. The presence of four or

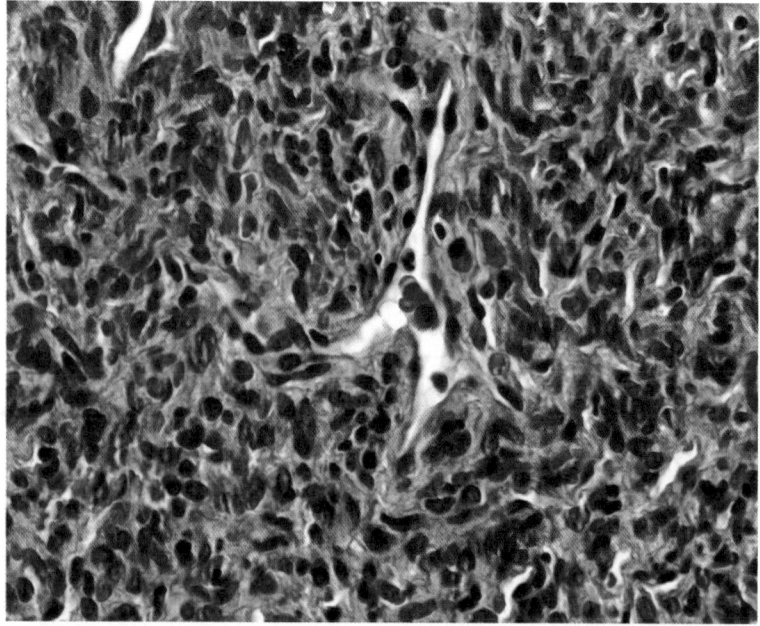

▲ **FIGURE 20-33** Hemangiopericytoma. Compact growth of a round stag horn-shaped lumina.

more mitotic figures per 10 high-power fields has been associated with recurrence and metastasis, whereas benign hemangiopericytomas generally show fewer than two or three mitoses per 10 high-power field. Recurrent or metastatic hemangiopericytoma in one study was associated with a trabecular pattern, necrosis, mitoses, vascular invasion, and cellular pleomorphism.[211]

Being derived from the pericyte, the hemangiopericytoma is generally negative for endothelial markers. Reactivity for Ulex europaeus I is absent, and factor VIII-related antigen is negative or only weakly positive. Conversely, the endothelial cells of the accompanying vasculature are richly stained by both markers. Hemangiopericytomas stain for vimentin and laminin, often stain for CD34, and rarely show focal staining for smooth muscle actin but are generally negative for CD31, desmin, cytokeratin, and S-100. Ultrastructurally, basal lamina-like material is present and either partially or completely surrounds tumor cells. This feature, along with the presence of myogenic filaments and pinocytotic vessels, serves to support a diagnosis of hemangiopericytoma in a histologically compatible tumor.

Differential diagnosis: Other soft-tissue tumors with a hemangiopericytoma-like pattern must be considered before rendering a diagnosis of hemangiopericytoma. Among these tumors are solitary fibrous tumor of the skin, solitary myofibromatosis, synovial sarcoma, extraskeletal mesenchymal chondrosarcoma, malignant schwannoma, and malignant fibrous histiocytoma. Immunohistochemical staining and ultrastructural examination are important adjuncts to diagnosis.[212,213] Finally, tumors with features between those of hemangiopericytoma and glomus tumor (glomangiopericytoma) have been described.[214]

Endovascular Papillary Angioendothelioma (EPA)

BOX 20-33   Summary

- EPA has a generally good prognosis despite local invasion and regional lymph node metastasis. It is regarded as one of the "borderline" vascular tumors.
- Clinically, it presents with enlarging cutaneous lesions, 4 to 9 cm in diameter, occurring as either a diffuse swelling or an intradermal tumor on the head, neck, and extremities.
- The most characteristic feature of EPA is the presence of intraluminal papillary struc-

tures lined by endothelial cells showing pleomorphism, hyperchromatism, mitotic activity, and multilayered endothelium.

Also known as malignant endovascular papillary angioendothelioma, Dabska tumor, and papillary intralymphatic angioendothlioma, this exceedingly rare vascular lesion was first reported by Dabska in 1969 as malignant endovascular papillary angioendothelioma of the skin in childhood.[215] However, the cumulative experience in the literature indicates that endovascular papillary angioendothelioma (EPA) has a generally good prognosis despite local invasion and regional lymph node metastasis. It is regarded as one of the "borderline" vascular tumors.

Clinical features: Dabska reported six children, 4 months to 15 years of age, who presented with enlarging cutaneous lesions, 4 to 9 cm in diameter, occurring as either a diffuse swelling or an intradermal tumor on the head, neck, and extremities. Few additional cases were reported[215–218] until 1998 when a review of 12 cases indicated a wider age range (mean age: 30 years; oldest individual was a 59-year-old woman).[219] Two of Dabska's cases displayed regional lymphadenopathy, and another had tumor penetration through the frontal bone and into the cranial vault. Treatment consisted of wide excision supplemented in individual cases by radiotherapy or regional lymphadenectomy.

Local recurrence was observed only once but resolved with a second surgical procedure. Lymph node metastasis was seen in two children, one of which showed involvement of eight axillary lymph nodes. All the children were well without evidence of disease on follow-up examinations 4 to 16 years later. A more recent series indicated no morbidity after excision for 8 of 12 cases with known follow-up (mean: 9 years).[219] Acknowledging the favorable prognosis but recognizing the capability of tumor for both local invasion and regional lymph node metastasis, Dabska viewed EPA as a variant of malignant angioendothelioma in childhood, possessing a limited degree of malignancy. It has been proposed that the lymph node inclusions might occur as a manifestation of regional endothelial proliferation rather than as an evidence of metastatic disease.

Histopathological features: The most characteristic feature of EPA is the presence of intraluminal papillary structures lined by endothelial cells showing pleomorphism, hyperchromatism, mitotic activity, and multilayered endothelium.[215–217] Tumor cells appear to float free in the lumina either in clumps or as single cells. The central framework of the papillations can appear eosinophilic and hyalinized. Papillary formations resembling renal glomeruli may be seen. More cellular lesions reveal hemorrhage, cholesterol clefts, and areas of necrosis. Dabska reported a moderate degree of mitotic activity in EPA; however, later reports have described only rare mitoses and only mild cellular pleomorphism.

Vascular channels may show a cuboidal- to columnar-appearing endothelial lining, at times, with a hobnail or matchstick-like appearance. Intravascular proliferations of endothelial cells may be arranged about hyaline globules, a feature interpreted as the earliest form of fibrovascular stalk formation. The globules have the staining characteristics of basement membrane, and ultrastructurally appear to be comprising basal lamina-like material. Collagen type IV can be demonstrated.[219] A lymphocytic infiltrate may be prominent and may frequently intermingle with the endothelial cells. The latter association suggests that the endothelial cells of EPA show differentiation toward "high" endothelial cells of postcapillary venules with attraction of lymphocytes mediated by intercellular adhesion molecule (ICAM-1).

Differential diagnosis: Grossly, upon sectioning, and on low-power microscopic examination, EPA may have cystic spaces resembling a cavernous lymphangioma. The presence of the lymphocytic infiltrate supports this impression, but confusion in diagnosis is unlikely as soon as the proliferative endothelial nature of EPA is appreciated. In contrast to EPA, IPEH has a generally flattened endothelial lining and an underlying thrombotic matrix. Both IPEH and angiosarcoma lack the hyaline globules and lymphocytic infiltrate of EPA. Finally, retiform hemangioendothelioma (RH) may focally have features similar to EPA; however, EPA typically lacks the rete testis-like appearance of retiform hemangioendothelioma.[219] However, in further support of a relationship between these two entities is one remarkable case of RH, occurring intradermally on the toe of a child that showed diffuse endovascular papillae similar to EPA.[220]

Retiform Hemangioendothelioma (RH)

BOX 20-34   Summary

- RH is a recently described vascular tumor that is considered a well-differentiated and low-grade form of angiosarcoma.
- The tumor usually presents on the extremities of young adults, has a tendency to recur, and uncommonly metastatize.
- The tumor has a predominantly subcutaneous location and is composed of ill-defined arborizing thin-walled vessels lined by a monotonous population of small protuberant hobnail endothelial cells.

Retiform hemangioendothelioma (RH) is a recently described vascular tumor that is considered a well-differentiated and low-grade form of angiosarcoma.[221] This tumor usually presents on the extremities of young adults. Although this tumor has a tendency for recurrence, metastatic spread appears to be very uncommon. Only one case with lymph node metastasis has been reported, and no deaths have occurred. In fact, one case of multiple cutaneous tumors of RH arising over a 10-year period and excised from the trunk and extremities of a 30-year-old woman without evidence of metastasis or death has been reported.[222] Detection of human herpesvirus type 8 was recently reported in one case of RH[223]; however, additional studies are necessary to confirm any etiologic role.

Histopathological features: The tumor has a predominantly subcutaneous location and is composed of ill-defined arborizing thin-walled vessels lined by a monotonous population of small protuberant hobnail endothelial cells.[221] The vascular architecture is reminiscent of rete testis (Fig. 20-34). Frequently, the tumor is surrounded by a lymphocytic infiltrate, and in some cases lymphocytes are present within lumina of the neoplastic vessels. Solid areas of more epithelioid or spindled endothelial cells may be present.

Differential diagnosis: Retiform hemangioendothelioma and endovascular papillary angioendothelioma (EPA) are considered together in the same section because they share clinical and histopathologic features; indeed, it has been recently proposed that these tumors represent the adult (retiform hemangioendothelioma) and pediatric (endovascular papillary angioendothelioma) counterparts of the same tumor. Moreover, an 11-year-old boy with a neoplasm sharing features of both RH and EPA has been reported.[220] However, some histologic differences between RH and EPA are recognized, these include papillary tufts, which are a striking feature in endovascular papillary endothelioma, are typically a focal finding when present in retiform hemangioendothelioma. In addition, the striking arborizing vascular channels that characterize retiform hemangioendothelioma are not usually present in endovascular papillary angioendothelioma.

Kaposiform Hemangioendothelioma (KH)

BOX 20-35   Summary

- KH is an exceedingly rare vascular tumor occurring almost exclusively in childhood and involving the deep soft tissues and skin.
- The tumor most commonly presents as a soft-tissue mass, but the skin may be the initial site of involvement.
- KH when involving the skin and subcutis usually presents as a multinodular tumor composed of sheets of spindle cells often connected and surrounded by dense hyalinized fibrous tissue.

Kaposiform hemangioendothelioma is also known as Kaposi-like infantile hemangoendothelioma, hemangioma with KS-like features, and Kaposi-like infantile hemangioendothelioma. KH is an exceedingly rare vascular tumor occurring almost exclusively in childhood and involving the deep soft tissues and skin.[224]

Clinical features: Most patients reported thus far have been under the age of 10 years with males and females equally affected.[224] Rarely, KH presents at birth[225] and in adults.[76] The tumor most commonly presents as a soft-tissue mass, but the skin may be the initial site of involvement. The deep soft tissues of the upper extremities or the retroperitoneum are commonly involved, but KH can present in diverse anatomic sites. Some tumors have developed in the context of a lymphangiomatosis or have been associated with the Kasabach–Merritt phenomenon. Lesions can exhibit locally aggressive behavior, but no patients have developed distant metastases. Because of the potential for locally aggressive disease, these tumors have been considered to be borderline malignancies. However, this can be questioned, given the lack of metastasis; the generally benign behavior of KH localized to the skin, with cure by complete excision; and the prognosis of noncutaneous KH, particularly retroperitoneal or visceral disease, seeming to relate to tumor site, extent, and possible delay in diagnosis. Two patients have died from complications not directly related to the tumor.

Histopathological features: KH when involving the skin and subcutis usually

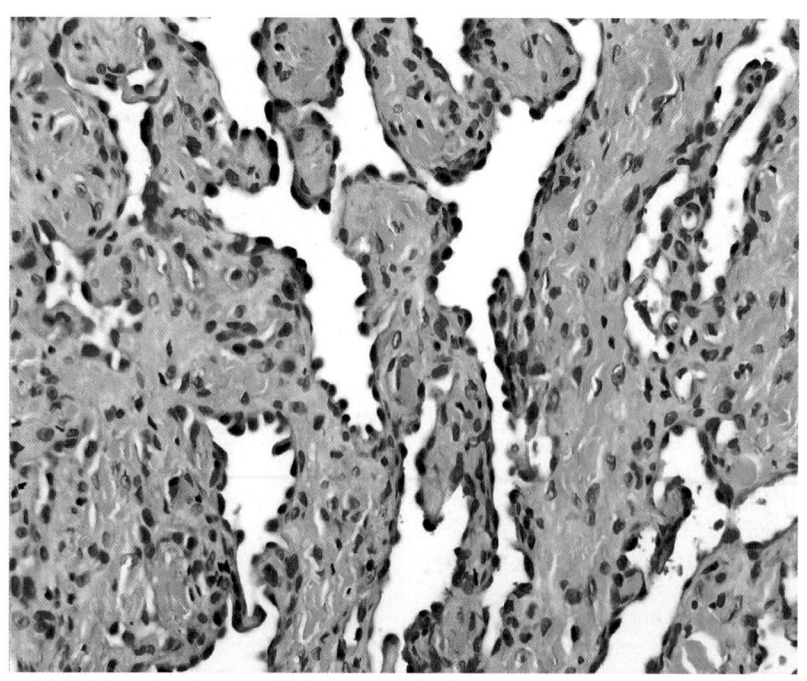

▲ **FIGURE 20-34** Retiform hemangioendothelioma. Note the close resemblance to the rete testis. Endothelial cells protrude into the vascular lumina.

presents as a multinodular tumor composed of sheets of spindle cells often connected and surrounded by dense hyalinized fibrous tissue. The spindle cells comprising such nodules have elongated or crescent-shaped vascular spaces and exhibit minimal cytological atypia.[224] Occasionally, rounded vascular lumina may also be observed. Among such spindle cell areas, one may encounter fairly discrete aggregates of cytologically bland epithelioid endothelial cells (glomeruloid clusters). The latter cells often contain hemosiderin and hyaline globules. Well-formed vascular channels are often nested at the periphery of tumor nodules. In general, the mitotic rate is low (commonly fewer than three per 10 high-power field). Inflammatory cell infiltrates containing lymphocytes and plasma cells are usually absent. The spindle cells comprising the tumor are positive for CD34 and generally negative for factor VIII-related antigen, Ulex europaeus lectin, and actin.

Differential diagnosis: The differential diagnosis includes KS, capillary hemangioma, spindle cell hemangioma, and acquired tufted angioma. KH generally affects younger individuals, presents as a deep solitary mass, and shows no association with HIV or immunodeficiency to date. The clinical differential diagnosis of congenital or neonatal lesions of KH includes neonatal hemangiomatosis, lesions that are differentiated from KH by being capillary-type hemangiomas.[225] Also, cutaneous KH generally presents at a later age than does capillary hemangioma of infancy.[226]

Composite Hemangioendothelioma (CH)

BOX 20-36   Summary

- CH is a recently described vascular tumor considered to be a low-grade malignancy mimicking conventional angiosarcoma, but with a better prognosis.
- CH usually presents as a poorly circumscribed uni- or multinodular lesions with individual nodules ranging from 0.7 to 6 cm.
- Histologically, the tumor is centered in the dermis and subcutis and shows complex histology that varies within individual tumors and between patients.

Composite hemangioendothelioma (CH) is a recently described vascular tumor considered to be a low-grade malignancy mimicking but behaving better than conventional angiosarcoma.[227] The

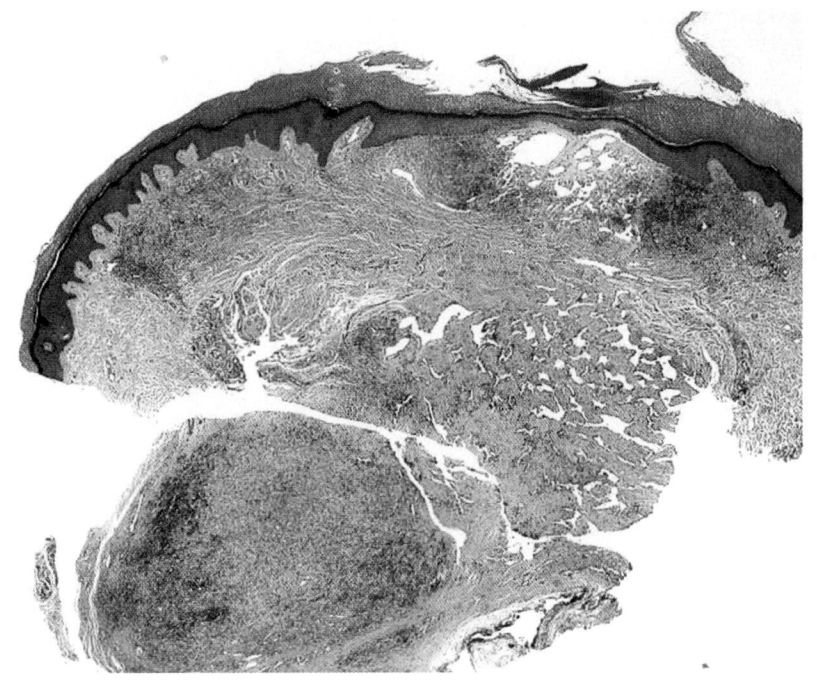

▲ **FIGURE 20-35** Composite hemangioendothelioma. The lesion combines a superficial lymphatic components, with central retiform and a deeper epithelioid hemangioendothelioma areas.

reported eight cases have usually presented on the hands and feet of adults (median age, 39.5 years; range 21 to 71 years) as poorly circumscribed uni- or multinodular lesions with individual nodules ranging from 0.7 to 6 cm. CH may recur locally and has the ability to metastasize. Follow-up of six patients (median duration, 6.5 years) identified local recurrence in three patients, and one of these patients, with an unusual primary site of the tongue, developed local lymph node metastasis and then two years later, metastasis as solid-type epithelioid hemangioendothelioma to the thigh.

Histopathological features: The tumor is centered in the dermis and subcutis and shows complex histology that varies within individual tumors and between patients (Fig. 20-35). Typical components, imperceptibly merging with one another, are epithelioid hemangioendothelioma, retiform hemangioendothelioma, and well-differentiated angiosarcoma-like areas (each in seven of eight cases), and less often, spindle cell hemangioma (four of eight cases). High-grade angiosarcoma was present in one case. In separate cases, one focus of arteriovenous malformation and another of lymphangioma circumscriptum were identified.

Differential diagnosis: Diagnosis of CH is dependent upon extensive sampling of the tumor. Small specimens may result in diagnosis of but one of the histologic components of CH and, in the

event of sampling an angiosarcoma-like area, could foster inappropriately aggressive therapy. The differential diagnosis of each individual component is described elsewhere in this chapter. Finally, polymorphous hemangioendothelioma (PH) is a grammatically similar but a distinct entity not to be confused with CE. Although one case of extranodal soft-tissue involvement has been reported, PH is a rare borderline malignant tumor of lymph nodes that is composed of varying proportions, hence the name polymorphous, of solid, primitive vascular and ectatic angiomatous elements.

MALIGNANT VASCULAR NEOPLASMS

Angiosarcoma (AS)

BOX 20-37   Summary

- AS is a rare, malignant endothelial tumor that arises in skin, soft tissue, breast, bones, liver, and other viscera. Cutaneous AS is the most common form of angiosarcoma.
- AS generally appears as ill-defined, asymptomatic, red to violaceous patches, plaques, or nodules.
- Cutaneous AS most commonly arise in the scalp and face of the elderly, with men affected more frequently than are women.
- Histologically, cutaneous AS extensively infiltrates the dermis, with microscopic involvement extending well beyond the clinically apparent boundaries.

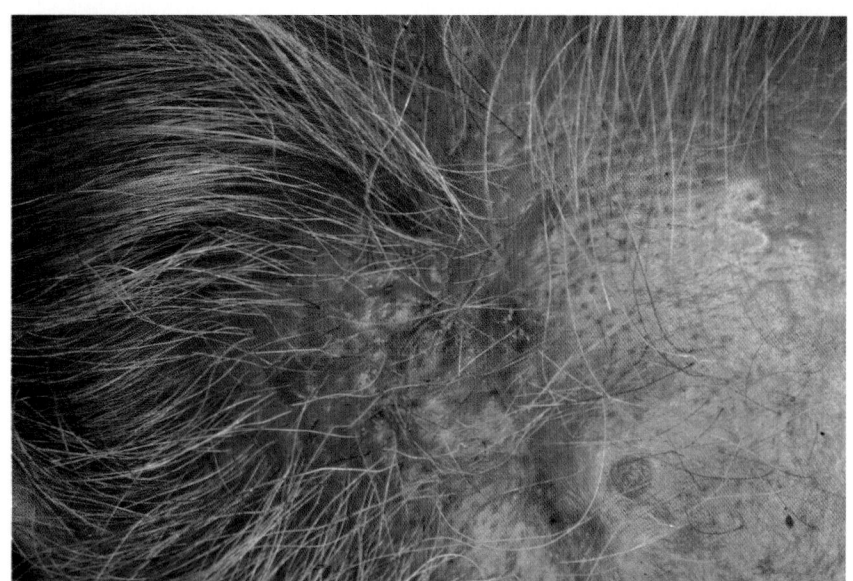

▲ **FIGURE 20-36** Cutaneous angiosarcoma. There are infiltrated plaques in the scalp.

Also known as malignant hemangioen-dothelioma or lymphangiosarcoma, angiosarcoma (AS) is a rare, malignant endothelial tumor that arises in skin, soft tissue, breast, bones, liver, and other viscera.[194,228–234] Cutaneous AS is the most common form of angiosarcoma. The prognosis for AS is poor. In one series of 72 patients with angiosarcoma of the face and scalp, one-half of the individuals died within 15 months of presentation.

Clinical features: In the skin, AS most commonly arises in the scalp and face of the elderly, with men affected more frequently than are women (Fig. 20-36).[228] AS may also occur in the setting of chronic lymphedema, often developing in a lymphedematous upper extremity as a late sequel of radical mastectomy, as described by Stewart and Treves.[194] Other causes of lymphedema—idiopathic, filarial, traumatic, congenital hereditary lymphedema (Milroy disease),[229] and morbid obesity—have also been implicated. Ionizing radiation has been linked to the development of AS with cases developing in the breast after radiation for breast cancer, in the abdominal region after irradiation of pelvic tumors, and in the face after irradiation of a congenital hemangioma.[235] Rarely, AS arises in association with foreign material (bullets, shrapnel, retained surgical sponges, and a gouty tophus) and with arteriovenous fistulae and vascular grafts.[236,237] Angiosarcoma metastatic to the skin is exceedingly rare but can herald the presence of occult tumor of an internal site such as the heart and the aorta.[238,239]

AS generally appears as ill-defined, asymptomatic, red to violaceous patches, plaques, or nodules.[228,230–234] Satellite lesions are frequent. AS frequently presents with multifocal disease, and there is a tendency toward both local recurrence and distant metastasis. The clinical appearance of AS varies somewhat according to the degree of histologic differentiation. Histologically more undifferentiated AS lesions may grow rapidly, with fungating and ulcerative appearances. Undifferentiated AS lesions may appear epithelioid and are high-grade neoplasms that generally affect deep, usually intramuscular, soft tissue, and rapidly develop metastases. Cutaneous occurrence has been reported, although a few cases that have been described had a distinctly better prognosis than does other undifferentiated AS. Such cutaneous tumors perhaps may fall into the spectrum of epithelioid hemangioendothelioma.

Histopathological features: Cutaneous AS extensively infiltrates the dermis, with microscopic involvement extending well beyond the clinically apparent boundaries.[194,228–234] The epidermis may be normal, atrophic, or ulcerated (Fig. 20-37). Direct epidermal invasion or involvement of the papillary dermis usually does not occur. Three distinct patterns of proliferation have been described: angiomatous, spindled, and undifferentiated. Individual tumors are composed of varying proportions of each pattern.

In angiomatous areas, vascular spaces that are distinctly individual or widely anastomosing are dispersed between dermal collagen bundles in a dissecting fashion (Fig. 20-38). The endothelium may be one to several cell layers in thickness and shows variable degrees of cytologic atypia. A mixed inflammatory response, often containing plasma cells, is usual. Hemosiderin deposition is variable. Some lymphedema-associated tumors have a lymphangiomatous appearance with irregular vascular channels devoid of erythrocytes dissecting dermal collagen bundles. The endothelium in these areas may be attenuated and show only subtle cytologic atypia. These foci are usually interspersed with more classic angiosarcomatous areas.

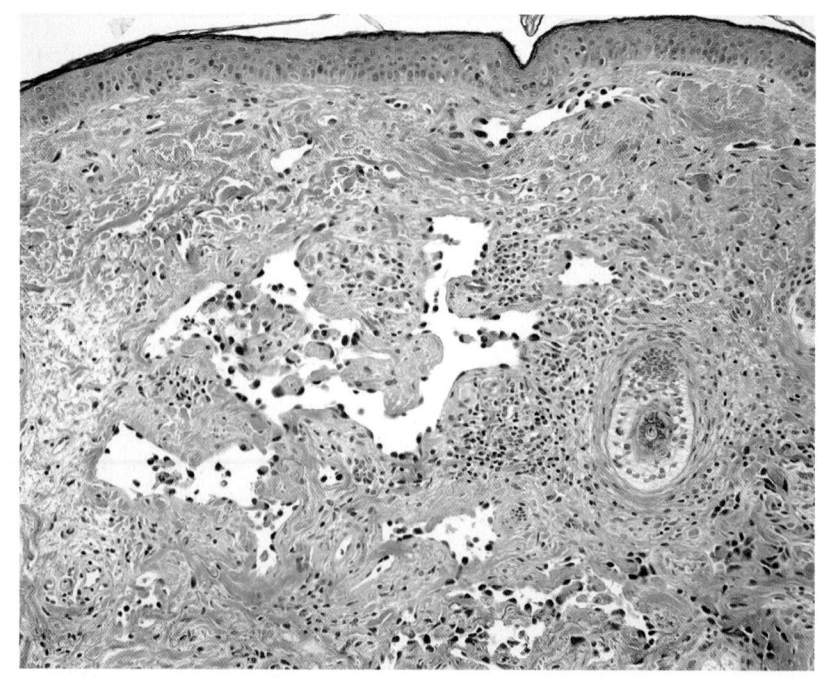

▲ **FIGURE 20-37** Cutaneous angiosarcoma. Well-differentiated neoplasm with angulated lumina and prominent pleomorphic endothelial cells.

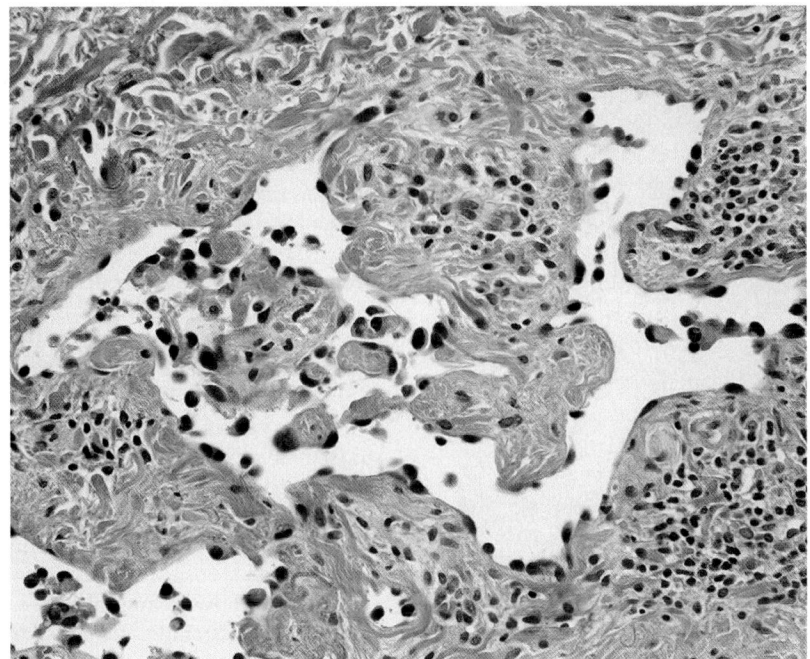

▲ **FIGURE 20-38** Cutaneous angiosarcoma. The neoplasm shows endothelial cell pleomorphism.

In spindle cell areas, spindled tumor cells are arranged in bundles that traverse the dermis in multiple directions, often enveloping adnexal structures. Cleft-like spaces and cracks containing erythrocytes are formed. The tumor may appear as a syncytium of cells without significant blood vessel formation. Undifferentiated areas are usually encountered as circumscribed nodules within more characteristic areas of AS (Fig. 20-39). Solid sheets of "epithelioid"

tumor cells with abundant acidophilic cytoplasm and large, atypical nuclei expand the dermis (Fig. 20-40). Lumen formation is usually only evident at the intracytoplasmic level. Intralesional hemorrhage may be prominent; this may not only obscure the diagnosis of AS, but with the addition of endothelial papillary hyperplasia, can appear as an organizing hematoma. A starry sky histologic pattern was noted in a subgroup of epithelioid angiosarcomas.[240]

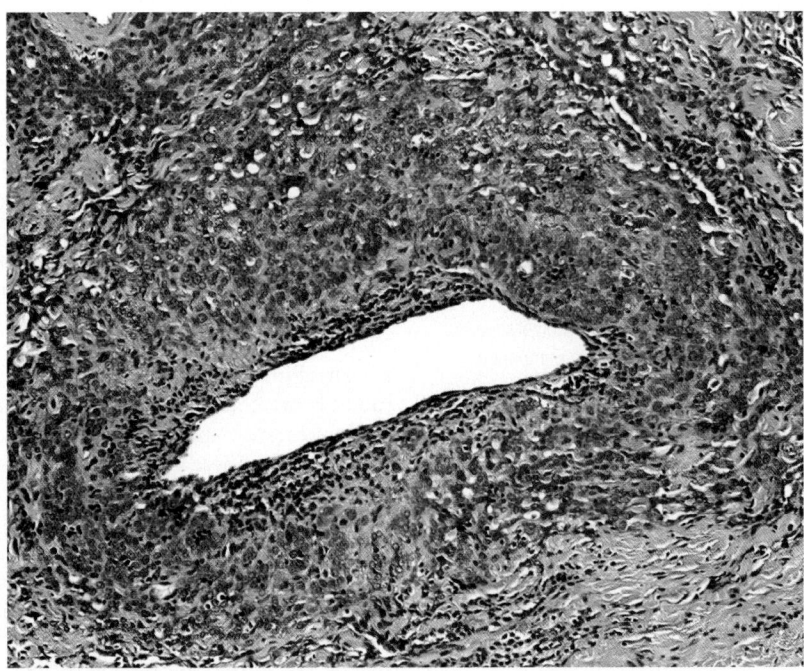

▲ **FIGURE 20-39** Cutaneous angiosarcoma. This is largely undifferentiated neoplasm with scant lumen formation.

Unusual variants of AS have been reported. An AS of the face contained many tumor cells with the appearance of granular cells. The newly described retiform hemangioendothelioma has a distinct retiform pattern of long arborizing vessels with a monomorphic hobnail endothelial lining. A lymphocytic infiltrate is usually present, and there are focal papillations similar to those of endovascular papillary angioendothelioma (Dabska tumor). Moreover, such papillations as well as features of epithelioid hemangioendothelioma, spindle cell hemangioma, and caverous and capillary hemangioma have been identified within AS of soft tissues.[241] Superimposed infection of a cutaneous angiosarcoma mimicked an inflammatory process, thereby delaying the diagnosis of AS in one case report.[242]

Studies of AS have variably indicated blood vessel or lymphatic differentiation; therefore, the histogenesis of AS is controversial. Ultrastructurally, AS generally shows features of endothelial cells, and cases often suggest blood vessel differentiation. Immunohistochemical analysis requires a broad panel of antibodies. AS may react with Ulex europaeus lectin 1, vimentin, and laminin (a constituent of basal lamina). Factor VIII-related antigen, the most sensitive marker in one study,[241] is variable, often stains only focally, and in some tumors is absent. CD31 and CD34 may react weakly and favor areas with better vascular differentiation. Furthermore, the immunohistochemical pattern of AS can vary within tumors, suggesting mixed differentiation of both blood vascular and lymphatic endothelium. Further clarification of the histogenesis must await the development of additional endothelial markers.

Differential diagnosis: KS displays dissection of dermal collagen by newly formed vascular channels similar to that of angiomatous- and lymphangiomatous-appearing areas of AS. An important feature to be identified within AS is endothelial "layering," associated with cytologic atypia. In contrast, the endothelial lining of KS is usually inconspicuous and almost always one cell layer in thickness. Particular confusion, however, may still arise between the lymphangiomatous pattern of AS and the lymphangiomatous variant of KS. The clinical setting associated with each entity is very helpful as are areas of more typical AS identified in lymphedema-associated AS. In general, AS displays more intralesional variation than does KS. In contrast to KS and

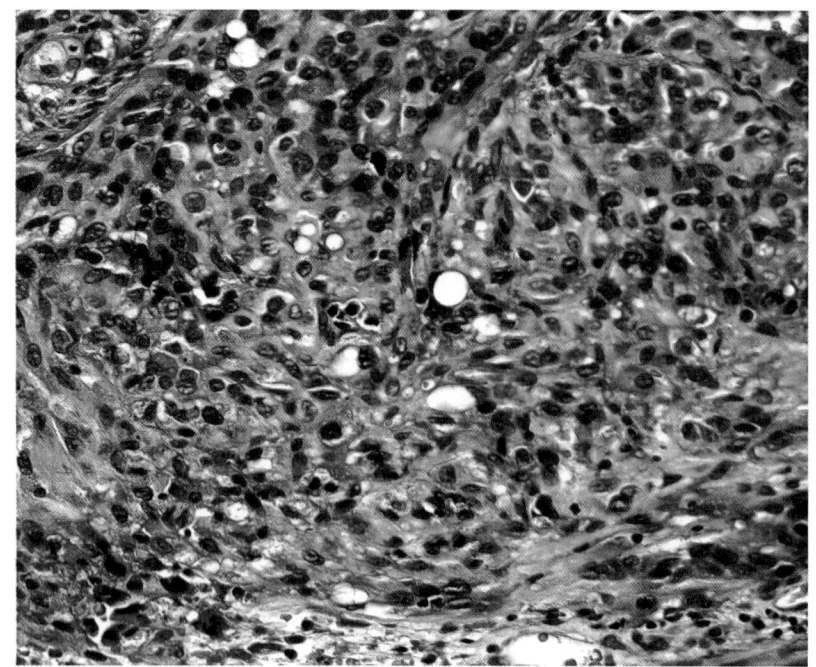

▲ FIGURE 20-40 Cutaneous angiosarcoma. This neoplasm contains pleomorphic epithelioid endothelial cells closely resembling a carcinoma. Note the numerous intracellular lumina.

despite some contradictory data, human herpesvirus 8 does not appear to be closely linked to AS.[243]

AS with a predominant spindle cell pattern may mimic plaques and nodules of KS. Features of distinction include the identification of more angiomatous areas in AS and a degree of cytologic atypia exceeding that observed in even florid nodules of KS. The clinical situation is also helpful, since AS is often confined to the head and neck of elderly individuals or unilaterally to a lymphedematous upper extremity. KS often does not involve such anatomic sites in older individuals. In contrast to AS, hemangiopericytomas contain dilated sinusoidal spaces with a characteristic antler-like or staghorn configuration lined by a single layer of flattened endothelial cells. A reticulin stain will further highlight differences between these two entities. In AS, the delicate reticulin sheath will be present peripheral to the inner lining of atypical endothelial cells, whereas in hemangiopericytoma the tumor cells will lie outside this reticulin sheath.

Epithelioid AS may be mistaken for poorly differentiated carcinoma or melanoma. Compounding the difficulty in distinction from carcinoma is the coexpression of cytokeratin and endothelial markers by epithelioid angiosarcoma.[232] This emphasizes the need for a broad panel of antibodies when such tumors are being evaluated. Finally, some squamous cell carcinomas

have an intense acantholytic pattern, closely resembling the histology of well-differentiated angiosarcoma. The demonstration of keratins and the absence of endothelial markers by immunohistochemistry are diagnostic, with the caveat of the rare keratin positive angiosarcoma.

Vascular Proliferation Associated With Mastectomy, Lumpectomy, and Adjuvant Radiation Therapy

BOX 20-38   Summary

- Cutaneous angiosarcomas, the first form of vascular proliferation, are aggressive angiosarcomas appearing in the setting of mammary carcinoma, radical mastectomy, and adjuvant therapy, as well as radiation therapy or chemotherapy.
- A second form of vascular proliferation has a more florid lymphatic component with features nearly indistinguishable from lymphangioma circumscriptum of infancy.
- The third form of the vascular proliferation is more disturbing for its histological appearance and potential biological implications. These lesions have complex histological features, with substantial variation from field to field. The lesion has some lymphatic appearance with lumina devoid of erythrocytes and containing proteinaceous material, alternating with frankly angiomatous areas.

Cutaneous angiosarcomas of the breast are neoplasms with a well-defined clinicopathological profile. These aggressive angiosarcomas appear in the setting of mammary carcinoma, radical mastectomy, and adjuvant therapy, as well as radiation therapy or chemotherapy. The tumors arise after a lengthy "incubation" period, usually 10 years or longer, in association with chronic lymphedema. By the time of diagnosis, the neoplasm is fully developed and the diagnosis is relatively straightforward. These have been known as Stewart–Treves syndrome.[194]

In recent times, less radical forms of surgery have been developed with the goal of reducing the morbidity of the surgical procedure. Thus, modified and limited mastectomies, lumpectomies, sentinel node biopsies, and postsurgical radiation are now commonly used. In spite of the less traumatic procedure, cases of vascular neoplasms arising in this clinical setting have been observed. In these closely managed patients, suspicious skin lesions are often biopsied, largely to evaluate for metastatic mammary carcinoma. In these circumstances, a complex group of vascular proliferations have also been biopsied. These lesions have a much shorter "incubation" period, often 2 to 3 years, and pose a serious diagnostic dilemma.[244-247] Some vascular proliferations seem to represent simple lymphangiectasias. This may likely have originated due to disruption of the lymphatic drainage, secondary to the surgical procedure or posterior radiation therapy. The lesions often arise without a background of major arm lymphedema.

A second form of vascular proliferation has a more florid lymphatic component with features nearly indistinguishable from lymphangioma circumscriptum of infancy. The thinwalled vascular lumina abut the epidermis, and the lesion is largely localized to the papillary dermis. Deeper lymphatics can be present in the reticular dermis. No cytological pleomorphism is seen (Fig. 20-41).

The third form of the vascular proliferation is more disturbing for its histological appearance and potential biological implications. These lesions have complex histological features, with substantial variation from field to field (Fig. 20-42). The lesion has some lymphatic appearance with lumina devoid of erythrocytes and containing proteinaceous material, alternating with frankly angiomatous areas. The lumina are rounded or jagged with certain staghorn quality (Fig. 20-43). There is a considerable variation of

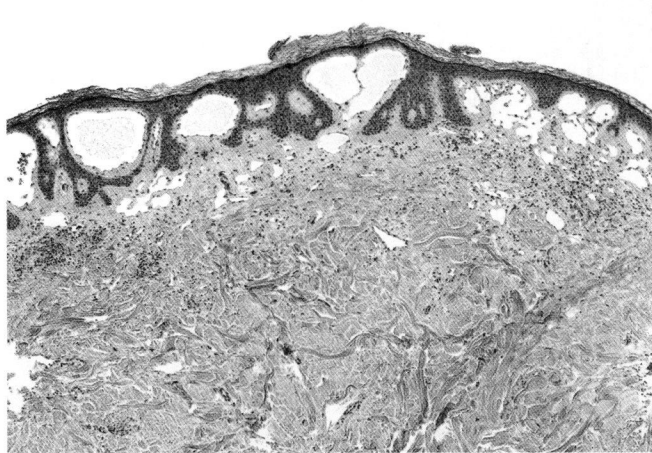

▲ **FIGURE 20-41** Lymphangiomatous proliferation in an irradiated breast. Note the close similarity with lymphangioma circumscriptum.

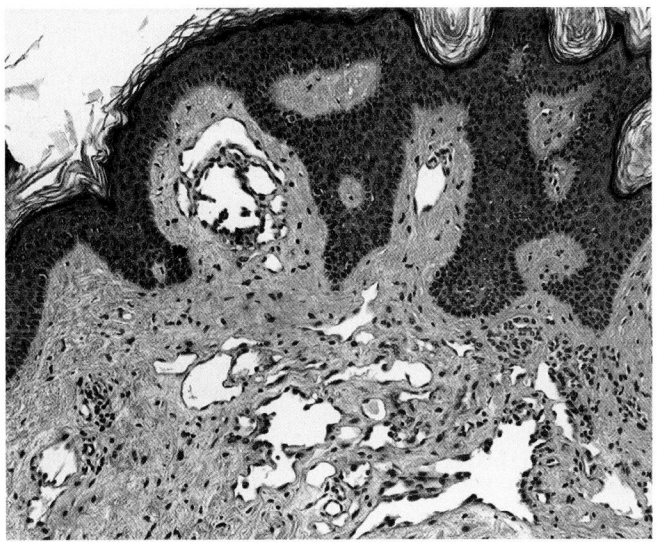

▲ **FIGURE 20-42** Atypical vascular proliferation in an irradiated breast. Some may classify this lesion as angiosarcoma while others may use the term atypical vascular proliferation.

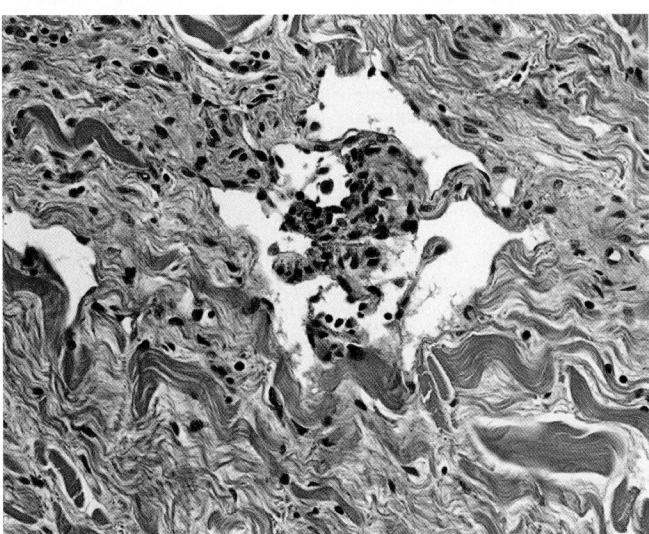

▲ **FIGURE 20-43** Atypical vascular proliferation in an irradiated breast. Higher power view. An infiltrative growth and moderate pleomorphism.

endothelial lining from flat and inconspicuous to prominent and epithelioid. The endothelial lining of the vessels can be irregular, with areas seemingly devoid of nuclei, to cellular clustering. The epithelioid component closely resembles the cytological features of epithelioid hemangiomas and hemangioendotheliomas. Solid clusters of epithelioid endothelial cells without lumen formation have a remarkable cytological similarity to melanocytic theques. The lesion is superficial, although it also involves the reticular dermis and it is relatively circumscribed. The biological potential of this proliferation is unknown. While it is tempting to regard it as a precursor lesion of angiosarcoma or actually its earlier manifestation, its nature is not understood at this time. Its pathogenesis is also poorly understood. It is not clear whether these proliferations are induced by lymphatic obstruction or radiation. Nevertheless, given the common clinicopathological setting, it is likely that all these vascular and lymphatic lesions are somehow related. To draw the conclusion that these lesions follow an evolutionary sequence, tempting as it may be, is speculatory at this time. Similar lesions related to therapeutic radiotherapy have been reported in other parts of the body, particularly the vulva. Further studies, hopefully, will elucidate many of these questions.

■ FINAL THOUGHTS

Vascular tumors of the skin comprise a heterogeneous group of lesions that offer a complex and overlapping histological spectrum, as well as different clinical courses and treatment options. They are of interest clinically because of their ability to mimic aggressive tumors and they may cause pain and cosmetic disfigurement. These lesions range from hamartomas to hyperplasias and benign, as well as malignant tumors. Only a thorough knowledge of the different clinicopathological entities assures an accurate diagnosis.

REFERENCES

1. Hunt S, Santa Cruz DJ. Acquired benign and "borderline" vascular lesions. *Dermatol Clin.* 1992;10:97–115.
2. Wassef M. Cervico-cephalic hemangiomas and vascular malformations. Histopathological appearance and classification. *J Mal Vasc.* 1992;17:20–25.
3. Mulliken JB. A biologic classification of vascular birthmarks. In: Boccalon H, ed. *Vascular Medicine.* 1993, Amsterdam: Elsevier Science; 1993:603–614.

4. Takahashi K, Mulliken J, Kozakewich H, et al. Cellular markers that distinguish the phases of hemangioma during infancy and childhood. *J Clin Invest.* 1994;93:2357–2364.

5. Cecchi R, Giomi A. Pyogenic granuloma as a complication of cryosurgery for venous lake. *Br J Dermatol.* 1999;140: 373–374.

6. Alcalay J, Sandbank M. The ultrastructure of cutaneous venous lakes. *Int J Dermatol.* 1987;26:645–646.

7. Epstein E, Novy FG, Jr, Allington HV. Capillary aneurysms of the skin. *Arch Dermatol.* 1965;91:335.

8. Bean WB. *Vascular Spiders and Related Lesions of the Skin.* Springfield, IL: CC Thomas; 1958.

9. Wenzl JE, Burgert EO. The spider nevus in infancy and childhood. *Pediatrics.* 1964;33:227–232.

10. Jessen R, Thompson S, Smith E. Cobb syndrome. *Arch Dermatol.* 1977;113: 1587–1590.

11. Uram M, Zubillaga C. The cutaneous manifestations of Sturge–Weber syndrome. *J Clin Neuroophthalmol.* 1982;2: 245–248.

12. Mullins JF, Naylor D, Redetsky J. The Klippel–Trenaunay–Weber syndrome. *Arch Dermatol.* 1982;85:120–124.

13. Viljoen D, Saxe N, Pearn J, et al. The cutaneous manifestations of the Klippel–Trenaunay–Weber syndrome. *Clin Exp Dermatol.* 1987;12:12–17.

14. Stevenson J, Lincoln C. Angioma serpiginosum. *Arch Dermatol.* 1967;95:16–22, 32.

15. Marriott P, Munro D, Ryan T. Angioma serpiginosum—familial incidence. *Br J Dermatol.* 1975;93:701–706.

16. Katta R, Wagner A. Angioma serpiginosum with extensive cutaneous involvement. *J Am Acad Dermatol.* 2000; 42:384–385.

17. Suzuki Y, Nakamura N, Fukuoka K, et al. beta-Galactosidase deficiency in juvenile and adult patients. Report of six Japanese cases and review of literature. *Hum Genet.* 1977;36:219–229.

18. Ishibashi A, Tsuboi R, Shinmei M. beta-Galactosidase and neuraminidase deficiency associated with angiokeratoma corporis diffusum. *Arch Dermatol.* 1984; 120:1344–1346.

19. Imperial R, Helwig E. Angiokeratoma. A clinicopathological study. *Arch Dermatol.* 1967;95:166–175.

20. Rossi A, Bozzi M, Barra E. Verrucous hemangioma and angiokeratoma circumscriptum: clinical and histologic differential characteristics. *J Dermatol Surg Oncol.* 1989;15:88–91.

21. Fleming C, Rennie A, Fallowfield M, et al. Cutaneous manifestations of fucosidosis. *Br J Dermatol.* 1997;136:594–597.

22. Shannon P, Ford M. Angiokeratomas in juvenile dermatomyositis. *Pediatr Dermatol.* 1999;16:448–451.

23. Kraus M, Lind A, Alder S, et al. Angiomatosis with angiokeratoma-like features in children: a light microscopic and immunophenotypic examination of four cases. *Am J Dermatopathol.* 1999;21:350–355.

24. Imperial R, Helwig E. Verrucous hemangioma. A clinicopathologic study of 21 cases. *Arch Dermatol.* 1967;96:247–253.

25. Klein J, Barr R. Verrucous hemangioma. *Pediatr Dermatol.* 1985;2:191–193, 43.

26. Wong D, Hunt S, Inserra D, et al. Unilateral keratotic vascular lesion on the leg. Verrucous hemangioma. *Arch Dermatol.* 1996;132:705, 708.

27. Wentscher U, Happle R. Linear verrucous hemangioma. *J Am Acad Dermatol.* 2000;42:516–518.

28. Rice JS, Fischer DS. Blue rubber-bleb nevus syndrome. *Arch Dermatol.* 1962; 86:503.

29. Jorizzo J, Amparo E. MR imaging of blue rubber bleb nevus syndrome. *J Comput Assist Tomogr.* 1986;10:686–688.

30. Bean WB. Dyschondroplasia and hemangiomata. *Arch Intern Med.* 1955;95:767.

31. Kunkeler A, Uitdehaag B, Stoof T. Familial cavernous haemangiomas. *Br J Dermatol.* 1998;139:166–167.

32. Watabe H, Kashima M, Baba T, et al. A case of unilateral dermatomal cavernous haemangiomatosis. *Br J Dermatol.* 2000;143:888–891.

33. Calonje E, Fletcher C. Sinusoidal hemangioma. A distinctive benign vascular neoplasm within the group of cavernous hemangiomas. *Am J Surg Pathol.* 1991;15:1130–1135.

34. Enjolras O, Herbreteau D, Lemarchand F, et al. Hemangiomas and superficial vascular malformations: classification. *J Mal Vasc.* 1992;17:2–19.

35. Mulliken JB, Young AE. *Vascular Birthmarks: Hemangiomas and Malformations.* Philadelphia, PA: Saunders; 1988:63–76.

36. Kasabach HH, Merritt KK. Capillary hemangioma with extensive purpura: report of a case. *Am J Dis Child.* 1940;59:1063.

37. Mills S, Cooper P, Fechner R. Lobular capillary hemangioma: the underlying lesion of pyogenic granuloma. A study of 73 cases from the oral and nasal mucous membranes. *Am J Surg Pathol.* 1980;4:470–479.

38. Cooper P, Mills S. Subcutaneous granuloma pyogenicum. Lobular capillary hemangioma. *Arch Dermatol.* 1982;118: 30–33.

39. Wilson B, Greer K, Cooper P. Eruptive disseminated lobular capillary hemangioma (pyogenic granuloma). *J Am Acad Dermatol.* 1989;21:391–394.

40. Strohal R, Gillitzer R, Zonzits E, et al. Localized vs. generalized pyogenic granuloma. A clinicopathologic study. *Arch Dermatol.* 1991;127:856–861.

41. Tosti A, Piraccini B, Camacho-Martinez F. Onychomadesis and pyogenic granuloma following cast immobilization. *Arch Dermatol.* 2001;137:231–232.

42. Katta R, Bickle K, Hwang L. Pyogenic granuloma arising in port-wine stain during pregnancy. *Br J Dermatol.* 2001; 144:644–645.

43. Bouscarat F, Bouchard C, Bouhour D. Paronychia and pyogenic granuloma of the great toes in patients treated with indinavir. *N Engl J Med.* 1998;338:1776–1777.

44. Harris M, Desai R, Chuang T, et al. Lobular capillary hemangiomas: An epidemiologic report, with emphasis on cutaneous lesions. *J Am Acad Dermatol.* 2000;42:1012–1016.

45. Valentic J, Barr R, Weinstein G. Inflammatory neovascular nodules associated with oral isotretinoin treatment of severe acne. *Arch Dermatol.* 1983;119:871–872.

46. Cooper P, McAllister H, Helwig E. Intravenous pyogenic granuloma. A study of 18 cases. *Am J Surg Pathol.* 1979;3:221–228.

47. Pierson J, Owens N. Pyogenic granuloma-like lesions associated with topical retinoid therapy. *J Am Acad Dermatol.* 2001;45:967–968.

48. Nakamura T. Apoptosis and expression of Bax/Bcl-2 proteins in pyogenic granuloma: a comparative study with granulation tissue and capillary hemangioma. *J Cutan Pathol.* 2000;27:400–405.

49. Rowlands C, Rapson D, Morell T. Extramedullary hematopoiesis in a pyogenic granuloma. *Am J Dermatopathol.* 2000;22:434–438.

50. Padilla R, Orkin M, Rosai J. Acquired "tufted" angioma (progressive capillary hemangioma). A distinctive clinicopathologic entity related to lobular capillary hemangioma. *Am J Dermatopathol.* 1987;9:292–300.

51. Jones E, Orkin M. Tufted angioma (angioblastoma). A benign progressive angioma, not to be confused with Kaposi's sarcoma or low-grade angiosarcoma. *J Am Acad Dermatol.* 1989;20:214–225.

52. Cho K, Kim S, Park K, et al. Angioblastoma (Nakagawa)—is it the same as tufted angioma? *Clin Exp Dermatol.* 1991;16:110–113.

53. Nakamura E, Ohnishi T, Watanabe S, et al. Kasabach–Merritt syndrome associated with angioblastoma. *Br J Dermatol (England).* 1998;139:164–166.

54. Kleinegger C, Hammond H, Vincent S, et al. Acquired tufted angioma: a unique vascular lesion not previously reported in the oral mucosa. *Br J Dermatol.* 2000;142:794–799.

55. Ishikawa O, Nihei Y, Ishikawa H. The skin changes of POEMS syndrome. *Br J Dermatol.* 1987;117:523–526.

56. Chan J, Fletcher C, Hicklin G, et al. Glomeruloid hemangioma. A distinctive cutaneous lesion of multicentric Castleman's disease associated with POEMS syndrome. *Am J Surg Pathol.* 1990;14:1036–1046.

57. Yang S, Cho K, Bang Y, et al. A case of glomeruloid hemangioma associated with multicentric Castleman's disease. *Am J Dermatopathol.* 1998;20:266–270.

58. Kishimoto S, Takenaka H, Shibagaki R, et al. Glomeruloid hemangioma in POEMS syndrome shows two different immunophenotypic endothelial cells. *J Cutan Pathol.* 2000;27:87–92.

59. Rosai J, Gold J, Landy R. The histiocytoid hemangiomas. A unifying concept embracing several previously described entities of skin, soft tissue, large vessels, bone, and heart. *Hum Pathol.* 1979;10: 707–730.

60. Rosai J. Angiolymphoid hyperplasia with eosinophilia of the skin. Its nosological position in the spectrum of histiocytoid hemangioma. *Am J Dermatopathol.* 1982;4:175–184.

61. Googe P, Harris N, Mihm M. Kimura's disease and angiolymphoid hyperplasia with eosinophilia: two distinct histopathological entities. *J Cutan Pathol.* 1987; 14:263–271.

62. Urabe A, Tsuneyoshi M, Enjoji M. Epithelioid hemangioma versus Kimura's disease. A comparative clinicopathologic

study. *Am J Surg Pathol.* 1987;11:758–766.

63. Chan J, Hui P, Ng C, et al. Epithelioid haemangioma (angiolymphoid hyperplasia with eosinophilia) and Kimura's disease in Chinese. *Histopathology.* 1989;15:557–574.

64. Olsen T, Helwig E. Angiolymphoid hyperplasia with eosinophilia. A clinicopathologic study of 116 patients. *J Am Acad Dermatol.* 1985;12:781–796.

65. Jang K, Ahn S, Choi J, et al. Polymerase chain reaction (PCR) for human herpesvirus 8 and heteroduplex PCR for clonality assessment in angiolymphoid hyperplasia with eosinophilia and Kimura's disease. *J Cutan Pathol.* 2001;28:363–367.

66. Kanik A, Oh C, Bhawan J. Disseminated cutaneous epithelioid hemangioma. *J Am Acad Dermatol.* 1996;35:851–853.

67. Tsuboi H, Fujimura T, Katsuoka K. Angiolymphoid hyperplasia with eosinophilia in the oral mucosa. *Br J Dermatol.* 2001;145:365–366.

68. Sakamoto F, Hashimoto T, Takenouchi T, et al. Angiolymphoid hyperplasia with eosinophilia presenting multinucleated cells in histology: an ultrastructural study. *J Cutan Pathol.* 1998;25:322–326.

69. Vadlamudi G, Schinella R. Traumatic pseudoaneurysm: a possible early lesion in the spectrum of epithelioid hemangioma/angiolymphoid hyperplasia with eosinophilia. *Am J Dermatopathol.* 1998;20:113–117.

70. Wong K, Shamsol S. Quantitative study of mast cells in Kimura's disease. *J Cutan Pathol.* 1999;26:13–16.

71. Watanabe C, Koga M, Honda Y, et al. Juvenile temporal arteritis is a manifestation of kimura disease. *Am J Dermatopathol.* 2002;24:43–49.

72. Hunt S, Santa CD, Barr R. Microvenular hemangioma. *J Cutan Pathol.* 1991;18:235–240.

73. Aloi F, Tomasini C, Pippione M. Microvenular hemangioma. *Am J Dermatopathol.* 1993;15:534–538.

74. Rikihisa W, Yamamoto O, Kohda F, et al. Microvenular haemangioma in a patient with Wiskott–Aldrich syndrome. *Br J Dermatol.* 1999;141:752–754.

75. Santa Cruz D, Aronberg J. Targetoid hemosiderotic hemangioma. *J Am Acad Dermatol.* 1988;19:550–558.

76. Mentzel T, Partanen T, Kutzner H. Hobnail hemangioma ("targetoid hemosiderotic hemangioma"): clinicopathologic and immunohistochemical analysis of 62 cases. *J Cutan Pathol.* 1999;26:279–286.

77. Guillou L, Calonje E, Speight P, et al. Hobnail hemangioma: a pseudomalignant vascular lesion with a reappraisal of targetoid hemosiderotic hemangioma. *Am J Surg Pathol.* 1999;23:97–105.

78. Carlson J, Daulat S, Goodheart H. Targetoid hemosiderotic hemangioma—a dynamic vascular tumor: report of 3 cases with episodic and cyclic changes and comparison with solitary angiokeratomas. *J Am Acad Dermatol.* 1999;41:215–224.

79. Christenson L, Stone M. Trauma-induced simulator of targetoid hemosiderotic hemangioma. *Am J Dermatopathol.* 2001;23:221–223.

80. Strutton G, Weedon D. Acro-angiodermatitis. A simulant of Kaposi's sarcoma. *Am J Dermatopathol.* 1987;9:85–89.

81. Kolde G, Worheide J, Baumgartner R, et al. Kaposi-like acroangiodermatitis in an above-knee amputation stump. *Br J Dermatol.* 1989;120:575–580.

82. LeBoit P. Lobular capillary proliferation: the underlying process in diverse benign cutaneous vascular neoplasms and reactive conditions. *Semin Dermatol.* 1989;8:298–310.

83. Marshall M, Hatfield S, Hatfield D. Arteriovenous malformation simulating Kaposi's sarcoma (pseudo-Kaposi's sarcoma). *Arch Dermatol.* 1985;121:99–101.

84. Larralde M, Gonzalez V, Marietti R, et al. Pseudo-Kaposi sarcoma with arteriovenous malformation. *Pediatr Dermatol.* 2001;18:325–327.

85. Kapdagli H, Gunduz K, Ozturk G, et al. Pseudo-Kaposi's sarcoma (Mali type). *Int J Dermatol.* 1998;37:223–225.

86. Clearkin K, Enzinger F. Intravascular papillary endothelial hyperplasia. *Arch Pathol Lab Med.* 1976;100:441–444.

87. Kuo T, Sayers C, Rosai J. Masson's "vegetant intravascular hemangioendothelioma:" a lesion often mistaken for angiosarcoma: study of seventeen cases located in the skin and soft tissues. *Cancer.* 1976;38:1227–1236.

88. Barr R, Graham J, Sherwin L. Intravascular papillary endothelial hyperplasia. A benign lesion mimicking angiosarcoma. *Arch Dermatol.* 1978;114:723–726.

89. Albrecht S, Kahn H. Immunohistochemistry of intravascular papillary endothelial hyperplasia. *J Cutan Pathol.* 1990;17:16–21.

90. Moon W, Chung G, Hong K. Intra vascular papillary endothelial hyperplasia in a vascular lesion of the paranasal sinus. *Arch Pathol Lab Med.* 2000;124:1224–1227.

91. Romani J, Puig L, Costa I, et al. Masson's intravascular papillary endothelial hyperplasia mimicking Stewart–Treves syndrome: report of a case. *Cutis.* 1997;59:148–150.

92. Rao V, Weiss S. Angiomatosis of soft tissue. An analysis of the histologic features and clinical outcome in 51 cases. *Am J Surg Pathol.* 1992;16:764–771.

93. Cockerell C, Le BP. Bacillary angiomatosis: a newly characterized, pseudoneoplastic, infectious, cutaneous vascular disorder. *J Am Acad Dermatol.* 1990;22:501–512.

94. Koehler J, Quinn F, Berger T, et al. Isolation of Rochalimaea species from cutaneous and osseous lesions of bacillary angiomatosis. *N Engl J Med.* 1992;327:1625–1631.

95. Koehler J, Glaser C, Tappero J. *Rochalimaea henselae* infection. A new zoonosis with the domestic cat as reservoir. *JAMA.* 1994;271:531–535.

96. Pfleger L, Tappeiner J. Zur Kenntnis der systemisierten Endotheliomatose der cutan theliose. *Hautarzt.* 1959;10:359–363.

97. Tappeiner J, Pfleger L. Angioendotheliomatosis proliferans systematisata. *Hautarzt.* 1963;14:67–70.

98. Wick M, Mills S, Scheithauer B, et al. Reassessment of malignant "angioendotheliomatosis". Evidence in favor of its reclassification as "intravascular lymphomatosis". *Am J Surg Pathol.* 1986;10:112–123.

99. Sheibani K, Battifora H, Winberg C, et al. Further evidence that "malignant angioendotheliomatosis" is an angiotropic large-cell lymphoma. *N Engl J Med.* 1986;314:943–948.

100. Bhawan J, Wolff S, Ucci A, et al. Malignant lymphoma and malignant angioendotheliomatosis: one disease. *Cancer.* 1985;55:570–576.

101. Lin B, Weiss L, Battifora H. Intravascularly disseminated angiosarcoma: true neoplastic angioendotheliomatosis? Report of two cases. *Am J Surg Pathol.* 1997;21:1138–1143.

102. Martin S, Pitcher D, Tschen J, et al. Reactive angioendotheliomatosis. *J Am Acad Dermatol.* 1980;2:117–123.

103. Eisert J. Skin manifestations of subacute bacterial endocarditis. Case report of subacute bacterial endocarditis mimicking Tappeiner's angioendotheliomatosis. *Cutis.* 1980;25:394–395, 400.

104. Lazova R, Slater C, Scott G. Reactive angioendotheliomatosis. Case report and review of the literature. *Am J Dermatopathol.* 1996;18:63–69.

105. LeBoit P, Solomon A, Santa CD, et al. Angiomatosis with luminal cryoprotein deposition. *J Am Acad Dermatol.* 1992;27:969–973.

106. Porras-Luque J, Fernandez-Herrera J, Dauden E, et al. Cutaneous necrosis by cold agglutinins associated with glomeruloid reactive angioendotheliomatosis. *Br J Dermatol.* 1998;139:1068–1072.

107. Salama S, Jenkin P. Angiomatosis of skin with local intravascular immunoglobulin deposits, associated with monoclonal gammopathy. A potential cutaneous marker for B-chronic lymphocytic leukemia. A report of unusual case with immunohistochemical and immunofluorescence correlation and review of the literature. *J Cutan Pathol.* 1999;26:206–212.

108. Creamer D, Black M, Calonje E. Reactive angioendotheliomatosis in association with the antiphospholipid syndrome. *J Am Acad Dermatol.* 2000;42:903–906.

109. Tomasini C, Soro E, Pippione M. Angioendotheliomatosis in a woman with rheumatoid arthritis. *Am J Dermatopathol.* 2000;22:334–338.

110. Requena L, Farina M, Renedo G, et al. Intravascular and diffuse dermal reactive angioendotheliomatosis secondary to iatrogenic arteriovenous fistulas. *J Cutan Pathol.* 1999;26:159–164.

111. Ortonne N, Vignon-Pennamen M, Majdalani G, et al. Reactive angioendotheliomatosis secondary to dermal amyloid angiopathy. *Am J Dermatopathol.* 2001;23:315–319.

112. Quinn T, Alora M, Momtaz K, et al. Reactive angioendotheliomatosis with underlying hepatopathy and hypertensive portal gastropathy. *Int J Dermatol.* 1998;37:382–385.

113. Krell J, Sanchez R, Solomon A. Diffuse dermal angiomatosis: a variant of reactive cutaneous angioendotheliomatosis. *J Cutan Pathol.* 1994;21:363–370.

114. Kimyai-Asadi A, Nousari H, Ketabchi N, et al. Diffuse dermal angiomatosis: a variant of reactive angioendotheliomatosis associated with atherosclerosis. *J Am Acad Dermatol.* 1999;40:257–259.

115. McLaughlin E, Morris R, Weiss S, et al. Diffuse dermal angiomatosis of the

breast: response to isotretinoin. *J Am Acad Dermatol.* 2001;45:462–465.

116. Biberstein HH, Jessner M. A cirsoid aneurysm in the skin. *Dermatologica.* 1956;113:129.

117. Girard C, Graham J, Johnson W. Arteriovenous hemangioma (arteriovenous shunt). A clinicopathological and histochemical study. *J Cutan Pathol.* 1974;1:73–87.

118. Carapeto F, Garcia-Perez A, Winkelmann R. Acral arteriovenous tumor. *Acta Derm Venereol.* 1977;57:155–158.

119. Connelly M, Winkelmann R. Acral arteriovenous tumor. A clinicopathologic review. *Am J Surg Pathol.* 1985;9:15–21.

120. Kadono T, Kishi A, Onishi Y, et al. Acquired digital arteriovenous malformation: a report of six cases. *Br J Dermatol.* 2000;142:362–365.

121. Onishi Y, Ohara K. Angiolymphoid hyperplasia with eosinophilia associated with arteriovenous malformation: a clinicopathological correlation with angiography and serial estimation of serum levels of renin, eosinophil cationic protein and interleukin 5. *Br J Dermatol.* 1999;140:1153–1156.

122. Kishimoto S, Takenaka H, Shibagaki R, et al. Verruciform xanthoma arising in an arteriovenous haemangioma. *Br J Dermatol.* 1998;139:546–548.

123. Feinmesser M, Taube E, Badani E, et al. Basal cell carcinomas arising over arteriovenous malformations: some speculations on the theme. *Am J Dermatopathol.* 1997;19:575–579.

124. Carroll R, Berman A. Glomus tumors of the hand: review of the literature and report on twenty-eight cases. *J Bone Joint Surg Am.* 1972;54:691–703.

125. Beham A, Fletcher C. Intravascular glomus tumour: a previously undescribed phenomenon. *Virchows Arch A Pathol Anat Histopathol.* 1991;418:175–177.

126. Landthaler M, Braun-Falco O, Eckert F, et al. Congenital multiple plaquelike glomus tumors. *Arch Dermatol.* 1990;126:1203–1207.

127. Aiba M, Hirayama A, Kuramochi S. Glomangiosarcoma in a glomus tumor. An immunohistochemical and ultrastructural study. *Cancer.* 1988;61:1467–1471.

128. Gould E, Manivel J, Albores-Saavedra J, et al. Locally infiltrative glomus tumors and glomangiosarcomas. A clinical, ultrastructural, and immunohistochemical study. *Cancer.* 1990;65:310–318.

129. Kaye V, Dehner L. Cutaneous glomus tumor. A comparative immunohistochemical study with pseudoangiomatous intradermal melanocytic nevi. *Am J Dermatopathol.* 1991;13:2–6.

130. Murray MR, Stout AP. The glomus tumor: investigation of its distribution and behavior, and the identity of its "epithelioid" cell. *Am J Pathol.* 1942;18:183–203.

131. Acebo E, Val-Bernal J, Arce F. Giant intravenous glomus tumor. *J Cutan Pathol.* 1997;24:384–389.

132. Yang J, Ko J, Suh K, et al. Congenital multiple plaque-like glomangiomyoma. *Am J Dermatopathol.* 1999;21:454–457.

133. Yoon T, Lee H, Chang S. Giant congenital multiple patch-like glomus tumors. *J Am Acad Dermatol.* 1999;40:826–828.

134. Hiruta N, Kameda N, Tokudome T, et al. Malignant glomus tumor: a case report and review of the literature. *Am J Surg Pathol.* 1997;21:1096–1103.

135. Lopez-Rios F, Rodriguez-Peralto J, Castano E, et al. Glomangiosarcoma of the lower limb: a case report with a literature review. *J Cutan Pathol.* 1997;24:571–574.

136. Brathwaite C, Poppiti R. Malignant glomus tumor. A case report of widespread metastases in a patient with multiple glomus body hamartomas. *Am J Surg Pathol.* 1996;20:233–238.

137. Folpe A, Fanburg-Smith J, Miettinen M, et al. Atypical and malignant glomus tumors: analysis of 52 cases, with a proposal for the reclassification of glomus tumors. *Am J Surg Pathol.* 2001;25: 1–12.

138. Watanabe K, Sugino T, Saito A, et al. Glomangiosarcoma of the hip: report of a highly aggressive tumour with widespread distant metastases. *Br J Dermatol.* 1998;139:1097–1101.

139. Weiss S, Enzinger F. Spindle cell hemangioendothelioma. A low-grade angiosarcoma resembling a cavernous hemangioma and Kaposi's sarcoma. *Am J Surg Pathol.* 1986;10:521–530.

140. Scott G, Rosai J. Spindle cell hemangioendothelioma. Report of seven additional cases of a recently described vascular neoplasm. *Am J Dermatopathol.* 1988;10:281–288.

141. Fletcher C, Beham A, Schmid C. Spindle cell haemangioendothelioma: a clinicopathological and immunohistochemical study indicative of a non-neoplastic lesion. *Histopathology.* 1991;18:291–301.

142. Pellegrini A, Drake R, Qualman S. Spindle cell hemangioendothelioma: a neoplasm associated with Maffucci's syndrome. *J Cutan Pathol.* 1995;22:173–176.

143. Perkins P, Weiss S. Spindle cell hemangioendothelioma. An analysis of 78 cases with reassessment of its pathogenesis and biologic behavior. *Am J Surg Pathol.* 1996;20:1196–1204.

144. Gardner T, Elston D. Multiple lower extremity and penile spindle cell hemangioendotheliomas. *Cutis.* 1998;62:23–26.

145. Hisaoka M, Hashimoto H, Iwamasa T. Diagnostic implication of Kaposi's sarcoma-associated herpesvirus with special reference to the distinction between spindle cell hemangioendothelioma and Kaposi's sarcoma. *Arch Pathol Lab Med.* 1998;122:72–76.

146. Whimster I. The pathology of lymphangioma circumscriptum. *Br J Dermatol.* 1976;94:473–486.

147. Flanagan B, Helwig E. Cutaneous lymphangioma. *Arch Dermatol.* 1977;113:24–30.

148. Dutheil P, Leraillez J, Guillemette J, et al. Generalized lymphangiomatosis with chylothorax and skin lymphangiomas in a neonate. *Pediatr Dermatol.* 1998;15:296–298.

149. Mu X, Tran T, Dupree M, et al. Acquired vulvar lymphangioma mimicking genital warts. A case report and review of the literature. *J Cutan Pathol.* 1999;26:150–154.

150. Oyler R, Davis D, Woosley J. Lymphangioma associated with Becker's nevus: a report of coincident hamartomas in a child. *Pediatr Dermatol.* 1997;14:376–379.

151. Jones E, Winkelmann R, Zachary C, et al. Benign lymphangioendothelioma. *J Am Acad Dermatol.* 1990;23:229–235.

152. Mehregan D, Mehregan A, Mehregan D. Benign lymphangioendothelioma: report of 2 cases. *J Cutan Pathol.* 1992; 19:502–505.

153. Guillou L, Fletcher C. Benign lymphangioendothelioma (acquired progressive lymphangioma): a lesion not to be confused with well-differentiated angiosarcoma and patch stage Kaposi's sarcoma: clinicopathologic analysis of a series. *Am J Surg Pathol.* 2000;24:1047–1057.

154. Tadaki T, Aiba S, Masu S, et al. Acquired progressive lymphangioma as a flat erythematous patch on the abdominal wall of a child. *Arch Dermatol.* 1988;124:699–701.

155. Sevila A, Botella-Estrada R, Sanmartin O, et al. Benign lymphangioendothelioma of the thigh simulating a low-grade angiosarcoma. *Am J Dermatopathol.* 2000;22:151–154.

156. Wilmer A, Kaatz M, Mentzel T, et al. Lymphangioendothelioma after a tick bite. *J Am Acad Dermatol.* 1998;39:126–128.

157. Weiss S, Enzinger F. Epithelioid hemangioendothelioma: a vascular tumor often mistaken for a carcinoma. *Cancer.* 1982;50:970–981.

158. Weiss S, Ishak K, Dail D, et al. Epithelioid hemangioendothelioma and related lesions. *Semin Diagn Pathol.* 1986;3:259–287.

159. Bollinger B, Laskin W, Knight C. Epithelioid hemangioendothelioma with multiple site involvement. Literature review and observations. *Cancer.* 1994; 73:610–615.

160. Marrogi A, Hunt S, Cruz D. Cutaneous epithelioid angiosarcoma. *Am J Dermatopathol.* 1990;12:350–356.

161. Polk P, Webb J. Isolated cutaneous epithelioid hemangioendothelioma. *J Am Acad Dermatol.* 1997;36:1026–1028.

162. Mentzel T, Beham A, Calonje E, et al. Epithelioid hemangioendothelioma of skin and soft tissues: clinicopathologic and immunohistochemical study of 30 cases. *Am J Surg Pathol.* 1997;21:363–374.

163. Quante M, Patel N, Hill S, et al. Epithelioid hemangioendothelioma presenting in the skin: a clinicopathologic study of eight cases. *Am J Dermatopathol.* 1998;20:541–546.

164. Roh H, Kim Y, Suhr K, et al. A case of childhood epithelioid hemangioendothelioma. *J Am Acad Dermatol.* 2000;42:897–899.

165. Kiryu H, Hashimoto H, Hori Y. Ossifying epithelioid hemangioendothelioma. *J Cutan Pathol.* 1996;23:558–561.

166. Mendlick M, Nelson M, Pickering D, et al. Translocation t(1; 3)(p36.3; q25) is a nonrandom aberration in epithelioid hemangioendothelioma. *Am J Surg Pathol.* 2001;25:684–687.

167. Cox FH, Helwig EB. Kaposi's sarcoma. *Cancer.* 1959;12:289–298.

168. O'Brien P, Brasfield R. Kaposi's sarcoma. *Cancer.* 1966;19:1497–1502.

169. Rothman S. Remarks on sex, age, and racial distribution of Kaposi's sarcoma and on possible pathogenetic factors. *Acta Un Int Cancer.* 1962;18:326.

170. DiGiovanna J, Safai B. Kaposi's sarcoma. Retrospective study of 90 cases

with particular emphasis on the familial occurrence, ethnic background and prevalence of other diseases. *Am J Med.* 1981;71:779–783.

171. Safai B, Mike V, Giraldo G, et al. Association of Kaposi's sarcoma with second primary malignancies: possible etiopathogenic implications. *Cancer.* 1980;45:1472–1479.

172. O'Connell K. Kaposi's sarcoma: histopathological study of 159 cases from Malawi. *J Clin Pathol.* 1977;30:687–695.

173. Templeton A. Kaposi's sarcoma. *Pathol Annu.* 1981;16:315–336.

174. Dorfman R. Kaposi's sarcoma. With special reference to its manifestations in infants and children and to the concepts of Arthur Purdy Stout. *Am J Surg Pathol.* 1986;10(suppl 1):68–77.

175. Friedman-Kien A, Saltzman B. Clinical manifestations of classical, endemic African, and epidemic AIDS-associated Kaposi's sarcoma. *J Am Acad Dermatol.* 1990;22:1237–1250.

176. Garcia-Muret M, Pujol R, Puig L, et al. Disseminated Kaposi's sarcoma not associated with HIV infection in a bisexual man. *J Am Acad Dermatol.* 1990;23:1035–1038.

177. Harwood A, Osoba D, Hofstader S, et al. Kaposi's sarcoma in recipients of renal transplants. *Am J Med.* 1979;67: 759–765.

178. Shmueli D, Shapira Z, Yussim A, et al. The incidence of Kaposi sarcoma in renal transplant patients and its relation to immunosuppression. *Transplant Proc.* 1989;21:3209–3210.

179. Chor P, Santa CD. Kaposi's sarcoma. A clinicopathologic review and differential diagnosis. *J Cutan Pathol.* 1992;19:6–20.

180. Francis N, Parkin J, Weber J, et al. Kaposi's sarcoma in acquired immune deficiency syndrome (AIDS). *J Clin Pathol.* 1986;39:469–474.

181. Santucci M, Pimpinelli N, Moretti S, et al. Classic and immunodeficiency-associated Kaposi's sarcoma. Clinical, histologic, and immunologic correlations. *Arch Pathol Lab Med.* 1988;112:1214–1220.

182. Niedt G, Myskowski P, Urmacher C, et al. Histology of early lesions of AIDS-associated Kaposi's sarcoma. *Mod Pathol.* 1990;3:64–70.

183. Ackerman A. Subtle clues to diagnosis by conventional microscopy. The patch stage of Kaposi's sarcoma. *Am J Dermatopathol.* 1979;1:165–172.

184. Blumenfeld W, Egbert B, Sagebiel R. Differential diagnosis of Kaposi's sarcoma. *Arch Pathol Lab Med.* 1985;109: 123–127.

185. Gottlieb G, Ackerman A. Kaposi's sarcoma: an extensively disseminated form in young homosexual men. *Hum Pathol.* 1982;13:882–892.

186. Kao G, Johnson F, Sulica V. The nature of hyaline (eosinophilic) globules and vascular slits of Kaposi's sarcoma. *Am J Dermatopathol.* 1990;12:256–267.

187. Fukunaga M, Silverberg S. Hyaline globules in Kaposi's sarcoma: a light microscopic and immunohistochemical study. *Mod Pathol.* 1991;4:187–190.

188. Gange R, Jones E. Lymphangioma-like Kaposi's sarcoma. A report of three cases. *Br J Dermatol.* 1979;100:327–334.

189. Holden C. Histogenesis of Kaposi's sarcoma and angiosarcoma of the face and the scalp. *J Invest Dermatol.* 1989;93: 119S–124S.

190. Chang Y, Cesarman E, Pessin M, et al. Identification of herpesvirus-like DNA sequences in AIDS-associated Kaposi's sarcoma. *Science.* 1994;266:1865–1869.

191. Dupin N, Grandadam M, Calvez V, et al. Herpesvirus-like DNA sequences in patients with Mediterranean Kaposi's sarcoma. *Lancet.* 1995;345:761–762.

192. Levy J. A new human herpesvirus: KSHV or HHV8? *Lancet.* 1995;346:786.

193. Sachsenberg-Studer E, Dobrynski N, Sheldon J, et al. Human herpes-virus 8 seropositive patient with skin and graft Kaposi's sarcoma after lung transplantation. *J Am Acad Dermatol.* 1999;40: 308–311.

194. Stewart FW, Treves N. Lymphangiosarcoma in postmastectomy lymphedema: a report of six cases in elephantiasis chirurgica. *Cancer.* 1948;1:64.

195. Allan A, Shoji T, Li N, et al. Two cases of Kaposi's sarcoma mimicking Stewart–Treves syndrome found to be human herpesvirus-8 positive. *Am J Dermatopathol.* 2001;23:431–436.

196. Cossu S, Satta R, Cottoni F, et al. Lymphangioma-like variant of Kaposi's sarcoma: clinicopathologic study of seven cases with review of the literature. *Am J Dermatopathol.* 1997;19:16–22.

197. Davis D, Scott D. Lymphangioma-like Kaposi's sarcoma: etiology and literature review. *J Am Acad Dermatol.* 2000; 43:123–127.

198. Borroni G, Brazzelli V, Vignoli G, et al. Bullous lesions in Kaposi's sarcoma: case report. *Am J Dermatopathol.* 1997;19:379–383.

199. Folpe A, Veikkola T, Valtola R, et al. Vascular endothelial growth factor receptor-3 (VEGFR-3): a marker of vascular tumors with presumed lymphatic differentiation, including Kaposi's sarcoma, kaposiform and Dabska-type hemangioendotheliomas, and a subset of angiosarcomas. *Mod Pathol.* 2000;13: 180–185.

200. Herman P, Shogreen M, White W. The evaluation of human herpesvirus 8 (Kaposi's sarcoma-associated herpesvirus) in cutaneous lesions of Kaposi's sarcoma: a study of formalin-fixed paraffin-embedded tissue. *Am J Dermatopathol.* 1998;20:7–11.

201. Nuovo M, Nuovo G. Utility of HHV8 RNA detection for differentiating Kaposi's sarcoma from its mimics. *J Cutan Pathol.* 2001;28:248–255.

202. Enzinger F, Smith B. Hemangiopericytoma. An analysis of 106 cases. *Hum Pathol.* 1976;7:61–82.

203. Hultberg B, Daugaard S, Johansen H, et al. Malignant haemangiopericytomas and haemangioendotheliosarcomas: an immunohistochemical study. *Histopathology.* 1988;12:405–414.

204. Schurch W, Skalli O, Lagace R, et al. Intermediate filament proteins and actin isoforms as markers for soft-tissue tumor differentiation and origin. III. Hemangiopericytomas and glomus tumors. *Am J Pathol.* 1990;136:771–786.

205. Porter P, Bigler S, McNutt M, et al. The immunophenotype of hemangiopericytomas and glomus tumors, with special reference to muscle protein expression: an immunohistochemical study and review of the literature. *Mod Pathol.* 1991;4:46–52.

206. Nunnery E, Kahn L, Reddick R, et al. Hemangiopericytoma: a light microscopic and ultrastructural study. *Cancer.* 1981;47:906–914.

207. Pollock A, Sweeney E. Polypoid dermal hemangiopericytoma: a case report. *Am J Dermatopathol.* 1998;20:506–508.

208. Zelger B, Zelger B. Polypoid dermal hemangiopericytoma? An alternative point of view. *Am J Dermatopathol.* 1999; 21:588–589.

209. Folpe A, Devaney K, Weiss S. Lipomatous hemangiopericytoma: a rare variant of hemangiopericytoma that may be confused with liposarcoma. *Am J Surg Pathol.* 1999;23:1201–1207.

210. Guillou L, Gebhard S, Coindre J. Lipomatous hemangiopericytoma: a fat-containing variant of solitary fibrous tumor? Clinicopathologic, immunohistochemical, and ultrastructural analysis of a series in favor of a unifying concept. *Hum Pathol.* 2000;31:1108–1115.

211. Middleton L, Duray P, Merino M. The histological spectrum of hemangiopericytoma: application of immunohistochemical analysis including proliferative markers to facilitate diagnosis and predict prognosis. *Hum Pathol.* 1998;29: 636–640.

212. Okamura J, Barr R, Battifora H. Solitary fibrous tumor of the skin. *Am J Dermatopathol.* 1997;19:515–518.

213. Hardisson D, Cuevas-Santos J, Contreras F. Solitary fibrous tumor of the skin. *J Am Acad Dermatol.* 2002;46:S37–S40.

214. Granter S, Badizadegan K, Fletcher C. Myofibromatosis in adults, glomangiopericytoma, and myopericytoma: a spectrum of tumors showing perivascular myoid differentiation. *Am J Surg Pathol.* 1998;22:513–525.

215. Dabska M. Malignant endovascular papillary angioendothelioma of the skin in childhood. Clinicopathologic study of 6 cases. *Cancer.* 1969;24:503–510.

216. Manivel J, Wick M, Swanson P, et al. Endovascular papillary angioendothelioma of childhood: a vascular lesion possibly characterized by "high" endothelial cell differentiation. *Hum Pathol.* 1986;17:1240–1244.

217. Morgan J, Robinson M, Rosen L, et al. Malignant endovascular papillary angioendothelioma (Dabska tumor). A case report and review of the literature. *Am J Dermatopathol.* 1989;11:64–68.

218. Argani P, Athanasian E. Malignant endovascular papillary angioendothelioma (Dabska tumor) arising within a deep intramuscular hemangioma. *Arch Pathol Lab Med.* 1997;121:992–995.

219. Fanburg-Smith J, Michal M, Partanen T, et al. Papillary intralymphatic angioendothelioma (PILA): a report of twelve cases of a distinctive vascular tumor with phenotypic features of lymphatic vessels. *Am J Surg Pathol.* 1999;23:1004–1010.

220. Sanz-Trelles A, Rodrigo-Fernandez I, Ayala-Carbonero A, et al. Retiform hemangioendothelioma. A new case in a child with diffuse endovascular papillary endothelial proliferation. *J Cutan Pathol.* 1997;24:440–444.

221. Calonje E, Fletcher C, Wilson-Jones E, et al. Retiform hemangioendothelioma. A

distinctive form of low-grade angiosarcoma delineated in a series of 15 cases. *Am J Surg Pathol.* 1994;18:115–125.

222. Duke D, Dvorak A, Harris T, et al. Multiple retiform hemangioendotheliomas. A low-grade angiosarcoma. *Am J Dermatopathol.* 1996;18:606–610.

223. Schommer M, Herbst R, Brodersen J, et al. Retiform hemangioendothelioma: another tumor associated with human herpesvirus type 8? *J Am Acad Dermatol.* 2000;42:290–292.

224. Zukerberg L, Nickoloff B, Weiss S. Kaposiform hemangioendothelioma of infancy and childhood. An aggressive neoplasm associated with Kasabach–Merritt syndrome and lymphangiomatosis. *Am J Surg Pathol.* 1993;17:321–328.

225. Gianotti R, Gelmetti C, Alessi E. Congenital cutaneous multifocal kaposiform hemangioendothelioma. *Am J Dermatopathol.* 1999;21:557–561.

226. Vin-Christian K, McCalmont T, Frieden I. Kaposiform hemangioendothelioma. An aggressive, locally invasive vascular tumor that can mimic hemangioma of infancy. *Arch Dermatol.* 1997;133:1573–1578.

227. Nayler S, Rubin B, Calonje E, et al. Composite hemangioendothelioma: a complex, low-grade vascular lesion mimicking angiosarcoma. *Am J Surg Pathol.* 2000;24:352–361.

228. Holden C, Spittle M, Jones E. Angiosarcoma of the face and scalp, prognosis and treatment. *Cancer.* 1987;59:1046–1057.

229. Offori T, Platt C, Stephens M, et al. Angiosarcoma in congenital hereditary lymphoedema (Milroy's disease)–diagnostic beacons and a review of the literature. *Clin Exp Dermatol.* 1993;18:174–177.

230. Mark R, Tran L, Sercarz J, et al. Angiosarcoma of the head and neck. The UCLA experience 1955 through 1990. *Arch Otolaryngol Head Neck Surg.* 1993;119:973–978.

231. Girard C, Johnson W, Graham J. Cutaneous angiosarcoma. *Cancer.* 1970;26:868–883.

232. Fletcher C, Beham A, Bekir S, et al. Epithelioid angiosarcoma of deep soft tissue: a distinctive tumor readily mistaken for an epithelial neoplasm. *Am J Surg Pathol.* 1991;15:915–924.

233. Rosai J, Sumner H, Kostianovsky M, et al. Angiosarcoma of the skin. A clinicopathologic and fine structural study. *Hum Pathol.* 1976;7:83–109.

234. McWilliam L, Harris M. Granular cell angiosarcoma of the skin: histology, electron microscopy and immunohistochemistry of a newly recognized tumor. *Histopathology.* 1985;9:1205–1216.

235. Cabo H, Cohen E, Casas G, et al. Cutaneous angiosarcoma arising on the radiation site of a congenital facial hemangioma. *Int J Dermatol.* 1998;37:638–639.

236. Ben-Izhak O, Vlodavsky E, Ofer A, et al. Epithelioid angiosarcoma associated with a Dacron vascular graft. *Am J Surg Pathol.* 1999;23:1418–1422.

237. Folpe A, Johnston C, Weiss S. Cutaneous angiosarcoma arising in a gouty tophus: report of a unique case and a review of foreign material-associated angiosarcomas. *Am J Dermatopathol.* 2000;22:418–421.

238. Val-Bernal J, Figols J, Arce F, et al. Cardiac epithelioid angiosarcoma presenting as cutaneous metastases. *J Cutan Pathol.* 2001;28:265–270.

239. Rudd R, Fair K, Patterson J. Aortic angiosarcoma presenting with cutaneous metastasis: case report and review of the literature. *J Am Acad Dermatol.* 2000;43:930–933.

240. Smith K, Lupton G, Skelton H. Cutaneous angiosarcomas with a starry-sky pattern. *Arch Pathol Lab Med.* 1997;121:980–984.

241. Meis-Kindblom J, Kindblom L. Angiosarcoma of soft tissue: a study of 80 cases. *Am J Surg Pathol.* 1998;22:683–697.

242. Diaz-Cascajo C, de la Vega M, Rey-Lopez A. Superinfected cutaneous angiosarcoma: a highly malignant neoplasm simulating an inflammatory process. *J Cutan Pathol.* 1997;24:56–60.

243. Fink-Puches R, Zochling N, Wolf P, et al. No detection of human herpesvirus 8 in different types of cutaneous angiosarcoma. *Arch Dermatol.* 2002;138:131–132.

244. Hoda SA, Cranor ML, Rosen PP. Hemangiomas of the breast with atypical histological features. Further analysis of histological subtypes confirming their benign character. *Am J Surg Pathol.* 1992;16:53–60.

245. Fineberg S, Rosen PP. Cutaneous angiosarcoma and atypical vascular lesions of the skin and breast after radiation therapy for breast carcinoma. *Am J Clin Pathol (United States).* Dec 1994;102:757–763.

246. Sener SF, Milos S, Feldman JL, et al. The spectrum of vascular lesions in the mammary skin, including angiosarcoma, after breast conservation treatment for breast cancer. *J Am Coll Surg (United States).* Jul 2001;193:22–28.

247. Requena L, Kutzner H, Mentzel T, Duran R, Rodriguez-Peralto JL. Benign vascular proliferations in irradiated skin. *Am J Surg Pathol.* 2002;26:328–337.

CHAPTER 21

Kaposi Sarcoma

Reuven Bergman, M.D.
Emma Guttman-Yassky, M.D.
Ronit Sarid, Ph.D.

BOX 21-1 Overview

- There are four clinical and epidemiological forms of Kaposi sarcoma (KS): classic KS (CKS), African (endemic) KS, epidemic AIDS-related KS, and KS in iatrogenically immunosuppressed patients.
- CKS is usually the most indolent form of KS.
- All forms of KS share similar histological findings.
- Human herpesvirus 8 (HHV-8) is the primary etiologic agent of KS; yet, HHV-8 is not sufficient by itself for the development of KS in seropositive individuals.
- Seropositive rates for HHV-8 show geographic variations strongly correlated with the risk of KS in the general population.
- In homosexual individuals, HHV-8 may be sexually transmitted by anal and/or oral contacts. In other forms of KS, nonsexual horizontal mode of transmission seems to play a major role.
- There has been a dramatic decline in epidemic, AIDS-related KS since the introduction of HAART chemotherapy.
- Most treatments for KS, especially CKS are palliative.
- KS in iatrogenically immunosuppressed patients may regress following the cessation of immunosuppressive therapy and Sirolimus may cause regression of kidney-transplant-associated KS.
- The newly approved agents for AIDS-related KS include alitretiroxin gel for topical administration, and liposomal doxorubicin, liposomal daunorubicin, palcitaxel, and interferon alpha for systemic treatment.

INTRODUCTION

In 1872, Moritz Kaposi first described "idiopatisches multiples pigmentsarkom der Haut" (idiopathic, multiple, pigment sarcoma), later designated Kaposi sarcoma (KS).[1] KS is a locally aggressive, vascular tumor that typically presents with cutaneous lesions in the form of multiple patches, plaques, or nodules; but, may also involve mucosal sites, lymph nodes, and visceral organs. The disease is uniformly associated with human herpesvirus 8 (HHV-8) infection.[2]

CLINICAL MANIFESTATIONS

BOX 21-2 Summary

- CKS arises mainly in patients over the age of 50 with a slow development of angiomatous patches, plaques, and nodules, most frequently on the lower extremities.
- CKS usually runs a relatively benign course, although it may spread extracutaneously and it is associated with an increased rate of reticuloendothelial malignancies.
- African (endemic) KS has been one of the most common neoplastic diseases in Africa.
- Four clinically distinct types of African (endemic) KS have been observed:
  - a benign nodular type, similar to CKS,
  - an infiltrative (aggressive) localized form,
  - a widely disseminated florid form with mucocutaneous and visceral involvement,
  - an unusually virulent lymphadenopathic type seen mostly in prepubescent African children.
- Epidemic, AIDS-related KS is one of the most common neoplasms in homosexual and bisexual men with AIDS, although its frequency has declined dramatically since the introduction of HAART chemotherapy.
- In contrast to CKS, the lesions in epidemic, AIDS-related KS are multiple, more widespread, and tend more to involve mucosal surfaces and internal organs such as the lungs, gastrointestinal tract, and lymph nodes.
- Immunosuppressive therapy for organ transplant recipients, especially kidney transplants, and long-term corticosteroid treatment for a variety of dermatological and other conditions may induce KS iatrogenically.
- KS in iatrogenically immunosuppressed patients may have a more aggressive clinical course than does CKS, and more frequent dissemination and internal organ involvement.
- Iatrogenically induced KS may regress following the cessation of the immunosuppressive therapy.

There are four clinical and epidemiological forms of KS that are recognized.

Classic KS

The disease mainly arises in patients over the age of 50 with a slow develop-

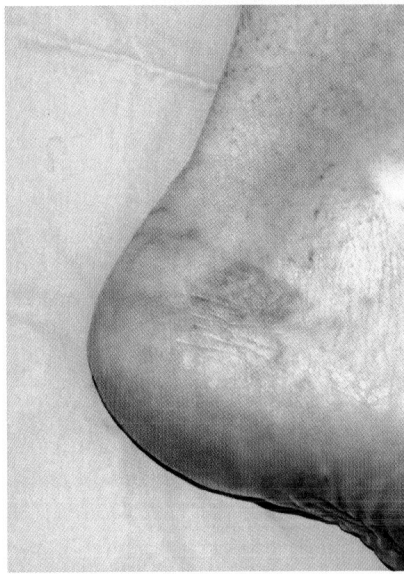

▲ **FIGURE 21-1** Early erythematous patch of CKS.

ment of angiomatous patches (Fig. 21-1), plaques, and nodules (Fig. 21-2), most frequently on the lower extremities.[3] The disease runs a protracted course, and those affected usually die of unrelated causes.[3] There is a distinct preponderance of people of either Jewish or Mediterranean descent and a preponderance of males over females.[3,4] Although KS has been reported in siblings and other members of the same family,[5] familial occurrences are rare. Classic KS

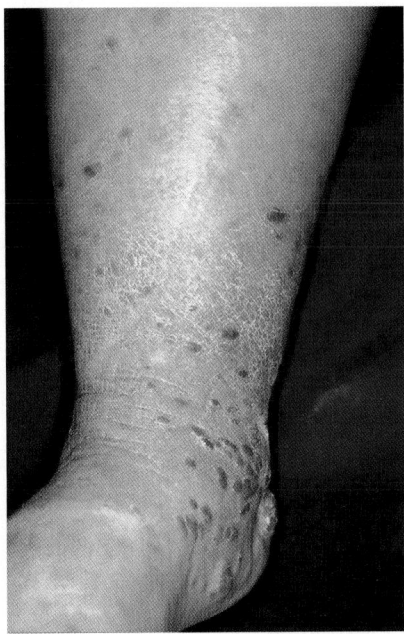

▲ **FIGURE 21-2** Numerous red nodules of CKS along with lymphedema.

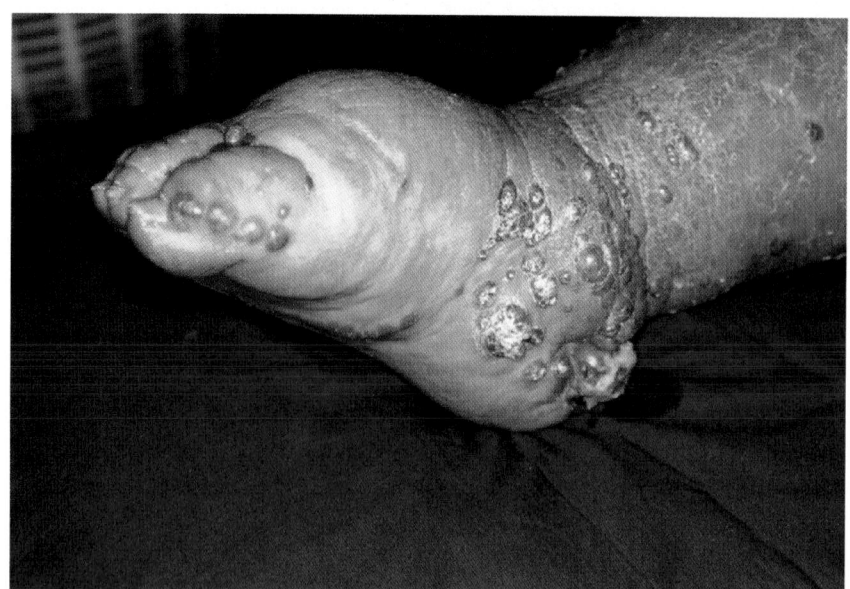

▲ **FIGURE 21-3** Marked lymphedematous lower extremity covered by numerous bluish red nodules and tumors of CKS. Some of the tumors display verrucous and hyperkeratotic surfaces.

(CKS) has been infrequently reported in children and young adults.[6]

CKS may present with single or multiple tumor lesions. The lesions often start as single or multiple bluish red nodules (Fig. 21-2) on the distal portions of the lower extremities. In most instances, the lesions progress very slowly and may coalesce to form large plaques, and subsequently nodules and tumors (Fig. 21-3).[7] As the lesions age, they become brownish in color, and may display a verrucous and hyperkeratotic surface (Fig. 21-3). Eczematous changes, erosions, and ulcerations may occur. Occasionally, individual lesions regress spontaneously, while new lesions continue to appear.[3] Unilateral involvement, seen at the onset of the disease, changes to bilateral and later to a more disseminated, multicentric pattern spreading in a centripetal fashion. An initial pitting edema may evolve fibrotic swelling of the limb that causes considerable discomfort (Fig. 21-3).[7]

CKS usually develops very slowly and therefore runs a rather benign course; however, rapid course with the development of disseminated mucocutaneous (Fig. 21-4) and visceral lesions may occur.[3,7] CKS may be in the skin alone or with involvement of the lymph nodes, oral cavity, gastrointestinal tract, liver, lungs, kidneys, or spleen of patients with longstanding disease.[3] Lesions of the brain or testes have rarely been reported.[6] Visceral lesions are frequently asymptomatic and may be discovered only at autopsy.[8,9] Rarely, KS has been detected within lymph nodes or visceral organs in the absence of skin lesions. An increased incidence of primary malignancies of reticuloendothelial origin, such as a non-Hodgkin's or other B-cell lymphomas, has been reported in CKS patients.[3,10]

African Endemic KS

Before the appearance of the human immunodeficiency virus (HIV), African KS was largely an endemic disease.[11] Its endemic occurrence was first noted in the 1950s, thus antedating the outbreak of the AIDS pandemic by several decades.[12] KS was soon recognized to be one of the most common neoplastic diseases in the black population in equatorial Africa and has been reported to account for 9% of all cancers in Uganda.[12,13]

Before the recognition of AIDS, four clinically distinct types of endemic KS in black Africans had been seen[3,7]:

1. Benign *nodular type*, similar to the "classical" localized disease

2. *Infiltrative* (*aggressive*) localized form, characterized by large, sometimes fungating, locally infiltrative lesions in which the tumors invade the underlying soft tissues and bone

3. A widely disseminated *florid form* with a widespread mucocutaneous and visceral involvement

4. An unusually virulent *lymphadenopathic* type

Nodular endemic KS runs a rather benign course, and resembles CKS. *The infiltrative (aggressive)* variants are characterized by a more aggressive biologic behavior and may extend deeply into the dermis, subcutis, muscle, and bone. All three forms occur in African adults with a male-to-female ratio of about 7:1 and patients' age ranging between 25 and 40 years. *Lymphadenopathic KS* is seen almost exclusively in prepubescent black African children between ages of 1 and 15 years (mean, 3 years) with a male-to-female ratio of 3:1.[8,12–16] In these children, the disease is characterized by rapidly disseminated tumors most often limited to the lymph nodes with occasional visceral organ involvement, and the absence of cutaneous lesions.[3] It is generally fatal within 1 to 3 years.[3,17]

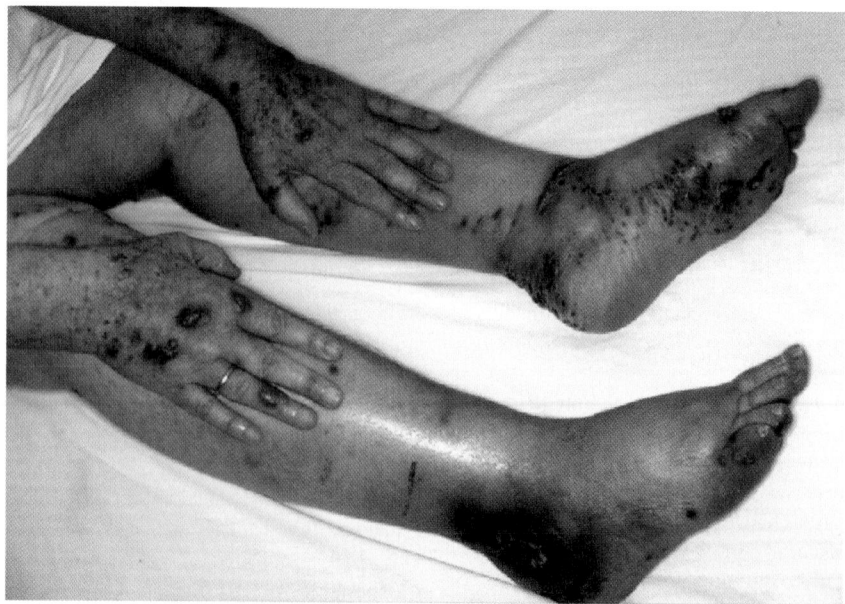

▲ **FIGURE 21-4** Numerous dark and hemorrhagic nodules of CKS that have spread rapidly to involve the lower and upper extremities.

KS in Africa has now reached epidemic proportions because of the explosive spread of AIDS.[11] The level of HHV-8 viremia has been shown to be significantly lower in patients with true endemic KS compared to those with AIDS who had similar tumor burdens.[18] This finding supports the premise that HIV-1 infection augments HHV-8 replication.

Epidemic, AIDS-Related KS

KS is one of the most common neoplasms in homosexual and bisexual men with AIDS.[19] Originally about 40% of patients with AIDS had concomitant KS, but this high percentage has later fallen to around 20% in the United States[20–22] and Europe.[23] KS is much more common in patients with AIDS than in the general population[20] and the risk to develop KS is much higher in homosexual males than in heterosexual males or females; such as hemophiliacs who receive contaminated blood products or drug abusers who share needles.[24]

The distribution of lesions in AIDS-related KS differs from that in CKS. The trunk, arms, head, and neck are frequently involved while lesions are usually multiple. There is frequent involvement of mucosal surfaces and internal organs such as the lungs, gastrointestinal tract, and lymph nodes, while about one-third of the patients may have evidence of visceral lesions without skin lesions.[7,25] The extent of cutaneous involvement does not correlate with the extent of visceral disease. Compared with the slow-growing, usually round tumors of CKS, the widespread skin and mucosal lesions of AIDS-related KS are highly varied in configuration (round, oval, elongated, fusiform, or irregular in shape) and tend to develop rapidly in a bilateral symmetric pattern of distribution along the lines of cleavage.[3] The diagnosis of AIDS has frequently been made by the chance discovery of one or more painless pink, deep purple, or brown skin lesions of KS in an otherwise seemingly healthy HIV-infected person.[3]

The clinical course ranges from chronic to rapidly progressive. Most patients die from opportunistic infections or other complications of AIDS rather than from KS.[3,7] The introduction of highly active antiretroviral therapy (HAART) aimed at controlling HIV has been associated with a dramatic decrease in the incidence of AIDS-KS and the clinical manifestations of KS appear to be less aggressive.[26–28] This has been associated with persistent reduction in circulating HHV-8-infected cells.[28]

KS in Iatrogenically Immunosuppressed Patients

Immunosuppressive therapy for organ transplant recipients is complicated by relatively high rates of malignant diseases, one of which is KS. KS may also be induced by chemotherapy for tumors and long-term corticosteroid treatment for a variety of dermatological and other conditions.[29–35] The induction of KS by immunosuppressive therapy and its subsequent regression on removal of such treatments provided some of the earlier clinical recognition of the reversibility of KS.[19] Iatrogenic KS may have a more aggressive clinical course than that of CKS with more frequent involvement of the gastrointestinal tract and disseminated disease.[29]

In the transplant setting, HHV-8 infection may be associated with fatal KS.[11,36,37] Most studies have supported the presumption that iatrogenic KS patients are HHV-8-positive before transplantation, implying that activation of latent viral infection leads to KS.[38,39] However, it has been recently proven that infected cells from organ donors themselves may also contribute to the development of post-transplant KS.[37,40]

The prevalence of KS in renal transplant patients is reported to be 0.4 to 5.3%.[29,38,39,41–43] It has been recently shown that conversion from cyclosporine to sirolimus, a new immunosuppressive agent with potent antitumor activity in renal transplant patients with KS, resulted in complete regression of the KS lesions without increasing the risk of graft rejection.[44]

■ HISTOPATHOLOGY

BOX 21-3   Summary

- The microscopic features of all four different epidemiological, clinical types of KS do not differ.
- The early macular stage (patch stage, early type) is characterized by proliferation of dilated, thin-walled, irregularly shaped blood vessels in the dermis, and a patchy, sparse perivascular infiltrate consisting of lymphocytes and plasma cells. A few spindle cells, red blood cell extravasation, and siderophages may also be present between the blood vessels.
- A lymphangiomatous type is a variant of the early type characterized by bloodless lymphatic-like spaces that dissect out collagen to give an appearance resembling lymphatic vessels.

- The plaque stage (mixed pattern type) is characterized by more or less equal mixture of spindle cells, and jagged vascular spaces and slits. Intracytoplasmic hyaline globules that represent destroyed red blood vessels are frequently found within spindle cells and macrophages.
- The nodular stage (spindle cell type) is formed by interlacing bundles of monomorphic spindle cells and vascular slits resulting in a honeycomb-like network of blood-filled spaces or slits associated with interweaving spindle cells.
- A pleomorphic (anaplastic form) exhibits greater cellularity, nuclear pleomorphism, and more frequent mitotic figures.
- Practically all cases, irrespective of epidemiologic subgroups, stain with an antibody to HHV-8 latency-associated nuclear antigen-1 (LANA-1). This may be used as the main tool to differentiate KS from its histological simulants.

The microscopic features of all four different epidemiological–clinical types of KS do not differ.[2] The histopathology of fully developed nodules of KS in all types of the disease is distinctive and should rarely cause problems in the diagnosis. The diagnostic pitfalls lie mainly in the early macular lesions and in the late lesions with marked cytologic atypia.[24] There is a rough correspondence between the clinical type of lesion and the histological stage, although, in reality, there is an overlap between stages; multiple biopsies taken at the same time or even a single biopsy may show features of different histologic stages.[24] The following are the main histologic subtypes:

Macular stage (patch stage, early type) (Figs. 21-1 and 21-5 to 21-7): It is characterized by proliferation of dilated, thin-walled, irregularly shaped blood vessels, around preexisting normal blood vessels in the dermis and/or aggregation of these vessels in close association with sweat glands, pilosebaceous structures, dermal nerves, and/or dissection of collagen by dilated or compressed thin-walled "jagged" vessels.[45,46] Normal adnexal structures and preexisting blood vessels often protrude into newly formed blood vessels, known as the "promontory sign." A few spindle cells, red blood cell extravasation, and siderophages may also be present in between the blood vessels. There is also usually a patchy, sparse, dermal perivascular infiltrate consisting of lymphocytes and plasma cells.[24] In some cases, the lesions are characterized by bloodless lymphatic-like spaces

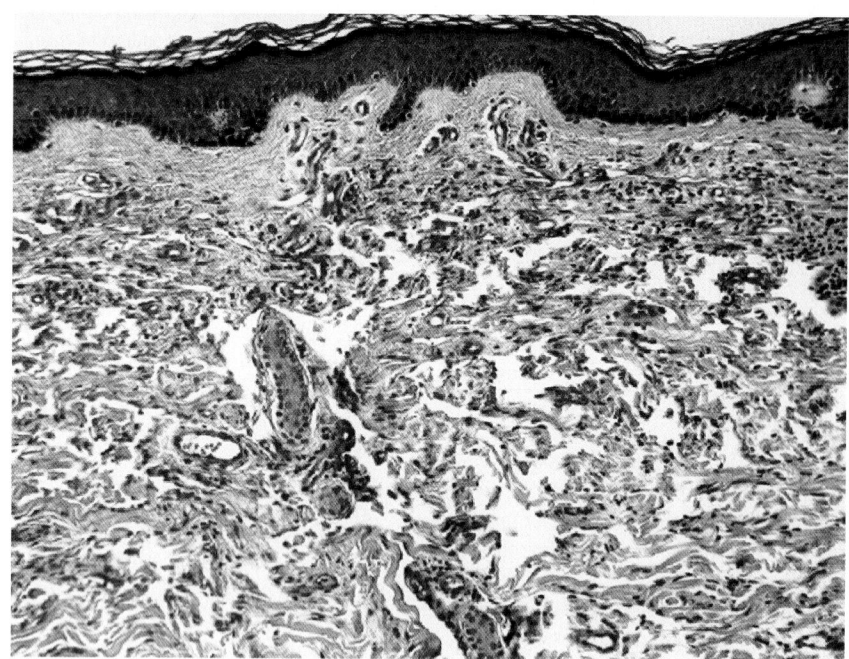

▲ **FIGURE 21-5** Patch-stage KS characterized by proliferation of irregularly shaped blood vessels around preexisting normal blood vessels and in between the dermal collagen bundles (hematoxylin–eosin (H&E), 200×).

that dissect out collagen to give an appearance resembling lymphatic vessels or a lymphangioma. This has also been designated as a *lymphangiomatous* type.[45,46]

Plaque stage (mixed pattern type): It has more or less equal mixtures of spindle cells and jagged vascular spaces and slits. The haphazard dispersal of the erythrocytes between the tumor cells may impart a distinctive low-power appearance described as "blood sponge." In the areas where the bundles of spindle cells are cut in cross section, a sieve-like appearance results in which the red blood cells seem to be lying in empty spaces.[45,46] The inflammatory infiltrates are more dense often with numerous siderophages.[2] Intracytoplasmic hyaline globules that represent destroyed red blood cells are frequently found.[2,24] They may be seen within spindle cells and macrophages or in an extracellular location; they also resemble Russel bodies and are PAS-positive.[47]

Nodular stage (spindle cell type) (Figs. 21-2, 21-3, 21-8, and 21-9): It is formed by interlacing bundles of monomorphic spindle cells and vascular slits.[45,46] The characteristic feature is a honeycomb-like network of blood-filled spaces or slits associated with interweaving spindle cells.[24] Either element can focally predominate.[45,46] The spindle-cell component shows variable nuclear pleomorphism and mitotic figures are usually infrequent.[47] Epidermal changes vary with the lesion, and include atrophy and ulceration over raised lesions, along with a peripheral epidermal collaret about papules and nodules resembling a pyogenic granuloma. A *pleomorphic (anaplastic form)* exhibits greater cellularity, nuclear pleomorphism, and more frequent mitotic figures; it may be difficult to differentiate from angiosarcoma, fibrosarcoma, and other pleomorphic and anaplastic malignant neoplasms.[45–47]

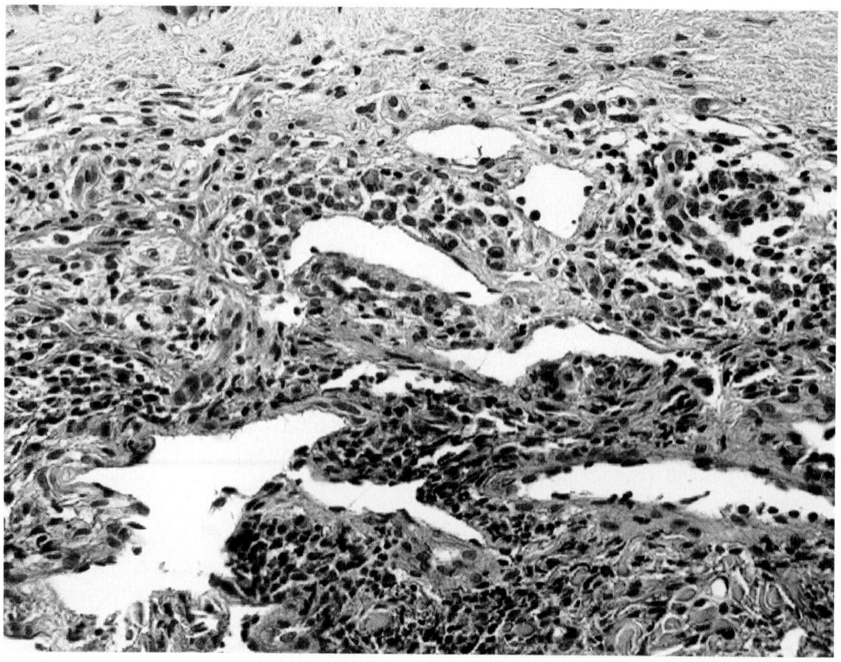

Immunohistochemistry

The lining cells of clearly developed vascular structures are usually positive for vascular markers (Fig. 21-7), while the spindle cells consistently show positive reaction for CD34 and commonly for CD31, but are factor VIII-negative.[2] Practically all cases, irrespective of epidemiologic subgroup, stain positively with an antibody to HHV-8 latency-associated nuclear antigen-1 (LANA-1) (Fig. 21-10).[2,48,49]

Differential Diagnosis

There are numerous conditions that either simulate KS or may be simulated by it, histologically.[50] Early lesions may be exceedingly subtle and may simulate closely a superficial perivascular or lichenoid dermatitis. Stasis changes and its exaggerated form acroangiodermatitis may also cause difficulty in the differential diagnosis. In more advanced lesions, the list of lesions to differentiate histologically include progressive lymphangioma, hemangiomas, pyogenic granuloma, angiosarcoma, scars, dermatofibromas, spindle-cell squamous cell carcinoma, spindle-cell malignant melanoma, leiomyosarcoma, glomus tumor, intravascular endothelial hyperplasia (Masson), angiolymphoid hyperplasia with eosinophilia,[50] Kaposiform hemangioendothelioma, spindle-cell hemangioma, reactive angioendotheliomatosis,

▲ **FIGURE 21-6** Patch-stage KS. The irregularly shaped blood vessels are surrounded by mononuclear cell infiltrates containing many plasma cells (H&E, 400×).

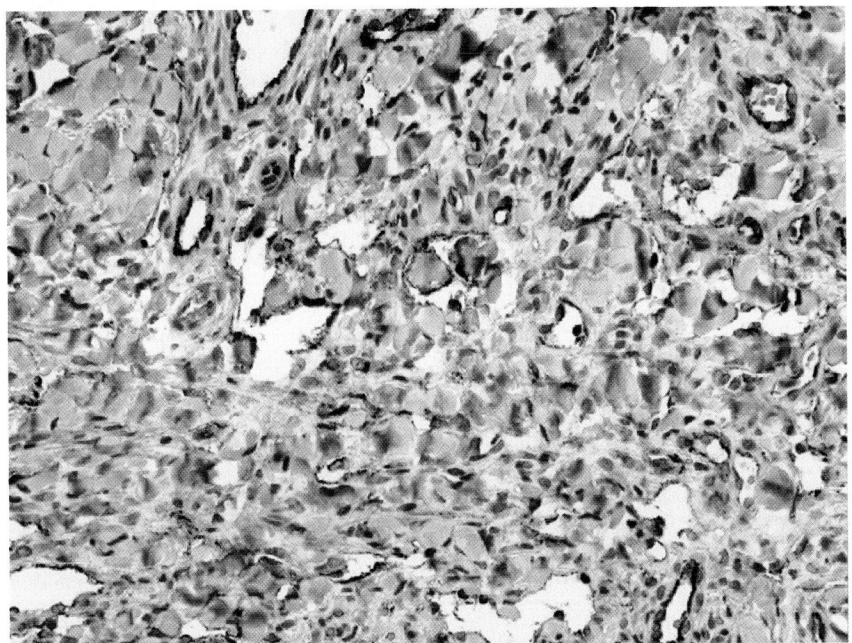

▲ **FIGURE 21-7** Patch-stage KS. CD31 immunostaining delineates the thin walls of the irregularly shaped blood vessels dissecting the dermal collagen bundles (immunoperoxidase, 400×).

bacillary angiomatosis, microvenular hemangioma, hobnail hemangioma, arteriovenous hemangioma,[49] and dermatofibrosarcoma protruberans.[51]

The differential diagnosis of KS from its simulants has become much easier with the immunohistochemical demonstration of HHV-8 LANA-1 (Fig. 21-10). Practically all cases of KS are associated with this virus and stain positively, whereas all the vascular and nonvascular simulants stain negatively.[48,49,51]

■ ETIOLOGY AND PATHOGENESIS
Human Herpesvirus 8 (HHV-8)

BOX 21-4 Summary

- HHV-8 is the primary etiologic agent of KS; yet, HHV-8 infection is not sufficient for KS.
- Among human herpesviruses, HHV-8 is most closely related to EBV.
- HHV-8 persists for the lifetime of an infected individual and exhibits two divergent phases of infection: latent and lytic.
- The lytic cycle is crucial for virus spread between cells and hosts, and is also likely to play an important role in the tumorigenesis induced by HHV-8.
- The signaling pathways that operate in the transition between latent and lytic phase are not completely understood.

HHV-8, also known as KS-associated herpesvirus (KSHV), is the primary etiologic agent of KS.[52]

This, now a widely accepted notion, is based on the following observations: (i) the common detection of viral DNA in KS lesions, but not in adjacent tissue of patients with all forms of the disease; (ii) the presence of HHV-8 in critical cellular components of KS, namely endothelial and spindle cells; (iii) the general correlation between HHV-8 prevalence and population risk to develop KS; and (iv) the strong predictive value of antibodies directed against HHV-8 antigens in the blood of HIV-infected subjects for their future development of KS. Yet, HHV-8 infection is not sufficient for KS, and the majority of infected individuals will never develop the disease.[38,53]

HHV-8 is classified as a gamma-2-herpesvirus, or rhadinovirus, and shares close homology with several primate and nonprimate mammalian viruses.[54,55] Among human herpesviruses, it is most closely related to the Epstein–Barr virus, known as a ubiquitous lymphotrophic virus that is associated causally with several human cancers, including certain types of lymphomas. Likely, HHV-8 has also been associated with two lymphoproliferative diseases, namely primary effusion lymphoma[56] and some forms of multicentric Castleman disease.[57] Rare cases presenting a concomitant occurrence of two or three HHV-8-related diseases have been reported in the literature.[58,59]

Natural Host Infection by HHV-8

Primary infection with HHV-8 persists for life.[38,53] In the host cell, infection with HHV-8 displays two distinct cycles: latent and lytic. During latency, the viral genome persists as a circular DNA (mini-chromosome), only few viral genes are expressed, and no viral particles are produced. The cellular site of HHV-8 latency and the mechanisms by which the latent virus escapes elimination by the hosts' immune system are not fully understood. In contrast to the latent cycle, extensive viral DNA replication and a well-controlled array of viral gene expression characterize the

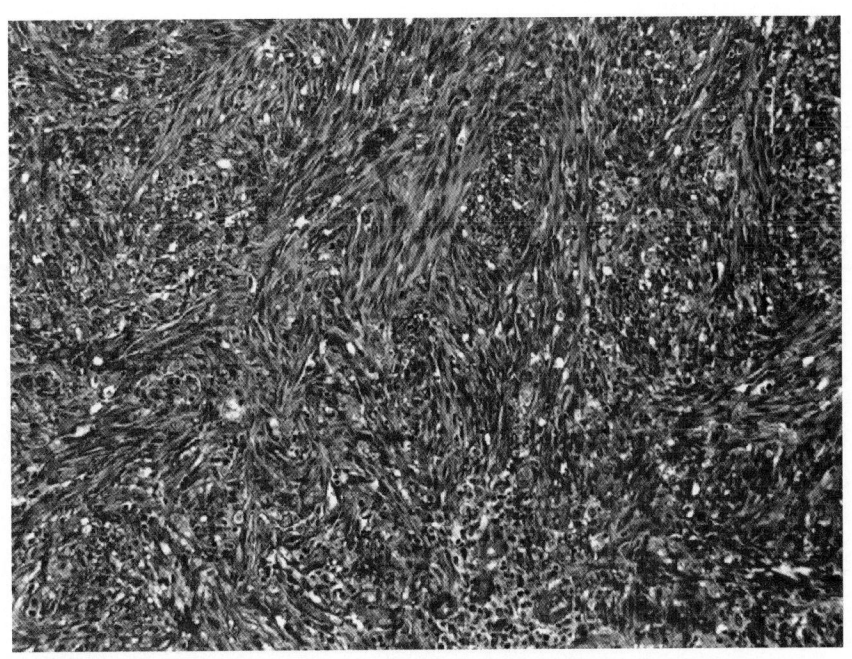

▲ **FIGURE 21-8** Nodular KS characterized by interlacing bundles of monomorphic spindle cells and vascular slits containing numerous erythrocytes (H&E, 200×).

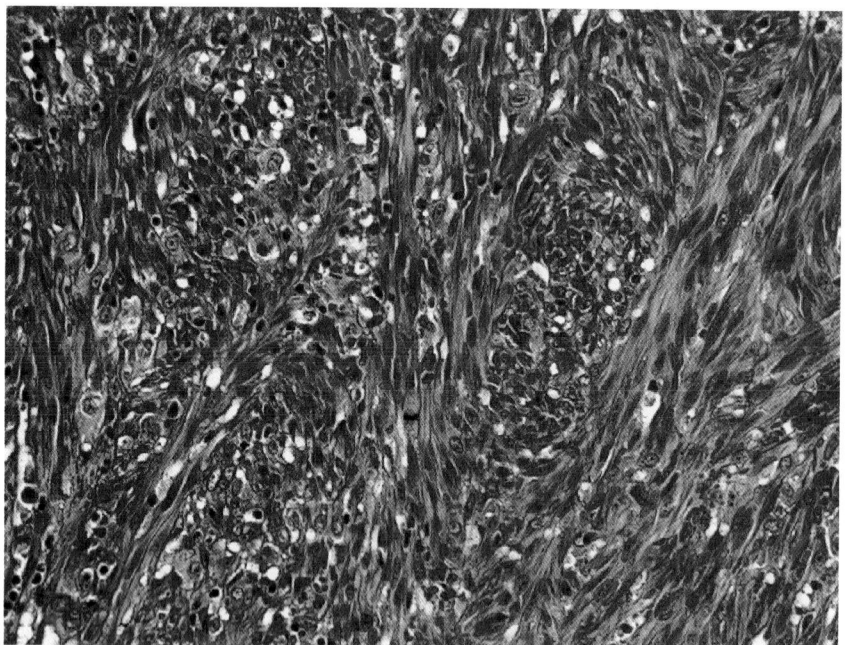

▲ **FIGURE 21-9** Higher magnification of Fig. 21-8 showing the interlacing bundles of spindle cells forming vascular slits engorged with erythrocytes (H&E, 400×).

lytic cycle, which may culminate in the production of infectious progeny virus and host cell death. This cycle is crucial for virus spread between cells and hosts, and is also likely to play an important role in the tumorigenesis induced by HHV-8. Certain physiologic conditions periodically reactivate the hidden latent virus in most asymptomatic carriers, increasing the risk for disease onset. Only some of the variables involved in this switch are known, and the interplay

between such variables is even less understood. The role of host immunodeficiency and the impact of the HIV-encoded TAT protein on HHV-8 activation and pathogenicity are well established. Accordingly, the use of HAART has led to decreased incidence rates of KS in AIDS patients,[60] and to the remission of clinical KS.[61] However, additional important factors and host signal transduction pathways that must operate in the transition between latent

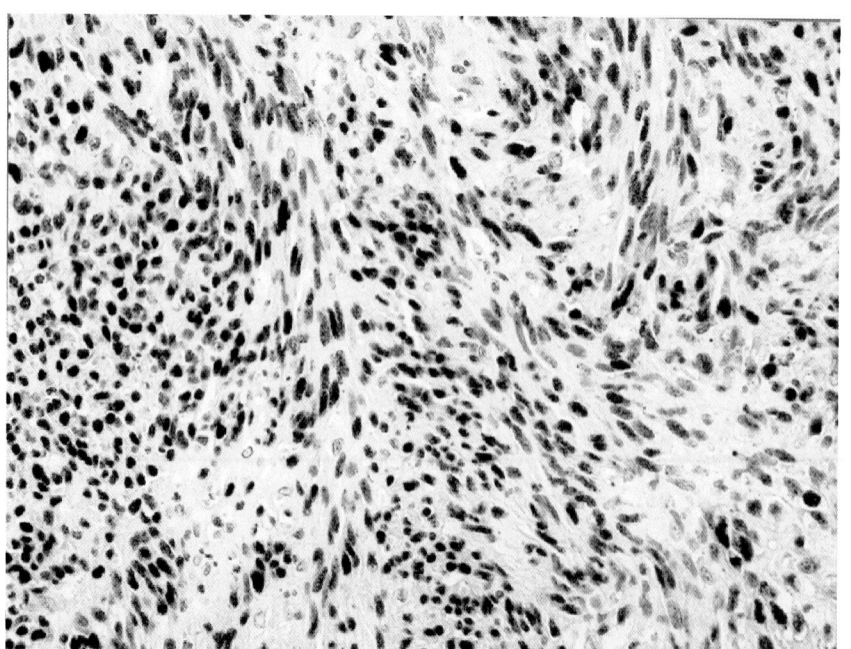

▲ **FIGURE 21-10** Nodular KS. The nuclei of most of the spindle cells stain positively for LANA-1 (immunoperoxidase, 400×).

asymptomatic viral carriage and the development of HHV-8-associated diseases remain to be elucidated.

Molecular Mechanisms of HHV-8 Pathogenesis

BOX 21-5 Summary

- HHV-8 genome encodes at least 12 candidate microRNAs and over 85 genes, including several cellular homologs.
- HHV-8 encodes an array of proteins that could potentially modify host cellular functions and immune responses.
- A number of viral genes are potentially tumorigenic.

The HHV-8 genome is a large linear double-stranded DNA encoding at least 12 candidate microRNAs[62] and over 85 genes, including a number of cellular homologs.[54] These viral homologs, along with other various virally encoded proteins, participate and subvert key cellular pathways by acting as cell cycle controllers, cytokines, chemokines, and G-protein-coupled receptors. This led to the "molecular pirate" epithet for HHV-8.

Like other oncogenic viruses, HHV-8 appears to have evolved a plethora of mechanisms for immortalizing and transforming cells, each of which may contribute to its tumorigenicity.[38,53,63] The tumorigenic potential of several protein encoded by HHV-8, such as ORF K1, Kaposin, viral interferon regulatory factor homolog (vIRF) 1, and viral G-protein-coupled receptor homolog (vGPCR), has been revealed using *in vitro* assays, whereby their individual expression in rodent cells induces tumorigenic transformation. For some virally encoded proteins, such as the viral FLICE-inhibitory protein homolog (vFLIP) and the LANA-1, transformation requires coexpression in this assay with another cellular or viral oncogene. Detailed studies of the molecular mechanisms of transformation has indicated that certain viral proteins, for example viral interleukin 6 homolog (vIL-6), vBcl-2, viral inhibitor-of-apoptosis protein (vIAP), LANA-1, viral cyclin D homolog (vCYC), and vFLIP, act as proliferative, anti-apoptotic or survival factors; thus, these genes probably contribute to HHV-8-induced tumorigenesis by extending the lifespan of virus-infected cells. HHV-8 infection causes alterations in the cellular gene expression profile, both at the level of transcription[64–66] and at the level of stability of mRNAs. Degradation of certain short-living cytokine transcripts can be blocked through activation of the p38-MK2 pathway by Kaposin B.[67] This may lead to a cellular environment more compatible with transformation. Notably, a subset of virally encoded proteins are secreted, or induce secretion of growth factors, and function as paracrine signaling molecules that mediate chemotaxis, angiogenesis, cell proliferation, and survival. Examples include viral chemokines (vCCL-1, 2, and 3), vOX2, vIL-6, and vGPCR.

On top of the capability of HHV-8 to actively induce tumorigenesis, it can block the activity of key cellular tumor suppressor genes that control cell cycle checkpoints. A viral homolog of cyclin D, vCYC, is capable of phosphorylating a wide range of targets including the retinoblastoma tumor suppressor protein (pRB), p27, histone H1, and CDC25a, mimicking the effect of both G1/S and S-phase mitotic cyclins.[68,69] Moreover, the cellular inhibitors of this pathway (p16, p21, and p27) fall short in inhibiting vCYC activities. Concomitantly, other viral proteins, such as LANA-1 and vIRFs,[70–72] interfere with the p53 tumor suppressor pathways to avoid host growth surveillance and to facilitate uncontrolled cell proliferation. LANA-1, a unique multifunctional viral protein, can also inactivate the pRB tumor-suppressive function,[73] and enable accumulation of the β-catenin protein toward stimulating a proliferative program of gene expression.[74]

In addition to its capacity to transform host cells, HHV-8 has evolved the ability to evade recognition and attack by host's innate and adaptive immune response. HHV-8 encodes two unique gene products, MIR-1 and MIR-2, which downregulate the expression of cellular immune response genes, such as those involved in class I MHC expression. MIR-2 also downregulates ICAM-1 and B7.2 gene expression, which encode accessory proteins required for T-cell stimulation. Another viral gene product, Rta, functions as a ubiquitin E3 ligase that targets the ubiquitination of a key mediator of type I interferon induction.[75] Immune evasion is also predicted to happen by viral chemokines that can bind chemokine receptors as natural ligands and reduce the recruitment of antiviral Th-1 cells by host chemokines.[76] Furthermore, by means of procaspase-8 inhibition and NFκB activation, vFLIP protects cells from apoptosis induced by T- and NK-cells, and promotes growth of HHV-8-infected cells.[77,78]

Paradoxically, in spite of this wide array of HHV-8-encoded proteins that could potentially influence host cellular functions and immune responses, most HHV-8-infected individuals never develop a disease. However, it is notable that several other viruses, which manipulate infected cells in a similar fashion to HHV-8, also seldom cause disease. This implies that tumorigenesis represents an exceptional consequence of the natural life cycle of these viruses.

HHV-8 Gene Expression in Kaposi Sarcoma Lesions

BOX 21-6   Summary

- HHV-8 genes can be classified according to their expression patterns.
- In KS lesions, HHV-8 infection is localized principally to spindle cells.
- Most HHV-8-positive cells in KS lesions exhibit latent infection, while a small fraction exhibits lytic infection.
- HHV-8 infection is restricted in early lesions and abundant in nodular lesions.
- KS spindle cells express certain lymphatic endothelium genes.
- Several inflammatory cytokines, chemokines, and angiogenic factors are being expressed in KS lesions.

Extensive studies concerning patterns of viral gene expression have begun to shed light on the biology of KS. These studies provided valuable insights into the complexity of the dynamic HHV-8 infection during lifelong latent infection and upon disease onset. HHV-8 genes have been classified into two groups: those expressed in latent infection and those expressed in lytic infection. Yet, it is clear that the pathogenicity of HHV-8 is far more intricate from this explicit dual gene-expression categorization.[79] This complexity is highlighted further by the finding that there are distinct viral expression patterns in each of the three HHV-8-associated diseases.

In KS tissues, HHV-8 infection is localized principally to spindle cells with most cells infected latently, demonstrating a highly restricted pattern of viral gene expression that includes LANA-1, vCYC, vFLIP, and Kaposin. Generally, in early KS lesions, only a small proportion (<10%) of spindle cells are positive for HHV-8 and the mature endothelial cells surrounding normal vessels are HHV-8-negative. In nodular lesions, however, virtually all (>90%) spindle cells are infected with HHV-8.[80–85] This observation supports the premise that HHV-8 latent proteins provide some growth advantage. Within the infected spindle cell population, a small subpopulation exhibits HHV-8 lytic infection to varying extents in lesions from different KS stages.

Cellular Gene Expression in Kaposi Sarcoma Lesions

The current view of the origin of KS spindle cells is that they emerge from a cell type capable of undergoing lymphatic endothelium differentiation. This notion has been suggested based on the transcriptional profile of KS,[86] and on the transcriptome comparison between noninfected and HHV-8-infected endothelial cells.[87–90]

Experimentally, the ability of HHV-8 to induce the expression of lymphatic lineage-specific genes on the one hand and to downregulate blood vascular genes on the other hand has been demonstrated in human dermal microvascular endothelial cells.[87,88,90] Thus, transcriptional reprogramming of immature uncharacterized progenitor cells by HHV-8 toward a lymphatic endothelium phenotype and away from a blood vascular endothelium phenotype may be at the center of KS pathogenesis.

Like the lymphatic endothelial cells (LECs), KS spindle cells are characterized by the expression of several specific lymphatic endothelium genes, including Prox1, vascular endothelial growth factor receptor (VEGFR) 3 (also known as Flt-4), podoplanin, and LYVE-1. In line, D2-40, a monoclonal antibody that stains specifically the lymphatic endothelium, positively stains KS.[91] Since the cognate VEGFR-3 ligand, VEGF-C, is also expressed highly in KS spindle cells, stimulation of migration and proliferation via VEGFR-3 is likely to be important for the phenotype of KS cells.[92,93] Although in nodular KS, cells expressing VEGFR-3 are infected with HHV-8, in early KS, this correlation is less strict, with more cells expressing VEGFR-3 than are infected with HHV-8.[81,94] This observation implies that viral infection neither induces the expression of VEGFR-3 nor promotes the proliferation of VEGFR-3-positive cells directly. Rather, it is possible that VEGFR-3 functions in early lesions of KS as a paracrine regulator of virus replication or as a recruitment factor for HHV-8-infected cells.

Several additional cellular genes have shown to be induced after HHV-8 infection in vitro, and their expression in the KS spindle cells was confirmed. This includes neuritin, RDC1, PDGF-1, and c-kit, shown to be required for the proliferative phenotype of cells infected by HHV-8.[95] In accordance, a partial regression of clinical and histological cutaneous

KS lesions was reported in AIDS-KS patients treated with the c-kit inhibitor imatinib mesylate (Gleevec).[96]

Another important parameter in the pathogenesis of KS lesions concerns interactions between infected cells and other cell types. Several inflammatory cellular cytokines (IFNγ, TNF, IL-1, IL-6, GM-CSF), chemokines (MCP-1, IL-8, SDF-1), and angiogenic factors (βFGF, VEGF, PDGF, angiopoietin 2) are expressed in KS lesions.[97–99] These molecules are produced by inflammatory cells (monocytes/macrophages and infiltrating lymphocytes) and/or by the spindle cells. Such molecules are essential for spindle cell viability in culture, and are also considered important for the pathogenesis of KS.

Current Understanding of the Pathogenesis of KS

BOX 21-7 Summary

- KS represents a consequence of a multistep process involving viral, cellular, and inflammatory factors.
- Current view suggests that KS begins as a polyclonal hyperplasia with a potential subsequent evolution to monoclonality.
- Lack of an animal model for KS limits our current understanding of the evolution of KS.
- Expression of lytic viral genes, such as the vGPCR, is required for KS development, persistence, and progression.

Despite over a century since its initial description, KS remains a poorly understood disease, even following the discovery of the involvement of HHV-8's in its etiology. In fact, several questions remain, such as why there is a large male predominance in classic and endemic KS, and more generally, what are the triggers and risk factors for KS onset apart from HHV-8 infection. Even the debate whether KS is a reactive process or a true malignant proliferation of spindle cells remains unsettled. As elaborated above, HHV-8 infection is essential for the development of KS; however, additional cofactors appear to be necessary and the exact role of HHV-8 in disease onset and progression is still puzzling.

The current model suggests that KS represents a consequence of a multistep process involving both viral and cellular factors that initiate reactive and inflammatory processes. Subsequently, some selective pressures or genetic alteration that are promoted in latently infected cells could give rise to the neoplastic monoclonal form of KS. This view is supported by studies showing that KS

lesions display all patterns of clonality (mono-, oligo-, and polyclonal), suggesting that KS begins as a polyclonal hyperplasia with a potential subsequent evolution to a monoclonality.[100–102] It should be noted that KS-like spindle cells can be cultured from peripheral blood mononuclear cell (PBMCs) of patients with KS,[103–105] and mesenchymal stem cells from bone marrow have shown to be susceptible to HHV-8 infection.[106] Therefore, it is possible that these progenitor cells serve as reservoir for HHV-8, or influence hematopoietic neighboring cells by paracrine mechanisms. Finally, a quite hypothetical model, though conceivable, envisions a rare event of hematopoietic stem cell infection by HHV-8 that leads to the establishment of a cancer stem cell harboring a potential to initiate KS. Unfortunately, the lack of suitable animal models to study KS pathogenesis *in vivo* has hindered evaluation of these hypotheses.

HHV-8 encodes an array of genes that allows the virus to assault and manipulate its host cell with many strategies; only a few of these genes are being expressed in KS spindle cells that principally possess latent infection. Founded on the observation that lytic virus replication causes cell death, it was assumed that cell transformation occurs only during the virus latency. Recent studies, however, indicate that the expression of latent proteins may not be sufficient to initiate and sustain KS, and therefore, reveal a requirement for the lytic cycle for tumorigenesis. Accordingly, increasing quantities of viral DNA in PBMCs, reflecting active virus replication, are strongly predictive of the onset of KS among HIV patients. Thus, it has been suggested that lytic activity is necessary for the development of the KS tumor, as it produces new viral particles for *de novo* infection. In line with this model, Martin et al[107] reported that treatment of AIDS patients with ganciclovir, a drug that inhibits lytic virus replication, but does not affect latent virus, resulted in a decline in the incidence of KS, supporting a role for lytic replication in the onset of KS.

Further support for the importance of the lytic cycle in the pathogenesis of KS comes from experiments comparing the tumor load in mice injected with various types of endothelial cells. When endothelial cells expressing viral latent genes are injected, they display weak tumorigenicity; when such cells are coinjected with a small number of endothelial cells stably expressing the lytic cycle gene vGPCR (at a ratio that approximates the proportion in KS), enhanced tumorigenicity is observed. Regression of such KS-like

tumors is elicited by selective depletion of vGPCR-expressing cells.[108] In addition, vGPCR induces the secretion of cellular KS cytokines, which in turn influence neighboring cells and may promote the tumorigenic potential of latently infected spindle cells. Yet, the implied role of vGPCR in the initiation of KS is unconfirmed, as all the experimental models do not incorporate virus infection and therefore the appearance of KS-like lesions may represent a similar, but distinct process.[76,108–111]

Overall, it is suggested that viral (e.g., vGPCR, viral chemokines, and/or vIL-6) and cellular (e.g., VEGF, SDF-1) paracrine functions are important in early KS development. These factors could contribute to the maintenance and expansion of the latently infected cell population, which own privileged growth characteristics, resulting in the subsequent development of a clonal malignant tissue. A similar function has been attributed previously to Reed–Sternberg cells in Hodgkin's lymphoma.[112] Importantly, it was shown recently that viral latent mini-chromosomes are lost rapidly from HHV-8-infected cultured cells, and LANA-1-mediated retention of viral mini-chromosomes appears to be an inefficient process.[113] This observation raises the possibility that the latent infection stage, observed in the majority of KS cells, may not persist in lesions over long periods and might explain the continuous need for lytic cycles to maintain HHV-8 infection of KS lesions. All in all, if long-term virus latency and tumor progression are indeed dependent on lytic HHV-8 replication, then there is a belief that remission of KS lesions should occur after continued treatment with ganciclovir or other targeted therapy to viral lytic proteins such as the vGPCR.

EPIDEMIOLOGY OF KAPOSI SARCOMA AND KAPOSI-SARCOMA-ASSOCIATED HERPESVIRUS

Seroepidemiology of Kaposi-Sarcoma-Associated Herpesvirus (KSHV)

BOX 21-8 Summary

- Seropositivity rates for HHV-8 show geographic variations strongly correlated with the risk of KS in the general population.
- Although most HHV-8 infections are asymptomatic, untreated HIV patients that acquire HHV-8 infection after HIV-seroconversion are highly likely to develop KS.

Multiple studies were conducted to assess the prevalence of HHV-8 antibodies, using a variety of techniques, but without an accepted reference for efficacy measurement of the various approaches. Nevertheless, the relative prevalence rates of HHV-8 among different populations can still be reliably compared, provided that the same assay is employed, and even if different assays are used, certain trends are evident.[114] Unlike other human herpesviruses, HHV-8 is not ubiquitous worldwide. Seropositivity rates for HHV-8 show remarkable racial and geographic variations, strongly correlated with the population's risk of KS. Almost all patients with KS have antibodies to HHV-8, independent of ethnicity and geography.[53,115] Overall, the infection rates with HHV-8 parallel the incidence of KS, being lower in northern Europe, the United States, and Asia; intermediate in southern Italy and other Mediterranean countries; and the highest in central Africa. Most HHV-8 infections appear to be asymptomatic, with the majority of infected individuals never developing a virally associated disease.[19,116] However, untreated HIV patients that acquire HHV-8 infection after HIV-seroconversion are highly likely to develop KS.[37]

Although the prevalence rates of infection with HHV-8 are low in the general population of the United States and the United Kingdom, it is common among high-risk populations such as HIV-negative and HIV-positive homosexual men in these countries.[117–119]

Kaposi Sarcoma (KS) and HHV-8

BOX 21-9   Summary

- Infection with HHV-8 is a prerequisite for KS development.
- The seroprevalence of HHV-8 correlates with KS incidence rates.
- In HIV-related KS, the risk for acquiring KS varies significantly between different HIV risk groups, being as high as 21% for homosexual men.
- The increasing and successful use of HAART chemotherapy in HIV-infected patients is associated with a dramatic decline in the incidence of KS.
- HHV-8 disease after organ transplantation, especially kidney transplants is an increasing concern for the transplant physician.
- KS is surprisingly uncommon in some populations despite high HHV-8 seroprevalence.

There is a strong epidemiological and molecular evidence that infection with HHV-8 is a prerequisite for KS development, and plays a critical role in its pathogenesis.[53] Seroepidemiologic studies identified HHV-8 antibodies in patients with all the pathogenic forms of KS disease.[53] Furthermore, seroconversion of HHV-8 precedes progression to KS and is a strong predictor of disease development.[117,118,120] Generally, the seroprevalence of HHV-8 correlates with KS incidence rates.[115,121,122] CKS presents medium-high incidence rates in Italy, Greece, Turkey, and Israel, and relatively low incidence rates in Northern Europe and United States.[116,121,123–125] In HIV-related KS, the risk for acquiring KS varies significantly between different HIV risk groups, ranging from as high as 21% for homosexual men to as low as 1% for men with hemophilia and 0.85% in Ethiopian Immigrants to Israel.[20,126] In this study, only 0.85% of Ethiopians with HIV who had immigrated to Israel developed KS, as compared with 12.5% of non-Ethiopian HIV patients. The low risk of KS exists in spite of high HHV-8 seroprevalence rates (above 39%) in HIV+ and HIV− Ethiopian populations.[126] The risk of KS in HIV patients was estimated to be 300 times that of other immunosuppressed patients, suggesting that HIV contributes more than merely by being an immunodeficiency state.[20] However, overrepresentation of HHV-8-seropositive gay men among HIV patients as opposed to immunosuppressed transplant patients, as well as differences in the degree of immunosuppression in these disorders may account for this discrepancy. In HIV-associated KS, the time from virus acquisition to the onset of disease is 2 to 10 years,[127–129] as opposed to decades in CKS. The increasing and successful use of HAART has been associated with a dramatic decline in the incidence of KS from 4.8 cases per 100 persons per year in 1990 to 1.5 cases per 100 persons per year in 1997,[130] so that in the HAART era, HIV-associated KS is only sporadically seen in the Western world.[60,130] As for endemic KS, prior to the emergence of HIV, KS was manifested in localized geographic areas throughout sub-Saharan Africa, with particularly high rates in northeastern Zaire, western Uganda, and Tanzania.[131] With the AIDS epidemic, the incidence of KS in Africa rose abruptly between 1988 and 1996 to an epidemic magnitude, so that in certain African countries, it is now the most common cancer in adult men, and the second most common cancer in adult women. In parallel, the male-to-female ratio has declined from 7:1 in 1988 to 2:1

in 1996.[132] Clinically, KS in Africa is more frequent in children and females than anywhere else worldwide.[133,134] The epidemiologic and clinical studies of endemic KS are now confounded by the AIDS epidemic in Africa. While in the HAART era, the incidence of HIV-associated KS has substantially declined in the Western world and the prevalence of KS in Africa has remained high, particularly in children, most probably due to the rising incidence of untreated HIV infection.[134]

HHV-8 disease after organ transplantation is an increasing concern for the transplant physician.[135] KS has been described in organ transplant recipients and in patients receiving chronic immunosuppressive therapy. The incidence of KS among transplant recipients is proportional to the ethnogeographic prevalence of HHV-8, ranging from 0.5% in most Western countries to 5.3% in Saudi Arabia.[136–140] KS represents more than 80% of posttransplantation cancers in high-prevalence countries, such as Saudi Arabia.[141] It usually appears early (mean interval, 13 months), but has been documented as late as 18 years after transplantation.[43,142] Interestingly, iatrogenic KS is seen predominantly in kidney allograft recipients, less frequently among other solid organ transplant recipients, and rarely in bone marrow transplant recipients.[143,144] It has been proposed that the transplanted kidney may be a site of latent HHV-8 infection.[40,145]

KS seems unexpectedly uncommon in some populations despite high HHV-8 seroprevalence.[126,146,147] Unique cases of familial clustering of KS have also been reported.[5,148] These suggest that unknown cofactors may modify the clinical expression of viral infection. Genetic factors, concurrent infections, environmental effects, and possibly molecular variants of HHV-8 probably play an important part in the establishment of HHV-8-associated diseases.

The Transmission Routes of HHV-8

BOX 21-10   Summary

- In homosexual individuals, HHV-8 may be sexually transmitted by anal and/or oral contacts. Parental HHV-8 transmission is unusual in these populations.
- Certain living conditions (close contact, crowding, etc.) predispose to HHV-8 infection by enhancing horizontal HHV-8 transmission.

- Horizontal transmission probably accounts for the largest proportion of HHV-8 infection in early childhood.
- A possible mode of transmission from mother to child is through saliva.
- There is still no clear evidence for KSHV transmission through blood products.
- KS may be a serious complication after renal transplantation.

Patterns of transmission for HHV-8 are being better defined as our understanding of the pathogenesis of this virus is increasing and testing methods are being used strategically. The virus, first thought as transmitted only sexually, is now also considered transmissible through low-risk or more casual behaviors.

Seroepidemiological studies of HHV-8 documented a transmission of HHV-8 through sexual activities, with a high prevalence of infection among homosexual and bisexual HIV carriers, as compared with other HIV carrier groups (hemophiliacs, drug users, and women) that generally present an infection rate that is close to the general population.[149] In a cohort of Danish homosexual men, a linear association was reported between the prevalence of anti-KSHV antibodies and the duration of homosexual lifestyle, the number of male partners, and the frequency of receptive anal intercourses in the homosexual community.[150] Similarly, among United States, homosexual/bisexual men, a strong correlation was found between HHV-8 infection and homosexual activity, the number of homosexual partners, and the presence of sexually transmitted diseases (STDs).[127] Additional studies demonstrated an association between the presence of HHV-8 antibodies and unprotected receptive anal sex, oral–anal sex, and deep kissing with an HIV-1-positive partner.[151,152] These findings have inferred that in homosexual individuals, HHV-8 may be sexually transmitted by anal/oral contacts and that parental HHV-8 transmission is unusual in those populations. KS is less common in bisexual men compared to men who were exclusively homosexual.[153] A simultaneous spread of HHV-8 along with HIV through a similar mode of transmission has been suggested,[150,154] though a high prevalence of HHV-8 among homosexual men in San Francisco has been documented prior to the HIV epidemic.[155]

Sexual transmission of HHV-8 may occur as a consequence of its presence in seminal fluid. Contrary to early reports,[156] HHV-8 does not appear to be a common infection of urogenital and prostatic tissue in healthy men.[157,158] However, HHV-8 DNA was found in the semen from a fraction of KS patients.[159] HHV-8 DNA has not yet been found in fecal matter,[160] although sexual practices involving oral–anal contact may be a risk factor for homosexual transmission.[161] HHV-8 DNA has been detected by PCR in oral KS lesions, oral tissues, and saliva implying that oral and/or nasal secretions can be a source of infectious virus.[162–164] The low prevalence of infection in heterosexuals in the United States and Europe suggests that infection from oral secretions is uncommon. It could be that virus transmission through saliva is inefficient and occurs only during intimate contact, whereas the low virus prevalence among certain populations may result in limited carriers that are able to spread the virus.

Detailed studies are still necessary to demonstrate the transmission routes of HHV-8 among heterosexual populations. Two recent studies from Africa have found HHV-8 infections to be correlated with risky heterosexual sex, suggesting that heterosexual transmission of the virus occurs in endemic populations.[165,166] The presence of HHV-8 infection in children in Africa suggests it may be acquired early in life through routes other than sexual transmission.[167] High seroprevalence rates, ranged from 27.5% in early childhood to 58% in children over 6 years old, were reported in endemic African areas.[168] This pattern of age-dependent seroprevalence is indicative of horizontal transmission of HHV-8 among children in endemic areas and is reminiscent of the pattern known from other herpesviruses, in particular EBV. This differs from HIV infection that peaks among the 20- to 30-year-old group, as expected for a sexually transmitted agent. It has been found that the presence of antibodies to two HHV-8 antigens was independently associated with hepatitis B virus (HBV) infection, which is known to be transmitted horizontally among young children in Africa.[169] This could suggest that certain living conditions predisposing to HHV-8 infection (close contact, crowding, etc.) may enhance horizontal HHV-8 transmission. In Italian children, evidence for horizontal transmission was also found, whereas crowded living conditions and poor hygiene associated with HBV transmission in Africa apparently did not play a major role in this population.[170] The presence of HHV-8 in saliva may account for horizontal transmission among young children, along the lines suggested for EBV.[171–173] Poor hygienic practices, lower socioeconomic status, and the use of surface water were lately associated with HHV-8 infection in Ugandan children.[174] Another hypothesis was provided lately, suggesting that blood-feeding arthropods (e.g., mosquitoes) play a role in the epidemiology of HHV-8 infection. According to this hypothesis, the conditions for HHV-8 transmission are met when a child shows a response to the bites of blood-feeding arthropods and an HHV-8-seropositive mother applies her infected saliva to the bite sites, attempting to cleanse the spots and relieve the child's itchiness.[175–177]

A significant familial correlation in HHV-8 seropositivity was seen between mother and child and between siblings, whereas a less significant dependence was found between father and child, supporting the occurrence of mother–child and sib–sib HHV-8 transmission in endemic populations.[171,174,178,179] This correlation does not necessarily represent transmission during pregnancy, delivery, or breast-feeding, and could reflect a greater role of the mother in intimate care. A possible mode of transmission from mother to child is through saliva while close interpersonal contacts (e.g., contact of nonintact skin or mucous membranes with body secretions or blood, premastication of food) could also have an important role in HHV-8 transmission in the endemic areas.[168,179,180] In addition, children may also be exposed during play and by sharing utensils with siblings.[178,180] Strong evidence for vertical transmission was presented by Mantina et al, who identified two Zambian neonates who had tested positive for HHV-8 DNA in their PBMCs at birth, suggesting *in utero* infection.[181] Although children born to HHV-8-infected mothers can be congenitally infected, the frequency of such transmission is apparently low.[182,183] The rarity of virus transmission during pregnancy or at delivery has been recently illustrated in an Italian population.[184] Perinatal transmission of HHV-8 may formally occur during breast-feeding, but it fails to account for the continued acquisition of HHV-8 after breast-feeding has ceased; while the lack of detection of HHV-8 DNA in breast milk further weakens the likelihood for this mode of HHV-8 transmission.[182] Therefore, horizontal transmission probably accounts for the largest proportion of HHV-8 infections that occurs in early childhood.

Among populations with a high incidence of classical KS, as in Sardinia, a threefold higher HHV-8 seroprevalence rate was reported among family members of CKS patients in comparison to the general population.[185] The clustering of HHV-8 among family members suggested possible vertical, or more likely horizontal transmission within a family. Another Italian study from Milan reported a much higher seroprevalence rate of HHV-8 among 27 partners of CKS patients, as compared with a control group of 25 individuals (44% versus 8%), supporting a sexual transmission route,[186] but little evidence was found for an association with sexual behavior in heterosexuals.[186] Studies from Israel, Italy, and Thailand reported conflicting findings on the association of HHV-8 status among spouses.[186–188] In a number of countries, HHV-8 seroprevalence in prostitutes was higher than that in nonprostitute women, suggesting that the former are a high-risk population.[165,189] However, other studies found no evidence for a significantly higher rate of seropositivity to HHV-8 among female sex workers.[165,190] Correlation of HHV-8 with a history of other STDs, such as gonorrhea, syphilis, chlamydia infection, and condyloma have also been reported.[166,191,192]

Iatrogenic transmission of HHV-8 is of particular concern, although KS rates among persons infected with HIV through blood products are generally low.[20] Most blood donors from the United States and Europe are not infected with the virus, yet infectious virus has been recovered from the blood of a healthy individual.[193] HHV-8 DNA was found in the PBMCs of up to 50% of individuals with AIDS-KS[160] and in 11% of healthy HHV-8 carriers in Italy.[194] These suggest that HHV-8 could potentially be transmitted by blood transfusion. In countries or populations that are highly endemic for HHV-8, transmission by blood transfusion could play a role, but is not believed to be a major modality.[195] Although syringe sharing is a common means of transmitting HIV-1, HBV, and hepatitis C virus among intravenous drug users, it does not result in a similar spread of HHV-8.[196] Lennette et al reported comparable rates of HHV-8 seroprevalence among hemophilia patients, intravenous drug users, and general adult population suggesting that parenteral HHV-8 transmission through blood or blood products is unusual.[197] In contrast, a longer duration of injection drug use has been associated with increased risk of HHV-8 infection that could not be explained by sexual behavior or demographic differences.[198] Recently, in a historical United States cohort, it was reported that HHV-8 might be transmitted via blood components, as evidenced by seroconversion.[199] An indirect evidence for a lack of transmission through blood products was provided by a Greek study demonstrating that HHV-8 transmission is uncommon in the hemodialysis setting.[200] Further surveys in countries with intermediate and high infection rates of HHV-8 are needed to better assess the risk for acquisition of HHV-8 infection through blood transfusion, while the outcome of such surveys could call for the screening of blood donations.

In contrast to blood transfusion, HHV-8 has been more clearly linked to transplantation-related immunosuppression and organ donation. KS is a serious complication after renal transplantation and its higher incidence among the transplant population has been repeatedly confirmed.[137,140,144,201,202] The tumor tends to occur more commonly in certain geographic areas and racial groups. Parravicini et al found that most (10/11) Italian patients developing KS after transplantation were infected prior to receiving organ allograft, suggesting virus reactivation.[203] One case of organ-related transmission has also been identified by this group, suggesting that clinical disease resulted predominantly from viral reactivation, but may also have occurred following a primary virus infection. The risk of posttransplant KS among patients who are HHV-8-seropositive before renal transplantation is 23 to 28%, as compared to a risk of 0.7% in patients who are seronegative.[202,204,205] These studies suggest that in endemic countries for HHV-8, most transplant patients develop KS as a consequence of the reactivation of a preexisting latent HHV-8 infection, but transmission of HHV-8 to the transplant recipient from the organ donor can occur and may play a role in the onset of KS.[142,206] A case of a primary HHV-8 infection was discovered, which had been acquired from an infected transplanted kidney and was associated with severe disseminated disease and fatal outcome.[145] Another study reported the presence of HHV-8-infected neoplastic cells in posttransplant KS from five of eight renal transplant patients harboring either genetic or antigenic markers of their matched donors.[40] Screening organ donors and recipients for infection, particularly in high prevalence areas is a prudent measure.

In summary, the understanding of HHV-8 transmission routes is increasing, although it is still to be elucidated and far from being fully resolved. The implications for the clinical management of associated diseases and public health have to be further evaluated in coming years.

KS THERAPY

BOX 21-11 Summary

- No definitive cure exists for KS and most treatments are palliative.
- Local treatments are the most common modality for the treatment of classical KS (CKS) including surgical excision, cryotherapy, radiotherapy, laser, and intralesional therapy.
- Intralesional cytotoxic chemotherapy, primarily vinblastine, is effective for both cutaneous and oral lesions.
- Low-dose interferon alpha (3 to 9 million U three times a week) therapy of CKS showed encouraging results.
- Systemic therapy for CKS includes liposomal anthracyclines (doxorubicin and daunorubicin), single-agent chemotherapy (vinblastine, bleomycin, etoposide, etc.), and low-dose subcutaneous IFN alpha treatment.
- For HIV-related KS, HAART regimens are equally effective in protecting against KS and are also associated with regression in the size and number of existing KS lesions.
- Currently, the five agents approved by the U.S. Food and Drug Administration for the treatment of HIV-induced KS are alitretinoin gel for topical administration and liposomal doxorubicin, liposomal daunorubicin, paclitaxel, and interferon-alpha for systemic administration.
- In patients with rapidly progressive cutaneous disease and/or with visceral involvement, cytotoxic chemotherapy is indicated. The "gold standard" for the treatment of systemic KS is currently liposomal anthracyclines.
- Sirolimus may cause regression of kidney-transplant-associated KS.
- Angiogenesis inhibitors are one of the promising agents currently studied.

A definitive cure for KS is usually unavailable, and most treatments are palliative and with a temporary benefit.[207] Most studies deal with the treatment of HIV-related KS, and those relating to the other forms of KS are relatively scarce. The outcome of KS varies from a slow evolution requiring no treatment (predominantly in CKS) to a fulminate course demanding intensive treatment.

Classic KS

Due to a highly variable clinical evolution of the disease, it is often difficult to decide whether or not to treat elderly patients with CKS. Local treatments are the most common modality for the treatment of CKS. These include simple excision, cryotherapy, radiotherapy, laser, and intralesional therapy, all aiming to remove and destroy tumor masses or to induce an inflammatory response that will assist in resolving the KS lesions.

KS is considered a radiosensitive tumor. Palliation to relieve pain and cosmetic and physical discomfort can be achieved with local radiotherapy.[208–210] A complete remission was achieved in up to 85% of the lesions, with minor side effects, including a residual hypopigmentation, as well as radiodermatitis and ulceration.[207]

Cryotherapy leads to more than 70% cosmetic improvement, but it may cause hypopigmentation, and can be used for small lesions only. Laser therapy (including argon laser, carbon dioxide laser, and pulsed-dye laser) has a limited use because of a high recurrence rate, and a possible risk of dissemination of viral particles.[207] Photodynamic therapy may also be used, although it has been used mainly for HIV-related KS.[211]

Intralesional cytotoxic chemotherapy, most commonly vinblastine, is effective for both cutaneous and oral lesions, but there are several disadvantages: possible skin ulceration, short duration of remission, and only individual lesions can be treated.[207,212] A beneficial effect of intralesional low-dose interferon (IFN) alpha was reported for CKS.[213–215] Low-dose interferon alpha (3 to 9 million U three times a week) treatment of CKS showed encouraging results. Moreover, unlike HIV-related KS, continuous treatment is not needed, and relapses are delayed and often limited.[214]

Recently, a new staging system for CKS was proposed, based on objective criteria that more closely follow the clinical variability of CKS and make the therapeutic choices easier. It comprises four stages, each divided further according to the speed of disease evolution and presence of complications.[216] The stages are as follows: stage I (maculo-nodular)—small isolated angiomatous macules and/or nodules, localized to lower limbs; stage II (infiltrative)—violet gray plaque lesions involving wide areas of lower limbs, sometimes associated with few nodules; stage III (florid)—exuberant angiomatous plaques and nodules, often ulcerated, involving one or more limbs; and stage IV (disseminated)—presence of a significant number of angiomatous plaques and nodules involving other skin districts in addition to the limbs. The application of this staging system to CKS patients has shown that evolution is slow in the maculo-nodular and infiltrative stages I and II, and faster during the florid and disseminated stages III and IV.[216] Systemic treatment is recommended for stages III and IV, and for stage II disease only if the growth was rapid (i.e., IIB) or accompanied by complications.[216]

Systemic therapy for CKS includes liposomal anthracyclines (doxorubicin and daunorubicin), single agent chemotherapy (vinblastine, bleomycin, etoposide, etc.), and low-dose subcutaneous IFN alpha treatment.[217] Single-agent chemotherapy with vinblastine and bleomycin is an effective, cheap, and relatively nontoxic treatment for advanced CKS.[19,217–219] Several studies report effectiveness of pegylated liposomal doxorubicin (PLD) in the treatment of CKS.[207,217,219] A recent report confirmed the efficacy and safety of PLD 20 mg/m^2 monthly and found it to be superior to subcutaneous IFN alpha for advanced CKS.[217] PLD consists of doxorubicin encapsulated in small unilamellar vesicles. It has the same efficacy and less toxicity than that of conventional doxorubicin.[217]

HIV-Related KS

Because KS is not considered curable with standard therapies, treatment decisions are guided by the presence and extent of symptomatic and extracutaneous KS. It is now accepted that most, if not all, patients with HIV-related KS should be treated with antiretroviral drugs.[220,221] The benefits of HAART include the inhibition of HIV replication, diminished production of Tat protein, amelioration of the host's immune response to HHV-8, and the direct antiangiogenic activity of some protease inhibitors.[220] There is data demonstrating that effective antiretroviral regimens alone are associated with regression in the size and number of existing KS lesions.[61,222] More recently, it has been shown that both protease inhibitor- and nonnucleoside reverse transcriptase inhibitor-based HAART regimens are equally effective in protecting against KS.[223]

Currently, there are five agents approved by the U.S. Food and Drug Administration for the treatment of HIV-induced KS. These include alitretinoin gel for topical administration, liposomal doxorubicin, liposomal daunorubicin, paclitaxel, and interferon-alpha for systemic administration.[220]

Local therapy is most useful for localized bulky KS lesions and/or cosmesis, but will not prevent the development of new lesions in untreated sites. Alitretinoin gel 0.1% (Panretin; Ligand Pharmaceuticals, Inc., San Diego, CA) is the only topical, patient-administered therapy approved for the treatment of KS.[224] Alitretinoin has been shown as effective after 4 to 8 weeks of therapy, with responses in up to 50% of patients.[225] Alternative local therapies include intralesional chemotherapy, radiation therapy, laser therapy, and cryotherapy.[226] Another optional treatment for HIV-related KS is photodynamic therapy that utilizes the activation by light of a photosensitizing drug that preferentially accumulates in tumor tissue such as KS. This treatment was demonstrated as an effective palliative measure for HIV-associated KS.[227]

Vinblastine is the most widely used intralesional agent and has a response rate of approximately 70%.[220] Although treated lesions may fade and regress, they do not resolve completely. In the setting of KS that is too extensive to be treated with intralesional chemotherapy, but not extensive enough to warrant a systemic therapy, radiation therapy can be employed to palliate symptoms. Complete responses to radiation therapy are found in up to 80% of patients.[220,226]

Individuals with more progressive disease may warrant systemic treatment. Cytotoxic chemotherapy is indicated in patients who have rapidly progressive cutaneous disease and in patients with visceral involvement. The "gold standard" for the treatment of systemic KS is now liposomal anthracyclines. Two new formulations, liposomal daunorubicin and liposomal doxorubicin, have been used as monotherapy in the treatment of HIV-related KS, with favorable response rates and durations compared to combination regimens.[222,226] Paclitaxel is the most recent systemic chemotherapeutic agent approved for KS. This agent has demonstrated striking efficacy, even for patients resistant to anthracyclines, with responses rates of 60 to 70% and a long duration (approximately 10 months) of sustained response. Although paclitaxel is well tolerated, it is less desirable than are the liposomal anthracyclines as first line therapy because of the need for a 3-h infusion and the increased risks of alopecia, myalgia, arthralgia, and bone marrow suppression.

For patients who have attained appropriate immune reconstitution with HAART therapy (CD4 counts >150 to 200/μL), but have residual cutaneous KS, systemic interferon-alpha can also be considered, with responses detected in 20 to 40% of patients. Interferon-alpha is the only immunomodulatory agent to have shown a therapeutic effect for HIV-related KS. Unfortunately, high-dose interferon-alpha (up to 8 million U subcutaneously daily) therapy is often associated with significant side effects,[228] including fever, chills neutropenia, hepatotoxicity, alopecia, and cognitive impairment. Recent advances in the understanding of KS pathogenesis have uncovered many potential targets for KS therapies, which are now the focus of several trials. Angiogenesis inhibitors are one group of investigational agents currently being tested in HIV-related KS. These include thalidomide, fumagiline, the MMP inhibitor COL-3, and imatinib mesylate.[220]

Thalidomide-induced regression of KS has been documented in several trials, showing an overall response rate of 40%.[229] The antiangiogenic properties of thalidomide may be responsible for the clinical efficacy in KS. In phase I, clinical trial of the MMP inhibitor COL-3, the tumor response rate was encouraging (44%) and correlated with decreased angiogenesis.[230] The administration of imatinib mesilate, a c-kit, and PDGF receptor inhibitor resulted in regression of HIV-related KS lesions.[96] This is not surprising, considering the role of PDGF and c-kit signaling in KS tumorigenesis.

Another therapeutic target involves antiviral therapy to target HHV-8. It seemed plausible that antiherpetic drugs might be effective against KS. This notion is reinforced by reports of KS responding to antiherpetic drugs, and from studies showing that treatment of AIDS patients with cytomegalovirus (CMV) infection with ganciclovir or foscarnet reduced the risk of KS.[231] Cidofovir was found to be one of the most active drugs against HHV-8.[232,233] Cidofovir is a potent nucleoside analog antiviral drug approved for the treatment of CMV retinitis in patients with HIV. It is currently available only for intravenous infusion. Its routine use in dermatology is hampered by its high cost, lack of continued interest by the manufacturer, and nagging concerns regarding carcinogenicity.[232]

Several investigational agents are being currently tested for HIV-related KS, including iron chelators such as desferrioxamine (DFO) and other iron withdrawal strategies,[234] as well as oral retinoids[235]; so far with limited therapeutic benefits, but further studies should evaluate those therapies.

Iatrogenic KS

Treatment of transplant-related KS consists mainly of reduction of, or withholding of, immunosuppression, often with deleterious effects on both graft and patient survival. Recent experimental evidence demonstrated that sirolimus, an immunosuppressive agent used in kidney transplantation, inhibits the progression of dermal KS when given at the usual immunosuppressive doses.[236] It was demonstrated that after conversion to sirolimus, patients showed continuous regression of their KS lesions, with only hyperpigmented atrophic cutaneous lesions remaining after 2 to 18 months.[237] Sirolimus seems to inhibit the growth of established vascularized tumors and this effect is best realized with relatively low immunosuppressive doses of drug.[136]

Endemic KS

Therapy for endemic KS is difficult and remains palliative. Different therapeutic options may be considered, including cryotherapy, multiple excisions, laser therapy (argon laser for smaller lesions and carbon dioxide laser for bigger lesions), intralesional interferon alpha, vinblastine sulfate, radiation therapy, and photochemotherapy.[238] However, the rate of local recurrences remains high after topically targeted therapies.[115] Dissemination of the tumor or systemic involvement requires a systemic therapeutic approach. The current options consist of interferon alpha, liposomal daunorubicin hydrochloride, vinblastine, vincristine sulfate, and dacarbazine.[115] The clinical outcomes of these treatments are relatively poor, and the long-term palliative treatment of these patients is frequently limited by hematologic and/or cardiological (e.g., anthracyclines) toxic effects. The antiangiogenic potential of protease inhibitors in HIV-seropositive or HIV-seronegative individuals with KS has been recently suggested as an additional treatment option.[115] A novel therapeutic approach based on the paradigm of antiangiogenic therapy was recently demonstrated, showing a partial remission that remained stable for 18 months. This consisted of the biomodulators pioglitazone hydrochloride and rofecoxib combined with metronomic low-dose daily chemotherapy with trofosfamide.[239]

In the near future, RNA interference (referred to as posttranscriptional gene silencing), a conserved cellular function known to control viral infection, will be exploited to prevent or treat HHV-8 infection,[240] and the role of gene therapy for KS may be closer than what we currently thought. Gene therapy using antiangiogenic cytokines or TIMPs has already been shown *in vitro* to inhibit KS-related angiogenesis effectively.[241,242]

■ FINAL THOUGHTS

KS has been known for more than 130 years since its original description by Moritz Kaposi. Besides the originally described classic form, other forms such as AIDS-related KS, African endemic KS, and iatrogenically induced KS have been recognized subsequently. The main breakthrough in recent years has been the association of KS with HHV-8 infection. New data has suggested different modes of transmission of KS including horizontal spread. The reason why only some individuals with HHV-8 infection develop KS and the mechanism by which HHV-8 participates in the induction of KS are still to be elucidated. Current treatments for KS are palliative, although HAART therapy has dramatically reduced the incidence of KS in AIDS patients, and the administration of sirolimus has been associated with improved prognosis of kidney transplant KS. The cessation of immunosuppressive agents in iatrogenically induced KS may cause KS to regress altogether. The newly approved agents for AIDS-related KS including alitretirxoin gel for topical administration, and lipsomal doxorubicin, lipsosomal daunorubicin, palcitaxel, and interferon alpha for systemic treatment, have improved the therapy of KS. Currently, investigational therapies such as angiogenic inhibitors show promising results.

REFERENCES

1. Kaposi M. Idiopathisches multiples pigmentsarkom der haut. *Arch Dermatol Syph.* 1872;3:265–273.
2. Lamovec J, Knuutila S. Kaposi's sarcoma. In: Fletcher CDM, Unni KK, Mertens F, eds. *World Health Organization Classification of Tumors. Pathology & Genetics, Tumors of Soft Tissue and Bone.* Lyon, France: IARC Press; 2002:170–172.

3. Friedman-Kien AE, Saltzman BR. Clinical manifestations of classical, endemic African, and epidemic AIDS-associated Kaposi's sarcoma. *J Am Acad Dermatol.* 1990;22:1237–1250.

4. Safai B. Kaposi's sarcoma: an overview of classical and epidemic forms. In: Broder S, ed. *AIDS, Modern Concepts and Therapeutic Challenges.* New York: Marcel Dekker; 1987:205.

5. Weissmann-Brenner A, Friedman-Birnbaum R, Brenner B. Familial Kaposi's sarcoma: a cluster of five Israeli cases. *Clin Oncol (R Coll Radiol).* 2004;16:125–128.

6. Krigel RL, Friedman-Kien A. Kaposi's sarcoma. In: DeVita VTJ, Hellman S, Rosenberg SA, eds. *AIDS: Etiology, Diagnosis, Treatment and Prevention.* Philadelphia, PA: Lippincott; 1985:185–211.

7. Rappersberger K, Stingl G, Wolff K. Kaposi's sarcoma. In: Freedberg IM, Eisen AZ, Wolff K, Austen KF, Goldsmith LA, Katz SI, eds. *Fitzpatrick's Dermatology in General Medicine.* New York: McGraw-Hill; 2003:1020–1026.

8. Templeton AC. Kaposi's sarcoma. In: Andrade R, Gumport SL, Popkin GL, et al, eds. *Cancer of the Skin: Biology, Diagnosis and Management.* Philadelphia, PA: WB Saunders; 1976:1183–1225.

9. Horowitz L, Stern JO, Segarra S. Gastrointestinal manifestations of Kaposi's sarcoma and AIDS. In: Friedman-Kien A, Laubenstein LJ, eds. *AIDS: The Epidemic of Kaposi's Sarcoma and Opportunistic Infections.* New York: Masson Publishing; 1984:235–239.

10. Safai B, Mike V, Giraldo G, Beth E, Good RA. Association of Kaposi's sarcoma with second primary malignancies: possible etiopathogenic implications. *Cancer.* 1980;45:1472–1479.

11. Pantanowitz L, Dezube BJ. Advances in the pathobiology and treatment of Kaposi sarcoma. *Curr Opin Oncol.* 2004;16:443–449.

12. Oettle AG. Geographical and racial differences in the frequency of Kaposi's sarcoma as evidence of environmental or genetic causes. *Acta Unio Int Contra Cancrum.* 1962;18:330–363.

13. Lothe F, Murray JF. Kaposi's sarcoma: autopsy findings in the African. *Acta Unio Int Contra Cancrum.* 1962;18:429–452.

14. Hood AF, Farmer ER, Weiss RA. Clinical conferences at the Johns Hopkins Hospital: Kaposi's sarcoma. *Johns Hopkins Med J.* 1982;151:222–230.

15. Slavin G, Cameron HM, Forbes C, Mitchell RM. Kaposi's sarcoma in East African children: a report of 51 cases. *J Pathol.* 1970;100:187–199.

16. Davies JN, Lothe F. Kaposi's sarcoma in African children. *Acta Unio Int Contra Cancrum.* 1962;18:394–399.

17. Olweny CLM. Epidemiology and clinical features of Kaposi's sarcoma in tropical Africa. In: Friedman-Kien A, Laubenstein LJ, eds. *AIDS: The Epidemic of Kaposi's Sarcoma and Opportunistic Infections.* New York: Masson Publishing; 1984:35–40.

18. Campbell TB, Borok M, White IE, et al. Relationship of Kaposi sarcoma (KS)-associated herpesvirus viremia and KS disease in Zimbabwe. *Clin Infect Dis.* 2003;36:1144–1151.

19. Schwartz RA. Kaposi's sarcoma: an update. *J Surg Oncol.* 2004;87:146–151.

20. Beral V, Peterman TA, Berkelman RL, Jaffe HW. Kaposi's sarcoma among persons with AIDS: a sexually transmitted infection? *Lancet.* 1990;335:123–128.

21. Tappero JW, Conant MA, Wolfe SF, Berger TG. Kaposi's sarcoma. Epidemiology, pathogenesis, histology, clinical spectrum, staging criteria and therapy. *J Am Acad Dermatol.* 1993;28: 371–395.

22. Roth WK. HIV-associated Kaposi's sarcoma: new developments in epidemiology and molecular pathology. *J Cancer Res Clin Oncol.* 1991;117:186–191.

23. Casabona J, Melbye M, Biggar RJ. Kaposi's sarcoma and non-Hodgkin's lymphoma in European AIDS cases. No excess risk of Kaposi's sarcoma in Mediterranean countries. *Int J Cancer.* 1991;47:49–53.

24. Calonje E, Wilson-Jones E. Vascular tumors and tumor-like conditions of blood vessels and lymphatics. In: Elder DE, Elenitsas R, Johnson B, eds. *Lever's Histopathology of the Skin.* Philadelphia, PA: Lippincott; 2005:1015–1059.

25. Lemlich G, Schwam L, Lebwohl M. Kaposi's sarcoma and acquired immunodeficiency syndrome. Postmortem findings in twenty-four cases. *J Am Acad Dermatol.* 1987;16:319–325.

26. Cheung TW. AIDS-related cancer in the era of highly active antiretroviral therapy (HAART): a model of the interplay of the immune system, virus, and cancer. "On the offensive—the Trojan Horse is being destroyed"—Part A: Kaposi's sarcoma. *Cancer Invest.* 2004;22:774–786.

27. Aversa SM, Cattelan AM, Salvagno L, et al. Treatments of AIDS-related Kaposi's sarcoma. *Crit Rev Oncol Hematol.* 2005;53:253–265.

28. Cattelan AM, Calabro ML, De Rossi A, et al. Long-term clinical outcome of AIDS-related Kaposi's sarcoma during highly active antiretroviral therapy. *Int J Oncol.* 2005;27:779–785.

29. Moray G, Basaran O, Yagmurdur MC, Emiroglu R, Bilgin N, Haberal M. Immunosuppressive therapy and Kaposi's sarcoma after kidney transplantation. *Transplant Proc.* 2004;36:168–170.

30. Piette WW. The incidence of second malignancies in subsets of Kaposi's sarcoma. *J Am Acad Dermatol.* 1987;16:855–861.

31. Gange RW, Jones EW. Kaposi's sarcoma and immunosuppressive therapy: an appraisal. *Clin Exp Dermatol.* 1978;3:135–146.

32. Harwood AR, Osoba D, Hofstader SL, et al. Kaposi's sarcoma in recipients of renal transplants. *Am J Med.* 1979;67:759–765.

33. Micali G, Gasparri O, Nasca MR, Sapuppo A. Kaposi's sarcoma occurring de novo in the surgical scar in a heart transplant recipient. *J Am Acad Dermatol.* 1992;27:273–274.

34. Trattner A, Hodak E, David M, Neeman A, Sandbank M. Kaposi's sarcoma with visceral involvement after intraarticular and epidural injections of corticosteroids. *J Am Acad Dermatol.* 1993;29:890–894.

35. Halpern SM, Parslew R, Cerio R, Kirby JT, Sharpe GR. Kaposi's sarcoma associated with immunosuppression for bullous pemphigoid. *Br J Dermatol.* 1997;137:140–143.

36. Garcia-Sesma A, Jimenez C, Loinaz C, et al. Kaposi's visceral sarcoma in liver transplant recipients. *Transplant Proc.* 2003;35:1898–1899.

37. Marcelin AG, Roque-Afonso AM, Hurtova M, et al. Fatal disseminated Kaposi's sarcoma following human herpesvirus 8 primary infections in liver-transplant recipients. *Liver Transpl.* 2004;10:295–300.

38. Dourmishev LA, Dourmishev AL, Palmeri D, Schwartz RA, Lukac DM. Molecular genetics of Kaposi's sarcoma-associated herpesvirus (human herpesvirus-8) epidemiology and pathogenesis. *Microbiol Mol Biol Rev.* 2003;67:175–212.

39. Weigert AL, Pires A, Adragao T, et al. Human herpes virus-8 serology and DNA analysis in recipients of renal allografts showing Kaposi's sarcoma and their respective donors. *Transplant Proc.* 2004;36:902–904.

40. Barozzi P, Luppi M, Facchetti F, et al. Post-transplant Kaposi sarcoma originates from the seeding of donor-derived progenitors. *Nat Med.* 2003;9:554–561.

41. Fenig E, Brenner B, Rakowsky E, Lapidoth M, Katz A, Sulkes A. Classic Kaposi sarcoma: experience at Rabin Medical Center in Israel. *Am J Clin Oncol.* 1998;21:498–500.

42. Pedagogos E, Nicholls K, Dowling J, Becker G. Kaposi's sarcoma post renal transplantation. *Aust N Z J Med.* 1994;24:722–723.

43. Montagnino G, Bencini PL, Tarantino A, Caputo R, Ponticelli C. Clinical features and course of Kaposi's sarcoma in kidney transplant patients: report of 13 cases. *Am J Nephrol.* 1994;14:121–126.

44. Campistol JM, Gutierrez-Dalmau A, Torregrosa JV. Conversion to sirolimus: a successful treatment for posttransplantation Kaposi's sarcoma. *Transplantation.* 2004;77:760–762.

45. Friedman-Birnbaum R, Bergman R, Bitterman-Deutsch O, Weltfriend S, Lichtig C. Classic and iatrogenic Kaposi's sarcoma. Histopathological patterns as related to clinical course. *Am J Dermatopathol.* 1993;15:523–527.

46. Harawi S. Kaposi's sarcoma. In: Harawi SJ, O'Hara CJ, eds. *Pathology and Pathophysiology of AIDS and HIV-Related Diseases.* St. Louis, MO: Mosby; 1989:83–131.

47. Weedon D. *Skin Pathology.* 2nd ed. London: Churchill Livingstone; 2002:1021–1025.

48. Robin YM, Guillou L, Michels JJ, Coindre JM. Human herpesvirus 8 immunostaining: a sensitive and specific method for diagnosing Kaposi sarcoma in paraffin-embedded sections. *Am J Clin Pathol.* 2004;121:330–334.

49. Cheuk W, Wong KO, Wong CS, Dinkel JE, Ben Dor D, Chan JK. Immunostaining for human herpesvirus 8 latent nuclear antigen-1 helps distinguish Kaposi sarcoma from its mimickers. *Am J Clin Pathol.* 2004;121:335–342.

50. Gottlieb, GB, Ackerman AB. *Kaposi's Sarcoma: A Text and Atlas.* Philadelphia, PA: Lea & Febiger; 1988:73–112.

51. Patel RM, Goldblum JR, Hsi ED. Immunohistochemical detection of

human herpes virus-8 latent nuclear antigen-1 is useful in the diagnosis of Kaposi sarcoma. *Mod Pathol.* 2004;17: 456–460.

52. Chang Y, Cesarman E, Pessin MS, et al. Identification of herpesvirus-like DNA sequences in AIDS-associated Kaposi's sarcoma. *Science.* 1994;266:1865–1869.

53. Sarid R, Olsen SJ, Moore PS. Kaposi's sarcoma-associated herpesvirus epidemiology, virology, and molecular biology. *Adv Virus Res.* 1999;52:139–232.

54. Russo JJ, Bohenzky RA, Chien MC, et al. Nucleotide sequence of the Kaposi sarcoma-associated herpesvirus (HHV8). *Proc Natl Acad Sci USA.* 1996;93:14862–14867.

55. Whitby D, Stossel A, Gamache C, et al. Novel Kaposi's sarcoma-associated herpesvirus homolog in baboons. *J Virol.* 2003;77:8159–8165.

56. Cesarman E, Chang Y, Moore PS, Said JW, Knowles DM. Kaposi's sarcoma-associated herpesvirus-like DNA sequences in AIDS-related body-cavity-based lymphomas. *N Engl J Med.* 1995;332:1186–1191.

57. Soulier J, Grollet L, Oksenhendler E, et al. Kaposi's sarcoma-associated herpesvirus-like DNA sequences in multicentric Castleman's disease. *Blood.* 1995;86:1276–1280.

58. Codish S, Abu-Shakra M, Ariad S, et al. Manifestations of three HHV-8-related diseases in an HIV-negative patient: immunoblastic variant multicentric Castleman's disease, primary effusion lymphoma, and Kaposi's sarcoma. *Am J Hematol.* 2000;65:310–314.

59. Ascoli V, Signoretti S, Onetti-Muda A, et al. Primary effusion lymphoma in HIV-infected patients with multicentric Castleman's disease. *J Pathol.* 2001;193:200–209.

60. Mocroft A, Kirk O, Clumeck N, et al. The changing pattern of Kaposi sarcoma in patients with HIV, 1994–2003: the EuroSIDA Study. *Cancer.* 2004;100:2644–2654.

61. Lebbe C, Blum L, Pellet C, et al. Clinical and biological impact of antiretroviral therapy with protease inhibitors on HIV-related Kaposi's sarcoma. *AIDS.* 1998;12:F45–F49.

62. Grundhoff A, Sullivan CS, Ganem D. A combined computational and microarray-based approach identifies novel microRNAs encoded by human gamma-herpesviruses. *RNA* 2006;12:733–750.

63. Moore PS, Chang Y. Kaposi's sarcoma-associated herpesvirus immunoevasion and tumorigenesis: two sides of the same coin? *Annu Rev Microbiol.* 2003;57:609–639.

64. An FQ, Compitello N, Horwitz E, Sramkoski M, Knudsen ES, Renne R. The latency-associated nuclear antigen of Kaposi's sarcoma-associated herpesvirus modulates cellular gene expression and protects lymphoid cells from p16 INK4A-induced cell cycle arrest. *J Biol Chem.* 2005;280:3862–3874.

65. Chang H, Gwack Y, Kingston D, et al. Activation of CD21 and CD23 gene expression by Kaposi's sarcoma-associated herpesvirus RTA. *J Virol.* 2005;79:4651–4663.

66. Nakamura H, Lu M, Gwack Y, Souvlis J, Zeichner SL, Jung JU. Global changes in Kaposi's sarcoma-associated virus gene expression patterns following expression of a tetracycline-inducible Rta transactivator. *J Virol.* 2003;77:4205–4220.

67. McCormick C, Ganem D. The kaposin B protein of KSHV activates the p38/MK2 pathway and stabilizes cytokine mRNAs. *Science.* 2005;307:739–741.

68. Godden-Kent D, Talbot SJ, Boshoff C, et al. The cyclin encoded by Kaposi's sarcoma-associated herpesvirus stimulates cdk6 to phosphorylate the retinoblastoma protein and histone H1. *J Virol.* 1997;71:4193–4198.

69. Verschuren EW, Jones N, Evan GI. The cell cycle and how it is steered by Kaposi's sarcoma-associated herpesvirus cyclin. *J Gen Virol.* 2004;85:1347–1361.

70. Nakamura H, Li M, Zarycki J, Jung JU. Inhibition of p53 tumor suppressor by viral interferon regulatory factor. *J Virol.* 2001;75:7572–7582.

71. Shin YC, Nakamura H, Liang X, et al. Inhibition of the ATM/p53 signal transduction pathway by Kaposi's sarcoma-associated herpesvirus interferon regulatory factor 1. *J Virol.* 2006;80:2257–2266.

72. Friborg JJ, Kong W, Hottiger MO, Nabel GJ. p53 inhibition by the LANA protein of KSHV protects against cell death. *Nature.* 1999;402:889–894.

73. Radkov SA, Kellam P, Boshoff C. The latent nuclear antigen of Kaposi sarcoma-associated herpesvirus targets the retinoblastoma-E2F pathway and with the oncogene Hras transforms primary rat cells. *Nat Med.* 2000;6:1121–1127.

74. Fujimuro M, Wu FY, ApRhys C, et al. A novel viral mechanism for dysregulation of beta-catenin in Kaposi's sarcoma-associated herpesvirus latency. *Nat Med.* 2003;9:300–306.

75. Yu Y, Wang SE, Hayward GS. The KSHV immediate-early transcription factor RTA encodes ubiquitin E3 ligase activity that targets IRF7 for proteosome-mediated degradation. *Immunity.* 2005;22:59–70.

76. Nicholas J. Human gammaherpesvirus cytokines and chemokine receptors. *J Interferon Cytokine Res.* 2005;25:373–383.

77. Matta H, Sun Q, Moses G, Chaudhary PM. Molecular genetic analysis of human herpes virus 8-encoded viral FLICE inhibitory protein-induced NF-kappaB activation. *J Biol Chem.* 2003;278:52406–52411.

78. Guasparri I, Wu H, Cesarman E. The KSHV oncoprotein vFLIP contains a TRAF-interacting motif and requires TRAF2 and TRAF3 for signalling. *EMBO Rep.* 2006;7:114–119.

79. Krishnan HH, Naranatt PP, Smith MS, Zeng L, Bloomer C, Chandran B. Concurrent expression of latent and a limited number of lytic genes with immune modulation and antiapoptotic function by Kaposi's sarcoma-associated herpesvirus early during infection of primary endothelial and fibroblast cells and subsequent decline of lytic gene expression. *J Virol.* 2004;78:3601–3620.

80. Staskus KA, Zhong W, Gebhard K, et al. Kaposi's sarcoma-associated herpesvirus gene expression in endothelial (spindle) tumor cells. *J Virol.* 1997;71:715–719.

81. Dupin N, Fisher C, Kellam P, et al. Distribution of human herpesvirus-8 latently infected cells in Kaposi's sarcoma, multicentric Castleman's disease, and primary effusion lymphoma. *Proc Natl Acad Sci USA.* 1999;96:4546–4551.

82. Sturzl M, Blasig C, Schreier A, et al. Expression of HHV-8 latency-associated T0.7 RNA in spindle cells and endothelial cells of AIDS-associated, classical and African Kaposi's sarcoma. *Int J Cancer.* 1997;72:68–71.

83. Katano H, Sato Y, Kurata T, Mori S, Sata T. Expression and localization of human herpesvirus 8-encoded proteins in primary effusion lymphoma, Kaposi's sarcoma, and multicentric Castleman's disease. *Virology.* 2000;269:335–344.

84. Parravicini C, Chandran B, Corbellino M, et al. Differential viral protein expression in Kaposi's sarcoma-associated herpesvirus-infected diseases: Kaposi's sarcoma, primary effusion lymphoma, and multicentric Castleman's disease. *Am J Pathol.* 2000;156:743–749.

85. Gessain A, Duprez R. Spindle cells and their role in Kaposi's sarcoma. *Int J Biochem Cell Biol.* 2005;37:2457–2465.

86. Wang HW, Trotter MW, Lagos D, et al. Kaposi sarcoma herpesvirus-induced cellular reprogramming contributes to the lymphatic endothelial gene expression in Kaposi sarcoma. *Nat Genet.* 2004;36:687–693.

87. Hong YK, Foreman K, Shin JW, et al. Lymphatic reprogramming of blood vascular endothelium by Kaposi sarcoma-associated herpesvirus. *Nat Genet.* 2004;36:683–685.

88. Carroll PA, Brazeau E, Lagunoff M. Kaposi's sarcoma-associated herpesvirus infection of blood endothelial cells induces lymphatic differentiation. *Virology.* 2004;328:7–18.

89. Cheung L, Rockson SG. The lymphatic biology of Kaposi's sarcoma. *Lymphat Res Biol.* 2005;3:25–35.

90. Naranatt PP, Krishnan HH, Svojanovsky SR, Bloomer C, Mathur S, Chandran B. Host gene induction and transcriptional reprogramming in Kaposi's sarcoma-associated herpesvirus (KSHV/HHV-8)-infected endothelial, fibroblast, and B cells: insights into modulation events early during infection. *Cancer Res.* 2004;64:72–84.

91. Kahn HJ, Bailey D, Marks A. Monoclonal antibody D2-40, a new marker of lymphatic endothelium, reacts with Kaposi's sarcoma and a subset of angiosarcomas. *Mod Pathol.* 2002;15:434–440.

92. Jussila L, Valtola R, Partanen TA, et al. Lymphatic endothelium and Kaposi's sarcoma spindle cells detected by antibodies against the vascular endothelial growth factor receptor-3. *Cancer Res.* 1998;58:1599–1604.

93. Marchio S, Primo L, Pagano M, et al. Vascular endothelial growth factor-C stimulates the migration and proliferation of Kaposi's sarcoma cells. *J Biol Chem.* 1999;274:27617–27622.

94. Ford PW, Hamden KE, Whitman AG, McCubrey JA, Akula SM. Vascular endothelial growth factor augments human herpesvirus-8 (HHV-8/KSHV) infection. *Cancer Biol Ther.* 2004;3:876–881.

95. Raggo C, Ruhl R, McAllister S, et al. Novel cellular genes essential for transformation of endothelial cells by Kaposi's sarcoma-associated herpesvirus. *Cancer Res.* 2005;65:5084–5095.

96. Koon HB, Bubley GJ, Pantanowitz L, et al. Imatinib-induced regression of AIDS-related Kaposi's sarcoma. *J Clin Oncol.* 2005;23:982–989.

97. Ensoli B, Sturzl M, Monini P. Cytokine-mediated growth promotion of Kaposi's sarcoma and primary effusion lymphoma. *Semin Cancer Biol.* 2000;10: 367–381.

98. Wang HW, Boshoff C. Linking Kaposi virus to cancer-associated cytokines. *Trends Mol Med.* 2005;11:309–312.

99. Yao L, Salvucci O, Cardones AR, et al. Selective expression of stromal-derived factor-1 in the capillary vascular endothelium plays a role in Kaposi sarcoma pathogenesis. *Blood.* 2003;102: 3900–3905.

100. Delabesse E, Oksenhendler E, Lebbe C, Verola O, Varet B, Turhan AG. Molecular analysis of clonality in Kaposi's sarcoma. *J Clin Pathol.* 1997;50: 664–668.

101. Judde JG, Lacoste V, Briere J, et al. Monoclonality or oligoclonality of human herpesvirus 8 terminal repeat sequences in Kaposi's sarcoma and other diseases. *J Natl Cancer Inst.* 2000; 92:729–736.

102. Gill PS, Tsai YC, Rao AP, et al. Evidence for multiclonality in multicentric Kaposi's sarcoma. *Proc Natl Acad Sci USA.* 1998; 95:8257–8261.

103. Browning PJ, Sechler JM, Kaplan M, et al. Identification and culture of Kaposi's sarcoma-like spindle cells from the peripheral blood of human immunodeficiency virus-1-infected individuals and normal controls. *Blood.* 1994;84:2711–2720.

104. Monini P, Colombini S, Sturzl M, et al. Reactivation and persistence of human herpesvirus-8 infection in B cells and monocytes by Th-1 cytokines increased in Kaposi's sarcoma. *Blood.* 1999;93: 4044–4058.

105. Uccini S, Sirianni MC, Vincenzi L, et al. Kaposi's sarcoma cells express the macrophage-associated antigen mannose receptor and develop in peripheral blood cultures of Kaposi's sarcoma patients. *Am J Pathol.* 1997;150:929–938.

106. Parsons CH, Szomju B, Kedes DH. Susceptibility of human fetal mesenchymal stem cells to Kaposi sarcoma-associated herpesvirus. *Blood.* 2004;104: 2736–2738.

107. Martin DF, Kuppermann BD, Wolitz RA, Palestine AG, Li H, Robinson CA. Oral ganciclovir for patients with cytomegalovirus retinitis treated with a ganciclovir implant. Roche Ganciclovir Study Group. *N Engl J Med.* 1999;340: 1063–1070.

108. Montaner S, Sodhi A, Ramsdell AK, et al. The Kaposi's sarcoma-associated herpesvirus G protein-coupled receptor as a therapeutic target for the treatment of Kaposi's sarcoma. *Cancer Res.* 2006; 66:168–174.

109. Montaner S, Sodhi A, Molinolo A, et al. Endothelial infection with KSHV genes in vivo reveals that vGPCR initiates Kaposi's sarcomagenesis and can promote the tumorigenic potential of viral latent genes. *Cancer Cell.* 2003;3:23–36.

110. Yang TY, Chen SC, Leach MW, et al. Transgenic expression of the chemokine receptor encoded by human herpesvirus 8 induces an angioproliferative disease resembling Kaposi's sarcoma. *J Exp Med.* 2000;191:445–454.

111. Guo HG, Sadowska M, Reid W, Tschachler E, Hayward G, Reitz M. Kaposi's sarcoma-like tumors in a human herpesvirus 8 ORF74 transgenic mouse. *J Virol.* 2003;77:2631–2639.

112. Thomas RK, Re D, Wolf J, Diehl V. Part I: Hodgkin's lymphoma—molecular biology of Hodgkin and Reed–Sternberg cells. *Lancet Oncol.* 2004;5:11–18.

113. Grundhoff A, Ganem D. Inefficient establishment of KSHV latency suggests an additional role for continued lytic replication in Kaposi sarcoma pathogenesis. *J Clin Invest.* 2004;113:124–136.

114. Ablashi D, Chatlynne L, Cooper H, et al. Seroprevalence of human herpesvirus-8 (HHV-8) in countries of southeast Asia compared to the USA, the Caribbean and Africa. *Br J Cancer.* 1999;81:893–897.

115. Antman K, Chang Y. Kaposi's sarcoma. *N Engl J Med.* 2000;342:1027–1038.

116. Cohen A, Wolf DG, Guttman-Yassky E, Sarid R. Kaposi's sarcoma-associated herpesvirus: clinical, diagnostic, and epidemiological aspects. *Crit Rev Clin Lab Sci.* 2005;42:101–153.

117. Kedes DH, Operskalski E, Busch M, Kohn R, Flood J, Ganem D. The seroepidemiology of human herpesvirus 8 (Kaposi's sarcoma-associated herpesvirus): distribution of infection in KS risk groups and evidence for sexual transmission. *Nat Med.* 1996;2:918–924.

118. Gao SJ, Kingsley L, Li M, et al. KSHV antibodies among Americans, Italians and Ugandans with and without Kaposi's sarcoma. *Nat Med.* 1996;2: 925–928.

119. Simpson GR, Schulz TF, Whitby D, et al. Prevalence of Kaposi's sarcoma associated herpesvirus infection measured by antibodies to recombinant capsid protein and latent immunofluorescence antigen. *Lancet.* 1996;348: 1133–1138.

120. Renwick N, Weverling GJ, Brouwer J, Bakker M, Schulz TF, Goudsmit J. Vascular endothelial growth factor levels in serum do not increase following HIV type 1 and HHV8 seroconversion and lack correlation with AIDS-related Kaposi's sarcoma. *AIDS Res Hum Retroviruses.* 2002;18:695–698.

121. Atzori L, Fadda D, Ferreli C, et al. Classic Kaposi's sarcoma in southern Sardinia, Italy. *Br J Cancer.* 2004;91: 1261–1262.

122. Dukers NH, Rezza G. Human herpesvirus 8 epidemiology: what we do and do not know. *AIDS.* 2003;17: 1717–1730.

123. Hengge UR, Ruzicka T, Tyring SK, et al. Update on Kaposi's sarcoma and other HHV8 associated diseases. Part 2: Pathogenesis, Castleman's disease, and pleural effusion lymphoma. *Lancet Infect Dis.* 2002;2:344–352.

124. Levi F, Randimbison L, Te VC, Franceschi S, La Vecchia C. Kaposi's sarcoma in Vaud and Neuchatel, Switzerland, 1978–2002. *Eur J Cancer.* 2004;40:1630–1633.

125. Iscovich J, Boffetta P, Franceschi S, Azizi E, Sarid R. Classic Kaposi sarcoma: epidemiology and risk factors. *Cancer.* 2000;88:500–517.

126. Grossman Z, Iscovich J, Schwartz F, et al. Absence of Kaposi sarcoma among Ethiopian immigrants to Israel despite high seroprevalence of human herpesvirus 8. *Mayo Clin Proc.* 2002;77:905–909.

127. Martin JN, Ganem DE, Osmond DH, Page-Shafer KA, Macrae D, Kedes DH. Sexual transmission and the natural history of human herpesvirus 8 infection. *N Engl J Med.* 1998;338:948–954.

128. Gao SJ, Kingsley L, Hoover DR, et al. Seroconversion to antibodies against Kaposi's sarcoma-associated herpesvirus-related latent nuclear antigens before the development of Kaposi's sarcoma. *N Engl J Med.* 1996;335: 233–241.

129. Renwick N, Halaby T, Weverling GJ, et al. Seroconversion for human herpesvirus 8 during HIV infection is highly predictive of Kaposi's sarcoma. *AIDS.* 1998;12:2481–2488.

130. Jones JL, Hanson DL, Dworkin MS, Ward JW, Jaffe HW. Effect of antiretroviral therapy on recent trends in selected cancers among HIV-infected persons. Adult/Adolescent Spectrum of HIV Disease Project Group. *J Acquir Immune Defic Syndr.* 1999;21(suppl 1):S11–S17.

131. Cook-Mozaffari P, Newton R, Beral V, Burkitt DP. The geographical distribution of Kaposi's sarcoma and of lymphomas in Africa before the AIDS epidemic. *Br J Cancer.* 1998;78:1521–1528.

132. Sitas F, Newton R. Kaposi's sarcoma in South Africa. *J Natl Cancer Inst Monogr.* 2001;28:1–4.

133. Kasolo FC, Mpabalwani E, Gompels UA. Infection with AIDS-related herpesviruses in human immunodeficiency virus-negative infants and endemic childhood Kaposi's sarcoma in Africa. *J Gen Virol.* 1997;78:847–855.

134. Mwanda OW, Fu P, Collea R, Whalen C, Remick SC. Kaposi's sarcoma in patients with and without human immunodeficiency virus infection, in a tertiary referral centre in Kenya. *Ann Trop Med Parasitol.* 2005;99:81–91.

135. von Muller L, Schliep C, Storck M, et al. Severe graft rejection, increased immunosuppression, and active CMV infection in renal transplantation. *J Med Virol.* 2006;78:394–399.

136. Zmonarski SC, Boratynska M, Puziewicz-Zmonarska A, Kazimierczak K, Klinger M. Kaposi's sarcoma in renal transplant recipients. *Ann Transplant.* 2005;10:59–65.

137. Alzahrani AJ, El Harith E, Milzer J, et al. Increased seroprevalence of human herpes virus-8 in renal transplant recipients in Saudi Arabia. *Nephrol Dial Transplant.* 2005;20:2532–2536.

138. Serraino D, Piselli P, Scuderi M, et al. Screening for human herpesvirus 8 antibodies in Italian organ transplantation centers. *Clin Infect Dis.* 2005;40: 203–205.

139. Stein L, Carrara H, Norman R, Alagiozoglou L, Morris L, Sitas F. Antibodies against human herpesvirus 8 in South African renal transplant recipients and blood donors. *Transpl Infect Dis.* 2004;6:69–73.

140. Huang JY, Chiang YJ, Lai PC, et al. Posttransplant Kaposi's sarcoma: report from a single center. *Transplant Proc.* 2004;36:2145–2147.

141. Almuneef M, Nimjee S, Khoshnood K, Miller G, Rigsby MO. Prevalence of antibodies to human herpesvirus 8 (HHV-8) in Saudi Arabian patients with and without renal failure. *Transplantation.* 2001;71: 1120–1124.

142. Regamey N, Tamm M, Wernli M, et al. Transmission of human herpesvirus 8 infection from renal-transplant donors to recipients. *N Engl J Med.* 1998;339: 1358–1363.

143. Verucchi G, Calza L, Trevisani F, et al. Human herpesvirus-8-related Kaposi's sarcoma after liver transplantation successfully treated with cidofovir and liposomal daunorubicin. *Transpl Infect Dis.* 2005;7:34–37.

144. Boeckle E, Boesmueller C, Wiesmayr S, et al. Kaposi sarcoma in solid organ transplant recipients: a single center report. *Transplant Proc.* 2005;37:1905– 1909.

145. Sarid R, Pizov G, Rubinger D, et al. Early detection of Kaposi's sarcoma-associated herpesvirus DNA in kidney allografts of transplant recipients who developed Kaposi's sarcoma. *Clin Infect Dis.* 2001;32:1502–1505.

146. Ariyoshi K, Schim van der Loeff M, Cook P, et al. Kaposi's sarcoma in the Gambia, West Africa is less frequent in human immunodeficiency virus type 2 than in human immunodeficiency virus type 1 infection despite a high prevalence of human herpesvirus 8. *J Hum Virol.* 1998; 1:193–199.

147. Biggar RJ, Whitby D, Marshall V, Linhares AC, Black F. Human herpesvirus 8 in Brazilian Amerindians: a hyperendemic population with a new subtype. *J Infect Dis.* 2000;181:1562– 1568.

148. Guttman-Yassky E, Cohen A, Kra-Oz Z, et al. Familial clustering of classic Kaposi sarcoma. *J Infect Dis.* 2004;189:2023–2026.

149. Gnann JW, Jr, Pellett PE, Jaffe HW. Human herpesvirus 8 and Kaposi's sarcoma in persons infected with human immunodeficiency virus. *Clin Infect Dis.* 2000;30(suppl 1):S72–S76.

150. Melbye M, Cook PM, Hjalgrim H, et al. Risk factors for Kaposi's-sarcoma-associated herpesvirus (KSHV/HHV-8) seropositivity in a cohort of homosexual men, 1981–1996. *Int J Cancer.* 1998;77: 543–548.

151. Pauk J, Huang ML, Brodie SJ, et al. Mucosal shedding of human herpesvirus 8 in men. *N Engl J Med.* 2000; 343:1369–1377.

152. Grulich AE, Cunningham P, Munier ML, et al. Sexual behaviour and human herpesvirus 8 infection in homosexual men in Australia. *Sex Health.* 2005;2: 13–18.

153. Nawar E, Mbulaiteye SM, Gallant JE, et al. Risk factors for Kaposi's sarcoma among HHV-8 seropositive homosexual men with AIDS. *Int J Cancer.* 2005;115: 296–300.

154. Dukers NH, Renwick N, Prins M, et al. Risk factors for human herpesvirus 8 seropositivity and seroconversion in a cohort of homosexual men. *Am J Epidemiol.* 2000;151:213–224.

155. Osmond DH, Buchbinder S, Cheng A, et al. Prevalence of Kaposi sarcoma-associated herpesvirus infection in homosexual men at beginning of and during the HIV epidemic. *JAMA.* 2002;287:221–225.

156. Monini P, de Lellis L, Fabris M, Rigolin F, Cassai E. Kaposi's sarcoma-associated herpesvirus DNA sequences in prostate tissue and human semen. *N Engl J Med.* 1996;334:1168–1172.

157. Blackbourn DJ, Levy JA. Human herpesvirus 8 in semen and prostate. *AIDS.* 1997;11:249–250.

158. Pellett PE, Spira TJ, Bagasra O, et al. Multicenter comparison of PCR assays for detection of human herpesvirus 8 DNA in semen. *J Clin Microbiol.* 1999;37: 1298–1301.

159. Howard MR, Whitby D, Bahadur G, et al. Detection of human herpesvirus 8 DNA in semen from HIV-infected individuals but not healthy semen donors. *AIDS.* 1997;11:F15–F19.

160. Whitby D, Howard MR, Tenant-Flowers M, et al. Detection of Kaposi sarcoma associated herpesvirus in peripheral blood of HIV-infected individuals and progression to Kaposi's sarcoma. *Lancet.* 1995;346:799–802.

161. Grulich AE, Kaldor JM, Hendry O, Luo K, Bodsworth NJ, Cooper DA. Risk of Kaposi's sarcoma and oroanal sexual contact. *Am J Epidemiol.* 1997;145: 673–679.

162. Taylor MM, Chohan B, Lavreys L, et al. Shedding of human herpesvirus 8 in oral and genital secretions from HIV-1-seropositive and -seronegative Kenyan women. *J Infect Dis.* 2004;190:484–488.

163. Triantos D, Horefti E, Paximadi E, et al. Presence of human herpes virus-8 in saliva and non-lesional oral mucosa in HIV-infected and oncologic immunocompromised patients. *Oral Microbiol Immunol.* 2004;19:201–204.

164. Cattani P, Capuano M, Cerimele F, et al. Human herpesvirus 8 seroprevalence and evaluation of nonsexual transmission routes by detection of DNA in clinical specimens from human immunodeficiency virus-seronegative patients from central and southern Italy, with and without Kaposi's sarcoma. *J Clin Microbiol.* 1999;37:1150–1153.

165. Lavreys L, Chohan B, Ashley R, et al. Human herpesvirus 8: seroprevalence and correlates in prostitutes in Mombasa, Kenya. *J Infect Dis.* 2003;187: 359–363.

166. Eltom MA, Mbulaiteye SM, Dada AJ, Whitby D, Biggar RJ. Transmission of human herpesvirus 8 by sexual activity among adults in Lagos, Nigeria. *AIDS.* 2002;16:2473–2478.

167. Andreoni M, El-Sawaf G, Rezza G, et al. High seroprevalence of antibodies to human herpesvirus-8 in Egyptian children: evidence of nonsexual transmission. *J Natl Cancer Inst.* 1999;91:465–469.

168. Sarmati L. HHV-8 infection in African children. *Herpes.* 2004;11:50–53.

169. Mayama S, Cuevas LE, Sheldon J, et al. Prevalence and transmission of Kaposi's sarcoma-associated herpesvirus (human herpesvirus 8) in Ugandan children and adolescents. *Int J Cancer.* 1998;77:817– 820.

170. Whitby D, Luppi M, Sabin C, et al. Detection of antibodies to human herpesvirus 8 in Italian children: evidence for horizontal transmission. *Br J Cancer.* 2000;82:702–704.

171. Plancoulaine S, Abel L, van Beveren M, et al. Human herpesvirus 8 transmission from mother to child and between siblings in an endemic population. *Lancet.* 2000;356:1062–1065.

172. Mbulaiteye SM, Pfeiffer RM, Engels EA, et al. Detection of Kaposi sarcoma-associated herpesvirus DNA in saliva and buffy-coat samples from children with sickle cell disease in Uganda. *J Infect Dis.* 2004;190:1382–1386.

173. Dedicoat M, Newton R, Alkharsah KR, et al. Mother-to-child transmission of human herpesvirus-8 infection in South Africa. *J Infect Dis.* 2004;190:1068–1075.

174. Mbulaiteye SM, Biggar RJ, Pfeiffer RM, et al. Water, socioeconomic factors, and human herpesvirus 8 infection in Ugandan children and their mothers. *J Acquir Immune Defic Syndr.* 2005;38:474– 479.

175. Coluzzi M, Calabro ML, Manno D, Chieco-Bianchi L, Schulz TF, Ascoli V. Saliva and the transmission of human herpesvirus 8: potential role of promoter-arthropod bites. *J Infect Dis.* 2004;190:199–200.

176. Coluzzi M, Calabro ML, Manno D, Chieco-Bianchi L, Schulz TF, Ascoli V. Reduced seroprevalence of Kaposi's sarcoma-associated herpesvirus (KSHV), human herpesvirus 8 (HHV8), related to suppression of Anopheles density in Italy. *Med Vet Entomol.* 2003;17:461–464.

177. Coluzzi M, Manno D, Guzzinati S, et al. The bloodsucking arthropod bite as possible cofactor in the transmission of human herpesvirus-8 infection and in the expression of Kaposi's sarcoma disease. *Parassitologia.* 2002;44:123–129.

178. Mbulaiteye SM, Pfeiffer RM, Whitby D, Brubaker GR, Shao J, Biggar RJ. Human herpesvirus 8 infection within families in rural Tanzania. *J Infect Dis.* 2003;187: 1780–1785.

179. Guttman-Yassky E, Kra-Oz Z, Dubnov J, et al. Transmission of Kaposi's sarcoma-associated herpes virus within families of classic Kaposi's sarcoma patients. *Arch Dermatol.* 2005;141:1424– 1434.

180. Plancoulaine S, Abel L, Tregouet D, et al. Respective roles of serological status and blood specific antihuman herpesvirus 8 antibody levels in human herpesvirus 8 intrafamilial transmission in a highly endemic area. *Cancer Res.* 2004; 64:8782–8787.

181. Mantina H, Kankasa C, Klaskala W, et al. Vertical transmission of Kaposi's sarcoma-associated herpesvirus. *Int J Cancer.* 2001;94:749–752.

182. Brayfield BP, Kankasa C, West JT, et al. Distribution of Kaposi sarcoma-associated herpesvirus/human herpesvirus 8 in maternal saliva and breast milk in Zambia: implications for transmission. *J Infect Dis.* 2004;189:2260–2270.

183. Brayfield BP, Phiri S, Kankasa C, et al. Postnatal human herpesvirus 8 and human immunodeficiency virus type 1 infection in mothers and infants from Zambia. *J Infect Dis.* 2003;187:559–568.

184. Sarmati L, Carlo T, Rossella S, et al. Human herpesvirus-8 infection in pregnancy and labor: lack of evidence of

vertical transmission. *J Med Virol.* 2004;72: 462–466.

185. Angeloni A, Heston L, Uccini S, et al. High prevalence of antibodies to human herpesvirus 8 in relatives of patients with classic Kaposi's sarcoma from Sardinia. *J Infect Dis.* 1998;177:1715–1718.

186. Brambilla L, Boneschi V, Ferrucci S, Taglioni M, Berti E. Human herpesvirus-8 infection among heterosexual partners of patients with classical Kaposi's sarcoma. *Br J Dermatol.* 2000;143:1021–1025.

187. Davidovici B, Karakis I, Bourboulia D, et al. Seroepidemiology and molecular epidemiology of Kaposi's sarcoma-associated herpesvirus among Jewish population groups in Israel. *J Natl Cancer Inst.* 2001;93:194–202.

188. Chen N, Nelson KE, Jenkins FJ, et al. Seroprevalence of human herpesvirus 8 infection in northern Thailand. *Clin Infect Dis.* 2004;39:1052–1058.

189. Bestetti G, Renon G, Mauclere P, et al. High seroprevalence of human herpesvirus-8 in pregnant women and prostitutes from Cameroon. *AIDS.* 1998;12: 541–543.

190. Marcelin AG, Grandadam M, Flandre P, et al. Kaposi's sarcoma herpesvirus and HIV-1 seroprevalences in prostitutes in Djibouti. *J Med Virol.* 2002;68:164–167.

191. Smith NA, Sabin CA, Gopal R, et al. Serologic evidence of human herpesvirus 8 transmission by homosexual but not heterosexual sex. *J Infect Dis.* 1999;180:600–606.

192. Tedeschi R, Caggiari L, Silins I, et al. Seropositivity to human herpesvirus 8 in relation to sexual history and risk of sexually transmitted infections among women. *Int J Cancer.* 2000;87:232–235.

193. Blackbourn DJ, Ambroziak J, Lennette E, Adams M, Ramachandran B, Levy JA. Infectious human herpesvirus 8 in a healthy North American blood donor. *Lancet.* 1997;349:609–611.

194. Cattani P, Capuano M, Lesnoni LP, et al. Human herpesvirus 8 in Italian HIV-seronegative patients with Kaposi sarcoma. *Arch Dermatol.* 1998;134: 695–699.

195. Mbulaiteye SM, Biggar RJ, Bakaki PM, et al. Human herpesvirus 8 infection and transfusion history in children with sickle-cell disease in Uganda. *J Natl Cancer Inst.* 2003;95:1330–1335.

196. Renwick N, Dukers NH, Weverling GJ, et al. Risk factors for human herpesvirus 8 infection in a cohort of drug users in the Netherlands, 1985–1996. *J Infect Dis.* 2002;185:1808–1812.

197. Lennette ET, Blackbourn DJ, Levy JA. Antibodies to human herpesvirus type 8 in the general population and in Kaposi's sarcoma patients. *Lancet.* 1996; 348:858–861.

198. Atkinson J, Edlin BR, Engels EA, et al. Seroprevalence of human herpesvirus 8 among injection drug users in San Francisco. *J Infect Dis.* 2003;187:974–981.

199. Dollard SC, Nelson KE, Ness PM, et al. Possible transmission of human herpesvirus-8 by blood transfusion in a historical United States cohort. *Transfusion.* 2005;45:500–503.

200. Zavitsanou A, Sypsa V, Petrodaskalaki M, et al. Human herpesvirus 8 infection in hemodialysis patients. *Am J Kidney Dis.* 2006;47:167–170.

201. Hoshida Y, Aozasa K. Malignancies in organ transplant recipients. *Pathol Int.* 2004;54:649–658.

202. Samhan M, Al Mousawi M, Donia F, Fathi T, Nasim J, Nampoory MR. Malignancy in renal recipients. *Transplant Proc.* 2005;37:3068–3070.

203. Parravicini C, Olsen SJ, Capra M, et al. Risk of Kaposi's sarcoma-associated herpes virus transmission from donor allografts among Italian posttransplant Kaposi's sarcoma patients. *Blood.* 1997;90:2826–2829.

204. Frances C, Mouquet C, Marcelin AG, et al. Outcome of kidney transplant recipients with previous human herpesvirus-8 infection. *Transplantation.* 2000;69: 1776–1779.

205. Farge D, Lebbe C, Marjanovic Z, et al. Human herpes virus-8 and other risk factors for Kaposi's sarcoma in kidney transplant recipients. Groupe Cooperatif de Transplantation d' Ile de France (GCIF). *Transplantation.* 1999;67:1236–1242.

206. Sabeel AI, Qunibi WY, Alfurayh OA, Al Meshari K. Kaposi's sarcoma in Sudanese renal transplant recipients: a report from a single center. *J Nephrol.* 2003;16:412–416.

207. Tur E, Brenner S. Treatment of Kaposi's sarcoma. *Arch Dermatol.* 1996;132:327–331.

208. Tombolini V, Osti MF, Bonanni A, et al. Radiotherapy in classic Kaposi's sarcoma (CKS): experience of the Institute of Radiology of University "La Sapienza" of Rome. *Anticancer Res.* 1999;19:4539–4544.

209. Brenner B, Rakowsky E, Katz A, et al. Tailoring treatment for classical Kaposi's sarcoma: comprehensive clinical guidelines. *Int J Oncol.* 1999;14:1097–1102.

210. Chang LF, Reddy S, Shidnia H. Comparison of radiation therapy of classic and epidemic Kaposi's sarcoma. *Am J Clin Oncol.* 1992;15:200–206.

211. Mitsuyasu RT. Update on the pathogenesis and treatment of Kaposi sarcoma. *Curr Opin Oncol.* 2000;12:174–180.

212. Klein E, Schwartz RA, Laor Y, Milgrom H, Burgess GH, Holtermann OA. Treatment of Kaposi's sarcoma with vinblastine. *Cancer.* 1980;45:427–431.

213. Pfrommer C, Tebbe B, Tidona CA, et al. Progressive HHV-8-positive classic Kaposi's sarcoma: rapid response to interferon alpha-2a but persistence of HHV-8 DNA sequences in lesional skin. *Br J Dermatol.* 1998;139:516–519.

214. Tur E, Brenner S. Classic Kaposi's sarcoma: low-dose interferon alfa treatment. *Dermatology.* 1998;197:37–42.

215. Costa da Cunha CS, Lebbe C, Rybojad M, et al. Long-term follow-up of non-HIV Kaposi's sarcoma treated with low-dose recombinant interferon alfa-2b. *Arch Dermatol.* 1996;132:285–290.

216. Brambilla L, Boneschi V, Taglioni M, Ferrucci S. Staging of classic Kaposi's sarcoma: a useful tool for therapeutic choices. *Eur J Dermatol.* 2003;13:83–86.

217. Kreuter A, Rasokat H, Klouche M, et al. Liposomal pegylated doxorubicin versus low-dose recombinant interferon Alfa-2a in the treatment of advanced classic Kaposi's sarcoma; retrospective analysis of three German centers. *Cancer Invest.* 2005;23:653–659.

218. Turk HM, Buyukberber S, Camci C, et al. Chemotherapy of disseminated cutaneous classic Kaposi's sarcoma with vinblastine. *J Dermatol.* 2002;29:657–660.

219. Azzarelli A, Mazzaferro V, Quagliuolo V, et al. Kaposi's sarcoma: malignant tumor or proliferative disorder? *Eur J Cancer Clin Oncol.* 1988;24:973–978.

220. Cheung MC, Pantanowitz L, Dezube BJ. AIDS-related malignancies: emerging challenges in the era of highly active antiretroviral therapy. *Oncologist.* 2005; 10:412–426.

221. Scadden DT. AIDS-related malignancies. *Annu Rev Med.* 2003;54:285–303.

222. Levine AM, Tulpule A. Clinical aspects and management of AIDS-related Kaposi's sarcoma. *Eur J Cancer.* 2001;37: 1288–1295.

223. Portsmouth S, Stebbing J, Gill J, et al. A comparison of regimens based on non-nucleoside reverse transcriptase inhibitors or protease inhibitors in preventing Kaposi's sarcoma. *AIDS.* 2003;17: F17–F22.

224. Dezube BJ, Pantanowitz L, Aboulafia DM. Management of AIDS-related Kaposi sarcoma: advances in target discovery and treatment. *AIDS Read.* 2004;14:236–244, 251.

225. Walmsley S, Northfelt DW, Melosky B, Conant M, Friedman-Kien AE, Wagner B. Treatment of AIDS-related cutaneous Kaposi's sarcoma with topical alitretinoin (9-cis-retinoic acid) gel. Panretin Gel North American Study Group. *J Acquir Immune Defic Syndr.* 1999;22:235–246.

226. Lynen L, Zolfo M, Huyst V, et al. Management of Kaposi's sarcoma in resource-limited settings in the era of HAART. *AIDS Rev.* 2005;7:13–21.

227. Abels C. Targeting of the vascular system of solid tumours by photodynamic therapy (PDT). *Photochem Photobiol Sci.* 2004;3:765–771.

228. Krown SE. Management of Kaposi sarcoma: the role of interferon and thalidomide. *Curr Opin Oncol.* 2001;13: 374–381.

229. Wu JJ, Huang DB, Pang KR, Hsu S, Tyring SK. Thalidomide: dermatological indications, mechanisms of action and side-effects. *Br J Dermatol.* 2005;153: 254–273.

230. Cianfrocca M, Cooley TP, Lee JY, et al. Matrix metalloproteinase inhibitor COL-3 in the treatment of AIDS-related Kaposi's sarcoma: a phase I AIDS malignancy consortium study. *J Clin Oncol.* 2002;20:153–159.

231. Glesby MJ, Hoover DR, Weng S, et al. Use of antiherpes drugs and the risk of Kaposi's sarcoma: data from the Multicenter AIDS Cohort Study. *J Infect Dis.* 1996;173:1477–1480.

232. Zabawski EJ, Jr. A review of topical and intralesional cidofovir. *Dermatol Online J.* 2000;6:3.

233. Robles R, Lugo D, Gee L, Jacobson MA. Effect of antiviral drugs used to treat cytomegalovirus end-organ disease on subsequent course of previously diagnosed Kaposi's sarcoma in patients with AIDS. *J Acquir Immune Defic Syndr Hum Retrovirol.* 1999;20:34–38.

234. Simonart T. Iron: a target for the management of Kaposi's sarcoma? *BMC Cancer.* 2004;4:1.

235. Aboulafia DM, Norris D, Henry D, et al. 9-cis-Retinoic acid capsules in the treatment of AIDS-related Kaposi sarcoma: results of a phase 2 multicenter clinical trial. *Arch Dermatol.* 2003;139:178–186.

236. Stallone G, Schena A, Infante B, et al. Sirolimus for Kaposi's sarcoma in renal-transplant recipients. *N Engl J Med.* 2005;352:1317–1323.

237. Gutierrez-Dalmau A, Sanchez-Fructuoso A, Sanz-Guajardo A, et al. Efficacy of conversion to sirolimus in posttransplantation Kaposi's sarcoma. *Transplant Proc.* 2005;37:3836–3838.

238. Aboulafia DM. Kaposi's sarcoma. *Clin Dermatol.* 2001;19:269–283.

239. Coras B, Hafner C, Reichle A, et al. Antiangiogenic therapy with pioglitazone, rofecoxib, and trofosfamide in a patient with endemic Kaposi sarcoma. *Arch Dermatol.* 2004;140:1504–1507.

240. Godfrey A, Laman H, Boshoff C. RNA interference: a potential tool against Kaposi's sarcoma-associated herpesvirus. *Curr Opin Infect Dis.* 2003;16:593–600.

241. Morini M, Albini A, Lorusso G, et al. Prevention of angiogenesis by naked DNA IL-12 gene transfer: angioprevention by immunogene therapy. *Gene Ther.* 2004;11:284–291.

242. Zacchigna S, Zentilin L, Morini M, et al. AAV-mediated gene transfer of tissue inhibitor of metalloproteinases-1 inhibits vascular tumor growth and angiogenesis in vivo. *Cancer Gene Ther.* 2004;11:73–80.

CHAPTER 22

Eyelid Cancers

Mahnaz Nouri, M.D.
Anita Singh, M.S.
Shalu S. Patel, B.S.
Keyvan Nouri, M.D.

BOX 22-1 Overview

- The incidence of eyelid malignancies has increased in recent years.
- The eyelid's main function is to shield the eyes from the external environment and allow them to remain moist.
- The major cancers that are found on the eyelids include basal cell carcinoma (BCC), squamous cell carcinoma (SCC), sebaceous gland carcinoma (SGC), and malignant melanoma (MM).
- Basal cell carcinoma (BCC) accounts for 90% of eyelid cancers in the United States and Western countries.
- Squamous cell carcinoma (SCC) is the second most common eyelid cancer, accounting for 5 to 10% of all eyelid malignancies.
- Sebaceous gland carcinoma (SGC) is the third most common eyelid tumor, accounting for 1 to 5% of all eyelid malignancies.
- Malignant melanoma (MM) of the skin near the eye is rare, constituting 1% or less of all malignant eyelid tumors.
- Ultraviolet radiation (UVR) is the main risk factor for BCC, SCC, and MM. SGC is independent of sun exposure.
- Eyelid malignancies are initially diagnosed with the slit lamp microscope, but a biopsy is necessary to confirm the diagnosis.
- BCC and SCC have an excellent prognosis.
- SGC has a high rate of recurrence, a significant risk of metastasizing, and a 5-year mortality rate as high as 30%.
- The metastatic potential and prognosis of MM depends on the depth of tumor invasion and the thickness of the tumor.
- Eyelid malignancies can be treated by a variety of ways; these include surgery, radiotherapy, cryotherapy, curettage and electrodessication, chemotherapy, and photodynamic therapy.
- Prevention is important in reducing eyelid malignancies.

INTRODUCTION

Along with the rise in skin cancer rates in recent years, the incidence of eyelid cancers has increased tremendously.

The eyelids are prone to various skin cancers because they often remain unprotected from UV radiation throughout a person's lifetime. The limited anatomical area is of significance because lesions can disrupt the functions of the eyelid, as well as create cosmetic concerns for the patient.

Eyelids are composed of an outer layer of skin, a middle layer of muscle and tissue that gives them the form, and an inner layer of moist conjunctival tissue. They serve to protect the anterior surface of the eye from foreign matter and local injury; they aid in regulation of light reaching the eye; they help spread tears over the eye to maintain the tear film that keeps the eye moist and comfortable; and they help with tear flow through their actions on the conjunctival sac and lacrimal sac.[1] Therefore, the eyelid's main function is to shield the eye from the external environment and to allow it to remain moist.[2]

The eyelids have several external landmarks that are important when examining the eye. The palpebral fissure is the space between the upper and lower eyelid margins when the eyelids are open.[3] The points at which the upper and lower eyelids come together are called the commissures. The medial commissure is the point nearest to the nose and the lateral commissure is on the side closest to the temple. The openings for the tear drainage system are called the lacrimal puncta, and are located on the eyelid margin just before the medial commissure.[3] The small red portion located at the inner corner of the eyelids, on the side nearest to the nose, is the caruncle. The areas of soft tissue just beyond the commissures are called the canthi. The medial canthus starts at the medial commissure and extends about half an inch toward the nose, whereas the lateral canthus starts at the lateral commissure and extends about half an inch toward the temple. The tarsus or tarsal plate is a thin cartilage-like structure that gives shape to the lower eyelid.[3] Eyelid cancers can develop on the upper or lower lids or the medial or lateral canthus. The medial canthus is of particular importance because this area is especially at risk of deep infiltration.[4]

The eyelid color in humans is due to cutaneous carotenoids and melanin, as well as the ratio of "oxygenated as well as reduced hemoglobin in capillaries and venules."[5] One of the most important factors is the "amount and distribution

of melanin." Melanin is a complex biopolymer shaped by tyrosin oxidation and polymerization. The color of the skin is due to the "number, size, and distribution of melanosomes, the cytoplasmic organelles devoted to the production of melanin." Melanin absorbs energy in the range of 200 to 2400 nm of the electromagnetic spectrum, giving it its black color that protects against the effects of the ultraviolet radiation (UVR). It lessens the carcinogenic effect of the sun, as well as its effects on aging.

Melanin is made in the melanosomes of the epidermal melanocytes, which are then transferred to the "neighboring keratinocytes in a complex series of steps." The number of melanocytes varies in different anatomical locations: 2000 melanocytes/mm^2 in the face, with less density in the eyelid compared to that in the face. Racial differences are due to qualitative and quantitative differences in melanin within the keratinocyte. Melanosomes in blacks are larger and individually packed, whereas in whites and Asians, there are small melanosomes. Eyelid melanocytes are modified by environmental factors.

The major cancers that are found on the eyelids include basal cell carcinoma (BCC), squamous cell carcinoma (SCC), sebaceous gland carcinoma (SGC), and malignant melanoma (MM).[6] BCC can be found in many areas of the body, though it is predominant in the head and neck region. It is the most common eyelid malignancy, usually appearing in the lower lid and medial canthal region as a firm, pearly nodule. Twenty to twenty-five percent of BCCs develop on the eyelids.[4] Dr. Arthur Jacob, an Irish ophthalmologist and surgeon, is credited for first describing the eyelid BCC in 1827.[4,7,8] His report noted "an ulcer of peculiar character which attacks the eyelids and other parts of the face." In the early 1800s, this disease was known as Jacob's ulcer.

SCC is the second most common skin cancer that usually appears on sun-exposed areas of the body. It can occur on all areas of the body, including the mucous membranes in the mouth and genitals; however, it most commonly arises on sun-exposed areas such as the face, arms, ears, hands, lips, neck, and scalp. Therefore, sun exposure is the most important cause of SCC.[5]

Though SGC is considered to be rare in non-eyelid skin, it is commonly found on the eyelid because there is an abundance of sebaceous glands in the tarsus (meibomian glands), eyelashes (Zeis glands), and the caruncle.[9,10] SGC typically arises from the Zeis glands or the meibomian glands of the upper eyelid.[10] SGC is known as the "the great masquerader" because it is commonly misdiagnosed as other benign and malignant lesions, often resulting in delayed diagnosis.[11]

Finally, MM can also occur on the eyelids. Cutaneous MMs can be classified into four groups—nodular melanoma (NM), superficial spreading melanoma, lentigo maligna melanoma (LMM), and acral lentiginous melanoma.[12] The two most common melanomas for the eyelids are LMM and NM.[13] Acral lentiginous melanoma occurs exclusively on the hands and feet, and does not affect the eyelids.

There are many premalignant lesions (such as actinic keratoses) that occur on the eyelid, but this chapter will delve into the epidemiology, pathogenesis, diagnosis, and treatment of the four major types of eyelid cancers: BCCs, SCCs, SGCs, and MM.

EPIDEMIOLOGY

BOX 22-2   Summary of Epidemiology

- Individuals with fair skin and a significant history of sun exposure are at risk of developing eyelid malignancies.
- BCC accounts for 90% of eyelid cancers in the United States and Western countries.
- Most eyelid BCCs occur on the lower eyelids and are due to chronic sun exposure.
- SCC is the second most common eyelid cancer, accounting for 5 to 10% of all eyelid malignancies.
- Most SCCs occur on the lower eyelids and are due to chronic sun exposure.
- SGC is the third most common eyelid tumor, accounting for 1 to 5% of all eyelid malignancies.
- SGC is most commonly found on the upper eyelid, and mostly independent of sun exposure.
- MM of the skin near the eye is rare, constituting 1% or less of all malignant eyelid tumors.
- A history of severe sunburns is a major risk factor for developing MM.

There is a vast difference in the incidence of various eyelid cancers worldwide. In general, those at greatest risk of developing skin cancer are the people with fair skin who have spent their childhood or the majority of their life in the sun.[4] Therefore, eyelid cancer is

expected to develop in older patients, especially those in the latter half of their lives. The epidemiology of eyelid cancers can be very useful in diagnosing these tumors. Knowing which cancers occur in certain world populations better enables physicians to make correct diagnoses.

In the United States and other Western countries, BCC accounts for the majority (about 90%) of the eyelid cancers.[4,14,15] The occurrence is more likely in the Irish or Scandinavian, fair-skinned population. The predominance of BCC over other eyelid skin cancers in Western populations is expected because people with fair skin, especially Europeans, have little natural protection from the sun. Because the incidence of BCC is increasing in these nations, it is sometimes referred to as the "quiet epidemic."[4]

BCC on the eyelid is often nodular and found on the lower eyelid, while BCC on the trunk or extremities is mostly superficial.[14,15] Furthermore, the eyelids tend to receive constant sun exposure, as opposed to the trunk or extremities that may receive intermittent and often intense exposure to UV radiation. Thus, the type of exposure correlates with the type of BCC, in that chronic exposure yields nodular BCCs. Though most BCCs occur on the lower eyelid, they have also been found to occur in the medial canthus, upper eyelid, and lateral canthus, in decreasing order of frequency.[15] These tumors can be seen in all age groups, but mostly in the older population with a history of exposure to actinic radiation.

SCC is the second most common eyelid cancer, accounting for 5 to 10% of all eyelid malignancies.[16] Like BCC, it occurs mostly on the lower eyelid, and has also been found to occur in the medial canthus, upper eyelid, and lateral canthus, in decreasing order of frequency.[17] This tumor is more common in fair-skinned individuals, especially those who have been chronically exposed to sunlight. It may be slightly more common in males than in females, but this may be due to certain occupations that involve more significant exposure to sunlight or other occupational hazards. The incidence of SCC increases significantly with age, especially in those individuals who are 60 years or older, and with increased proximity to the equator.[18,19]

SGC is mostly independent of sun exposure. It is the third most common eyelid tumor, accounting for 1 to 5% of all the eyelid malignancies.[6,10] In many

studies, it has been noted that SGC is more commonly found in women.[9,20,21] Those at greatest risk of developing SGC include women over 60 years of age and younger people who have had radiation therapy to the face.[22,23] SGC is most commonly found in the upper eyelid, followed in order of frequency by the lower eyelid, the bulbar conjunctiva, and the caruncle.[24] Because it is well known for masquerading as other benign or malignant lesions, there may be a delayed diagnosis and this may lead to higher morbidity and mortality. Interestingly, the frequency of SGC and SCC is much higher in Asian countries. For example, in Japan, SGC and SCC combined contribute to almost 50% of malignant eyelid cancers, while BCC represents about 40%.[9] So, in most Asian countries, BCC is marginally the most common eyelid cancer, closely followed by SGC and then SCC and MM.[9]

Primary MM of the skin near the eye is rare, constituting 1% or less of all the malignant eyelid tumors, but it is the leading cause of death from primary skin tumors.[10] Risk factors for developing MM include excessive sun exposure, Caucasian race, and an age greater than 20 years. MM is 12 times more common in Caucasians than in African Americans and individuals from the Caribbean. In contrast to BCC, a history of severe sunburns, rather than cumulative sun exposure is thought to be a major risk factor for developing MM.[25]

PATHOGENESIS

BOX 22-3   Summary

- BCC is derived from the germinal cells in the basal layer.
- There are many risk factors in the pathogenesis of BCC but UVR is the main risk factor.
- SCC arises from the prickle-squamous cell layer of the epidermis.
- There are many risk factors in the pathogenesis of SCC but UVR is the main risk factor.
- SGC is derived from cells that comprise sebaceous glands.
- SCG appear to arise *de novo*; however, there are several risk factors that are thought to be associated with the development of SGC.
- MM is a neoplasm arising from the proliferation of melanocytes.
- Sun exposure and UV exposure are major risk factors for MM; however, there are other known risk factors.

Basal Cell Carcinoma (BCC)

BCC is a malignant tumor derived from germinal cells in the basal layer of the epidermis. A tumor forms when basal cells increase in size and extend into the dermis as bulbous nodules or invasive strands. The margins of the lesion become more pronounced as the center suffers a loss of blood supply resulting in necrosis with a crusted umbilicated center, which may bleed episodically.[10]

Exposure to UVR is the main causative factor in the pathogenesis of BCC. However, susceptibility to BCC seems to be determined by an interaction between UVR and polymorphic genes. It has been shown that skin type 1 (skin that always burns and never tans), red or blonde hair, and blue or green eyes have been shown to be risk factors for the development of BCC. In addition, recreational sun exposure in childhood seems to be an important risk factor. Development of BCC is found to be more frequent after freckling in childhood and also after frequent or severe sunburn in childhood, as opposed to a history of sunburn as an adult.[26]

Patients on immunosuppressive treatment also have an increased risk of BCC. Psoralens plus ultraviolet A radiation (PUVA), which is a treatment for psoriasis, modestly increases the risk of BCC. Mutations in the *p53* gene and other tumor suppressor genes, such as the human patched gene, have been found in hereditary and sporadic BCCs. A family history of skin cancers also seems to be a predictor of development of BCC. Several genetic conditions are associated with the risk of developing BCC. These include albinism, xeroderma pigmentosa, Bazex's syndrome, and the nevoid BCC syndrome. Finally, other non-ultraviolet environmental exposures that have been associated with the increased risk of BCC include ionizing radiation, high dietary energy (especially fat), low intake of vitamins, arsenic exposure, and various other chemicals and dust.[26]

Squamous Cell Carcinoma (SCC)

SCC arises from the prickle-squamous cell layer of the epidermis and extends into the underlying dermis. SCC begins when atypical keratinocytes breach the dermal basement membrane and invade the dermis.[10] The most important risk factor for the development of SCC is the exposure to UVR. Other risk factors include infection with human papillomavirus, chronic degenerative and chronic inflammatory skin changes, chemical carcinogens, long-term heat exposure, genetic factors (light-skin, fair or red hair, light eyes, and people affected by xeroderma pigmentosum or albinism), and immunosuppression with the use of immunosuppressive treatments, patients with AIDS, and congenital immune defects.[27–31]

Sebaceous Gland Carcinoma (SGC)

SGC is a malignant neoplasm that originates from cells comprising sebaceous glands. There is a large quantity of sebaceous glands in the periorbital region, particularly in the tarsus where there are meibomian glands, and in association with the eyelashes where the Zeis glands are common. Other structures that have an abundance of sebaceous glands are the caruncles and the eyebrow region.[32]

SCG appear to arise *de novo*; however, there are several risk factors that are thought to be associated with the development of SGC. These include patient of older age (57 to 72 years), female sex, Asian race, prior irradiation, Muir–Torre syndrome (MTS), prolonged use of diurectics, infection with human papillomavirus, and immunosuppression. However, there is not enough evidence supporting the relationship between prolonged use of thiazide diurectics and the development of SGC.[32]

Sebaceous gland neoplasms are associated with visceral malignancies in patients with MTS. MTS is a rare autosomal-dominant inherited disorder characterized by the predisposition to both sebaceous skin tumors and internal malignancies. The majority of the MTS-associated tumors have mutations in DNA mismatch repair (MMR) genes (most often MSH-2 and MLH-1) and microsatellite instability.[33] It has also been thought that diminished expression of retinoid X receptors (RXR) beta and gamma might be related to the development of sebaceous cell carcinoma.[34]

Malignant Melanoma (MM)

MM is a neoplasm arising from the proliferation of melanocytes. The risk factors for developing melanoma are both environmental and genetic. Sun exposure and UV exposure are the major risk factors for melanoma, especially intense, intermittent sun exposure and sunburns. Ultraviolet B radiation (UV-B) appears more closely associated with the development of melanoma than is ultraviolet A radiation (UV-A); however, PUVA therapy for psoriasis is associated with a delayed increase in the risk of melanoma. Additional factors include the presence of atypical and congenital nevi, personal or family history of melanoma, presence of nonmelanoma skin cancers, immunosuppression, and familial syndromes (e.g., familial atypical multiple mole melanoma (FAMMM) syndrome).[25,35,36]

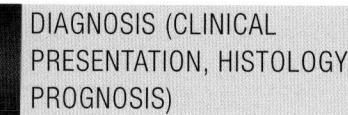

DIAGNOSIS (CLINICAL PRESENTATION, HISTOLOGY, PROGNOSIS)

BOX 22-4 Summary

- Eyelid malignancies are initially diagnosed with the slit lamp microscope.
- A biopsy is used to confirm the diagnosis of an eyelid malignancy.
- Conjunctival map biopsies are useful in determining the extent of the disease.
- Approximately 75% of eyelid malignancies are nodular and nodulo-ulcerative BCC. These lesions are small, translucent, telangiectatic nodules or papules with a pearly border, sometimes with a central ulcerated crater.
- There is an overall 5-year cure rate of 98 to 100% for primary BCC.
- SCC may be difficult to diagnose in the periocular region because there are no pathognomonic features to distinguish it from other lesions.
- Treatment of primary SCCs results in an overall 5-year cure rate of greater than 90%.
- SGC tumors may appear as a firm, painless, yellowish nodule due to its fat content.
- SGC has a high rate of recurrence, a significant risk of metastasis, and a 5-year mortality rate as high as 30%.
- The three types of melanoma that can be found on the eyelid region include NM, superficial spreading melanoma, and LMM.
- The metastatic potential and prognosis of these melanomas depends on the depth of tumor invasion and the thickness of the tumor. Tumor thicknesses less than 0.75 mm have a 100% five-year survival rate, and tumors thicker than 3 mm have a poorer prognosis.

Eyelid cancers are initially diagnosed after an examination with a slit lamp microscope. The slit lamp microscope is an instrument consisting of a high-intensity light source that can be focused to shine as a slit beam. The slit lamp examination provides a magnified view of the eye structures, enabling diagnoses to be made for a variety of eye conditions.[37] However, the slit lamp microscope alone is not enough to make a complete diagnosis. Often, a biopsy of suspicious

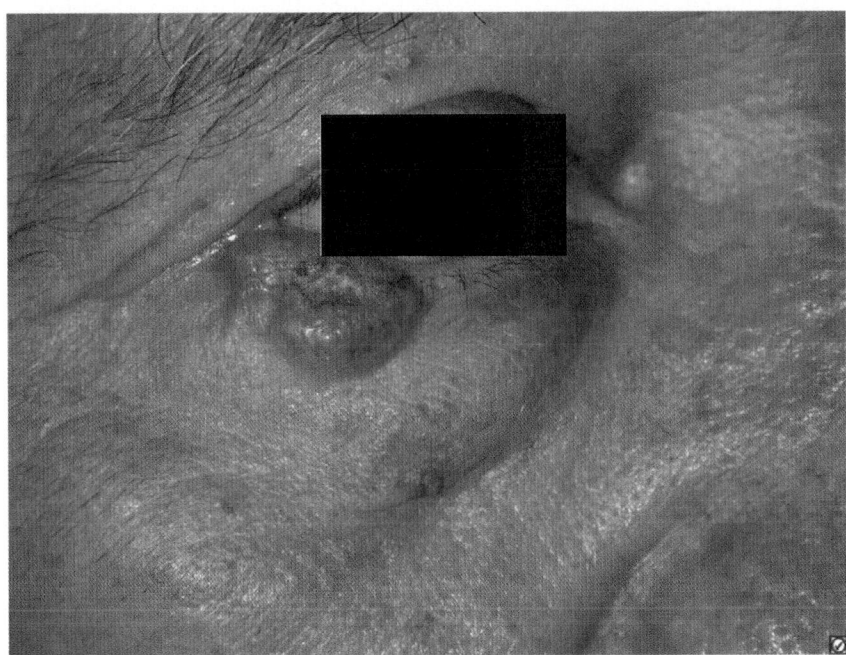

▲ **FIGURE 22-1** Nodular BCC on right lower lid.

lesions confirms the diagnosis, and the appropriate prognosis can be determined.

In certain cases, conjunctival map biopsies are important to determine the extent of the disease and to plan treatment. This technique involves taking biopsies from different areas of the eye (e.g., palpebral conjunctiva, bulbar conjunctiva, and tarsus). It is very important to keep a diagram labeling and numbering of each biopsy site for histopathologic study, and the biopsy specimens should be submitted for permanent sections. The routine for map biopsies may need to be modified according to the clinical and surgical findings.[38]

Basal Cell Carcinoma

The majority of the eyelid BCC occurs on the lower eyelid.[14,17] BCC of the eyelid can be divided into three groups: localized (nodular, ulcerative, cystic), diffuse (morpheaform, sclerosing), and superficial, multifocal BCC.[39]

The most common clinical subtype of eyelid BCC is nodular and noduloulcerative, accounting for almost 75% of all BCCs in this region (see Figs. 22-1 and 22-3).[14,15] The nodular form is a small, translucent, telangiectatic nodule or papule with a pearly border. As the tumor grows, central ulceration may occur, leading to a lesion with a central ulcerated crater and pearly raised and rolled border. The lesion may become darkly pigmented and may be misdiagnosed as melanoma. These neoplasms may progressively enlarge over months

to years.[6,10] Histologically, nodular BCC appears as large lobules with cystic pseudo cavitations or as numerous small cavities that look glandular in structure.[4]

Approximately 15% of all BCCs are morpheaform or sclerosing.[6,10] These appear as white-pink to yellow plaques with indistinct margins. This subtype of BCC tends to invade deeply into the dermis. Additionally, morpheaform tumors in the medial canthus may extend into the orbit or paranasal sinuses.[6,10]

Histologically, they are characterized by an intense stromal proliferation that encloses cellular areas. The fibrous stroma consists of fibrocytic proliferation and dense collagen fibers. The tumor may extend deeply to involve fat or muscle.[4]

Superficial, multifocal BCCs present as a bright pink, shiny, well-defined erythematous lesion, but with a more irregular surface than do nodular BCCs. These lesions can sometimes be itchy and progressively enlarge over months. This subtype has a diffuse multicentric involvement of the epidermis and superficial dermis.[6,10] Histologically, there is a multicentric and superficial extension of the tumor without invasion of the reticular dermis.[4]

There is an overall 5-year cure rate of 98 to 100% for primary BCC and 93% for recurrent BCC after Mohs' micrographic surgery (MMS).[40] The rate of recurrence of BCC depends on the location of the lesion, with the medial canthus being the most frequent location for recurrence. Recurrence can also be seen in lesions greater than 2 cm in size, morpheaform subtype, infiltrative growth pattern, and an increased number of re-excisions.[4,15] Metastasis is rare, but these lesions need to be treated.[15]

Squamous Cell Carcinoma

SCCs frequently occur on the lower eyelid, like BCCs. It is difficult to diagnose SCC of the periocular region because

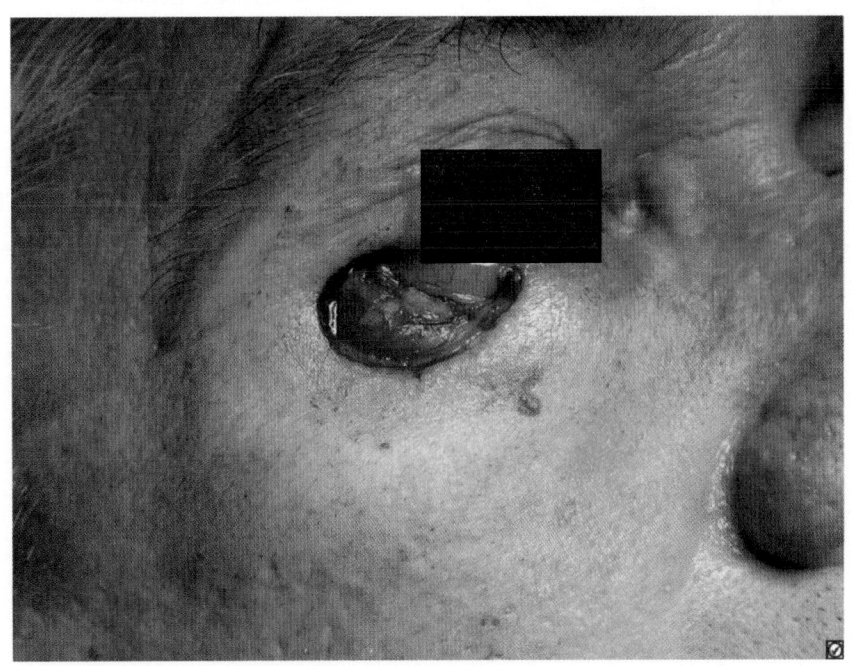

▲ **FIGURE 22-2** Nodular BCC removed by MMS.

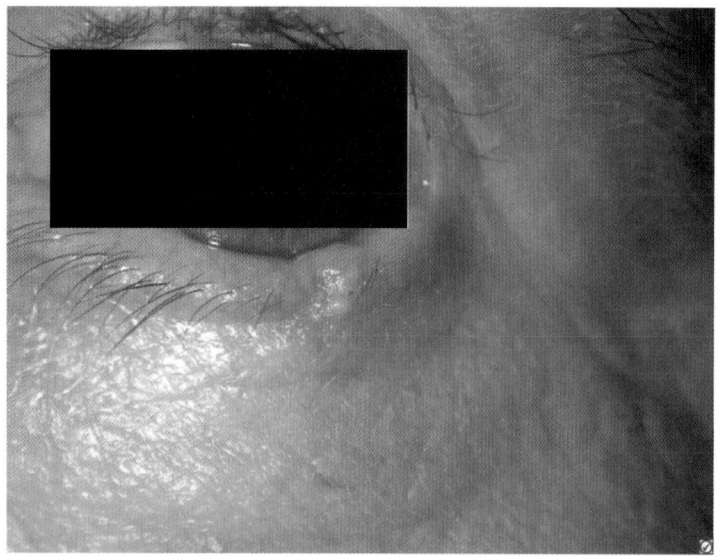

▲ **FIGURE 22-3** BCC located on patients' left lower lid.

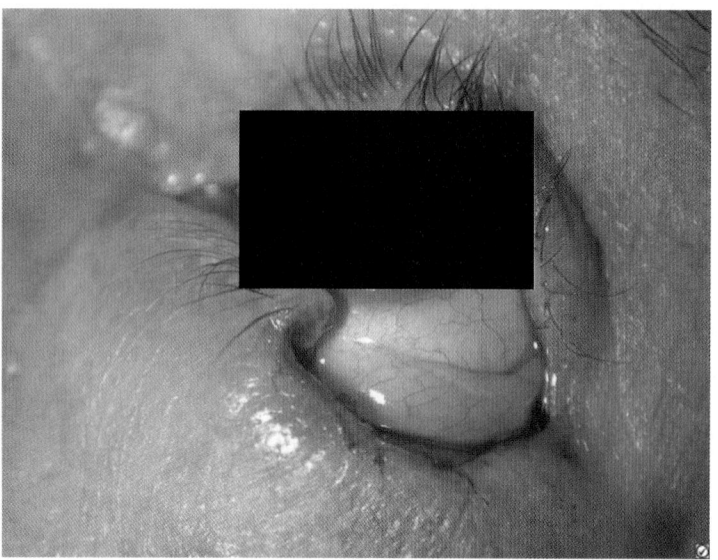

▲ **FIGURE 22-4** BCC removed by MMS.

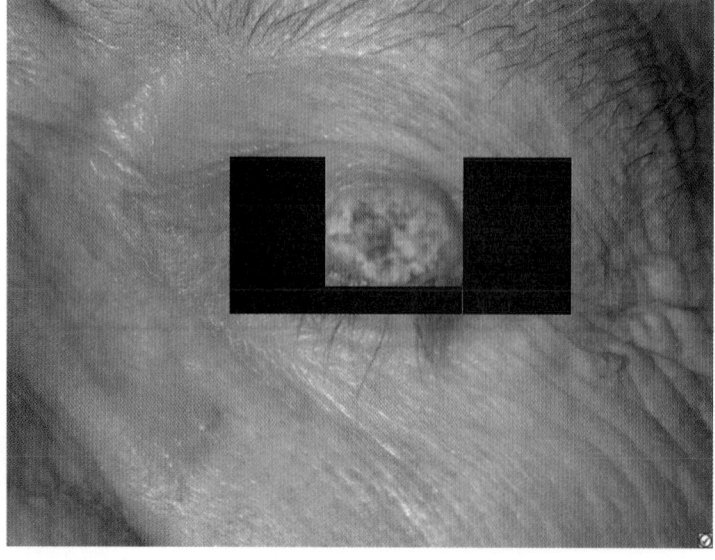

▲ **FIGURE 22-5** SCC located on the left upper lid of a patient.

there are no pathognomonic features to distinguish it from other lesions. SCC of the eyelid region may appear as a nodular or plaque-like lesion (see Figs. 22-5 and 22-7). The edges of the lesion may appear irregular and rolled, or may even have a pearly border. Scaling, fissuring, central ulceration, and telangiectasias may also be present.[6,10] Other characteristics that may be seen are papillomatous growths, cutaneous horns, or cystic lesions along the lid margin. Another variant of SCC is adenoid SCC. These lesions appear raised, with a scaly patch of reddened skin. They may bleed or drain pus, and metastasis is rare but possible.

Histologically, SCC begins when atypical keratinocytes invade the dermis. The cells of SCC vary from large, well-differentiated, polygonal cells with vesicular nuclei to completely anaplastic cells with basophilic cytoplasm. Most tumors invade as strands and columns, and reproduce the same pattern in their metastases.[41]

SCC has a tendency to metastasize to regional lymph nodes and distant sites through hematogenous and lymphatic pathways.[10] Invasion of the dermis in the eyelids results in an extension into the superficial orbicularis muscle. Deeper penetration results in the spread along fascial and embryologic fusion planes, periosteum, lymphatic vessels, blood vessels, and nerve sheaths. The likelihood of metastasis is related to inciting cause or origin, degree of differentiation, tumor size, and depth of dermal invasion. Since SCCs can look like benign and malignant lesions, a biopsy is necessary to confirm the diagnosis. It is important to identify any suspicious lesions in the sun-exposed areas, as individuals with SCC of the periocular region frequently have additional actinic-related lesions on the face, neck, scalp, and dorsum of the hands.

The overall prognosis of patients with SCC is excellent and mortality is rare. Treatment of primary SCCs results in an overall 5-year cure rate of greater than 90%. When the initial treatment is unsuccessful, recurrence can occur either locally or in regional lymph nodes.[42] Both regional lymph node and distant metastases are associated with a drastic increase of disease-related mortality. Overall survival rates for patients with regional lymph node metastases are about 25 to 35% at 5 years and less than 20% at 10 years. In patients with distant metastases, the 5-year survival rate is less than 10%.[10,16,42]

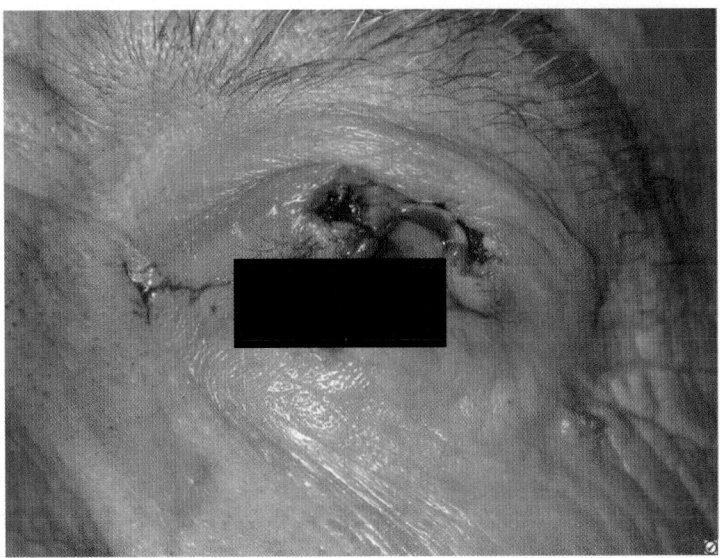

▲ **FIGURE 22-6** SCC removed by MMS.

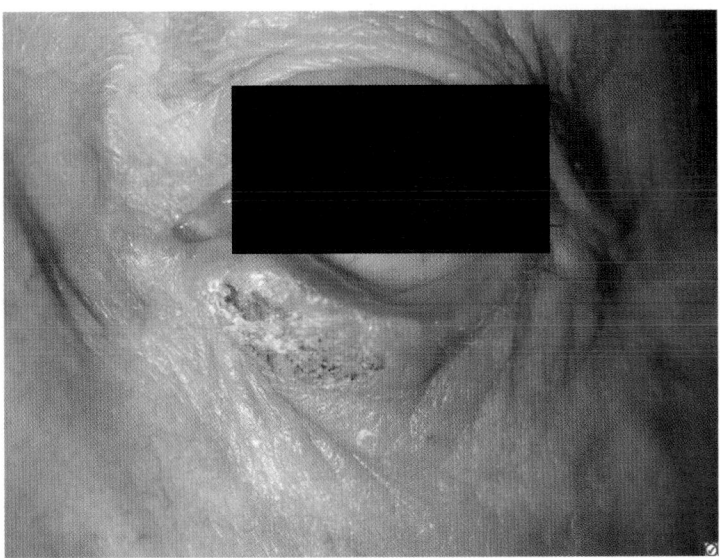

▲ **FIGURE 22-7** SCC located on patients' left lower lid.

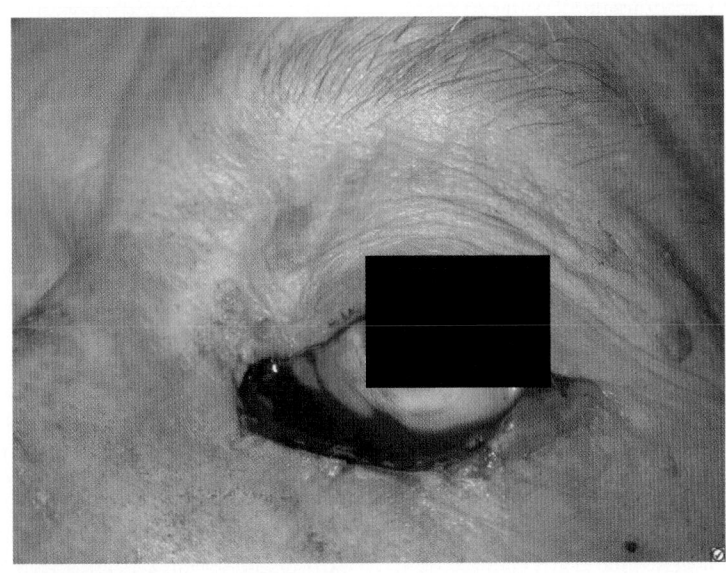

▲ **FIGURE 22-8** SCC removed by MMS.

Sebaceous Gland Carcinoma

SGC most commonly occurs on the upper eyelid because this is where majority of the meibomian glands are found (see Fig. 22-9). There are two forms of SGC, the nodular type and the non-nodular type. The nodular type is minimally infiltrative, while the non-nodular type is moderately to highly infiltrative. SGC tumors may appear as a firm, painless, yellowish nodule due to its fat content. They usually present with diffuse eyelid thickening associated with inflammation, or as an eyelid nodule or mass. Since SGC is known as the great masquerader, it can often be misdiagnosed as chronic chalazion, chronic blepharitis, cutaneous horn, BCC or SCC, etc.[6,10] Histologically, the nodular type of SGC appears as compact lobules organized into nodules with only minimal extensions into the stroma. The nonnodular variant appears as infiltrating cords of malignant cells, with little or no areas of lobule formation.[10]

SGC has a high rate of recurrence, a significant risk of metastasizing, and a 5-year mortality rate as high as 30%. Because it can mimic many benign lesions, SGC can be diagnosed late.[6] SGC can spread by a direct extension into the orbit, paranasal sinuses, and other nearby structures. Orbital invasion is usually associated with a poorer prognosis. SGC can also spread through lymphatic channels in the upper and lower eyelids to the regional lymph nodes. Various other factors are associated with a worse prognosis. These include vascular and lymphatic invasion, involvement of both upper and lower eyelids, tumor diameter greater than 10 mm, symptom duration of greater than 6 months, etc.[32]

Malignant Melanoma

The three types of melanoma that can be found on the eyelid region include NM, superficial spreading melanoma, and LMM. LMM is thought to be the most common type found in the eyelid region.[13,43] It has a very slow, progressive growth. This type of melanoma is thought to evolve from the noninvasive lentigo maligna. Lentigo maligna can be found on the sun-damaged face of elderly patients. It usually appears as an irregularly pigmented macule. LMM can evolve from a lentigo maligna that has been present on the skin of a patient for about 10 to 15 years. Malignant transformation of a lentigo maligna into an LMM can involve elevation or nodule formation of the previous lentigo maligna. This type of

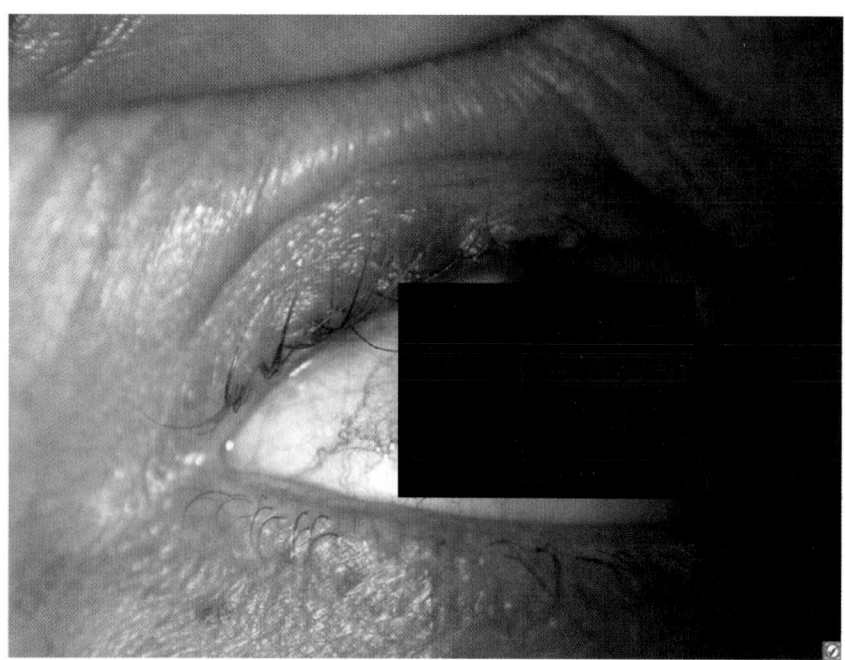

▲ **FIGURE 22-9** Sebaceous carcinoma located on the patients' right upper lid.

lesion is commonly found on the lower eyelids and medial canthus.[13,43]

NM is a blue-black, slightly elevated lesion that may look like a blood blister. It has an irregular surface and may increase in size rapidly, with bleeding and ulceration. NM is the most aggressive type with a higher rate of systemic metastasis than are BCC and SCC. These lesions are usually fully invasive when diagnosed.[44,45] Superficial spreading melanomas have a wide range of colors. They may appear tan, black, gray, pink, or rose colored. This variant of melanoma is typically elevated with a distinct border. As the tumor progresses, the borders may become irregular.[44]

The metastatic potential and prognosis of these melanomas depend on the depth of tumor invasion and the thickness of the tumor. Tumor thicknesses less than 0.75 mm have a 100% five-year survival rate; on the other hand, tumors thicker than 3 mm have a poorer prognosis. Cure rates for LMM are between 97 and 100% using Mohs micrographic surgery (MMS).[46] MMs involving the eyelid margin have poorer prognosis, and this is due to conjunctival involvement.

TREATMENT

BOX 22-5 Summary

- Eyelid malignancies can be treated by a variety of ways; these include surgery, radiotherapy, cryotherapy, chemotherapy, and photodynamic therapy.

- BCC and SCC are preferentially treated by MMS and surgical excision.
- Eyelid SGC is best treated by the use of conjunctival map biopsy combined with MMS, or excision with frozen- or paraffin-section control.
- There are many recommendations for treatment of MM. Treatment options include MMS and surgical excision, with varying margins of excision depending on the thickness of the tumor; and the use of lymph node dissection and adjuvant inferferon for more advanced stages of melanomas.

The major forms of effective treatment for eyelid cancers are surgery, radiotherapy, and cryotherapy.[14] Surgery seems to be the treatment of choice because it provides assurance of complete tumor removal, while most other therapies do not. In 2001, Cook and Bartley stated in a review of treatment options that MMS and surgical excision provided optimal results.[15] Hamada et al define surgical excision as the "gold standard for treatment among oculoplastic surgeons," and they also note that a 4-mm safety margin allows for the most tissue conservation while also reducing the chance of recurrence. Surgical complications that were noted in the follow-up include granuloma formation for 4.1% of the patients and trichiasis for 2.7%.[14] Though the Australian MMS database found MMS to be the treatment of choice for periocular BCC, Hamada et al feel that surgical excision provides a

"reliable and cost-effective surgical treatment."[14] Allali et al noted that MMS has the lowest 5-year recurrence rate compared to exeresis, curettage-electrodessication, cryotherapy, and radiotherapy.[4] MMS has also been found to be useful in distinguishing between sebaceous carcinoma and SCC *in situ*. These cases indicate that SGC was confirmed during the Mohs' procedure, though histopathology revealed SCC *in situ*.[16] For eyelid SGCs, treatment is primarily surgical, for example wide local excision with a 5-mm margin or MMS, though radiotherapy or exenteration may be used as well.[16,21] When comparing MMS and wide local excision, it was determined by several studies that MMS offered a lower recurrence rate.[21] Exenteration is the treatment of choice for SGC when there is orbital invasion or extensive bulbar conjuctival involvement.[21]

Radiotherapy has been considered as an option for adjuvant treatment to surgery for eyelid BCC.[4] This has mostly been effective for cases with a high risk of recurrence. It has also been used as an alternative if patients refuse or cannot tolerate surgical treatment.[4] However, Allali et al caution that this technique should not be used in patients with genetic cutaneous tumor predisposition syndrome. There are also a few possible complications of this therapy, including stenosis of the lacrimal passages, cataract, or retinal attacks, and severe dryness syndrome.[4] For patients with SGC, radiotherapy can be used if there is orbital invasion and exenteration is refused.[21,47]

Cryotherapy for periocular BCC is usually indicated for tumors less than 3 mm in size. A benefit of this therapy, especially for the lid margin and the canthi, is that occlusion of the lacrimal passages is less likely.[4] It can also be used as a supporting therapy.[9] However, scarring can occur as a side effect and the rate of recurrence is higher than with other therapies.[4] For patients with SGC and conjunctival pagetoid involvement, cryotherapy may be used in treatment. For cryotherapy, there is no guarantee of complete removal.

Other treatments that are less often used are chemotherapy using 5-fluorouracil or curettage-electrodessication.[4] Systemic chemotherapy may be necessary for cases in which metastasis has occurred. However, side effects involving the gastrointestinal tract and other skin disorders have been documented. For superficial lesions, a laser or photo-

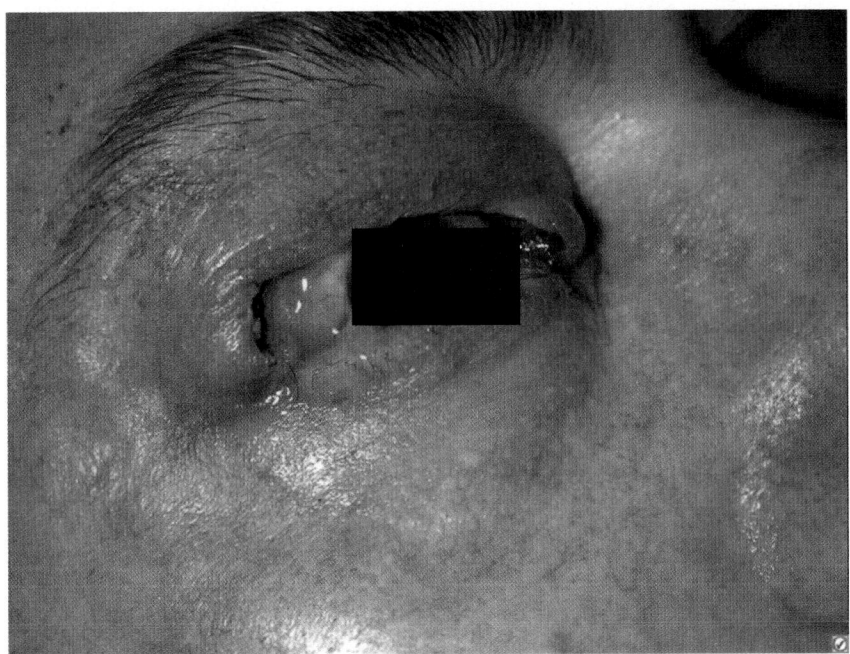

▲ **FIGURE 22-10** Sebaceous carcinoma removed by MMS.

dynamic therapy can be used to burn the lesion off. This treatment has been successful for BCCs and SCCs that are not deep. However, this may not be appropriate for eyelid cancers because of location.

In conclusion, BCC and SCC are preferentially treated by MMS and surgical excision (see Figs. 22-1 to 22-8), even though other nonsurgical treatments such as cryotherapy, radiation, and photodynamic therapy have been suggested.[6,10,39] Eyelid SGC is best treated by the use of conjunctival map biopsy combined with MMS, or excision with frozen- or paraffin-section control (see Figs. 22-9 and 22-10).[6,10] There are many recommendations for treatment of MM, and many of these are conflicting. LMM has been treated by a variety of ways. These include surgical excision, cryotherapy, and radiotherapy.[48] The treatment of NMs is more difficult, and therefore, there is currently no ideal way to manage these lesions. Treatment options include MMS and surgical excision, with varying margins depending on the thickness of the tumor; and the use of lymph node dissection and adjuvant interferon for more advanced stages of melanomas. There is no clear evidence as to the ideal adjuvant therapy to be used with surgery. The adjuvant therapy that is currently available include immunotherapy with melanoma vaccines or monoclonal antibodies, interleukin-2, dacarbazine, and interferon alpha-2b therapy.[6,10]

PREVENTION

BOX 22-6 Summary

- Prevention is important in reducing eyelid malignancies.
- Individuals who plan to go outside should protect their eyes by wearing hats with wide brims, sunglasses, and stay out of the sun between the hours of 10 am and 4 pm.

Prevention is the key in reducing eyelid cancer rates. Individuals should keep in mind that the peak levels of UVR are present between the hours of 10 am and 4 pm. When going outside, hats with a wide brim are helpful in reducing direct exposure to sunlight. In addition, adults and children should wear sunglasses when outside. Sunglasses are helpful in decreasing exposure to solar radiation. Individuals taking drugs that make them more photosensitive (e.g., psoralens, tetracycline, doxycycline) are also at an increased risk from solar radiation.[49] Minimizing exposure to direct sunlight and shielding the eyes with sunglasses can help prevent eyelid cancers, as well as other disorders affecting the eye. Patients should be aware of lesions around the eye and how they progress. Even small tumors can destroy the structure and function, not to mention, the appearance of the eye.

FINAL THOUGHTS

Eyelid malignancies are increasing in incidence. Many of these malignancies are induced by sun exposure or develop from benign lesions. Of the eyelid malignancies, BCC is the most frequent malignant eyelid tumor, followed by SCC, SGC, and MM. It is important to be aware of the clinical features of each of these malignancies and to protect the eyes from prolonged sun exposure.

REFERENCES

1. Doxanas MT, Anderson RL. *Clinical Orbital Anatomy*. Baltimore, MD: Lippincott Williams and Wilkins; 1984.
2. Salomon J, Bieniek A, Baran E, Szepietowski J. Basal cell carcinoma on the eyelids: own experience. *Dermatol Surg.* 2004;30:257–263.
3. Warwick R, ed. *Eugene Wolff's Anatomy of the Eye and Orbit*. Philadelphia, PA: WB Saunders; 1977.
4. Allali J, D'Hermies F, Renard G. Basal cell carcinomas of the eyelids. *Ophthalmologica.* 2005;219:57–71.
5. Albert DM, Jakobiec FA, Azar DT, et al. *Principles and Practice of Ophthalmology.* 2nd ed. Philadelphia, PA: WB Saunders; 2000:3430–3446.
6. Fong K, Malhotra R. Common eyelid malignancies: Clinical features and management options. *Optom Today.* November 2005:30–34.
7. Jacob A. Observations respecting an ulcer of peculiar character, which attacks the eye lids and other parts of the face. *Dublin Hosp Rep.* 1827;4:232–239.
8. Netscher DT, Spira M. Basal cell carcinoma: an overview of tumor biology and treatment. *Plast Reconstr Surg.* 2004;113(5):74–94.
9. Takamura H, Yamashita H. Clinicopathological analysis of malignant eyelid tumor cases at Yamaguta University Hospital: statistical comparison of tumor incidence in Japan and other countries. *Jpn J Ophthalmol.* 2005;49:349–354.
10. Cook BE, Bartley GB. Treatment options and future prospects for the management of eyelid malignancies: an evidence-based update. *Ophthalmology.* 2001;108(11):2088–2098.
11. Yeats RP, Waller RR. Sebaceous carcinoma of the eyelid: Pitfalls in diagnosis. *Ophthal Plast Reconstr Surg.* 1985;1:35–42.
12. Mihm MC, Clark WH, From L. The clinical diagnosis, classification, and histogenetic concepts of the early stages of cutaneous malignant melanomas. *N Engl J Med.* 1981;284:1078–1083.
13. Vaziri M, Buffan FV, Martinka M, et al. Clinicopathological features and behaviour of cutaneous eyelid melanoma. *Ophthalmology.* 2002;109:901–908.
14. Hamada S, Kersy T, Thaller VT. Eyelid basal cell carcinoma: non-Mohs excision, repair, and outcome. *Br J Ophthalmol.* 2005;89:992–994.
15. Chatterjee S, Moore S, Kumar B. Punch biopsy in the management of periocular basal cell carcinomas. *Orbit.* 2004;23:87–92.
16. Donaldson MJ, Sullivan TJ, Whitehead KJ, Williamson RM. Squamous cell carcinoma of the eyelids. *Br J Ophthalmol.* 2002;86:1161–1165.
17. Cook BE, Bartley GB. Epidemiologic characteristics and clinical course of patients with malignant eyelid tumors in

an incidence cohort in Olmsted County, Minnesota. *Ophthalmology.* 1999;106:746–750.

18. Vitaliano PP, Urbach F. The relative importance of risk factors in non-melanoma carcinoma. *Arch Dermatol.* 1980;116:454–456.

19. Doxanas MT, Iliff WJ, Iliff NT, et al. Squamous cell carcinoma of the eyelids. *Ophthalmology.* 1987;94(5):538–541.

20. Lai TF, Huilgol SC, Selva D, et al. Eyelid sebaceous carcinoma masquerading as in situ squamous cell carcinoma. *Dermatol Surg.* 2004;30:222–225.

21. Callahan EF, Appert DL, Roenigk RK, et al. Sebaceous carcinoma of the eyelid: a review of 14 cases. *Dermatol Surg.* 2004;30:1164–1168.

22. Doxanas MT, Green WR. Sebaceous gland carcinoma: Review of 40 cases. *Arch Ophthalmol.* 1984;102:245–249.

23. Howrey RP, Lipham WJ, Schultz WH, et al. Sebaceous gland carcinoma: A subtle second malignancy following radiation therapy in patients with bilateral retinoblastoma. *Cancer.* 1998;83:767–771.

24. Shields JA, Demirci H, Marr BP, et al. Sebaceous carcinoma of the eyelids: personal experience with 60 cases. *Ophthalmology.* 2004;111(12):2151–2157.

25. Rhodes AR, Weinstock MA, Fitzpatrick TB, et al. Risk factors for cutaneous melanoma: A practical method for recognizing predisposed individuals. *JAMA.* 1987;258:3146–3154.

26. Wong CS, Strange RC, Lear JT. Basal cell carcinoma. *BMJ.* 2003;327(7418):794–798.

27. Armstrong BK, Kricker A. The epidemiology of UV induced skin cancer. *J Photochem Photobiol B.* 2001;63(1–3):8–18.

28. Nijsten TE, Stern RS. The increased risk of skin cancer is persistent after discontinuation of psoralen + ultraviolet A: a cohort study. *J Invest Dermatol.* 2003;121(2):252–258.

29. Jensen P, Hansen S, Moller B, et al. Skin cancer in kidney and heart transplant recipients and different long-term immunosuppressive therapy regimens. *J Am Acad Dermatol.* 1999;40(2, Pt 1):177–186.

30. Jellouli-Elloumi A, Kochbati L, Dhraief S, et al. Cancers arising from burn scars: 62 cases. *Ann Dermatol Venereol.* 2003;130(4):413–416.

31. Cleaver JE, Thompson LH, Richardson AS, et al. A summary of mutations in the UV-sensitive disorders: xeroderma pigmentosum, Cockayne syndrome, and trichothiodystrophy. *Hum Mutat.* 1999;14(1):9–22.

32. Shields JA, Demirci H, Marr BP, et al. Sebaceous carcinoma of the ocular region: A review. *Surv Ophthalmol.* 2005;50(2):103–122.

33. Popnikolov NK, Gatalica Z, Colome-Grimmer MI, et al. Loss of mismatch repair proteins in sebaceous gland tumors. *J Cutan Pathol.* 2003;30(3):178–184.

34. Chakravarti N, El-Naggar AK, Lotan R, et al. Expression of retinoid receptors in sebaceous cell carcinoma. *J Cutan Pathol.* 2006;33(1):10–17.

35. Rivers JK. Melanoma. *Lancet.* 1996;347(9004):803–806.

36. Stern RS. The risk of melanoma in association with long-term exposure to PUVA. *J Am Acad Dermatol.* 2001;44(5):755–761.

37. Miller D, Thall EH, Atebara NH. Ophthalmic instrumentation. In: M Yanoff and JS Duker, eds. *Ophthalmology.* 2nd ed. St. Louis, MO: Mosby; 2004:87–89 (chapter 13).

38. Putterman AM. Conjunctival map biopsy to determine pagetoid spread. *Am J Ophthalmol.* 1986;102:87–90.

39. Riedel KG, Beyer-Machule CK. *Basal Cell Carcinoma. Principles and Practices of Ophthalmology.* 2nd ed. Philadelphia, PA: WB Saunders; 2000:3361–3365.

40. Rowe DE, Carroll RJ, Day CL. Mohs surgery is the treatment of choice for recurrent (previously treated) basal cell carcinoma. *J Dermatol Surg Oncol.* 1989;15:424–431.

41. Cassarino DS, Derienzo DP, Barr RJ. Cutaneous squamous cell carcinoma: A comprehensive clinicopathologic classification—Part II. *J Cutan Pathol.* 2006;33(4):267–279.

42. Rowe DE, Carroll RJ, Day CL. Prognostic factors for local recurrence, metastasis, and survival rates in squamous cell carcinoma of the skin, ear, and lip. Implications for treatment modality selection. *J Am Acad Dermatol.* 1992;26(6):976–990.

43. Wayte DM, Helwig EB. Melanotic freckle of Hutchinson. *Cancer.* 1968;21:893–911.

44. Margo CE. *Pigmented Lesions of the Eyelid. Principles and Practices of Ophthalmology.* 2nd ed. Philadelphia, PA: WB Saunders; 2000:3430–3446.

45. Garner A, Koorneef L, Levene A, et al. Malignant melanoma of the eyelid skin: Histopathology and behaviour. *Br J Opthalmol.* 1985;69:180–186.

46. Breslow A. Thickness, cross-sectional areas and depth of invasion in the prognosis of cutaneous melanoma. *Ann Surg.* 1970;172:902–908.

47. Gardetto A, Rainer C, Ensinger C, Baldissera E, Piza-Katzer H. Sebaceous carcinoma of the eyelid: a rarity worth considering. *Br J Ophthalmol.* 2002;86:243–244.

48. Mahendran RM, Newton-Bishop JA. Survey of UK current practice in treatment of lentigo maligna. *Br J Dermatol.* 2001;144:71–76.

49. Young S, Sands J. Sun and the eye: Prevention and detection of light-induced disease. *Clin Dermatol.* 1998;16(4):477–485.

CHAPTER 23

Oral Cancer

Robert A. Ord, D.D.S, M.D.,
F.R.C.S., F.A.C.S.

Andrew R. Salama, D.D.S., M.D.

BOX 23-1   Overview

- Squamous cell carcinoma of the mouth is the sixth most common cancer worldwide.
- Tobacco and alcohol use are the strongest etiologic risk factors and their use accounts for approximately 75% of oral squamas cell carcinoma (OSCCs).
- The gender incidence disparity in OSCC has narrowed over the past 50 years, the current male:female ratio is 3:2.
- Early stage disease (Stages I and II) may be treated with either surgery or radiation alone; however, surgery is preferred as it allows comprehensive pathologic staging and permits later use of adjuvant therapy in the event of recurrence.
- Primary surgery and adjuvant simultaneous chemo/radiotherapy offers a survival advantage in advanced stage disease.
- Pathologic staging of the neck is recommended in Stage II disease or greater, or in tumors in excess of 3-mm depth.
- The 5-year survival approaches 60% and is inversely correlated to advanced stage, nodal metastasis, and the presence of extracapsular spread in the lymphatics.
- Survival amongst African American is less than amongst whites.
- Regional nodal metastasis reduces survival by 50%.
- Distant metastasis at presentation are rare; however, this occurs in up to 25% of patients with advanced nodal disease with extracapsular spread.

INTRODUCTION

The term "oral cancer" is usually used synonymously with oral squamous cell carcinoma (OSCC) that comprises the majority of malignant neoplasms of the oral cavity. However, although some published series show 90 to 95% of oral cancers to consist of OSCC, this has not been the case in the author's series (Table 23-1). As can be seen in this series of 1157 consecutive cases of cancer of the mouth and jaws seen at the Department of Oral and

TABLE 23-1
Cancer of the Oral Cavity/Jaws[a] 1991–2005

Epidemoid carcinoma	873
CIS	51
Salivary	124
Sarcomas	41
Lymphomas	32
Metastatic	25
Other	11
Total	1157

[a]Oral cancer diversity among 1157 patients treated at the Department of Oral and Maxillofacial Surgery, University of Maryland Medical Center.

Maxillofacial Surgery, University of Maryland, only 873 (75.5%) were epidermoid carcinomas. Even within this group, some rare histologic variants from typical OSCC, e.g., verrucous carcinoma are seen (Table 23-2). This chapter will primarily discuss the current management of squamous cell carcinoma of the oral cavity with some comments on rare variants and oral mucosal melanoma (OMM). The term oral cavity will be defined as the region extending from the external lip to the retro molar region according to the *AJCC Staging Manual*.[1] Tumors of the oropharynx and paranasal sinuses will not be discussed.

EPIDEMIOLOGY

BOX 23-2   Summary

- The demographics of OSCC are changing and although the older male smoker who is a heavy drinker remains the stereotype, there is a significant increase in women, patients under 40 years, and nonsmokers/nondrinkers.
- OMM is a rare clinical entity that demonstrates aggressive clinical behavior.
- There are profound racial differences in the frequency of OMM, it being more common in populations of African and Japanese decent.
- OMM can present a diagnostic challenge due to its variable clinical and histologic characteristics.

Oral Squamous Cell Carcinoma

Estimated new cases of oral cancer were 20,010 in 2004, with 5160 deaths and an approximate 3:2 male to female ratio.[2]

TABLE 23-2
Histologic Variants of Epidermoid Carcinoma[a]

Squamous cell carcinoma	784
Verrucous carcinoma	22
Papillary carcinoma	7
Spindle cell carcinoma	6
Basaloid carcinoma	3
Total	822

[a]Histologic variants of OSCC seen at the Department of Oral and Maxillofacial Surgery, University of Maryland Medical Center (1991–2005)

Oral cancer represents 3% of all cancers in males and is the seventh most common cancer in men in the United States. There is a marked racial difference with 37 and 46% of white patients presenting with localized or regional disease while the figures for African American patients are 19% localized and 57% regional disease. In terms of survival, even when stratified for stage, white patients have a survival for localized and regional disease of 83 and 50%, respectively, while for African American patients, the figures are 69 and 31%. The relative 5-year survival (1992–1999) for white patients was 60% compared to 36% for blacks. The increase in the number of women with oral cancer may be a result of the gender difference in susceptibility to carcinogens, and an unexplained increase in patients without the traditional risk factors (see below) for oral cancer, most of whom are females.[3,4] Although OSCC is regarded as a disease of the elderly with the highest incidence in the sixth decade, there has been a marked increase in affected patients under the age of 40 in recent years, particularly in young males with tongue cancer. In one series from the MD Anderson Hospital, an increase from 4 to 18% was seen between 1971 and 1993.[5] In reviewing 63,000 head and neck cancer patients using the SEER database, Schantz and Yu found a 60% increase in tongue cancer in patients aged less than 40 years in the cohorts between 1973 and 1984 compared to that between 1985 and 1997.[6] This increase in young patients with OSCC has been documented worldwide, and although initially thought to represent a very aggressive cancer, it is now thought to have a similar prognosis to OSCC in older patients. Overall for OSCC, tongue is the most common site followed by floor of mouth cancer in patients who smoke and drink. In nonsmokers, floor of mouth cancer is rare.

Oral Mucosal Melanoma

Mucosal melanoma constitutes less than 1% of all melanomas and is less well understood than is cutaneous melanoma because of its relative rarity. OMMs occur at rates of 1.2 cases per 10 million.[7,8] While rare in the West, there is a racial predilection for OMM to occur in Japanese and Africans.[9] OMM occurs more commonly in males over a broad range of age (20 to 90 years), the median age is 60 years.[10] There is no formal staging system for OMM; however, the Ballantyne system is commonly referenced: Stage I, disease confined to the primary site; Stage II, the primary lesion with regional metastasis; Stage III, systemic metastasis.[11] An alternative staging system from the Memorial Sloan-Kettering Cancer Center uses reproducible histologic parameters and microanatomic compartments to stage OMM.[12]

▮ PATHOGENESIS

BOX 23-3 Summary

- Tobacco and alcohol abuse are independent risk factors for OSCC. The overall risk is multiplied in patients who use both.
- Chewing tobacco or "spit" tobacco confers less risk than do cigarettes/cigars.
- Immunosuppressed patients (e.g. renal transplant patients) have increased risk of lip and intraoral SCC.
- SCC of the lower lip is associated with sun exposure and behaves like a skin SCC rather than a mucosal OSCC.
- Intraoral melanosis confers an increased risk for OMM.

Oral Squamous Cell Carcinoma

OSCC is associated with tobacco and alcohol abuse, the highest risk for developing this cancer is in patients who both smoke and drink. Although snuff dipping is a well-documented risk factor for verrucous carcinoma, the overall risk of developing OSCC is much less with the use of chewing tobacco than with cigarettes.[13] Other risk factors important in cancer pathogenesis in general, e.g., poor diet and environmental factors are less well documented for oral cancer, although a diet deficient in fruits and vegetables may be a risk factor.[14,15] Patients who have no risk factors, i.e., never smokers and never drinkers are more likely to be women, be

very young or very old, and have tongue or gingival cancer.[16] Recent interest in these patients has focused around the possible role of human papillomavirus (HPV; particularly HPV16). Although there appears to be a cohort of patients with oropharyngeal cancer that are associated with HPV infection, the evidence is less clear for oral cancer. Despite reviews that have shown 23.5% of OSCC to have HPV present, many authors caution that the case for causality has not yet been established and that further studies are necessary to define any role HPV may have in pathogenesis.[17,18] Immunosuppression plays a role in OSCC and there is an increased incidence especially of tongue cancer in renal transplant patients.[19] Although the lip vermillion is classified as being a part of the oral cavity, squamous carcinoma of the vermillion behaves more like a true skin cancer than does a mucosal OSCC. The pathogenesis is related to sun exposure and this cancer is more common in fair-skinned individuals of Celtic origin. Cigarette smoking, pipe smoking, and alcohol have all been implicated as contributing factors. The causative role of herpes simplex virus is controversial. Pharmacologic immunosuppression secondary to renal transplantation is important, with nonmelanoma skin cancers and lip cancer being the most common post-transplant malignancies.[20]

Oral Mucosal Melanoma

The risk factors for OMM are less clearly defined than for cutaneous melanoma and OSSC. There are no known environmental agents that have conclusively shown causality in the development of OMM. OMM is believed to arise from mucosal melanocytes that are deposited embryologically from neuroectodermal derivatives. Intraepithelial melanocytes are more common in darkly pigmented individuals.[8] Racial or benign pigmentation has been found to be associated with OMM and melanotic pigmentation is present in one-third of the patients prior to the diagnosis of OMM.[9] The highest incidence of OMM occurs in the regions of oral racial pigmentation.[21]

▮ DIAGNOSIS

BOX 23-4 Summary

- Diagnosis and management of premalignant lesions that are at high risk for malignant change is important.

- Any lesion present in the mouth for 3 weeks, which has not responded to therapy and is undiagnosed, requires biopsy.
- The most important determinate for survival is the presence of a metastatic node.
- Red lesions have a much higher rate of change to OSCC than that of white lesions among PET malignant theory.
- Although CT, MR, PET, and ultrasound have all improved the diagnosis of metastatic cervical nodes, there is currently no way to reliably diagnose micrometastases (<3 mm) by imaging.
- Biopsy should be deep enough to display the maximum depth of invasion of OSCC, which is important in treatment planning.

Clinical Presentation

PREMALIGNANT LESIONS Clinically premalignant/potentially malignant lesions are seen in the oral cavity most commonly as white lesions (leukoplakias), which represent 85% of all precancerous lesions, or red lesions (erythroplasias).[22] Leukoplakias are simply defined as white patches of the mucosa of unknown etiology and that cannot be rubbed off. In Western civilization, it is usually said that 3 to 6% of leukoplakias will transform to OSCC; however, rates vary widely in different reports according to the geographic location, and the percentage of transformation rises as the length of follow-up increases. Site is a very important factor in assessing the risk of carcinomatous change with rates of 50% for floor of mouth, 24% for tongue, and 20% for lower lip vermillion being reported, and these sites account for 93% of all severe dysplasias or cancers.[23] Clinical signs that raise suspicion for higher risk of malignant change include ulceration, thickening of the leukoplakia, bleeding, or a "speckled" appearance, i.e., a mixture of red and white areas within the lesion (Fig. 23-1). Verrucous leukoplakia or proliferative verrucous leukoplakia has a warty fernlike appearance (Fig. 23-2) and has a high likelihood of malignant transformation, as first documented by Hansen et al[24] This type of leukoplakia is particularly aggressive and tends to recur, often multifocally, despite treatment. The presence of dysplasia, particularly severe or high-grade dysplasia, seen on biopsy is concerning for a higher malignant potential. The incidence of carcinomatous change in dysplastic leukoplakia appears to be 13 to 16%.[25] The histologic diagnosis of dysplasia, however, is a subjective one and will vary between pathologists.[26] As the average time from the

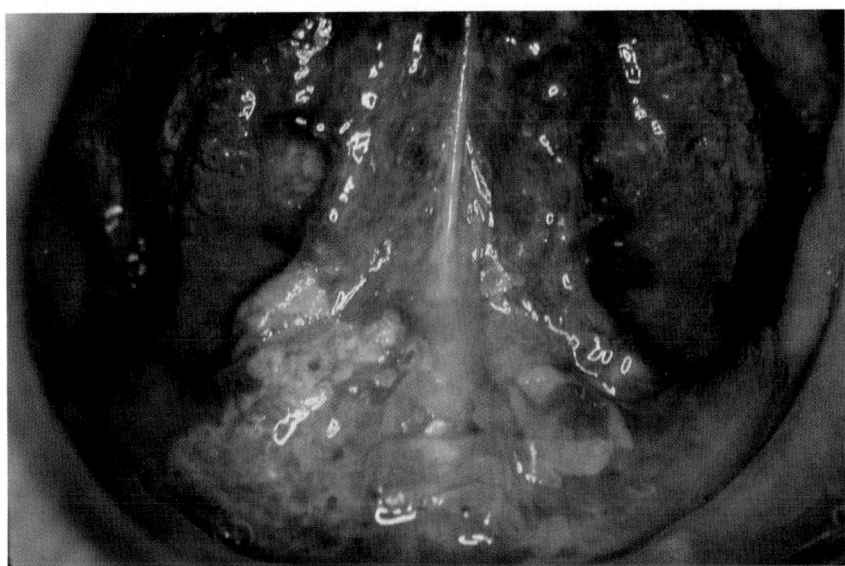

▲ **FIGURE 23-1** Leukoplakia floor of mouth. Note the irregular margin, different thickness, and the red speckled areas within the lesion. This is a leukoplakia that has >50% chances of transforming to a carcinoma.

diagnosis of a leukoplakia to the development of OSCC is 2.5 years, in theory, many cases of OSCC should be preventable by treating the premalignant lesion correctly.[27] However, it is still impossible to predict exactly which leukoplakias will transform and the widespread nature of some of these lesions and tendency to recur can make this a challenging exercise. Available treatment options include retinoids, laser ablation, cryotherapy, topical chemotherapy, and surgical excision, and the success rates for these different modalities are nicely reviewed by Clayman.[28] Another alternative for dysplastic lesions

is photodynamic therapy that should, in theory, be able to ablate dysplastic cells but leave normal cells intact minimizing the damage to the normal structures.[29,30] Certainly, for very-high-risk lesions, e.g., leukoplakias of the floor of mouth with severe dysplasia, we would favor excision with 5-mm margins. Erythroplasias are a very concerning group of lesions as the vast majority will represent either invasive OSCC, carcinoma *in situ*, or severe dysplasia at presentation. They have a red velvety appearance and are most common in the floor of mouth (Fig. 23-3) or the soft palate/retromolar region. These lesions are best treated sur-

gically as if they were all cancers. Whether oral lichen planus is a potentially malignant lesion is a controversial subject. The scientific evidence for and against is debated in the two papers referenced.[31,32] Although the debate continues, both the published literature and experience in clinical practice suggest that OSCC occurring in conjunction with oral lichen planus is a rare event. When it is seen, it appears to be related to erosive lichen planus, which is often longstanding.

ORAL SQUAMOUS CELL CARCINOMA Clinical presentation of OSCC varies and the diagnosis can be difficult in early stages. Approximately 6% of leukoplakias will be invasive cancers on biopsy and the majority of red patches, even those that are small, will represent early cancers. As the disease process progresses, the lesions will develop as a granular ulcer with rolled edges that are indurated to palpation (Fig. 23-4). The most common site is the lateral border of the tongue in its middle third, cancers of the dorsum of the tongue being very rare. Most OSCCs are painless initially; however, about one-third of our cases present with pain. If left undiagnosed, the tongue muscles will become fixed by infiltrating tumor with slurring of the speech and difficulty in swallowing. Involvement of the lingual nerve causes otalgia and, of course, with advanced disease, a mass in the neck due to regional metastasis may be the presenting sign. The second most common site is the floor of mouth, particularly in smokers. The vast majority of these cancers occur anteriorly within 1 cm of the

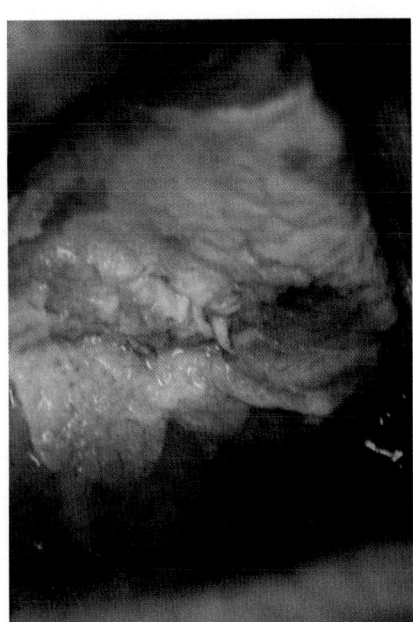

▲ **FIGURE 23-2** Verrucous leukoplakia of the palate. Note the frond-like appearance in the center.

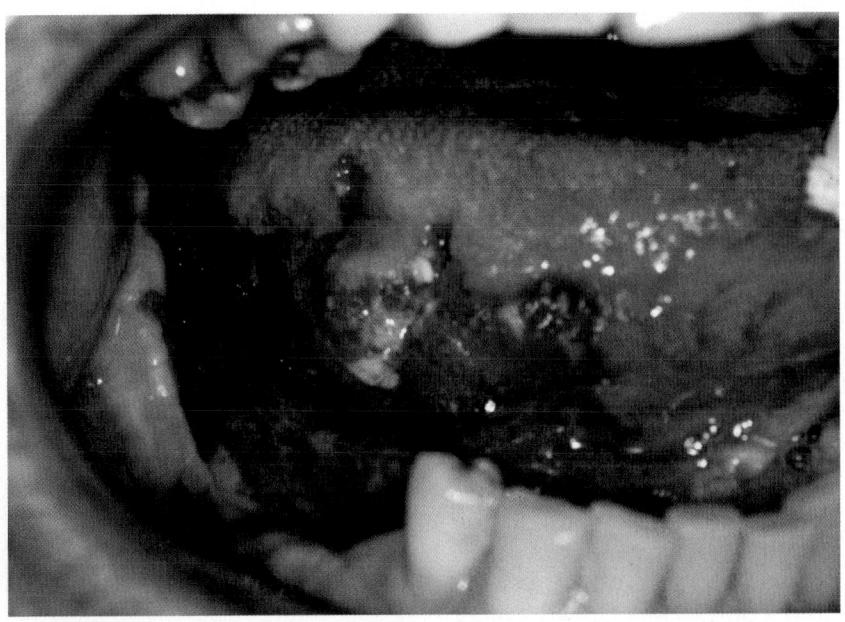

▲ **FIGURE 23-3** Erythroplasia of the floor of mouth and tongue. Note the invasive nature of the margins, on biopsy this was a squamous cell carcinoma.

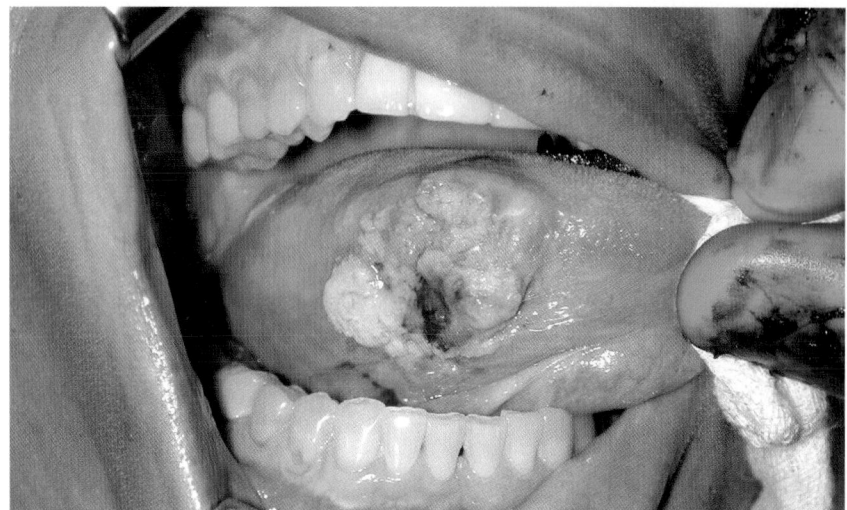

▲ **FIGURE 23-4** Typical squamous cell carcinoma of the tongue in the mid-third of the lateral border. Note the raised rolled edges and the central ulceration.

lingual frenum and frequently involving Wharton's duct. These ulcers may be involved with leukoplakias and lymph node metastases occur early. Involvement of the mandible with loosening of teeth is seen at a later stage and invasion of the inferior alveolar nerve will cause anesthesia of the ipsilateral lower lip. OSCC of the gingiva, retromolar fossa, and buccal mucosa is less common, although gingival cancer is seen in female nonsmokers and buccal mucosal cancer among Indians who chew betel nut. OSCC of the hard palate is rare in the West. Lymph node metastases are usually rounded and hard to palpation. As extracapsular spread occurs, lymph nodes become fixed to adjacent muscles and the overlying skin that becomes shiny and erythematous.

Obviously, not all cancers look the same; sometimes OSCC may have a very small surface component but burrows deeply into tongue muscles with a large submucosal component that is not visible but very obvious as a hard mass on palpation. Conversely, papillary exophytic tumors that are very superficial with little deep infiltration are also seen. There is also a wide variability in metastatic potential not only by site (tongue being at high risk) but by size also. Despite the fact that, as a general rule, the larger the primary tumor, the greater the incidence of metastases, some small cancers can involve multiple nodes while large T4 lesions may occasionally have N0 necks.

There are histologic variants of OSCC with different clinical presentations that are important to recognize. Verrucous carcinoma is exophytic, papillary, and fern-like, and does not metastasize to lymph nodes (Fig. 23-5). Spindle cell carcinoma may be polypoid and

pedunculated. In the lower lip, OSCC usually appears as a crusted lesion that keeps reappearing when "picked off" (Fig. 23-6); however, with time a more typical ulcer with a rolled edge is seen.

ORAL MUCOSAL MELANOMA OMM commonly presents as a pigmented lesion of the hard palate, gingiva, or buccal mucosa. The soft palate, tongue, and floor of mouth are less common sites.[8] Lesions typically manifest as a painless, progressively enlarging irregularly shaped macule arising in a preexisting region of pigmented mucosa, although lesions may also arise *de novo*. Clinically, the color may assume combinations of black, gray, purple, or red (Fig. 23-7). Morphologically

they may appear flat, elevated, nodular, or multifocal. Advanced tumors typically appear as ulcerated, fleshy lesions that bleed easily. Barker et al suggested that irregular or heterogeneous macules in high-risk sites (palate and gingiva) warrant suspicion and further investigation.[33] Because of the relative rarity of OMM and low level of clinical suspicion among numerous pigmented oral lesions, the time to diagnosis may be delayed. The amelanotic variant may be difficult to distinguish from other oral soft lesions. The differential diagnosis should include pyogenic granuloma, giant cell granuloma, lymphoma, soft tissue sarcomas, as well benign pigmented lesions. Most patients present with stage I disease, confined locally without regional or distant metastasis. A review of head and neck mucosal melanoma performed by Manolidis et al, including 547 patients, summarized that two-thirds present with stage I disease, and the remainder with evidence of regional or distant disease.[8] Among head and neck melanomas, OMM is more likely to demonstrate regional metastasis. Less than 10% present with distant metastasis.

Histology

ORAL SQUAMOUS CELL CARCINOMA The gold standard for diagnosis is, of course, histopathology and any undiagnosed ulcer or lesion in the mouth present for 3 weeks or more that has not responded to primary treatment (e.g., antibiotics, topical steroids, antifungal) should be biopsied. Because of the difficulty in identify-

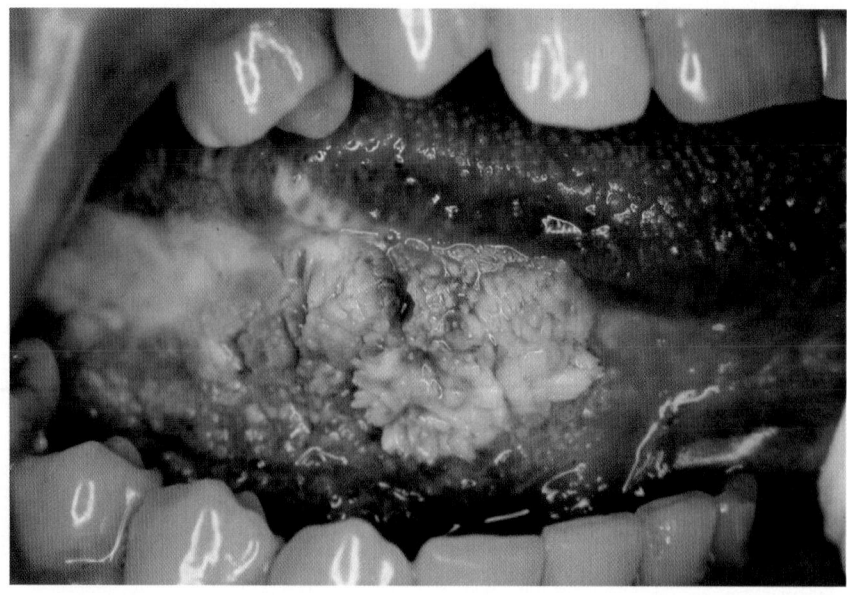

▲ **FIGURE 23-5** Verrucous carcinoma of the tongue. Note the warty, fern-like appearance in the background of leukoplakia.

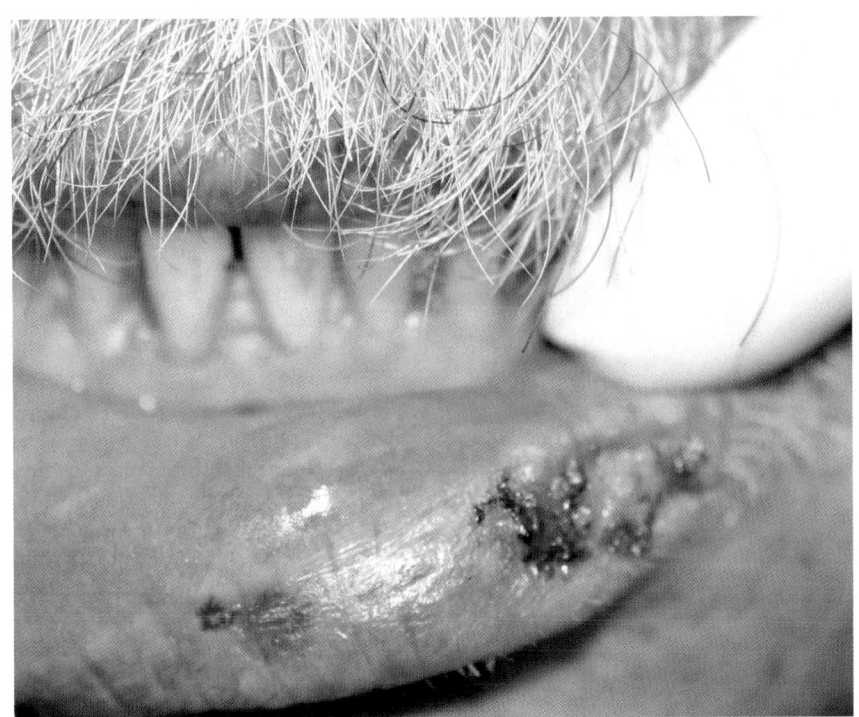

▲ **FIGURE 23-6** Squamous cell carcinoma of the lower lip, presenting as recurrent, nonhealing ulcer.

ing early lesions, a number of adjunctive techniques have been suggested. These include the use of Toluidene blue vital dye and the Oral CDX cytology brush. Toluidene blue has been used to help diagnose dysplasia and cancer for more than 40 years. The dye can be placed topically on the lesion with a cotton swab or used as a rinse in more extensive or multiple lesions and after decolorizing with dilute acetic acid. Severe dysplasia and cancer stain a dark blue color. Much of the pioneering work on this technique was undertaken by Mashberg, who showed false positive rates of 5.7% and false negative rates of 2.5% using the topical application.[34] The author finds this technique most helpful when a patient presents with widespread leukoplakia and it is not clear which area(s) to biopsy. The Oral CDX biopsy brush is basically a stiff brush that, unlike conventional brushes, can sample the whole thickness of the epithelium including the basal cells. It has been promoted as an easy, quick way to sample lesions that are not obviously cancers. The initial published study claimed a false negative rate of 0 with a statistical sensitivity of 97% and specificity of 97% for positive CDx results and 90% for atypical CDx results.[35] However, more recent publications have questioned these findings; Poate et al found a sensitivity of 71.4% and a specificity of 32% with a PPV of 44.1% and NPV of 60%.[36] A 2005 Cochrane systematic review found no robust evidence for the use of clinical oral cancer screening, the use of Toluidene

blue or brush biopsy.[37] Scalpel biopsy remains the method of choice for definitive diagnosis. Although biopsy at the periphery of the lesion including normal oral mucosa has been advocated, it is not essential to include normal tissue. Biopsy should not be taken in the center of a necrotic ulcer that would not give a representative diagnostic sample. Biopsy should be deep enough to show the depth of invasion of the tumor into the underlying tissue. The histologic appearance is that of a typical squamous cell carcinoma with abnormal epithelial cells invading through the basement membrane. By reviewing the cytologic and nuclear abnormalities of the cells along with their differentiation and number of mitotic figures, the pathologist can classify the OSCC into well, moderately, and poorly differentiated carcinomas. Well-differentiated tumors tend to form keratin nests while poorly differentiated cancers show little keratinisation and have a spindle cell appearance, and may require special stains to rule out melanoma and other anaplastic tumors. Histologic grade does not seem to be an important prognostic factor in OSCC except for fast-growing poorly differentiated tumors that behave aggressively. When dealing with a suspected verrucous carcinoma, it is important to obtain an adequate sample particularly to show the entire depth of the tumor including the invasive front. These tumors are cytologically bland and an inadequate sample will lead to a spurious benign diagnosis. Besides their deep

parakeratin clefts and their thickened acanthotic epithelium, the invasive front shows a bulbous-broad-based pushing front. When there is a mixture of verrucous and squamous cell elements (hybrid tumor), the tumor will behave like a conventional OSCC. In spindle cell carcinomas, a deep biopsy is important as the surface epithelium shows only dysplasia with the malignant spindle cells found in the underlying submucosa. Special stains may or may not show cytokeratins, which prove the diagnosis.[38]

ORAL MUCOSAL MELANOMA Pigmented, heterogeneous lesions that exhibit progressive growth or change over time in high-risk locations should be subjected to histologic examination. Two general microscopic patterns appear prevalent: *in situ* and invasive; however, it is more common for both patterns to exist simultaneously. Tumors show varied histologic features including spindle-like, plasmacytoid, and epitheloid cells arranged in sheets or organoid/alveolar forms[33] (Fig. 23-8). Melanin is present in 50 to 70% of lesions. Amelanotic varieties may microscopically resemble poorly differentiated carcinomas, lymphomas, or sarcomas. Poorly differentiated tumors may histologically appear as small, round blue cells tumors suggestive of lymphoma. Immunohistochemical markers specific for HMB-45 and S-100 show intense staining patterns. The desmoplastic variant of OMM demonstrates marked neurotropism. Additional features include angiolymphatic invasion and reactive lymphoblastic proliferations.[8] As in OSSC, a biopsy specimen should be of adequate depth (into connective tissue), as superficial biopsies may lead to a misdiagnosis.

Prognosis

ORAL SQUAMOUS CELL CARCINOMA The prognosis for OSCC is related to TNM classification (Table 23-3) and Staging (Table 23-4).[1] Five-year survival is 82% for localized disease, 51% for regional disease, and 28% for distant disease for all races. Trends in 5-year survival rates for all stages and all races were 54% between 1974 and 1976, and 59% between 1995 and 2001, and this difference is statistically significant.[39] Whether this improvement is due to improvements in treatment, earlier diagnosis or change in the pattern of disease is not clear. Although the TNM system is the most important way of stratifying OSCCs, determining treatment and prognosis, there are many other useful factors

349

SKIN CANCER

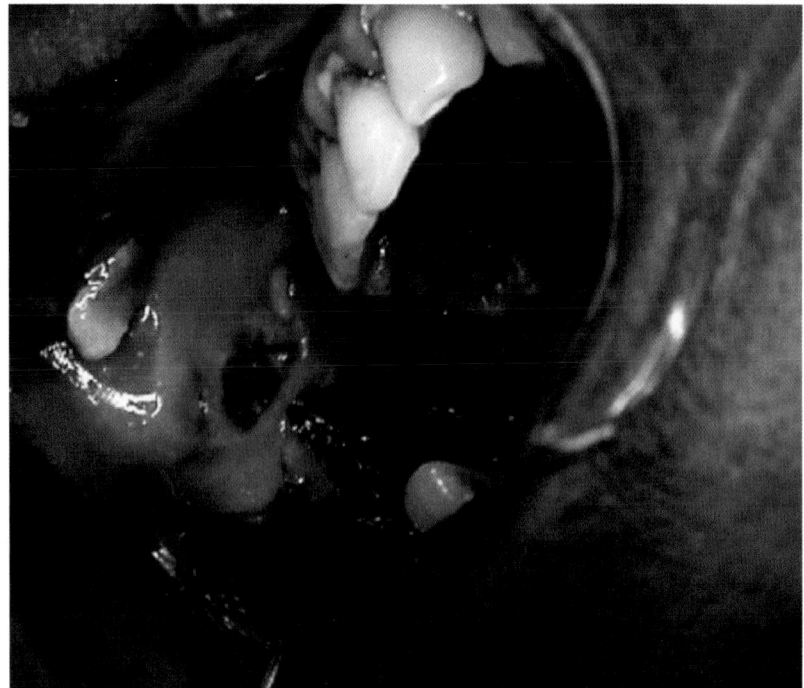

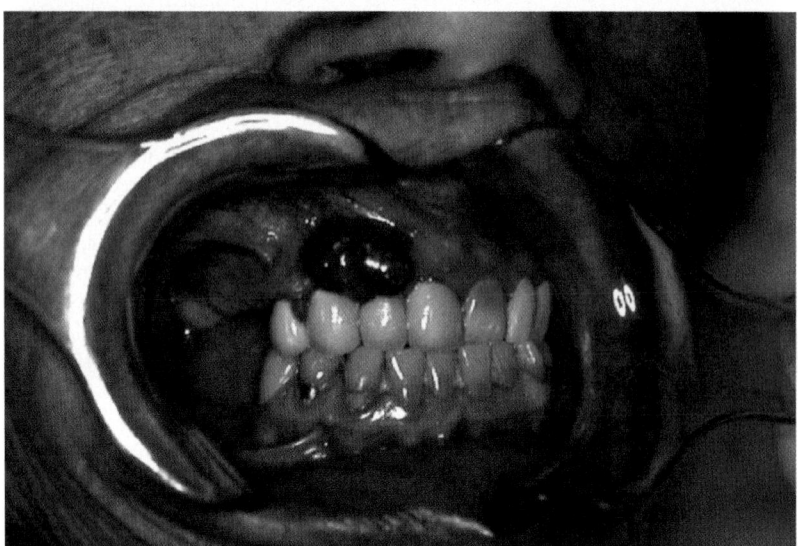

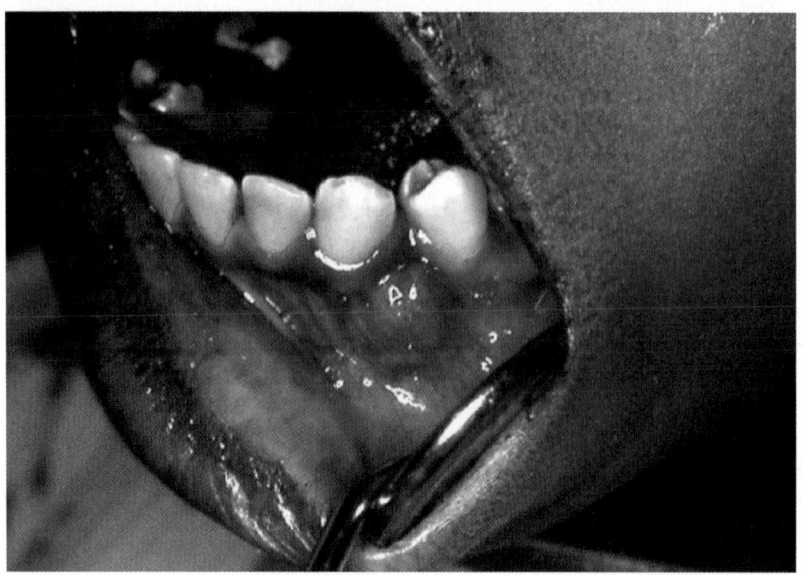

that predict prognosis that the clinician can utilize. It has become clear that tumor thickness is very important in squamous cell carcinoma in predicting lymph node metastasis and the need for therapy to address the neck.[40] In a similar manner to melanoma, the thicker the tumor, the worse the prognosis. Other predictive factors related to the primary site are the presence of perineural spread, the mode of invasion, and positive margins after surgery. The presence of one positive node reduces survival by 50% and this has always been said to be the single most important factor in survival. However, there is sufficient data to implicate extracapsular spread as the most significant finding in lymph node metastasis.[41,42] In addition, the level of lymph node involvement may be important, yet is not reflected in the current TNM system. The system of separating the neck nodes into five levels was first introduced by the Sloane Kettering Hospital in New York (Table 23-5) and, more recently, sublevels have been introduced.[43,44] In addition, cancers at different sites in the oral cavity, e.g., lower lip versus oral tongue behave very differently in their aggressiveness and ability to metastasize. In the lower lip, the differentiation of the carcinoma is important in outcomes. Different histologic variants will also have a different prognosis. Verrucous carcinoma in the oral cavity has a 5-year survival of 73.7% and an 85.7% survival if surgery alone is the primary treatment, which is much better than for OSCC, presumably due its lack of nodal metastases.[45] At the current time, there is much interest in identifying molecular markers for cancer that can be used for diagnosis, prognostic markers, and for possible novel therapies; these will be discussed in a later section.[46]

ORAL MUCOSAL MELANOMA In contrast to cutaneous melanoma, OMM collectively is known to carry an ominously poor clinical prognosis. Histologic parameters predictive of poor survival include angiolymphatic invasion, necrosis, and cellular polymorphism.[47] Clinical harbingers include the presence of regional and distant metastasis, reducing survival by 50%.[7] Tumor thickness, depth of invasion, and mitotic index have not been uniformly shown to predict clinical behavior. Prasad et al showed an associated decrease in survival with increasing level of invasion, and notably less survival in patients with poorly differentiated tumors; tumors >5-mm depth behaving more poorly.[12] The 5-year survival of OMM is dismal and is generally noted to be less

▲ **FIGURE 23-7** Typical presentation of an OMM as a gingival submucosal pigmented lesion.

TABLE 23-3
AJCC Staging for Lip and Oral Cavity Tumors[1]

PRIMARY TUMOR (T)

TX	Primary tumor cannot be assessed
T0	No evidence of primary tumor
Ta	Carcinoma *in situ*
T1	Tumor 2 cm or less in greatest dimension
T2	Tumor more than 2 cm but not more than 4 cm in greatest dimension
T3	Tumor more than 4 cm in greatest dimension
T4	(Lip) tumor invades through cortical bone, inferior alveolar nerve, floor of mouth, or skin of face, i.e., chin or nose
T4a	(Oral cavity) tumor invades through cortical bone, into deep [estrinsic] muscle of tongue (genioglossus, hyoglossus, palatoglossus, and styloglossus), maxillary sinus, or skin of face
T4b	Tumor involves masticator space, pterygoid plates, or skull base and/or encases internal carotid artery

REGIONAL LYMPH NODES (N)

NX	Regional lymph nodes cannot be assessed
N0	No regional lymph node metastasis
N1	Metastasis in a single ipsilateral lymph node, 3 cm or less in greatest dimension
N2	Metastasis an a single ipsilateral lymph node, more than 3 cm but not more than 6 cm in greatest dimension; or in multiple ipsilateral lymph nodes, none more than 6 cm in greatest dimension; or in bilateral or contralateral lymph nodes, none more than 6 cm in greatest dimension
N2a	Metastasis in single ipsilateral lymph node more than 3 cm but not more than 6 cm in greatest dimension
N2b	Metastasis in multiple ipsilateral lymph nodes, none more than 6 cm in greatest dimension
N2c	Metastasis in bilateral or contralateral lymph nodes, none more than 6 cm in greatest dimension
N3	Metastasis in a lymph node more than 6 cm in greatest dimension

DISTANT METASTASIS (M)

MX	Distant metastasis cannot be assessed
M0	No distant metastasis
M1	Distant metastasis

than 15% with a median survival of 25 months.[7,8] The 5-year survival is slightly worse for patients with palatal lesions.

TABLE 23-4
AJCC Stage Grouping for Lip and Oral Cavity Tumors[1]

0	Tis	N0	M0
I	T1	N0	M0
II	T2	N0	M0
III	T3	N0	M0
	T1	N1	M0
	T2	N1	M0
	T3	N1	M0
IVA	T4a	N0	M0
	T4a	N1	M0
	T1	N2	M0
	T2	N2	M0
	T3	N2	M0
	T4a	N2	M0
IVB	Any T	N3	M0
	T4b	Any N	M0
IVC	Any T	Any N	M0

Imaging

SQUAMOUS CELL CARCINOMA The TNM classification is a clinical staging system, and clinical stage is based on information available to the clinician prior to the first definitive treatment that includes physical examination, imaging, endoscopy, biopsy, and surgical exploration.[1]

The oral cavity is easily examined without special instrumentation in most cases unless trismus is present due to invasion of the masticatory muscles or secondary to submucous fibrosis in betel nut chewers. Early lesions can be misdiagnosed, the extent of deep invasion can be difficult to quantify by palpation alone, and whether true bone invasion has occurred in OSCC close to or fixed to the jaws is frequently impossible to assess clinically. With regards to the neck, clinical palpation is about 70% accurate and lymph nodes <1 cm are not easily felt. Patients who are obese, very muscular, or those who have had previous radiation therapy (RT) to the neck are more challenging to assess. Imaging has improved the accuracy of staging and allowed better pretreatment planning. Frequently, a combination of different imaging modalities will give the optimum information. In assessing soft tissue invasion, MRI gives the best information, e.g., OSCC of the tongue invading to the midline. Bony invasion, e.g., maxillary sinus or skull base involvement is best delineated by CT (bone windows); however, CT is often limited in assessing the oral cavity due to dental artifact. It is challenging to assess early mandibular invasion, and may make the difference between a marginal or segmental resection for the patient. CT seems best for early cortical involvement while MR shows marrow spread better. The isotope bone scan has a high percentage of false positives but, when negative, rules out any bone involvement. The final decision is sometimes made at surgery when periosteal stripping allows the surgeon to view directly whether invasion through the periosteal barrier has occurred ("peek and

TABLE 23-5
Cervical Node Levels[a]

Level I	Submandibular triangle between the anterior and posterior belly of the digastric muscle (includes the submental triangle)
Level II	Extends from skull base to carotid artery bifurcation (surgical landmark), or the hyoid bone (surface anatomical landmark) posteriorly is the posterior border of the sternocleidomastoid muscle
Level III	Extends from the carotid bifurcation to the point where the omohyoid muscle covers the internal jugular vein (surgical landmark) or the cricoid cartilage (surface anatomical landmark
Level IV	Extends from the point where the omohyoid crosses the internal jugular vein to the clavicle
Level V	Posterior triangle from posterior sternocleidomastoid muscle to the trapezius with the clavicle inferiorly

[a]Cervical lymph node by anatomic levels.[43]

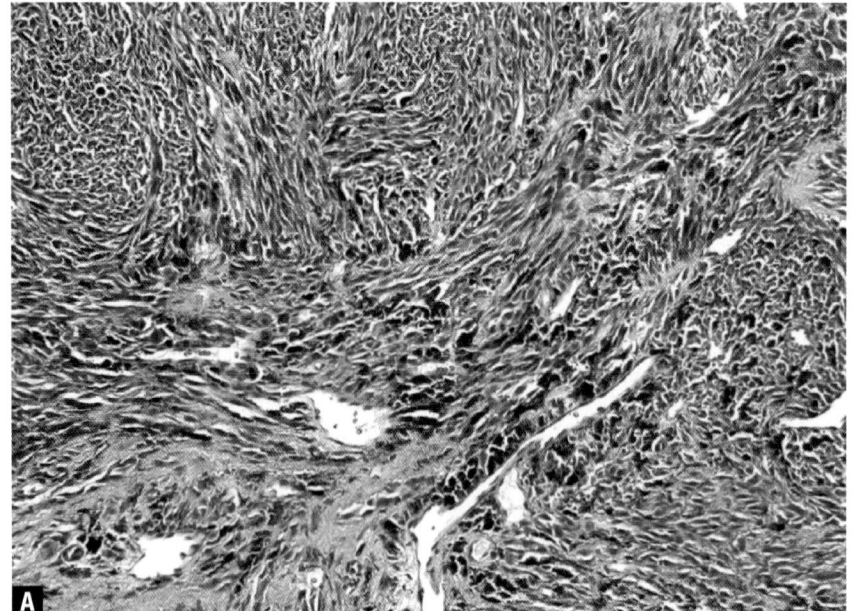

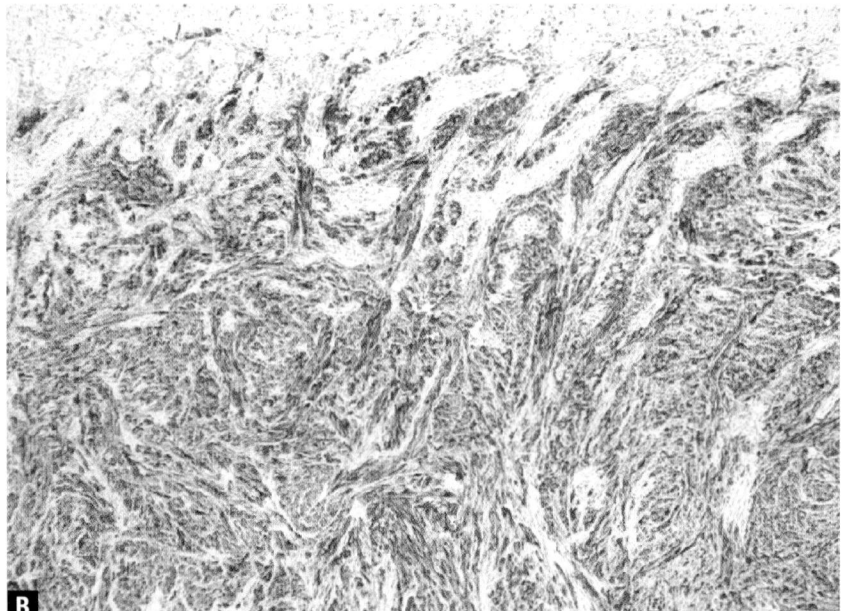

▲ **FIGURE 23-8** A. Histomicrograph of a palatal OMM of the hard palate demonstrating pleomorphic spindle cells with the presence of melanin (H/E, 200×). B. HMB-45 immunohistochemical stain of an OMM showing intense reactivity (HMB-45, 100×).

formed, chest radiograph or CT is an essential part of the work up.[56]

ORAL MUCOSAL MELANOMA Currently, available imaging modalities for OSCC can be used in the evaluation of OMM. CT and MRI are both valuable in assessing the size, extent, and involvement of adjacent structures as well as regional lymphatic basins. MRI excels in delineation of soft tissues, and CT in determining bone invasion. Early stage lesions of the gingiva and palate may be difficult to interpret secondary to radiation scatter from dental restorations. Although fluorodeoxyglucose (FDG)-PET has limited value in assessing early-stage cutaneous melanoma, and is an insensitive tool for detecting occult metastatic disease, it does have some utility in mucosal melanoma.[57] Large exophytic tumors or those exhibiting nodular growth are better visualized than are small, thin, or superficial lesions.[58]

▮ MOLECULAR ASPECTS

BOX 23-5 Summary

- A greater understanding of the molecular events involved in OSCC provides opportunity to develop novel therapeutics and interventions.
- Developing molecular techniques may allow for more precise risk stratification among oral cancer patients, allowing directed use of adjuvant therapy in high-risk patients.
- p53 is the most common gene mutation occurring in >50% of cases of OSCC in smokers and drinkers. p53 mutations are much less frequent in nonsmokers and nondrinkers.
- Development of OSCC involves "multiple hits" with progressive changes in oncogenes/suppressor genes and chromosomal loss of heterozygosity (LOH), leading eventually to invasive cancer.
- Recent novel therapies developed from molecular biology include the use of Cetuximab, an EGFR inhibitor in conjunction with radiation therapy (RT).

Oral Squamous Cell Carcinoma

At a molecular level, OSCC essentially stems from a derangement of cellular events that occur in the life cycle of oral epithelia. The role of tumor-suppressor genes and oncogenes revealed in the pioneering research of Fearon and Vogelstein revolutionized cancer research and spawned a new generation of

shriek"), and the complex problem of diagnosing mandibular invasion is well reviewed by Brown and Lewis-Jones.[48] Newer modalities such as SPECT scan and Dentascans (GE Healthcare) may play a role in this area.[49,50]

In reviewing imaging for neck nodes, both CT and MR give increased accuracy compared to palpation. CT features of malignancy include the size of the node, its shape, and the presence of central necrosis. However, comparative studies have shown little difference between CT and MR's ability to detect central necrosis or extracapsular spread.[51] Some authorities claim ultrasound with fine needle aspiration

biopsy (FNAB) to be a superior technique in imaging and diagnosing cervical nodes.[52] In the last few years, positron emission tomography (PET) and fused PET/CT scanning has become increasingly popular for head and neck cancer imaging and although this does not solve the problem of micrometastasis in the N0 neck, it is very sensitive for nodes of size 8 mm or more.[53] The present major use for PET scanning is in the detection of recurrent disease postsurgery or chemotherapy/RT and the detection of distant metastases or second primary cancers and these additional findings may be present in up to 22% of cases.[54,55] If PET scan is not per-

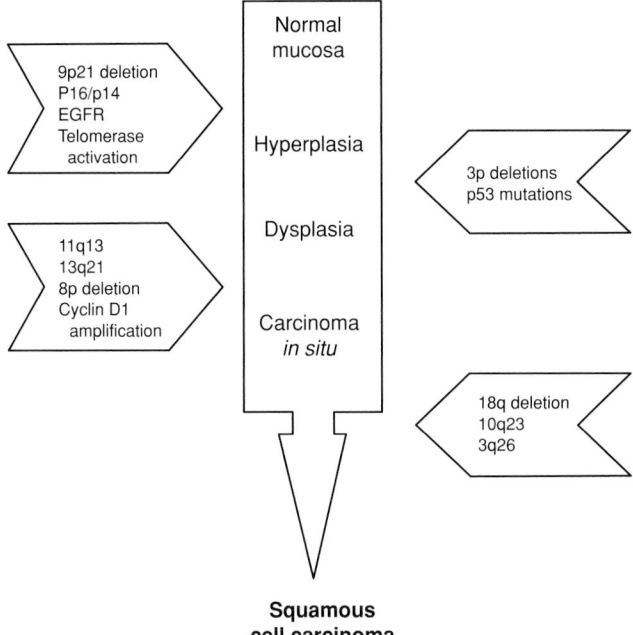

FIGURE 23-9 Proposed genetic progression model in head and neck squamous cell carcinoma (adapted from Califano et al[60]).

investigations focused on diagnostics and biologically directed therapy.[59]

The dominant theories in the origins of OSCC focus on clonal evolution, the molecular progression model, and field cancerization. The chronic exposure of oral epithelia to mutagens such as tobacco and alcohol exerts selective pressure on cellular populations. This process selects certain cells for preferential growth under adverse conditions whereby some are able to evade cell death or injury through native or acquired genetic differences. A natural selection process occurs, resulting in a subpopulation of cells with accumulated genetic alterations favoring survival in a "hostile" environment. Cancer ensues with the acquired ability for invasion and clonal proliferation within a cell line.

The malignant potential of oral leukoplakia/erythroplakia is a commonly accepted principle in OSCC. The molecular progression model links phenotypic and genetic changes in the progression from normal/wild-type cells through dysplasia to cancer. Microsatellite marker analysis has assisted in identifying mutation patterns that occur in the process of developing dysplasia and cancer (Fig. 23-9). A head and neck model proposed by Califano et al suggests that a finite number of accumulated genetic mutations are required in the formation of cancer and emphasizes that the sum of genetic mutations are more important than is the sequence in which they occur chronologically.[60] Field cancerization, a concept proposed by Slaughter nearly 50 years ago, implies that tissues of the aerodigestive tract develop premalignant change or dysplasia under mutagenic pressure.[61] These multicentric regions of at-risk tissue are therefore susceptible to develop distinct polyclonal lesions, giving rise to recurrence and second primary tumors. Contemporary interpretations of this theory have illustrated that some, but not all, OSCC in a field are clonally related.

The exquisite control of cell growth, apoptosis, and detection of genetic errors fall under autonomous control to prevent cancer and regulate the fate of aging cell populations. These complex systems include tumor-suppressor genes, oncogenes, and other stabilizing genes.[62] The detection of loss of heterozygosity (LOH), allelic imbalance, telomerase activation, and DNA promoter hypermethylation are among the first changes recognized in the transition from dysplasia to cancer.[63] These findings alone do not specifically identify mutations, but localize regions of interest among the thousands of genes in the human genome.

LOH and allelic imbalance are indicative of genetic alterations and are commonly the result of point mutations, amplifications, deletions, and rearrangements.[64] Comparative genomic hybridization studies have shown that well-differentiated tumors undergo changes in regions 3p, 3q, 5q, 9p, with LOH in the specific region of 9p21–22 being reported in over 70% of head and neck squamous cell carcinoma.[65] These changes have also been demonstrated in premalignant lesions.[66] LOH at 9p21, 3p, and 17p13 have been demonstrated to be early events in the progression from dysplasia to carcinoma.[67]

Tumor-suppressor genes are complex regulatory genes responsible for limiting uncontrolled cell growth. The *p53* gene located on 17p13 encodes a 53-kDa protein responsible for cell-cycle coordination, DNA repair, and apoptosis.[68] Mutations occur in albeit predictable different regions within the gene, and are found in approximately 50% of all OSCC. The prevalence of p53 mutations increases through stages of disease progression, being far more common in carcinoma than in dysplasia. p53 expression indirectly controls a cyclin-dependant kinase inhibitor, p21 that induces cell-cycle arrest, allowing gene repair and preventing propagation of genetic errors. The *p21* gene may also function as a tumor-suppressor gene.[69] Alterations in p53 activity are not limited to mutations. Gene products from human *mdm2* forms complexes with both mutant and wild-type p53, inhibiting transcriptional activation. Normally functioning in symbiotic fashion, when amplified or overexpresed, *mdm2* can inhibit wild-type p53.[70] A viral protein product of the HPV16, E6 has been shown to form inhibitor complexes that promote the rapid degradation of p53, implicating viral infection in oncogenesis.[71] LOH at 9p21 inhibits p16 and the cyclin-dependant kinase activity of its gene product that serves as a cell-cycle arrest signal contributing to oncogenesis.[64] Cyclin D1 is a regulatory protein involved in cell-cycle transitions, overexpression, and amplification in oropharyngeal cancer, and has been associated with unfavorable outcomes.[68]

Oncogenes are growth-promoting regulatory genes that govern cellular signal transduction pathways, and mutations resulting in overexpression are initiators in the development of OSCC.[72] In contrast to tumor-suppressor genes, oncogenes act to initiate cancer with a singly altered copy in the genome. The epidermal growth factor receptor (EGFR) proto-oncogene encodes a growth factor receptor, and mutations induce growth-signal autonomy that affects the expression of a number of oncogenic processes leading to cell survival and proliferation. Overexpression of EGFR is observed in nearly 90% of OSCC.[62]

The ability of tumors to invade and metastasize are fundamental characteristics of malignancy. Cadherins are epithelial-specific proteins that maintain intracellular adhesion and their loss of function or downregulation occurs in OSCC.[62] Altered expression of metalloproteinases

TABLE 23-6
Molecular Abnormalities in OSCC[63]

LOH 9p	70–80%
LOH 3p	60–70%
LOH 17p	50–70%
LOH 11q	30%
LOH 13q	30%
p16 inactivation	80%
p53 mutation	50–80%
Cyclin D1 amplification	30%

have been implicated in aggressive tumor behavior and metastasis.

Considerable efforts have been made to identify potential biomarkers predictive of outcomes (Table 23-6). It appears that most of the genetic changes responsible for cancer occur early, and are therefore detectable. Several potential biomarkers have been shown to correlate with reduced survival and lymph node metastasis.[73] The aberrations in cellular processes that lead to cancer affect several housekeeping regulatory genes, including those responsible for cellular adhesion, apoptosis, and cell signaling. Profiling cancers and specific mutation patterns can be determined by DNA microarray analysis and allows one to develop a cancer-specific signature that can be used to predict outcomes in the research setting.[73]

The analysis of DNA ploidy, which roughly estimates cellular DNA content in premalignant lesions, has been used to evaluate the risk of malignant transformation. Aneuploid and tetraploid dysplastic lesions have been shown to have greater potential to develop into cancer; this relationship is even stronger with erythroplakia. Although this data has come under criticism, it is likely to hold some clinical value.[74]

Brennan et al used patient-specific p53 PCR primers to analyze surgical margins and lymph node metastasis in patients with OSCC. Among specimens with histologically negative margins, patients with p53 mutations in adjacent, phenotypically benign tissue had substantially increased risk for local recurrence.[75] Although time-consuming, this technique may play a supportive role in the determination of surgical margins and need for adjuvant therapy.

Cetuximab (Erbitux, ImClone Systems) is an EGFR monoclonal antibody that binds the receptor and subsequently inhibits growth, and survival has been used either alone or in combination with cisplatin and/or radiation and demonstrated significant rates of tumor regression. Bonner et al demonstrated prolonged progression-free survival in nonsurgically treated patients with radiation and Cetuximab.[76] Phase III trials are currently in progress to investigate the value of Cetuximab combined with traditional chemotherapy and radiation in patients with high-risk pathologic features following surgery.

HPV has been implicated in a number of head and neck cancers, notably oropharyngeal tumors; moreover, HPV positivity portends a more favorable outcome. The HPV oncogenic proteins E6 and E7 are potential future therapeutic targets. An HPV16 vaccine targeted against viral capsid proteins has been shown to affect the development of cervical cancer and phase I clinical trials specific for oral cancer show therapeutic potential.[77]

MANAGEMENT/TREATMENT

BOX 23-6   Summary

- Wide margins are essential to prevent local recurrence, and the best chance of cure is with initial radical therapy as salvage therapy gives poor cure rates.
- In the N0 neck with a >20% chance of occult metastasis, an elective selective neck dissection should be performed.
- OSCC is a multidisciplinary and multimodality disease, especially for Stages III and IV.
- Radical surgery is the preferred treatment for OMM.
- Radiation and chemotherapy may be used in the adjuvant setting.
- The role of sentinel lymph node biopsy has not been proven in OMM.

Oral Squamous Cell Carcinoma

OSCC is a cancer that demonstrates aggressive local invasion and cervical metastases, with the development of distant metastases being rare and occurring usually in advanced cases. Treatment is therefore directed at loco/regional control and cure as there is currently no curative option for distant metastases. Standard of care involves review of cases by an inter displinary tumor board. Treatment and prognosis are related to staging of the tumor with Stages I and II being early stage and Stages III and IV the late stage. Despite the fact that most OSCCs have a preceding premalignant lesion, and take months or years to transform and develop at a site (the oral cavity) that is easy to screen clinically, the majority of OSCCs still present at a late stage. In early Stages I and II, OSCC can be adequately man-

aged by one modality, i.e., either surgery or radiation therapy (RT). In the United States, primary surgery is the standard of care for oral cavity tumors, and is particularly indicated for tumors adjacent to the jaw bones. The survival rate from RT is equivalent to surgery for small early tumors but morbidity is significant and also RT may be required later for recurrent disease or a second primary cancer. Recent advances in RT have been directed toward reducing morbidity by selectively targeting the tumor using 3D planning, conformal therapy, and intensity modulated radiation therapy (IMRT), and reducing the dose of radiation to the surrounding normal tissues.[78,79] Another method of achieving this is the use of brachytherapy as many oral sites, e.g., the anterior tongue are easy to implant. The hope with these techniques is to reduce the problems of mucositis, xerostomia, osteoradionecrosis, and radiation fibrosis causing trismus and dysphagia. Other advances have been in hyperfractionation techniques to improve patient benefit.[80] The principles of surgery for OSCC primary tumor dictate excision with 1 to 2 cm margins in order to obtain histologically negative margins. Margins <5 mm from the cancer, involved by dysplasia or invasive carcinoma are regarded as positive, giving a high risk of local recurrence. In these cases, reexcision is required, where this is not possible, adjuvant RT is given. Cases with histologic evidence of perineural invasion, vascular invasion, and close/positive margins are also candidates for postoperative RT. Most oral cancers are amenable to transoral excision, although retromolar fossa and posterior tongue tumors may need a cervical approach. Tongue cancer has a sinister reputation for deep infiltration and 1.5- to 2-cm margins can be justified. OSCC of the lower lip behaves more like a conventional skin cancer and 3- to 5-mm margins may be adequate.[81] In squamous cell carcinoma of the lower lip, consideration should always be given to treating the remaining sun-damaged vermillion by vermillionectomy.

Although Stage I and II patients are, by definition, N0 clinically and by imaging (CT/MR/PET), about 33% of these patients will have occult microscopic neck disease, and for many years, the benefits of an elective neck dissection versus observation of the neck and performing a neck dissection only when a node develops" was debated. Two initial prospective randomized studies showed no difference in outcomes between these two treatments; however, a more recent study showed a survival advan-

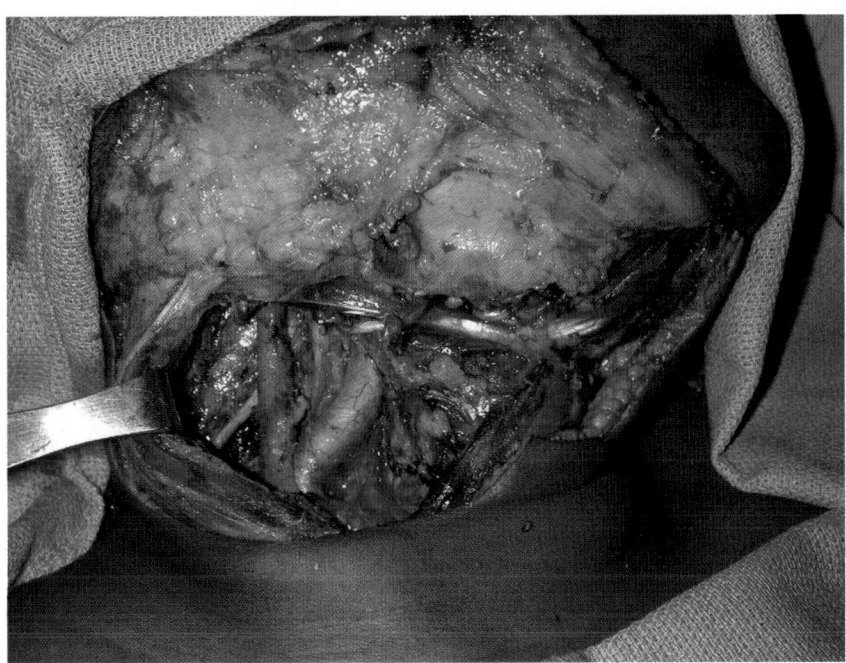

▲ **FIGURE 23-10** Selective neck dissection. The retractor is holding the sternocleidomastoid muscle to reveal the accessory nerve passing diagonally posteriorly from under the internal jugular vein. The carotid artery lies more anteriorly.

tage for elective neck dissection for early stage tongue cancer especially in T2 and tumors thicker than 4 mm.[82–84] Current standard of care in the United States mandates an elective neck dissection when the risk of occult metastasis is greater than 20%, which will include all T2 tumors and above, and all primary tumors thicker than 3 to 4 mm (includes T1) especially of the tongue and floor of mouth. In cancer of the lower lip, although T stage and thickness are important, histologic differentiation plays a major role in determining metastasis.[85] The elective neck dissection indicated for OSCC encompasses the nodes most likely to be involved by metastatic spread, i.e., those at Levels I–III (Table 23-5), the supraomohyoid neck dissection (Fig. 23-10). This dissection spares all muscles and nerves removing only the adipose tissues and nodes. Although some have advocated the removal of Level IV for tongue cancer, the evidence for this is weak.[86] Sentinel node biopsy, although well established for head and neck melanoma, is not currently established for OSCC.[87] Following elective neck dissection, if more than one positive node is found or extracapsular spread is present, adjuvant RT or chemotherapy/RT is recommended. There is not sufficient evidence whether micrometastases (<3 mm) influences outcomes in OSCC or whether adjuvant therapy is required.[88,89] In advanced Stages III and IV disease, multimodality

treatment is indicated with primary surgery for resectable cases. In unresectable or non operable cases, a chemotherapy/RT combination is used, but is usually palliative and not curative in Stage IV OSCC. In these advanced cases, the primary tumor frequently cannot be resected via a transoral approach, and a mandibular swing procedure

(Fig. 23-11) or a pull-through operation (Fig. 23-12a and b) is necessary. In the N0 neck, selective neck dissection is required and where palpable nodes are present, modified radical or true radical neck dissection is utilized encompassing Levels I–V. These patients require adjuvant therapy and two recent large randomized prospective trials have shown an advantage for the combination of chemotherapy and RT for patients at high risk of recurrence.[90,91]

Recent advances in microvascular reconstruction has allowed the surgeon to accomplish larger resections with the knowledge that free flap reconstruction for both hard and soft tissue is available with the restoration of function such as speech and swallowing. Most commonly, the free radial forearm flap (Fig. 23-13a and b), rectus abdominis flap, and anterolateral thigh flap are used for soft tissue reconstruction with the fibular and DCIA flap for bony reconstruction of the jaws. Intraosseous titanium dental implants are ideal for replacing teeth and restoring a functional occlusion in the oral cancer patient.

Future directions in the management of OSCC will be linked to research discoveries at a molecular level. Although much work has been done on oncogenes and tumor-suppressor genes, with research on chromosomal deletions and angiogenesis, little of this work has made an impact on therapy. Currently, there is much interest in anti-EGFR

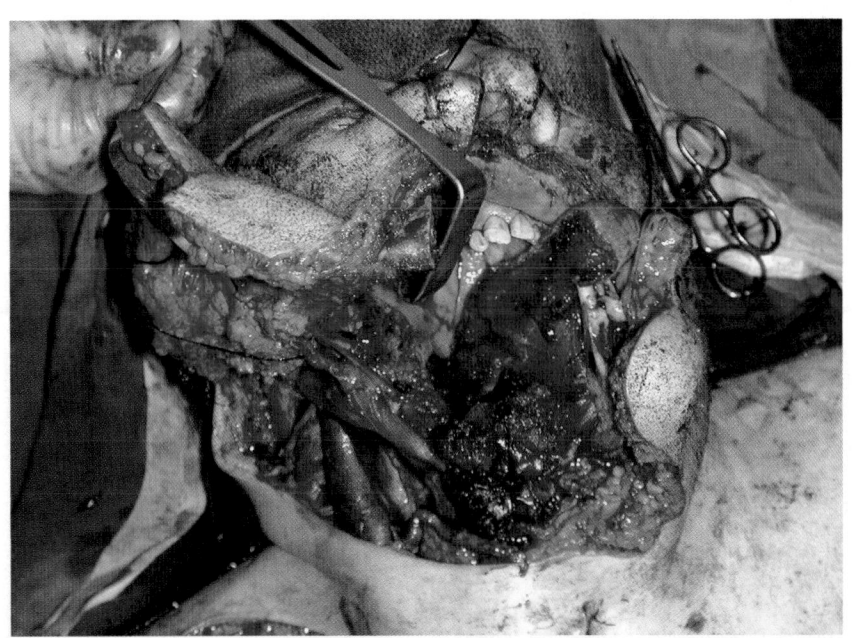

▲ **FIGURE 23-11** Lip split and mandibulotomy for access to the posterior tongue. The lip has been split in continuity with the neck dissection incision and the mandible has been osteotomized. The retractor is holding the sectioned mandible laterally to show the tongue following right hemiglossectomy and selective neck dissection. The right internal jugular vein is seen in the posterior neck.

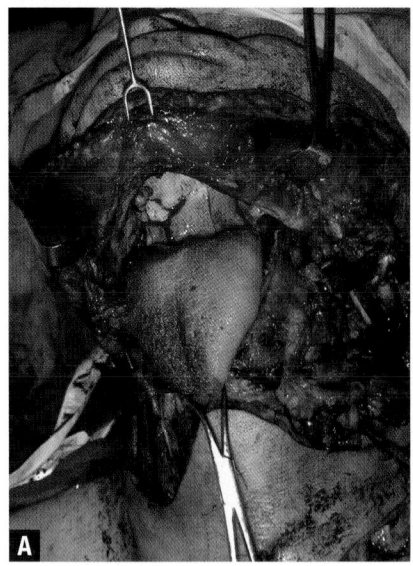 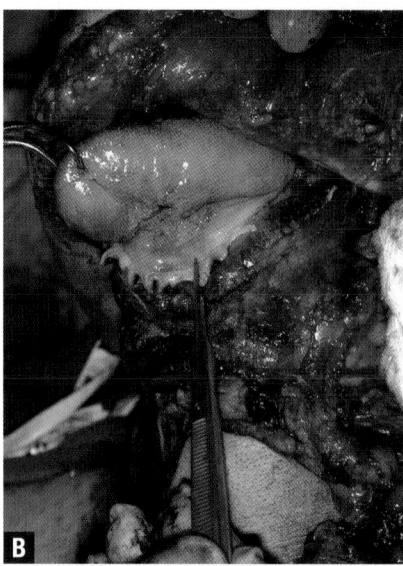

▲ **FIGURE 23-12** **A.** In this pull-through technique, the tongue and contents of the oral cavity have been released from the mandible and pulled through into the neck for better access and resection outside the mouth. **B.** By lifting the tongue tip, the floor of mouth is seen with a carcinoma invading into the under side of the tongue.

therapy and combinations of this with chemotherapy and RT.[76,92]

Oral Mucosal Melanoma

Radical surgical resection is the preferred treatment modality in OMM and offers the best chance for local control and survival.[93] Complete tumor extirpation is important for both local and regional disease control, and while there is no general consensus on the required surgical margins, a 1.5-cm margin is desirable. Achieving adequate margins is made difficult by the multifocality of some tumors, the depth of invasion, and the required resection of vital structures. Although many patients succumb to disease, control of disease and relief of symptoms are optimized with a radical surgical approach. Treatment of the N0 neck is controversial, but frequently performed for lesions within the oral cavity. Therapeutic neck should be performed in the presence of clinical or radiographic

signs of regional metastasis, and in most cases, a comprehensive neck dissection is undertaken. OMM is generally considered to be radio-resistant, but external beam radiotherapy is commonly recommended in the adjuvant setting and said to provide some degree of disease control. In advanced unresectable disease, radiation may be used palliatively as a sole treatment modality. Definitive radiotherapy may achieve cure in a small subset of patients, but local/regional control is optimized with a combined approach.[10] There is little evidence to support the use of chemotherapy or immunotherapy. To date, the value of sentinel lymph node biopsy in OMM has not been substantiated in the literature.

■ PREVENTION

The single best means of preventing OSCC would be an effective patient education program to discuss the health

problems of nicotine and alcohol abuse, and encourage tobacco cessation. In the head and neck cancer, the premalignant stage is potentially reversible as is the "field change" that occurs in this disease and so research into therapies for chemoprevention has been active. Trials have been undertaken both in patients with leukoplakia and to try and prevent the development of second primary cancers. The most popular drugs have been vitamin A and the retinoid analogues. Several of these studies have shown response to the drug and remission of the leukoplakias; however, relapse following cessation of therapy, retinoid toxicity, and the lack of large-scale randomized prospective trials have so far prevented chemoprevention from becoming standard of care.[94,95] The interest in EGFR inhibitors (Cetuximab) in head and neck cancers and its comparative low toxicity profile other than the common acneform skin rash has led to interest in this agent as a possible chemopreventive agent and trials have started to assess its role.

■ FINAL THOUGHTS

Oral cancer remains a therapeutic challenge in spite of the medical advances over the past 50 years. Primary surgery is the preferred treatment modality, with surgical margins of 1 cm offering optimal rates of local control. The survival advantage of pathologically staging the relevant lymphatic basins in N0 patients is controversial. However, elective neck dissection more accurately stages patients, and permits targeted therapy in patients with lymph node metastasis. Therapeutic neck dissection, radical or modified radical neck dissection, is recommended for patients who present with clinical or radiographic lymph node metastasis. Adjuvant radiotherapy or chemo/radiotherapy is reserved for patients with high-risk features (close margins, angiolymphatic invasion, perineural invasion, and greater than one lymph node metastasis). Chemotherapy alone has a limited role in the treatment of OSCC; however, it may be used in the palliative setting. Developing novel therapeutics and diagnostics hold potential in the treatment of OSCC. PET/CT imaging has prognostic promise in the evaluation of primary and recurrent disease as well as distant metastasis.

REFERENCES

1. Greene FL, Page DL, Fleming ID, et al. *AJCC Cancer Staging Manual.* 6th ed. New York: Springer; 2002.

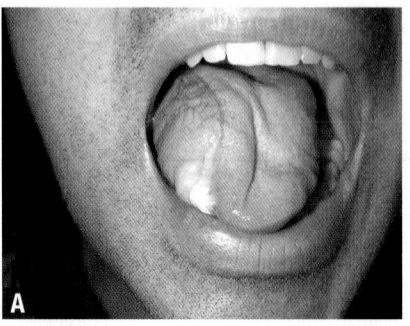 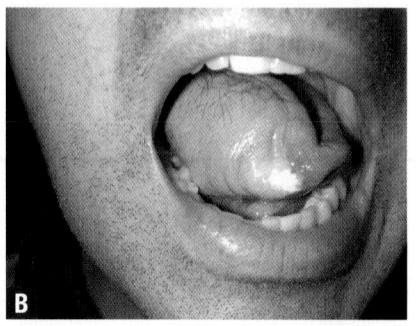

▲ **FIGURE 23-13** **A.** Free radial forearm flap reconstructing the shape and volume of the right tongue for speech and swallowing. **B.** Patient shows good protrusion and left lateral movement with this thin pliable flap.

2. Jemal A, et al. Cancer statistics. *CA Cancer J Clin.* 2004;54(1):8–29.

3. Muscat JE, et al. Gender differences in smoking and risk for oral cancer. *Cancer Res.* 1996;56(22):5192–5197.

4. Talamini R, et al. Cancer of the oral cavity and pharynx in nonsmokers who drink alcohol and in nondrinkers who smoke tobacco. *J Natl Cancer Inst.* 1998; 90(24):1901–1903.

5. Myers JN, et al. Squamous cell carcinoma of the tongue in young adults: increasing incidence and factors that predict treatment outcomes. *Otolaryngol Head Neck Surg.* 2000;122(1):44–51.

6. Schantz SP, Yu GP. Head and neck cancer incidence trends in young Americans, 1973–1997, with a special analysis for tongue cancer. *Arch Otolaryngol Head Neck Surg.* 2002;128(3):268–274.

7. Hicks MJ, Flaitz CM. Oral mucosal melanoma: epidemiology and pathobiology. *Oral Oncol.* 2000;36(2):152–169.

8. Manolidis S, Donald PJ. Malignant mucosal melanoma of the head and neck: review of the literature and report of 14 patients. *Cancer.* 1997;80(8):1373–1386.

9. Garzino-Demo P, et al. Oral mucosal melanoma: a series of case reports. *J Craniomaxillofac Surg.* 2004;32(4):251–257.

10. Mendenhall WM, et al. Head and neck mucosal melanoma. *Am J Clin Oncol.* 2005;28(6):626–630.

11. Ballantyne AJ. Malignant melanoma of the skin of the head and neck. An analysis of 405 cases. *Am J Surg.* 1970;120(4):425–431.

12. Prasad ML, et al. Primary mucosal melanoma of the head and neck: a proposal for microstaging localized, Stage I (lymph node-negative) tumors. *Cancer.* 2004; 100(8):1657–1664.

13. Accortt NA, et al. Cancer incidence among a cohort of smokeless tobacco users (United States). *Cancer Causes Control.* 2005;16(9):1107–1115.

14. Llewellyn CD, et al. An analysis of risk factors for oral cancer in young people: a case–control study. *Oral Oncol.* 2004; 40(3):304–313.

15. Rodriguez T, et al. Risk factors for oral and pharyngeal cancer in young adults. *Oral Oncol.* 2004;40(2):207–213.

16. Koch WM, et al. Head and neck cancer in nonsmokers: a distinct clinical and molecular entity. *Laryngoscope.* 1999;109(10): 1544–1551.

17. Ha PK, Califano JA. The role of human papillomavirus in oral carcinogenesis. *Crit Rev Oral Biol Med.* 2004;15(4):188–196.

18. Kreimer AR, et al. Human papillomavirus types in head and neck squamous cell carcinomas worldwide: a systematic review. *Cancer Epidemiol Biomarkers Prev.* 2005;14(2):467–475.

19. Meng S, Jiamei L. Management of tongue cancer in the patient who is systemically immunosuppressed: a preliminary report. *Oral Surg Oral Med Oral Pathol Oral Radiol Endod.* 2000;90(6):689–693.

20. de Visscher JG, Bouwes Bavinck JN, van der Waal I. Squamous cell carcinoma of the lower lip in renal-transplant recipients. Report of six cases. *Int J Oral Maxillofac Surg.* 1997;26(2):120–123.

21. Cove H. Melanosis, melanocytic hyperlasia, and primary malignant melanoma of the nasal cavity. *Cancer.* 1979;44(4): 1424–1433.

22. Bouquot JE. Reviewing oral leukoplakia: clinical concepts for the 1990s. *J Am Dent Assoc.* 1991;122(6):80–82.

23. Bouquot JE. Common oral lesions found during a mass screening examination. *J Am Dent Assoc.* 1986;112(1):50–57.

24. Hansen LS, Olson JA, Silverman S Jr. Proliferative verrucous leukoplakia. A long-term study of thirty patients. *Oral Surg Oral Med Oral Pathol.* 1985;60(3): 285–298.

25. Lumerman H, Freedman P, Kerpel S. Oral epithelial dysplasia and the development of invasive squamous cell carcinoma. *Oral Surg Oral Med Oral Pathol Oral Radiol Endod.* 1995;79(3):321–329.

26. Abbey LM, et al. Intraexaminer and interexaminer reliability in the diagnosis of oral epithelial dysplasia. *Oral Surg Oral Med Oral Pathol Oral Radiol Endod.* 1995;80(2):188–191.

27. Bouquot JE, Weiland LH, Kurland LT. Leukoplakia and carcinoma in situ synchronously associated with invasive oral/oropharyngeal carcinoma in Rochester, Minn., 1935–1984. *Oral Surg Oral Med Oral Pathol.* 1988;65(2):199–207.

28. Clayman L. Management of mucosal premalignant lesions. *Oral Maxillofac Clin North Am.* 1994;6(3):431.

29. Tsai JC, et al. Photodynamic therapy of oral dysplasia with topical 5-aminolevulinic acid and light-emitting diode array. *Lasers Surg Med.* 2004;34(1):18–24.

30. Fan KF, et al. Photodynamic therapy using 5-aminolevulinic acid for premalignant and malignant lesions of the oral cavity. *Cancer.* 1996;78(7):1374–1383.

31. Eisenberg E. Oral lichen planus: a benign lesion. *J Oral Maxillofac Surg.* 2000;58(11):1278–1285.

32. Silverman S Jr. Oral lichen planus: a potentially premalignant lesion. *J Oral Maxillofac Surg.* 2000;58(11):1286–1288.

33. Barker BF, et al. Oral mucosal melanomas: the WESTOP Banff workshop proceedings. Western Society of Teachers of Oral Pathology. *Oral Surg Oral Med Oral Pathol Oral Radiol Endod.* 1997; 83(6):672–679.

34. Mashberg A. Final evaluation of tolonium chloride rinse for screening of high-risk patients with asymptomatic squamous carcinoma. *J Am Dent Assoc.* 1983; 106(3):319–323.

35. Sciubba JJ. Improving detection of precancerous and cancerous oral lesions. Computer-assisted analysis of the oral brush biopsy. U.S. Collaborative OralCDx Study Group. *J Am Dent Assoc.* 1999;130 (10):1445–1457.

36. Poate TW, et al. An audit of the efficacy of the oral brush biopsy technique in a specialist Oral Medicine unit. *Oral Oncol.* 2004;40(8):829–834.

37. Kujan O, et al. Evaluation of screening strategies for improving oral cancer mortality: a Cochrane systematic review. *J Dent Educ.* 2005;69(2):255–265.

38. Slootweg PJ, et al. Spindle-cell carcinoma of the oral cavity and larynx. Immunohistochemical aspects. *J Craniomaxillofac Surg.* 1989;17(5):234–236.

39. Jemal A, et al. Cancer statistics, 2006. *CA Cancer J Clin.* 2006;56(2):106–130.

40. Pentenero M, Gandolfo S, Carrozzo M. Importance of tumor thickness and depth of invasion in nodal involvement and prognosis of oral squamous cell carcinoma: a review of the literature. *Head Neck.* 2005;27(12):1080–1091.

41. Woolgar JA, et al. Cervical lymph node metastasis in oral cancer: the importance of even microscopic extracapsular spread. *Oral Oncol.* 2003;39(2):130–137.

42. Myers EN, Gastman BR. Neck dissection: an operation in evolution: Hayes Martin lecture. *Arch Otolaryngol Head Neck Surg.* 2003;129(1):14–25.

43. Robbins KT, et al. Neck dissection classification update: revisions proposed by the American Head and Neck Society and the American Academy of Otolaryngology—Head and Neck Surgery. *Arch Otolaryngol Head Neck Surg.* 2002;128(7):751–758.

44. Spiro RH. The management of neck nodes in head and neck cancer: a surgeon's view. *Bull N Y Acad Med.* 1985; 61(7):629–637.

45. Koch BB, et al. National survey of head and neck verrucous carcinoma: patterns of presentation, care, and outcome. *Cancer.* 2001;92(1):110–120.

46. Salesiotis AN, Cullen KJ. Molecular markers predictive of response and prognosis in the patient with advanced squamous cell carcinoma of the head and neck: evolution of a model beyond TNM staging. *Curr Opin Oncol.* 2000;12(3):229–239.

47. Bradley PJ. Primary malignant mucosal melanoma of the head and neck. *Curr Opin Otolaryngol Head Neck Surg.* 2006; 14(2):100–104.

48. Brown JS, Lewis-Jones H. Evidence for imaging the mandible in the management of oral squamous cell carcinoma: a review. *Br J Oral Maxillofac Surg.* 2001; 39(6):411–418.

49. Brockenbrough JM, Petruzzelli GJ, Lomasney L. DentaScan as an accurate method of predicting mandibular invasion in patients with squamous cell carcinoma of the oral cavity. *Arch Otolaryngol Head Neck Surg.* 2003;129(1): 113–117.

50. Van Cann EM, et al. Bone SPECT reduces the number of unnecessary mandibular resections in patients with squamous cell carcinoma. *Oral Oncol.* 2006;42(4):409–414.

51. King AD, et al. Necrosis in metastatic neck nodes: diagnostic accuracy of CT, MR imaging, and US. *Radiology.* 2004; 230(3):720–726.

52. van den Brekel MW, et al. Modern imaging techniques and ultrasound-guided aspiration cytology for the assessment of neck node metastases: a prospective comparative study. *Eur Arch Otorhinolaryngol.* 1993;250(1):11–17.

53. Rumboldt Z, et al. Imaging in head and neck cancer. *Curr Treat Options Oncol.* 2006;7(1):23–34.

54. Lonneux M, et al. Positron emission tomography with fluorodeoxyglucose for suspected head and neck tumor recurrence in the symptomatic patient. *Laryngoscope.* 2000;110(9):1493–1497.

55. Canning CA, et al. Positron emission tomography scan to determine the need for neck dissection after chemoradiation for head and neck cancer: timing is everything. *Laryngoscope.* 2005;115(12):2206–2208.

56. Ong TK, et al. The role of thorax imaging in staging head and neck squamous cell carcinoma. *J Craniomaxillofac Surg.* 1999; 27(6):339–344.

57. Clark PB, et al. Futility of fluorodeoxyglucose F 18 positron emission tomography in initial evaluation of patients with T2 to T4 melanoma. *Arch Surg.* 2006;141(3): 284–288.

58. Goerres GW, et al. FDG PET for mucosal malignant melanoma of the head and neck. *Laryngoscope.* 2002;112(2):381–385.

59. Fearon ER, Vogelstein B. A genetic model for colorectal tumorigenesis. *Cell.* 1990; 61(5):759–767.

60. Califano J, et al. Genetic progression model for head and neck cancer: implications for field cancerization. *Cancer Res.* 1996;56(11):2488–2492.

61. Slaughter DP, Southwick HW, Smejkal W. Field cancerization in oral stratified squamous epithelium: clinical implications of multicentric origin. *Cancer.* 1953; 6(5):963–968.

62. Kupferman ME, Myers JN. Molecular biology of oral cavity squamous cell carcinoma. *Otolaryngol Clin North Am.* 2006; 39(2):229–247.

63. Perez-Ordonez B, Beauchemin M, Jordan RC. Molecular biology of squamous cell carcinoma of the head and neck. *J Clin Pathol.* 2006;59(5):445–453.

64. Williams HK. Molecular pathogenesis of oral squamous carcinoma. *Mol Pathol.* 2000;53(4):165–172.

65. Bockmuhl U, et al. Genomic alterations associated with malignancy in head and neck cancer. *Head Neck.* 1998;20(2):145–151.

66. Zhang L, et al. Increased genetic damage in oral leukoplakia from high risk sites: potential impact on staging and clinical management. *Cancer.* 2001;91(11):2148–2155.

67. Califano J, et al. Genetic progression and clonal relationship of recurrent premalignant head and neck lesions. *Clin Cancer Res.* 2000;6(2):347–352.

68. Quon H, Liu FF, Cummings BJ. Potential molecular prognostic markers in head and neck squamous cell carcinomas. *Head Neck.* 2001;23(2):147–159.

69. Yanamoto S, et al. p53, mdm2, and p21 expression in oral squamous cell carcinomas: relationship with clinicopathologic factors. *Oral Surg Oral Med Oral Pathol Oral Radiol Endod.* 2002;94(5):593–600.

70. Agarwal S, et al. MDM2/p53 co-expression in oral premalignant and malignant lesions: potential prognostic implications. *Oral Oncol.* 1999;35(2):209–216.

71. Mao L, Hong WK. How does human papillomavirus contribute to head and neck cancer development? *J Natl Cancer Inst.* 2004;96(13):978–980.

72. Partridge M, et al. Patient-specific mutation databases for oral cancer. *Int J Cancer.* 1999;84(3):284–292.

73. Wreesmann VB, et al. Identification of novel prognosticators of outcome in squamous cell carcinoma of the head and neck. *J Clin Oncol.* 2004;22(19):3965–3972.

74. Lippman SM, Sudbo J, Hong WK. Oral cancer prevention and the evolution of molecular-targeted drug development. *J Clin Oncol.* 2005;23(2):346–356.

75. Brennan JA, et al. Molecular assessment of histopathological staging in squamous-cell carcinoma of the head and neck. *N Engl J Med.* 1995;332(7):429–435.

76. Bonner JA, et al. Radiotherapy plus cetuximab for squamous-cell carcinoma of the head and neck. *N Engl J Med.* 2006;354(6):567–578.

77. Fakhry C, Gillison ML. Clinical implications of human papillomavirus in head and neck cancers. *J Clin Oncol.* 2006; 24(17):2606–2611.

78. Chao KS, et al. A prospective study of salivary function sparing in patients with head-and-neck cancers receiving intensity-modulated or three-dimensional radiation therapy: initial results. *Int J Radat Oncol Biol Phys.* 2001;49(4):907–916.

79. Lin A, et al. Quality of life after parotid-sparing IMRT for head-and-neck cancer: a prospective longitudinal study. *Int J Radiat Oncol Biol Phys.* 2003;57(1):61–70.

80. Fu KK, et al. A Radiation Therapy Oncology Group (RTOG) phase III randomized study to compare hyperfractionation and two variants of accelerated fractionation to standard fractionation radiotherapy for head and neck squamous cell carcinomas: first report of RTOG 9003. *Int J Radiat Oncol Biol Phys.* 2000;48(1):7–16.

81. Hjortdal O, Naess A, Berner A. Squamous cell carcinomas of the lower lip. *J Craniomaxillofac Surg.* 1995;23(1):34–37.

82. Kligerman J, et al. Supraomohyoid neck dissection in the treatment of T1/T2 squamous cell carcinoma of oral cavity. *Am J Surg.* 1994;168(5):391–394.

83. Vandenbrouck C, et al. Elective versus therapeutic radical neck dissection in epidermoid carcinoma of the oral cavity: results of a randomized clinical trial. *Cancer.* 1980;46(2):386–390.

84. Fakih AR, et al. Elective versus therapeutic neck dissection in early carcinoma of the oral tongue. *Am J Surg.* 1989;158(4): 309–313.

85. Weiss MH, Harrison LB, Isaacs RS. Use of decision analysis in planning a management strategy for the stage N0 neck. *Arch Otolaryngol Head Neck Surg.* 1994; 120(7):699–702.

86. Khafif A, Lopez-Garza JR, Medina JE. Is dissection of level IV necessary in patients with T1–T3 N0 tongue cancer? *Laryngoscope.* 2001;111(6):1088–1090.

87. Pitman KT, et al. Sentinel lymph node biopsy in head and neck cancer. *Oral Oncol.* 2003;39(4):343–349.

88. Woolgar JA. Micrometastasis in oral/oropharyngeal squamous cell carcinoma: incidence, histopathological features and clinical implications. *Br J Oral Maxillofac Surg.* 1999;37(3):181–186.

89. Nieuwenhuis EJ, et al. Assessment and clinical significance of micrometastases in lymph nodes of head and neck cancer patients detected by E48 (Ly-6D) quantitative reverse transcription-polymerase chain reaction. *Lab Invest.* 2003;83(8):1233–1240.

90. Cooper JS, et al. Postoperative concurrent radiotherapy and chemotherapy for high-risk squamous-cell carcinoma of the head and neck. *N Engl J Med.* 2004;350(19):1937–1944.

91. Bernier J, et al. Postoperative irradiation with or without concomitant chemotherapy for locally advanced head and neck cancer. *N Engl J Med.* 2004;350(19): 1945–1952.

92. Posner MR, Wirth LJ. Cetuximab and radiotherapy for head and neck cancer. *N Engl J Med.* 2006;354(6):634–636.

93. Medina JE, et al. Current management of mucosal melanoma of the head and neck. *J Surg Oncol.* 2003;83(2):116–122.

94. Hong WK, et al. 13-*cis*-Retinoic acid in the treatment of oral leukoplakia. *N Engl J Med.* 1986;315(24):1501–1505.

95. Lippman SM, et al. Comparison of low-dose isotretinoin with beta carotene to prevent oral carcinogenesis. *N Engl J Med.* 1993;328(1):15–20.

CHAPTER 24

Genital Cancers

Wolfgang H. Cerwinka, M.D.
Norman L. Block, M.D.

BOX 24-1 Overview

- Tumors of the penis
  - Neurofibromas
  - Angiokeratoma of Fordyce
  - Granular cell tumor
  - Glomus tumor
  - Hemangiomas
  - Leiomyomas
  - Verruciform xanthoma
  - Cutaneous horns
  - Balanitis xerotica obliterans
  - Pseudoepitheliomatous hyperplasia
  - Condylomata
  - Giant condyloma
  - Intraepithelial neoplasia
  - Bowen's disease
  - Erythroplasia of Queyrat
  - Extra-mammary Paget's disease
  - Carcinoma
- Tumors of the scrotum
- Tumors of the vulva
- Extra-mammary Paget's disease of genital skin

INTRODUCTION

Cancers of the genital skin are similar in nature to those occurring elsewhere on the skin. What differentiates these tumors from their analogs in other areas is the tremendous psychological overlay complicating their presence. This may be more evident or of greater extent in males, but certainly exists in both sexes.

This quality, which distinguishes genital skin tumors from other skin tumors, plays a major role in discovery, diagnosis, and treatment. It is extremely important that the clinician takes this quality into account when dealing with such patients.

As an example of the impact of psychological overlay on these diseases, one of the authors (Block) is reminded of an occurrence early in his career. A patient with a penile lesion was seen in consultation in a hospital room. History and physical exam were completed and biopsy of a very suspicious lesion was recommended. The patient asked for information on what the biopsy result might lead to, and upon being advised that a penile cancer might lead to partial penectomy, calmly climbed out of bed and leapt through his hospital room window to his death!! Be judicious in your comments!

TUMORS OF THE PENIS

BOX 24-2 Summary

- May arise from any tissue of the penis.
- Benign tumors are underreported and treated by local excision.
- Hemangiomas are treated by vascular laser.
- Verruciform xanthoma resembles squamous cell cancer; foam cells are pathognomonic.
- Cutaneous horns: one third is associated with squamous cell cancer.
- Balanitis xerotica obliterans is associated with squamous cell cancer.
- Pseudoepitheliomatous hyperplasia is related to inflammation.
- Condylomata are benign and treated locally.
- Giant condyloma often recur and are treated by wide excision.
- Intraepithelial neoplasia is associated with HPV infection.
- Bowen's disease is carcinoma *in situ* on the skin.
- Erythroplasia of Queyrat is carcinoma *in situ* on the glans.

The most common site of genital neoplasms is the penis. Neoplasms of this organ may arise from its overlying skin or may originate from tissues lying within the penile shaft and involve the skin. These may include sarcomas of connective tissue, carcinomas of urethra, extra-mammary Paget's disease (EMPD), and will be discussed separately (see below).

Numerous benign tumors have been described on penile skin. Pigmented penile macules seem to be unusual but are probably greatly underreported (Fig. 24-1). They must be distinguished clinically from malignant melanomas. Only 0.1% of all nevi occur on the genitals while 2.8% of malignant melanomas occur here. It is considered that 65 to 80% of malignant melanomas arise from preexisting nevi.[1–3]

Neurofibromas

BOX 24-3 Summary

- Neurofibromas of the penis are rare, but may be underreported.
- Neurofibromas are most likely due to abnormalities of the *NF1* gene.

Neurofibromas of the penis are said to be rare but are likely underreported (Fig. 24-2); they are likely related to abnormalities of the *NF1* gene. Treatment is related to specifics of organ distortion. Penile schwannoma is thought to be related to abnormalities of *NF2* gene, and may cause elephantiasis of penis, which is even more rare.[4–6]

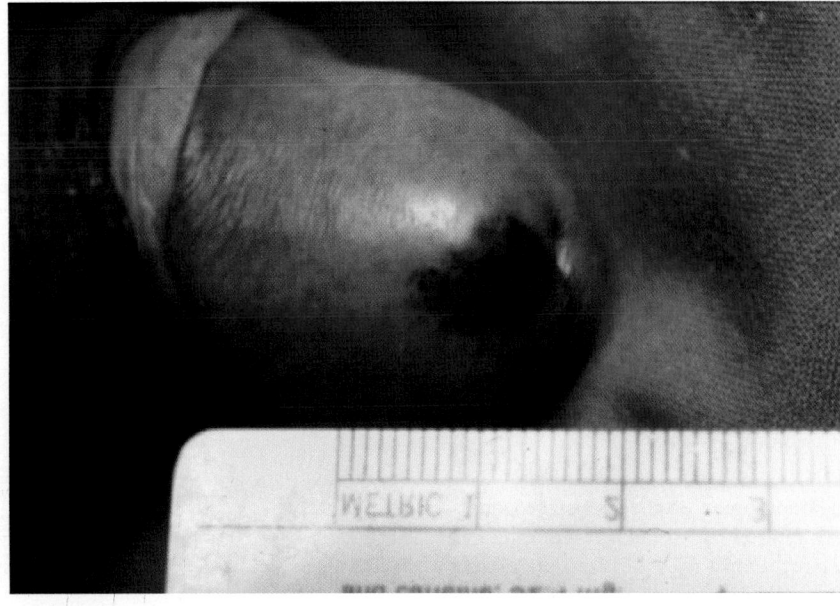

▲ **FIGURE 24-1** Pigmented penile lesion—benign (biopsy proven).

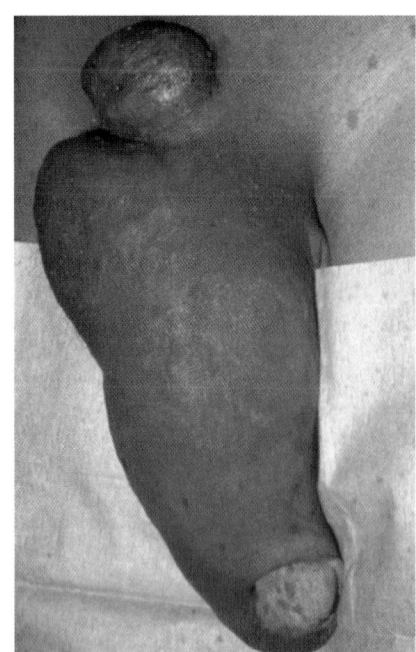

▲ **FIGURE 24-2** Neurofibroma of penis. Three pounds of tumor were removed from penis and adjacent area.

Angiokeratoma of Fordyce, Granular Cell Tumor, and Glomus Tumor

BOX 24-4   Summary

- Angiokeratoma of Fordyce can be found on the penis.
- Granular cell tumor is a soft tissue tumor, rarely found on the penis.
- Glomus tumor is a specialized arteriovenous structure that may be found on the penis.

Angiokeratoma of Fordyce has been reported on the penis.[7] Granular cell tumor is a soft tissue tumor, probably of neural sheath origin, rarely reported on the penis. It may be treated by local excision or Mohs' micrographic surgery.[8–10] Glomus tumor of penis, a specialized arteriovenous structure, has been reported nine times, and is treated by excision.[11]

Hemangiomas and Leiomyomas

BOX 24-5   Summary

- Hemangiomas of the penis are treated with vascular lasers.
- Leiomyoma of the penis is rare and arises from smooth muscle.

Hemangiomas of the penis are generally treated by vascular lasers whereas sclerotherapy may be used at institutions where laser equipment is not available.[12] Leiomyoma of penis, rarely re-

ported, arises from smooth muscle, may grow rapidly, and should be treated by excision.[13]

Verruciform Xanthoma

BOX 24-6   Summary

- Verruciform xanthoma is a rare lesion that may occur in the anogenital region.
- The histologic pathognomonic feature is large foam cells limited to the dermal papillae.

Verruciform xanthoma, another rare lesion, may resemble a wide variety of benign and malignant lesions. The majority of these lesions occurs on oral mucosa but may occur in the anogenital region. Its significance lies in its simulation of verrucous or invasive squamous cell carcinoma (SCC). The histologic pathognomonic feature is large foam cells limited to the dermal papillae. It may be treated by shave biopsy for diagnosis or by excisional biopsy.[14]

Cutaneous Horns

BOX 24-7   Summary

- Cutaneous horns on the penis are mostly benign but can be associated with malignancy.

Cutaneous horns can be seen on the penis. They are typically benign but as many as one-third are associated with underlying malignancy. They should be

managed by surgical excision with histologic examination of the base.[15,16]

Balanitis Xerotica Obliterans

BOX 24-8   Summary

- BXO is a chronic inflammatory lesion of unknown etiology.
- BXO can cause the penile skin to manifest dysplastic changes that may be difficult to differentiate from cancer clinically and/or pathologically.

Balanitis xerotica obliterans (lichen sclerosus, BXO) is a chronic inflammatory lesion of unknown etiology (Fig. 24-3). First described by Stühmer in 1928, its relationship to SCC was soon noted.[17,18] Its incidence is unknown but probably more common than usually thought. Its premalignant potential has been debated through the years but recent papers have noted a 2.6 to 5.8% incidence of penile cancer in patients with BXO.[19,20] Conversely, a recent report shows 28% of patients with SCC had BXO.[21] BXO may be treated by steroids, laser vaporization, or surgery.[22]

In addition to frank carcinoma, the penile skin may manifest dysplastic changes that may be difficult to differentiate from cancer clinically and/or pathologically. The spectrum of these lesions may begin with pseudoepitheliomatous hyperplasia and continue through condylomata to borderline lesions such as Buschke–Löwenstein tumor (giant condyloma) and on to actual SCC.

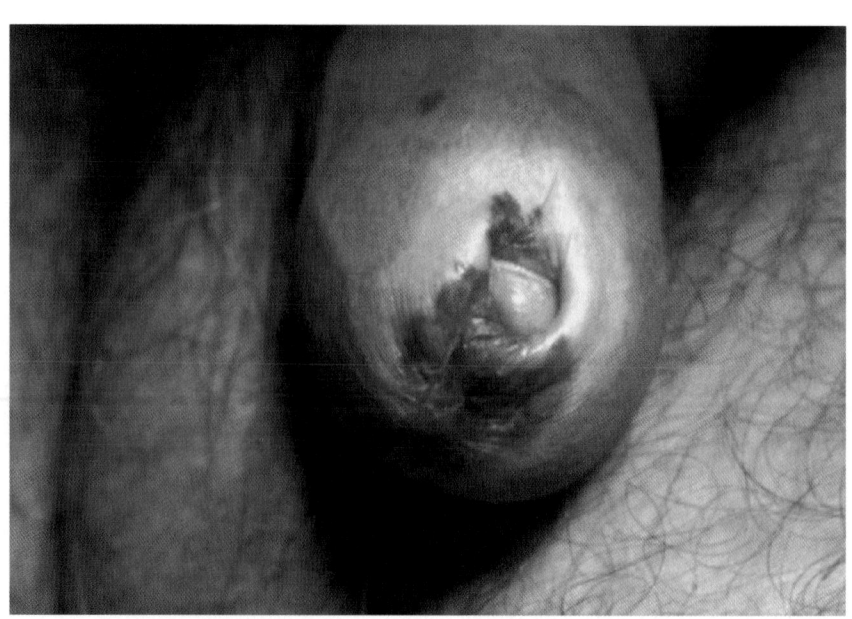

▲ **FIGURE 24-3** BXO (biopsy proven).

Pseudoepitheliomatous Hyperplasia

BOX 24-9   Summary

- Pseudoepitheliomatous hyperplasia is a lesion of proliferating epithelium that may occur at the edge of a chronic ulcer.
- The epithelium appears thickened, lighter in color, and moist to touch or appearance.

Pseudoepitheliomatous hyperplasia is a lesion of proliferating epithelium usually related to an inflammatory process and may occur at the edge of a chronic ulcer. The gross appearance is that of a thickened epithelium, frequently lighter in color than surrounding epithelium and moist to touch or appearance. Histologically, the epidermis is thickened, acanthotic, and with irregular rete ridges. The cells are highly differentiated with little or no pleomorphism, and maintain their continuity with the epidermis. The underlying dermis may contain a chronic inflammatory infiltrate and/or fibrosis.

Condylomata

BOX 24-10   Summary

- Condylomata frequently occur on the moist mucocutaneous regions of male and female genitalia.
- Histologically, condylomata exhibit acanthosis and hyperplasia of the prickle cell layer.

Condylomata (synonyms: squamous papillomas, venereal warts) are closely related to verruca vulgaris and occur most frequently on the moist mucocutaneous regions of male and female genitalia. In males, they have been found most often in the preputial sac, the coronal sulcus surrounding the glans, and rarely on the penile shaft. More recently, patients seen with HIV infection may manifest these with a more extensive distribution and number. They are aggravated by the presence of a prepuce, warmth, moisture, and irritating discharges (Fig. 24-4).[23] Treatment options for these include podophyllotoxin, trichloroacetic acid, cryotherapy, electrocoagulation, CO_2 laser, and imiquimod.[24]

Histologically, condylomata exhibit acanthosis and hyperplasia of the prickle cell layer. The rete ridges are elongated and rounded; the bases of the acanthotic papillae extend approximately to the same depth; there is no hyperplasia of the basal cell layer; the overall picture is of an orderly proliferation of the epithelium with maintenance of the stratifica-

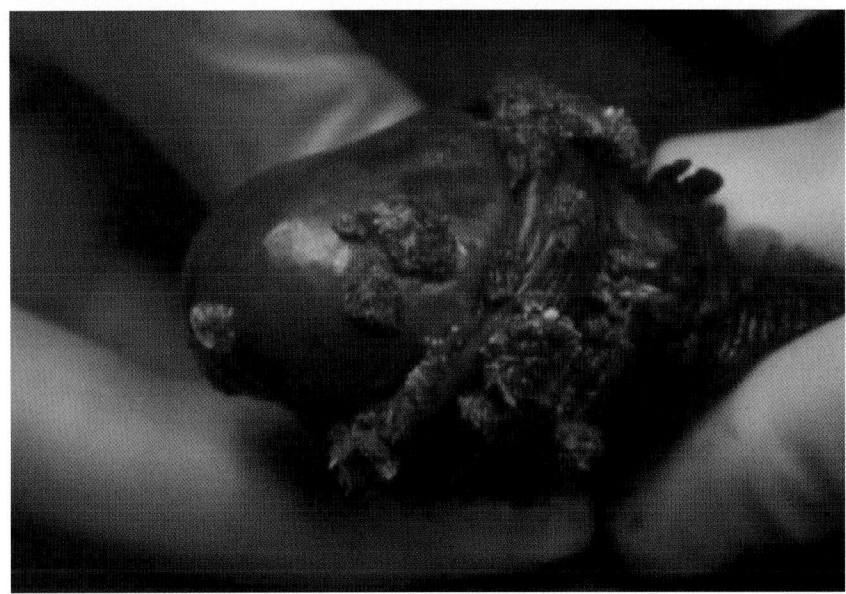

▲ **FIGURE 24-4** Condylomata of penis (patient was HIV positive).

tion of skin/mucosa. The underlying dermis is usually edematous and may have a chronic inflammatory infiltrate. The lesion is distinguished from giant condyloma by its remaining superficial without extension into underlying tissue.

Giant Condyloma

BOX 24-11   Summary

- Giant condyloma typically arises in the preputial cavity of uncircumcised middle-aged men, and forms an extensive cauliflower-like warty mass.
- Histologically, giant condyloma has a similar appearance to typical condyloma. There is acanthosis, thickened stratum corneum, and hyperplasia of the prickle cell layer.

Giant condyloma (synonyms: giant condyloma acuminatum, condylomatoid carcinoma, carcinoma-like condyloma, Buschke–Löwenstein tumor) has been separated from typical condyloma because of a progressive recurrent invasive growth. The lesion typically arises in the preputial cavity of uncircumcised middle-aged men. It forms extensive cauliflower-like warty masses (Fig. 24-5). Secondary infection and ulceration may occur. A characteristic feature is the downward growth of the lesion into underlying tissues, in addition to the upward growth seen in simpler condylomata. This growth appears to be an expansion rather than a true invasion. The tissues underlying the giant condyloma are compressed and may be destroyed by pressure necrosis. The

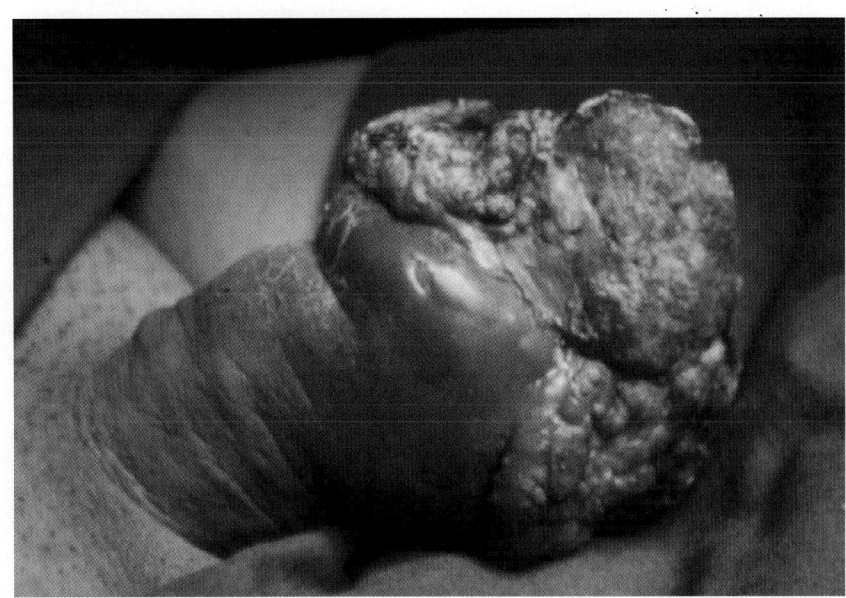

▲ **FIGURE 24-5** Buschke–Löwenstein tumor of penis.

lesion may then perforate the glans or prepuce and extend onto or beneath the shaft skin. Multiple fistulae may then form. The prepuce and glans can be extensively involved and may be destroyed. Giant condyloma does not respond to podophyllotoxin or radiation. Surgical excision or amputation may be necessary; recurrence is common; the lesion does not metastasize.[23]

Giant condyloma has a similar histologic appearance to typical condyloma. There is acanthosis, thickened stratum corneum, and hyperplasia of the prickle cell layer. In contrast to typical condyloma, however, the papillae extend deeper into underlying tissue; mitoses are present but not numerous; cells maintain their normal stratification and polarity. When fistulae are present, secondary inflammatory reaction is evident.[23]

Dysplastic Lesions

Continuing the spectrum toward actual carcinoma takes us now to the several dysplastic lesions: intraepithelial neoplasia, Bowen's disease, erythroplasia of Queyrat, and EMPD.

INTRAEPITHELIAL NEOPLASIA

> **BOX 24-12** Summary
>
> - Intraepithelial neoplasia is thought to develop from human papillomaviruses.
> - Most patients with intraepithelial neoplasia are asymptomatic but may have pruritus, pain, tenderness, bleeding, crusting, scaling, and difficulty in prepuce retraction.

Intraepithelial neoplasia (IN) is felt to develop from 1 or more of 30 sexually transmitted human papillomaviruses (HPVs).[25,26] These are of variable oncogenic potential and may lead to one of three levels of precursor IN. In grade I, the epithelial change in transformed basaloid cells involves the lower third of epithelium; in grade II, the lower two thirds; and in grade III, the full epithelial thickness. At this point, it can be called Bowen's atypia or *in situ* SCC. The basaloid cell nuclei are hyperchromatic, pleomorphic, and accompanied by a loss of cellular polarity. Most patients with IN are asymptomatic but may have pruritus, pain, tenderness, bleeding, crusting, scaling, and difficulty in prepuce retraction. Bowenoid papulosis (BP) is IN grade III. It cannot be distinguished histopathologically from Bowen's disease (BD).

BOWEN'S DISEASE, ERYTHROPLASIA OF QUEYRAT, EXTRA-MAMMARY PAGET'S DISEASE

> **BOX 24-13** Summary
>
> - Bowenoid papulosis (BP) and Bowen's disease (BD) are very similar in appearance.
> - The typical clinical appearance of BD is a well-demarcated reddish papule or plaque.
> - When BD is found on the penis, it is known as Erythroplasia of Queyrat.
> - Many people consider extra-mammary Paget's disease to be premalignant.

Clinically, BP and BD overlap in appearance. The lesions manifest increased pigmentation and vary from reddish-brown to red or grayish white or, even, brownish-black. They may be 2 to 10 mm maculopapular or coalesce into larger plaques, then being indistinguishable from BD. Both may simulate lichen sclerosus, psoriasis, or eczema. BP is generally clinically benign but may progress to BD. Transformation of BD to SCC has been reported in 5 to 33% of uncircumcised men. The typical clinical appearance of BD is a well-demarcated reddish papule or plaque (Fig. 24-6). When this is on the glans penis, it is traditionally called erythroplasia of Queyrat (EQ). Lesions may occasionally ulcerate or develop hyperkeratosis (called "cutaneous horn," see above). BD/EQ tend to occur in older patients than does BP; the average age for BP is 28 years and for BD/EQ 51 years.[15,27]

Treatment of these dysplastic lesions may be topical 5-fluorouracil (5-FU), circumcision, electrosurgery, or Mohs' micrographic surgery.[10] In older or immunosuppressed patients, these lesions should be dealt with as the premalignant lesions that they are and managed surgically if not quickly responsive to topical agents. Patients then continue to be at risk for new or recurrent lesions and should be followed closely.

Many consider EMPD to be premalignant. This will be discussed below.

CARCINOMA

> **BOX 24-14** Summary
>
> - Most common type is squamous cell carcinoma
> - Occurs almost exclusively in uncircumcised men
> - Delayed presentation
> - Metastasizes to inguinal lymph nodes
> - Treatment is related to stage of disease
> - Melanomas and sarcomas are very rare
> - Metastatic lesions are most commonly of bladder/prostatic origin

Carcinoma of the penis accounts for 1% of male malignancies in the United States. The tumor typically is found in the seventh decade of life but may occur at either extreme. The disease seems to be most common in geographic areas where genital cleanliness is least, and is least common in those groups that practice circumcision.

The definite etiology is indeterminate but HPV and retained preputial secretions are felt to be significant. The specific role of venereal disease is unclear

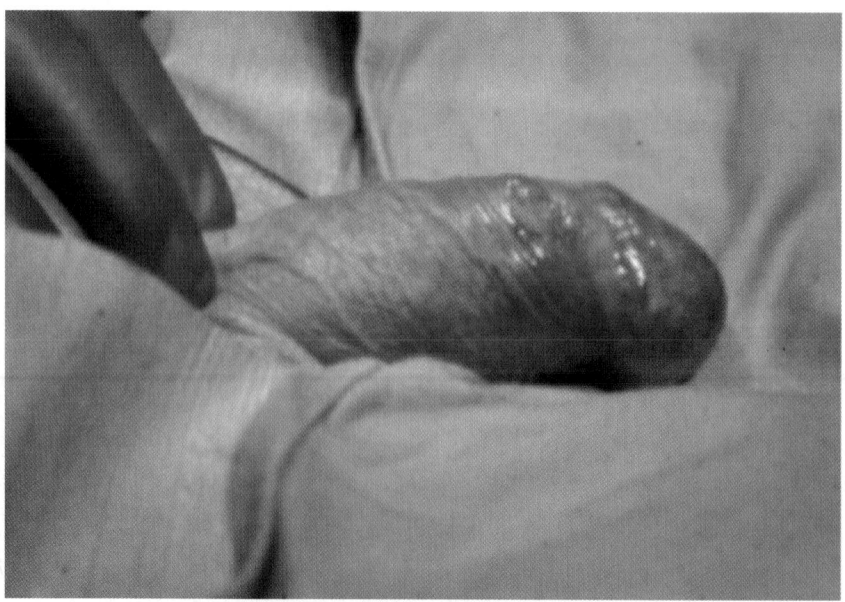

▲ **FIGURE 24-6** Erythroplasia of Queyrat (biopsy proven).

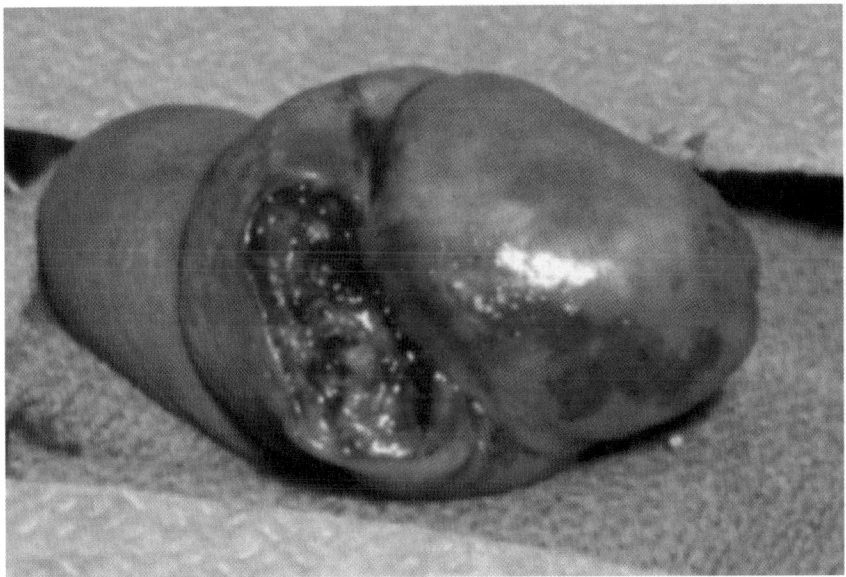

▲ **FIGURE 24-7** Ulcerating carcinoma of penis: 47-year-old Latin male.

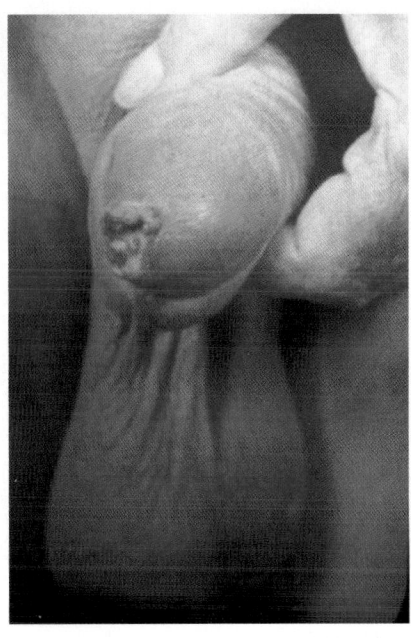

▲ **FIGURE 24-8** Nodular carcinoma of penis: 68-year-old Caucasian male gave a history of catching tip in zipper.

but may be related to increased HPV inoculation. The precancerous conditions of penile dysplasia, Bowen's disease, and erythroplasia of Queyrat have been noted (see above).[27]

Carcinoma of the penis typically develops as an ulcer, nodule, or verruca on the glans or prepuce. As the tumor progresses, it may become large, fungating, and ulcerated (Figs. 24-7 to 24-12). It may involve or destroy an extensive area of the penis before being diagnosed (Figs. 24-13 and 24-14). Penile SCC infrequently involves the skin of the shaft. Tumors appearing to involve only the

shaft must be distinguished from Kaposi sarcoma (KS), other sarcomas (generally perforate from deeper tissues), and urethral cancers perforating the skin of the shaft. Ulcerating lesions, which in recent years have been more commonly seen because of HIV or other immunosuppression, must be distinguished from bacterial infective ulceration.[27]

Typically, penile cancers are associated with a foul, purulent, or bloodstained discharge. Pain, voiding difficulty, and lymphadenopathy may also be present. Patients whose prepuce becomes unaccountably and recurrently nonretractile should be examined with a high level of suspicion for cancer con-

tained in the preputial cavity. Related to emotional issues noted above, these lesions may be discovered very late in their development. In addition, patients who have an SCC of penis may be much less likely to accept treatment than would a patient with SCC elsewhere on the body.[27]

These tumors tend to spread by the lymphatic rather than by the hematogenous route. Patients presenting with primary lesions often have inguinal lymphadenopathy (Figs. 24-15 and 24-16).

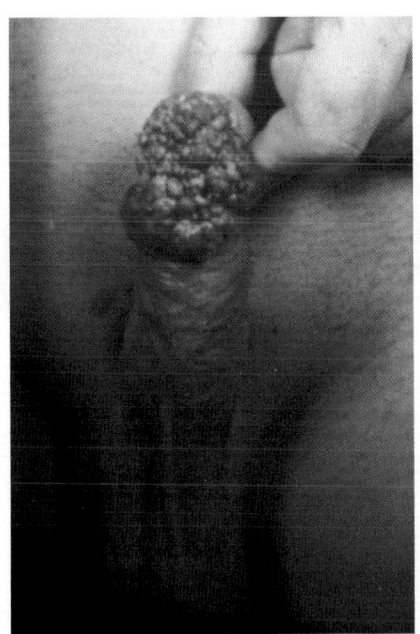

▲ **FIGURE 24-9** Verrucous carcinoma of penis: 38-year-old Latin male with 2-year history of condylomata.

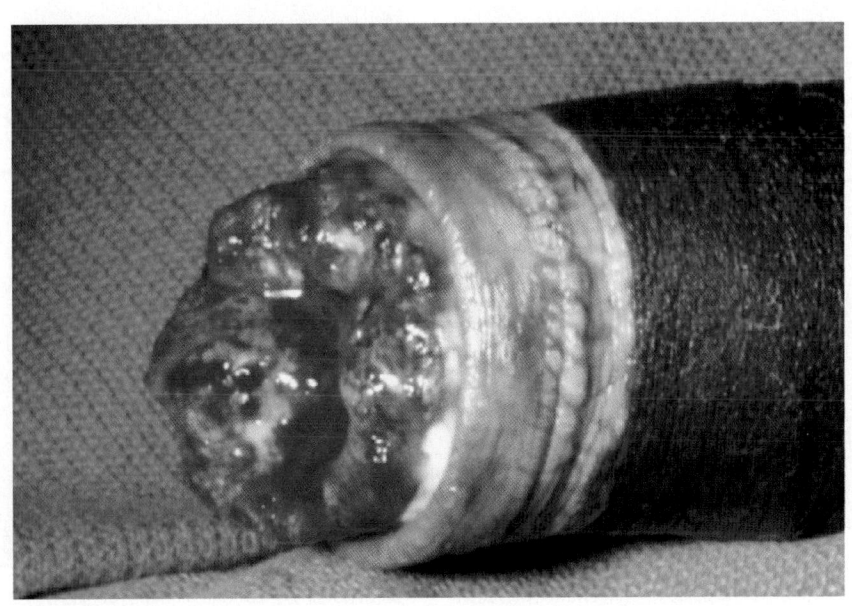

▲ **FIGURE 24-10** Carcinoma of penis: 34-year-old African American male.

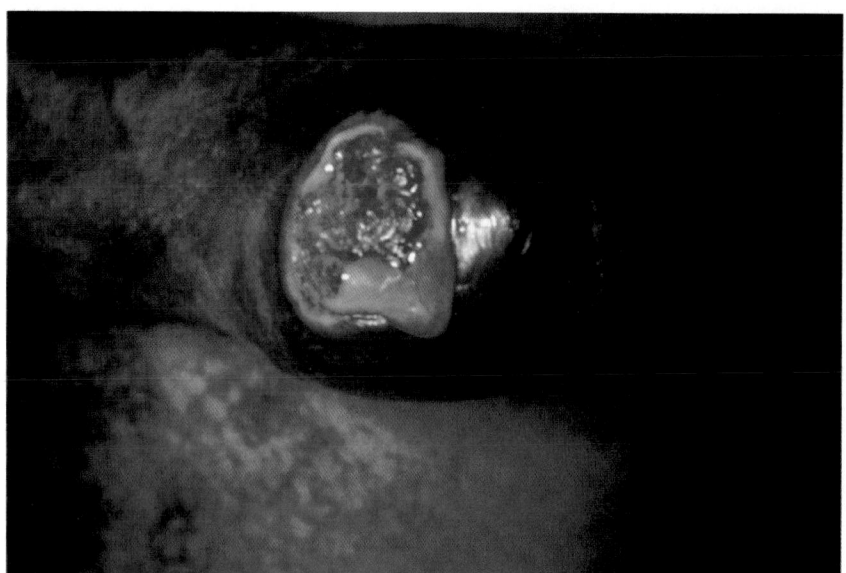

▲ **FIGURE 24-11** Carcinoma of inner prepuce eroding to outer prepuce: 40-year-old African American male.

mis and deeper tissues in an irregular pattern.[23]

The treatment of SCC of the penis depends on the stage and extent of the malignancy. Intraepithelial penile carcinoma can be treated by excision, Mohs' micrographic surgery, cryotherapy, CO_2-laser therapy, and topical 5-FU.[28] Recently, treatment with an immune response modifier, imiquimod, has been successful.[28–31] Imiquimod has an antiviral and antitumor activity *in vivo*, and is also approved for the treatment of anogenital warts.[30,32] More extensive and/or deeper carcinomas involving only the prepuce may be treated by circumcision alone.

Those tumors of limited size involving the glans or coronal sulcus may be treated by Mohs' micrographic surgery (see Chapter 40) or by limited local surgical excision (Fig. 24-17). These approaches can be useful in preserving sexual stimulation. Unfortunately, most penile tumors, when first seen by a physician, already involve more of the penile structure than would allow such limited approaches to treatment.

The majority of penile cancers seen by a urologic surgeon involve enough of the penis to require partial penectomy. This approach removes not only the cancer but also most erogenous sensibility. A lesser percentage of cancers require total penectomy. This procedure removes all of the penile shaft and its internal structures (corpora, pendulous urethra), and requires the proximal urethra to be redirected to the perineum to form a perineal

This may be reactive or metastatic. The larger, nontender lymph nodes are generally metastatic; the smaller tender lymph nodes, generally reactive. In the majority of cases, distinguishing one from the other is difficult and may be resolved only after treatment of the primary tumor, followed by a 6- to 8-week course of antibiotics and, if then necessary, lymph node biopsy.[27]

Carcinomas of the penis are almost always squamous cell histologically. They may be well- to poorly differentiated, and they resemble SCC occurring elsewhere on the skin. Papillary or verrucous tumors typically show marked acanthosis, hyperkeratosis, parakeratosis, and papillomatosis. In well-differentiated tumors, the cells may be orderly as those of giant condyloma but multiple sections will reveal areas of cellular disorganization, loss of maturation and polarity, and increased numbers of mitoses. Infiltration of dermis is present but may be difficult to demonstrate. The solid or nodular tumors tend to be of higher grade than are verrucous types. They invade der-

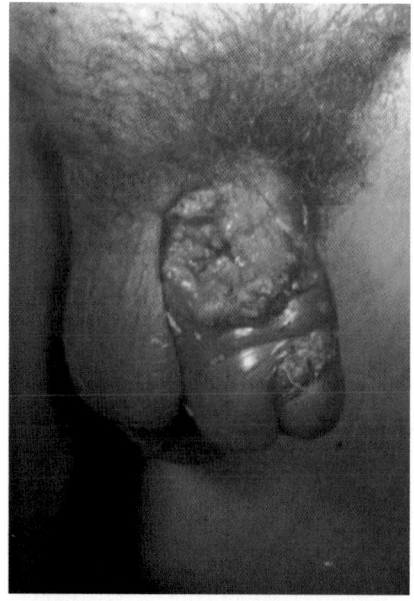

▲ **FIGURE 24-12** Carcinoma of penis: 61-year-old Caucasian male, started on glans and extended down shaft to reappear near the base of shaft.

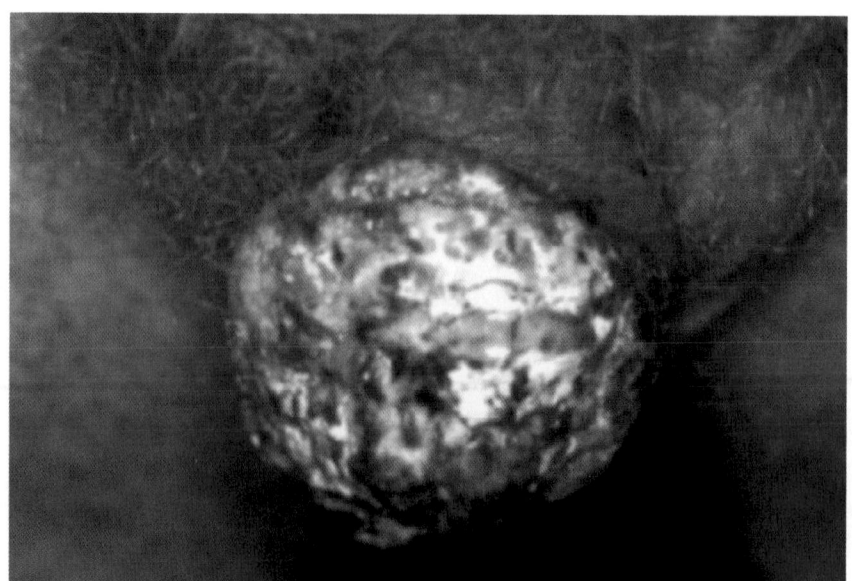

▲ **FIGURE 24-13** Carcinoma of penis: 47-year-old Caucasian male, all of penile shaft is involved or destroyed.

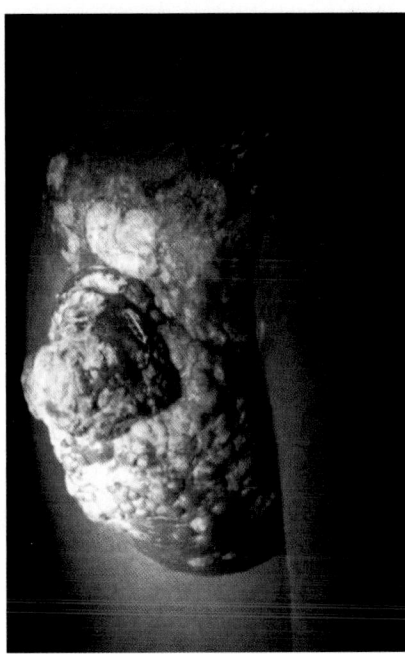

▲ **FIGURE 24-14** Carcinoma of penis: 53-year-old African American male. At presentation, the tumor had involved penis, scrotum, perineum, pubic escutcheon, and superficial skin of groins (plus lymph nodes).

nodes. Small high-grade tumors may produce metastatic lymph nodes, as well as more extensive tumors. Clinical evaluation of the inguinal lymph nodes is thus critical to the treatment plan for a penile malignancy. The reader is directed to urologic surgical texts for further details of treatments of the primary tumor and lymph node metastasis.[33]

Other cancers that may occur on the penis are basal cell carcinoma, sarcomas, metastatic lesions, perforating urethral lesions, and Paget's disease (see below). Basal cell carcinomas of penis are rare, usually limited to the penile shaft and can be successfully treated by local excision. Less than 20 cases have been reported.[34,35] Basal cell carcinoma may be preceded by the premalignant fibroepithelioma of Pinkus.[36]

Most of the various potential sarcomas have been reported to occur on or in the penis. They are extremely rare; a recent review from the Armed Forces Institute of Pathology noted just over 100 primary mesenchymal tumors; an equal number were benign or malignant.[27] Malignant lesions tended to be more proximal, and benign more distal.[37]

Epithelioid sarcoma has been reported to mimic Peyronie's disease, a benign pathological fibrosis of the penile tunica albuginea. Any case of Peyronie's disease enlarging significantly should, therefore, be considered for biopsy.[38–42] Other sarcomas reported to occur on penis are rhabdomyosarcoma,[43] Ewing's sarcoma,[44] leiomyosarcoma,[45] mesothelioma,[46] synovial sarcoma,[47] and lymphoma.[27]

urethrostomy. This procedure removes all sexual sensibility. Reconstructive procedures are available to deal with the effects of both partial and total penectomy but are not satisfactory due to complex urethral reconstruction, as well as the lack of reconstituted erogenous sensibility. A further consideration in the treatment of penile carcinoma is the presence or absence of metastatic inguinal lymph

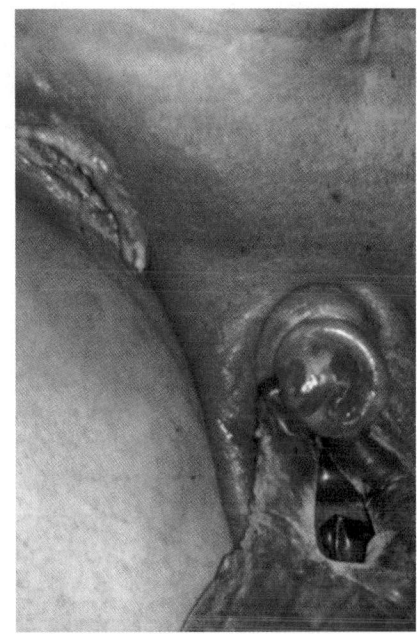

▲ **FIGURE 24-16** Carcinoma of penis on glans: 55-year-old Latin male. Tumor is too small to distort apparent shape of prepuce but presented with ulcerated inguinal lymph node metastasis.

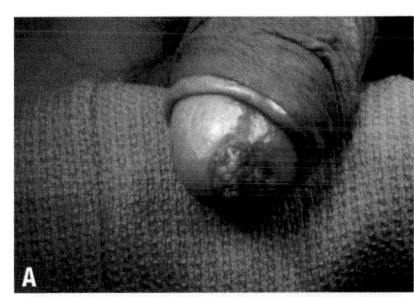

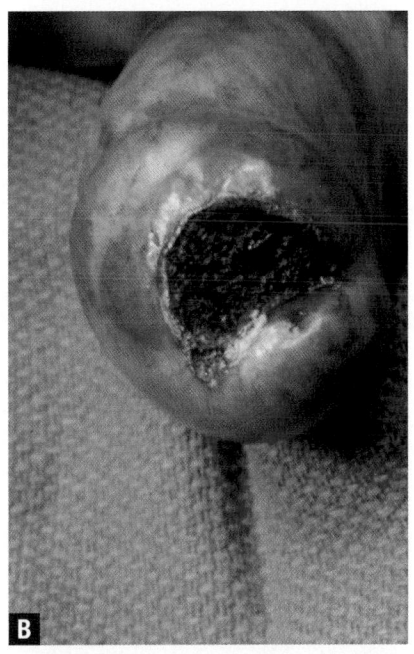

▲ **FIGURE 24-17** Carcinoma of penis involving glans only, treated successfully by limited local surgical excision. **A.** Before surgery. **B.** After surface is heavily cauterized.

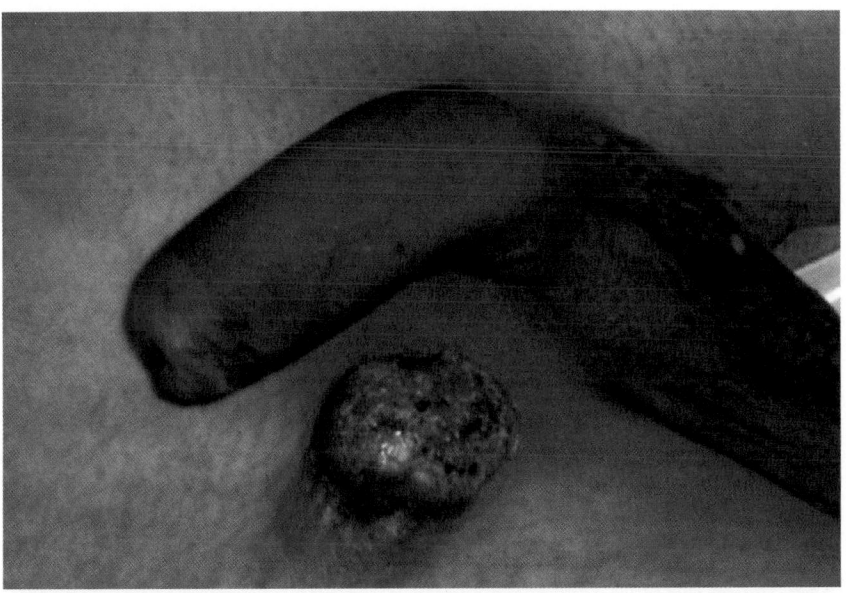

▲ **FIGURE 24-15** Carcinoma of penis with ulcerating inguinal lymph node metastasis: 52-year-old Caucasian male. The tumor starting in coronal sulcus was still small, but pathologically of high grade.

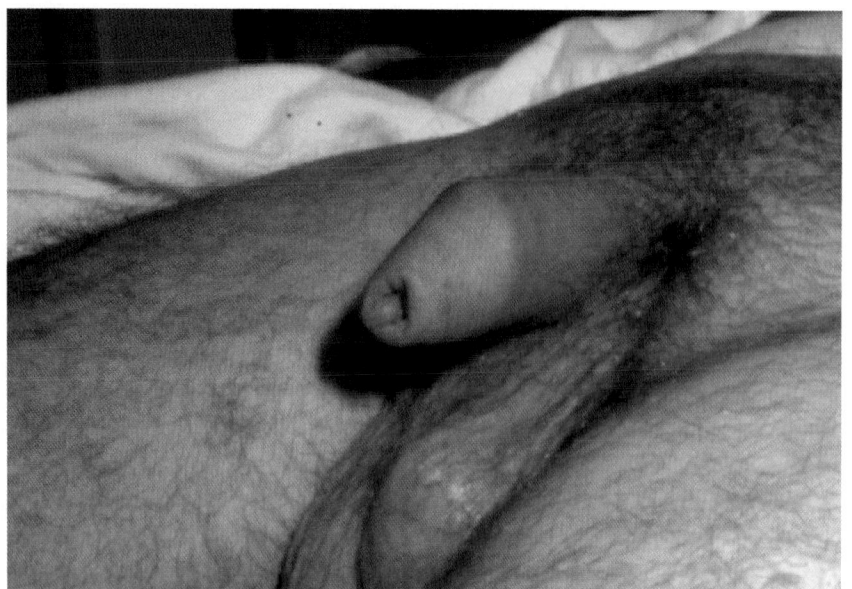

▲ **FIGURE 24-18** Malignant priapism—metastatic bladder carcinoma: 67-year-old Latin male.

retrograde venous flow, retrograde lymphatic flow, arterial embolization, and instrumental spread.[54] The primary tumor is bladder in 30 to 35% of cases, prostate in 30%, rectosigmoid in 13%, kidney in 10%, and testes in 5%. In the remaining cases, the primary tumor is gastrointestinal or respiratory in origin; few primary sites are elsewhere.[55] Only two cases of metastatic melanoma have been reported.[56] Treatment is related to that of the primary lesion; metastasis to penis occurs late in the patient's course and prognosis is poor, less than a year.[57]

Primary urethral cancers can involve the skin of the penis. This may occur either by their breaking through the skin, typically along the shaft, or by infiltrating the glanular or shaft skin simulating an infiltrating lesion of skin when, in fact, the source is deeper (Fig. 24-19).

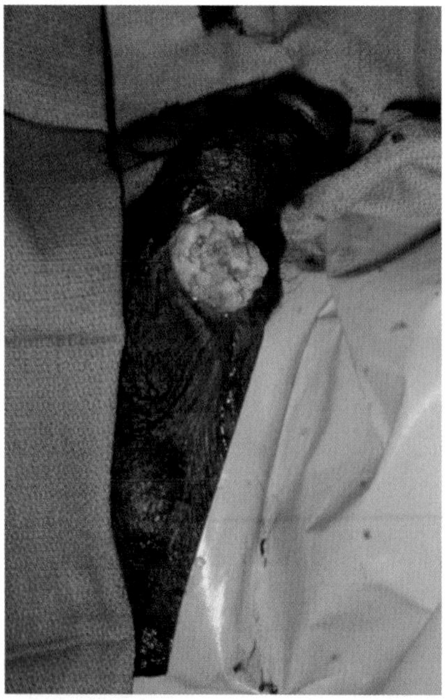

Malignant melanocytic lesions of the penis are rare; just over 100 cases are reported. Most penile melanomas occur on the glans; the remainder on prepuce and shaft. Management is the same as those of other regions. Other melanocytic lesions include penile melanosis, genital lentiginosis, lentiginous hyperplasia, and melanocytic nevi.[27,48–50]

KS of penis was rare, but with the advent of acquired immunodeficiency syndrome (AIDS), it has become the most common mesenchymal tumor of the penis.[27,51] KS of penis is rare, nevertheless, and is usually a sign of generalized disease. It usually presents as a patch, plaque, or nodule often with a purplish or erythematous surface.[27] Treatment can be by a local or wide excision, radiation, or chemotherapy. KS involving the glans penis may obstruct the urethral meatus and require dilation or meatotomy.[52]

Metastatic cancer to penis is rare. Since first described in 1870, approximately 300 cases were reported by 2004.[53] The presenting symptoms of the penile lesion are typically malignant priapism or penile pain (Fig. 24-18). The corpora cavernosa are the usual metastatic site but penile skin, corpus spongiosum, or urethra may be involved.[27] The mechanisms by which the penis may become involved with primary tumors of other sites include direct extension,

TUMORS OF THE SCROTUM

BOX 24-15 Summary

- May arise from any tissue of the scrotum
- Most common malignancy is squamous cell carcinoma
- Metastasizes to inguinal lymph nodes
- Treatment is related to stage of disease

The scrotum is composed of pigmented skin and dermis that contains hair follicles, sebaceous glands, and sweat glands. The scrotum may, therefore, be the primary site of any neoplasm originating from the epidermis or these underlying structures. Tumors of the scrotum are quite rare; nevi and inclusion cysts are occasional (Figs. 24-20 and 24-21). Mela-

▲ **FIGURE 24-19** SCC of urethra eroding to skin of penile shaft: 61-year-old African American male.

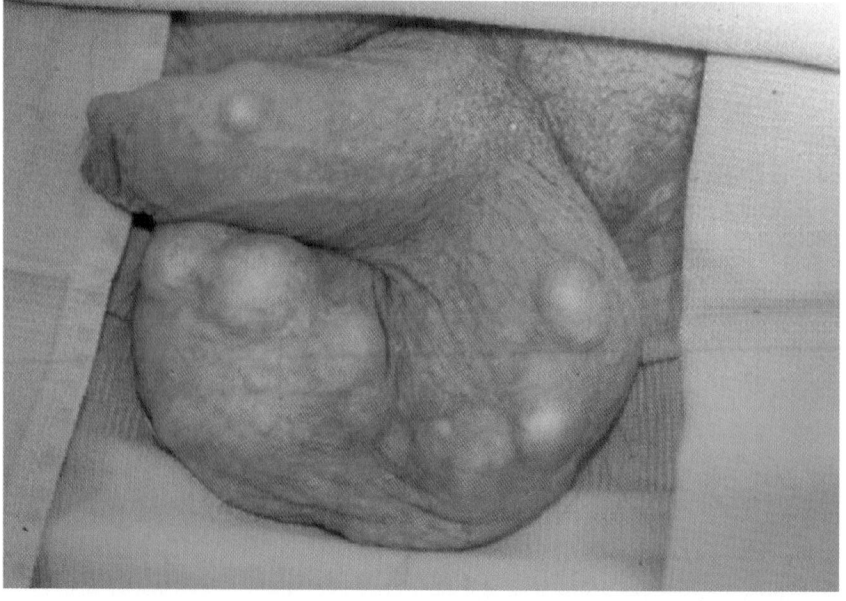

▲ **FIGURE 24-20** Multiple sebaceous cysts of scrotum/penis: 46-year-old Latin male.

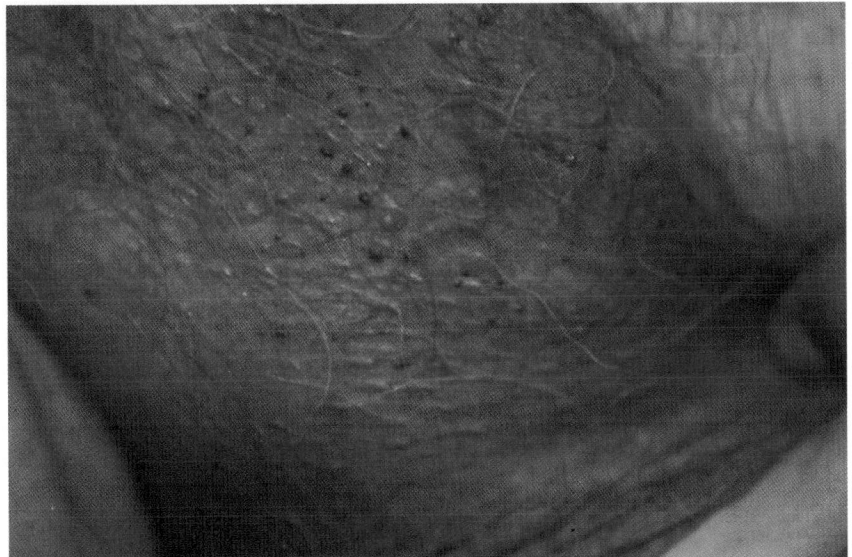

▲ **FIGURE 24-21** Angiokeratomas of Fordyce: 68-year-old Caucasian male.

noma has been reported six times.[58] Granular cell tumor and verruciform xanthoma have also been reported.[14,59]

Carcinoma of the scrotum was the first cancer associated with a specific carcinogen.[60] With the elimination of such industrial hazards, scrotal cancer has become rare and is still declining over the last three decades. A clinical impression of recent increasing occurrence (Block, personal observation) may be related to AIDS. Mesenchymal tumors are very rare. Lipoma, hemangioma, and leiomyoma (the last arising from dartos muscle or vascular structures) are seen occasionally.[23] Metastatic lesions from the GI tract have been reported.[15] In addition, carcinoma of Cowper's gland has been seen extending to scrotal skin.[2]

Scrotal carcinoma occurs in the fifth and sixth decades of life usually. The reported incidence is high in Caucasians and low in African Americans.[61] The average age-adjusted incidence rate of epithelial scrotal cancer is 1.32 per million males.[33] Scrotal carcinoma usually starts as a verrucous lesion or an area of hyperkeratosis. Early cases seen recently have been ulcerated (Block, personal observation). Pruritus is an early symptom but as the usual lesion enlarges and ulcerates, and becomes secondarily infected and pain manifests. As with penile cancer, inguinal lymphadenopathy may be inflammatory, metastatic, or both. Differentiation is similar to that of penile cancer (see above) (Fig. 24-22).

Scrotal carcinoma is almost always squamous cell type. Histologic appearance and manner of growth is similar to that of SCC in other areas of skin. Extensive local invasion may occur; per-

foration of the scrotal tunical layers is rare. Metastasis is primarily due to inguinal lymph nodes, and is frequently bilateral. Distant metastasis is rare.[23]

Carcinoma of scrotum has a 5-year mortality of 50 to 60%. Death usually has been a result of infection or hemorrhage from large, ulcerated lesions. Improving modern surgical therapy should produce a better outcome.

Scrotal basal cell carcinoma (BCC) has been reported less than 40 times by 2001.[34,62–64] As with SCC, BCC of the scrotum can be treated by a wide excision, fulguration, CO_2 laser, or Mohs' micrographic surgery. A recent report indicated that only 1 of 30 genital BCC cases recurred; no metastases occurred.[34]

TUMORS OF THE VULVA

BOX 24-16 Summary

- May arise from any tissue of the vulva
- Most common malignancy is squamous cell carcinoma
- Metastasizes to inguinal lymph nodes
- Treatment is related to stage of disease

Vulvar malignancies are relatively rare, accounting for 3 to 5% of gynecologic cancers. These occur usually in the older population; the mean age is in the late sixties. As the population ages, these cancers are expected to be more common.

As previously described for penile and scrotal skin, the usual range of cell types plus malignant and premalignant variations can be seen. The primary cell type accounting for 85% of these malignancies is SCC. The remaining 15% are the less common or rare tumors.[64]

There is a consistent association between cervical, vaginal, and vulvar malignancies. This has been ascribed to HPV, herpes, smoking, and some of those premalignant lesions also seen on penile skin. Twenty percent of women with vulvar carcinoma *in situ* eventually develop invasive disease.[64] Vulvar cancer may present with pruritus, bleeding, or a growth. A delay in diagnosis may occur because patients avoid or deny the recognition of symptoms or the physician may attempt trivial treatment before biopsy.[64]

Diagnosis is made by biopsy. The most efficient method is the use of a dermal punch biopsy with local anesthesia. Treatment of premalignant vulvar lesions

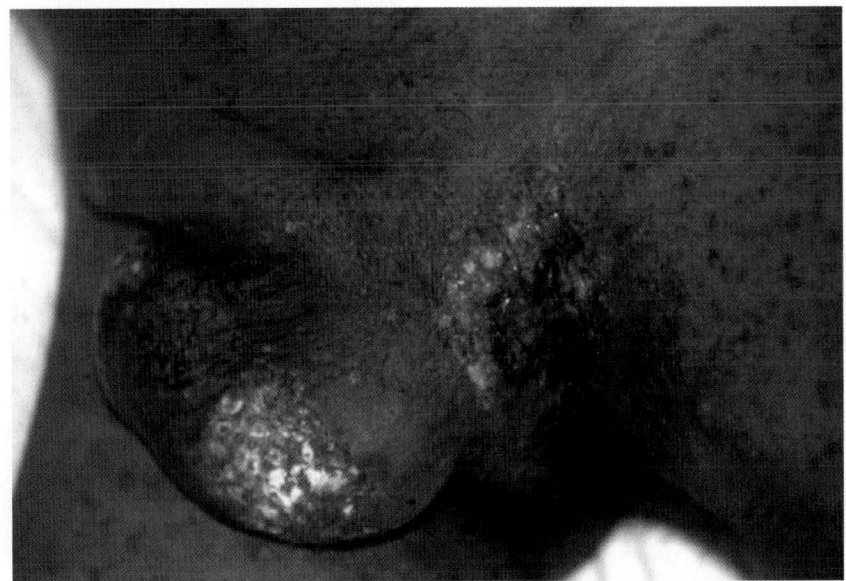

▲ **FIGURE 24-22** Carcinoma of scrotum: 41-year-old African American male with AIDS, multiple ulcerated, and nodular lesions are present.

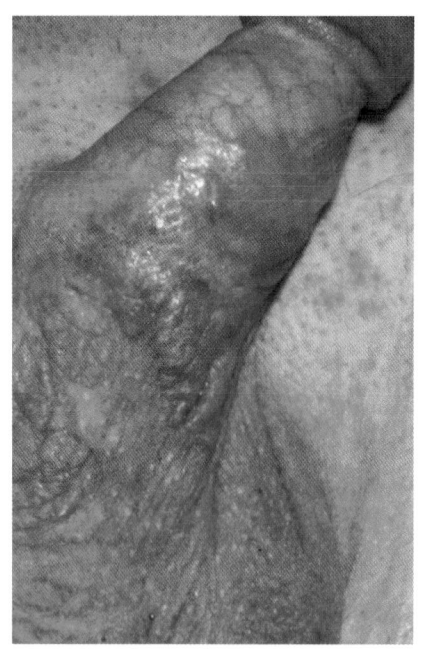

▲ **FIGURE 24-23** Extra-mammary Paget's disease of penis: 75-year-old Caucasian male with bladder cancer, lesion treated by wide excision.

(including carcinoma *in situ*, dysplasia, and vulvar intraepithelial neoplasia) can be carried out by local destruction or excisional biopsy. When margins are negative, the recurrence rate is 20%; when positive, the rate is 40%. In areas around the clitoris or anus, and in patients in whom sexual function is important, laser vaporization or Cavitron ultrasonic aspiration (CUSA) is preferred and produces less cicatrisation. The treatment of choice for invasive SCC of vulva is radical vulvectomy, with treatment of inguinal lymph nodes by lymph node dissection or local radiation.

Other lesions occurring on the vulvar skin including BCC, Bartholin's gland carcinoma, verrucous carcinoma, melanoma, sarcoma, and adenocarcinoma can be treated in a similar manner with a wide local excision, radical vulvectomy, and possible inguinal lymph node dissection.[64,65]

EXTRA-MAMMARY PAGET'S DISEASE OF GENITAL SKIN (SEE CHAPTER 25)

BOX 24-17   Summary

- More common in women
- Resembles dermatitis
- Association with malignancy in 20%

EMPD in men most frequently involves the penoscrotal skin.[66] In women, EMPD occurs on the vulva, typically in

postmenopausal Caucasians.[65] The lesions are more common in women.[67] In both sexes, the lesions present as crusty, erythematous, pruritic, pink/red eczematous patches (Fig. 24-23). In both sexes, EMPD may be misdiagnosed as eczema or other forms of dermatitis, and treated locally and unsuccessfully. Cutaneous Crohn's disease may also mimic EMPD.[68] Biopsy is diagnostic. Histologically, Paget cells have malignant appearing nuclei and nucleoli. They occur singly or in nests distributed through the epithelium. In both sexes, 10 to 20% cases have an underlying adnexal tumor of dermis and up to 22% have associated internal malignancies.[66]

Therapeutic modalities include local laser treatment, radiotherapy, chemotherapy, and topical cytotoxic agents such as 5-FU. A wider local excision with negative margins seems to be best. Local recurrence (occurs up to 20%) may be successfully treated by repeat wide excision.[66] When large amounts of penoscrotal skin must be excised, split-thickness skin grafts provide the best result (Fig. 24-24). Full-thickness grafts and pedicle grafts have been reported.[65] Those female patients having an underlying occult adenocarcinoma should have radical vulvectomy and inguinal lymphadenectomy.[69] Recurrences are common in both sexes, and the patients should be carefully followed for the long term.[65,66]

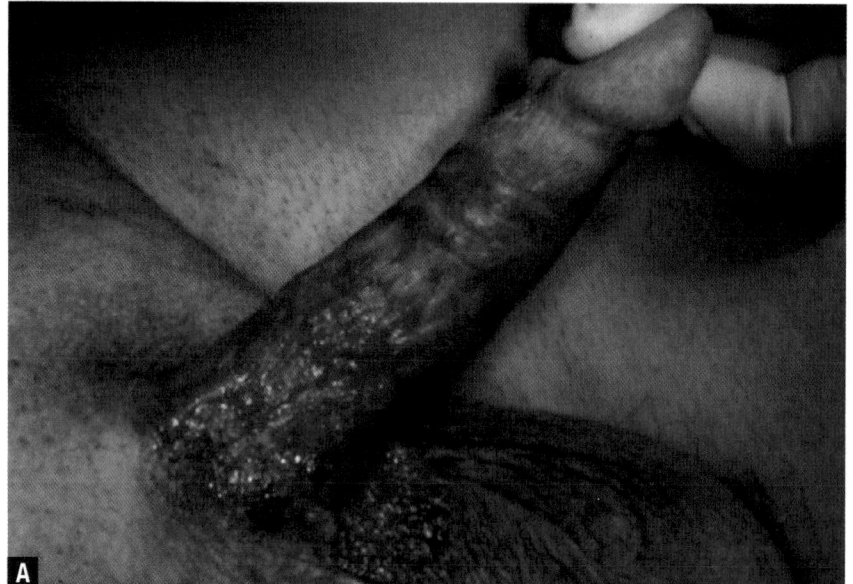

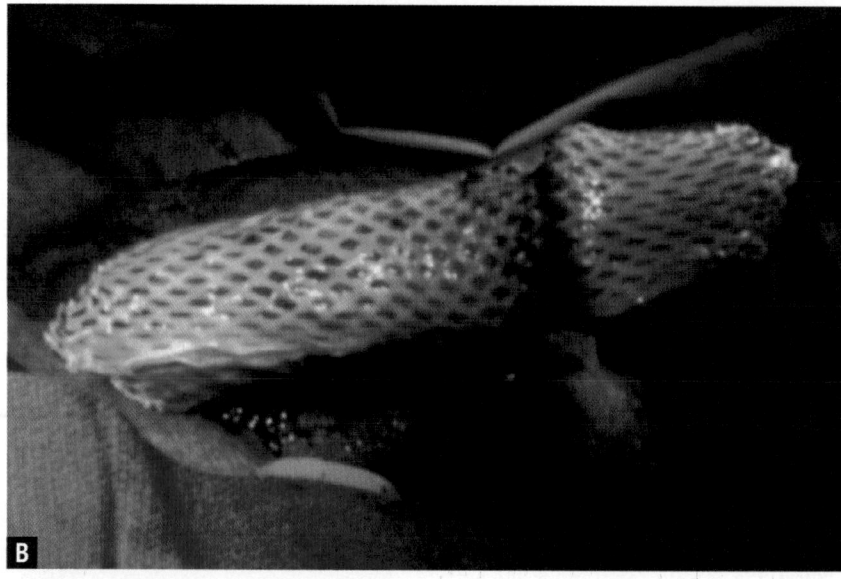

▲ **FIGURE 24-24** Extra-mammary Paget's disease of penis and adjacent scrotum: 67-year-old Latin male. The entire penile skin was resected and treated by split-thickness skin graft. The patient was subsequently diagnosed with carcinoma of prostate. **A.** Pretreatment. **B.** Skin graft in place.

FINAL THOUGHTS

In conclusion, any neoplasm occurring on the skin may be diagnosed in the genital area. The most common genital malignancy is squamous cell cancer, which often presents at an advanced stage. Such delayed diagnosis is mainly due to the patient's emotional barrier to seek professional care and to accept treatment. While genital cancer at early stages may be treated locally with excellent cosmetic results and preserved organ function, more advanced stages require radical surgery, and if indicated, adjuvant treatment.

REFERENCES

1. Mahto M, Woolley PD, Ashworth J. Pigmented penile macules. *Int J STD AIDS.* 2004;15:717.
2. Wilkinson TS, Paletta GX. Malignant melanoma: current concepts. *Am Surg.* 1969;35:301.
3. Pack GT, Lenson N, Gerber DM. Regional distribution of moles and melanomas. *AMA Arch Surg.* 1952;65:862.
4. Kousseff BG, Hoover DL. Penile neurofibromas. *Am J Med Genet.* 1999;87:1.
5. Fethiere W, Carter HW, Sturim HS. Elephantiasis neuromatosa of the penis. Light and electron microscopical studies. *Arch Pathol.* 1974;97:326.
6. Sato D, Kase T, Tajima M, et al. Penile schwannoma. *Int J Urol.* 2001;8:87.
7. Bechara FG, Huesmann M, Stücker M, et al. An exceptional localization of angiokeratoma of Fordyce on the glans penis. *Dermatology.* 2002;205:187.
8. Carver BS, Venable DD, Eastham JA. Large granular cell tumor of the penis in a 53-year-old man with coexisting prostate cancer. *Urology.* 2002;59:602.
9. Gardner ES, Goldberg LH. Granular cell tumor treated with Mohs micrographic surgery: report of a case and review of the literature. *Dermatol Surg.* 2001;27:772.
10. Mohs FE, Snow SN, Larson PO. Mohs micrographic surgery for penile tumors. *Urol Clin North Am.* 1992;19:291.
11. Saito T. Glomus tumor of the penis. *Int J Urol.* 2000;7:115.
12. Hemal AK, Aron M, Wadhwa SN. Intralesional sclerotherapy in the management of hemangiomas of the glans penis. *J Urol.* 1998;159:415.
13. Bartoletti R, Gacci M, Nesi G, et al. Leiomyoma of the corona glans penis. *Urology.* 2002;59:445.
14. Cuozzo DW, Vachher P, Sau P, et al. Verruciform xanthoma: a benign penile growth. *J Urol.* 1995;153:1625.
15. Schellhammer PF, Jordan GH, Robey EL, et al. Premalignant lesions and nonsquamous malignancy of the penis and carcinoma of the scrotum. *Urol Clin North Am.* 1992;19:131.
16. Solivan GA, Smith KJ, James WD. Cutaneous horn of the penis: its association with squamous cell carcinoma and HPV-16 infection. *J Am Acad Dermatol.* 1990;23:969.
17. Stühmer A. Balanitis xerotica obiterans und ihre Beziehungen zur "Kraurosis glandis et praeputii penis". *Arch Dermatol Syph.* 1928;156:613.
18. Grutz O. Beiträge zur Klinik der Balanitis xerotica obliterans. *Dermat Wochenschr.* 1937;105:1206.
19. Nasca MR, Innocenzi D, Micali G. Penile cancer among patients with genital lichen sclerosus. *J Am Acad Dermatol.* 1999;41:911.
20. Depasquale I, Park AJ, Bracka A. The treatment of balanitis xerotica obliterans. *BJU Int.* 2000;86:459.
21. Pietrzak P, Hadway P, Corbishley CM, et al. Is the association between balanitis xerotica obliterans and penile carcinoma underestimated? *BJU Int.* 2006;98:74.
22. Das S, Tunuguntla HS. Balanitis xerotica obliterans—a review. *World J Urol.* 2000;18:382.
23. Mostofi FK, Price EB Jr. Tumors and tumor-like lesions of the penis. In: *Tumors of the Male Genital System—Atlas of Tumor Pathology.* Fascicle 8. Washington, DC: Armed Forces Institute of Pathology; 1973:277.
24. Buechner SA. Common skin disorders of the penis. *BJU Int.* 2002;90:498.
25. de Villiers EM. Taxonomic classification of papillomaviruses. *Papillomavirus Rep.* 2001;12:57.
26. Dillner J, Meijer CJ, von Krogh G, et al. Epidemiology of human papillomavirus infection. *Scand J Urol Nephrol.* 2000;205(suppl):194.
27. Cubilla AL, Dillner J, Schellhammer PF, et al. Malignant epithelial tumors. In: Eble JN, Sauter G, Epstein JI, et al, eds. *Tumours of the Urinary System and Male Genital Organs.* Lyon, France: IARC Press; 2004:280.
28. Micali G, Nasca MR, Tedeschi A. Topical treatment of intraepithelial penile carcinoma with imiquimod. *Clin Exp Dermatol.* 2003;28(suppl):4.
29. Thai KE, Sinclair RD. Treatment of Bowen's disease of the penis with imiquimod. *J Am Acad Dermatol.* 2002;46:470.
30. Edwards L, Ferenczy A, Eron L, et al. Self-administered topical 5% imiquimod cream for external anogenital warts. HPV Study Group. Human Papilloma Virus. *Arch Dermatol.* 1998;134:25.
31. Hengge UR, Esser S, Schultewolter T, et al. Self-administered topical 5% imiquimod for the treatment of common warts and molluscum contagiosum. *Br J Dermatol.* 2000;143:1026.
32. Workowski KA, Berman SM. Centers for Disease Control and Prevention: sexually transmitted diseases treatment guidelines. *MMWR Recomm Rep.* 2006;55:1.
33. Grossman HB. Premalignant and early carcinomas of the penis and scrotum. *Urol Clin North Am.* 1992;19:221.
34. Gibson GE, Ahmed I. Perianal and genital basal cell carcinoma: a clinicopathologic review of 51 cases. *J Am Acad Dermatol.* 2001;45:68.
35. Kim ED, Kroft S, Dalton DP. Basal cell carcinoma of the penis: case report and review of the literature. *J Urol.* 1994;152:1557.
36. Heymann WR, Soifer I, Burk PG. Penile premalignant fibroephithelioma of Pinkus. *Cutis.* 1983;31:519.
37. Ashley DJ, Edwards EC. Sarcoma of the penis; leiomyosarcoma of the penis: report of a case with a review of the literature of sarcoma of the penis. *Br J Surg.* 1957;45:170.
38. Usta MF, Adams DM, Zhang JW, et al. Penile epithelioid sarcoma and the case for a histopathological diagnosis in Peyronie's disease. *BJU Int.* 2003;91:519.
39. Ormsby AH, Liou LS, Oriba HA, et al. Epithelioid sarcoma of the penis: report of an unusual case and review of the literature. *Ann Diagn Pathol.* 2000;4:88.
40. Rossi G, Ferrari G, Longo L, et al. Epithelioid sarcoma of the penis: a case report and review of the literature. *Pathol Int.* 2000;50:579.
41. Huang DJ, Stanisic TH, Hansen KK. Epithelioid sarcoma of the penis. *J Urol.* 1992;147:1370.
42. Moore SW, Wheeler JE, Hefter LG. Epithelioid sarcoma masquerading as Peyronie's disease. *Cancer.* 1975;35:1706.
43. Antoneli CB, Novaes PE, Alves AC, et al. Rhabdomyosarcoma of the penis in a 15-month-old boy. *J Urol.* 1998;160:2200.
44. Toh KL, Tan PH, Cheng WS. Primary extraskeletal Ewing's sarcoma of the external genitalia. *J Urol.* 1999;162:159.
45. Fetsch JF, Davis CJ, Miettinen M, et al. Leiomyosarcoma of the penis: a clinicopathologic study of 14 cases with review of the literature and discussion of the differential diagnosis. *Am J Surg Pathol.* 2004;28:115.
46. Polsky EG, Lele SM, Holley P, et al. Primary malignant mesothelioma of the penis: case report and review of the literature. *Urology.* 2003;62:551.
47. Al-Rikabi AC, Diab AR, Buckai A, et al. Primary synovial sarcoma of the penis—case report and literature review. *Scand J Urol Nephrol.* 1999;33:413.
48. El Shabrawi-Caelen L, Soyer HP, Schaeppi H, et al. Genital lentigines and melanocytic nevi with superimposed lichen sclerosus: a diagnostic challenge. *J Am Acad Dermatol.* 2004;50:690.
49. Bundrick WS, Culkin DJ, Mata JA, et al. Penile malignant melanoma in association with squamous cell carcinoma of the penis. *J Urol.* 1991;146:1364.
50. Demitsu T, Nagato H, Nishimaki K, et al. Melanoma in situ of the penis. *J Am Acad Dermatol.* 2000;42:386.
51. Kavak A, Akman RY, Alper M, et al. Penile Kaposi's sarcoma in a human immunodeficiency virus-seronegative patient. *Br J Dermatol.* 2001;144:207.
52. Swierzewski SJ III, Wan J, Boffini A, et al. The management of meatal obstruction due to Kaposi's sarcoma of the glans penis. *J Urol.* 1993;150:193.
53. Bordeau KP, Lynch DF. Transitional cell carcinoma of the bladder metastatic to the penis. *Urology.* 2004;63:981.
54. Paquin AJ, Roland SI. Secondary carcinoma of the penis: a review of the literature and a report of nine new cases. *Cancer.* 1956;9:626.
55. Berger AP, Rogatsch H, Hoeltl L, et al. Late penile metastasis from primary bladder carcinoma. *Urology.* 2003;62:145.
56. Sagar SM, Retsas S. Metastasis to the penis from malignant melanoma: case report and review of the literature. *Clin Oncol.* 1992;4:130.
57. Haddad FS. Penile metastases secondary to bladder cancer. Review of the literature. *Urol Int.* 1984;39:125.
58. Konstadoulakis MM, Ricaniadis N, Karakousis CP. Malignant melanoma of the scrotum: report of 2 cases. *J Urol.* 1994;151:161.

59. Bryant J. Granular cell tumor of penis and scrotum. *Urology.* 1995;45:332.

60. Melicow MM. Percivall Pott (1713–1788): 200th anniversary of first report of occupation-induced cancer of scrotum in chimney sweepers (1775). *Urology.* 1975;6:745.

61. Tucci P, Haralambidis G. Carcinoma of the scrotum: review of literature and presentation of 2 cases. *J Urol.* 1963;89:585.

62. Nahass GT, Blauvelt A, Leonardi CL, et al. Basal cell carcinoma of the scrotum. Report of three cases and review of the literature. *J Am Acad Dermatol.* 1992;26:574.

63. Schleicher SM, Milstein HJ, Ilowite R. Basal cell carcinoma of the scrotum. *Cutis* 1997;59:116.

64. Hopkins MP, Nemunaitis-Keller J. Carcinoma of the vulva. *Obstet Gynecol Clin North Am.* 2001;28:791.

65. Finan MA, Barre G. Bartholin's gland carcinoma, malignant melanoma and other rare tumours of the vulva. *Best Pract Res Clin Obstet Gynaecol.* 2003;17:609.

66. Lai YL, Yang WG, Tsay PK, et al. Penoscrotal extramammary Paget's disease: a review of 33 cases in a 20-year experience. *Plast Reconstr Surg.* 2003;112: 1017.

67. Salamanca J, Benito A, Garcia-Penalver C, et al. Paget's disease of the glans penis secondary to transitional cell carcinoma of the bladder: a report of two cases and review of the literature. *J Cutan Pathol.* 2004;31:341.

68. Shum DT, Guenther L. Metastatic Crohn's disease. Case report and review of the literature. *Arch Dermatol.* 1990;126:645.

69. Lai CS, Lin SD, Yang CC, et al. Surgical treatment of the penoscrotal Paget's disease. *Ann Plast Surg.* 1989;23:141.

CHAPTER 25

Paget's Disease

Zeina Tannous, M.D.

BOX 25-1   Overview

- Paget's disease is uncommon.
- Large rounded clear-staining Paget's cells are found at varying levels of the epidermis.
- There are mammary and extramammary variants.
- Extramammary Paget's disease (EMPD) can be primary or secondary.
- Secondary EMPD is associated with underlying adnexal or internal carcinoma.

INTRODUCTION

Paget's disease of the skin includes both mammary and extramammary variants. Mammary Paget's disease (MPD) was described by Sir James Paget in 1874.[1] He described 15 women with chronic eruption of the nipple and the areola and associated breast cancer that developed within 2 years. MPD has been reported in 1 to 3% of diagnosed breast cancer.[2] Extramammary Paget's disease (EMPD) is very rare. EMPD constitutes less than 1% of vulvar cancer.[3]

MAMMARY PAGET'S DISEASE

BOX 25-2   Summary

- Predominantly affects the nipple and areola of women.
- Worse prognosis in men.
- 1 to 3% of diagnosed breast cancer.
- Cutaneous epidermotropic metastasis from an underlying breast ductal carcinoma.
- Paget's cells do not invade the dermis, unlike EMPD.
- Mastectomy is recommended for MPD with palpable masses or mammographic abnormalities.
- Breast conservative surgery, with or without radiotherapy, is recommended for MPD with no palpable mass or mammographic density.

MPD is also referred to as Paget's disease of the nipple and the areola. It is a relatively rare disease that predominantly affects women in their fifties or sixties. It can rarely affect men where it carries a worse prognosis.[4]

Pathogenesis

MPD represents a form of cutaneous metastasis from an underlying ductal carcinoma of the breast. It results from the epidermotropism of the malignant cells that reach the epidermis through the lactiferous ducts.

Clinical Features

MPD usually presents as a unilateral, pruritic, well-demarcated, erythematous, crusted, and scaly eczematous patch or plaque on the nipple or the areola. It can be mistaken for acute or chronic dermatitis and psoriasis. Bilateral and symmetric involvement has been rarely described. With advanced disease, it may become ulcerated and the nipple may be retracted. In later stages, it can also become indurated and infiltrated, and an underlying nodule might be palpated. Regional lymphadenopathy is rarely present in early disease.[5]

Histopathology

Both MPD and EMPD show identical histological findings. The epidermis is usually acanthotic with hyper or parakeratosis. The Paget's cells are large and rounded with abundant, clear-staining cytoplasm and large pleomorphic and vesicular nuclei. They can be distributed in single cells or in groups or clusters between the keratinocytes at varying levels of epidermis. Unlike keratinocytes, the Paget's cells have no intercellular bridges. They also stain much lighter than the surrounding keratinocytes. Usually the Paget's cells are separated from the underlying dermis by flattened basal cells, in contrast to melanoma that replaces the basal cell layer. Paget's cells can also be seen in the epithelium of hair follicles extending from the epidermis.

Unlike EMPD, Paget's cells in MPD do not invade the dermis. Furthermore, in contrast to EMPD, the periodic acid-Schiff (PAS) stain is only occasionally positive and the PAS-positive Paget's cells are usually few in number.[6] Paget's cells in MPD are usually positive for carcinoembryogenic antigen (CEA) as well as cytokeratins of the glandular epithelium, such as CAM 5.2 and Cytokeratin 7.[7]

Diagnosis

Persistent unilateral eczematous plaque on the nipple or the areola should be biopsied to exclude MPD.

Differential Diagnosis

MPD can be mistaken for eczematous dermatitis, psoriasis, tinea corporis, Bowen's disease, superficial basal cell carcinoma, and erosive adenomatosis of the nipple.[8]

Treatment and Prognosis

MPD is almost always associated with underlying breast carcinoma. Mastectomy has been considered the standard of care for MPD. Recent studies have shown that breast conserving surgery (BCS) provides similar local control and survival rates to those achieved with mastectomy.[9] It is generally approved that mastectomy is the treatment of choice for patients diagnosed with MPD associated with palpable masses or mammographic abnormalities. In patients presenting with MPD, but with no associated palpable mass or mammographic density, BCS with or without radiotherapy is recommended.[10–12] Prognosis is related to the underlying carcinoma.

EXTRAMAMMARY PAGET'S DISEASE (EMPD)

BOX 25-3   Summary

- Predominantly in the elderly, more common in women.
- Commonly involves the anogenital area, the vulva being the most common site.
- Very rare, less than 1% of vulvar cancer.
- Can be primary or secondary.
- Primary EMPD is limited to the epidermis with no underlying malignancy.
- Secondary EMPD is associated with underlying adnexal carcinoma (25% of EMPD cases) or adjacent internal carcinoma (12% of EMPD cases).
- The treatment of choice is wide local excision or Mohs' micrographic surgery.

EMPD is a very rare disease that affects areas of the skin rich in apocrine glands. It occurs predominantly in the elderly, and is more common in women.

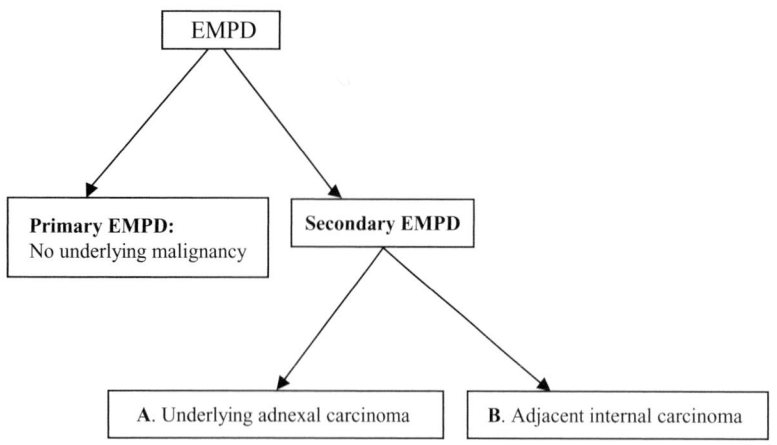

▲ **FIGURE 25-1** Pathogenesis of EMPD: primary and secondary forms.

Pathogenesis

The pathogenesis of EMPD is still controversial. It can be divided into two forms: primary and secondary forms (Fig. 25-1). Primary form is defined as EMPD limited to the epidermis where no underlying malignancy could be demonstrated. The origin of Paget's cells in the primary form could be from the poral portion of the apocrine duct[13] or from epidermal pluripotential stem cells that can differentiate into apocrine structures.[14,15] Secondary EMPD is associated with an underlying adnexal carcinoma or a local adjacent internal carcinoma. Approximately 25% of EMPD cases are associated with an underlying adnexal carcinoma of the skin, mostly of apocrine origin.[16] Furthermore, approximately 12% of EMPD cases are associated with a visceral carcinoma; where they represent an extension of an adenocarcinoma of the rectum, prostate, cervix, or bladder to the perianal area, vulvar region, urethra, glans penis or the groin.[17–20]

Clinical Features

EMPD lesions are clinically similar to MPD lesions. EMPD commonly presents as an intensely pruritic, erythematous, and exudative eczematous patch or plaque with scaling and crusting (Fig. 25-2). It is usually well demarcated, slowly expanding, and may exhibit bleeding, ulceration, and regional lymphadenopathy in later stages. EMPD usually involves the anogenital area with the vulva being the most common site, in addition to the anal, perianal and perineal areas, urethra, penis, and scrotum. Less common sites include the axillae, chest, and umbilicus, as well as sites of ceruminal and Moll's glands.[21–24]

Histopathology

Both MPD and EMPD show identical histological findings that were discussed in the previous section (Fig. 25-3a and b). However, in contrast to MPD, EMPD can invade the dermis from the epidermis.[25] Unlike MPD, abundant sialomucin is present in Paget's cells of EMPD in almost all cases. They stain positively with PAS, mucicarmine (Fig. 25-3c), colloidal iron, and alcian blue at pH 2.5.[6] Paget's cells also show positive staining for carcinoembryogenic antigen (CEA), epithelial membrane antigen (EMA), gross cystic disease fluid protein (GCDFP), CAM 5.2, and Cytokeratin 7.[7,26]

Diagnosis

Persistent eczematous plaque in the anogenital area should be biopsied to exclude EMPD.

Differential Diagnosis

EMPD can be mistaken for eczematous dermatitis, inverse psoriasis, tinea corporis, candidal infection, erythrasma, lichen simplex chronicus, Bowen's disease, invasive squamous cell carcinoma, basal cell carcinoma, amelanotic melanoma, and HPV-induced intraepithelial neoplasia when present on the vulvar area or the penis.

Treatment

Once the diagnosis is confirmed with a biopsy, an adequate search for an underlying malignancy should be performed. The anogenital area including the cervix, rectum, and urethra should be carefully examined for any sign of malignancy. The treatment of choice is wide local excision or Mohs' micrographic surgery (MMS). In a retrospective review of 95 patients with EMPD, MMS compared very well with wide local excision.[27] The use of intraoperative immunostaining with Cytokeratin 7 or carcinoembryonic antigen (CEA), as well as preoperative scouting biopsies can help in delineating tumor margins in MMS.[28,29] Other treatment modalities include topical 5-fluorouracil, topical imiquimod, photodynamic therapy with 5-aminolevulinic acid, radiotherapy, and CO_2 laser ablation.[30,31] Recurrence rates are high due to the multifocality and the clinically nonapparent spread of EMPD. Close long-term follow-up is advised.

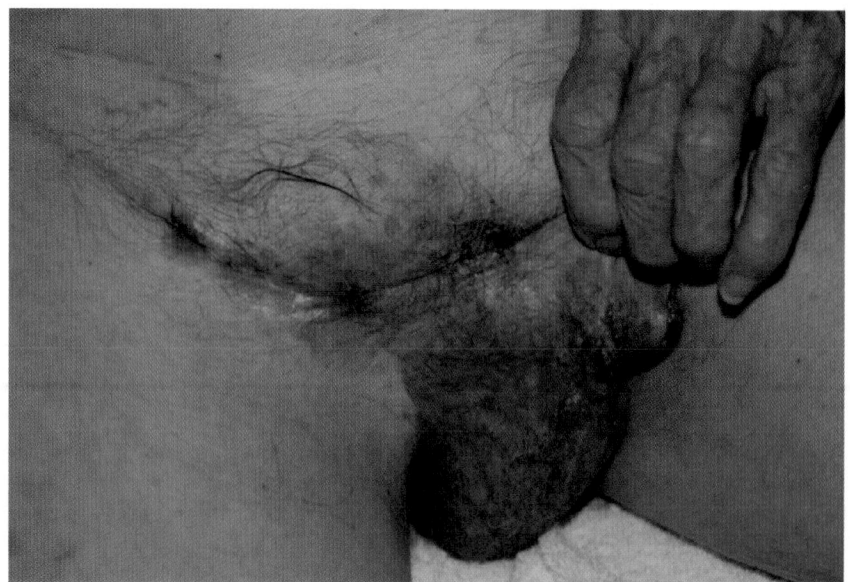

▲ **FIGURE 25-2** A unilateral erythematous eczematous patches of primary EMPD in the genital area of a male patient (courtesy of Richard Johnson, M.D.).

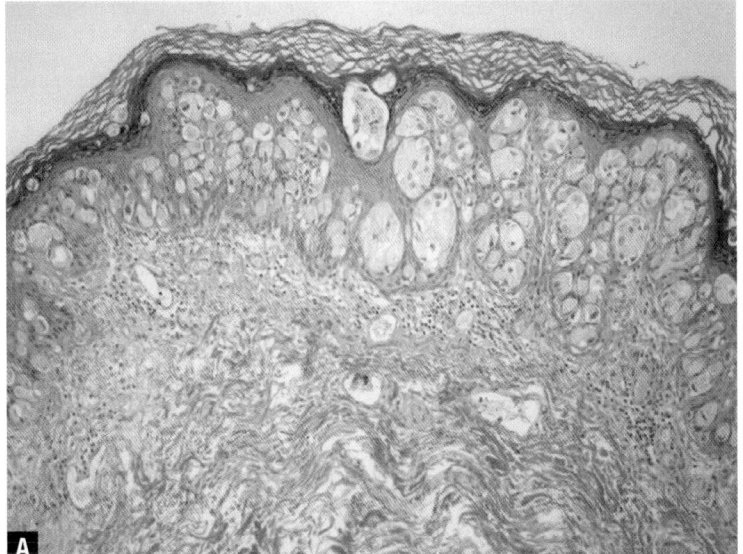

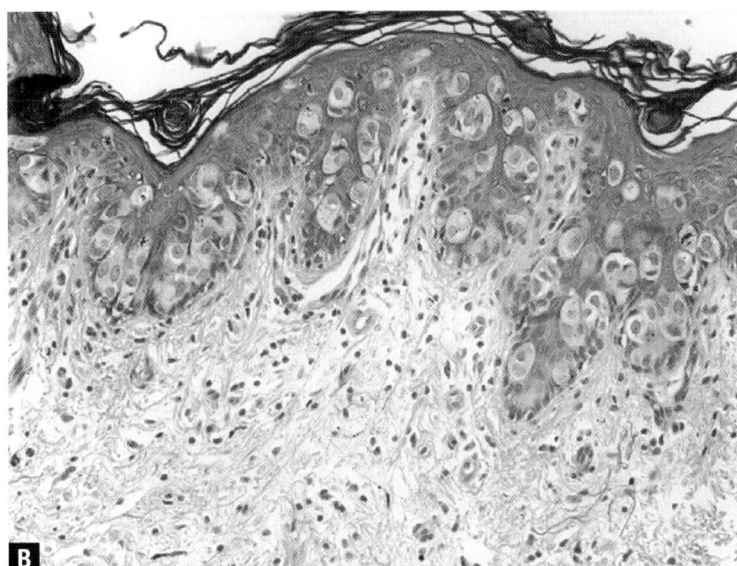

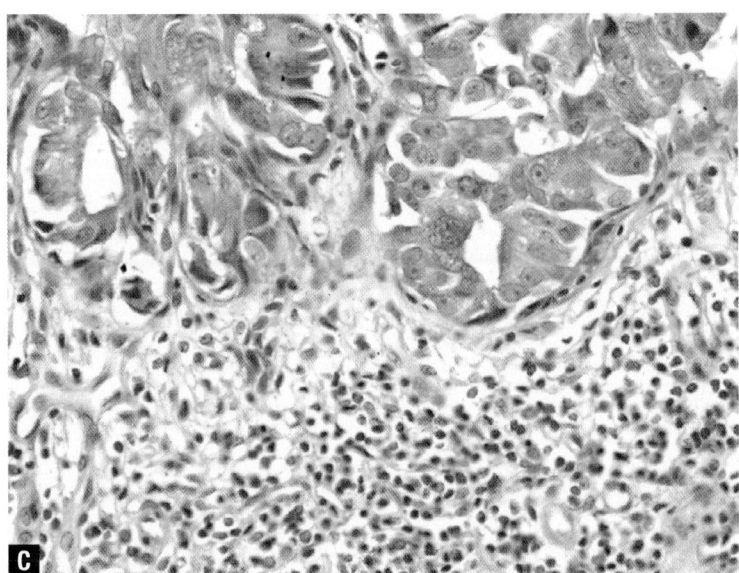

▲ **FIGURE 25-3** (**A, B**) Histology of EMPD showing large rounded neoplastic Paget's cells with abundant pale-staining cytoplasm and large hyperchromatic and vesicular nuclei distributed in single cells or in groups at different levels of epidermis. **C.** Mucicarmine stain highlights the intracellular mucin (courtesy of Lyn Duncan, M.D.).

FINAL THOUGHTS

Paget's disease is an uncommon cutaneous disease. It includes both MPD and EMPD variants. Both variants are characterized histologically by the presence of enlarged round pale-staining Paget's cells at different levels of the epidermis. MPD is almost always associated with underlying ductal breast carcinoma. Treatment options of MPD include mastectomy or breast conservative surgery, with or without radiotherapy. EMPD can be primary or secondary: primary EMPD is not associated with underlying malignancy; secondary EMPD is associated with underlying adnexal carcinoma or adjacent internal carcinoma. Treatment options include wide local excision or Mohs' micrographic surgery. In addition, adequate treatment is necessary for the underlying cancer in secondary EMPD.

REFERENCES

1. Paget J. On disease of the mammary areola preceding cancer of the mammary gland. *St. Bartholomew's Hosp Rep.* 1874;10:87.
2. Jemal A, Siegel R, Ward E, et al. Cancer statistics, 2006. *CA Cancer J Clin.* Mar/Apr 2006;56(2):106–130.
3. Parker LP, Parker JR, Bodurka-Bevers D, et al. Paget's disease of the vulva: pathology, pattern of involvement and prognosis. *Gynecol Oncol.* Apr 2000;77(1):183–189.
4. Jaiyesimi A, et al. Carcinoma of the male breast. *Ann Intern Med.* 1992;117:771.
5. Paone JF, Baker RR. Pathogenesis and treatment of Paget's disease of the breast. *Cancer.* Aug 1981;48(3):825–829.
6. Sitakalin C, Ackerman AB. Mammary and extramammary Paget's disease. *Am J Dermatopathol.* Aug 1985;7(4):335–340.
7. Lau J, Kohler S. Keratin profile of intraepidermal cells in Paget's disease, extramammary Paget's disease, and pagetoid squamous cell carcinoma in situ. *J Cutan Pathol.* Aug 2003;30(7):449–454.
8. Lewis HM, Ovitz ML, Golitz LE. Erosive adenomatosis of the nipple. *Arch Dermatol.* Oct 1976;112(10):1427–1428.
9. Kawase K, Dimaio DJ, Tucker SL, et al. Paget's disease of the breast: there is a role for breast-conserving therapy. *Ann Surg Oncol.* May 2005;12(5):391–397.
10. Marcus E. The management of Paget's disease of the breast. *Curr Treat Options Oncol.* Apr 2004;5(2):153–160.
11. Pierce LJ, Haffty BG, Solin LJ, et al. The conservative management of Paget's disease of the breast with radiotherapy. *Cancer.* Sep 1997;80(6):1065–1072.
12. Marshall JK, Griffith KA, Haffty BG, et al. Conservative management of Paget disease of the breast with radiotherapy: 10- and 15-year results. *Cancer.* May 2003; 97(9):2142–2149.
13. Pinkus H, Mehregan AH. *A Guide to Dermatopathology.* 3rd ed. New York: Appleton-Century-Crofts; 1981:471.
14. Murrell TW, Jr, Mcmullan FH. Extramammary Paget's disease. A report of

two cases. *Arch Dermatol.* May 1962;85:600–613.

15. Jones RE, Jr, Austin C, Ackerman AB. Extramammary Paget's disease. A critical reexamination. *Am J Dermatopathol.* Summer 1979;1(2):101–132.

16. Piura B, Zirkin HJ. Vulvar Paget's disease with an underlying sweat gland adenocarcinoma. *J Dermatol Surg Oncol.* May 1988;14(5):533–537.

17. Jones RE, Jr, Austin C, Ackerman AB. Extramammary Paget's disease. A critical reexamination. *Am J Dermatopathol.* Summer 1979;1(2):101–132.

18. McKee PH, Hertogs KT. Endocervical adenocarcinoma and vulval Paget's disease: a significant association. *Br J Dermatol.* Oct 1980;103(4):443–448.

19. Metcalf JS, Lee RE, Maize JC. Epidermotropic urothelial carcinoma involving the glans penis. *Arch Dermatol.* Apr 1985;121(4):532–534.

20. Ojeda VJ, Heenan PJ, Watson SH. Paget's disease of the groin associated with adenocarcinoma of the urinary bladder. *J Cutan Pathol.* Aug 1987;14(4):227–231.

21. Saida T, Iwata M. "Ectopic" extramammary Paget's disease affecting the lower anterior aspect of the chest. *J Am Acad Dermatol.* Nov 1987;17(5, Pt 2):910–913.

22. Remond B, Aractingi S, Blanc F, et al. Umbilical Paget's disease and prostatic carcinoma. *Br J Dermatol.* Apr 1993;128(4):448–450.

23. Fligiel Z, Kaneko M. Extramammary Paget's disease of the external ear canal in association with ceruminous gland carcinoma. A case report. *Cancer.* Sep 1975;36(3):1072–1076.

24. Whorton CM, Patterson JB. Carcinoma of Moll's glands with extramammary Paget's disease of the eyelid. *Cancer.* Sep/Oct 1955;8(5):1009–1015.

25. Orr JW, Parish DJ. The nature of the nipple changes in Paget's disease. *J Pathol Bacteriol.* Jul 1962;84:201–208.

26. Merot Y, Mazoujian G, Pinkus G, et al. Extramammary Paget's disease of perianal and perineal regions: evidence of apocrine derivation. *Arch Dermatol.* 1985;121:750.

27. O'Connor WJ, Lim KK, Zalla MJ, et al. Comparison of Mohs micrographic surgery and wide excision for extramammary Paget's disease. *Dermatol Surg.* Jul 2003;29(7):723–727.

28. Battles OE, Page DL, Johnson JE. Cytokeratin, CEA and mucin histochemistry in the diagnosis and characterization of extramammary Paget's disease. *Am J Clin Pathol.* Jul 1997;108(1):6–12.

29. Appert DL, Otley CC, Phillips PK, Roenigk RK. Role of multiple scouting biopsies before Mohs micrographic surgery for extramammary Paget's disease. *Dermatol Surg.* Nov 2005;31(11, Pt 1):1417–1422.

30. Cohen PR, Schulze KE, Tschen JA, Hetherington GW, Nelson BR. Treatment of extramammary Paget disease with topical imiquimod cream: case report and literature review. *South Med J.* Apr 2006;99(4):396–402.

31. Mikasa K, Watanabe D, Kondo C, Kobayashi M, Nakaseko H, Yokoo K, Tamada Y. Matsumoto Y5-aminolevulinic acid-based photodynamic therapy for the treatment of two patients with extramammary Paget's disease. *J Dermatol.* Feb 2005;32(2):97.

CHAPTER 26

HPV-Associated
Skin Cancers

Ammar M. Ahmed, M.D.
Brenda Chrastil, M.D.
Vandana Madkan, M.D.
Stephen K. Tyring, M.D., Ph.D.
Oliver A. Perez, M.D.
Brian Berman, M.D., Ph.D.

> **BOX 26-1   Overview**
>
> - There is a clear association between persistent infection with certain human papillomaviruses (HPVs) and development of squamous cell carcinomas in patients with epidermodysplasia verruciformis (EV).
> - These EV-related HPVs are also found in a large proportion of skin tumors in non-EV patients, and to a lesser extent in normal skin.
> - The E6 and E7 proteins of EV-related HPVs appear to be involved in the process of early skin carcinogenesis; precise mechanisms are not fully understood.
> - HPV infection alone is insufficient for carcinogenesis. UV irradiation works as a co-carcinogen with HPV infection.
> - Assessment of certain genetic polymorphisms may have a future role in predicting which patients are susceptible to HPV-related carcinogenesis.

INTRODUCTION

Human papillomaviruses (HPVs) have long been associated with epithelial cancers of the genital tract and have been proven to be a necessary causative factor in the development of cervical cancer.[1] More recently, certain types of HPVs have been implicated in the development of cutaneous cancers, especially squamous cell carcinoma (SCC) and its precursor lesions. While the precise relationship between HPV infection and cutaneous malignancy is still largely undefined, emerging evidence suggests that HPV infection, likely in concert with other factors such as UV radiation, plays an important role in skin carcinogenesis. The first evidence of an association of HPV infection with skin cancer was seen in patients with epidermodysplasia verruciformis (EV); since then,

numerous studies have suggested a role of HPV infection in skin cancer development in non-EV patients, both among immunosuppressed and immunocompetent populations.

EPIDERMODYSPLASIA VERRUCIFORMIS

> **BOX 26-2   Summary**
>
> - Patients with EV develop a variety of benign skin lesions and multiple squamous cell carcinomas on sun-exposed skin.
> - HPV-5 and HPV-8 are detected in over 90% of skin cancers in EV patients; numerous other HPV types are detected in the benign lesions.
> - EV patients have an undefined defect in cell-mediated immunity that prevents normal rejection of EV-harboring keratinocytes.
> - Specific polymorphisms of the interleukin-10 gene promoter and codon 72 of the p53 tumor-suppressor gene are associated with the development of skin cancers in EV patients.
> - Two susceptibility loci have been identified for EV, and at one of these loci, specific mutations in the *EVER1* and *EVER2* genes have been detected.

First described by Lewandowsky and Lutz in 1922,[2] EV is a rare, lifelong, autosomal recessive disease,[3] characterized by a predisposition to persistent infection by certain HPV types (termed EV-HPV types or beta-HPV types). Starting in childhood, affected persons develop skin-colored papules resembling plane warts and scaly, red macules and plaques, which predominate on sun-exposed areas of the skin (brown plaques, pityriasis versicolor-like lesions, papillomas, and seborrheic keratosis-like lesions are also seen less commonly). Roughly 50% of patients develop, multiple SCCs or SCCs *in situ* in the same distribution, mostly in the fourth and fifth decades. Fig. 26-1 depicts the progression of premalignant lesions to metastatic SCC in an EV patient. Approximately 20 HPV types are associated with EV, and these types are different from those seen in other HPV-associated lesions such as condyloma acuminata and cervical cancers. About 90% of the SCCs in EV patients contain HPV-5 or -8, and less commonly types 14, 17, 20, and 47; noncancerous lesions contain any of these genotypes or a number

of other HPV types (types 9, 12, 15, 19, 21–25, 36–39, 49).[4]

Despite the rarity of the disease, the pathogenic mechanisms of EV have received a considerable amount of interest because EV serves as a model of cutaneous HPV oncogenesis. It has been determined that individuals with EV have a mild but demonstrable defect in cell-mediated immunity, including inhibition of natural killer cell[5] and cytotoxic T cell[6] activity and are unable to reject EV-HPV-harboring keratinocytes. However, a persistent HPV infection alone likely does not result in skin cancer. Interaction with other factors, particularly UV radiation, is needed to induce neoplasia.[7] The precise immunogenetic defect is not known, but two susceptibility loci on chromosomes 17 and 2 have been identified.[8,9] At the first of these loci two specific genes (named *EVER1* and *EVER2*) with EV-associated mutations have been discovered.[10,11] Among individuals with EV, genetic differences regarding specific polymorphisms of the interleukin-10 gene promoter and codon 72 of the p53 tumor-suppressor gene are associated with whether patients do or do not develop skin cancers.[12,13] Further research into the function of the EVER proteins and into the molecular mechanisms of skin cancer development in EV patients may provide new perspectives on HPV-associated cutaneous oncogenesis in the broader population.

EPIDEMIOLOGICAL RELATIONSHIP OF HPV AND SKIN CANCER

> **BOX 26-3   Summary**
>
> - EV-related HPV types are found in a variety of malignant and benign skin lesions in non-EV patients, as well as in normal skin.
> - Numerous EV-related HPV types are detected in nonmelanoma skin cancers in non-EV patients; there is no preponderance of infection with HPV-5 or -8.
> - High-risk genital HPV types such as HPV-16 have also been detected in a large proportion of skin cancers, especially in verrucous carcinomas, and digital and periungual squamous cell carcinomas.
> - There is a limited and conflicting serological evidence supporting a role for HPV in skin cancer development.

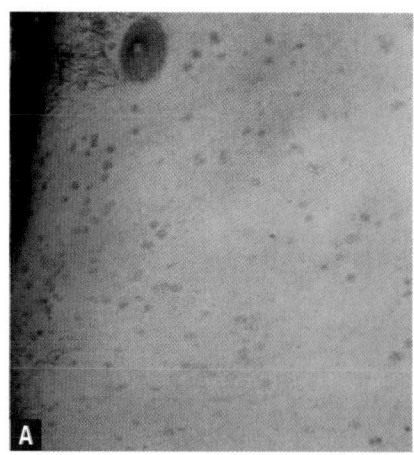
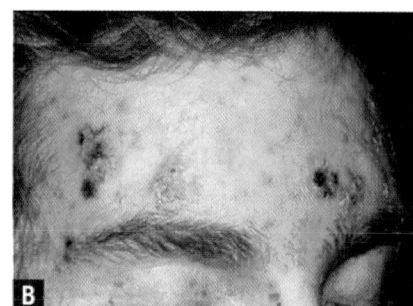
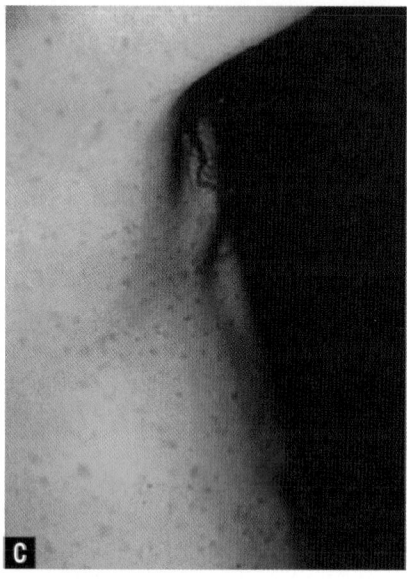
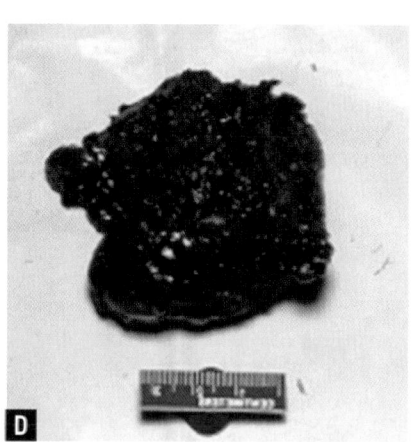

▲ **FIGURE 26-1** Progression of HPV infection to metastatic SCC in an EV patient. **A.** Premalignant macules containing episomal HPV-8 DNA. **B.** The same patient after development of multiple SCCs. (**C, D**) Metastatic SCC containing HPV-8 DNA integrated into the host genome.

With more sensitive polymerase chain reaction (PCR) assays, it was discovered that the so-called EV-HPV types were not limited to patients with EV. Rather, these HPV types and phylogenetically closely related types were found in skin lesions in a broad spectrum of patients, both immunocompromised and immunocompetent. In certain immunocompromised, non-EV patients infected with EV associated HPVs, the patients developed lesions that were clinically and histologically consistent with EV.[14] While various studies using different primers and amplification protocols have found widely diverging rates of HPV DNA, it is clear that a significant percentage of nonmelanoma skin cancers (NMSCs) and their precursor lesions contain HPV. The detection rate of EV-related HPV types in SCCs and actinic keratoses (AKs) of immunosup-

pressed patients is around 80%.[15] In immunocompetent patients, HPV detection rates have been reported at 30% in SCCs and 60% in AKs.[4] There is also evidence that patients with NMSC have a significantly higher rate of EV-related HPV DNA in normal skin, compared with control patients.[16] However, a high rate of HPV detection in skin tumors alone does not imply causation. EV-related HPV DNA is also found in a significant percentage of normal skin samples and hair follicles, both in immunocompromised and immunocompetent patients, and asymptomatic EV and cutaneous HPV infections of normal skin occur in early infancy.[4,17] Furthermore, the cutaneous HPV DNA found in NMSCs spans numerous types (and often multiple types in one tumor) with no preponderance of HPV-5 or -8, as seen in EV patients.[14] It has also been

reported that the prevalence of HPV DNA resting on top of skin tumors, detected by skin swab, is higher than that found in the tumor biopsies themselves.[18]

As the genotypes most commonly identified in cancerous lesions, EV-related HPV types have received much attention. There is also, however, an epidemiological association between certain cutaneous malignancies and genital HPV types. High-risk genital HPV types (e.g., HPV-16) have been detected in over 60% of SCCs and precancerous lesions in immunocompetent patients[19]; the significance of this finding is still unknown.

There are two HPV-associated lesions that do have a particularly strong connection with genital HPV types: verrucous carcinoma, and digital and periungual carcinoma. Verrucous carcinoma, also known as carcinoma cuniculatum when it occurs extragenitally, most often on the sole of the foot, is a low-grade SCC that is thought to arise from plantar warts. These tumors are slow-growing but can develop into large, fungating, deeply invasive cancers. The tumors commonly harbor either high-risk HPV such as HPV-16 or HPV types 6 and 11, those generally found in genital warts. SCCs of the digits also have a distinctly elevated rate of genital HPV presence, with one review reporting HPV-16 in 94% of HPV-positive digital SCCs.[20] Bowen's disease (BD) and Bowenoid papulosis (BP) have also been associated with HPV-16 infection. A recent study by Hama et al examined the presence of mucosal HPV DNA, including HPV-16 and -31, in normal skin, BD, BP, and SCC skin specimens. HPV DNA was detected with PCR, and the HPV type was identified by DNA sequencing. Mucosal HPV DNA was not detected in the 17 normal controls examined; however, HPV-16, -31, and/or -34 DNA was detected in 4.8% (1/21) of BD, 66.7% (2/3) of BP, and 23.0% (6/26) of SCC specimens examined (HPV-34 was found only in 1 of the 26 SCC specimens examined). HPV occurrence was significantly elevated in BP and SCC specimens when compared to normal controls ($P < 0.01$ and $P < 0.01$, respectively), as well as in BP when compared to BD specimens ($P < 0.05$).[21]

There is limited immunological evidence that supports or refutes a role of HPV in skin carcinogenesis in the general population. Several studies have found increased seroreactivity to certain EV- and non-EV-related HPV types in patients with cutaneous SCCs compared to controls; however, this finding has not been consistent across all studies.[21–23]

PROPOSED MECHANISMS OF HPV-RELATED SKIN CARCINOGENESIS

BOX 26-4   Summary

- The E6 protein of EV-related HPVs does not appear to degrade p53 protein.
- The E6 and E7 viral oncogenes are transcriptionally active in squamous cell carcinomas and precursor lesions.
- There is *in vivo* and *in vitro* evidence supporting a role for the transforming capability of E6 and E7 proteins from EV-related HPVs.
- E6 protein from EV-related HPVs degrades the proapoptotic protein Bak and delays DNA repair in cells mutated by UV irradiation.
- Further work is required to clarify the role of genetic heterogeneity in determining the susceptibility to HPV-induced carcinogenesis.

It has been well established that the E6 and E7 proteins of high-risk genital HPV types induce carcinogenesis by directly inactivating cellular p53 and retinoblastoma (Rb) proteins, respectively. The situation is more complex with regards to the EV-related HPV types. Specifically, it has been shown that E6 protein of several of these HPVs (including types 5, 8, and 38) does not degrade p53.[24] However, transcriptional activity of the E6 and E7 oncogenes from EV-HPV types is very frequent in EV tumors, and has been detected in AKs and SCCs from organ transplant recipients.[25] Additionally a substantial amount of *in vitro*, and some *in vivo*, work has demonstrated that these oncogenes from EV-related types do have transforming capabilities. Early studies showed that the E6 genes of EV-related HPVs were sufficient to induce anchorage-independent growth and morphological transformation in certain established rodent cell lines.[15] While some evidence suggests that this effect may be through inhibition of downstream transcriptional targets of p53 activation,[26] the bulk of evidence points toward alteration of p53-independent pathways as the oncogenic stimulus. *In vitro* studies have shown that the E6 protein of HPV-5 and -8 inhibits apoptosis in response to damage by UV light through degradation of the proapoptotic Bak protein.[27] EV-HPV E6 also appears to delay DNA repair in cells mutated by irradiation, thus promoting retention of DNA damage. Together, this evidence points to a role for the E6 oncoprotein of EV-related HPV types in the early stages of skin carcinogenesis. These findings are further supported by the detection of higher levels of EV HPV DNA in AKs than in SCCs.[28]

The E7 oncoprotein of EV-related HPV types differs substantially in its ability to bind to Rb protein, but it appears that the oncogenic EV-related HPV types as a whole do possess the ability to degrade Rb protein.[15] E7 from HPV-5 and -8 has been shown to transform cell lines in conjunction with the activated Ha-ras gene.[29] In organotypic keratinocytes cultures, HPV-8 E7 induces epithelial hyperproliferation and invasion of keratinocytes into the dermis.[30] EV HPV E6 and E7 proteins thus appear to effect different functions in the oncogenic pathway, but both appear to be involved in the development of skin cancer. Schaper et al reported that integrating the entire early region of the HPV-8 genome (including the E2, E6, and E7 genes) into mice caused the development of benign skin tumors in a large majority of transgenic mice, and SCCs in 6% of the transgenic mice, proving the carcinogenic potential of EV HPV gene products in a non-EV animal.[31] HPV-16 transgenic mice, under the same promoter, developed only hyperplasia associated with hyperkeratosis.[32] While these experiments were done with integration of the viral DNA into the mouse genome, it is interesting to note that in tumors in EV patients, there is rarely an integration of HPV DNA into host DNA, except in cases of metastatic disease.

The role of UV light (especially UV-B) in skin carcinogenesis is widely accepted; potential mechanisms include mutation of p53, and local and systemic immunosuppression. HPV infection alone is thought to be insufficient for skin carcinogenesis, but by stimulating cellular proliferation and altering DNA repair and cellular apoptotic ability, infection with certain HPV types works as a cocarcinogen with UV radiation. A model of the proposed roles of UV light and HPV infection in skin carcinogenesis is shown in Fig. 26-2. It is currently unknown whether there is a genetic variation in the susceptibility to HPV-associated skin cancer in the non-EV population. Several groups have looked at polymorphisms of codon 72 of the p53 gene in immunocompetent and immunosuppressed non-EV patients to determine if Arg/Arg homozygosity is associated with a higher risk of skin cancers, as has been shown in EV patients.[13] Results are conflicting, and further work is required to determine if genotypic differences may have a role in predicting which individuals are most susceptible to HPV-associated skin cancers.

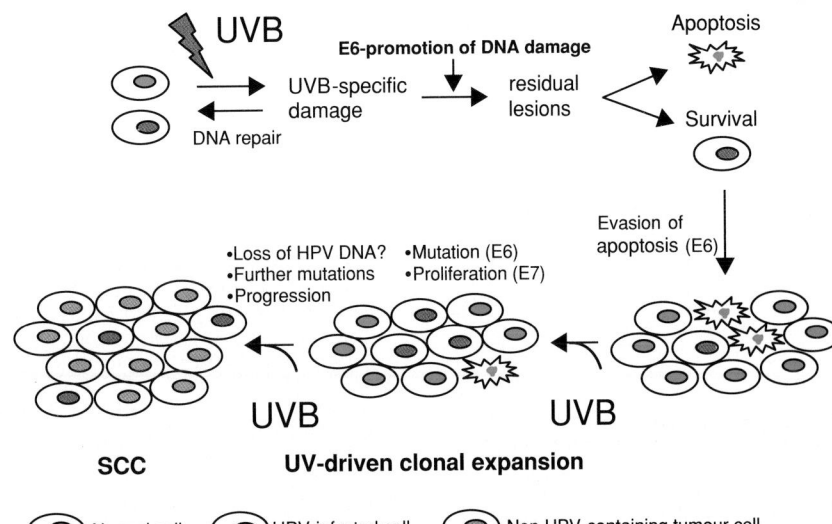

▲ **FIGURE 26-2** Role of UV irradiation and HPV infection in skin cancer development. HPV infection acts as an initiator mechanism for SCC development, in combination with UV light, on sun-exposed body sites. Exposure to UV light leads to DNA damage in skin cells. In HPV-infected cells, E6 promotes retention of DNA damage and protects cells from UV-mediated apoptosis. Normal cells that are fully competent for apoptosis are preferentially deleted following UV damage, allowing clonal expansion of HPV-containing cells. Accumulation of mutations/genetic damage allows cells to progress to SCC independently of the proliferative and mutagenic effects of HPV infection. From Akgul B, Cooke JC, Storey A. HPV-associated skin disease. *J Pathol.* 2006;208:165–175, Copyright Pathological Society of Great Britain and Ireland. Reproduced with permission. Permission is granted by John Wiley & Sons, Ltd., on behalf of PathSoc.

TREATMENT

BOX 26-5 Summary

- There are no current therapies specific for HPV-associated skin cancers.
- Squamous cell carcinomas should generally be treated surgically.
- It is often impossible to remove all malignant and premalignant lesions in EV patients; prophylactic skin grafting may have a role.
- There is no current vaccine for EV-related HPV types.

The various modes of treatment for cutaneous SCCs and precursor lesions are discussed in detail in other chapters of this book. There are currently no therapies specific for HPV-associated skin tumors. Surgical excision is the mainstay of therapy, and topical therapies such as imiquimod and 5-flourouracil can be used for premalignant lesions. For patients with EV, it is often not possible to remove all individual premalignant and malignant lesions, and prophylactic skin grafting has been used with some success in areas of the skin most susceptible to malignant transformation.[14] Retinoids have been tried experimentally in EV patients, without much success. Although a recent study demonstrated that interferon regulatory factor 5.2 acts as a transcription repressor of EV-related HPV, clinical results in EV patients have varied.[3,33,34] For both EV and non-EV patients, proper sun protection remains paramount, as UV irradiation is a major etiological factor in development of NMSC in all subsets of patients. To date, no vaccine exists against EV-related HPV types, but the future may see the development of such vaccines, paralleling the recent development of vaccines against HPV types associated with cervical cancer and genital warts.

FINAL THOUGHTS

BOX 26-6 Summary

- Additional research is required to clarify the mechanisms of HPV-induced carcinogenesis.
- HPV may also be associated with primary melanoma and other skin tumors.
- Work in animal models, as was performed with HPV-16, will be useful in studying the mechanisms of HPV-associated oncogenesis.

With the exception of EV tumors, the etiopathologic relationship between HPV and other cutaneous cancers is still largely unclear. While a large body of epidemiological and some pathogenic evidence points to a role for EV-related HPV types as cocarcinogens in the development of SCCs, the precise mechanisms have yet to be described. A relationship between HPV and other skin tumors may also be proven in the future. Associations between HPV infection and tumors ranging from large-cell acanthomas of the skin[35] to primary melanomas[36] have been reported, and time will tell if these associations are reproducible and important clinically. For the near future, more work in animal models, as has been done with HPV-16, is needed to examine the specific role of EV-related HPVs in the development of skin cancer. Further knowledge of the mechanisms of carcinogenesis will lead to novel methods of preventing and treating these cancers.

REFERENCES

1. Ahmed AM, Madkan V, Tyring SK. Human papillomaviruses and genital disease. *Dermatol Clin.* 2006;24(vi):157–165.
2. Lewandowsky F, Lutz W. Ein fall einer bisher nicht beschriebenen hauterkrankungen (epidermodysplasia verruciformis). *Arch Dermatol Syphilol.* 1922;141:193–203.
3. Anadolu R, Oskay T, Erdem C, Boyvat A, Terzi E, Gurgey E. Treatment of epidermodysplasia verruciformis with a combination of acitretin and interferon alfa-2a. *J Am Acad Dermatol.* 2001;45:296–299.
4. Sterling JC. Human papillomaviruses and skin cancer. *J Clin Virol.* 2005;32(suppl 1):S67–S71.
5. Majewski S, Malejczyk J, Jablonska S, et al. Natural cell-mediated cytotoxicity against various target cells in patients with epidermodysplasia verruciformis. *J Am Acad Dermatol.* 1990;22:423–427.
6. Cooper KD, Androphy EJ, Lowy D, Katz SI. Antigen presentation and T-cell activation in epidermodysplasia verruciformis. *J Invest Dermatol.* 1990;94:769–776.
7. Majewski S, Jablonska S. Epidermodysplasia verruciformis as a model of human papillomavirus-induced genetic cancer of the skin. *Arch Dermatol.* 1995;131:1312–1318.
8. Ramoz N, Rueda LA, Bouadjar B, Favre M, Orth G. A susceptibility locus for epidermodysplasia verruciformis, an abnormal predisposition to infection with the oncogenic human papillomavirus type 5, maps to chromosome 17qter in a region containing a psoriasis locus. *J Invest Dermatol.* 1999;112:259–263.
9. Ramoz N, Taieb A, Rueda LA, et al. Evidence for a nonallelic heterogeneity of epidermodysplasia verruciformis with two susceptibility loci mapped to chromosome regions 2p21–p24 and 17q25. *J Invest Dermatol.* 2000;114:1148–1153.
10. Ramoz N, Rueda LA, Bouadjar B, Montoya LS, Orth G, Favre M. Mutations in two adjacent novel genes are associated with epidermodysplasia verruciformis. *Nat Genet.* 2002;32:579–581.
11. Tate G, Suzuki T, Kishimoto K, Mitsuya T. Novel mutations of EVER1/TMC6 gene in a Japanese patient with epidermodysplasia verruciformis. *J Hum Genet.* 2004;49:223–225.
12. de Oliveira WR, Rady PL, Grady J, et al. Polymorphisms of the interleukin 10 gene promoter in patients from Brazil with epidermodysplasia verruciformis. *J Am Acad Dermatol.* 2003;49:639–643.
13. de Oliveira WR, Rady PL, Grady J, et al. Association of p53 arginine polymorphism with skin cancer. *Int J Dermatol.* 2004;43:489–493.
14. Majewski S, Jablonska S. Epidermodysplasia verruciformis in human papillomaviruses: clinical and scientific advances. In: *Human Papillomaviruses: Clinical and Scientific Advances.* Sterling JC, Tyring SK, eds. London: Oxford Press; 2001:90–101.
15. Akgul B, Cooke JC, Storey A. HPV-associated skin disease. *J Pathol.* 2006;208:165–175.
16. Harwood CA, Surentheran T, Sasieni P, et al. Increased risk of skin cancer associated with the presence of epidermodysplasia verruciformis human papillomavirus types in normal skin. *Br J Dermatol.* 2004;150:949–957.
17. Antonsson A, Karanfilovska S, Lindqvist PG, Hansson BG. General acquisition of human papillomavirus infections of skin occurs in early infancy. *J Clin Microbiol.* 2003;41:2509–2514.
18. Forslund O, Lindelof B, Hradil E, et al. High prevalence of cutaneous human papillomavirus DNA on the top of skin tumors but not in "stripped" biopsies from the same tumors. *J Invest Dermatol.* 2004;123:388–394.
19. Iftner A, Klug SJ, Garbe C, et al. The prevalence of human papillomavirus genotypes in nonmelanoma skin cancers of nonimmunosuppressed individuals identifies high-risk genital types as possible risk factors. *Cancer Res.* 2003;63:7515–7519.
20. Alam M, Caldwell JB, Eliezri YD. Human papillomavirus-associated digital squamous cell carcinoma: literature review and report of 21 new cases. *J Am Acad Dermatol.* 2003;48:385–393.
21. Hama N, Ohtsuka T, Yamazaki S. Detection of mucosal human papilloma virus DNA in Bowenoid papulosis, Bowen's disease and squamous cell carcinoma of the skin. *J Dermatol.* 2006;33:331–337.
22. Feltkamp MC, Broer R, di Summa FM, et al. Seroreactivity to epidermodysplasia verruciformis-related human papillomavirus types is associated with nonmelanoma skin cancer. *Cancer Res.* 2003;63:2695–2700.
23. Masini C, Fuchs PG, Gabrielli F, et al. Evidence for the association of human papillomavirus infection and cutaneous squamous cell carcinoma in immunocompetent individuals. *Arch Dermatol.* 2003;139:890–894.
24. Steger G, Pfister H. In vitro expressed HPV 8 E6 protein does not bind p53. *Arch Virol.* 1992;125:355–360.

25. Dang C, Koehler A, Forschner T, et al. E6/E7 expression of human papillomavirus types in cutaneous squamous cell dysplasia and carcinoma in immunosuppressed organ transplant recipients. *Br J Dermatol.* 2006;155:129–136.

26. Giampieri S, Garcia-Escudero R, Green J, Storey A. Human papillomavirus type 77 E6 protein selectively inhibits p53-dependent transcription of proapoptotic genes following UV-B irradiation. *Oncogene.* 2004;23:5864–5870.

27. Jackson S, Storey A. E6 proteins from diverse cutaneous HPV types inhibit apoptosis in response to UV damage. *Oncogene.* 2000;19:592–598.

28. Weissenborn SJ, Nindl I, Purdie K, et al. Human papillomavirus-DNA loads in actinic keratoses exceed those in non-melanoma skin cancers. *J Invest Dermatol.* 2005;125:93–97.

29. Yamashita T, Segawa K, Fujinaga Y, Nishikawa T, Fujinaga K. Biological and biochemical activity of E7 genes of the cutaneous human papillomavirus type 5 and 8. *Oncogene.* 1993;8:2433–2441.

30. Akgul B, Garcia-Escudero R, Ghali L, et al. The E7 protein of cutaneous human papillomavirus type 8 causes invasion of human keratinocytes into the dermis in organotypic cultures of skin. *Cancer Res.* 2005;65:2216–2223.

31. Schaper ID, Marcuzzi GP, Weissenborn SJ, et al. Development of skin tumors in mice transgenic for early genes of human papillomavirus type 8. *Cancer Res.* 2005;65:1394–1400.

32. Kim SH, Kim KS, Lee EJ, et al. Human keratin 14 driven HPV 16 E6/E7 transgenic mice exhibit hyperkeratinosis. *Life Sci.* 2004;75:3035–3042.

33. Akgul B, Curten M, Haigis H, Rogosz I, Pfister H. Interferon regulatory factor 5.2 acts as a transcription repressor of epidermodysplasia verruciformis-associated human papillomaviruses. *Arch Virol.* 2006;151:2461–2473.

34. Gubinelli E, Posteraro P, Cocuroccia B, Girolomoni G. Epidermodysplasia verruciformis with multiple mucosal carcinomas treated with pegylated interferon alfa and acitretin. *J Dermatol Treat.* 2003;14:184–188.

35. Berger T, Stockfleth E, Meyer T, Kiesewetter F, Funk JO. Multiple disseminated large-cell acanthomas of the skin associated with human papillomavirus type 6. *J Am Acad Dermatol.* 2005;53:335–337.

36. La Placa M, Ambretti S, Bonvicini F, et al. Presence of high-risk mucosal human papillomavirus genotypes in primary melanoma and in acquired dysplastic melanocytic naevi. *Br J Dermatol.* 2005;152:909–914

CHAPTER 27

Cutaneous Metastases

Daniel G. Federman, M.D., F.A.C.P.
Jeffrey D. Kravetz, M.D.
Robert S. Kirsner, M.D., Ph.D.
Peter W. Heald, M.D.

BOX 27-1 Overview

- Cancer is the second leading cause of death in the United States.
- Cutaneous metastases can be a sign of failure of the ongoing therapy or recurrence of a previously diagnosed malignancy as well as a sign of an undiagnosed cancer.
- Skin metastases have been reported to occur between 0.7 and 9% of all malignancies.
- Classically, metastases are discrete, firm or rubbery, dermal or subcutaneous masses, from several millimeters to many centimeters in diameter. However, there are a myriad of presentations.
- In general, treatment should be aimed at the underlying malignancy and consultation with an oncologist is imperative.
- In selected patients, skin metastases may respond to systemic treatment, intralesional chemotherapy, surgical excision, and radiotherapy. Photodynamic therapy, local chemotherapy, and immunotherapy can be considered.
- With notable exceptions, the prognosis for affected individuals is poor.

INTRODUCTION

Cancer is the second leading cause of death in the United States, and is estimated to account for over 550,000 deaths in 2006.[1] Afflicted patients may not succumb to complications only from the primary cancer, but also from the metastatic spread to distant sites. While prevention of cancer holds the most promise in prolonging life, earlier detection of malignancy has the potential to improve survival if successful, targeted therapy can be employed. Cutaneous metastases, though often occurring late in the course of a known malignancy, can serve as a clue to an astute clinician to the failure of the ongoing therapy, the recurrence of a malignancy thought to be treated successfully, or even the presence of an unsuspected, undiagnosed malignancy.

HISTORY

BOX 27-2 Summary

- Cutaneous metastases were first described in 1838 by Velpeau, who described "cancer en cuirasse" in patients with metastatic breast cancer.
- Early case series of cutaneous metastases highlighted their poor prognosis.

Cutaneous metastatic disease has long been recognized as an unfortunate and a disfiguring complication of internal malignancy. In fact, the incidence of cutaneous metastases was likely higher historically given the inability to effectively treat primary malignancies. Given the relatively high rate of cutaneous metastases from breast cancer, the early history of cutaneous metastases centers on the cases of untreated breast cancer.

In 1838, Velpeau first described a form of metastatic breast cancer as "cancer en cuirasse," literally portraying the cancer as appearing like a metal breastplate (see Fig. 27-1) of a soldier.[2] In 1874, Paget described eczema of the breast associated with metastatic breast cancer, now known as Paget's disease.[3] Inflammatory breast cancer was first described by Hutchinson in 1893 as "erythema-scirrhus of the skin in association with cancer of the breast."[4] As shown in Fig. 27-2, this presentation may mimic cellulitis, and is often referred to as *carcinoma erysipeloides*. Over time, other physicians described other presentations of cutaneous breast cancer metastases, including nodular metastatic carcinoma and carcinoma telangiectaticum.[5,6] The earliest case series of patients with cutaneous metastases was reported by Kaufmann-Wolf in 1913, followed by Suzuki in 1918.[7,8] Both case series observed a poor prognosis of patients presenting with cutaneous metastases. Thus, though cutaneous metastases are relatively uncommon, their appearance has been noted for well over a century.

ETIOLOGY

BOX 27-3 Summary

- Cutaneous metastases can arise from hematologic or lymphatic spread or from direct invasion or tracking of a tumor after intervention.
- Metastases to the skin can be random or site-specific, depending on factors such as lymphatic drainage, vascular supply, and body temperature.

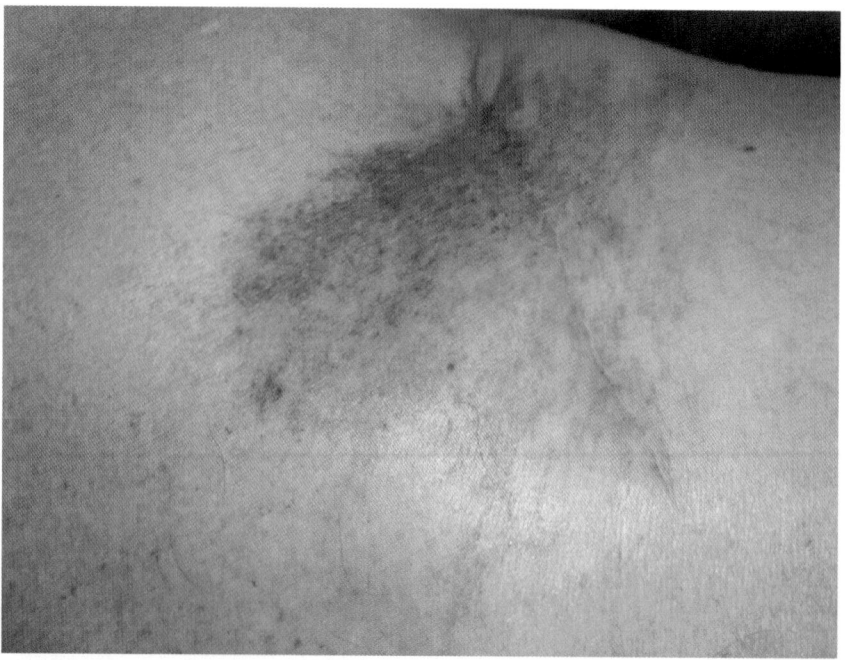

▲ **FIGURE 27-1** *Carcinoma en cuirasse* is the firm infiltration of the skin with carcinoma, typically from the original site of the tumor as in the chest of this patient postmastectomy for ductal carcinoma.

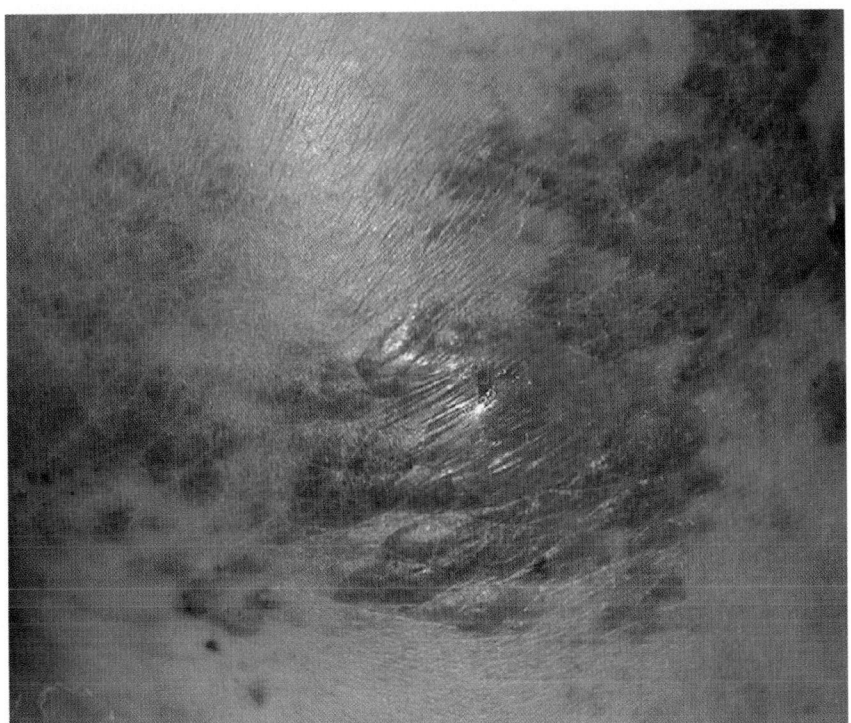

▲ **FIGURE 27-2** Carcinoma erysipeloides is the inflammatory dermal extension or metastasis of cancer. Breast cancer is the most common cause with involvement, as in this patient on the upper abdomen and lower chest, as a local recurrence.

graph distinguishes the entities discussed in this chapter from the multifocal malignancies of the skin such as Kaposi sarcoma, Langerhans cell histiocytoses, and cutaneous lymphomas.

◼ FREQUENCY

BOX 27-4 Summary

- Autopsy series identify cutaneous metastases in 0.7 to 9% of cancer patients.
- Breast cancer is the most common cause of cutaneous metastases in women, while lung cancer is the most common primary cancer identified in men.

The frequency of skin metastases comes largely from autopsy series, which report a frequency of 0.7 to 9.0%.[11–16] However, in a retrospective study of 7316 cancer patients enrolled in a tumor registry from a single institution, 5.0% had skin involvement. Skin involvement was present in 1.3% of all patients at the time of presentation, and was the initial sign of cancer in 0.8%.[17] In this study, breast cancer accounted for 65% of cases of cutaneous involvement in all patients and 82% of cases in women.

In an older report by Brownstein and Helwig,[18] high rates of cutaneous metastases from those with lung and kidney carcinoma were noted at initial presentation. They reported that skin metastases were present *at presentation* in 60% of patients with lung cancer and in 53% of

A metastasis, which can be defined as "a neoplastic lesion arising from another neoplasm that is no longer in continuity,"[9] can be thought of as occurring in a sequence of events. Initially, neoplastic cells detach from the primary malignancy and invade either blood or lymphatic vessels. These cells circulate, and with some stasis, extravasate from circulation, and invade tissue. At this metastatic site, these cells proliferate.[10] Schwartz postulates that this sequence accounts for the "three basic patterns of distribution of metastases": mechanical stasis from the tumor (with anatomic proximity and lymphatic drainage), site-specific disease (wherein tumor cells selectively attach to a specific organ), and nonselective spread (spread that is neither due to mechanical factors or organ-specific factors).[10] Other factors, such as minor differences in body temperature in different anatomic regions as well as vascular or lymphatic drainage characteristics may also play a role in determining the site of spread. An example can be seen in the terminology of melanoma metastases. Melanoma excisions are often accompanied by sentinel lymph node sampling. In Fig. 27-3, a patient had a complete excision with a negative sentinel node. However, a metastasis arose between the primary site and the draining lymph node. This is termed an *in transit* metastasis. Cutaneous involvement by malignancy can be caused by several pos-

sible mechanisms. The primary tumor may extend directly to the skin, either through its own inherent growth or through "tracking" after intervention. Furthermore, skin involvement may occur through metastatic spread, which can be local or distant, and occur via the blood or lymphatic systems. The concept of the metastasis presented in this para-

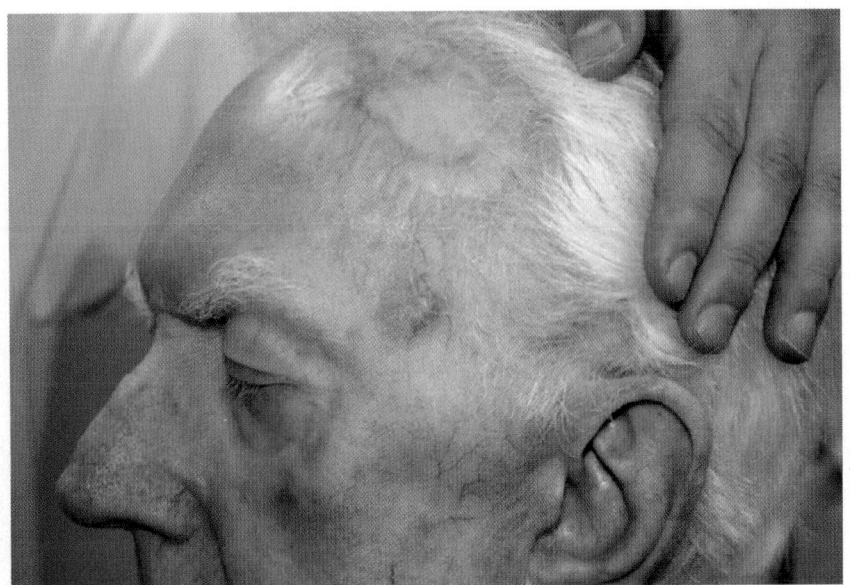

▲ **FIGURE 27-3** Erythematous nodule arising between the excision site of the primary melanoma (scar on the left side of the photograph) and the draining lymph nodes in the cervical chain. Metastases in this region are often referred to as *in transit*.

those with kidney cancer. The most frequent primary tumors associated with skin metastases in men were carcinoma of the lung (24%), colon cancer (19%), melanoma (13%), and squamous cell cancer of the oral cavity (12%). In women, the most common primary tumors were breast cancer (69%), colon cancer (9%), melanoma (5%), and ovarian cancer (4%). Lookingbill et al,[17] however, found lower rates of patients with lung and kidney cancers presenting with cutaneous metastases. In their series, only 4 of 21 (19%) patients with lung cancer and cutaneous metastases had evidence of the cutaneous metastases at presentation, and no patients with renal cell cancer had evidence of cutaneous metastases at presentation. Changes in cancer epidemiology, early detection, and advances in oncology leading to prolonged survival time may account for some of the differences found between earlier and more recent studies.[19]

More recently, Bansal and Naik in a study from India found that, in men, the GI tract was primary site in nearly half of the patients with cutaneous metastases, while in women, the breast was the most common primary site, accounting for nearly one-third of the cutaneous metastases. These GI tract cancers in men were most likely to metastasize to the abdominal skin while the breast cancers were more likely to metastasize to the anterior chest wall. In women, thyroid and ovarian malignancies were the next most common primary sites (12% each), while in men, lung and oral cavity accounted for 16 and 9% of cutaneous metastases, respectively.[20]

CLINICAL FEATURES

BOX 27-5   Summary

- Most cutaneous metastases are painless, firm, or rubbery, but vary in appearance and number.
- A new nodule developing in an existing scar can be a sign of a cutaneous metastasis.
- Subungual involvement from a metastasis is usually painful and associated with a poorer prognosis.

Since cutaneous metastases may assume a plethora of clinical appearances, there is no clear pathognomonic gross appearance that is completely diagnostic. Classically, metastases are discrete, firm or rubbery, dermal, or subcutaneous masses, ranging from several millimeters to many cen-

timeters in diameter. Metastatic lesions may be single or multiple, and may even number more than 100.[11] When multiple, lesions may be localized or scattered diffusely. Ulceration or erosion of metastatic nodules may also occur. In general, lesions are painless, moveable, and skin-colored, although may be of various shades of red, blue, purple, brown, or black.[21] Metastases may be hyperkeratotic, and even resemble a cutaneous horn[22] or keratoacanthoma,[23] or even mimic pyogenic granuloma.[24]

Metastases to the scalp can induce a localized area of cicatricial alopecia, known as alopecia neoplastica. As exemplified in Fig. 27-4, these lesions are usually painless, well-demarcated, round, or oval, non-pruritic pink plaques with a smooth surface. Scalp metastases are sometimes confused with epidermal and pilar cysts, benign appendage tumors, as well as malignant sweat gland neoplasms.

Another distinctive form, inflammatory metastatic carcinoma, known as carcinoma erysipeloides, can present with an ill-defined warm, tender, erythematous, edematous area that resembles erysipelas or cellulitis. While carcinoma erysipelatoides is most commonly associated with breast cancer,[25] it may also be seen in primary cancer of the vulva,[26] pancreas,[27] stomach,[28] lung,[29] uterus,[30] rectum,[31] and ovary.[32]

Another common site for metastatic disease is the periumbilical region, where lesions commonly arise from primary gastric (see Fig. 27-5), pancreatic, or ovarian adenocarcinomas. The term "Sister

Mary Joseph's nodule" was named after a scrub nurse of Dr. Mayo who associated these lesions she encountered while prepping patients for surgery with primary malignant disease in the abdomen.[33]

Scars may be sites for metastatic disease to the skin, either at the site of surgery or other iatrogenic cutaneous insult, often in or near the procedure, usually appearing within a year of the surgery.[34] Scar involvement at a site distant to the primary cancer has been observed. It would therefore be prudent to consider metastatic disease when someone is noted to have a new nodule in an existing scar. These are sometimes confused with a foreign body reaction, a hypertrophic scar, the development of squamous cell carcinoma within a scar, calcification, or a traumatic neuroma.[34]

Cancer may also spread to the nail unit. Subungual metastases usually portend an extremely poor prognosis and most commonly arise from primary lung cancers, tumors of the genitourinary tract (especially kidney), and breast cancer. These lesions are often painful, are more common in the upper extremities, and may take the appearance as an erythematous swelling of the distal digit or a red-purple nodule that has the potential to distort the nail plate and soft tissue of the distal digit.[35]

Given the multitude of possible clinical presentations, cutaneous metastatic disease should be considered in any cancer patient with a suspected new skin tumor or any patient providing a history or physical examination suspicious for an

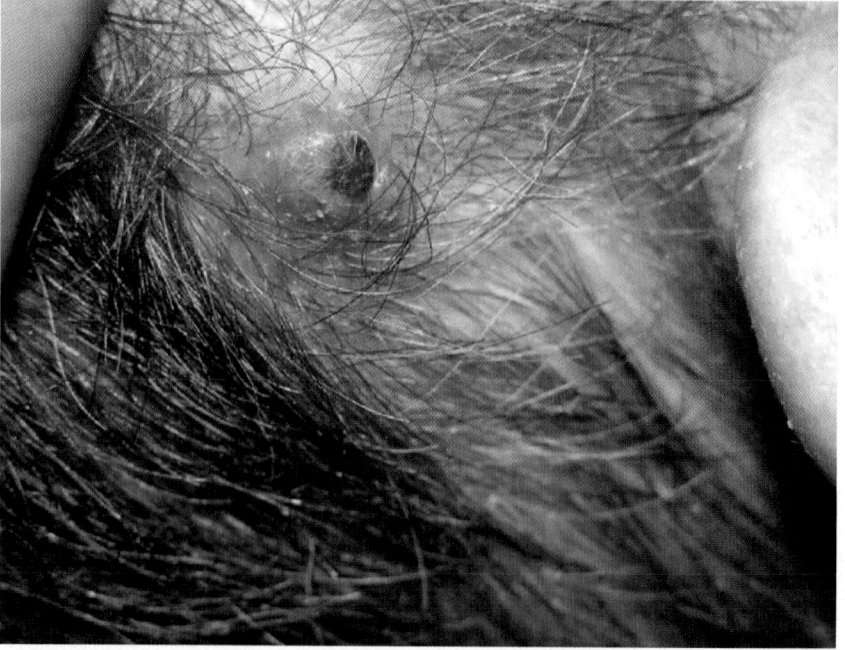

▲ **FIGURE 27-4** Pink ulcerated asymptomatic scalp nodule of metastatic lung cancer.

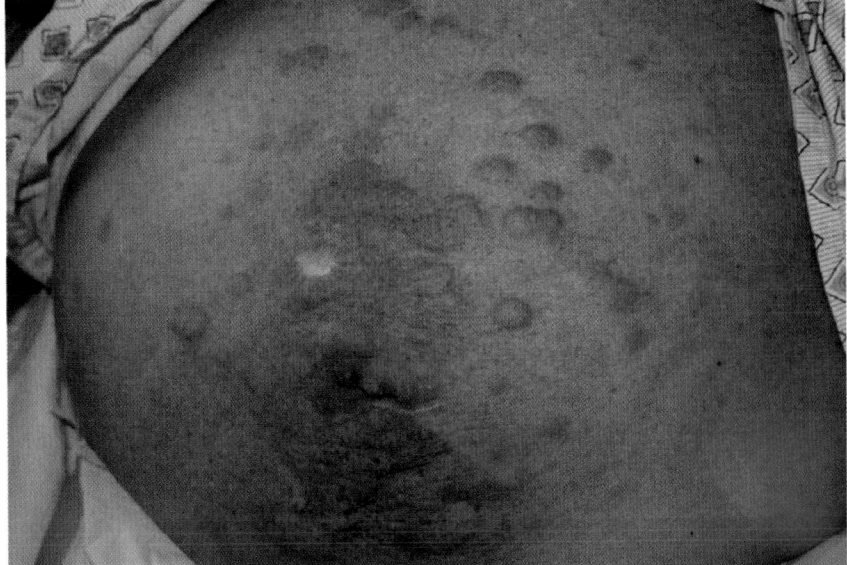

▲ **FIGURE 27-5** Umbilical nodules of metastatic gastric lymphoma, the "Sister Mary Joseph Sign." This patient expired within 4 weeks of the photograph.

internal malignancy who has such a skin lesion. It is important to be familiar with some of the more common malignancies to present with cutaneous metastases. For a more comprehensive review of specific malignancies, readers are directed to the review of Schwartz.[10]

BREAST CANCER

BOX 27-6 Summary

- Cutaneous metastases from breast cancer can present in multiple different forms, including inflammatory, en cuirasse, telangiectatic, and nodular carcinoma, as well as Paget's disease.
- Lung cancer most frequently metastasizes to the chest wall and abdomen.
- Colon carcinoma cutis usually occurs on the abdominal wall, most commonly at the site of resection of the underlying tumor.
- Genitourinary tumors (prostate, bladder, kidney, and testicular) most frequently are identified on the head and neck, as well as the trunk.

Breast cancer is the most commonly diagnosed malignancy in women in the United States and the second leading cause of cancer death.[1] As previously mentioned, breast cancer may present with an inflammatory metastatic form that may mimic erysipelas, inflammatory metastatic carcinoma, or as shown in Fig. 27-2, *carcinoma erysipelatoides*. The inflammatory appearance is thought to be due to capillary congestion; malignant cells are within dilated lymphatic vessels.[10]

The chest wall may take on the appearance of a leather shield in the carcinoma en cuirasse variant. Lymphatic permeation by malignant cells leads to fibrosis, and thickening of the dermis and subcutaneous tissue, as shown in Fig. 27-1. This can be severe enough to lead to a restrictive ventilatory defect.

Metastatic breast cancer may also present with nodular and telangiectatic variants, as well as in the inframammary crease, where it can be overlooked.[10] Paget's disease of the breast, in which there is a migration of the underlying breast cancer to the nipple or areolar region, can present with a sharply demarcated, occasionally weepy, erythematous plaque or patch that simulates eczema.

LUNG CANCER

Lung cancer is the leading cause of cancer death in men and women. An older study found skin metastases in 1.5% of more than 2000 cases of lung cancer.[36] Lookingbill et al[17] found that nearly half of the patients with cutaneous metastases from lung cancer had the skin as the first site of extranodal metastases, while another study found that 7% of those with skin metastases from lung cancer had the nodule found before the lung cancer while they were diagnosed concurrently in 16%.[37] While skin metastases from lung cancer can occur throughout the body, including the scrotum,[38] the most common sites are the abdomen and chest wall.

COLON CANCER

Colorectal cancer is the third most common malignancy in men and women.[1] Cutaneous metastases from colon cancer, referred to as colon carcinoma cutis,[39] occurs in approximately 2% of patients with colonic malignancies.[17] Lookingbill et al reported cutaneous metastases to be the presenting feature in 0.5% of patients with underlying colon carcinoma.[17] Though the relative incidence of colon carcinoma cutis is low, it is still one of the most common causes of cutaneous metastases, given the overall high incidence of underlying colon cancer. Colon carcinoma was the second most common cause of cutaneous metastases in a 1972 study, accounting for 19% of all cutaneous metastases in men and 9% of all cutaneous metastases in women.[18] A more recent review suggests an increasing prevalence of metastatic melanoma, now replacing cutaneous colon cancer as the second most common cause of cutaneous metastasis in men. However, this 2004 retrospective study still identified colon carcinoma as the underlying etiology in 6.5% of patients with cutaneous metastases.[40]

The most common site of cutaneous metastasis from colon carcinoma is the abdominal wall, usually occurring following surgery for resection of the underlying malignancy. Brownstein and Helwig identified colon cancer as the cause of abdominal wall metastases in 37% of the patients, with an equal frequency in both men and women.[18] Though umbilical metastases, also known as Sister Mary Joseph's nodule, have classically been reported to occur with underlying gastric cancer, colon cancer is the second most common cause of umbilical metastasis, accounting for approximately 15% of all umbilical metastases.[41] Various other locations have been less frequently reported to be the site of colon carcinoma cutis, including the scalp,[42,43] face,[44] buttocks,[45] and perianal region, appearing as hidradenitis suppurativa.[17]

GENITOURINARY MALIGNANCIES

Genitourinary malignancies account for nearly one in four cancer diagnoses and commonly metastasize to lymph nodes, bones, liver, and lungs.[46] In a large review, dermatologic spread from a primary urologic malignancy occurred in 2.9% of cases.[46] Cutaneous metastases from primary kidney, bladder, prostate, and testicular cancers were found in 3.4, 0.84, 0.36, and 0.4% of cases. The most common site of involvement is the trunk, and head and neck; lesions are often multiple and nodular. Metastases from renal cell cancer may present a decade after the original diagnosis.[47]

DIAGNOSIS

While the history and clinical findings are often suggestive of metastatic disease, adequate surgical sampling for histopathology is recommended for more definitive diagnosis.

PROGNOSIS

> **BOX 27-7 Summary**
>
> • Most patients with cutaneous metastases have an extremely poor prognosis.
> • There are a few scenarios where the prognosis for patients with cutaneous metastases is not poor, including placental choriocarcinoma and solitary cutaneous hypernephroma.

With several notable exceptions, the prognosis for patient with cutaneous metastases is generally poor, especially for those with primary cancers of the lung, ovary, upper respiratory tract, or upper digestive tract.[17,48–50] For example, the median survival of patients with ovarian carcinoma and skin metastases is 12 months.[51] Other primary malignancies with cutaneous metastatic involvement also have a poor prognosis. Patients with primary malignancies of the genitourinary system survived an average of less than 6 months after their cutaneous metastases.[46] Similarly, leukemia cutis (leukemic skin infiltrates),[52] secondary cutaneous CD30+ lymphoma, and non-Hodgkin's B-cell lymphoma do not have a good prognosis.[53–55] Similarly, those with umbilical metastases usually die within a few months.[10]

While the overall prognosis for most patients is poor, some patients with cutaneous metastases may have a prolonged survival.[56] For example, patients with cutaneous involvement from placental choriocarcinoma may derive benefit from the treatment of their primary malignancy,[57] and rarely, spontaneous regression or cure in those with metastatic cutaneous hypernephroma has been seen.[58] Additionally, patients with a solitary metastatic cutaneous hypernephroma undergoing resection of the primary malignancy and metastatic skin

lesion have a 5-year survival rate of 35%.[59] Clearly, with advances in oncology, many patients may live longer than they would have previously.

TREATMENT

Patients with primary malignancies and skin metastases should be considered for systemic treatment aimed at their underlying cancers. While the actual skin metastases may respond to systemic treatment, intralesional chemotherapy, surgical excision, and radiotherapy can be beneficial in selected cases.[10] Similarly, photodynamic therapy,[60] local chemotherapy, and immunotherapy[61] can be considered. Afflicted patients should also receive symptomatic therapy. Consultation with an oncologist is imperative.

FINAL THOUGHTS

Given the prevalence of cancer and its propensity to metastasize, clinicians should be aware of the plethora of clinical presentations of cutaneous metastases. Diagnosis of metastases to the skin can inform both the clinician and patient about the failure of the ongoing therapy, the recurrence of previously diagnosed cancer, or even the presence of an undiagnosed malignancy. While the prognosis for affected individuals is generally poor, there are some notable exceptions.

REFERENCES

1. Jemal A, Siegel R, Ward E, Murray T, et al. Cancer statistics, 2006. *CA Cancer J Clin*. 2006;56:106–130.
2. Hyde JN. Disseminated lenticular cancer of the skin: "cancer en cuirasse." *Am J Med Sci*. 1892;103:235–245.
3. Paget J. On disease of the mammary areola preceding cancer of the mammary gland. *St Bartholomew's Hosp Rep*. 1874;10:87–89.
4. Hutchinson J. Notes from congresses and continental hospitals: erythema-scirrhus of the skin in association with cancer of the breast. *Arch Surg (London)*. 1893;4:220–222.
5. Crocker HR. *Diseases of the Skin: Their Description, Pathology, Diagnosis, and Treatment with Special Reference to the Skin Eruptions of Children*. 2nd ed. Philadelphia, PA: Blakiston; 1893:658–660.
6. Parkes Weber F. Bilateral thoracic zosteroid spreading marginate telangiectasia—probably a variety of "carcinoma erysipelatodes" (C. Rasch)—associated with unilateral mammary carcinoma, and better termed "carcinoma telangiectaticum." *Br J Dermatol Syphilol*. 1933;45:418–423.
7. Kaufmann-Wolf M. Klinische und histologische Beobachtungen bei Hautmetastasen im Anschluss an Karzinon innerer Organe.

Arch Dermatol Syphilol (Wien). 1913;114:709–744.
8. Suzuki N. Multiple skin metastases from cancer of internal organs. *J Cancer Res*. 1918;3:357–388.
9. Brodland DG, Zitelli JA. Mechanisms of metastases. *J Am Acad Dermatol*. 1992;27:1–10.
10. Schwartz RA. Cutaneous metastatic disease. *J Am Acad Dermatol*. 1995;33:161–182.
11. Gates O. Cutaneous metastases of malignant disease. *Am J Cancer*. 1937;30:718–730.
12. Abrams HL, Siro R, Goldstein N. Metastases in carcinoma: analysis of 1000 autopsied cases. *Cancer*. 1950;3:74–85.
13. Enticknap JB. An analysis of 1000 cases of cancer with special reference to metastasis. *Guy's Hosp Rep*. 1952;101:273–279.
14. Reingold IM. Cutaneous metastases from internal carcinoma. *Cancer*. 1966 Feb;19(2):162–168.
15. McWhorter JE, Cloud AW. Malignant tumors and their metastases: a summary of the necropsies on eight hundred sixty-five cases performed at the Bellevue Hospital of New York. *Am Surg*. 1930;92:434–443.
16. Spencer PS, Helm TN. Skin metastases in cancer patients. *Cutis*. 1987;39:119–121.
17. Lookingbill DP, Spangler N, Sexton FM. Skin involvement as the presenting sign of internal carcinoma. A retrospective study of 7316 cancer patients. *J Am Acad Dermatol*. 1990;22:19–26.
18. Brownstein MH, Helwig EB. Patterns of cutaneous metastasis. *Arch Dermatol*. 1972;105:862–868.
19. Sgambati SA, Barrows GH. Cutaneous metastases of colon carcinoma: a case report. *Conn Med*. 1993;57:665–667.
20. Bansal R, Naik R. A study of 70 cases of cutaneous metastases from internal carcinoma. *J Indian Med Assoc*. 1998;96:10–12.
21. Rosen T. Cutaneous metastases. *Med Clin North Am*. 1980;64:885–900.
22. Peterson JL, McMartin SL. Metasatic renal-cell carcinoma presenting as a cutaneous horn. *J Dermatol Surg Oncol*. 1983;9:815–818.
23. Cotton DWK, Fairris GM. Metasatic breast carcinoma on the lip: case report. *Dermatologica*. 1985;171:362–365.
24. Hager CM, Cohen PR. Cutaneous lesions of metastatic visceral malignancy mimicking pyogenic granuloma. *Cancer Invest*. 1999;17:385–390.
25. Taylor GW, Meltzer A. Inflammatory carcinoma of the breast. *Am J Cancer*. 1938;33:33–49.
26. Cianfrani T, Smith JS. Inflammatory diffuse cutaneous metastatic carcinoma from epidermal carcinoma of the vulva. *Obstet Gynecol*. 1956;8:500–503.
27. Edelstein JM. Pancreatic carcinoma with unusual metastasis to the skin and subcutaneous tissue stimulating cellulitis. *N Engl J Med*. 1950;242:779–781.
28. Harvey G, Cocharane T. Carcinoma en cuirasses: primary lesion in the stomach. *Arch Dermatol*. 1950;62:651–654.
29. Hazelrigg DE, Rudolph AH. Inflammatory metastatic carcinoma: carcinoma erysipelatoides. *Arch Dermatol*. 1977;113:69–70.
30. Ingram JT. Carcinoma erysipelatoides and carcinoma telangiectaticum. *Arch Dermatol*. 1938;77:227–231.

31. Reuter MJ, Nomland R. Inflammatory cutaneous metastatic carcinoma. *Wisc Med.* 1941;40:196–201.

32. Urbach E, Waldow I, Stamm C. Diffuse cutaneous metastatic lesions from an ovarian carcinoma. *Arch Dermatol Syphilol.* 1941;43:962–970.

33. Flynn VT, Spurrett BR. Sister Joseph's nodule. *Med J Aust.* 1969;1:728–730.

34. Brownstein MH, Helwig EB. Spread of tumors to the skin. *Arch Dermatol.* 1973; 107:80–86.

35. Cohen PR. Metastatic tumors to the nail unit: subungual metastases. *Dermatol Surg.* 2001;27:280–293.

36. Ask-Upmark E. On the location of malignant metastases with special regard to the behavior of the primary malignant tumors of the lung. *Acta Pathol Microbiol Scand.* 1932;9:239–248.

37. Brady LW, O'Neill EA, Farber SH. Unusual sites of metastases. *Semin Oncol.* 1977;4:59–64.

38. Weitzner S. Cutanoeus metastasis confined to the scrotum. *Rocky Mountain Med J.* 1970;67:40–42.

39. Proffer LH, Czarnik KL, Sartori CR. Colon carcinoma cutis: a case report. *Cutis.* 1999;63:301–302.

40. Saeed S, Keehn CA, Morgan MB. Cutaneous metastasis: a clinical, pathological, and immunohistochemical appraisal. *J Cutan Pathol.* 2004;31:419–430.

41. Galvan VG. Sister Mary Joseph's nodule. *Ann Int Med.* 1998;128:410.

42. Lee M, Duke E, Munoz J, Holaday L. Colorectal cancer presenting with a cutaneous metastatic lesion on the scalp. *Cutis.* 1995;55:37–38.

43. Luh JY, Han ES, Simmons JR, Whitehead RP. Poorly differentiated colon carcinoma with neuroendocrine features presenting with hypercalcemia and cutaneous metastases. *Am J Clin Oncol.* 2002;25:160–163.

44. Gmitter TL, Dhawan SS, Phillips MG, Wiszniak J. Cutaneous metastases of colonic adenocarcinoma. *Cutis.* 1990 July;46(1):66–68.

45. Wiener K. Skin manifestations of internal disorders (dermadromes). St. Louis, MO: CV Mosby; 1947:565–569.

46. Mueller TJ, Wu H, Greenberg RE, et al. Cutaneous metastases from genitourinary malignancies. *Urology.* 2004;63:1021–1026.

47. Menter A, Boyd AS, McCaffree DM. Recurrent renal cell carcinoma presenting as skin nodules: two case reports and review of the literature. *Cutis.* 1989;44:305–308.

48. Terashima T, Kanazawa M. Lung cancer with skin metastsis. *Chest.* 1994;106: 1448–1450.

49. Lucas FV, Perez-Mesa C. Inflammatory carcinoma of the breast. *Cancer.* 1978;41:1595–1605.

50. Bozzetti F, Saccozzi R, DeLena M, et al. Inflammatory cancer of the breast: analysis of 114 cases. *J Surg Oncol.* 1981;18: 355–361.

51. Dauplat J, Hacker NF, Nieberg RK, et al. Distant metastases in epithelial ovarian carcinoma. *Cancer.* 1987;60:1561–1566.

52. Su WPD, Buechner SA, Li C-Y. Clinicopathologic correlations in leukemia cutis. *J Am Acad Dermatol.* 1984;11:121–128.

53. Willemze R, Kaudewitz P, Berti E, et al. Primary CD30 (Ki-1) positive large cell lymphomas: definition and differential diagnostic aspects. In: Lambert WC,

Giannotti B, van Vloten WA, eds. *Basic Mechanisms of Physiologic and Aberrant Lymphoproliferation in the Skin.* New York: Plenum Press; 1994:265–273.

54. Santucci M, Pimpinelli N. Cutaneous B-cell lymphoma: a SALT-related tumor? In: Lambert WC, Giannotti B, van Vloten WA, eds. *Basic Mechanisms of Physiologic and Aberrant Lymphoproliferation in the Skin.* New York: Plenum Press; 1994:301–315.

55. Rijlaarsdam U, Bakels V, van Oostveen JW, et al. Changing concepts in cutaneous pseudo-B-cell lymphomas and their relationship to cutaneous B-cell lymphomas. In: Lambert WC, Giannotti B, van Vloten WA, eds. *Basic Mechanisms of Physiologic and Aberrant Lymphoproliferation in the Skin.* New York: Plenum Press; 1994:355–361.

56. Kanitakis J. Les metastases cutanees des cancers profonds. *Presse Med.* 1993;22: 631–636.

57. Cosnow I, Fretzin DF. Choriocarcinoma metatatic to skin. *Arch Dermatol.* 1974; 109:551–553.

58. Holland JM. Cancer of the kidney: natural history and staging. *Cancer.* 1973;32: 1030–1042.

59. Lumpkin LR III, Tschen JA. Renal cell carcinoma metastatic to skin. *Cutis.* 1984;34: 143–144.

60. Cairnduff F, Stringer MR, Hudson EJ, et al. Superficial photodynamic therapy with topical 5-aminolaevulinic acid for superficial primary and secondary skin cancer. *Br J Cancer.* 1994;69:605–608.

61. Klein E, Schwartz RA, Solomon J, et al. Accessible tumors. In: LoBuglio AF, ed. *Clinical Immunotherapy.* New York: Marcel Dekker; 1980:31–71.

CHAPTER 28

Skin Cancer in Transplant Patients

John A. Carucci, M.D., Ph.D.

BOX 28-1 Overview

- SCC is more common in transplant recipients, and has higher morbidity and mortality in this group of patients.
- The aggressive nature of SCC in transplant patients is due to a number of factors including UV exposure, HPV infection, and antirejection drugs.
- Immune suppressive medications play both direct and indirect roles in aggressive carcinogenesis in transplant patients.
- Treatment options include Mohs' surgery, standard excision, oral retinoids, and in some cases, modified immune suppressive medications.
- Transplant patients are predisposed to higher rates of recurrence and metastasis, and must be followed more frequently for relapse.

INTRODUCTION

Squamous cell carcinoma (SCC) is the second most common human cancer with over 300,000 cases expected in the United States in 2007.[1] While prognosis is favorable for most cases of primary cutaneous SCC, there is a subset of patients in whom SCC can become catastrophic and in whom the consequences of skin cancer may be devastating. Catastrophic outcome following primary nonmelanoma skin cancer is most often seen in transplant recipients. Iatrogenic immunosuppression after solid organ transplantation was identified as a risk factor for aggressive cutaneous SCC by Rowe et al.[2] Many subsequent studies have supported that skin cancers occur more frequently and with potentially devastating results in organ transplant recipients.[3]

Currently, over 92,000 patients are awaiting transplantation. Over 25,000 organ transplantations were performed in the United States in 2005, with nearly 7000 performed in the first quarter of 2006.[4] Patients' survival continues to increase after organ transplant, as does graft survival, with the half-life of kidney

grafts doubling over the last 25 years.[5,6] Survival rates are increasing for all transplants, and with increased longevity comes an increased incidence of aggressive skin cancer (Fig. 28-1).

In this chapter, the etiology, pathogenesis, and treatment options for SCC solid organ transplant recipients will be discussed.

EPIDEMIOLOGY

BOX 28-2 Summary

- Transplant patients are at a 65-fold increased risk to develop cutaneous SCC.

- Risk for SCC correlates with age, time since transplant, fair skin, and long-term immune suppression.

Transplant recipients are at significantly increased risk for developing skin cancers, particularly SCC. SCC is a cause of significant morbidity and even mortality in transplant patients. In general, as many as 40 to 70% of transplant patients may eventually develop skin cancer with increased rates of SCC compared with basal cell carcinoma (BCC).[7] A series of 5356 consecutive patients receiving organ transplants between 1970 and 1994 was reviewed by Lindelof et al.[8]

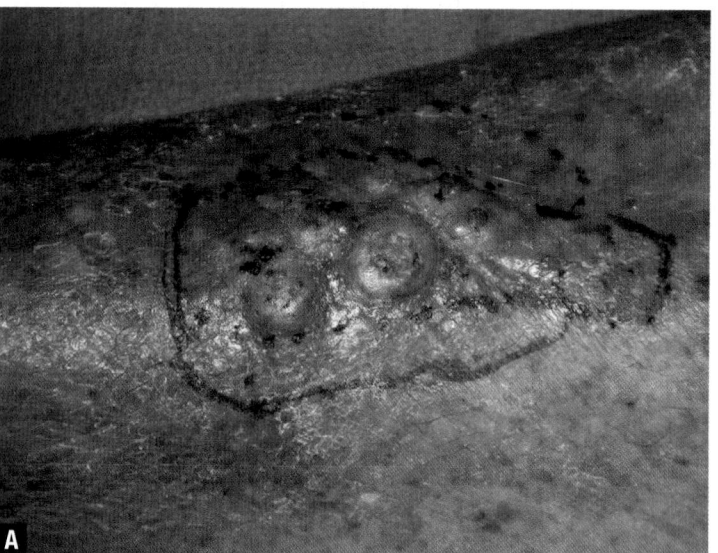

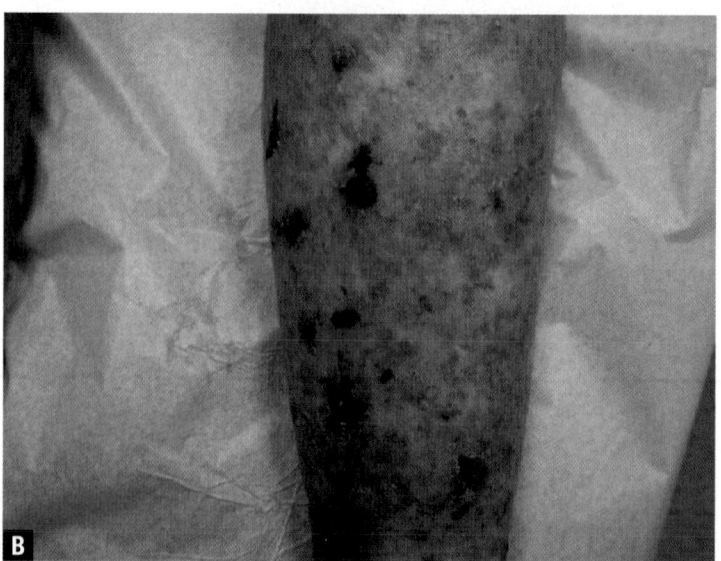

▲ **FIGURE 28-1 A.** Aggressive recurrent skin cancer in a transplant patient. **B.** Extensive field disease is more common in transplant patients.

They found that 325 nonmelanoma skin cancers excluding BCC occurred in 172 patients. Risk of skin cancer was increased on sun-exposed skin. The relative risk for transplant recipients was 108.6 for men and 92.8 for women. Naldi et al reviewed 1329 transplant patients (1062 kidney and 267 heart), and showed a cumulative incidence of 5.85% at 5 years and 10.8% after 10 years.[9] Age at transplantation and male sex favored the development of skin cancer. In contrast to other studies, there was no difference in risk between kidney and heart transplant recipients. The SCC:BCC ratio was 1:1.1 for heart transplant recipients and 1:2.6 for kidney transplant patients. Jensen et al studied skin cancer in a Norwegian cohort of more than 2500 kidney and heart transplant recipients.[10,11] In this study, transplant recipients had increased risk for cutaneous SCC (65-fold), malignant melanoma (3-fold), and SCC of the lip (20-fold). After adjusting for age, kidney transplant recipients on cyclosporine, azathioprine, and prednisolone had a 2.8-fold increased risk for developing cutaneous SCC relative to those receiving azathioprine and prednisolone without cyclosporine. Heart transplant recipients had an increased risk of developing SCC (2.9-fold) compared with kidney transplant recipients. Increased risk for skin cancer correlated with increased age at transplantation (19.8:1) for patients over age 60 compared with patients under age 60, triple immunosuppression, and in heart transplant recipients (2.9:1) when compared with kidney transplant recipients. There was no correlation between SCC and HLA haplotypes or HLA-B mismatch in recipients.

In 1999, Ong et al reviewed skin cancers in 455 heart transplant patients in Australia and found a cumulative incidence of 31% at 5 years and 43% at 10 years.[12] In this study, skin cancer accounted for 27% of 41 deaths after the fourth year following transplantation. Fair skin, increased age at transplant, increased length of time after transplant, and HLA-DR homozygosity were associated with skin cancer. HLA-DR7, HLA-A1, and HLA-A11 seemed to be protective. SCCs were the most common cancers in this group outnumbering BCCs by a ratio of 3:1. The development of aggressive cutaneous malignancy after cardiothoracic transplant (CTT) was addressed by Veness et al in a study of 619 patients who received heart, lung, or heart–lung transplants between 1984 and 1995.[13] In their study, aggressive cutaneous malignancy defined as locally invasive SCC, poorly differentiated SCC, regionally metastatic SCC, recurrent SCC, or malignant melanoma was seen in 27 of 66 (~41%) patients diagnosed with a major malignancy. Out of 27 patients, 13 died, of which 10 deaths (37%) were attributable to metastases. Metastases or residual disease was noted in 11 of 19 patients (57.8%) with aggressive SCC, with a mean time to death of 20 months.

In a study by Lampros et al, 248 heart transplant patients were followed between 1985 and 1996.[14] Forty-one patients (17%) developed 192 SCCs or BCCs. SCC accounted for ~90% of the skin malignancies with a SCC:BCC ratio of 8.6:1. Cumulative risk of skin cancer increased with time and with use of OKT3. Risk factors included male sex (19.5:1), fair skin (59% of patients), and blue eyes (59% of patients). In this study, two patients (4.8%) developed metastases from primary cutaneous SCC. Euvrard et al reviewed the development of skin cancer in 580 kidney and 150 heart transplant patients.[15] They found a twofold increase in premalignant and malignant lesions in heart transplant patients compared with kidney transplant patients. In this study, heart transplant patients were older at transplantation, received more intense immunosuppression, and had a shorter delay from transplantation to development of the first lesion. The SCC:BCC ratio was 2.37:1 in kidney and 1.08:1 in heart transplant recipients.

In a study of heart transplant patients from Spain by Espana et al, skin cancer was diagnosed in 14 of 92 patients between 1984 and 1993.[16] The risk for skin cancer rose from 4.8% in the first year after transplantation, to 43.8% at 7 years. Skin cancers occurred primarily in patients with skin types II and III. The SCC:BCC ratio was 1.3:1. Out of 14 patients, 4 developed SCC of the lip and 1 died of metastatic disease.

There was no association with haplotype HLA-A3, HLAA11, HLA-DR, and mismatches for HLA-B. In one large series by Levy et al, liver transplant recipients showed a 4.5% incidence of malignancy with a 1.6% mortality rate.[17] The incidence of skin cancer was 1.6% with one metastatic SCC.

In a study by Frezza et al, 50 of 1657 adult patients undergoing liver transplantation developed tumors.[18] Skin cancers were most common with the following distribution: BCC (25%), SCC (20.3%), Bowen's (6.2%), and melanoma (6.2%). A higher incidence of overall tumors was observed in patients treated with cyclosporine as opposed to tacrolimus.

PATHOGENESIS

BOX 28-3 Summary

- Immune suppressive agents including calcineuin inhibitors may have direct carcinogenic effects.
- HPV is more prevalent in transplant-associated SCC, and may accelerate carcinogenesis via proteins E6 and E7.

Immunosuppression

Immunosuppression is a key to preventing graft rejection and optimizing graft survival. However, most immunosuppressive regimens have been associated with increased rates of cancer, particularly skin cancer. There remains debate as to which particular agent brings with it the highest risk of increased incidence of cancer. Calcineurin inhibitors, including cyclosporin, remain a mainstay of posttransplant regimens, and may contribute accelerated development of skin cancer through nonimmune-mediated mechanisms.

Cyclosporine inhibits IL-2 transcription and, thus, inhibits T cell function.[19,20] Animal studies support direct carcinogenesis by cyclosporine. In one study, cyclosporine was associated with tumor growth in SCID mice.[21] Since these mice were without functioning immune systems, a direct carcinogenic mechanism was supported. The carcinogenic effects of cyclosporine were blocked by antibody against transforming growth factor beta (TGF-β), implicating TGF-β in cyclosporine-induced carcinogenesis. Cyclosporine has been shown to enhance invasive tumors in vitro and to promote the growth of transplanted UV-induced tumors in mice.[22]

Yarosh et al showed that cyclosporine inhibited removal of cyclobutane dimers and UV-mediated apoptosis.[23] Takahashi and Kamimura demonstrated that cyclosporine enhanced proliferation of murine epidermal keratinocytes over a wide range of doses.[24] Das et al further demonstrated a twofold increase in keratinocyte growth factor attributable to cyclosporine.[25,26]

In contrast, Karashima et al[27] reported cell cycle blockade by cyclosporine in cultured human keratinocytes. They found that cyclosporine inhibited keratinocyte proliferation induced by EGF, TGF-α, or IL-6. The antiproliferative effects of cyclosporine directly correlated with the blockade of the keratinocyte cell cycle at the G0/G1 phases. These findings might indicate that the effects of FK506 and cyclosporine on proliferation of cultured normal human keratinocytes are probably related to direct effects on growth regulation of keratinocytes via EGF, TGF-α, or IL-6 stimulation.

Santini et al showed that the treatment of primary mouse keratinocytes with cyclosporine suppressed the expression of terminal differentiation markers p21 (WAF1/Cip1) and p27 (KIP1).[28] In parallel, with down-modulation of the endogenous genes, suppression of calcineurin function blocks induction of the promoters for the p21 (WAF1/Cip1) and loricrin differentiation marker genes, whereas, activity of these promoters is enhanced by calcineurin overexpression.

Human Papillomavirus

The role of human papillomavirus (HPV) in the development of skin cancer has been described.[29–31] HPV types 6, 11, 16, and 18 have been associated with cervical cancers, while HPV types 5 and 8 associated with epidermodysplasia verruciformis (EDV).[32,33] HPV 16 has been implicated in digital SCC.[34] HPV 16 and 18 have been associated with E6 and E7, which inhibit tumor suppressor p53.[30] In addition, it has been shown that E6 may inhibit UV-induced apoptosis by a p53-independent mechanism, thus acting as a p53-independent tumor promoter by allowing propagation of atypical keratinocytes. Furthermore, it has been shown that EDV-associated HPV types are found in SCCs from transplant recipients.[35]

In a large study by Euvrard et al, warts, actinic keratoses (AKs), and SCCs from renal transplant recipients were examined for the presence of HPV types 1a, 2a, 5, 16, and 18.[36] Overall, HPV DNA was detected in 44 of 86 specimens, including 14 of 17 warts, 4 of 17 AKs, and 14 of 30 SCC. Benign types 1 and 2 were detected in five SCC.

MANAGEMENT OF SQUAMOUS CELL CARCINOMA IN TRANSPLANT RECIPIENTS

BOX 28-4   Summary

- Mohs' surgery
- Standard excisional surgery with postoperative margin assessment
- Oral retinoids
- Reduction of immune suppression
- Radiation treatment

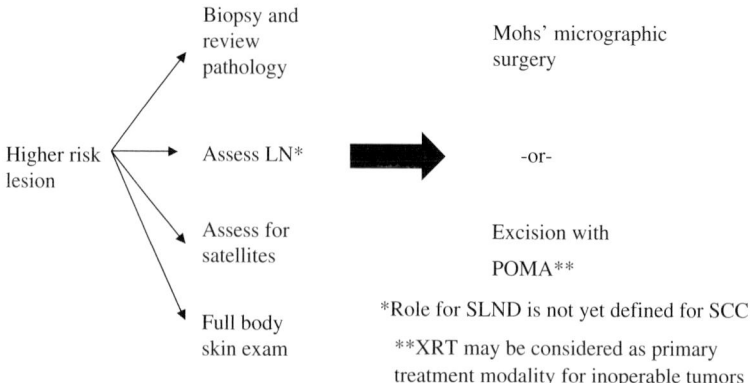

Management of otherwise uncomplicated higher risk cutaneous SCC in OTRs

Higher risk lesion → Biopsy and review pathology

→ Assess LN*

→ Assess for satellites

→ Full body skin exam

→ Mohs' micrographic surgery

-or-

Excision with POMA**

*Role for SLND is not yet defined for SCC

**XRT may be considered as primary treatment modality for inoperable tumors

▲ **FIGURE 28-2** Management of highest risk SCC in transplant patients.

It is crucial to remember that SCC in an immune-suppressed transplant recipient is considered to be a high-risk lesion, as defined by Rowe et al.[2] When managing SCC in a transplant recipient, it is important to differentiate those lesions that are the "highest risk" for recurrence or metastasis. An expert panel from the International Transplant Skin Cancer Collaborative was convened to identify those factors that correlated with highest risk for recurrence and metastasis in transplant recipients.[37] Increased risk was found to be most likely associated with factors including rapid growth, large diameter, location on scalp, aggressive histology, history of local recurrence, and presence of satellite lesions. Careful inspection of the surrounding skin to exclude the presence of satellite lesions is necessary, as is examination of the draining lymph nodes. SCC in organ transplant recipients is managed by standard modalities including Mohs' surgery, standard excision, destruction, and radiation therapy. Other strategies may include the use of retinoids and reduction of immunosuppression. Managing SCC in transplant recipients may also include diagnosis and treatment of in transit, nodal, or distant metastases.[38]

Management of Highest Risk Lesions

Rapidly growing, poorly differentiated, large lesions, and scalp lesions represent considerable risk in transplant recipients.[37] All attempts should be made to obtain a tumor-free plane by Mohs' surgery or standard excision with postoperative margin control. Patients with perineural invasions should be evaluated for postoperative radiation treatment. Patients with highest risk lesions should be followed frequently for local recurrence or development of in-transit metastasis. It is imperative that these patients be reeducated on photoprotection. Management is summarized in Fig. 28-2.

Management of Moderate Risk Lesions

Moderate risk lesions include thin (*in situ*) lesions and well-differentiated superficial lesions located on the trunk and extremities.[37] These lesions may be managed by standard excision or destruction (Fig. 28-3). For patients with hundreds of lesions or with numerous lesions occurring on a background of severe field disease, it may be reasonable to tangentially excise the lesions prior to destruction and hold decisions on further therapy pending histologic confirmation of the superficial nature of the lesion. These patients in particular would likely benefit from adjunctive field treatment, with either topical 5-FU or imiquimod. In one study, SCC *in situ* in five transplant patients was effectively managed by using these agents in combination.[39] In a recent study by Brown et al, skin dysplasia was improved in patients using imiquimod and fewer SCC developed in treated areas.[40] There was no effect on renal function. The treatment area in this study measured 60 cm². Management of moderate risk lesions is summarized in Fig. 28-3.

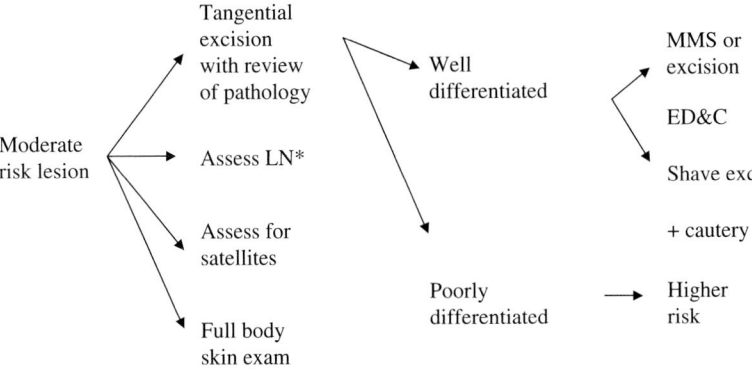

Management of moderate risk
cutaneous SCC in OTRs

▲ FIGURE 28-3 Management of moderate risk SCC in transplant patients.

Management of In-Transit Metastatic SCC

In some cases of SCC, satellite lesions appear either with the primary lesion or as recurrent disease.[3,7,38] These lesions are usually clinically nondescript subcutaneous papules that are histologically similar to the primary lesion but are not contiguous with it (Fig. 28-4). The presence of in-transit metastatic disease is a poor prognostic indicator and represents a therapeutic challenge. In one study, in-transit metastases from primary cutaneous SCC resulted in 33% mortality at 2 years.[38] Management of in-transit metastasis is usually multidisciplinary by nature and must proceed on a case-by-case basis.

The following should be considered in the approach to in-transit metastases: (1) complete examination, and work up to exclude nodal and distant metastases; (2) excision of the lesion where feasible; (3) wide field adjunctive radiation therapy; (4) alteration of immune suppression; and (5) oral retinoids. Management is summarized in Fig. 28-5.

Oral Retinoids in Transplant Recipients

Retinoids have been used as chemoprophylaxis against skin cancers in transplant patients. Previous studies favor the use of acitretin over isotretinoin due to a better side effect profile. The first report of acitretin chemoprophylaxis was by

Vandeghinste et al, who reported the cessation of new dysplastic skin lesions during acitretin treatment.[41] Since that time, several series and controlled studies have been published.[42] One patient temporarily discontinued the drug due to side effects. No laboratory abnormalities including hyperlipidemia were observed. Bavinck et al enrolled 44 renal transplant recipients with more than 10 keratotic skin lesions on the hands and forearms into a randomized, double-blind, placebo-controlled trial to evaluate chemoprevention with acitretin (30 mg/day).[43] During the 6-month treatment period, 2 of 19 patients (11%) in the acitretin group reported a total of two new SCCs compared with 9 of 19 patients (47%) in the placebo group who developed a total of 18 new carcinomas. Side effects included dry mucous membranes, mild hair loss, elevated cholesterol, and increased serum triglycerides. Yuan et al treated 15 renal transplant recipients with progressive AKs, widespread warts, or recurrent skin cancers with acitretin (10 to 50 mg/day).[44] A reduction of warts and AKs was seen in all patients while a reduction in the number of skin malignancies was seen in four of six patients treated for 12 months or more. Cutaneous side effects were seen in nine patients, while decreased kidney function was not observed in any patient. Most recently, Harwood et al showed the effectiveness of low-dose retinoids in chemoprophylaxis.[45] In a 16-year retrospective study, 28 renal transplant recipients were treated for at least 12 months at doses ranging from 0.2 to 0.4 mg/kg. The results showed a reduction in the number of posttreatment SCCs. They also showed that an interruption in the treatment lead to return to pretreatment rates of development of SCCs.

Reduction of Immunosuppression

Reduction of immunosuppressive therapy may be considered in cases of severe life-threatening skin cancer.[46] In one study of six patients in whom skin immunosuppressive therapy was discontinued, four patients experienced decreased development of skin cancers.[47] Moloney et al reported increased metastasis-free survival in nine renal transplant recipients with aggressive disease in whom immunosuppression was reduced.[48] In a recent consensus study, it was determined that mild reduction would most likely be considered in patients with multiple carcinomas or a single high-risk lesion, while drastic reduction or discontinuation would be reserved for patients

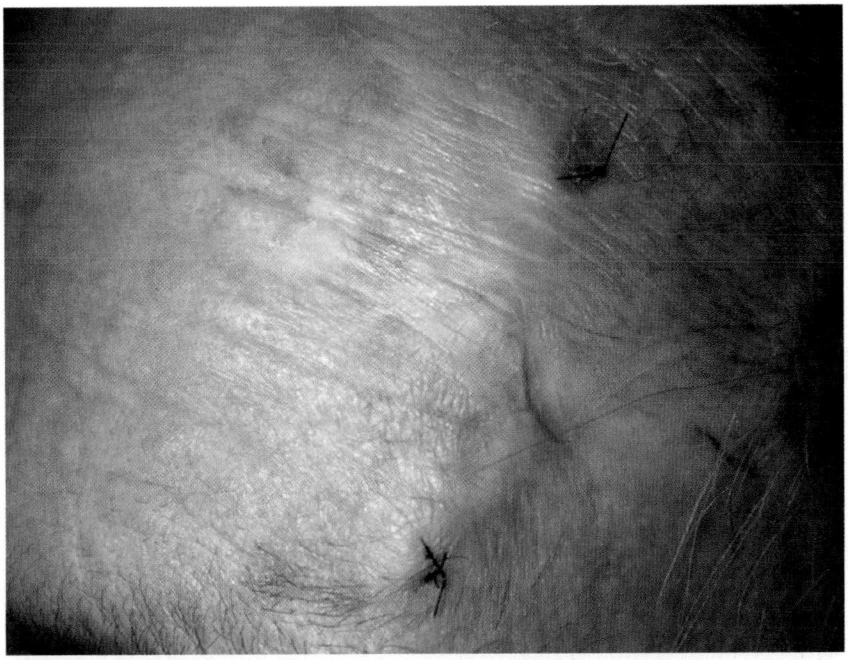

▲ FIGURE 28-4 In-transit metastases form primary cutaneous characteristically present with subcutaneous papule (inferior) or nodules discontiguous form the original site (superior).

Management of in-transit metastatic
SCC in OTRs

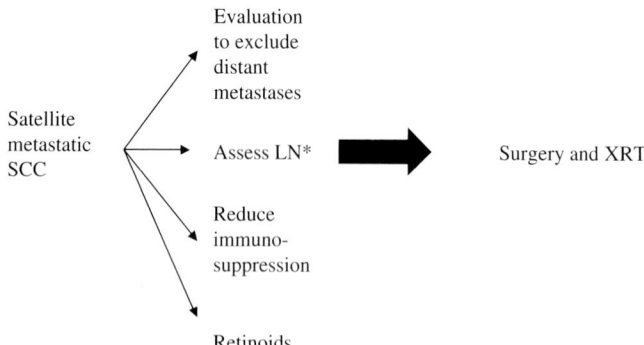

*Role for SLND is not yet defined for SCC

▲ **FIGURE 28-5** Management strategy for in-transit metastatic SCC.

with life-threatening lesions.[46] It must be remembered that reducing immunosuppression may predispose to rejection and, therefore, any decisions regarding alteration of immunosuppression must be reached in cooperation with the primary transplant physician.

Other Skin Cancers in Transplant Patients

BCC is approximately 10-fold more common in transplant recipients, particularly superficial BCC on the trunk and extremities.[7] BCC in this population is thought to be a result of sun exposure as in the general population and less related to immune suppression. However, regression of BCC following withdrawal of immune suppression was recently reported.[49] BCC in transplant patients is best managed by standard therapies including destruction, excision, and Mohs' micrographic surgery.

Melanoma is ~3.4-fold more common in transplant patients.[7] Melanoma in transplant patients should be managed by a complete removal with consideration for sentinel lymph node biopsy where appropriate. In one study, Le Mire et al[50] reported excellent outcomes in 9 of 10 renal transplant recipients with melanoma. In all cases that did not recur, the tumors were <1 mm in Breslow depth. This reinforces the need for early detection in transplant population as well as in the general population.

Other skin cancers may occur and should be treated by standard modalities including excision and Mohs' micrographic surgery. Management decisions should be guided by factors including

location, size, histologic nature, and potential biological aggressiveness of the tumor.

Follow-Up

There are several practical models for providing comprehensive dermatologic care for transplant recipients described by Christensen et al.[51] These include multidisciplinary transplant clinics, designated dermatology transplant subspecialty clinics, and integration of transplant patients into existing dermatology practices. Regardless of the design, an organized and firmly established clinic model facilitates longitudinal care and promotes education, prevention, and early intervention. Transplant recipients usually need more frequent dermatologic follow-up.[7] Patients with multiple or severe life-threatening cancers may need to be followed as frequently as every 1 to 2 months, while those with skin type greater than III or patients with no history of AKs, or skin cancers may be evaluated annually. Follow-up should include evaluation of previously treated areas for signs of recurrence and careful examination of draining lymph nodes.

■ FINAL THOUGHTS

As the number of solid organ transplant patients continues to rise, dermatologists and dermatologic surgeons will be called upon to rationally manage skin cancers in this group of patients. Reduction of the morbidity and potential mortality from skin cancer in this group will require education of both transplant physicians and patients regarding the need for periodic evaluation by a dermatologist.

REFERENCES

1. Halpern AC, Kopp LJ. Awareness, knowledge and attitudes to non-melanoma skin cancer and actinic keratosis among the general public. *Int J Dermatol.* 2005;44: 107–111.
2. Rowe DE, Carroll RJ, Day CL Jr. Prognostic factors for local recurrence, metastasis, and survival rates in squamous cell carcinoma of the skin, ear, and lip. Implications for treatment modality selection. *J Am Acad Dermatol.* 1992;26:976–990.
3. Carucci JA. Squamous cell carcinoma in organ transplant recipients: approach to management. *Skin Therapy Lett.* 2004;9: 5–7.
4. Available at: www.UNOS.org, u.d.
5. Ojo AO, Hanson JA, Wolfe RA, Leichtman AB, Agodoa LY, Port FK. Long-term survival in renal transplant recipients with graft function. *Kidney Int.* 2000;57:307–313.
6. Seikaly M, Ho PL, Emmett L, Tejani A. The 12th Annual Report of the North American Pediatric Renal Transplant Cooperative Study: renal transplantation from 1987 through 1998. *Pediatr Transplant.* 2001;5:215–231.
7. Berg D, Otley CC. Skin cancer in organ transplant recipients: epidemiology, pathogenesis, and management. *J Am Acad Dermatol.* 2002;47:1–17; quiz 18–20.
8. Lindelof B, Dal H, Wolk K, Malmborg N. Cutaneous squamous cell carcinoma in organ transplant recipients: a study of the Swedish cohort with regard to tumor site. *Arch Dermatol.* 2005;141:447–451.
9. Naldi L, Fortina AB, Lovati S, et al. Risk of nonmelanoma skin cancer in Italian organ transplant recipients. A registry-based study. *Transplantation.* 2000;70:1479–1484.
10. Jensen P, Hansen S, Moller B, et al. Skin cancer in kidney and heart transplant recipients and different long-term immunosuppressive therapy regimens. *J Am Acad Dermatol.* 1999;40:177–186.
11. Jensen P, Moller B, Hansen S. Skin cancer in kidney and heart transplant recipients and different long-term immunosuppressive therapy regimens. *J Am Acad Dermatol.* 2000;42:307.
12. Ong CS, Keogh AM, Kossard S, Macdonald PS, Spratt PM. Skin cancer in Australian heart transplant recipients. *J Am Acad Dermatol.* 1999;40:27–34.
13. Veness MJ, Quinn DI, Ong CS, et al. Aggressive cutaneous malignancies following cardiothoracic transplantation: the Australian experience. *Cancer.* 1999;85: 1758–1764.
14. Lampros TD, Cobanoglu A, Parker F, Ratkovec R, Norman DJ, Hershberger R. Squamous and basal cell carcinoma in heart transplant recipients. *J Heart Lung Transplant.* 1998;17:586–591.
15. Euvrard S, Kanitakis J, Pouteil-Noble C, et al. Comparative epidemiologic study of premalignant and malignant epithelial cutaneous lesions developing after kidney and heart transplantation. *J Am Acad Dermatol.* 1995;33:222–229.
16. Espana A, Martinez-Gonzalez MA, Garcia-Granero M, Sanchez-Carpintero I, Rabago G, Herreros J. A prospective study of incident nonmelanoma skin cancer in heart transplant recipients. *J Invest Dermatol.* 2000;115:1158–1160.
17. Levy M, Backman L, Husberg B, et al. De novo malignancy following liver trans-

plantation: a single-center study. *Transplant Proc.* 1993;25:1397–1399.

18. Frezza EE, Fung JJ, van Thiel DH. Non-lymphoid cancer after liver transplantation. *Hepatogastroenterology.* 1997;44:1172–1181.

19. Matsuda S, Koyasu S. Mechanisms of action of cyclosporine. *Immunopharmacology.* 2000;47:119–125.

20. Nickel T, Schlichting CL, Weis M. Drugs modulating endothelial function after transplantation. *Transplantation.* 2006;82:S41–S46.

21. Hojo M, Morimoto T, Maluccio M, et al. Cyclosporine induces cancer progression by a cell-autonomous mechanism. *Nature.* 1999;397:530–534.

22. Sugie N, Fujii N, Danno K. Cyclosporin-A suppresses p53-dependent repair DNA synthesis and apoptosis following ultraviolet-B irradiation. *Photodermatol Photoimmunol Photomed.* 2002;18:163–168.

23. Yarosh DB, Pena AV, Nay SL, Canning MT, Brown DA. Calcineurin inhibitors decrease DNA repair and apoptosis in human keratinocytes following ultraviolet B irradiation. *J Invest Dermatol.* 2005;125:1020–1025.

24. Takahashi T, Kamimura A. Cyclosporin a promotes hair epithelial cell proliferation and modulates protein kinase C expression and translocation in hair epithelial cells. *J Invest Dermatol.* 2001;117:605–611.

25. Das SJ, Newman HN, Olsen I. Keratinocyte growth factor receptor is up-regulated in cyclosporin A-induced gingival hyperplasia. *J Dent Res.* 2002;81:683–687.

26. Das SJ, Parkar MH, Olsen I. Upregulation of keratinocyte growth factor in cyclosporin A-induced gingival overgrowth. *J Periodontol.* 2001;72:745–752.

27. Karashima T, Hachisuka H, Sasai Y. FK506 and cyclosporin A inhibit growth factor-stimulated human keratinocyte proliferation by blocking cells in the G0/G1 phases of the cell cycle. *J Dermatol Sci.* 1996;12:246–254.

28. Santini MP, Talora C, Seki T, Bolgan L, Dotto GP. Cross talk among calcineurin, Sp1/Sp3, and NFAT in control of p21 (WAF1/CIP1) expression in keratinocyte differentiation. *Proc Natl Acad Sci USA.* 2001;98:9575–9580.

29. Cassarino DS, Derienzo DP, Barr RJ. Cutaneous squamous cell carcinoma: a comprehensive clinicopathologic classification—part two. *J Cutan Pathol.* 2006;33:261–279.

30. Dang C, Koehler A, Forschner T, et al. E6/E7 expression of human papillomavirus types in cutaneous squamous cell dysplasia and carcinoma in immunosuppressed organ transplant recipients. *Br J Dermatol.* 2006;155:129–136.

31. Karagas MR, Nelson HH, Sehr P, et al. Human papillomavirus infection and incidence of squamous cell and basal cell carcinomas of the skin. *J Natl Cancer Inst.* 2006;98:389–395.

32. Guilhou JJ, Malbos S, Barneon S, Habib A, Baldet P, Meynadier J. Epidermodysplasia verruciformis (2 cases) Immunological study [author's translation]. *Ann Dermatol Venereol.* 1980;107:611–619.

33. Matsukura T, Sugase M. Human papillomavirus genomes in squamous cell carcinomas of the uterine cervix. *Virology.* 2004;324:439–449.

34. Alam M, Caldwell JB, Eliezri YD. Human papillomavirus-associated digital squamous cell carcinoma: literature review and report of 21 new cases. *J Am Acad Dermatol.* 2003;48:385–393.

35. Stockfleth E, Nindl I, Sterry W, Ulrich C, Schmook T, Meyer T. Human papillomaviruses in transplant-associated skin cancers. *Dermatol Surg.* 2004;30:604–609.

36. Euvrard S, Chardonnet Y, Pouteil-Noble C, et al. Association of skin malignancies with various and multiple carcinogenic and noncarcinogenic human papillomaviruses in renal transplant recipients. *Cancer.* 1993;72:2198–2206.

37. Stasko T, Brown MD, Carucci JA, et al. Guidelines for the management of squamous cell carcinoma in organ transplant recipients. *Dermatol Surg.* 2004;30:642–650.

38. Carucci JA, Martinez JC, Zeitouni NC, et al. In-transit metastasis from primary cutaneous squamous cell carcinoma in organ transplant recipients and nonimmunosuppressed patients: clinical characteristics, management, and outcome in a series of 21 patients. *Dermatol Surg.* 2004;30:651–655.

39. Smith KJ, Germain M, Skelton H. Squamous cell carcinoma in situ (Bowen's disease) in renal transplant patients treated with 5% imiquimod and 5% 5-fluorouracil therapy. *Dermatol Surg.* 2001;27:561–564.

40. Brown VL, Atkins CL, Ghali L, Cerio R, Harwood CA, Proby CM. Safety and efficacy of 5% imiquimod cream for the treatment of skin dysplasia in high-risk renal transplant recipients: randomized, double-blind, placebo-controlled trial. *Arch Dermatol.* 2005;141:985–993.

41. Vandeghinste N, De Bersaques J, Geerts ML, Kint A. Acitretin as cancer chemoprophylaxis in a renal transplant recipient. *Dermatology.* 1992;185:307–308.

42. McNamara IR, Muir J, Galbraith AJ. Acitretin for prophylaxis of cutaneous malignancies after cardiac transplantation. *J Heart Lung Transplant.* 2002;21:1201–1205.

43. Bavinck JN, Tieben LM, Van der Woude FJ, et al. Prevention of skin cancer and reduction of keratotic skin lesions during acitretin therapy in renal transplant recipients: a double-blind, placebo-controlled study. *J Clin Oncol.* 1995;13:1933–1938.

44. Yuan ZF, Davis A, Macdonald K, Bailey RR. Use of acitretin for the skin complications in renal transplant recipients. *N Z Med J.* 1995;108:255–256.

45. Harwood CA, Leedham-Green M, Leigh IM, Proby CM. Low-dose retinoids in the prevention of cutaneous squamous cell carcinomas in organ transplant recipients: a 16-year retrospective study. *Arch Dermatol.* 2005;141:456–464.

46. Otley CC, Berg D, Ulrich C, et al. Reduction of immunosuppression for transplant-associated skin cancer: expert consensus survey. *Br J Dermatol.* 2006;154:395–400.

47. Otley CC, Coldiron BM, Stasko T, Goldman GD. Decreased skin cancer after cessation of therapy with transplant-associated immunosuppressants. *Arch Dermatol.* 2001;137:459–463.

48. Moloney FJ, Kelly PO, Kay EW, Conlon P, Murphy GM. Maintenance versus reduction of immunosuppression in renal transplant recipients with aggressive squamous cell carcinoma. *Dermatol Surg.* 2004;30:674–678.

49. Rawlins J, Platt A, Gowda, P. Regression of BCC following immune suppression withdrawal in a renal transplant recipient. *Clin Exp Dermatol.* 2006;31(5):717–718.

50. Le Mire L, Hollowood K, Gray D, Bordea C, Wojnarowska F. Melanomas in renal transplant patients. *Br J Dermatol.* 2006;154(3):472–477.

51. Christenson LJ, Geusau A, Ferrandiz C, et al. Specialty clinics for the dermatologic care of solid-organ transplant recipients. *Dermatol Surg.* 2004;30:598–603.

CHAPTER 29

Skin Cancers in HIV Patients

Julie K. Karen, M.D.
Miguel R. Sanchez, M.D.

SKIN CANCER

BOX 29-1   Overview

- Both the incidence and clinical course of cutaneous malignancies are altered in the context of HIV infection.
- The mechanisms responsible for the observed increased rate of cancer in persons with HIV are poorly understood; however, such features as impaired cell-mediated immunity, increased susceptibility to certain oncogenic viruses, preferential expression of TH_2 cytokines, and the presence of HIV proteins known to promote oncogenesis are thought to contribute.
- Epidemic Kaposi sarcoma (KS) remains the most common cancer associated with HIV infection in the United States despite dramatically declining incidence rates since the advent of HAART.
- In HIV-infected persons, lymphohematopoietic malignancies occur in great excess. These malignancies are typically more aggressive, diagnosed at more advanced stages, respond less favorably to treatment, and are classically of T-cell phenotype.
- Malignant melanoma appears to occur with an increased frequency, at an earlier age, and behaves more aggressively in HIV-infected persons than in the general population.
- The risk of nonmelanoma skin cancers is approximately three- to fivefold elevated among patients with AIDS relative to the general population.
- Bowenoid papulosis, generally regarded as a transitional state between condyloma and Bowen's disease that is induced by oncogenic HPV, occurs in excess in HIV-seropositive individuals.
- Anal carcinoma and its precursor lesions are associated with infection with certain oncogenic HPV subtypes, and occur with great excess among HIV-infected individuals. These lesions are oftentimes asymptomatic, but may manifest as pruritic, bleeding, or painful, perianal masses.
- In HIV-infected patients, sebaceous carcinoma may deviate from its classic presentation, and present in extraocular locations or achieve unusually large size.

- Guidelines for prevention and management of each of these malignancies should be tailored to the particular needs of the HIV-infected population.

INTRODUCTION

BOX 29-2   Summary

- Both the incidence and clinical course of cutaneous malignancies are altered in the context of HIV infection.
- Despite some gains, the advent of HAART has not normalized the excess rate of malignancy in HIV-seropositive individuals.
- The clinical findings and course of cutaneous malignancies in HIV-positive patients may differ markedly from those seen in the general population.
- Several cutaneous malignancies tend to behave more aggressively in the context of HIV-induced immunosuppression.

The immune suppression that results from infection with the human immunodeficiency virus (HIV) appears to alter both the incidence and clinical course of several malignant neoplasms. The mechanisms behind this altered behavior remain poorly understood. Notably, certain cancers, such as Kaposi sarcoma (KS), primary central nervous system lymphoma, non-Hodgkin lymphoma (NHL), and invasive cervical cancer, occur at such increased rates among HIV-infected persons that these malignancies are termed "AIDS-defining." Other non-AIDS-defining malignancies that occur more frequently in the setting of HIV infection include anal carcinoma, nonmelanoma skin cancer, and lung cancer, among others.

The emergence of two novel classes of antiretroviral agents in the past decade led to the introduction of combination highly active antiretroviral therapy (HAART). The availability of this treatment regimen has resulted in dramatic decreases in HIV-related morbidity and mortality, as well as striking declines in the incidences of two AIDS-defining malignancies, KS and NHL. On the other hand, the impact of HAART on the epidemiology and outcome of other cancer types and sites remains unclear.[1]

Several malignancies known to occur more commonly in HIV-infected individuals involve the skin. Additionally,

the physical findings and course of these neoplasms may be different from those observed in the general population. Thus, it is imperative for dermatologists to be aware of the diverse presentations, course, and management of cutaneous cancers in the context of HIV.

MECHANISMS OF INCREASED RISK

BOX 29-3   Summary

- The precise mechanisms responsible for the increased risk of malignancy in HIV-seropositive persons are ill-defined.
- HIV-associated immune dysfunction is characterized by impaired cell-mediated immune (CMI) responses, increased susceptibility to certain oncogenic viruses, and preferential expression of TH_2 cytokines, all of which likely contribute to the observed increased risk.
- Certain viral proteins, such as tat and nef, are suspected to favor oncogenesis, and thus, further contribute to the increased risk of malignancy in this population.

The mechanisms responsible for the observed increased risk of cancer in persons with HIV are poorly understood. The characteristic immune dysfunction associated with HIV infection consists of impairment of cell-mediated immune (CMI) responses coupled with a predominance of humoral responses. Specifically, HIV infection causes progressive depletion of CD4+ lymphocytes, a key player in CMI responses. The availability of HAART has dramatically extended the life expectancy of this population, despite the persistence of low-grade CD4-lymphopenia. Impaired CMI response is known to be a feature of many malignancies in immunocompetent individuals, and is generally considered to be responsible for the increased risk of malignancy in the HIV-seropositive population.[2,3]

During HIV infection, shifts in cytokine profile expression lead to preferential expression of T_H2 cytokines (IL-4, IL-5, IL-6, and IL-10). Whereas T_H1 (or CMI-associated) cytokines are antiangiogenic, T_H2 cytokines promote angiogenesis. Additionally, these cytokines are associated with decreased apoptosis and abet HIV proliferation, immune evasion, and transcription of certain oncogenes. Malignant disease flourishes in

392

this environment of suppressed CMI, increased angiogenesis, and reduced apoptosis.[2]

Furthermore, certain HIV proteins may promote oncogenesis. Though a comprehensive discussion of these mechanisms is beyond the scope of this chapter, we will briefly review the proposed mechanisms by which two viral proteins, tat and nef, are suspected to favor oncogenesis. Upon release by HIV-infected cells, tat enters uninfected cells. Tat regulates expression of cytokines, chemokine receptors, and cellular proliferation genes, thereby promoting inappropriate angiogenesis. Additionally, tat induces the expression of heterologous viral promoters, thereby facilitating the development of opportunistic infections with potentially oncogenic viruses. In mice, anti-tat antibodies inhibit the formation of KS-like lesions, corroborating a pathogenic role for this protein in the development of this malignancy.[4] Another HIV protein, nef, decreases cell-surface expression of major histocompatibility complex class 1 (MHC-1). This, in turn, hinders the detection of altered self-cells.[5]

Observed increased rates of certain cancers without established links to immunosuppression in persons living with HIV are likely attributable to HIV-unrelated exposures such as smoking, which is common among this population.[5] Several cohort studies evaluating HIV-associated malignancy have failed to find an increased risk for certain age-related cancers (i.e., colon, breast, and prostate).[6] This finding suggests that immune surveillance does not play a role in eliminating the genetically altered cells that represent the precursors of these cancers.

EPIDEMIC KAPOSI SARCOMA

BOX 29-4 Summary

- In the United States, epidemic KS remains the most common cancer associated with HIV infection.
- The advent of HAART has dramatically decreased the prevalence of KS.
- HHV-8, a gamma herpesvirus, is the causative agent of KS.
- Clinically, KS manifests with nontender, violaceous, mucocutaneous lesions that may ulcerate.
- Visceral involvement most commonly involves the lymphatics and gastrointestinal tract.
- Multiple therapeutic options exist and should be selected based on the response

of the tumors to antiretroviral agents, the aggressiveness of the lesions, the degree of immunosuppression, extent of KS involvement, and the presence of concurrent morbidities.

Epidemiology

An outbreak of KS among young homosexual men residing in metropolitan areas during the early 1980s heralded the onset of the HIV epidemic. KS was then the AIDS-defining diagnosis in nearly half of all AIDS patients. So much so, this fulminant and disseminated form of the disease became known as epidemic KS to differentiate it from the classic KS with a more benign course seen predominantly in HIV-seronegative middle age or elderly men, the African KS endemic to native populations in the equatorial nations of the continent, and the immunosuppressive treatment-induced KS. A few years later, a rare, cutaneous form of KS with scarce lesions characterized by an indolent course was reported in HIV-seronegative gay men.[7]

At the zenith of the HIV epidemic, approximately 26% of HIV-infected men who have sex with men (MSM) but only 3% of intravenous HIV-infected heterosexual intravenous drug abusers presented with, or eventually developed, KS. Although its prevalence has substantially diminished with the advent of HAART, epidemic KS remains the most common cancer associated with HIV infection in the United States, and is the initial presentation of approximately 10% of patients.

Pathogenesis

In 1994, Chang et al employed representational difference analysis to identify the long-sought agent responsible for KS, a gamma herpesvirus, now known as human herpesvirus 8 (HHV-8) or KS-associated herpesvirus (KSHV). This virus is shed from oral mucosal surfaces and may be transmitted vertically, or through casual or sexual contact. Risk factors include receptive anal intercourse, and for gay men, an increased number of male sexual partners. Homosexual contact appears to more efficiently transmit the virus than does heterosexual activity. The risk of transmission through blood is unknown. Viremia appears uncommon as standard polymerase chain reaction (PCR) detects KSHV DNA in the peripheral blood of only one-half of infected persons. However, essentially all KS lesions contain detectable KSHV DNA.

Clinical Evaluation

Epidemic KS presents with generally asymptomatic, mucocutaneous lesions that may comprise any combination of nontender, violaceous macules, patches, papules, plaques, and nodules. Lesions are often multiple, multifocal, and in a symmetrical distribution. The lesions grow larger and more numerous, especially in profoundly immunosuppressed patients. Large lesions uncommonly ulcerate. Less typical presentations with bullae have been reported. Sites of predilection include the oral mucosa, head, trunk, penis, lower extremities, palms, and soles (Fig. 29-1).

Prognosis

Involvement of the extremities may result in profound lymphedema. The disease can be so disfiguring that it has been reported to be the most feared manifestation of HIV infection. However, in the past, patients who presented with KS had

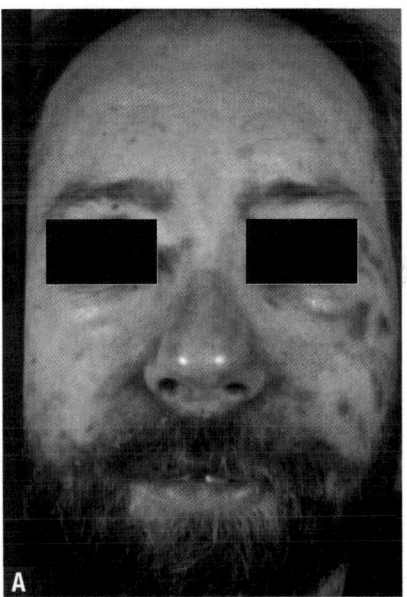

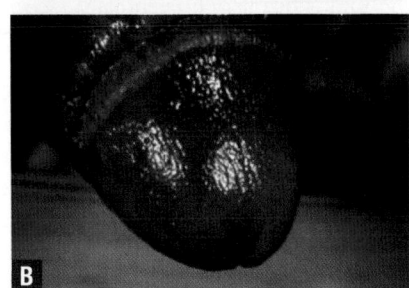

▲ **FIGURE 29-1** Kaposi sarcoma. **A.** Multiple violaceous papules, plaques, and nodules are distributed over the face, accompanied by marked facial edema. **B.** A glistening, reddish purple patch is localized to the glans and distal shaft of the penis, a site of predilection in epidemic KS.

a far better prognosis than did those whose initial manifestation was a systemic opportunistic infection. Visceral involvement occurs in the majority of patients with epidemic KS. Without treatment, approximately 60% develop lymph node and 45% gastrointestinal tract involvement.[8] Pulmonary KS, though far less common, confers a grim prognosis.

Treatment

The widespread use of HAART has dramatically reduced the incidence of KS, and a role for combination antiretroviral agents as monotherapy in the management of early KS is well-established. It is unclear whether the therapeutic effect stems from improved immune function that interferes with HHV-8 replication, or from reduced HIV titers, and consequently lowered production of HIV-induced growth factors known to stimulate tumor growth.

Insofar as the response of KS to HAART is unpredictable, concomitant targeted local or systemic therapy is often employed. The tumors are exquisitely sensitive to localized radiation delivered in single doses (8 to 12 Gy) to an extended field and to total skin electron-beam therapy. However, these modalities are less commonly used today due to concerns about the eventual development of radiation dermatitis given prolonged patient survival. Radiotherapy is not an option for mucosal lesions, as it causes severe mucositis.

For localized lesions, cryotherapy with two 30-s freeze–thaw cycles with 3-mm margins every 4 weeks has been recommended, but the ensuing ulcer can take long to heal so this treatment is reserved for small and superficial lesions. Most dermatologists spray in cycles of shorter duration. Cosmetic improvement can be achieved in larger plaques as the cryotherapy will destroy the top portion of the tumor but it will eventually recur. Intralesional vinca alkaloids, usually vinblastine sulfate injected at a concentration of 0.2 to 0.3 mg/cc, reduce the size of the lesions but may produce pain, ulceration, and pigmentation. The combination of intralesional vinblastine and cryotherapy has been proposed since the former tends to hyperpigment while the latter reduces pigmentation, and because vinblastine is more effective than is cryotherapy alone in reducing the deeper portions of the tumor. Intralesional hyaluronic acid previous to the vinblastine injection has been reported to increase the efficacy of the intralesional chemotherapeutic agent in the treatment of

tumor lesions. Intralesional injections of interferon-alpha-2b (IFN-α2b) at a dose of 1 to 3 million U may also be effective. Topical 9-*cis*-retinoic acid gel is effective in early superficial macules or patches only.[9]

Systemic cytotoxic therapy is usually employed for the treatment of patients with extensive mucocutaneous, lymph node, or visceral disease. Liposomal anthracyclines (doxorubicin and daunorubicin) are first line therapy for patients with advanced-stage KS. When these fail, paclitaxel and etoposide provide better results than do other standard chemotherapeutic agents.[3] Additional modalities are currently under investigation. Please see Chapter 21 for a more comprehensive discussion of this entity.

◼ LEUKEMIA AND LYMPHOMA

BOX 29-5   Summary

- Lymphohematopoietic malignancies occur in great excess in HIV-infected persons.
- Cutaneous lymphomas in HIV-infected persons are typically of T-cell phenotype.
- In the context of HIV, cutaneous lymphomas tend to be more aggressive, diagnosed at more advanced stages, and respond less favorably to treatment.
- Most HIV-associated cutaneous lymphomas comprise two distinct forms: the first, an indolent, epidermotropic, CD30-lymphoma resembling MF; and the second, a more aggressive lymphoma of large, CD30+ cells that classically harbor EBV.
- Atypical cutaneous lymphoproliferative disorder (ACLD) refers to an inflammatory, pruritic, lymphoproliferative eruption in HIV-seropositive individuals that histologically mimics MF.

Lymphohematopoietic malignancies are diagnosed at greatly increased rates among HIV-seropositive versus HIV-seronegative persons. Of special notice, HIV-infected persons have a 100-fold higher risk of developing NHL than that expected in the general population.[6] The majority of AIDS-associated lymphomas are of B-cell lineage with a predilection for such extranodal sites as the central nervous system and gastrointestinal tract. In contrast, cutaneous NHLs are rare in patients with HIV infection and are typically of T-cell phenotype. In HIV disease, cutaneous lymphomas are characteristically more aggressive, diagnosed at more advanced stages, and less responsive to therapy.[10]

Kerschmann et al discerned two forms of HIV-associated cutaneous lymphomas: the first an indolent, epidermotropic, CD30-lymphoma resembling mycosis fungoides (MF) or Sézary syndrome, and the second, a lymphoma composed of large, CD30+ cells that classically harbor the Epstein–Barr virus (EBV), with a typically grave prognosis.[11] This chapter will briefly review the altered behaviors induced by HIV on cutaneous lymphomas, and the reader is referred to Chapter 12 for a more detailed discussion of these malignancies.

Mycosis Fungoides (MF)

MF rarely complicates HIV disease and tends to occur in individuals with a relatively intact immune system. The etiopathogenesis of MF in HIV-seropositive patients is poorly understood. The clinical and histopathological manifestations are similar to those in the general population (Fig. 29-2). Features of MF include epidermotropism, EBV negativity, and an indolent course. Diagnosis is achieved by combined histopathology and immunohistochemistry. However, a careful review of all biopsy specimens is essential as certain other dermatoses characterized by lymphocyte-rich infiltrates (i.e., seborrheic dermatitis, contact dermatitis, atopic dermatitis, and drug eruptions) may be misdiagnosed as MF in HIV-infected individuals.[11]

HAART should be instituted if appropriate, and existing algorithms for the treatment of MF in immunocompetent individuals should be followed. Special consideration is warranted for the use of certain agents such as denileukin diftitox (Ontak) and total skin electron beam therapy, which have unknown safety in this population. Bexarotene, a retinoid, approved for the topical treatment of KS patches, is currently under study for the treatment of HIV-associated cutaneous T-cell lymphoma (CTCL).[3]

Atypical Cutaneous Lymphoproliferative Disorder (ACLD)

An inflammatory, pruritic, lymphoproliferative eruption that histologically mimics MF has been described in HIV-seropositive individuals. The terms *pseudo-Sézary*, *pseudo-CTCL*, *CTCL-simulant*, and *atypical cutaneous lymphoproliferative disorder* (ACLD) are synonymous for this entity. The descriptive term ACLD is most appropriate as the dermatosis does not clinically resemble MF, the relationship between this entity and

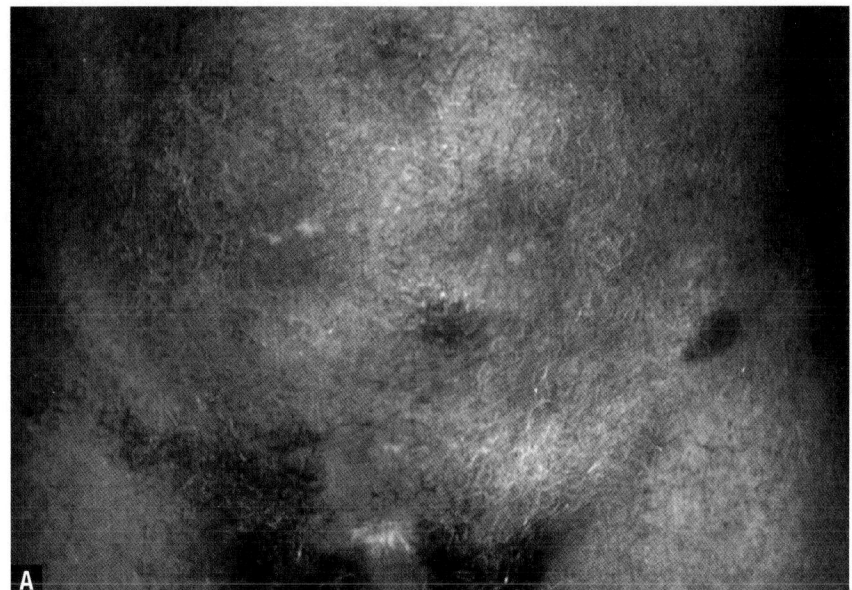

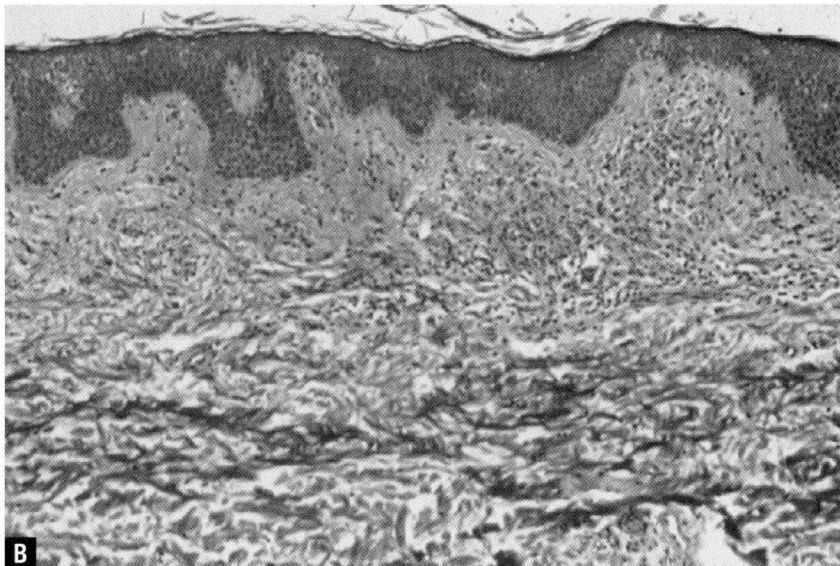

▲ **FIGURE 29-2** Mycosis fungoides. **A.** Ill-defined, erythematous, scaly patches and infiltrated plaques are present over the trunk and genitals. This patient had similar lesions on his extremities and buttocks. **B.** Histopathological examination reveals a mildly hyperkeratotic and focally parakeratotic epidermis with little spongiosis. A superficial, perivascular, lymphoid infiltrate is present in the dermis. Epidermotropism is present, resulting in scattered intraepidermal clusters of lymphocytes. High-power examination would reveal atypical features of the lymphocytes, including scant cytoplasm and hyperchromatic, convoluted nuclei. These features are indistinguishable from those seen in mycosis fungoides of immunocompetent individuals.

MF is not clear, and the potential for malignant transformation is not known.

ACLD classically manifests with an intensely pruritic, generalized, persistent eruption of poorly circumscribed erythematous papules and plaques. Less commonly, ACLD may present with nodules, pustules, hyperpigmentation, or lichenification (Fig. 29-3). There are also reports of ACLD occurring as a morbilliform drug-like eruption and as a photodistributed eruption.[3] In contradistinction to MF, ACLD typically occurs in patients with advanced HIV disease as evidenced by their low CD4+ lymphocyte counts.

Histology alone does not routinely distinguish between ACLD and authentic MF. Similarly to MF, the histopathologic changes of ACLD may consist of a psoriasiform lichenoid infiltrate with exocytosis of lymphocytes and minimal spongiosis. More characteristically, however, the lesions show a superficial and deep perivascular and perifollicular infiltrate of atypical mononuclear cells admixed with eosinophils, plasma cells,

and rare neutrophils. Atypical lymphocytes possess enlarged (and sometimes cerebriform) nuclei with prominent nucleoli, further complicating distinction from MF.[12]

Immunohistochemistry demonstrates a predominance of CD8+ cells, whereas the vast majority of MF lesions have a CD4+ phenotype. T-cell receptor gene rearrangement studies may be employed to demonstrate whether the infiltrate is monoclonal or polyclonal. The clinical significance of these findings, however, has been questioned by recent evidence demonstrating that MF is not simply a clonal expansion of a single malignant T cell, as was traditionally believed.

Since ACLD is not a true lymphoma, chemotherapy is not required. There is, however, one report of a patient who developed frank MF 4 years after the initial presentation of ACLD. Treatment with potent topical steroids or phototherapy is usually effective. However, as we await full understanding of the potential for malignant transformation, careful clinicopathologic correlation and regular follow-up of these patients is of utmost importance.[3]

CD30+ Large-Cell Lymphoma

CD30+ large-cell lymphoma may occur as either a visceral or a primary cutaneous malignancy. Whereas visceral CD30+ lymphomas are classically of B-cell lineage, the preponderance of cutaneous CD30+ large-cell lymphomas in HIV disease originate from T-lymphocytes. Patients classically present with one to several rapidly growing nodule(s) (Fig. 29-4). These lymphomas develop in patients with profound HIV immunosuppression. As with HIV-seronegative individuals, the diagnosis is confirmed with a combination of routine histology and immunohistochemistry. Histopathological features include dermal collections of cells with abundant, pale eosinophilic cytoplasm, and large, pleomorphic, vesicular nuclei with prominent nucleoli. Common additional features include multinucleate cells and occasionally bizaare mitotic figures. Epidermal involvement is variable. Epidermotropism is absent. The denomination *pyogenic cutaneous lymphoma* denotes a neutrophil-rich variant of CD30+ large-cell lymphoma, described in some patients with HIV. Immunohistochemistry typically reveals a CD3+ lineage and CD30 positivity. Additionally, the presence of the EBV genome is demonstrable either by staining with EVA latent membrane protein

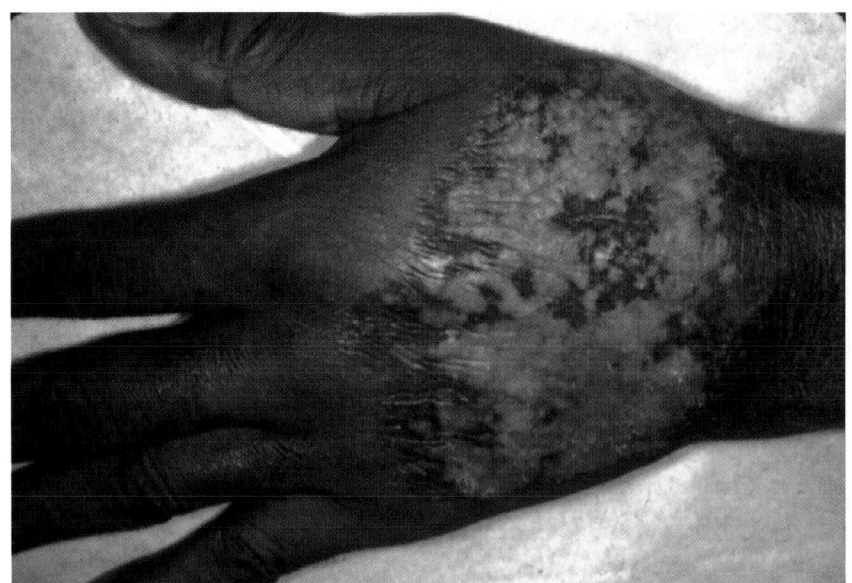

▲ **FIGURE 29-3** Atypical cutaneous lymphoproliferative disease. A large, exophytic, hyper- and hypopigmented, lichenified nodule is localized to the dorsal hand. Histopathological examination revealed a predominance of CD8+ T cells.

antiserum or *in situ* hybridization for EBV-encoded RNA (EBER-1).

In immunocompetent persons, the term "primary cutaneous" lymphoma denotes cutaneous lymphoma that has been present for at least 6 months without an evidence of nodal or visceral involvement. This designation is clouded in patients with HIV disease. Thus, metastatic disease should be fervently sought at the time of diagnosis with lymph node palpation, imaging, and bone marrow biopsy in all patients with AIDS-associated CD30+ large-cell lymphoma. Although there are rare reports of spontaneous regression of both solitary and multiple lesions, AIDS-associated CD30+ large-cell lymphoma generally carries a grave prognosis.[3] Survival in one study was only 6.7 months.[11]

CD30+ large-cell lymphoma in association with HIV appears to be more aggressive than in immunocompetent hosts. However, in existing reports, very few patients died of metastatic lymphoma, while the majority died of opportunistic infections. It, therefore, remains possible that CD30+ large-cell lymphomas are not intrinsically more aggressive in this population, but rather, that they represent a marker for more advanced immunosuppression.

Localized disease without systemic involvement may be treated with such destructive modalities as surgical excision and radiation therapy, either alone or in combination. More advanced, multifocal disease mandates multidrug chemotherapy.

MELANOMA

BOX 29-6   Summary

- In HIV-infected individuals, malignant melanoma appears to occur with a higher frequency and at a younger age than in the general population.
- Malignant melanoma often presents atypically and behaves more aggressively in HIV-infected persons.
- Formal guidelines are lacking for the management of HIV-seropositive melanoma patients.

Epidemiology

Malignant melanoma appears to occur with higher frequency among HIV-infected individuals. The literature contains more than 22 reports of concurrent melanoma and HIV infection.[13] Melanoma patients who are HIV-seropositive are typically younger (with a median age of approximately 38 years) than those in the general population.[14]

Pathogenesis

The reason for the altered behavior of malignant melanoma in persons with HIV has not yet been elucidated. As is the case with the previously discussed neoplasms, depressed CMI response appears to be important, but there are also other contributing factors.

Clinical Evaluation

Malignant melanoma in persons living with HIV may present atypically but it is not clear if the rate of uncharacteristic appearance is elevated. In the literature, there are reports of melanoma in this population mimicking normal nevi, benign pigmented macules, or multiple nevoid lesions. HIV-infected cases of melanoma are more likely to present with multiple lesions and more likely to have metastatic disease at presentation.[3]

Prognosis

The behavior of malignant melanoma in HIV-infected persons is more aggressive.

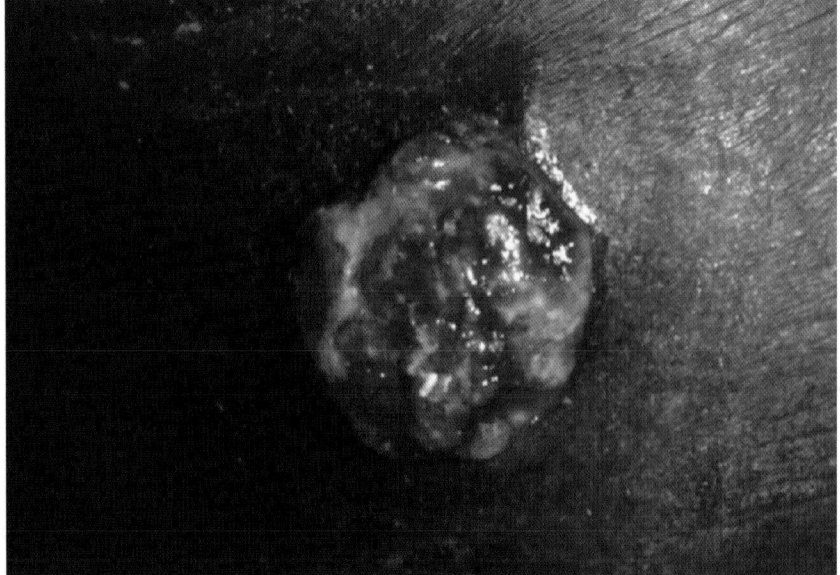

▲ **FIGURE 29-4** CD30+ lymphoma. A rapidly growing, erythematous, exophytic, eroded nodule is present on the buttocks of this HIV-infected man.

In a case–control study, 17 HIV-infected persons with melanoma were matched for melanoma subtype, tumor thickness, Clark level, tumor location, sex, and age. The HIV-seropositive patients experienced significantly shorter disease-free and overall survival relative to the HIV-seronegative controls. Of interest, the majority of melanoma fatalities in the HIV-seropositive group were in patients who either were not receiving treatment for their HIV disease or receiving only single-agent antiretroviral therapy. In general, HIV-infected patients with lower CD4+ lymphocyte counts experienced shorter disease-free survival; however, the authors detected no relationship between absolute CD4 count and tumor depth at presentation.[13] Staging at presentation has been shown to correlate inversely with CD4+ T-cell counts in several other small cases series.[15,16]

Treatment and Follow-Up

Wilkins et al propose annual complete skin examination for all high-risk individuals (positive family history, history of blistering sunburns , >50 typical nevi, and >5 atypical nevi). Physicians should maintain a high index of suspicion, and have a low threshold for biopsy irrespective of CD4 count. No formal guidelines exist for the management of primary cutaneous melanoma in persons with HIV. Therefore, the current recommendations of excision with margins depending on the depth, as discussed in Chapter 11, continues to be the recommended management. Some authors propose an expansion of the existing criteria for sentinel lymph node biopsy so as to incorporate tumors of lesser thickness among persons with HIV.[3] Prospective studies investigating this theory are lacking. Metastatic disease should be fervently sought at the time of diagnosis.

Current guidelines regarding the frequency and content of follow-up fail to include infection with HIV as a factor to consider.[17] Wilkins et al recommend follow-up every 3 months for the first 2 years subsequent to diagnosis and twice annually thereafter.[3] Follow-up visits should include a comprehensive history and physical examination, including palpation for enlarged lymph nodes and hepatosplenomegaly. The appropriateness of such testing as chest radiography and routine serology (i.e., lactate dehydrogenase) awaits formal investigation.

Because of evidence suggesting improved outcomes among patients treated with HAART,[13] initiation of combination antiretroviral agents is recom-mended unless contraindicated. Such immunotherapeutic interventions as IFN-α2b and interleukin 2 (IL-2) warrant exploration in this population. Though not yet studied for melanoma, the relative safety of IFN-α2b in this population for the treatment of unrelated conditions has been reported.[18] IL-2 is not contraindicated in HIV-infected persons, and has surfaced as an agent of interest in the treatment of HIV infection itself. HIV-infected individuals are not currently candidates for most existing vaccine trials.[3]

◼ OTHER NONMELANOMA SKIN CANCERS

BOX 29-7   Summary

- The risk of developing a BCC or SCC is elevated three- to fivefold among patients with AIDS relative to the general population.
- As in the general population, risk factors for developing nonmelanoma skin cancer in HIV-seropositive patients include fair skin, actinic damage, and family history.
- BCCs and SCCs tend to be more aggressive in the context of HIV-induced immunosuppression.
- Most BCCs occurring in HIV-positive patients are superficial type, multifocal, and located on the trunk.
- SCC in the context of HIV is clinically indistinguishable from that which occurs in the general population.
- A pathogenic role for HPV in the development of cutaneous SCC in HIV-seropositive persons is plausible, but remains speculative.
- Primary and secondary prevention are critical, especially in patients with fair skin types.

Patients with AIDS have a three- to fivefold increased risk of developing a basal cell carcinoma (BCC) or a squamous cell carcinoma (SCC). Whereas the number of SCCs exceeds that of BCCs among other well-defined immunocompromised groups such as transplant patients, the ratio of SCC to BCC in HIV-seropositive patients approximates 1:7.[3]

Risk factors for developing nonmelanoma skin cancer in HIV-seropositive patients mimic those in immunocompetent, HIV-seronegative individuals, and include fair skin, actinic damage, and family history.[10] The incidence of these ultraviolet-induced skin cancers will expectedly increase, as survival in this population is prolonged by current and emerging antiretroviral agents.

Basal Cell Carcinoma (BCC)

EPIDEMIOLOGY Persons living with HIV are at greatly increased risk for developing BCCs. This increased risk appears to be independent of CD4+ lymphocyte counts.[14] In a prospective study involving 724 HIV-infected members of the military followed for 3 years with skin exams, BCC, with an incidence of 1.8%, ranked second only to KS.[19] A multicenter retrospective study of hemophiliacs demonstrated an 11.4-fold higher incidence of BCCs among HIV-seropositive hemophiliacs than that expected in the general population. In this study, BCCs developed at a lower mean age among HIV-infected than among HIV-seronegative hemophiliacs (40 years versus 55 years).[20]

CLINICAL MANIFESTATIONS In immunocompetent persons and HIV-infected persons with relatively intact immunity, BCC characteristically presents as a dome-shaped, pearly papule or nodule with prominent telangiectasia and a tendency toward central ulceration, the so-called nodular BCC (Fig. 29-5). In immunocompromised patients who do not seek health care, the tumors can grow rapidly and can reach sizeable dimensions. A less common subtype in the general population is the superficial spreading BCC, which manifests as an erythematous sometimes atrophic patch with thin pearly borders. Most BCCs occurring in HIV-immunocompromised patients are superficial type, multifocal, and located on the trunk[3] (Fig. 29-6).

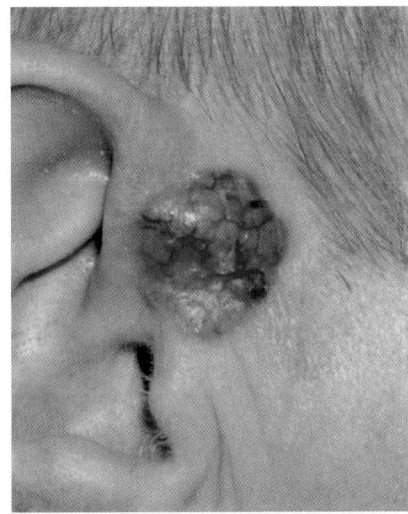

▲ **FIGURE 29-5** Nodular BCC. A large, well-circumscribed, pearly nodule with prominent telangiectasia is present on the preauricular cheek.

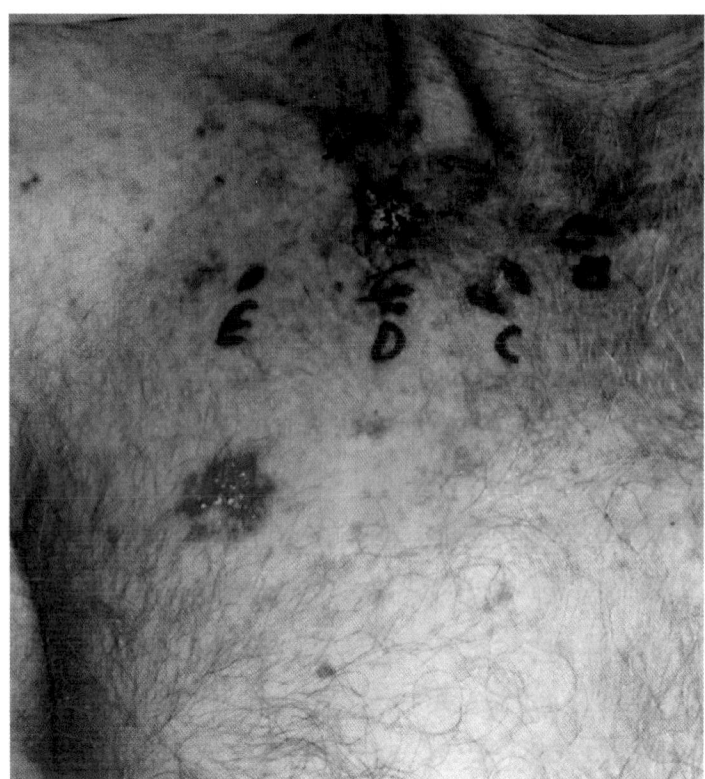

▲ **FIGURE 29-6** Multiple superficial BCCs. HIV-seropositive man with multiple ill-defined, variably sized, erythematous, atrophic, scaly patches distributed over the upper chest. Several lesions are eroded. This patient also had lesions on his head, neck, and extremities.

PROGNOSIS BCC tends to be more aggressive in the context of HIV-induced immunosuppression. Aggressive subtypes, including multiple infundibulocystic BCC,[21] metastatic BCC,[22] and aggressive morpheaform BCC arising within a scar have been reported within this population.[23]

TREATMENT AND FOLLOW-UP Both primary prevention, including diligent sunscreen use and sun avoidance, and secondary prevention, with regular, careful skin examination by a dermatologist, are critical, especially in patients with light skin types. Biopsy of any suspicious lesion should not be delayed. Adherence to standard treatment protocols for BCC achieves cure rates comparable with those achieved in the general population.[19,24] Use of the topical immunomodulator, imiquimod, for superficial tumors warrants further investigation in these patients.[25] Chemoprevention with acitretin (dosed 25 to 50 mg daily, as tolerated) for cases with multiple lesions may be considered, but the medication needs to be continued indefinitely as its beneficial effect ceases 2 to 3 months after treatment discontinuation. Following treatment, regular, semiannual follow-up is recommended.[26] Physical examination should include a search for both local and nodal recurrence.

Squamous Cell Carcinoma (SCC)

EPIDEMIOLOGY HIV-infected individuals have an elevated risk of developing mucocutaneous SCC. In a published report, the median age at which patients developed a cutaneous SCC was 44 years, compared with 70 years in the general population.[27]

PATHOGENESIS Specific high-risk HPV genotypes have been implicated in the development of anogenital, cervical, oral, and some nail unit SCCs. Epidermodysplasia verruciformis (EV)-type HPV refers to those subtypes, including HPV-5 and -8, whose DNA has been detected by PCR in SCC occurring in individuals with this rare disorder.[28]

Suppressed CMI, as occurs with advancing HIV disease, alters susceptibility to viral infection. HPV is chief among the pathogenic viruses that infect the immunosuppressed host. Between 5 and 27% of HIV-infected persons develop HPV-associated mucocutaneous lesions. Additionally, the prevalence of common and plantar warts is increased in this population, and histopathological review of these lesions more commonly demonstrates atypia.[29] A pathogenic role for HPV in the development of cutaneous SCC in HIV-seropositive persons is certainly plausible, but awaits elucidation.

CLINICAL MANIFESTATIONS SCC in the context of HIV is clinically indistinguishable from that which occurs in the general population. The typical presentation is an erythematous, scaly, and sometimes ulcerated plaque or nodule (Fig. 29-7).

PROGNOSIS Cutaneous SCCs appear to be more aggressive in HIV-seropositive persons. One retrospective series of 10 aggressive SCCs in HIV-infected persons demonstrated high rates of local recurrence and metastasis, and 50% mortality (6 months to 7 years). Poor outcomes did not correlate with the patients' histories of opportunistic infections or CD4+ lymphocyte counts. Rather, morbidity and mortality were most closely linked to the initial control of local and metastatic disease.[27]

TREATMENT AND FOLLOW-UP Primary and secondary prevention, including early biopsy of suspicious lesions, is essential in this population. A low threshold for biopsy of anogenital, periungual, or otherwise persistent verrucous lesions, particularly in those patients with a history of genital warts or of dysplasia, is prudent. Insofar as initial control of local and metastatic disease has been demonstrated to be the principal predictor of morbidity and mortality, all tumors should be treated aggressively, irrespective of CD4+ T-cell count. Evaluation for metastasis with high-resolution scans should be considered. Resection with margin control (i.e., Mohs' micrographic surgery) represents the most prudent approach, whereas ablative therapy without histologic control should be discouraged.[27] Sentinel lymph node procedures and local or regional adjuvant therapy should be considered for all high-risk tumors. Regular, careful follow-up including a search for local and metastatic recurrence should be conducted twice annually after treatment.

BOWENOID PAPULOSIS

BOX 29-8 Summary

- Bowenoid papulosis occurs in excess in HIV-seropositive individuals.
- Bowenoid papulosis is generally regarded as a transitional state between condyloma

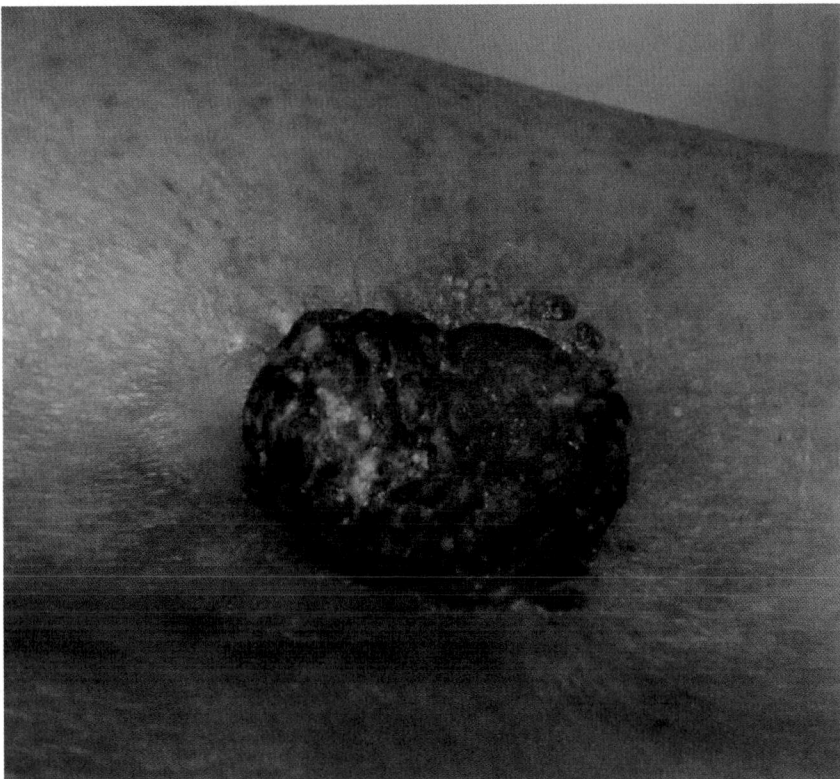

▲ **FIGURE 29-7** Nodular SCC. Exophytic, crusted and eroded, erythematous nodule localized to the right lateral thigh in this HIV-positive male. Patchy erythema extends peripherally from the lesion.

excision, elctrodessication and curettage, laser therapy, aggressive cryotherapy, and topical fluorouracil. More recently, topical imiquimod (alone or in combination with other therapies) and topical 1% cidofovir formulated in beler base[31] have been reported to be effective.

ANAL CARCINOMA

BOX 29-9 Summary

- The incidence of anal cancer is significantly higher in HIV-infected individuals (particularly among homosexual men) than in the general population.
- Anal cancer and its precursor, squamous intraepithelial lesions, are associated with infection with certain oncogenic HPV subtypes (i.e., HPV-16, -18, -31, -35).
- HIV-seropositive individuals are at increased risk for infection with multiple different and high-risk HPV types.
- Among HIV-infected patients, the incidence of anal SCC has risen since the advent of HAART.
- Lesions of anal cancer are oftentimes asymptomatic, but may manifest as pruritic, bleeding, or painful, perianal masses.
- Insofar as anal SCC is potentially preventable, anal cytologic screening for all HIV-seropositive homosexual men is prudent.

and Bowen's disease that is induced by oncogenic HPV.
- Classic lesions are flesh-colored, reddish, or pigmented papules with a flat or verrucous surface on the anogenital (and less often oral) areas.
- Therapeutic options include destructive modalities and topical immunotherapy.

The incidence of bowenoid papulosis appears to be increased in men and women with HIV infection. The typical lesions are flesh-colored, reddish, or pigmented papules with a flat or verrucous surface on the anogenital (and less often oral) areas and resemble condyloma accuminata. Individual papules often coalesce into larger plaques (Fig. 29-8). The neoplasm is considered to represent a transitional state between condyloma and Bowen's disease that is induced by oncogenic HPV (predominantly HPV-16). The neoplasm is assumed to have a nonaggressive nature; however, data regarding the course in HIV-immunocompromised persons is scant. A case of orolabial bowenoid papulosis was caused by HPV-32.[30] The lesions respond poorly to treatment and tend to recur after the use of superficial treatments of warts, such as podophyllin or trichloroacetic acid. Therapeutic options include

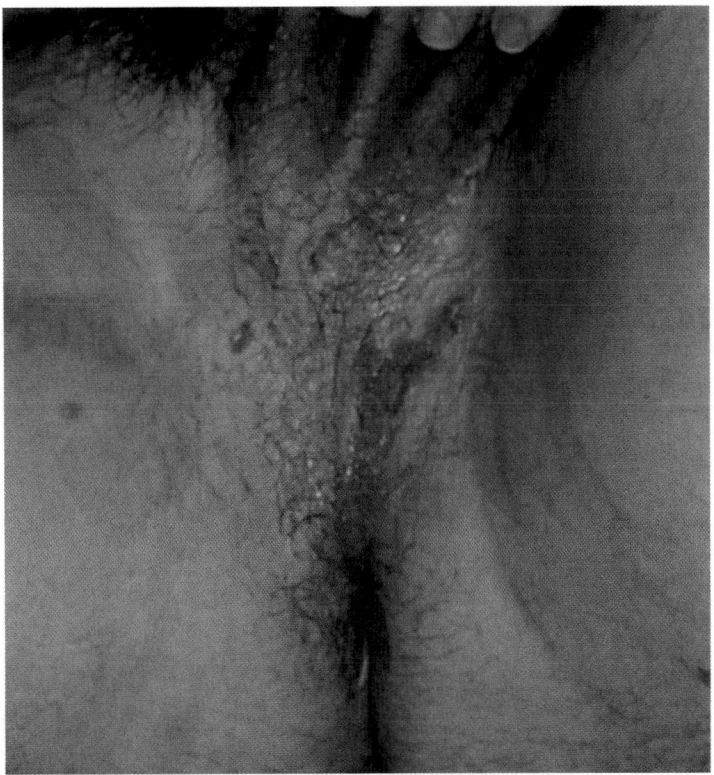

▲ **FIGURE 29-8** Bowenoid papulosis of the perineum. Smooth and verrucous hyperpigmented-to-flesh colored papules are scattered over the perineum. Several smaller papules coalesce into plaques.

Epidemiology

Before the HIV epidemic, the incidence of anal cancer among men who have sex with men (MSM) was estimated to be as high as 35 per 100,000, which is similar to that of cervical carcinoma before screening with PAP smears. Recent studies have estimated a twofold higher incidence among MSM who are HIV-infected than among those who are HIV-seronegative.[32] The majority of anal carcinomas in this country stem from squamous epithelium but tumors arising from columnar cells predominate in certain nations such as Japan. Perianal cancers are SCCs.

Frisch et al reported that in contrast to the general population, the relative risk for developing invasive anal cancer among HIV-seropositive men and women is approximately 38- and 7-fold higher, respectively. For *in situ* anal cancers, the relative risk is 60- and 8-fold higher among HIV-infected men and women, respectively. Men with HIV infection and a history of anal intercourse have a 60-fold higher risk of invasive and 100-fold higher risk of *in situ* anal SCC compared to the general population. Though diminished, an elevated risk remains for those who deny anal intercourse. For example, HIV-positive men with a history of intravenous drug use have a sixfold higher risk of developing invasive or *in situ* anal SCC compared with the general population.[33]

The terms *anal dysplasia, anal intraepithelial neoplasia,* and *squamous intraepithelial lesions* (SIL) are synonymous. Anal SIL may be subdivided into low-grade squamous intraepithelial lesions (LSIL) and high-grade squamous intraepithelial lesions (HSIL). Anal HSIL represents the precursor lesion to anal cancer. Though not typically regarded as a direct precursor to anal cancer, LSIL may progress to HSIL.[34] The prevalence of SIL among HIV-seropositive MSM and women is reported to be 36 and 14%, respectively.[3] Risk factors include lower absolute T-cell counts, history of an AIDS-defining event, infection with high-risk HPV types, and infection with multiple HPV types.[32]

Pathogenesis

Anal SCC and its precursor lesion, SIL, are associated with HPV infection by strains with high risk for oncogenicity (i.e., HPV-16, -18, -31, and -33).[3] An etiologic role for HPV infection in the pathogenesis of anal SCC is strongly suggested by the detection of HPV DNA in anal cancer and SIL tissues. High-risk HPV-16

is detected in most cases of anal HSIL, whereas LSIL more commonly contains HPV-6 and -11, types known to have a low risk of oncogenicity in the cervix.

Among HIV-seropositive persons, irrespective of sexual practices, the rate of anal HPV infection is elevated two- to sixfold. HIV-infected persons are at increased risk for infection with multiple different and high-risk HPV types. Utilizing PCR, Palefsky et al detected anal HPV DNA in the lesions of 93% of HIV-infected and 61% of HIV-seronegative homosexual men. Multiple HPV types were detected in 73% of HIV-infected and 23% of HIV-seronegative cases. Both groups demonstrated a similar spectrum of HPV type, with HPV-16 representing the most common type. An apparent association between advanced immunosuppression and increased replication of more oncogenic HPV types was suggested by higher levels of group B HPV types, (including high-risk types HPV-16, -18, -31, and -33) among HIV-infected individuals with lower CD4 counts.[35]

Reservoirs for HPV include persons with clinical and subclinical infection, and rarely the environment. The HPV life cycle is only completed in fully differentiated squamous epithelia. HPV does not encode the machinery required for transcription or replication, and is therefore entirely dependent on co-opting the cellular machinery of the host. Productive infection is initiated when the virus enters its primary target, the proliferating basal epithelial cells. Within the mid-epidermis, viral DNA is incorporated into host cells and viral proteins are expressed by host cells.[36]

Early HIV disease is characterized by a nearly intact host immune response, and thus, low levels of HPV infection and anal SIL. Declining CD4+ T-cell counts, and consequently, compromised CMI responses result in higher levels of HPV, increased risk for development of SIL, and subsequent progression to more advanced disease.

An improved understanding of the molecular biology of HPV has helped to elucidate a mechanism for its oncogenicity. Two viral oncoproteins, *early (E) genes 6 and 7*, have been identified and are expressed at high levels in HSIL. *E6* facilitates destruction of p53, and thus, eliminates a brake on cell-cycling. *E7* binds the tumor suppressor gene *Rb*, thereby liberating growth factor E2F from its typical cell-cycle inhibition.[36] Integration of viral DNA into host chromosomes induces chromosomal instability and cellular proliferation. Within this unchecked environment, other

cocarcinogens may exert a deleterious effect, thereby promoting progression from dysplasia to invasive cancer.[37]

Thus far, evidence to suggest that the introduction of HAART has led to a decreased incidence of SIL is lacking.[38] Conversely, several recent population-based analyses have demonstrated increased rates of anal SCC among HIV-seropositive persons during the past decade. Some investigators posit that high mortality rates prior to the advent of HAART may have masked rising rates of anal SCC or its precursor lesions.[39]

Clinical Evaluation

Anal dysplasia is generally asymptomatic and therefore identified only by targeted screening with cytologic anal smears and colposcopically guided biopsy. Occasionally, anal cancer is readily visible as an erythematous, verrucous, and sometimes eroded perianal plaque (Fig. 29-9). Patients may complain of such nonspecific symptoms as pruritus, discomfort, bleeding, or a perianal mass; however, these symptoms more commonly herald the presence of exophytic condylomata typical of infection with low-risk HPV subtypes.

Prevention and Treatment

Anal SCC is potentially preventable. Insofar as anal dysplasia is generally asymptomatic, anal cytologic screening is critical to the early detection of this cancer. Screening comprises regular cytologic (Papanicolaou) smears of the lower rectum, squamocolumnar junction, and anal canal. Several experts have recommended anal cytologic screening irrespective of sexual history in all HIV-seropositive men, especially those with CD4+ T-cell counts below 500×10^6 cells/L.[32] Abnormal Pap smear results warrant further investigation with high-resolution anoscopy (analogous to colposcopy) and biopsy of all visualized lesions.[25] Any lesion observed should be biopsied and HSIL lesions should be destroyed.

Treatment depends on staging (Fig. 29-10). Published guidelines for the treatment of SIL and anal cancer, including both surgical and nonsurgical modalities, should guide treatment once dysplasia is documented. Treatment of *in situ* lesions with topical 5-fluorouracil and/or imiquimod remains investigational.[40] Carcinoma *in situ* or small, well-differentiated anal cancers that have not invaded into the anal sphincter can be surgically resected. Radiation

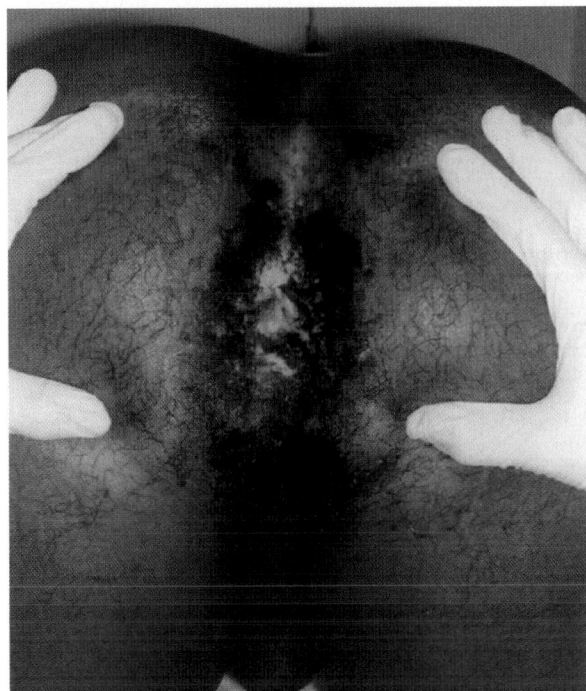

▲ **FIGURE 29-9** Anal carcinoma. A hypopigmented-to-pink, nonulcerated, smooth plaque extends from the anus. A large, hyperpigmented, verrucous plaque surrounds the lesion and extends onto the buttocks.

with or without chemotherapy is the mainstay of treatment for other tumors. A potential role for HPV vaccines (designed for cervical cancer-associated HPV infection) in the prevention of anal cancer in this population is under investigation.[3]

■ **SEBACEOUS CARCINOMA**

BOX 29-10 Summary

- Sebaceous carcinoma classically presents as a firm, skin colored-to-yellowish,

- slowly enlarging papule on the upper eyelid.
- In HIV-infected patients, lesions may present in extraocular locations or achieve unusually large size.

There are a few reports of sebaceous carcinomas in HIV-infected persons with or without the Muir–Torre syndrome (characterized by sebaceous neoplasms and/or keratoacanthomas with internal malignancy). However, the scarcity of these reports argues against an increased incidence of this neoplasm in this group. Characteristically, sebaceous carcinomas are present in the periocular region, specifically the upper eyelid. Only 25% are extraocular and the majority of these appear on the head and neck. One-half of periocular tumors arise from Meibomian glands. The neoplasm appears as a firm, skin-colored, or yellowish papule that slowly grows into a nodule. Metastasis occurs in 14 to 25% of patients. Several cases reported in HIV-infected patients achieved unusually large sizes and were not present on the face. The treatment of choice is complete surgical excision with Mohs' microscopically guided surgery being the preferred technique. Other destructive modalities such as cryotherapy are less definitive.[41]

■ **FINAL THOUGHTS**

Several malignancies that are more prevalent in HIV-infected individuals involve the skin. The mechanisms underlying the observed increased rate of malignancy in HIV-infected individuals remain poorly understood. Depressed cell-mediated immunity and increased susceptibility to certain oncogenic viruses (i.e., HHV-8 and HPV) are responsible in part. The clinical findings and course of several neoplasms differ dramatically in HIV-seropositive individuals. The introduction of effective antiretroviral therapy has led to marked reductions in the incidence of and mortality from certain malignancies, such as KS; however, the excess malignancy rate in this population has not normalized. It is essential for dermatologists to be aware of the diverse presentations, course, and management of cutaneous cancers in the context of HIV. Moreover, it is imperative to recognize that the standard of care for prevention, treatment, and follow-up of certain malignancies in HIV-infected individuals differ substantially from that set forth for immunocompetent populations.

T Stage

- Tis Carcinoma *in situ*
- T0 No evidence of primary tumor
- T1 Tumor <2 cm in greatest dimension
- T2 Tumor >2 cm but <5 cm in greatest dimension
- T3 Tumor >5 cm in greatest dimension
- T4 Tumor of any size that invades adjacent organs including the vagina, urethra, or bladder. Tumors that invade the anal sphincter only do not qualify as T4 tumors

N Stage

- N0 No evidence of spread to the lymph node
- N1 Spread of cancer to the lymph nodes directly adjacent to the rectum (perirectal lymph nodes)
- N2 Spread of the cancer to lymph nodes of the inguinal or internal iliac lymph node chains on one side
- N3 Spread of the cancer to lymph nodes of the inguinal or internal iliac lymph node chains on both sides OR cancer involvement of both the perirectal lymph nodes

M Stage

- M0 No evidence of distant spread of the cancer
- M1 Evidence of distant spread of the cancer including spread to lymph node chains other than the ones listed under "N Stage"

▲ **FIGURE 29-10** Staging for anal carcinoma.

REFERENCES

1. International Collaboration on HIV and Cancer. Highly active antiretroviral therapy and incidence of cancer in human immunodeficiency virus-infected adults. *J Natl Cancer Inst.* 2000;92:1823.

2. Dalgleish AG, O'Byrne KJ. Chronic immune activation and inflammation in the pathogenesis of AIDS and cancer. *Adv Cancer Res.* 2002;84:231.

3. Wilkins K, Turner R, Dolev JC, et al. Cutaneous malignancy and human immunodeficiency virus disease. *J Am Acad Dermatol.* 2006;54:189.

4. Giordano GG, Sigalotti L, Maio M. New dimensions in cancer biology and therapy. *J Cell Physiol.* 2000;183:284.

5. Frisch M, Biggar RJ, Engels EA, et al. Association of cancer with AIDS-related immunosuppression in adults. *JAMA.* 2000;285:1736.

6. Dal Maso L, Franceschi S, Polesel J, et al. Risk of cancer in persons with AIDS in Italy, 1985–1998. *Br J Dermatol.* 2003;89:94.

7. Friedman-Kien AE, Saltzman BR, Cao YZ, et al. Kaposi's sarcoma in HIV-negative homosexual men. *Lancet.* 1990;335:168.

8. Krigel RL, Laubenstein LJ, Muggia FM. Kaposi's sarcoma: a new staging classification. *Cancer Treat Rep.* 1983;67:531.

9. Antman K, Chang Y. Kaposi's sarcoma. *N Engl J Med.* 2000;342:1027.

10. Sanchez M, Friedman-Kien AE. Skin manifestations of HIV infection. In: Wormser GP, ed. *AIDS and Other Manifestations of HIV Infection.* 4th ed. Philadelphia, PA: Lippincott-Raven; 2004:663.

11. Kerschmann RL, Berger TG, Weiss LM, et al. Cutaneous presentations of lymphoma in human immunodeficiency virus disease: predominance of T-cell lineage. *Arch Dermatol.* 1999;131:1281.

12. Friedler S, Parisi MT, Waldo E, et al. Atypical cutaneous lymphoproliferative disorder in patients with HIV infection. *Int J Dermatol.* 1999;39:111.

13. Rodriques LKE, Klencke BJ, Vin-Christian K, et al. Altered clinical course of malignant melanoma in HIV-seropositive patients. *Arch Dermatol.* 2002;138:765.

14. Cooley TP. Non-AIDS-defining cancer in HIV-infected people. *Hematol Oncol Clin North Am.* 2003;17:889.

15. McGregor JM, Newell M, Ross J, et al. Cutaneous malignant melanoma and human immunodeficiency virus (HIV) infection: a report of three cases. *Br J Dermatol.* 1992;126:516.

16. Aboulafia DM. Malignancy melanoma in an HIV-infected man: a case report and literature review. *Cancer Invest.* 1998;16:217.

17. Tsao H, Atkins MB, Sober AJ. Management of cutaneous melanoma. *N Engl J Med.* 2004;351:998.

18. Myers RP, Benhamou Y, Bochet M, et al. Pegylated interferon alpha 2b and ribavirin in HIV/hepatitis C virus-co-infected non-responders and relapsers to IFN-based therapy. *AIDS.* 2004;18:75.

19. Smith KJ, Skelton HG, Yeager J, et al. Cutaneous neoplasms in a military population of HIV-1-positive patients. *J Am Acad Dermatol.* 1993;29:400.

20. Ragni MV, Belle SH, Jaffe RA, et al. Acquired immunodeficiency syndrome-associated non-Hodgkin's lymphomas and other malignancies in patients with hemophilia. *Blood.* 1993;81:1889.

21. Kagen MH, Hirsch RJ, Chu P, et al. Multiple infundibulocystic basal cell carcinomas in association with human immunodeficiency virus. *J Cutan Pathol.* 2000;27:316.

22. Sitz KV, Keppen M, Johnson DF. Metastatic basal cell carcinoma in acquired immunodeficiency syndrome-related complex. *JAMA.* 1987;257:340.

23. Rahimizadeh A, Shelton R, Weinberg H, et al. The development of a Marjolin's cancer in a human immunodeficiency virus-positive hemophilic man and review of the literature. *Dermatol Surg.* 1997;23:560.

24. Lobo DV, Chu P, Grekin RC, et al. Non-melanoma skin cancers and infection with the human immunodeficiency virus. *Arch Dermatol.* 1992;128:623.

25. Wilkins K, Dolev HC, Turner R, et al. Approach to the treatment of cutaneous malignancy in HIV-infected patients. *Dermatol Ther.* 2005;18:77.

26. Cameiro RV, Sotto MN, Azevedo LS, et al. Acitretin and skin cancer in kidney transplanted patients. Clinical and histological evaluation and immunohistochemical analysis of lymphocytes, natural killer cells and Langerhans' cells in sun exposed and sun protected skin. *Clin Transplant.* 2005;19:115.

27. Nguyen P, Vin-Christian K, Ming ME, et al. Aggressive squamous cell carcinomas in persons infected with the human immunodeficiency virus. *Arch Dermatol.* 2002;138:758.

28. Purdie KJ, Surentheran T, Sterling JC, et al. Human papillomavirus gene expression in cutaneous squamous cell carcinomas from immunosuppressed and immunocompetent individuals. *J Invest Dermatol.* 2005;125:98.

29. Harwood CA, McGregor JM, Proby CM, et al. Human papillomavirus and the development of non-melanoma skin cancer. *J Clin Pathol.* 1999;52:249.

30. Degener AM, Laino L, Pierangeli A, et al. Human papillomavirus-32-positive extragenital Bowenoid papulosis (BP) in a HIV patient with typical genital BP localization. *Sexually Transmitted Dis.* 2004;31:619.

31. Snoeck R, Van Laethem Y, De Clercq E, et al. Treatment of a bowenoid papulosis of the penis with local applications of cidofovir in a patient with acquired immunodeficiency syndrome. *Arch Intern Med.* 2001;161;2382.

32. Piketty C, Darragh TM, Da Costa M, et al. High prevalence of anal human papillomavirus infection and anal cancer precursors among HIV-infected persons in the absence of anal intercourse. *Ann Intern Med.* 2003;183:453.

33. Frisch M, Biggar RJ, Goedert JJ. Human papillomavirus-associated cancers in patients with human immunodeficiency virus infection and acquired immunodeficiency syndrome. *J Natl Cancer Inst.* 2000;92:1500.

34. Chiao EY, Giordano TP, Palefsky JM, et al. Screening HIV-infected individuals for anal cancer precursor lesions: a systematic review. *Clin Infect Dis.* 2006;43:223.

35. Palefsky JM. Biology of HPV in HIV infection. *Adv Dent Res.* 2006;19:99.

36. Lowy DR, Schiller JT. HPV infection: future prospects. *Clin Dermatol.* 1997;15:299.

37. Palefsky JM, Holly EA, Efird JT, et al. Anal intraepithelial neoplasia in the highly active antiretroviral therapy era among HIV-positive men who have sex with men. *AIDS.* 2005;19:1407.

38. Chin-Hong PV, Palefsky JM. Natural history and clinical management of anal human papillomavirus disease in men and women infected with human immunodeficiency virus. *Clin Infect Dis.* 2002;35:1127.

39. Chiao EY, Krown SE, Stier EA, et al. A population-based analysis of temporal trends in the incidence of squamous anal canal cancer in relation to the HIV epidemic. *J Acquir Immune Defic Syndr.* 2005;40:451.

40. Pehoushek J, Smith KJ. Imiquimod and 5% fluorouracil therapy for anal and perianal squamous cell carcinoma in situ in an HIV-1-positive man. *Arch Dermatol.* 2001;137:14.

41. Kuwahara RT, Rudolph TM, Skinner RB, Jr, et al. A large ulcerated tumor on the back. Diagnosis: solitary giant sebaceous carcinoma in a human immunodeficiency virus-positive patient. *Arch Dermatol.* 2001;137:1367.

CHAPTER 30

Nonmelanoma Skin Cancers in Non-White Populations

Panta Rouhani, M.P.H.
Shasa Hu, M.D.
Robert S. Kirsner, M.D., Ph.D.

BOX 30-1   Overview

- Despite the global prevalence of basal and squamous cell carcinoma, nonmelanoma skin cancer (NMSC) is significantly less common among non-white populations.
- Malignant skin lesions in darker-skinned individuals often occur with atypical presentations.
- Clinicians should include NMSC in their differential diagnoses and maintain a high index of suspicion when examining patients with darker skin to avoid the morbidity and mortality that is associated with a delay in diagnosis.

INTRODUCTION

Basal cell carcinoma (BCC) and squamous cell carcinoma (SCC) of the skin, collectively known as nonmelanoma skin cancer (NMSC), are the most common cancers worldwide and their incidence collectively are reported to be increasing.[1-4] Over one million cases of NMSC are expected to be newly diagnosed in 2006.[5] For this reason, NMSC ranks as the eighth health priority among the Healthy People 2010 objectives.[6] Despite their global prevalence, NMSC is significantly less common among non-white populations.[7,8] Skin cancers account for less than 2% of all malignancies in blacks.[9] An analysis of NMSC data from the Southeastern Arizona Skin Cancer Registry between 1985 and 1996 reported incidence rates of SCC and BCC for the non-Hispanic white population approximately 11 and 14 times greater than rates for Hispanics, respectively.[10]

EPIDEMIOLOGY

BOX 30-2   Summary

- Despite its global prevalence, NMSC is significantly less common among non-white populations.

- There is little information systematically collected regarding NMSC in ethnic populations.
- The exact incidence of NMSC is not known, as NMSCs are not uniformly captured in a representative national database.

There is little information systematically collected regarding NMSC in ethnic populations. In general, among NMSC, BCC is the more common of the two. Among blacks and Indians, however, SCC is more frequently encountered.[9,11,12] The exact incidence of NMSC is not known, as NMSCs are not uniformly captured in a representative national database. Dhir et al report that incidence rates of skin cancers in Asian Indians closely parallel those of blacks in the United States.[11] In Europe, NMSC rates are higher among adults from southern European countries and lower among adults from Nordic countries.[13]

In Kauai, HI, the incidence rate of SCC is among the highest documented in the United States.[14] The average annual incidence of SCC for Kauai Caucasian residents is 118 per 100,000.[14] A 5-year (1983–1987) study of NMSC among Filipinos from the island of Kauai found the incidence of BCC and SCC to be 12.3 per 100,000 and 1.8 per 100,000, respectively.[15] When standardized to the Japanese population in Japan, a similar prospective 5-year population-based incidence study of NMSC among Japanese residents of Kauai reported the annual BCC and SCC incidence rates to be 30 per 100,000 and 23 per 100,000, respectively.[16]

In general, there are many challenges in obtaining data on NMSC, especially for ethnic or racial minority populations from cancer registries. First, NMSC is not consistently reported to most cancer registries.[10] Population-based surveillance of NMSC is not conducted in the United States because cases are mainly diagnosed in (dermatology) offices and clinics rather than in hospitals.[17] Often times, especially in light-skin/high-risk populations, precursor lesions such as actinic keratoses are treated, and either all or some of these might represent SCC. Secondly, distinctions between geographic areas with higher UV radiation exposure are not made, thereby underestimating the projections of probable experiences in regions of the United States with greater environmental UV dose.[10,18] Lastly, most registries do not directly collect race-eth-

nicity information. As a result, many researchers must make assumptions using census population data or match probable ethnic surnames.[10]

PATHOGENESIS

BOX 30-3   Summary

- The rare occurrence of NMSC in populations of darker-skinned individuals and in atypical locations of the body such as sun-protected areas led researchers to hypothesize that NMSC may have occurred as a result of an alteration in tumor surveillance or impaired cellular immunity.
- Future work is needed to elucidate the role of sun exposure in the development of NMSC among non-white populations.

Risk factors implicated in the development of NMSC include sun exposure, albinism, preexisting pigmented lesions, nevus sebaceous, trauma, arsenic ingestion, chronic inflammation, human papillomavirus exposure, burn scars, prior radiation exposure, basal cell nevus syndrome and other genetic syndromes, immunosuppression, and chronic discoid lupus erythematous.[18,19] Although many etiologic factors in the pathogenesis of NMSC have been described, UV radiation (either acute or chronic—depending on the type of NMSC) from the sun is thought to be the most important risk factor, especially for SCC that predominantly presents on sun-exposed areas of the head, neck, arms, and hands.[18-20] Among darker-skinned populations, melanin pigment was thought to be protective against NMSC.[21] In a retrospective study of 276 patients with BCC, BCC occurred more frequently in sun-protected areas of the body among black patients when compared to lighter-skinned patients.[22] In a retrospective case–control study of 215 patients with either SCC or BCC, the ratio of BCC to SCC in non-sun-exposed areas was 1:8.5 for black patients compared with 1:1 for the control group ($P < 0.001$).[23] Additionally, the presence of BCC was postulated to be associated with a concomitant second primary malignancy.[22] The rare occurrence of NMSC in populations of darker-skinned individuals and in atypical locations of the body such as sun-protected areas led researchers to hypothesize that NMSC may have occurred as a result of an alteration in tumor surveillance or impaired cellular immunity (which may be induced by UV radiation exposure in some cases).[22,24] In a retrospective case–control study that compared age-adjusted DNA repair capacity (DRC) in Puerto Rican patients with and without NMSC, the authors found the risk of developing NMSC increased 21% with every 1% decrease in DRC. As a result, the authors concluded that a low DRC was a susceptibility factor for NMSC, even in darker-pigmented individuals.[25]

Case reports and case series of NMSC among darker-skinned individuals in sun-exposed areas have been reported.[18,24] Using data from the state as well as from the Surveillance, Epidemiology, and End Results Program (SEER), Pennello et al suggested that sunlight exposure increased skin cancer risk in blacks.[26] In another large-scale population study recently conducted in Puerto Rico, all participants, both Caucasian and non-Caucasian of all Fitzpatrick skin types, were classified into three environmental UV dose groups.[18] The authors found that UV dose influenced the BCC/SCC ratio, the number of tumors, as well as the tumor location. There were 254 cases of BCC (53% males) and 72 cases of SCC ratio (58% males).[18] On average, each patient had more than one tumor (2.1 tumors) and, interestingly, those with low and high exposure to UV levels were not found to differ ($P > 0.05$) by number of tumors.[18] The proportion of tumors that occurred in sun-exposed or sun-protected areas was equally distributed among the three groups of environmental UV doses. There were 17 participants that had tumors in both sun-exposed as well as sun-protected locations, and they were not considered for statistical analyses. Despite this study and earlier case series, future work is needed to elucidate the role of sun exposure in the development of NMSC among non-white populations.

CLINICAL EVALUATION

BOX 30-4   Summary

- Malignant skin lesions in African Americans often have atypical presentations.
- In darker-pigmented populations, the majority of BCCs was reported to occur in sun-protected areas: the back, extremities, and groin.
- Of the various subtypes of NMSC, pigmented basal cell carcinoma (PBCC) has been reported to occur more frequently among black and Hispanic populations.

- Histopathologic features of BCC and SCC in darker-pigmented populations are similar to their counterparts in lighter-pigmented populations.
- Halder et al suggest that higher mortality rates may be due to either more advanced stage of disease at time of diagnosis and/or the more aggressive course of disease in African Americans that occur for unknown reasons.

Clinical Presentation

Malignant skin lesions in African Americans often have atypical presentations. In a case series of BCC in blacks, only 2 of the 15 patients had a typical presentation: a central depression and elevated pearly borders.[21] The remaining patients had atypical presentations of their BCCs that appeared more like nevus, melanoma, or an epidermal inclusion cyst.[21] Additionally, features that assist in clinical diagnosis of BCC in lighter-skinned patients, such as erythema and pearly transluency, may be easily overlooked in darker-skinned individuals.[9]

In a case report of a 50-year-old black man with a 7-year history of discoid lupus erythematosus (DLE), multifocal SCCs in addition to an actinic keratosis were found.[27] The initial lesion on a discoid plaque proved to be an SCC and was treated with electrodessication. While SCC of the skin infrequently metastasizes, this patient experienced recurring SCCs as well as left axillary adenopathy.[27] Previous reports in the literature postulated that DLE predisposes blacks to SCC of the skin, which can metastasize. An altered immune status or previous treatments were offered as potential contributing factors by the authors. Clinicians should be suspicious of hyperkeratotic or poor healing lesions in patients with DLE, and those patients with proven SCC should be closely monitored for potential metastasis.[27]

In a case series of 19 black patients with Bowen's disease, a total of 21 lesions of Bowen's disease were reported.[28] Over three-fourths of the lesions (76.1%) occurred on sun-protected areas of the body. The most common site was the lower extremity. Bowen's disease is often overlooked or misdiagnosed in blacks. In addition to the low index of suspicion of skin cancer among blacks, Bowen's lesions closely resemble other benign lesions and do not incur as many symptoms among patients.[28] Nevertheless, the inclusion of Bowen's disease in the differential diagnosis may provide the opportu-

nity to prevent invasion, metastases, and possible secondary internal neoplastic disease.

In darker-pigmented populations, the majority of BCCs were reported to occur in sun-protected areas: the back, extremities, and groin.[12,21,22] In a case report of a darkly pigmented Indian woman, BCC was found on her photo-protected hairy scalp in an area of previous trauma.[11] These findings have led researchers to question whether there is a subgroup of BCC that arises from factors unrelated to UV radiation.

Of the various subtypes of NMSC, pigmented basal cell carcinoma (PBCC) has been reported to occur more frequently among black and Hispanic populations.[29-31] In a prospective clinical study of patients with suspected BCC, 66% of clinically diagnosed PBCC was found in Hispanic patients where only 11% of nonpigmented BCC were reported in non-Hispanic patients ($P <$ 0.01).[32] It is therefore important to include PBCC in the differential diagnosis of suspicious pigmented lesions among darker-skinned populations.[29,32] Overall, clinicians should include NMSC in their differential diagnosis of any suspicious lesion among darker-skinned populations to avoid the morbidity and mortality that is associated with a delay in diagnosis.[22,24]

Histology

Histopathologic features of BCC and SCC in darker-pigmented populations are similar to their counterparts in lighter-pigmented populations.[33] BCC on microscopic examination commonly demonstrates a downward proliferation of basaloid cells extending from epidermis. The basaloid cells have uniform, hyperchromic, large oval to round nuclei, and relatively little cytoplasm. There is a variable degree of cytologic atypia and mitosis, although typically uncommon. Peripheral palisading within the nests or cords of basaloid cells and clefting artifact from a reactive stroma are other common features of BCC. Central necrosis of cystic changes within the tumor masses can also be seen. The architectural arrangement of tumor cells, degree of differentiation, and stroma reaction vary with subtypes of BCC that include superficial spreading BCC, nodular (or solid type) BCC, micronodular BCC, pigmented BCC, morpheaform (or infiltrative) BCC, BCC with sebaceous differentiation, adenoid BCC, and basosquamous carcinoma (see Chapter 6 for further discussion on histology and histological differential diagnosis of BCC). Pigmented BCC has either large amounts of melanin within melanocytes in the tumor or melanophages in the connective tissue stroma surrounding the basaloid tumor mass. In a large-scale retrospective analysis of 234 Japanese patients with BCC, researchers found a high incidence of hyperpigmentation as the most characteristic feature of BCCs in Japanese patients.[34] Although most of BCC in black patients are of pigmented type, morpheaform subtype have also been reported in black patients.[35,36]

Histopathological examinations of SCC typically show an invasive proliferation of abnormal keratinocytes into the dermis. Cytologic atypia (i.e., hyperchromatish, nuclei pleomorphism, mitosis) and degree of differentiation toward keratinization vary considerably. Well-differentiated SCC contain mostly mature squamous cells and evidence of differentiation toward keratinzation such as keratin pearls, while poorly differentiated SCC has markedly anaplastic cells with a significant amount of pleomorphism and high mitotic figures. In addition to histological classification based on the degree of squamoid differentiation, other variants of SCC include SCC with horn formation, spindle cell SCC, acantholytic (adenoid) SCC, mucin-producing SCC, desmoplastic SCC, and verrucous carcinoma (see Chapter 7 for further discussion of histology and histologic differential diagnosis of SCC). In a study of 35 SCCs in African Americans[37] and another study of 176 SCCs in African Americans,[38] no specific subtypes of SCCs were identified.

Prognosis

Among NMSC, mortality from SCC is higher than from BCC and the risk of SCC is strongly associated with cumulative lifetime sun exposure.[39] African Americans do not do as well as their white counterparts in terms of prognosis. Halder and Bridgman-Shah suggest that higher mortality rates may be due to either a more advanced stage of disease at the time of diagnosis and/or the more aggressive course of disease in African Americans that occur for unknown reasons.[9] Although not life-threatening, BCC is an important public health concern because of its incidence as well as its financial expenditures from national health resources.[40]

TREATMENT

BOX 30-5 Summary

- Treatment of NMSC is the same for patients regardless of skin color or ethnicity.
- Once the NMSC is treated, the guidelines for follow-up and surveillance for future skin cancers should be the same as for Caucasian patients.

Treatment of NMSC is the same for patients regardless of the skin color or ethnicity. The mainstay of BCCs and SCCs include electrodessication and curettage, excision with margin, Mohs' micrographic surgery, radiation therapy, or cryosurgery. Alternative therapies for superficial lesions may be utilized, such as topical imiquimod,[41] topical chemotherapy with 5-fluorouracil, photodynamic therapy, and CO_2 laser.[42,43] Chapters 6 and 7 present a more detailed discussion on the treatment of BCC and SCC. When deciding the treatment modality for NMSC in a darker-skinned patient, one should take into consideration the higher risk of hypo- or hyperpigment from topical chemotherapy, cryosurgery, or laser treatment, and the higher risk of keloid formation in darker-skinned populations. Once the NMSC is treated, the guidelines for follow-up and surveillance for future skin cancers should be the same as for Caucasian patients.

PREVENTION

BOX 30-6 Summary

- While the financial feasibility from implementation of a widespread public health campaign directed at non-white populations in the United States may be debated, clinicians should consider NMSC in the differential diagnosis of suspicious lesions in ethnic populations.
- Emphasis should be placed on earlier diagnoses by physicians to reduce morbidity and mortality.

There is a need for heightened awareness of NMSC among non-white populations by physicians. In the absence of intervention today, skin cancer is one form of cancer that will increasingly become a greater public health concern.[40] A widespread public health initiative to reduce NMSC incidence in Australia has proven to be successful and beneficial.[44] While the financial fea-

sibility from the implementation of a widespread public health campaign directed at non-white populations in the United States may be debated, clinicians should consider NMSC in the differential diagnosis of suspicious lesions in ethnic populations. Additionally, clinicians may elect to screen the patient for coexisting malignancies.[21] Emphasis should be placed on earlier diagnoses by physicians to reduce morbidity and mortality.

REFERENCES

1. Scotto J, Fears TR, Fraumeni JF. *Incidence of Nonmelanoma Skin Cancer in the United States* (NIH Publication no. 83–2433). Washington, DC: Public Health Service; 1983.
2. Glass AG, Hoover RN. The emerging epidemic of melanoma and squamous cell skin cancer. *JAMA.* 1989;262:2097–2100.
3. Gloster HM, Jr, Brodland DG. The epidemiology of skin cancer. *Dermatol Surg.* 1996;22:217–226.
4. Karagas MR, Greenberg ER, Spencer SK, Stukel TA, Mott LA. Increase in incidence rates of basal cell and squamous cell skin cancer in New Hampshire, USA. New Hampshire Skin Cancer Study Group. *Int J Cancer.* 1999;81:555–559.
5. Jemal A, Siegel R, Ward E, et al. Cancer statistics, 2006. *CA Cancer J Clin.* 2006;56: 106–130.
6. U.S. Department of Health and Human Services. Healthy People 2010. 2nd ed. *With Understanding and Improving Health and Objectives for Improving Health.* 2 vols. Washington, DC: U.S. Government Printing Office, November 2000.
7. Boring CC, Squires TS, Tong T. Cancer statistics 1992. *Cancer J Clin.* 1993;43:7–26.
8. Preston DS, Stern RS. Nonmelanoma cancers of the skin. *N Engl J Med.* 1992;327: 1649–1662.
9. Halder RM, Bridgman-Shah S. Skin cancer in African Americans. *Cancer.* 1995;75 (2, suppl):667–673.
10. Harris RB, Griffith K, Moon TE. Trends in the incidence of nonmelanoma skin cancers in southeastern Arizona. *J Am Acad Dermatol.* 2001;45(4):528–536.
11. Dhir A, Orengo I, Bruce S, Kolbusz RV, Alford E, Goldberg L. Basal cell carcinoma on the scalp of an Indian patient. *Dermatol Surg.* 1995;21:247–250.
12. Bang KM, Halder RM, White JE, Sampson CC, Wilson J. Skin cancer in black Americans: a review of 126 cases. *J Natl Med Assoc.* 1987;79(1):51–58.
13. Boyle P, Smans M. *Cancer Mortality Atlas of European Union, 1993–1997.* Oxford, UK: Oxford University Press; 2003.
14. Chuang TY, Reizner GT, Elpern DJ, Stone JL, Framer ER. Squamous cell carcinoma in Kauai, Hawaii. *Int J Dermatol.* 1995;34:393–397.
15. Chuang TY, Reizner GT, Elpern DJ, Stone JL, Farmer ER. Non-melanoma skin cancer and keratoacanthoma in Filipinos: an incidence report from Kauai, Hawaii. *Int J Dermatol.* 1993;32:717–718.
16. Chuang TY, Reizner GT, Elpern DJ, Stone JL, Farmer ER. Non-melanoma skin

cancer in Japanese ethnic Hawaiians in Kauai, Hawaii: an incidence report. *J Am Acad Dermatol.* 1995;33:422–426.

17. Athas WF, Hunt WC, Key CR. Changes in nonmelanoma skin cancer incidence between 1977–1978 and 1998–1999 in northcentral New Mexico. *Cancer Epidemiol Biomarkers Prev.* 2003;12:1105–1108.

18. Ramos J, Villa J, Ruiz A, Armstrong R, Matta J. UV dose determines key characteristics of nonmelanoma skin cancer. *Cancer Epidemiol Biomarkers Prev.* 2004;13(12):2006–2011.

19. Woods SG. Basal cell carcinoma in the black population. *Int J Dermatol.* 1995;34:517–518.

20. Buettner PG, Raasch BA. Incidence rates of skin cancer in Townsville, Australia. *Int J Cancer.* 1998;78:587–593.

21. Chorun L, Norris JE, Gupta M. Basal cell carcinoma in blacks: a report of 15 cases. *Ann Plast Surg.* 1994;33(1):90–95.

22. Beckenstein MS, Windle BH. Basal cell carcinoma in black patients: the need to it in the differential diagnosis. *Ann Plast Surg.* 1995;35:546–548.

23. Singh B, Bhaya M, Shaha A, Har-El G, Lucente FE. Presentation, course, and outcome of head and neck skin cancer in African-Americans: a case–control study. *Laryngoscope.* 1998;108:1159–1163.

24. Nouri K, Romanelli P, Trent JT, Javid R, Jimenez G. Rare presentations of basal cell carcinoma. *J Cutan Med Surg.* 2002;6(3):226–228.

25. Matta JL, Villa JL, Ramos JM, Sanchez J, Chompre G, Ruiz A, Grossman L. DNA repair and nonmelanoma skin cancer in Puerto Rican populations. *J Am Acad Dermatol.* 2003;49:433–439.

26. Pennello G, Devesa S, Gail M. Association of surface ultraviolet B radiation levels with melanoma and nonmelanoma skin cancer in United States blacks. *Cancer Epidemiol Biomarkers Prev.* 2000;9:291–297.

27. Presser SE, Taylor JR. Squamous cell carcinoma in blacks with discoid lupus erythematosus. *J Am Acad Dermatol.* 1981;4(6):667–669.

28. Mora RG, Perniciaro C, Lee B. Cancer of the skin in blacks. III. A review of nineteen black patients with Bowen's disease. *J Am Acad Dermatol.* 1984;11(4, Pt 1):557–562.

29. Abreo F, Sanusi ID. Basal cell carcinoma in North American blacks. *J Am Acad Dermatol.* 1991;25:1005–1011.

30. Smith LM, Garrett HD, Hart MS. Pigmented basal cell epithelioma. *Arch Dermatol.* 1960;81:95–102.

31. Kalter DC, Goldberg LH, Rosen T. Darkly pigmented lesions in dark-skinned patients. *J Dermatol Surg Oncol.* 1984;10:876–881.

32. Bigler C, Feldman J, Hall E, Padilla RS. Pigmented basal cell carcinomas in Hispanics. *J Am Acad Dermatol.* 1996;34:751–752.

33. Matsuoko LY, Schauer PK, Sordillo PP. Basal cell carcinoma in black patients. *J Am Acad Dermatol.* 1981;4(6):670–672.

34. Kikuchi A, Shimizu H, Nishikawa T. Clinical and histopathological characteristics of basal cell carcinoma in Japanese patients. *Arch Dermatol.* 1996;132:320–324.

35. Lesher JL, Jr, d'Aubermont PC, Brown VM. Morpheaform basal cell carcinoma in a young black woman *J Dermatol Surg Oncol.* 1988;14(2):200–203.

36. Nadiminti U, Rakkhit T, Washington C. Morpheaform basal cell carcinoma in African Americans. *Dermatol Surg.* 2004;30(12, Pt 2):1550–1552.

37. McCall CO, Chen SC. Squamous cell carcinoma of the legs in African Americans. *J Am Acad Dermatol.* 2002;47(4):524–529.

38. Mora RG, Perniciaro C. Cancer of the skin in blacks. I. A review of 163 black patients with cutaneous squamous cell carcinoma. *J Am Acad Dermatol.* 1981;5(5):535–543.

39. Rosso S, Zanetti R, Martinez C. The multicentre south European study 'Helios.' II: Different sun exposure patterns in the aetiology of basal cell and squamous cell carcinomas of the skin. *Br J Cancer.* 1996;73:1447–1454.

40. Boyle P, Dore JF, Autier P, Ringborg U. Cancer of the skin: a forgotten problem in Europe. *Ann Oncol.* 2004;15:5–6.

41. Naylor M. Imiquimod and superficial skin cancers. *J Drugs Dermatol.* 2005;4(5):598–606.

42. McGillis ST, Fein H. Topical treatment strategies for non-melanoma skin cancer and precursor lesions. *Semin Cutan Med Surg.* 2004;23(3):174–183.

43. Iyer S, Bowes L, Kricorian G, Friedli A, Fitzpatrick RE. Treatment of basal cell carcinoma with the pulsed carbon dioxide laser: a retrospective analysis. *Dermatol Surg.* 2004;30(9):1214–1218.

44. Staples M, Marks R, Giles G. Trends in the incidence of non-melanocytic skin cancer (NMSC) treated in Australia 1985–1995: are primary prevention programs starting to have an effect? *Int J Cancer.* 1998;78:144–148.

CHAPTER 31

Melanoma in Non-White Populations

Panta Rouhani, M.P.H.
Shasa Hu, M.D.
Robert S. Kirsner, M.D., Ph.D.

BOX 31-1 Overview

- Although incidence rates for melanoma are lower among Hispanics and blacks compared to that among whites, melanomas among darker-skinned populations present at more advanced stages, are more likely to metastasize, and have poorer outcomes.
- Risk factors for melanoma among non-whites have not been elucidated. Recent evidence suggests a positive association between UV radiation and melanoma development in non-whites, but some results are inconclusive.
- Clinicians should include melanoma in their differential diagnosis and maintain a high index of suspicion when examining patients with darker skin to yield an earlier diagnosis at a more favorable stage with the ultimate hope of increasing survival.

INTRODUCTION

Cutaneous melanoma is increasing at an alarming rate. In the past several decades, the incidence of melanoma has increased more rapidly than any other cancer. It has doubled over the last 25 years in the United States, rising at an average of 6% annually during the 1970s and 2.4% annually in the last decade.[1] As a result, melanoma has earned its rank among the top 10 leading new cancer diagnoses in American men and women.[2] Melanoma currently ranks as the sixth most common cancer and is a leading cause of cancer deaths among young adults.[3] It is predicted that 1 in 70 Americans will develop melanoma over their lifetime,[4] and of these, 1 in 53 men and 1 in 78 women will develop melanoma. Early detection can alter the clinical outcome; when melanoma is detected early, lesions are thin allowing for a 99% cure rate. When detected later, lesions may be thicker, yielding more than a 50% mortality rate.[3,5] Screening and early detection is therefore essential in optimizing patient outcomes. The overall melanoma mortality, which has risen at a slower rate than incidence, has stabilized over the last decade and has even begun to fall in younger cohorts. The decline in mortality has likely resulted from heightened awareness and surveillance leading to earlier detection.[6]

EPIDEMIOLOGY

BOX 31-2 Summary

- Age-adjusted melanoma incidence rates: Hispanics, 4.3 per 100,000; blacks, 1.0 per 100,000; whites, 20.8 per 100,000.
- Over the past 15 years, the incidence of melanoma has increased at an annual rate of 2.9% among Hispanics and 3.0% among non-Hispanic whites ($P < 0.05$).
- Melanomas among darker-skinned populations are more likely to metastasize and have poor outcomes compared to those among whites.

Although age-adjusted incidence rates (per 100,000) for melanoma are lower among Hispanics and blacks (4.3 and 1.0, respectively) compared to whites (20.8),[1] melanomas among darker-skinned populations are more likely to metastasize and have poorer outcomes than among whites.[7,8] Among Hispanics in the United States, the incidence of melanoma has increased at an annual rate of 2.9% in the last 15 years ($P < 0.05$) comparable to the 3.0% annual increase among white non-Hispanics.[1] An analysis of melanoma data from the California Cancer Registry between 1988 and 2001 found that the incidence of invasive melanoma increased markedly among Hispanics in California compared to that among non-Hispanics, and that thicker melanomas (associated with worse prognosis) account for most of such increases, highlighting an emerging public health concern.[9]

PATHOGENESIS

BOX 31-3 Summary

- While it is known that melanoma is diagnosed at a more advanced stage in dark-skinned populations, the etiology is poorly understood. Risk factors among darker-skinned populations have not been elucidated.

Risk Factors for Melanoma

More than 95% of melanomas are diagnosed in white or light-skinned populations.[1] As a result, most of the epidemiologic evidence is drawn from the observations of these populations and most of the public education efforts have addressed these populations since they are at higher risk of developing melanoma. White or light-skinned individuals are thought to be more susceptible to the mutagenic activities of UV radiation because they lack protective melanin pigments.[10] Numerous epidemiologic studies have consistently reported UV radiation as the paramount risk factor for melanoma in white or light-skinned populations.[11–15] Other risk factors include evolving nevus/nevi, adulthood, the presence of a large number of common acquired and dysplastic melanocytic nevi, large congenital nevus/nevi, Caucasian race, personal or family history of melanoma, immunosuppression, tendency to burn rather than to tan, and a genetic predisposition such as xeroderma pigmentosa or albinism.[16,17]

Melanoma Risk Factors in Non-White Populations

While it is known that melanoma is diagnosed at a more advanced stage in dark-skinned populations, the etiology is poorly understood.[1] Risk factors for melanoma among non-whites have not been elucidated. Sun exposure was previously thought to play little role in melanoma development in darker-pigmented populations.[18,19]

Counterintuitive to this argument is the fact that the lower incidence of melanoma in Hispanics and blacks had been attributed to the protective effects of darker skin.[7] Recent studies have suggested a positive association between UV radiation and melanoma development in non-whites, but some results are inconclusive.[20–23] For example, by correlating melanoma incidence rates in six states in varying regions in the United States with inclusion of three-fourths of the U.S. black and Hispanic population, with estimated UV index and latitude of residency for each state, Hu et al reported that melanoma incidence is associated with UV radiation exposure in both blacks and Hispanics in the United States.[20] Using similar methodology, Eide and Weinstock extracted data from the SEER database (which contained smaller population), and did not find significant association of UV exposure and melanoma incidence in black or Hispanic populations.[23] Overall, the analysis of melanoma incidence data in Hispanics and blacks is limited by the low incidence in these populations and the lack of readily available cancer data in Hispanics as many state cancer registries still do not have Hispanic ethnicity as a variable.[24,25]

CLINICAL EVALUATION

BOX 31-4 Summary

- The paucity of studies on melanoma among Hispanics partly reflects the small number of cases in many areas of the United States, as well as limitations of ethnicity information in cancer registries.
- The disparity in melanoma at stage of diagnosis likely contributes to the poorer survival rates among Hispanics and blacks.
- Despite similar trends in melanoma incidence, melanoma survival in Hispanics has not improved to the same degree as that in whites.

Clinical Presentation: Stage at Diagnosis in White and Non-White Populations

Several studies have reported advanced melanoma presentation in association with worse survival rates among U.S. blacks.[7,8,26–29] A recent review of 649 melanoma cases (36 in blacks and 613 in whites) at the Washington Hospital Center between 1981 and 2000 reported that blacks were more likely to present with stage III/IV disease (32.1%) compared with white patients (12.7%), and that the 5-year survival rate was also poorer among blacks (58.8%) compared to whites (84.8%).[9] Using data from the Florida Cancer Data System, Hu et al reported a similarly higher percentage of late-stage diagnosis of melanoma among blacks residing in Miami-Dade County, FL; from 1997 to 2001, almost half (48%) of the black patients presented with regional or distant stage melanoma compared to 22% of white patients ($P = 0.015$).[26]

Data on stage at diagnosis among Hispanics is sparse, with only three published reports in the United States to date.[7,24,30] A study using California Cancer Registry data, 1988–1993, evaluated 361 cases of invasive melanoma diagnosed in Hispanics, found that Hispanics (23%) were twice as likely to present with

regional or distant stage than were non-Hispanic whites ($P < 0.01$).[7] An analysis of 81 melanoma cases from the New Mexico Melanoma Registry and New Mexico Tumor Registry between 1970 and 1986 found that a greater percentage (36%) of Hispanics had melanoma 2 mm or thicker in depth than that of non-Hispanic whites (16%).[24] The gap in melanoma stage at diagnosis likely contributes to differences in survival.

The paucity of studies on melanoma among Hispanics partly reflects the small number of cases in many areas of the United States, as well as limitations of ethnicity information in cancer registries.[25,31] Most published studies on skin cancer incidence and mortality describe data for whites only. Some include blacks, but very few include other racial groups such as Asian Americans or Hispanics.[32] Despite inherent limitations of classifying Hispanic race/ethnicity within all registry-based cancer data,[7,31] the consistent findings of more advanced melanoma presentation from large registry data support the validity of this trend.

Prognosis

Improved secondary prevention measures with earlier detection of thin (early stage) melanoma may account for the improvement in melanoma survival in white populations from 68% in the early 1970s to 92% in recent years.[1] The disparity in melanoma stage at diagnosis likely contributes to the poorer survival rates among Hispanics and blacks, since melanoma prognosis is intimately related to the stage at diagnosis. The 5-year relative survival rate for localized melanoma (98%) falls to 64 and 16% for regional and distant stage, respectively.[1]

Unlike the similar trends in melanoma incidence, melanoma survival in Hispanics has not improved to the same degree as that in whites. The 5-year survival rate of melanoma is 77.1% for white Hispanic males, 86.8% for white Hispanic females, compared to 86.5% in non-Hispanic white males and 92.2% in non-Hispanic white females.[2] The 5-year relative survival rate for blacks has changed little from 67% in 1974–1976 to 78% in 1995–2001 (not a statistically significant difference).[1]

PREVENTION

BOX 31-5 Summary

- While prevention measures with earlier detection may account for improved survival rates in white populations, such

advances have not occurred in other segments of the population.
- Evidence suggests that secondary prevention efforts such as skin cancer screenings are suboptimal in Hispanics and blacks.
- Understandably, darker-skinned individuals perceive themselves at either low or nil risk for melanoma, as much of the public education efforts have targeted white populations.

Much of the current literature and most public health efforts have targeted melanoma in white populations. While prevention measures with earlier detection may account for improved survival rates in white populations, such advances have not occurred in other segments of the population. Hispanics and blacks continue to have poorer survival rates.[2] The more advanced stage of melanoma in Hispanics and blacks highlight the disparity in secondary prevention of melanoma in minority populations.

Evidence suggests that secondary prevention efforts such as skin cancer screenings are suboptimal in Hispanics and blacks. Using the National Health Interview Surveys, among U.S. adults, both Hispanics and blacks are screened for skin cancer less frequently than are white non-Hispanics.[33] In 2000, only 3.7% of white Hispanics and 6.2% of blacks had a recent skin examination by physicians, compared to 8.9% white non-Hispanics surveyed. Hispanic ethnicity is additionally correlated with decreased likelihood of having a recent skin cancer exam (odds ratio 0.61, $P = 0.001$). As the incidence of skin cancer is lower among minorities, better understanding of risk factors among these populations would aid in identifying more cost-effective screening efforts. Hispanic ethnicity is also consistently associated with deficits in the use of other major cancer screening tests such as Pap tests, mammography, prostate-specific antigen (PSA) screening, and colorectal screening.[34] Socioeconomic status, sociocultural values, and skin cancer awareness are likely factors that account for differences in the delivery and utilization of healthcare resources among minority populations.[35,36] Among socioeconomic factors, poverty and lack of health insurance influence access and utilization of cancer-screening services and treatment, thus contributing to current disparities in cancer burden among minority groups.[2,34,37,38] Ineffective or insufficient public education efforts may also affect utilization of skin-cancer-screening resources. A recent study on U.S. media coverage from 1979 to 2003 found overall suboptimal media attention on skin cancer education; the amount of coverage on skin cancer has not increased since 1986. With only 6.6% of stories on dermatologic detection and 5.5% of stories on self-detection of skin cancer, the media pays little attention to skin cancer education.[39]

Lastly, the delayed diagnosis of melanoma among Hispanics and blacks could also reflect lower skin cancer awareness. Understandably, darker-skinned individuals perceive themselves at either low or nil risk for melanoma, as much of the public education efforts have targeted the white populations, especially those with blue eyes and blond or red hair. Lower skin cancer awareness could thereby influence an individual's decision to seek timely medical care for suspicious skin lesions. Byrd et al had commented that the lack of public education on melanoma risk and prevention in black communities may be a major factor in its advanced presentation.[27] In a recent study comparing skin cancer awareness among Hispanics to non-Hispanics with similar access to health care, awareness of melanoma and non-melanoma skin cancers as well as perceived risk were less among Hispanics than among non-Hispanics. Hispanics also performed less-frequent self-skin exams, and were unaware of the clinical signs of skin cancer.[32]

■ FINAL THOUGHTS

The delayed presentation of melanoma among Hispanics and blacks along with worse survival in these populations highlights an increasingly significant public health concern. The lowest survival rate and highest proportion of advanced presentation of melanoma are seen in blacks. Disparity in melanoma stage at diagnosis between Hispanics and whites also deserves attention since both the Hispanic population and melanoma incidence in this population are on the rise. Hispanics are among the fastest growing minority groups in the United States; the Hispanic population increased more than 50% since 1990, and is projected to reach 17% of total U.S. population by 2020.[40] The fast-growing Hispanic population in the United States warrants closer examination of melanoma epidemiology in this group.

Recent public health education and prevention efforts on melanoma in Caucasians have led to a trend toward earlier detection of melanoma at localized stage (which is more treatable) in the white population[41]; however, such improvement in melanoma diagnosis has not been seen in U.S. blacks or Hispanics. Hispanics and blacks are the two largest racial/ethnic groups in the United States after non-Hispanic white, comprising 12.5 and 12.3% of total U.S. populations, respectively.[42] While the cost-effectiveness of implementing primary prevention of melanoma with photoprotection may be debated in darker-skinned population, public education regarding melanoma risk in blacks and Hispanics, and delivery of skin cancer screening and exams represent the main potential areas of intervention to improve the stage at diagnosis in minorities. It is hopeful that an earlier diagnosis of melanoma at a more favorable stage will ultimately improve melanoma survival rate in minority populations.

REFERENCES

1. Ries LAG, Eisner MP, Kosary CL, et al. *SEER Cancer Statistics Review, 1975–2001.* Bethesda, MD: National Cancer Institute. Available at: http://seer.cancer.gov/csr/1975_2001. Accessed March 5, 2006.
2. Jemal A, Clegg LX, Ward E, et al. Annual report to the nation on the status of cancer, 1975–2001, with a special feature regarding survival. *Cancer.* 2004;101:3–27.
3. Greenlee RT, Murray T, Bolden S, Wingo PA. Cancer statistics, 2000. *CA Cancer J Clin.* 2000;50(1):7–33.
4. Marks R. An overview of skin cancers. Incidence and causation. *Cancer.* 1995;75 (2, suppl):607–612.
5. Almahroos M, Kurban AK. Ultraviolet carcinogenesis in nonmelanoma skin cancer. Part II: review and update on epidemiologic correlations. *Skinmed.* 2004;3 (3):132–139.
6. Schaffer JV, Rigel DS, Kopf AW, Bolognia JL. Cutaneous melanoma—past, present, and future. *J Am Acad Dermatol.* 2004;51 (1, suppl):S65–S69.
7. Cress RD, Holly EA. Incidence of cutaneous melanoma among non-Hispanic whites, Hispanics, Asians, and blacks: an analysis of California cancer registry data, 1988–93. *Cancer Causes Control.* 1997; 8:246–252.
8. Bellows CF, Belafsky P, Fortgang IS, Beech DJ. Melanoma in African-Americans: trends in biological behavior and clinical characteristics over two decades. *J Surg Oncol.* 2001;78:10–16.
9. Cockburn MG, Zadnick J, Deapen D. Developing epidemic of melanoma in the Hispanic population of California. *Cancer.* 2006;106:1162–1168.
10. Tsai T, Vu C, Henson DE. Cutaneous, ocular and visceral melanoma in African Americans and Caucasians. *Melanoma Res.* 2005;15(3):213–217.

11. IARC. IARC monographs on the evaluation of carcinogenic risks to humans: solar and ultraviolet radiation. *IARC Monogr Eval Carcinog Risks Hum.* 1992;55:1–316.
12. Lee JA, Scotto J. Melanoma: linked temporal and latitude changes in the United States. *Cancer Causes Control.* 1993;4: 413–418.
13. Lee JA. Latitude, coastal or interior location and the evaluation of the melanoma epidemic in the United States. *Melanoma Res.* 1997;7:179–188.
14. Bulliard JL, Cox B, Elwood JM. Latitude gradients in melanoma incidence and mortality in the non-Maori population of New Zealand. *Cancer Causes Control.* 1994; 5:234–240.
15. Armstrong BK, Kricker A. The epidemiology of UV induced skin cancer. *J Photochem Photobiol B.* 2001;63:8–18.
16. Rhodes AR, Weinstock MA, Fitzpatrick TB, Mihm MC, Jr, Sober AJ. Risk factors for cutaneous melanoma. A practical method for recognizing predisposed individuals. *JAMA.* 1987;258(21):3146–3154.
17. Marks R. Epidemiology of melanoma. *Clin Exp Dermatol.* 2000;25:459–463.
18. Elder DE. Skin cancer: melanoma and other specific non-melanoma skin cancers. *Cancer.* 1995;75:245–256.
19. Armstrong B, Kricker A. How much melanoma is caused by sun exposure? *Melanoma Res.* 1993;3:395–401.
20. Hu S, Ma F, Collado-Mesa F, Kirsner RS. UV radiation, latitude, and melanoma in US Hispanics and blacks. *Arch Dermatol.* 2004;140:819–824.
21. Krishnamurthy S. The geography of nonocular malignant melanoma in India: its association with latitude, ozone levels and UV light exposure. *Int J Cancer.* 1992; 51:169–172.
22. Pennello G, Devesa S, Gail M. Association of surface ultraviolet B radiation levels with melanoma and nonmelanoma skin cancer in United States blacks. *Cancer Epidemiol Biomarkers Prev.* 2000;9: 291–297.
23. Eide MJ, Weinstock MA. Association of UV index, latitude, and melanoma incidence in nonwhite populations—US Surveillance, Epidemiology, and End Results (SEER) Program, 1992–2001. *Arch Dermatol.* 2005;141:477–481.
24. Black WC, Goldhahn RT, Jr, Wiggins C. Melanoma within a southwestern Hispanic population. *Arch Dermatol.* 1987;123 (10):1331–1334.
25. Poe GS, Powell-Griner E, McLaughlin JK, Placek PJ, Thompson GB, Robinson K. Comparability of the death certificate and the 1986 National Mortality Followback Survey. *Vital Health Stat 2.* 1993:1–53.
26. Hu S, Parker DF, Thomas AG, Kirsner RS. Advanced presentation of melanoma in African Americans: the Miami-Dade County experience. *J Am Acad Dermatol.* 2004;51(6):1031–1032.
27. Byrd KM, Wilson DC, Hoyler SS, Peck GL. Advanced presentation of melanoma in African Americans. *J Am Acad Dermatol.* 2004;50(1):21–24.
28. Crowley NJ, Dodge R, Vollmer RT, Seigler HF. Malignant melanoma in black Americans. A trend toward improved survival. *Arch Surg.* 1991;126(11):1359–1364.
29. Reintgen DS, McCarty KM, Jr, Cox E, Seigler HF. Malignant melanoma in black American and white American

populations. A comparative review. *JAMA.* 1982;248(15):1856–1859.

30. Feun LG, Raub WA, Jr, Duncan RC, et al. Melanoma in a southeastern Hispanic population. *Cancer Detect Prev.* 1994; 18(2):145–152.

31. Rosenberg HM, Maurer JD, Sorlie PD, et al. Quality of death rates by race and Hispanic origin: a summary of current research, 1999. *Vital Health Stat 2.* 1999:1–13.

32. Pipitone M, Robinson JK, Camara C, Chittineni B, Fisher SG. Skin cancer awareness in suburban employees: a Hispanic perspective. *J Am Acad Dermatol.* 2002;47:118–123.

33. Saraiya M, Hall HI, Thompson T, et al. Skin cancer screening among U.S. adults from 1992, 1998, and 2000 National Health Interview Surveys. *Prev Med.* 2004;39:308–314.

34. Swan J, Breen N, Coates RJ, Rimer BK, Lee NC. Progress in cancer screening practices in the United States: results from the 2000 National Health Interview Survey. *Cancer.* 2003;97:1528–1540.

35. Freeman HP. Poverty, culture, and social injustice: determinants of cancer disparities. *CA Cancer J Clin.* 2004;54:72–77.

36. Margolis ML, Christie JD, Silvestri GA, Kaiser L, Santiago S, Hansen-Flaschen J. Racial differences pertaining to a belief about lung cancer surgery: results of a multicenter survey. *Ann Intern Med.* 2003;139:558–563.

37. Ward E, Jemal A, Cokkinides V, et al. Cancer disparities by race/ethnicity and socioeconomic status. *CA Cancer J Clin.* 2004;54:78–93.

38. Jemal A, Murray T, Ward E, et al. Cancer statistics, 2005. *CA Cancer J Clin.* 2005;55:10–30.

39. Stryker JE, Solky BA, Emmons KM. A content analysis of news coverage of skin cancer prevention and detection, 1979 to 2003. *Arch Dermatol.* 2005;141:491–496.

40. Ramirez R, De la Cruz G. *The Hispanic Population the United States: March 2002.* Washington, DC: U.S. Census Bureau; 2003.

41. Dennis LK. Analysis of the melanoma epidemic, both apparent and real: data from the 1973 through 1994 surveillance, epidemiology, and end results program registry. *Arch Dermatol.* 1999;135(3):275–280.

42. U.S. Census Bureau. *Census 2000.* Washington, DC: U.S. Census Bureau, Population Division; 2002.

CHAPTER 32

Skin Cancer and Pregnancy

Mercedes E. Gonzalez, M.D.
Elizabeth Alvarez Connelly, M.D.

BOX 32-1 Overview

- During pregnancy, many women will seek medical attention for the growth of old skin lesions and the new appearance of benign skin lesions.
- Changing nevi should be evaluated as they would be in a nonpregnant patient.
- Malignant melanoma is one of the most frequently diagnosed primary cancers during pregnancy.
- Pregnancy in itself is not a prognostic factor in the course of malignant melanoma.
- Excision, sentinel lymph node mapping, and biopsy can be safely performed in pregnancy for stage I and stage II melanoma.
- The evidence suggests that there is no association between exogenous hormone use and an increased risk of malignant melanoma.
- The uncommon tumor, dermatofibrosarcoma protuberans (DFSP) can present or rapidly enlarge during pregnancy.

INTRODUCTION

Pregnancy represents a unique hormonal and metabolic milieu. The well-known cutaneous changes associated with pregnancy have led to the hypothesis of hormonal mediators. However, the specific influences that pregnancy and exogenous hormones have on skin physiology are incompletely understood.

The incidence of malignancies during pregnancy has increased to approximately 1 in 1000 cases, likely as a result of delaying pregnancy into the later reproductive years.[1] The most common malignancies seen during pregnancy are those generally seen in younger individuals such as breast, cervix, leukemia, lymphoma—including Hodgkin's, and malignant melanoma (MM). MM is the second most common cancer in women of childbearing age. As a result, the diagnosis, management, and prognosis of MM during pregnancy have been the subject of much investigation.

This chapter will present the physiologic skin changes and growth of benign skin lesions in pregnancy (Fig. 32-1). Secondly, it will provide the latest information on the incidence, prognosis, and management of MM during pregnancy and with exogenous hormone use. The implications of malignant melanoma on the developing fetus and subsequent pregnancies will also be discussed. Lastly, dermatofibrosarcoma protuberans (DFSP), a rare malignant tumor, known to enlarge during pregnancy will be presented.

SKIN CHANGES IN PREGNANCY

BOX 32-2 Summary

- While there are many physiologic skin changes that occur during pregnancy, darkening or enlarging melanocytic nevi are not physiologic changes in pregnancy.

Nevi

Hyperpigmentation is one of the most common cutaneous changes during pregnancy, occurring mostly on the linea alba, the areolae, axillae, and genitalia. Melasma, a pregnancy-associated darkening of the skin on the face, occurs in more than 50% of women during pregnancy, and in almost one third of women taking oral contraceptives. These changes occur so frequently that they are considered physiologic skin changes.[2]

In contrast to the melanocytes throughout the body, these "physiologic changes" are not seen in melanocytic nevi. The classic teaching that preexisting nevi darken during pregnancy has led to delays in diagnosis and mismanagement of MM.[3] There is a paucity of studies that have followed the changes in melanocytic nevi during pregnancy.[4] Early studies that report nevi enlarge or darken in pregnancy were based on self-reported color and size change by patients. In one of these studies, most of the patient-reported changes were actually skin tags or dermatofibromas.[5] Evidence from case-controlled studies has discredited this idea and suggest rather that changing nevi should always be suspect.[6,7] Pennoyer et al followed 129 nevi in pregnant women with photographs, and all changing lesions were biopsied. Only 6.2% of nevi showed any change and no lesions demonstrated malignant degeneration.[7] In another study, self-reported changing nevi were histologically evaluated. The investigators found no differences in the histopathologic features of the pigmented lesions from pregnant women and their age-matched nonpregnant controls.[6]

Nevi in patients with the dysplastic nevus syndrome (aka atypical mole syndrome) may represent an exception. One study used photos to evaluate changes in nevi of 17 pregnant patients with dysplastic nevus syndrome (DNS). The patients served as their own controls. Nevi in patients with DNS were 3.9 times more likely to change clinically and two times more likely to have histologic changes during pregnancy.[8] The same increased rate of change was not seen in women with DNS taking hormonal supplements. However, DNS is characterized by atypical nevi that have an increased risk for MM and the observed changes may

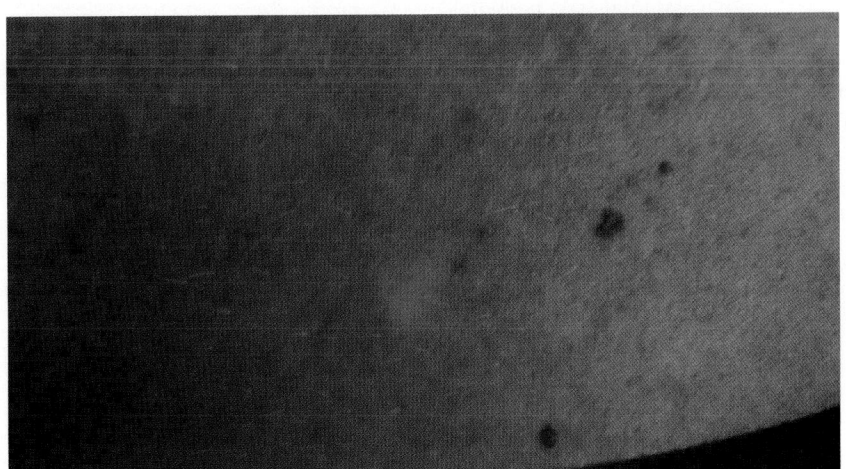

▲ FIGURE 32-1 Numerous cherry angiomas and melanocytic nevi on the abdomen of a woman in her second trimester of pregnancy.

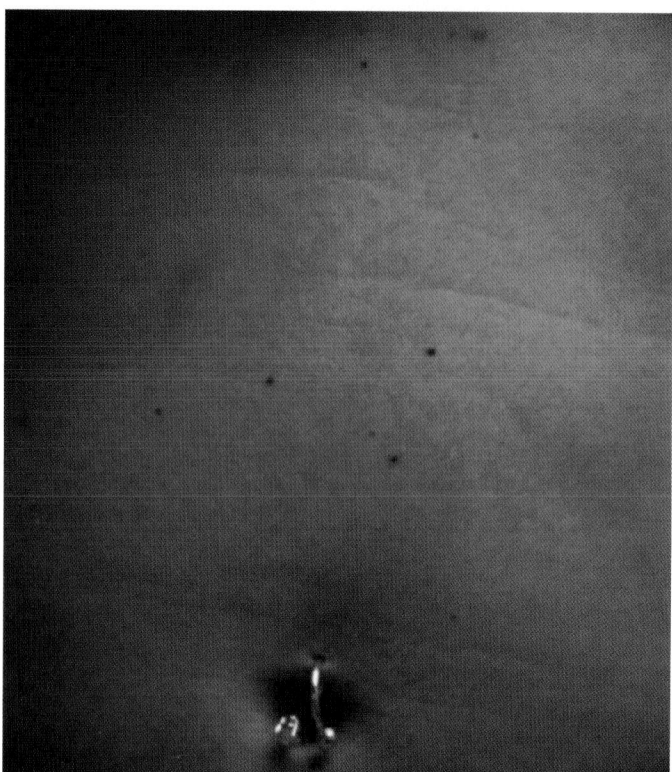

▲ **FIGURE 32-2** Atypical nevus in a woman at 5-month gestation. The two cherry angiomas flanking the nevus were present prior to the onset of pregnancy.

simply be the natural course of the syndrome and not an effect of pregnancy. More studies are necessary to confirm this finding. Fig. 32-2 demonstrates an atypical nevus in a pregnant woman during her fifth month of gestation.

Benign Growths

During pregnancy, many women seek medical attention for the growth of old skin lesions or the new appearance of benign skin lesions (see Table 32-1). Some experience the growth of skin tags (aka molluscum fibrosum gravidarum) on the lateral portions of the neck and axillae or vascular tumors such as glomus tumors or cherry angiomas (Fig. 32-1). Other women develop palmar erythema and/or spider angiomas during pregnancy. Less frequently, a pyogenic granuloma of the gingiva (aka granuloma gravidarum) may appear in the second or third trimester of pregnancy and resolves shortly thereafter.[2]

Neurofibromas, benign tumors of the peripheral nerve sheath, occur sporadically and in association with neurofibromatosis type 1. In both situations, neurofibromas are known to increase in number and size during pregnancy, and become smaller after delivery. A recent study found progesterone receptors on neurofibroma cells and suggests that this phenomenon may be directly mediated by progesterone.[9] Plexiform neurofibromas have also been reported to enlarge with pregnancy and shrink after birth.[10]

The growth of seborrheic keratoses, dermatofibromas, mild to moderate hirsutism, and the development of striae distensae are also commonly noted changes in pregnant patients.

▌MELANOMA AND PREGNANCY

BOX 32-3   Summary

- The exact role of hormones on malignant melanoma (MM) remains unclear.
- Clinically, results from several large studies indicate that pregnancy has no effect on disease-free interval or on overall survival.
- There are no standard guidelines on how long to wait after the diagnosis and/or treatment of an MM to become pregnant.
- Stage I and stage II MM in a pregnant patient should be treated as it would be in a nonpregnant patient.
- Stage III and IV MM requires individualized management optimizing both fetal well-being and maternal outcome.
- Metastatic melanoma to the placenta or fetus is extremely rare. When it does occur, the prognosis is poor.
- Several large studies suggest no increased risk of malignant melanoma in supplemental hormone users.

Background

The effect of pregnancy and exogenous hormones on MM has been the subject of controversy for over 50 years. The hypothesis that the hormonal changes of pregnancy may influence malignant degeneration of nevi arises largely from clinical observations that MMs are rare prior to puberty.[11] Secondly, men have a more aggressive course of MM than do females; lastly, older reports link MM in pregnant women with a grave prognosis.[12] Nevertheless, biochemical evidence to support the hypothesis of a hormonal mediator in MM cell proliferation and the induction of angiogenesis is lacking. Although early reports point to a hormone receptor on some MM cells,[13] recent studies using monoclonal antibody techniques have failed to detect estrogen receptors on benign nevi, primary MM, metastatic MM, or pregnancy-associated MM.[14]

Epidemiology

Most cases of MM in the United States occur among men, but the age-specific incidence rates are higher among females rather than among males in the first four decades of life. Melanoma is the second most common primary cancer in white women in the United States (ages 15 to 44 years) and consequently one of the most frequently diagnosed during pregnancy. In the United States, the age-specific incidence rate in women aged 25 to 34 years is 15.8 per 100,000.[15] Population-based studies report that the incident number of melanoma cases in pregnant women does not exceed the number for the corresponding age group expected based on current incident rates.[16]

In several European countries, the incidence of melanoma is higher in women of all ages.[17] Australia, like the United States, reports a higher incidence in men. Nonetheless, Australian incidence rates for both sexes are the highest in the world with a lifetime risk of 1 in 16 for men and 1 in 24 for women.[18]

Table 32-1
Benign Growths Associated With Pregnancy

Skin tags	Spider angiomas
Dermatofibromas	Pyogenic granuloma
Seborrheic keratoses	Striae distensae
Glomus tumors	Hirsutism
Cherry angiomas	Neurofibromas (incl. plexiform)

Prognosis

Reports from the 1950s paint a poor prognosis for melanoma diagnosed in pregnancy.[19,20] Many of these studies have been criticized for failing to adjust for other prognostic determinants, the lack of an appropriate control group, and a relatively small number of cases.[21]

In 1985, the WHO conducted a retrospective study of patients with melanoma that showed no survival differences between pregnant and non-pregnant women with stage I melanoma after correcting for tumor thickness, which remains the strongest predictor of mortality in melanoma.[22] There are several other well-controlled studies that have compared survival rates and disease-free interval (DFI) in pregnant versus age-matched nonpregnant controls. A recent review by Driscoll and Grant-Kels lists these studies in table format.[4] In all of the studies reviewed, there was no significant difference in overall survival (OS) rates between the two groups. Only two of the studies reported a significantly shorter DFI in pregnant patients.[23,24] A third study trended toward a longer DFI in the pregnant group, but this difference was not statistically significant.[25]

Other studies have assessed prognosis of MM by looking at large populations over time from state and national registries.[26] One of these reported on the prognosis of "pregnancy-associated MM" that referred to MM diagnosed during or within 1 year of pregnancy, and found no differences in overall survival in 9 years of follow-up.[27] However, in both studies, tumor thickness data was missing for a percentage of patients.

Two reports indicate that pregnancy may be associated with worse prognostic factors such as increased thickness.[22,28] However, this difference has not been consistently reported. The traditional belief that changing nevi is normal in pregnancy may have contributed to this finding.

Otherwise, there may in fact be a selective growth advantage during pregnancy. Larger case-controlled studies using objectively monitored enlarging nevi in pregnancy and newer laboratory techniques to histologically study melanoma cells are needed.

Management

Results from the most recent studies indicate that pregnancy in itself is not a prognostic factor in MM. Thus, recommendations for the management of changing nevi during pregnancy are identical to those in the nonpregnant patient. All pregnant patients should have a full skin exam and changing nevi that are clinically suspicious should be biopsied. Several studies have demonstrated the effectiveness of dermatoscopic evaluation during pregnancy.[29] Wide excision around the melanoma site adhering to current guidelines is standard of care for all patients with stage I and stage II melanoma. This can be safely performed during pregnancy.[30] Sentinel lymph node mapping and biopsy, if necessary, may also be safely performed in pregnancy.[31] It may be prudent however to consult with the patient's obstetrician and to monitor the fetus before and after the surgery.

The management of advanced or metastatic melanoma in pregnancy is more challenging. Each case is individual and no broad guidelines exist. Interdisciplinary care is necessary to assure proper management and the discussion of treatment should include optimal maternal therapy and fetal well-being. Imaging studies should be limited to those that have the lowest amount of exposure to ionizing radiation.

Patients who have had a melanoma often ask about becoming pregnant after treatment and about the risk for recurrence. There are no standard guidelines on the length of time to wait after the diagnosis of melanoma before getting pregnant. Studies that have assessed this relationship have revealed that pregnancy following a diagnosis and treatment of melanoma does not change prognosis.[21,24] How long to wait before getting pregnant should be based on the risk of recurrence weighed against the age of the patient and the desire to get pregnant. There are no set guidelines, but patients typically wait 0 to 5 years. Most recurrences happen within 3 years.[32]

Effects on the Fetus

Melanoma metastasizing to the placenta or the fetus is an exceedingly rare event. Despite this, of all malignant tumors in pregnancy, MM is the tumor that most frequently metastasizes to the placenta or fetus, and accounts for >50% of all tumors with fetal involvement.[33] An extensive review of the literature in 2003 by Alexander et al found 27 cases of placental or fetal metastasis of MM; 6 of the 27 cases had fetal metastasis. All cases occurred with stage IV melanoma and involvement of other viscera.[34] With placental involvement the fetal risk of melanoma is estimated at 22%. Both the infant and the mother fair poorly in this situation; five out of six infants with metastatic melanoma died in infancy and the life expectancy of women with placental metastasis is 6 months. If there has been placental metastasis, the pediatrician must be notified in order to regularly evaluate the infant for skin nodules and other signs of metastatic lesions.

Supplemental Hormones and Malignant Melanoma

The influence of exogenous hormones such as oral contraceptive pills and hormone replacement therapy (HRT) on MM has also been the focus of extensive study.

Early studies discovered that a proportion of melanoma cells carry a type II estrogen receptor; however, the absence or presence of this receptor did affect the outcome of an individual patient.[35] Newer techniques have failed to confirm the presence of an estrogen receptor on melanoma cells. Placental growth factor, a member of the platelet-derived growth factor family, has recently been found to be secreted from human melanoma cell lines; however, only one group was able to show MM cell proliferation in response to placental growth factor.[36]

Regardless of the conflicting laboratory findings, clinical data from a systematic review of 18 case-controlled studies that collectively evaluated 3796 cases and 9442 controls failed to identify an increased risk of MM in oral contraceptive users.[37] In 2003, Karagas et al pooled data from 10 case-controlled studies; and again found no relationship between melanoma incidence and duration of oral contraceptive use.[38] However, in a 1999 prospective study of the Nurses Health Study cohort, there was a twofold increased risk of MM in current oral contraceptive users when compared to never users and a further increase in current users of greater than 10 years.[39] This study was limited by lack of information on confounding variables such as sunbathing habits.

There has been less study on the topic of HRT. Two recent reports indicate that HRT after a melanoma does not adversely affect prognosis.[40,41] Currently, there is no data to contraindicate the use of HRT after a melanoma.

DERMATOFIBROSARCOMA PROTUBERANS IN PREGNANCY

BOX 32-4   Summary

- Dermatofibrosarcoma protuberans (DFSP) is a rare tumor that may first present or rapidly enlarge during pregnancy.

Dermatofibrosarcoma protuberans (DFSP) is an uncommon tumor of the dermis that has a high rate of local recurrence, but rarely metastasizes, occurring in only 5% of cases. DFSP usually presents as a slow-growing tumor that can clinically mimic a keloid. It may first appear, or rapidly enlarge, during pregnancy.[42] However, there is no evidence to suggest that pregnancy is associated with the fibrosarcomatous changes that are associated with a more aggressive tumor. DFSP is known to be responsive to platelet-derived growth factor and possibly progesterone, which may explain its rapid growth during pregnancy.[43] Levels of both PDGF and progesterone are increased during pregnancy. Nonetheless, patients with a history of DFSP should be monitored for recurrences and rapidly enlarging tumors should be followed during pregnancy.

FINAL THOUGHTS

There are a number of physiologic cutaneous changes and benign cutaneous growths that are associated with pregnancy. However, changing pigmented lesions are not a normal part of pregnancy and a suspicious lesion should be evaluated as it would in any other individual.

Pregnancy or hormone use before, during, or after a diagnosis of melanoma does not influence survival. Breslow thickness, site, and the presence of ulceration are still the key determinants of prognosis. Patients should be counseled on these factors and not on the prognostic significance of pregnancy. Dermatologic surgery, including sentinel lymph node biopsy can be safely performed in pregnancy.

More studies are needed to evaluate the hormone responsiveness of melanoma cells and on the relationship of HRT and MM. Patients with a history of DFSP should be monitored especially closely during pregnancy.

REFERENCES

1. Pavlidis NA. Coexistence of pregnancy and malignancy. *Oncologist.* 2002;7:279–287.
2. Lawley TJ, Yancey KB. Skin changes across the span of life: skin changes and diseases in pregnancy. In: *Fitzpatrick's Dermatology in General Medicine.* 6th edn. New York: McGraw-Hill Medical Publishing Division; 2003.
3. Lewis KD, Gonzalez R, Robinson WA, et al. A young woman with melanoma diagnosed during pregnancy. *Oncology.* 2004;18(7):794–799.
4. Driscoll MS, Grant-Kels JM. Nevi and melanoma in pregnancy. *Dermatol Clin.* 2006;24:199–204.
5. Foucar E, Bentley TJ, Laube DW, et al. A histopathologic evaluation of nevocellular nevi in pregnancy. *Arch Dermatol.* 1985;121:350–354.
6. Sanchez JL, Figueroa LD, Rodriguez E. Behavior of melanocytic nevi during pregnancy. *Am J Dermatopathol.* 1984;6(suppl 1): 89–91.
7. Pennoyer JW, Grin CM, Driscoll MS, et al. Changes in the size of melanocytic nevi in pregnancy. *J Am Acad Dermatol.* 1997;36:378-382.
8. Ellis DL. Pregnancy and sex steroid hormone effects on nevi of patients with the dysplastic nevus syndrome. *J Am Acad Dermatol.* 1991;25:467–482.
9. McLaughlin ME, Jacks T. Progesterone receptor expression in neurofibromas. *Cancer Res.* 2003;63:752–755.
10. Isikoglu M, Has R, Korkmaz D, et al. Plexiform neurofibroma during and after pregnancy. *Arch Gynecol Obstet.* 2002;267: 41–42.
11. Sober AJ, Lew RA, Koh HK, et al. Epidemiology of cutaneous melanoma: an update. *Dermatol Clin.* 1991;9:617–629.
12. Riberti C, Marola G, Bertani A. Malignant melanoma: the adverse effect of pregnancy. *Br J Plast Surg.* 1981;34:338–339.
13. Grill HJ, Benes P, Manz B, et al. Steroid hormone receptor analysis in human melanoma and non-malignant human skin. *Br J Dermatol.* 1982;107(suppl 23): 64–65.
14. Duncan LM, Travers RL, Koerner FC, et al. Estrogen and progesterone receptor analysis in pregnancy-associated melanoma: absence of immunohistochemically detectable hormone receptors. *Hum Pathol.* 1994;25:36–41.
15. Available at: http://seer.cancer.gov/fast-stats/sites.php?site=Melanoma+of+the+Skin&stat=Mortality. Accessed July 30, 2006.
16. Lambe M, Ekbom A. Cancers coinciding with child bearing: delayed diagnosis during pregnancy? *BMJ.* 1995;311:1607–1608.
17. Reis LAG, Eisner MP, Kosary CL, et al, eds. *SEER Cancer Statistics Review, 1975–2002.* Bethesda, MD: National Cancer Institute. Available at: http://seer.cancer.gov/csr/1975_2002/. Accessed July 31, 2006.
18. McPherson M, Elwood M, English DR, et al. Presentation and detection of invasive melanoma in a high-risk population. *J Am Acad Dermatol.* 2006;54:783–792.
19. Byrd FJ, Jr, McGanity WJ. Effect of pregnancy on the clinical course of malignant melanoma. *South Med J.* 1954;47:196–200.
20. Pack GT, Scharnagel IM. The prognosis for malignant melanoma in the pregnant women. *Cancer.* 1951;4324–4334.
21. Wiggins CL, Berwick M, Newton Bishop JA. Malignant melanoma in pregnancy. *Obstet Gynecol Clin N Am.* 2005;32: 559–568.
22. MacKie RM, Bufalino R, Morabito A, et al. Lack of effect on outcome of melanoma. For the World Health Organization Programme. *Lancet.* 1991;337:653–655.
23. Slingluff CL, Jr, Reintgen DS, Vollmer RT, et al. Malignant melanoma arising during pregnancy: a study of 100 patients. *Ann Surg.* 1990;21:552–559.
24. Reintgen DS, McCarty KS, Vollmer R, et al. Malignant melanoma and pregnancy. *Cancer.* 1985;55:1340–1344.
25. Daryanani D, Plukker JT, De Hullu JA, et al. Pregnancy and early-stage melanoma. *Cancer.* 2003;97(9):2248–2253.
26. O'Meara AT, Cress R, Xing G, et al. Malignant melanoma in pregnancy: a population based study. *Cancer.* 2005;103: 1217–1226.
27. Lens MB, Rosdehl I, Ahlbom A, et al. Effect of pregnancy on survival in women with cutaneous malignant melanoma. *J Clin Oncol.* 2004;22:4369–4375.
28. Travers RL, Sober AJ, Berwick M, et al. Increased thickness of pregnancy-associated melanoma. *Br J Dermatol.* 1995;132: 876–883.
29. Zalaudek I, Wolf IH, Hofmann-Wellenhof R, et al. Dermatoscopic follow-up of a changing pigmented melanocytic skin lesion during pregnancy: from nevus to melanoma? *Melanoma Res.* 2004;14:323–325.
30. Richards KA, Stasko T. Dermatologic surgery and the pregnant patient. *Dermatol Surg.* 2002;28(3):248–256.
31. Schwartz JL, Mozurkewich EL, Johnson TM. Current management of patients with melanoma who are pregnant, want to get pregnant or do not want to get pregnant. *Cancer.* 2003;97(9):2130–2133.
32. Gamel JW, George SL, Edwards MJ, et al. The long term clinical course of patients with cutaneous melanoma. *Cancer.* 2002; 95:1286–1293.
33. Altman JF, Lowe L, Redman B, et al. Placental metastasis of maternal melanoma. *J Am Acad Dermatol.* 2003;49(6):1150–1154.
34. Alexander A, Samlowski WE, Grossman D, et al. Metastatic melanoma in pregnancy: risk of transplancental metastases in the infant. *J Clin Oncol.* 2003;21(11): 2179–2186.
35. Neifeld JP, Lippman MC. Steroid hormone receptors and melanoma. *J Invest Dermatol.* 1980;74:379–381.
36. Lacal PM, Failla CM, Pagani E, et al. Human melanoma cells secrete and respond to placenta growth factor and vascular endothelial growth factor. *J Invest Dermatol.* 2000;115(6):1000–1007.
37. Gefeller O, Hassan K, Wille L. Cutaneous malignant melanoma in women and the role of oral contraceptives. *Br J Dermatol.* 1998;138:122–124.
38. Karagas MR, Stukel TA, Dykes J, et al. A pooled analysis of 10 case–control studies of melanoma and oral contraceptive use. *Br J Cancer.* 2002;86:1085–1092.
39. Feskanich D, Hunter DJ, Willett WC, et al. Oral contraceptive use and risk of melanoma in premenopausal women. *Br J Cancer.* 1999;81:918–923.
40. Jeffery SL, Lewis JS. Malignant melanoma and hormone replacement therapy. *Br J Plast Surg.* 2000;53(6):539.
41. MacKie RM, Bray CA. Hormone replacement therapy after surgery for stage 1 or 2 cutaneous melanoma. *Br J Cancer.* 2004; 90(4):770–772.
42. Parlette E, Smith KJ, Germain M, et al. Accelerated growth of dermatofibrosarcoma protuberans during pregnancy. *J Am Acad Dermatol.* 1999;41:778–783.
43. Kikuchi K, Soma Y, Fujimoto M, et al. DFSP: increased growth response to platelet-derived growth factor BB in cell culture. *Biochem Biophys Res Commun.* 1993;196:409–415.

CHAPTER 33

Skin Cancer in the Pediatric Population

Cheryl G. Aber, M.D.
Elizabeth Alvarez Connelly, M.D.
Lawrence Schachner, M.D.

BOX 33-1   Overview

- Skin cancer in the pediatric population is rare, occurring between 1 and 3% of pediatric tumors.
- There is a rising incidence of skin cancer worldwide, particularly in the adolescent population.
- Predisposing conditions of cutaneous malignancy include light pigment skin type, congenital melanocytic nevi, atypical nevi, underlying syndromes, immunosuppression, infection and chronic wound trauma, and genetic susceptibility.
- Environmental factors, especially exposure to sunlight, exacerbate any underlying condition and considerably increase the risk of developing skin cancer.

INTRODUCTION

Skin cancer is a rare occurrence in children. However, there is an overall rising incidence of melanoma, basal cell carcinoma (BCC), and squamous cell carcinoma (SCC) in the pediatric population worldwide. Although sun exposure has been shown to be a predominate risk factor in the development of each of these skin cancers in adults, additional underlying factors or diseases are more common in children. Predisposing conditions such as light pigmentary phenotype, congenital melanocytic nevi (CMN), atypical nevi, an underlying syndrome, immunosuppression, infection, or chronic wound trauma have all been associated with the development of cutaneous malignant tumors. Melanoma represents the most common type of skin cancer in children accounting for 1 to 3% of pediatric tumors.

This chapter will provide a comprehensive review of the incidence, pathogenesis, clinical presentation, and treatment of melanoma in youth. Nonmelanoma skin cancer, although considerably more rare, is also described in the pediatric population and is usually associated with an underlying genetic mutation or syndrome. Prevention strategies discussed at the end of this chapter emphasize the importance of limiting sun exposure and learning protective behaviors at an early age.

MELANOMA

BOX 33-2   Summary

- Overall incidence of melanoma is increasing worldwide.
- Prepubertal melanoma (congenital, infantile, and childhood) accounts for only 0.3 to 0.4% of malignancies in children.
- Adolescents account for the most dramatic increase in incidence, accounting for up to 7% of pediatric cancers.
- The population at risk can be characterized as individuals with light pigmentary phenotype living in latitudes with increased cumulative ultraviolet exposure (e.g., Australia).

Epidemiology

There is an increasing evidence of the rising incidence of melanoma in the pediatric population, particularly adolescents.[1,2] Childhood melanoma or prepubertal melanoma can be categorized into congenital (from utero to birth), infantile (birth to 1 year), and childhood (1 year to puberty).[3] Congenital and infantile melanomas are extremely rare. Melanoma accounts for 2 to 3% of malignancies in pediatric patients.[4] Only 0.3 to 0.4% of the reported melanoma occurs in prepubertal children. The greater part occurs in the adolescent population, as evidenced by a rising incidence of melanoma that has practically doubled in a 10-year period.[5] In the United States, the Surveillance, Epidemiology and End Results Section (SEER) of the National Cancer Institute recorded the newly diagnosed cases of cutaneous melanoma from 1973 to 1996 in patients of all ages. In patients younger than 15 years of age, melanoma accounts for 0.9% of cancers, but increases substantially to 7% in patients aged 15 to 19 years. Patients aged 15 to 19 years carry an annual incidence rate of 14.1 per million, representing the most dramatic increase in melanoma incidence rate compared to any other age group.[6] Epidemiologic data from Australian,[7] Scottish,[8] and British[9] melanoma studies exhibit similar trends of rising rates of melanoma with increasing age in the white population.

Pathogenesis

Understanding which factors cause or contribute to the development of melanoma is complicated. Congenital malignant melanoma, an extremely rare entity, may develop *in utero* by one of three mechanisms: (1) transplacental transmission to a fetus from a mother with metastatic melanoma, (2) primary melanoma arising from giant CMN, or (3) *de novo* cutaneous melanoma without maternal melanoma.[10] Childhood melanoma typically arises from giant CMNs, accounting for at least one-third of prepubertal melanomas. Understanding the natural history of melanoma in childhood and adolescence requires identifying the multiple risk factors that influence the development of this skin malignancy. Interaction of predisposing determinants include CMN, increased density of acquired melanocytic nevi, pigmentary phenotype, sun exposure, numerous or atypical nevi, a family history of melanoma, underlying syndromes, and immunosuppression.

CONGENITAL MELANOCYTIC NEVI

BOX 33-3   Summary

- Congenital melanoma may arise from a giant congenital melanocytic nevi (CMN), *de novo* or via transplacental transmission from a mother with metastatic melanoma.
- Multiple interacting risk factors influence the development of melanoma.
- Large or giant CMNs carry a 4.5 to 10% lifetime risk of developing into melanoma.
- High density of acquired nevi serve as a risk factor and possible precursor for melanoma.
- Lightly pigmented skin types coupled with high cumulative sun exposure correlate with increased nevi and increased incidence of melanoma.
- Atypical nevi confer an increased risk of melanoma.
- Positive family history of atypical nevi and/or melanoma and susceptibility genes play an important role in the development of nevi and melanoma.

Congenital melanocytic nevi (CMNs) are present in approximately 1% of newborns or 1 in 20,000 newborns.[10] CMNs are classified according to the predictive size they will attain in adulthood. Small nevi are less than 1.5 cm in greatest diameter, medium are between 1.5 cm and less than 20 cm, large are at least 20 cm or greater, and giant nevi are greater than 50 cm in diameter. Patients with large or giant CMNs are at greatest risk of developing melanoma.[11] These individuals carry a 4.5 to 10% lifetime risk of developing a cutaneous or extracutaneous melanoma,[12] although recent studies reveal that the risk is at the low end of these estimates.[13] The incidence of melanoma arising from giant CMNs is highest in the first decade of life, more specifically in the first 5 years of life. Patients with large or giant CMNs are additionally at risk of developing neurocutaneous melanosis (NCM). NCM is a rare nonhereditary condition characterized by a large and/or multiple (>3) congenital melanocytic nevi associated wtih a melanocytic proliferation within the leptomeninges.[14] Malignant transformation of these melanocytes into primary central nervous system melanomas may result in serious neurologic sequelae or death.[15] Studies have shown that the presence of many satellite nevi (>20) significantly increase the relative risk of NCM.[16]

In contrast to the earlier prepubertal onset of melanoma in large CMN, small and medium CMNs carry a lifetime risk of less than 1%, with almost no risk before puberty.[17] However, there continues to be much debate regarding the malignant potential of small- and medium-sized nevi since various studies fail to demonstrate any malignant transformation at all.[18]

ACQUIRED MELANOCYTIC NEVI, PHENOTYPE, AND ENVIRONMENTAL INFLUENCES

The onset of acquired melanocytic nevi occurs after infancy in sun-exposed areas and typically increases in size yearly, especially after puberty.[19] Preadolescent children should have less than 15 acquired nevi. Multiple epidemiologic studies have demonstrated that there is a relationship between the development of these nevi and melanoma during childhood and adolescence.[20] The relevance of melanocytic nevi serving as risk factors and precursors of melanoma underlies the importance of understanding the associated factors in the development of melanocytic nevi. The combined affects of both pigmentary phenotype and exposure to ultraviolet light influence the development of nevus. Multiple studies have shown that

the presence of lightly pigmented skin types (fair skin color, red hair, blue eyes, freckles) and propensity to burn are associated with higher nevus counts.[21,22]

Much of the Australian scientific literature has focused on examining factors associated with melanoma in children and adolescents. A prevalence survey of melanocytic nevi among young children (aged 1 to 3 years) attending childcare centers in Brisbane, Australia, demonstrated high total nevus counts associated with heavy facial freckling, sun exposure, and Caucasian ethnicity.[23] In a retrospective study, Youl et al examined the Queensland Cancer Registry from 1987 to 1994 and identified factors associated with the development of melanoma in adolescents aged 15 to 19 years.[24] Patients with melanoma in this study demonstrated a greater density of nevi (2 mm or greater) versus the control group, and a greater nevi count larger than 5 mm. Both of these variables are associated with a higher prevalence of melanoma. In addition, greater than 50% of patients diagnosed with melanoma had more than 100 nevi on their body compared to 13% of the control group. Additional determinants associated with melanoma included light pigmented skin type, propensity to sunburn, degree of facial freckling, increased number of blistering sunburns, lack of sunscreen use, and family history of melanoma. In addition, a growing body of evidence has demonstrated that intense sun exposure during childhood is associated with increased nevi counts. A majority of sunburn studies suggest that ultraviolet radiation from sun exposure and sunburns early in life is associated with an increased rate of melanoma in adulthood.[25,26]

ATYPICAL NEVI

Atypical nevi, replacing the term dysplastic nevi, are lesions irregular in size, color, and texture or contour. Atypical nevi do not typically appear until puberty and have a predilection for sun-exposed sites. Presence of these nevi confers an increased risk for early onset of melanoma. In a case-controlled study, 1 nevi corresponded to a 2-fold risk, and 10 atypical nevi conferred a 12-fold increased risk of melanoma.[27] An increased number of atypical nevi is also seen subsequent to chemotherapy for childhood malignancy, suggesting that immunosuppression may play a role in the development of nevi.

FAMILIAL ATYPICAL MOLE/MELANOMA (FAMM) SYNDROME

Children or adolescents with multiple atypical nevi and a family member with atypical nevi or melanoma may be affected by the hereditary syndrome, Familial Atypical Mole and Melanoma (FAMM) Syndrome. Characterized by early onset cutaneous melanomas and multiple atypical melanocytic nevi (often exceeding 100), this syndrome has a probable polygenic inheritance pattern. Germline mutations of *CDKN2A* were demonstrated by Hussussian et al[28] in 92% of melanoma-prone patients, with linkage to the 9p21 chromosome. The *CDKN2A* gene is composed of the p16 and p14ARF exons. p16 is necessary to arrest the cellular proliferation, while p14ARF is involved in enhancing a separate tumor suppressor, p53. Mutations of these components contribute to tumorigenesis.[29] Individuals with FAMM develop a higher rate of melanomas at earlier ages of onset with an increased risk of developing multiple primary melanomas compared to the general population.[30] Ten percent of affected persons experience their first melanoma in childhood.[31] An increased prevalence of atypical nevi is noted to occur in sun-exposed sites[32] and after chemotherapy for childhood malignancy,[33] suggesting that environmental factors such as ultraviolet radiation and immunosuppression play a role in the development of these nevi and melanoma.

CLINICAL EVALUATION

BOX 33-4 Summary

- Underestimation of melanoma in children leads to delay or underdiagnosis.
- There is a variability in clinical signs when diagnosing melanoma in children.
- Common features of melanoma include color change (including amelanotic), bleeding, itching, and a palpable subcutaneous mass.
- Superficial spreading melanoma is the most common subtype of pediatric melanoma.
- A melanoma with a nodular focal area signifies deeper penetration of cancer.
- Primary determinants of prognosis of localized disease is based on tumor thickness and depth of invasion.

Clinical Presentation

Diagnosing melanoma in children can be particularly challenging given that the growth of a nevi or increase in the number of acquired nevi may represent a physiologic, as opposed to a malignant change. As a rule of thumb, melanomas are often larger than benign nevi. As in adults, the "ABCD" mnemonic is a useful guideline when assessing a suspicious lesion. However, in children, a tumor can appear amelanotic or simulate a pyogenic granuloma.[34] Common clinical features observed in pediatric and adolescent melanoma include color change, recent increase in the size of a lesion, bleeding, itching, palpable subcutaneous mass, and adenopathy.[35] Irregularities in pigmentation with shades ranging from brown black to red purple and borders can help make the diagnosis. In a SEER report[5] (National Cancer report), 89% of affected patients less than 20 years of age had localized melanoma, most commonly on the trunk. A separate study found that primary melanoma in children most commonly presented on the extremities followed by the trunk, and head and neck.

Histology

Of the four clinical subtypes of melanoma, superficial spreading melanoma is the most common in children. These malignancies tend to grow laterally for a longer phase before piercing deeper into the dermal layer. Clinically, it may appear as a wide melanotic plaque with possible nodular or papular focal areas signifying deeper penetration. In contrast, the nodular subtype of melanoma has a comparatively shorter lateral growth period with a deeper vertical infiltration. This nodular subtype typically develops from CMNs. Acral lentiginous melanomas, which are rare in children, develop in deeply pigmented individuals typically on the palms, soles, and mucosa. Lentigo maligna, the fourth subtype does not develop in children. The same pathologic criteria used to diagnose melanoma in adults are used for children.

Prognosis

Although comprehensive staging guidelines have not been established for children, progression of tumor growth can be categorized into three stages: localized disease, lymphatic invasion, and distant metastases.[2] Similar to the adult population, primary determinants of prognosis of localized disease are based on tumor thickness (Breslow thickness) and anatomic depth of invasion (Clark levels). Clark defined the level of tumor invasion (I to V) and correlated it with

survival rates.[36] Breslow quantified tumor thickness and its prognostic relationship to survival. Tumors less than 0.76 mm in thickness are curable, melanomas of size 0.76 to 3.65 mm carry an intermediate prognosis, and tumors thicker than 3.65 mm portend the poorest outcome.[37] The American Joint Committee on Cancer has developed a revised (adult) staging system that provides detailed information on prognostic variables that influence clinical outcome and survival. Emphasis on the prognostic significance of ulceration of the lesion, sentinel node biopsy results, number of lymph nodes involved, and sites of metastases are taken into account in this staging system. The mortality rate for pediatric melanoma is comparable to the adult data, varying between 14 and 67%, and is dependent on the stage of the tumor.[38] Some studies report a poorer prognosis of childhood melanoma, presumably due to a delay in the diagnosis of such a rare childhood entity.[39] Brain metastasis affects approximately 18% of children diagnosed with melanoma and carries a very poor prognosis.[40]

Treatment

BOX 33-5 Summary

- Surgical excision is the mainstay of therapy for localized disease.
- Staging with sentinel lymph node biopsy is indicated in lesions >1 mm, the presence of ulceration, or Clark level of IV or V.
- There is a limited pediatric research on the treatment of disseminated disease.

The mainstay of therapy is excisional biopsy of any suspicious lesions and subsequent prompt surgical resection. Management guidelines for resection of *in situ* melanoma are taken from the adult literature. Resection of lesions thinner than 1 mm in depth requires a 1 cm margin. Lesions greater than 1 mm in thickness require at least a 2-cm margin. Staging with a sentinel lymph node biopsy is indicated in lesions thicker than 1 mm, the presence of ulceration, or a Clark level of IV or V.[41] Although there is a lack of pediatric data regarding microscopic involvement of the sentinel node and its therapeutic implications, lymphadenectomy of the involved area is recommended with a positive sentinel node biopsy. Adjuvant therapy with interferon alpha-2b has been shown to improve relapse-free survival in survival in patients with high-risk melanoma in the adult population[42] and two small

pediatric series.[43] No large trials of this medication have been studied in the pediatric population. Treatment of disseminated advanced melanoma may involve chemotherapy, radiotherapy, and immunotherapy.[2]

NONMELANOMA SKIN CANCER (NMSC)

NMSC has increasingly become more common in many population throughout the world.[44] BSC and SCC represent the two most common types of NMSC. Children more susceptible to these malignancies are those with underlying syndromes or immunosuppressive states due to various causes. Certain syndromes are associated with increased photosensitivity, placing affected individuals more at risk for the development of these cancers. In addition, secondary NMSC in childhood cancer survivors as a long-term adverse effect of cancer therapy (radiation, immunosuppressive medication) is increasing in incidence.[45] Similarly, lifelong immunosuppression following pediatric organ transplantation poses a risk for skin cancer development.[46] Ionizing radiation is also a well-established risk factor of NMSC,[47] as observed in individuals with radiation therapy during childhood[48] and in survivors of the atomic bombing.[49]

Squamous Cell Carcinoma

Squamous cell carcinoma (SCC), accounting for less than 5% of childhood skin cancers and less than 0.10% of all childhood malignancies, is extremely uncommon.[50] Often those affected harbor significant risk factors that include intense exposure to ultraviolet or ionizing radiation, a predisposing genetic syndrome, immunosuppression, human papillomavirus (HPV) infection, or a combination of these factors. Syndromes such as xeroderma pigmentosum, a degenerative disorder resulting from defective DNA nucleotide excision repair mechanisms, is characterized by exquisite photosensitivity to ultraviolet radiation and early onset of cutaneous malignancies, including SCCs.[51] Rothmund–Thomson syndrome is associated with an increased incidence of SCCs.[52] Chronic wounds in individuals suffering from dystrophic epidermolysis bullosa are also at risk for developing SCCs.[53]

Basal Cell Carcinoma

Basal cell carcinoma (BCC), comprising approximately 0.24% of pediatric tumors and accounting for 13% of pediatric cutaneous skin cancers,[54] often has a delayed diagnosis secondary to a low index of suspicion. Due to the rarity of BCC in children, underlying disease or condition is often investigated. Nevoid BCC syndrome (NBCCS), an autosomal dominant disease, is characterized by multiple BCCs that typically develop by a median age of 20 years.[55] BCCs appear as skin color to tan, dome-shaped papules or skin tags predominantly distributed on the face (mostly on periorbital areas, eyelids, nose, malar region, and upper lip), neck, back, chest, and upper limbs.[56] These basal cell nevi often increase in number after puberty. However, most of these BCCs remain localized within the epidermis for many years before becoming locally aggressive, invading the dermis. Rombo and Basex syndromes are associated with BCCs.

PREVENTION

BOX 33-6   Summary

- Strategies that limit sun exposure include sun avoidance during peak hours, protective clothing, and application of sunblock.
- Sun safety programs through the media and school programs can influence the knowledge, attitudes, and behaviors of children.
- Rising use of tanning beds among the teenage population is a growing concern.
- Secondary prevention includes full-body skin examination during routine office visits by the primary care physician and the dermatologist.

The risk of melanoma and non-melanoma skin cancers (BCCs and SCCs) is markedly increased with excessive sun exposure and sunburns. Studies have shown that exposure to high levels of sunlight in childhood is a strong risk factor for the development of melanoma,[57] BCC,[58] and SCC.[59] Primary prevention strategies that limit sun exposure, such as avoidance during peak sunlight hours, protective clothing, and use of broad-spectrum (UVA and UVB) sunscreen and sun block, are important steps in limiting the risk of developing skin cancer. Behavioral modification learned during the early years can have long-lasting effects into adulthood. Sun safety education learned in schools and through the media have the potential to improve the knowledge, attitudes, and behaviors of children at a pivotal time in their lives. Influencing the behavior of

adolescent youth presents a unique challenge to health educators given the increased tendency toward high-risk behaviors. The rising use of tanning beds among adolescents, especially females aged 15 to 18 years,[60] underscores the need to educate the public regarding the risks of sun exposure and the need to create legislation that discourages use of tanning beds. Much can be learned from the Australian national public health skin cancer prevention program whose policy guidelines have translated into decreased incidence of sunburn, skin cancer, and mortality.[61]

Secondary prevention through regular screening for skin cancer by the pediatrician, general practitioner, or dermatologist is essential in detecting any suspicious lesions. Performing full-body skin examinations during routine office visits is a vital screening practice that can have a life-saving outcome. Familiarity with known high-risk populations (patients with lightly pigmented features, dysplastic nevi, a family history, or syndrome associated with skin cancer), should alert a clinician to have a higher index of suspicion when screening.

FINAL THOUGHTS

Although skin cancer accounts for a small percentage of pediatric cancers, its rising occurrence and its underdiagnosis warrant more attention to be focused on this condition. An awareness of factors that place an individual at risk coupled along with preventative behavior strategies will hopefully limit the increasing incidence of cutaneous malignancies in the pediatric population.

REFERENCES

1. Desmond RA, Soong SJ. Epidemiology of malignant melanoma. *Surg Clin North Am.* 2003;83:1–29.
2. Pappo AS. Melanoma in children and adolescents. *Eur J Cancer.* 2003;39:2651–2661.
3. Richardson SK, Tannous ZS, Mihm MC. Congenital and infantile melanoma: a review of the literature and report of an uncommon variant, pigment-synthesizing melanoma. *J Acad Dermatol.* 2002;47:77–90.
4. Young JL, Percy CL, Asire AJ, et al. Cancer incidence and mortality in the United States, 1973–77. *Natl Cancer Inst Monogr.* 1981;57:1–187.
5. Berg P, Lindelof B. Differences in malignant melanoma between children and adolescents. *Arch Dermatol.* 1997;133:295.
6. Gloecker RL, Smith LA, Gurney JG, et al. Cancer incidence and survival among children and adolescents: United States

SEER program 1975–1995. SEER program pub. no. 99-4649, National Cancer Institute, Bethesda, MD; 1999.
7. MacLennan R, Green AC, McLeod GRC, et al. Increasing incidence of cutaneous melanoma in Queensland, Australia. *J Natl Cancer Inst.* 1992;84:1427–1432.
8. Mackie RM, Bray CA, Hole DJ. Incidence and survival from malignant melanoma in Scotland: an epidemiological study. *Lancet.* 2002;360:587–591.
9. Stiller C. Epidemiology of cancer in adolescents. *Med Pediatr Oncol.* 1997;39:139–155.
10. Fishman C, Mihm MC, Sober AJ. Diagnosis and management of nevi and cutaneous melanoma in infants and children. *Clin Dermatol.* 2002;20:44–50.
11. Marghoob AA. Congenital melanocytic nevi. In: Rigel D, et al, eds. *Cancer of the Skin.* Philadelphia, PA: Saunders; 2004:1–22.
12. Watt AJ, Kotsis SV, Chung KC. Risk of melanoma arising in large congenital melanocytic nevi: a systemic review. *Plast Reconstr Surg.* 2004;113:1968–1974.
13. Berg P, Lindelof B. Congenital nevocytic nevi: follow-up of a Swedish birth register sample regarding etiologic factors, discomfort and removal rate. *Pediatr. Dermatol.* 2002;19:293–297.
14. Kadonaga N, Frieden J. Neurocutaneous melanosis: definition and review of the literature. *J Am Acad Dermatol.* 1997;24:747–755.
15. Hale EK, Stein J, Ben-Porat L, et al. Association of melanoma and neurocutaneous melanocytosis with large congenital melanocytic nevi—results from the NYU-LCMN registry. *Br J Dermatol.* 2005;152:512–517.
16. Bittencourt FV, Marghoob AA, Kopf AW. Large congenital melanocytic nevi and the risk for development of malignant melanoma and neurocutaneous melanocytosis. *Pediatrics* 2000;106(4):736–741.
17. Morelli JG, Weston WL. Sun, kids, moles and melanoma. *Contemp Pediatr.* 1999.
18. Swerdlow AJ, English JSC, Qiao Z. The risk of melanoma in patients with congenital nevi: a cohort study. *J Am Acad Dermatol.* 1995;32:595–599.
19. McLean DI, Gallagher MA. "sunburn" freckles, café-av-lait macules, and other pigmented lesions of schoolchildren: The Vancouver Mole Study. *J Am Acad Derm* 1995;32:565–70.
20. Holly EA, Kelly JW, Shpall SN, Chiu SH. Number of melanocytic nevi as a major risk factor for malignant melanoma. *J Am Acad Dermatol.* 1987;17:459–468.
21. Carli P, Biggeri A, Giannotti B. Malignant melanoma in Italy: risks associated with common and clinically atypical melanocytic nevi. *J Am Acad Dermatol.* 1995;32:734–739.
22. Harrison SL, MacLennan R, Speare R, Wronski I. Sun exposure and melanocytic nevi in young Australian children. *Lancet.* 1994;344:1529–1532.
23. Whiteman DC, Brown RM, Purdie DM, Hughes MC. Melanocytic nevi in very young children: the role of phenotype, sun exposure, and sun protection. *J Am Acad Dermatol.* 2005;52:40–47.
24. Youl P, Aitken J, Hayward N, et al. Melanoma in adolescents: a case–control study of risk factors in Queensland, Australia. *Int J Cancer.* 2002;98:92–98.

25. Oliveria SA, Saraiya M, Geller AC, Heneghan MK, Jorgensen C. Sun exposure and risk of melanoma. *Arch Dis Child.* 2006;91:131–138.
26. English DR, Armstrong DK, Kricker A, Fleming C. Sunlight and cancer. *Cancer Causes Control.* 1997;8:271–283.
27. Tucker MA, Halpern A, Holly EA, et al. Clinically recognised dysplastic nevi. A central risk factor for cutaneous melanoma. *JAMA.* 1997;277:1439–1444.
28. Hussussian CJ, Struewing JP, Goldstein AM, et al. Germline p16 mutations in familial melanoma. *Nat Genet.* 1994;8:15–21.
29. Piepkorn M. Melanoma genetics: an update with focus on the CDKN2A(p16)/ARF tumor suppressors. *J Am Acad Dermatol.* 2000;42:705–722.
30. Goldstein AM, Fraser MC, Clark WHJ, Tucker MA. Age at diagnosis and transmission of invasive melanoma in 23 families with cutaneous malignant melanoma/dysplastic nevi. *J Natl Cancer Inst.* 1994; 86:1385–1390.
31. Greene MH, Tucker WH, Jr., Tucker MA, et al. High risk of malignant melanoma in melanoma prone families with dysplastic nevi. *Ann Intern Med.* 1985;102: 458.
32. Kopf AW, Lindsay AC, Rogers GS, et al. Relationship of nevocytic nevi to sun exposure in dysplastic nevus syndrome. *J Am Acad Dermatol.* 1985;12: 656–662.
33. Green A, Smith P, McWhorter W, et al. Melanocytic nevi and melanoma in survivors of childhood cancer. *Br J Cancer.* 1993;67:1053–1057.
34. Ferrari A, Bono A, Collini P, et al. What do we know about cutaneous melanoma of childhood? *Contemp Pediatr.* 2006;23(9): 42–48.
35. Bodie AW, Jr., Smith JL, Jr., McBride CM. Malignant melanoma in children and young adults: effect of diagnostic criteria on staging and end results. *South Med J.* 1978;17:1074–1078.
36. Clark WH, Jr., From L, Bernardino EA, et al. The histogenesis and biologic behavior of primary human malignant melanomas of the skin. *Cancer Res.* 1969;29:705.

37. Breslow A. Tumor thickness, level of invasion and node dissection in stage I cutaneous melanoma. *Ann Surg.* 1975;182:572.
38. Williams ML, Pennella R. Melanoma, melanocytic nevi and other melanoma risk factors. *J Pediatr.* 1994;124(6):833–845.
39. Handfield-Jones SE, Smith NP. Malignant melanoma in childhood. *Br J Dermatol.* 1996;34:607.
40. Rodriguez-Galindo C, Pappo AS, Kaste SC, et al. Brain metastasis in children with melanoma. *Cancer.* 1997;79:2440.
41. Balch CM, Ross MI. Final version of the American Joint Committee of Cancer staging system for cutaneous melanoma. *J Clin Oncol.* 2001;19:3635–3648.
42. Agarwala SS, Kirkwood JM. Update on adjuvant interferon therapy for high-risk melanoma. *Oncology.* 2002;16:1177–1187.
43. Navid F, Furnam WL, Fleming M, et al. The feasibility of adjuvant interferon alpha-2b in children with high risk melanoma. *Cancer.* 2005;103:780.
44. Diepgen TL, Mahler V. The epidemiology of skin cancer. *Br J Dermatol.* 2002; 146(suppl):1–6.
45. Karagas MR, Greenberg ER, Spencer SK. Increase in incidence rates of basal cell and squamous cell skin cancer in New Hampshire, USA. *Int J Cancer.* 1999;81: 555–559.
46. Euvrard S, Kanitakis J, Cochat P, Claudy A. Skin cancers following pediatric organ transplantation. *Dermatol Surg.* 2004;30: 616–621.
47. Shore RE. Radiation-induced skin cancer in humans. *Med Pediatr Oncol.* 2001;36: 549–554.
48. Ron E, Modan B, Preston D, et al. Radiation-induced skin carcinomas of the head and neck. *Radiat Res.* 1991;125: 318–325.
49. Ron E, Preston DL, Kishikawa M, et al. Skin tumor risk among atomic-bomb survivors in Japan. *Cancer Causes Control.* 1998;9:393–401.
50. Burggorf WHC, Ruiz-Maldonado R. In: Schachner LA, Hansen RC, eds. *Benign and Malignant Tumors in Pediatric Dermatology.* 3rd ed. Amsterdam, The Netherlands: Elsevier; 2003:880.

51. Kraemer KH, Lee MM, Scotto J. Xeroderma pigmentosum. Cutaneous, ocular and neurologic abnormalities in 830 published cases. *Arch Dermatol.* 1987; 123:241–250.
52. Piquero-Casals J, Okubo AY, Nico MM. Rothmund–Thomson syndrome in three siblings and the development of cutaneous squamous cell carcinoma. *Pediatr Dermatol.* 2002;19(4):312–316.
53. Bosch RJ, Gallardo MA, Ruiz del Portal G, et al. Squamous cell carcinoma secondary to recessive dystrophic epidermolysis bullosa: report of eight tumours in four patients. *J Eur Acad Dermatol Venereol.* 1999;13(3):198–204.
54. Burggorf WHC, Ruiz-Maldonado R. In: Schachner LA, Hansen RC, eds. *Benign and Malignant Tumors in Pediatric Dermatology.* 3rd ed. Amsterdam, The Netherlands: Elsevier; 2003:881.
55. Shanley S, Ratcliffe J, Hockey A. Nevoid basal cell carcinoma syndrome: review of 118 affected individuals. *Am J Hum Genet.* 1994;50:282–290.
56. Tsao H. Update on familial cancer syndromes and the skin. *J Am Acad Dermatol.* 2000;42:939–969.
57. Whiteman DC, Whiteman CA, Green AC. Childhood sun exposure as a risk factor for melanoma: a systematic review of epidemiologic studies. *Cancer Causes Control.* 2001;12:69–82.
58. Armstrong BK, Kricker A. The epidemiology of UV induced skin cancer. *J Photochem Photobiol B.* 2001;63:8–18.
59. Gallagher RP, Hill GB, Bajdik CD, et al. Sunlight exposure, pigmentation factors, and risk of nonmelanocytic skin cancer. II. Squamous cell carcinoma. *Arch Dermatol.* 1995;131:164–169.
60. Geller AC, Colditz G, Oliveria S, et al. Use of sunscreens, sun burning rates, and tanning bed use among more than 10,000 US children and adolescents. *Pediatrics.* 2002;109:1009–1014.
61. Marks R. Two decades of the public health approach to skin cancer control in Australia: why, how and where are we now? *Australas J Dermatol.* 1999;40: 1–5.

CHAPTER 34

Syndromes Associated With Skin Cancers

Cheryl Aber, M.D.

Elizabeth Alvarez Connelly, M.D.

Lawrence A. Schachner, M.D.

BOX 34-1   Overview

- Genodermatosis is a disease that is genetically based with cutaneous findings as a primary feature.
- Primary cutaneous malignancies at early ages of onset are suggestive of an inherited disorder.
- Cutaneous skin cancer associated with many syndromes are exacerbated by environmental conditions such as sun exposure.
- Increased identification of affected gene loci has enabled greater understanding and diagnosis of many of these syndromes.

INTRODUCTION

Skin cancer is at times one of the primary findings associated with several syndromes affecting multisystems of the body. Cancer is fundamentally a genetic disorder of a cell's ability to proliferate; therefore, it stands to reason that there are many skin cancers associated with genetic diseases. These genetic disorders predispose an individual to both malignant and nonmalignant tumors. Genodermatoses is a term used to describe a genetically based disease in which one of the primary features includes cutaneous findings. Many of these disorders clearly have a hereditary component. Some of these hereditary genodermatoses follow a mendelian genetic pattern, but most familial diseases follow a more complex pattern of inheritance. This chapter will review syndromes associated with skin cancers both with a known and unknown familial hereditary pattern.

FAMILIAL ATYPICAL MOLE AND MELANOMA SYNDROME

BOX 34-2   Summary

- Higher rate of cutaneous melanoma and atypical nevi at an early age

---

- Increased incidence of multiple primary melanomas
- Positive family history of melanoma
- Inheritance pattern is of polygenic etiology
- Affected gene loci of the *CDKN2A* region with linkage to the 9p21 site
- Require regular dermatologic screening exams
- Sun protection and avoidance recommended

Familial atypical mole and melanoma syndrome (FAMM), also known as dysplastic nevus syndrome (DNS), represents a group of disorders characterized by multiple cutaneous melanomas and atypical nevi associated with a probable polygenic inheritance pattern.

Epidemiology and Genetics

Although melanoma and atypical nevi have demonstrated an autosomal dominant hereditary pattern, inheritance of familial melanoma syndrome (FMS) is complex and most likely of polygenic etiology.[1] Prevalence of FMS is difficult to assess due to an absence of standardized diagnostic criteria and a lack of a reproducible clinical pattern.[1] Identification of the affected gene loci was localized to chromosome 9p21.[2] Germline mutations of *CDKN2A* were demonstrated by Hussussian et al[3] in 92% of melanoma-prone patients with linkage to the 9p21 chromosome. However, only 30% of persons with dysplastic nevi had mutations in the *CDKN2A* region, suggesting a related but diverse etiology. The *CDKN2A* gene is composed of the P16 and p14ARF exons. P16 is necessary to arrest the cellular proliferation, while p14ARF is involved in enhancing a separate tumor suppressor, p53. Mutations of these components contribute to tumorigenesis.[4] A recent study demonstrated that the phenotypic expression of melanoma in *CDKN2A* mutation carriers was dependent on geographic location: 58% in Europe, 76% in the United States, and 91% in Australia,[5] demonstrating a genetic and environmental influence on expression. Studies demonstrate approximately a 50% risk of developing a cutaneous melanoma by 50 years of age among individuals with a positive family history of melanoma.[6]

Cutaneous Findings

Hallmark features of FAMM are atypical nevus, defined as a macular papular mole >5 to 10 mm and melanomas, exhibiting border and color irregularities. Individuals with FAMM develop a higher rate of melanomas at earlier ages of onset with an increased risk of developing multiple primary melanomas compared to the general population.[7]

Extracutaneous Findings Diagnosis

Earlier studies suggest a link between familial melanoma and pancreatic cancer. Goldstein et al reported a 22-fold increased risk of pancreatic cancer in melanoma-prone families with defective *CDKN2A*.[8] Some reports of squamous cell carcinomas of the head and neck have also been described in patients with FAMM.

Diagnosis

Clinical diagnosis of atypical nevi and melanomas with a family history of melanoma contributes to the diagnosis of FAMM. Genetic *CDKN2A* testing, although commercially available, is usually performed in academic settings.

Therapeutics and Prognosis

Regular dermatologic screening exams with emphasis on sun avoidance and sunscreen use are essential components of care in individuals with FAMM. Genetic screening or therapeutic interventions are currently not recommended for relatives of affected family members at this time; although, a lower tolerance for removal of suspicious lesions is warranted.

Specific therapeutic care of atypical nevi and melanomas are discussed in earlier chapters.

NEVOID BASAL CELL CARCINOMA (GORLIN SYNDROME)

BOX 34-3   Summary

- Multiple basal cell nevi, benign dermal cysts, palmar/plantar pits, odontogenic keratocysts, vertebral and ophthalmologic anomalies, and ectopic calcifications
- Autosomal dominant inheritance pattern
- Germline mutations in the *PATCHED (PTC)* gene linked to 9q22–31 chromosome
- 60% of nevoid basal cell carcinoma syndrome (NBCCS) are sporadic cases

---

- Prevalence 1:60,000; mostly in Caucasian population
- Require regular dermatologic screening for basal cell carcinomas (BCC)
- Children less than 8 years require baseline head MRI screening for medulloblastomas.
- Dental X-rays screening for jaw cysts starting at 8 years of age
- Range of medical and surgical treatment options depending on location and nature of lesion

Nevoid basal cell carcinoma syndrome (NBCCS), also referred to as basal cell nevus syndrome or Gorlin–Goltz syndrome, typically demonstrates an autosomal dominance inheritance pattern with high penetration and variable expression. The main characteristics of this disease include multiple basal cell nevi, benign dermal cysts, palmer or planter pits, odontogenic keratocysts, vertebral anomalies, ectopic calcifications, and ophthalmologic anomalies.

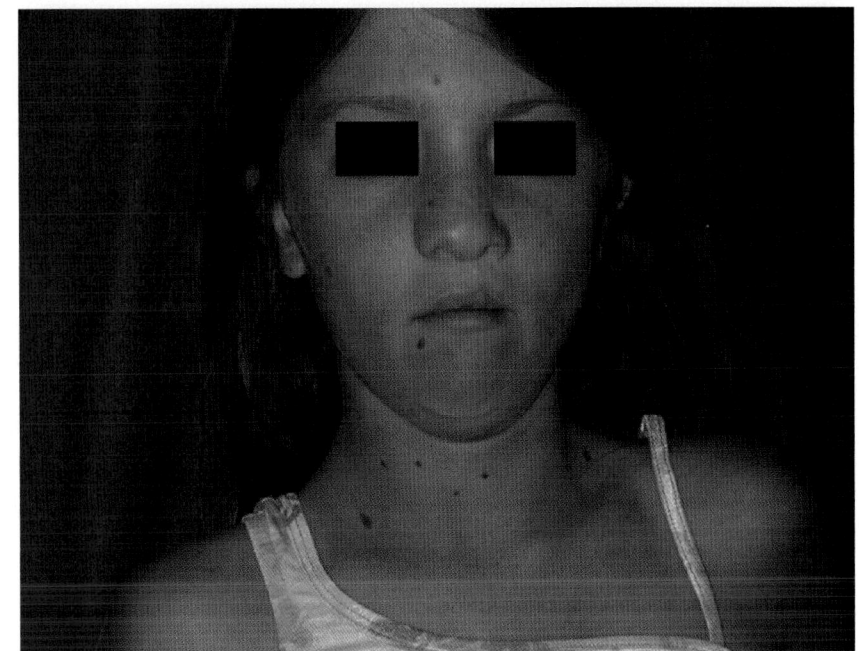

▲ **FIGURE 34-1** Basal cell nevus syndrome. Facial features of NBCCS include a broad nasal bridge, ocular hypertelorism, mandibular hyperplasia, frontal and biparietal bossing, and palate abnormalities. Courtesy Dr. Bari Cunningham.

Epidemiology and Genetics

The prevalence of this syndrome is estimated to be 1 per 60,000. This syndrome arises in most ethnic groups but is more prevalent in the European Caucasian population, and has no sex predilection.[9] The lower frequency of basal cell carcinomas (BCCs) in the African American population probably reflects the inherent protection of melanotic pigment from ultraviolet light. Typically, the clinical features of NBCCS arise during the 1st[10] to 3rd decade of life.[11] Although this syndrome demonstrates an autosomal dominant hereditary pattern with high penetration and variable expression, it may also arise spontaneously. Almost 60% of patients with NBCCS are sporadic cases with no known affected family members and 35 to 50% of these demonstrate new mutations.[12]

Linkage analysis has enabled the gene for NBCCS to be mapped to chromosome 9q22–31.[13] Johnson et al[14] and Hahn et al[15] demonstrated germline mutations of the *PATCHED (PTC)* gene from patients with NBCCS and in somatic DNA from sporadic BCCs. Further studies revealed that 15 to 39% of probands of NBCCs families possessed mutations in the *PTC* gene.[16] The *PTC* gene is involved in the SONIC HEDGEHOG (HH) signaling pathway. HH, a soluble protein, binds and thereby inhibits PTC. In the absence of this inhibition, PTC binds and inhibits a transmembrane protein SMOOTHENED

(SMO), which is essential for tumor suppression. As a result, mutations that increase SMO signaling have shown to be associated with human cancers, specifically BCCs.[17]

Cutaneous Findings

The most prominent skin lesions in NBCCS are the multiple BCCs that typically develop by a median age of 20 years.[18] BCCs appear as skin color to tan, dome-shaped papules predominantly distributed on the face (mostly on periorbital areas, eyelids, nose, malar region, and upper lip), neck, back, chest, and upper limbs[19] (Fig. 34-1). These basal cell nevi often increase in number after puberty. However, most of these BCCs remain localized within the epidermis for many years before becoming locally aggressive, invading the dermis. This transition is usually preceded by an increase in size, and the development of ulceration, bleeding, and crusting.[20] The malignant predisposition in the skin of patients with NBCCS make it extremely sensitive to X-radiation and hundreds of tumors can develop in a given radiation field.

Palmer and plantar pits, occurring in 65 to 80% of patients, are another cutaneous manifestation of NBCCS. These pits measuring 1 to 3 mm in depth by 2 to 3 mm in diameter are defective areas of keratinization that become more evident after immersion in water. They typically develop during the second decade of life and increase in number with age.

Extracutaneous Findings

Facial features often seen in NBCCS are a broad nasal bridge, fused eyebrows, ocular hypertelorism, mandibular hyperplasia, frontal and biparietal bone bossing, and palate anomalies[21] (Fig. 34-2). Jaw cysts (odontogenic keratocysts) develop in over 70% of patients with NBCCS predominately in the mandible with average age of onset between 15 and 20 years. Additional extracutaneous findings include skeletal anomalies (bifid ribs and vertebral malformations) and ectopic calcifications of brain structures (falx cerebri and sella turcica), uterine or ovarian fibromas, cardiac fibromas, and intracranial anomalies, such as medulloblastomas (greatest risk between 2 and 3 years of age).[22]

Diagnosis

NBCCS is a clinical diagnosis that is made by following the major and minor criteria proposed by Evans et al. The finding of any two major criteria or one major criterion plus two minor criteria reaches a diagnosis[23] (Table 34-1).

Therapeutics and Prognosis

The lifespan of a patient diagnosed with NBCCS is equal to the general population but is dependent on the surveillance and management of aggressive BCCs. Due to the autosomal dominant inheritance pattern of NBCCS, all family

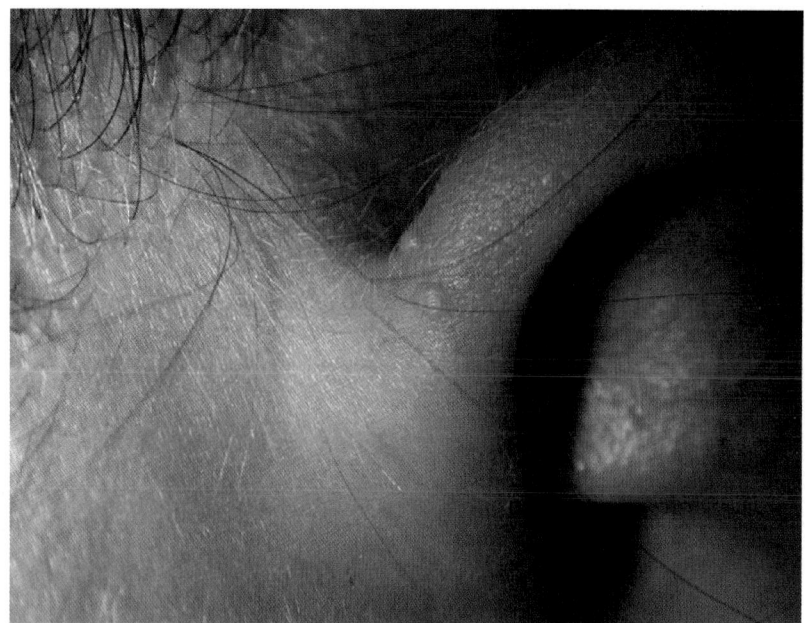

▲ **FIGURE 34-2** Basal cell carcinoma in NBCCS.

Table 34-1

Diagnostic Criteria of Nevoid Basal Cell Carcinoma Syndrome

MAJOR CRITERIA

1. More than two basal cell carcinomas (BCC) or one BCC under the age of 20 years

2. Histologically proven odontogenic keratocysts of the jaw

3. Three or more cutaneous palmar or plantar pits

4. Bifid, fused, or markedly splayed ribs

5. First degree relative with NBCCS

MINOR CRITERIA

Any one of the following features

1. Proven macrocephaly, after adjustment for height

2. One of several orofacial congenital malformations: cleft lip or palate, frontal bossing, "coarse face," moderate or severe hypertelorism

3. Other skeletal abnormalities: Sprengel deformity, marked pectus deformity, marked syndactyly of the digits

4. Radiological abnormalities: bridging of the sella turcica, vertebral anomalies such as hemivertebrae, fusion, or elongation of the vertebral bodies, modeling defects of the hands and feet, or flame-shaped lucencies or the hands or feet

5. Ovarian fibroma

6. Medulloblastoma

The diagnosis of NBCCS requires the presence of two major, or one major and two minor criteria.

members of patients with NBCCS require clinical and genetic evaluation. All children under 8 years that may be carrying the causative gene require yearly neurological screenings and a baseline head magnetic resonance imaging screening for medulloblastomas.[24] Dental X-rays screening for jaw cysts should be performed yearly starting at 8 years. These patients should have regular dermatological visits evaluating for BCCs and associated signs of NBCCS. Preventative measures such as sun avoidance and sunscreen use are essential components of counseling.

The treatment of BCCs in NBCCS is challenging due to the large number of lesions. Small, well-defined primary BCCs that are not located in high-risk locations (nasolabial, periorbital sites) may be treated with curettage and electrodessication. Nonrecurrent BCCs present in high-risk zones may be treated with cryosurgery. Mohs' micrographic surgery is a better option for conservative removal of recurrent and aggressive BCCs. Given the aggressive nature of some BCCs, laser radiotherapy is contraindicated.

Superficial, more benign BCCs without hair follicles may be managed with topical 0.1% 5-fluorouracil. Recent studies applying 5% imiquimod cream on superficial and nodular BCCs from 8 to 14 weeks have demonstrated clearance of the treated BCC and clinical resolution.[25,26] Another therapeutic alternative for these lesions is the use of photodynamic therapy using the topical application of a photodynamically active dye, 5-aminolevulinic acid. Intralesionally

administered interferon alpha-2b has been proposed for the removal of small papular lesions. Prophylactic oral retinoids can prevent early BCCs but it is a difficult drug to monitor for long-term use.

The clinical course of NBCCS varies widely. Some patients have a mild presentation while others suffer a more severe form of this syndrome. It is imperative to screen and diagnose these patients early to prevent any life-threatening consequences. Care of affected patients should include regular genetic, dermatologic, and dental follow-up with referral to additional subspecialties based on clinical findings.

■ BASEX SYNDROME

BOX 34-4   Summary

- Characterized by follicular atrophoderma, hypotrichosis, facial milia, and early onset of BCCs
- Probable X-linked inheritance; Xq24–q27
- Treatment of BCCs similar to NBCCS

Bazex syndrome, also known as Basex–Dupré–Christol (BDC) syndrome, was initially described by Bazex et al in 1964.[27] This inherited disorder with a skin cancer predisposition is characterized by follicular atrophoderma, hypotrichosis, and early onset of BCCs.

Epidemiology and Genetics

Early reports suggest an X-linked mode of inheritance[28] based on the absence of documented male to male transmission in familial cases. In addition, phenotypic differences in gender are consistent with the lionization phenomenon.[29] Linkage analysis has identified the defective gene to Xq24–q27, a site considered to be involved in hair follicle development and differentiation.[30] Up until the year 2000, 18 families with 77 affected individuals have been identified with BDC syndrome worldwide.

Cutaneous Findings

The main skin findings of BDC syndrome are follicular atrophoderma, congenital generalized hypotrichosis, and early-onset BCCs (Fig. 34-3). BCCs often occur in the 2nd and 3rd decades of life, and typically have an aggressive course. Follicular atrophoderma, follicular depressions resembling multiple ice-pick marks, is most frequently localized

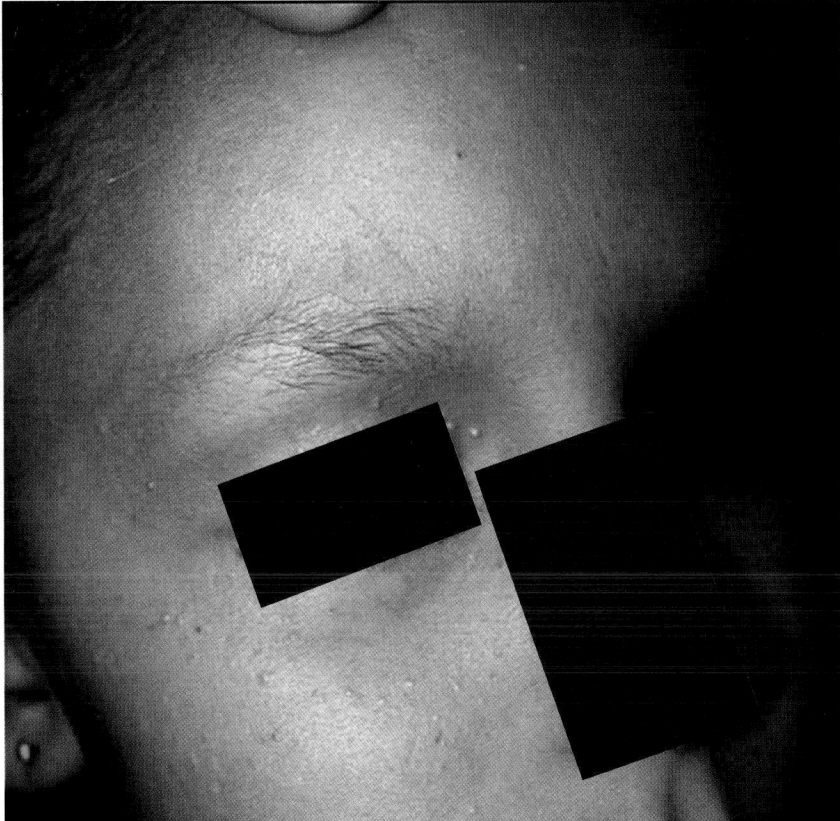

▲ **FIGURE 34-3** Bazex syndrome. Main features of Bazex syndrome include follicular atrophoderma, congenital generalized hypotrichosis, and early onset basal cell carcinomas. Courtesy Dr. Bari Cunningham.

- Dermatologic cancer screenings every 3 months
- Ocular protection and ophthalmologic follow-up
- Cutaneous cancers treated by excision, chemosurgery, cryosurgery, IL IFN-α
- Oral retinoids may play a preventative role against cutaneous malignancies
- Severely shortened lifespans

on the dorsa of hands and feet, on the face, and on the extensor surfaces of the elbows and knees.[31] Additional reported features include generalized hypotrichosis with hair shaft abnormalities (pili torti, trichorrhexis nodosa),[31] facial milia, and hypohidrosis. Fewer associated findings include atopic diathesis, comedos, keratosis pilaris, lingua plicata, joint hyperflexibility, and forehead hyperpigmentation.[32]

Diagnosis

Diagnosis of BDC is based on triad of clinical findings: follicular atrophoderma, hypotrichosis, and early onset of BCCs.

Therapeutics and Prognosis

Treatment of BCCs is the same as described for NBCCS. Prognosis is related to surveillance and treatment of BCCs.

Differential Diagnosis

Rombo syndrome is an autosomal dominantly inherited disorder characterized by multiple BCCs, multiple facial milia, vermiculate atrophoderma, hypotrichosis, and trichoepitheliomas. Distinguishing features are the absence of follicular atrophoderma and the onset of these findings in late childhood.[33]

XERODERMA PIGMENTOSUM (XP)

BOX 34-5 Summary

- Autosomal dominant inherited disorder
- Defective DNA nucleotide excision repair mechanism
- Photosensitivity to UV radiation, early onset of cutaneous malignancies (basal cell carcinomas (BCC), squamous cell carcinomas (SCC), melanomas), ocular complications
- More than seven different XP complementation groups (A–G)
- Subtypes A, B, D, G may develop progressive neurologic degeneration
- Subtypes A and D associated with sensorineural hearing loss, ataxia, and spasticity.
- Western countries: subtype C most prevalent
- Increased risk of developing internal organ malignancy
- Sun protection and avoidance are imperative

Xeroderma pigmentosum (XP) is an autosomal recessive syndrome characterized by a group of degenerative disorders resulting from defective DNA nucleotide excision repair mechanisms. Main features of this disorder include exquisite photosensitivity to UV radiation, early onset of cutaneous malignancies, ocular complications, and in certain subtypes, progressive neurological degeneration.

Epidemiology and Genetics

The prevalence of XP has been estimated at 1 in 1,000,000 people in the United States and Europe, with a much higher frequency in Japan (1 in 40,000). Males and females are equally affected. Various XP genes have been mapped and cloned. Cell fusion technique has elucidated at least seven different XP complementation groups (A, B, C, D, E, F, or G) with impaired excision repair type and one XP variant form with deficient postreplication repair. Each complementation group corresponds to different gene defects that in turn codes for different enzymes involved in the DNA nucleotide excision repair process. Among these eight types of XP, patients with type A, B, D, and G may develop neurodegenerative symptoms as well. Most people affected in Western countries belong to XPC, which typically manifests with extreme cutaneous findings, but without neurologic symptoms. In Japan, XPA is the prevailing form, manifesting with a more severe clinical presentation. XPD mutations have also been associated with other neurologic disorders (trichothiodystrophy, Cockayne syndrome) in patients who display similar clinical features to XP.[34]

PIBIDS, an inherited genetic disorder that shares the same XPD mutation seen in XP, is characterized by photosensitivity, mild noncongenital ichthyosis, brittle sulfur-deficient hair, impaired intelligence, occasional decreased fertility, and short stature. PIBIDS is associated with severe photosensitivity with defective repair of UV-induced lesions, rendering

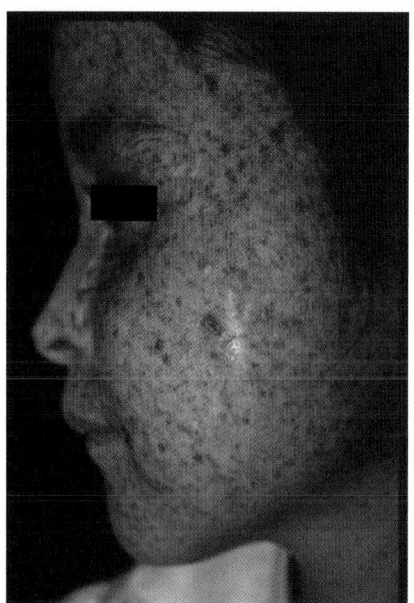

▲ **FIGURE 34-4** Xeroderma pigmentosum. Skin findings include poikiloderma: epidermal thinning, telangiectasias, patchy hyperpigmented macules. Courtesy Dr. Bari Cunningham.

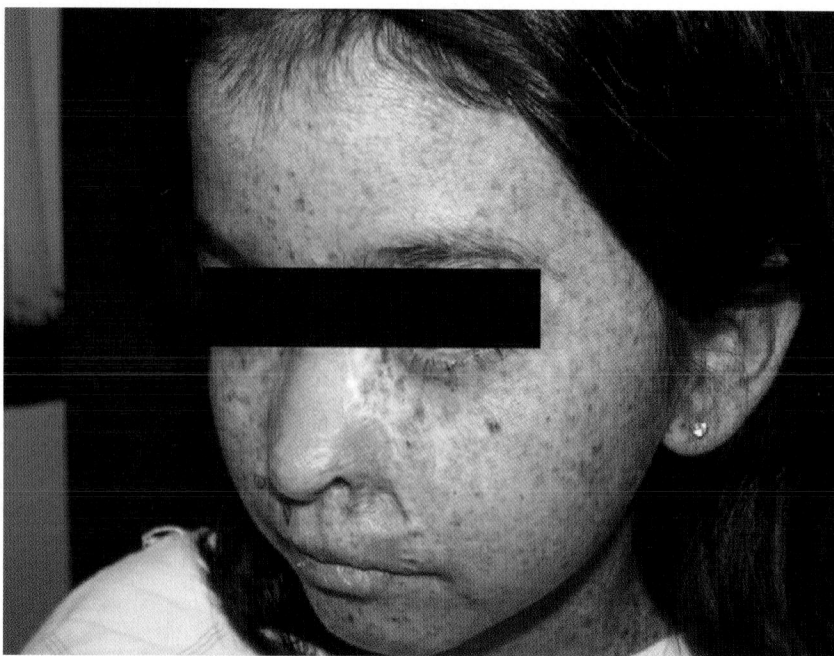

▲ **FIGURE 34-5** Xeroderma pigmentosum. Facial disfigurement and scarring due to the cumulative effect of numerous cancers. Courtesy Dr. Bari Cunningham.

them more susceptible to squamous cell carcinomas.

Cutaneous Findings

The initial age of onset of cutaneous symptoms typically appears at 1 to 2 years of age. At the outset, patients develop a severe prolonged erythematous reaction to minimal sun exposure (abnormal sunburn) and photodistributed actinic lentigines. At an early age, signs of premature aging (dermatoheliosis) become apparent such as epidermal thinning, telangiectasias, patchy hyper/hypopigmentation, macules; collectively termed poikiloderma[35] (Fig. 34-4). These skin changes are more typical in older adults after many years of sun exposure.

Skin malignancies such as keratoacanthomas, BCCs, SCCs, and melanomas start presenting at an early age primarily in photodistributed areas and often result in significant disfigurement of facial features. More than 95% of SCCs and BCCs are located in the head and neck region.[35] The median age of onset of a nonmelanoma skin cancer is 8 years. Lentigo melanomas, a common type of cutaneous cancer in XP, develop at a median age of 17.5 years.[24] There is also a very high propensity to develop SCC at the apex of the tongue, a site vulnerable to much sun exposure.[36] Less common skin tumors include sarcomas, fibromas, histocytomas, and angiomas. Compared with age-matched controls, affected XP patients are 2000 times

more likely to develop a cutaneous skin malignancy.[36] The cumulative effect of numerous cancers and surgical scars over time result in severe facial disfigurement. Patient survival is severely compromised by the course of these malignancies (Fig. 34-5).

Extracutaneous Findings

Patients with XP have a 10 to 20 times increased risk of developing an internal malignancies compared to age-matched controls, with an increased incidence of lung, breast, pancreatic, stomach, brain, and testicular cancer as well as leukemia. Ocular findings are usually confined to the anterior portion of the eye (eyelids, cornea, conjunctiva), vulnerable to greatest exposure of UV radiation. Complications at this site include photophobia, conjunctivitis, keratitis, ectropian, corneal vascularization, BCCs, SCCs, and melanomas. In addition, neurologic degeneration, including mental deterioration, sensorineural hearing loss, ataxia, and spasticity occur more frequently in certain complementation groups (XPA and XPD).

Diagnosis

Identifying a patient's specific subtype of XP is done through complementation studies using cultured skin fibroblasts from affected individuals. Cultured cells from affected patients demonstrate intense hypersensitivity to UV radiation,

impaired DNA repair mechanism, and a high rate of UV-induced mutations.[37] Once the affected XP gene is identified, direct mutation analysis allows for carrier detection and prenatal diagnosis of family members.[38]

Therapeutics and Prognosis

Counseling XP patients must include a rigorous protection program against UV light from infancy. Sun avoidance, physical block sunscreens, wide brimmed hats, appropriate long-sleeved clothing, and UV blocking sunglasses with side shields are some measures that require adherence. Dermatological cancer screenings should occur every 3 months with prompt removal of suspicious lesions. Premalignant lesions can be treated with cryosurgery, topical 5-fluorouracil, or imiquimod. Neoplasms should be removed by excision, chemosurgery, cryosurgery, or intralesional IFN-α. Topical use of a prokaryotic DNA repair enzyme, T4 endonuclease V, has been shown to initiate repair of UV-induced DNA damage, thereby preventing the development of skin cancers.[24,37] Certain XP patients may benefit from oral isotretinoin that plays a role in the prevention of new skin cancers. However, the xerotic side affect of isotretinoin may exacerbate the xerosis associated with the underlying condition. In those patients with severe destructive carcinomas, procedures such as resurfacing, dermabrasion, and skin grafts may improve skin appearance. Referral to an ophthalmologist is essential for regular screenings. If a patient displays neurological symptoms, close follow-up with a neurologist is recommended.

Given the inherent propensity to develop multiple cutaneous and internal malignancies, the lifespan of those affected with XP is shortened by almost 30 years. The mortality rate is 30% at 40 years of age.[35] Due to the severe psychosocial impact of this disease, professional counseling and support groups are recommended.

MUIR–TORRE SYNDROME

BOX 34-6 Summary

- Autosomal dominant inherited disorder
- Mutation in *MLH 1* or *MSH 2*; DNA mismatch repair genes
- Characterized by sebaceous gland tumors associated with internal malignancies
- Most common visceral malignancy: gastrointestinal cancer, followed by genitourinary cancer.
- Muir–Torre syndrome (MTS) is probably a clinical variant of hereditary nonpolyposis colorectal cancer (HNPCC)
- Regular dermatologic screening for sebaceous gland tumors is needed

Muir–Torre syndrome (MTS) is an autosomal dominant genetic disorder, characterized by tumors of the sebaceous gland or multiple keratoacanthomas that are associated with internal malignancies. MTS may represent a clinical variant of hereditary nonpolyposis colorectal cancer (HNPCC). However, the hallmark distinguishing features of MTS, which differentiates it from HNPCC, are the cutaneous sebaceous tumors.

Epidemiology and Genetics

MTS was independently described by Muir in 1967[39] and subsequently by Torre in 1968.[40] In a review done by Akhtar et al, 205 reported cases of MTS in whom 399 internal malignancies were identified from the scientific literature. However, most case reports of MTS describe Caucasian patients living in developed countries. Epidemiological data is lacking in the Asian and African populations. Defining features of inclusion in this epidemiologic study were a combination of sebaceous gland tumors with at least one primary visceral malignancy.[41] The most common internal malignancies are gastrointestinal cancers (61%) followed by

cancers affecting the genitourinary apparatus (22%). Fifteen percent of women with MTS develop endometrial cancer.[42] This syndrome presents in both sexes with a male to female ratio of 3:2, presenting at a mean age of 55 years.

The genetic disorder of MTS is an inherited mutation in one of the DNA mismatch repair genes, MLH 1 and MSH 2. In patients with MTS, reports of 39 different constitutional mutations have been identified, 36 in human MSH2 and 3 in human MLH 1.[43] Patients with MTS demonstrate microsatellite instability in sebaceous gland tumors and colorectal carcinomas. Microsatellites are repetitive sequences prone to replication errors that are scattered in a given genome. Therefore, microsatellite instability reflects a defect of the mismatch repair genes. The autosomal dominant transmission of this mutation has a high degree of penetrance and variable expression. Offspring of an affected parent carry a 50% risk of inheriting this cancer predisposition.[44] A variant, sporadic form of MTS exists that does not have a familial inheritance pattern nor microsatellite instability.

Research has elucidated that MTS is likely a clinical variant of HNPCC due to their shared genetic mutations. The MTS phenotype appears to represent a fuller expression of the genetic abnormality. HNPCC tumors exhibit microsatellite instability at 86% versus 15% of sporadic tumors. In addition, patients with this genetic abnormality demonstrate a greater number of visceral malignancies with a significantly earlier onset.[45] Overall, the clinical similarities between MTS and HNPCC and the shared autosomal dominant inheritance pattern support genetic overlap.

Cutaneous Findings

The principal skin lesions characterizing MTS are tumors (benign or malignant) of the sebaceous gland. Usually presenting in the fifth decade of life, these solitary or multiple lesions present as firm, yellow papules or nodules, arising predominately on the face, scalp, and eyelids. Cutaneous findings include sebaceous adenomas, epitheliomas, carcinomas, and multiple keratoacanthomas (Fig. 34-6). Sebaceous carcinomas most commonly occur on the eyelids, typically arising from the meibomian or Zeiss glands. This tumor presents as a firm yellow nodule with a propensity to ulcerate and extend into the adipose

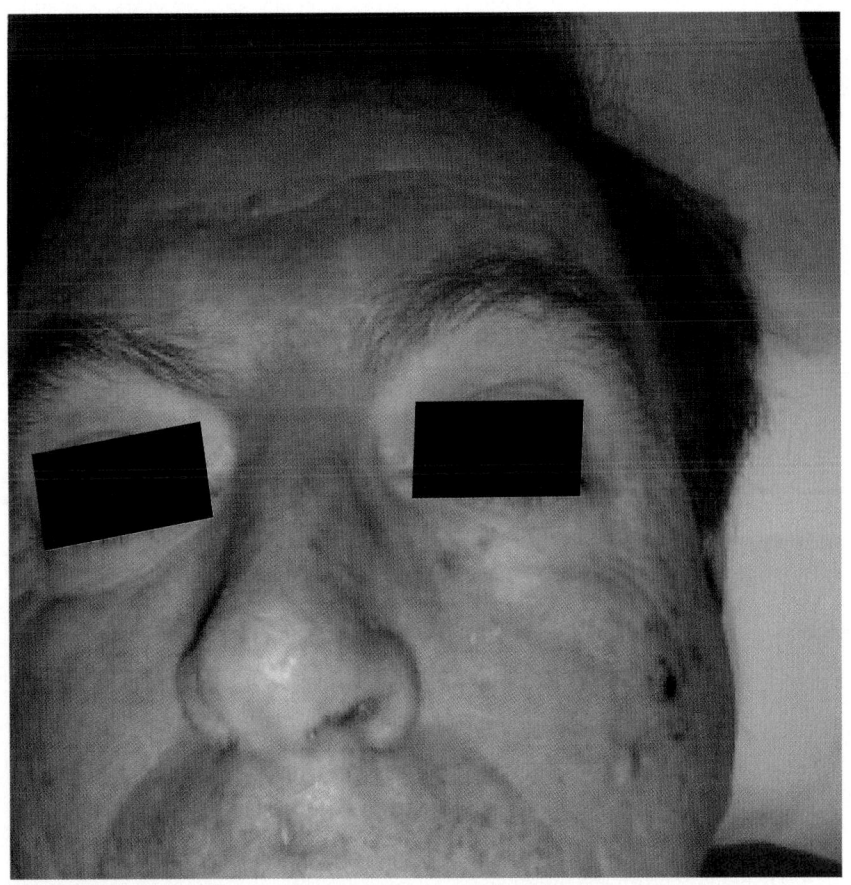

▲ **FIGURE 34-6** Muir–Torre syndrome. Cutaneous findings include sebaceous adenomas, epitheliomas, carcinomas, and keratoacanthomas. Courtesy Dr. Paolo Romanelli.

tissue of the eye orbit. Keratoacanthomas appear as dome-shaped nodules, with keratin-filled centers, achieving a 1 to 2.5 cm diameter within 1 to 2 months.

A statistical review by Cohen et al revealed that among 120 patients with MTS, 143 sebaceous tumors were diagnosed. Of these tumors, 68% were adenomas, 30% carcinomas, and 27% epitheliomas. Approximately 20% of patients had at least one keratoacanthoma. In this study, 59% of these patients were diagnosed with a visceral malignancy before the diagnosis of a sebaceous tumor. Other studies have shown that in 22% of patients with MTS, skin lesions precede an internal cancer and 6% occur concomitantly.[41]

Extracutaneous Findings

Colorectal cancer is the most common internal malignancy that occurs in patients with MTS with a median age of onset at 50 years (10 to 20 years younger than the general population). Cancers are most frequently located in the proximal colon with limited colonic polyposis (similar to HNPCC syndrome). An extensive review by Cohen et al identified 235 visceral malignancies on 120 patients diagnosed with MTS. Of these internal cancers, 119 (51%) were colorectal, 59 (25%) were genitourinary, 14 (6%) were breast, 12 (5%) were hematologic, 11 (4.7%) were head and neck, and 8 (3.4%) were small intestinal carcinomas.

Diagnosis

The diagnosis of MTS is based on clinical findings of at least one sebaceous gland tumor associated with at least one primary visceral malignancy. Diagnosis can also be made if a patient presents with multiple keratoacanthomas with multiple internal malignancies plus a family history of MTS. Genetic testing via mutation analysis of hMSH2 and hMLH1 is also available. In addition, analysis of most skin and visceral tumors from MTS patients demonstrate microsatellite instability, as discussed earlier.

Management and Prognosis

A multidisciplinary approach is required in the management of MTS that includes primary care physicians, dermatologists, geneticists, gastroenterologists, and surgeons. Initially, creating an extended pedigree using extensive clinical history of the proband and family members helps confirm the diagnosis of MTS. Genetic analysis of affected family members enables identification of the

inherited mutation, distinguishing between carrier and noncarrier relatives. This in turn screens that family members require more extensive workup.

Regular dermatologic exams are imperative for early detection of sebaceous gland tumors with expedient removal. Benign sebaceous gland tumors and keratoacanthomas can be removed via excision or cryotherapy. Excision of a sebaceous carcinoma requires wide local margins as well as fine needle aspiration of suspicious lymph nodes. Preliminary research on chemoprevention of sebaceous tumors has shown oral isotretinoin to have a limited effect.[46] However, the combination of retinoids with interferon is yielding more promising results in the prevention of tumor development.[47]

Cohen et al suggest that the workup searching for internal malignant disease be undertaken in patients diagnosed with MTS, patients with an MTS-associated tumor, or any family member of an MTS patient. A surveillance program that includes annual physical exams, carcinogenic embryonic antigen, cervical smear, chest radiography, urine cytology, and colonoscopy at least every 3 to 5 years starting at 25 to 30 years of age. In female patients, mammography every 1 to 2 years, annually after 50 years, and endometrial biopsy every 3 to 5 years starting at age 50 years.

There have been limited studies assessing prognosis and survival of patients with MTS. Both cutaneous and visceral tumors of MTS tend to follow an indolent course with a prolonged survival if treated appropriately.[42] This underlies the importance of early diagnosis and proper management.

DYSKERATOSIS CONGENITA

BOX 34-7   Summary

- Autosomal dominant and recessive inheritance patterns
- Most cases caused by mutation in dyskerin gene *DKC1* on Xq28 chromosome
- Cutaneous features: reticular pigmentation, nail dystrophy and mucosal leukoplakia, and palmar–plantar hyperkeratosis
- Premalignant leukoplakia may develop into SCC
- Hair abnormalities: alopecia of scalp, eyebrows, and eyelashes
- Hematological abnormalities: anemia and ultimately pancytopenia secondary to bone marrow failure
- Shortened lifespan

Dyskeratosis congenita (DC) is a hereditary disorder characterized by a triad of abnormal cutaneous pigmentation, nail dystrophy, and mucosal leukoplakia.[48–50]

Although this syndrome is accompanied by a variety of multisystemic abnormalities (dental, gastrointestinal, genitourinary, neurologic, ophthalmic, pulmonary, skeletal), bone marrow failure is the leading cause of early mortality.

Epidemiology and Genetics

Several different genetic patterns of inheritance exist in DC that manifest with varying clinical presentations. Most cases of DC are X-linked and caused by a mutation on the dyskerin gene of *DKC1* at Xq28.[51] This gene encodes the protein dyskerin, which is integral to ribosome biogenesis and telomerase ribonucleoproteins (RNPs) assembly. In peripheral hematopoietic cells, this results in reduced telomere lengths, but normal levels of activity.[52] This mutation may be inherited or occur by spontaneous mutation during early embryogenesis. Typically, most affected individuals are males. Female carriers of the mutation may exhibit subtle symptoms.[53]

Autosomal dominant and recessive forms have also been identified. The dominant form also encodes an RNA component of the telomerase complex. These patients generally present with a milder variant of the disease. Recent studies suggest that anticipation occurs with an earlier age of onset and increasing severity of the disease with each subsequent generation. Epidemiologic data has been summarized most recently by Dokal[54] and Knight et al.[55] Much of the prevalence and physical finding data is based on 92 families (148 affected individuals) enrolled in a DC registry established at the Hammersmith Hospital (London) in 1995.

Cutaneous Findings

DC is characterized by the classic triad of cutaneous features: reticular pigmentation of the skin, nail dystrophy, and mucosal leukoplakia. These dermatologic findings typically present between 5 and 10 years of age. Significant variability in clinical presentation exists amongst those affected in different families.

Abnormal skin pigmentation appears as a reticulated gray-brown hyperpigmentation and occasional hypopigmentation on the neck, face, trunk, upper arms, and thighs typically associated with atrophy and telangiectasias (Fig. 34-7). Characteristic hair abnormalities

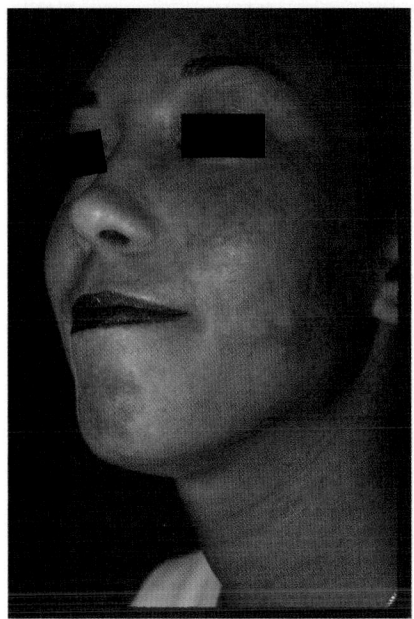

▲ **FIGURE 34-7** Dyskeratosis congenita. Abnormal skin pigmentation appears as a reticulated gray-brown hyperpigmentation on the neck, face, trunk, and extremities, typically associated with telangiectasisas and atrophy. Courtesy Dr. Bari Cunningham.

are a thinning alopecia of the scalp, eyelashes, and eyebrows. Nail dystrophy presents as longitudinal ridging, thinning, or complete atrophy of nails with pterygium formation[56] (Fig. 34-8).

Mucosal abnormalities affect 98% patients and demonstrate a premalignant leukoplakia of any mucosal surface. These findings that present later than other cutaneous findings, appear on the tongue, buccal mucosa, pharynx, con-junctiva, vagina, rectum, gastrointestinal, or genitourinary tract.[24] These leukoplastic sites may develop into aggressive squamous cell carcinomas.[57] Additional cutaneous findings include palmar–plantar hyperkeratosis and hyperhydrosis friction bullae and acrocyanosis (SPITZ, genodermatosis).

Extracutaneous Findings

Extracutaneous findings associated with DC are highly variable and include epiphoria, peridontitis, osteoporosis, short stature, hair loss, underdeveloped testes, combined immunodeficiency, pulmonary fibrosis, liver cirrhosis, esophageal stricture, and mental retardation. Hematologic abnormalities develop in up to 80% of patients during the 1st to 3rd decade of life. Early signs include anemia, typically appearing during adolescence, and ultimately pancytopenia due to bone marrow failure presenting during the 2nd and 3rd decades of life. Knight et al found that in 71% of affected individuals, bone marrow failure was the leading cause of death. Additional findings associated with a high mortality rate include pulmonary fibrosis and gastrointestinal carcinomas. Hoyeraal–Hreidarsson syndrome, a severe variant form of DC associated with cerebellar hypoplasia, presents with ataxia, bone marrow failure, immunodeficiency, growth retardation, and gastrointestinal abnormalities.

Diagnosis

DC is typically diagnosed by the triad of cutaneous findings. However, this can be challenging due to the clinical and genetic heterogeneity of DC. DC shares clinical features associated with other bone marrow failure syndromes (Fanconi's anemia, aplastic anemia). Affected individuals may die before cutaneous findings present. Genetic testing can be done on patients with inherited forms of DC. Optimal methods of screening for excessive telomere shortening have not been established but may represent a future diagnostic tool in the evaluation of a person with suspected DC.[53]

Management and Prognosis

The overall management of these patients requires a multidisciplinary approach involving dermatology, genetics, hematology–oncology, transplant, and additional specialties based on clinical findings. As these patients carry an increased risk of mucosal and cutaneous malignancy, surveillance of leukoplasias and hematologic counts is important in the care of these patients. Routine screenings for malignant transformation and preventative counseling against excessive sun exposure and smoking are essential. Current treatments for DC are symptomatic and very limited. Pancytopenia can be treated with transfusions and anabolic steroids. However, the benefits are temporary and carry significant side effects. Patients undergoing hematopoietic stem cell transplantation (HSCT) from an allogeneic donor fare poorly due to all the transplant related complications. Treatment with granulocyte-macrophage colony-stimulating factor has yielded mixed results.[58] Gastrointestinal and genitourinary surveillance for malignancies (endoscopies) should begin in the third decade of life.[53]

Due to increased malignant susceptibility, affected individuals have a severely shortened lifespan. The development of bone marrow failure by the third decade of life carries a high rate of morbidity and mortality early in life.

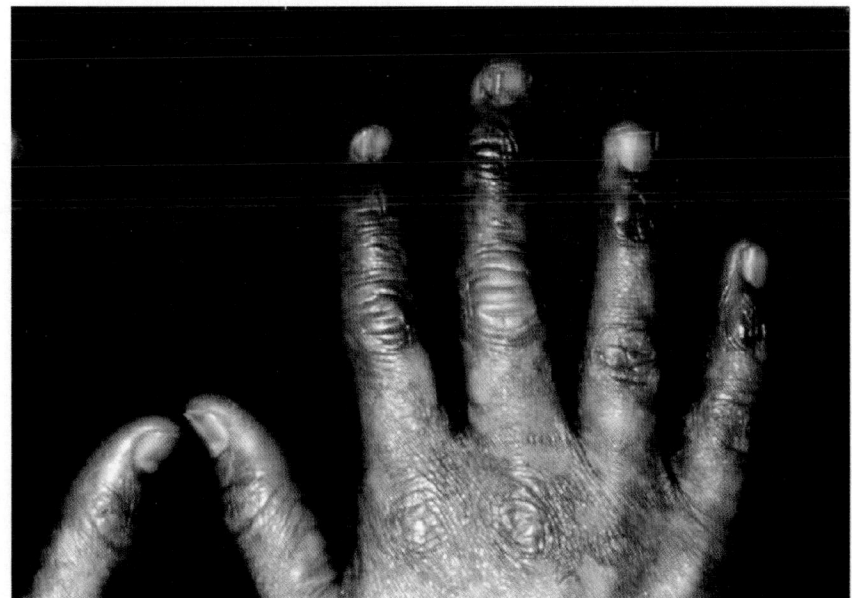

▲ **FIGURE 34-8** Dyskeratosis congenita. Nail dystrophy presents as longitudinal ridging, thinning, or complete atrophy of nail. Courtesy Dr. Bari Cunningham.

ROTHMUND THOMSON SYNDROME

BOX 34-8   Summary

- Autosomal recessive inheritance
- Mutation in *RECQL4* gene coding the DNA helicase-impaired DNA repair
- Hallmark feature: Poiklioderma
- Associated findings: alopecia, keratosis, nail and teeth dystrophy, skeletal abnormalities, and juvenile cataracts

- Increased incidence of cutaneous malignancies (squamous cell carcinoma, SCC) at young age of onset
- Facial features: frontal bossing, saddle nose, prognathism
- Sun protection and avoidance recommended

Rothmund Thomson disorder (RTS) is a rare, autosomal recessive genodermatosis with the predominant feature of poikiloderma of the face and extremities early in life. Variable additional features include alopecia, keratosis, nail and teeth dystrophy, juvenile cataracts, skeletal abnormalities. RTS is associated with a higher rate of cutaneous and extracutaneous malignancies.[59]

Epidemiology and Genetics

A prominent finding of RTS, rapidly progressive juvenile cataracts, was initially described in 1868 by German ophthalmologist, Rothmund.[60] Subsequently in 1936, an English dermatologist, Thomson[61] described the hallmark features of poikiloderma and associated bony abnormalities. At that time, only 300 cases of this rare syndrome had been reported in the medical literature.[62] Epidemiologic analysis supports an autosomal recessive inheritance pattern with no sex predilection. In a study by Venus et al, 28 out of 105 patients (27%) were born from consanguineous unaffected parents and 60% had family members with similar findings.

Cytogenetic analysis of peripheral lymphocytes and fibroblasts of affected individuals reveals chromosome 8 abnormalities, including trisomy 8.[63] Mutations in the *RECQL4* gene have been identified in a subset of RTA patients. This gene codes for DNA helicase contributing to chromosomal instability syndrome and ultimately a predisposition to malignancies.[64] Kitao et al recently cloned and mapped RECQL4 to chromosome 8q24.3.[65] Mutations of DNA helicases have already been identified for Bloom and Werner syndrome.

Cutaneous Findings

The hallmark skin finding of this disorder is the poikilodermatous skin changes that begin on the face and neck during the first 2 years of life (89% of patients during first year). Initially, these skin changes present as red edematous plaques with rare blistering that start on the cheeks, forehead, ears, and extend to the extensor surface of the arms, forearms and hands, legs and buttocks, sparing the palms and soles. This progression may occur over months to years. Ultimately, the affected skin becomes atrophic telangiectatic and hyper and hypopigmented (poikiloderma). These changes primarily occur in sun-exposed areas (Figs. 34-9 and 34-10).

Acral and diffuse keratosis may develop after puberty appearing verrucous-like. Progressive hair thinning, initially of the brows and eyelashes and eventually including the scalp, facial and pubic hair may continue into the 3rd decade of life. Nail thinning also occurs in a third of those affected.

A significantly greater incidence of cutaneous malignancies occurs in those affected at a young age of onset (most less than 32 years). Although squamous

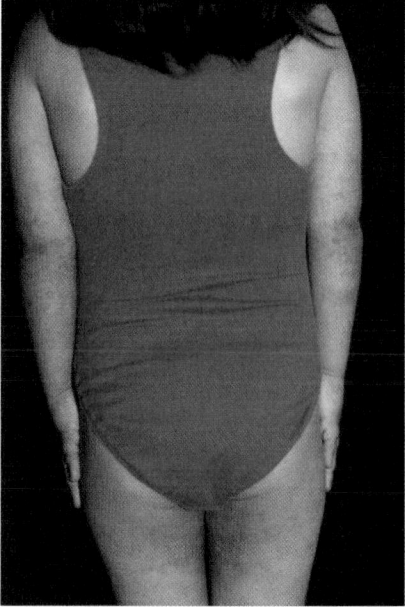

▲ **FIGURE 34-10** Rothmund Thomson syndrome. Poikilodermatous skin changes of extensor surfaces of arms, forearms, legs, and buttocks.

cell carcinoma is most common, Bowen's disease, BCC, and spindle cell carcinoma have also been reported in RTS patients. This may be explained by the impaired capacity of DNA repair following oncogenic stimuli.

Extracutaneous Findings

Skeletal abnormalities including short stature and varying dysplastic lesions are common in RTS. Characteristic facial features include frontal bossing, saddle nose, and prognathism. RTS individuals have proportionately smaller hands and feet, and long bone abnormalities such as deformed or absent radii and malformed thumbs. A greater frequency and earlier age of onset of osteosarcoma is associated with RTS. Again, this predisposition of bone and skin cancer probably relates to faulty DNA repair.[66]

Ocular abnormalities, including rapidly progressive juvenile cataracts are diagnosed in over 70% of patients by 6 years of age.[59,62] Hypogonadism and delayed sexual development occurs in close to a third of patients with RTS, with many cases of infertility.

Diagnosis

RTS is a clinical diagnosis of poikiloderma and additional variable findings.

Management and Prognosis

Medical care of a patient with RTS requires a multidisciplinary approach

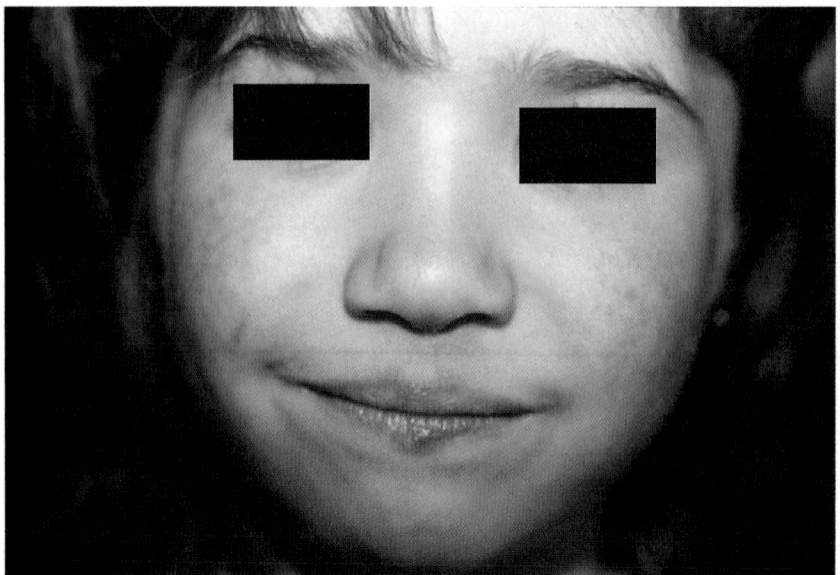

▲ **FIGURE 34-9** Rothmund Thomson syndrome. Poikilodermatous skin changes of cheeks and forehead.

involving a dermatologist, geneticist, and orthopedist based on clinical findings. Sun avoidance and adequate sun protection is strongly recommended due to the photodistribution of skin findings and increased risk of squamous cell carcinoma. However, no conclusive evidence exists that ultraviolet radiation causes the skin findings characteristic of RTS. Laser therapy has been successful in treating telangiectases.[67] Dermatologic treatments for hyperkeratosis include dermabrasion, topical dinitrochlorobenzene, etretinate, and keratolytics that have yielded limited results.[59,62] Due to the increased risk of bone findings and osteosarcoma, a baseline long bone radiologic survey is recommended before 3 years of age with annual follow-up of any dysplastic findings. Prenatal counseling to explain risk of affected subsequent pregnancies is recommended.

■ FINAL THOUGHTS

Skin cancer diagnosed at either an early age or in the setting of a positive family history should alert a clinician to investigate further for a systemic inherited disorder. Careful attention to both cutaneous and extracutaneous findings can provide diagnostic clues in identifying a genodermatoses. Earlier diagnosis of these syndromes allows for earlier protective behavior and surveillance for any emerging external or internal malignancies or associated abnormalities. Although many gene loci associated with these syndromes have been identified, continued research will enable a better understanding of the genetic predisposition of each of these diseases and its interaction with the environment.

REFERENCES

1. Somoano B, Niendorf KB, Tsao H. Hereditary cancer syndromes of the skin. *Clin Dermatol.* 2005;23:85–106.
2. Cannon-Albright LA, Goldgar DE, Meyer LJ, et al. Assignment of a locus for familial melanoma, MLM, to chromosome 9p13–p22. *Science.* 1992;258:1148–1152.
3. Hussussian CJ, Struewing JP, Goldstein AM, et al. Germline p16 mutations in familial melanoma. *Nat Genet.* 1994;8:15–21.
4. Piepkorn M. Melanoma genetics: an update with focus on the CDKN2A(p16)/ARF tumor suppressors. *J Am Acad Dermatol.* 2000;42:705–722.
5. Bishop DT, Demenais F, Goldstein AM, et al. Geographical variation in the penetrance of CDKN2A mutations for melanoma. *J Natl Cancer Inst.* 2002;94:894–903.
6. Tucker MA, Fraser MC, Goldstein AM, et al. Risk of melanoma and other cancers in melanoma-prone families. *J Invest Dermatol.* 1993;100(suppl):350s–355s.
7. Goldstein AM, Fraser MC, Clark WHJ, Tucker MA. Age at diagnosis and transmission of invasive melanoma in 23 families with cutaneous malignant melanoma/dysplastic nevi. *J Natl Cancer Inst.* 1994;86:1385–1390.
8. Goldstein AM, Fraser MC, Struewing JP, et al. Increased risk of pancreatic cancer in melanoma-prone kindreds with p16 mutations. *N Engl J Med.* 1995;333:970–974.
9. Gorlin RJ. Nevoid basal cell carcinoma (Gorlin) syndrome: unanswered issues. *Lab Clin Med.* 1999;134:551–552.
10. Veenstra-Knol HE, Scheewe JH, Vlist GJ, et al. Early recognition of basal cell naevus syndrome. *Eur J Pediatr.* 2005;164:126–130.
11. Kimonis VE, Golstein AM, Pastakia B, et al. Clinical manifestations in 105 persons with nevoid basal cell carcinoma syndrome. *Am J Med Genet.* 1997;69:299–308.
12. Gorlin RJ. Nevoid basal cell carcinoma syndrome. *Dermatol Clin.* 1995;13:113–125.
13. Goldstein AM, Stewart C, Bale AE, et al. Localization of the gene for the nevoid basal cell carcinoma syndrome. *Am J Hum Genet.* 1994;54:765–773.
14. Johnson RL, Rothman AL, Xie J, et al. Human homolog of patched, a candidate gene for the basal cell nevus syndrome. *Science.* 1996;272:1668–1671.
15. Hahn H, Wicking C, Zaphiropoulous PG, et al. Mutations of the human homolog of *Drosophila* patched in the nevoid basal cell carcinoma syndrome. *Cell.* 1996;85:841–851.
16. Aszterbaum M, Rothman A, Johnson RL, et al. Identification of mutations of the human PATCHED gene in sporadic basal cell carcinomas and in patients with the basal cell nevus syndrome. *J Invest Dermatol.* 1998;11:885–888.
17. Bale AE, Kuan-Ping Y. The hedgehog pathway and basal cell carcinomas. *Hum Mol Genet.* 2001;10(7):757–762.
18. Shanley S, Ratcliffe J, Hockey A. Nevoid basal cell carcinoma syndrome: review of 118 affected individuals. *Am J Hum Genet.* 1994;50:282–290.
19. Tsao H. Update on familial cancer syndromes and the skin. *J Am Acad Dermatol.* 2000;42:939–969.
20. Manfredi M, Vescovi P, Bonanini M. Nevois basal cell carcinoma syndrome: a review of the literature. *Int J Oral Maxillofac Surg.* 2004;33:117–124.
21. Gorlin RJ, Cohen MM, Lewis LS. *Syndromes of the Head and Neck*, 3rd ed. Oxford, UK: Oxford University Press; 1990.
22. Bakaeen G, Rajab AD, Sawair FA, et al. Nevoid basal cell carcinoma syndrome: a review of the literature and report of a case. *Int J Paediatr Dent.* 2004;14:279–287.
23. Evans DG, Ladusans EJ, Rimmer S, et al. Complications of the naevoid basal cell carcinoma syndrome: results of a population based study. *J Med Genet.* 1993;30:460–464.
24. Itin PH, et al. Genodermatoses. In: Schachner LA, Hansen RC, eds. *Pediatric Dermatology*, 3rd ed. Philadelphia, PA: Elsevier; 2003:346.
25. Micali G, Lacarruba F, Nasca MR, De Pasquale R. The use of imiquimod 5% cream for the treatment of basal cell carcinoma as observed in Gorlin's syndrome. *Clin Exp Dermatol.* 2003;28(S1):19–23.
26. Stockfleth E, Ulrich C, Hauschild A, et al. Successful treatment of basal cell carcinomas in a nevoid basal cell carcinoma syndrome with topical 5% imiquimod. *Eur J Dermatol.* 2002;12(6):569–572.
27. Bazex A, Dupré A, Christol B. Génodermatose complexe de type indétermineé associant une hypotrichose, un état atrophodermique generalize et des dégénérescences cutanées multiples (epitheliomas-basocellulaires). *Bull Soc Franc Syph.* 1964;71:206.
28. Viksnins P, Berlin A. Follicular atrophoderma and basal cell carcinomas: the Bazex syndrome. *Arch Dermatol.* 1977;113:948–951.
29. Goeteyn M, Geerts ML, Kint AK, et al. The Bazex–Dupré–Christol syndrome. *Arch Dermatol.* 1994;130:337–342.
30. Vabres P, Lacombe D, Rabinowitz LG, et al. The gene for Bazex–Dupré–Christol syndrome maps to chromosome Xq. *J Invest Dermatol.* 1995;105:87–91.
31. Glaessl A, Hohenlautner U, Landthaler M, Vogt T. Sporadic Bazex–Dupré–Christol syndrome: early onset basal cell carcinoma, hypohidrosis, hypotrchosis, and prominent milia. *Dermatol Surg.* 2000;26:152–154.
32. Herges A, Stieler W, Stadler R. Das Bazex–Dupré–Christol syndrome. *Hautarzt.* 1993;44:385–391.
33. Michaelsson G, Olsson E, Westermark P. The Rombo syndrome: a familial disorder with vermiculate atrophoderma, milia, hypotrichosis, trichoepithelioma, basal cell carcinomas and peripheral vasodilation with cyanosis. *Acta Derm Venerol.* 1981;61:497–503.
34. Mallory S. Disorders with malignant potential. In: Spitz J, ed. *Genodermatosis.* Baltimore, MD: Williams and Wilkins.
35. Kraemer KH, Lee MM, Scotto J. Xeroderma pigmentosum. Cutaneous, ocular and neurologic abnormalities in 830 published cases. *Arch Dermatol.* 1987;123:241–250.
36. Bootsma D, Kraemer KH, Cleaver JE, et al. Nucleotide excision repair syndromes: xeroderma pigmentosum, Cocakyne syndrome and trichothiodystrophy. In: Vogelstein B, Kinzler KW, eds. The Genetic Basis of Human Cancer. New York: McGraw-Hill; 1998:245–274.
37. Moriwaki SI, Kraemer KH. Xeroderma pigmentosum—bridging a gap between clinic and laboratory. *Photodermatol Photoimmunol Photomed.* 2001;17:47–54.
38. Bale SJ, Digiovanna JJ. Cancer-associated genodermatosis and familial cancer syndromes with cutaneous manifestations. *Clin Dermatol.* 2001;19:284–289.
39. Muir EG, Bell AJY, Barlow KA. Multiple primary carcinoma of the colon, duodenum and larynx associated with keratoacanthoma of the face. *Br J Surg.* 1967;54:191–195.
40. Torre D. Multiple sebaceous tumors. *Arch Dermatol.* 1968;98:549–551.
41. Akhtar S, Oza KK, Khan SS, Wright J. Muir–Torre syndrome: case report of a patient with concurrent jejunal and ureteral cancer and a review of the literature. *J Am Acad Dermatol.* 1999;41:681–686.
42. Cohen PR, Kohn SR, Kurzrock R. Association of sebaceous gland and internal malignancy: the Muir–Torre syndrome. *Am J Med.* 1991;90:606–613.

43. Ponti G, Ponz de Leon M. Muir–Torre syndrome. *Lancet.* 2005;6:980–987.

44. Tsalis K, Blouhos K, Vasiliadis K. Sebaceous gland tumors and internal malignancy in the context of Muir–Torre syndrome. A case report and review of the literature. *World J Surg Oncol.* 2006;4:8.

45. Honchel R, Halling KC, Schald DJ. Microsatellite instability in Muir–Torre syndrome. *Cancer Res.* 1994;54:1159–1163.

46. Spielvogel RL, De Villez RL, Roberts LC. Oral isotretinoin therapy for familial Muir–Torre syndrome. *J Am Acad Dermatol.* 1985;12:475–478.

47. Graefe T, Wollina U, Schulz H, et al. Muir–Torre syndrome with isotretinoin and interferon alpha-2a can prevent tumor development. *Dematology.* 2000;200:331–333.

48. Zinsser F. Atrophia cutis reticularis cum pigmentatione, dystrophia unguium et leukoplakia oris (poikliodermia atrophicans vascularis Jacobi). *Ikonogr. Derm (Kyoto).* 1906;fas 5:219–223.

49. Cole H, Rauschkolb J, Toomey J. Dyskeratosis congenital with pigmentation, dystrophia unguis and leukokeratosis. *Arch Drem Syph.* 1930;21:71–95.

50. Engman M. A unique case of reticular pigmentation of the skin with atrophy. *Arch Derm Syph.* 1926;13(suppl):685–687.

51. Heiss NS, Knight SW, Vulliamy TJ, Klauck SM, et al. X-linked dyskeratosis congenita is caused by mutations in a highly conserved gene with putative nucleolar functions. *Nat Genet.* 1998;19:32–38.

52. Marrone A, Mason PJ. Human genome and diseases: review dyskeratosis congenita. *Cell Mol Life Sci.* 2003;60:507–517.

53. Mason PJ, Wilson DB, Bessler M. Dyskeratosis congenita—a disease of dysfunctional telomere maintenance. *Curr Mol Med.* 2005;5:159–170.

54. Dokal I. Review: dyskeratosis congenita in all its forms. *Br J Haemotol.* 2000;110:768–779.

55. Knight S, Vulliany T, Copplestone A, et al. Dyskeratosis Congenita Registry: identification of new genes of DC. *Br J Haematol.* 103:990–996.

56. Genodermatosis text.

57. Moretti S, Spallanzani A, Chiarugi A. Oral carcinoma in a young man: a case of dyskeratosis congenital. *JEADV.* 2000;14:123–125.

58. Erduran E, Hacisalihoglu S, Ozoran Y. Treatment of dyskeratosis congenital with granulocyte macrophage colony-stimulating factor and erythropoietin. *J Pediatr Hem Oncol.* 2003;25(4):333–335.

59. Vennos EM, Collins M, James WD. Rothmund Thomson syndrome. *Dermatol Clin.* 1995;13(1):143–150.

60. Rothmund A. Uber Cataracten in Verbindung mit einer eigentumlichen hautgeneration. *Arch Klein Exp Opthalmol.* 1868;4:159–182.

61. Thomson MS. Poikilioderma congenitale. *Br J Dermatol.* 1936;4:221–234.

62. Vennos EM, Collins M, James WD. Rothmund Thomson syndrome--review of the world literature. *J Am Acad Dermatol.* 1992;27:750–762.

63. Ying KL, Oizumi J, Curry CJR. Rothmund–Thomson syndrome associated with trisomy 8 mosaicism. *J Med Genet.* 1990;27:258–260.

64. Larizza L, Magnani I, Roversi G. Rothmond–Thomson syndrome and RECQL4 defect: splitting and lumping. *Cancer Lett.* 2006;232:107–120.

65. Kitao KL, Shimamoto A, Goto M, et al. Mutations in RECQL4 cause a subset of cases of Rothmond–Thomson syndrome. *Nat Genet.* 1999;22:82–84.

66. El Khoury JM, Haddad SN, Atallah NG. Osteosarcomatosis with Rothmund–Thomson syndrome. *Br J Radiol.* 1997;70:215–218.

67. Potozskin JR, Geronemus RG. Treatment of the poikilodermatous component of the Rothmund–Thomson syndrome with the flashlamp-pumped pulsed dye laser: a case report. *PediatrDermatol.* 1991;8:162–165.

CHAPTER 35

Dermatologic Manifestations of Internal Malignancy

Cindy England Owen, M.D.
Jeffrey P. Callen, M.D.

BOX 35-1 Overview

- Skin lesions may serve as a marker of internal malignancy.
- The strongest support for a link between a skin condition and an internal malignancy is when the manifestation occurs at the same time as the internal cancer is discovered, there is a distinct type or site of cancer, and the course of the skin follows that of the cancer.
- Some of the conditions are statistically associated with a greater prevalence of malignancy, but do not follow the course listed earlier.

INTRODUCTION

Paraneoplastic dermatoses are those disorders in which the skin serves as a marker for an internal malignancy. In the original text, *Cancer of the Skin*, Curth outlined a set of criteria that could be used to analyze the relationship between an internal malignancy and a cutaneous disorder.[1] Curth's postulates (Table 35-1), as Callen has subsequently labeled them, consist of five characteristics: (1) a concurrent onset—the malignancy is discovered concurrently with the diagnosis of the dermatosis, (2) a parallel course—if the malignancy is removed or successfully treated, the dermatosis remits, and when the malignancy recurs, the cutaneous disease also recurs, (3) a uniform site or type of malignancy—there is a specific tumor cell type or specific organ associated with the skin disease, (4) a statistical association—evidence-based, population, or case-control studies demonstrate a statistically significant more frequent occurrence of malignancy in a patient with a cutaneous disease, and/or (5) a genetic association. These criteria are extremely useful in the analysis of the relationship between skin diseases and malignancy. However, often not all

Table 35-1
Criteria Used to Associate a Dermatosis with Malignancy

- Concurrent onset
- Parallel course
- Specific cell type or site of malignancy
- Statistical association
- Genetic association

of these criteria are met, yet there remains a strong belief that a relationship exists. In its truest sense, the meaning of paraneoplastic requires that there be a direct and often parallel course of the dermatosis and the malignancy. Most of the conditions that are discussed in this chapter do not have such a course and yet their presence serves as an important marker of a potential malignancy. A wide spectrum of inflammatory, proliferative, metabolic, and neoplastic diseases may affect the skin in association with an underlying malignancy. Hereditary syndromes with associated skin manifestations and increased risk of cancer are covered in Chapter 34. Metastases to the skin, which are clearly a skin sign that is reflective of an internal malignancy, are covered in Chapter 27.

SKIN CHANGES RESULTING FROM HORMONE-SECRETING TUMORS

BOX 35-2 Summary

- Ectopic production of ACTH results in signs of Cushing disease.
  - This condition is most often associated with small cell carcinoma of the lung, but other tumors that are associated include carcinoid tumors, islet cell tumors of the pancreas, medullary carcinoma of the thyroid, ovarian and uterine carcinoma, and prostate cancer.
- Carcinoid syndrome is due to carcinoid tumors that have metastasized to the liver or are primary to the lungs.
  - This syndrome is characterized by episodic flushing, wheezing, diarrhea, and abdominal cramping.
- The glucagonoma syndrome is due to a glucagon-secreting tumor of the pancreas.
  - It is characterized by diabetes mellitus, necrolytic migratory erythema, weight loss, glossitis, and angular cheilitis.

Ectopic ACTH-Producing Tumors

Ectopic ACTH (corticotropin)-producing tumors cause many of the typical signs and symptoms of Cushing's syndrome. The etiologies of Cushing's syndrome include excessive corticotropin production from the pituitary gland, ectopic corticotropin secretion by a nonpituitary tumor, or excessive secretion of cortisol from an adrenal tumor. Corticotropin, a protein derived from pituitary proopiomelanocortin (POMC), is the major hormone that regulates glucocorticoid and adrenal androgen secretion. Ectopic corticotropin syndrome has been characterized as a unique disorder of POMC gene expression in nonendocrine tumors. Ectopic POMC production may actually represent cancer-induced amplification of POMC normally present in cells from which the cancer originated, given the widespread expression of POMC peptides in a large number of normal tissues.[2] The primary extra-adrenal effect of excessive POMC peptides in ectopic Cushing's syndrome is hyperpigmentation, which occurs over a relatively short period of time. While the hyperpigmentation has been attributed to the α-MSH secreted by tumors, it has also been demonstrated that corticotropin itself can increase skin pigmentation, induce melanogenesis in cultured human melanocytes, and be a potent agonist of the MC-1 receptor, the principal melanocortin receptor in the skin.[3–5] At diagnosis, a high proportion of patients also show weakness and proximal myopathy, moon facies, truncal obesity, or weight gain.[2] Clinical signs with predictive value for ectopic POMC production include the presence of abnormal glucose tolerance, which is more abundant in patients with ectopic POMC syndrome, as well as hypokalemia and metabolic alkalosis which are rarely seen in patients with Cushing's disease, but are common in ectopic POMC syndrome.[2]

The lung is by far the most likely organ to harbor an ectopic POMC-secreting tumor, most commonly small cell carcinomas of the lung, followed by carcinoid tumors of the lung, then other bronchial tumors. The next most frequently reported tumors that cause ectopic POMC syndrome include (in decreasing order of frequency): islet cell tumors of the pancreas, carcinoid tumors of the thymus, medullary thyroid carcinomas, adrenal pheochromocytomas, ovarian carcinomas, uterine cervix carcinomas, and prostate cancers.[2] The endocrine workup of a patient with suspected ectopic POMC syndrome includes the establishment of pathologic hypercortisolism (elevated 24-hour urine for urinary free cortisol), diagnosis of corticotropin dependency (elevated plasma corticotropin levels), and the differential diagnosis of corticotropin-dependent Cushing's syndrome (multiple dynamic endocrine tests including high-dose dexamethasone suppression test). If ectopic POMC-syndrome is confirmed, then conventional diagnostic imaging and/or somatostatin receptor scintigraphy should be used to localize the source of ectopic POMC production.

Carcinoid Syndrome

The malignant *carcinoid syndrome* is caused by circulating neuroendocrine mediators produced by carcinoid tumors. Carcinoid tumors are neoplasms of peptide- and amine-producing neuroendocrine cells with variable hormone production based on the site of origin. These tumors have been found to secrete serotonin, corticotropin, histamine, dopamine, substance P, prostaglandins, and kallikrein.[6] One of the best-characterized of these substances is serotonin. Serotonin is synthesized from its precursor, 5-hydroxytryptophan, and is subsequently metabolized to 5-hydroxyindoleacetic acid (5-HIAA), which is excreted in the urine. The release of serotonin and other vasoactive substances into the systemic circulation causes the carcinoid syndrome, the manifestations of which are episodic flushing, diarrhea, and abdominal cramping, and less often, wheezing and valvular heart disease. The vasoactive substances produced by carcinoid tumors are normally metabolized by the liver; however, in cases of liver metastases, extra-abdominal tumors, or overwhelming production by large abdominal tumors, the substances can escape into the systemic circulation. Flushing is a nearly universal symptom of the carcinoid syndrome and generally occurs over the face, neck, and upper trunk. It lasts from 2 to 10 minutes usually, but can last for up to 2 days. It can be difficult to distinguish from physiologic flushing as it is similar in distribution and shares similar triggers including emotional stress, alcohol, and certain foods. Wheezing may occur concurrently with carcinoid syndrome flushing, as well as abdominal cramping and diarrhea. The character of the flush varies from bright salmon pink to violaceous in color. If the episodic flushing occurs for many years, features of rosacea may develop. The flushing reaction of the carcinoid syndrome is

thought to be related to tachykinins and is, therefore, not controlled by serotonin antagonists.[7] Severe, extensive flushing coexistent with hypotension occurs in carcinoid crisis caused by the massive release of catecholamines from the neoplasm. A late skin finding of carcinoid tumors is a pellagra-like dermatitis. In patients with carcinoid tumors, it is hypothesized that as much as 60% of the body's tryptophan is shunted to the 5-hydroxylation pathway to make 5-HTP instead of being oxidized into nicotinic acid (in the normal state, only 1% of tryptophan goes to the 5-hydroxylation pathway).[7]

The incidence of carcinoid syndrome varies according to the extent of disease from 10 to 18% in localized or incidental tumors, to 40 to 50% in more extensive disease. Carcinoid tumors have traditionally been classified according to their presumed derivation from different embryonic divisions of the gut. Foregut carcinoid tumors most commonly originate in the lungs, bronchi, or stomach; midgut carcinoid tumors in the small intestine, appendix, and proximal large bowel; and hindgut carcinoid tumors in the distal colon and rectum. The midgut carcinoid tumors have high serotonin content and are therefore most strongly associated with the classical carcinoid syndrome. On the other hand, foregut and hindgut carcinoid tumors have lower serotonin contents and are therefore more frequently associated with absent or atypical carcinoid syndrome.[7] Somatostatin analogs are highly effective in relieving the symptoms of the carcinoid syndrome. Diagnosis of carcinoid

tumors is based on clinical symptoms of flushing and diarrhea and is supported by elevated 24-hour urine 5-HIAA levels. Localization of the tumor and metastases should be undertaken by a radiolabeled octreotide scan or a positron emission tomography (PET) scan.

Glucagonoma Syndrome

The *glucagonoma syndrome* is characterized by the triad of (1) glucagon-secreting pancreatic alpha-cell tumor, (2) diabetes mellitus, and (3) necrolytic migratory erythema. Other common associations include anemia, weight loss, stomatitis, neuropsychiatric disorders, gastrointestinal disturbances, hypoaminoacidemia, and thromboembolic phenomena. Necrolytic migratory erythema (NME) consists of intense erythematous macules and patches with superficial epidermal necrosis leading to vesicles and bullae that unroof to form erosions (Fig. 35-1). Central healing occurs, leading to an annular appearance. The margins spread centrifugally and progress from erythema to vesicles to erosions and resolution. NME most often affects the perineum and other intertriginous areas. The trunk, distal extremities, and perioral skin can be involved, as can sites of minor trauma. The progression is characterized by remissions and spontaneous exacerbations. NME will develop in nearly all patients with glucagonoma at some time during the course of the disease, and it is the presenting symptom in 67 to 72% of patients.[8] The pathogenesis of NME in glucagonoma is not well understood. Theoretical causes include epidermal nec-

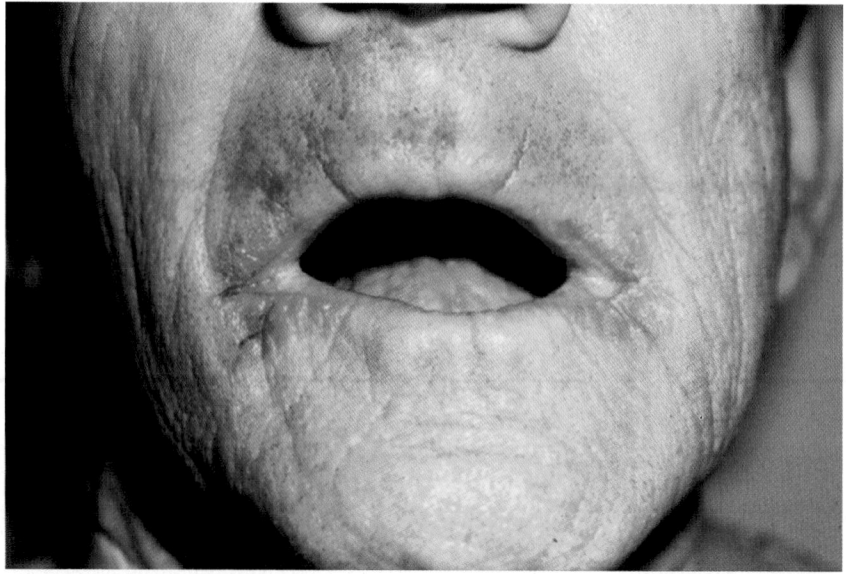

▲ **FIGURE 35-1** Angular cheilitis in a patient with glucagonoma syndrome—Courtesy of Kenneth E. Greer, M.D., Charlottesville, VA.

rosis secondary to hypoaminoacidemia and other deficiency states (e.g., zinc and fatty acid deficiencies). Diagnosis of glucagonoma is made by the presence of the characteristic clinical features, an elevated serum glucagon level by radioimmunoassay, and radiographic or histologic demonstration of a neuroendocrine tumor. Contrast-enhanced computed tomography (CT) scan is the most common radiographic diagnostic modality, but visceral angiography is more sensitive due to the hypervascularity of glucagonomas.[8] NME responds rapidly and completely following definitive treatment of the glucagonoma, when possible. Octreotide administration is very effective in controlling the NME, with resolution within 1 to 2 weeks of the initiation of therapy.[8] However, with recurrence, NME reappears.

PROLIFERATIVE AND INFLAMMATORY DERMATOSES ASSOCIATED WITH CANCER

Many of the conditions to be discussed in this section are nonspecific and have been reported both in association with and in the absence of underlying malignant disease. Malignancy is most often only one of a number of possible etiological or associated factors.

Hypertrichosis Lanuginosa Acquisita

> **BOX 35-3 Summary**
>
> - Hypertrichosis lanuginosa, aka malignant Down, is manifested by the excessive growth of fine lanugo hair.
> - Lung cancer is the most frequently associated malignancy.

Hypertrichosis lanuginosa acquisita is a rare syndrome consisting of the development of excessive amounts of lanugo hair (Fig. 35-2). The hair can grow to great length and is easily pulled out. Typical distribution is on the forehead, ears, nose, and less commonly the axillae, limbs, and trunk.[9] This syndrome has also been referred to as "malignant down." The syndrome should be distinguished from hirsutism (in which the hair is not of the lanugo type), from congenital hypertrichosis lanuginosa, and from other causes of hypertrichosis, such as porphyria and endocrinopathies. Also, a number of medications can cause hypertrichosis including testosterone, DHEA, phenytoin, minoxidil, diazoxide, cyclosporine, streptomycin, pso-

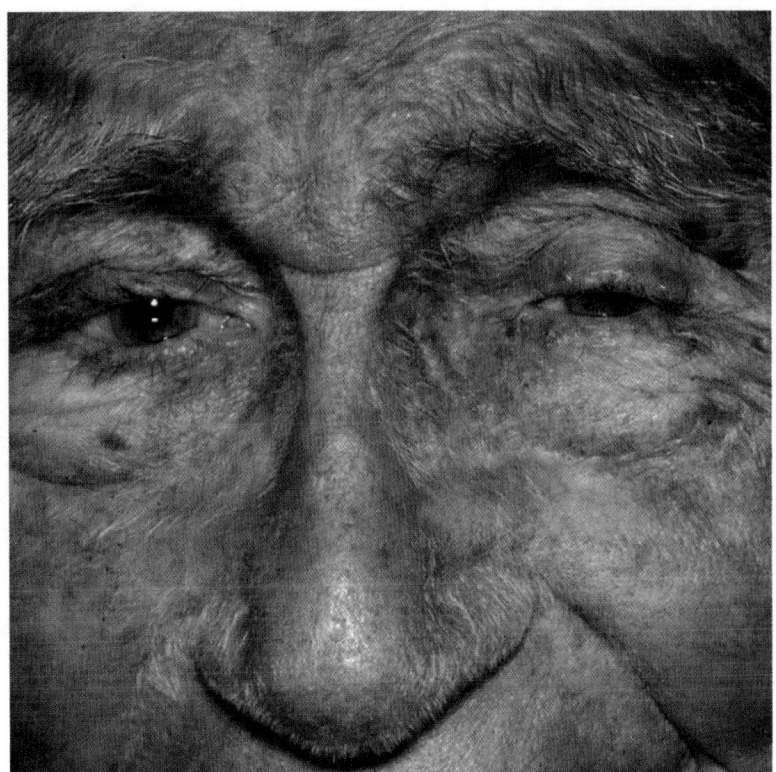

▲ **FIGURE 35-2** Hypertrichosis lanuginosa acquisita associated with cancer of the lung— Courtesy of Kenneth E. Greer, M.D., Charlottesville, VA.

ralen, penicillamine, high-dose corticosteroids, metyrapone, phenothiazines, acetazolamide, and hexachlorobenzene; however, usually this is terminal hair and not lanugo hair. Histopathology will demonstrate unmedullated hair with an elevated anagen/telogen ratio.[9] A painful glossitis, angular cheilitis, and swollen red fungiform papillae on the anterior half of the tongue often accompany the cutaneous changes.

The most common malignancy associated with hypertrichosis lanuginosa acquisita is lung cancer, followed by colorectal cancer.[10] Other reportedly associated malignancies include cancers of the kidney, breast, uterus, ovaries, parotid gland, pancreas, liver, gallbladder, lymphoma, and acute myeloid leukemia.[11] In women, hypertrichosis lanuginosa is most frequently associated with colorectal cancer, followed by lung, and breast cancers; whereas in men, lung cancer is the most common followed by colorectal cancer.[10] The pathogenesis of hypertrichosis lanuginosa acquisita is unknown. Patients who present with this finding in the absence of offending medications should be evaluated for underlying malignancy. Evaluation should include a full history and physical, complete blood count (CBC) with peripheral smear, and a CT of the chest, abdomen, and pelvis. In women, a mammogram and pelvic

examination are warranted. Additional studies should be guided by the patient's combination of risk factors, signs, and symptoms.

Acanthosis Nigricans

> **BOX 35-4 Summary**
>
> - AN in association with weight loss should be considered a potential sign of internal malignancy, particularly when an endocrinopathy is excluded.
> - The most frequent sites of malignancy are intra-abdominal, with gastric adenocarcinoma being most frequent.
> - Concurrent onset and parallel course for malignancy-associated AN are common.
> - Patients with AN, may also have multiple, eruptive seborrheic keratoses or may have tripe palms.

Acanthosis nigricans (AN) is a common disorder usually associated with underlying endocrinopathies (especially insulin resistance), obesity, and various syndromes, as well as underlying neoplasia. Clinically, AN appears as hyperpigmented, velvety patches and plaques in intertriginous areas (Fig. 35-3) and areas of trauma (knuckles, elbows, and knees). It is most commonly seen on the posterior and lateral neck, axillae, and inguinal folds.

433

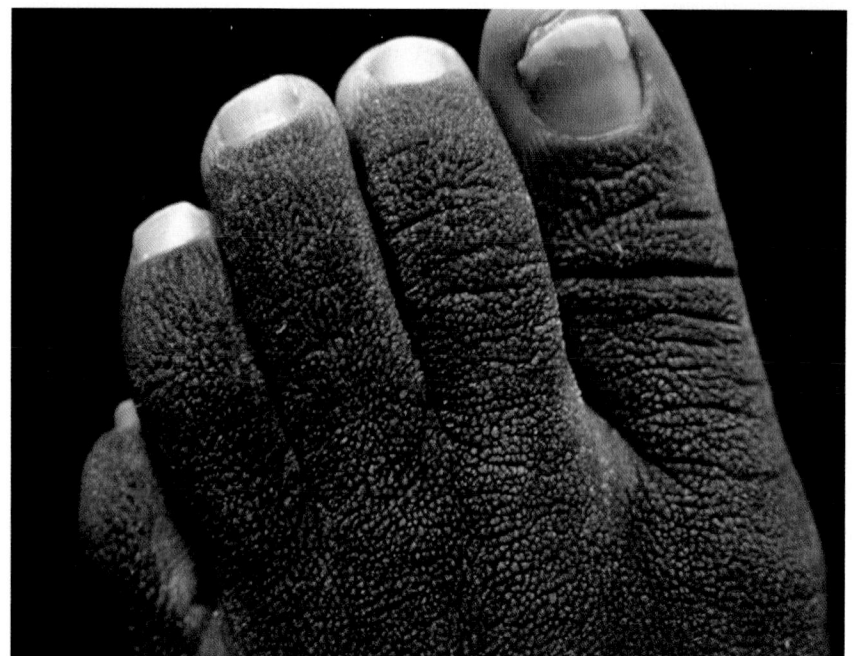

▲ **FIGURE 35-3** AN—this patient developed generalized lesions in addition to the traditional intertriginous involvement.

Malignant AN is characterized by a rapid onset with possible involvement of the palms, soles, and mucosal surfaces, not commonly seen in other types of AN.[12] Mucosal findings may present as papillomatous thickening or hyperpigmentation without associated thickening. Other findings may include tripe palms, acrochordons, multiple seborrheic keratoses (see Sign of Leser–Trélat), and multiple verrucous or papillary lesions (see florid cutaneous papillomatosis). Malignant AN may become generalized. While other types of AN show racial predilections (occurring more commonly in black and Hispanic patients), malignant AN does not.[13]

The most common underlying malignancy associated with AN is an adenocarcinoma, most frequently of the gastrointestinal or genitourinary tracts. The single most common association is with adenocarcinoma of the stomach.[14] The histology of malignant AN does not differ from other types of AN. The skin has overlying hyperkeratosis with a papillomatous and occasionally acantholytic epidermis, and an unremarkable dermis. The dermal papillae are elongated with upward projections into the thinned epidermis giving a papillomatous appearance. There may be increased melanin in the basal keratinocytes, but with no associated increase in the number of melanocytes.[15] The pathogenesis of malignant AN is thought to be secondary to increased levels of circulating epidermal growth factors that stimulate both keratinocytes and dermal fibroblasts.[13]

A diagnosis of malignant AN should be considered in patients when other more frequent causes of AN are ruled out; especially in older patients who complain of weight loss. In suspicious cases, workup should include a CT of the chest, abdomen, and pelvis, complete endoscopic examination of the gastrointestinal tract, as well as a mammogram and cervical cytologic examination in women and prostate-specific antigen in men. The course of malignant AN generally parallels that of the underlying malignancy, with treatment of the underlying malignancy resulting in improvement or resolution of the AN. A return of AN following remission usually heralds a relapse of the underlying malignancy.

The Sign of Leser–Trélat

Leser–Trélat is a syndrome characterized by the abrupt appearance and rapid increase in size of multiple seborrheic keratoses (Fig. 35-4) associated with an underlying malignancy. It is most frequently associated with adenocarcinoma, particularly of the gastrointestinal tract. Patients with Leser–Trélat syndrome very often also have AN and florid cutaneous papillomatosis.[16] The association of eruptive seborrheic keratoses and internal malignancy is controversial.[17] The difficulty lies in the lack of a strict definition for what constitutes an "eruption" of lesions, and in the fact that both seborrheic keratoses and cancer are common findings in the elderly, raising the question of a spurious relationship. Several case control studies and a retrospective review have called into question its validity.[18–20] Further studies, however, are required to determine the relative risk of developing cancer in patients with eruptive seborrheic keratoses. Reports of resolution of eruptive seborrheic keratoses following treatment of underlying malignancy support the argument that the sign of Leser–Trélat fits the criteria as a paraneoplastic phenomenon.[16]

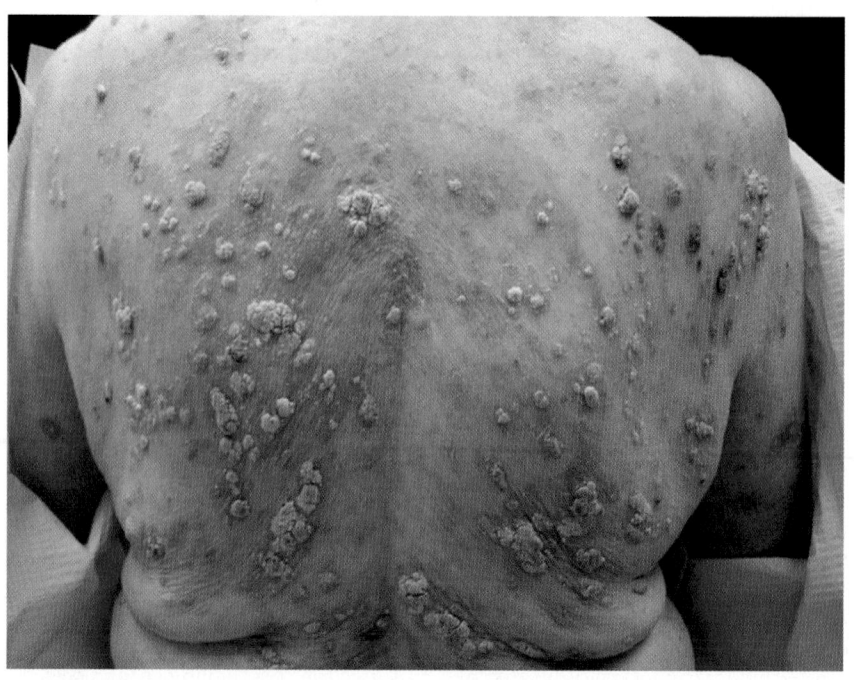

▲ **FIGURE 35-4** Sign of Leser–Trélat—this patient did not harbor an internal malignancy.

Clinically, the lesions appear as exophytic, "stuck-on" appearing tumors covered with a thick, greasy scale. They are mainly seen on the trunk (but may occur anywhere) and follow skin lines. Pigmentation varies from minimal to dense. The lesions of Leser–Trélat syndrome are clinically indistinguishable from sporadically occurring seborrheic keratoses, though there may be increased pruritus and/or inflammation. Histologically, the lesions are characterized by hyperkeratosis overlying a thickened, papillomatous epidermis. Increased melanin may be seen within basal keratinocytes. Pathogenesis is uncertain, but appears to be related to a tumor-secreted growth factor similar to malignant AN.

In considering a diagnosis of Leser–Trélat syndrome, the appearance of the seborrheic keratoses should be strikingly abrupt. There are no diagnostic criteria, however, for the length of the eruptive period or for the number of seborrheic keratoses. Although the relationship with malignancy has been called into question, it is not unreasonable to consider an evaluation for malignancy in patients with eruptive seborrheic keratoses, especially if they occur in conjunction with AN or florid cutaneous papillomatosis (or other paraneoplastic dermatoses) or in patients also complaining of weight loss. The sign is most commonly associated with adenocarcinoma of the gastrointestinal tract, but breast cancer is also frequently reported, as well as lymphoma or leukemia.[16,21] Patients should undergo a CT scan of the chest, abdomen, and pelvis, complete endoscopic examination of the gastrointestinal tract, as well as mammogram and cervical cytologic examination in women and prostate-specific antigen in men. Additional evaluation may be considered, but should be guided by the signs and symptoms in a given patient.

Tripe Palms

Tripe palms are characterized by thickened, velvet- or moss-textured palms, which may appear cobbled or honeycombed, with pronounced skin ridging. The term "tripe" refers to a food prepared from the bovine foregut which has a rugose surface said to resemble the ridging of the palms in this condition. Several other names have been used for the same condition, such as acanthosis palmaris, palmar hyperkeratosis, palmar keratoderma, and AN of the palms. Tripe palms may simply represent the manifestation of AN on the palms. It is dealt with separately, however, because it sometimes occurs in patients with no other manifestations of AN, and it has a different neoplastic association than malignant AN. Tripe palms are usually seen in patients with an underlying malignancy and its presentation often precedes the diagnosis of the neoplasm.

In a review by Cohen of 87 reported cases of tripe palms, 79 patients had an associated malignancy.[22] AN was also seen in 57 of the 79 patients with malignancy-associated tripe palms. In 69% of the patients with associated malignancy, the onset of tripe palms preceded the diagnosis of the cancer or occurred within 1 month of the diagnosis. Pulmonary (25.6%) and gastric (25.6%) carcinomas were the most common neoplasms.[22] When tripe palms presents alone, the incidence of pulmonary carcinoma is greater than when tripe palms presents in conjunction with AN. In patients with tripe palms and no associated AN, pulmonary cancer accounted for 56% of malignancies. Bladder, breast, cervical, ovarian, and renal carcinomas were also associated with tripe palms. In one-third of the cases, the tripe palms resolved following treatment of the underlying neoplasm.[22] Histology of tripe palms lesions demonstrates hyperkeratosis and acanthosis of the epidermis. All patients with tripe palms should undergo diagnostic evaluation for an associated cancer, especially gastric and pulmonary types. Workup should include CT of the chest and abdomen, along with endoscopic evaluation of the upper gastrointestinal tract.

Additional workup should be based on the patient's risk factors, medical history, symptoms, and laboratory findings.

Acrokeratosis Paraneoplastica (Bazex Syndrome)

BOX 35-5 Summary

- Acrokeratosis paraneoplastica manifests as psoriasiform dermatitis on acral surfaces.
- Malignancies associated with AP are generally in the upper airways, proximal esophagus, or nasopharyngeal.

Acrokeratosis paraneoplastica (Bazex syndrome) is a rare finding that is almost always associated with carcinomas of the upper "aerodigestive" tract. This syndrome is seen primarily in white males over 40 years of age.[23] Bazex syndrome is a psoriasiform eruption that changes appearance as it progresses. The first stage consists of erythema with a fine scale that occur on the fingers and toes (Fig. 35-5), spreading to the aural helices of the ears, and a violaceous erythema and scaling of the nose. Nail changes can be seen at this stage consisting of dystrophy with subungual hyperkeratosis progressing to onycholysis.[23] In the second stage, a keratoderma with violaceous color develops affecting the entirety of the hands and feet. At this stage, the entire pinna is scaly and erythematous, and the nasal eruption spreads to involve the malar areas of the face and the philtrum.[23] If the neoplasm is not treated at the second stage, the rash spreads

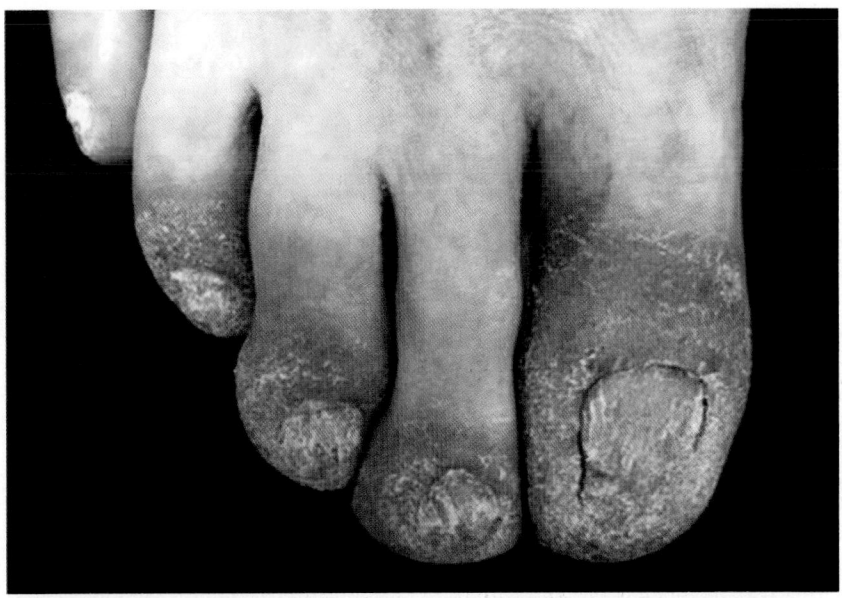

▲ **FIGURE 35-5** Acrokeratosis paraneoplastica (Bazex syndrome)—this patient presents with cutaneous findings prior to his diagnosis of squamous cell carcinoma of the tonsillar pillar.

centripetally and begins to appear at new sites such as legs, knees, thighs, and arms (comprising the third stage).[23]

An analytic review of Bazex syndrome by Bolognia et al. demonstrated an association with malignancy in all of the 93 cases reviewed.[24] Squamous cell carcinomas of the head and neck and squamous cell carcinomas of unknown primary found in cervical lymph nodes were the most commonly associated malignancies. In 91% of patients in the Bolognia series, the rash improved significantly following treatment of the underlying cancer with the exception of nail dystrophy, which persisted.[24] Biopsy findings in Bazex syndrome include hyperkeratosis, parakeratosis, spongiosis, dyskeratotic keratinocytes, vacuolar degeneration, and incontinent pigment. Direct immunofluorescence studies are nonspecific. Pathogenesis is unknown, but theories include a paraneoplastic autoimmune phenomenon as well as possible tumor-produced or induced growth factors. In patients with findings suspicious for Bazex syndrome, workup should be undertaken to diagnose head and neck cancer. This should include triple endoscopy (bronchoscopy, laryngoscopy, and esophagoscopy) in addition to a CT of the head, neck, and chest. If the search for cancer of the head and neck is negative, then evaluation for cancers of other sites based on risk factors, signs, and symptoms should be considered.

Acquired Ichthyosis

BOX 35-6 Summary

- Acquired ichthyosis usually follows the diagnosis of malignancy.
- It is most often observed in lymphoreticular malignancies or premalignant conditions.

Ichthyosis is characterized by the accumulation of visible scales on the skin, predominately affecting the trunk and extensor surfaces of the limbs. The scales are white to brown in color, rhomboid in shape, and have a free edge (Fig. 35-6). Palms, soles, and flexural areas are usually spared. The histologic pattern is characterized by epidermal narrowing, a thinned or absent granular layer, and no dermal infiltrate.[25] The condition can be genetic or acquired, with the genetic forms presenting in childhood and the acquired form generally seen in adulthood. *Acquired ichthyosis (AI)* is seen in conjunction with various chronic diseases, infectious causes, and underlying malignancies; it is clinically

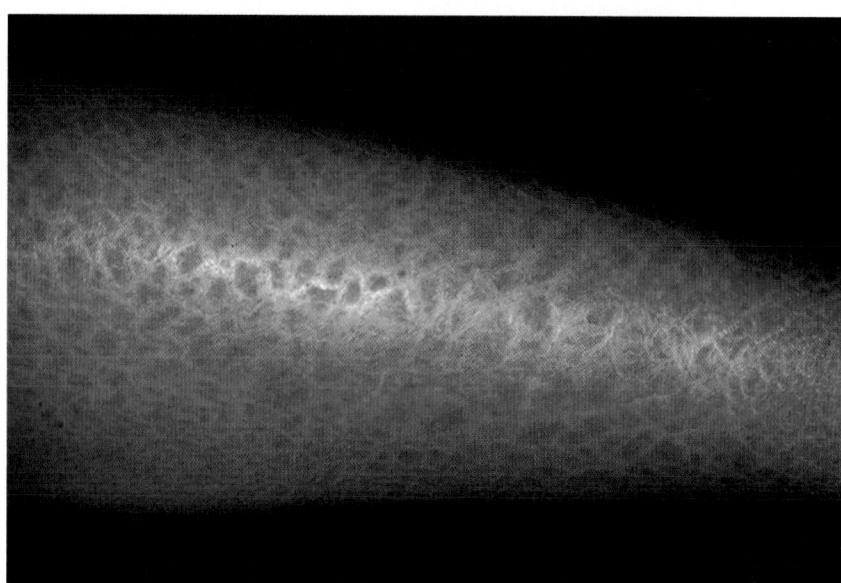

▲ **FIGURE 35-6** Acquired ichthyosis in a patient with uterine cancer.

and histologically similar to genetic ichthyosis.

Hodgkin's lymphoma is the most common malignancy associated with AI. Information on the incidence of AI is lacking, but in one small series of 32 cases, Hodgkin's lymphoma was noted in roughly 75% of the patients with AI.[26] Other AI-associated lymphoreticular malignancies have been reported, including T-cell lymphoma, small bowel lymphoma, various types of leukemia, and multiple myeloma. Also reported are non-lymphoproliferative disorders, especially sarcomas, and solid tumors of the breast, lung, and cervix. AI usually occurs after the onset of symptoms of the underlying malignancy. The course of AI generally varies with the severity of the disease.[26] Currently, the most common setting for AI is in patients with acquired immunodeficiency syndrome. Other known associations with AI are endocrine and metabolic disorders, connective tissue diseases, sarcoidosis, human T-lymphotrophic virus 1 and 2, leprosy, polycythemia rubra vera, and malnutrition.[26,27] Various medications can also cause AI, including, but not exclusively, cholesterol-lowering agents (triparanol, azacosterol, benzophene, and niacin).[27]

Because AI usually presents after the underlying disease has been diagnosed, evaluation is not generally an issue. However, in the patient who presents with AI without a history of an existing malignancy, a thorough history (including medication history) and physical examination with basic laboratory studies will be necessary to guide the diagnostic approach.

Amyloidosis

BOX 35-7 Summary

- There are multiple forms of amyloid that can affect the skin, including some that are local.
- Systemic amyloidosis occurs in two forms—AL type and AA type.
- The AL type is associated with paraproteinemia and occasionally with myeloma.
- AL amyloidosis manifests as purpura with or without waxy changes.
- High-dose chemotherapy with or without autologous stem cell transplantation is the therapy of choice.

Amyloidosis refers to the extracellular deposition of insoluble fibrillar proteins in organs and tissues. Amyloidosis can be classified according to the nature of the proteins that form the fibrillar deposits. The major classes are primary amyloidosis (AL type), secondary amyloidosis (AA type), and familial amyloidoses (multiple types, including ATTR). The amyloid fibrils in primary amyloidosis are fragments of immunoglobulin light chains that stain with Congo red, demonstrating apple green birefringence under polarized light. Electron microscopy reveals rigid nonbranching fibrils. The AL type occurs in the setting of a plasma cell dyscrasia such as multiple myeloma.[28] Up to 40% of multiple myeloma-associated amyloidoses present with mucocutaneous findings and these findings may be the presenting signs.[29] The most common findings are purpura, petechiae, and ecchymoses

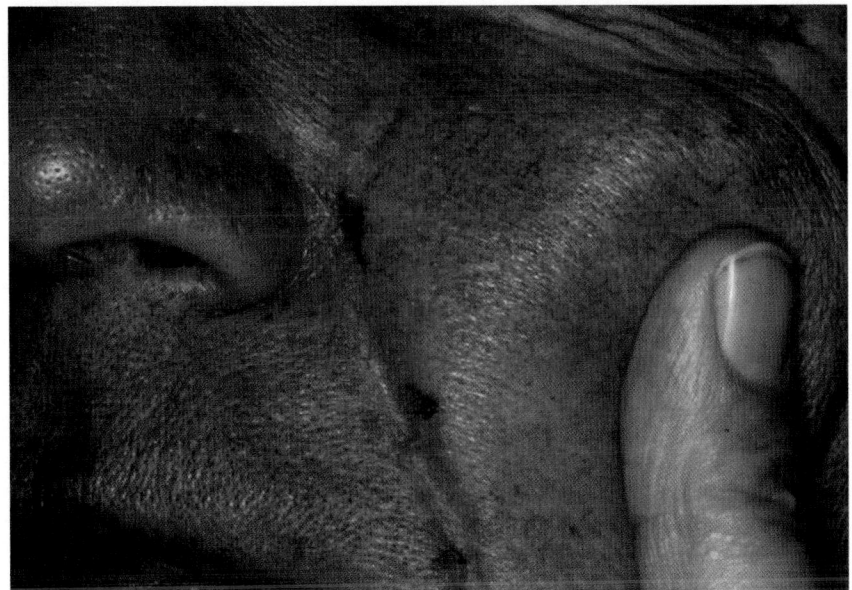

▲ **FIGURE 35-7** Amyloidosis—subtle "pinch purpura" in the nasolabial fold.

(Fig. 35-7). These manifestations are thought to result from amyloid infiltration of the dermal vasculature causing problems with hemostasis and easy bruising ("pinch purpura") following minor trauma (though major bleeding may be due to an interaction between amyloid and calcium-dependent clotting factors and should prompt an evaluation for clotting disorders). Periorbital purpura can be seen following Valsalva-like maneuvers or dependent positioning of the head. Other common presentations include papules, plaques, and nodules. Papules and plaques are frequently hemorrhagic, but may be yellow or flesh-colored with a characteristic waxy appearance. These are most commonly seen on the face, neck, and intertriginous areas. Nodules are commonly shiny and wax-like and found on the extremities, head, and trunk. Additionally reported mucocutaneous presentations of AL amyloidosis include bullous eruptions, scleroderma-like changes, macroglossia, shoulder pad enlargement, nail dystrophies, and alopecia.

The diagnosis of amyloidosis is established by tissue biopsy. Masses of amyloid are present in the dermis (with corresponding loss of rete ridges), the subcutaneous fat, and in blood vessel walls. Amyloid deposits around individual fat cells ("amyloid rings") are a distinctive finding. On hematoxylin- and eosin-stained specimens, amyloid deposits appear as homogenous eosinophilic masses with a fissured appearance ("cracked pavement").[29] As mentioned earlier, amyloid can be demonstrated in tissue using Congo red stain and examination under polarized light for apple-green birefringence, or using crystal violet stain. Distinction between primary and secondary amyloidosis was classically made by pretreating the specimen with potassium permanganate, as secondary amyloidosis will not stain with Congo red following this treatment, but primary amyloidosis will. Immunohistochemical studies are more sensitive, however, in determining the clonality of the plasma cell population. Commercial antisera are available for κ and λ immunoglobulin light chains (as well as for TTR and AA).[30] These immunohistochemical studies are important to confirm the clinical diagnosis. Patients with biopsy-proven amyloidosis must undergo a workup for plasma cell dyscrasia by protein electrophoresis of serum and urine with immunofixation. If the skin biopsy suggests AL-type amyloidosis, but electrophoresis is negative, a bone marrow biopsy with immunohistochemical staining is recommended because in most of these patients a clonal dominance of plasma cells will be identified. If both tests are negative, a workup for familial ATTR amyloidosis should be undertaken.[28]

AL amyloidosis can affect every organ except the brain and the prognosis is poor, especially with cardiac or visceral involvement. Radiolabeled serum amyloid P (SAP) component scintigraphy is a noninvasive means of determining the extent of disease, though this test is not universally available. Systemic chemotherapy, particularly with alkylating agents, is used to suppress the plasma cell clone in the bone marrow. The most common regimen is melphalan with or without prednisone or colchicine. More patients are being offered high-dose chemotherapy with stem cell reconstitution, though evidence as to the superiority of this treatment is lacking.[30]

Scleromyxedema, Lichen Myxedematosus, and Papular Mucinosis

> **BOX 35-8   Summary**
>
> - These disorders are characterized by cutaneous infiltration by mucopolysaccharides.
> - Paraproteinemia is common, but myeloma is rare in these patients.
> - Autologous stem cell transplantation combined with melphalan chemotherapy seems to offer a viable therapy for these patients.

Scleromyxedema (also known as generalized lichen myxedematosus) includes the following: (1) generalized papular and sclerodermoid eruption, (2) mucin deposition, fibrosis, and fibroblast proliferation, (3) monoclonal gammopathy, and (4) absence of thyroid disease. Scleromyxedema usually affects middle-aged adults and presents with a widespread eruption of small (2 to 3 mm), hard, waxy papules often arranged in a linear fashion (Fig. 35-8) and occurring most commonly on the face, neck, forearms, and hands, but with sparing of the palms and mucous membranes. The affected areas may exhibit erythema, edema, and brownish discoloration. Sparse eyebrow, axillary, and pubic hair is an associated finding. Leonine facies may develop. The presenting complaint is often that of limited range of motion and skin stiffness around joints and the mouth. There are multiple associated systemic symptoms including peripheral neuropathies, dysphagia, and proximal muscle weakness, among others. The paraproteinemia associated with scleromyxedema is IgG lambda in most cases; however, this paraproteinemia is usually of uncertain significance with few cases of associated multiple myeloma.[31] Treatment options are limited and have traditionally included corticosteroids and low-dose melphalan with mixed results. Improved outcomes have been reported with high-dose melphalan followed by autologous stem cell transplantation.[32,33]

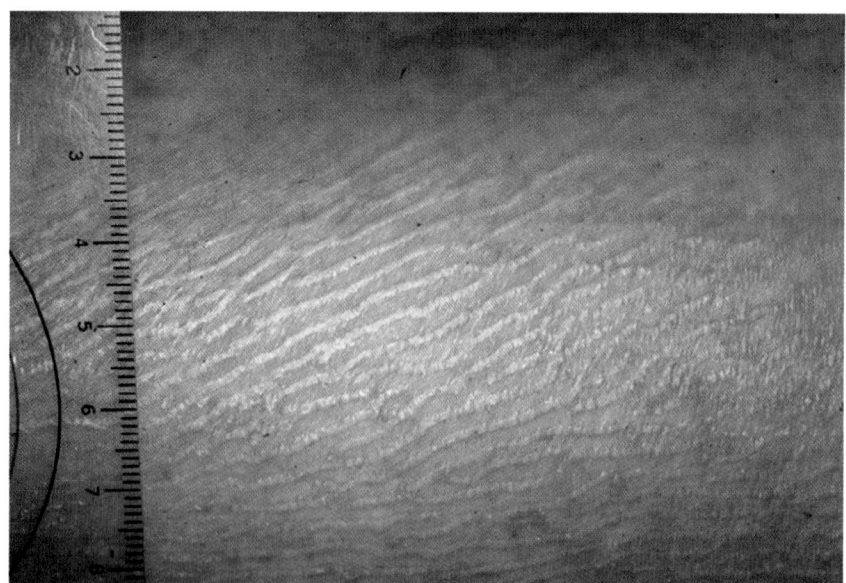

▲ **FIGURE 35-8** Scleromyxedema—linear papules.

POEMS Syndrome

> **BOX 35-9 Summary**
>
> - There are many cutaneous changes that occur in patients with POEMS syndrome, but the glomeruloid hemangioma appears to be highly specific for the disorder even though it occurs in a minority of patients.
> - POEMS syndrome patients most often have an osteoclastic myeloma or Castleman's disease.

POEMS syndrome (also known as Crow–Fukase syndrome) is a rare multisystem disorder that complicates plasma cell dyscrasia, especially osteosclerotic myeloma and solitary plasmacytoma. POEMS is an acronym for the constellation of findings in the syndrome: *p*olyneuropathy, *o*rganomegaly, *e*ndocrinopathy, *m*onoclonal gammopathy, and *s*kin changes.[34] The most common skin change seen is hyperpigmentation, but numerous other skin changes have been reported including sclerodermatous thickening, acrocyanosis, plethora, hypertrichosis, hyperhidrosis, clubbing, and hemangiomas (Fig. 35-9). Multiple seborrheic keratoses, ichthyosis, livedo reticularis, and vasculitis have also been reported.[34–37] Tsai et al. proposed that glomeruloid hemangiomas, while a rare finding, are a specific cutaneous marker of POEMS syndrome when present.[38] Various other clinical signs can be seen in association with POEMS syndrome, such as sclerotic bone lesions, multicentric Castleman's disease, papilledema, edema, pleural effusions and ascites, fatigue, weight loss, and thrombocyto-

sis. Less frequently reported phenomena include pulmonary hypertension, restrictive lung disease, cardiomyopathy, and venous thrombosis.[35]

The pathogenesis of POEMS syndrome is not completely understood, but an imbalance of proinflammatory cytokines along with a derangement of vascular endothelial growth factor (VEGF) production have been proposed.[39,40] The monoclonal protein present in POEMS syndrome is nearly always a λ light chain (IgA, IgG, or IgM). The monoclonal protein is present in the serum by immunofixation in 75 to 85% of patients, and the remaining percentage will have a clonal λ

plasmaproliferative disorder demonstrated by immunohistochemical staining of bone marrow.[34,35] Patients with unexplained peripheral neuropathy and skin findings noted earlier (especially hyperpigmentation) should raise clinical suspicion for POEMS syndrome. If clinical suspicion is high, serum and urine electrophoresis with immunofixation should be performed. Immunofixation is required because monoclonal protein is nearly always present in low concentration and many cases would be missed by electrophoresis alone.[35] Bone marrow biopsy with immunofixation may be required in cases of high clinical suspicion, but without findings on serum or urine electrophoresis. All patients should have a metastatic bone survey done to look for osteosclerotic lesions. Dispenzieri et al. proposed that a diagnosis of POEMS should require satisfaction of two major criteria–polyneuropathy and a clonal plasmaproliferative disorder, and one minor criterion—osteosclerotic bone lesions; Castleman's disease; papilledema; organomegaly (including lymphadenopathy); edema, pleural effusion, or ascites; endocrinopathy; and skin changes.[35]

Prognosis for patients with POEMS syndrome is generally better than that for patients with classical multiple myeloma. In a study of 99 patients with POEMS syndrome, median survival was 165 months regardless of how many features were present at diagnosis.[35] Chemotherapy or radiation (for solitary plasmacytoma) are the most common treatment modalities.

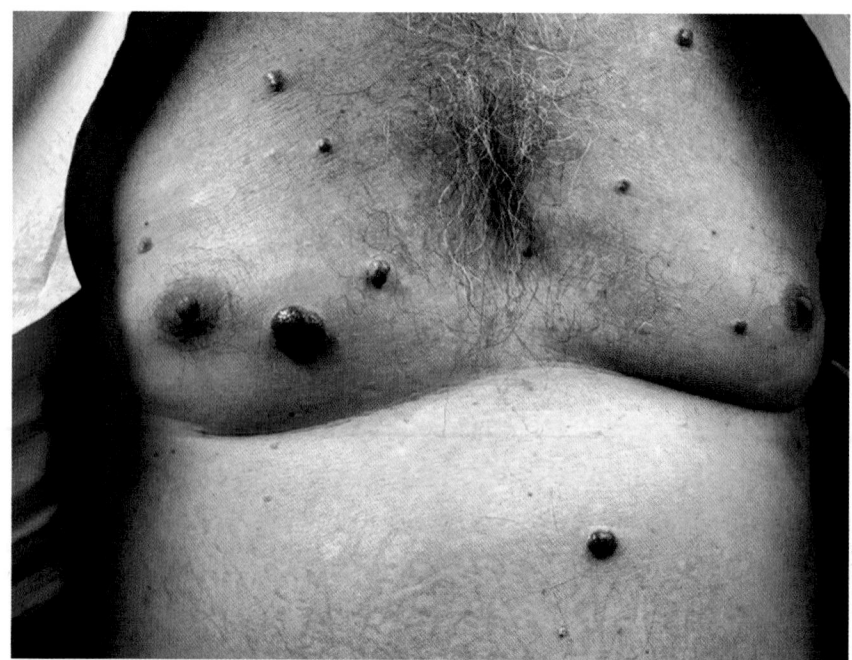

▲ **FIGURE 35-9** POEMS syndrome in a patient with an osteosclerotic myeloma.

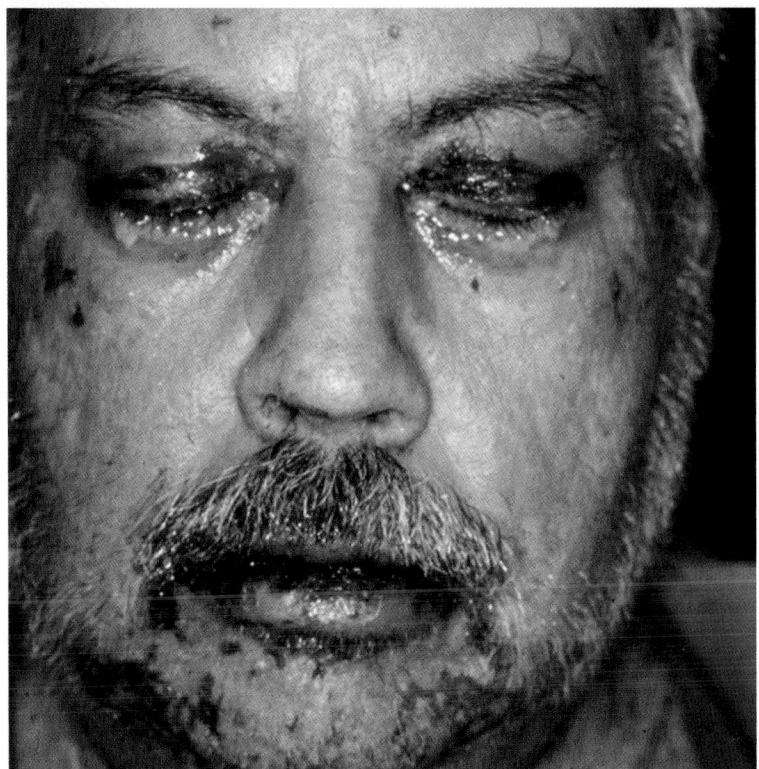

▲ FIGURE 35-10 Paraneoplastic pemphigus—marked crusting of multiple mucosal surfaces.

Paraneoplastic Pemphigus

BOX 35-10   Summary

- Paraneoplastic pemphigus is a distinct immunologic disease characterized by mucousal erosions and polymorphic skin lesions that resemble lichen planus, bullous pemphigoid, or pemphigus vulgaris.
- PNP is associated with a variety of lymphoproliferative diseases, but Castleman's disease appears to be particularly prevalent.
- Bronchiolitis obliterans is a severe life-threatening complication of PNP.
- Treatment with traditional immunosuppressive agents with or without rituximab is useful in some patients.

A variety of *blistering diseases* have been reported in patients with cancer. *Paraneoplastic pemphigus* (PNP) is an autoimmune mucocutaneous disease associated with neoplasia, most commonly a lymphoproliferative disorder. The most common associations are with non-Hodgkin's B-cell lymphoma, chronic lymphocytic leukemia, and Castleman's disease.[41–43] Even in the absence of obvious lymphoproliferative malignancy, a small nidus of Castleman's disease may exist and cause PNP. The clinical presentation is extremely variable, but the most consistent feature is the development of painful stomatitis (Fig. 35-10). This is

often the presenting sign and is the most resistant to therapy. The erosions and ulcerations of PNP stomatitis can affect all surfaces of the oropharynx, but most often affect the lateral borders of the tongue and frequently extend onto the lips up to and including the vermillion border. Stomatitis lesions in PNP differ from those of pemphigus vulgaris in that they are more necrotic and have lichenoid changes. The finding of stomatitis is so uniform that the diagnosis of

PNP should rarely be considered in its absence.[44] Cutaneous lesion morphology varies between patients and in individual patients over time. Blisters may be tense, resembling those of bullous pemphigoid, or they can resemble erythema multiforme with surrounding erythema (Fig. 35-11). When the blisters rupture leaving an erosion, the eroded areas can become confluent, especially on the trunk. Because of these findings, the most common differential for PNP is erythema multiforme/toxic epidermal necrolysis. Cutaneous lichenoid lesions are also common in PNP and consist of erythematous papules and plaques. Both the blisters and lichenoid lesions can be seen on the palms, soles, and paronychium. This is a distinguishing feature of PNP in that the blisters of pemphigus vulgaris rarely involve these sites. It is important to note that PNP can affect the bronchial and alveolar airways leading to airflow obstruction and ultimately to functional changes characteristic of bronchiolitis obliterans.[45]

The immunopathology of PNP involves both autoantibodies similar to classical pemphigus and a coexistent cell-mediated cytotoxicity. The pathogenesis of PNP has not been well-characterized, but a leading hypothesis involves the dysregulation of cytokines, particularly IL-6, driving autoantibody production.[46] Histology of PNP reflects the variability of clinical lesions, with findings dependent on the nature of lesion biopsied. Acantholysis is often present similar to that of classical pemphigus, but a marked lichenoid inflammatory infiltrate at the dermal–epithelial junction is also frequently evident. Biopsies of stomatitis

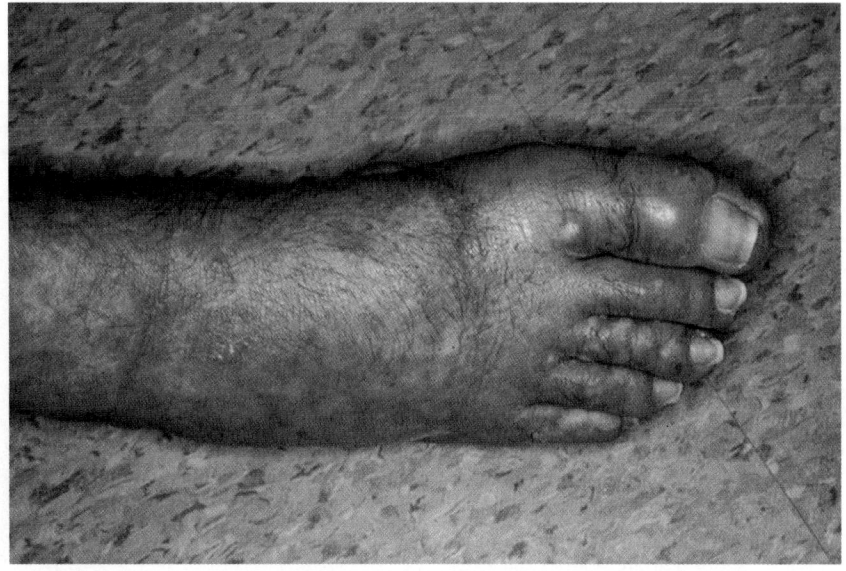

▲ FIGURE 35-11 Paraneoplastic pemphigus—bullous lesions on the dorsum of the foot.

lesions may demonstrate only ulceration and inflammation, but suprabasilar acantholysis can be seen if perilesional epithelium is also sampled.[47] Intact cutaneous blisters demonstrate suprabasilar acantholysis, sometimes with an associated inflammatory cell infiltrate. Nonblistering lesions may show individual keratinocyte necrosis with lymphocytic infiltrate in the upper dermis and occasionally within the epidermis.[47] Direct immunofluorescence (DIF) reveals deposition of IgG antibodies in intercellular spaces of epithelium and often at the dermal–epithelial junction as well.[48] DIF is frequently negative in PNP, however, and is therefore not essential for diagnosis. Serological findings of antiplakin autoantibodies can be very specific for PNP, however, and are required for the diagnosis. The plakins are proteins that mediate the attachment of cytoskeletal intermediate filaments to transmembrane adhesion molecules like desmogleins. The autoantibodies are directed against (in decreasing order of frequency): envoplakin, periplakin, and desmoplakin I and II. Almost all PNP patients have autoantibodies against desmoglein as well. Screening for these autoantibodies can be done by indirect immunoflouresence (IF) reactive with rodent urinary bladder epithelium, but immunochemical techniques are much more precise.[44]

Given the clinical and histopathological variability of PNP, diagnosis can be difficult. Anhalt has proposed four minimal criteria for diagnosing PNP: (1) painful progressive stomatitis with preferential involvement of the tongue, (2) histologic features of acantholysis, lichenoid, or interface dermatitis, (3) demonstration of antiplakin autoantibodies (immunochemistry demonstrating periplakin and envoplakin at the least), and (4) demonstration of an underlying lymphoproliferative neoplasm.[44] The frequency of PNP-associated neoplasms is non-Hodgkin's lymphoma (42%), chronic lymphocytic leukemia (29%), Castleman's disease (10%), thymoma, sarcoma, and Waldenstrom's macroglobulinemia (all 6% each). These frequencies are different in children, with Castleman's disease as the underlying malignancy for almost all pediatric PNP cases.[44] Occult malignancies presenting with PNP account for one-third of cases (usually secondary to Castleman's disease, abdominal lymphoma, thymoma, or retroperitoneal sarcomas).[42–44] In a patient diagnosed with PNP without known malignancy, computerized tomography of the chest, abdomen, and pelvis will usually reveal the neoplasm.

PNP is generally progressive despite treatment of the underlying neoplasm, though remission is possible after removal of benign thymomas or encapsulated Castleman's tumors. Treatment with oral corticosteroids at a dose of 0.5 to 1 mg/kg may lead to improvement in lesions. Cutaneous lesions are the most responsive. Stomatitis and pulmonary involvement are more refractory to treatment. Other agents such as cyclosporine, cyclophosphamide, and rituximab have been tried in combination with prednisone.[44] A recognized complication of PNP is respiratory failure with features of bronchiolitis obliterans, which continues to progress even after the resolution of cutaneous and mucosal lesions on immunosuppressive therapy.[45]

Anti-Epiligrin Cicatricial Pemphigoid

BOX 35-11 Summary

- Anti-epiligrin cicatricial pemphigoid is characterized by severe mucosal disease with antibodies directed against laminin 5.
- Roughly one-third of the patients have a malignancy, usually a solid tumor.
- The discovery of a malignancy may precede, follow, or occur concurrently with diagnosis.

Anti-epiligrin cicatricial pemphigoid (AECP) is a rare subset (~5%) of cicatricial pemphigoid (CP) that shows IgG antibodies to laminin 5. AECP is a chronic autoimmune subepidermal blistering disease characterized by severe, painful lesions of the oral mucosa and evidence of skin involvement. Mucosal findings consist of erosive and/or vesiculobullous lesions. Skin lesions consist of tense blisters and erosions on an erythematous base (Fig. 35-12). In a series of 35 patients, mucosal involvement was noted at the following sites and percentages: oral (100%), ocular (66%), laryngeal (51%), nasal (46%), pharyngeal (46%), esophageal (20%), genital (31%), and anal (11%).[49] Sequelae of these lesions can be severe with gingival destruction, loss of teeth, restricted mobility of the tongue or pharynx, blindness, dysphonia, airway compromise, and esophageal strictures noted as potential complications. In the series of 35 patients noted earlier, skin involvement was seen in 86%, but lesions were few in number and mild in severity. Skin lesions most frequently involved the extremities and trunk, but were also noted on the scalp, chest, buttocks, and face.[49]

Diagnostic criteria for AECP require: (1) the presence of erosive and/or blistering lesions of mucous membranes, (2) *in situ* deposits of IgG autoantibodies in epidermal basement membranes, or circulating IgG autoantibodies that bind the dermal side of 1-M NaCl split human skin, and (3) circulating IgG that immunoprecipitates laminin 5 on extracts or conditioned media of radiolabeled human keratinocytes.[49] It is important to distinguish this subset of CP because of the severity of mucosal lesions and sequelae, in addition to an

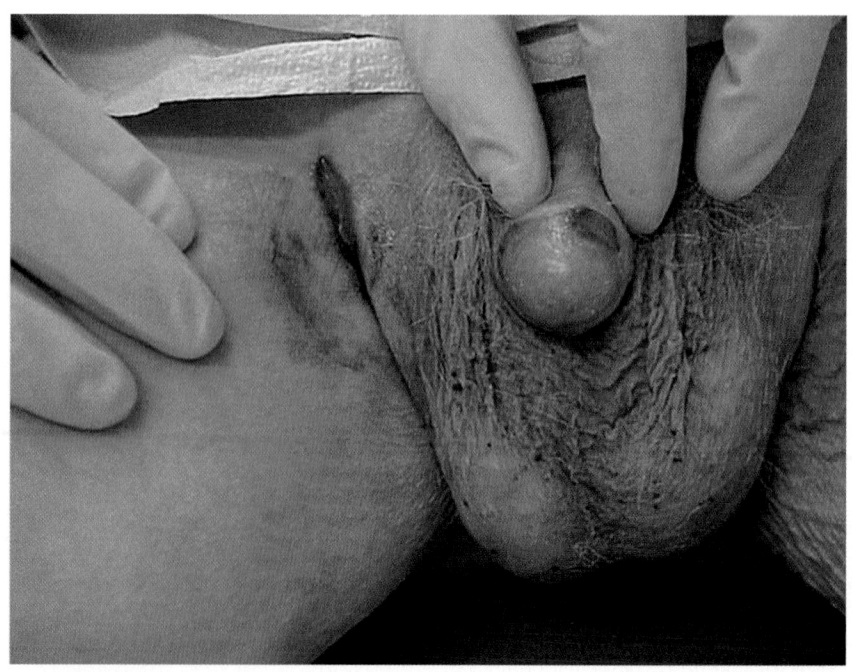

▲ **FIGURE 35-12** Anti-epiligrin cicatricial pemphigoid.

association with cancer. In a series of 35 patients, 10 (29%) developed an associated cancer, all adenocarcinomas (three lung, three stomach, two colon, two endometrial).[50] The time between blister onset and cancer diagnosis ranged between 14 months prior to and 14 months after diagnosis of AECP.[39] In the year following blister onset, the relative risk for cancer in AECP patients was 15.4 (95% CI 5.7 to 33.6) when compared to age- and sex-matched rates for all cancers in the National Cancer Institute's Surveillance, Epidemiology, and End Results Registry.[50] Common treatments for AECP include systemic corticosteroids alone or with cyclophosphamide, azathioprine, or other immunosuppressive therapy. AECP appears to be a progressive disease with a high mortality rate. In two patients, however, AECP clinically improved or resolved after complete resection of the associated cancer.[49] In patients diagnosed with AECP, a diagnostic workup for cancer should be considered in those patients with risk factors (e.g., tobacco use) or other causes for a high index of suspicion for cancer.

Dermatitis Herpetiformis

BOX 35-12 Summary

- Dermatitis herpetiformis is only indirectly associated with malignancy by virtue of its association with gluten-sensitive enteropathy.
- A gluten-free diet most likely decreases the risk of lymphoma in patients with DH.

Dermatitis herpetiformis (DH) is a chronic gluten-sensitive bullous disease characterized by pathognomonic granular IgA deposits in the basement membrane zone of uninvolved skin areas.[51] DH is characterized by intensely pruritic papules and vesicles on the extensor surface of the extremities, the trunk, and the buttocks. While gastrointestinal symptoms are rare in patients with DH, roughly 80% will have a gluten-sensitive enteropathy characterized by villous atrophy and/or an increased number of gamma/delta receptor-bearing T lymphocytes in the jejunal mucosa.[52] The DH and the enteropathy (i.e., celiac disease) clear with a gluten-free diet and relapse when the diet is withdrawn.[53] An increased incidence of malignancy, especially lymphoma, in DH patients has been reported in several studies.[54–56] One recent series of

305 patients with DH in Finland followed for a mean of 9.9 years demonstrated a significant increase in relative risk for non-Hodgkin's lymphoma.[57] A larger series of 1354 patients with DH from Sweden, however, failed to detect any significantly increased risk of lymphoma or other malignancies.[58] In a recent study by Hervonen et al. of 1100 patients with DH, 1% developed lymphoma.[59] A 30-year population-based study of 1147 patients with DH and celiac disease demonstrated no increased risk for malignancy relative to the population, but an incidence ratio of 6.0 for development of non-Hodgkin's lymphoma in patients with DH.[60] It is not clear, therefore, whether a truly increased risk of developing lymphoma is associated with DH. There is evidence, however, that the risk of lymphoma in patients with DH can be lowered by adherence to a gluten-free diet.[59,61,62] Studies show a statistical difference in lymphoma rates between patients who have adhered to a gluten-free diet for more than 5 years, and those patients who do not take a gluten-free diet or who have been on the diet for less than 5 years.[61,62] In patients diagnosed with DH, therefore, a need to workup for lymphoma is not suggested by the data. While DH can be treated successfully with dapsone, a gluten-free diet should be encouraged based on the protective effect of such a diet against lymphoma development.

Sweet's Syndrome

BOX 35-13 Summary

- Sweet's syndrome and its related condition, atypical pyoderma gangrenosum have been associated with leukemia or preleukemic states.
- Paraneoplastic Sweet's syndrome patients frequently have anemia and more often have mucosal involvement.
- Treatment of the leukemia or preleukemic process will effectively control the dermatosis.

Sweet's syndrome (acute febrile neutrophilic dermatosis) is classically associated with infections of the upper respiratory or gastrointestinal tracts, inflammatory bowel disease, and pregnancy, but can also be paraneoplastic or drug-induced (most commonly secondary to administration of granulocyte colony-stimulating factor).[63] The syndrome consists of fever, elevated neutrophil count, and painful, red papules, nodules, and plaques (Fig. 35-13). Other symptoms can include arthralgia, malaise, headache, and myalgia. Pathology demonstrates mature neutrophils diffusely distributed in the upper dermis. Perivascular infiltrates may be seen, but with classic sparing of the vessel walls. In patients with leukemia, some atypical cells may be seen within the infiltrate.[64] Lesions typically occur on the upper extremities, face, and neck. Cutaneous pathergy is often seen, with lesions

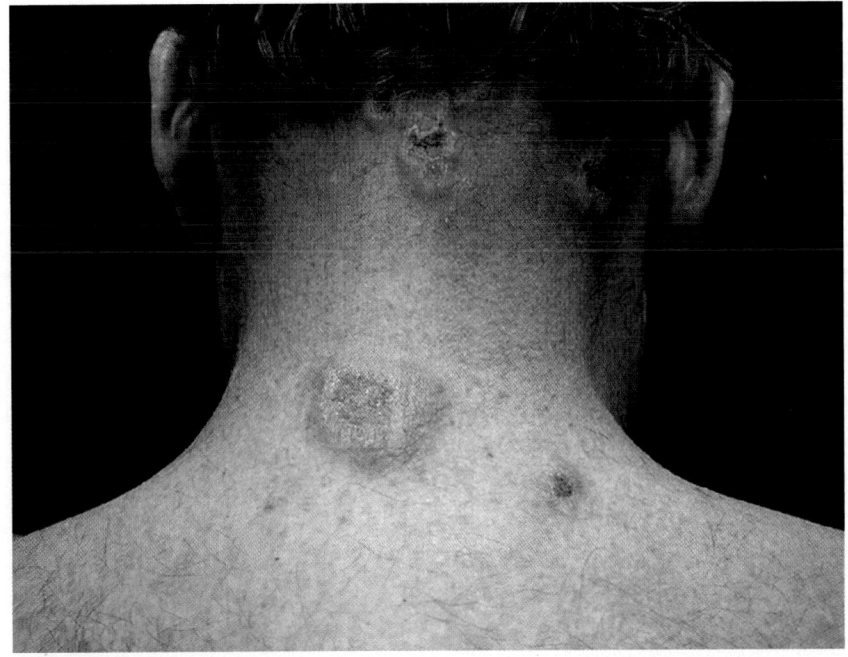

▲ **FIGURE 35-13** Sweet's syndrome in a patient with leukemia—Courtesy of Kenneth E. Greer, M.D., Charlottesville, VA.

developing at sites of needle sticks, biopsies, scratches, or insect bites.[64] Lesions can appear vesicular as a result of underlying upper dermis edema, but palpation confirms that the lesions are solid. The attacks can be recurrent (especially when associated with hematologic malignancy) and resolve with the use of systemic corticosteroids. The lesions usually heal without scarring. While classical Sweet's syndrome is most commonly seen in females between the ages of 30 and 70, malignancy-associated Sweet's does not have a female predominance.[63] The associated malignancies are often hematologic, most commonly acute myeloid leukemia. When associated with solid tumors, the most frequently reported are genitourinary, breast, and gastrointestinal carcinomas.[63] In paraneoplastic Sweet's syndrome, lesions of the oral mucosa are somewhat more frequent than in the classical syndrome (especially when associated with hematologic malignancies), as are lesions of the lower extremities.[63] The pathogenesis of Sweet's syndrome is unknown, but cytokines appear to play a role in lesion development and other symptomatology. Treatment with systemic corticosteroids results in prompt improvement and rapid resolution of both lesions and symptoms. In patients with malignancy-associated Sweet's syndrome, effective therapy results in a remission and relapse occurs with recurrence of the malignancy. For treatment of localized lesions, high-potency topical corticosteroids or intralesional corticosteroids have proven useful.[64]

Pyoderma Gangrenosum

Pyoderma gangrenosum (PG) is a neutrophilic dermatosis characterized by ulcerations and has an association with systemic disease, particularly inflammatory bowel disease, hematologic malignancies, and arthritis. The characteristic lesions of PG are painful ulcerations with well-defined dusky, violaceous borders that overhang the ulcerations. Lesions typically begin as tender pustules or fluctuant nodules with surrounding erythema, then expand peripherally to form central ulcerations surrounded by rolled borders that may be studded with pustules. The lesions most frequently occur on the lower extremities, especially on the anterior tibial surface, and, as in Sweet's syndrome, can be pathergic with occurrence at sites of trauma. PG lesions heal with scarring often described as cribriform. There are four types of PG: ulcerative, pustular, bullous, and vegetative. Bullous and ulcerative types have the

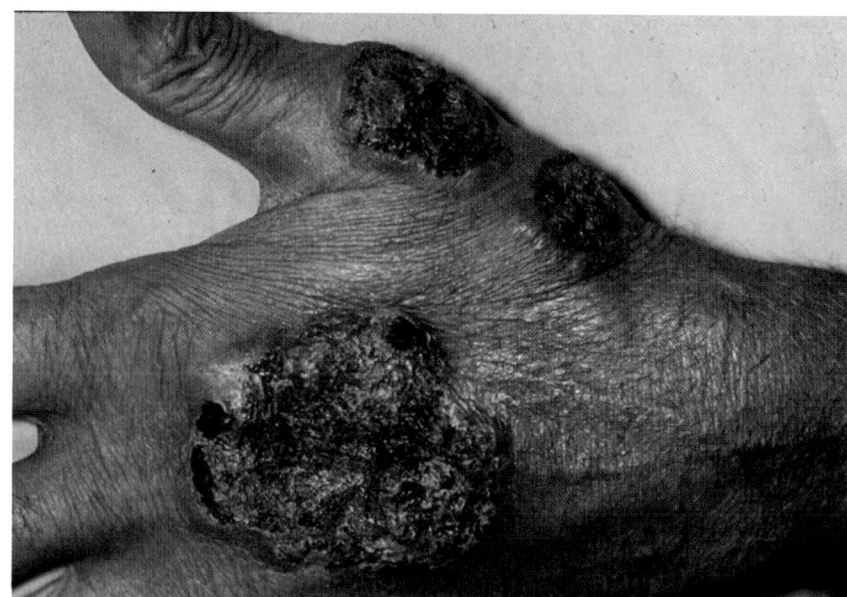

▲ **FIGURE 35-14** Atypical pyoderma gangrenosum in a patient with leukemia preceded by polycythemia vera.

strongest association with underlying malignancy. Bullous PG, in particular, is strongly associated with underlying hematologic malignancies.[65] This type of PG shows clinical overlap with Sweet's syndrome and the two may exist on a spectrum of neutrophilic dermatoses associated with myeloproliferative disease. Bullous PG is characterized by rapidly enlarging painful vesicles and coalescing grouped bullae (Fig. 35-14). Central necrosis occurs, but is more superficial than in ulcerative PG. The periphery of the erosion is gray in color with blisters. Bullous PG may occur on the face as well as the extremities. This variant is a poor prognostic indicator in patients with hematologic malignancy.[66] To diagnose PG, it is necessary to take a biopsy for histopathology and culture to rule out other causes of the lesions. A new diagnosis of PG should prompt an evaluation of the gastrointestinal tract and an analysis of serum proteins and other hematologic studies to rule out hematologic malignancy or paraproteinemia, as well as coagulation studies to rule out thrombosis as the cause of ulceration.[67]

Erythema Gyratum Repens

> **BOX 35-14   Summary**
>
> - Erythema gyratum repens is a very rare process that almost always occurs in association with an internal malignancy.
> - Carcinoma of the lung, esophagus, or breast is most frequent.
> - Effective therapy of an associated malignancy results in a resolution of this dermatosis.

Erythema gyratum repens is a reactive erythema that is characterized by multiple scaly serpiginous bands arranged in parallel configuration, often described as having a wood-grain appearance (Fig. 35-15). The rings are typically macular, but can be papular and may contain bullae. The rapid rate of migration of the lesions adds to the dramatic presentation of this dermatosis. Erythema gyratum repens can cover any body surface, but normally involves the trunk and proximal extremities with sparing of the palmar and plantar surfaces. Pruritus is a nearly universal symptom and can be severe. Erythema gyratum repens is one of the most specific skin signs of internal malignancy as greater than 80% of patients with this sign have an associated cancer. The most common associated malignancy is lung cancer (in one-third of patients), followed by esophageal, and breast cancers.[68] The majority of patients develop erythema gyratum repens prior to the diagnosis of the internal malignancy, 4 to 9 months prior to cancer diagnosis on average. With treatment of the underlying malignancy, erythema gyratum repens will resolve rapidly along with the associated pruritus. Other treatment options have not proven useful to date. In patients whose cancers prove fatal, it has been noted that the lesions of erythema gyratum repens resolve spontaneously in the days preceding death. Patients diagnosed with erythema gyratum repens should undergo a thorough workup for underlying malignancy.

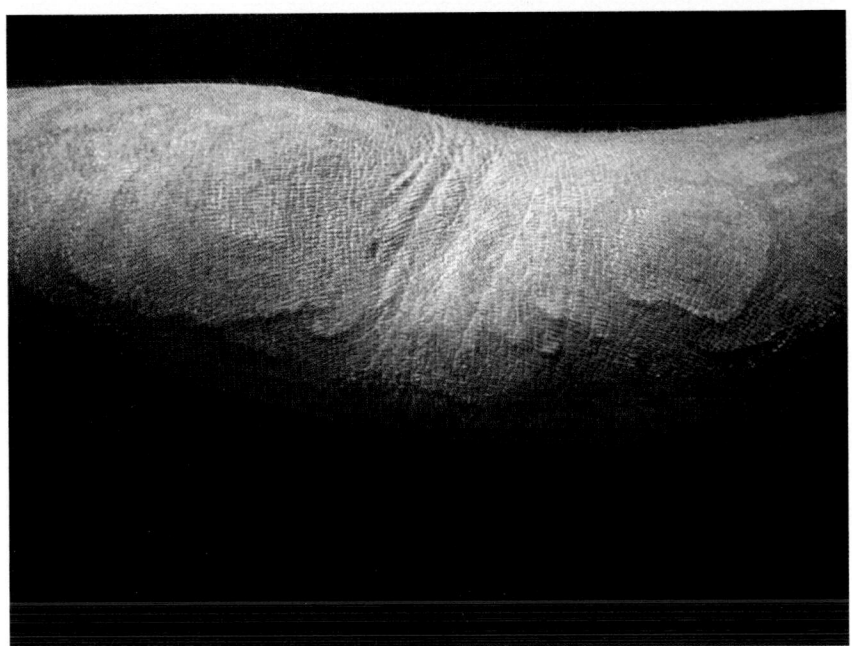

▲ **FIGURE 35-15** Erythema gyratum repens.

Dermatomyositis

BOX 35-15   Summary

- Dermatomyositis is manifested by characteristic skin lesions; most often with proximal muscle weakness and elevated muscle-derived enzymes.
- Patients with DM are statistically more likely to have a malignancy than age-sex-race matched controls.
- Ovarian cancer is overrepresented, but malignancy may occur in any organ system.
- Malignancy risk is greatest within the first 3 years following onset.
- A parallel course is possible, but is not usual.

Dermatomyositis (DM) is an idiopathic inflammatory myopathy characterized by progressive, symmetrical, proximal weakness and accompanying cutaneous findings. The pathognomonic cutaneous findings are a heliotrope rash (erythematous rash involving periorbital skin) and Gottron's papules (scaly violaceous papules and plaques over bony prominences, especially of the hands [Fig. 35-16]). Additional cutaneous findings include a photodistributed poikiloderma (Fig. 35-17), malar erythema, periungual telangiectases, and photosensitivity. Other criteria for diagnosis include elevated muscle enzymes, abnormal electromyogram, and abnormal muscle biopsy. DM is associated with an increased risk of malignancy, especially in males over 50 years of age.[69] A wide range of tumor types have been associated with DM, but ovarian, breast, uterine, lung, gastric, colorectal, and pancreatic cancers seem to have more frequent associations.[70,71] In paraneoplastic DM, the malignancy is usually detected within 3 years of the diagnosis of DM, and the majority are detected within 1 year.[69] While cutaneous vasculitis, and the presence or absence of Raynaud syndrome were once thought to be useful in differentiating between idiopathic and paraneoplastic DM, data from larger studies have called into question the predictive value of these clinical signs.[71] Similarly, the comparison of creatine kinase (CK) levels between patients with idiopathic and paraneoplastic DM has been made; however, the number of patients in these studies is too small to firmly conclude that normal CK levels are a marker of malignancy risk in patients with DM.[72] Lastly, there are patients with skin disease characteristic for DM who do not have muscle weakness or elevated levels of muscle enzymes. Patients with this presentation, known as amyopathic DM, also may have an associated malignancy.[73,74] The suggested malignancy workup for a patient with DM should begin with a thorough history and physical examination, complete blood count, comprehensive metabolic panel, chest X-ray, and test of the stool for occult blood. Any abnormalities discovered in this basic workup should be investigated with additional testing as indicated. The remaining workup should be based on age-based health maintenance guidelines (e.g., colonoscopy for patients over 50). CT scan of the chest and abdomen in all patients with DM may be considered. For women with DM, a CT scan and/or ultrasound of the pelvis, in addition to mammography can be justified based on the current data regarding cancer types in DM.[72]

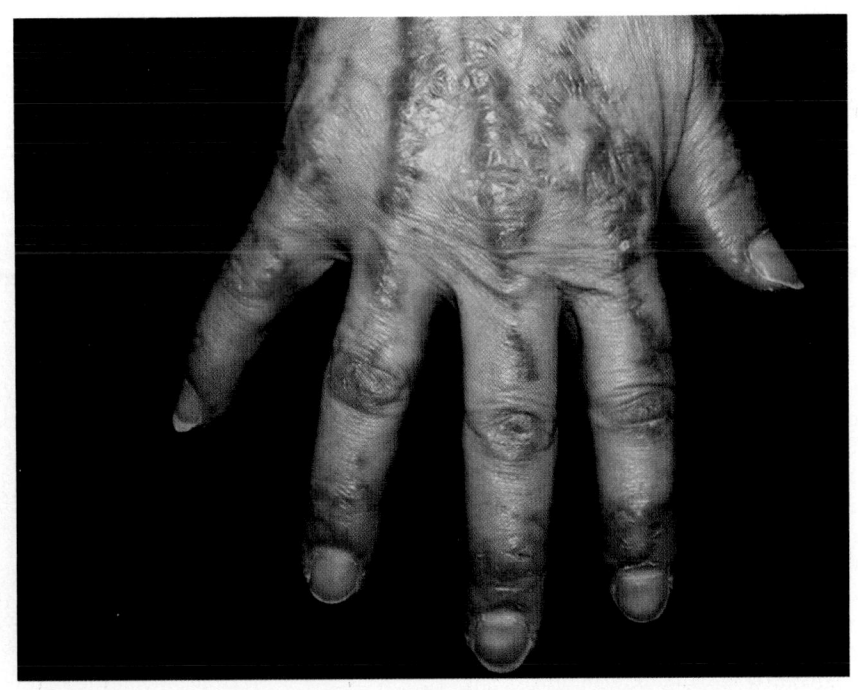

▲ **FIGURE 35-16** Dermatomyositis—Gottron's papules.

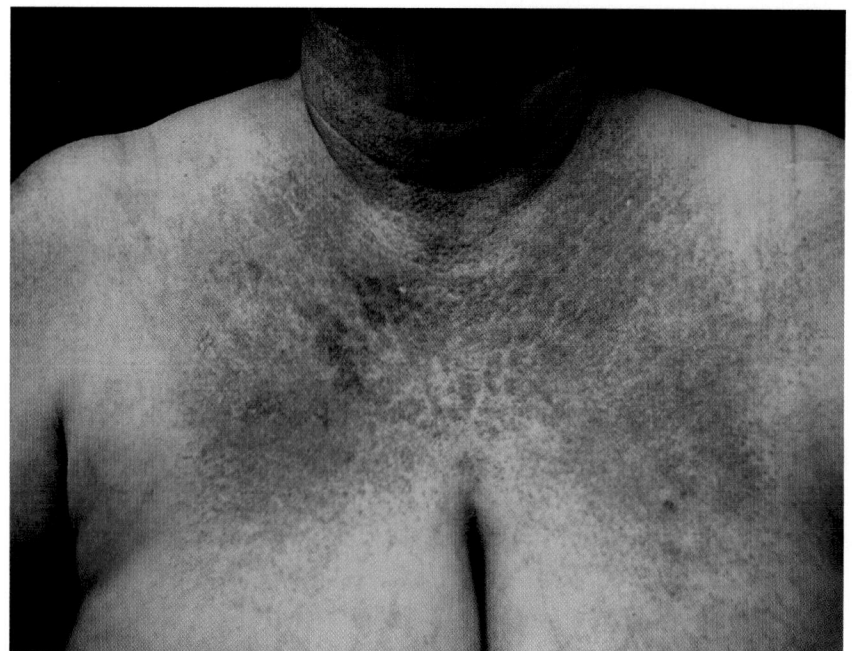

▲ **FIGURE 35-17** Dermatomyositis in a patient with B-cell lymphoma.

Extramammary Paget's Disease

BOX 35-16 Summary

- Extramammary Paget's disease is a neoplastic process that occurs most often on the genitalia or in a perineal or perianal location.
- Roughly 25% of patients with EMPD will have a malignancy in tissue near the site of the dermatosis, but the EMPD is not contiguous with the underlying malignancy.
- Treatment of EMPD involves an appropriate excision.

Extramammary Paget's disease (EMPD) is a neoplastic condition with intraepithelial infiltration of cells showing glandular differentiation. EMPD manifests as a nonhealing dermatitis of apocrine-gland bearing areas. The vulva is the most common location, followed by perineal, perianal, scrotal, and penile skin. Patients present with a well-demarcated erythematous plaque that is often pruritic (Fig. 35-18). Other commonly associated symptoms include burning, irritation, pain, swelling, or bleeding. The presentation is nonspecific and therefore EMPD is often originally misdiagnosed as an inflammatory or infective condition. Diagnosis eventually hinges on the identification of intraepidermal, infiltrating Paget's cells by histopathology. Immunohistochemistry is used to differentiate EMPD from other diseases that are characterized by pagetoid spread on histology (especially Bowen disease and superficial spreading melanoma), and is useful in helping to identify the cell of origin in EMPD associated with internal malignancy.[75]

Roughly 25% of EMPD cases are associated with an underlying *in situ* or invasive neoplasm (a neoplasm of local internal organs with contiguous epithelial linings), though actual rates vary by the site involved. Vulvar EMPD most commonly arises in the epidermis and is not usually associated with underlying neoplasm, though associations have been described with endometrial, endocervical, vaginal, urethral, and bladder cancers. EMPD of the male genitalia, on the other hand, is thought to be more commonly associated with underlying neoplasms of the urethra, bladder, prostate, or testicle. Perianal EMPD is rare, but has a strong association with underlying invasive malignancy of the anus, rectum, or colon.[75] The malignancy workup, therefore, should be directed by the site of involvement and immunohistochemical findings. Treatment depends on whether the EMPD is primary or associated with an underlying neoplasm. Primary EMPD that is localized to the epidermis is managed with local excision with 1-cm margins of uninvolved skin. In primary EMPD that has spread into the dermis, combination chemoradiotherapy modalities are common, though the prognosis is poor. When associated with an underlying carcinoma, treatment is aimed at the internal disease. Long-term follow-up is required in cases of primary EMPD to monitor for recurrence and for the development of an associated neoplasm.

Digital Clubbing

BOX 35-17 Summary

- Clubbing is most often reflective of cardiopulmonary disease and in some instances a pulmonary malignancy.
- Hypertrophic osteoarthropathy is a syndrome that involves clubbing with polyarthralgia and periostosis. A vast majority of such patients have an associated pulmonary neoplasm.

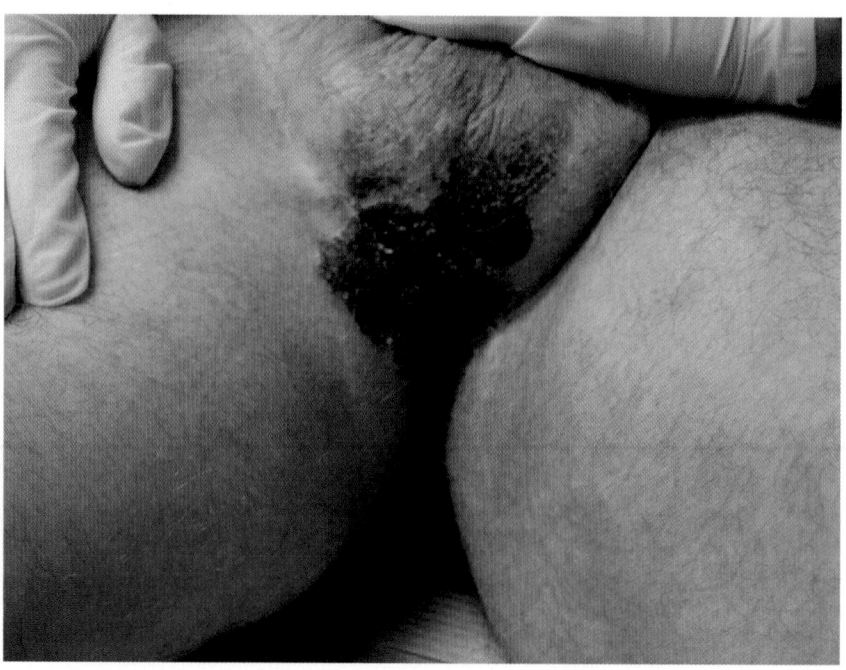

▲ **FIGURE 35-18** Extramammary Paget's disease.

Digital clubbing is characterized by enlargement of the terminal aspects of the fingers and/or toes along with increased convexity of the nails, with loss of the normal 15 to 20° angle between the proximal nail and the cuticle. These changes result from the proliferation of connective tissue and accompanying subungual edema. Clubbing is most commonly associated with chronic lung disease, but other causes include cyanotic heart disease, infective endocarditis, inflammatory bowel disease, hepatic cirrhosis, and hyperthyroidism. The most common underlying malignancies are bronchogenic carcinoma and mesothelioma.[76] Hypertrophic osteoarthropathy (HOA) is a syndrome defined by digital clubbing, polyarthralgias, and periostosis. The causes of HOA are similar to those of digital clubbing, with pulmonary neoplasm as the most common underlying disorder (occurring in about 90% of HOA cases). It is more commonly associated with non–small cell lung cancer than small cell lung cancer, and with peripheral pulmonary lesions rather than central.[77] In cases associated with metastatic disease to the lung, sarcoma is the most common primary tumor type. Patients with HOA should receive a thorough workup for pulmonary neoplasm.

Migratory Superficial Thrombophlebitis

BOX 35-18 Summary

- Migratory superficial thrombophlebitis is reflective of a hypercoagulable state that might be due to an associated malignancy.

Migratory superficial thrombophlebitis (also known as Trousseau syndrome) is frequently associated with mucin-producing adenocarcinomas and consists of disseminated microangiopathy. Pancreatic cancer is the most commonly associated neoplasm. Other associated malignancies include those of the lung, prostate, stomach, and colon.[78] The diagnosis of migratory superficial thrombophlebitis often precedes that of the underlying malignancy. In patients with migratory superficial thrombophlebitis, therefore, a search for underlying malignancy is warranted and should include a CT of the chest and abdomen, and other workup as indicated by associated signs and symptoms.

Cutaneous Vasculitis

BOX 35-19 Summary

- Cutaneous vasculitis is only rarely associated with an internal malignancy; however when it is, there is often a paraneoplastic course.

Cutaneous vasculitis has been associated with underlying malignancy, especially hematologic malignancies, though underlying solid tumors have also been reported.[79] The most common solid tumors reported are non–small cell lung, colon, prostate, renal, breast, head and neck squamous, and endometrial cancers.[80] In patients with hematologic malignancies, the vasculitis was most frequently leukocytoclastic or small vessel vasculitis, manifesting as palpable purpura (Fig. 35-19). The associated hematologic malignancies are typically lymphoproliferative or, less frequently, myelodysplastic syndrome. Solid tumors are associated with many types of vasculitis, including polyarteritis nodosa and Henoch–Schönlein purpura.[80] The proportion of patients with cutaneous vasculitis who harbor an associated malignancy has not been well characterized, but appears to be relatively small. Therefore, the need to begin a workup for underlying malignancy in patients with vasculitis should be based on other associated factors, especially decline in general health, or abnormalities of the CBC.

Multicentric Reticulohistiocytosis

BOX 35-20 Summary

- Multicentric reticulohistiocytosis is manifested by flesh colored or yellow–brown colored nodules and a destructive polyarthritis.
- One quarter of the patients with MRH will have an associated malignancy.
- Treatment of MRH is difficult, but often immunosuppressive agents are utilized.

Multicentric reticulohistiocytosis (MRH) is a rare multisystem disease that consists of a histiocytic dermatosis in combination with a disabling, destructive polyarthritis. MRH exists on a spectrum of histiocytic dermatoses, along with isolated reticulohistiocytoma, and diffuse cutaneous reticulohistiocytosis.[81] All three dermatoses are similar in appearance, both clinically and histopathologically; however, MRH is the only one associated with systemic disease. MRH involves skin and joints primarily, but can involve any organ system. Skin lesions are flesh-colored to yellow–brown papules and nodules. The lesions have a predilection for the upper half of the body, seen most frequently on the face, hands, forearms, and ears. Periungual lesions may have a "coral bead" appearance.[82] Mucosal lesions can be seen as well. About one-third of patients have coexisting xanthelasma.[83] Skin lesions of MRH are generally asymptomatic and have a tendency to regress spontaneously. Histologically, they

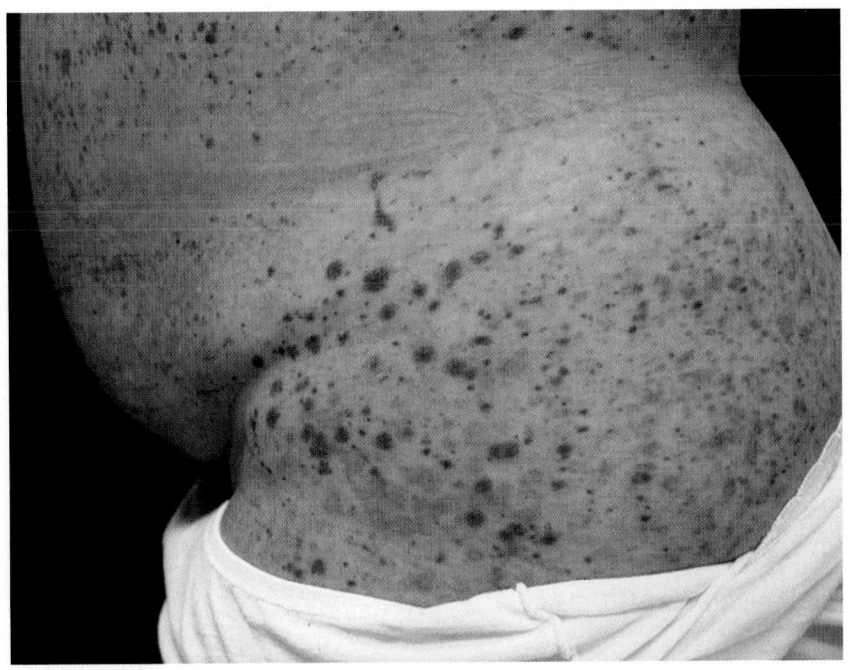

▲ **FIGURE 35-19** Vasculitis—palpable purpura in a patient with a history of B-cell lymphoma.

demonstrate circumscribed, nonencapsulated dermal infiltrates of mononuclear and multinucleate giant cells with eosinophilic "ground glass" cytoplasm.[81] The cells comprising the dermal infiltrate stain with monocyte-macrophage markers, most reliably CD68. The arthritis associated with MRH can involve a wide variety of joints and normally presents after the skin lesions. While its severity varies over time, the arthritis of MRH can be rapidly destructive and progresses to arthritis mutilans in roughly half of patients.[83] One-third of patients also complain of weakness, weight loss, and fever.

MRH is associated with underlying malignancy in one-quarter of patients.[81,83,84] The associated malignancies vary widely in type with hematological, breast, and gastric cancer as the most common. Cancers of the cervix, pleura, lung, ovary, colon, endometrium, and pancreas have also been reported, as have melanoma and metastases with unknown primary.[81,82] MRH presents before the diagnosis of malignancy in 70 to 75% of patients. The skin findings and arthritis of MRH do not appear to follow a parallel course with the underlying malignancy. As with many rare disorders, furthermore, the literature consists primarily of case reports and not prospective studies; therefore, the bias toward reporting of those cases associated with cancer may exaggerate the association of MRH with malignancy. Nevertheless, given the apparent association and lack of prospective studies, patients with MRH warrant an evaluation for underlying malignancy. The type of evaluation will need to be determined based on the patient's history, physical exam, review of systems, and laboratory findings. MRH itself tends to resolve spontaneously after an average of 8 years, but the extent of joint destruction prior to disease resolution can be severe.[83]

■ FINAL THOUGHTS

Skin lesions may serve as a marker of internal malignancy, but most of the conditions discussed in this chapter are relatively uncommon. The strongest support for a link between a skin condition and an internal malignancy is when the cutaneous disease is noted at the same time as the internal cancer is discovered, there is a distinct type or site of cancer, and the course of the skin disease follows that of the cancer. In addition, there are some conditions that are statistically associated with a greater prevalence of malignancy, but do not follow a parallel course

with the malignancy. In many instances, a careful and directed assessment of the patient will lead to an early discovery of an underlying malignancy and hopefully to an improved clinical outcome.

REFERENCES

1. Curth HO. Skin lesions and internal carcinoma. In: Andrade R, Gumport SL, Popkin GL, et al, eds. *Cancer of the Skin.* Philadelphia, PA: WB Saunders; 1976: 1308–1309.
2. Beuschlein F, Hammer GD. Ectopic pro-opiomelanocortin syndrome. *Endocrinol Metab Clin North Am.* 2002;31(1):191–234.
3. Lerner AB, McQuire JS. Melanocyte stimulating hormone and adrenocorticotrophic hormone: Their relation to skin pigmentation. *N Engl J Med.* 1964;270: 539–546.
4. Hunt G, Todd C, Kyne S, et al. ACTH stimulates melanogenesis in cultured human melanocytes. *J Endocrinol.* 1994; 140:R1–R3.
5. Wakamatsu K, Graham A, Cook D, et al. Characterisation of ACTH peptides in human skin and their activation of the melanocortin-1 receptor. *Pigment Cell Res.* 1997;10:288–297.
6. Kulke MH, Mayer RJ. Medical progress: Carcinoid tumors. *N Engl J Med.* 1999; 340(11):858–868.
7. Schnirer II, Yao JC, Ajani JA. Carcinoid: A comprehensive review. *Acta Oncol.* 2003; 42(7):672–692.
8. Chastain MA. The glucagonoma syndrome: A review of its features and discussion of new perspectives. *Am J Med Sci.* 2001;321(5):306–320.
9. Hovenden AL. Hypertrichosis lanuginosa acquisita associated with malignancy. *Clin Dermatol.* 1993;11:99–106.
10. Hovenden AL. Acquired hypertrichosis lanuginosa associated with malignancy. *Arch Intern Med.* 1987;147:2013–2018.
11. Farina MC, Tarin N, Grilli R, et al. Acquired hypertrichosis lanuginosa: Case report and review of the literature. *J Surg Oncol.* 1998;68:199–203.
12. Curth HO. Malignant acanthosis nigricans. *Arch Dermatol.* 1970;102:479–481.
13. Schwartz RA. Acanthosis nigricans. *J Am Acad Dermatol.* 1994;31:1–19.
14. Curth HO, Hillberg AW, Machacek GF. The site and histology of the cancer associated with malignant acanthosis nigricans. *Cancer.* 1962;15:364–382.
15. Hall JM, Moreland A, Cox CJ, Wade TR. Oral acanthosis nigricans: Report of a case and comparison of oral and cutaneous pathology. *Am J Dermatopathol.* 1988; 10:68–73.
16. Schwartz RA. Sign of Leser–Trélat. *J Am Acad Dermatol.* 1996;35:88–95.
17. Rampen HJ, Schwengle LE. The sign of Leser–Trélat: Does it exist? *J Am Acad Dermatol.* 1989;21:50–55.
18. Grob JJ, Rava MC, Gouvernet J, et al. The relation between seborrheic keratoses and malignant solid tumors. A case-controlled study. *Acta Derm Venereol.* 1991; 71:166–169.
19. Lindelöf B, Sigurgeirsson B, Melander S. Seborrheic keratosis and cancer. *J Am Acad Dermatol.* 1992;26:947–950.
20. Schwengle LEM, Rampen FHJ, Wobbes T. Seborrheic keratoses and internal malignancies: A case control study. *Clin Exp Dermatol.* 1988;13:177–179.
21. Dantzig PI. Sign of Leser–Trélat. *Arch Dermatol.* 1973;108:700–701.
22. Cohen PR, Grossman ME, Almeida L, Kurzrock R. Tripe palms and cancer. *Clin Dermatol.* 1993;11:165–173.
23. Bazex A, Griffiths A. Acrokeratosis paraneoplastica—a new cutaneous marker for malignancy. *Br J Dermatol.* 1980;102: 301–306.
24. Bolognia JL, Brewer YP, Cooper DL. Bazex syndrome (acroekeratosis paraneoplastica): An analytic review. *Medicine.* 1991; 70:269–280.
25. Schwartz RA, Williams ML. Acquired ichthyosis: A marker for internal disease. *Am Fam Physician.* 1984;29:181–184.
26. Griffin LJ, Massa MC. Acquired ichthyosis and pityriasis rotunda. *Clin Dermatol.* 1993;11:27–32.
27. DiGiovanna JJ, Robinson-Bostom L. Ichthyosis: Etiology, diagnosis, and management. *Am J Clin Dermatol.* 2003;4:81–95.
28. Falk RH, Comenzo RL, Skinner M. The systemic amyloidoses. *N Engl J Med.* 1997; 337:898–909.
29. Touart DM, Sau P. Cutaneous deposition diseases. Part I. *J Am Acad Dermatol.* 1998; 39:149–171.
30. Gertz MA, Lacy MQ, Dispenzieri A. Therapy for immunoglobulin light chain amyloidosis: The new and the old. *Blood Rev.* 2004;18:17–37.
31. Jackson EM, English JC. Diffuse cutaneous mucinoses. *Dermatol Clin.* 2002;20: 493–501.
32. Lacy MQ, Hogan WJ, Gertz MA, et al. Successful treatment of scleromyxedema with autologous peripheral blood stem cell transplantation. *Arch Dermatol.* 2005; 141:1277–1282.
33. Donato ML, Feasel AM, Weber DM, et al. Scleromyxedema: Role of high-dose melphalan with autologous stem cell transplantation. *Blood.* 2006;107:463–466.
34. Nakanishi T, Sobue I, Toyokura Y, et al. The Crow–Fusake syndrome: A study of 102 cases in Japan. *Neurology.* 1984;34: 712–720.
35. Dispenzieri A, Kyle RA, Lacy MQ, et al. POEMS syndrome: Definitions and long-term outcome. *Blood.* 2003;101:2496–2506.
36. Longo G, Emilia G, Torelli U. Skin changes in POEMS syndrome. *Haematologica.* 1999;84:86.
37. Fishel B, Brenner S, Weiss S, Yaron M. POEMS syndrome associated with cryoglobulinemia, lymphoma, multiple seborrheic keratoses, and ichthyosis. *J Am Acad Dermatol.* 1988;19:979–982.
38. Tsai CY, Lai CH, Chang HL, Kuo T. Glomeruloid hemangioma—a specific cutaneous marker of POEMS syndrome. *Int J Dermatol.* 2001;40:403–406.
39. Gherardi RK, Bélec L, Soubrier M, et al. Overproduction of proinflammatory cytokines imbalanced by their antagonists in POEMS syndrome. *Blood.* 1996; 87:1458–1465.
40. Soubrier M, Dubost JJ, Serre AF, et al. Growth factors in POEMS syndrome: Evidence for a marked increase in circulating vascular endothelial growth factor. *Arthritis Rheum.* 1997;40:786–787.

41. Anhalt GJ, Kim SC, Stanley JR, et al. Paraneoplastic pemphigus. An autoimmune mucocutaneous disease associated with neoplasia. *N Engl J Med*. 1990;323:1729–1735.
42. Wang L, Bu D, Yang Y, Chen X, Zhu X. Castleman's tumours and production of autoantibody in paraneoplastic pemphigus. *Lancet*. 2004;363:525–531.
43. Wang J, Zhu X, Li R, et al. Paraneoplastic pemphigus associated with Castleman tumor. *Arch Dermatol*. 2005;141:1285–1293.
44. Anhalt GJ. Paraneoplastic pemphigus. *J Investig Dermatol Symp Proc*. 2004;9:29–33.
45. Nousari HC, Deterding R, Wojtczack H, et al. The mechanism of respiratory failure in paraneoplastic pemphigus. *N Engl J Med*. 1999;340:1406–1410.
46. Nousari HC, Kimyai-Asadi A, Anhalt GJ. Elevated levels of IL-6 in paraneoplastic pemphigus. *J Invest Dermatol*. 1999;112:396–398.
47. Horn TD, Anhalt GJ. Histologic features of paraneoplastic pemphigus. *Arch Dermatol*. 1991;128:1091–1095.
48. Nguyen VT, Ndoye A, Bassler KD, et al. Classification, clinical manifestations, and immunopathological mechanisms of the epithelial variant of paraneoplastic autoimmune multiorgan syndrome: A reappraisal of paraneoplastic pemphigus. *Arch Dermatol*. 2001;137:193–206.
49. Egan CA, Lazarova Z, Darling TN, Yee C, Yancey KB. Anti-epiligrin cicatricial pemphigoid: Clinical findings, immunopathogenesis, and significant associations. *Medicine*. 2003;82:177–186.
50. Egan CA, Lazarova Z, Darling TN, Yee C, Coté T, Yancey KB. Anti-epiligrin cicatricial pemphigoid and relative risk for cancer. *Lancet*. 2001;57:1850–1851.
51. van der Meer JB. Granular deposits of immunoglobulins in the skin of patients with dermatitis herpetiformis. *Br J Dermatol*. 1969;81:493–503.
52. Savilahti E, Reunala T, Mäki M. Increase in lymphocytes bearing the (//(T-cell receptor in the jejunum of patients with dermatitis herpetiformis. *Gut*. 1992;33:206–211.
53. Reunal T, Blomqvist K, Tarpila S, Halme H, Kangas K. Gluten-free diet in dermatitis herpetiformis. I. Clinical response of skin lesions in 81 patients. *Br J Dermatol*. 1977;97:473–480.
54. Swerdlow AJ, Whittaker S, Carpenter LM, English JSC. Mortality and cancer incidence in patients with dermatitis herpetiformis: A cohort study. *Br J Dermatol*. 1993;129:140–144.
55. Leonard JN, Tucker WFG, Fry JS, et al. Increased incidence of malignancy in dermatitis herpetiformis. *BMJ*. 1983;286:16–18.
56. Sigurgeirson B, Agnarsson BA, Lindelof B. Risk of lymphoma in patients with dermatitis herpetiformis. *BMJ*. 1994;308:13–15.
57. Colin P, Pukkala E, Reunala T. Malignancy and survival in dermatitis herpetiformis: A comparison with coeliac disease. *Gut*. 1996;38:528–530.
58. Askling J, Linet M, Gridley G, Halstensen TS, Ekström K, Ekbom A. Cancer incidence in a population-based cohort of individuals hospitalized with celiac disease or dermatitis herpetiformis. *Gastroenterology*. 2002;123:1428–1435.
59. Hernoven K, Vornanen M, Kautiainen H, Collin P, Reunala T. Lymphoma in patients with dermatitis herpetiformis and their first-degree relatives. *Br J Dermatol*. 2005;152:82–86.
60. Viljamaa M, Kaukinen K, Pukkala E, Hervonen K, Reunala T, Collin P. Malignancies and mortality in patients with coeliac disease and dermatitis herpetiformis: 30-year population-based study. *Dig Liver Dis*. June 2006;38(6):374–380.
61. Holmes GKT, Prior P, Lane MR, Pope D, Allan RN. Malignancy in Coeliac disease—effect of a gluten-free diet. *Gut*. 1989;30:333–338.
62. Lewis HM, Renaula TL, Garioch JJ, et al. Protective effect of gluten-free diet against development of lymphoma in dermatitis herpetiformis. *Br J Dermatol*. 1996;135:363–367.
63. Cohen PR, Kurzrock R. Sweet's syndrome: A neutrophilic dermatosis classically associated with acute onset and fever. *Clin Dermatol*. 2000;18:265–282.
64. Cohen PR, Kurzrock R. Sweet's syndrome revisited: A review of disease concepts. *Int J Dermatol*. 2003;42:761–778.
65. Crowson AM, Mihm AC, Magro C. Pyoderma gangrenosum: A review. *J Cutan Pathol*. 2003;30:97–107.
66. Hensley CD, Caughman SW. Neutrophilic dermatoses associated with hematologic disorders. *Clin Dermatol*. 2000;18:355–367.
67. Callen JP. Neutrophilic dermatoses. *Dermatol Clin*. 2002;20:409–419.
68. Boyd AS, Neldner KH, Menter A. Erythema gyratum repens: A paraneoplastic eruption. *J Am Acad Dermatol*. 1992;26:757–762.
69. Wakata N, Kurihara T, Saito E, Kinoshita M. Polymyositis and dermatomyositis associated with malignancy: A 30-year retrospective study. *Int J Dermatol*. 2002;41:729–734.
70. Hill CL, Zhang Y, Sigurgeirsson B, et al. Frequency of specific cancer types in dermatomyositis and polymyositis: A population-based study. *Lancet*. 2001;357:96–100.
71. Parodi A, Caproni M, Marzano AV, et al. Dermatomyositis in 132 patients with different clinical subtypes: Cutaneous signs, constitutional symptoms, and circulating antibodies. *Acta Derm Venereol*. 2002;82:48–51.
72. Callen JP. When and how should the patient with dermatomyositis and amyopathic dermatomyositis be assessed for possible cancer? *Arch Dermatol*. 2002;138:969–971.
73. el-Azhary RA, Pakzadsy SY. Amyopathic dermatomyositis: Retrospective review of 37 cases. *J Am Acad Dermatol*. 2002;46:560–565.
74. Gerami P, Schope JM, McDonald L, Walling HW, Sontheimer RD. A systematic review of adult-onset, clinically amyopathic dermatomyositis (dermatomyositis sine myositis): A missing link within the spectrum of the idiopathic inflammatory myopathies. *J Am Acad Dermatol*. 2006;54:597–613.
75. Shepherd B, Davidson EJ, Davies-Humphreys J. Extramammary Paget's disease. *BJOG*. 2005;112:273–279.
76. Myers KA, Farquhar DR. The rational clinical examination. Does this patient have clubbing? *JAMA*. 2001;286:341–347.
77. Landrum ML, Ornstein DL. Hypertrophic osteoarthropathy associated with metastatic phylloides tumor. *Am J Clin Oncol*. 2003;26:146–150.
78. Pinzon R, Drewinko JM, Trujillo V, et al. Pancreatic carcinoma and Trousseau's syndrome: Experience at a large cancer center. *J Clin Oncol*. 1986;4:509–514.
79. Kurzrock R, Cohen PR. Vasculitis and cancer. *Clin Dermatol*. 1993;11:175–187.
80. Kurzrock R, Cohen PR, Markowitz A. Clinical manifestations of vasculitis in patients with solid tumors. *Arch Intern Med*. 1994;154:334–340.
81. Snow JL, Muller SA. Malignancy-associated multicentric reticulohistiocytosis: A clinical, histological, and immunophenotypic study. *Br J Dermatol*. 1995;133:71–76.
82. Malik MK, Regan L, Robinson-Bostom L, Pan TD, McDonald CJ. Proliferating multicentric reticulohistiocytosis associated with papillary serous carcinoma of the endometrium. *J Am Acad Dermatol*. 2005;53:1075–1079.
83. Rapini RP. Multicentric histiocytosis. *Clin Dermatol*. 1993;11:107–111.
84. Worm M, Kleine-Tebbe A, von Stebut E, Haas N, Kolde G. Multicentric reticulohistiocytosis indicating metastasis of an unknown primary tumor. *Acta Derm Venereol*. 1998;78:67–79.

CHAPTER 36

Biopsy Techniques

Keyvan Nouri, M.D.
Shalu S. Patel, B.S.
Voraphol Vejjabhinanta, M.D.

Table 36-1
Summary of Biopsy Techniques

Biopsy Type	Lesion Examples
Shave	BCC, AK, SCC
Saucerization	SCC, pigmented lesions
Punch	DFSP
Incisional	Large congenital nevus
Wedge	Ulcers
Excisional	Melanoma, atypical nevi

BOX 36-1   Overview

- Biopsies are mostly used for accurate diagnosis of cutaneous lesions.
- Shave biopsies are ideal for epidermal tumors.
- A saucerization biopsy is a variation of a shave biopsy used for deeper lesions.
- Punch biopsies are used for deep lesions such as DFSP. Sutures may be required depending on the size of the punch.
- Incisional biopsies are recommended for larger and deeply located diseases involving fascia, such as giant congenital nevi.
- Wedge biopsies are pie-shaped samples taken for lesions such as suspicious ulcerative SCCs.
- Excisional biopsies are ideal for atypical pigmented lesions such as melanoma.
- For any hardened or firm lesion, obtaining a full-thickness will allow for the most accurate diagnosis.
- Each biopsy is examined under a microscope to determine or confirm the disease process.

INTRODUCTION

A biopsy is a diagnostic and sometimes therapeutic method by which cutaneous lesions can be examined microscopically. It is used to determine if a lesion is benign or malignant. For melanoma specifically, it can determine the depth of the lesion. In fact, in 1970, Breslow suggested that a biopsy is the most important prognostic factor for melanoma.[1] An excisional biopsy is also useful to check margins of neoplastic lesions to ensure that complete removal has been achieved.

There are various techniques by which a biopsy can be performed, and each is tailored for specific indications. These allow the physician to obtain samples from different skin layers, and each depends on both the site and the size of the lesion. Also, cosmetic outcomes must be taken into account. The different types discussed in this chapter are those used most commonly for skin cancers:

shave, saucerization, punch, incisional, excisional, and wedge biopsies. Other techniques such as fine needle aspiration and sentinel lymph node biopsy are discussed in other related chapters.

It is important that the cutaneous surgeon understand not only the various techniques discussed in this chapter, but also the disease processes for which each is best indicated (Table 36-1).

PREOPERATIVE CARE

BOX 36-2   Summary

- Obtain full history, perform a physical exam, and obtain consent.
- Cleanse biopsy site with an antiseptic.
- Local anesthesia is beneficial not only to diminish pain but also to raise the lesion for certain biopsies.

Prior to any biopsy, a complete history and physical exam must be taken. The physician must assess potential coagulation problems, drug allergies, and inquire about any artificial heart valves or joints due to an increased risk of infection. Then, the potential risks, benefits, and other options of the procedure must be explained prior to obtaining consent. Sterilized equipment and other materials necessary for each procedure should be placed on the table for easy access. The biopsy site should be cleansed in two cycles with an antiseptic, for example, chlorhexidine, isopropyl alcohol, or povidone iodine for 10 to 15 s prior to anesthetic injection. Local anesthesia is most commonly achieved between 30 s and 5 minutes depending on the level of injection and can last up to 2 hours. A 30-gauge needle with slow injection can be used to minimize the pain of the injection. Also, the distraction technique in which the surgeon vibrates or pinches the adjacent skin can ease the pain.

SHAVE BIOPSY

BOX 36-3   Summary

- Shave biopsies are used for superficial cutaneous lesions.
- Anesthesia, when injected, raises the lesion to make the shave easier.
- A blade is used to shave a sample of the lesion in a sawing motion.
- Chemical or electrical cautery can be used for hemostasis.
- No sutures are required.

Shave biopsies are usually preferred because they are minimally invasive and thereby offer better cosmetic results. Because this technique only removes the upper layer of the skin, it is indicated for superficial skin cancers such as basal cell carcinoma (BCC), actinic keratosis (AK), and squamous cell carcinoma (SCC), and other epidermal tumor lesions. Tumor regression is common after this procedure, especially for BCCs.[2] A disadvantage of this technique is that it may lead to an inaccurate measurement of tumor thickness.[2]

Equipment and other materials needed for this procedure are: a #15 blade, Adson toothed forceps, a hemostatic agent, cotton swabs, gauze, and a bandage.

After prepping with an antiseptic as described earlier, local anesthesia is injected to provide a small wheal under the lesion. This elevation provides a level horizontal surface for the surgeon, thereby making the biopsy easier to perform.

The shave biopsy procedure is rather quick and simple (Fig. 36-1). First, using the thumb and index finger, stretch the skin in opposite directions around the lesion to stabilize it. Then, gently use the tip of the blade to outline the border of the lesion. While holding the belly of blade parallel to the skin, slowly advance the blade in a sawing motion. As most of the lesion is separated from the skin's surface, a gentle use of forceps or the tip of a needle may be helpful to hold the specimen while the final cuts are being made. After the specimen is removed, electrical or chemical cautery can be used for hemostasis. Generally, electrocautery is optimal for larger wounds. For other wounds, chemical cautery with aluminum chloride solution at 20% concentration in ethyl alcohol is commonly applied with a cotton swab after the biopsy. Monsel's solution

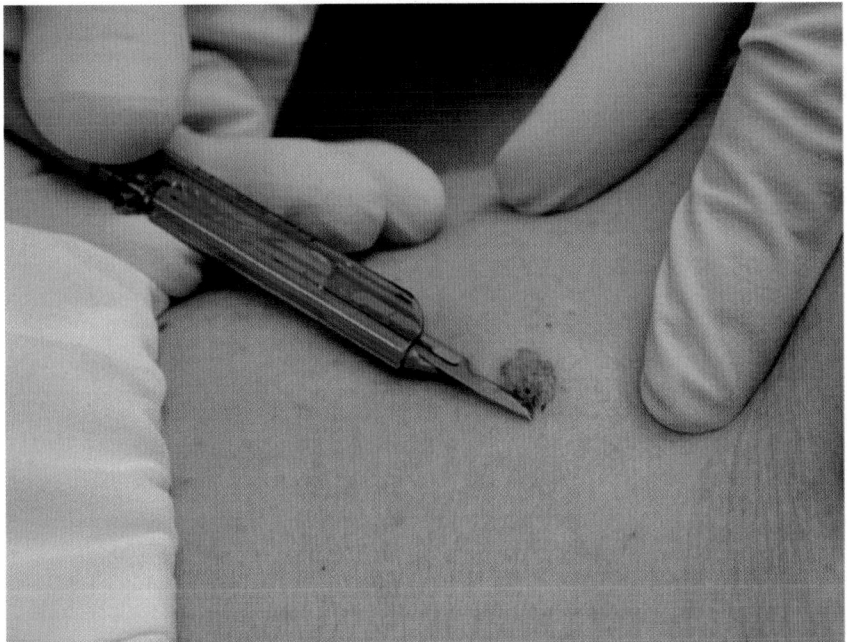

▲ **FIGURE 36-1** Shave biopsy.

(ferric subsulfate), which is also used for chemical cautery, is not recommended initially because pigmentation may occur due to iron deposition and because the solution may be counterproductive to wound healing.

Postoperative care is relatively easy after a shave biopsy. The wound should be washed once or twice daily with water or a mild soap and kept moist with white petroleum jelly under a bandage until it has healed (often within 7 to 10 days). This biopsy does not render significant cosmetic defects, though short-term hypopigmentation and cutaneous depression have been noted.

SAUCERIZATION BIOPSY

BOX 36-4   Summary

- Saucerization biopsies are used to reach deeper lesions by using a blade bent into a U-shape to match the depth desired.
- Chemical or electrical cautery is used to achieve hemostasis.

A saucerization biopsy is a deep shave biopsy recommended for the diagnosis and treatment of deeper-seated lesions reaching the upper to middermis such as SCC, atypical nevi, and melanoma. It is beneficial because it rarely results in residual disease.

Using the thumb and index finger, bend a Gillette Super Blue razor blade into a concave shape according to the depth desired (Fig. 36-2). This will form

an equally concave incision reaching down to the dermal tissue. Use a sawing motion similar to a shave biopsy to obtain the specimen. Hemostasis can then be achieved using the same method as for a shave biopsy.

PUNCH BIOPSY

BOX 36-5   Summary

- A punch biopsy is useful for determining the depth of a lesion because it can reach

subcutaneous tissue, depending on the punch size used.
- The punch is made vertically through the lesion, and the specimen is removed with forceps.
- If the punch is less than 3 mm, the wound can be healed without sutures.
- If the punch is 3 mm or greater, sutures may be needed.

A punch biopsy is primarily obtained for inflammatory or neoplastic conditions such as dermatofibrosarcoma protuberans (DFSP). It is a relatively quick and simple procedure and is ideal for reaching subcutaneous tissue, thereby providing more information about the depth of tumor invasion. The technique can be incisional or excisional depending on the size of the lesion and the diameter of the instrument. For deep lesions, a 6-mm punch may be necessary. Generally, a 3 to 4-mm punch is recommended, though sutures will be needed after the procedure. To avoid this, a 2-mm punch can be used.[3] Limitation for a 2-mm punch biopsy, however, is that the tissue may shrink during tissue processing, making it difficult for the dermatopathologist to interpret results.

Equipment and material needed include: a sterile punch, scissors, a skin hook, Adson toothed forceps, nonabsorbable (and absorbable for larger punches) sutures, and gauze.

The punch biopsy preparation and anesthesia is similar to that for a shave

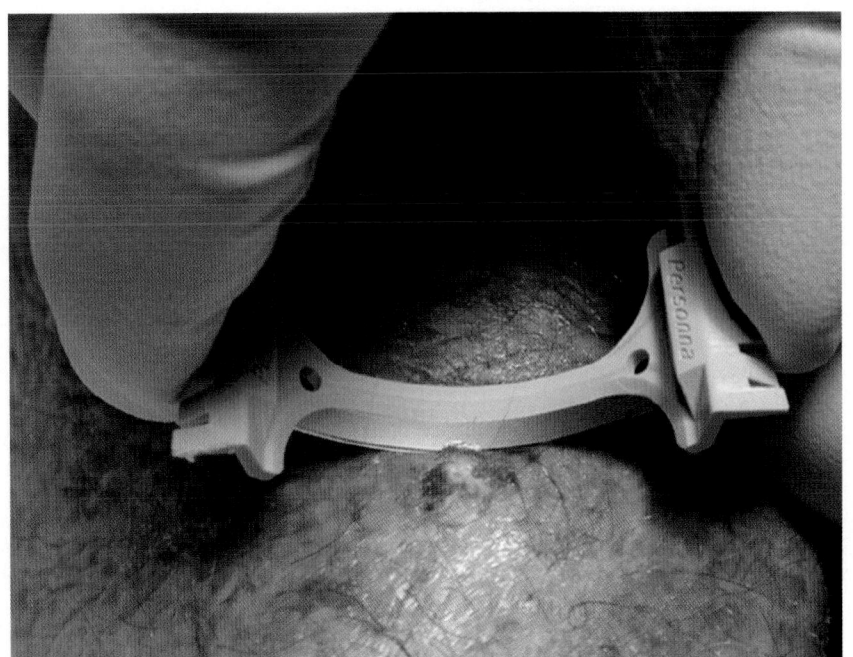

▲ **FIGURE 36-2** Saucerization biopsy.

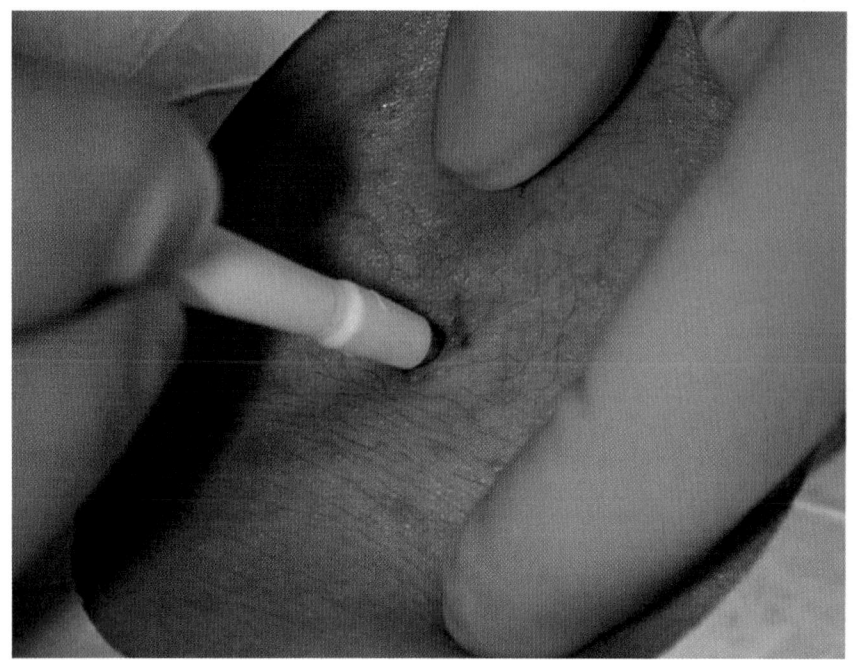

▲ **FIGURE 36-3** Punch biopsy.

biopsy. Though both disposable and reusable punches are available, it is optimal to use disposable ones because the reusable ones tend to get dull, affecting the histological evaluation of the specimen.

Before beginning the procedure, stabilize the area of the lesion by pulling the skin taut and perpendicular to the relaxed skin tension lines with the opposite hand (Fig. 36-3). This will allow for a more oval defect to be created when the punch is done, yielding a better cosmetic outcome. The punch is held between the thumb and index finger, and the edge of the cylinder is vertically pressed gently against the lesion and rotated to pierce the layers of the skin. The punch is then removed carefully with the same vertical direction used to pierce the skin, thereby leaving the specimen intact. Forceps, a skin hook, or tip of the needle can be used to gently lift the specimen, making sure not to damage it for appropriate microscopic examination. Chemical cautery will achieve hemostasis, or sutures may be applied depending on the size of the wound. Generally, only a wound greater than 3 mm requires sutures, mostly for cosmetic purposes.

The punch biopsy site should be cleaned once or twice daily and kept moist with white petroleum jelly. Certain antibiotic ointments are not recommended because they may cause allergic contact dermatitis.[4] Sutures should be removed between 1 and 2 weeks, depending on location.

INCISIONAL BIOPSY

BOX 36-6   Summary

- Incisional biopsies are performed when larger specimens are needed for examination.
- The sample is taken from the middle of the lesion in a fusiform fashion, and then it is removed with forceps.
- The wound is sutured after the biopsy.
- Adverse effects include infection or hematoma formation.

The incisional biopsy is used when a wider or deeper portion of the skin is needed for examination. Often, both skin from the lesion and normal skin are taken for analysis. This biopsy is especially useful for examining inflammatory processes involving the subcutaneous tissue or fascia. Incisional biopsies are also done on pigmented lesions that are large, and on difficult sites or elderly patients.[3]

The biopsy site should be prepped in a similar fashion to the punch biopsy site as described earlier. The instruments need to be sterilized and include: a #15 scalpel, Adson toothed forceps, a skin hook, scissors, suture material, and gauze.

An incisional biopsy is best accomplished with the scalpel held perpendicularly to the skin's surface. The incision then is made in a fusiform fashion in the middle of the lesion to reach the subcutaneous tissue, and the depth of the cut should remain the same throughout.

The specimen can then be removed carefully, and the wound is sutured.

Incisional biopsies may have adverse effects, such as wound infection, dehiscence, scar and/or hematoma formation, and pigmentary alterations.

WEDGE BIOPSY

BOX 36-7   Summary

- Wedge biopsies are used to examine ulcers.
- Normal skin and a part of the lesion are taken in the biopsy.
- Electrical cautery is used for hemostasis, and then the wound may be sutured.
- Adverse effects include bleeding, pigmentation, and scarring.

A wedge biopsy is performed primarily for ulcers. It allows a larger specimen to be obtained and analyzed. The depth of the cut should include subcutaneous fascia and sometimes muscle, depending on the nature of the lesion.

The shape of the incision is evident in the name. The incisions should be made from the normal skin toward the center of the lesion to form a pie-shaped specimen that can then be removed with a forceps.

The wound or defect can either be sutured or hemostasis can be achieved for healing.

Adverse effects of wedge biopsies can include bleeding, infection, pigmentary alterations, and scarring.

EXCISIONAL BIOPSY

BOX 36-8   Summary

- Excisional biopsies are primarily used for suspected melanoma.
- It is performed with a scalpel held at an angle following the markings bordering the lesion.
- Fusiform excision is preferred for better cosmetic results.
- Adverse effects include infection, scarring, and hematoma formation.

Excisional biopsies are used when a larger specimen is needed for examination, especially of deep lesions reaching the subcutaneous tissue. This is important when determining melanoma because it allows for a complete histological assessment.[5] When an atypical nevus is present or melanoma is suspected, a

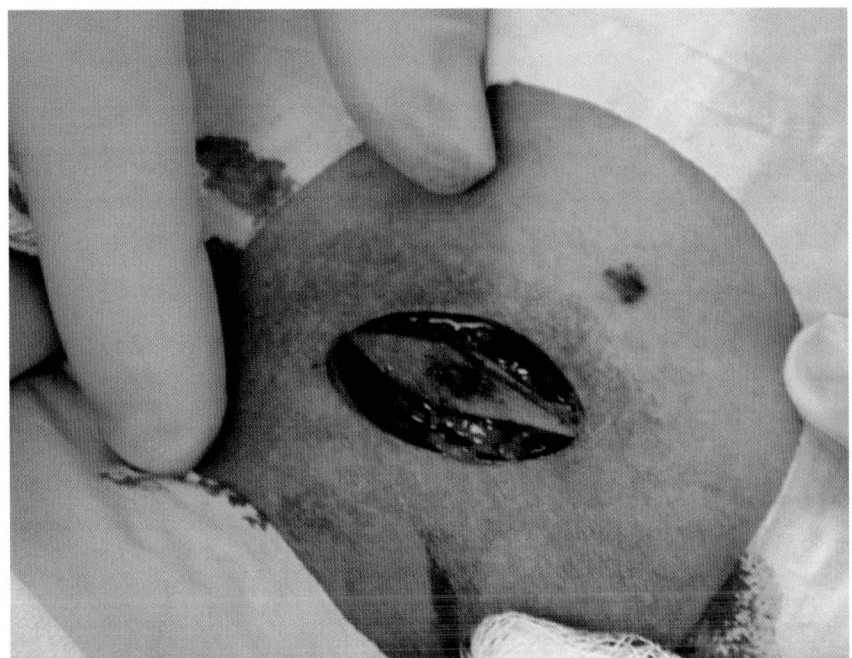

▲ **FIGURE 36-4** Excisional biopsy.

all cells that are part of the lesion are removed.

Adverse side effects of excisional biopsies are possible. Wound infection, dehiscence, scar and/or hematoma formation, are some examples. Also, compared to incisional biopsies, excisional biopsies are more costly and require more postoperative management.

FINAL THOUGHTS

Biopsies are extremely important in diagnosing cutaneous lesions. The physician must be aware of the various types and determine which would provide the most accurate information with the best cosmetic outcome. Also, margins of normal skin that are taken with the lesion depend on the type of lesion suspected, and this should be evaluated upon clinical and histological exam.

full-thickness excisional biopsy is preferred over others.[1,2,5] It is preferable to use this technique to rule out malignancy, rather than using it for diagnostic or analytical purposes.

In a full-thickness excision, the lesion is completely removed using a scalpel, and then the wound is sutured (Fig. 36-4). Prior to anesthesia and excision, the surgeon should mark the borders of the lesion with a skin marker. The excisional biopsy can be performed in a fusiform approach at 30° angles or in a more circular manner requiring a cone or dog-ear repair. With a circular excision, less skin is removed and thus can yield a better cosmetic outcome.

It is advisable to put a suture at the 12 o'clock position of the specimen to orient the position of the lesion and the patient's body for the dermatopathologist.

Margins of normal skin are also excised to histologically guarantee that

REFERENCES

1. Martin RCG II, Scoggins CR, Rozz MI, et al. Is incisional biopsy of melanoma harmful? *Am J Surg.* 2005;190:913–917.
2. Bong JL, Herd RM, Hunter JA. Incisional biopsy and melanoma prognosis. *J Am Acad Dermatol.* 2002;46:690–694.
3. Lorusso GD, Sarma DP, Sarwar SF. Punch biopsies of melanoma: A diagnostic peril. *Dermatol Online J.* 2005;11:7.
4. Jacob SE, James WD. From road rash to top allergen in a flash: Bacitracin. *Dermatol Surg.* 2004;30:521–524.
5. Rice JC, Zaragoza P, Waheed K, et al. Efficacy of incisional vs. punch biopsy in the histological diagnosis of periocular tumors. *Nature.* 2003;17:478–481.

CHAPTER 37

Dermoscopy and Mole Mapping

Ralph P. Braun, M.D.
Olivier Gaide, M.D., Ph.D.
A. Marghoob, M.D.
Margaret Oliviero, A.R.N.P.
Alfred W. Kopf, M.D.
L.E. French, M.D.
J.-H. Saurat, M.D.
Harold S. Rabinovitz, M.D.

> **BOX 37-1   Overview**
>
> - Dermoscopy is a noninvasive method for the *in vivo* diagnosis of melanoma and the differential diagnosis of pigmented lesions of the skin.
> - As immersion liquid, we recommend the use of 60% alcohol, which should be used in an eye dropper bottle. For nail dermoscopy and in areas close to the mucosa, we recommend the use of a gel.
> - Polarized light dermoscopy allows the examination without contact and shows best the vascular architecture of a lesion. This is particularly important for nonpigmented lesions.
> - Colors are very important for the diagnosis because the color enables the clinician to identify the corresponding chromophore as to see where it is located in the skin.
> - The inspection of blood vessels has gained more importance in dermoscopy over the last few years.
> - In the first step, one has to differentiate between melanocytic and nonmelanocytic lesions.
> - In the second step, one has to determine whether the lesion is benign, suspect, or malignant.
> - Digital dermoscopy adds additional features such as computer-assisted diagnosis and digital monitoring.
> - Total body photography allows the identification of lesions that appear *de novo* or which change in color, size, and/or shape.

INTRODUCTION

Dermoscopy (also known as epiluminescence microscopy, dermatoscopy, and amplified surface microscopy) is an *in vivo* method that has been reported to be a useful tool for the early recognition of malignant melanoma and the differential diagnosis of pigmented lesions of the skin. Its use increases diagnostic accuracy between 5 and 30% over clinical visual inspection, depending on the type of skin lesion and experience of the physician. This was confirmed by two recent evidence-based publications from a meta-analysis of the literature.[1,2]

INDICATIONS AND CONTRAINDICATIONS

As a noninvasive method, dermoscopy can be used on every skin lesion pigmented or nonpigmented, melanocytic or nonmelanocytic. Initially, it has been used for pigmented lesions, but since recent publications on dermoscopy of blood vessels, the use on nonpigmented lesions is getting more popular, as more diagnostic criteria become available.

There is theoretically no contraindication for the use of dermoscopy. However, we do not recommend using the dermatoscope on open wounds or bleeding tumors in order to avoid contamination.

PHYSICAL ASPECTS

Light is either reflected, dispersed, or absorbed by the stratum corneum due to its refraction index and its optical density, which is different from air. Thus, deeper underlying structures cannot be adequately visualized. The use of immersion fluid renders the skin surface translucent and reduces reflections, so that the underlying structures will become visible and optical magnification can be used for examination. Taken together, these optical means allow for the visualization of certain epidermal, dermoepidermal, and dermal structures. As immersion fluid, we recommend the use of 60% alcohol (ethanol) that can be applied directly on the skin using an eye dropper bottle.[3] The advantages are that ethanol results in the best image quality and the least air inclusions. It evaporates immediately, does not have to be wiped off, and does not stain the patient clothing or underwear. Alcohol in higher concentrations can be used but it has a strong odor. In areas close to the eyes or to the mucosa as well as for the examination of the nail apparatus, we rather recommend the use of a gel (ultrasound gel, cosmetic gel, etc.). The latter does not burn the eyes, and most importantly it fills out the gap between the convex nail surface and the handheld device nicely.[4] Some devices use polarized light in order to reduce the surface reflections. This technique allows a faster examination of the patient, but if the patient has a dry skin the use of immersion liquid is still required.

Dermoscopy is most often performed with relatively inexpensive handheld devices with 10 to 20× magnification [Dermatoscope Delta 20®, (Heine AG); DermoGenius Basic® (Biocam), Dermlite® (3GenLLC)] (Fig. 37-1). All listed devices are devices of the second generation that

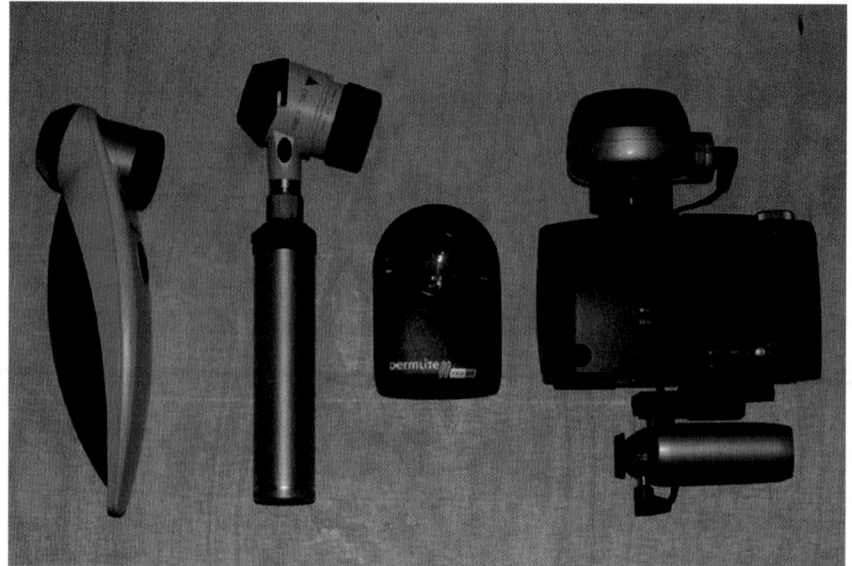

▲ **FIGURE 37-1** Selection of handheld devices for dermoscopy. From *left* to *right*: Dermogenius basic, Heine Delta 20, Dermlite II pro HR, and Dermlite Foto for documentation and digital dermoscopy.

have improved optics and illumination (LED). The optics is designed such that a lesion can be examined at a distance from the skin. This is an advantage because the examination is much faster and more convenient for both the physician and the patient if the lesion is, for example, on the face or in the genital area.

DERMOSCOPY CRITERIA

BOX 37-2   Summary

- Black color in dermoscopy corresponds to melanin in the upper parts of the epidermis or the stratum corneum.
- Blue color in dermoscopy corresponds to melanin in the dermis.
- The interpretation of blood vessels has gained more and more importance.
- The use of ultrasound gel or instruments that use polarized light for dermoscopy is important for the evaluation of the blood vessels that are very sensitive to pressure.

Dermoscopy is used for the identification of many different structures, colors, as well as blood vessels not seen by the naked eye. The correlation of these structures with histology is well established.

Colors

Colors play an important role in Dermoscopy. Common colors are light brown, dark brown, black, blue, blue-gray, red, yellow, and white. The most important chromophore of the skin and especially in melanocytic neoplasms is melanin. The color of melanin as seen with dermoscopy depends on its localization in the skin. For example: Melanin appears black if located in the stratum corneum and the upper epidermis, light to dark brown in the epidermis, gray to gray-blue in the papillary dermis, and steel blue in the reticular dermis.[5,6] Melanin appears to be blue when it is localized within the deeper parts of the skin because the portions of the visible light with shorter wavelengths (blue-violet end of the spectrum) are more dispersed than the portions with longer wavelengths (red end of the visible spectrum). The color red is either associated with an increased number or dilatation of blood vessels, trauma, or neovascularization (see "Vascular Architecture"). The color *white* is often due to regression and/or scarring (see "Regression").

Vascular Architecture

At the beginning of dermoscopy, this technique was mainly used for the evaluation of pigmentation. In recent years, the interpretation of blood vessels has gained much more importance, and their morphological aspect enables the clinician in many cases to make the diagnosis, especially in nonpigmented lesions and lesions of nonmelanocytic origin. For the evaluation of blood vessels, there has to be as little pressure as possible on the lesion during the examination, otherwise the vessels are simply compressed and will not be visible.[5] The use of ultrasound gel for immersion helps to reduce the pressure. An excellent alternative is the use of noncontact polarized light examination as used in some handheld dermatoscopes. Devices such as the Dermlite allow the evaluation of blood vessels without contact.

The following types of blood vessels have been described: red lagoons, hairpin vessels, dotted vessels, comma-like vessels, glomerular vessels, string of pearls, crown vessels, cork screw vessels, and arborizing vessels. Atypical vascular patterns, also called irregular (polymorphous) vessels, may include linear, dotted, or globular red vessels irregularly distributed within the lesion.

DERMOSCOPIC STRUCTURES

BOX 37-3   Summary

- Regular pigment network; dots, globules, and blotches can be currently found in melanocytic nevi.
- Irregular pigment network; irregular dots, globules, as well as irregular blotches are commonly found in dysplastic nevi or melanoma.
- Radial streaming, pseudopods, regression structures, and blue-white veil are common dermoscopy criteria for melanoma and should be considered as malignant criteria.

This chapter is based on the nomenclature as proposed by the Consensus Netmeeting on Dermoscopy with some revisions.

Pigment Network

The pigment network is a honeycomb-like network consisting of pigmented "lines" and hypopigmented "holes" (Fig. 37-2). The reticulation (network)

represents the rete ridge pattern of the epidermis. Its histopathological correlation is either melanin pigment in keratinocytes, or in melanocytes along the dermo-epidermal junction. The hypopigmented holes in the network correspond to tips of the dermal papillae and the overlying suprapapillary plates of the epidermis.

The pigment network can be either typical or atypical. The typical network is relatively uniform, regularly meshed, homogeneous in color, and usually thinning out at the periphery. An atypical network is nonuniform, with darker and/or broadened lines and "holes" that are heterogeneous in diameter and shape. The lines are often hyperpigmented and may end abruptly at the periphery.

Dots

Dots are small, round structures of less than 0.1 mm in diameter, which may be black, brown, gray, or blue-gray. According to what has been said before, black dots are due to pigment accumulation in the stratum corneum and the upper part of the epidermis (see "Colors"). Brown dots represent focal melanin accumulations at the dermo-epidermal junction. Gray-blue granules are due to tiny melanin structures in the papillary dermis. Gray-blue or blue granules are due to loose melanin, fine melanin particles, or melanin "dust" in melanophages or free in the deep papillary or reticular dermis.

Globules

Globules are round to oval, well-demarcated structures that may be brown, black, or red (Fig. 37-3). They have a diameter larger than 0.1 mm and correspond to nests of pigmented melanocytes, clumps of melanin, and/or melanophages situated usually in the lower epidermis, at the dermo-epidermal junction or in the papillary dermis.

Both dots and globules may occur in benign, as well as in malignant melanocytic proliferations. In benign lesions, they are rather regular in size, shape, and distribution (frequently in the center of a lesion). In melanomas, they tend to vary in size, color, and shape and are frequently found irregularly distributed at the periphery of lesions.

Branched Streaks

Branched streaks are an expression of an altered, perturbed pigment network in which the network becomes broken

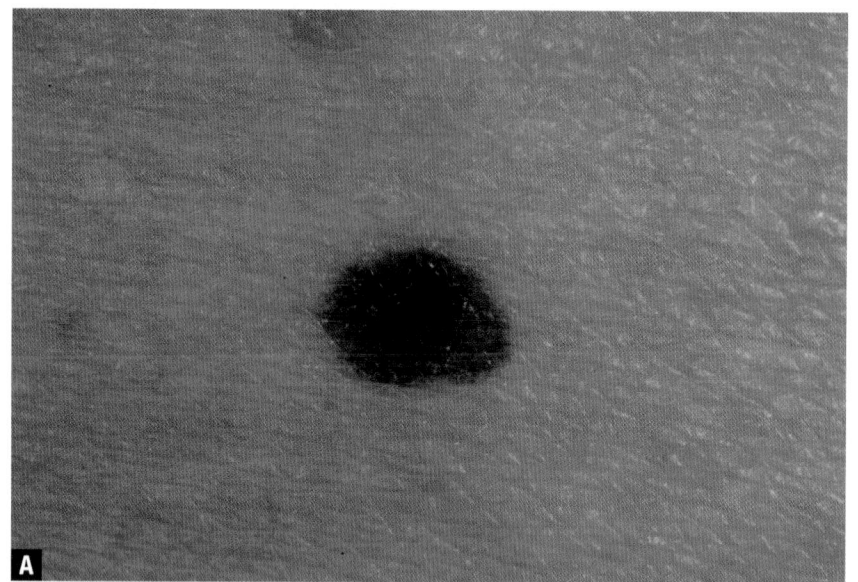

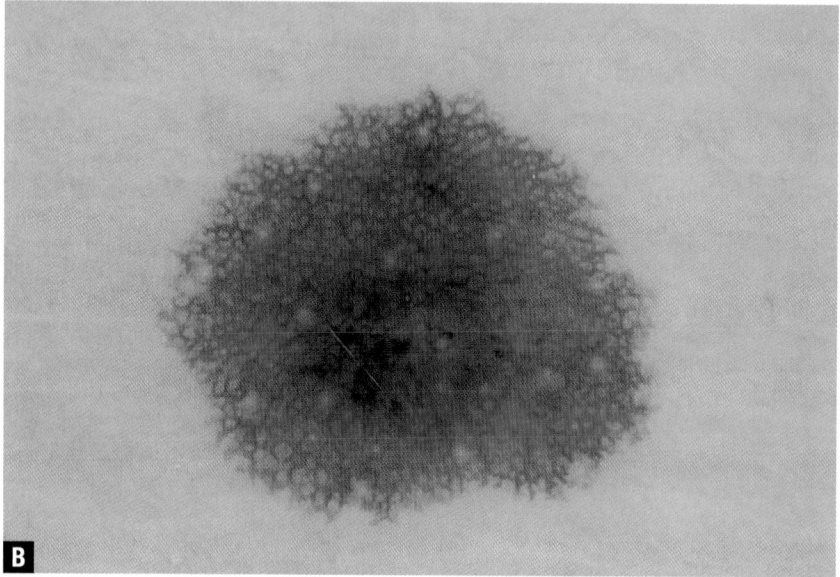

▲ **FIGURE 37-2** **A.** Clinical image of a junctional nevus. **B.** Dermoscopy of (**A**) showing a typical regular pigment network.

up (see Fig. 37-4). Their pathological correlations are remnants of pigmented rete ridges and bridging nests of melanocytic cells within the epidermis and papillary dermis. This term is exclusively used in the ABCD rule of dermoscopy and should not be confounded with the term "streaks," as used in the "7-point checklist."

Streaks

Both radial streaming and pseudopods correspond histopathologically to intraepidermal or junctional confluent radial nests of melanocytes. This is why some authors prefer using the term "streaks" interchangeably with radial streaming or pseudopods (Fig. 37-5). Streaks can be irregular when unevenly distributed (malignant melanoma), or regular (symmetrical radial arrangement over the entire lesion). The latter is particularly found in the pigmented spindle cell nevi (Reed's nevi).

Radial Streaming

Radial streaming appears as radially and asymmetrically arranged, parallel linear extensions at the periphery of a lesion (Fig. 37-5).

Pseudopods

Pseudopods represent finger-like projections of dark pigment (brown to black) at the periphery of the lesion.

They may have small knobs at their tips, and are either connected to the pigment network or directly to the tumor body (Fig. 37-5).

Structureless Areas

Structureless areas represent areas devoid of any dermoscopy structures (globules, network, etc.). They tend to be hypopigmented due to the absence of pigment or diminution of pigment intensity within a lesion. A structureless or hypopigmented area cannot be lighter than the surrounding skin and does not have signs of granularity (peppering) in its periphery.

Blotches

A blotch (black lamella) is a diffuse pigmentation of black to dark brown color that obscures underlying structures. It is due to a large concentration of melanin pigment localized throughout the epidermis and/or dermis visually. A blotch can be regular, often in the center of a lesion (junctional nevus), or irregular (melanoma).

Regression

Regression appears either as a white scar-like depigmentation (lighter than the surrounding skin) or "peppering" (speckled multiple blue-gray granules within a hypopigmented area). Histologically, regression shows fibrosis, loss of pigmentation, epidermal thinning, effacement of the rete ridges, and melanin granules free in the dermis or in melanophages scattered in the papillary dermis. If areas of peppering are confluent, they might have a bluish appearance, which can be virtually indistinguishable from blue-white veil (Fig. 37-4).

Blue-White Veil

Blue-white veil is an irregular, indistinct, confluent blue pigmentation with an overlying white ground glass haze (Fig. 37-5). The pigmentation cannot occupy the entire lesion and is mainly found in the papular part of the lesion. Histopathologically, this corresponds to an aggregation of heavily pigmented cells or melanin in the dermis (blue color) in combination with a compact orthokeratosis. Blue-white veil should not be confused with confluent peppering (granularity) in regression areas of melanomas, which is the dermoscopy criterion for (histopatho-

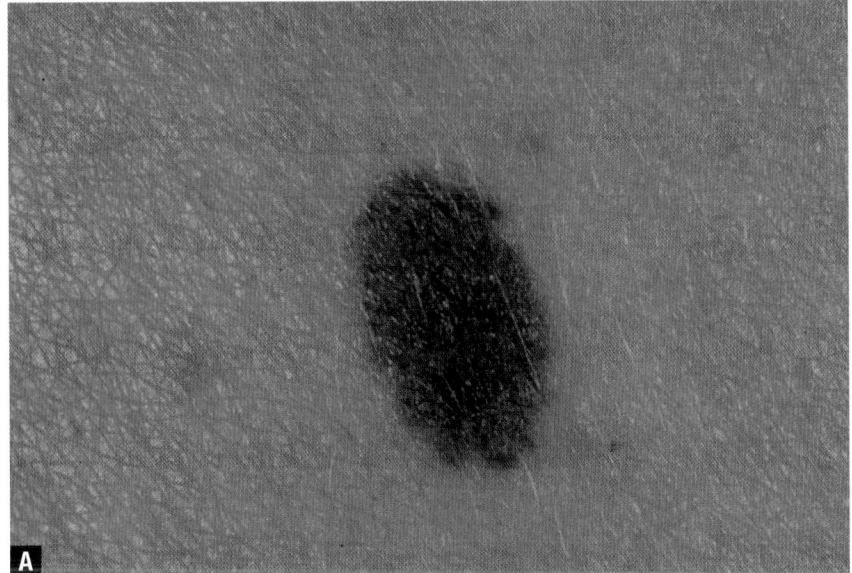

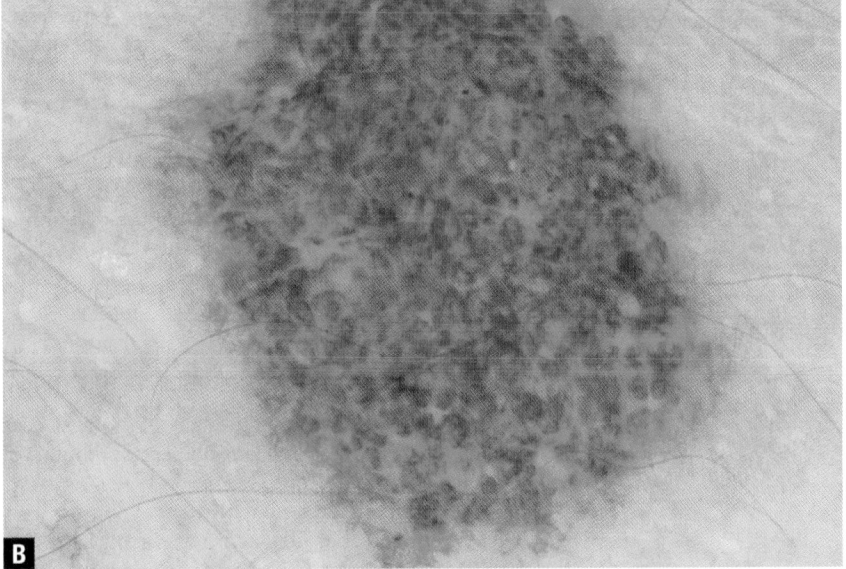

▲ **FIGURE 37-3 A.** Clinical image of a compound nevus. **B.** Dermoscopy of (**A**) showing multiple regular globules.

logic) melanosis. Both entities might have a similar dermoscopy aspect but do not have the same histopathologic correlation.

Milia-Like Cysts

Milia-like cysts are round whitish or yellowish structures that are mainly seen in seborrheic keratosis (Fig. 37-6). They correspond to intraepidermal keratin-filled cysts and may also be seen in congenital nevi, as well as in some papillomatous melanocytic nevi.[5,7]

Comedo-Like Openings (Crypts, Pseudofollicular Openings)

Comedo-like openings (pseudocomedos) are mainly seen in seborrheic ker-atosis or in some rare cases in papillomatous melanocytic nevi (Fig. 37-6).[5,7] Histopathologically, they correspond to keratin-filled invaginations of the epidermis.

FISSURES AND RIDGES ("BRAIN-LIKE APPEARANCE") Fissures are irregular, linear keratin-filled depressions, commonly seen in seborrheic keratosis (Fig. 37-6). They may also be seen in melanocytic nevi with congenital patterns and in some dermal melanocytic nevi. Multiple fissures might give a "brain-like appearance" to the lesion. This pattern has also been named "gyri and sulci" by some authors. The only difference from comedo-like openings is that fissures are not round but rather linear.[5,7]

Fingerprint-Like Structures

Some flat seborrheic keratoses (also known as solar lentigines) can show tiny ridges running in parallel and producing a pattern that resembles the parallel lines that are seen in the fingerprints (Fig. 37-7).

Moth-Eaten Border

Some flat seborrheic keratoses (mainly on the face) have a concave border so that the pigment ends with a curved structure (Fig. 37-7). This has been compared to a moth-eaten garment.

Leaf-Like Areas

Leaf-like areas (maple-leaf-like areas) are seen as brown to gray-blue discrete bulbous blobs, sometimes forming a leaf-like pattern (Fig. 37-8).[8] Their distribution reminds one of the shapes of a hand. In absence of a pigment network, they are suggestive of pigmented basal cell carcinomas.

Spoke-Wheel-Like Structures

Spoke-wheel-like structures are well circumscribed brown to gray-blue-brown radial projections meeting at a darker brown central hub.[8] In the absence of a pigment network, they are highly suggestive of basal cell carcinoma.

Large Blue-Gray Ovoid Nests

Ovoid nests are large, well-circumscribed, confluent or near-confluent pigmented ovoid areas, larger than globules, and not intimately connected to a pigmented tumor body. When a network is absent, ovoid nests are highly suggestive of basal cell carcinoma.

Multiple Blue-Gray Globules

Multiple blue-gray globules are round well-circumscribed structures, which in the absence of a pigment network are highly suggestive of basal cell carcinoma (Fig. 37-8). They have to be differentiated from multiple blue-gray dots (which correspond to melanophages and melanin dust).[8]

■ DIFFERENTIAL DIAGNOSIS OF PIGMENTED LESIONS OF THE SKIN

BOX 37-4 Summary

• In the first step, one has to look for dermoscopy criteria of a melanocytic lesion.

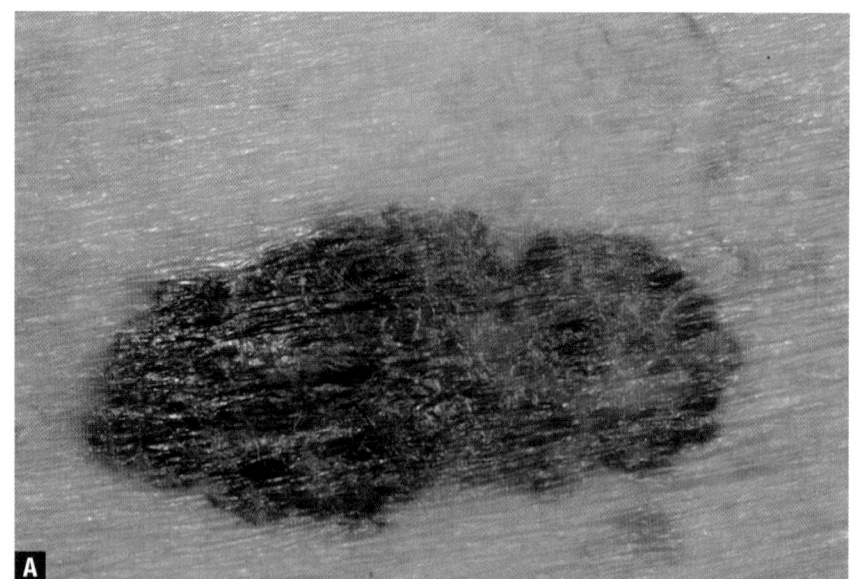

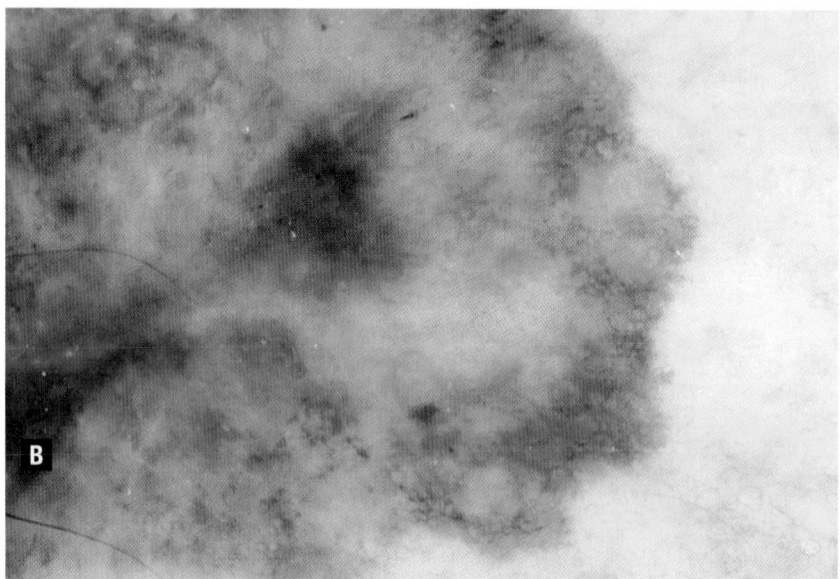

▲ **FIGURE 37-4** **A.** Clinical image of a melanoma (Breslow 0.4 mm). **B.** Dermoscopy of (**A**) showing branched streaks (remnants of pigment network), blue-white veil, and regression (scar-like depigmentation).

- In the second step, one should specifically search for dermoscopy criteria for seborrheic keratosis.
- In the third step, one has to look for dermoscopy criteria for pigmented basal cell carcinoma.
- In the fourth step, one should try to find specific dermoscopy criteria for vascular lesions.
- If none of the previous criteria were found, the lesion should still be considered to be melanoma in order not to miss melanoma.

The Board of the Consensus Netmeeting agreed on a two-step procedure for the classification of pigmented lesions of the skin (Fig. 37-9).[9]

The first step is the differentiation between a melanocytic and a nonmelanocytic lesion. Once a lesion has been identified to be of melanocytic origin, it has to be determined in a second step whether the lesion is benign, suspicious or malignant. This can be done with the help of different algorithms that will be discussed later.

For the first decision (melanocytic vs. nonmelanocytic), the following algorithm is used (Fig. 37-10):

Step 1: Are aggregated globules, pigment network, branched streaks, and homogenous blue pigmentation or a parallel pattern (palms, soles, and mucosa) visualized? If this is the case, the lesion should be considered as a melanocytic lesion.

Step 2: If not, the lesion should be evaluated for the specific morphologic criteria for seborrheic keratoses such as the presence of comedo-like plugs, multiple milia-like cysts, and comedo-like openings, irregular crypts, light brown fingerprint-like structures, or "fissures and ridges" (brain-like appearance) pattern. If so, the lesion is suggestive of seborrheic keratosis.

Step 3: If not, the lesion has to be evaluated for the presence of arborizing blood vessels (telangiectasias), leaf-like areas, large blue-gray ovoid nests, multiple blue-gray globules, spoke-wheel areas, or ulceration. If present, the lesion is suggestive of basal cell carcinoma.

Step 4: If not, one has to look for red or red-blue (to black) lagoons. If these structures are present, the lesion should be considered as hemangioma or an angiokeratoma.

Step 5: If all the preceding questions were answered with "no," the lesion should still be considered as a melanocytic lesion in order not to miss a melanoma.

Once the lesion is identified to be of melanocytic origin, the decision has to be made if the melanocytic lesion is benign, suspect, or malignant. To accomplish this, the following different algorithms are the most commonly used.

Pattern Analysis (Pehamberger et al.)

Pattern recognition has in the past been used by clinicians and histopathologists to differentiate benign lesions from malignant neoplasms.[10] A similar process has been found useful with dermoscopy and has been termed "pattern analysis." It allows distinction between benign and malignant growth features. It was described by Pehamberger and colleagues based on the analysis of more than 7000 pigmented skin lesions. Table 37-1 shows the typical patterns of some common, pigmented skin lesions using pattern analysis.

Revised Pattern Analysis

The revised pattern analysis distinguished between global patterns and local features. The general appearance of *C*olor, *A*rchitectural order, *S*ymmetry of pattern, and *H*omogeneity (CASH) are important components in distinguishing benign lesions from melanoma.[11,12] Benign melanocytic lesions tend to have few colors, architectural order, symmetry of pattern, and homogeneity. Malignant melanoma often has many colors, architectural disorder, asymmetry of pattern, and heterogeneity.

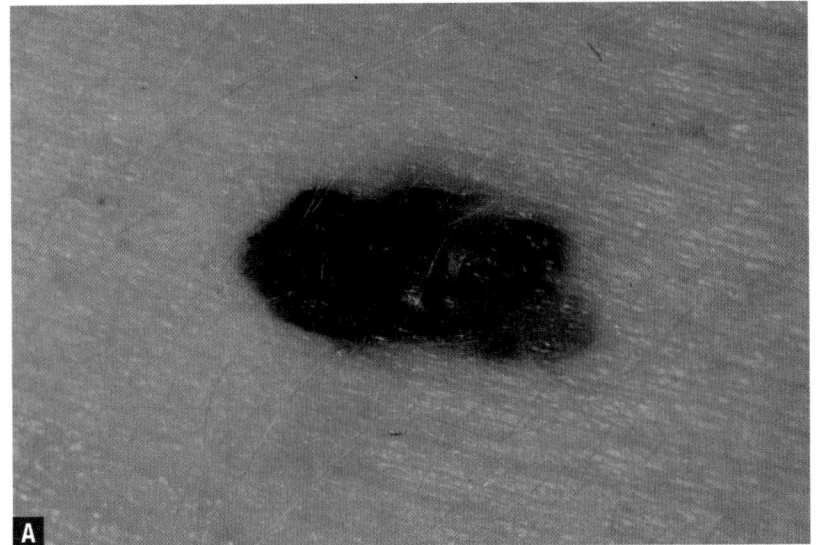

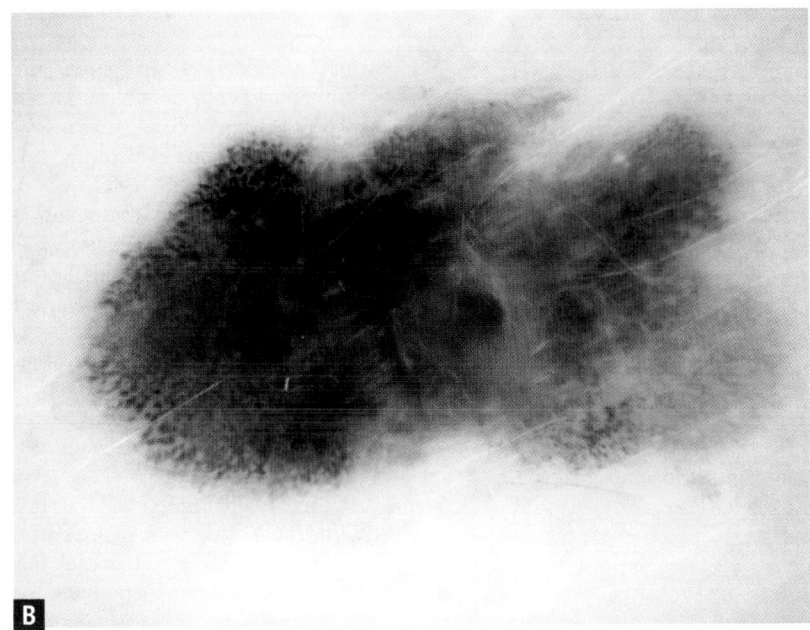

▲ **FIGURE 37-5 A.** Clinical image of a melanoma (Breslow 0.5 mm) **B.** Dermoscopy of (**A**) showing an irregular pigment network, irregular dots, pseudopods, radial streaming, and a central blue-white veil.

ABCD Rule of Dermatoscopy (Stolz et al.)

The ABCD rule of dermatoscopy, described by Stolz et al. in 1993, was based on an analysis of 157 pigmented skin lesions.[13] It is based on a scoring system for melanocytic neoplasms that differentiates them into benign, suspicious, and malignant categories. This is accomplished by calculating a total dermoscopy score (Table 37-2).

ASYMMETRY The lesion is bisected by two lines that are placed 90° to each other. The first line attempts to bisect the lesion at the division of most symmetry and the other one is placed 90° to it. Symmetry takes into account the contour, colors, and structures within the lesion. Lesions that are symmetric in both axes are given zero points.

BORDER First, the lesion is divided into eight equal pie-shaped pieces. Next, one counts the number of segments that have an abrupt perimeter cutoff. Thus the points range from 0 to 8.

Colors

Number the following colors present: light brown, dark brown, black, red, white, blue, and grey. The points will range from 1 to 6.

Dermoscopic Structures

Number the following five structures: dots, globules, structureless areas, network, and branched streaks. The points range from 1 to 6. The individual points are multiplied with a weighting factor, which is specific for each criterion. The

Table 37-1
Pattern of Benign and Malignant Melanocytic Lesions

	BENIGN MELANOCYTIC LESIONS	MALIGNANT MELANOCYTIC LESIONS
Dots	Centrally located or situated right on the network	Unevenly distributed and scattered focally at the periphery
Globules	Uniform in size, shape, and color, symmetrically located at the periphery, centrally located, or uniform throughout the lesion as in a cobblestone pattern	Globules, which are unevenly distributed and when reddish in color are highly suggestive of melanoma
Streaks	Radial streaming or pseudopods tend to be symmetrical and uniform at the periphery	Radial streaming or pseudopods tend to be focal and irregular at the periphery
Blue-white veil	Tends to be centrally located	Tends to be asymmetrically located or diffuse almost over the entire lesion
Blotch	Centrally located or may be a diffuse hyperpigmented area that extends almost to the periphery of the lesion	Asymmetrically located or there are often multiple asymmetrical blotches
Network	Typical network that consists of light to dark uniform pigmented lines and hypopigmented holes	Atypical network that may be nonuniform with black/brown or gray thickened lines and holes of different sizes and shapes
Network borders	Either fades into the periphery or is symmetrically sharp	Focally sharp

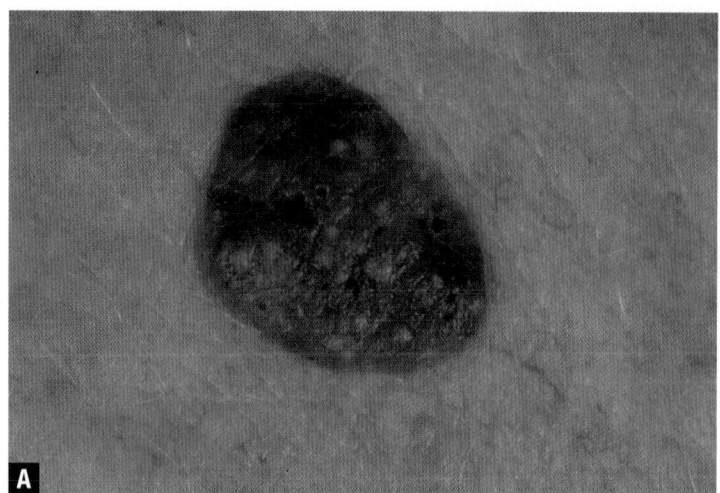

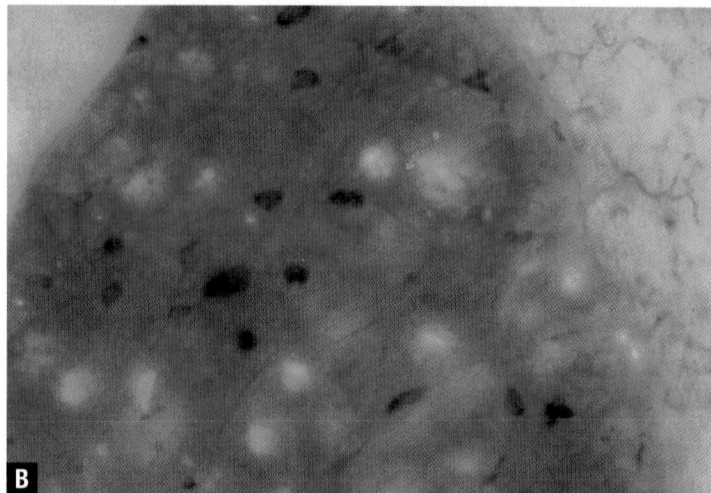

▲ **FIGURE 37-6 A.** Clinical image of a pigmented seborrheic keratosis **B.** Dermoscopy of (**A**) showing multiple milia like cysts, comedo like openings, some fissures, as well as a sharp demarcation of the border.

Table 37-2
ABCD Rule of Dermoscopy (Stolz et al.)

		POINTS	WEIGHT FACTOR	SUBSCORE RANGE
ASYMMETRY	• Complete symmetry	0	1.3	0–2.6
	• Asymmetry in one axis	1		
	• Asymmetry in two axes	2		
BORDER	• Eight segments, 1 point for abrupt cutoff of pigment	0–8	0.1	0–0.8
COLOR	1 point for each color	1–6	0.5	0.5–3.0
	• White			
	• Red			
	• Light brown			
	• Dark brown			
	• Black			
	• Blue-gray			
DIFFERENTIAL STRUCTURES	1 point for every structure	1–5	0.5	0.5–2.5
	• Pigment network			
	• Structureless areas			
	• Dots			
	• Globules			
	• Branched streaks			
	Total score range			1.0–8.9

Table 37-3
7-Point Checklist (Argenziano et al.)

CRITERIA	7-POINT SCORE
MAJOR CRITERIA	
• Atypical pigment network	2
• Blue-white veil	2
• Atypical vascular pattern	2
• Dotted vessels	
• Linear irregular vessels	
MINOR CRITERIA	
• Irregular streaks	1
• Pseudopods	
• Radial streaming	
• Irregular pigmentation	1
• Irregular dots/globules	1
• Regression structures	1

different subscores are then added together in order to obtain the total dermoscopy score (TDS). A lesion with a TDS < 4.75 can be considered to be benign. A lesion with a TDS > 5.45 should be considered malignant and should be removed. Lesions with a TDS between 4.75 and 5.45 should be considered suspicious and should be either removed or monitored.

7-POINT CHECKLIST In 1998, Argenziano and colleagues described a 7-point checklist based on the analysis of 342 pigmented skin lesions.[14] They distinguish three major criteria and four minor criteria (Table 37-3). Each major criterion has a score of 2 points, while each minor criterion has a score of 1 point. A minimum total score of 3 is required for the diagnosis of malignant melanoma. The 7-point checklist was the first algorithm that included the vascular architecture of a lesion.

Menzies Method

This algorithm has been descibed by Menzies et al.[15] The authors distinguish between negative features that must both be absent and positive criteria of which at least one must be found. Negative features are the following: A single color (tan, dark brown, grey, black, blue, and red, but white is not considered) and "point and axial symmetry of pigmentation" (refers to symmetry of pattern around any axis through the center of the lesion). This does not require the lesion to have symmetry of shape.

In addition, at least one or more of the positive features has to be found (Table 37-4).

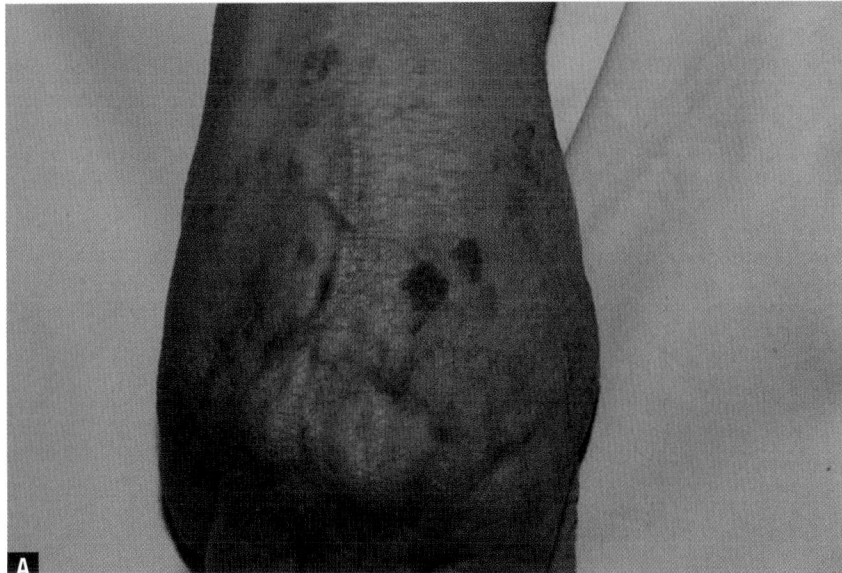

▲ **FIGURE 37-7** **A.** Clinical picture of solar lentigines, **B.** Dermoscopy of 37-(**A**) showing fingerprinting and moth-eaten border.

Table 37-4
Menzies Method

NEGATIVE FEATURES
- Symmetry of pattern
- Presence of a single color

POSITIVE FEATURES
- Blue-white veil
- Multiple brown dots
- Broadened network
- Peripheral black dots-globules
- Pseudopods
- Multiple colors (five or six)
- Radial streaming
- Scar-like depigmentation
- Multiple blue/gray dots

Digital Dermoscopy

BOX 37-5 Summary

- Handheld dermatoscopes are the easiest way to perform dermoscopy in the daily routine.
- Special coupling adapters can be used to take dermoscopy images of reasonably good quality with a handheld dermatoscope.
- Dermoscopy attachments (lenses) are more expensive but offer a superior image quality and are more user-friendly.
- Systems for digital dermoscopy are the most expensive, but are as well the most user-friendly and offer maximum comfort to the user, as well as many important

features such as digital monitoring and teledermoscopy.

Digital dermoscopy is further development of conventional dermoscopy using digital or digitized dermoscopy images. Digital dermoscopy images can be performed in many different ways:

1. The digital camera can be directly attached to a handheld dermatoscope (coupling adapters are available for most handheld devices). In this case, the camera uses the optics and the illumination of the handheld device. This is the most inexpensive way of taking dermoscopy images, but because the optics of the handheld devices is not designed to fit a camera, the images are always a bit blurred toward the periphery.

2. Dermoscopy attachments (lenses) are directly attached to digital cameras. They provide currently the best image quality, which is important, for example, for telemedicine purposes. There are many different attachments available, but we mainly use the Dermlite Foto attachment (3GEN) and recommend this for physicians who send us cases for telemedicine purposes. Of course, the image quality depends on the digital camera used.

3. Systems for digital dermoscopy consist of a video camera that is linked directly to a computer. The lesion can be examined "live" on the computer screen and most of these systems offer other features such as follow up, teledermoscopy, or computer-assisted diagnosis. Though they can make your life much easier, their disadvantage remains their high cost and their lack of portability.

The main applications for digital dermoscopy are the following.

***IN VIVO* MICROSCOPY** Handheld dermatoscopes provide images of excellent quality, but in some conditions the physician would like to see more details, especially of small and dark lesions. Some systems of digital dermoscopy use cameras with optical zooms that allow further enhancement of details. It enables the physician to see the lesion larger and thus in greater detail.

TELEDERMOSCOPY Digital dermoscopy images that have been taken with today's equipment are of excellent quality.

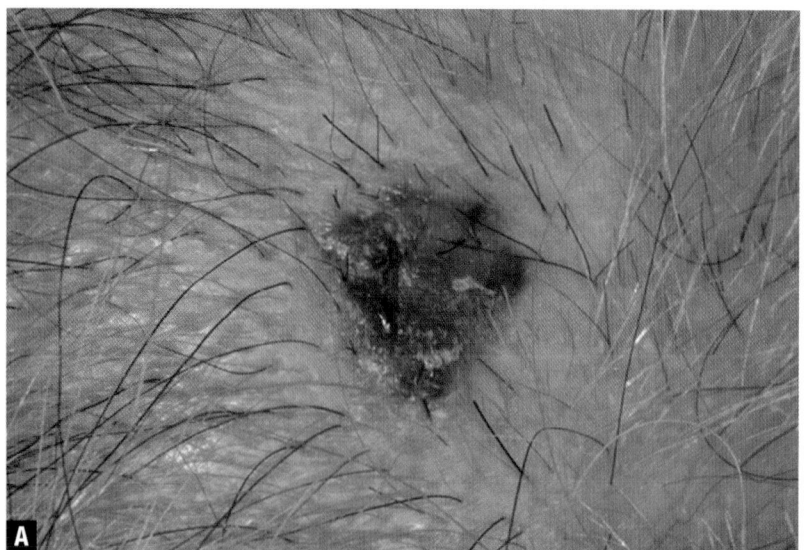

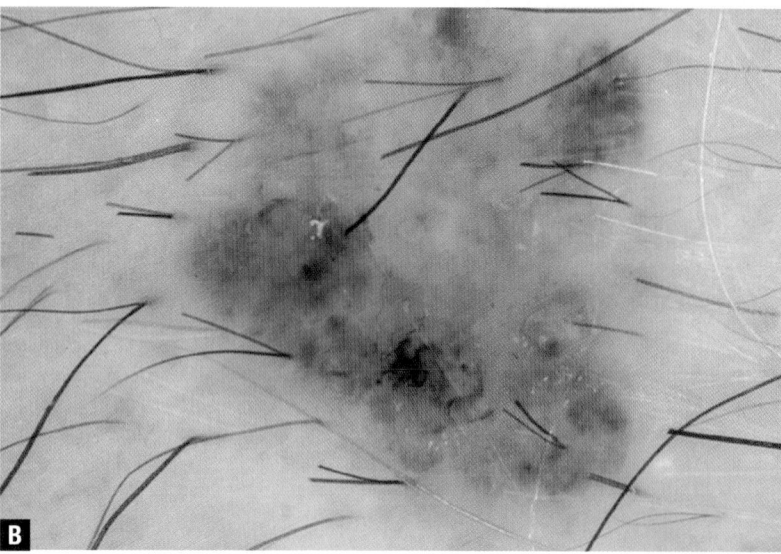

▲ **FIGURE 37-8** A. Dermoscopy of a pigmented basal cell carcinoma, **B.** Dermoscopy of (**A**) showing ulceration, arborizing telangiectasia, leaf-like areas, and multiple blue-gray dots and globules.

the lesion is not sent together with the patient information, which could theoretically allow the identification of the patient. We recommend sending this information in a separate e-mail referring to the name of the image file to avoid any confusion.

COMPUTER-ASSISTED DIAGNOSIS A digital image contains image information that can be used by a computer to try to make the diagnosis of melanoma. Several machines offering this feature are commercially available in Europe. For the moment, this feature should be considered with precaution, though it might be an important issue in the future.

FOLLOW UP OF PIGMENTED LESIONS Digital dermoscopy can be used for the follow up of pigmented lesions over time. For this purpose, the digital dermoscopy image has to be taken and stored in a way that at the next patient visit, the lesion can be easily identified and compared to the baseline image. This can be performed with any type of digital dermoscopy image, but is very convenient and comfortable with systems for digital dermoscopy. The problem is that this procedure is very time-consuming, and in patients with many pigmented lesions, it is virtually impossible to store and follow up every lesion using dermoscopy.

TOTAL BODY PHOTOGRAPHY (BODY MAPPING) It is a known fact that melanoma can either appear *de novo* or develop within a preexisting mole. Thus, the challenge is to identify new lesions or lesions that have changed in their color, size, and shape. This may pose a dilemma to the attending physician as dysplastic nevi often present as widespread lesions that may easily reach into the hundreds. For this high-risk melanoma population, total body photography is the most adequate method for identifying high-risk lesions, which can then be examined with dermoscopy and either be monitored or surgically removed. Total body photography is a routine technique in specialized centers in the United States. In fact, this technique uses a series of overview images of the skin covering the maximal surface of the skin (Fig. 37-11). To be as reproducible as possible, the images have to be taken under identical conditions (distance, illumination, etc.). At the next patient visit, the images can then be directly compared to the patient or another set of photographs of the patient (baseline image of the patient). Digital total body photography uses high-

They easily can be sent to an expert at distance for a second opinion or interpretation. This can be done by simply sending the dermoscopy picture via e-mail or using systems for digital dermoscopy, which have the built-in telemedicine module.[16] Since the patient cannot be recognized on the dermoscopy image, the issue of confidentiality is not of major concern as long as

pigmented skin lesions

Step I

melanocytic → non-melanocytic

algorithm

Step II

benign → malignant

Pattern analysis
ABCD–rule
7 point checklist
Menzies m ethod
etc.

▲ **FIGURE 37-9** Algorithm for the classification of pigmented lesions.

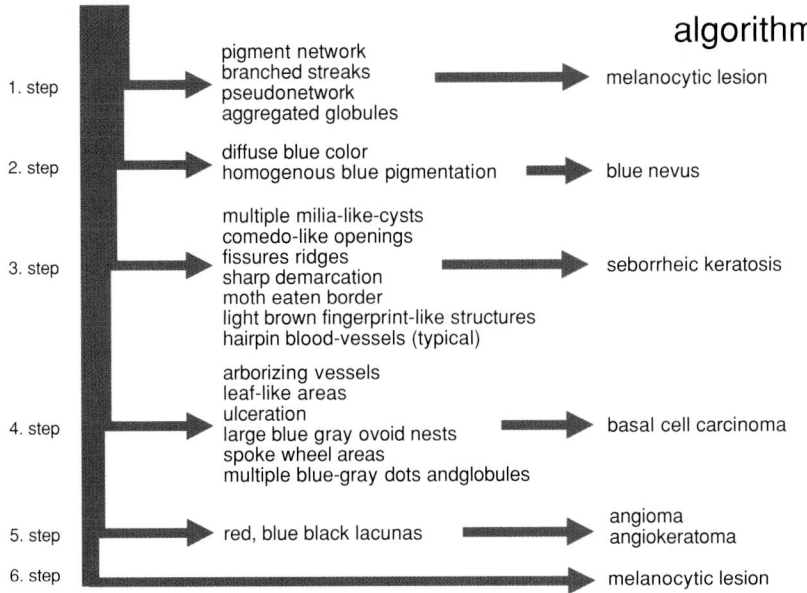

algorithm

1. step	pigment network branched streaks pseudonetwork aggregated globules	→ melanocytic lesion
2. step	diffuse blue color homogenous blue pigmentation	→ blue nevus
3. step	multiple milia-like-cysts comedo-like openings fissures ridges sharp demarcation moth eaten border light brown fingerprint-like structures hairpin blood-vessels (typical)	→ seborrheic keratosis
4. step	arborizing vessels leaf-like areas ulceration large blue gray ovoid nests spoke wheel areas multiple blue-gray dots andglobules	→ basal cell carcinoma
5. step	red, blue black lacunas	→ angioma angiokeratoma
6. step		→ melanocytic lesion

▲ **FIGURE 37-10** Algorithm for the differentiation of melanocytic and nonmelanocytic lesions.

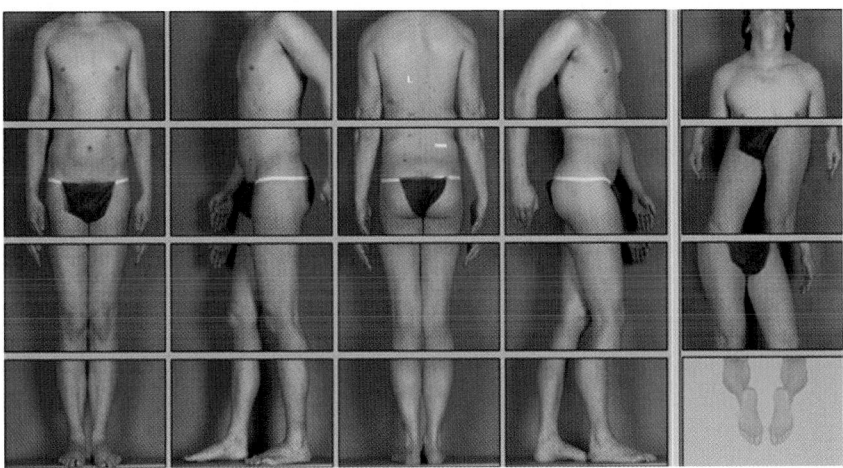

▲ **FIGURE 37-11** Screenshot of a system for digital total body photography (Dermagraphix Canfield).

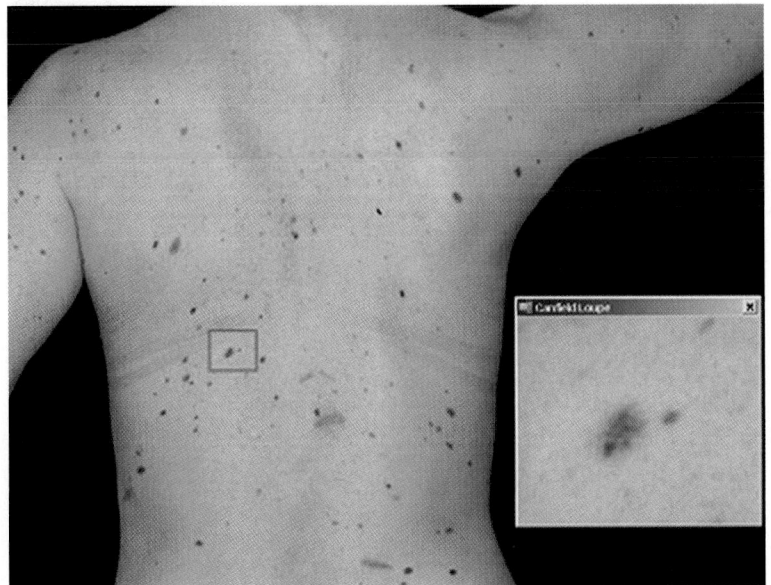

▲ **FIGURE 37-12** Back of a patient with a dysplastic nevus syndrome as well as the possibility of digital enhancement of suspect lesions.

resolution digital images of the patient. The advantages are that the images can be easily accessed during the patient visit and suspicious lesions can be compared side-by-side on the computer screen. An important advantage of digital total body photography is the fact that suspect lesions can be digitally enhanced on the screen (Fig. 37-12).

■ FINAL THOUGHTS

Dermoscopy is a great tool for every clinician who has to deal with skin cancers of all kinds. After an initial training period, it will definitively increase the diagnostic performance of the physician. The best way to learn dermoscopy is to see the patients the way you are used to and to make your biopsy decisions at the beginning the way you used to do this. Every suspicious lesion should then be examined using dermoscopy and lesions that are biopsied should be documented so that once the biopsy result is available, one can go back to the dermoscopy image. In our opinion, this is the best way to improve quickly in dermoscopy and to become familiar with the method. Digital dermoscopy with the possibility of digital monitoring of pigmented lesions brings the method to the next level. A combination with total body photography is recommended in high-risk patients as the monitoring using digital dermoscopy only allows the identification of some isolated lesions and does not allow the surveillance of the total skin surface of the patients.

Dermoscopy provides a way of avoiding unnecessary surgery and makes the diagnosis of melanoma at the earliest possible stages. This might result in important savings for health systems around the world.

REFERENCES

1. Bafounta ML, Beauchet A, Aegerter P, et al. Is dermoscopy (epiluminescence microscopy) useful for the diagnosis of melanoma? Results of a meta-analysis using techniques adapted to the evaluation of diagnostic tests. *Arch Dermatol.* 2001;137:1343–1350.
2. Kittler H, Pehamberger H, Wolff K, et al. Diagnostic accuracy of dermoscopy. *Lancet Oncol.* 2002;3:159–165.
3. Gewirtzman AJ, Saurat JH, Braun RP. An evaluation of dermoscopy fluids and application techniques. *Br J Dermatol.* 2003;149:59–63.
4. Ronger S, Touzet S, Ligeron C, et al. Dermoscopic examination of nail pigmentation. *Arch Dermatol.* 2002;138:1327–1333.
5. Malvehy J, Puig S, Braun RP, et al. *Handbook of Dermoscopy.* 1st ed. London and New York: Taylor & Francis; 2006.

6. Marghoob AA, Braun RP, Kopf AW. *Atlas of Dermoscopy*. New York: Taylor & Francis; 2004.

7. Braun RP, Rabinovitz H, Krischer J, et al. Dermoscopy of pigmented seborrheic keratosis. *Arch Dermatol*. 2002;138:1556–1560.

8. Menzies SW. Dermoscopy of pigmented basal cell carcinoma. *Clin Dermatol*. 2002;20:268–269.

9. Argenziano G, Soyer HP, Chimenti S, et al. Dermoscopy of pigmented skin lesions: Results of a consensus meeting via the Internet. *J Am Acad Dermatol*. 2003;48:679–693.

10. Pehamberger H, Steiner A, Wolff K. *In vivo* epiluminescence microscopy of pigmented skin lesions. I. Pattern analysis of pigmented skin lesions. *J Am Acad Dermatol*. 1987;17:571–583.

11. Argenziano G, Bauer J, Blum A, et al. In: Malvehy J, Puig S, eds. *Principles of Dermoscopy*; Barcelona: CEGE Editors, 2002.

12. Braun RP, Rabinovitz HS, Oliviero M, et al. Pattern analysis: A two-step procedure for the dermoscopic diagnosis of melanoma. *Clin Dermatol*. 2002;20:236–269.

13. Stolz W, Braun-Falco O, Bilek P, et al. *Color Atlas of Dermatoscopy*. 2nd ed. Berlin: Blackwell Wissenschafts-Verlag; 2002.

14. Argenziano G, Fabbrocini G, Carli P, et al. Epiluminescence microscopy for the diagnosis of doubtful melanocytic skin lesions. Comparison of the ABCD rule of dermatoscopy and a new 7-point checklist based on pattern analysis. *Arch Dermatol*. 1998;134:1563–1570.

15. Menzies SW, Crotty KA, Ingvar C, et al. *An Atlas of Surface Microscopy of Pigmented Skin Lesions*. 2nd ed. Sydney, Australia: McGraw-Hill; 2003.

16. Braun RP, Meier M, Pelloni F, et al. Teledermatoscopy in Switzerland: A preliminary evaluation. *J Am Acad Dermatol*. 2000;42:770–775.

CHAPTER 38

The Role of Sentinel Lymph-Node Biopsy in Skin Cancer Management

Frederick L. Moffat, Jr., M.D.
Carol P.R. Bowen-Wells, M.D.
Francisco J. Civantos, M.D.
M. Baris Karakullukcu, M.D.

BOX 38-1   Overview

- Assessing the lymphatics for the presence of subclinical metastases is important for certain subgroups of skin malignancies, and can allow for better treatment and determination of prognosis.
- For melanoma, SLNB has replaced conventional regional lymphadenectomies which are associated with a higher morbidity and cost.
- The sensitivity of SLNB is equal to regional lymphadenectomy in identifying involved lymph nodes, and actually superior to the conventional lymphadenectomy in identifying lymph nodes in anatomically unexpected lymphatic basins.
- The FN rate of SLNB is around 5%.
- Although not as well established as for MM, SLNB has promising results for identifying lymphatic metastasis for a certain group of patients with aggressive squamous cell carcinomas and Merkel cell carcinomas.

INTRODUCTION

BOX 38-2   Summary

- Surgical resection is the only curative treatment for early and intermediate-stage MM, and SLNB should be considered for lesions of intermediate thickness.
- Accurate nodal staging can help to select candidates for experimental adjunctive therapies.
- Formal lymphadenectomy, including the highest risk lymphatic basins, is advisable in patients known to have nodal disease.

Surgery is the sole curative treatment modality for patients with melanoma in its locoregional stages. It is therefore important that both the primary tumor and regional nodal metastases, if present, be resected at the time of initial treatment. Although in breast cancer, nodal metastases are thought to "indicate" rather than "instigate" disseminated disease, in melanoma, the available evidence strongly suggests the opposite. Untreated occult regional melanoma metastases will almost invariably progress and prejudice the prospects for cure. However, even when palpable nodal disease is present, therapeutic radical lymphadenectomy still offers the possibility of cure and long-term survival, and is essential for a favorable outcome.

The advent of effective adjuvant systemic therapy for node-positive melanoma has heightened the importance of accurate nodal staging at the time of diagnosis and initial treatment. In 1996, an Eastern Cooperative Oncology Group (ECOG) prospective randomized double-blind study of interferon α2b (IFNα2b) as adjuvant therapy in node-positive and high-risk primary melanoma demonstrated a 10% increase in 5-year survival in favor of the immunotherapy arm in node-positive patients.[1] The findings of this and subsequent studies, published in parallel with those of sentinel lymph-node biopsy (SLNB), hold forth a real hope that significant improvements in treatment outcome for cutaneous melanoma may be realized over the next decade.

Formal lymph-node dissections are expensive, morbid procedures that can disfigure and disable to the point of becoming unemployable. While assumption of such risks can be justified in melanoma patients with documented nodal metastases, doing so for nodal staging only is another matter entirely. These operations can only be of benefit if the nodal basin in question harbors metastatic melanoma. It is highly desirable that these operations be performed only in patients known to have node-positive disease.

ELECTIVE NODE DISSECTION VERSUS OBSERVATION

BOX 38-3   Summary

- ELND for management of a certain group of patients with MM provides survival benefit.
- ELND has not been shown to be superior to observation and salvage lymphadenectomy in terms of overall survival.

A decades-long debate over surgical management strategy for clinical node-negative melanoma has remained unresolved. The two competing strategies at issue were immediate "elective lymph-node dissection" (ELND) and "watchful waiting," with delayed therapeutic lymphadenectomy only if nodal metastases developed in the course of follow-up. Each strategy has been articulately and energetically advocated by its partisans in the absence of decisive evidence for either.

Retrospective data suggested a survival advantage might be conferred by ELND. Patients found to have micrometastatic nodal disease at ELND had a 44 to 61% probability of long-term survival. This compares to only 21 to 38% survival among patients undergoing resection of the primary only, of who subsequently developed clinical nodal metastases during follow-up and required salvage radical lymphadenectomy.[2-4] A recent report from a large prospective database showed a similar difference in survival in favor of patients who underwent ELND revealing occult nodal metastases.[5]

Although four of the five prospective randomized trials published to date have demonstrated survival benefit with ELND in certain subgroups of patients (Table 38-1), no overall survival advantage for ELND as compared to clinical follow-up and salvage lymphadenectomy for clinical progression was observed in any of them.[7-13] That said, one of these studies[13] demonstrated that 5-year survival of patients with micrometastases in their ELND specimens was 48% as compared to 27% for patients in the observation group who required delayed lymph-node dissection for interval development of palpable nodal disease ($p = 0.04$). These data, tantalizing though they are, are inconclusive on the question of superior outcome associated with resection of regional nodal disease when clinically occult rather than palpable.

The advent of SLNB, in affording surgeons a powerful tool with which to identify micrometastatic nodal disease in clinical node-negative melanoma patients, has sidelined the ELND controversy. This procedure permits surgeons to avoid formal lymphadenectomy in patients who do not have nodal metastases.

Table 38-1

Subsets Showing Survival Benefit in Four Prospective Randomized Trials of ELND in Clinical Node-Negative Melanoma

	PATIENT SUBSET INTERMEDIATE-THICKNESS MM	SURVIVAL BENEFIT 22% 10-YEAR SURVIVAL ADVANTAGE
WHO melanoma trial #16,[7]	• Nonulcerated MM	• 10-year survival 84% versus 77% ($p = 0.03$)
Intergroup melanoma trial[8,11,12]	• MM 1.0–2.0-mm thick	• 10-year survival 86% versus 80% ($p = 0.03$)
	• Extremity melanoma	• 10-year survival 84% versus 70% ($p = 0.05$)
Mayo Clinic trial[9]	None	—
WHO melanoma trial #15[10,13]	• Males, MM < 4 mm	• $p = 0.03$
	• Males, trunk MM	• $p = 0.04$

EXTERNAL LYMPHOSCINTIGRAPHY

BOX 38-4   Summary

- Lymphatic drainage in the head, neck, and truncal regions is unpredictable.
- Elective nodal dissections based on traditional anatomical guidelines are not likely to address the lymph nodes involved in MM.
- Preoperative LS imaging is essential in patients undergoing SLNB for melanoma because of the unpredictability and complexity of lymphatic drainage patterns, especially in truncal and head and neck sites.

Traditional concepts of lymphatic drainage in the head and neck and truncal regions, the so-called "zones of ambiguity," have been challenged and substantially discredited by lymphoscintigraphy (LS) studies in melanoma patients.[14–19] A higher than expected incidence of bilateral drainage, "skip" drainage to a more distal node in a group than might be anticipated from the location of the primary melanoma, drainage to multiple lymph-node groups, and patterns of lymphatic drainage thus far considered "unorthodox" have been documented.

In a prospective study of LS in 82 patients with clinical node-negative melanomas of the trunk and head and neck, Norman et al.[17] found that elective nodal dissections based on traditional anatomical guidelines rather than LS would not have removed all the lymphatics at risk for occult metastasis in 48 patients (59%). In this study, only one patient (1.2%) developed a metastasis in a lymphatic basin that was not predicted by LS. Berman et al[18] documented discordance between lymphoscintigraphic and clinical prediction of regional lymphatic melanoma metastasis in 24 of 36 patients (67%) with head and neck lesions. Moreover, in this series, the melanoma primary was shown to drain to a single cervical lymphatic zone or basin in only

eight patients (22%); in nine patients (25%), the drainage was to three or more zones or basins. O'Brien et al.,[19] in an LS study of 97 patients with melanoma of the head and neck, found discordance between clinical and lymphoscintigraphic prediction of lymphatic drainage in 34% of patients and multiple sentinel nodes in 85%. In 21 patients, sentinel nodes were found outside the parotid and the five main neck zones (postauricular nodes in 13 of these patients). Wells et al[20] reported discordance between LS and clinical prediction of lymphatic drainage in 21 of 25 patients with head and neck melanoma. LS definitively showed that historical concepts of lymphatic anatomy and surgical experience do not reliably predict either lymphatic drainage patterns or distribution of melanoma metastases.

Lymphatic mapping has led to a complete rethinking of cutaneous lymphatic drainage patterns in the management of melanoma and other cancers. Preoperative LS imaging is essential in patients undergoing SLNB for melanoma because of the unpredictability and complexity of lymphatic drainage patterns, especially in truncal and head and neck sites.

SENTINEL-NODE BIOPSY (SLNB) FOR CLINICALLY NODE-NEGATIVE (CN-) MALIGNANT MELANOMA

BOX 38-5   Summary

- The SLNs are the one, two, or few lymph nodes that the lymphatic vessels draining a tumor reach first in their course to that of those regional lymph-node basins.
- The ELND debate has been resolved by SLNB, and is now of historical interest only.
- Patients with negative sentinel nodes can be spared the expense and morbidity of radical surgery.
- Sentinel-node identification started with blue dye injections and evolved into the radionuclide injection techniques.

The SLNs are the one, two, or few lymph nodes that the lymphatic vessels draining a tumor reach first in their course to that or those regional lymph-node basins. The sentinel-node hypothesis is that cancer cells metastasizing through the lymphatics should seed out in the sentinel node(s) before spreading to other nodes in the affected lymph-node basins. Thus, in patients who have all SLNs free of tumor, no further regional nodal surgery is indicated. In those with positive SLNs, subsequent formal lymphadenectomy yields residual nodal metastases in 30 to 70% of cases.

The ELND debate has been overtaken by SLNB, and is now of historical interest only. The presence or absence of occult metastatic melanoma in regional nodes can be determined very accurately with this new minimally invasive technique. Thus, patients with negative sentinel nodes can be spared the expense and morbidity of radical surgery from which they could not possibly benefit, while radical lymphadenectomy and postoperative adjuvant immunotherapy would clearly be indicated in those with positive sentinel nodes.

Cabanas[21] was the first to describe SLFNB as a method of triage of patients with penile carcinoma for radical inguinal lymphadenectomy. Morton et al[22] explored this concept in a prospective study in patients with clinical node-negative (cN-) cutaneous melanoma. The sentinel node is defined as the first lymph node in a given lymphatic basin that receives lymph flow from a primary tumor site. This node is the first lymph node encountered by tumor cells metastasizing through lymphatic channels; the histological status of this node should, therefore, be highly predictive of the status of the regional lymph-node basin in which it is found.[23]

In the studies by Morton et al,[22,24] vital blue dye (isosulfan blue or patent blue-V) was injected into the dermis immediately surrounding the primary melanoma or biopsy site, and an incision was then

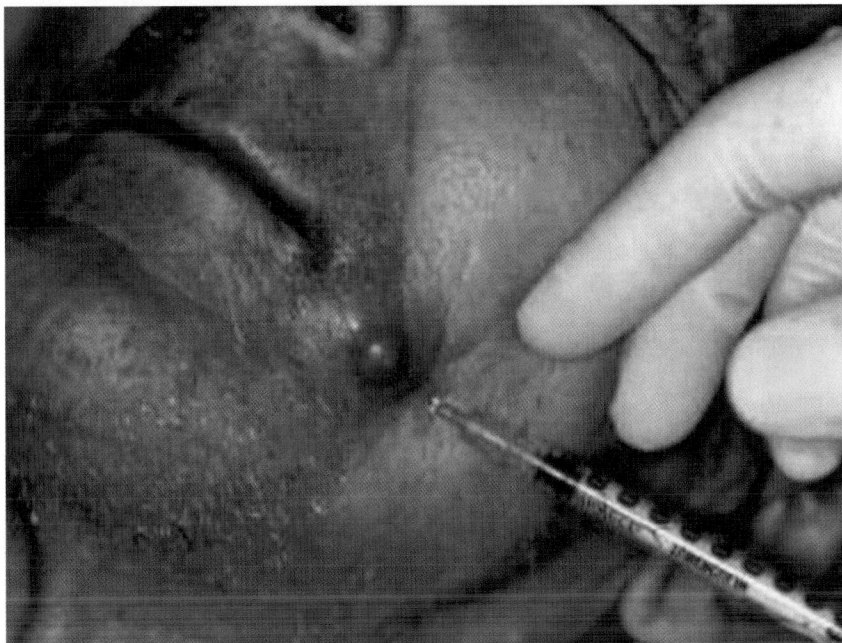

▲ **FIGURE 38-1** Radiocolloid is injected to four quadrants of the lesion in the intradermal plane.

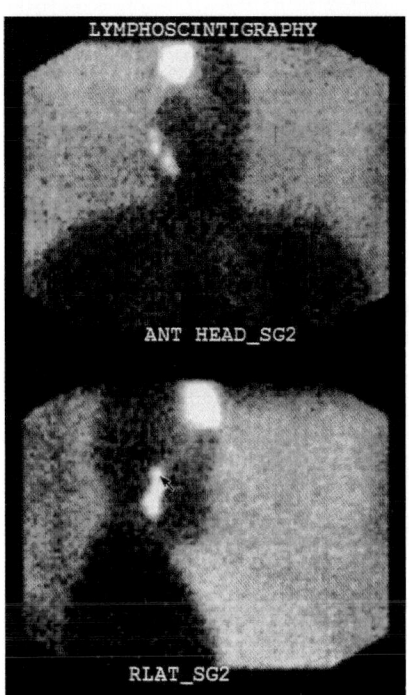

▲ **FIGURE 38-2** LS of a scalp melanoma. The scintigraphy shows uptake in the scalp where the primary skin melanoma is and two lymph nodes, one in the right parotid gland and the other in the upper neck.

made over the regional lymphatic basin at risk for metastasis. After dissection of skin flaps, one or more blue-stained lymphatics were identified and followed to one or more blue-stained nodes (the sentinel or "blue node(s)"), which were then removed for histopathologic evaluation. The biopsy was preceded by LS in ambiguous situations in which there were several possible at-risk nodal groups (i.e., melanomas located in the trunk or head and neck) to define patterns of lymphatic drainage in individual cases. Using this technique, 259 sentinel nodes were identified in 194 of 237 lymphatic nodal basins, and the incidence of false-negative (FN) sentinel nodes (that is, the identified sentinel node is found to be disease-free when metastatic disease is present in the regional lymphatics) was less than 1%. In patients with head and neck melanoma, there were no FN sentinel nodes.[24]

The innovation of using radionuclide injection instead of blue dye was introduced by Alex and Krag in 1993.[25,26] Sentinel-node biopsy has most recently been performed using peritumoral intradermal injections of 99mtechnetium sulfur colloid (99mTcSC), nuclear imaging, and intraoperative gamma detection probes (GDP)[14,15,23,25–34] (Figs. 38-1 to 38-4). This approach was developed as the blue-node technique is prone to wound infection and slough of skin edges due to the need to develop extensive skin flaps to locate blue-stained lymphatic vessels. Morton et al[22] reported wound

seromas in 5.5% of their 223 patients, wound infections in 4.8%, and wound edge necrosis in 4%. In addition, the extent of dissection in search of the blue node can be quite significant especially in the axilla, occasionally approaching that of therapeutic lymphadenectomy. The use of 99mTcSC and the GDP allows placement of the biopsy incision directly over the radiolabeled sentinel node(s), and the probe directs dissection straight to the node without disturbance of surrounding tissues.

Sentinel-node localization rates with blue dye as compared to radiocolloid and GDP, with or without blue dye, are shown in Table 38-2. Sentinel-node biopsy using the gamma probe in combination with blue dye or alone results in retrieval of sentinel nodes in 82 to 100% of cases, with a very modest incidence of FNs.[29,30]

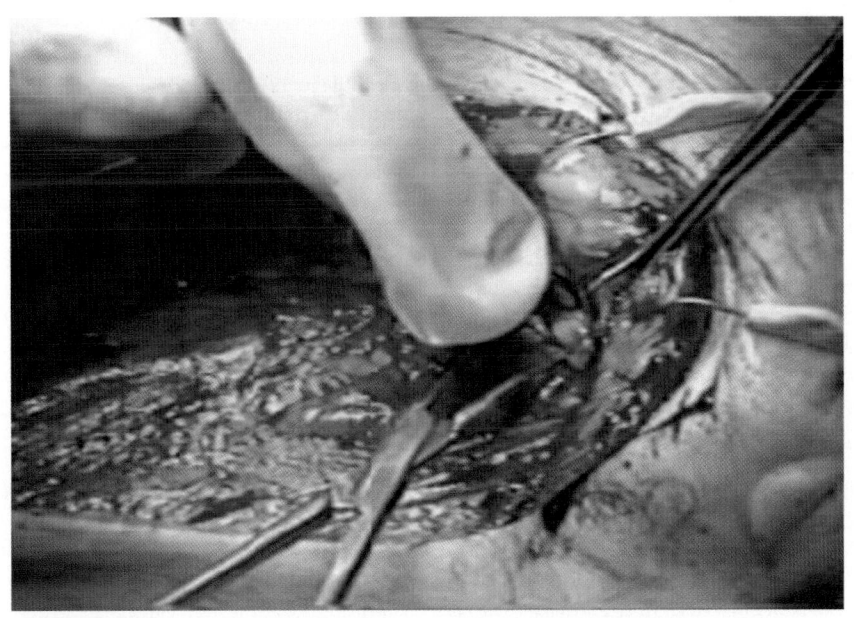

▲ **FIGURE 38-3** Dissection and removal of an upper neck (level 2) lymph node.

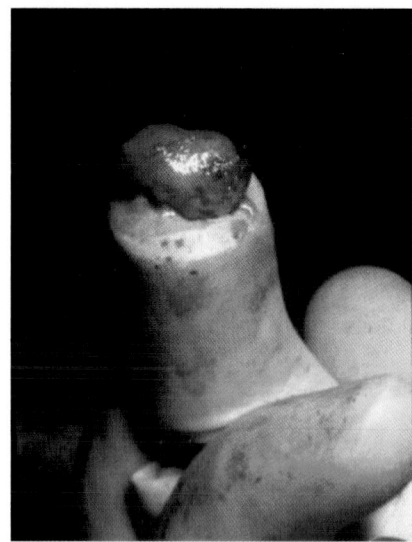

▲ **FIGURE 38-4** "Hot" lymph node has been excised and placed on the gamma probe for counting.

SELECTION OF PATIENTS FOR LYMPHOSCINTIGRAPHY AND SLNB

BOX 38-6   Summary

- For clinical node-negative (cN-) melanomas of 1 to 4 mm in thickness, there is a consensus that the incidence of occult nodal disease is sufficiently high, and that of occult systemic disease sufficiently low, to justify LS and SLNB.
- In patients with cN- melanomas of over 4 mm in thickness, SLNB has prognostic value.

The probability of regional lymph-node metastases varies by tumor site (extremities, trunk, and head and neck) and correlates directly with primary tumor microstage (Clark's levels and Breslow's depth, especially the latter), American Joint Committee on Cancer (AJCC) T category, and AJCC stages I and II subcategory.[5,39–41] In general, the risk of occult nodal metastases in patients with melanomas of less than 1 mm in thickness ("thin melanomas") is very low. Stratification of risk for nodal disease among patients with these lesions has been attempted, but a consensus as to when LS and SLNB should be offered to patients with thin melanomas has yet to be reached. Factors suggesting higher risk for nodal disease include Clark's levels III and IV lesions,[42,43] lesions of over 0.5 mm,[44] 0.76 mm,[45–47] or 0.8 mm[43,48] (depending on authors' cutoff preference) in thickness, young age, high mitotic rate, substantial

regression, and presence of vertical growth phase.[49]

For cN- melanomas of 1 to 4 mm in thickness, there is a consensus that the incidence of occult nodal disease is sufficiently high, and that of occult systemic disease sufficiently low, to justify LS and SLNB.

In patients with cN- melanomas of over 4 mm in thickness, SLNB has prognostic value. In a series of 131 such patients, Gershenwald et al[50] showed that those with negative sentinel nodes had significantly higher disease-free and overall survival as compared to those who were node-positive.

FAILURE RATES AND COMPLICATIONS OF SLNB IN MELANOMA

BOX 38-7   Summary

- Overall FN rate of SLNB is 5.5%.
- Complications associated with SLNB are less frequent than those associated with selective lymphadenectomy.

SLNB selects out pathological node-positive (pN+) patients among those with cN- melanoma, thus sparing node-negative patients the expense and morbidity of formal lymphadenectomy.

Failure of SLNB to identify node-positive disease has been documented in three studies of a total of 383 patients in

whom concurrent confirmatory ELND was performed (Table 38-3). The overall FN rate (the proportion of pN+ patients in whom SLNB yielded nodes that did not harbor metastatic disease) was 5.5%. Follow-up studies of patients in whom all identified and resected SLNs were negative have documented a clinical relapse rate in the affected nodal basin(s) of about 1% per year over the first 5 years of follow-up (Table 38-4). This figure is concordant with that reported in the studies in which confirmatory ELND was performed. These data attest to the precision of current SLNB techniques when used in melanoma patients and validate the clinical utility of the SLN hypothesis.

Although the incidence of complications with therapeutic lymphadenectomy is well documented, those of SLNB are less well defined. The Melanoma Sunbelt Trial[56] has shown that complications with SLNB are less common and significant than those of lymphadenectomy. Incidence of complications and lymphedema of patients undergoing SLNB only, with negative SLNs, were compared to those of patients with positive SLNs who then underwent complete lymph-node dissection (CLND) of the affected nodal basin(s). For those with cervical SLNs, the complication rate for SLNB alone was 2.4% as compared to 10% in those requiring neck dissections ($p = 0.008$). For patients with axillary SLNs, complication rates were 4.4% and 19%, respectively ($p < 0.0001$), and for inguinal

Table 38-2

Localization Rates for SLNB for Melanoma Blue Dye Alone Versus Radiocolloid/GDP

	BLUE DYE (%)	GDP ± BLUE DYE (%)
Krag (1995)[29]	91	100
Glass (1996)[30]	75	97
Albertini (1996)[31]	70	96
Thompson (1996)[33]	89	99
Kapteijn (1997)[35]	84	99.5
Leong (1997)[36]	73	99.2
Morton (1999)[37]	95.2	99.1
Ariyan (2004)[38]	51	100

Table 38-3

FN Rates with SLNB in cN- Melanoma Patients

	TOTAL NO. PATIENTS	NO. pN+ PATIENTS	SLN LOCALIZATION RATE (%)	FN RATE (%)
Morton (1992)[22]	223	40	82	5
Reintgen (1994)[51]	42	8	100	0
Thompson (1995)[33]	118	25	87	8
Total	383	73	85	5.5

Table 38-4
Nodal Relapse After Negative SLNB

	NO. PATIENTS	NO. NEGATIVE SLNs	MEDIAN FOLLOW-UP (MONTHS)	NODAL RELAPSE (%)	ISOLATED NODAL RELAPSE (%)
Gershenwald (1998)[52]	322	243	35	4.1	2.8
Morton (1999)[37]	584	—	45	5.0	—
Essner (1999)[53]	—	267	45	4.8	—
Cascinelli (2000)[54]	710	569	29	5.6	—
Statius Muller (2000)[55]	204	162	42	3.0	1.8
Ariyan (2004)[38]	263	235	32	1.3	—

SLNs, 8.1% and 51.2%, respectively ($p < 0.0001$). Lymphedema rates for axillary SLNB alone as compared to SLNB plus CLND were 0.3% and 4.6%, respectively ($p < 0.0001$), and the figures for inguinal procedures were 1.5% and 31.5%, respectively ($p < 0.0001$). SLNB is clearly less morbid than therapeutic lymphadenectomy in any of these three major lymph-node basins, and one can reasonably infer a similar advantage over ELND.

INTERVAL AND UNEXPECTED SLNs IN MELANOMA PATIENTS

BOX 38-8   Summary

- SLNB enables the surgeon to identify lymphatic drainage to unexpected sites that might have been missed by conventional lymphadenectomy
- Unexpected sites can include unusual patterns of drainage, or interval nodes between the primary tumor and the usual lymphatic basin.

The findings of LS in melanoma patients have refuted many of our traditional notions about lymphatic drainage of the skin. One of the most startling observations in earlier reports was drainage to "interval" lymph nodes outside any of the expected lymph-node basins in 19 to 26% of melanoma patients.[19,57–59] For extremity melanomas, drainage to epitrochlear, popliteal, or supraclavicular nodes has been documented. In head and neck melanomas, sentinel lymphatic drainage to occipital, retroauricular, facial artery, or even axillary nodes has been observed (Fig. 38-5). Truncal melanoma sites have been shown to drain directly to intermuscular, internal mammary, rectus sheath, mediastinal, para-aortic, or retroperitoneal lymph nodes. In the case of the latter three sites, excision of such nodes would be a very major undertaking, and clinical discretion is appropriate.

In three more recent studies (Table 38-5),[60–62] interval SLNs were resected in 4.7 to 7.2% of patients and 13 to 20% of these SLNs were positive for tumor. Moreover, the interval SLNs were not infrequently the only positive SLN.

SLNB AFTER DEFINITIVE RESECTION OF THE PRIMARY LESION

Concerns about alteration of lymphatic drainage patterns by wide local excision (WLE) of the primary melanoma with clear margins have been addressed and substantially allayed by a number of studies. At issue is whether prior WLE of the primary tumor would increase the FN rate of SLNB because of disruption of lymphatic vessels proximate to the tumor that metastasizing cells would normally traverse. Studies to date suggest that wide excision with closure by skin graft or rotational flap may increase the probability of an FN SLNB. However, WLE with primary closure simply increases the number of sentinel nodes, and may increase the number of lymph-node basins that have to be biopsied. However, the FN rate does not appear to be affected adversely.

Evans et al[63] reported a meta-analysis comparing 1440 patients in seven series (follow-up 15 to 36 months) in which SLNB was performed at the time of WLE to 149 patients in four series (followed for 36 to 38 months) in which SLNB was performed after WLE. SLN localization rate was not adversely affected in the 149 patients in whom SLNB was delayed and the mean number of SLNs retrieved was only slightly increased (2.0 vs. 1.7). The FN rate was slightly lower (6.0% as compared to 9.6%) in the 149 patients in whom SLNB was delayed, as was the nodal recurrence rate (2.0% vs. 2.8%).

SLNB IN THE HEAD AND NECK REGION

BOX 38-9   Summary

- Lymphatic drainage of the head and neck region has complicated patterns and anatomy.

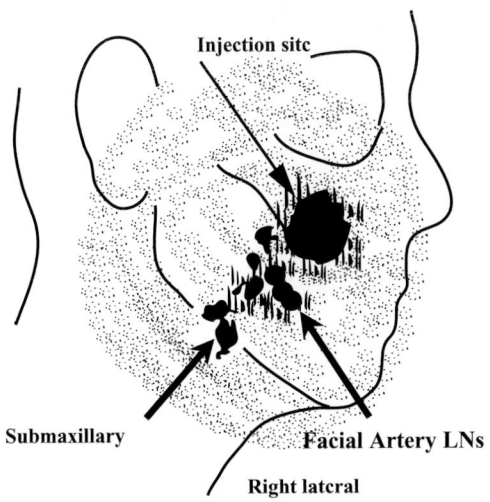

▲ FIGURE 38-5 Interval nodes imaged around the facial artery after injection of a left-cheek skin cancer.

Table 38-5
Interval Sentinel Nodes in Melanoma Patients

	NO. PATIENTS	PATIENTS WITH INTERVAL SLNs	POSITIVE INTERVAL SLNs	ONLY INTERVAL SLN(S) POSITIVE
Uren (2000)[60]	2045	148 (7.2%)	3/21 (14%)[a]	3 (100%)
Thelmo (2001)[61]	557	30 (5%)	6 (20%)	3 (10%)
Sumner (2002)[62]	1145	54 (4.7%)	7 (13%)	4 (57%)

[a]Only 21 of 148 interval SLNs were resected.

- SLNB obviates the need for elective lymphadenectomies that are associated with a high risk of morbidity.
- Several head and neck surgical teams have confirmed that sentinel-node biopsy can be performed accurately in the head and neck region.
- The FN rate of SLNB in the head and neck region is around 5%
- Although not as well established as for MM, SLNB has promising results for identifying lymphatic metastasis for a certain group of patients with squamous cell carcinomas and Merkel cell carcinomas in this anatomic region

Sentinel-node biopsy for cutaneous malignancy of the head and neck poses greater difficulty than sentinel-node biopsy of trunk or extremity cutaneous carcinomas. Melanomas in the head and neck have a higher risk of recurrence as evidenced in the Intergroup Melanoma Trial[64] and a higher incidence of nodal relapse; especially, if not all SLNs predicted on preoperative LS are accounted for at the operating table. It is possible that subspecialization and increased experience in the head and neck region may allow more complete evaluation of the head and neck region using the sentinel-node technology, and that the results may eventually approach that of other sites. In contrast to the lymphatics of the trunk and extremities, the head and neck area has a dense and complicated network of lymphatics (Fig. 38-6). Lymph nodes of the head and neck account for one-third of all the lymph nodes in the body and reach an astounding number of 200 to 300. These lymph nodes are organized into superficial and deep networks with connections at unpredictable sites. Lymphatic pathways often cross each other adding to the complexity of the lymphatic drainage of head and neck sites.[65]

The superficial lymphatic system is located within the subcutaneous fatty tissue plane. Deep to this plane is the superficial fascia of the head and neck. Lymph nodes accompany vessels and especially veins located in this plane. Major lymphatic pathways in the face and scalp accompany the facial vein at the anterior portion of the face, the superficial temporal vein at the lateral scalp and face, and the retroauricular and occipital veins at the posterior scalp and posterior to the ear. Thus, the scalp and upper facial skin will often drain to SLNs in the parotid, mastoid, and occipital regions, superior to the well-described cervical lymphatics. These superficial pathways eventually join deep lymphatic pathways to reach the neck. The superficial lymphatic pathway accompanying the facial vein drains into submandibular nodes and joins the deep lymphatic pathway. The superficial temporal pathway enters the superficial parotid gland, and later joins to the facial lymph nodes or directly to the deep lymphatic system. Retroauricular and occipital pathways join the lymphatics accompanying the internal jugular vein high in the neck. Lymphatic drainage of the lower lip has a different pattern than the other parts of the face and scalp. The lower lip drains immediately into the deep lymphatic system via the sublingual lymph nodes.[65]

The deep cervical lymphatic system is located within the fibrofatty tissue between two layers of the deep cervical fascia. These nodes are located in a large area deep to the sternocleidomastoid muscle accompanying the internal jugular vein. The deep lymphatic system is subdivided into levels. Level I comprises

VII. Lymphatic system

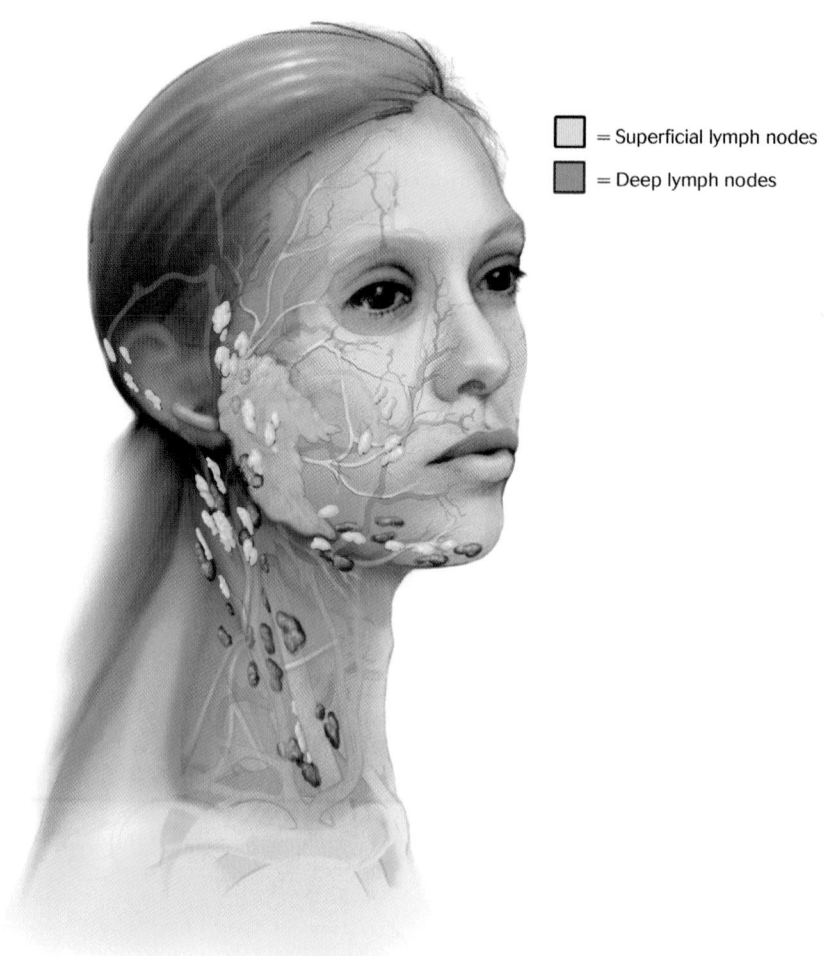

= Superficial lymph nodes

= Deep lymph nodes

▲ **FIGURE 38-6** Lymphatic drainage patterns of the head and neck area.

the submental and submandibular areas bound by the inferior border of the mandible, hyoid bone, and posterior belly of the digastric muscle. The submandibular salivary gland is located in this level and contains lymph nodes within the gland. Levels II to IV run along the internal jugular vein from the level of the digastric muscle to the level of the clavicle. Level V comprises the lymph nodes located in the posterior cervical triangle bound by the posterior margin of the sternocleidomastoid muscle, anterior border of the trapezius muscle, and the clavicle. Level V usually receives lymphatics from the areas posterior to the ear and sometimes from lymphatics running in the parotid gland. Anterior areas of the neck and scalp usually drain into Levels I to IV. Level VI includes paratracheal nodes that very rarely receive metastasis from skin cancer (Fig. 38-5).

Lymphatic patterns are well described for the head and neck. By knowing the location of the cancer, one can roughly predict which areas are under risk of lymphatic metastasis. This principle dictated that certain types of lymphatic dissections were required for tumors located in certain areas. Several kinds of neck dissections are described, based on the location of the tumors and observed patterns of clinical cervical metastases. One should keep in mind that classic neck dissections are primarily described for mucosal tumors of the upper aerodigestive tract that drain into the deep lymphatic system directly. Skin tumors of the head and neck usually first drain to the superficial lymphatic system, which is not included in the classical neck dissections. A lateral lobe parotidectomy, and careful consideration regarding the potential for preauricular, mastoid, and occipital nodes, which essentially represent so-called "in transit"

nodes, need to be considered. Performing a classical neck dissection will miss the superficial lymph nodes, especially of the face and parotid, and result in leaving tumor behind and understaging of the tumor. SLNB techniques overcome this difficulty in sampling lymph nodes for skin cancers of the face and neck. LS detects superficial lymph nodes that drain the skin area of concern.

Another advantage of sentinel-node biopsy is that it compensates for the great variability of lymphatic drainage patterns. The vast number of lymph nodes and complicated communications between them result in difficult to predict lymphatic patterns of drainage that may not follow a chain of lymph nodes classically described.[17,18] Without using the LS, adequate sampling of a lymphatic subsystem entails resection of the whole lymphatic area resulting in increased morbidity and longer operation time. Histopathologic evaluation of such a large resection specimen can lead to missed micrometastases. Looking for micrometastasis in a small number of selected sentinel nodes could be a simpler job and more precise for the pathologist.

Our experience specific to the head and neck region was published in 2006.[66] In our experience, 14 out of 103 cases (13.6%) had SLNs outside of expected lymph-node basins. These lymph nodes probably would not have been dissected with standard planned lymphadenectomy. These cases include three well-lateralized face lesions draining to the contralateral lymphatic system as well as ipsilateral drainage outside the expected subregion.

The most important feature of sentinel-node biopsy technique is its sensitivity. Several studies report an FN rate of

5% for detecting micrometastasis from malignant melanomas (MMs).[22,31,33] However, there has been some debate as to whether or not we could anticipate the same level of accuracy in the head and neck region. There can be little doubt that sentinel-node biopsy should only be performed in the head and neck region by surgeons familiar with the neurovascular anatomy and well versed in the techniques of parotidectomy and modified radical neck dissection. In our experience with 35 head and neck melanomas, we encountered one FN SLN.[66] The subsequent recurrence was in the dissected lymphatic basin. This could be the result of missed micrometastasis in pathologic analysis of the sentinel node, uneven injection of radiocolloid, or a failure to excise all hot nodes. Two additional patients with negative sentinel-node biopsies developed distant metastasis, reminding us that a negative sentinel node is not necessarily a guarantee of the absence of distant metastasis.

Other head and neck surgical teams have confirmed that sentinel-node biopsy can be performed accurately in the head and neck region. Seven reports of SLNB in head and neck melanoma are summarized in a table (see Table 38-6). The number of patients per series is modest, which may account for the disparity between them in FN rates. The initial concerning number of FNs has given way to improved experience at experienced centers. In aggregate, they echo the early experience reported by O'Brien et al.[19]

In our experience, we were able to identify sentinel nodes in 98% of the head and neck patients; a value parallel to the global success rate. Injection of blue dye has not been proven to add additional value to the overall success. In our practice, we prefer to use radiocolloid

Table 38-6
SLNB for Head and Neck Melanomatable

	NUMBER OF PATIENTS	SLN LOCALIZATION RATE	SLNs IN MULTIPLE ZONES	PATIENTS WITH POSITIVE SLNs	F/U (MONTHS)	LN RECURRENCE	FN RATE
Morton (1993)[24]	70	90%	10+%	12	—	0	0 (0%)
Bostick (1997)[67]	117	92.2%	10%	14	48	0	0 (0%)
Wells (1997)[68]	58	95%	36%	6	13	0	0 (0%)
Alex (1998)[69]	23	96%	—	3	17	1	1 (25%)
Ollila (1999)[70]	39	95%	—	4	33	1	1 (20%)
Jansen (2000)[71]	30	90%	—	8	23	3	2 (20%)
Medina-Franco (2001)[72]	38	92%	40%	4	18	2	1 (20%)
Smallbach (2003)[73]	80	96.3%	—	14	25	8	3 (4.5%)
Fincher (2004)[74]	51	—	30%	8	35	7	5 (14%)
McNeill (2005)[75]	44	94%	22.4%	7	22.4	5	0 (0%)
Civantos (2006)[66]	35	100%	13.6%	2	23	2	1 (3%)
Total	585			94		29	14 (2%)

and avoid dye injection. Avoiding dye injection also prevents possible blue staining of tissue planes that would make dissection harder, and eliminates the rare risk of anaphylaxis related to the dye. Many authors prefer to use blue dye, but all agree that the radiocolloid injection is crucial.

Although accuracy and reduced invasiveness make sentinel-node biopsy a reasonable option, there are challenges associated with this technique. The sheer complexity of the lymphatic system can result in numerous sentinel nodes in different lymphatic basins. Excisional biopsy of all of the "hot" lymph nodes may not be possible from a single small incision. Furthermore, the lymph nodes are smaller and usually either deep to, or in close contact with vital or important structures in the neck or face. Excision of perifacial lymph nodes puts distal inferior branches of the facial nerve in danger. Blunt dissection in level II deep neck nodes may result in injury to the spinal accessory nerve. Any trauma to the major vessels of the neck can cause a bleeding difficult to control from the small incision. Sentinel nodes located within the parotid gland require an extensive surgical approach to protect facial nerve function. Superficial parotidectomy may be necessary to sample parotid lymph nodes. Performing a superficial parotidectomy may seem against the principles of shorter operation time and low morbidity with sentinel-node biopsy, but will provide information that would not have been available with conventional approaches. In our series, 36 sentinel nodes were identified in the periparotid region. The main trunk of the facial nerve was identified in 10 (28%), while peripheral branches of the facial nerve were identified in 13 (36%). Facial nerve identification was not necessary in 12 (33%). No facial injury or weakness occurred in any of the patients.[66] Clearly, in the hands of an inexperienced surgeon, the risk might be higher. Our experience with sentinel biopsies performed in 106 cases in the head and neck region does not include any major complications. Thus, this method is safe when performed by surgeons with significant experience in the head and neck region.

When sentinel-node biopsy shows lymph node positive for melanoma or other cutaneous malignancy, the general principle is to perform a completion lymphadenectomy. For anterior face and neck lesions, a lateral selective neck dissection is appropriate. This dissection would include levels I to IV of the neck lymphatics. For tumors located posterior to the ear and positive lymph nodes in the parotid area, level IV should be included in the dissection.[76,77] If gross involvement of neck nodes is identified, the patient may go on to systemic therapy and/or radiation depending on the extent of disease, presence of extracapsular extension, and other details.

Sentinel-node biopsy for melanoma is currently widely practiced. In contrast to the experience with MM, sentinel-node biopsy experience with other kinds of cutaneous malignancies are limited. Head and neck surgeons encounter parotid and cervical metastases from cutaneous squamous cell carcinomas. However, these represent a small percentage of the many squamous cell carcinomas that never develop metastases. The rate of cervical metastases from cutaneous squamous cell carcinomas reportedly ranges from 0.3 to 16%. Squamous cell carcinomas are slower to invade the deeper tissues compared to MMs. Superficial dermis and epidermis is devoid of lymphatic drainage making squamous cell carcinoma less likely to spread via lymphatics. Sentinel-node biopsy of high-risk cutaneous squamous cell carcinomas is currently under investigation; however, the number of cases reported to date is not adequate to draw a conclusion.[78–80] We attempted to do sentinel node biopsies for a subgroup of high-risk cutaneous squamous cell carcinomas.[81] Table 38-7 lists the risk factors we considered to be significant. We identified one micrometastasis in 10 patients. Nine patients with negative sentinel-node biopsies were disease-free. The number is not adequate to draw any conclusions. We will be able to comment better as the experience in literature grows. In the

Table 38-7

Suggested High-Risk Criteria for Sentinel-Node Study of Squamous Cell Carcinomas of the Skin of the Head and Neck

Size greater than 2 cm;

Clinical evidence of deep invasion (over 8 mm or Clark's level IV);

Immunosupression;

Auricula, nasal vestibule, or lip carcinomas where skin is thinner;

Cancer developing in a scar from burns or trauma;

High-grade pathologic features including, perivascular, perilymphatic, or perineural invasion, single-cell invasion pattern at tumor–host interface, poor differentiation, rapid growth pattern over a short-time interval.

future, better selection criteria, including possible use of biomarkers or DNA hybridization via microarrays, might allow us to narrow our focus to those carcinomas truly at highest risk of metastasizing. This would allow us to identify a population truly at risk who might benefit from SLNB biopsy versus the current practice of waiting for clinically-evident metastases to become clinically evident.

Sentinel-node biopsy has also been studied for Merkel cell carcinoma, given its propensity to spread progressively to regional lymph nodes and distant sites. Regional nodal metastases range from 31 to 75%,[82–84] necessitating management of regional lymph nodes. A recent meta-analysis of the role of SLN studies of merkel cell carcinoma reports 40 of 60 patients (67%) with biopsy-negative SLNs had 97% locoregional control at 7.3 months median follow-up.[85] Twenty patients (33%) had a biopsy-positive SLN and 33% of this group experienced local, regional, or systemic recurrence at 12 months median follow-up. Risk of recurrence or metastasis was 19-fold greater in biopsy-positive patients. None of the 15 biopsy-positive patients who underwent therapeutic lymph-node dissection experienced a regional recurrence; three of four who did not receive therapeutic lymphadenectomy experienced regional recurrence. The meta-analysis concludes that SLN studies have an important role for management of the regional lymph nodes.[85] Other series of sentinel-node biopsies for N0 Merkel cell carcinoma report similar micrometastases rates.[82–84]

Our own experience at the University of Miami with 15 patients with Merkel cell carcinoma of the head and neck region who underwent sentinel-node biopsy resulted in seven positives after step sectioning and immunohistochemistry (IHC). Two of these positives were found only with extensive step sectioning of the sentinel node and IHC for cytokeratin. This group of patients had a median age of 62 years (range: 54 to 85 years). Follow up ranged from 5 to 84 months (median: 24 months). Patients with negative sentinel nodes were radiated to the primary site, but not to the lymphatic basin. None of the patients who underwent SLNB had any evidence of regional lymphatic or distant metastases at presentation (clinical N0 neck) by clinical and radiological staging. There were 8 T1 lesions (less than 2 cm) one T2 lesion, and five T3 lesions. Two of the 15 have recurred locally after the initial treatment and were treated again, while one patient developed distant metastases and died (7% mortality). No patient with a negative sentinel node developed regional recurrence in the lymphatic basin. The patient who developed distant metastases was immune suppressed due to the additional diagnosis of multiple myeloma. He developed local and distant metastases and died after 4 years. The remaining patients are disease-free with a median follow-up of 24 months. Given the modest period of follow-up, it is likely that additional cases have developed distant metastases years later, and were cared for elsewhere. Sentinel-node biopsy helps to determine the patients who need further lymphatic basin management in Merkel cell carcinoma. Considering the high micrometastases rate, watchful waiting is not an acceptable approach for these patients. It is reasonable to debate whether sentinel-node biopsy is enough or whether formal lymphadenectomy should be performed in all patients with Merkel cell carcinoma, particularly with significant depth of invasion. Even in this setting, lymphatic mapping and gamma probe guidance allow for a superior, gamma-probe-guided lymphadenectomy, in order to avoid missing unusual lymphatic drainage patterns or nodes outside the usual dissection.[66,86]

We conclude that LS and SLNB can be used safely and with technical success in the head and neck region, despite complex anatomy. Our data adds to the body of data supporting this approach as valid for melanoma in the head and neck region. It also adds to the early data exploring this approach as an alternative to more extensive lymphadenectomies for Merkel cell carcinoma. It offers the potential for more anatomically accurate surgery based on each patient's unique lymphatic drainage pattern.

For cutaneous squamous cell carcinoma, this represents a more aggressive approach than the standard watchful waiting approach to the lymphatics for these patients. Therefore, by showing that the risks of the procedure are low in the head and neck region, we feel justified to continue to study these procedures in this population, and other populations previously considered borderline for SLNB, after appropriate informed consent, in patients who prefer an exhaustive search for lymphatic metastases over the standard observational approach.

■ FINAL THOUGHTS

It is likely that a high-risk subgroup of patients with various types of skin malignancy can be identified that will benefit from evaluation of the sentinel node. This has been studied most for high-risk melanomas, and the depth of invasion of

1 to 4 mm is becoming a standard criterion for this procedure. Squamous cell carcinomas with certain invasive features and Merkel cell carcinomas are known to spread to regional lymph nodes, and it is possible that sentinel-node biopsy will ultimately have a role in this group. Addressing the lymphatic basins in an appropriately selected group of patients results in more accurate staging, and hopefully this will ultimately result in demonstrable survival benefits. SLNB has advantages over elective regional lymphadenectomies as a staging procedure. SLNB is associated with fewer complications, and shorter operating room times and hospital stays. SLNB is as effective as conventional lymphadenectomy in identifying microscopically involved lymph nodes and more effective in identifying lymph nodes located in unexpected regions of the body. The technique is a definite option as a less invasive alternative to formal lymphadenctomy, within the standard of care, for melanoma. Furthermore, the potential benefits in terms of more accurate excision of lymph nodes at risk and more accurate staging, can be realized in conjunction with formal lymphadenectomy, and are independent of the use of these techniques to minimize surgery. Hence, the gamma-probe-guided lymphadenectomy for higher risk situations with unpredictable lymphatic drainage, as encountered, for example, in Merkel cell carcinoma, may prove to be an option. Thus, the sentinel-node biopsy technique may ultimately improve the quality of formal lymphadenectomies, in situations where a sentinel-node biopsy alone is not advisable. In the final analysis, the role of this technology will certainly continue to evolve and may allow for better surgical care in multiple situations.

REFERENCES

1. Kirkwood JM, Strawderman MH, Ernsthoff MS, et al. Interferon α2b adjuvant therapy of high-risk resected cutaneous melanoma: The Eastern Cooperative Oncology Group Trial 1684. *J Clin Oncol*. 1996;14:7–17.
2. Cohen MH, Ketcham AS, Felix EL, et al. Prognostic factors in patients undergoing lymphadenectomy for malignant melanoma. *Ann Surg*. 1977;186:635–642.
3. Milton GW, Shaw HM, McCarthy WH, Pearson L, Balch CM, Soong S-J. Prophylactic lymph node dissection in clinical stage I cutaneous malignant melanoma: Results of surgical treatment in 1319 patients. *Br J Surg*. 1982;69:108–111.
4. Roses DF, Provet JA, Harris MN, Gumport SL, Dubin N. Prognosis of patients with pathologic stage II cutaneous malignant melanoma. *Ann Surg*. 1985;201:103–107.

5. Balch CM, Soong S-J, Gershenwald JE, et al. Prognostic factors analysis in 17,600 melanoma patients: Validation of the American Joint Committee on Cancer melanoma staging system. *J Clin Oncol*. 2001;19:3622–3634.
6. Cruse CW, Reintgen D. Treatment of the primary melanoma: A review. *Semin Surg Oncol*. 1993;9:215–218.
7. Veronesi U, Adamus J, Bandiera DC, et al. Inefficacy of immediate node dissection in stage I melanoma of the limb. *N Engl J Med*. 1977;297:627–630.
8. Balch CM, Soong S-J, Bartolucci A, et al. Efficacy of an elective regional lymph node dissection of 1 to 4 mm thick melanomas for patients 60 years of age or younger. *Ann Surg*. 1996;224:255–266.
9. Sim FH, Taylor WF, Pritchard DJ, et al. Lymphadenectomy in the management of stage I malignant melanoma: A prospective randomized study. *Mayo Clin Proc*. 1986;61:697–705.
10. Veronesi U, Adamus J, Bandiera DC, et al. Delayed regional lymph node dissection in stage I melanoma of the skin of the lower extremities. *Cancer*. 1982;49:2420–2430.
11. Balch CM, Soong S-J, Ross MI, et al. Long-term results of a multi-institutional randomized trial comparing prognostic factors and surgical results for intermediate thickness melanomas (1.0 to 4.0 mm). *Ann Surg Oncol*. 2000;7:87–97.
12. Balch CM. The role of elective lymph node dissection in melanoma: Rationale, results, and controversies. *J Clin Oncol*. 1988;6:163–172.
13. Cascinelli N, Morabito A, Santinami M, et al. Immediate or delayed dissection of regional nodes in patients with melanoma of the trunk: A randomized trial. *Lancet*. 1998;351:793–796.
14. Pijpers R, Collet GJ, Meijer S, Hoekstra OS. The impact of dynamic lymphoscintigraphy and gamma probe guidance on sentinel node biopsy in melanoma. *Eur J Nucl Med*. 1995;22:1238–1241.
15. Uren RF, Howman-Giles R, Thompson JF. Lymphoscintigraphy to identify sentinel lymph nodes in patients with melanoma. *Melanoma Res*. 1994;4:395–399.
16. Ross MI, Reintgen D, Balch CM. Selective lymphadenectomy: Emerging role for lymphatic mapping and sentinel node biopsy in the management of early stage melanoma. *Semin Surg Oncol*. 1993;9:219–223.
17. Norman J, Cruse CW, Espinosa C, et al. Redefinition of cutaneous lymphatic drainage with the use of lymphoscintigraphy for malignant melanoma. *Am J Surg*. 1991;162:432–437.
18. Berman CG, Norman J, Cruse CW, et al. Lymphoscintigraphy in malignant melanoma. *Ann Plast Surg*. 1992;28:29–32.
19. O'Brien CJ, Uren RF, Thompson JF. Prediction of potential metastatic sites in cutaneous head and neck melanoma using lymphoscintigraphy. *Am J Surg*. 1995;170:461–466.
20. Wells KE, Cruse CW, Daniels S, Berman C, Norman J, Reintgen DS. The use of lymphoscintigraphy in melanoma of the head and neck. *Plast Reconstr Surg*. 1994;93:757–761.
21. Cabanas R. An approach for the treatment of penile carcinoma. *Cancer*. 1977;39:456–466.

22. Morton DL, Wen D-R, Wong JH, et al. Technical details of intraoperative lymphatic mapping for early stage melanoma. *Arch Surg.* 1992;27:392–399.

23. Gulec SA, Moffat FL, Carroll RG. The expanding clinical role of intraoperative gamma probes. In: Freeman LM, ed. *Nuclear Medicine Annual 1997.* Philadelphia, PA: Lippincott-Raven; 1997:209–237.

24. Morton DL, Wen D-R, Foshag LJ, Essner R, Cochran A. Intraoperative lymphatic mapping and selective cervical lymphadenectomy for early-stage melanomas of the head and neck. *J Clin Oncol.* 1993;11:1751–1756.

25. North JH Jr, Spellman JE. Role of sentinel node biopsy in the management of malignant melanoma. *Oncology.* 1996;10:1237–1242.

26. Alex JC, Krag DN. Gamma-probe guided localization of lymph nodes. *Surg Oncol.* 1993;2:137–143.

27. Alex JC, Weaver DL, Fairbanks JT, Rankin BS, Krag DN. Gamma probe-guided lymph node localization in malignant melanoma. *Surg Oncol.* 1993;2:303–308.

28. Krag DN, Weaver DL, Alex JC, Fairbank JT. Surgical resection and radiolocalization of the sentinel node in breast cancer using a gamma probe. *Surg Oncol.* 1993;2:335–340.

29. Krag DN, Meijer SJ, Weaver DL, et al. Minimal-access surgery for staging of malignant melanoma. *Arch Surg.* 1995;130:654–658.

30. Glass LF, Messina JL, Cruse W, et al. The use of intraoperative radiolymphoscintigraphy for sentinel node biopsy in patients with malignant melanoma. *Dermatol Surg.* 1996;22:715–720.

31. Albertini JJ, Cruse CW, Rapaport D, et al. Intraoperative radiolymphoscintigraphy improves sentinel node identification in patients with melanoma. *Ann Surg.* 1996;223:217–224.

32. Godellas CV, Berman CG, Lyman G, et al. The identification and mapping of melanoma regional nodal metastases: Minimally invasive surgery for the diagnosis of nodal metastases. *Am Surg.* 1995;61:97–101.

33. Thompson JF, McCarthy WH, Bosch CMJ. Sentinel node status as an indicator of the presence of metastatic melanoma in regional lymph nodes. *Melanoma Res.* 1995;5:255–260.

34. Reintgen D, Albertini J, Miliotes G, et al. The accurate staging and modern day treatment of malignant melanoma. *Cancer Res Ther Control.* 1995;4:183–197.

35. Kapteijn BAE, Nieweg OE, Liem IH, Mooi WJ, Balm AJM, Muller SH. Localizing the sentinel node in cutaneous melanoma: Gamma probe detection versus blue dye. *Ann Surg Oncol.* 1997;4:156–160.

36. Leong SPL, Steinmetz I, Habib FA, et al. Optimal selective sentinel lymph node dissection in primary malignant melanoma. *Arch Surg.* 1997;132:666–673.

37. Morton DL, Thompson JF, Essner R, et al. Validation of the accuracy of intraoperative lymphatic mapping and sentinel lymphadenectomy for early-stage melanoma. A multicenter trial. *Ann Surg.* 1999;230:453–465.

38. Ariyan S, Ariyan C, Farber LR, Fischer DS, Flynn SD, Truini C. Reliability of identification of 655 sentinel lymph nodes in 263 consecutive patients with malignant melanoma. *J Am Coll Surg.* 2004;198:924–932.

39. Rousseau DL, Ross MI, Johnson MM, et al. Revised American Joint Committee on Cancer. Staging criteria accurately predict sentinel lymph node positivity in clinically node-negative melanoma patients. *Ann Surg Oncol.* 2003;10:569–574.

40. Slingluff CL, Stidham KR, Ricci WM, Stanley WE, Seigler HF. Surgical management of regional nodes in patients with melanoma. Experience with 4682 patients. *Ann Surg.* 1994;219:120–130.

41. Doubrovsky A, De Wilt JH, Scolyer RA, McCarthy WH, Thompson JF. Sentinel node biopsy is more accurate than elective lymph node dissection in determining the regional node status of patients with cutaneous melanoma. *Ann Surg Oncol.* 2004;11:S122–S123.

42. Corsetti RL, Allen HM, Wanebo HJ. Thin ≤ 1 mm level II and IV melanomas are higher risk lesions for regional failure and warrant sentinel lymph node biopsy. *Ann Surg Oncol.* 2003;7:456–460.

43. Zapas JL, Coley HC, Beam SL, Brown SD, Jablonski KA, Elias EG. The risk of regional lymph node metastases in patients with melanoma less than 1.0 mm thick: Recommendations for sentinel lymph node biopsy. *J Am Coll Surg.* 2003;197:403–407.

44. Ranieri JM, Wagner JD, Wenck SD, Calley C, Coleman JJ III. The prognostic relevance of sentinel lymph node biopsy in thin melanoma patients. *Ann Surg Oncol.* 2004;11:S122.

45. Bleicher RJ, Essner R, Foshag LJ, Wanek LA, Morton DL. Role of sentinel lymphadenectomy in tin invasive melanomas. *J Clin Oncol.* 2003;21:1326–1331.

46. Jacobs IA, Chang CK, DasGupta TK, Salti GI. Role of sentinel lymph node biopsy in patients with thin (<1 mm) primary melanoma. *Ann Surg Oncol.* 2003;10:558–561.

47. Bedrosian I, Gershenwald JE. Surgical clinical trials in melanoma. *Surg Clin N Am.* April 2003;83(2):385–403.

48. Vacquerano J, Kraybill W, Cheney R, Kane JM. Indications for sentinel lymph node biopsy in thin melanomas. *Ann Surg Oncol.* 2004;11:S77–S78.

49. Bedrosian I, Faries MB, Guerry DuPont IV, et al. Incidence of sentinel node metastasis in patients with thin primary melanoma (≤1 mm) with vertical growth phase. *Ann Surg Oncol.* 2000;7:262–267.

50. Gershenwald JE, Mansfield PF, Lee JE, Ross MI. Role for lymphatic mapping and sentinel lymph node biopsy in patients with thick (≥4 mm) primary melanoma. *Ann Surg Oncol.* 2000;7:160–165.

51. Reintgen DS, Cruse CW, Wells K, et al. The orderly progression of melanoma nodal metastases. *Ann Surg.* 1994;220:759–767.

52. Gershenwald JE, Colome MI, Lee JE, et al. Patterns of recurrence following a negative sentinel lymph node biopsy in 243 patients with stage I or II melanoma. *J Clin Oncol.* 1998;16:2253–2260.

53. Essner R, Conforti A, Kelley MC, et al. Efficacy of lymphatic mapping, sentinel lymphadenectomy, and selective complete node dissection as a therapeutic procedure for early-stage melanoma. *Ann Surg Oncol.* 1999;6:442–449.

54. Cascinelli N, Belli F, Santinami M, et al. Sentinel lymph node biopsy in cutaneous melanoma: The WHO Melanoma Program experience. *Ann Surg Oncol.* 2000;7:467–474.

55. Statius Muller MG, Borgstein PJ, Pijpers R, et al. Reliability of the sentinel node procedure in melanoma patients: Analysis of failures after long-term follow-up. *Ann Surg Oncol.* 2000;7:461–468.

56. Wrightson WR, Wong SL, Edwards MJ, et al. Complications associated with sentinel lymph node biopsy for melanoma. *Ann Surg Oncol.* 2003;10:676–680.

57. Norman J, Wells K, Kearney R, Cruse CW, Berman C, Reintgen D. Identification of lymphatic drainage basins in patients with cutaneous melanoma. *Semin Surg Oncol.* 1993;9:224–227.

58. McCarthy WH, Shaw HM, McCarthy SW, Rivers JK, Thompson JF. Cutaneous melanomas which defy conventional prognostic indicators. *Semin Oncol.* 1996;23:709–713.

59. Uren RF, Howman-Giles RB, Shaw HM, Thompson JF, McCarthy WH. Lymphoscintigraphy in high-risk melanoma of the trunk: Predicting draining node groups, defining lymphatic channels, and locating the sentinel node. *J Nucl Med.* 1993;34:1435–1440.

60. Uren RF, Howman-Giles R, Thompson JF, et al. Interval nodes: The forgotten sentinel nodes in patients with melanoma. *Arch Surg.* 2000;135:1168–1172.

61. Thelmo MC, Morita ET, Treseler PA, et al. Micrometastasis to in-transit lymph nodes from extremity and truncal malignant melanoma. *Ann Surg Oncol.* 2001;8:444–448.

62. Sumner WE III, Ross MI, Mansfield PF, et al. Implications of lymphatic drainage to unusual sentinel lymph node sites in patients with primary cutaneous melanoma. *Cancer.* 2002;95:354–360.

63. Evans HL, Krag DN, Teates CD, et al. Lymphoscintigraphy and sentinel node biopsy accurately stage melanoma in patients presenting after wide local excision. *Ann Surg Oncol.* 2003;10:416–425.

64. Balch CM, Soong SJ, Smith T, et al. Long-term results of a prospective surgical trial comparing 2 cm vs. 4 cm excision margins for 740 patients with 1 to 4 mm melanomas. *Ann Surg Oncol.* 2001;8:101–108.

65. Alex JC. The application of sentinel node radiolocalization to solid tumors of the head and neck: A 10-year experience. *Laryngoscope.* 2004;114:2–19.

66. Civanto FJ, Moffat FI, Goodwin WJ. Lymphatic mapping and sentinel lymphadenectomy for 106 head and neck lesions: Contrasts between oral cavity and cutaneous malignancy. *Laryngoscpe.* 2006;16:1–15.

67. Bostick P, Essner R, Sarantou T, et al. Intraoperative lymphatic mapping for early-stage melanoma of the head and neck. *Am J Surg.* 1997;174:536–553.

68. Wells KE, Rapaport DP, Cruse CW, et al. Sentinel lymph node biopsy in melanoma of the head and neck. *Plast Reconstr Surg.* 1997;100:591–594.

69. Alex JC, Krag DN, Harlow SP, et al. Localization of regional lymph nodes in melanomas of the head and neck. *Arch Otolaryngol Head Neck Surg.* 1998;124:135–140.

70. Ollila DW, Foshag LJ, Essner R, Stern SL, Morton DL. Parotid region lymphatic mapping and sentinel lymphadenectomy for cutaneous melanoma. *Ann Surg Oncol.* 1999;6:150–154.

71. Jansen L, Koops HS, Nieweg OE, et al. Sentinel node biopsy for melanoma in the head and neck region. *Head Neck.* 2000;22:27–33.

72. Medina-Franco H, Beenken SW, Heslin MJ, Urist MM. Sentinel node biopsy for cutaneous melanoma in the head and neck. *Ann Surg Oncol.* 2001;8:716–719.

73. Schmalbach CE, Nussenbaum B, Rees RS, Schwartz J, Johnson TM, Bradford CR. Reliability of sentinel lymph node mapping with biopsy for head and neck cutaneous melanoma. *Arch Otolaryngol Head Neck Surg.* 2003;129(1): 61–65.

74. Fincher TR, O'Brien JC, McCarty TM, et al. Patterns of drainage and recurrence following sentinel lymph node biopsy for cutaneous melanoma of the head and neck. *Arch Otolaryngol Head Neck Surg.* 2004;130(7):844–848.

75. MacNeill KN, Ghazarian D, McCready D, Rotstein L. Sentinel lymph node biopsy for cutaneous melanoma of the head and neck. *Ann Surg Oncol.* 2005; 12(9):726–732.

76. Shah JP, Kraus DH, Dubner S, Sarkar S. Patterns of regional lymph node metastases from cutaneous melanomas of the head and neck. *Am J Surg.* 1991;162:320–323.

77. Shah JP, Andersen PE. The impact of patterns of nodal metastases on modifications of neck dissection. *Ann Surg Oncol.* 1994;1:521–532.

78. Weisberg NK, Bertagnolli MM, Becker DS. Combined sentinel lymphadenectomy and Mohs micrographic surgery for high-risk cutaneous squamous cell carcinoma. *J Am Acad Dermatol.* 2000; 43(3):483–488.

79. Reschly MJ, Messina J, Zaulyanov LL, Cruse W, Fenske NA. Utility of sentinel lymphadenectomy in the management of patients with high-risk cutaneous squamous cell carcinoma. *Dermatol Surg.* 2003; 29(2):135–140.

80. Altinyollar H, Berberoglu U, Celen O. Lymphatic mapping and sentinel node biopsy in squamous cell carcinoma of the lower lip. *Eur J Surg Oncol.* 2002;28: 72–74.

81. Veness MJ, Palme ME, Morgan GC. High-risk cutaneous squamous cell carcinoma of the head and neck: Results from 266 treated patients with metastatic lymph node disease. *Cancer.* 2006;106(11): 2389–2396.

82. Gupta SG, Wang LC, Penas PF, Gellenthin M, Lee SJ, Nghiem P. Sentinel lymph node biopsy for evaluation and treatment of patients with Merkel cell carcinoma: The Dana–Farber experience and meta-analysis of the literature. *Arch Dermatol.* 2006;142(6):685–690.

83. Schmalbach CE, Loewe L, Teknos TN, Johnson TM, Bradford CR. Reliability of sentinel lymph node biopsy for regional staging of head and neck Merkel cell carcinoma. *Arch Otolaryngol Head Neck Surg.* 2005;131(7):610–614.

84. Maza S, Trefzer U, Hofmann M, et al. Impact of sentinel lymph node biopsy in patients with Merkel cell carcinoma: Results of a prospective study and review of the literature. *Eur J Nucl Med Mol Imaging.* 2006;33(4):433–440.

85. Mehrany K, Otley CC, Weenig RH, Phillips PK, Roenigk RK, Nguyen TH. A meta-analysis of the prognostic significance of sentinel lymph node status in Merkel cell carcinoma. *Dermatol Surg.* February 2002;28(2):113–117.

86. Civantos F, Shnayder Y, Bared A, et al. Lymphoscintigraphy and Sentinel Node Biopsy for Merkel Cell Carcinoma of the Head and Neck. In: *Presentation at the American Head and Neck Society*, August 17–20, 2006. Chicago, IL; In press.

CHAPTER 39

Surgical Excision

Ivan D. Camacho, M.D.
Keyvan Nouri, M.D.

BOX 39-1   Overview

- Surgical excision is the most common and accepted treatment for melanoma and nonmelanoma skin cancer.
- Most authors recommend a 4-mm surgical margin in the treatment of nonmelanoma skin cancers.
- Mohs micrographic surgery is currently considered the treatment of choice for skin cancers, under the following indications: recurrent BCCs and SCCs, poorly differentiated tumors and aggressive histological types, large tumors, tumors in areas of high risk of recurrence, tumors with poorly defined clinical margins, tumors with positive margins after conventional excision, tumors located in areas where tissue sparing is required, tumors arising at sites of chronic scarring and in immuno-compromised patients, and those causing perineural invasion.
- Based on multiple clinical trials, current recommendations regarding the optimal surgical management of the primary cutaneous melanoma are as follows: a 5-mm surgical resection margin for melanoma *in situ* lesions, a 1-cm surgical margin for melanoma lesions less than 2 mm in thickness (by Breslow microstaging), and a 2-cm surgical margin for melanoma lesions equal or greater than 2 mm in thickness.
- Sentinel-node biopsy and dissection is mostly recommended in patients with tumors between 1 and 4 mm in thickness, where positive nodes can be expected in up to 25% of cases and lymphadenectomy will reveal another 15 to 20% of nodal metastases.
- Nodal staging also helps to identify appropriate candidates for adjuvant immunotherapy with interferon alpha-2b, improving the overall 5-year disease-free survival of patients with positive regional nodes.

INTRODUCTION

Surgical excision of melanoma and nonmelanoma skin cancer (NMSC) is the most common and accepted method for treating these cutaneous malignancies. The effective surgical resection of skin cancer requires considerable skills in identifying the clinical margins of the tumor and avoiding unnecessary surgical resection of uninvolved skin, while preserving the greatest possibility of complete surgical removal.[1]

NONMELANOMA SKIN CANCER

BOX 39-2   Summary

- A 4-mm surgical margin is generally acceptable for all types of nonmelanoma skin cancers.
- Well-demarcated tumors such as nodular BCC may be excised with a smaller 3-mm surgical margin.
- The mean interval between excision and recurrence is on average 2 years.
- For some particular indications, Mohs micrographic surgery is currently considered the treatment of choice: recurrent BCCs and SCCs, poorly differentiated tumors and aggressive histological types, large tumors, tumors in areas of high risk of recurrence, tumors with poorly defined clinical margins, tumors with positive margins after conventional excision, tumors located in areas where tissue sparing is required, tumors arising at sites of chronic scarring and in immuno-compromised patients and those causing perineural invasion.

Nonmelanoma skin cancer (NMSC), primarily basal cell carcinoma (BCC) and squamous cell carcinoma (SCC), is the most common malignancy of white populations[2] with increasing incidence rates of 3% and 8% per year for BCC and SCC, respectively.[3] Because the microscopic margin is often considered to extend beyond the macroscopic margin, surgical excision of basal cell and squamous cell carcinomas should include a margin of healthy skin. In the past, the suggested excision margins for nonmelanotic skin cancers were based mostly on the surgeon's experience rather than scientific evidence, and ranged from 2 to 10 mm for BCC and 4 to 15 mm for SCC. The likelihood of recurrence is directly related to the adequacy of the excision and the main goal is to completely excise the tumor, thereby preventing recurrence and metastases. However, excessively wide skin margins should be avoided as this sacrifices normal tissue.[4,5]

A prospective study performed on 150 primary nonmelanotic skin lesions, clinically diagnosed as either BCC (nodular, superficial, infiltrating, or sclerosing) or SCC (well, moderately, or poorly differentiated), were excised over a 9-month period in an outpatient facility. After completing the histopathologic analysis of the macroscopically assessed and excised lesions, the authors recommend a 4-mm surgical margin as the optimal margin in the treatment of nonmelanotic skin cancers up to 2 cm in diameter, achieving a microscopic free lateral margin beyond one microscopic high-power field (0.5 mm) in 96% of cases of BCC and in 97% of cases of SCC. No incomplete excisions were found at the deep margin. If the borders of the tumor are well demarcated, such as a nodular BCC, then an excision margin of 3 mm may be appropriate.

Several other studies were developed aiming to establish the most appropriate surgical excision margins for BCC and SCC. Pascal et al.,[6] examined 143 primary nonmultifocal BCCs over a 5-year follow-up period and correlated the recurrence rate to the microscopic margin taken. They found that BCCs excised beyond 0.5 mm of normal tissue, or one microscopic high-power field ($\times 400$), had a recurrence rate of 1.2%. The recurrence rate was 12% when the tumor was within 0.5 mm or one microscopic high-power field of the surgical margin and 33% when the tumor involved the margin itself. The mean interval between excision and recurrence was 24 months; there was no significant difference between the frequency of recurrent tumors involving the lateral edge of excisions and those involving the deep surface. Liu et al.,[7] showed a 5-year recurrence rate of 17% when the lateral margin was positive and 33% when the deep margin was positive. Those findings were contradicted by Pearl et al.,[8] who showed a 100% recurrence rate in a 4-year follow-up of a small series of BCC excisions with positive margins.

Most authors advised re-excising all lesions having marginal involvement as soon as the wound has healed. Patients who do not undergo re-excision and those who have had two or more previous BCCs should be followed up every 3 to 4 months during the first year and annually thereafter for a minimum of 5 years, as they are at an increased risk of tumor recurrence, new lesions, or both.

Based on an analysis of 141 SCCs, Brodland and Zitelli[9] concluded that for SCCs smaller than 20 mm in diameter, a 95% clearance was achieved with a 4-mm margin, whereas a 6-mm margin was required for 95% clearance of lesions 20 mm or larger, or lesions with the following characteristics: histologic grades 2, 3, and 4; location on the scalp, ears, eyelids, nose, and lips; and invasion to the level of the subcutaneous tissue.

Mohs micrographic surgery is currently considered the treatment of choice in certain indications, where a higher cure rate along with lower recurrence and metastases rates are documented, compared to conventional surgical excision: recurrent BCCs and SCCs, because of their unpredictable growth pattern along the surgical scar and through low-resistance planes; poorly differentiated tumors and aggressive histological types such as the morpheaform, micronodular, infiltrative, and metatypical BCC; large tumors, defined as tumors larger than 2 cm on the trunk and extremities or 1 cm on the face and neck; tumors in areas of high risk of recurrence such as the H-zone of the face and skin overlying cartilage and bony structures like in the preauricular area, retroauricular sulcus, nasolabial fold, inner canthus, philtrum, temple, upper lip, columella, nose, and lower eyelids; tumors with poorly defined clinical margins; incompletely excised tumors and tumors with positive margins after conventional excision, as the scar becomes a low-resistance pathway to deep infiltration of malignant cells; tumors located in areas where tissue sparing is required such as the fingers, toes, eyelids, and genitalia; tumors arising at sites of chronic scarring due to radiodermatitis, osteomyelitis, and ulcers; tumors in immunocompromised patients, either by medications or infection; tumors with a high risk of metastases such as those invading the dermis to a depth of 4 mm or more (Clark level IV and V); tumors causing perineural invasion, often asymptomatic or manifested by pain or paresthesias; and other rare tumors such as dermatofibrosarcoma protuberans (DFSC) and microcystic adnexal carcinoma.[10–15]

PRIMARY CUTANEOUS MELANOMA

BOX 39-3 Summary

- Breslow thickness is the most accepted method for assessing melanoma lesions and determining prognosis.
- Based on multiple studies, the current recommendations on the surgical management of the primary cutaneous melanoma favor a 5-mm surgical margin for melanoma *in situ* lesions; a 1-cm surgical margin for thin melanoma lesions (<2 mm in thickness); and a 2-cm surgical margin for melanoma lesions greater than 2 mm in thickness.
- The presence of ulceration of the primary melanoma was reported to be a significant prognostic factor, indicating a 6 to 8-fold increased risk of local recurrence and metastatic disease.
- Melanomas of the head and neck have a higher risk of local recurrence whereas thin melanomas of the hands and feet have a lower incidence of nodal metastases.

Malignant melanoma is currently the malignancy with most rapidly rising incidence in the United States and an estimated 60,000 new cases of cutaneous melanoma will be diagnosed in 2007.[16] As the incidence of malignant melanoma is increasing and surgical excision of the lesion remains the mainstay of treatment for primary cutaneous melanoma, it becomes necessary to optimize the surgical management of these patients.

However, how much of the normal skin should be excised around the primary melanoma is controversial. For decades, a wide local excision with a perilesional margin as large as 5 cm was the standard surgical treatment, with the conviction that a large excision would provide optimal outcomes in terms of local recurrence rate and overall survival; resulting in significant morbidity and cosmetic disfiguring that required extensive skin grafting and therefore the use of additional resources and more intensive wound care.[17]

Some studies supported an extensive excision: increased numbers of melanocytes were found in the clinically normal skin surrounding many melanomas, and melanocytic activation was reported up to 4 cm from the primary tumor in clinically normal skin.[18,19] In some cases, extremely wide excisions were recommended because recurrences were found up to 15 cm from the original site of primary tumor excision.[20]

In 1975, Dr. Alexander Breslow described a method for determining the prognosis of melanoma patients, based on his observations that the thickness of a melanoma is related to the 5-year survival rate after the surgical removal of the tumor (see Fig. 39-1). The Breslow thickness (Table 39-1) is currently in wider use than an older system, the Clark level of

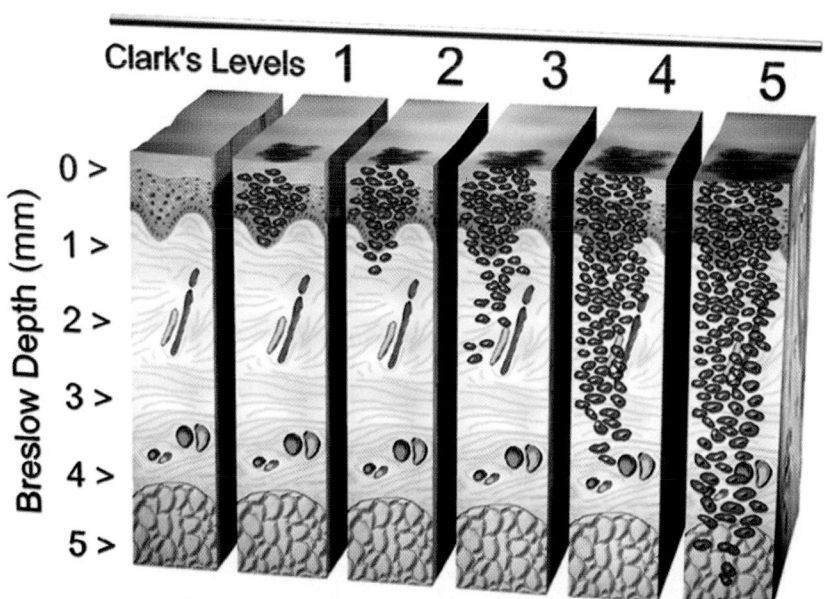

▲ **FIGURE 39-1** Breslow thickness and Clark levels. (with permission from Med-Art~www.med-ars.it).

Table 39-1

Breslow Thickness and 5-Year Survival

LESION THICKNESS (-mm)	5-YEAR SURVIVAL
<0.75	99%
0.76–1.5	94%
1.51–3.99	78%
>4.00	42%

Modified from Skin Cancer Unit, www.kcl.ac.uk

invasion (Table 39-2)—a method described by the pathologist Wallace Clark for measuring the depth of penetration of a melanoma into the skin according to the anatomic layers: epidermis, dermis, and subcutaneous tissue. The Clark level adds little additional information except for the level-I tumors.

Several large multicentric studies have illustrated the importance of tumor thickness in predicting local disease recurrence and have suggested that a moderate conservative approach in the surgical excision margin size would be sufficient for thin lesions.[21]

The World Health Organization (WHO) Melanoma Program led by Veronesi et al.[22,23] studied 612 patients with malignant melanoma of 2 mm or less in thickness with a mean follow-up of 90 months; concluding that a 1-cm radial margin for thin melanoma (<1 mm) was as safe as a 3-cm margin or more, with no evidence of difference in the overall survival rates, disease-free survival rates, and local recurrence rates. In patients with lesions thicker than 1 mm who underwent a 1-cm excision margin, 4 of 307 lesions metastasized, confirming that

Table 39-2

Clark Levels of Invasion

	DESCRIPTION
Level I	Melanomas confined to the epidermis or melanoma *in situ*
Level II	The melanoma penetrates to the layer immediately under the epidermis, the papillary dermis
Level III	The melanoma fills the papillary dermis and impinges on the reticular dermis
Level IV	The melanoma penetrates into the reticular or deep dermis
Level V	The melanoma invades the subcutaneous fat

Modified from www.SkinCancer.org

lesions of 1-mm thick or thinner have better overall and disease-free survival rates compared with lesions of 1 to 2 mm.

Balch et al.,[24–26] in a prospective study of 486 patients with a median follow-up of 8 years, evaluated the effectiveness of 2-cm versus 4-cm margins in the surgical excision of malignant melanoma lesions 1 to 4-mm thick. There were two local tumor recurrences in the 2-cm margin group, both with a thickness of 2.1 mm or less, and there were three local tumor recurrences in the 4-cm margin group, all with thicknesses greater than 2.3 mm; concluding that a 2-cm or 4-cm margin demonstrated no statistical difference with regard to overall survival rates and local tumor recurrence rates. However, the presence of ulceration of the primary melanoma was reported to be a significant prognostic factor, indicating a 6-fold to 8-fold increased risk for local recurrence and metastatic disease. Anatomic site and tumor thickness were also found to be independent predictors of outcome; melanomas of the head and neck have a worse prognosis compared with other anatomical sites and melanoma thickness from 1 mm to 4 mm increase the risk of local recurrence by 4-fold to 6-fold. There was a significant reduction in the need for skin grafting with narrow excisions compared with wide excisions: for every three patients who underwent a wide excision, one patient required a skin graft that would not have been necessary if a narrower excision had been performed. This study also demonstrated the high mortality rate associated with local recurrence: the 10-year survival for patients with a local recurrence, either as a first relapse or at anytime in the course of metastatic disease, was only 5%, evidencing the presence of retained primary melanoma cells or neighboring intralymphatic satellites.

The Swedish Melanoma Study Group published a trial of 989 patients with a tumor thickness of 0.8 to 2.0 mm and a long-term follow-up for survival (median of 11 years). They found no advantage of performing a 5-cm margin excision over a 2-cm margin in this group of melanoma patients.[27,28]

Haigh et al.,[29] compared the three previously mentioned studies and their follow-up (including a total of 2087 patients), with the primary goal of establishing the optimal margin of surgical excision that achieves the highest disease-free survival rate, overall survival rate, and the lowest local recurrence rate in adult patients with primary cutaneous melanoma of the trunk or extremities, without evidence of metastatic disease. They concluded that

there are not statistically significant differences between wide surgical excisions (with margins ranging from 3 to 5 cm) and narrower surgical excisions (with margins ranging from 1 to 2 cm with respect to local recurrence rates, disease-free survival rates, and overall mortality; therefore, surgical excision margins of 2 cm or less are adequate for this group of melanoma patients.

Khayat et al.,[30] in a large multicentric prospective study, where margins of 2 cm versus 5 cm were compared in patients who underwent surgical excision of primary malignant melanomas less than 2.1-mm thick, showed that there was no significant statistical difference in either the rate and time of local tumor recurrence or on 10-year overall survival rates between the two margins; hence, excision margins larger than 2 cm for lesions of these characteristics are unnecessary. They also agreed that for lesions measuring less than 1 mm, a more conservative 1-cm margin may be used.

Other studies distinguished the importance of the primary tumor location in the preoperative assessment. Tseng et al.,[31] showed that melanomas of the hands and feet <1.5-mm thick have a low incidence of nodal metastases; whereas thicker melanomas are associated with a more than 50% rate of regional or systemic involvement. In the absence of metastatic disease, they recommended that these individuals undergo local excision with a 2-cm margin and intraoperative lymphatic mapping followed by lymphadenectomy should the sentinel node be positive.

Zitelli et al., in a prospectively collected series of 535 patients with primary cutaneous melanoma, where all melanomas were excised by means of Mohs micrographic surgery with frozen section, showed on examination of the margin that 83% of melanomas were successfully excised with a 6-mm margin, 95% of the melanomas were removed with a 9-mm margin, and 97% of melanomas were removed with a 1.2-cm margin. Margins to remove melanomas on the head, neck, hands, and feet were wider than those on the trunk and extremities as well as margins to remove melanomas that were more than 2 to 3 cm in diameter. Therefore, they recommended that predetermined surgical margins for excision of melanoma or melanoma *in situ* by standard surgical techniques should include 1 cm of normal-appearing skin for melanomas on the trunk and proximal extremities that are smaller than 2 cm in diameter, or a 1.5-cm margin for tumors larger than 2 cm in diameter. For melanomas on the head, neck, hands, and feet, the recommendation was a minimum surgical margin of 1.5 cm or a margin of 2.5 cm for melanomas larger than 3 cm in diameter. Mohs micrographic surgery is a useful alternative to standard surgery when narrower margins are desired, particularly for melanomas on the head, neck, hands, and feet; for melanomas larger than 2.5 cm in diameter; and for melanomas without distinct clinical margins such as lentigo maligna melanoma.[32]

Since tumors 4-mm thick or more have a particularly high recurrence rate, some authors still recommend a wider safety margin based on the hypothesis that a better local control is achieved.[33,34] However, given the high likelihood that metastatic activity had already occurred in this group of patients, the survival rates may not change whether a narrow or a wide excision is performed.

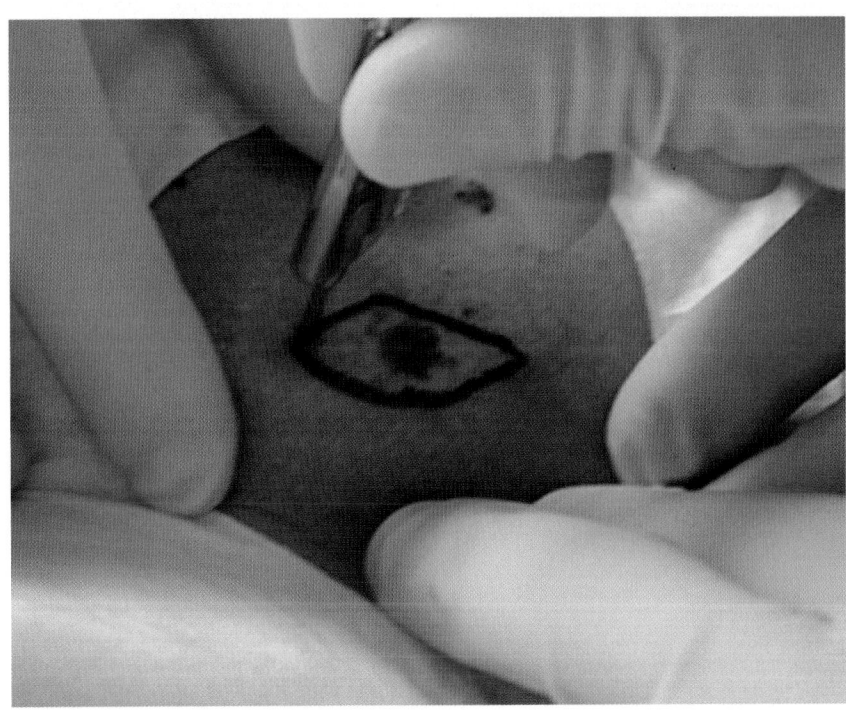

▲ **FIGURE 39-2** Elliptical excision.

■ BIOPSY/SURGICAL TECHNIQUE

BOX 39-4 Summary

- Biopsy of the primary suspicious lesion by a punch biopsy or preferably an excisional biopsy should first be performed, with the longitudinal axis of the excision directed toward the regional nodes. Also, during the definitive resection, an elliptical incision should be made around the primary site, with the long axis of the ellipse directed toward the regional nodal basin.
- A deep excision down to the fascia, or to the underlying muscle if the fascia is absent, is generally recommended.

Biopsy of the primary suspicious lesion by a punch biopsy or preferably an excisional biopsy should first be performed. The longitudinal axis of the excisional biopsy should be directed toward the regional nodes. Moreover, during the definitive resection, an elliptical incision should be made around the primary site, with the long axis of the ellipse directed toward the regional nodal basin, where the surgical margins recommended are the lateral margins of the short axis of the ellipse. The long axis of the ellipse is estimated such that primary closure can be performed adequately. The rationale for the long axis of the ellipse to be directed toward the nodal basin is biologic in nature: melanoma cells in the lymphatics are coursing toward the regional nodes and would more likely be captured through a longitudinal incision. A transverse incision is less likely to

extirpate in-transit cells and more lymphatics would be interrupted, possibly contributing to lymphedema. Following the outline of the incision, the dissection is carried vertically through the subcutaneous fat to the fascia or to the underlying muscle if the fascia is absent (see Fig. 39-2). Some authors recommend beveling the scalpel in a way that when the fascia is reached a wider circle of subcutaneous fat has been removed from the level of the skin to the fascia.[35] Due to the provoked skin tension, the closure with sutures or staples is usually left for 2 to 3 weeks to allow proper healing.[36]

In cases where tumors involve acral areas or those of the head and neck, a special plan needs to be made considering anatomical and functional requirements, and often Mohs micrographic surgery is the most appropriate approach to manage these lesions.[37,38]

Elective Lymph-Node Dissection and Sentinel Lymph-Node Biopsy

BOX 39-5 Summary

- Sentinel-node biopsy and further lymph-node dissection is mostly recommended in patients with tumors between 1 and 4 mm in thickness, where positive nodes can be expected in up to 25% of cases and lymphadenectomy will reveal another 15 to 20% of nodal metastases.

- Nodal staging also helps to identify appropriate candidates for adjuvant immunotherapy with interferon alpha-2b, improving the overall 5-year disease-free survival of patients with positive regional nodes.

Malignant melanomas can disseminate through both the lymphatic and hematogenous routes. For intermediate-thickness lesions, the proportion of lymphogenous spread is higher than for thicker lesions, in which the hematogenous spread predominates.[39] However, even under the hypothesis that cutaneous melanomas metastasize predominantly via the lymphatics, the role of elective lymph-node dissection (ELND) to improve survival in patients with clinically localized primary malignant melanoma remains controversial (see Fig. 39-3).

Generally, the 5-year survival rate for melanoma patients with only microscopic involvement of the regional nodes is reported to be about 53%, whereas that of patients with clinically palpable positive nodes is about 26%. As shown in this study, in patients with intermediate-thickness melanoma (1 to 4 mm), the incidence of microscopic involvement of the regional nodes is about 20% and improvement in survival by elective dissection of microscopically involved nodes is about 30%. Therefore, ELND may be expected to affect the survival of only about 6% of the patients undergoing ELND. Further attempts for a better

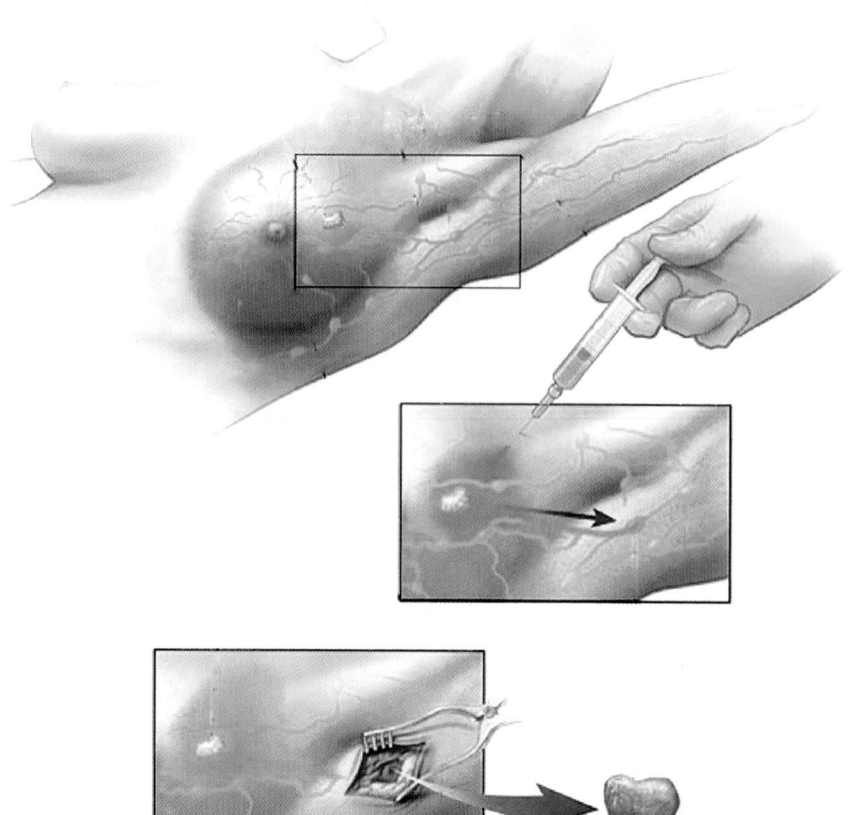

▲ **FIGURE 39-3** Diagram of sentinel lymph-node biopsy. From www.mayoclinic.org.

selection of patients with possible occult metastases undergoing ELND is essential in order to minimize needless morbidity and costs associated with the procedure.

Morton et al., introduced the concept of sentinel lymph-node biopsy with the purpose of mapping and detecting potential micrometastases in the first nodes of the lymphatic basin draining the primary cutaneous site at the time of the melanoma surgery, and restricting regional lymphadenectomy only to cases with positive sentinel micrometastases. The technique originally involved the intradermal injection of a vital blue dye or isosulfan blue dye and subsequent regional lymph basin dissection to identify the blue-stained lymphatic channel coming from the primary site and followed by the sentinel node(s); all blue-stained lymph nodes should be removed and then subjected to frozen section. When the sentinel node is positive, about 37% probability exists that additional nodes are positive, and therefore, a complete regional node dissection is required. Negative sentinel node provides 99% assurance that the remaining regional nodes are indeed negative and no ELND is necessary.[40] In the series by

Morton et al., the sentinel node was identified in 82% of patients overall.

The technique developed later to the peritumoral intradermal injection of a 99-Technetium antimony trisulfide colloid with subsequent lymphoscintigraphy, gamma-ray probe detection, and radio-guided biopsy.[41] This method successfully detected up to 97% of sentinel nodes as demonstrated by Morton et al. in a multicentric study.[42]

The evidence suggests that the benefit in survival conferred by sentinel-node biopsy and ELND is only significant when performed in patients with lesions 1 to 4 mm in thickness, where positive nodes can be expected in up to 25% of cases and lymphadenectomy will also reveal another 15 to 20% of nodal metastases.[43–46] In patients with thin (<1 mm) melanoma lesions, ELND is not recommended, and risks probably outweighs the benefits, unless lymph nodes are clinically palpable and suspicious for tumor. For melanoma lesions more than 4 mm in thickness, elective nodal dissection is not recommended but therapeutic nodal dissection is performed if the lymph nodes are clinically suspicious for tumor and no evidence of metastases is present.[47,48]

Nodal staging also helps in identifying appropriate candidates for immunotherapy.[49] Prospective randomized trials have shown that adjuvant treatment with interferon alpha-2b increases the 5-year disease-free survival of patients with positive regional nodes and no evidence of distant disease, from 26% for the observation group to 37% for the treated group.[50] Although interferon alfa-2b has been shown to increase disease-free survival of melanoma patients at high risk for disseminated disease, the effect of interferon alfa-2b on overall survival has been mixed according to recently published trials and meta-analysis, failing to reveal a statistically significant overall survival advantage.

Other diagnostic techniques using reverse transcription polymerase chain reactions with tyrosinase-specific primers have contributed to enhance the micrometastases detection rates, but further studies will have to determine the clinical significance and effect in survival of these tests.

Resection of Distant Metastases

Only patients with a relatively small number of lesions (e.g., one to four) and a disease-free interval of 1 to 2 years after the resection of the primary lesion are likely to benefit from resection of distant metastases. Using these criteria, about 25% of the patients with distant disease may become candidates for surgical resection. However, location and ease of resection may be even more important factors than the number of metastatic lesions. In some studies, the 5-year survival rate following resection of distant subcutaneous metastases has been as high as 33% and following resection of pulmonary metastases 23%.[51–53]

Surgery for distant metastatic disease is also indicated for the palliation of symptoms such as compressing brain masses or gastrointestinal metastases causing obstructive symptoms or bleeding.[54,55]

◾ OTHER RARE TUMORS

BOX 39-6 Summary

- Although BCC, SCC, and melanoma are the most common cutaneous malignancies, other rare malignancies are also encountered and usually become a diagnostic and therapeutic challenge.
- MCC, a neuroendocrine tumor, is generally treated with a wide-margin (3 cm)

surgical resection and adjuvant radiotherapy to control the tumor's nature to spread via lymphatics. Mohs surgery has also been an effective alternative to wide excision.

- MAC is a locally invading tumor with high risk of recurrence and tendency for perineural involvement. Wide surgical excision has been performed with high recurrence rates, and Mohs surgery may be the most adequate approach.
- DFSP is a locally aggressive malignant spindle-cell tumor, with pseudopod-like projections and tendency for local recurrence. Surgical resection with wide surgical margins is the mainstay of treatment and adjuvant radiotherapy may be beneficial. Mohs micrographic surgery provides an optimal outcome, with low incidence of local recurrence.
- Angiosarcoma is a rare vascular tumor with tendency to recur and metastasize and difficult to treat.
- Superficial leiomyosarcoma is a rare malignant tumor derived from smooth muscle cells. Wide surgical excision with 3 to 5-cm surgical margins is the accepted approach for both cutaneous and subcutaneous leiomyosarcomas.
- Defined recommendations for the surgical excision of these rare tumors have not been established due to the few reported cases and limited studies performed.

BCC, SCC, and melanoma are the most commonly occurring cutaneous malignancies, but other rare malignancies are also encountered and impose a challenge for the clinician in terms of diagnosis and management.

Merkel Cell Carcinoma

Merkel cell carcinoma (MCC), an uncommon type of neuroendocrine tumor, is derived from poorly differentiated epidermal stem cell that acquired the ability to produce neurosecretory granules.[56]

MCC is managed depending on the clinical stage: stage I or localized disease, when the tumor is confined to the primary site at diagnosis; stage II or regional disease, when the tumor has spread to local lymph nodes; and stage III or systemic disease, when there is evidence of distant metastases.

For stages I and II, the mainstays of treatment are surgery and radiotherapy; however, there is controversy as to the best margins of excision, and no controlled trials have been done comparing different margins of excision with outcomes. Given the tumor's nature to spread via the dermal lymphatics, most

authors emphasize the importance of a wide clearance, with recommended surgical margins of 3 cm. [57,58] The excision should include the skin and subcutaneous tissue, as well as the underlying fascia when the tumor is close to it. Excision margins of less than 3 cm were associated with a higher incidence of local failure in a large retrospective analysis of a single institution experience.[59] Even when a wide local excision of 3 cm is performed as recommended, some studies showed local recurrence rates of 12 to 16% with this surgical margin.

Mohs micrographic surgery is also reported as an effective alternative to wide excision for MCC, and studies showed low local recurrence rates.[60] Given the ability for MCC to disseminate in a noncontiguous fashion via the dermal lymphatics, there is no advantage of Mohs surgery alone in the management of primary MCC. As shown by O'Connor et al.,[61] and later by Boyer et al.,[62] Mohs micrographic surgery combined with adjuvant radiotherapy appears to be the most effective approach for stage-I lesions, with remarkable advantage in the local and regional recurrence rates when compared to Mohs micrographic surgery alone.

Despite improvements in regional control, there is no survival advantage with prophylactic lymph-node dissection, and therefore, this procedure is generally not recommended on a routine basis.[63] However, some surgeons recommended prophylactic node dissection for tumors at high risk of recurrence: tumors larger than 2 cm, mitotic rate higher than 10 mitoses per high-power field, histological evidence of lymphatic permeation, and small-cell histological pattern.[64] Unfortunately, Stage-III disease carries a poor prognosis, with median survival of 9 months and only palliative treatment is recommended.[65]

Microcystic Adnexal Carcinoma

Microcystic adnexal carcinoma (MAC) is an often underdiagnosed, slow growing, locally destructive, and aggressive neoplasm, with a high rate of recurrence. This mixed tumor, displays both keratinous-cystic and ductal differentiation resembling the hair matrix and sweat glands, respectively. Although MAC is usually asymptomatic, some characteristic features of this tumor are the indurated, cyst-like consistency and its tendency to produce perineural invasion, reported in 60 to 80% of documented cases.[66]

Different treatment options for MAC have been considered, including wide excision and Mohs surgery, but final recommendations have not been defined because of the few reported cases. Before considering all possible treatment options, the physician should anticipate tumor spread far beyond the clinically apparent lesion. Likely due to deep tissue and perineural invasion, MAC has a tendency to recur later in time, even when treated with wide (5-cm margin) local excision and even in cases with reported negative margins.[67,68] Adjuvant radiotherapy has not prevented recurrence, and the tumor is considered radioresistant.

With the aggressive nature and deep involvement of this tumor, usually several centimeters beyond the clinical margin, Mohs surgery may be the most viable treatment modality, combined with lateral permanent sections to enhance local tumor control. Recurrence of MAC after Mohs micrographic surgery has been reported and some authors recommend an additional 0.5 to 1.5-cm margin resection, beyond the final Mohs stage.[69]

Dermatofibrosarcoma Protuberans

DFSP is a relatively uncommon, locally aggressive malignant spindle cell tumor, with approximately 50% predisposition for local recurrence.

Surgical resection is the mainstay of treatment for DFSP, and wide surgical margins are necessary to achieve complete resection of the pseudopod-like projections that usually arise from the tumor mass. Although a 3-cm surgical margin has been established as a standard for the surgical resection of DFSP, retrospective studies suggested that a 2.5-cm surgical margin, taken through deep fascia or periosteum may be adequate.[70] Even with margins of 3 cm beyond the tumor border, recurrence rates of up to 10% are reported. Regional lymph-node involvement and distant metastasis are rare and elective-node dissection is not recommended.[71] Several studies demonstrated that Mohs micrographic surgery provides an optimal outcome in the management of DFSP, with low incidence of local tumor recurrence, suggesting that Mohs surgery should be considered when treating DFSP.[72–74] Radiotherapy may also have a role in the treatment of DFSP, as an effective adjunct therapy to surgery for primary or recurrent DFSP; or even a sole option in nonsurgical candidates.[75] Chemotherapy is reserved for metastatic disease.[76]

Angiosarcoma

Angiosarcoma (AS) is a rare subset of vascular tumors that tends to recur and metastasize, with 5-year survival rates of 10 to 20% as described in the literature. Sixty percent of these neoplasms are found within the skin and soft tissues, and usually arise in one of the following clinical settings: AS of the scalp and face in older individuals, AS of lymphedematous extremities, AS of previously irradiated sites, and AS of renal transplant patients.[77]

Surgical protocols for the treatment of AS are not being defined because of the rarity of this type of tumor. The aggressive nature, extension beyond apparent clinical margins, as well as early metastases, make complete surgical resection a challenge, especially in areas where wide-margin resections are not desirable for cosmetic or functional reason.[78]

Some series showed that even when taking wide surgical margins, the margins were still positive in 50% of cases.[79] No overall survival benefits were found with the use of radiotherapy or chemotherapy for AS.

Superficial Leiomyosarcoma

Superficial leiomyosarcoma is a rare malignant tumor derived from smooth muscle cells, subdivided in two types: cutaneous (or dermal) and subcutaneous.[80] Cutaneous leiomyosarcomas derive from the smooth muscle of the arrectores pilorum and are generally considered of better prognosis than subcutaneous tumors that arise from smooth muscle in the walls of arterioles and veins, dartos of the scrotum, the areola, or the female external genitalia. Leiomyosarcomas have the tendency to develop clinically undetectable extensions from the main tumor mass.

The generally accepted treatment for both cutaneous and subcutaneous leiomyosarcomas is wide surgical excision with 3 to 5-cm surgical margins, through deep fascia or periosteum.[81] Use of Mohs surgery has been reported with positive results and the benefit of strict margin control and tissue conservation.[82]

FINAL THOUGHTS

Surgical excision continues to be the most common and accepted method in the treatment of nonmelanoma and melanoma skin cancer, although Mohs micrographic surgery became the surgical approach of preference for nonmelanoma lesions. The size of the surgical margin to be excised around nonmelanoma and melanoma lesions is an important consideration for the surgeon, and is based primarily on the tumor thickness for melanoma skin cancer. Most surgeons agree on the standard surgical resection margins for nonmelanoma and melanoma lesions, but further studies are necessary to better establish the clinical significance of such recommendations. The benefit of the sentinel-node biopsy and ELND in the overall survival remains controversial and additional trials will be necessary to clarify the impact of this procedure. Defined recommendations for the surgical excision of rare tumors such as MCC, MAC, DFSP, etc, have not been fully established, and further studies will elucidate better answers for the management of these tumors.

ACKNOWLEDGMENTS

Asha R. Patel for her contribution with the photograph presented in this chapter.

REFERENCES

1. Cook J. Delivery of dermatologic care in different health care systems. *Dermatol Clin.* 2000;12:251–259.
2. Manternach T, Housman T, Williford P, et al. Surgical treatment of nonmelanoma skin cancer in the medicare population. *Dermatol Surg.* 2003;29:1167–1169.
3. Gloster HM, Brodland DG. The epidemiology of skin cancer. *Dermatol Surg.* 1996; 22:217–226.
4. Rippey JJ, Rippey E. Characteristics of incompletely excised basal cell carcinomas of the skin. *Med J Aust.* 1997;166: 581–586.
5. Brodland DG, Zitelli JA. Surgical margins for excision of primary cutaneous squamous cell carcinoma. *J Am Acad Dermatol.* 1992;27:241–248.
6. Pascal RR, Hobby LW, Lattes R, Crikelair GF. Prognosis of "incompletely excised" versus "completely excised" basal cell carcinoma. *Plast Reconstr Surg.* 1968;41: 328–332.
7. Liu F, Maki E, Warde P, et al. A management approach to incompletely excised basal cell carcinoma of skin. *Int J Radiat Oncol Biol Phys.* 1991;20:423–428.
8. Pearl RM, McAllister H, Pruzansky J. An economic analysis of health-care reform and its implications for plastic surgery. *Plast Reconstr Surg.* 1997;99:1–9.
9. Brodland DG, Zitelli JA. Surgical margins for excision of primary cutaneous squamous cell carcinoma. *J Am Acad Dermatol.* 1992;27:241–248.
10. Nouri K. What you need to know about Mohs micrographic surgery. *Skin Aging.* 2000;8:68–70.
11. Shriner D, McCoy DK, Goldberg DJ, et al. Mohs micrographic surgery. *J Am Acad Dermatol.* 1998;39:79–97.
12. Tulli A. Mohs micrographic surgery. In: Chu T, Chu AC, Edelson RL, eds. *Malignant Tumors of the Skin.* London, UK: Arnold; 1999:381–395.
13. Telfer NR. Mohs micrographic surgery for nonmelanoma skin cancer. *Clin Dermatol.* 1995;13:593–600.
14. Drake LA, Dinehart SM, Goltz RW, et al. Guidelines of care for Mohs micrographic surgery. *J Am Acad Dermatol.* 1995; 33:271–278.
15. Steinman HK. Indications for Mohs surgery. In: Gross KG, Steinman HK, Rapini RP, eds. *Mohs Surgery Fundamentals and Techniques.* St. Louis, MO: Mosby; 1999:9–14.
16. Jemal A, Siegel R, Ward E, et al. Cancer statistics. *CA Cancer J Clin.* 2007;57: 43–66.
17. Haigh P, DiFronzo L, McCready D. Optimal excision margins for primary cutaneous melanoma: A systematic review and meta-analysis. *Can J Surg.* 2003; 46:419–426.
18. Cochran AJ. Studies of the melanocytes of the epidermis adjacent to tumors. *J Invest Dermatol.* 1971;57:38–43.
19. Wong CK. A study of the melanocytes in the normal skin surrounding malignant melanoma. *Dermatologica.* 1970;141: 215–225.
20. Peterson NC, Bodenham DC, Lloyd OC. Malignant melanomas of the skin: A study of the origin, development, etiology, spread, treatment, and prognosis. *Br J Plast Surg.* 1962;15:49–94.
21. Balch CM, Murad TM, Soong S-J, et al. Tumor thickness as a guide to surgical management of clinical stage I melanoma patients. *Cancer.* 1979;43:883–888.
22. Veronesi U, Cascinelli N. Narrow excision (1-cm margin) a safe procedure for thin cutaneous melanoma. *Arch Surg.* 1991;126:438–441.
23. Veronesi U, Cascinelli N, Adamus J, et al. Thin stage I primary cutaneous malignant melanoma. Comparison of excision with margins of 1 or 3 cm. *N Engl J Med.* 1988;318:1159–1162.
24. Balch CM, Urist MM, Constantine P, et al. Efficacy of a 2 cm surgical margin for intermediate thickness melanomas (1 to 4 mm). Results of a multi-institutional randomized surgical trial. *Ann Surg.* 1993;218:262–269.
25. Balch CM, Soong SJ, Smith T, et al. Long-term results of a prospective surgical trial comparing 2-cm vs. 4-cm excision margins for 740 patients with 1 to 4-mm melanomas. *Ann Surg Oncol.* 2001;8: 101–108.
26. Balch CM, Urist MM, Karakousis CP, et al. Efficacy of 2-cm surgical margins for intermediate-thickness melanomas (1 to 4 mm). *Ann Surg.* 1993;218:262–269.
27. Cohn-Cedermark G, Rutqvist LE, Andersoson R, et al. Long-term results of a randomized study by the Swedish Melanoma Study Group on 2-cm versus 5-cm resection margins for patients with cutaneous melanoma with a tumor thickness of 0.8 to 2.0 mm. *Cancer.* 2000: 89:1495–1501.
28. Ringborg U, Andersson R, Eldh J, et al. Resection margins of 2 versus 5 cm for cutaneous malignant melanoma with a tumor thickness of 0.8 to 2.0 mm. A randomized study by the Swedish Melanoma Study Group. *Cancer.* 1996;77:1809–1814.

29. Haigh P, DiFronzo L, McCready D. Optimal excision margins for primary cutaneous melanoma: A systematic review and meta-analysis. *Can J Surg*. 2003;46: 419–426.

30. Khayat D, Rixe O, Martin G, et al. Surgical margins in cutaneous melanoma (2 cm versus 5 cm for lesions measuring less than 2.1-mm thick). Long-term results of a large European multicentric phase III study. *Cancer*. 2003;97:1941–1946.

31. Tseng J, Tanabe K, Gadd M, et al. Surgical management of primary cutaneous melanomas of the hands and feet. *Ann Surg*. 1997;225:544–553.

32. Zitelli JA, Brown CD, Hanusa BH. Surgical margins for excision of cutaneous melanoma. *J Am Acad Dermatol*. 1997;37:422–426.

33. Heaton KM, Sussman JJ, Gershenwald JE, et al. Surgical margins and prognostic factors in patients with thick (>4 mm) primary melanoma. *Ann Surg Oncol*. 1998;5:322–328.

34. Karakousis CP, Balch CM, Urist MM, Ross MM, Smith TJ, Bartolucci AA. Local recurrence in malignant melanoma: Long-term results of the multiinstitutional randomized surgical trial. *Ann Surg Oncol*. 1996;3:446–452.

35. Karakousis CP. Surgical treatment of malignant melanoma. *Surg Clin North Am*. 1996;76:1299–1312.

36. Kaufmann R. Surgical approaches to melanoma treatment. *Dermatol Ther*. 1999;10:8–18.

37. Hudson DA, Krige JE, Grobbelaar AO, Morgan B, Grover R. Melanoma of the face: The safety of narrow excision margins. *Scand J Plast Reconstr Surg Hand Surg*. 1998;32:97–104.

38. Kaufmann R. Surgical management of primary melanoma. *Clin Exp Dermatol*. 2000;25:476–481.

39. Balch CM. Surgical management of regional lymph nodes in cutaneous melanoma. *J Am Acad Dermatol*. 1980;3: 511–524.

40. Morton DL, Wen D-R, Wong JH, et al. Technical details of intraoperative mapping for early stage melanoma. *Arch Surg*. 1992;127:392–399.

41. Nieweg OE, Jansen L, Kroon BB. Technique of lymphatic mapping and sentinel node biopsy for melanoma. *Eur J Surg Oncol*. 1998;24:520–524.

42. Morton DL, Thompson JF, Essner R, et al. Validation of the accuracy of intraoperative lymphatic mapping and sentinel lymphadenectomy for early stage melanoma: A multicenter trial. Multicenter Selective Lymphadenectomy Trial Group. *Ann Surg*. 1999;230:453–463.

43. Balch CM, Soong SJ, Bartolucci AA, et al. Efficacy of an elective regional lymph node dissection of 1 to 4-mm thick melanomas for patients 60 years of age and younger. *Ann Surg*. September 1996; 224(3):255–263.

44. Lyons JH, Cockerell CJ. Elective lymph node dissection for melanoma. *J Am Acad Dermatol*. 1994;30:467–480.

45. Lenisa L, Santinami M, Belli F, et al. Sentinel node biopsy and selective lymph node dissection in cutaneous melanoma patients. *J Exp Clin Cancer Res*. 1999;18: 69–74.

46. Essner R, Conforti A, Kelley MC, et al. Efficacy of lymphatic mapping, sentinel lymphadenectomy, and selective complete lymph node dissection as a therapeutic procedure for early-stage melanoma. *Ann Surg Oncol*. 1999;6:442–449.

47. Harris MN, Shapiro RL, Roses DF. Malignant melanoma. Primary surgical management (excision and node dissection) based on pathology and staging. *Cancer*. 1995;75:715–725.

48. Landi G, Polverelli M, Moscatelli G, et al. Sentinel lymph node biopsy in patients with primary cutaneous melanoma: Study of 455 cases. *J Eur Acad Dermatol Venereol*. 2000;14:35–45.

49. Gershenwald TE, Thompson W, Mansfield PF, et al. Multiinstitutional melanoma lymphatic mapping experience: The prognostic value of sentinel lymph node status in 612 stage I and II melanoma patients. *J Clin Oncol*. 1999;17:976–983.

50. Kirkwood JM, Strawderman MH, Ernstoff MS, et al. Interferon alfa-2b adjuvant therapy of high-risk resected cutaneous melanoma: The Eastern Cooperative Oncology Group Trial EST 1684. *J Clin Oncol*. 1996;14:7–17.

51. Feun LG, Gutterman J, Burgess A, et al. The natural history of resectable metastatic melanoma (stage IVA melanoma). *Cancer*. 1982;50:1656–1683.

52. Karakousis CP, Velez A, Driscoll DL, Takita H. Metastasectomy in malignant melanoma. *Surgery*. 1994;115:295–302.

53. Wornom IL III, Soong S-j, Urist MM, et al. Surgery as palliative treatment for distant metastases of melanoma. *Ann Surg*. 1986;204:181–185.

54. Madajewicz S, Karakousis CP, West CR, et al. Malignant melanoma brain metastases. Review of Roswell Park Memorial Institute experience. *Cancer*. 1984;53: 2550–2552.

55. Goodman PL, Karakousis CP. Symptomatic gastrointestinal metastases from malignant melanoma. *Cancer*. 1981;48: 1058–1059.

56. Puolsen M. Merkel-cell carcinoma of the skin. *Lancet Oncol*. 2004;5:593–599.

57. Haag M, Glass LF, Fenske NA. Merkel cell carcinoma: Diagnosis and treatment. *Dermatol Surg*. 1995;21:669–683.

58. Krasagakis K, Tosca A. Overview of Merkel cell carcinoma and recent advances in research. *Int J Dermatol*. 2003;42:669–676.

59. Yiengpruksawan A, Coit D, Thaler H, et al. Merkel cell carcinoma: Prognosis and management. *Arch Surg*. 1991;126:1514–1519.

60. Roenigk R, Goltz R. Merkel cell carcinoma: A problem with micrographically controlled surgery. *J Dermatol Surg Oncol*. 1986;12:332–336.

61. O'Connor WJ, Roenigk RK, Brodland DG. Merkel cell carcinoma: Comparison of Mohs micrographic surgery and wide excision in eighty-six patients. *Dermatol Surg*. 1997;23:929–933

62. Boyer JD, Ziltelli JA, Brodland DG, D'Angelo G. Local control of primary Merkel cell carcinoma: Review of 45 cases treated. *J Am Acad Dermatol*. 2002; 47:885–892.

63. Ratner D, Nelson BR, Brown M, Johnson T. Merkel cell carcinoma. *J Am Acad Dermatol*. 1993;29:143–156.

64. Allen PJ, Zhang ZF, Coit DG. Surgical management of Merkel cell carcinoma. *Ann Surg*. 1999;229:97–105.

65. Voog E, Biron P, Martin JP, Blay JY. Chemotherapy for patients with locally advanced or metastatic Merkel cell carcinoma. *Cancer*. 1999;85:2589–2595.

66. Cook T, Fosko S. Unusual cutaneous malignancies. *Semin Cutan Med Surg*. 1998;17:114–132.

67. Sebastien TS, Nelson BR, Lowe L, et al. Microcystic adnexal carcinoma. *J Am Acad Dermatol*. 1993;29:840–845.

68. Hazen PG, Bass J. Microcystic adnexal carcinoma: Successful management using Mohs' micrographically-controlled surgery. *Int J Dermatol*. 1994;133:801–802.

69. Sebastien TS, Nelson BR, Lowe L, et al. Microcysticadnexal carcinoma. *J Am Acad Dermatol*. 1993;29:840–845.

70. Parker TL, Zitelli JA. Surgical margins for excision of dermatofibrosarcoma protuberans. *J Am Acad Dermatol*. 1995;32: 233–236.

71. Bendix-Hansen K, Myhre-Jensen O, Kaae S. Dermatofibrosarcoma protuberans: A clinicopathological study of nineteen cases and a review of the world literature. *Scand J Plast Reconstr Surg Hand Surg*. 1983;17:247–252.

72. Wacker J, Khan-Durani B, Hartschuh W. Modified Mohs micrographic surgery in the therapy of dermatofibrosarcoma protuberans: Analysis of 22 patients. *Ann Surg Oncol*. 2004;11:438–444.

73. Nouri K, Lodha R, Jimenez G, Robins P. Micrographic surgery for dermatofibrosarcoma protuberans: University of Miami and NYU experience. *Dermatol Surg*. 2002;28:1060–1064.

74. Loss L, Zeitouni NC. Management of scalp dermatofibrosarcoma protuberans. *Dermatol Surg*. November 2005;31(11 pt 1): 1428–1433.

75. O'Sullivan B, Catton C, Bell R, et al. Treatment outcome in dermatofibrosarcoma protuberans referred to a radiation oncology practice. *Int J Radiat Oncol Biol Phys*. 1995;32(suppl 1):289.

76. Gloster HM. Dermatofibrosarcoma protuberans. *J Am Acad Dermatol*. 1996;35: 355–374.

77. Cook T, Fosko S. Unusual cutaneous malignancies. *Semin Cutan Med Surg*. 1998;17:114–132.

78. Mark RJ, Tran LM, Sercarz J, et at. Angiosarcoma of the head and neck. *Arch Otolaryngol Head Neck Surg*. 1993;119: 973–978.

79. Farhood AL, Hajdu SI, Shiu MH, et al. Soft tissue sarcomas of the head and neck in adults. *Am J Surg*. 1990;160:365–369.

80. Fish FS. Soft tissue sarcomas in dermatology. *Dermatol Surg*. 1996;22:268–273.

81. Davidson LL, Frost ML, Hanke CW, et al. Primary leiomyosarcoma of the skin. *J Am Acad Dermatol*. 1989;21:1156–1160.

82. Brown MD, Zachary CB, Grekin RC, et al. Genital tumors: Their management by micrographic surgery. *J Am Acad Dermatol*. 1988;18:115–122.

CHAPTER 40

Mohs Micrographic Surgery

Keyvan Nouri, M.D.
Asha R. Patel, B.S.
Voraphol Vejjabhinanta, M.D.

BOX 40-1 Overview

- Mohs micrographic surgery is an established and respected technique for the treatment of contiguous cutaneous lesions. Indications for surgery are most frequently nonmelanoma skin carcinoma. However, rare and aggressive tumors may also be excised in certain situations.
- Currently, Mohs micrographic surgery is the technique that offers patients the lowest cancer recurrence rates for BCC and SCC.
- Mohs micrographic surgery has a high cure rate, a superior tissue conservation record, exceptional cosmetic results, and can be performed in an outpatient setting.
- Dr. Frederic E. Mohs, the founder of this surgical technique, combined the fresh-tissue technique, reconstructive surgery, and the knowledge of cutaneous oncology and dermatopathology to establish Mohs surgery into mainstream medicine.
- Mohs micrographic surgery is recommended for locally invasive, aggressive, cutaneous tumors that have proven to be difficult to remove by traditional excisional techniques.
- Criteria that must be considered for Mohs micrographic surgery are lesion morphology, pathology, size, invasion, location, involvement of surrounding structures, patient immunity, and history of tumor recurrence.
- The basis of Mohs micrographic surgery is to follow extensions until tumor-free margins are attained. Therefore, tumors must be contiguous for this surgery to be efficacious.
- A multidisciplinary approach may be instituted if the tumor is at high risk for metastases. This type of approach may require contact between multiple specialties such as: Mohs surgeon, otolaryngoloist, oculoplastic specialist, ophthalmologist, facial plastic surgeon, surgical oncologist, oncologist, and radiation therapist.

INTRODUCTION

According to the World Health Organization, the incidence of skin cancer has been increasing at an alarming rate making skin cancer the most common type of cancer. Globally, it is estimated that 2 to 3 million nonmelanoma skin cancers (NMSC) and 132,000 melanoma cases will be diagnosed this year. Even more disturbing, at least one out of three cancers diagnosed will be a skin cancer.[1] Exclusively, in the United States for the year 2003, it was estimated that there were approximately 1 million cases of NMSC and 54,200 cases of melanoma.[2] Skin Cancer Foundation Statistics report that one in five Americans will develop a type of skin cancer in their lifetime.[1] In the year 2002, the United States reported that 9600 deaths were related to skin cancer. Melanoma caused 7400 of these deaths, and the remaining 2200 were related to other types of skin cancer.[2]

The two major skin cancers that comprise the group of NMSC are basal cell carcinoma (BCC) and squamous cell carcinoma (SCC).[3] Most statistics agree that BCC is held accountable for approximately 75% of NMSC cases; therefore, BCC being the most common malignancy in the United States[3,4] and the world.[3,5] SCC is the second most common form of cutaneous malignancy and accounts for approximately 20% of NMSCs.[3,6,7]

Skin cancer has been increasing at a rapid pace because of many controllable factors. For many years now, the incidence of skin cancer has been linked to one's exposure to the sun.[8] With the excessive recreational and occupational sun exposure at these times,[9] skin cancer has become rampant,[8,9] particularly due to the ultraviolet B (UVB) rays.[8] Our surroundings are also becoming a more conducive environment for skin cancer due to the decline of the protective ozone-layer thickness.[9] The general population's lack of education regarding skin cancer and their indifferent attitude toward liberal use of sunscreen and protective clothing has also had an impact on incidence rates of skin cancer. In the United States, this elevated rate of skin cancer has caused NMSCs to be the fifth most costly cancer for patients to manage.[10] Because of these excessive incidence rates, it is crucial to find a treatment that is effective and within the financial limitations of the patient. Morbidity and mortality can be drastically reduced with treatment suited to the patient's specific case.

Modalities that have been used in the treatment of cutaneous malignancies include: surgical excision, Mohs micrographic surgery, curettage and electrodesiccation, lasers, cryosurgery, radiotherapy, 5-fluorouracil, intralesional interferon treatment, and imiquimod.[11] Each method has its advantages and limitations. Of particular concern is the fact that cure rates and patient satisfaction can vary significantly among the various modalities of treatment.

To date, Mohs micrographic surgery is the sole technique that offers the patient the lowest cancer recurrence rates. Not only does it have a high cure rate, it also spares the most tissue, has a higher patient satisfaction rate, and can be performed in an outpatient setting. Nevertheless, there are disadvantages such as cost, length of procedure, necessary equipment and personnel, and the obvious requirement of a trained Mohs micrographic surgeon.[12] For the most part, Mohs micrographic surgery is for the treatment of aggressive BCCs and SCCs. Other aggressive, rare cutaneous neoplasms have also been treated by Mohs surgery.[13] A thorough review of Mohs micrographic surgery including background history, various techniques, indications, and limitations is imperative.

HISTORY

BOX 40-2 Summary

- Initially, Mohs had experimented with a zinc chloride paste perfecting the fixed-tissue surgical technique.
- In 1953, Mohs stumbled upon the fresh-tissue technique, which is now largely used.
- Dr. Theodore A. Tromovitch was a pioneer in chemosurgery and the fresh-tissue technique.
- "MOHS" is used as an acronym for Microscopically Oriented Histographic Surgery in honor of the founder, Dr. Frederick E. Mohs.

Dr. Frederic E. Mohs, the founder of this surgical technique, was born in 1910 and received his M.D. in 1934 from the University of Wisconsin. During his medical school years, Mohs was fortunate enough to work with Professor Michael F. Guyer. His time spent with Guyer proved to be most beneficial because that is when Mohs formulated his idea of micrographic surgery for skin lesions. In 1932, the discovery of fixation *in situ* was stumbled upon by accident when a 20% solution of zinc chloride was used as an alternative for an irritant in a rat cancer experiment. Mohs realized that the zinc chloride let tissue retain its normal architecture just as well as placing an actual piece of tissue in a bottle of fixative solution. This discovery inspired young Mohs to explore the possibility of excising skin cancer, using this newly discovered fixation *in situ* design, guided by a microscopic technique.[14–16] Eventually, the idea of excising horizontal layers of tissue evolved.[16] The horizontal technique was unique to the Mohs method, because pathologists examined tissue specimens vertically. By using a horizontal plane, one could visualize more of the surgical margin leading to a better curative outcome.[17] The undersurface of each layer was examined until cancer was no longer visualized. This was the foundation of all future advancements in this surgical procedure.[16,17]

Mohs experimented with different forms of zinc chloride and found that a paste was the best method of fixation with the least side effects. Along with zinc chloride, this paste consisted of four parts of stibnite and one part of *Sanguinaria canadensis*. When used on cancer covered with skin, a keratolytic was needed so the zinc chloride could penetrate the lesion. For this purpose, Mohs applied dichloroacetic acid so the paste could be efficacious. Although there were many alternatives for a fixative substance, zinc chloride was chosen because it was essentially nontoxic at doses used, preserved tissue architecture, penetrated tissue well, and was a controllable and convenient substance.[14–16]

In 1936, in Madison, Wisconsin, Mohs began treating skin cancer patients with his fixed-tissue surgical technique. His time there was well spent because he refined his technique of fixing, staining, mapping, excising, freezing, and examining skin lesions.[15,16] Complete microscopic control was found to be essential in this type of surgery because of the microextensions of tumor cells, invisible to the naked eye, that were causing recurrence. The fixed-tissue technique made it possible to follow and excise these silent outgrowths in a precise and conservative manner. Soon after, this technique of surgery was called "chemosurgery" because of the crucial component of chemical fixation prior to excision.[16,18]

Mohs published his first article on the clinical aspects of chemosurgery in 1941. Mohs stated that the absolute advantage of this technique of excision was the definite removal of a skin lesion

in a bloodless procedure, regardless of its irregularities and extensions, with minimal damage to normal tissue. At this time, the major steps of his technique were assessing and debulking the tumor, application of the dose-dependent fixative to the surface of the skin tumor, excisions of the fixed layer of tissue approximately 24 hours later, location and mapping of the tumor in association with body landmarks, staining and examining of the frozen tissue section, and daily repetition of this process until a microscopically noncancerous plane was achieved.[18–20] During this time, indications for such surgery were usually reserved for skin neoplasms in readily accessible surfaces of the skin. Areas of the body that were commonly treated at this time were the nose, ear, lower eyelid, temporal region, lip, and penis.[19] One of the early studies regarding primary lesions of the lip had a 97.7% eradication rate.[21] Another physician and pioneer in chemosurgery, Dr. Theodore A. Tromovitch, reported a 93% five-year cure rate for BCCs using Mohs zinc chloride paste.[22]

There were several disadvantages that did render this type of fixed-tissue technique unpopular in its early years. The striking disadvantage was the length of treatment; the formulated zinc chloride paste required at least 18 hours for full penetration and fixation of the lesion. This meant that only a layer of skin could be removed each day, requiring a tedious long-term daily commitment for removal.[19,21,23] In addition, postsurgery care required sloughing off the necrotic and fixed tissue attached to the tumor-free area, which delayed reconstructive surgery for weeks.[23] For the most part, healing by secondary intention was preferred for the fixed-tissue technique.[20] This was considered a drawback because secondary intention meant healing via granulation tissue, which was not always conducive to a proper cosmetic result, sometimes leaving contraction and depression of the remaining viable tissue.[24] Another disadvantage was that the paste was a foreign substance, causing most patients to have an intense inflammatory reaction to this irritant. Patients frequently complained of burning, stinging, fever, and pain. An analgesic was provided, but a better method of surgery was on the horizon.[19,21,25]

In 1953, Mohs was filming an instructional film on the chemosurgical excision of a neoplasm of the lower eyelid when he came across what is now called the fresh tissue technique. To reduce irritation of the eye and to avoid delay with

the filming process, Mohs decided to inject local anesthetic and remove layers of the tumor without prior chemical fixation.[15,16,26] Mohs color-coded the tumor edges and created maps as usual, with the only difference being the preparation of frozen sections of fresh tissue as opposed to fixed-tissue preparation for the microscopic examination.[26] Surprisingly, the technique was remarkably successful and was used for all eyelid margin skin cancers to follow. Since no prior fixative or preparation was done on the cancerous tissue, it was dubbed the fresh-tissue technique.[15,16,23,24] In 1969, Mohs presented a paper at the American College of Chemosurgery regarding his fresh-tissue technique for eyelid cancers. He reported a 100% five-year cure rate.[26] Regardless, Mohs had doubts regarding this new variation of surgery, primarily because it was a bloody, untidy procedure that was more difficult to control and orient oneself to.[16]

It was not until Tromovitch's successful series of 102 facial BCCs excised by the fresh-tissue technique[27] that Mohs dispelled his doubts.[16] Tromovitch rationalized that if Mohs could use this fresh-tissue technique on eyelid cancers, it could be done for any skin neoplasm. Tromovitch had felt restricted by the fixed-tissue technique because the zinc chloride paste was such an irritative agent and the duration of the procedure made his patients extremely anxious.[26,27] Nonetheless, Tromovitch was uncertain about utilizing the fresh-tissue technique because the concern at that time was that the fresh-tissue technique was mediocre compared to the fixed-tissue technique.[26] His results proved that notion to be untrue. Not only were tumors successfully removed, but there was less pain and anxiety for the patients.[26,27] After Tromovitch's presentation of 75 fresh-tissue cases to the College of Chemosurgery in 1970, the switch to the fresh-tissue technique began to transpire on a larger scale.[15,26,28] Tromovitch's and Mohs experimental fresh-tissue technique emphasized that for successful tumor removal, microscopic control was essential; not fixation of the tissue.[26]

The replacement of the fixed-tissue technique by the fresh-tissue technique brought many benefits toward the advancement of this type of surgery. The fresh-tissue technique made time-efficient, microscopically controlled surgery not only possible, but popular. A major advantage was the patient's satisfaction with the procedure, including less irritation, pain, and anxiety. An additional significance of this procedure was its much shorter duration. Reconstruction of the defect caused by surgery was more easily performed and could take place on the same day of the excision. Wounds could be healed via primary intention, leaving a smoother cosmetic result.[26,29] The art of combining the fresh-tissue technique, the science of reconstructive surgery, and the knowledge of cutaneous oncology and dermatopathology gained acceptance and popularity for Mohs surgery.[26]

In 1974, Dr. Daniel Jones created the name "micrographic surgery" to indicate the importance of the microscope and the drawing of color-coded maps for the surgery. At the American College of Chemosurgery meeting in 1985, the name of the specialty was officially changed to Mohs micrographic surgery.[26,28] Dr. Walter Shelley recommended using "MOHS" as an acronym spelling out *Microscopically Oriented Histographic Surgery* as well as honoring its founder.[28] Fellowship training requirements were developed and the American College of Mohs Micrographic Surgery and Cutaneous Oncology (ACMMSCO) was soon founded. Currently a 1-year fellowship is the minimum required length for training of Mohs micrographic surgery as accredited by ACMMSCO.[26]

With the advent of this procedure, skin neoplasms, the most common cancer afflicting Americans to date,[1,2] are being cured more efficiently and effectively. Mohs micrographic surgery is significant because it is a curative measure for skin tumors, especially on delicate facial locations. It has been reported to have a high cure rate, a superior tissue conservation record, and exceptional cosmetic results. Due to proper training and dedication to the field, Mohs micrographic surgery has become the standard of care.[26]

OPERATIVE MANAGEMENT AND CURRENT MOHS TECHNIQUE

BOX 40-3   Summary

- The majority of cutaneous surgeons today use the fresh-tissue technique with local anesthesia, allowing the surgery to be performed in an outpatient setting.
- The surgical technique consists of excision, color-coding, numbering, mapping, and microscopic examination; it is repeated for every subsequent layer until tumor-free margins are achieved.
- In certain situations, a surgeon might also utilize permanent or paraffin sections to analyze the specimen even further.

The great majority of Mohs surgeons use the fresh-tissue technique exclusively. This method has evolved into a tremendous asset for dermatologists. Mohs micrographic surgery is usually performed under local anesthesia in an outpatient setting; not only making Mohs surgery a more suitable choice in today's cost-effective world, but also allowing it to be performed in a safer environment for the patient. The use of local anesthesia is beneficial for those who are poor candidates for general anesthesia. Also, an outpatient setting enables a patient to remain awake throughout the entire procedure. Pre- or intraoperative sedation may be required in rare circumstances and postoperative pain is relatively uncommon. General anesthesia for Mohs micrographic surgery is only recommended when extensive surgery is anticipated or if there is a risk of hemorrhage.[30]

After the patient completes their informed consent process[31] and is comfortably positioned and draped, the area of surgical excision is prepped with a designated antiseptic treatment.[30,31] With the aid of surgical loupes, proper lighting, and manipulation of the skin,[30] the location of the lesion is confirmed and outlined by the surgeon with a surgical marking pen[30,31] or gentian violet.[31] This step is very important because the anesthesia may warp anatomic features and may misguide the surgeon on the extent of the tumor.[31] Outlining the tumor also gives the surgeon a baseline during the procedure and is useful for irregularly bordered lesions.[30] Local anesthetic is then administered, preferably 1% lidocaine solution combined with epinephrine 1:100000.[30,31] After administration, enough time should be allowed for the anesthesia to take effect.[30,31] After vasoconstriction is confirmed by visual skin blanching, the surgeon usually debulks the tumor.[30] The mode of debulkment is under the surgeon's discretion and preference. A curette or a scalpel are common tools used to debulk a lesion.[30,31] Some argue that a curette lets the surgeon "feel out" for subclinical extensions[30,31] and allows for thinner sections during excision.[31] Also, there has been a study revealing that use of curette before excision of BCCs offers a 24% reduction in surgical failure rates.[32] Others argue that a scalpel is better to "feel out" for recurrences and fibrotic stroma; also, a scalpel does not damage adjacent epidermis as a curette may sometimes do.[30]

Removal of the gross tumor requires a blade; the type of blade is up to the

Mohs surgeon's discretion, but usually it is a #15 for smaller tumors and thinner skin, or #10 Bard–Parker blade for larger tumors and thicker skin.[30,31] When a tumor is rather large and vascular, a CO_2 laser may be utilized to remove the tumor and to excise a layer for microscopic examination. The laser actually seals small vessels, thus facilitating the surgery by decreasing operative bleeding.[33] Surgical excision margins vary upon the aggressiveness of the lesion and the surgeon's judgment. After debulkment, excision is carried out achieving an average of 2 to 3 mm of margin around the debulked area.[30,31] With aggressive tumors capable of metastasis, several millimeters of surgical margins beyond the gross tumor may be advised to ensure complete removal.[30]

When one removes the gross tumor and its layers one at a time, the surgeon is recommended to hold the blade at a 45° angle to the skin. This angle is preferred because the tissue sample is better prepared and viewed during histologic sectioning and microscopic examination.[30,31] Along with angling the blade, the surgeon should go deeper than the estimated tumor level and then undercut the lesion parallel to the skin surface. This achieves a saucer-like or a shallow-bowl-shaped tissue specimen that is an ideal shape for the histotechnician to manipulate for visualization.[31]

After the initial excision of the lesion, a layer of tissue is removed in the saucer-shape manner, which should include the floor and the walls of the surgical wound. The depth and the width of the cut are determined by how large and aggressive the tumor is. The dimensions of the excision also depend upon vital structures and cosmetic features surrounding the surgical area. Again, the excision and its measurements are up to the surgeon's discretion, but layers of tissue must be of adequate thickness and width for proper histologic preparation to successfully assess tumor extension.[30]

The layer of tissue that is removed has to be microscopically examined to see if the surgical margins are clear of tumor cells. The technique of histologic preparation of a tissue sample varies from laboratory to laboratory. In most cases, the layer removed is excised into smaller subdivisions and asymmetric notches or hatch marks are made on adjacent skin for precise orientation and localization.[30,31] These asymmetric marks can be made with sutures, staples, temporary tattoos, or with superficial scalpel incisions, all depending on

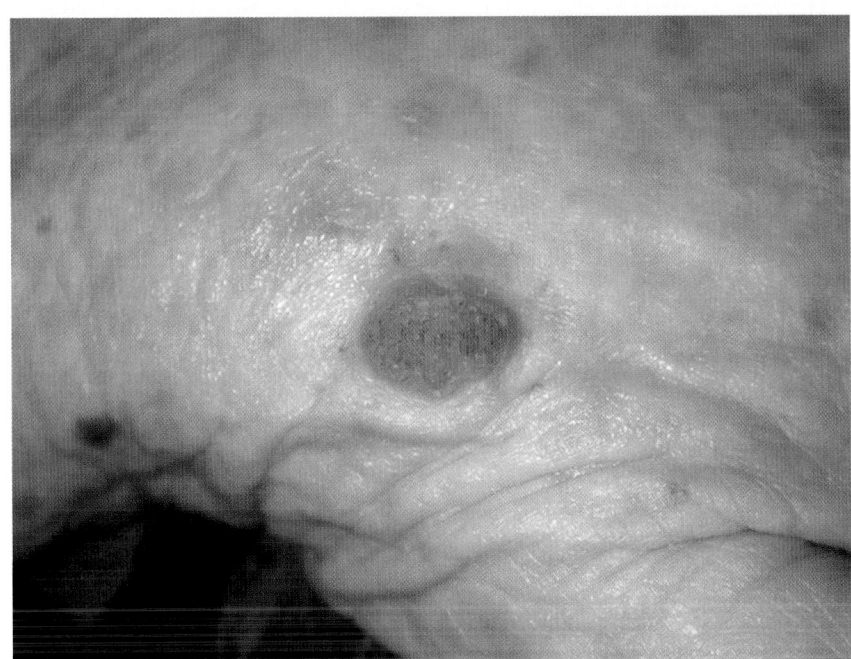

▲ **FIGURE 40-1** SCC on the dorsum of the left hand.

the preference of the surgeon.[23,31] Then, the fresh-tissue specimens are labeled with a mapping system that is consistent within the surgeon's laboratory. The tissue specimens are usually color-coded with an assortment of dyes and marking agents.

Popular stains used today are mercurochrome, tattoo dye, merbromin, ferrous ferrocyanide, and India ink.[30,31] To preserve orientation, a numbering system for each segment is also used to maintain an accurate map of the lesion.[31] The staining treatment and the numbering method localize the tumor in the specimen and allow the physician to determine if the tissue specimen is infiltrated with tumor cells. One at a time, layers of tissue are removed, color-coded, and examined. As the tissue specimens are excised, a map of the surgical wound is illustrated revealing the tumor, its colored location, and its extensions within the wound. A histotechnician then prepares the tissue specimens for the microscopic examination following proper laboratory specifications and guidelines.[30,31] The technician takes the fresh-tissue specimens to a cryostat and makes horizontal frozen sections approximately 5 to 7 μm in size. Numerous variations of this extensive process exist.[31] The surgeon then performs a histologic examination on each layer with the aid of a microscope to ensure there are no residual tumor cells or microextensions. This process of excision, color-coding, numbering, mapping, and microscopic examination is repeated for every subsequent

layer until tumor-free margins are achieved (Figs. 40-1 to 40-16).[30]

It should be mentioned that on rare occasions and on the surgeon's preference, a surgeon might also utilize permanent or paraffin sections. These permanent sections are only employed when further examination is needed or when personal preference presides by the surgeon. Some Mohs surgeons use permanent sections on cases that involve rare tumors. The permanent-section technique is usually utilized by taking the last section or an extra tissue section after negative margins are assessed by the fresh-tissue technique of Mohs micrographic surgery. After the frozen section has verified negative margins, a surgeon may take a last permanent section for double assurance of the negative margin. An entire procedure done by the permanent-section technique is unheard of nowadays. These permanent sections require overnight preparation by a pathology lab, therefore prolonging the final outcome.[30]

Hemostasis may be controlled with electrocautery and the surgical wound should be properly dressed with gauze, antibiotic ointment, and tape. While the patient is comfortably awaiting the last results in the waiting area, the final specimens are microscopically examined to ensure a complete removal of the tumor. If any tumor residue remains in the specimens, the patient is brought back to the operative table and the entire process is repeated that day.[30] Since the wound is fresh, reconstruction is an option if the area is amenable for immediate repair at that time.[31] When there is a minimum risk of recurrence, complex closures, flaps, and grafts may be taken into consideration. If the surgeon has a suspicion of recurrence, allowing the wound to heal via granulation or split-thickness skin graft is usually the treatment of choice. Secondary intention healing is ideal when dealing with concave areas as well as small defects. Split-thickness grafts have a lower nutritional requirement; therefore,

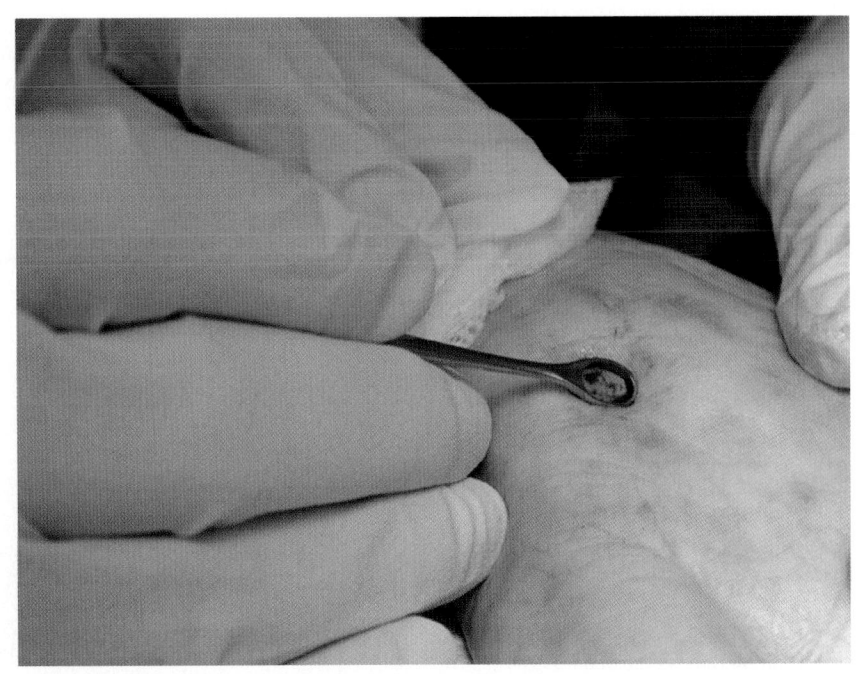

▲ **FIGURE 40-2** Debulking the tumor by curettage.

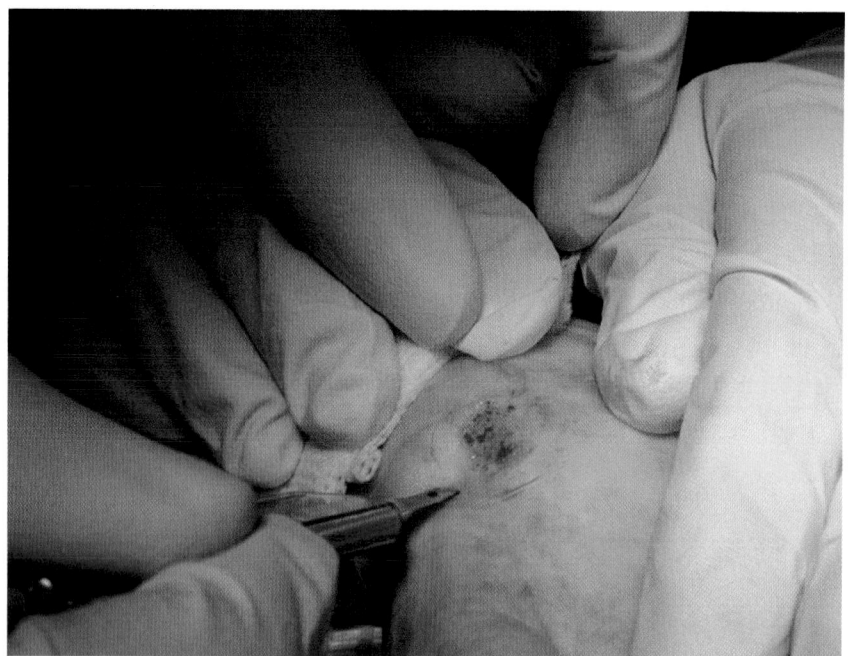

▲ **FIGURE 40-3** Pie-shaped excision is performed with a scalpel at a 45 degree angle.

BOX 40-4   Summary

- Minimal marginal surgery is the foundation of the Mohs surgical technique and method.
- Mohs micrographic surgery is generally recommended for locally invasive and aggressive tumors that have proven to be difficult to remove by other traditional means.
- Mohs micrographic surgery is suitable for tumors that have proven to be recurrent because its technique of detailed three-dimensional mapping is more successful than other established methods.
- Mohs micrographic surgery is indicated when positive margins are identified after standard surgical excision of a cutaneous neoplasm.
- Mohs offers the best chance for a successful excision in delicate areas such as eyelids and genital regions, because of its superior control over the tumor margins; thereby conserving maximum tissue for appropriate functional and cosmetic results.
- For cases with perineural invasion and involvement, Mohs micrographic surgery is an indicated procedure.

they have a higher rate of "take" than do full-thickness grafts.[34]

Indeed, there are many advantages that have already been discussed with the fresh-tissue technique over the older fixed-tissue technique; yet, some scenarios still require the surgeon to use chemical fixation.[30] This method has not changed significantly since its original introduction by Mohs. The zinc chloride fixation decreases the need for local anesthesia.[25] The obvious and major advantage of the fixed-tissue technique is the creation of a bloodless operative field.[18-20,25,30] Lesions or areas of the body that are highly vascular, such as the penis, are more amenable to chemical fixation excision.[30,35-37] As previously mentioned, a CO_2 laser in combination with the fresh-tissue technique may also be utilized for vascular lesions.[33] Another advantage of the fixed-tissue technique is that theoretically the surgeon does not need to worry about implantation of malignant cells as long as the surgery is within the fixed tissue.

Therefore, melanomas and aggressive SCCs may be removed by this technique upon the surgeon's discretion.[30,36,38,39] The fixed-tissue technique may also be indicated for surgical locations deep within a narrow cavity. This is because the chemical fixation allows for accurate mapping on the floor of the wound since lines are more easily drawn, due to the chemicals and clean operative field.[30,34] This fixative has even been known to be effective on tumor invasion of the bone; therefore, it allows the surgeon to accurately trace out the tumor in bone invasion.[25,35,40]

Although some may view Mohs micrographic surgery as a tedious process due to repetition of each step layer by layer, this technique of surgery is superior for maximum preservation of normal tissue.[30,31] Mohs micrographic surgery is also generally completed in one visit and done in an outpatient setting, resulting in a cost and time-effective surgical procedure.[30]

Mohs micrographic surgery is a specialized technique founded on the basis of minimal marginal surgery. There is maximum sparing of surrounding tissue due to the histologic mapping of the

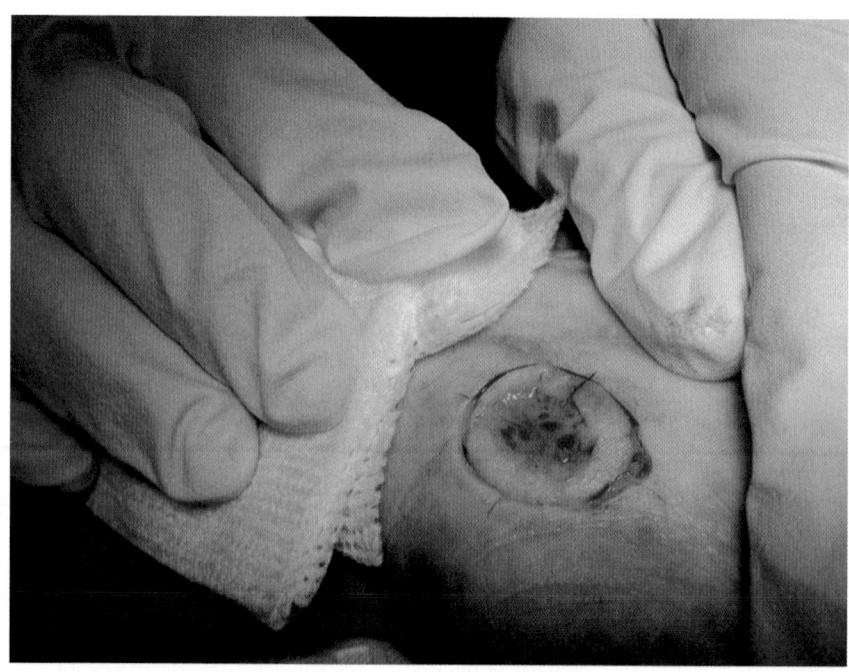

▲ **FIGURE 40-4** Hatch marks are done by a scalpel to orient tissue.

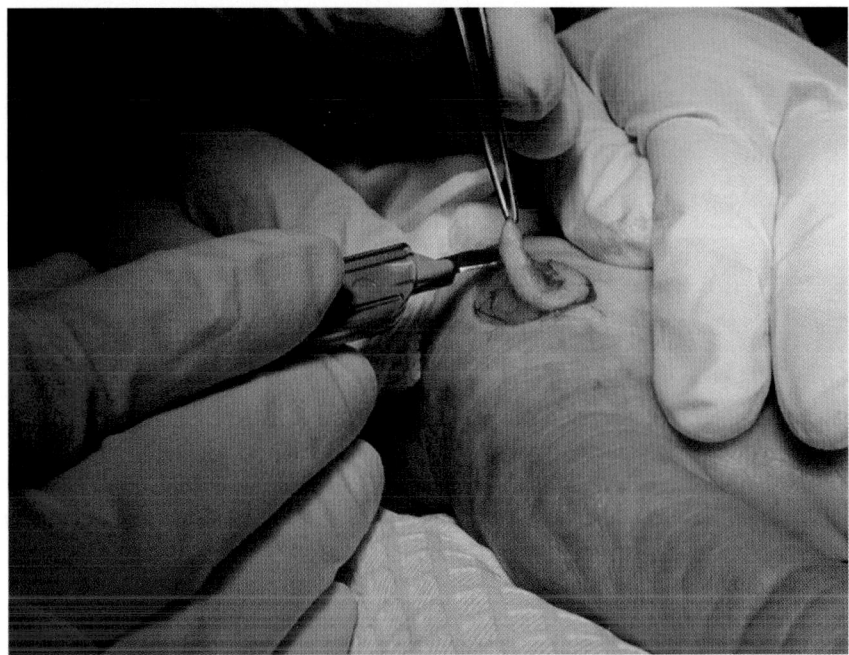

▲ **FIGURE 40-5** Tissue is removed.

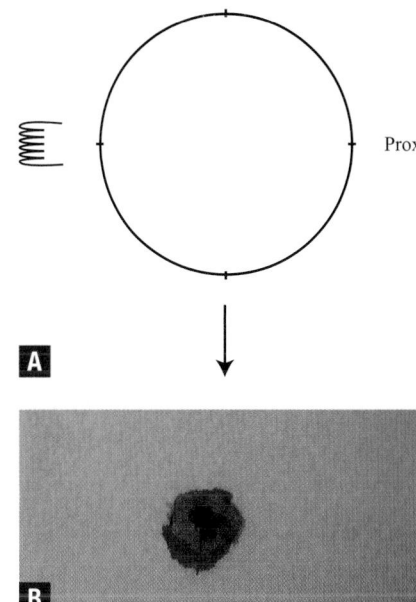

▲ **FIGURE 40-7** Magnified view of excised tumor and oriented card.

neoplasm boundaries; therefore, permitting immediate wound reconstruction in most cases.[31]

Malignant cutaneous neoplasms that are locally invasive are successfully treated by a variety of modalities.[11,31] Popular techniques, other than Mohs, that are used in the treatment and eradication of skin malignancies include: surgical excision, curettage and electrodesiccation, lasers, cryosurgery, radiotherapy, 5-fluorouracil, intralesional interferon treatment, and imiquimod.[11,31] Although these popular tech-

niques can offer excellent outcomes in certain cases, they are all missing the crucial step of the ability to accurately define and confirm a tumor's border that only Mohs offers.[31]

A recent randomized trial compared surgical excision and Mohs micrographic surgery for facial BCCs. The trial found that there were fewer, but not statistically significant, recurrences after Mohs than after surgical excision in the treatment of primary and recurrent facial BCCs. Although a 5-year follow-up period is yet to be completed, the initial

results suggest that the overall recurrence rates are lower after Mohs. Particularly, this study found an increased number of incomplete excisions and more complications after surgical excision. This study concluded that more operations were needed to eradicate tumors completely in surgical excision, therefore causing the risk of a complication per tumor to be higher. They also noted that defect size was significantly reduced with the Mohs treatment, leading to a more pleasant aesthetic outcome. This conclusion was due to the superior mapping technique that is unique to Mohs alone.[41] As regards the amount of tissue conservation, a study had found that conventional surgery removed 180% more tissue than Mohs surgery in primary skin

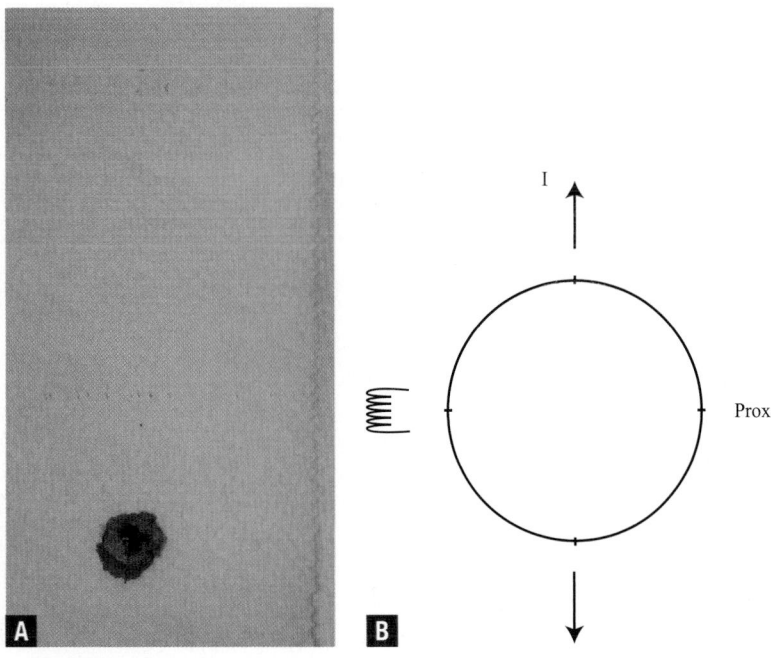

▲ **FIGURE 40-6** Tissue is placed on paper and oriented on the card.

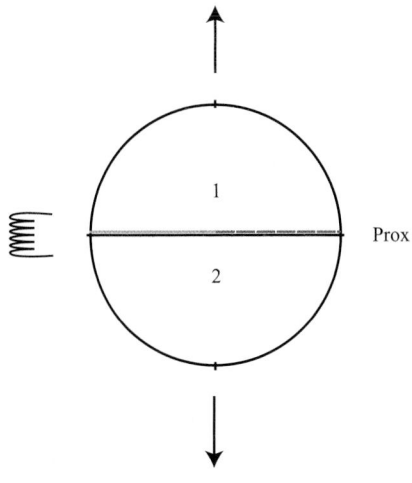

▲ **FIGURE 40-8** Card is marked with blue and yellow for orientation.

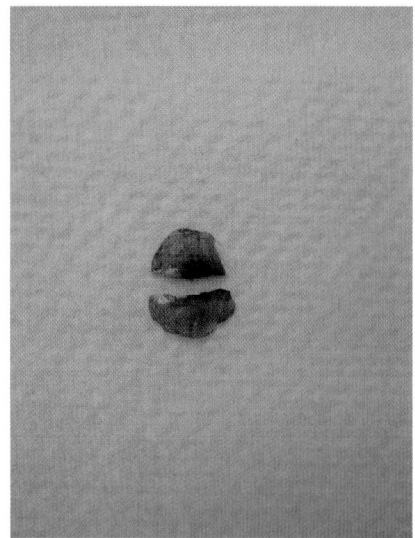

▲ **FIGURE 40-9** Tissue's margin is dyed blue and yellow for orientation.

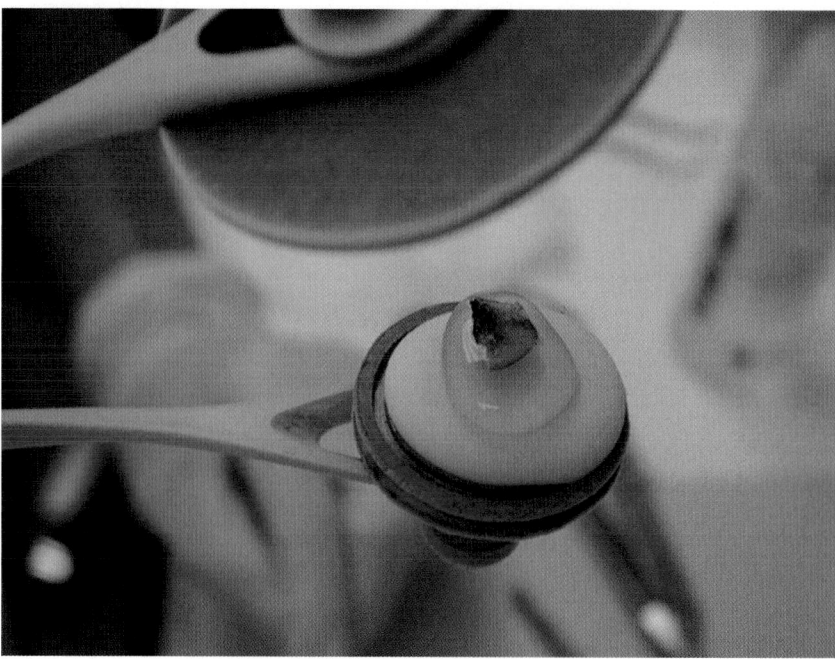

▲ **FIGURE 40-10** Tissue is embedded in OTC and frozen.

cancers, while surgical excision removed 347% more tissue than Mohs in recurrent tumors.[42]

Mohs micrographic surgery is recommended for locally invasive, aggressive, cutaneous tumors that have proven to be difficult to remove by other means. Several types of cutaneous malignancies and certain lesions that arise in specific anatomic locations have a higher rate of local recurrence because of asymmetry or unusual morphology. These recurrent tumors are amenable to Mohs micrographic surgery. Recurrence most commonly arises from microscopic finger-like extensions of tumor cells that grow in unpredictable patterns laterally and deep to the gross lesion. These extensions cannot be visualized by the naked eye or palpated.[31] Recurrent tumors tend to grow along pathways of least resistance and have intricate, irregular growth patterns. Usually, the complicated growth of a recurrent tumor is due to fibrosis or irradiation from past excisions and treatment. The fibrosis and irradiated skin prevents an even growth pattern; consequently, recurrent malignant cells flourish in unusual configurations in and around the existing scar tissue.[23,31,43–45] Another complication occurs when recurrent tumors grow within skin grafts or skin flaps that were used for prior surgical excision wound reconstruction. The grafts or flaps supply many pathways for recurrent tumors to extend into. These convoluted pathways within reconstruction sites present many challenges to the Mohs surgeon who is chasing the recurrent tumor's complex extensions.[25,31,46–48] Although the surgery may prove to be more delicate and difficult, Mohs micro-

graphic surgery, with its technique of detailed three-dimensional mapping, is successful in the removal of problematic recurrent neoplasms.[31,46–48]

In addition to recurrent tumors, those tumors that are found to be incompletely excised can be properly excised via the Mohs method. Mohs micrographic surgery is indicated when positive margins are identified after standard surgical excision of a tumor. These tumors may have significant subclinical extensions, resulting in the incomplete

resection during the original surgery. This may be found even with adequate surgical margins, indicating a considerable tumor size. Since it is likely that the first surgery may have created an irregular tumor growth pattern, Mohs micrographic surgery is indicated to ensure proper removal.[31,46–50]

Tumor extensions have been known to follow nerve tracts, which lead to perineural invasion and involvement. The perineural space is a conduit for tissue spreading and can result in the extension

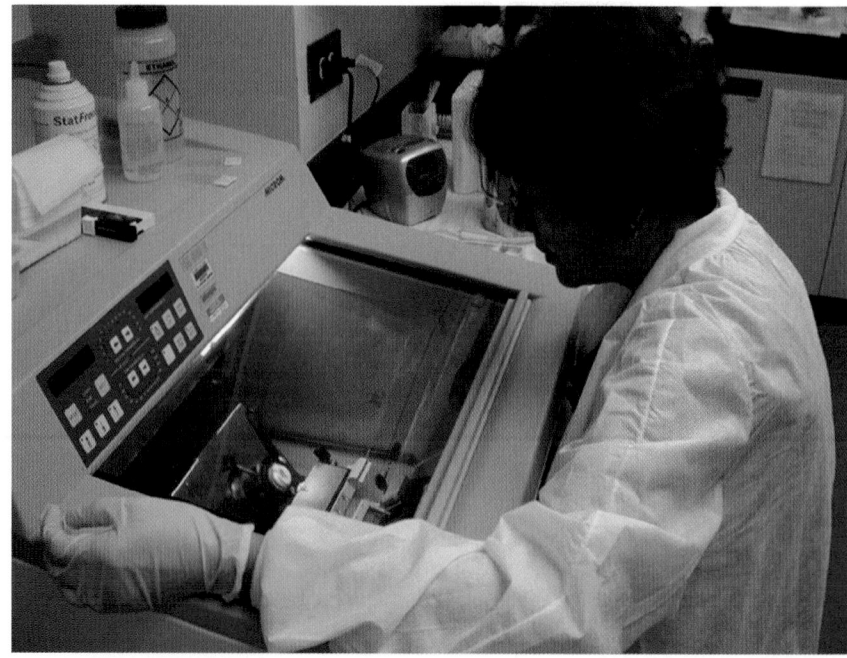

▲ **FIGURE 40-11** Cryostat is used to cut the tissue.

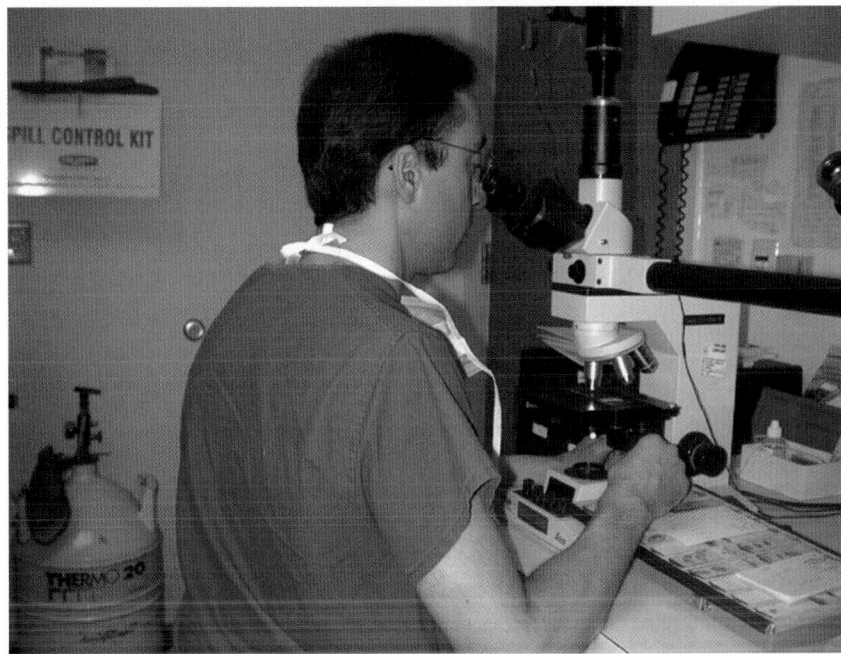

▲ **FIGURE 40-12** Slides are examined by Mohs surgeon to check the residual tumor, positive areas are marked on the card.

of tumor far beyond the clinical lesion. When perineural invasion occurs, not only can vital nerves be sacrificed, but recurrence and metastasis risks are significantly higher as well.[31,49,51–54] Mohs surgery is often modified when nerves are involved. The surgeon usually takes more "generous" biopsies for examination due to the risk of crucial nerve involvement. Postoperative irradiation may be considered after perineural invasion.[49] Advanced tumors may also extend toward bone and cartilage, especially critical in facial locations.[31,54] Tumors that arise in particular anatomic locations are correlated with greater silent spread and as a result have a higher risk of recurrence. In areas where skin is

overlying cartilage or bone, the tumor not only involves this underlying structure but spreads laterally along the pathway of least resistance. This causes a "tip of the iceberg" phenomenon because the tumor can be immensely larger compared to its gross appearance. As the Mohs surgeon progresses with the surgery, the excision in these cases may be much larger than anticipated. Examples of such areas that are extensively affected are the pinna of the ear, the scalp, the temple, upper nose, and fore-

head. On the nasal tip, a tumor may even dissect between the cartilage planes leading to deep penetration and massive damage.[23,31,49,55]

Another point to note is the penetration of embryonic fusion planes, which are common places for a tumor to extend into. These theoretical planes form during embryonic development by the fusion of certain epithelial surfaces. The theory of fusion planes is backed by evidence of deeper invasion in midfacial neoplasms, but these planes have not been demonstrated histologically.[31,56] Areas that are common facial embryonic fusion planes occur along the preauricular area, retroauricular sulcus, nasolabial fold, inner canthus, and philtrum.[45,49,57–61] The periocular area is especially sensitive to recurrence because the inner canthus is an embryonic fusion plane where subclinical spread can lead posteriorly into the periosteum along the medial wall of the orbit.[49,61]

Mohs micrographic surgery is also indicated for large or invasive tumors, regardless of its location. Tumors are considered large when they are greater than 1 cm on the face and greater than 2 cm on the trunk or extremities. These tumors tend to have a higher incidence of recurrence because of their association with substantial subclinical distribution.[31,34,46–49]

Tumors that are in critical locations, have a higher rate of recurrence, or are at a risk for metastasis are suitable candidates for Mohs micrographic surgery. Areas such as the ears or lips require

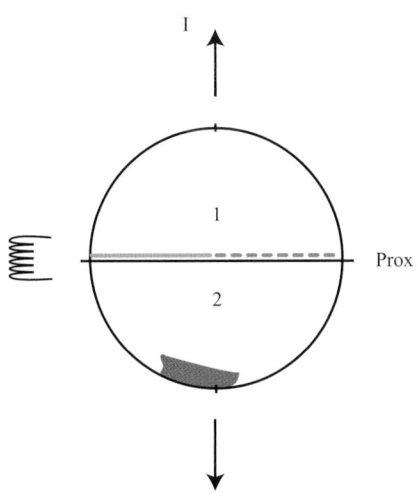

▲ **FIGURE 40-13** First stage's card indicating areas of positive margin.

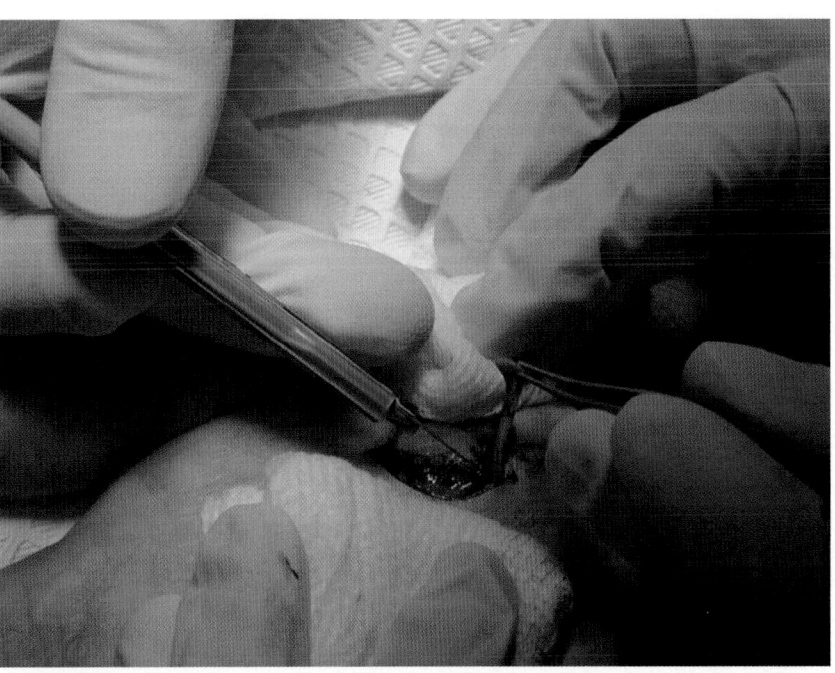

▲ **FIGURE 40-14** Residuals tumor is cleared with repeated Mohs procedure.

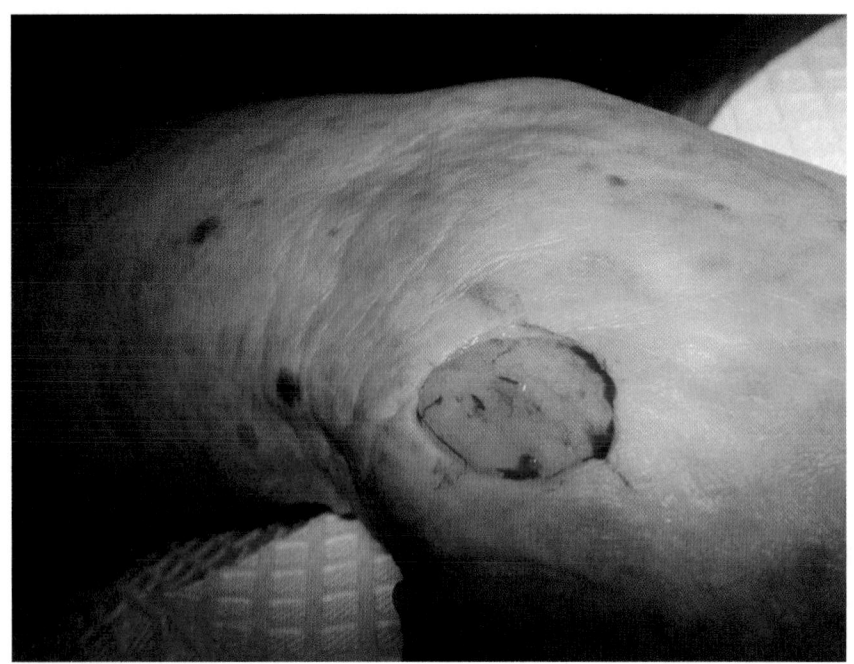

▲ **FIGURE 40-15** Defect after tumor removal.

will be discussed in detail. Melanoma will also be discussed; it has been effectively treated with the Mohs method, but still remains a hotly debated topic. Other tumors and lesions, that are rare compared to that discussed earlier, are also indicated for Mohs treatment and will be briefly discussed (Table 40-2).

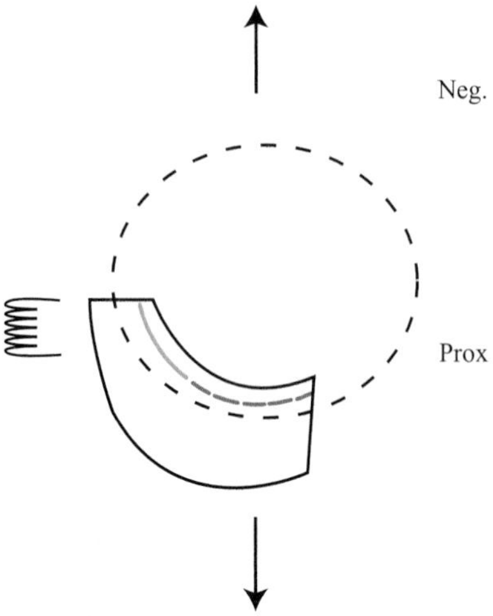

BASAL CELL CARCINOMA

BOX 40-5   Summary

- The most common and the most successful indication for Mohs micrographic surgery are BCC cases.
- Overall 5-year cure rates have been reported to be greater than 99% in primary BCC studies and 96% in recurrent tumors.
- Various subtypes of BCC exist; however, the more aggressive types are best suited for Mohs micrographic surgery as per previously mentioned indications.

ultimate tissue preservation and also are areas prone to metastasis. Other areas of concern are the nasal ala, nasal septum, medial and lateral canthi, preauricular and postauricular areas, philtrum, and the vermilion borders of the lip. These structures compose the "H-zone" of the face. The facial features of this zone need maximum tissue conservation not only for cosmetic reasons, but because they are important in function as well. Tumors can also occur on eyelids, digits, and the anogenital region, areas that obviously call for maximum tissue preservation as well.[23,25,34,49] The eyelids are prone to extensive subclinical spread, where tumor extensions can occur along the tarsal plate.[49,61] Surgery in the eyelid

region tends to be ultraconservative due to the necessity of conserving as much tissue as possible to maintain proper function. For the most part, conventional surgical excision is not adequate in these cases, because microscopic control is not as well managed with traditional techniques. Mohs offers the best chance for a successful excision in this delicate area because of superior control over the tumor margins, thereby conserving maximum tissue for proper cosmetic and function reasons.[49]

Criteria that must be considered for Mohs micrographic surgery are lesion morphology, pathology, size, invasion, location, involvement of surrounding structures, patient immunity, and history of tumor recurrence (Table 40-1).[31]

NMSCs, most commonly BCCs and SCCs, are most amenable to treatment via Mohs micrographic surgery and they

The majority of Mohs micrographic surgery cases are for BCC.[31,49] This is consequent to the fact that BCC is the most common type of skin malignancy in the United States.[3,4] With the Mohs method, overall 5-year cure rates of greater than 99 and 96% are achieved with primary BCC and recurrent BCC, respectively.[31,46,48,62] For perioral and periocular areas, the cure rate is slightly lower at 98%. Although the cure rates are exceptional for BCCs, the cure rate for BCCs greater than 3 cm in size declines to 93%.[31,36] Unpredictable subclinical spread has been found to be significant in BCCs greater than 2 cm in diameter.[49,63–65] Since Mohs micrographic surgery involves superior microscopic control, it is the best method to follow unusual patterns of spread for a successful excision.[31,49] In stark comparison,

▲ **FIGURE 40-16** Second stage with negative margins.

Table 40-1
General Indications for Mohs Micrographic Surgery

Size
- Tumors that are greater than 1 cm on the face and greater than 2 cm on the trunk or extremities

Perineural invasion and involvement
Aggressive pathology

History of tumor recurrence

Location:
- The "H-zone" of the face: nasal ala, nasal septum, medial and lateral canthi, eyelids, preauricular and postauricular areas, philtrum, the vermilion borders of the lip
- Digits
- Anogenital region
Lesion morphology
When positive margins are identified after standard surgical excision of a tumor
Patient immunity status

Table 40-2
Tumor treated with Mohs Micrographic Surgery

BCC	EMPD
SCC	MCC
Melanoma	Adenocystic carcinoma,
DFSP	Sebaceous gland carcinoma
MAC	Eccrine porocarcinoma
AFX	Leiomyosarcoma
MFH	Sweat gland carcinoma

5-year cure rates of primary and recurrent BCC achieved with other techniques are not as successful. Traditional surgical excision is 89.9% and 82.6%, curettage and electrodesiccation is 92.3% and 60.0%, and radiotherapy is 91.3% and 90.2%, respectively.[31,36,66] An intralesional injection of 5-fluorouracil and epinephrine combination gel was proven to have an overall 91% complete response rate for solely superficial and nodular BCC.[67] A topical cream, imiquimod 5%, was proven to have an overall 77.8% complete response rate for superficial BCCs.[68] Another recent study for Imiquimod 5% cream found complete response rates to be 75% and 73% for 5×/week and 7×/week, respectively, in superficial BCCs.[69] An evidence-based review of cryosurgery established cure rates to be greater than 90%, but only for BCCs that are of superficial or nodular types. There is no promising data for more aggressive forms of BCC; therefore, this study suggests that cryosurgery may be contraindicated for these difficult forms of BCC as it does not involve the analysis of tumor margins.[70] These routine techniques are less effective for recurrent BCCs than primary BCCs.[49,63]

Cure rates via the Mohs method depend upon criteria such as BCC subtype, location, size, and whether the lesion is primary or recurrent.[31] Various subtypes of BCC exist, but the more aggressive histologic types are best suited for Mohs micrographic surgery.[31,49,71] The more aggressive histologic subtypes of BCC include morpheaform, infiltrative, micronodular, metatypical, superficial, and field-fire. These are best treated with Mohs micrographic surgery.

The morpheaform or sclerosing BCC is a distinct clinicopathologic subtype that clinically presents as a cicatrix or a white indurated plaque-like lesion,[49,72,73] which has an appearance similar to scar tissue.[31,49] Upon microscopic examination, there appear to be small and elongated nests of tumor cells embedded in a dense fibrous stroma.[31,49] These elonga-tions of tumor cells often lead to extensive subclinical spread.[31,49,74] If a conventional surgical excision is performed, it is possible for one to miss these microscopic extensions of tumor cells, consequently leading to recurrence.[49] In a study of 51 morpheaform BCCs, 7.2 mm was the average length of subclinical spread from the gross tumor.[74]

Histologically, the infiltrative or aggressive subtype of BCC shows a narrow band of cells with elongated strands, but the stroma is neither dense nor fibrous. The tumor comprises of irregular nests of tumor cells, the nests having distinctive spiky projections.[31,49] Clinically, the lesion is ill-defined,[31,49] can present as a flat or plaque-like shape,[49] and is capable of deep tumor invasion.[31,49] Although it is not a common characteristic of BCCs to be involved in perineural invasion,[31,49,51,61,75,76] this subtype is capable of infiltration in and around nerves.[17,31,77]

The micronodular BCC is a subtype that clinically presents as a small plaque[31,78] as opposed to an actual nodule[31] and typically has marked subclinical tumor extension.[78] On histologic examination, palisading tumor cells are found in nests, approximately the size of follicular structures.[78] The tumor nests are smaller and more dispersed compared to the nodular BCC growth pattern.[31] After a simple surgical excision, micronodular BCCs are more likely to have positive tumor margins than nodular BCCs, 18.6% and 6.4%, respectively. When micronodular BCCs were compared with nodular BCCs in a retrospective study, the micronodular subtype was found to have considerably greater tumor extensions. The microinvasive nature of the tumor and substantial subclinical spread account for lower cure rates with standard surgical excision.[78] In a study of 51 recurrent BCCs, the histology of the original tumor was reviewed for subtypes. Out of the 51 recurrent tumors, 65% were found to have infiltrative and micronodular components.[71] Consequently, Mohs micrographic surgery is the treatment of choice for these unusually aggressive and recurrent tumors.

The metatypical or basosquamous BCC subtype is composed of typical BCC and SCC histologic features.[31,79] The metatypical subtype's behavior is more similar to SCCs,[79,80] and therefore is more locally aggressive and has a higher incidence of recurrence after conventional therapy.[23,31,49] Metastasis is also more likely to occur when compared to the more common variants of BCC.[31,49,79] Metatypical BCC has an approximate 9.7% incidence of metastasis.[79]

The superficial BCC variant is characteristically nonaggressive,[31] but the recurrence rate is higher than any other subtype of BCC.[81] This subtype is often referred to as superficial spreading or superficial multicentric BCC.[31,49] This subtype of BCC shows histologic broadbase tumor involvement in the epidermis and has horizontally arranged lobules of unusual basal cells in the papillary dermis.[31] These lobules may exhibit considerable subclinical spread well beyond the gross tumor border,[31,49] and may also present with follicular involvement.[49] In most cases, superficial BCC can be treated effectively with conventional methods such as Imiquimod, 5-fluorouracil (5-FU), cryosurgery, or curettage and electrodessication.[49] If this subtype presents with or is suspected of subclinical spread or follicular involvement, Mohs micrographic surgery is the method of choice because of the technique's precision.[49] However, these tumors can have discontinuous sites, and in such a case, one may want to treat the periphery with an adjunct treatment such as imiquimod or 5-FU.

The field-fire BCC subtype is challenging because it is a multicentric process with many discontinuous foci. Regarding the pathogenesis, theories suggest that this subtype may arise from a multifoci recurrence of a prior BCC that was not completely treated. Another theory suggests that it represents a carcinogenic field effect in which several primary tumors occur in an area that was once irradiated or exposed to a carcinogen. As one can imagine, it is difficult to clinically define tumor borders with such irregularity in growth pattern. Mohs micrographic surgery may be considered for treatment, but because of possible discontinuity of tumor cells, Mohs may fail. Mohs micrographic surgery in conjunction with an adjuvant therapy, such as imiquimod on the peripheral margins, may be considered.[23,31,49,82]

Regarding location, BCCs can appear almost anywhere on the body, more so on sun-exposed areas. Locations that are more amenable to Mohs are anatomic areas associated with high risk of recurrence as well as those requiring maximum tissue preservation. Areas that have a tendency to recur, as mentioned before, are the embryonic fusion planes, the nasal ala, periocular areas, ears, scalp, and the temple.[49] On the nasal ala, BCCs have been known to bud off of the pilosebaceous units, thus escaping therapy by curette.[83] BCCs on the scalp may also hide by budding off the follicles and hiding between them, thus escaping curette treatment.[49]

Mohs micrographic surgery should be seriously considered for all the aforementioned subtypes of BCC. These aggressive histologic variants of BCC have a dangerous potential because they tend to have significant subclinical involvement, high recurrence rates, and a risk for metastasis.

■ SQUAMOUS CELL CARCINOMA

BOX 40-6   Summary

- SCC is the second most common indication for treatment via Mohs micrographic surgery.
- SCC tends to be more discontiguous when compared to BCC; thereby, making a successful treatment with the Mohs technique more complicated.
- Overall five-year cure rates have been reported to be between 96 and 98% in primary SCC case studies, compared to approximately 16% in those patients with metastases.

SCC is the second most common type of skin cancer. It accounts for approximately 20% of all NMSCs,[3,6,7] with approximately 200,000 cases per year in the United States.[84] SCC is also the second most common tumor treated with Mohs micrographic surgery.[31] SCC proves to be more difficult to treat when compared to BCC. Overall, SCCs are more likely to present with local metastasis because some parts of the tumor tend to be discontiguous from the clinically apparent tumor. As previously mentioned, for Mohs micrographic surgery to be completely successful, the tumor must be contiguous; therefore, there is a reduced complete cure rate of SCCs with the Mohs procedure.[31] In a large trial treating SCCs with Mohs micrographic surgery, the 5-year cure rate of patients without SCC metastases was 98% compared to 16% in those patients with metastases.[31,36] Another report found 5-year cure rates of 96 to 98% for primary invasive SCCs.[85]

SCC metastasis depends upon anatomical location, tumor size, depth of invasion, degree of differentiation, perineural invasion, and underlying medical conditions such as immunosuppression.[31] In the case of SCCs, the risk of metastatic disease increases when the tumor invades the dermis to a depth of 4 mm or more.[48,85–87] With primary cutaneous SCCs, the metastatic rate is 2 to 3%.[88–90] If a SCC arises on the skin that was damaged by sun exposure, the metastasis rate

is estimated to be 0.5%.[91] An SCC that is of the mucocutaneous subtype is estimated to have an 11% metastasis rate.[90]

SCCs have also arisen in areas of chronic scarring due to ulcers or burns, chronic osteomyelitis, radiation dermatitis, and chronic skin disorders.[31,85,86,92] In one study, 18% of patients with a primary SCC in a burn scar had metastatic tumors, 31% of patients had SCC metastases in chronic osteomyelitis, 20% of patients had SCC metastases within a site that was once irradiated, and 30% of patients had SCC metastases within an area of discoid lupus erythematosus.[31,89] Normally, the route of metastasis is through the regional lymph nodes and lymphatic system;[31,89] however, as reported in the literature, SCC is quite capable of spreading to distant organs via the hematogenous route in as many as 5 to 10% of metastatic cases.[89]

Immunosuppressed patients have an increased risk for developing SCC. There are many etiologies for immune suppression, but the most common are transplant patients on immunosuppressive medications or infections such as human immunodeficiency virus (HIV). If the immune system is compromised, tumors may present in younger patients as multiple lesions. Lesions of SCC are more aggressive in the setting of immunosuppression as the body is not as capable in its immune defense mechanisms and DNA repair mechanisms.[17,31,48,86,92]

Perineural invasion is a more common feature of an advanced SCC as opposed to BCCs, where this occurrence is quite rare.[31,49,51,61,75,76] Nerve invasion is suggestive of an advanced and aggressive tumor that requires a more careful and detailed treatment approach. Tumors with perineural invasion not only damage nerves involved, but also put the patient at a high risk for recurrence and metastases.[31,49,51–54] SCC tumors that extend into the cranial foramina via a nerve tract may require a multidisciplinary approach if the tumor is at all resectable.[51,53,93–95] Mohs micrographic surgery is indicated for these complex situations. Its tight control over surgical margins and the superior tissue conservation record are undoubtedly crucial in this situation for saving nerves and functional tissue. Since tumor involvement in perineural invasion can be microscopic and unpredictable, it is recommended to use adjunctive therapy such as postoperative irradiation to enhance eradication of tumor cells and control metastases.[49] Perineural invasion has been reported in up to 36% of SCCs.[31,96,97] It has been found that 64% of SCC tumors that are 2.5 cm or greater

go on to metastasize while 11% of SCC tumors that have a diameter of less than 2.5 cm show evidence of metastasis.[93,96] The degree of differentiation also plays a role in the incidence of metastases.[31] Broders classified four histologic grades of SCC, which is based on the tumor's cellular differentiation. Grades 1 and 2 are more differentiated while grades 3 and 4 are poorly differentiated.[98] The less differentiated a SCC tumor, the more likely it will exhibit perineural invasion.[93,96] Mohs micrographic surgery holds the lowest rate of local recurrence in the management of SCC with perineural invasion.[85,96,99]

In a large review of 3299 SCCs, which included metastatic and extensive growth tumors, Mohs analyzed 5-year cure rates based on size and histologic grade. The 5-year cure rate for tumors less than 2 cm had more than 99% rate, tumors between 2 and 3 cm had an 82% rate, and tumors larger than 3 cm had a 59% rate. Regarding differentiation and histologic types, grade 1 was at 99%, grade 2 was at 94%, grade 3 was at 74%, and grade 4 was at 45% with respect to the 5-year cure rate. The trend of a larger and more poorly differentiated tumor having a lower 5-year cure rate was most commonly due to metastases and tumor damage via extension into crucial anatomic locations.[31,36]

SCC *in situ* (SCCIS) presents in two clinical forms: Bowen disease (cutaneous SCCIS) or erythroplasia of Querat.[31,55,100] Bowen disease is characterized by a slow-growing erythematous scaly patch or a sharply demarcated, irregular-bordered, pigmented plaque that develops on skin, nails, or mucous membranes.[31,100] Most commonly, it occurs on the skin that has suffered excessive sun exposure.[31] Erythroplasia of Querat presents as an erythematous velvety patch.[31,100] It most commonly occurs on the mucosa of the glans penis or on the inner side of the prepuce, usually in uncircumcised males.[31] Bowenoid papulosis is another variant that remains distinctive from the other two types of SCCIS. Bowenoid papulosis is considered by some to be a transitional state between a genital wart, commonly caused by human papillomavirus 16 (HPV-16), and Bowen disease. Bowenoid papulosis has a histologic tendency toward adenocarcinomatous differentiation and a clinical tendency toward spontaneous resolution.[100] Bowenoid papulosis presents as dome-shaped papules[100] that normally penetrate deeply.[31] In males, these papules appear on the glans or shaft of the penis and in females, perineal or vulvar areas are afflicted.[31] For treatment, traditional modalities are usually sufficient, except in cases where extensive and poorly defined margins are found. Tissue conservation is an important matter to take into consideration for the genitalia regions. Mohs micrographic surgery is recommended for these cases as penile amputation or other drastic treatments must be avoided.[31,101,102]

Another subtype of SCC that should be noted is verrucous carcinoma. It is a low-grade well-differentiated carcinoma that penetrates deeply. The mouth (oral florid papillomatosis), foot (epithelioma cuniculatum), and penis (giant condyloma of Buschke–Löwenstein) are more common presentations. Again, the goal is to conserve as much tissue as possible in these sensitive areas; therefore, Mohs is recommended to avoid a potential amputation.[102–104]

An additional tumor of note is the keratoacanthoma (KA). KAs are cutaneous tumors that have been described by some as a subtype of SCC. Others argue that it is a separate malignancy, but possesses a histologic similarity to SCC.[31,105] KAs commonly occur on sun-exposed areas and are thought to be derived from hair follicle cells.[105] Regardless, KAs are known to regress spontaneously in approximately 6 months, leaving a distinctive flattened scar. Rarely, a KA may transform into an invasive SCC, which will cause serious damage if not treated.[31,105] When KAs begin to express this aggressive and invasive behavior they are capable of perineural and vascular invasion, which is locally destructive.[106] Recurrent KAs have been documented to have a more aggressive growth pattern with a potential to metastasize.[17,31,55] Giant KAs are another variant that can grow as large as 9 cm or more. They are capable of deep penetration, and if they occur on delicate facial features they may incur significant damage.[31,55,105] Since KAs may acquire destructive behavior similar to SCCs, invasive KAs, recurrent KAs, and giant KAs are recommended for Mohs micrographic surgery if they pose any danger to delicate anatomic areas of functional or cosmetic importance.[31,107]

◼ MELANOMA

BOX 40-7 Summary

- Melanoma excision via the Mohs method is a highly controversial subject because of the potential mortality that melanoma may cause.
- Presently, there are no prospective randomized controlled trials comparing conventional surgical excision to Mohs micrographic surgery in the management of melanomas.
- Facial melanomas have been successfully treated with the Mohs technique, with 89 of the 92 available patients showing no local recurrence or evidence of melanoma over a 6-year period.
- Conventional surgical excision with recommended margins still remains the gold standard for melanoma treatment; however, more clinical trials with Mohs as the treatment are being further studied.

Melanoma is the deadliest form of skin cancer, with a rapidly increasing annual incidence. In 2003, there were an estimated 54,200 new cases of melanoma and 7600 deaths attributable to melanoma in the United States alone.[108] In 2005, it is estimated that 59,580 new cases of melanoma and 7770 deaths attributable to melanoma will occur in the United States. It is also predicted that in 2005, melanoma was the fifth leading type of new cancer in males and the sixth in females in the United States.[109] In the 1960s, the risk of acquiring melanoma was 1 in 600, in 1985 it was 1 in 150, and now the current projected lifetime risk of melanoma is 1 in 71.[110,111]

The subject of excising melanoma with Mohs micrographic surgery is highly debated. Despite the controversy, there have been studies reporting the success of melanoma removal by the Mohs method. Mohs himself published a study that reported 5-year cure rates that were comparable with traditional surgical excision.[36] Unfortunately, at this time, there are no prospective randomized controlled trials comparing conventional surgical excision to Mohs micrographic surgery regarding the management of melanoma.

Currently, conventional surgical excision with recommended margins is the gold standard for melanoma treatment. The prognosis of melanoma directly correlates with the depth of invasion (i.e., Clark levels or Breslow classification); therefore, the amount of surgical margins considered is dependent upon the depth of involvement.[112,113] Clark levels are: level I: tumor is confined to the epidermis with an intact basal lamina (also known as melanoma *in situ*), level II:

melanoma extends through the basal lamina into the papillary dermis, level III: tumor cells fill and expand the papillary dermis, level IV: tumor extension into the reticular dermis, and level V: tumor extension to the subcutaneous fat.[113,114] Breslow used an ocular micrometer to measure the vertical thickness of the melanoma tumor invasion from the granular layer or base of the ulcer to the deepest section of the melanoma tumor that is not contiguous with adjacent structures.[113,115]

It is suggested that for cutaneous melanomas less than 2-mm thick, a 1 cm margin is adequate without compromising overall survival.[112,116] In cutaneous melanomas that are greater than 2-mm thick, margins of 2 cm are recommended.[112,117,118] Prospective randomized trials have yet to be performed to verify the suggested margins. The surgical margins for melanoma *in situ* have not been researched, but the National Institutes of Health (NIH) consensus panel suggests that margins of 0.5 cm are generally appropriate.[112]

One recent retrospective study analyzed the efficacy of Mohs micrographic surgery on facial melanomas. Facial melanomas present a challenge to the surgeon as the face is an area where maximum tissue preservation is essential due to functional and cosmetic reasons. The accuracy of margin control by frozen tissue sections was assessed. Eighty-nine of the 92 available patients had no local recurrence or evidence of melanoma over a 6-year period. It was concluded in this study that Mohs micrographic surgery appears to be an effective treatment for facial melanomas. The study also revealed a complete correlation between frozen section tissue margins and permanent section controls.[119]

There is also a dispute over which technique of Mohs micrographic surgery to use, fresh-tissue or fixed-tissue.[31] Mohs as well as others supported the use of fixed-tissue sections when excising most melanomas as there is a small possibility of seeding the tumor cells in noncancerous areas.[30,31,36,38,39] However, studies in the literature show that this theoretical possibility is not supported by actual data.[31,120–122] Regardless of the risk of seeding, Mohs did encourage the use of fresh-tissue sections for periorbital melanomas and for small, thin melanomas combined with generous surgical margins.[31,123,124]

Mohs micrographic surgery has proven to be effective in certain cases of melanoma, being especially beneficial in delicate areas, but again, the premise of Mohs surgery is that the tumor must be contiguous. If a melanoma tumor has micrometastasized or has microsatellite tumors, there is a high probability that the tissue preserving Mohs procedure may miss these dangerous lesions. Therefore, most prefer to err on the side of caution and use wider surgical margins to excise a potentially silent metastatic cancer. The success of Mohs micrographic surgery for the management of melanoma relies mostly upon the skill of the histotechnician and the experience of the surgeon.[31]

DERMATOFIBROSARCOMA PROTUBERANS

BOX 40-8   Summary

- DFSP is a locally aggressive, rare malignant cutaneous tumor frequently found on nonsun-exposed areas of the body.
- Mohs micrographic surgery has promise of becoming an effective treatment for DFSP, with studies reporting recurrence rates of 0 to 2.4% in primary tumors and 4.8% for previously treated tumors.
- Some physicians prefer paraffin-embedded sections rather than the commonly used frozen sections to analyze samples during surgery, especially with the last stage to verify clear margins.

Dermatofibrosarcoma protuberans (DFSP) is a rare, malignant spindle cell tumor that typically arises in nonsun-exposed areas, such as the trunk and proximal extremities. This tumor is insidious in growth, locally aggressive, and tends to grow in an asymmetric pattern with microscopic extension into surrounding tissue. Consequently, there is often a significant subclinical component to a DFSP lesion. DFSP rarely metastasizes, only in approximately 3% of patients; but when metastases do occur, lung and lymph nodes are favored locations.[13,31,125–127]

DFSP characteristically presents as an indurated plaque with a nodular surface.[13,128] CD34 has been established as a useful marker, not only in the diagnosis of DFSP, but also when making the diagnosis of deep penetrating dermatofibroma.[128] Other markers that help narrow the differential diagnosis include S100, positive in neurofibromas, and factor XIIIa, positive in dermatofibro-

mas.[13,125,129–131] Progesterone receptors are also present in DFSP lesions, accounting for the accelerated growth noted during pregnancy.[132]

Inadequate resection is common and certainly contributes to the high recurrence rate observed with these tumors. In fact, with conventional excision, recurrence rates are estimated at up to 30%.[13] Some reports in the literature have recommended more radical measures, namely removing deep underlying fascia and taking 2.5 to 3-cm surgical margins.[133–135] However, employment of these radical measures has been estimated to leave residual tumor in up to 15.5% of cases.[136,137] Radiation therapy is used primarily as adjunctive therapy. When combined with wide resection of DFSP, it decreases recurrence rates, but it is associated with a risk of significant side effects, such as dermatitis and secondary malignancy.[138,139] Mohs micrographic surgery has been reported as an effective treatment option for DFSP, with recurrence rates of 0 to 2.4% in primary tumors and 4.8% for previously treated tumors.[137,140] In efforts to analyze the accuracy of Mohs surgery for this particular tumor, some authors have advocated the use of paraffin-embedded histologic sections rather than the typical frozen sections. This is because the tumor extensions may be subtle in some cases of DFSP and a paraffin section may help visualize the border more precisely.[31,141,142]

MICROCYSTIC ADNEXAL CARCINOMA

BOX 40-9   Summary

- MAC is a highly aggressive and rare cutaneous neoplasm.
- MAC is prone to deep penetration, following nerve tracts; however, it rarely causes metastases. Since it generally has a contiguous nature with delicate neural involvement, Mohs micrographic surgery is a possible option for successful treatment.
- Because of its destructive nature and large spread, some authors suggest sending the last stage of resected samples for permanent sections to further verify clear margins.

Microcystic adnexal carcinoma (MAC) is a rare and highly aggressive appendageal malignancy, which shows evidence of both eccrine and follicular differentiation.[143] It is associated with significant morbidity as well as frequent recur-

rences. Radiation and immunosupression are associated with increased incidence of this tumor.[144–146] Clinically, it presents as an indurated, ulcerated nodule or plaque, usually on the sun-exposed central facial area. It typically resembles a morpheaform BCC subtype clinically, but may also resemble a SCC, cyst, scar, or various adnexal tumors. Secondary to the tumor's predilection for perineural invasion, patients may experience pain, anesthesia, or paresthesia, but tumors are typically asymptomatic.[144–147] MAC is locally aggressive and deeply infiltrating with the capability of invading tissue far beyond its gross margins, but reports of metastases are rare.[146,148]

MAC may be easily confused with other entities because biopsy specimens are, at times, too small to reveal typical features. Therefore, immunohistochemical stains can be important in identifying MAC, for this tumor is easily misdiagnosed on pathology.[147,149] Such stains used to differentiate this tumor include cytokeratin, CEA, and epithelial membrane antigen.[150–152] If MAC is suspected, a history of radiation therapy or exposure should be assessed as a possible etiologic factor. Some believe there is a correlation between MAC occurrence and earlier irradiation to the affected skin.[144,145,153]

Treatment options for MAC include wide surgical excision and Mohs.[144,145] Studies are few, but it is reported that the cumulative recurrence rate with surgical excision, using surgical margins of up to 3 to 5 cm,[154] has been reported to be approximately 47%,[155,156] with most recurrences within a median of 3 years.[154] Thus far, results using Mohs micrographic surgery for MAC have been promising.[144,145,149,157–160] In a series of 13 MAC cases treated with Mohs surgery, Snow et al. reported an overall success rate to be 89% at 2-year follow-up.[144] Friedman et al. reported a recurrence rate of 0% at a 5-year follow up period in a series of 11 MAC patients treated with Mohs.[145] When using Mohs micrographic surgery for this indication, some authors recommend that the precision of margin control be further bolstered by sending the last stage of resected tissue for paraffin section; this is believed to verify margin control.[145,154] Chiller et al. have calculated that complete excision of this tumor results in a defect four times the size of the clinically defined lesion.[161]

Mohs micrographic surgery is showing promising results as a treatment for MAC. With the Mohs technique, subclinical tumor is better appreciated and results in lower recurrence rates than those realized with wide excision. Additionally, since

MAC is more commonly located in high-risk anatomical areas, tissue preservation is a key consideration.

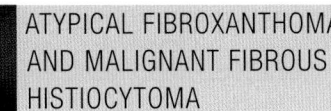

ATYPICAL FIBROXANTHOMA AND MALIGNANT FIBROUS HISTIOCYTOMA

BOX 40-10 Summary

- AFX and MFH are both malignant neoplasms that are rare and aggressive.
- The clinical appearances of both these neoplasms may be deceptive, histologically being much larger than how they appear to the naked eye.
- Tissue conservation and lower recurrence rates have been reported in small trials and the Mohs technique still needs to be studied largely in regards to these two neoplasms.

Atypical fibroxanthoma (AFX) is a rare, malignant spindle cell tumor that presents clinically as an indurated, eroded, or ulcerated nodule, usually less than 2 cm in size.[13,162–164] Malignant fibrous histiocytoma (MFH) is a high-grade sarcoma with pleomorphic characteristics. Clinical presentation varies, but generally it presents as a painless and enlarging nodule.[165] There is a theory that AFX represents a superficial or limited form of MFH.[13,162–164] AFX and MFH have been differentiated on the basis of CD74/LN-2 positivity; reduced immunoexpression for CD74/LN-2 in AFX distinguishes it from MFH.[166] AFX tends to occur in elderly patients and favors sun-exposed areas, particularly the ears, the cheeks, and the nose. It has also been reported to occur in previously irradiated areas.[13,162–164] One study found an increased incidence of this tumor in a population of immune-suppressed patients.[167] This tumor is locally aggressive and has limited metastatic potential.[13,162–164]

MFH is characterized by deceptive anatomic boundaries and diffusely infiltrative growth. Any location on the body may be involved, but skeletal muscles of the extremities and the retroperitoneum are favored sites. MFH is categorized as deep or superficial, deep being the most common. They extend from the subcutaneous tissue through fascia and into muscle, or may be isolated solely to muscle. Superficial MFH tumors develop in the subcutaneous tissue.[168]

Published treatment options include excision, cryosurgery, radiation, and Mohs micrographic surgery. AFX typically arises on the face, and recom-

mended margins for wide excision are at least 1 cm. The result is a relatively large defect in a cosmetically sensitive area.[169,170] The recurrence rate for wide surgical excision has been reported to be 12% after 73.6 months,[171] whereas the recurrence rate with Mohs micrographic surgery has been reported to be 0% after 29.6 months,[171] 6% after 3 years,[162] and 6.9% after 3.3 years.[172]

Thus far, the literature supports the use of Mohs micrographic surgery for the treatment of AFX. Low recurrence rates are undoubtedly a function of the careful microscopic assurance of tumor-free margins that is integral to the Mohs technique. However, another important factor that bolsters the role of Mohs in the treatment of AFX is the tissue sparing nature of the technique.[162,172] Some authors have recommended modification of the Mohs procedure for this indication by incorporating the use of tangential, paraffin-embedded sections, but again this is up to the surgeon's preference.[142,173]

The use of Mohs micrographic surgery for the treatment of MFH has reported a wide range of recurrence rates. Brown et al. reported a recurrence rate of 6% (average time for follow-up was 3 years),[162] while Huether et al. reported a recurrence rate of 43% (average time for follow-up was 3.8 years).[172] Both reports found no significant difference in recurrence rates between MMS and conventional excision; however, tissue conservation was noted as a significant advantage of MMS.[162,172]

EXTRAMAMMARY PAGET'S DISEASE

BOX 40-11 Summary

- EMPD is a cutaneous neoplasm that is generally in delicate areas of the body.
- Reported recurrence rates with Mohs micrographic surgery are lower than the standard surgical excisional techniques.
- Since a majority of these neoplasms are found in the genital region, Mohs micrographic surgery is a more significant option because of the superior tissue conservation record it offers.

Extramammary Paget's disease (EMPD) is an apocrine carcinoma. It presents clinically as a demarcated, erythematous, dermatitic patch or plaque over where apocrine glands normally exist. Oozing discharge, ulceration, tenderness, and pruritis are common. Elderly women are

most frequently affected. The most common location is the vulva; other typical locations include the perineum, perianal region, groin, buttocks, thighs, and nipple line.[13,31,174–177] Primary EMPD is usually insidious in growth and stays in a localized area for years; however, invasion and lethal metastasis have been reported in the literature.[31,174,175,177] When EMPD presents with dermal invasion, excision of the tumor itself and regional lymph-node dissection are recommended.[31,178] EMPD has also been known to be secondary to underlying adenocarcinomas of adnexal derivation.[31,178,179] This occurs in approximately 25% of EMPD cases.[179] The prognosis is poor in these situations where EMPD is associated with underlying malignancy.[31,178,179] The cells of EMPD can be distinguished from those of mammary Paget's disease, for they contain a significantly higher amount of mucin.[180] With paraffin sections of EMPD, cytokeratin 7 is the favored immunohistochemical stain. The lesions may also be CEA positive.[13,176,180,181]

Established treatment options for EMPD include wide excision and Mohs micrographic surgery.[13,31,182] Other, more recent treatments in the literature include the use of topical imiquimod, which has also been reported as an adjunctive treatment.[183,184] After standard surgical management, reported local recurrence rates are between 33 and 60%.[185] On the other hand, reported recurrence rates with Mohs micrographic surgery are between 23 and 33%.[31,178] A recent study directly compared the effectiveness of wide surgical excision and Mohs. After 65 months, there was a 22% recurrence rate in the surgically managed patients, and after 24 months, there was only an 8% recurrence rate in the Mohs-treated lesions.[186] An even more current study concluded Mohs recurrence rates for the following: 16% for primary EMPD and 50% for recurrent EMPD. The 5-year tumor-free rates were 80% for primary tumors and 56% for recurrent tumors.[185] If for some reason Mohs surgery cannot be offered, a 5-cm surgical margin of normal skin is recommended to compensate for potential and extensive subclinical lesion involvement.[185]

It has been proposed that the recurrences following Mohs may be secondary to the lack of contiguity that is evident in some lesions of EMPD. Some authors recommend perioperative tumor mapping to further bolster the effectiveness of Mohs. Suggested modalities have included scouting biopsies and photodynamic mapping with topical aminolevulinic acid (ALA-induced fluorescence). Additionally,

5-fluourouracil has been used to delineate lesions of EMPD prior to surgical excision.[31,176,178] These modifications of the Mohs micrographic surgery technique for this particular indication are debatable and may warrant further investigation in the future.

Mohs micrographic surgery appears to have a significant advantage over traditional excision in the treatment of EMPD, as regards to the recurrence rates. An additional advantage of Mohs is tissue conservation. This is a particularly significant factor in the treatment of EMPD, since a predominant number of these tumors are found in the genital region, where preservation of functional and structural integrity is of paramount importance.[31,182,185,186]

MERKEL CELL CARCINOMA

BOX 40-12 Summary

- MCC is a rare neoplasm often affecting the head and neck.
- The tumor is locally aggressive and appears histologically more widespread than what the clinical picture portrays.
- Mohs micrographic surgery has been associated with higher cure rates compared to surgical excision in smaller clinical trials, yet more studies are necessary to verify these results.
- Radiation postoperatively is a suggested adjunctive therapy to reduce recurrence rates.

Merkel cell carcinoma (MCC) is a rare, cutaneous tumor also known as trabecular carcinoma, neuroendocrine carcinoma of the skin, and "Murky cell carcinoma." MCCs are found primarily on the head and neck but may occur on the extremities. Patients are typically over 60 years old. Clinically, the tumor presents as a purple, indurated nodule, is known to be painless, and grows quickly. The tumor is also likely to be more extensive than what is clinically apparent.[13] The actual tumor is extremely aggressive and local recurrence is common. Local recurrence occurs in one-third of patients within 1 year. In an estimated 55% of cases, spread to regional lymph nodes is seen and in approximately 35% of cases, either multifocal skin satellites or distant metastases are seen.[13,187–189] MCC is said to have an estimated mortality rate of 25%, and is often more fatal than other malignancies, including melanoma.[190]

As regards immunohistochemical stains, cytokeratin 20 has proven to be specific to distinguish MCCs from metastatic small cell carcinomas, for example.[191] When stained for cytokeratin, cells exhibit a characteristic perinuclear dot-like pattern.[13,191] Most MCCs also express neuron-specific enolase, neurofilament, and epithelial membrane antigen.[13]

In the past, the standard treatment for MCC was wide local excision with 2 to 3-cm margins, but controversy now exists as regards treatment options.[192] Reported local recurrence rates for wide excision have been shown to range from 26 to 44%. O'Connor et al. reported a 31.7% local recurrence rate with surgical excision and a 48.8% rate of regional metastasis, after a 60-month follow-up. With the Mohs-treated lesions, only 8.3% reflected local persistence, after a 36-month follow-up.[193]

Since regional lymph-node metastases may be involved with this tumor, many authors advocate sentinel lymph-node mapping and sentinel lymph-node biopsy. The selective sentinel lymph-node dissection has been shown to be particularly useful in the staging of MCC invasion and is a practical technique with nominal procedural morbidity to detect clinically silent disease in patients with MCC.[194–199] Additionally, MCCs are sensitive to both chemotherapy and radiation. As adjunctive therapies, these modalities have been shown to reduce postoperative recurrence rates, but there is a wide range of opinion as regards the significance of these findings.[200–202] Additionally, immune suppression is associated with an increased incidence of MCC. This situation may warrant further study into possible immunological treatments for this tumor.[203] Complete removal of the MCC remains the mainstay of treatment to this day, and Mohs micrographic surgery has been associated with higher cure rates compared to surgical excision because of its basis of superior margin control.[193,200,202]

It is important to note that other neoplasms are also amenable to Mohs micrographic surgery, including: adenocystic carcinoma, sebaceous gland carcinoma, eccrine porocarcinoma, leiomyosarcoma, and sweat gland carcinoma.[13,31,49]

CRITICISMS AND LIMITATIONS

BOX 40-13 Summary

- Mohs micrographic surgery is a unique surgical technique that offers high cure rates and superior tissue conservation.

- A major limitation to the technique is that tumors must be contiguous for its complete removal to be successful.
- The duration of the procedure, although daunting, is necessary to ensure complete removal and finer cosmetic results.
- A multidisciplinary medical team is essential for the entire treatment of a patient with complicated lesions or a likelihood of metastatic disease.
- Mohs micrographic surgery has a higher fundamental value and an insignificant cost difference when compared to traditional surgical excision.

Mohs micrographic surgery is truly beneficial as regards its high cure rates and superior record of tissue preservation; however, drawbacks do exist. Since the basis of Mohs micrographic surgery is to follow extensions until tumor-free margins are achieved, it is important to reiterate that tumors must be contiguous for this surgery to be completely successful. If Mohs micrographic surgery is successfully performed and a new tumor arises or a primary tumor that was previously imperceptible occurs close to the surgical site, it is an indication that the excised tumor was most likely noncontiguous at the time of original surgery. Unfortunately, these cases of recurrent tumors are not preventable with Mohs micrographic surgery.[31,204]

Mohs micrographic surgery undoubtedly requires a skilled surgeon, trained office staff, and, of course, availability of a location that is convenient for the patient. A qualified histotechnician must also be on staff to prepare the tissue sections that are so essential to the Mohs technique.[205] An inconvenience to the patient might be the duration of the procedure because of the meticulous surgery and mandatory review of each tissue section. A compulsive examination of the removed tissue section and mapping of the surgical wound are critical for the basis of tissue conservation, but also increases operating time and may be tedious and exhausting for the surgeon, staff, and patient.[49] The duration of tissue examination might be even more prolonged if fat and cartilage sections are taken for preparation. These sections require further processing by modification of standard laboratory technique. Access and maintaining orientation within a deep surgical site may also prolong the procedure because sites involving muscle, fat, and cartilage are known to be complex and the surgeon must proceed with the utmost caution.[31,49] Most Mohs operations are performed with local anesthesia in a safe office environment, but extensive and high-risk lesions may require the patient to undergo general anesthesia. Duration and risks of the surgery are obviously increased with this addition of pain management.[49]

Review of the frozen and paraffin sections require scrutiny because many artifacts may lead the surgeon to misinterpret tumor margins. For instance, inflammatory infiltrate on a frozen specimen may be confused with cancer cells or may even be obscuring tumor infiltrate. Also, a BCC may appear to be a hair follicle or vice versa. A skilled Mohs surgeon must be aware of these types of misinterpretations so surgical error is reduced.[31,49] These types of technical errors have been reported to be the most common cause of local recurrence in Mohs surgery.[206]

A multidisciplinary approach may be instituted if the tumor is at high risk for metastases, there is a requirement for extensive reconstruction, or there is a need to preserve vital anatomic structures. This type of approach requires the utmost cooperation between many medical specialties including: Mohs surgeon, otolaryngoloist, oculoplastic specialist, ophthalmologist, facial plastic surgeon, surgical oncologist, oncologist, and radiation therapist. This interdisciplinary approach promises the best treatment for patients suffering from such extensive disease. Most importantly, for this approach to be successful, cooperation, communication, and a close working relationship are the key.[49]

As regards financial concerns, Mohs micrographic surgery has actually been proven to be cost-effective, in contrast to previous notions.[31] Compared to radiation therapy and full-thickness excision with frozen sections, Mohs micrographic surgery is usually less expensive.[207] The rationale behind the cost-effectiveness of Mohs surgery is debatable between authors, but the literature suggests Mohs micrographic surgery has a higher intrinsic value and a nominal cost difference when compared to traditional surgical excision.[208]

Although Mohs micrographic surgery is a quite popular technique to cure skin cancer, the majority of data comes from retrospective studies. Since there are hardly any prospective studies regarding Mohs surgery, large prospective studies are warranted to verify its cure rates and benefits to the patient population.

FINAL THOUGHTS

Mohs micrographic surgery is an established and respected technique for the treatment of contiguous cutaneous lesions, most commonly NMSCs. An increasing amount of literature supports its use for rare and aggressive tumors in specific situations. The utilization of microscopic surgical margin control achieves the high cure rates and incredible tissue conservation that is unique to Mohs surgery. Accordingly, for skin lesions located in crucial anatomic locations or that may have a potential recurrence rate with traditional treatment, Mohs micrographic surgery is recommended.

REFERENCES

1. World Health Organization. Health topics: Skin cancer, 2006. Available at: http://www.who.int.
2. American Cancer Society. *Cancer Facts and Figures 2003.* Atlanta, GA: American Caner Society; 2003. Available at: http://www.cancer.org.
3. Gloster HM, Broadland DG. The epidemiology of skin cancer. *Dermatol Surg.* 1996;22:217–226.
4. Silverberg E, Lubera JA. Cancer statistics, 1988. *CA Cancer J Clin.* 1988;38:14–15.
5. Waterhouse J, Muir C, Correa P, et al. *Cancer in Five Continents.* Vol 3. Lyon, France: International Agency for Research on Cancer, World Health Organization; 1976.
6. Shiffman NJ. Squamous cell carcinomas of the skin of the pinna. *Can J Surg.* 1975;18:279–283.
7. Ames FC, Hichey RC. Metastasis from squamous cell carcinoma of the extremities. *South Med J.* 1982;75:920–923.
8. Garner KL, Rodney WM. Basal and squamous cell carcinoma. *Dermatology.* 2000;27(2):447–458.
9. Diepgen TL, Mahler V. The epidemiology of skin cancer. *Br J Dermatol.* 2002; 146(suppl 61):1–6.
10. Housman TS, Feldman SR, Willford PM, et al. Skin cancer is among the most costly of all cancers to treat for the medicare population. *J Am Acad Dermatol.* 2003;48 (3):425–429.
11. Stockfleth E, Sterry W. New treatment modalities for basal cell carcinoma. *Recent Results Cancer Res.* 2002;160:259–265.
12. Anthony ML. Surgical treatment of non-melanoma skin cancer. *AORN J.* 2000; 71(3):552–564.
13. Rapini RP. Mohs surgery for unusual tumors. In: Gross KG, Steinman HK, Rapini RP, eds. *Mohs Surgery: Fundamentals and Techniques.* St Louis, MO: Mosby; 1999:193–208.
14. Mohs FE. *Chemosurgery in Cancer, Gangrene, and Infections.* Springfield, IL: Charles C Thomas; 1956:3–6.
15. Mohs FE. Mohs micrographic surgery: A historical perspective. *Dermatol Clin.* 1989;7(4):609–611.
16. Mohs FE. Contemporaries. Frederick E. Mohs, M.D. *J Am Acad Dermatol.* 1983; 9(5):806–814.
17. Bennett RG. Current concepts in Mohs micrographic surgery. *Dermatol Clin.* 1991;9(4):777–788.
18. Mohs FE. Chemosurgery for facial neoplasms. *Arch Otolaryngol.* 1972;95:62–67.
19. Mohs FE. Chemosurgical: A microscopically controlled method of cancer excision. *Arch Surg.* 1941;42:279–295.
20. Cottel WI, Proper S. Mohs' surgery, fresh-tissue technique. *J Dermatol Surg Oncol.* 1982;8(7):576–587.
21. Mohs FE. Chemosurgical treatment of cancer of the lip: A microscopically controlled method of excision. *Arch Surg.* 1944;48:478–488.
22. Tromovitch TA, Beirne G, Beirne C. Mohs' technique (cancer chemosurgery): Treatment of recurrent cutaneous carcinomas. *Cancer.* 1966;19(6):867–868.
23. Hruza GJ. Mohs micrographic surgery. *Otolaryngol Clin North Am.* 1990;23(5): 845–864.
24. Bailin PL, Bailin MD. Correction of depressed scars following Mohs' surgery: The role of collagen implantation. *J Dermatol Surg Oncol.* 1982;8(10):845–849.
25. Bennett RG. Mohs' surgery: New concepts and applications. *Dermatol Clin.* 1987;5(2):409–428.
26. Broadland DG, Amonette R, Hanke CW, Robins P. The history and evolution of Mohs micrographic surgery. *Dermatol Surg.* 2000;26(4):303–307.
27. Tromovitch TA, Stegeman SJ. Microscopically controlled excision of skin tumors. *Arch Dermatol.* 1974;110:231–232.
28. Tromovitch TA. Mohs' surgery, fresh-tissue technique. *J Dermatol Surg Oncol.* 1982;8(8):651–653.
29. Tromovitch TA. Microscopic-controlled excision of cutaneous tumors: Chemosurgery, fresh-tissue technique. *Cancer.* 1978;41:653–658.
30. Lang PG Jr. Mohs micrographic surgery. Fresh-tissue technique. *Dermatol Clin.* 1989;7(4):613–626.
31. Shriner DL, McCoy DK, Goldberg DJ, Wagner RF. Mohs micrographic surgery. *J Am Acad Dermatol.* 1998;39(1):79–97.
32. Chiller K, Passaro D, McCalmont T, Vin-Christian K. Efficacy of curettage before excision in clearing surgical margins of non-melanoma skin cancer. *Arch Dermatol.* 2000;136:1327–1332.
33. Bailin PL, Ratz JL, Lutz-Nagey L. CO_2 laser modification of Mohs surgery. *J Dermatol Surg Oncol.* 1981;7:621–623.
34. Nouri K. What you need to know about Mohs micrographic surgery. *Skin Aging.* 2000;8(3):68–70.
35. Braun M III. The case for Mohs surgery by the fixed-tissue technique. *J Dermatol Surg Oncol.* 1981;7(8):634–640.
36. Mohs FE. Chemosurgical techniques. In: *Chemosurgery. Microscopically Controlled Surgery for Skin Cancer.* Springfield, IL: Charles C Thomas; 1978:1–29, 153–164.
37. Mohs FE, Snow SN, Messing EM, Kuglitsch ME. Microscopically controlled surgery in the treatment of carcinoma of the penis. *J Urol.* 1985;133:961–966.
38. Mohs FE. Chemosurgery for melanoma. *Arch Dermatol.* 1977;113:285–291.
39. Mohs FE. Fixed tissue micrographic surgery for melanoma of the ear. *Arch Otolaryngol Head Neck Surg.* 1988;114: 625–631.

40. Mohs FE, Larson PO, Iriondo M. Micrographic surgery for the microscopically controlled excision of carcinoma of the external ear. *J Am Acad Dermatol.* 1988;19:729–737.

41. Smeets NWJ, Krekels GAM, Ostertag JU, et al. Surgical excision vs. Mohs' micrographic surgery for basal-cell carcinoma of the face: Randomised controlled trial. *Lancet.* 2004;364:1766–1772.

42. Bumstead RM, Ceilley RI. Auricular malignant neoplasms. *Arch Otolaryngol.* 1982;108:225–231.

43. Smith SP, Foley EH, Grande DJ. Use of Mohs micrographic surgery to establish quantitative proof of heightened tumor spread in basal cell carcinoma recurrent following radiotherapy. *J Dermatol Surg Oncol.* 1990;16:1012–1016.

44. Smith SP, Grande DJ. Basal cell carcinoma recurring after radiotherapy: A unique, difficult treatment subclass of recurrent basal cell carcinoma. *J Dermatol Surg Oncol.* 1991;17:26–30.

45. Mora RG, Robins P. Basal-cell carcinomas in the center of the face: Special diagnostic, prognostic, and therapeutic considerations. *J Dermatol Surg Oncol.* 1978;4:315–321.

46. Tulli A. Mohs' micrographic surgery. In: Chu AC, Edelson RL, eds. *Malignant Tumors of the Skin.* London: Arnold; 1999:381–395.

47. Steinman HK. Indications for Mohs' surgery. In: Gross KG, Steinman HK, Rapini RP, eds. *Mohs Surgery: Fundamentals and Techniques.* St Louis, MO: Mosby; 1999:9–14.

48. Martinez JC, Otley CC. The management of melanoma and non-melanoma skin cancer: A review for the primary care physician. *Mayo Clin Proc.* 2001; 76:1253–1265.

49. Lang PG Jr, Osguthorpe JD. Indications and limitations of Mohs micrographic surgery. *Dermatol Clin.* 1989;7:627–644.

50. Biely HC, Kirsner RS, Reyes BA, Garland LD. The use of Mohs' micrographic surgery for determination of residual tumor in incompletely excised basal cell carcinoma. *J Am Acad Dermatol.* 1992;26:754–756.

51. Ballantyne AJ, McCarter AB, Ibanez ML. The extension of cancer of the head and neck through peripheral nerves. *Am J Surg.* 1963;106:651–667.

52. Dandy DJ, Munro DD. Squamous cell carcinoma of the skin involving the median nerve. *Br J Dermatol.* 1973;89: 527–531.

53. Hanke CW, Wolf RL, Hochman SA, et al. Chemosurgical reports: Perineural spread of basal cell carcinoma. *J Dermatol Surg Oncol.* 1983;9:742–747.

54. Weimar VM, Ceilly RI, Babin RW, et al. Chemosurgical reports. Squamous cell carcinoma with invasion of the facial nerve and underlying bone and muscle. Report of a case. *J Dermatol Surg Oncol.* 1979;5:526–530.

55. Albom MJ, Swanson NA. Mohs micrographic surgery for the treatment of cutaneous neoplasms. In: Friedman RJ, Rigel DS, Kopf AW, Harris MN, Baker D, eds. *Cancer of the Skin.* Philadelphia, PA: WB Saunders; 1991:484–529.

56. Wentzell MJ, Robinson JK. Embryologic fusion planes and the spread of cutaneous carcinoma: A review and reassessment. *J Dermatol Surg Oncol.* 1990; 16:1000–1006.

57. Panje WR, Ceilley RI. The influence of embryology of the mid-face on the spread of epithelial malignancies. *Laryngoscope.* 1979;89:1914–1920.

58. Granstrom G, Aldenburg F, Jeppsson PH. Influence of embryonal fusion lines for recurrence of basal cell carcinoma in the head and neck. *Otolaryngol Head Neck Surg.* 1986;95:76–82.

59. Gullane PG. Extensive facial malignancies. Concepts and management. *J Otolaryngol.* 1986;15:44.

60. Levine HL, Bailin PL. Basal cell carcinoma of the head and neck. Identification of the high risk patient. *Laryngoscope.* 1980;90: 955–961.

61. Mohs FE. Modes of spread of cancer. In: *Chemosurgery. Microscopically Controlled Surgery for Skin Cancer.* Springfield, IL: Charles C Thomas; 1978:256–273.

62. Lawrence CM. Mohs micrographic surgery for basal cell carcinoma. *Clin Exp Dermatol.* 1999;24:130–133.

63. Spiller WF, Spiller RF. Cryosurgery and adjuvant surgical techniques for cutaneous carcinomas. In: Zacarian SA, ed. *Cryosurgery for Skin Cancer and Cutaneous Disorders.* St. Louis, MO: Mosby; 1985: 187.

64. Spiller WF, Spiller RF. Treatment of basal cell epithelioma by curettage and electrodesiccation. *J Am Acad Dermatol.* 1984;11:808–814.

65. Wolf DJ, Zitelli JA. Surgical margins for basal cell carcinoma. *Arch Dermatol.* 1987;123:340–344.

66. Leslie DF, Greenway HT. Mohs micrographic surgery for skin cancer. *Aust J Dermatol.* 1991;32:159–164.

67. Miller BH, Shavin JS, Coognetta A, et al. Nonsurgical treatment of basal cell carcinoma with interlesional 5-fluourouracil/epinephrine injectable gel. *J Am Acad Dermatol.* 1997;36:72–77.

68. Marks R, Gebauer K, Schumack S. Imiquimod 5% cream in the treatment of superficial basal cell carcinoma. Results of a multicenter 6-week dose response trial. *J Am Acad Dermatol.* 2001; 44:807–811.

69. Geisse J. Imiquimod 5% cream for the treatment of superficial basal cell carcinoma: Results from two phase III, randomized, vehicle-controlled studies. *J Am Acad Dermatol.* 2004;50(5):722–733.

70. Kokoszka A, Scheinfeld N. Evidence-based review of the use of cryosurgery in treatment of basal cell carcinoma. *Dermatol Surg.* 2003;29(6):566–571.

71. Lang PG, Maize JC. Histologic evolution of recurrent basal cell carcinoma and treatment implications. *J Am Acad Dermatol.* 1986;14:186–196.

72. Leffell DJ, Fitzgerald DA. Basal cell carcinoma. In: Freedberg IM, Eisen AZ, Wolff K, et al, eds. *Dermatology in General Medicine.* New York: McGraw-Hill; 1999:857–864.

73. Maloney ME. Histology of basal cell carcinoma. *Clin Dermatol.* 1995;13:545–549.

74. Salasche SJ, Ammonette RA. Morphea-form basal cell epitheliomas. A study of subclinical extensions in a series of 51 cases. *J Dermatol Surg Oncol.* 1981;7:387–393.

75. Goepfert H, Dichtel WJ, Medina JE, et al. Perineural invasion in squamous cell skin carcinoma of the head and neck. *Am J Surg.* 1984;148:542–547.

76. Mark GJ. Basal cell carcinoma with intraneural invasion. *Cancer.* 1977;40: 2181–2187.

77. Mehregan AH. Aggressive basal cell epithelioma on sunlight-protected skin: Report of eight cases, one with pulmonary and bone metastases. *Am J Dermatopathol.* 1983;5:221–229.

78. Hendrix JD, Parlette HL. Micronodular basal cell carcinoma: A deceptive histological subtype with frequently clinically undetected tumor extension. *Arch Dermatol.* 1996;132:295–298.

79. Borel DM. Cutaneous basosquamous carcinoma: Review of the literature and a report of 35 cases. *Arch Pathol.* 1973;95:293–297.

80. Stellmack RK, Rehrmann A, Koch H. Malignant degeneration of basal cell carcinomas of the face: Basal-squamous carcinoma. *Plast Reconstr Surg.* 1971;48: 471–473.

81. Sloane JP. The value of typing basal cell carcinomas in predicting recurrence after surgical excision. *Br J Dermatol.* 1977;96:127–132.

82. Wagner RF Jr, Cottel WI. Multifocal recurrent basal cell carcinoma following primary tumor treatment by electrodessication and curettage. *J Am Acad Dermatol.* 1987;17:1047–1049.

83. Salasche SJ. Curettage and electrodessication in the treatment of midfacial basal cell epithelioma. *J Am Acad Dermatol.* 1983;8:496–503.

84. Schwartz RA, Stoll HL. Squamous cell carcinoma. In: Freedberg IM, Eisen AZ, Wolff K, et al., eds. *Dermatology in General Medicine.* New York: McGraw-Hill; 1999:840–856.

85. Rowe DE, Carroll RJ, Day CL. Prognostic factors for local recurrence, metastasis, and survival rates in squamous cell carcinoma of the skin, ear, and lip. *J Am Acad Dermatol.* 1992;26:976–990.

86. Maguire B, Smith MP. Histopathology of cutaneous squamous cell carcinoma. *Clin Dermatol.* 1995;13:559–568.

87. Motley R, Kersey P, Lawrence C. Multiprofessional guidelines for the treatment of the patient with primary cutaneous squamous cell carcinoma. *Br J Dermatol.* 2002;146:18–25.

88. Katz AD, Urbach F, Lilienfeld AM. The frequency and risk metastases in squamous cell carcinoma of the skin. *Cancer.* 1957;10:1162–1166.

89. Epstein E, Epstein NN, Bragg K, Linden G. Metastases from squamous cell carcinomas of the skin. *Arch Dermatol.* 1968; 97:245–249.

90. Moller R, Reymann F, Hou-Jensen K. Metastases in dermatological patients with squamous cell carcinoma. *Arch Dermatol.* 1979;115:703–705.

91. Lund HZ. How often does squamous cell carcinoma of the skin metastasize? *Arch Dermatol.* 1965;92:635–637.

92. Drake LA, Dinehart SM, Goltz RW, et al. Guidelines for Mohs' micrographic surgery. *J Am Acad Dermatol.* 1995;33: 271–278.

93. Carter RL, Tanner NSB, Clifford P, et al. Perineural spread in squamous cell carcinoma of the head and neck: A clinico-

pathological study. *Clin Otolaryngol.* 1979;4:271–281.

94. Strauss M, Cohen C. Perineural invasion of the facial nerve: A case report with extension from cutaneous squamous cell carcinoma. *Otolaryngol Head Neck Surg.* 1981;89:831–835.

95. Trobe JD, Hood CI, Parsons JT, et al. Intracranial spread of squamous carcinoma along the trigeminal nerve. *Arch Opthalmol.* 1982;100:608–611.

96. Matorin PA, Wagner RF Jr. Mohs micrographic surgery: Technical difficulties posed by perineural invasion. *Int J Dermatol.* 1992;31:83–86.

97. Carter RL, Foster CS, Dinsdale EA, Pittam MR. Perineural spread by squamous cell carcinomas of the head and neck: A morphological study using anti-axonal and antimyelin monoclonal antibodies. *J Clin Pathol.* 1983;36:269–275.

98. Broders AC. Squamous-cell epithelioma of the skin. *Ann Surg.* 1921;73:141–160.

99. Cottel WI. Perineural invasion by squamous cell carcinoma. *J Dermatol Surg Oncol.* 1982;8:589–600.

100. Orengo I, Rosen T, Guill CK. Treatment of squamous cell carcinoma *in situ* of the penis with 5% imiquimod cream: A case report. *J Am Acad Dermatol.* 2002;47: S225–S228.

101. Mortiz DL, Lynch WS. Extensive Bowen's disease of the penile shaft treated with fresh tissue. Mohs micrographic surgery in two separate operations. *J Dermatol Surg Oncol.* 1991;17:374–378.

102. Mohs FE, Snow SN, Larson PO. Mohs micrographic surgery for penile tumors. *Urol Clin North Am.* 1992;19:291–304.

103. Dzubow L, Grossman D. Squamous cell carcinoma and verrucous carcinoma. In: Friedman RJ, Rigel DS, Kopf AW, Harris MN, Baker D, eds. *Cancer of the Skin.* Philadelphia, PA: WB Saunders; 1991: 74–84.

104. Mora RG. Microscopically controlled surgery (Mohs chemosurgery) for treatment of verrucous squamous cell carcinoma of the foot (epithelioma cuniculatum). *J Dermatol Surg Oncol.* 1978;8: 354–356.

105. Schwartz RA. Keratoacanthoma. *J Am Acad Dermatol.* 1994;30:157–165.

106. Janecka IP, Wolff M, Crikelair GF, Cosman B. Aggressive histological features of keratoacanthoma. *J Cutan Pathol.* 1978;4:342–348.

107. Larson PO. Keratoacanthomas treated with Mohs' micrographic surgery (chemosurgery). *J Am Acad Dermatol.* 1987;16:1040–1044.

108. Jemal A, Murray T, Samuels A, Ghafour A, Ward E, Thun MJ. Cancer Statistics, 2003. *CA Cancer J Clin.* 2003;53:5–26.

109. American Cancer Society. *Cancer facts and figures 2005.* Atlanta, GA: American Cancer Society; 2005.

110. Koh, HK. Cutaneous melanoma. *N Engl J Med.* 1991;325:171–182.

111. Weiner R, Anderson C, Edison K, Greer E. Melanoma reporting in Missouri. *Missouri Med.* 2004;101(6):598–602.

112. Day TA, Hornig JD, Sharma AK, Brescia F, Gillespie MB, Lathers D. Melanoma of the head and neck. *Curr Sci.* 2005;6: 19–30.

113. Kanzler M, Mraz-Gernhard S. Primary cutaneous malignant melanoma and its precursor lesions: Diagnostic and thera-

114. Clark WH Jr, From L, Bernardino EA, Mihm MC Jr. The histogenesis and biologic behavior of primary human malignant melanoma of the skin. *Cancer Res.* 1969;29:705–727.

115. Breslow A. Prognostic factors in the treatment of cutaneous melanoma. *J Cutan Pathol.* 1979;6:208–212.

116. Cascinelli N, Santinami M, Maurichi A, et al. World Health Organization experience in the treatment of melanoma. *Surg Clin North Am.* 2003;83:405–416.

117. Cascinelli N. Margin of resection in the management of primary melanoma. *Semin Surg Oncol.* 1998;14:272–275.

118. Piepkorn M. Melanoma resection margin recommendations, unconventionally based on available facts. *Semin Diagn Pathol.* 1998;15:230–234.

119. Bienert TN. Treatment of cutaneous melanoma of the face by Mohs micrographic surgery. *J Cutan Med Surg.* 2003; 7:25–30.

120. Epstein E. Thoughts on melanoma. In: Epstein E, ed. *Skin Surgery.* Philadelphia, PA: WB Saunders; 1987:554.

121. Zitelli JA, Mohs FE, Larson P, Snow S. Mohs micrographic surgery for melanoma. *Dermatol Clin.* 1989;7:833–843.

122. Zitelli JA. Mohs surgery for melanoma. In: Mikhail GR, ed. *Mohs micrographic surgery.* Philadelphia, PA: WB Saunders; 1991:275–288.

123. Mohs FE. Microscopically controlled surgery for periorbital melanoma: Fixed-tissue and fresh-tissue techniques. *J Dermatol Surg Oncol.* 1985;11:284–291.

124. Mohs FE. Micrographic surgery for the microscopically controlled excision of eyelid cancers. *Arch Opthalmol.* 1986;104: 901–909.

125. Nouri K, Lodha R, Jiminez G, Robins P. Mohs micrographic surgery for dermatofibrosarcoma protuberans: University of Miami and NYU experience. *Dermatol Surg.* 2002;28(11):1060–1064.

126. Lal P, Sharma R, Mohan H, Sekhon MS. Dermatofibrosarcoma protuberans metastasizing to lymph nodes: A case report and review of literature. *J Surg Oncol.* 1999;72(3):178–180.

127. Zorlu F, Yildiz F, Ertoy D, Atahan IL, Erden E. Dermatofibrosarcoma protuberans metastasizing to cavernous sinuses and lung: Case report. *Jpn J Clin Oncol.* 2001;31(11):557–561.

128. Garcia C, Clark RE, Buchanon M. Dermatofibrosarcoma protuberans. *Int J Dermatol.* 1996;35:867–871.

129. Wick MR, Ritter JH, Lind AC, Swanson PE. The pathological distinction between deep penetrating dermatofibroma and dermatofibrosarcoma protuberans. *Semin Cutan Med Surg.* 1999;18(1):91–98.

130. Checketts SR, Hamilton TK, Baughman RD. Congenital and childhood dermatofibrosarcoma protuberans: A case report and review of literature. *J Am Acad Dermatol.* 2000;42:907–913.

131. Gloster HM Jr, Harris KR, Roenigk RK. A comparison between Mohs' micrographic surgery and wide surgical excision for the treatment of dermatofibrosarcoma protuberans. *J Am Acad Dermatol.* 1996;35:82–87.

132. Parlette LE, Smith CK, Germain LM, Rolfe CA, Skelton H. Accelerated

growth of dermatofibrosarcoma protuberans during pregnancy. *J Am Acad Dermatol.* 1999;41:778–783.

133. Lidner NJ, Scarborough MT, Powel GJ, Spanier S, Enneking WF. Revision surgery in dermatofibrosarcoma protuberans of the trunk and extremities. *Eur J Surg Oncol.* 1999;25(4):392–397.

134. Gayner SM, Lewis JE, McAffrey TV. Effect of resection margins on dermatofibrosarcoma protuberans of the head and neck. *Arch Otolaryngol Head Neck Surg.* 1997;123:430–433.

135. Parker TL, Zitelli JA. Surgical margins for excision of dermatofibrosarcoma protuberans. *J Am Acad Dermatol.* 1995;32: 233–236.

136. Dawes KW, Hanke CW. Dermatofibrosarcoma protuberans treated with Mohs' micrographic surgery: Cure rates and surgical margins. *Dermatol Surg.* 1997;22:530–534.

137. Ratner D, Thomas CO, Johnson TM, et al. Mohs micrographic surgery for the treatment of dermatofibrosarcoma protuberans. Results of a multi-institutional series with an analysis of the extent of microscopic spread. *J Am Acad Dermatol.* 1997;37:600–613.

138. Ballo MT, Zaggars GK, Pisters P, Pollack A. The role of radiation therapy in the management of dermatofibrosarcoma protuberans. *Int J Radiat Oncol Biol Phys.* 1998;40:823–827.

139. Sun L, Wang CJ, Huang CC, et al. Dermatofibrosarcoma protuberans: Treatment results of thirty-five cases. *Radiother Oncol.* 2000;57:175–181.

140. Haycox CL, Odland PB, Olbricht SM, Casey B. Dermatofibrosarcoma protuberans (DFSP); growth characteristics based on tumor model and a review of cases treated with Mohs' micrographic surgery. *Ann Plast Surg.* 1997;38: 246–251.

141. Massey RA, Tok J, Strippoli BA, Szabolcs MJ, Silvers DN, Eliezri YD. A comparison of frozen and paraffin sections in dermatofibrosarcoma protuberans. *Dermatol Surg.* 1998;24(9):995–998.

142. Clayton BD, Leshin B, Hitchcock MG, Marks M, White WL. Utility of rush paraffin embedded sections in management of cutaneous neoplasms. *Dermatol Surg.* 2000;26:671–678.

143. Hodgson TA, Haricharan AK, Barrett AW, Porter SR. Microcystic adnexal carcinoma: An unusual cause of swelling and paresthesia of the lower lip. *Oral Oncol.* 2003;39:195–198.

144. Snow S, Madjar DD, Hardy S, et al. Microcystic adnexal carcinoma: Report of thirteen cases and review of literature. *Dermatol Surg.* 2001;27:401–408.

145. Friedman PM, Friedman RH, Jiang SB, Nouri K, Amonette R, Robins P. Microcystic adnexal carcinoma: A collaborative series review and update. *J Am Acad Dermatol.* 1999;41:225–231.

146. Carroll P, Goldstein GD, Brown CW. Metastatic microcystic adnexal carcinoma in an immunocompromised patient. *Dermatol Surg.* 2000;26:531–534.

147. Ongenae KC, Verhaegh MEJM, Vermeulen AHM, et al. Microcystic adnexal carcinoma: An uncommon tumor with debatable origin. *Dermatol Surg.* 2001;27:979–984.

148. Bier-Laning CM, Horn DB, Gapany M, et al. Microcystic adnexal carcinoma: Management options based on long-term follow-up. *Laryngoscope.* 1995;105: 1197–1201.

149. Billingsley EM, Fedok F, Maloney ME. Microcystic adnexal carcinoma. Case report and review of literature. *Arch Otolaryngol.* 1996;122:179–182.

150. Nickoloff BJ, Fleischman HE, Carmel J, Wood CC, Roth RJ. Microcystic adnexal carcinoma: An immunohistologic observation suggesting dual (pillar and eccrine) differentiation. *Arch Dermatol.* 1986;122:290–294.

151. Wick MR, Cooper PH, Swanson PE, Kaye VN, Sun TT. Microcystic adnexal carcinoma: An immunohistochemical comparison with other cutaneous appendage tumors. *Arch Dermatol.* 1990;126:189–194.

152. Swanson PE, Cherwitz DL, Neumann MP, Wick MR. Eccrine sweat gland carcinoma: A histologic and immunohistochemical study of 32 cases. *J Cutan Pathol.* 1987;14:65–86.

153. Antley CA, Carney M, Smoller BR. Microcystic adnexal carcinoma arising in the setting of previous radiation therapy. *J Cutan Pathol.* 1999;26:48–50.

154. Sebastien TS, Nelson BR, Lowe L, Baker S, Johnson TM. Microcystic adnexal carcinoma. *J Am Acad Dermatol.* 1993;29: 840–845.

155. Cooper PH, Headington JT, Mills SE, et al. Sclerosing sweat duct (syringomatous) carcinoma. *Am J Surg Pathol.* 1985;9:422–433.

156. Cooper PH. Sclerosing carcinomas of sweat ducts (microcystic adnexal carcinoma). *Arch Dermatol.* 1986;122:261–264.

157. Burns MK, Chen SP, Goldberg LH. Microcystic adnexal carcinoma. Ten cases treated by Mohs micrographic surgery. *J Dermatol Surg Oncol.* 1994;20:429–434.

158. McAlvany JP, Stonecipher MR, Leshin B, Prichard E, White W. Schlerosing sweat gland carcinoma in an 11-year-old boy. *J Dermatol Surg Oncol.* 1994;20: 767–768.

159. Callahan EF, Vidimos AT, Bergfeld WF. Microcystic adnexal carcinoma of the scalp with extensive pilar differentiation. *Dermatol Surg.* 2002;28:536–539.

160. Abbate M, Zeitouni NC, Seyler M, Hicks W, Loree T, Cheney RT. Clinical course, risk factors, and treatment of microcystic adnexal carcinoma: A short series report. *Dermatol Surg.* 2003;29:1035–1038.

161. Chiller K, Passaro D, Scheuller M, Singer M, McCalmont T, Grekin RC. Microcystic adnexal carcinoma: Fourty-eight cases, their treatment, and their outcome. *Arch Dermatol.* 2000;136:1355–1359.

162. Brown MD, Swanson NA. Treatment of malignant fibrous histiocytoma and atypical fibroxanthomas with micrographic surgery. *J Dermatol Surg Oncol.* 1989;15:1287–1292.

163. Stadler FJ, Scott GA, Brown MD. Malignant fibrous tumors. *Semin Cutan Med Surg.* 1998;17:141–152.

164. Rizzardi C, Angiero F, Melato M. Atypical fibroxanthoma and malignant fibrous histiocytoma of the skin. *Anticancer Res.* 2003;23:1847–1851.

165. Rothman AE, Lowitt MH, Pfau RG. Pediatric cutaneous malignant fibrous histiocytoma. *J Am Acad Dermatol.* 2000;42:371–373.

166. Ly H, Selva D, James CL, Huilgol SC. Superficial malignant fibrous histiocytoma presenting as recurrent atypical fibroxanthoma. *Aust J Dermatol.* 2004;45: 106–109.

167. Hafner J, Kunzi W, Weinreich T. Malignant fibrous histiocytoma and atypical fibroxanthoma in renal transplant recipients. *Dermatology.* 1999;198:29–32.

168. Mansoor A, White CR Jr. Myxofibrosarcoma presenting in the skin: Clinicopathological features and differential diagnosis with cutaneous myxoid neoplasms. *Am J Dermatopathol.* 2003;25: 281–286.

169. Hakim I. Atypical fibroxanthoma. *Ann Otol Rhinol Laryngol.* 2001;110:985–987.

170. Fish FS. Soft tissue sarcomas in dermatology. *Dermatol Surg.* 1996;22:268–273.

171. Davis JL, Randle HW, Zalla MJ, et al. A comparison of Mohs micrographic surgery and wide excision for the treatment of atypical fibroxanthoma. *Dermatol Surg.* 1997;23(2):105–110.

172. Huether MJ, Zitelli JA, Brodland DG. Mohs micrographic surgery for the treatment of spindle cell tumors of the skin. *J Am Acad Dermatol.* 2001;44:656–659.

173. Hafner J, Schutz K, Morgenthaler W, Steiger E, Meyer V, Burg G. Micrographic surgery ("slow Mohs") in cutaneous sarcomas. *Dermatology.* 1999;198(1):37–43.

174. Hart WR, Millman JB. Progression of intraepithelial Paget's disease of the vulva to invasive carcinoma. *Cancer.* 1977;40:2333–2337.

175. Hock WH. Adenocarcinoma of the scrotum (extramammary Paget's disease): Case report and review of the literature. *J Urol.* 1984;132:137–139.

176. Goltz R. Paget's disease, mammary and extramammary. In: Chu AC, Edelson RL, eds. *Malignant Tumors of the Skin.* London: Arnold; 1999:294–301.

177. Parmley TH, Woodruff JD, Julian CG. Invasive vulvar Paget's disease. *Obstet Gynecol.* 1975;46:341–346.

178. Coldiron MB, Goldsmith BA, Robinson JK. Surgical treatment of extramammary Paget's disease: A report of six cases and a reexamination of Mohs micrographic surgery compared with conventional surgical excision. *Cancer.* 1991;67:933–938.

179. Mazoujian G, Pinkus GS, Haagenson DE. Extramammary Paget's disease—evidence for an apocrine origin. An immunoperoxidase study of gross cystic disease fluid protein-15, CEA, and keratin proteins. *Am J Surg Pathol.* 1984;8:43–50.

180. Battles OE, Page DL, Johnson JE. Cytokeratins, CEA, and mucin histochemistry in the diagnosis and characterization of extramammary Paget's disease. *Am J Clin Pathol.* 1997;108:6–12.

181. Harris DW, Kist DA, Bloom K, Zachary CB. Rapid staining with carcinoembryonic antigen aids limited excision of extramammary Paget's disease treated by Mohs' surgery. *J Dermatol Surg Oncol.* 1994;20:260–264.

182. Mohs FE, Blanchard L. Microscopically controlled surgery for extramammary Paget's disease. *Arch Dermatol.* 1979;115: 706–708.

183. Zampogna JC, Flowers FP, Roth WI, et al. Treatment of primary limited cutaneous extramammary Paget's disease with topical imiquimod monotherapy: Two case reports. *J Am Acad Dermatol.* 2002;47:S229–S235.

184. Berman B, Poocheron VN, Villa AM. Novel dermatologic uses of immune response modifier imiquimod 5% cream. *Skin Ther Lett.* 2002;7:1–6.

185. Hendi A, Brodland DG, Zitelli JA. Extramammary Paget's disease: Surgical treatment with Mohs micrographic surgery. *J Am Acad Dermatol.* 2004;51(5): 767–773.

186. O'Connor WJ, Lim KK, Zalla MJ, et al. Comparison of Mohs' micrographic surgery and wide excision for extramammary Paget's disease. *Dermatol Surg.* 2003;29:723–727.

187. Al-Ghazal SK, Arora D, Simpson R, et al. Merkel cell carcinoma of the skin. *Br J Plast Surg.* 1996;49:491–496.

188. Herbst A, Haynes HA, Nghiem P. The standard of care for Merkel cell carcinoma should include adjuvant radiation and lymph node surgery. *J Am Acad Dermatol.* 2002;46:640–641.

189. Ott MJ, Tanabe KK, Gadd MA. Multimodality management of Merkel cell carcinoma. *Arch Surg.* 1999;134: 388–393.

190. Nghiem P, McKee P, Haynes H. Merkel cell (cutaneous neuroendocrine) carcinoma. In: Sober AJ, Haluska FG, eds. *Atlas of Clinical Oncology: Skin Cancer.* Hamilton, Ontario, Canada: BC Decker; 2001:127–141.

191. Leech SN, Kolar AJO, Barrett PD, Sinclair SA, Leonard N. Merkel cell carcinoma can be distinguished from metastatic small cell carcinoma using antibodies to cytokeratin 20 and thyroid transcription factor 1. *J Clin Pathol* 2001;54:727–729.

192. Chiarelli TG, Grant-Kels JM, Sporn JR, ezuke WN, Whalen JD. Unusual presentation of Merkel cell carcinoma. *J Am Acad Dermatol.* 2000;42:366–370.

193. O'Connor WJ, Roenigk RK, Brodland DG. Merkel cell carcinoma. Comparison of Mohs micrographic surgery and wide surgical excision in eighty-six patients. *Dermatol Surg.* 1997;23:929–933.

194. Duker I, Starz H, Bachter D, Balda BR. Prognostic and therapeutic implications of sentinel lymphnodectomy and S-staging in Merkel cell carcinoma. *Dermatology.* 2001;202(3):225–229.

195. Sian KU, Wagner JD, Sood R, Park HM, Havlick R, Coleman JJ. Lymphoscintigraphy with sentinel lymph node biopsy in cutaneous Merkel cell carcinoma. *Ann Plast Surg.* 1999;42:679–682.

196. Rodrigues LK, Leong SP, Kashani-Sabet M, Wong JH. Early experience with sentinel lymph node mapping for Merkel cell carcinoma. *J Am Acad Dermatol.* 2001;45:303–308.

197. Zeitouni NC, Cheney RT, Delacure MD. Lymphoscintigraphy, sentinel lymph node biopsy, and Mohs' micrographic surgery in the treatment of Merkel cell carcinoma. *Dermatol Surg.* 2000;26:12–18.

198. Wasserberg N, Schachter J, Fenig E, Feinmesser M, Gutman H. Applicability of sentinel node technique to Merkel cell carcinoma. *Dermatol Surg.* 2000;26: 138–141.

199. Hill ADK, Brady MS, Coit DG. Intraoperative lymphatic mapping and sentinel lymph node biopsy for Merkel cell carcinoma. *Br J Surg.* 1999;86:518–521.

200. Gollard R, Weber R, Kosty MP, Greenway HT, Massullo V, Humberson C. Merkel cell carcinoma; review of 22 cases with surgical, pathologic, and therapeutic considerations. *Cancer.* 2000;88:1842–1851.

201. Akhtar S, Oza KK, Wright J. Merkel cell carcinoma: Report of ten cases and review of literature. *J Am Acad Dermatol.* 2000;43:755–767.

202. Boyer JD, Zitelli JA, Brodland DG, D'Angelo G. Local control of primary Merkel cell carcinoma: Review of 45 cases treated with Mohs' micrographic surgery with and without adjuvant radiation. *J Am Acad Dermatol.* 2002;47:885–892.

203. An KP, Ratner D. Merkel cell carcinoma in the setting of HIV infection. *J Am Acad Dermatol.* 2001;45:309–312.

204. Morman MR. Mohs micrographic surgery. *N J Med.* 1989;86:369–373.

205. Finucane DJ, Parlette HL. Mohs surgery: Guidelines for technicians. *J Assoc Mil Dermatol.* 1991;17:3–9.

206. Hruza GJ. Mohs micrographic surgery. Local recurrences. *J Dermatol Surg Oncol.* 1994;20:573–577.

207. Miller PK, Roenigk RK, Broadland DG, Randle HW. Cutaneous micrographic surgery: Mohs procedure. *Mayo Clin Proc.* 1992;67:971–980.

208. Cook J, Zitelli JA. Mohs micrographic surgery: A cost analysis. *J Am Acad Dermatol.* 1998;39:698–703.

CHAPTER 41

Reconstructive Surgery of Eyelid Cancers

Jennifer I. Hui, M.D.
David T. Tse, M.D., F.A.C.S

BOX 41-1 Overview—Methods of Eyelid Reconstruction

- Anterior lamella defect, eyelid margin intact
  - Primary closure
  - Skin graft
  - Flap
- Full-thickness eyelid defect
  - Primary closure
  - Rotational flap
  - Replacement of posterior lamella plus flap
- Special circumstances
  - Medial canthal defect
  - Insufficient posterior lamella
  - Insufficient anterior lamella
  - Insufficient vascularized pedicle

■ INTRODUCTION

The most common malignancy in the United States is cutaneous carcinoma. Approximately 800,000 and 200,000 Americans annually receive treatment for basal cell and squamous cell carcinoma of the skin, respectively. In addition, 51,000 Americans are diagnosed with malignant cutaneous melanoma each year.[1] The eyelids account for 5 to 9% of all skin cancers with the most common malignancies being basal cell carcinoma, squamous cell carcinoma, sebaceous cell carcinoma, and malignant melanoma. Kaposi's sarcoma is being recognized with increasing frequency among immunosuppressed patients. Systemic diseases such as basal cell nevus syndrome, xeroderma pigmentosum, and Muir–Torre syndrome are also associated with periocular cutaneous tumors.

Early accurate diagnosis, preservation or restoration of eyelid function, and cosmesis are the most important factors in the management of malignant eyelid lesions. An eyelid lesion with clinical features suggestive of malignancy requires a definitive diagnosis. An excisional biopsy with at least a 2 to 3-mm margin of normal tissue should be considered if the lesion is small. If the lesion is sufficiently large such that the size of the anticipated excisional defect will induce eyelid malposition, an incisional biopsy should be undertaken before proceeding with further manipulation of the surgical site. The surgical margins require histologic confirmation of tumor eradication prior to any anticipated reconstruction with a graft or a flap.

A definitive excision of the malignant lesion is pursued once the histologic diagnosis is confirmed. Mohs micrographic surgery followed by immediate reconstruction is the authors' preferred treatment of primary periocular malignant eyelid lesions. This treatment provides for maximum tissue conservation as well as precise evaluation of surgical margins. A trained dermatologist best accomplishes the Mohs micrographic surgery resection.

The resection first involves bulk removal of the tumor along with a small peripheral margin of normal tissue.[2-6] A tissue layer approximately 2-mm thick is further removed from the entire base and edges of the wound. The specimen is divided and placed onto glass slides. The edges are then carefully marked with different colored dyes to preserve proper orientation. Frozen sections from the undersurface and skin edges of each specimen are then taken and the locations of residual tumor are marked on a map. These areas undergo further re-excision (Fig. 41-1). The exact location of residual tumor is determined systematically, thus ensuring tumor-free margins. The oculoplastic surgeon then reconstructs the eyelid defect on the same or following day. This interdisciplinary collaborative team approach allows two unbiased specialists to offer their shared expertise in achieving the optimum surgical outcome for the patient.

Careful palpation of preauricular and submandibular lymph nodes should be performed in patients with biopsy-proven malignant eyelid lesions with demonstrated biological tendencies for regional lymph-node metastasis. These entities include squamous cell carcinoma, sebaceous cell carcinoma, melanoma, and Merkel cell carcinoma. Wide surgical excision ensuring tumor-free margins of excision with subsequent, immediate reconstruction of the defect should be undertaken. Lymphatic mapping with sentinel lymph-node biopsy is an additional consideration for solid tumors with a propensity for regional nodal metastasis.[7] This procedure provides more accurate early staging of disease.

Technetium-labeled sulfur colloid and blue dye are two pharmaceuticals used in the most common method of detecting microscopic metastases in clinically negative regional lymph nodes. Two components are key to the identification of the sentinel lymph node: an intraoperative gamma-detecting probe and a vital blue dye.

The afferent lymphatics are initially mapped with preoperative lympho-

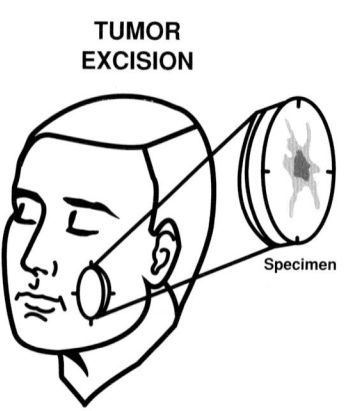
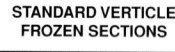
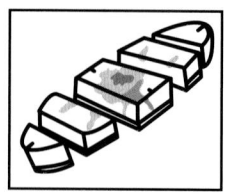
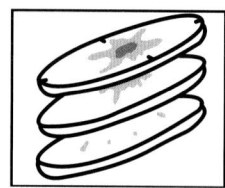

TUMOR EXCISION

Specimen

STANDARD VERTICLE FROZEN SECTIONS

HORIZONTAL FROZEN SECTIONS

▲ **FIGURE 41-1** During Mohs micrographic excision of a malignant lesion, frozen sections are obtained from the undersurface and skin edges. Areas of residual tumor are then marked on a map for subsequent excision. The process is repeated until the tumor margins are all negative.

scintigraphy. 0.3 mCi of technetium Tc 99m-labeled sulfur colloid in 0.2 mL of buffered saline is administered in the area of interest.[7] Fifteen to 30 minutes later, lymphoscintigrams of the ipsilateral neck region are taken. The radiopharmaceutical injection is repeated on the day of surgery. 0.2 mL of a second mapping agent, blue dye, is also administered around the lesion on this day. Five to 10 minutes after the second injection, the gamma detector probe is placed over the skin covering the draining lymphatics in search of the sentinel lymph node, which is represented by an area of increased radioactivity. A small incision is then made in this area. The course of the blue afferent lymphatics is followed in the subcutaneous tissue until the node is identified. Identification of the node is facilitated through the use of two localization methods: sound with the gamma detector probe and visually with the blue dye. It is then excised and sent for histologic evaluation. This enhanced method of sentinel lymph-node identification allows for improved staging of eyelid tumors and prevents unnecessary neck dissection.

▮ RECONSTRUCTION

The foundations of reconstructive surgery are preservation or restoration of both eyelid function as well as cosmesis.[2] Detailed knowledge of regional eyelid anatomy is a key factor in successful reconstructive strategy. The eyelid is a bilamellar structure: skin and orbicularis oculi muscle compose the anterior lamella while the tarsal plate and conjunctiva form the posterior lamella.

The following principles of eyelid reconstruction must be taken into consideration in order to achieve the optimum functional and cosmetic outcome. First and foremost, either the anterior or posterior lamella must have its own blood supply. Two free grafts without independent blood supplies will not survive. Other important principles include maximal horizontal stabilization with minimal vertical tension, proper canthal fixation and an epithelialized internal surface.[8] Finally, proper opening and closing functions of the reconstructed eyelid must be maintained through precise identification of both the transverse edge of the levator aponeurosis and the facial nerve. Proper opening and closing functions are necessary for protection of the globe and prevention of exposure.

Lower Eyelid Defects

ANTERIOR LAMELLA DEFICIT, LID MARGIN INTACT

Primary closure Anterior lamella defects without lid margin involvement are generally closed primarily if distortion is not induced. Closure should be directed along a horizontal tension line, not a vertical plane, to minimize lid-margin distortion. A vertical incision is needed for horizontal undermining and subsequent closure. The defect is closed with deep, interrupted 6-0 Vicryl sutures and interrupted, superficial 6-0 or 7-0 nylon or silk, being careful to avoid horizontal lid distortion. A full-thickness pentagonal wedge that includes the anterior lamella defect may be required if insufficient anterior lamella remains. The wedge is excised with Wescott's scissors. The tarsal borders must be sharp and perpendicular to the lid margin. This resulting full-thickness defect is then closed primarily as outlined later.

Skin graft Full-thickness skin graft is one option used to repair defects that are too large for primary closure. Split-thickness skin grafts are generally not recommended in eyelid reconstruction.[4] The ipsilateral upper eyelid and preauricular or retroauricular skin are excellent donor sites for full-thickness grafts. If there is insufficient tissue in these areas, other possible nonhair bearing donor sites include the supraclavicular fossa and the upper inner arm. Skin grafts must be thinned of subcutaneous fat and connective tissue prior to placement in the recipient site. The graft is then trimmed to size and sutured into the defect with superficial, interrupted 7-0 nylon or silk sutures.[9]

Ellipse sliding flap A second option for the closure of anterior lamella defects is the elliptical sliding flap.[9] The tissue surrounding a wound is undermined in the suborbicular fascial plane, advanced, and then closed primarily. The conversion of a circular or ovoid defect into an ellipse prevents a dog-ear formation. Orienting the ellipse parallel to the relaxed skin tension lines minimizes distortion of the surrounding tissue and the size of the resultant scar. Anterior lamella defects near the lid margin, however, should not be reconstructed with the elliptical flap because ectropion or retraction may be induced by excessive perpendicular tension.

The defect should be incorporated into the ellipse with its long axis parallel to wrinkle lines. The ellipse angle should be 30° with the long axis four times longer than the short axis. The skin and subcutaneous tissue are incised with a #15 blade and then undermined with Wescott's scissors along the edges of the flap. Undermining is performed until the edges of the elliptical defect are closed without tension. The subcutaneous tissue is closed with deep interrupted 6-0 or 7-0 Vicryl sutures and the skin with interrupted 6-0 or 7-0 nylon sutures.

Myocutaneous advancement flap A third option for the closure of an anterior lamella defect with an intact lid margin is the myocutaneous advancement flap. This method is ideal for larger defects as well as those that involve the medial canthal area as it provides the best tissue match and, most importantly, an autonomous blood supply (Fig. 41-2A). Incision lines should blend within naturally occurring skin creases. Additionally,

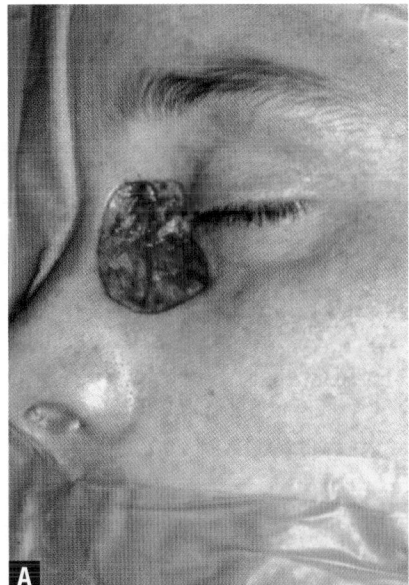

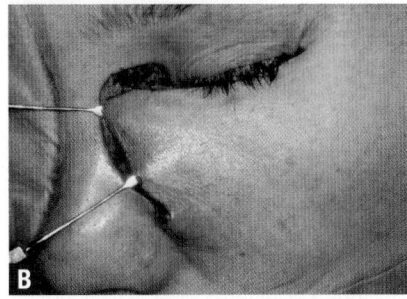

▲ **FIGURE 41-2 A.** A myocutaneous advancement flap allows for closure of a large anterior lamella defect involving the medial canthal area while providing a good tissue match with an inherent vascular supply. **B.** A flap of sufficient size provides for tension-free closure.

tension lines in the lower eyelid should be oriented horizontally, not vertically. The flap must be sufficiently large such that closure is achieved without tension (Fig. 41-2B). Ideally, planes of dissection should be determined prior to advancement of undermining past the lateral orbital rim.[9,10]

This skin and muscle flap is designed to advance medially to fill an anterior lamella defect. The creation of the flap begins with an infralash incision that extends laterally to the canthus and arches superiorly. The laxity of the periocular tissues determines the degree of lateral extension of the incision. The incision may be extended to the ear if necessary. The incision is made with a #15 blade and the skin-muscle flap is undermined with Steven's scissors anterior to the orbital septum in the lid. The undermining is extended into the temporal region and inferiorly toward the cheek. Undermining is continued until the temporal edge of the flap may be advanced nasally to the medial edge of the defect without tension. The most important step in the execution of a myocutaneous advancement flap is the strategic placement of a tension-bearing permanent suture (4-0 Prolene) at the zygoma or the lateral orbital rim. This technique provides an anterior lamella replacement with an inherent vascular supply. Closure begins at the tip of the advancement flap with deep, interrupted 6-0 Vicryl sutures followed by superficial, interrupted 6-0 nylon sutures through the skin.

Full-Thickness Eyelid Defect

PRIMARY CLOSURE Primary closure without lateral cantholysis is the best method of closing small defects involving less than one-third of the lower eyelid margin. A layered, primary closure provides the best tissue match, a smooth lid margin, and a continuous eyelash line. A lateral canthotomy may yield an additional 5 to 6 mm of medial advancement of the temporal eyelid margin if tension precludes proper lid-margin reapproximation.[8,9]

In a primary closure, the edges of the eyelid defect are trimmed so the borders are sharp and perpendicular to the lid margin. Tissue inferior to the tarsus is cut into a wedge to form a pentagonal-shaped defect. Direct closure is pursued if the borders of the defect may be reapproximated without excess tension.

A lateral cantholysis is needed if primary reapproximation of the edges induces tension. First, a 4 to 5-mm horizontal incision through the skin and orbicularis muscle is made with Steven's scissors from the lateral canthal angle and directed toward the orbital rim. The tip of the Wescott's scissors is used to identify the lateral attachment of the lower lid. The inferior crus of the lateral canthal tendon is cut with a vertical incision. The incision allows for medial mobilization of the wound without excess tension. The conjunctiva should not be disrupted during the cantholysis. The incision is then closed with interrupted 7-0 nylon sutures.

Precise approximation of the tarsal edges is the most important step in the primary closure of a pentagonal lid-margin defect. Accurate vertical alignment provides the majority of the tension-bearing support of the wound. First, three interrupted 5-0 Vicryl sutures are placed at partial thickness through the tarsal plate. Full-thickness sutures should not be used because they cause corneal irritation. Next, the lid margin is closed with a vertical mattress suture that provides anteroposterior alignment. A 6-0 silk suture is placed in the meibomian gland orifice 3 mm from the wound edge on one side and exits through the tarsal plate 3 mm from the lid margin on the same side. The suture is then placed through the tarsal edge on the opposite side to emerge from a meibomian gland orifice 3 mm from the wound edge on that side. The suture is then passed back through the lid margin in a near-to-near fashion, entering and exiting through a meibomian gland orifice 1 mm from the would edges. This vertical lid margin suture induces puckering of the wound edges, which prevents notching once the margin is healed. In addition, the tails of the suture should be on the side of the defect that is farther from the central cornea. If needed, the lid margin may be further aligned with two additional sutures, one posterior and another inferior to the lashes. The ends of the silk sutures are left long and secured away from the wound on the lower lid skin with a suture to prevent corneal irritation. The anterior lamella 7-0 nylon or silk sutures close the skin (Fig. 41-3).

SEMICIRCULAR ROTATIONAL FLAP Larger, more centralized defects involving up to two-thirds of the central lower lid may be reconstructed with a lateral semicircular rotational flap. This flap is only useful if there is sufficient temporal tarsal remnant as this remnant and the myocutaneous flap are moved as a unit.[9]

First, a semicircle, approximately 20 mm in diameter, starting at the lateral canthal angle, is outlined. The semicircle should arc superiorly and temporally but not pass the lateral extent of the brow. The skin is incised with a #15 blade and Wescott's scissors are used to bluntly dissect the skin and orbicularis from the orbital rim. The flap is undermined inferiorly so it may be moved medially.

A canthotomy is performed with the scissors extending to the inside of the orbital rim once the flap is retracted

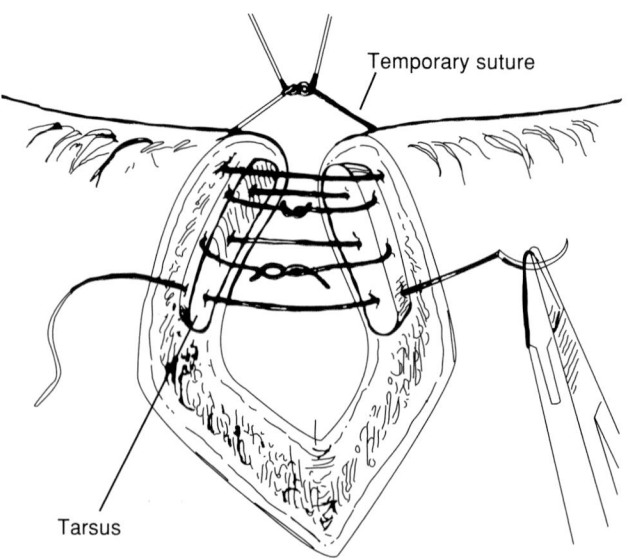

▲ **FIGURE 41-3** During closure of a full-thickness eyelid margin defect, the lid margin is aligned with a 6-0 silk vertical mattress suture. Partial thickness 5-0 Vicryl sutures reapproximate the edges of the tarsal plate and interrupted 7-0 nylon or silk sutures close the skin.

inferiorly. The inferior crus of the lateral canthal tendon is cut at the rim and the superior crus is left intact. The lateral lower lid and flap are moved medially until the lid-margin defect is closed and covered without tension. If the lateral lid is not rotated easily, scissors are placed under the inferior tarsal border between the conjunctiva and orbicularis muscle to separate it from the septum and retractors. The lateral canthus is reformed after the defect is closed. Posterior and lateral vector forces should be directed in a way that allows the reconstructed lower eyelid to lay in apposition with the globe. This requires fixation of the lateral edge of the flap. The flap's deep edge is secured to the inner aspect of the lateral orbital rim inferior to the superior crus with 4-0 Vicryl sutures. A running 7-0 Vicryl suture is used to attach the skin edge of the lateral lid margin to the conjunctival edge after the latter is advanced superiorly.

FREE TARSAL GRAFT PLUS MYOCUTANEOUS ADVANCEMENT FLAP

A free tarsal graft from the ipsilateral or contralateral upper eyelid may be used for posterior lamella replacement in larger defects for which primary closure is not possible.[9] The graft provides two important factors: posterior lamellar support and a mucous membrane lining for the reconstructed lower lid. A myocutaneous advancement flap that provides blood supply to the free graft is then designed (Fig. 41-4). This is the most appropriate option for patients whose involved eyelid is on the side of the only seeing eye.

First, a 4-0 silk traction suture is placed through the central upper lid margin. Everting the lid over a Desmarre's retractor or a lid plate exposes the tarsoconjunctival surface. The graft is outlined on the conjunctival surface with a marking pen. The inferior edge of the graft is parallel to and 4 mm or more from the lid margin. The vertical height of the graft is determined by the location of the superior tarsal border. A #15 blade is used to incise the conjunctiva and full-thickness tarsus along the inferior and vertical edges. The levator aponeurosis is dissected from the underlying tarsus while Mueller's muscle and conjunctiva are cut from the superior tarsal border with scissors, leaving 2 mm of conjunctiva attached to the graft. The donor site is allowed to heal by secondary intention.

The graft is secured to the defect with the conjunctival surface in contact with the globe and the superior edge of the graft in contact with the conjunctival remnant along the new lid margin. The medial edges are closed with partial thickness, interrupted 5-0 Vicryl sutures to minimize ocular irritation. Interrupted 7-0 Vicryl sutures around to secure the conjunctiva to the inferior tarsal graft as well as the skin to the anterior, superior tarsal graft. If necessary, the graft may be covered with a vascularized myocutaneous advancement flap.

The myocutaneous advancement flap is outlined with a marking pen in either a semicircular manner or as a cheek flap extending 1 to 2 cm beyond the lateral commissure. The skin is incised with a

#15 blade. Wescott's scissors are used to cut down to the orbital rim through the orbicularis muscle. Steven's scissors are used to undermine the temporal eyelid and skin and muscle of the cheek allowing for medial rotation of the myocutaneous flap. Buried, interrupted, tension-bearing 6-0 Vicryl sutures are placed in the muscular layer, while interrupted 7-0 nylon sutures close the skin.

PERIOSTEAL STRIP PLUS MYOCUTANEOUS ADVANCEMENT FLAP

The periosteal strip with myocutaneous advancement flap is an alternative method of reconstructing a larger defect not amenable to primary closure. It is especially useful in reconstruction of the lower lid when the lateral one-third of the tarsus is absent. It may also be used in combination with other procedures for larger defects.

First, the skin overlying the flap is outlined with a marking pen in a semicircular shape or as a cheek flap extending 1 to 2 cm past the lateral commissure. A #15 blade is used to incise the skin and orbicularis muscle down to orbital rim. The anterior lamella is then mobilized from the underlying tissue bed with blunt dissection. The lateral orbital rim is exposed once the flap is reflected. A rectangular strip of periosteum based at the inner aspect of the rim is fashioned. Ideally, the strip should be 1 cm in width and angled 45° to follow the contour of the lower lid. The distance from the lateral edge of the tarsal defect to the orbital rim determines the length of the strip. The fascia is undermined from the temporalis muscle and separated from the bony rim with a periosteal elevator. The strip is reflected medially to fill the tarsal defect so the anterior periosteum lies against the globe. The distal end of the strip is secured to the lateral border of the tarsal remnant with partial thickness 5-0 Vicryl sutures. The strip provides the posterior lamella support for the reconstructed lower eyelid. Rotating the myocutaneous advancement flap into place, as previously described, covers the anterior lamella defect.

FREE TARSAL GRAFT PLUS UNIPEDICLE FLAP FROM THE UPPER EYELID

A third method used to close full-thickness defects of the lower eyelid is the free tarsal graft with a unipedicle flap from the upper eyelid. The free tarsal graft is harvested as described earlier. The flap from excess upper lid skin and subcutaneous tissue is then harvested. First, a flap based at the lateral canthus is outlined with a marking pen (Fig. 41-5). The skin and subcuta-

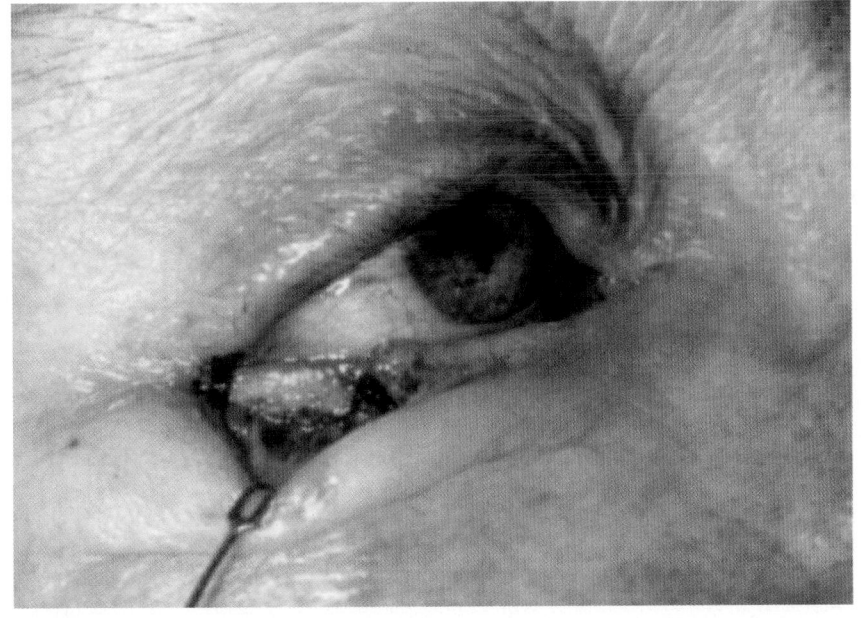

▲ **FIGURE 41-4** Myocutaneous advancement flap over a free tarsal graft.

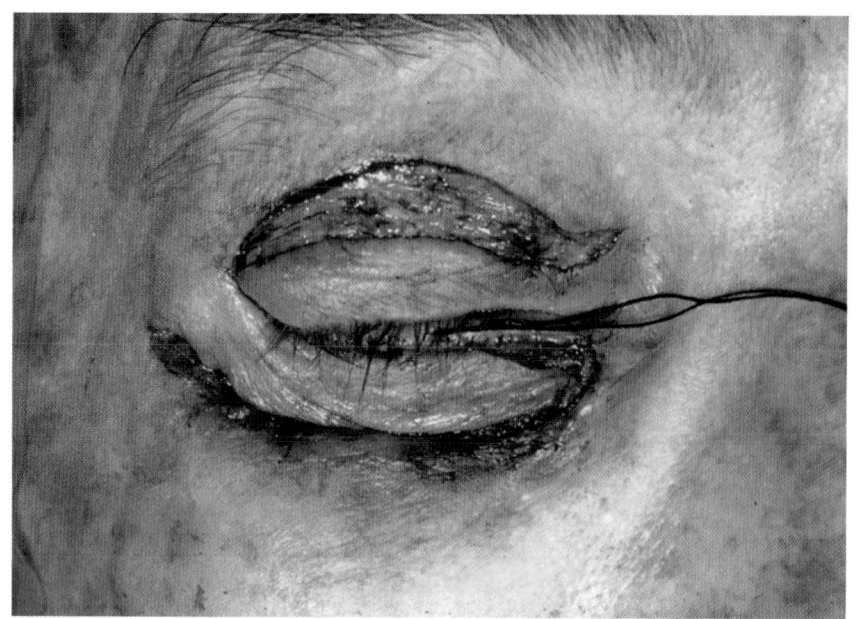

▲ **FIGURE 41-5** Lower eyelid anterior lamella defect may be closed with an unipedicle flap. The flap is taken from the anterior lamella of the upper eyelid and is based at the lateral canthus.

neous tissue are incised with a #15 blade and then undermined with Wescott's scissors temporally to the lateral orbital rim. The flap is rotated inferiorly to fill the lower anterior lamella defect once sufficient tissue has been undermined. It is secured with deep, interrupted 6-0 Vicryl sutures and superficial, interrupted 6-0 or 7-0 nylon or silk sutures. This unipedicle flap may leave the patient with a lump of tissue at the lateral canthus. If necessary, a second-stage procedure 6 to 8 weeks later is used to thin the base of the flap and remove this excess tissue.

TARSOCONJUNCTIVAL FLAP (HUGHES FLAP) PLUS FREE SKIN GRAFT OR MYOCUTANEOUS ADVANCEMENT FLAP A tarsoconjunctival flap (*Hughes flap*) with a free skin graft or myocutaneous advancement flap may be used for large defects involving more than 50% of the eyelid margin.[9] A tarsoconjunctival flap from the upper eyelid is passed behind the upper eyelid margin remnant and advanced into the posterior lamellar defect of the lower eyelid. A skin advancement flap or a free skin graft taken from the preauricular or retroauricular area replaces the anterior lamella of the lower eyelid. Obscuration of the pupil by the tarsoconjunctival bridge for 4 to 8 weeks is the main disadvantage of this procedure. Once the lower eyelid flap is revascularized, the vascularized pedicle is severed and released in a second procedure.

To begin the Hughes flap, the inferior border of the defect should be squared off to create a rectangular defect with the lateral and medial edges perpendicular to the lid margin. The edges are advanced centrally with forceps. The horizontal length of the tarsoconjunctival flap to be advanced is measured and the upper lid is everted over a lid plate or a Desmarre's retractor. A 4-0 silk traction suture placed through the central upper lid margin may facilitate this process. A three-sided flap is then outlined on the central tarsal conjunctival surface of the upper lid. A horizontal incision is made with a #15 blade. The incision should be at least 4 mm from the lid margin to minimize the incidence of entropion, contour deformities, loss of lashes, and trichiasis. The vertical incisions are directed toward the superior fornix perpendicular to the lid margin and are made through conjunctiva and tarsus (Fig. 41-6A). The flap is undermined from the overlying levator aponeurosis and orbicularis muscle with Wescott's scissors and the dissection is continued above the superior tarsal border between the conjunctiva and the Mueller's muscle toward the superior fornix. In the majority of cases, the conjunctiva provides sufficient blood supply to the flap. However, if necessary, the blood supply may be augmented with a myocutaneous advancement flap. If the blood supply is potentially marginal or a skin graft will be used to reconstruct the anterior lamella, Mueller's muscle should be incorporated into the flap.

Following mobilization of the tarsoconjunctival flap into the lower lid defect, the advanced upper lid superior

tarsal border should be aligned with the lower lid margin remnant (Fig. 41-6B). Interrupted 5-0 Vicryl sutures passed through the anterior two-thirds of the tarsus secure the lateral and medial edges of the flap to the tarsal stumps. The flap may be secured to the periosteum of the inner aspect of the lateral orbital rim with two 4-0 Polydek sutures if insufficient tarsal stump remains. If necessary, the flap is secured to the posterior limb of the medial canthal tendon. Finally, a running 7-0 Vicryl suture secures the inferior edge of the flap to the cut edge of the inferior forniceal conjunctiva and lower lid retractors. Once reconstruction of the posterior lamella is complete, the anterior lamella is reconstructed with a myocutaneous flap or full-thickness skin graft as previously described.

The second stage of the Hughes procedure is undertaken 4 to 8 weeks later. The second stage is delayed until the reconstructed lower lid has established a new blood supply and counteracted the downward contractile forces of scar maturation and gravity. The flap is incised 0.5 to 1.0 mm above the new lower lid margin with blunt Wescott's scissors while care is taken to avoid traumatizing the underlying cornea. The excess mucosa

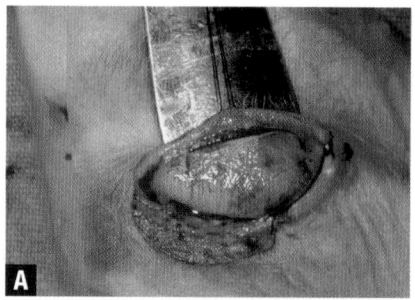

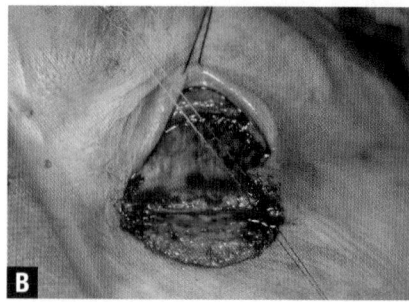

▲ **FIGURE 41-6 A.** Hughes flap is begun by everting the upper eyelid over a retractor. The horizontal incision should be at least 4 mm from the lid margin and the vertical incisions should be directed superiorly, perpendicular to the lid margin. **B.** The tarsoconjunctival flap should be mobilized into the lower eyelid defect to allow for alignment of the superior tarsal border of the donor upper lid with the lower, recipient lid margin remnant.

from the lower portion of the flap is left to retract or sutured to a skin incision made along the new lid margin with a running 7-0 Vicryl suture. This process establishes a new mucocutaneous border. The upper portion of the flap is allowed to retract under the upper lid and may be trimmed in the future if necessary. Undermining between Mueller's muscle and the levator aponeurosis should be performed if Mueller's muscle is incorporated into the flap. This is done in a stepwise fashion until the height and contour of the upper lid are sufficient to minimize postoperative lid retraction.

Upper Eyelid Defects

ANTERIOR LAMELLA DEFICIT, LID MARGIN INTACT

Primary closure As in the case of the lower eyelid, small defects may be closed primarily if lid distortion is not induced. To avoid lid margin distortion, closure should be directed along a horizontal tension line rather than in a vertical plane. A vertical incision is needed for subsequent undermining of the skin and subcutaneous tissues along the horizontal plane.

The anterior lamella may be undermined from the tarsal plate and then closed primarily with deep, interrupted 6-0 Vicryl sutures and interrupted, superficial 6-0 or 7-0 silk or nylon sutures if horizontal lid distortion is not induced. If insufficient anterior lamella remains, a full-thickness pentagonal wedge, including the anterior lamella defect, may be excised with Wescott's scissors. The tarsal border should be sharp and perpendicular to the lid margin. The resulting full-thickness defect may then be closed primarily as described earlier.

SKIN GRAFT For larger defects not involving the lid margin, a free full-thickness skin graft may be employed.[9,10] The graft may be harvested from the contralateral upper eyelid. If this is not possible, preauricular, retroauricular, supraclavicular, and upper inner arm skin grafts may be employed. Upper eyelid mobility, however, may be inhibited by the relative greater thickness of these grafts.

Once again, the skin graft must be thinned of subcutaneous fat and connective tissue. The graft is then trimmed to size and sutured to the edges of the defect with interrupted 7-0 nylon or silk sutures.

ELLIPSE SLIDING FLAP As described in the lower eyelid defect section, an elliptical sliding flap is one technique used to close some anterior lamella defects.[9] The anterior lamella may be reconstructed while preserving the maximal amount of normal tissue.

MYOCUTANEOUS ADVANCEMENT FLAP A myocutaneous advancement flap may also be used as in the case of lower lid defects. Flaps provide the best tissue match, cosmetic result, and an inherent vascular supply. To maximize cosmesis, incisions should be hidden in natural skin creases. Secondly, the flap should be of adequate size and be sufficiently anchored to minimize tension on the final closure.

Full-Thickness Eyelid Defect

PRIMARY CLOSURE Up to 30% of a central lid defect in younger patients, and up to 50% in older patients, may be closed using the technique described in the lower lid section. The primary distinction is that the vertical height of the tarsus should be two to three times longer than that of the lower lid. Even, uniform wound closure requires that the tarsal defect extend perpendicular to the lid margin for its full length. The levator aponeurotic attachments should be preserved to minimize postoperative ptosis.

If necessary, lateral cantholysis may be used to provide 3 to 5 mm of medial mobilization of the remaining lateral eyelid margin. The superior crus of the lateral canthal tendon may be incised with Wescott's scissors, similar to the procedure used on the inferior crus in lower eyelid reconstruction.

SEMICIRCULAR ROTATIONAL FLAP Primary closure with a lateral semicircular or myocutaneous flap, similar to that described for the lower lid, may be used to reconstruct up to one-half of the medial or central upper lid.[9] An inferiorly, rather than superiorly, arching semicircle flap is fashioned. The semicircle should be approximately 20 mm in diameter and arch inferiorly and temporally from the lateral canthal angle. The second difference is that the superior, not inferior, crus of the lateral canthal tendon is disrupted. The defect is also closed primarily, making sure to exactly approximate the tarsal edges and secure the myocutaneous flap as outlined in the lower lid section.

FREE TARSAL GRAFT PLUS MYOCUTANEOUS ADVANCEMENT FLAP Larger defects may require a free tarsal graft with a myocutaneous advancement flap.[9] As in the lower eyelid repair, a free tarsoconjunctival graft from the contralateral upper

eyelid may provide posterior lamella reconstructive tissue for an upper lid defect. First, a 4-0 silk traction suture is placed through the central lid margin. The lid is then everted over a Desmarre's retractor or lid plate to expose the tarsoconjunctival surface. A marking pen is used to outline a graft of appropriate length on the conjunctival surface. The inferior border should be parallel to and no more than 4 mm from the lid margin. The vertical height of the graft is determined by the vertical height of the tarsus. A #15 blade is used to incise the conjunctiva and full-thickness tarsal plate as well as the inferior and vertical borders. The anterior tarsal surface is then dissected free from the overlying levator aponeurosis. Conjunctiva and Mueller's muscle attachments are severed from the superior tarsal border with scissors so 2 mm of conjunctiva remains attached to the graft. The donor site is then allowed to heal spontaneously.

The graft is secured with the conjunctival surface in apposition to the globe, while the superior edge of the graft with the conjunctival remnant lies along the new lid margin. The lateral edge of the graft is sutured to the stump of the superior crus of the lateral canthal tendon, if present, or to the lateral orbital rim at the level of the lateral orbital tubercle with interrupted 4-0 Polydek sutures. The medial edges are then secured with interrupted 5-0 Vicryl sutures, which are passed at partial thickness to avoid ocular irritation. The superior edge is attached to the superior forniceal conjunctiva and edges of Mueller's muscle and levator aponeurosis with interrupted 7-0 Vicryl sutures.

Next, a myocutaneous flap from the upper lid or lateral canthal area is used to cover the tarsal graft. If there is sufficient upper lid skin and orbicularis muscle superior to the defect, this area may be undermined and advanced down over the graft. If the lateral canthal area is chosen to cover the graft, an advancement flap should be outlined and arched inferiorly and temporally. This myocutaneous flap is undermined and then rotated medially to fill the anterior lamella defect without tension.

Once the flap is in place, the deep orbicularis layer is closed with interrupted 5-0 Vicryl sutures while the skin edges are closed with interrupted or a running 7-0 Vicryl suture. The conjunctival remnant is then advanced anteriorly and secured to the inferior flap skin edge with a running 7-0 Vicryl suture. This step is needed to reestablish the mucocutaneous junction along the newly reconstructed eyelid margin. To minimize postoperative retraction, the superior eyelid must be immobilized and kept on stretch. This is best accomplished with a temporary 4-0 silk suture tied over bolsters with traction directed inferiorly.

TARSOCONJUNCTIVAL FLAP (CUTLER–BEARD FLAP) PLUS FREE SKIN GRAFT OR MYOCUTANEOUS ADVANCEMENT FLAP Large, full-thickness upper eyelid defects involving more than 50% of the lid margin may be reconstructed with the Cutler–Beard procedure. This is a two-staged method of closure. A lower eyelid flap of skin, muscle, and conjunctiva is advanced behind the remaining lower eyelid margin into the upper lid defect. The flap is then sutured to the levator aponeurosis at the superior border of the upper eyelid defect. Since the Cutler–Beard flap includes the anterior lamella, a thick, relatively immobile upper eyelid is created. Also, because tarsus is not included in the flap, the lid margin is relatively unstable. This procedure is therefore used when no there are no alternative methods of defect closure.[9,10]

First, the full-thickness eyelid defect is trimmed in a rectangular fashion so the borders are perpendicular to the lid margin. After pulling the edges together under slight tension, the width of the defect is measured. A marking pen is then used to outline the superior border of the flap 5 mm below and parallel to the lower lid margin. The outline should be 1 to 2 mm wider than the upper lid defect. The superior outline should be no less than 5 mm below the lid margin to prevent disruption of the latter's blood supply. The vertical outlines should extend 15 mm in length. Following marking, a 4-0 silk traction suture is placed in the central portion of the lower lid, through the gray line. Upward traction is applied with a lid plate inserted into the inferior fornix between the lid and the globe.

While this lid plate protects the globe, a #15 blade is used to make full-thickness incisions along the previously placed outlines. Using scissors, the incisions are extended horizontally and then vertically to the inferior fornix, from the conjunctival side of the flap. The skin and orbicularis are then undermined over the inferior orbital rim. After the lid plate and traction suture are removed, the inferior edge of the marginal bridge is allowed to granulate spontaneously.

The flap is then passed beneath the lower lid margin remnant and sutured into the upper eyelid defect in layers. If the full vertical height of tarsus is absent in the upper lid, the conjunctival edges of the flap and upper lid are sutured together with a running 6-0 plain gut suture. Then, the lower lid retractors are secured to the cut edge of the levator aponeurosis with interrupted 6-0 Vicryl sutures. Otherwise, the conjunctiva and lower lid retractors are sutured to the anterior tarsal edges with interrupted 6-0 Vicryl sutures at the medial and lateral borders of the flap. Sutures should only be passed at partial thickness through the tarsus to avoid corneal irritation. If there is a tarsal remnant along the superior border of the recipient bed, the conjunctiva and lower lid retractors are sutured to the lower edge of the tarsus with interrupted 6-0 Vicryl sutures.

The anterior lamella may then be reconstructed with a myocutaneous advancement flap from the lower lid. The deep muscular layer is closed with interrupted 7-0 Vicryl sutures and the skin with interrupted 7-0 nylon sutures. An alternative method of anterior lamella reconstruction is the use of a free skin graft. The same general principles as previously described apply in the repair of these defects.

After 6 to 8 weeks, the flap is separated during the second stage of the procedure. Sufficient time should be allowed for stretching of the advanced tissues and formation of new vasculature in the reconstructed upper lid. A marking pen is first used to outline the dividing incision 2 mm below the new upper lid margin. While retracting the lower lid margin inferiorly, a straight horizontal skin incision is made along the mark. A groove director is placed under the flap to tent it away from the globe. Steven's scissors are then used to make a full-thickness incision through the flap in a slightly beveled direction. The conjunctival edge should be left longer than the skin edge. This beveled edge gives the newly reconstructed lid margin a smooth conjunctival surface. The skin and muscle edges are trimmed by 1 mm so the conjunctival remnant may be sutured to the skin edge with a running 7-0 Vicryl suture. This creates a new mucous membrane-lined lid margin and is important in avoiding irritation of the cornea by keratinized skin or skin hair. Next, the inferior border of the lower lid margin bridge is deepithelialized with a blade or sharp Wescott's scissors. The conjunctiva and flap retractors are sutured to the inferior edge of the tarsus with running or interrupted 6-0 plain or 7-0 Vicryl sutures. Finally, the skin is closed with interrupted 7-0 nylon sutures.

Medial Canthal Defects

MEDIAN FOREHEAD FLAP Large anterior lamellar defects of the lower eyelid and medial canthus may be reconstructed with the median forehead flap.[10] This unipedicle flap may be combined with other rotational flaps for larger defects. The median forehead flap is first outlined on the axis of the contralateral supraorbital neurovascular bundle (Fig. 41-7A). A drape may be used as a model to ensure adequate flap size prior to skin incision. The length of the flap is determined by rotating the template while anchoring it at the contralateral supraorbital notch. Some flaps may even extend into the hairline.

After the incision is made with a #15 blade, the flap is dissected free from the underlying loose areolar tissue anterior to the periosteum of the frontal bone with Wescott's scissors. The forehead is then undermined extensively to allow for closure of the wound while minimizing

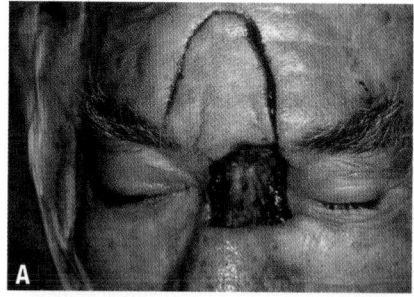

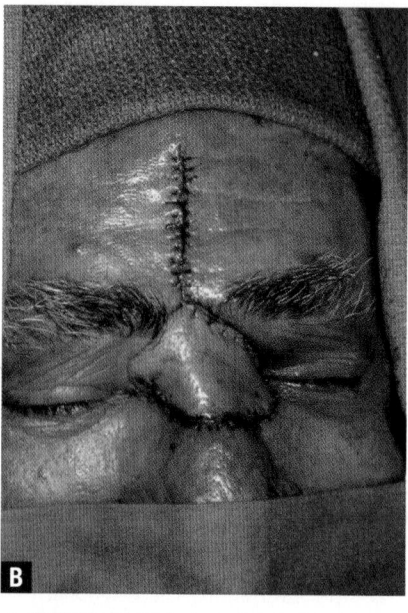

▲ **FIGURE 41-7 A.** A median forehead flap of sufficient size is created to allow for closure of this large medial canthal defect involving the bridge of the nose. **B.** Following adequate dissection, the flap is rotated and secured into the defect. The donor site is closed primarily.

tension. The flap tip is thinned to the subcutaneous plane. The flap is secured into place following 120 to 180° of rotation into the defect. Deep, interrupted 6-0 Vicryl sutures are used to close the subcutaneous tissue, while interrupted 6-0 nylon or silk sutures are used to close the skin (Fig. 41-7B).

Forehead closure follows placement of the flap. Aggressive subcutaneous dissection anterior to the periosteum of the frontal bone is needed to close the donor wound. Deep 3-0 Vicryl sutures should be placed to enhance wound stability. The subcutaneous tissue is then closed with interrupted 5-0 Vicryl sutures and the skin with interrupted 6-0 nylon sutures. The median forehead flap leaves the patient with a large lump of tissue at the bridge of the nose. If necessary, a second-stage procedure is implemented 6 to 8 weeks later to thin the base of the flap.

In patients who do not have sufficient forehead skin for primary closure, the forehead defect may be repaired with a free skin graft. Such patients may have undergone excision of a lesion in the forehead region leaving them with insufficient tissue for primary closure.

Glabellar flap The glabellar flap, a modified V to Y rotation flap, may also be used to repair medial canthal defects.[9] This flap may require secondary debulk-ing as the skin and subcutaneous tissue from the donor forehead glabellar region are thicker than that of the recipient medial canthus.

First, an inverted V is outlined from the midpoint of the glabella just above the brow with an angle less than 60°. Both segments of the flap should extend below the brow with the longer portion joining the lateral aspect of the defect. The previously outlined skin and subcutaneous tissue are incised with a #15 blade and then undermined extensively with Steven's scissors. The flap is then rotated into the defect. The apex of the flap should be placed at the lateral edge and the point at the inferior tip. Once the tip of the flap is trimmed to fit the defect, the flap is secured with buried anchoring, interrupted, subcutaneous 6-0 Vicryl sutures. The skin is then closed with interrupted 6-0 nylon or silk sutures. The donor site is sutured in a V to Y closure. This may induce a shortening of the interbrow distance and, occasionally, this flap requires a secondary debulking.

Rhombic flap Medial and lateral canthal defects may be repaired with the rhombic flap, which is a nontransposition flap.[9] Most defects may be converted to a rhombic configuration with angles of 60 and 120° and all sides of equal length, with minimal sacrifice of normal tissue.

As with all repairs, eyelid margin and brow distortion should not be induced and minimal tension should be placed on the reconstructed area. The latter is facilitated by closing donor lines with the proper orientation along lines of maximal tissue elasticity.

A rhombus is formed from the defect. First, two lines are marked parallel to the lines of maximum extensibility (LME). These LME should be perpendicular to the relaxed skin tension lines (RSTL). While sacrificing the minimum amount of normal tissue, the first rhombic flap is created with two additional, equally long parallel lines. This second set of lines should be tangential to the defect at either 60 or 120° from the first set of lines. A line connecting each end of the shorter diagonal that bisects the 120° angle is then drawn. This line must be equal in length to the sides of the rhombus. At the end of this previous mark, the last lines are drawn at 60° angle parallel to the sides of the rhombic defect (Fig. 41-8A).

Of the four possible flaps, only one that is near the donor site along LME is appropriate for reconstruction. After rotating medially, the flap is advanced into the defect so point B aligns with the medial point of the defect while point A is at the inferior apex (Fig. 41-8B). The deep, subcutaneous layer is closed with interrupted 6-0 Vicryl

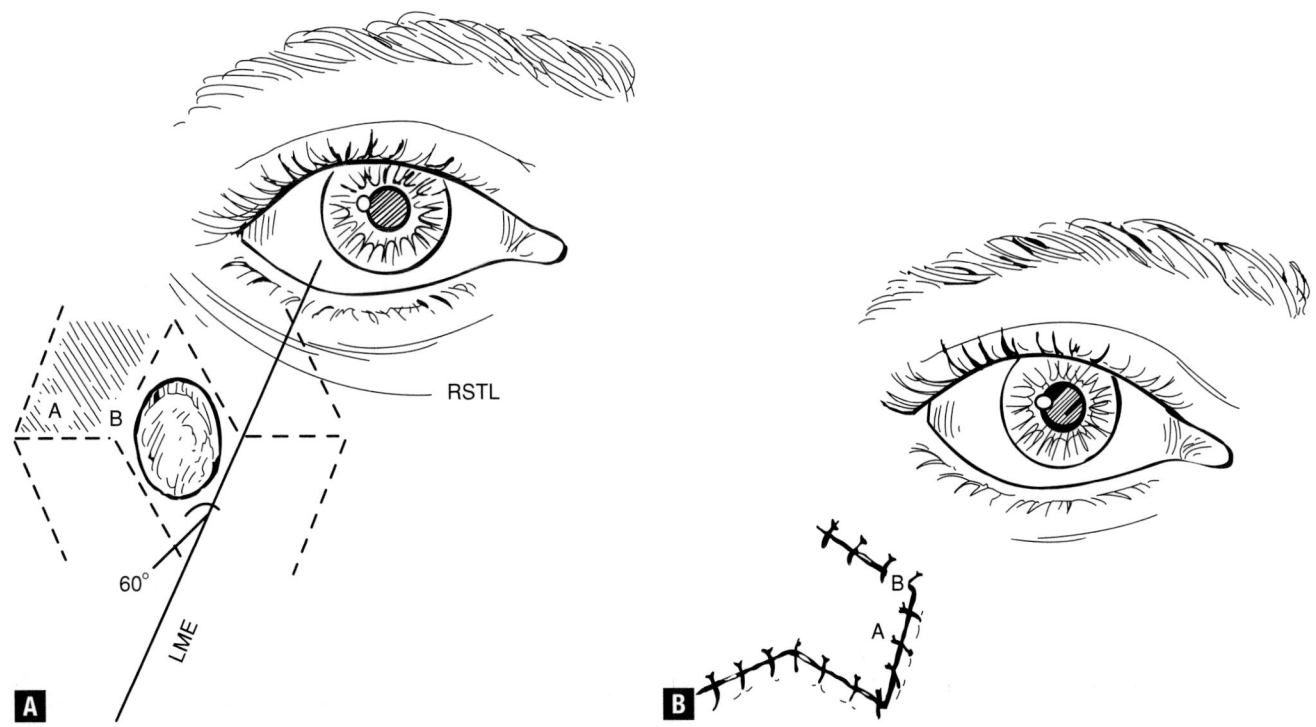

▲ **FIGURE 41-8** **A.** Defect is first converted into a rhombus. **B.** The flap that causes the least amount of distortion is chosen for final closure.

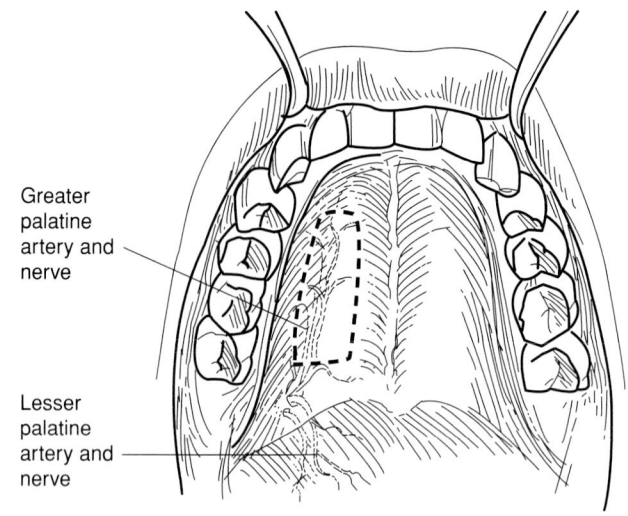

Greater
palatine
artery and
nerve

Lesser
palatine
artery and
nerve

A

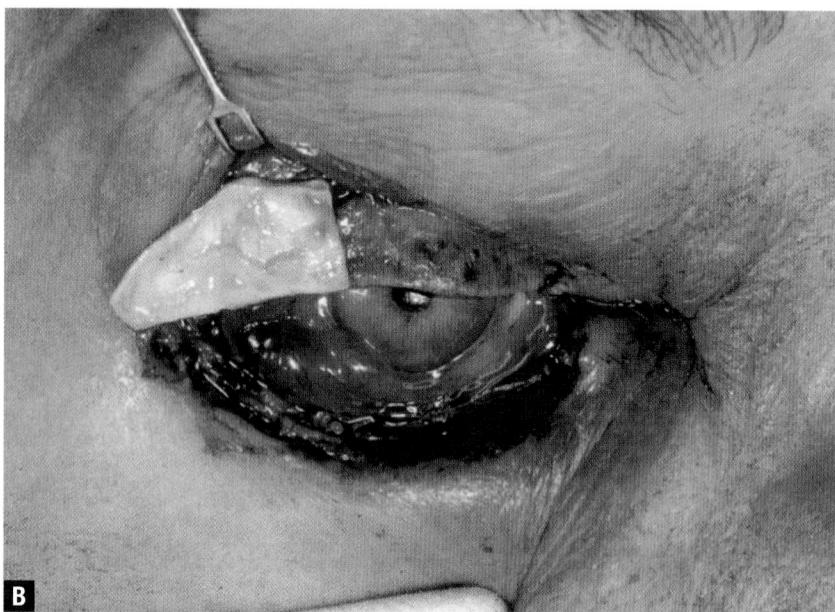

B

▲ **FIGURE 41-9** **A.** Hard palate graft is outlined on the gingival surface of the roof of the mouth while taking care to avoid the critical structures. **B.** Once the hard palate graft is harvested, it is placed into this upper eyelid defect.

achieve further hemostasis if cautery is inadequate.

The harvested hard palate graft is soaked in an antibiotic solution and trimmed to the proper size and shape. It is very difficult to thin the graft once it is free from the donor bed, thus the graft thickness should be taken into consideration during the initial dissection. The free graft is then used to fill the posterior lamella defect and sutured into place (Fig. 41-9B). A diamond burr is used to remove the keratinized surface of the hard palate graft.

INSUFFICIENT ANTERIOR LAMELLA More involved methods of repair may be required for larger defects of the anterior lamella. Tissue expansion has been used in periocular reconstruction in patients with more extensive defects.[13] The posterior lamella is reconstructed with a graft as described earlier. As previously emphasized, the anterior lamella must be reconstructed with a vascular flap if a free posterior graft is used. Tissue expanders provide vascularized skin that is similar in appearance, thickness, and texture to the skin adjacent to the defect while preserving the maximal amount of normal tissue. Furthermore, tissue expansion enhances the vascularity of the skin flap. This provides for more rapid vascularization of any free grafts beneath the flap. The nonhair bearing nature and pliability of the created tissue are additional advantages. The creation of temporary disfigurement, however, is the main disadvantage.

Reconstructive tissue is recruited from the adjacent skin, such as the forehead, temporalis and preauricular regions, and the lid. Care should be taken with expansion of the lid proper given the lack of information of the effects of tissue expansion on the underlying globe. During expansion, adequate tissue area is created in a staged procedure. First, a skin incision is made along the hairline, brow, or a preexisting incision line. The incision site should not be located over the subsequently placed expander or interfere with the vascular supply or subsequent rotation of the flap.

A recipient pocket is dissected in the subcutaneous tissue following skin incision. In the forehead region, a large pocket is dissected between the periosteum and the galea or deep fascia of the frontalis muscle. In the temporal region, a pocket is dissected in a plane between the subdermal fatty layer and the superficial temporal fascia. In the upper eyelid, the pocket is created between the preseptal orbicularis oculi and the levator

sutures. Thinner skin is closed with interrupted 6-0 nylon sutures and thicker skin with interrupted 5-0 nylon vertical mattress sutures.

Special Circumstances

INSUFFICIENT POSTERIOR LAMELLA Tarso-conjunctival grafts are preferred in defects with insufficient posterior lamella as they provide a smooth surface over the cornea. However, if such a graft is not available, other tissues must be considered. Hard palate grafts, nasal or ear cartilage grafts, and donor sclera have been used to reconstruct the deficient structure in these cases.

Hard palate grafts have been used with increasing frequency. The gingival surface of the roof of the mouth is the most commonly chosen donor site.[11,12] Structures to avoid include the central palatine raphé, the anterior palatine rugae, and the area overlying the greater palatine foramen where the anterior palatine artery exits. In most cases, rectangular-shaped grafts are harvested. A graft of appropriate size and shape is outlined either with a marking pen or using a surrogate marker, including paper. The midline of the hard palate should be avoided (Fig. 41-9A). A #15 blade may be used to harvest the graft. The palatal periosteum should be left intact in order to enhance healing of the donor site. Oxidized regenerated cellulose or microfibrillar collagen hemostat may be placed in the donor bed to

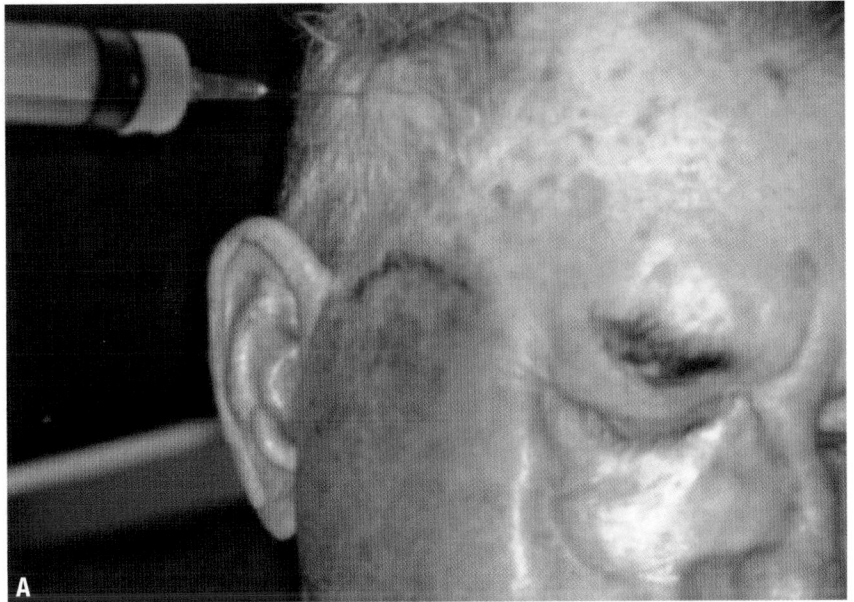

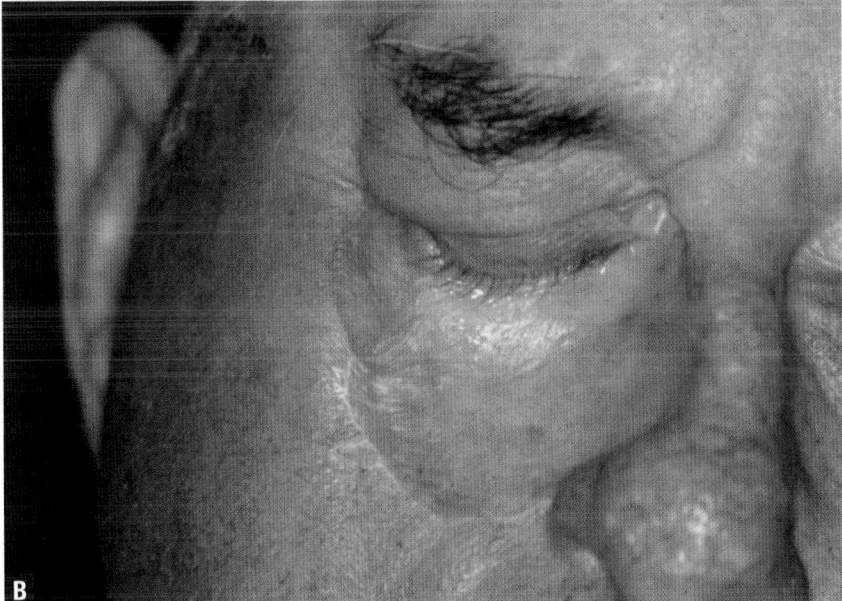

▲ **FIGURE 41-10** **A.** Tissue expander is inflated percutaneously with a 27-gauge needle. **B.** Inflation should be sufficient to cause skin overlying the expander to feel taut.

The newly created skin now provides a local skin flap for eyelid reconstruction. In most cases, serial expansion also allows for sufficient thinning of the dermal tissue such that the final flap is of appropriate thickness to fill the defect and match the adjacent tissue. Enough tissue should be created so the risk of marginal flap ischemia from tight sutures is minimized.

INSUFFICIENT VASCULARIZED PEDICLE

Galeal and pericranial flaps may be utilized for large defects with an insufficient vascularized pedicle.[14] These flaps have a reliable vascular supply for the recipient site, as well as underlying free tarsoconjunctival and free overlying skin grafts. Unlike the median forehead flap, skin is not transposed with a galeal or pericranial flap. Bunching over the nasal bridge is less of concern secondary to the thinner nature of these flaps. Of note, the galeopericranial flap is thought to be superior to the pericranial flap because of its increased vascularity.

The five layers of the soft tissue in the scalp are the skin, subcutaneous soft tissue, galea aponeurotica, subgaleal loose areolar tissue, and periosteum. The pericranium consists of the periosteum and the overlying subaponeurotic loose connective tissue. It is contiguous with the deep temporal fascia in the temporal region. The pericranium also has a dual blood supply, thus ensuring the viability of a pericranial flap. The galea aponeurotica is composed of dense fibrous tissue.

As described earlier, the posterior lamella is first reconstructed prior to the repair of large upper eyelid defects. The soft tissue defect is then filled with a galeopericranial or pericranial flap. A standard bicoronal incision is made over the vertex of the skull. A transcoronal incision is then made to access the pericranium of the forehead. The plane of dissection is between the subcutaneous tissue and the galea for a galeopericranial flap. The plane for pericranial flaps is subgaleal. The loose areolar tissue and periosteum adherent to the frontal bone are not disturbed. Dissection is carried toward the supraorbital rim. Care is taken to leave the supraorbital and supratrochlear vessels intact. Dissection is stopped where the vessels enter the base of the flap. The pericranium and galea are then incised and elevated off the frontal bone with a periosteal elevator. Once the entire flap is mobilized, it is turned down anteriorly through the skin defect. It may be turned to multiple arcs for reconstructive purposes. The length, width, angle, and shape can be tailored

aponeurosis. Complete hemostasis is an absolute requirement to prevent the formation of a hematoma.

Prior to placement, the expander is soaked in an antibiotic solution. The deflated device is subsequently tested for leaks and then placed subcutaneously into the recipient pocket. After any remaining air is expressed, the expander is filled with enough saline to flatten its folds and remove any dead space in the pocket. The expander is then deflated until the tension on the skin is sufficient to provide adequate hemostasis. A remote expander is then placed into the pocket through the same skin incision. The wound is closed in

two layers and systemic antibiotics are given for 1-week postoperatively.

Two to 3 weeks after placement, serial expansion is begun. Using a 27-gauge needle, the expander is inflated with saline percutaneously through the injection port (Fig. 41-10A). Inflation is ceased once the expander feels taut (Fig. 41-10B). In general, 10 to 15% of the total expander volume may be injected at any one time. Two times per week, the expander is reinjected with approximately 1 mL of saline in the remote expander and 10 mL in the larger expander. Expansion is usually complete in 6 to 8 weeks. The expander is removed once adequate tissue has been created.

Table 41-1
Methods of the Eyelid Reconstruction

ANTERIOR LAMELLA DEFECT, LOWER EYELID, EYELID MARGIN INTACT
- Primary closure
  - with lateral cantholysis
  - without lateral cantholysis
- Skin graft (of nonhair bearing skin)
  - ipsilateral upper eyelid
  - preauricular skin graft
  - retroauricular skin graft
  - supraclavicular skin graft
  - upper inner arm skin graft
- Ellipse sliding flap
- Myocutaneous advancement flap

FULL-THICKNESS EYELID DEFECT, LOWER EYELID
- Primary closure
  - with lateral cantholysis
  - without lateral cantholysis
- Semicircular rotational flap
  - temporal tarsal remnant plus myocutaneous advancement flap
  - only feasible if sufficient temporal tarsal remnant
- Free tarsal graft plus myocutaneous advancement flap
- Periosteal strip plus myocutaneous advancement flap
- Free tarsal graft plus unipedicle rotational flap from the upper eyelid
- Hughes tarsoconjunctival flap plus free skin graft or myocutaneous advancement flap

ANTERIOR LAMELLA DEFECT, UPPER EYELID, EYELID MARGIN INTACT
- Primary closure
  - with lateral cantholysis
  - without lateral cantholysis
- Skin graft (of nonhair bearing skin)
  - contralateral upper eyelid
  - preauricular skin graft
  - retroauricular skin graft
  - supraclavicular skin graft
  - upper inner arm skin graft
- Ellipse sliding flap
- Myocutaneous advancement flap

FULL-THICKNESS EYELID DEFECT, UPPER EYELID
- Primary closure
  - with lateral cantholysis
  - without lateral cantholysis
- Semicircular rotational flap
  - temporal tarsal remnant plus myocutaneous advancement flap
  - only feasible if sufficient temporal tarsal remnant
- Free tarsal graft plus myocutaneous advancement flap
- Cutler–Beard tarsoconjunctival flap plus free skin graft or myocutaneous advancement flap

MEDIAL CANTHAL DEFECT
- Median forehead flap
- Glabellar flap
- Rhombic flap

INSUFFICIENT POSTERIOR LAMELLA
- Tarsoconjunctival graft
- Hard palate graft
- Nasal cartilage graft
- Ear cartilage graft
- Donor sclera

INSUFFICIENT ANTERIOR LAMELLA
- Tissue expansion

INSUFFICIENT VASCULARIZED PEDICLE
- Galeopericranial flap
- Pericranial flap

for the specific deformity to allow for adequate rotation and coverage. It is important to avoid a transverse incision of the flap two fingerbreadths above the superior orbital rim as the frontalis nerve enters the frontalis muscle in this area. Once the flap is in place, it serves as a well-vascularized bed for a skin graft.

FINAL THOUGHTS

Total tumor excision is of utmost importance in the treatment of malignant eyelid lesions. Mohs micrographic surgery technique is the preferred method of excision of periocular malignancies because tumor margins are cleared with minimal sacrifice of normal tissue. Optimum function, globe protection, and aesthetics are then addressed during eyelid reconstruction. The chosen reconstructive method (see Table 41-1) is dependent upon the state of the eyelid margin. Defects involving the lid margin require reconstruction of both the anterior and posterior lamellae. However, the most important principle to remember is the need for either the reconstructed anterior or posterior lamella to have its own inherent blood supply (pedicle flap). An inherent vascular supply ensures tissue survival and, thus, the optimum surgical outcome for the patient.

REFERENCES

1. Scott J, Fears T, Fraumeni JJ. The incidence of nonmelanoma skin cancer in the United States. *Natl Inst Health.* 1981; 82:2433.
2. Tse DT, Gilberg SM. Malignant eyelid tumors. In: Krachmer JH, Mannis MJ, Holland EJ, eds. *Cornea: Surgery of the Cornea and Conjunctiva.* Vol 2. 2nd ed. Philadelphia, PA: Elsevier Mosby; 2005: 463–480.
3. Esmaeli B, Wang B, Deavers M, et al. Prognostic factors for survival in malignant melanoma of the eyelid skin. *Ophthal Plast Reconstr Surg.* 2000;16:250–257.
4. Cook BE Jr, Bartley GB. Treatment options and future prospects for the management of eyelid malignancies: An evidence-based update. *Ophthalmology.* 2001;108:2088–2098.
5. Coleman WP III, Davis RS, Reed RJ, Krementz ET. Treatment of lentigo maligna and lentigo maligna melanoma. *J Dermatol Surg Oncol.* 1980;6:476–479.
6. Zitelli JA, Mohs FE, Larson P, Snow S. Mohs micrographic surgery for melanoma. *Dermatol Clin.* 1989;7:833–842.
7. Esmaeli B. Sentinel lymph node mapping for patients with cutaneous and conjunctival melanoma. *Ophthal Plast Reconstr Surg.* 2000;16:170–172.
8. Kersten RC, Kodère F, Dailey RA, et al. Section 7: Orbit, eyelids, and lacrimal system. In: American Academy of Ophthalmology, ed. *Basic and Clinical Science*

Course. San Francisco, CA: American Academy of Ophthalmology; 2003:134–146.

9. Kronish J. Eyelid reconstruction. In: Tse DT, ed. *Color Atlas of Ophthalmic Surgery: Oculoplastic Surgery*. Philadelphia, PA: J.B. Lippincott; 1992:245–294.

10. Nerad JA. The requisites in ophthalmology oculoplastic surgery: Eyelid recon-struction. In: Krachmer JH, ed. *Requisites in Ophthalmology: Oculoplastic Surgery*. St. Louis, MO: Mosby; 2001:282.

11. Bartley GB, Kay PP. Posterior lamellar eyelid reconstruction with a hard palate mucosal graft. *Am J Ophthalmol.* 1989;107:609–612.

12. Beatty RL, Harris G, Bauman GR, et al. Intraoral palatal mucosal graft harvest. *Ophthal Plast Reconstr Surg.* 1993 Jun;9(2):120–124.

13. Tse DT, McCafferty LR. Controlled tissue expansion in periocular reconstructive surgery. *Ophthalmology.* 1993;100:260–268.

14. Tse DT, Goodwin WJ, Johnson T, et al. Use of galeal and pericranial flaps for recon-struction of orbital and eyelid defects. *Arch Ophthalmol.* 1997;115:932–937.

CHAPTER 42

Reconstructive Surgery of Skin Cancer Defects

Valencia D. Thomas, M.D.
Wendy Long Mitchell, M.D.
Neil A. Swanson, M.D.
Thomas Rohrer, M.D.
Ken K. Lee, M.D.

BOX 42-1   Overview

- Cutaneous reconstruction of the nose, lip, ear, cheek, scalp, and forehead requires an understanding of the anatomy, form, and function of each region. It is important to consider the relationship between an area to be reconstructed and its surrounding structures as well.

- Maximizing eversion is a common technique utilized to minimize scars on the face. This can be achieved by the careful placement of dermal and epidermal sutures. Tight approximation of deep tissues, such as muscle and fascia, may also aid in the final eversion of the wound.

- Undermining allows for increased tissue mobility and the formation of a plate-like scar that results in a more aesthetically-pleasing outcome. Knowledge of regional anatomy can help guide where to best undermine. Critical nerves or arteries should be avoided if possible. Undermining in planes that allow maximal tissue movement, such as in the subgaleal plane of the scalp or the submuscular plane of the dorsal nose, may be required to aid in approximation of superficial tissues.

- Tissue injury from overmanipulation, crush injury, and excessive use of cautery may impair healing, compromise the health of adjacent tissue, and affect the final outcome of the repair.

- Management of aggressive tumors or tumors with a high likelihood of recurrence may mandate repairs that facilitate tumor surveillance such as split-thickness skin grafts or healing via secondary intent.

- Secondary intention healing results in a good cosmetic outcome in areas of concavity, such as the alar groove, the temple, or the conchal bowl.

- Full-thickness and split-thickness skin graft donor sites should be chosen with texture, color, and thickness of the recipient tissue in mind. Regardless of donor site, however, graft viability is more likely if the defect is shallow or if the graft is not placed directly on cartilage.

INTRODUCTION

Surgery is the definitive treatment for the vast majority of skin cancers. Many of these tumors arise in the head and neck region resulting in defects in these cosmetically sensitive areas. Skillful repair of these defects are paramount in order to restore both the functional and aesthetic aspects. This chapter will provide a regional overview of the many reconstructive techniques that are used to repair skin cancer defects.

RECONSTRUCTION OF THE NOSE

BOX 42-2   Summary

- Undermining for a linear closure on the nose should be performed at the level of the perichondrium to increase tissue mobility and decrease the risk of tissue ischemia.

- Maintaining a length to width ratio of 4:1 will help in preventing the formation of standing cutaneous cones.

- The myocutaneous island pedicle flap is useful in the closure of defects on the nose.

- The bilobed flap is generally used for defects that are smaller than 1.5 cm in diameter and located on the nasal sidewall, tip, supratip, or medial alae. The Dufourmentel variant minimizes the standing cone redundancy that can occur at the point of rotation in the classic rhombic flap.

- Interpolation flaps, in general, require the surgeon to assess a patient's willingness to undergo a staged procedure that requires the formation of a pedicle that will protrude from the patient's face for approximately 3 weeks.

Defects on the nose can be challenging to repair for even the most seasoned cutaneous surgeon. The nose is made up of several cosmetic subunits, and although carcinomas have no regard for these borders, the surgeon must pay close attention to respecting these units when designing an aesthetically pleasing repair (Fig. 42-1). Every attempt to restore the natural intricate balance and symmetry of the many concavities and convexities of the nose should be made.

Surgeons must also keep in mind the variable thickness and mobility of the nasal skin in different subunits (nasal skin types as detailed by Burget).[1] The nasal dorsum, sidewalls, soft triangles, and columella are generally composed of more thin, more mobile, and less sebaceous skin. Skin of the nasal tip, supratip, and alae is generally much thicker, more sebaceous, and less mobile. The differences in skin thickness, texture, and mobility vary from patient to patient and must be recognized and identified individually for optimal cosmetic reconstruction. In addition, the free margins of the nose, the alae, can be grossly distorted by even subtle flaws in repair design and must be constantly watched even during the procedure to be sure they do not move. The underlying bony and cartilaginous structures must be restored to maintain proper nasal function. Another obstacle to repair on the nose is that one frequently finds that the nose has been operated on in the past for other carcinomas. This scarred tissue from previous repairs or treatment modalities even further limits skin mobility and decreases

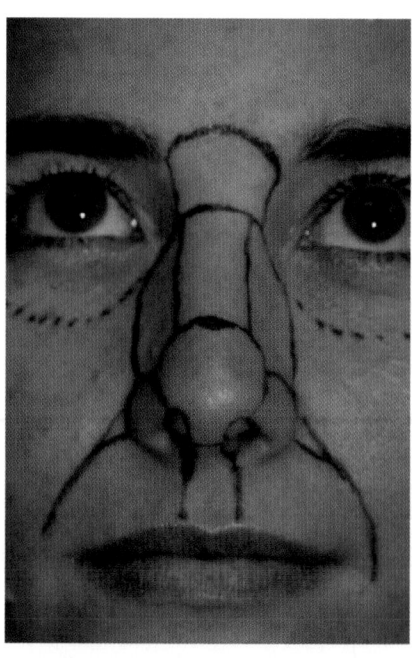

▲ **FIGURE 42-1** Cosmetic units of the nose.

normal tissue from which to draw for local flap repairs. While challenging, nasal defects present the surgeon with the gratifying opportunity to choose between a number of viable repair designs that maintain both the form and function of the nose.

Secondary Intention

Healing by secondary intention may be considered for smaller and more superficial defects located in concave areas of the nose, such as the nasal alar sulcus and crease, and the junction of the medial canthus and nasal sidewall. Conceptualizing the design in two parts may allow superior repair of defects that span two cosmetic units. Secondary intention healing can be used in combination with a local flap or graft when a portion of the defect lies in a concave aspect of one cosmetic unit and the remaining part of the defect in another unit.[2] Occasionally, very superficial defects on the sebaceous nasal tip or alae may be left to heal by second intention and the surrounding area buffed out with resurfacing lasers or dermabrasion (Fig. 42-2A to C).

Primary Closure

Linear repairs are often an excellent option for small defects on the nasal sidewalls, nasal dorsum, alar crease, and the center of the nasal tip. Simple linear closures typically leave an aesthetic linear or curvilinear scar, are easier to perform, and generally have lower complication rates than flaps and grafts. Tension should be oriented in such a manner that it does not make the nasal alae asymmetric or raise

the nasal tip so much that it creates a significant distortion. Since many of the patients that present with skin cancer are elderly and have some degree of nasal tip ptosis, it is often cosmetically beneficial to plan a reconstructive procedure that pleasantly elevates the nasal tip to a more youthful position.[3]

Dog-ears, or standing vertical cones, on the nose are cosmetically unacceptable. To avoid this outcome, it is advisable to design the length to defect width ratio of the ellipse closer to a 4:1 ratio, than the traditional 3:1 ratio, whenever the closure is going over a convex surface. Any linear closure on the nose undermining should be done at the level of the perichondrium to increase tissue mobility and decrease risk of tissue ischemia. Care to evert the wound edges should always be taken, but good wound eversion that reduces tension on the scar line is especially essential when closing thicker sebaceous skin on the nose.

Local Flaps

ADVANCEMENT Although traditional U-shaped advancement flaps are rarely used anymore in nasal reconstruction, A-to-L-type advancement flaps offer a reasonable reconstructive option for small to medium-sized defects on the nasal sidewall and supratip (Fig. 42-3A to C). Although they may be designed from either direction, they generally are created to have the Burow's triangle designed superiorly and the flap extending along the alar groove. A crescentic shape often must be excised along the lateral aspect of the ala to maintain its position and prevent distortion of the ala.

ISLAND PEDICLE ADVANCEMENT FLAP
The myocutaneous island pedicle is very useful in the closure of defects on the nasal sidewall, nasal tip, and supratip (Fig. 42-4A to C). They are generally designed and advanced down from an area just superior to the defect or from a lateral position if the inferior scar line may be placed along the alar groove. This flap has a rich vascular supply facilitating movement and viability. When used on the nasal tip, one can achieve a greater degree of flap movement without sacrificing vascular supply by creating a myocutaneous pedicle with bi-level undermining as described by Papadopolous.[4] Vertical tension on the nasal tip can occur with this flap, but can be utilized to improve the nasal tip ptosis that frequently occurs with age.

ROTATION FLAP
Dorsal nasal rotation flap This flap, as originally described by Rieger in 1967[5] is useful in the repair of large distal nasal defects. The level of undermining is at the periosteum or perichondrium. It is especially important that the area of the medial canthus is undermined fastidiously, as this is the main source of the flap's vascular supply. With the appropriate flap design and undermining, the flap can be easily rotated to fill the primary defect under minimal tension. The area harvested from the glabella should be thinned as it is brought into the medial canthal area. Likewise, the flap generally requires thinning distally to match the skin thickness of the nasal tip.

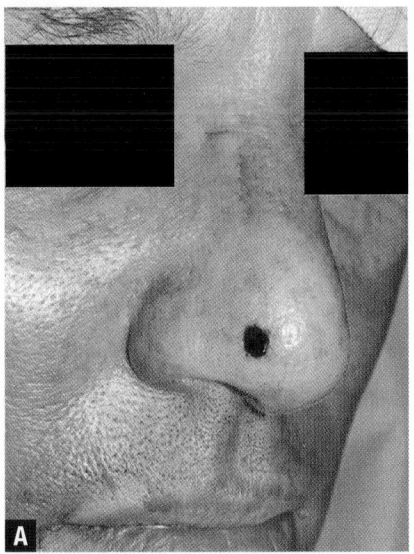
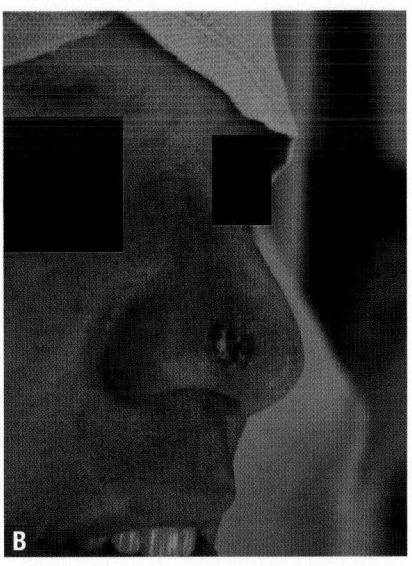
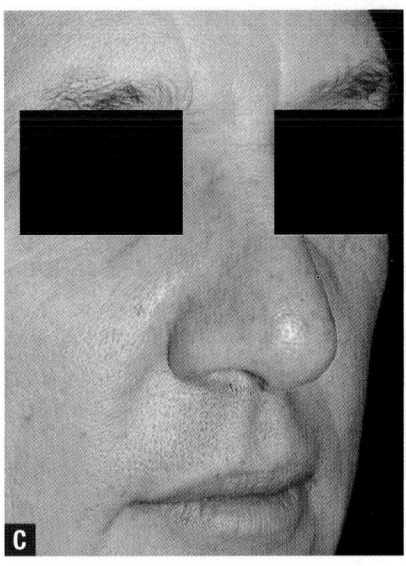

▲ **FIGURE 42-2** Improving second intent healing with dermarasion. **A.** Post-Mohs defect. **B.** Dermabrasion at the time of tumor excision. **C.** Long-term outcome.

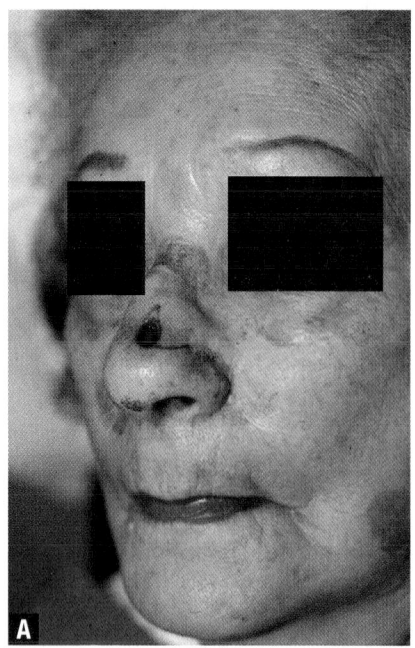
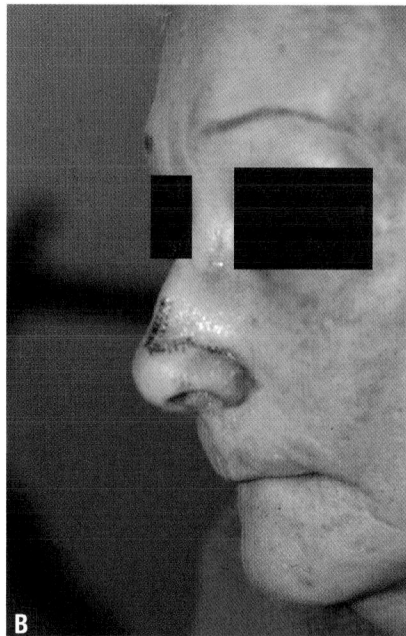
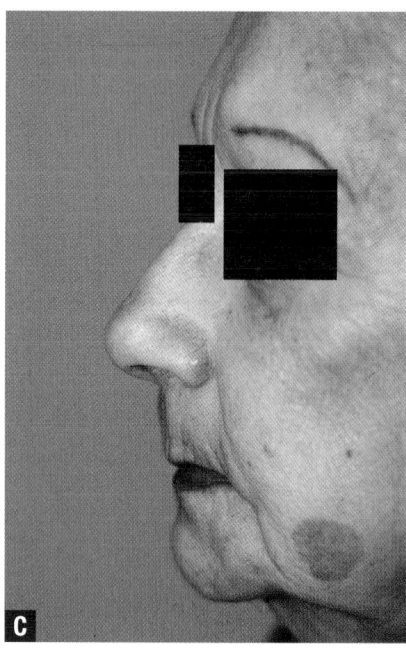

▲ **FIGURE 42-3** A to L advancement flap. **A.** Mohs defect on the dorsal nose. **B.** Repair immediately following surgery. **C.** Long-term outcome.

TRANSPOSITION FLAP

Rhombic transposition flap The rhombic transposition flap was first described in 1946 by Limberg as a repair technique to close a 60° rhombus-shaped defect. The rhombic flap is particularly useful to repair nasal sidewall and glabellar defects. The use of a rhombic flap on the distal nose or alae often produces unacceptable nasal contour distortion. While a full discussion of the rhombic flap variations is beyond the scope of this chapter, two will be mentioned briefly.

In 1962, Dufourmentel presented a modification to close defects with any acute angle. The obtuseness of the leading angle in this repair decreases the pivotal restraint leading to lateral tip tension versus the more vertical tip tension of the classic rhombic flap repair, and is therefore used when some sharing of the tension is acceptable. It also minimizes the standing cone redundancy that can occur at the origin of the flap in a classic rhombic repair. In 1977, Webster used a 30° distal flap end angle combined with an M-plasty closure of the defect base.[6]

BILOBED TRANSPOSITION FLAP Originally described by Esser, the bilobed flap is composed of two flaps of identical shape and diameter separated by an angle of 90°.[7] The bilobed flap became a mainstay in nasal reconstruction after it was modified by Zitelli. The original arc of rotation used in the bilobed flap was 180°. The Zitelli modification decreased this arc to between 90 and 110°, which

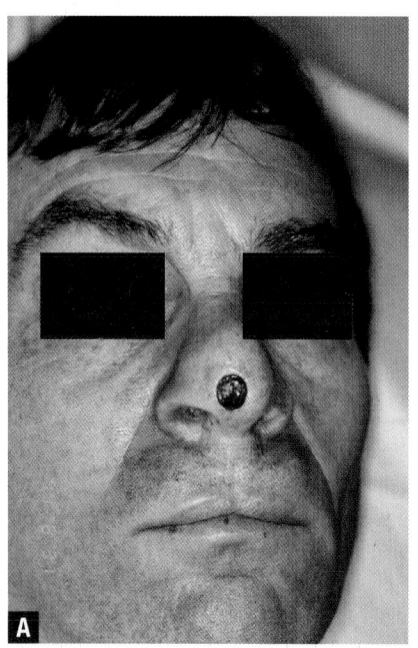
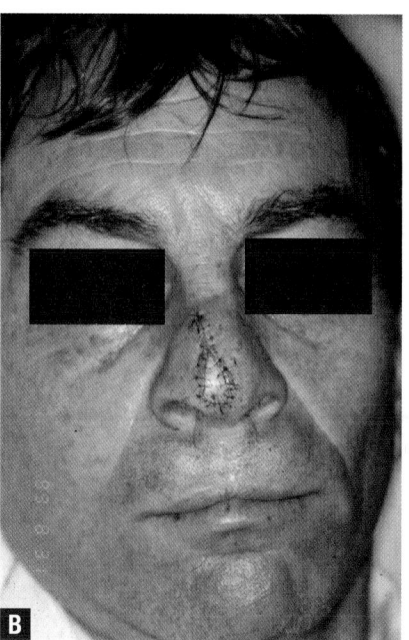
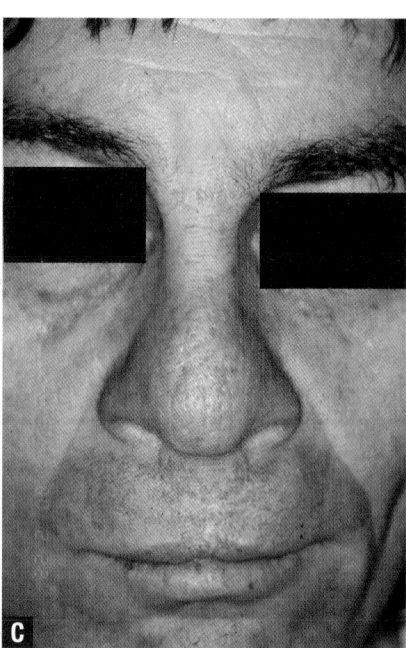

▲ **FIGURE 42-4** Myocutaneous island pedicle flap. **A.** Mohs defect on the nasal tip **B.** Repair immediately following surgery. **C.** Long-term outcome.

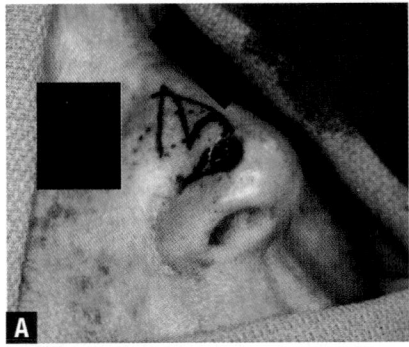 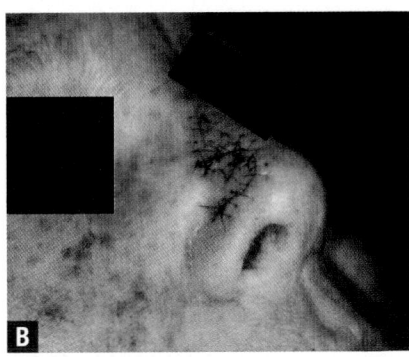 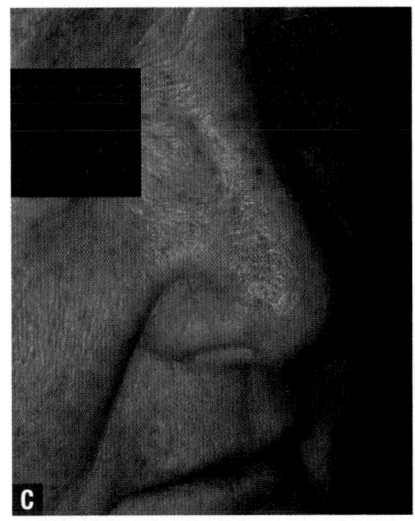

▲ **FIGURE 42-5** Zitelli modification of the bilobed flap. **A.** The design of the flap. Note that the flap will rotate between 90 and 110°. **B.** Repair immediately following surgery. **C.** Long-term outcome.

allows much greater mobility and significantly decreases the occurrences of trapdoor deformities and dog-ear formation.[8] The Zitelli modification of the original bilobed flap also provides more control over the orientation of the scar lines by taking a dog-ear at any orientation off of the circular defect. It also precludes the removal of the dog-ear that occurs at the point of rotation and facilitates better vascular supply of the flap by avoiding incising the base of the defect. This modification is a wonderful example of taking a repair that could "fill the hole" and by understanding flap dynamics, modifying it into a cosmetically elegant closure (Fig. 42-5A to C).

The bilobed flap is generally used for defects that are smaller than 1.5 cm in diameter and located on the nasal sidewall, tip, supratip, or medial alae. Medial defects are generally closed with a laterally based flap, while nasal ala defects with medially based flap.

Wide undermining in the submuscular plane improves flap viability and increases distance of movement. As with other flaps, the aesthetic of the outcome is optimized when the scar lines align with the nasal subunits. The design, if possible, should attempt to distribute the tension on the nasal tip equally in order to avoid distortion.[9] Keep in mind that the distal edge of the flap is at risk for necrosis, perhaps even more so than in other flap repairs, because it is frequently necessary to thin the lobe filling the primary defect. Thinning is essential to avoid pincushioning, but should be performed cautiously. Submuscular undermining can improve distal flap viability.[10]

INTERPOLATION FLAP The forehead or paramedian forehead flap is an axial interpolation flap based on supratrochlear artery vascular supply. The pedicled melolabial flap is based on the rich vascular supply of the melolabial area. These staged procedures are used to close large defects on the distal nose that cannot be repaired in an aesthetically pleasing manner with other repair methods. These defects usually involve at least two nasal subunits. A full discussion of the flap's design and execution is beyond the scope of this chapter, but a few general remarks follow.

The initial procedure of flap pedicle design and placement can be lengthy. While the length of this procedure has been used to support its use only under general anesthesia, in the hands of an experienced cutaneous surgeon, this procedure can be safely performed in an office setting with local anesthesia. The surgeon must also assess the patient's willingness to undergo a staged procedure that requires a pedicle of skin to protrude from the patient's face for 3 weeks and the patient's likely ability to comply with postoperative wound instructions prior to undertaking this procedure.

GRAFT

Full-thickness skin graft Full-thickness skin grafts (FTSG) are appropriate for shallow defects of the nasal tip and alae obviating the need for flap repairs that have a much higher potential for distorting nasal contour. Other modalities, including secondary intention, linear, and flap repair should all be considered prior to making the decision to use an FTSG. The donor site should be chosen with the texture and color of the nasal skin in mind.

Commonly reported donor sites include the pre- and postauricular, supraclavicular, clavicular, conchal bowl, forehead, and melolabial fold skin. The conchal bowl is an ideal harvest site based on clinical and histologic assessment[11] (Fig. 42-6). A less frequently reported, but useful donor site for repair of nasal defects with FTSG, is the forehead.[12]

Occasionally, regional FTSGs work well to repair nasal defects. This can be the case when an island pedicle flap is designed, but the mobility is suboptimal, in which case the pedicle can be severed, converting the repair from a local flap to a regional graft. Although the vascular supply is obviously less than an island pedicle flap, the mobility is increased, there is less superior pull and potential for nasal tip distortion, and the color and texture match is generally excellent.

Regardless of donor site, the recipient bed will promote graft viability best if the defect is shallow, electrocautery has been used only if absolutely necessary, and, in the case of the nasal tip, perichondrium is present. The authors do not routinely use bolster sutures.

Split-thickness skin graft While split-thickness skin grafts can be used to repair nasal defects, there is almost always a more functionally and aesthetically appropriate option. Split-thickness skin grafts have been appropriately used in a case of an extremely aggressive tumor in which case a complicated closure would preclude the ability to monitor for potential recurrence.

517

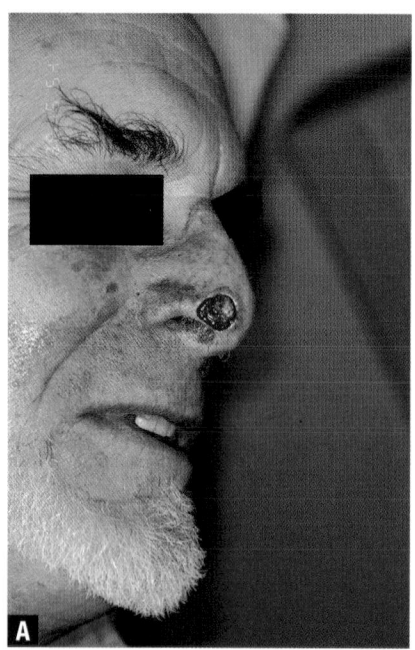 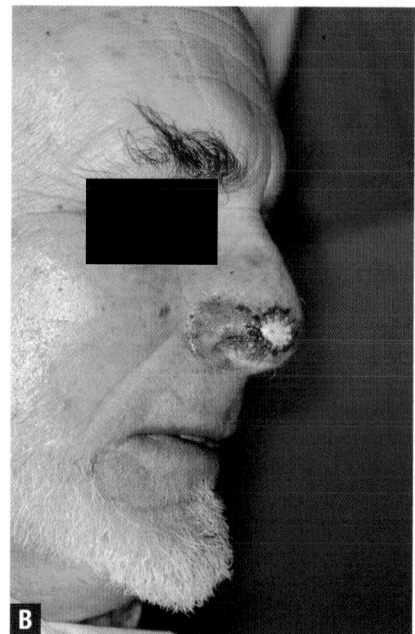 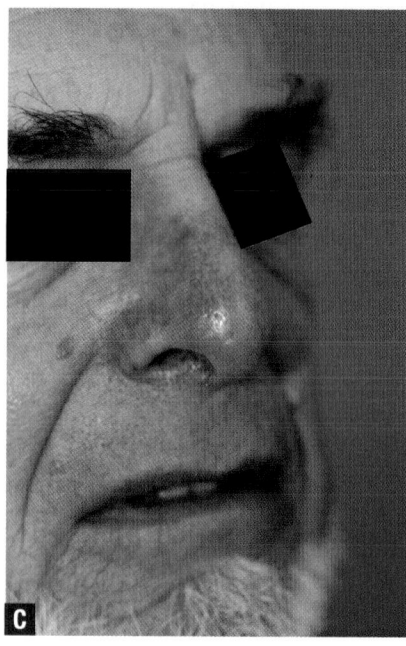

▲ **FIGURE 42-6** **A.** Mohs defect involving the soft triangle of the nose. **B.** An FTSG harvested from the conchal bowl is used to repair the defect. **C.** Long-term outcome.

SKIN CANCER

RECONSTRUCTION OF THE LIP

BOX 42-3 Summary

- It is advisable to mark out the vermilion border and the cosmetic subunits of the lip preoperatively, as these landmarks are essential in designing a repair and are often lost due to swelling from edema and local anesthesia.
- Lip defects with a diameter less than 30% of the lip can usually be closed primarily, while defects measuring up to 60% of the lip may be repaired with a flap.
- The island pedicle flap lends itself well to reconstruction of defects on the upper lateral lip and the scar line can be hidden along the melolabial fold.

The lips are the focal point of verbal and nonverbal human interaction. They are functionally essential for drinking, eating, and speaking. They are free margins, mobile and elastic. They do not have bony or cartilaginous underpinnings. All of the above challenges the reconstructive surgeon in a different way than any other part of the face. When considering how to repair the lips, one must keep in mind that the lip is made of cutaneous, vermilion, and mucosal components. The subunits of the upper cutaneous lip are two lateral units and one central, or philtral, unit. The lower lip is one aesthetic unit. Any asymmetry of the lip, the oral commis-

sure, or misalignment of the vermilion is readily apparent to passers-by, making lip reconstruction a challenge.

It is advisable to mark out the vermilion border and the cosmetic subunits of the lip preoperatively, as these landmarks are essential in designing a repair and are often lost due to swelling from edema and local anesthesia. The authors have found intraoperative botulinum toxin injection into the orbicularis oris directly surrounding the repair helpful by decreasing tension on the wound and, thereby, improving the functional and aesthetic outcome.

Secondary Intention

Larger defects in the perioral area do not lend themselves to healing by secondary intention because of the potential for contracture and resulting asymmetry and functional disability. Very superficial wounds on the vermilion lip, such as those resulting from laser resurfacing, heal well with secondary intention. Another area that heals very well secondarily is the lateral upper cutaneous lip at the junction between the ala and medial cheek.[13]

Primary Closure

Lip defects with a diameter less than 30% of the lip can usually be closed primarily. It is essential when closing a surgical defect on the lip primarily that standing vertical cones be avoided. The

resultant puckering is cosmetically unacceptable. With this in mind, the surgeon should not hesitate to take the triangle onto the vermilion lip[14] or to excise through underlying subcutaneous tissue and muscle to avoid any fullness or puckering. When closing the lower lip primarily, one can use an M-plasty on the cutaneous lip to decrease the length of the incision, to avoid crossing the mental crease onto the separate cosmetic unit, the chin.

Advancement Flap

Advancement flaps are very useful in the repair of defects of the lip measuring up to 60% of the lip. Advancement flaps allow the surgeon to mobilize medial cheek tissue to preserve the vermilion contour.

The unilateral Burow's advancement is commonly used to repair defects on the upper cutaneous lip that lie just lateral to the philtral column. Defects that are more laterally located in the upper cutaneous lip can be repaired well using an A to T or A to L advancement flap, in which the inferior limbs can hide along the vermilion border and the vertically oriented scar line can hide well in the "pucker" lines of the lip. Crescentic perialar cheek excision allows the surgeon to hide one scar line in the alar crease by excising a crescent of skin from the perialar skin along one limb of the advancement incision.[15] Likewise, a crescentic advancement flap may be designed around the corner of the mouth to pre-

518

vent distorting the corner of the mouth when repairing defects in the middle part of the cutaneous lip.

The island pedicle flap lends itself well to reconstruction of defects on the upper lateral lip. The pedicle's superior scar line and the secondary defect scar line can be hidden along the melolabial fold (Fig. 42-7A to C).

Rotation Flap

Lateral defects in the upper lip can be repaired with the use of inferiorly based rotation flaps. The incision line lies along the melolabial fold, so the scar is well hidden. It is important to pay attention to the oral commissure so that untoward upward displacement does not result from this rotational repair. The O to Z bilateral rotation flap fills defects on the lower lip quite well, leaving an incision line along the mental crease, the lower vermilion border, and a diagonal scar across the cutaneous lower lip.

For very large, full-thickness defects, one rotational flap that serves the cutaneous surgeon well, both functionally and aesthetically is the Karapandzic flap. This repair is used predominantly to close very large lower lip defects. Incisions are made along the mental crease and the bilateral melolabial folds and the flaps are rotated in and down resulting in intact vascular supply and innervation to a symmetric, if not smaller, oral aperture.[14]

Transposition Flap

Because transposition flaps are designed to allow transposition of tissue over stationary tissue, their use is challenging in the reconstruction of lip defects given the mobility of the lip. When used to repair the lip, they are usually used for medium-sized defects on the upper, lateral cutaneous lip utilizing tissue from the medial cheek or utilizing tissue from the inferior nasolabial fold to repair defects on the lateral lower cutaneous lip.

Interpolation Flap

Interpolation flaps are rarely used to repair lip defects.

Skin Graft

Skin grafts, full or split thickness are rarely used to repair lip defects due to their inability to adequately match the color, texture, and functionality of the lip tissue. However, defects in women that preclude excision of the entire philtrum may be aesthetically reconstructed with an FTSG (Fig. 42-8A to C).

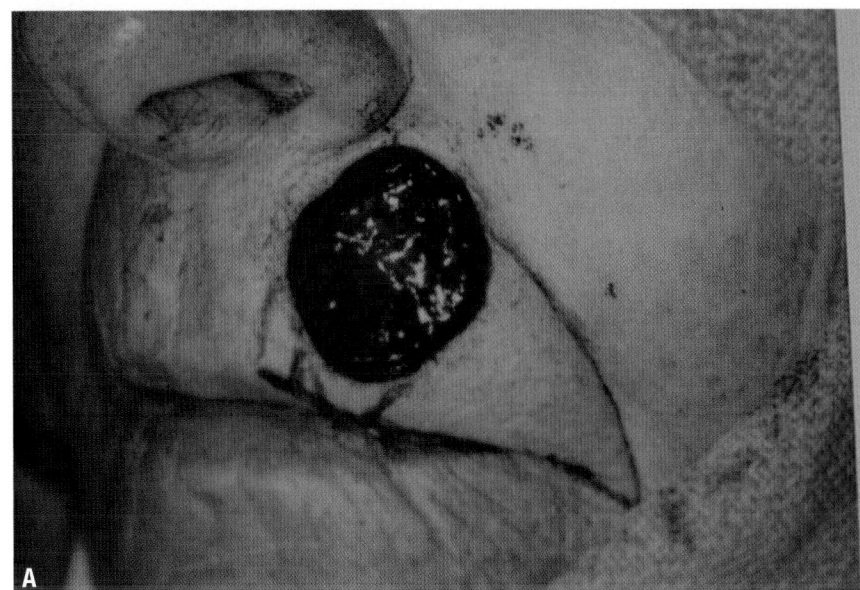
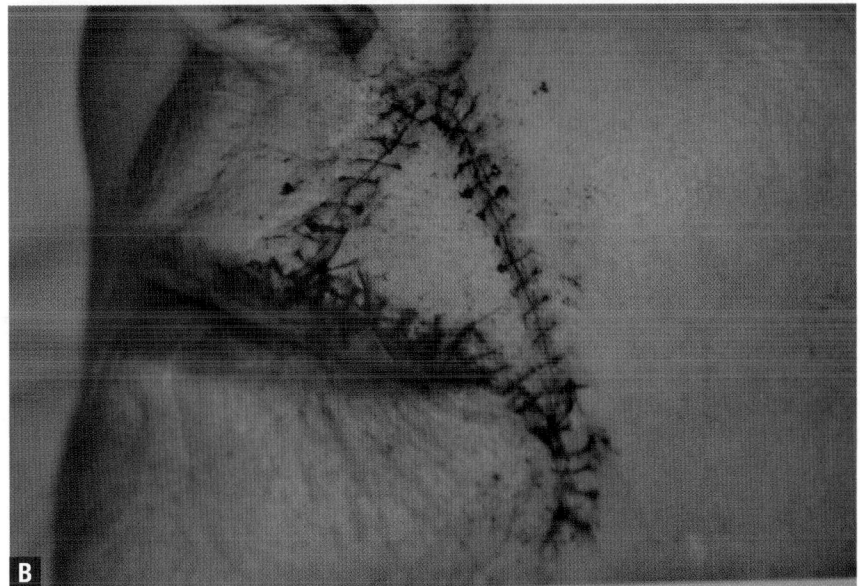
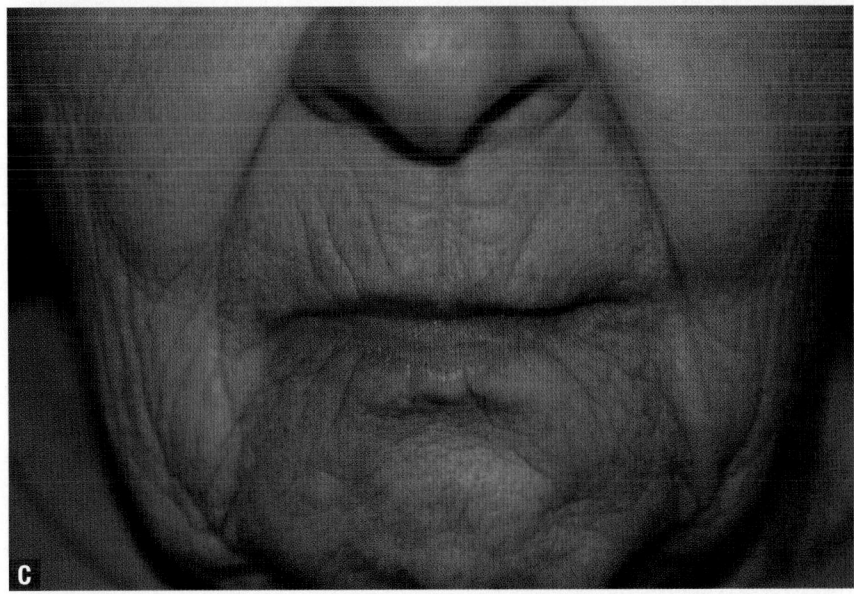

▲ **FIGURE 42-7 A.** Defect on the upper cutaneous lip. **B.** Repair immediately following surgery. **C.** Long-term outcome.

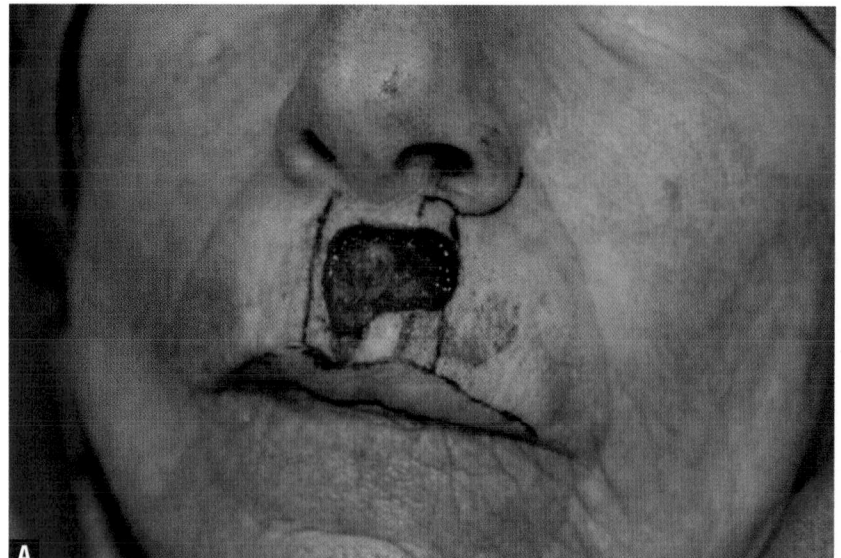

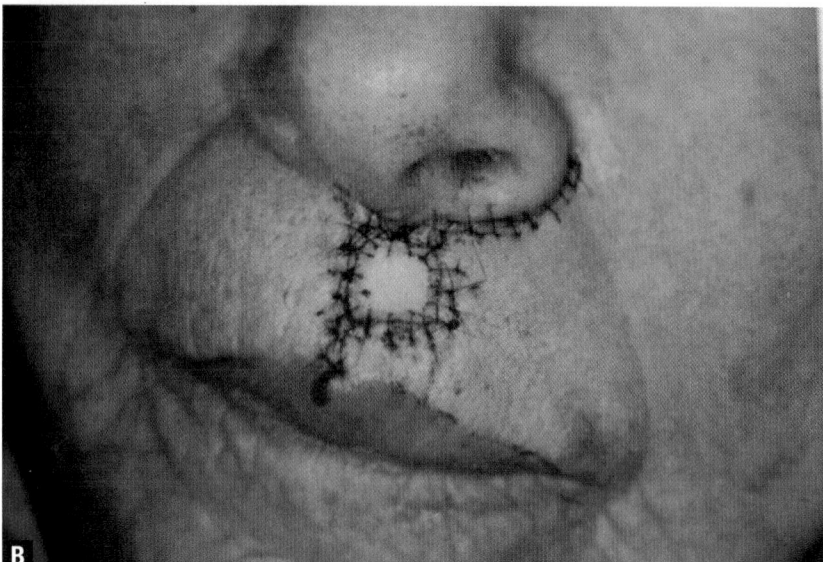

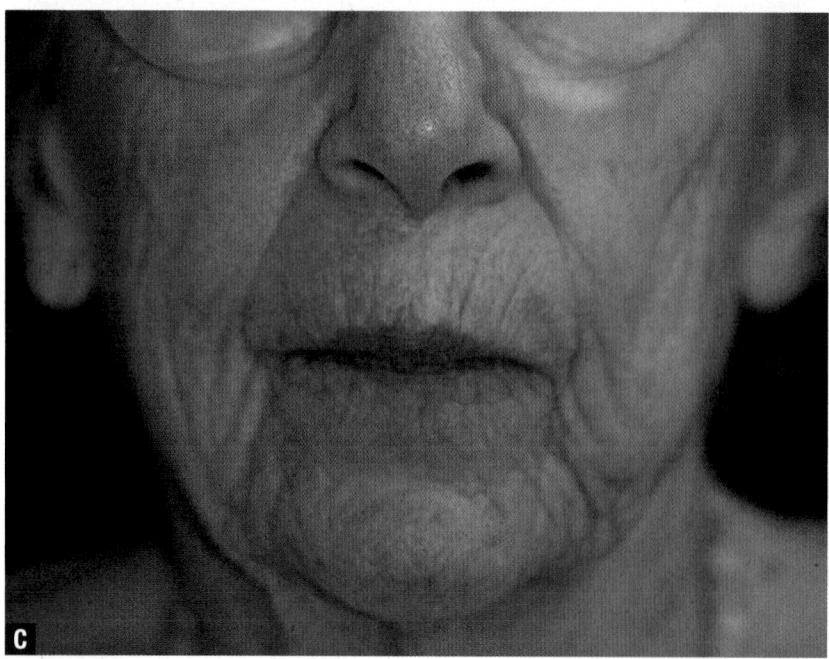

▲ **FIGURE 42-8** FTSG. **A.** Defect on the upper lip. **B.** Repair immediately following surgery. **C.** Long-term outcome.

The advantage of this repair is that it will not obliterate or distort the cupid's bow, while other options may. Occasionally, larger defects in women that involve an entire side of the upper cutaneous lip may be reconstructed with an FTSG.

RECONSTRUCTION OF THE EAR

BOX 42-4 Summary

- Defects located in a concavity of the ear can be allowed to heal via secondary intention if the perichondrium is intact.
- If there is no perichondrium on the ear, then 2 to 3-mm fenestrations through the cartilage made with a dermal punch can be made to facilitate granulation from the vascular perichondrium deep to the defect.
- Placing vertical mattress sutures on the helical rim can aid in the detailed restoration of the helical contour.
- Chondrocutaneous composite flaps, profused by the rich vascular supply surrounding the ear, can be used to address full-thickness defects of the ear.
- Rotation, advancement, and transposition flaps based on the posterior helix, postauricular scalp, or preauricular scalp can be used to repair defects on the helix without significant morbidity.
- For defects less than 1 cm, the simple wedge repair may be used.

The external ear is an important and complex specialized structure. Its collagen is supple, allowing for bending without losing its shape, while its concave structure acts as an amplifier of sound. The contour of the ears provides an important silhouette of the head aesthetically. The ear remains of great clinical importance because the embryologic fusion planes formed by the first and second branchial arches as well as the first branchial groove are potential paths along which malignancies can travel.[16] Reconstruction of this unique organ involves the repair of cutaneous, cartilaginous, or combined defects. Although differences in the ears can be tolerated because both ears are only viewed during a head-on view, effort must be made to maintain aesthetic similarities between the ears.[16]

The structural support of the ear is composed of type II collagen. This scaffold receives its nutrients from the perichondrium with its anastamosing network of vessels formed by the superficial temporal and posterior auricular arteries. The skin is directly adherent to this network of fascia laterally, while a layer of subcutis separates the skin and the cartilage medially. Innervation of the auricle is provided by the auriculotemporal nerve superiorly, the greater auricular nerve inferiorly, the lesser occipital nerve posteriorly, and branches of the vagus nerve, and cranial nerve IX centrally in the concha.[17,18]

The surface anatomy of the ear is complex, divided into various convexities and concavities. The helix, antihelix, tragus, and lobule represent some of the major projections of the ear while the triangular fossa, conchal bowl, scapha, postauricular sulcus, preauricular sulcus and external auditory meatus are the major concavities.[19]

Secondary Intention

Defects located in a concavity of the ear can be allowed to heal via secondary intention if the perichondrium is intact. This oftentimes results in a very pleasing cosmetic result without significant distortion of the anterior anatomy of the ear. If there is no perichondrium, then 2 to 3-mm fenestrations through the cartilage made with a dermal punch can be made to facilitate granulation from the vascular perichondrium deep to the anterior defect. Allowing granulation of the posterior helix is also an acceptable repair option. If a defect extends from the posterior helix onto the postauricular scalp, however, granulation may result in a pinned-back ear when one was not intended. In this case, primary repair of either the scalp or the posterior pinna will prevent this from occurring. Alternatively, a barrier of vaseline-impregnated gauze may also be used to cover the wounds until fully epithelialized.

Primary Linear Repair

Small defects of the helix can be closed by a linear closure. Extending the length of the incision far beyond the usual 3:1 or 4:1 length to width ratio may allow for a more gradual taper and thus less distortion of the helical rim. Placing vertical mattress sutures can aid in the detailed restoration of the helical contour. Defects on the lobule, the postauricular sulcus, or preauricular sulcus can have a very desirable cosmetic result with this type of repair. Directly in the postauricular sulcus, the skin on the postauricular scalp and the posterior helix can be reapproximated by placing a single layer of vertical mattress suture. If the width of the defect on the posterior helix is great, this repair will result in the pinning-back of the ear that can be undesirable, especially if the patient wears eyeglasses.

Wedge Repair

For defects less than 1 cm, the simple wedge repair can be used.[20] This is a type of repair based on making v-shaped incisions around the defect with subsequent side-to-side suturing. This chondrocutaneous flap is ideally designed with a 30° angle between the edges of the flap.[17] For defects greater than 1 cm in width, additional v-shaped incisions placed near the helical rim may help maintain the front and side contours of the pinna. Once any repair is designed, the cartilage must be reapproximated carefully so as not to tear the cartilage. Once the cartilage is sutured, the overlying skin can be manipulated in an anterior or posterior manner to restore a pleasing contour.

Chondrocutaneous Defect

It is not uncommon to have full-thickness cutaneous defects that involve the cartilage and the overlying soft tissue. Once the perichondrium is stripped, tissue must be rearranged to cover the exposed cartilage or risk cartilage necrosis. Random pedicle flaps are often reasonable options for repairing defects on the ear (Fig. 42-9A to E). Rotation, advancement, and transposition flaps based on the posterior helix, postauricular scalp, or preauricular scalp can be used to repair defects on the helix without significant morbidity. In these cases, flaps take advantage of the nutrient-rich, vascular supply of the skin surrounding the ear.

Many named flaps have been described to repair defects on the helix. Bilobed flaps based on mobile, posterior helix skin can be used to repair partial or full-thickness defects on the helical rim. The Banner transposition flap harvested from skin the preauricular fold is also a reasonable option for proximal defects of the helix.

Chondrocutaneous Advancement Flap

Various types of chondrocutaneous composite flaps can be used to address full-thickness defects of the ear. A common chondrocutaneous advancement flap is created by making an incision in the scapha. The lateral helical skin and attached cartilage is then rotated superiorly to close defects on the superior helix. Variations of this simple chondrocutaneous flap, including O to T flaps or bilateral advancement flaps can be designed with similar relocation of the skin and underlying cartilage.

Skin Graft

Skin grafts, either full or partial thickness, can be successfully used to repair defects on the ear. If naked cartilage is at the base of the defect, it can be removed prior to graft placement provided the cartilage is not providing essential structural support to the remainder of the ear. In these cases, the graft is placed directly on the perichondrium, thus increasing the likelihood of graft survival. Graft anchors, such as tie-over bolsters or basting sutures can also be used to immobilize the graft and increase the risk of survival.

RECONSTRUCTION OF THE CHEEK

BOX 42-5 Summary

- When repairing defects on the cheek, it is essential that the surgeon be comfortable with local anatomy, anatomic danger zones, and adjacent free margins.
- Cheek repairs may be best camouflaged by orienting scars to fall within relaxed skin tension lines.
- Grafts and secondary intention are not ideal repair options for cheek defects.
- Rotation flaps and transposition flaps lend themselves well to the repair of larger surgical defects on the cheek, taking advantage of skin laxity in the preauricular or neck area.

While defects on the cheek may seem less challenging to repair in an aesthetically pleasing manner than the nose, lip, or eyelids, reconstruction of the cheek can be rift with complications if the surgeon does not heed the anatomic variables of this facial region. The facial nerve branches, specifically the marginal mandibular and the temporal nerves, are at risk. When repairing defects close to the mandible or at the junction of the cheek and the temple, it is essential that the surgeon be comfortable with local anatomy. The reconstruction of cheek defects demands that attention be given to the free margins of the lower eyelid, oral commissure, and upper lip. It is advisable to be in the practice of asking the patient to gaze upward and even sit up intraoperatively after the initial sutures are placed, in order to assess for tension on the lid margin after adjusting for gravity and dynamic movement.

Secondary Intention

The cheek rarely lends itself to healing by secondary intention since this facial region is concave, for the most part.

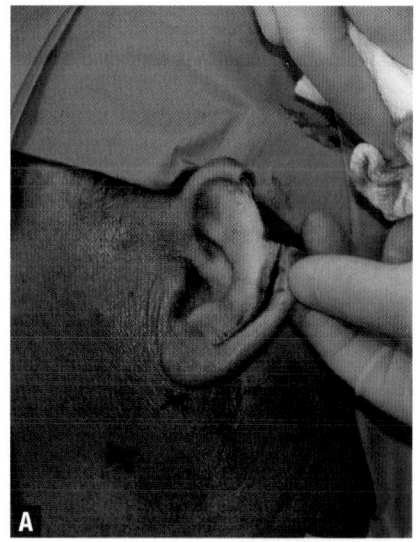
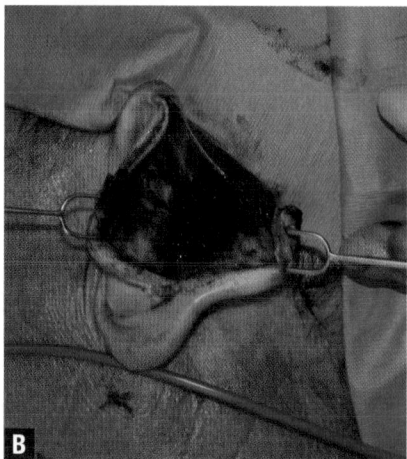
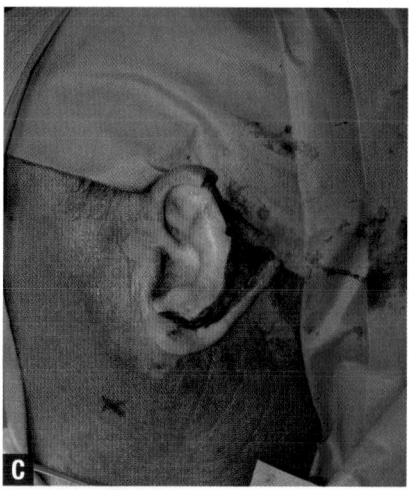
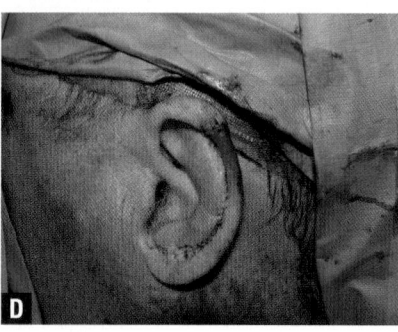
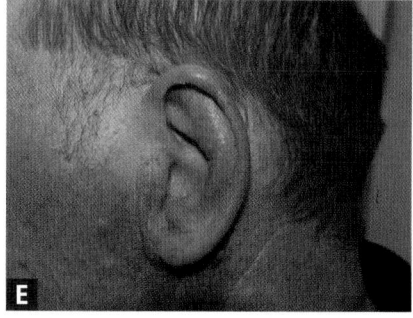

▲ **FIGURE 42-9** Chondrocutaneous advancement flap following a sentinel lymph-node biopsy (lymphoscintigraphy). **A.** A left helix defect immediately following a sentinel lymph-node biopsy (lymphoscintigraphy) and a wide local excision of an invasive melanoma. Note the residual blue dye in the skin from the lymphoscintigraphy. An incision inferior to the defect was made in the helical groove through anterior helical skin and cartilage. **B.** Wide undermining was performed medial to the defect at the level between the posterior helical perichondrium and subcutis. **C.** The flap is resting in place. **D.** The chondrocutaneous flap is rotated superiorly to cover the defect. **E.** Repair at 2 months.

Primary Closure

A linear or crescentic primary closure is often the repair of choice for defects on the cheek. These scars are usually camouflaged in relaxed skin tension lines on the lateral cheeks, the preauricular regions, and along the nasofacial sulcus and the melolabial groove. Linear repairs on the upper cheek should not necessarily be avoided because of the proximity of the lower lid and concern over this free margin. If linear closure can be designed so that the final scar line is perpendicular to the free margin, there should not be tension resulting in ectropion. Since natural lines of skin tension are slightly curvilinear, the repair design should be as well.

Advancement Flap

The Burow's advancement flap is a viable option for the reconstruction of certain cheek defects. It can be combined with a slight rotation to facilitate hiding the scars in relaxed skin tension lines, which are arciform in nature.

The island pedicle flap can be a very useful repair on the cheek and can be easily camouflaged in the melolabial fold. When designed to repair a defect on the upper cheek, the island pedicle's lateral incisions can be made in a curvilinear fashion, creating a slight rotation and minimizing tension on the lower eyelid.

Rotation Flap

Large defects on the cheek often lend themselves to closure via a rotation flap, using adjacent cheek, preauricular, or neck skin. They are usually laterally or inferiorly based. The curvilinear borders of rotation flaps frequently hide well in relaxed skin tension lines and in the melolabial and nasofacial folds. Tacking sutures into the periosteum are generally required to prevent the weight of a large rotation flap from pulling the eyelid downward and creating an ectropion. Rotation flaps may be combined with a transposition flap for large cheek defects extending superiorly onto the lower eyelid.[21]

Transposition Flaps

Rhombic transposition flaps lend themselves well to the repair of larger surgical defects on the cheek. Lateral and inferiorly based rhombic transposition flaps allow the surgeon to hide scar lines along the lateral face and to take advantage of the skin laxity of the preauricular region.

Skin Grafts

Other options for closure are preferred to the use of a graft on the cheek because of aesthetic concerns. It is difficult to match graft texture, thickness, and color to adjacent cheek skin. Graft contracture is also a concern given the convex contour of the cheek, making contracture an obviously unacceptable aesthetic outcome. Grafts are appropriate for the closure of cheek defects that are too large for primary or flap repair or when the resected tumor has a significantly high local tumor recurrence potential. The use of a graft, especially split-thickness, allows for closer monitoring for tumor recurrence.

RECONSTRUCTION OF THE SCALP AND FOREHEAD

BOX 42-6   Summary

- Care must be taken regarding the reconstruction of surgical defects on the scalp and forehead in order to maintain the contour of the head, create cosmetically pleasing scars, and prevent brow asymmetry.
- Achieving maximal eversion of linear repairs of the scalp and forehead maximally everts and tightly reapproximates the skin, thus, preventing a widened or fish-mouth scar.
- The primary linear repair is often one of the simplest options for repairing small defects on the scalp.
- Transposition flaps can also be of great utility in the scalp, providing repairs that can rearrange hairs without creating large areas of alopecia.
- When considering reconstruction options for the forehead, it is important to consider the contraction of the scar and the possible distortion of the brow line, the free margin of the eyelid, and the temporal hairline.

The scalp and forehead are areas of great aesthetic importance. Care must be taken regarding the reconstruction of surgical defects in this region to maintain the contour of the head, to create cosmetically pleasing scars, and to prevent brow asymmetry. Understanding the anatomy of the scalp and forehead is of utmost importance in designing and executing repairs in this region. The anterior–posterior anatomic boundaries of the scalp are the supraorbital ridge and the nuchal line. Laterally, the temporal fossae and the zygomatic arches define the boundaries of the scalp. The nonhair bearing scalp areas are divided into separate cosmetic units of the forehead and the posterior neck.[20,22]

In the hair-bearing scalp, five layers of tissue overlie the cranium: the skin, the subcutis, the galea aponeurotica, the subgaleal alveolar tissue, and the periosteum. The scalp, rich in adnexal structures, is profused by the supraorbital, supratrochlear, and the anterior branches of the temporal arteries. The temperoparietalis and the occipitofrontalis muscles are the major muscle groups of the scalp. The occipitofrontalis muscle, divided into occipitalis and frontalis muscles bellies, is connected by a thick layer of fascia named the galea aponeurotica. The subgaleal alveolar tissue plane provides a low-resistance, avascular plane ideal for undermining. Sensory innervation of the scalp and forehead is provided by the ophthalmic branch of the trigeminal nerve and cervical plexus, while motor innervation is provided through the facial nerve.[20,22]

The cosmetic unit of the forehead is bounded laterally by the zygoma, superiorly by the frontal and temporal hairlines, and inferiorly by the glabella and eyebrows. The musculature of the forehead overlaps the anterior musculature of the scalp. The occipitofrontalis, procerus, and corrugator muscles are contained in the forehead unit with their major motor innervation provided by the temporal branch of cranial nerve VII. This nerve lies deep to the frontalis muscle and the superficial muscular aponeurotic system (SMAS) in the midforehead. Over the zygoma, however, the temporal branch of the facial nerve is not protected by an overlying muscle. Care should be taken when undermining over the zygoma and in the temple region to prevent transection of this nerve. The forehead is profused by the left and right supraorbital, supratrochlear, and anterior branches of the temporal artery. Coursing with these arteries are the similarly named nerves that provide sensory innervation to the tissues of the forehead and anterior scalp. These sensory nerves, which arise from the opthalmic branch of the trigeminal nerve, lie in the subcutaneous fat.

RECONSTRUCTION OF THE HAIR-BEARING SCALP

Secondary Intention

Many partial or full-thickness defects on the scalp can be allowed to heal via secondary intention if the periosteum is intact. This option is reasonable for those who cannot tolerate a repair procedure or for individuals whose defect lies in an area of alopecia. The limitation of this closure is alopecia in the scar and the size of the scar.

Primary Linear Repairs

The primary linear repair is often one of the simplest options for repairing small defects on the scalp. Considerations must be made, however, to respect the natural contours of the scalp and forehead while minimizing distortion of adjacent structures. On the scalp, defects less than 3 cm can usually be closed primarily.[20] Care must be taken to maximally evert and tightly reapproximate the skin to prevent a widened or fish-mouth scar. Such scars remain prominent because they persist as well-demarcated areas of alopecia that can be particularly noticeable on short-haired individuals. To achieve strong wound edge eversion, wide undermining in the subgaleal plane followed by the reapproximation of the galea with buried vertical mattress sutures can result in immediate hypereversion and, ultimately, a cosmetically pleasing scar.[23] When necessary, galeotomies on either side of the wound placed parallel to the incision line and at least 1 cm laterally can offer additional movement for difficult to approximate wound edges. Epidermal eversion can be completed by the placement of staples or percutaneous epidermal sutures. The removal of standing cutaneous cones is imperative in the scalp to maintain the contour of the head.

Random-Pedicle Flaps

Random-pedicle advancement, rotation, and transposition flaps can be ideal for the closure of defects greater than 3 cm on the scalp.[20,24] Once the area around the defect is widely undermined in the subgaleal plane, an advancement or rotation flap can be designed to close the wound while respecting the anatomic boundaries of the adjacent cosmetic units. To avoid the extension of a linear repair onto the forehead, an A to T flap can be designed such that the "T" of the incision lies within the hairline of the scalp. Rotation flaps can be an ideal closure technique as well, taking on dimensions much larger than those seen on other areas of the face. These flaps take advantage of the spherical shape of the calvarium, ensuring closure along the natural arcs of the underlying structure. When designing a single rotation flap on the scalp, the incision must be at least four times the width of the defect width.[24] Multiple rotation flaps, also known as "pinwheel" flaps, do not need to adhere to this length to width ratio. Transposition flaps can also be of great utility in the scalp, providing repairs that can rearrange hairs without creating large areas of alopecia (Fig. 42-10A to D).

Skin Grafts

Partial or FTSGs on the scalp are oftentimes cosmetically inferior to the repairs achieved with flap repairs due to the areas of alopecia created with grafted skin. In some cases, however, grafting may be the best option to close large defects. Patient selection remains very

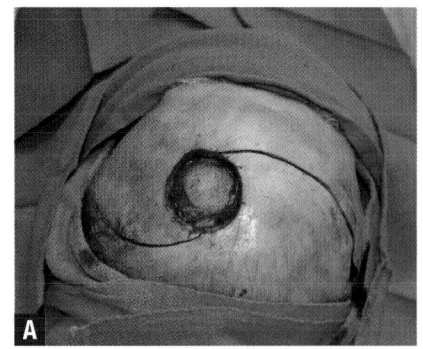
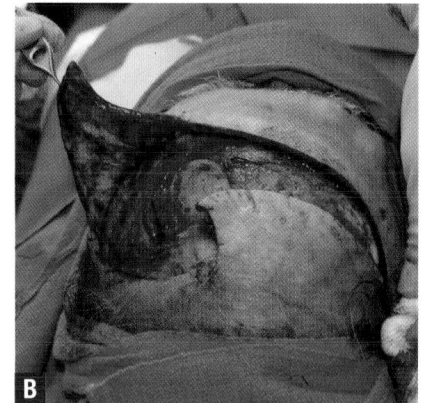
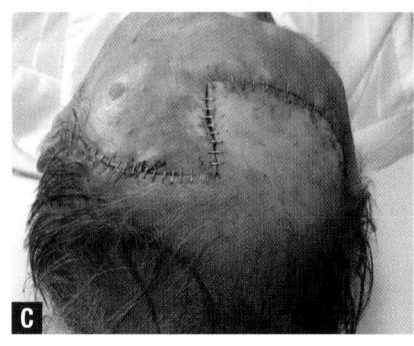
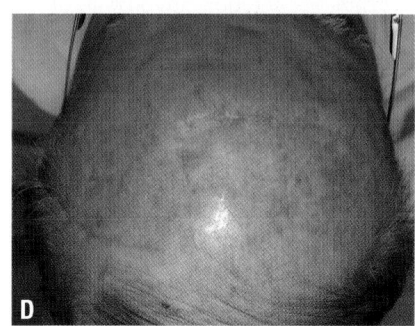

▲ **FIGURE 42-10** An O to Z random pedicle flap on the scalp. **A.** A scalp defect after a Mohs-assisted excision of a nonmelanoma skin cancer. The defect extends to the level of the periosteum. **B.** Wide undermining around the defect in the subgaleal plane is performed. Note the galeotomies made to increase tissue mobility. **C.** The flap is rotated into place and fixed with sutures and staples. **D.** Repair at 3 months.

important when considering split- or full-thickness skin grafts. The harvested skin for an FTSG should be matched for color and texture when possible. Excised Burow's triangles from partial closure of the wound can serve in this capacity.

RECONSTRUCTION OF THE FOREHEAD

Secondary Intention

Granulation of forehead wounds is ideal in the concavities of the temples when the periosteum is intact. When weighing this option, it is important to consider the contraction of the scar and the possible distortion of the brow line, the free margin of the eyelid, and the temporal hairline. This option is reasonable for those who cannot tolerate a repair procedure.

Primary Linear Repairs

Midline forehead defects can, at times, be easily repaired with a vertically-oriented linear repair. Due to the absence of frontalis muscle fibers in midline forehead, scars in this area heal extremely well. In general, efforts should be made to orient primary linear repairs on the forehead in the direction of relaxed skin

tension lines. Standing cutaneous cones must be removed to prevent deformity of the forehead. Finally, eversion of the epidermis is very important on the convexity of the forehead to prevent prominent, indented scars. Percutaneous, vertical or horizontal mattress sutures can be used to reapproximate the epidermis to allow for ideal completion of eversion.[25,26]

Random Pedicle Flaps

Due to important motor and sensory nerves coursing through the forehead, careful undermining and flap design are imperative to prevent brow ptosis and sensory deficits that extend to the parietal scalp.

O to T Advancement Flap

On the forehead, flaps must be designed to respect the anatomic boundaries of the adjacent cosmetic units of the eyelid and the scalp. O to T flaps can be oriented to avoid involvement of these adjacent units while allowing for closure of the defect in relaxed skin tension lines.

Island Pedicle Flap

The island pedicle flap can be of great use on the lateral forehead, borrowing

from skin laxity in the superior forehead or lateral cheek. Because of the rich vascular supply of the lateral face, island pedicle flaps can be designed to repair both small and large defects without significant distortion to adjacent structures.

Transposition Flaps

Transposition flaps that result in lateral facial incisions result in scars that are difficult to see from a head-on view of the patient. In many older patients, redundant tissue in the preauricular cheek can be utilized to close forehead defects. Rhombic, bilobed, and other random pedicle flaps can be used to successfully repair defects that would otherwise result in significant tissue distortion. Additionally, anatomic landmarks such as the preauricular sulcus and the boundaries between the forehead and cheek can be exploited in the design of such flaps.

Skin Grafts

Ideally, skin for an FTSG repair should be harvested from the same cosmetic unit to give the best cosmetic match of skin tone and texture. If part of the defect can be closed primarily, excised Burow's triangle can be used to repair the remaining defect. In general, however, full- or split-thickness skin grafts harvested from any location carry a risk of being quite conspicuous on the forehead. Every case requires assessment of the various benefits and drawbacks with the ultimate choice of repair being what is best for the patient.

FINAL THOUGHTS

The successful reconstruction of skin cancer defects requires the consideration of the defect, the location, and most importantly, the patient. Elegant reconstruction of skin cancer defects that restore or maintain the local anatomy, aesthetics, and functional workings of an area may be possible. However, if the patient will not tolerate or does not desire to undergo a reconstructive procedure, the surgeon must respect their patient's wishes. Communication of the risks, benefits, and alternatives to reconstructive procedures is fundamental to the successful practice of reconstructive surgery. This informed consent process also requires the physician to help the patient set realistic expectations for their reconstruction. Ultimately, physician–patient communication will allow for the best patient care and the highest level of patient satisfaction.

REFERENCES

1. Burget GC. Aesthetic reconstruction of the tip of the nose. *Dermatol Surg.* 2005; 21(5):419–429.
2. Zitelli JA. Secondary intention healing: An alternative to surgical repair. *Clin Dermatol.* 1984;2(3):92–106.
3. Cook J, Zitelli JA. Primary closure for midline defects of the nose: A simple approach for reconstruction. *J Am Acad Dermatol.* 2000;43(3):508–510.
4. Papadopoulos DJ, Trinei FA. Superiorly based nasalis myocutaneous island pedicle flap with bilevel undermining for nasal tip and supratip reconstruction. *Dermatol Surg.* 1999;25(7):530–536.
5. Rieger RA. A local flap for repair of the nasal tip. *Plast Reconstr Surg.* 1967;40(2): 147–149.
6. Webster RC, Davidson TM, Smith RC. The thirty-degree transposition flap. *Laryngoscope.* 1978;88(1 Pt 1):85–94.
7. Esser JFS. Gestielte loakle Nasenplastik mit zweizipfligen Lappen, Deckung des sekundaren Defektes vom ersten Zipfel durch den Zweiten. *Dtsch Zschr Chir.* 1918;143:385.
8. Zitelli JA. The bilobed flap for nasal reconstruction. *Arch Dermatol.* 1989;125(7): 957–959.
9. Cook JL. A review of the bilobed flap's design with particular emphasis on the minimization of alar displacement. *Dermatol Surg.* 2000;26(4):354–362.
10. Moy RL, Grossfeld JS, Baum M. Reconstruction of the nose utilizing a bilobed flap. *Int J Dermatol.* 1994;33(9): 657–660.
11. Rohrer TE, Dzubow LM. Conchal bowl skin grafting in nasal tip reconstruction: Clinical and histologic evaluation. *J Am Acad Dermatol.* 1995;33(3):476–481.
12. Dimitropoulos V, Bichakjian CK, Johnson T. Forehead donor site full-thickness skin graft. *Dermatol Surg.* 2005; 31(3):324–326.
13. Zitelli JA, Brodland DG. A regional approach to reconstruction of the upper lip. *J Dermatol Surg Oncol.* 1991;17(2):143–148.
14. Jabaley ME, Clement RL, Orcutt TW. Myocutaneous flaps in lip reconstruction. Applications of the Karapandzic principle. *Plast Reconstr Surg.* 1997;59(5): 680–688.
15. Webster JP. Crescentic peri-alar cheek excision for upper lip flap advancement with a short history of lip repair. *Plast Reconstr Surg.* 1955;16:434–464.
16. Roenigk RK, Roenigk HH. *Dermatologic Surgery: Principles and Practice.* New York: Marcel Dekker; 1989.
17. Tromovich TA, Stegman SJ, Glogau RG. *Flaps and Grafts in Dermatologic Surgery.* Chicago, IL: Tearbook Medical; 1989.
18. Salache SJ, Bernstein G, Senkarik M. *Surgical Anatomy of the Skin.* Norwalk, CT: Appleton & Lange; 1988.
19. Lee KK. Ear reconstruction. Emedicine. com. Available at: http://www.emedicine.com/derm/topic881.htm, September 22, 2005. Accessed January 28, 2005.
20. Panje WR, Minor LB. Reconstruction of the Scalp. In: Baker SR, Swanson NA, eds. *Local Flaps in Facial Reconstruction.* St Louis, MO: Mosby-Year Book; 1995:481–514.
21. Boutros S, Zide B. Cheek and eyelid reconstruction: The resurrection of the angle rotation flap. *Plast Reconstr Surg.* 2005;16(5): 1425–1430; discussion 1431–1433.
22. Salasche SJ, Bernstein G, Senkarik M, eds. *Surgical Anatomy of the Skin.* Norwalk, CT: Appleton & Lange; 1988:151–162.
23. Zide MF. Scar revision with hypereversion. *J Oral Maxillofac Surg.* 1996;54(9): 1061–1067.
24. Leedy JE, Janis JE, Rohrich RJ. Reconstruction of acquired scalp defects: An algorithmic approach. *Plast Reconstr Surg.* September 15, 1995;116(4):54e–72e.
25. Moody BR, McCarthy JE, Linder J, Hruza GJ. Enhanced cosmetic outcome with running horizontal mattress sutures. *Dermatol Surg.* 2005;31(10):1313–1316.
26. Krunic AL, Weitzul S, Taylor RS. Running combined simple and vertical mattress suture: A rapid skin-everting stitch. *Dermatol Surg.* 2005;31(10):1325–1329.

CHAPTER 43

Cryosurgery

Christopher M. Scott, M.D.
Gloria F. Graham, M.D.

BOX 43-1 Overview

- Cryosurgery depresses the temperature of the targeted tissue below its cold-resistance threshold.
- A "heat sink" draws warmth from target tissue.
- The cryogen of choice is liquid nitrogen, with its boiling point at −195.8°C.
- Rate of freezing, the rate of rewarming, solute concentration, the duration of freeze, and the coldest temperature reached in the target tissue determine the degree of tissue destruction.
- Patient selection and education are important. Education should include a discussion on the possibility of pain, hypopigmentation, alopecia, hemorrhage, and uncommon numbness or scarring. Adequate informed consent is essential.
- Most large cryosurgery treatment series report basal cell carcinoma cure rates between 95 to 98%.
- Cryosurgery may be a useful adjunct to other skin cancer treatments, including excision, curettage, electrosurgery, chemosurgery, laser surgery, and radiation therapy.

INTRODUCTION

In broadest terms, cutaneous neoplasms are treated by either excision or destruction. The appropriate course of action is determined by the tumor type and physical characteristics, the anatomic site, patient expectations, overall health of the patient, and cost. Many small benign or premalignant lesions are treated by cryosurgery. In a survey of the International Transplant-Skin Cancer Collaborative and the Association of Academic Dermatologic Surgeons, 95% of respondents used cryosurgery for actinic keratoses and verrucae, where 24% also used liquid nitrogen for early cancer or *in situ* or superficial nonmelanoma skin cancers.[1] In truth, cryosurgery, however, may be used by those appropriately trained for a large variety of skin cancers. This chapter will address the theory behind the action of cold on the skin, as well as basic techniques for treating malignant and premalignant lesions that have provided high cure rates and satisfactory cosmetic results in an efficient manner.

Cryosurgery is the introduction of an element that depresses the temperature of the targeted tissue below its cold-resistance threshold. Localized frostbite ensues, producing necrosis and tissue destruction. The term "cryotherapy" is often inappropriately used where cryosurgery, cryoablation, cryogenic surgery, and cryocoagulation are more accurate descriptions of the destructive process required to treat malignancies. Basal cell carcinoma, squamous cell carcinoma, Bowen disease (squamous cell carcinoma *in situ*), and Kaposi's sarcoma may be treated by cryosurgery. There are numerous reports of successful treatment of lentigo maligna, but cryosurgery may not be the treatment of choice for lesions amenable to simple excision or Mohs surgery when these options are readily available. Cryogen application may be used for palliation in several metastatic cancers including those of the skin and liver.

Cryosurgery has been recognized as the treatment of choice for many cutaneous conditions, and has supplemented the use of various other modalities, such as excision, curettage, electrosurgery, chemosurgery, laser surgery, and radiation therapy. Benefits of cryosurgery include cost effectiveness, good cosmetic results, and high cure rates.[2] Cryosurgery seems to fit into the gap where other procedures have shortcomings.

HISTORY

BOX 43-2 Summary

- Numerous skin conditions have been treated with various liquefied gases.
- Current cryosurgical modalities have been guided by 150 years of medical research.

The destructive effects of extreme cold have been known for thousands of years, as described in ancient manuscripts. Egyptians used medical cryogens for topical anesthesia over 4000 years ago. More recently, the anesthetic effects of cold were exploited in Napoleon's time, as snow and ice were used to aid amputations during the retreat of Napoleon's armies from Moscow.[3] In 1855, James Arnott performed palliative treatment of cancerous tumors with a brine solution, achieving temperatures around −10°C.[4] Liquefied air, reaching temperatures around −180°C, replaced application of saline slurries in the late eighteenth century. Dr. A. Campbell White described treatment of nevi, warts, varicose leg ulcers, chancroid, boils, carbuncles, herpes zoster, and epitheliomas with liquid air.[5] Whitehouse engineered the first spray device to deliver cryogen.[6] Liquid nitrogen became widely available in the 1940s. However, it was not until Irving Cooper developed a closed system apparatus in 1961 that cryosurgery as we know it was born.[7] Modern cutaneous cryosurgery was further pioneered by Douglas Torre and Setrag Zacarian, by working with engineers to develop more effective and efficient cryogen delivery devices. These advances enabled cryosurgery to become widely used, and recognized as an effective and inexpensive surgical modality. For a more detailed history of cryosurgery, the reader is directed to an excellent recent review.[8]

BIOLOGY OF CRYOSURGERY

BOX 43-3 Summary

- Tissue injury is a function of the absolute temperature achieved and the duration of exposure.
- Tissue cryoablation is caused by at least three distinct processes: extracellular and intracellular ice crystallization, intracellular dehydration, and arterial insufficiency with intermittent spasm.
- Microcirculatory failure occurs in the thawing period.
- Rapid cooling rate enhances formation of intracellular ice crystals. Slower thaw times form damaging solute gradients and cause tumor killing by oxidative stress.
- Tumor cure rates are predictably better with a target temperature of −50°C.

Cryosurgery is described to patients as "localized frostbite." As seen in frostbite, subsequent tissue injury is a function of the absolute temperature achieved and the duration of exposure. This section offers an overview of basic cryobiology as it applies to cryosurgery. For additional details, the reader is directed to an expert review of the molecular basis of cryosurgery by Baust and Gage.[9]

Heat moves from warm to cold objects. A cold element is considered a "heat sink," drawing warmth from target tissue. As tissue is frozen, further thermal conduction is facilitated by formation of an ice-ball. Thermal gradients develop within the ice-ball, enhancing tissue freezing. Tissue cryoablation is caused by at least three distinct processes: extracellular and intracellular ice crystallization, intracellular dehydration, and arterial insufficiency with intermittent spasm.[10] First, ice crystals form in the extracellular matrix. Intracellular water shifts to the relatively dehydrated extracellular matrix, increasing intracellular osmolarity, which promotes intracellular ice crystal formation. Intracellular ice crystals are particularly destructive, as they can shear cellular membranes. Loss of blood flow due to vascular stasis adds to tissue destruction. Microcirculatory failure occurs in the thawing period. Loss of oxygen and nutrients ensures cell death. Cycles of freezing and thawing release prostaglandin F2 and thromboxane A2, promoting further vasoconstriction, platelet aggregation, and thrombosis.

More recently, the role of apoptosis in cryosurgery has become better understood. Apoptosis is programmed cell death, recognized by nonrandom DNA cleavage, caspase activation, and membrane blebbing. Caspases are cysteine proteases that are essential in apoptosis, amplifying programmed cell death via cascade reactions. Apoptotic cells are most prominent in the peripheral zone, where the cold injury is not great enough to rapidly ablate the tissue. These changes may be elicited by modest temperatures, such as −6 to −36°C.[11]

Destructive effects are determined by the rate of temperature fall, the rate of rewarming, solute concentration, the duration of freeze, and the coldest temperature reached in the target tissue. The cooling rate should be rapid, enhancing formation of intracellular ice crystals. Frozen tissue should thaw slowly, forming damaging solute gradients within the tissue. Slower thaw times augment tumor killing by high solute concentrations, prolonged oxidative stress, and recrystallization. Effective tumoricidal dosing requires achieving a lethal temperature throughout the lesion. Temperatures should reach −40 to −50°C to kill malignant tumors. Between −20 and −30°C, cancer cells are not reliably destroyed.[9] In the 1960s and 1970s, most tumors were treated with a target of −25 to −35°C, until research elucidated that not all target tissue was destroyed at these higher temperatures.

Experimental simulations of heat transfer are very arduous, due to the complexity of biological models. Treatment of visceral malignancies has propagated further research. Intrinsic physical properties (i.e., specific heat, density), biologic parameters (i.e., perfusion, metabolic activity, core temperature), geometric parameters, and parameters of the cryogen present major challenges in predicting cryokinetics. Bioheat transfer may be estimated by mathematical models that allow estimations of each area of uncertainty, as proposed by Rabin.[12]

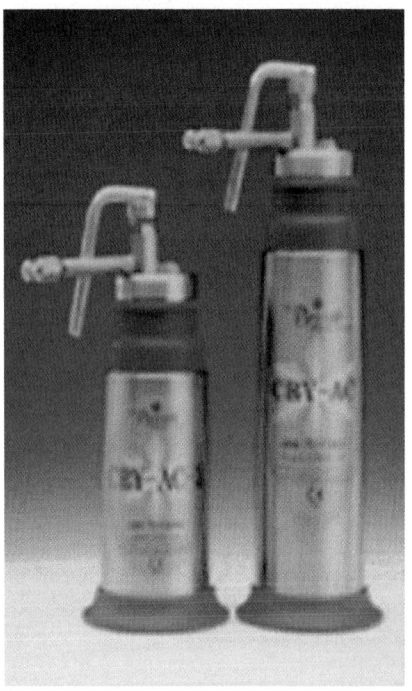

▲ **FIGURE 43-1** Two cryosurgical units. The static holding time is 24 hours. (Photograph courtesy of Brymill Cryogenic Systems, Ellington, CT).

APPLICATIONS AND CONSIDERATIONS

BOX 43-4 Summary

- The delivery device application tip should be tailored to the lesion size.
- Intermittent spray is often more useful than continuous application, to avoid excessive lateral spread of freeze.
- Contraindications to cryosurgery include previous adverse reaction, cold anaphylaxis, or severe cold urticaria.
- Freezing time, extent of halo formation, halo thaw time, and lesional thaw time are clinical parameters in cryosurgery.
- Multiple freeze–thaw cycles increase efficacy when treating malignancies.

Equipment

In simplest terms, all you need to perform cryosurgery is something that is cold, a delivery device for the cold substance, and a patient.

CRYOGEN The coldest and most efficient medical cryogen is liquid nitrogen, with a boiling point of −195.8°C. Liquid nitrogen cannot be used in probes less than 3 mm, a practical limitation when treating prostate and kidney cancers, but not significant in cutaneous cryosurgery where smaller tips may be useful. Liquid nitrogen storage dewars are made from high-strength aluminum, with significant insulation. It is critical that any liquid nitrogen reservoir should be vented to prevent excess pressure accumulation.

Although not widely used by dermatologists today, nitrous oxide and nonflammable liquefied gases (i.e., tetrafluoroethane, pentafluoroethane, and trifluoroethane) should be included in this discussion for completeness. Verruca-Freeze (Cryosurgery, Inc., Nashville, TN) is a chemical refrigerant, available in small spray canisters. This product contains the latter three gases listed earlier. This treatment is approved for benign, but not malignant, lesions. These liquefied gases do not routinely achieve temperatures effective to treat malignancies, with nitrous oxide at −90°C, and Verruca-Freeze at −70°C. The delivery devices used for liquid nitrogen are not compatible for nitrous oxide delivery (Fig. 43-1). Nitrous oxide requires a pressurized closed system with pressure gauge and regulator. Verruca-Freeze is an inexpensive cryosurgical modality that may be effective for warts, seborrheic keratoses, and actinic keratoses, but is not indicated for malignancies.

DELIVERY DEVICE Swabs, sprays, and cryoprobes (Fig. 43-2) are the preferred cryogen modalities in use today. Deeper freezes are achieved with sprays and probes, but larger swabs, with extra cotton as a reservoir, may approach the potential depth of these modalities. However, swabs are impractical for use with deeper malignancies. With any delivery device, the treatment tip should be tailored to the lesion. If pinpoint accuracy is desired, use either a point–point cotton swab, a small aperture spray, or a small probe tip.

If a swab technique is used, portable insulated hot–cold containers are extremely useful. Liquid nitrogen is not sterile,[13] so single-use foam cups should be used with swab application. Burke et al. showed that herpes simplex virus may survive on a swab 12 hours in liquid nitrogen, confirmed by culture growth.[14] It is recommended that cryogen should be dispensed individually, and discarded after each patient.

All tumors may be treated with spray application of cryogen, including malignancies. Depth of penetration depends on spray velocity and duration of application. Cryogen is propelled from a reservoir, through an aperture selected for the target tissue. Possible spray patterns include central direct spray for tumors less than 6 mm, spiral pattern for 5 to 10 mm, and a side-to-side "paint-brush" pattern for larger or irregularly shaped lesions (Fig. 43-3). Intermittent spray is more often used than continuous application to avoid excessive lateral spread of freeze. When treating malignancies, an insulating cone may focus the cryogen, resulting in deeper freezing (Fig. 43-4). Neoprene or plastic cones are useful, but metal cones should be avoided.

Cryoprobes operate as a heat sink, with circulating liquid nitrogen through the tip. Use of cryoprobes requires more time than sprays, but probes may achieve a deeper depth-of-freeze to lateral spread ratio.[15] Probes are cooled by circulating liquid nitrogen through the hollow center, indirectly exposing the target tissue to cryogen. The tumor dictates the probe size and shape to be used.

Protective shields should be utilized when treating near sensitive areas on the face, such as periocular lesions. The current trend in cryosurgery is use of sprays, rather than swabs, in both dermatology and primary care clinics. Very few studies have evaluated efficacy of spray versus swabs. Ahmed et al. treated palmar and plantar warts biweekly with cryospray or cotton wool bud, with clinical measure of 2-mm frozen margin, and evaluated cure rate after 3 months. Cure rates were 47% in the cotton swab group and 44% in the cryospray group ($P = 0.8$, not significant).[16]

METHODS

Considerations Before Treatment

All patients should be warned of discomfort, both during treatment and up to an hour posttreatment. Due to longer freezing times, local anesthesia may be used if malignancies are to be treated, but anesthesia usually is not needed for benign or precancerous lesions. Vasovagal reactions are possible, so position the patient accordingly. Resultant bullae may be painful due to distension or

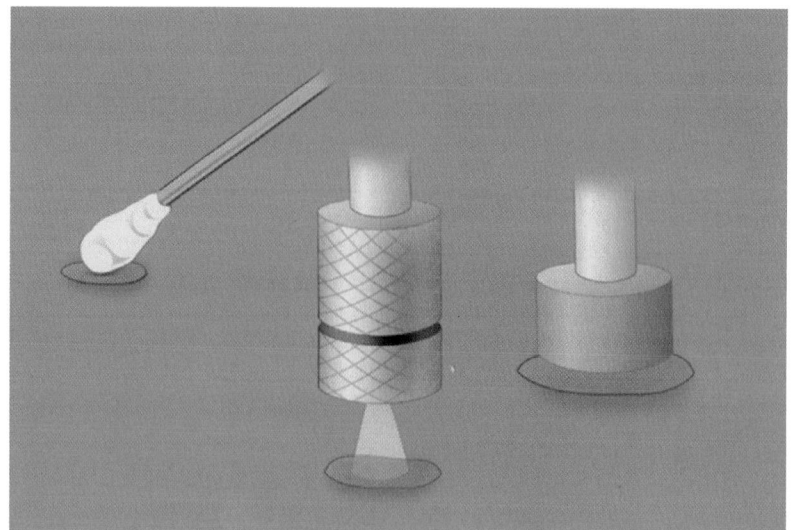

▲ **FIGURE 43-2** Cotton swab, spray nozzle, and probe tip are all commonly used techniques in cryosurgery. (Permission requested from Elsevier Saunders. *Current Problems In Dermatology.* Vol 15. 2003:223–250).

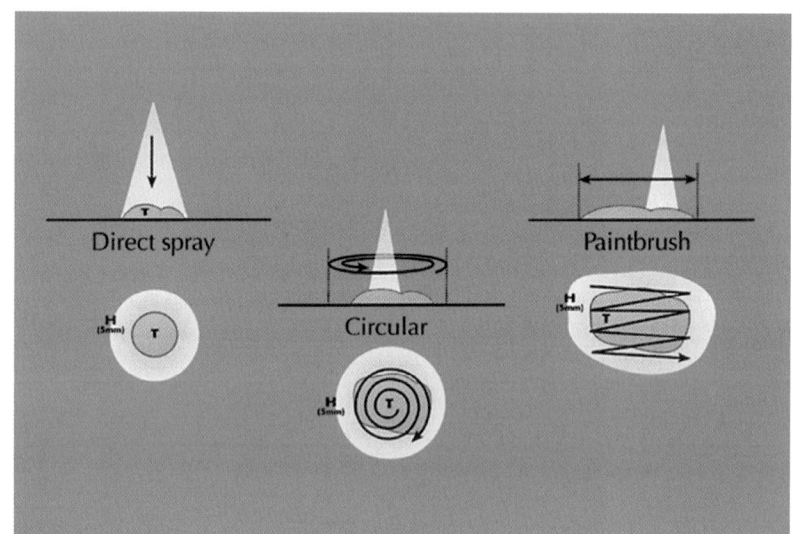

▲ **FIGURE 43-3** Central direct, spiral, and paintbrush techniques are all commonly used with spraying of cryogen. T = target; H = halo. (Permission requested from Elsevier Saunders. *Current Problems In Dermatology.* Vol 15. 2003:223–250).

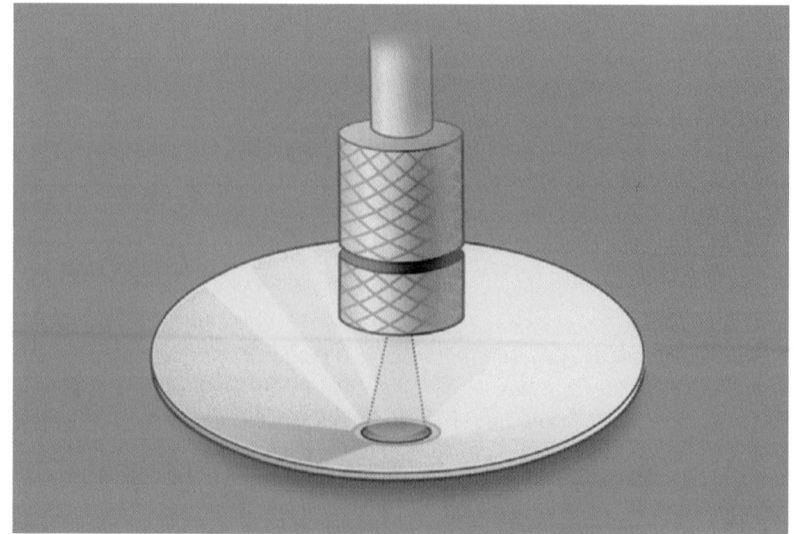

▲ **FIGURE 43-4** Plastic cone may be used with spraying of cryogen on the lesion. (Permission requested from Elsevier Saunders. *Current Problems In Dermatology.* Vol 15. 2003:223–250).

external pressure, and may require mild analgesics.

Patient selection is important and appropriate education desirable. Patients should also be aware of potential hypopigmentation, uncommon numbness that is usually transient, and increased risk of sunburn in the treated area. If treating darkly pigmented areas, hypopigmentation is a greater risk. Scarring is more likely when treating malignancies, especially hypertrophic or atrophic scars. While written consent forms are not usually required, adequate informed consent is essential.

A contraindication to cryosurgery includes treatment of any neoplasm of undetermined malignant potential. If any undiagnosed lesion is suspicious for malignancy, it is often preferable to obtain tissue for diagnosis prior to treatment. While benign melanocytic nevi have been effectively treated with cryosurgery, the primary histopathology is lost with cryosurgery. A clear understanding of the need for follow-up must be stressed. Another contraindication to cryosurgery is previous adverse reaction, such as cold anaphylaxis or severe cold urticaria. Special care is advised when treating patients with cold urticaria, especially cryosurgery on a large tumor on the head or neck. Small lesions have been treated without problems in patients with cold urticaria. If potential scar contracture may lead to severe sequelae, such as larger periorbital or perioral tumors, consideration should be given to other techniques. There are numerous reports of very satisfactory results in treating such tumors (personal reports from Turjansky, Pasquali, and others).

Many recurrent basal cell carcinomas and sclerosing basal cell carcinomas are best treated by Mohs surgery, but have been treated quite successfully by cryosurgery where Mohs is not available or when patient comorbidities prohibit other large procedures. Breitbart[17] has studied cryosurgery of melanoma, and freezing can be effective for satellites, recurrent tumors, and lentigo maligna. However, cryosurgery is not the first-line treatment modality for melanoma in general.

Relative contraindications include cryoglobulinemia, cryofibrinogenemia, and pyoderma gangrenosum, Patients with myleoma, lymphoma, autoimmune disorders such as Raynaud disease, concurrent treatment with immunosuppressive drugs, and areas of vascular compromise should be given special consideration. Hemorrhagic bullae were a complication after minimal cryosurgery

for verruca vulgaris in a patient with hemophilia A.[18] Also, special care must be taken when treating eyelids or areas with more superficial cutaneous nerves, such as the elbow or fingers. Treating glabrous hair-bearing areas, such as eyebrow or scalp, may result in hair loss if freeze time is over 20 to 30 s.

Clinical Techniques

Accurate assessment of freeze depth is critical in cryosurgery. An experienced clinician relies on freezing time, extent of halo formation, halo thaw time, and lesional thaw time to determine success. When treating a lesion centrally, the freezing will spread peripherally. An ice halo may be observed around the frozen tumor (Fig. 43-5). Larger halos are the clinical result of colder tumor temperatures and deeper freezing. The lateral progression of the halo correlates to the freezing depth. A 6-mm diameter spread on the surface approximates a freezing depth of 6 mm (Fig. 43-5). When freezing a nodular tumor, cryogen is delivered to a central point, reducing risk of false halo effect. Malignancies require a 5-mm freeze halo, while actinic keratoses and verrucae only require a 1 or 2-mm halo of frozen normal skin for destruction. Large, superficial basal cell carcinomas may require treatment in sections over several applications.

Halo thaw time is the period required to thaw the region extending from the outer halo edge in to the tumor. Malignancies should achieve a halo thaw time

between 60 and 90 s. If repeated freeze–thaw cycles are used, it is best if the halo and the tumor thaw completely before subsequent freezes. As stated earlier, a slower thaw time is more tumorcidal than fast thaw time, so do not hasten thaw times with exogenous heat sources. One to 2 minutes of halo thaw times and 3 to 5 minutes of complete thaw times are the rule.

Another method to monitor freezing depth is thermocoupling, where the temperature at a given depth is quantified. Treatment of many lesions may be monitored clinically. However, deeper lesions may benefit from more accurate assessment of depth and quality of freeze, as measured by thermocouple needles. The standard instrument-aided assessment involves one or more thermocouples attached to a pyrometer. Thermocouple needles may be inserted at the borders or underneath the tumor. This technique may assist the novice cryosurgeon in terms of tumor treatment, but experience is required to place the thermocouple needle accurately.

Lesions in very sensitive areas may be accurately targeted by grasping small exophytic lesions with forceps, followed by swab or spray application of cryogen.[19] The depth of freeze will be limited, precluding use of this technique in treating malignancies.

Multiple freeze–thaw cycles increase efficacy when treating malignancies, especially if preceded by curettage or deep shave excision. One freeze may adequately treat actinic keratoses and superfi-

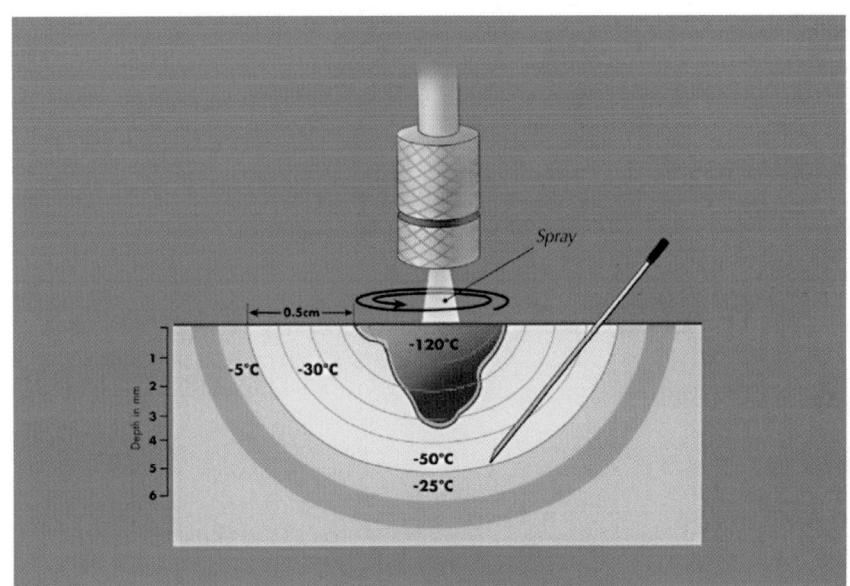

▲ **FIGURE 43-5** Use of thermocouple needle allows clinician to monitor the area and degree of freeze around the lesion. (Permission requested from Elsevier Saunders. *Current Problems In Dermatology* Vol 15. 2003:223–250).

cial basal cell carcinomas, but many tumors greater that 2 to 3-mm deep benefit from two cycles of freezing. The double-freeze, or freeze–thaw–freeze, cryosurgical technique facilitates tumor destruction by direct freezing, and by reperfusion injury via inflammatory cytokines.[9] Preliminary debulking of the tumor effectively reduces tumor depth, and curettage may better demonstrate the lateral extent of the tumor. Freezing may immediately follow debulking. Tumor debulking may incorporate other modalities. Goncalves described debulking of skin tumors with radiosurgery,[20] as well as using "fractional cryosurgery" to progressively treat skin cancers.[21] Fractional cryosurgery may effectively debulk large tumors by freezing, followed by staged cryosurgery with possible improved cosmesis, compared to single-stage cryosurgery. There are no studies that prospectively evaluate effects of curettage on cryosurgical cure rates, but it is the experience of numerous cryosurgeons that debulking leads to a higher cure rate.[22]

The "cryoblast" technique has been suggested for treating thicker actinic keratoses, verrucae, and possibly small squamous cell carcinomas. Cryoblasting removes the standard spray tip from the handheld cryosurgery canister, allowing full flow of liquid nitrogen from device to target. Authors reported reduced patient discomfort and equivalent scarring and hypopigmentation to traditional cryosurgery.[23] Cryoblasting does not match the lesion to the cryogen delivery, so patient selection is extremely important.

Local anesthesia may aid treatment of malignancies, allowing longer treatment and prolonging thaw times. Epinephrine in injected anesthetics will cause vasoconstriction, decreasing warming effect from perfusion. Cryosurgery may immediately follow debulking or biopsy. Treating at the time of the debulking or biopsy may be more effective, since there is no scar formation at the bed of the tumor. However, as previously discussed, cryosurgery is best performed when the diagnosis is certain.

POSTOPERATIVE CARE

BOX 43-5 Summary

- Patients may gently cleanse the surgical site with soap and water, and resume activities as tolerated.
- Oral vitamins, topical vitamins, and topical steroid treatments have *not* been proven to be beneficial postsurgically.

Patients should gently cleanse the cryosurgical site daily with soap and water. The patient may resume all normal activities, including bathing and swimming. After the initial bulla resolves, a natural biologic dressing will remain in the form of an eschar, minimizing risk of infection. The dry covering will separate naturally within 3 to 6 weeks, except on the back and lower legs where final separation of the eschar may take up to 3 months. Should trauma precipitate earlier to removal of the eschar, topical antibiotics may be applied. Lesions treated on the back or lower leg may take up to 3 months to heal completely.

Other adjunctive measures have been assessed, but none have added therapeutic benefit. Clobetasol propionate ointment was shown to reduce inflammation after cryosurgery in a double-blind, placebo-controlled trial.[24] However, postsurgical clobetasol is not broadly recommended by the authors due to the theoretical increased risk-of-infection susceptibility. In another prospective, randomized, double-blind, placebo-controlled study design, Gach et al. examined the effects of orally administered free radical scavengers, vitamin C (ascorbic acid) and vitamin E (D-alpha-tocopherol), starting 7 days prior to cryosurgery. There were no differences in presence or absence of blistering, edema volume, erythema level, or pain intensity.[25]

RESULTS

BOX 43-6 Summary

- Cure rates for actinic keratoses are as high as 98.8%.
- Large clinical trials have demonstrated basal cell carcinoma cure rates as high as 98.4%, but usually between 95 to 97% in retrospective series.
- Nodular basal cell carcinomas on the face require two freeze–thaw cycles of open-spray cryosurgery.
- Superficial basal cell carcinomas on the trunk may be adequately treated with one 30-s freeze–thaw cycle of open-spray cryosurgery.
- Much fewer data exist for treatment of other cutaneous carcinomas.
- Patients treated with cryosurgery should be followed carefully for 2 years postoperatively.

Actinic keratoses are the most common premalignant lesions treated cryosurgically, but there is a paucity of trials that

evaluate efficacy. Historically reported cure rates are as high as 98.8%.[26] Feldman et al. reviewed 540,000 new patient visits for actinic keratoses, finding that destructive procedures were performed during 80.9% of visits.[27] A prospective, multicenter trial evaluated untreated 421 actinic keratoses treated with a single-spray liquid nitrogen freeze–thaw cycle. Lesions were greater than 5 mm in diameter, located on the face and scalp. No freeze time was specified in the study protocol, but 1-mm treatment rim was required. At 3 months posttreatment, the overall individual complete response rate was only 67.2%. Complete response varied with freeze time, from 39% for less than 5 s, to 69% greater than 5 s, and 83% for freeze times greater than 20 s. Among complete responders, cosmesis was good to excellent in 94%.[28]

One nonrandomized study compared curettage and electrocautery versus two freeze–thaw cycles with liquid nitrogen for 80 cases of Bowen disease.[29] However, only 5 to 10-s freezes were applied to the lesions. As expected, curettage and electrocautery demonstrated better efficacy versus the attenuated cryosurgery. Bowen disease frequently involves adnexal structures, requiring more substantial freezing.

Most large cryosurgery treatment series are retrospective, reporting basal cell carcinoma cure rates between 95 and 97%, as determined by the presence or absence of recurrence.[30] Two freeze–thaw cycles, applied to 225 basal cell carcinomas, demonstrated 97.3% clearance in one series.[31] Kuflik and Gage reported a cure rate of 98.4% in a series of 3540 primary skin cancers, most of which were basal cell carcinomas, treated by open-spray technique with two freeze–thaw cycles.[32] Zacarian reported a basal cell carcinoma cure rate between 96 and 97%, retrospectively analyzing more than 4000 tumors.[33] Mallon and Dawber evaluated the efficacy of one versus two freeze–thaw cycles, with basal cell carcinomas on the face versus the trunk, in a prospective randomized posttreatment follow-up study.[34] Regarding nodular basal cell carcinomas on the face, two freeze–thaw cycles of open-spray cryosurgery were more effective than one cycle (95.3% vs. 79.4% cure) (Fig. 43-6). One 30-s freeze–thaw cycle was sufficient on the trunk (95.5% cure), where most lesions were superficial basal cell carcinomas. The benefit of one versus two freeze–thaw cycles appears to be important in treating malignancies, but

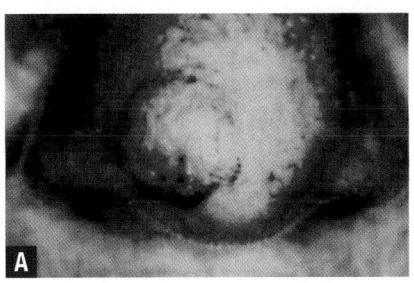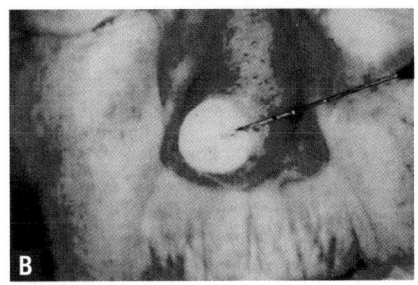
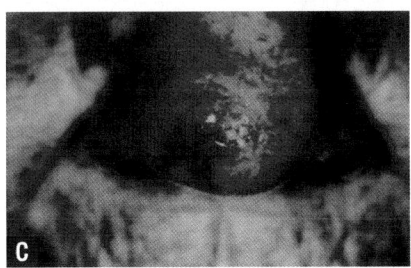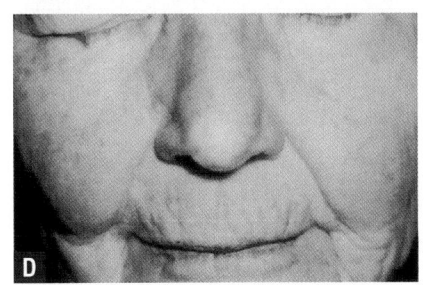

▲ **FIGURE 43-6** **A.** A recurrent basal cell carcinoma on the tip of the nose of a 73-year-old woman who has multiple health problems. Patient chose to have cryosurgery after careful consideration of her options. **B.** Thermocouple needle is implanted to the cartilage and double freeze-thaw cycles to −50°C. Freeze time was about 1 minute and halo thaw 1.5 minutes. **C.** Typical edema, erythema, and vesiculation are noted a few minutes after freezing. **D.** The site is well-healed 21 months after freezing. Hypopigmentation is observed. (Permission requested from Elsevier Saunders. *Cancer of the Skin* 2005:487–498).

not verrucae (Fig. 43-7). A randomized, parallel-group study evaluated the influence of a second freeze–thaw cycle on cure rate. At 3 months, hand and foot warts demonstrated a cure rate of 57% with a single freeze, versus 62% with two freeze–thaw cycles.[35]

Recently, Giuffrida et al. evaluated histologic cure for 12 noduloulcerative basal cell carcinomas, treated with a single freeze–thaw cryoprobe application of liquid nitrogen. A thermocouple needle was used to attempt freezing between −50 and −60°C. Lesions were located on the trunk and proximal upper extremities, and measured less than 1 cm. After 1 to 2 months, treatment sites were excised and horizontally sectioned throughout the entire block. There was no histologic evidence of tumor, but all patients demonstrated noticeable hypopigmentation.[36]

Much fewer data exist for squamous cell carcinomas and verrucous carcinomas. Graham and Clark reported a cure rate of 97.3% for 563 primary squamous cell carcinomas, with recurrences generally becoming evident within 2 years (Fig. 43-8).[37] Seventeen cases of oral verrucous hyperplasia and nine cases of oral verrucous carcinoma were treated by shave debulking and cryospray.[38] Three consecutive freeze–thaw cycles were used, where verrucous hyperplasia was treated for 25 to 30 s per cycle and 40 to 50 s for verrucous carcinoma. Twenty of 26 lesions responded well, with complete resolution reported for 11 lesions. Recurrence was reported in three cases, with mean follow-up of 2 years. It was unclear from the report whether verrucous hyperplasia or verrucous carcinoma was more likely to fail to resolve or recur.

Patients treated with cryosurgery should be followed carefully for 2 years postoperatively. Remote recurrences are rare, but have been reported.

■ **COMPLICATIONS**

BOX 43-7   Summary

- Pain, blistering, and edema should be expected in the acute period.
- Immediate reactions also include syncope, hemorrhage, headache, and nitrogen gas insufflation.
- Short-term reactions (days to weeks) include bullae, infection, delayed hemorrhage, pyogenic granuloma, and systemic febrile reaction.
- Delayed healing may be observed in lower extremity cryosurgery.
- Common long-term reactions (weeks to months) include pigmentary alterations and alopecia.
- Uncommon long-term reactions include nerve dysfunction, pseudoepitheliomatous hyperplasia, scarring, milia formation, and cartilage necrosis.

Cryosurgery is generally a safe, well-tolerated treatment with several well-defined effects and side effects. Most adverse effects are direct results of normal physiologic events. The surgeon must be able to delineate normal reactions to cutaneous freezing versus sequellae that require intervention.

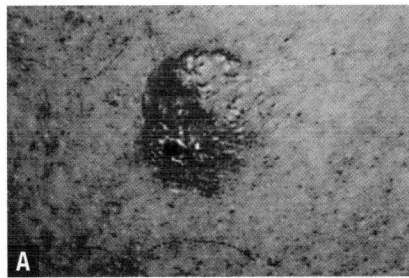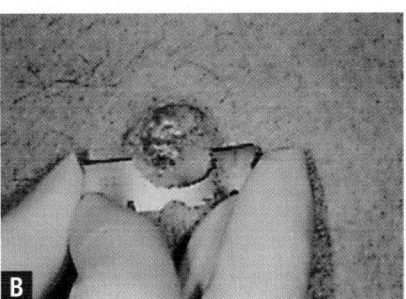
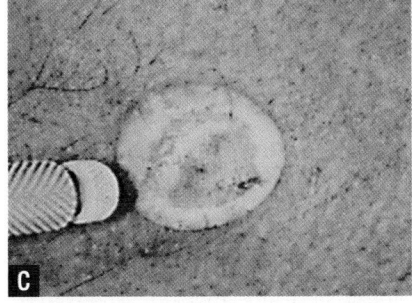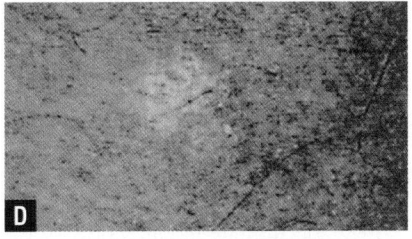

▲ **FIGURE 43-7** **A.** Basal cell carcinoma 1.5 cm on the back. **B.** Tangential shave excision of the exophytic portion of the tumor. **C.** Freeze until a 0.5-cm halo. **D.** Hypopigmentation is noted 1 month later. (Permission requested from Elsevier Saunders. *Cancer of the Skin* 2005:487–498).

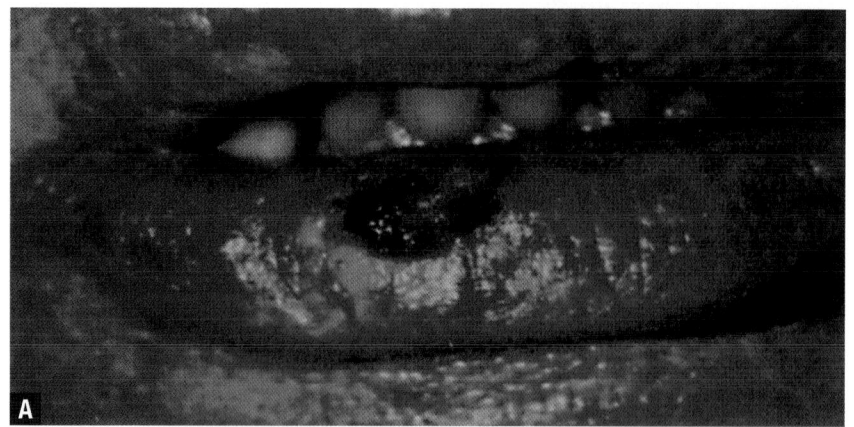

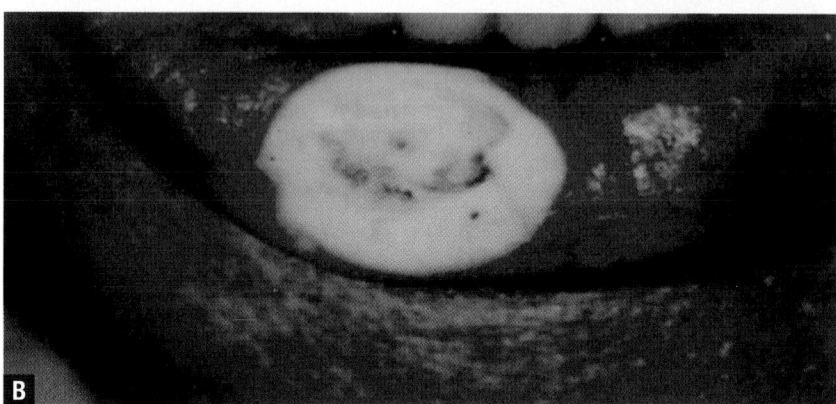

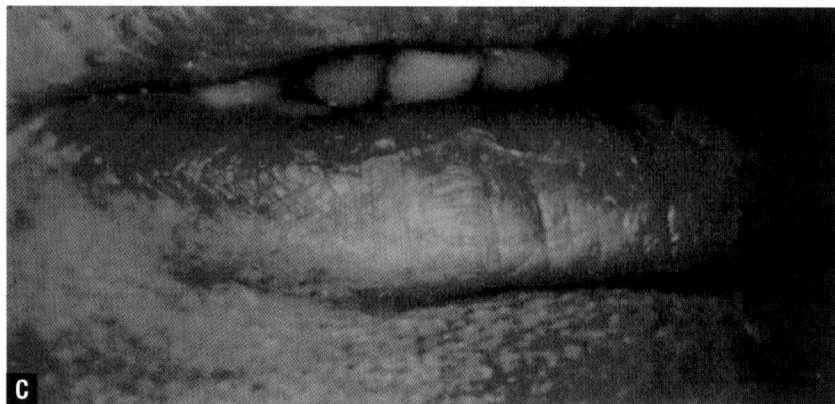

▲ **FIGURE 43-8** Squamous cell carcinoma (2.0 cm) on the patient's lip. **A.** Before cryosurgery and after biopsy. **B.** During cryosurgery. Note the size of the halo. **C.** Two months after cryosurgical treatment on the patient's lip. The site is well healed. (Permission requested from Elsevier Saunders. *Current Problems In Dermatology.* Vol 15. 2003:223–250).

Immediate Clinical Effects

Pain, blistering, and edema should be expected in the acute period (Fig. 43-6C). Immediate intense pain usually remits after 30 minutes. Edema is more pronounced after freezing loose skin, such as periorbital tumors, the forehead, the mandibular area, and around the ears. Periorbital edema may be prolonged, up to 5 days, but systemic steroids may suppress this edema. Deeper freezing, as required to treat malignancies, may cause hemorrhage, but may lack bulla formation. When treating the scalp or forehead, patients may experience headache symptoms. As discussed earlier, syncope is possible, so all patients should be treated at rest. Special consideration should be given to elderly patients or when freezing is especially uncomfortable.

As discussed earlier, treating skin cancers may benefit from debulking the tumor prior to cryosurgery (Fig. 43-7B). Hemorrhage may occur if debulking or biopsy occurs in conjunction with cryosurgery. Aluminum chloride, Monsel solution, or electrocautery should be sufficient to control bleeding. Local anes-

thetic and pretreatment with acetaminophen may assist deeper ablation. Nonsteroidal anti-inflammatory drugs may slightly increase the risk of hemorrhage. Analgesic may be continued up to 24 to 48 hours postoperatively. Nitrogen gas insufflation rarely occurs, but may be precipitated by antecedent biopsy or tumor debulking. Cryogen spray may enter an opening in the skin surface, especially in loose tissues, such as the periorbital area and the dorsal hand. Probe tips may freeze to treated skin. This side effect is diminished by coating the probe tip with lubricating jelly or by prechilling the probe.

Short-Term Reactions

The surgical site evolves in the days to weeks following cryosurgery. Bullae indicate successful treatment of superficial epidermal lesions, but may not be seen with deeper freezing. A bulla may be evacuated due to pain from large size or hemorrhage. Otherwise, bullae should not be disturbed, to serve as a sterile dressing. Topical antibiotics may be indicated after penetrating this barrier to prevent infection.

Venous stasis and diabetes mellitus may cause delayed wound healing, which promotes infection. Lower extremity cryosurgery should be cautiously approached in these patients. Immunocompromised and diabetic patients at high risk for infections may benefit from prophylactic systemic antibiotics. Blister fluid culture may help determine whether fluid accumulation is due to normal exudation or infection.

Delayed hemorrhage due to a persistent vascular supply may become evident after the eschar breaks away. Manual pressure to the surgical site is usually sufficient to achieve hemostasis. A pressure dressing or suture may be required in extreme cases.

Pyogenic granulomas have been described as a delayed side effect at cryosurgical sites. This tumor has been described after combined cryoablation and salicylic acid treatment of verruca vulgaris,[39] and with cryosurgery alone.[40] In addition, this uncommon complication was noted to appear after cryogen was applied to a venous lake.[41] Electrodesiccation and curettage or silver nitrate therapy should adequately treat this benign vascular tumor. If the diagnosis is in question, maintain a low threshold to biopsy, since amelanotic melanoma may mimic pyogenic granuloma.

A systemic, febrile reaction may occur if the patient receives widespread cryosurgery, whether to an especially large lesion or multiple treatments during one session. The patient may experience flu-like symptoms or a fever that usually resolves within 24 hours. Antipyrectics may be used for relief.

Long-Term Reactions

Pigmentation changes, both hypopigmentation (Fig. 43-9) and hyperpigmentation, are very common and should be considered a probability in all patients.

Pigment-producing cells do not survive below −4 to −7°C.[42] Better cosmetic results may be achieved with multiple brief freeze–thaw applications, but this regimen is not sufficient for cancer cryosurgery. Since treatment of malignant tumors demands freezing to −40 to −60°C, some degree of hypopigmentation is observed universally in these patients. Dark-skinned individuals and patients with freckles or telangiectasias within the cryosurgical site must be advised of cosmetics side effects.

Postinflammatory hyperpigmentation usually resolves over time, but may persist more than 12 months. Metal cones should not be used since they promote peripheral hyperpigmentation.

Any glabrous hair-bearing skin is susceptible to alopecia with deeper freezing. Fifteen to 20 s of treatment may lead to local permanent alopecia. Malignancies require greater than 30 s of freezing and the tumor may extend into the hair follicle. Therefore, local hair loss is expected after treating cutaneous malignancies.

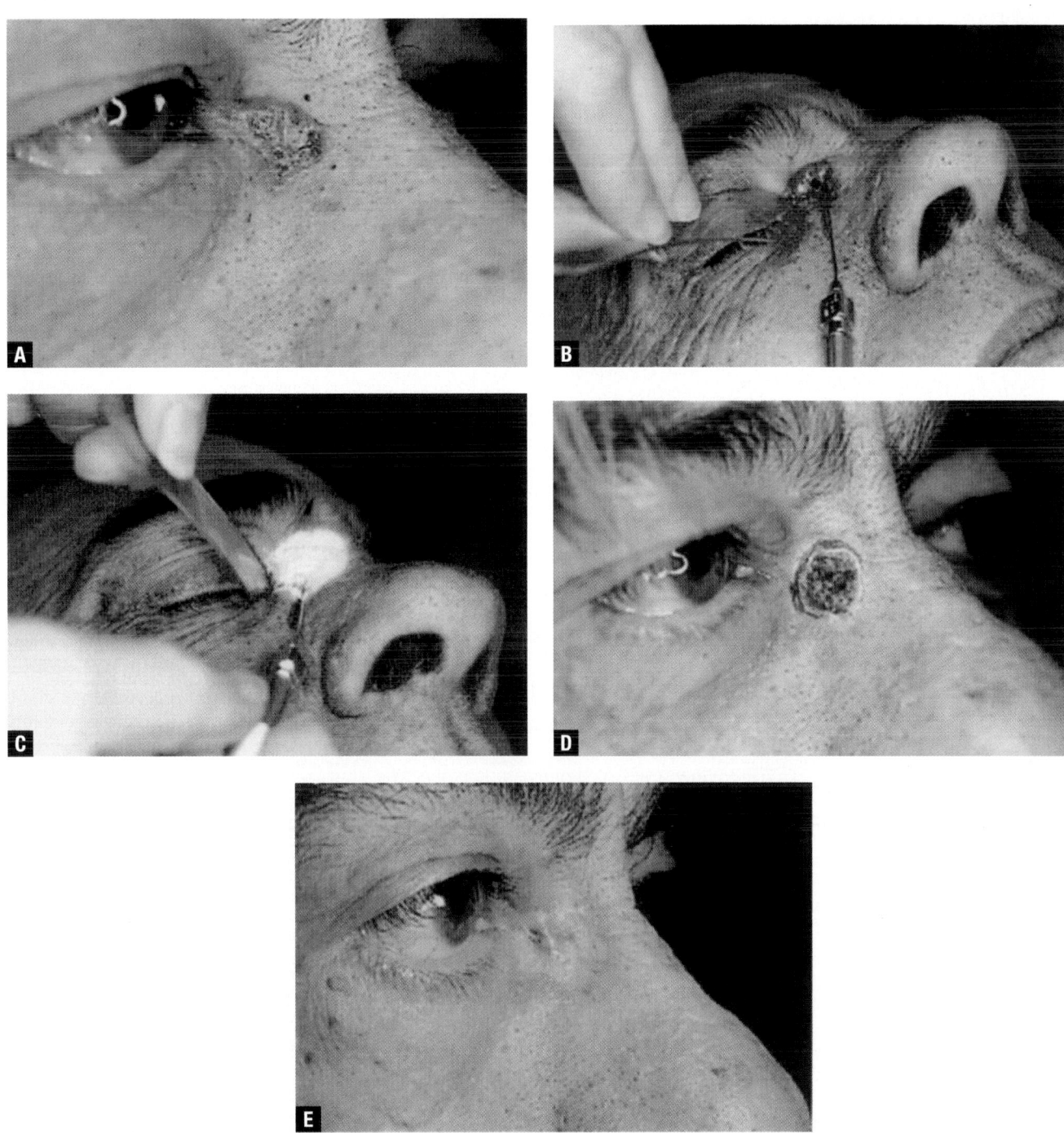

▲ **FIGURE 43-9** **A.** Pigmented basal cell carcinoma. **B.** Monitoring with thermocouple needle. **C.** During cryosurgery. **D.** 3 weeks postcryosurgery. **E.** 6 weeks postcryosurgery.

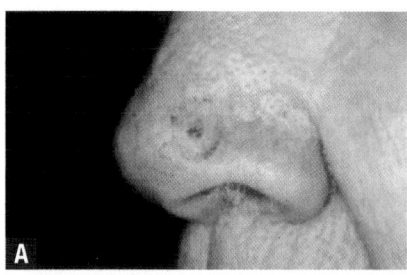
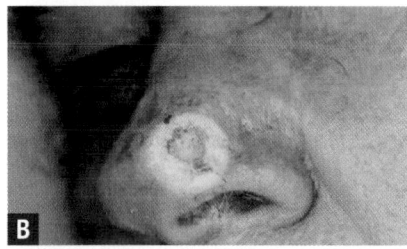
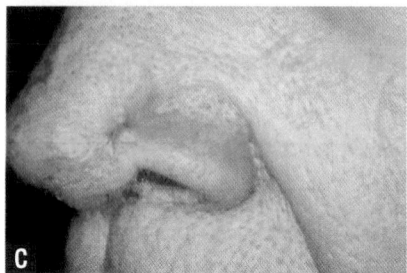

▲ **FIGURE 43-10** A. Basal cell carcinoma on the nose. **B.** Basal cell carcinoma during cryosurgery. (Note the size of the halo). **C.** 1-month postcryosurgery.

Pseudoepitheliomatous hyperplasia is an inflammatory reaction, which may be confused with persistent neoplasm. The hyperplasia may mimic tumor recurrence, but no treatment is required since improvement is usually noted within 3 months. If in doubt, a biopsy is prudent.

Superficial nerves, especially unmyelinated C-fibers, may be affected during cryosurgery. However, permanent nerve dysfunction is rare. Extra care should be taken when treating pre- and postauricular areas, fingers, lateral regions of the tongue, and the ulnar fossa, since nerves are more superficial in these locations. As long as the neural sheath is not damaged extensively, the neural function may be spared.

Other potential side effects include scarring and milia formation. The helix of the ear and the rim of the ala nasi are more sensitive to cryosurgery and demonstrate an increased tendency toward scar and atrophy. Hypertrophic scarring may develop 4 to 6 weeks postsurgery, more frequently on the back, chest, side of the nose (Fig. 43-10), and upper lip. Scarring may improve over the following 6 months. Deeper freezing may cause milia to develop, and may be seen more often with the cone spray technique. Cartilage necrosis, notching, and, in extremely rare cases, perforation may be caused by full-thickness freezing over nasal and otic cartilage.

FRONTIERS IN CRYOSURGERY

Future applications and adjuncts for cryosurgery are substantial and exciting. Optical coherence tomography, a light-based analog of ultrasound imaging, may be used to monitor depth of freeze in cutaneous cryosurgery.[43] Cryosurgery is gaining importance as a method of treating liver and prostate cancer.[44] Significant research efforts are exploring electrical impedance tomography as an inexpensive and noninvasive intraoperative assessment during cryosurgery.[45,46]

Thermal injury thresholds for various cell types and tissues, as well as improved understanding of cryobiology, may be elucidated by engineered tissue equivalents. By seeding and culturing target cells within a type-I collagen matrix, one group was able to simulate *in vivo* prostate cancer. The tissue equivalents produced kinetic data to evaluate thermal thresholds of cryoinjury for these cell types.[47] Future tissue equivalents may allow better understanding of cutaneous thermal thresholds, cell death mechanisms, and extracellular matrix structural damage in response to cold injury.

Adjunctive therapeutic agents may enhance tumoricidal effects of cryosurgery, introducing the field of cryochemotherapy. After 5-fluorouracil pretreatment, cultured prostate cells were rendered nonviable with mild temperatures.[48] Bleomycin demonstrates significant tumor cytotoxicity, but is limited by poor cell penetration. Mir and Rubinsky exposed melanoma cells to −20°C temperatures, in the presence of low levels of bleomycin. Exposed cells were killed at a significantly higher degree to a bleomycin concentration of 10 nM.[49] Tumoral cryosurgery with adjunctive intralesional or low-dose systemic chemotherapy may present many new cancer therapeutic options.

FINAL THOUGHTS

Overall, cryosurgery is a well-tolerated surgical modality with a proven track record. Common premalignant and malignant lesions are treated every day in dermatologists' offices across the globe. The science of cryobiology is ever expanding. Cryosurgery also provides good cosmesis, ease of administration, minimal cost, and good patient tolerance. This modality may be used in patients with multiple medical problems, of advanced age, and in geographically remote areas. With proper patient education, the versatility of cryosurgery is exceptionally useful in treatment of cutaneous malignancies.

REFERENCES

1. Clayton AS, Stasko T. Treatment of nonmelanoma skin cancer in organ transplant recipients: Review of responses to a survey. *J Am Acad Dermatol.* 2003;49:413–416.
2. Graham GF. Chair's summary: Cryosurgery. In: *Dermatology: Progress & Perspectives: Proceedings of the Eighteenth World Congress of Dermatology,* New York; June 12–18, 1992;1146–1148.
3. Schecter D, Sarot I. Historical accounts of injury due to cold. *Surgery.* 1968;63:527–535.
4. Arnott J. *On the Treatment of Cancers by Regulated Application of an Anaesthetic Temperature.* London: Churchill Livingstone; 1855.
5. White AC. Liquid air: Its application in medicine and surgery. *Med Rec.* 1899;56:109–112.
6. Whitehouse HH. Liquid air in dermatology: Its indications and limitations. *JAMA.* 1907;49:371–377.
7. Kuflik E. Cryosurgery for cutaneous malignancy: An update. *Dermatol Surg.* 1997;23:1081–1087.
8. Kuflik EG, Gage AA, Lubritz RR, et al. Millenium paper: History of dermatologic cryosurgery. *Dermatol Surg.* 2000;26:715–722.
9. Baust JG, Gage AA. The molecular basis of cryosurgery. *BJU Int.* 2005;95:1187–1191.
10. Hoffman NE, Bischof JC. The cryobiology of cryosurgical injury. *Urology.* 2002;60(suppl 2A):40–49.
11. Hanai A, Yang WL, Ravikumar TS, et al. Induction of apoptosis in human colon carcinoma cells HT29 by sublethal cryoinjury: Medication by cytochrome C release. *Int J Cancer.* 2001;93:26–33.
12. Rabin Y. A general model for the propagation of uncertainty in measurements into heat transfer simulations and its application to cryosurgery. *Cryobiology.* 2003;46:109–120.
13. Morris GJ. The origin, ultrastructure, and microbiology of the sediment accumulating in liquid nitrogen storage vessels. *Cryobiology.* 2005;50:231–238.
14. Burke WA, Baden TJ, Wheeler CE, et al. Survival of herpes simplex virus during cryosurgery with liquid nitrogen. *J Dermatol Surg Oncol.* 1986;12:1033–1035.
15. Torre D, Lubritz RR, Kuflik EG, eds. Cryobiology. In: *Practical Cutaneous Cryosurgery.* Norwalk, CT: Appleton and Lange; 1988:17.
16. Ahmed I, Agrawal S, Ilchyshyn A, et al. Liquid nitrogen cryotherapy of common warts: Cryo-spray vs.cotton wool bud. *Br J Dermatol.* 2001;144:1006–1009.
17. Breitbart EW. Cryosurgery in the treatment of cutaneous malignant melanoma. *Clin Dermatol.* 1990;8:96–100.
18. Hancox JG, Graham GF, Yosipovitch G, et al. Hemorrhagic bullae after cryo-

surgery in a patient with hemophilia A. *Dermatol Surg.* 2003;29:1084–1086.

19. Kuwahara RT, Craig SR, Amonette RA, et al. Forceps and cotton applicator method of freezing benign lesions. *Dermatol Surg.* 2001;27:183–184.

20. Goncalves JC, Martins C. Debulking of skin cancers with radio frequency before cryosurgery. *Dermatol Surg.* 1997;23:253–256.

21. Goncalves JC. Fractional cryosurgery. A new technique for basal cell carcinoma of the eyelids and periorbital area. *Dermatol Surg.* 1997;23:475–481.

22. Graham GF, Clark LC. Statistical analysis in cryosurgery of skin cancer. *Clin Dermatol.* 1990;8:101–107.

23. Callaway SR, Ratz JL. Surgical pearl: Cryoblast, a modified cryosurgical technique for thick lesions. *J Am Acad Dermatol.* 2004;51:458–459.

24. Hindson TC, Spiro J, Scott LV, et al. Clobetasol propionate ointment reduces inflammation after cryotherapy. *Br J Dermatol.* 1985;112:599–602.

25. Gach JE, Humphreys F, Berth-Jones J, et al. Randomized, double-blind, placebo-controlled pilot study to assess the value of free radical scavengers in reducing inflammation induced by cryotherapy. *Clin Exp Dermatol.* 2005;30:14–16.

26. Lubritz RR. Cryosurgery cure rate of actinic keratoses. *J Am Acad Dermatol.* 1982;7:631–632.

27. Feldman SR, Fleisher AB, Williford PM, et al. Destructive procedures are the standard of care for treatment of actinic keratosis. *J Am Acad Dermatol.* 1999;40:43–47.

28. Thai KE, Fergin P, Freeman M, et al. A prospective study of the use of cryosurgery for the treatment of actinic keratoses. *Int J Dermatol.* 2004;43:687–692.

29. Ahmed I, Berth-Jones J, Charles-Holmes S, et al. Comparison of cryotherapy with curettage in the treatment of Bowen's disease: A prospective study. *Br J Dermatol.* 2000;143:759–766.

30. Torre D. Cryosurgery of basal cell carcinoma. *J Am Acad Dermatol.* 1986;15:917–929.

31. Holt P. Cryotherapy for skin cancer: Results over a 5-year period using liquid nitrogen spray cryotherapy. *Br J Dermatol.* 1988;119:231–240.

32. Kuflik EG, Gage AA. The five-year cure rate achieved by cryosurgery for skin cancer. *J Am Acad Dermatol.* 1991;24:1002–1004.

33. Zacarian SA. Cryosurgery of cutaneous carcinomas: An 18-year study of 3022 patients with 4228 carcinomas. *J Am Acad Dermatol.* 1983;9:947–956.

34. Mallon E, Dawber R. Cryosurgery in the treatment of basal cell carcinoma. *Dermatol Surg.* 1996;22:854–858.

35. Berth-Jones J, Bourke J, Eglitis H, et al. Value of a second freeze–thaw cycle in cryotherapy of common warts. *Br J Dermatol.* 1994;131:883–886.

36. Giuffrida TJ, Jimenez G, Nouri K, et al. Histologic cure of basal cell carcinoma treated with cryosurgery. *J Am Acad Dermatol.* 2003;49:483–486.

37. Graham GF, Clark LC. Statistical analysis in cryosurgery of skin cancer. *Clin Dermatol.* 1990;8:101–107.

38. Yeh CJ. Treatment of verrucous hyperplasia and verrucous carcinoma by shave excision and simple cryosurgery. *Int J Oral Maxillofac Surg.* 2003;32:280–283.

39. Kolbusz RV, O'Donoghue MN. Pyogenic granuloma following treatment of verruca vulgaris with cryotherapy and Duoplant. *Cutis.* 1991;47(3):204.

40. Greer KE, Bishop GE. Pyogenic granuloma as a complication of cutaneous cryosurgery. *Arch Dermatol.* 1975;111:1536–1537.

41. Cecchi R, Giomi A. Pyogenic granuloma as a complication of cryosurgery for venous lake. *Br J Dermatol.* 1999;140:373–374.

42. Gage AA, Meenaghan MA, Natiella JR, et al. Sensitivity of pigmented mucosa and skin to freezing injury. *Cryobiology.* 1979;16:348–361.

43. Choi B, Milner TE, Kim J, et al. Use of optical coherence tomography to monitor biological tissue freezing during cryosurgery. *J Biomed Opt.* 2004;9:282–286.

44. Rubinsky B. Cryosurgery. In: Yarmush ML, ed. *Annual Review of Biomedical Engineering.* Vol 2. Palo Alto, CA: Annual Reviews; 2000:157–187.

45. Otten DM, Rubinsky B. Cryosurgical monitoring using bioimpedance measurements—a feasibility study for electrical impedance tomography. *IEEE Trans Biomed Eng.* 2000;47:1376–1381.

46. Hartov A, LePivert P, Soni N, et al. Using multiple-electrode impedance measurements to monitor cryosurgery. *Med Phys.* 2002;29:2806–2814.

47. Han B, Grassl ED, Barocas VH, et al. A cryoinjury model using engineered tissue equivalents for cryosurgical applications. *Ann Biomed Eng.* 2005;33:972–982.

48. Clarke DM, Baust JM, Van Buskirk RG, et al. Chemo-cryo combination therapy. An adjunctive model for the treatment of prostate cancer. *Cryobiology.* 2001;42:274–285.

49. Mir LM, Rubinsky B. Treatment of cancer with cryochemosurgery. *Br J Cancer.* 2002;86:1658–1660.

CHAPTER 44

Curettage and Electrodesiccation

Voraphol Vejjabhinanta, M.D.
Anita Singh, M.S.
Shalu S. Patel, B.S.
Keyvan Nouri, M.D.

BOX 44-1 Overview

- Curettage and electrodesiccation is most commonly used for benign or low-risk lesions, such as superficial and nodular basal cell carcinomas (BCC).
- Tumor cells have a very soft, fragile texture that can be easily distinguished from healthy, normal skin.
- Curettage and electrodesiccation is recommended for small, well-defined, primary BCCs, but not for morpheaform, infiltrative, and recurrent BCCs.
- Curettage and electrodesiccation is contraindicated for malignant melanoma.
- There are several steps that are essential before curettage and electrodesiccation can be performed.
- Curettage removes the bulk of the tumor. The two widely used methods for curettage are the pen technique and the potato peeler technique, both named for the way the curette is held and maneuvered.
- Electrodesiccation helps to destroy the tumor cells that cannot be reached by the curette, in addition to, helping with hemostasis and sealing the lymphatic vessels.
- Modifications to the standard treatment include: using curettage alone, electrosurgery followed by curettage, curettage followed by excision, curettage followed by cryosurgery, curettage followed by imiquimod, or curettage and electrodesiccation followed by imiquimod.
- Wound care after curettage and electrodesiccation is very simple, and the wound should heal within 2 to 6 weeks with minimal scarring.

INTRODUCTION

Curettage alone or in combination with electrosurgery (C & ED) is an effective technique widely used in the destruction of many benign and some malignant cutaneous lesions. This technique involves the use of a curette. The curette was first developed in the 1870s, but it was not until 1876 that Wigglesworth[1] reported that the curette had multiple uses for a variety of skin lesions. Electrodesiccation of skin lesions was first noted in 1911 by Clark[2], when he applied a high-voltage, low-current electrode to the skin and noticed drying of superficial tissue.

Curettage and electrodesiccation is most commonly used for low-risk lesions, such as superficial and nodular basal cell carcinomas (BCC).[3,4] Curettage takes advantage of the soft texture of these lesions. These tumors become fragile due to a variety of reasons that include: impaired adherence between the tumor cells themselves, impaired adherence between the tumor cells with the basement membrane, and finally a mucinous stromal change that occurs in the environment of the tumor.[3] Some other lesions that can be treated by curettage and electrodesiccation include: molluscum contagiosum, warts,[5] syringoma,[6] cherry angiomas,[7] extramammary Paget's disease,[8] actinic keratosis,[9] and keratoacanthomas.[10]

The soft, fragile texture of these lesions can easily be differentiated from the healthy fibrous tissue of normal skin, which feels tough and gritty. Therefore, curettage may be used for defining the clinical border of cutaneous tumors.[3,4] It has been used in conjunction with other surgical treatments, such as excision and cryosurgery, to aid in debulking tumors and defining the borders of the lesion. In addition, it is commonly used prior to electrodessication or electrocautery for superficial or deep lesions, respectively.[3]

Curettage and electrodesiccation is recommended for small, well-defined, primary BCCs.[3] However, the location of the lesion is also very important in determining whether or not to use C & ED. Low-risk sites include the neck, trunk, and the extremities. Moderate-risk sites include the scalp, forehead, pre- and postauricular, and malar areas. High-risk sites include the nose, nasolabial folds, eyelids and periorbital areas, lips, chin, and ears.[11] BCCs that are less than or equal to 2 cm in diameter and in low-risk areas have cure rates reportedly of more than 90%; however, larger tumors, that are not superficial or in high-risk sites, need to be treated by other means.[3,4,12–15] In addition, morpheaform, infiltrative, and recurrent BCCs are not recommended to be treated by C & ED. Morpheaform BCCs tend to recur because they may extend into the stroma, where they may not be reached.[16] Infiltrative BCCs should not be treated with C & ED because they may be highly aggressive and tend to recur.[17] Recurrent BCCs tend to recur because they may be aggressive or hidden in scar tissue from previous treatment.[16]

Curettage and electrodesiccation is contraindicated for malignant melanoma, as well as, lentigo maligna and lentigo maligna melanoma.[3,18] The reason for this involves the characteristic nature of dysplastic melanocytes to extend down hair follicles. These dysplastic melanocytes are also often found at the dermoepidermal junction, which may be very far away from the border of the primary lesion.[18,19]

MECHANISM OF ACTION

Curettage grossly removes the majority of the tumor, whereas electrosurgery is a method that tries to kill remaining superficial cells by burning them off. There are four modes of electrosurgery, these include: electrodesiccation, electrofulguration, electrocautery, and electrosection. The two that are discussed in this chapter are electrodesiccation and electrocautery. The mechanism of action of electrodesiccation is by directing a spark of electricity from the tip of an electrode to the diseased tissue, without any actual contact between the tip of the electrode and the tissue. It acts almost like lightning. Electrodesiccation is used primarily for superficial tissue destruction. Electrocautery works by conducting electricity from the tip of an electrode to the damaged tissue and then to another electrode. It has the same mechanism of action as an electrical shock. Electrocautery is used for deep lesions, which require more intense tissue damage.

Both curettage and electrosurgery cause skin damage and initiate the wound healing process (inflammation, proliferation, and maturation). It is believed that the wound healing phases can induce a patient's immune system to help eliminate any residual tumor cells. However, in two studies,[20,21] it was demonstrated that inflammatory and proliferative phases have no effect on clearing the tumor.

PREOPERATIVE CARE

BOX 44-2 Summary

- The following steps are essential before curettage and electrodesiccation can be performed:
  - A thorough history must be taken, including use of pacemakers, anticoagulants, immunosuppressive drugs, and drug allergies.
  - The procedure, possible outcomes, complications, and other treatment modalities must be explained to the patient.
  - Informed consent from the patient is required prior to initiating treatment.
  - The borders of the lesion, with the appropriate margins, must be drawn out and then confirmed with the patient that this is the correct lesion.
  - The area of the lesion needs to be cleaned with an antiseptic solution that is nonflammable.
  - Local anesthesia is given prior to the procedure.

First, it is essential to obtain a history, specifically concerning pacemakers, anticoagulants, immunosuppressive drugs, or any potential drug allergies (e.g., anesthetic drugs, antiseptics, topical antibiotics). Modern pacemakers are very resistant to electrical interference; therefore, simple electrosurgery, with short contact time, of small lesions on relatively healthy patients who have pacemakers poses negligible risks. However, both cardiac pacemakers and defibrillators can be affected by electrosurgery and this factor must be taken into account.[22]

After the history is obtained, the physician should explain the procedure, the risks and benefits, complications, and other modalities of the treatment to the patient. Once the patient fully understands the procedure, consent should be obtained. Before starting the procedure, the physician must draw out the borders of the lesion with the appropriate margins and confirm with the patient that this is the correct lesion. For nonmorpheaform BCCs with a diameter less than 2 cm, a minimum safety margin of 4 mm normal skin is necessary.

The procedure begins by carefully cleaning the area with an antiseptic solution that is nonflammable (i.e., Povidone-iodine), to avoid inadvertent fires when electrodesiccation is done (see Fig. 44-1). Local anesthesia, which is always used prior to the procedure, is 1% lidocaine with epinephrine injected with a 27- or 30-gauge needle (see Fig. 44-2).[4] When

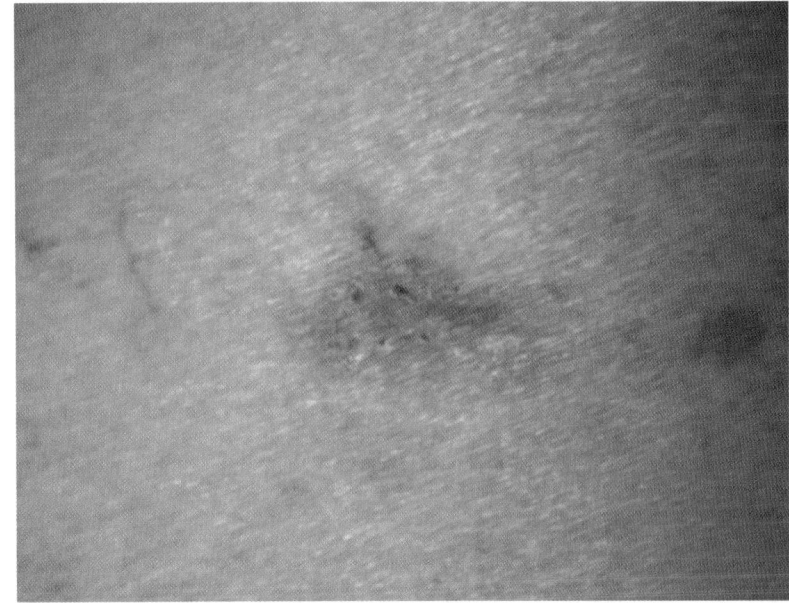

▲ **FIGURE 44-1** Superficial BCC before treatment.

directly injecting the lesion, care should be taken because this technique may transplant tumor into uninvolved skin.[3]

TECHNIQUES

Standard Treatment

BOX 44-3 Summary

- The curette removes the bulk of the lesion, while electrodesiccation removes residual cells at the base and rim of the lesion.
- The two widely used methods for curettage are the pen technique and the potato peeler technique, both named for the way the curette is held and maneuvered.

- Tumor cells have a very soft, fragile texture that can be easily distinguished from healthy, normal skin.
- There are several precautions that must be taken into account before electrodesiccation can begin.
- Electrodesiccation helps to destroy the tumor cells that cannot be reached by the curette, in addition to, helping with hemostasis and sealing the lymphatic vessels.
- Electrodesiccation should be done on the normal skin at least 2 mm around the rim of the initial lesion for small and benign lesions. Malignant tumors require a 4 to 6-mm margin.

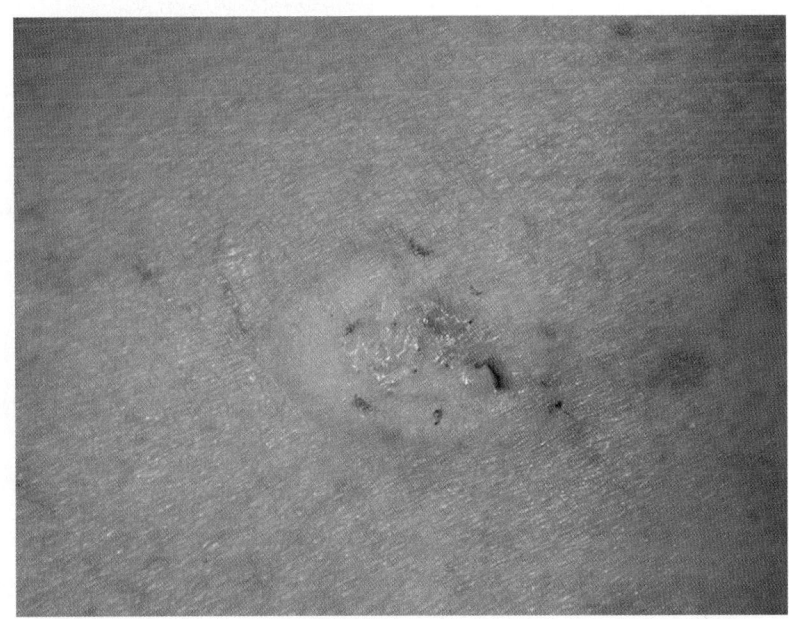

▲ **FIGURE 44-2** BCC lesion after anesthesia is applied.

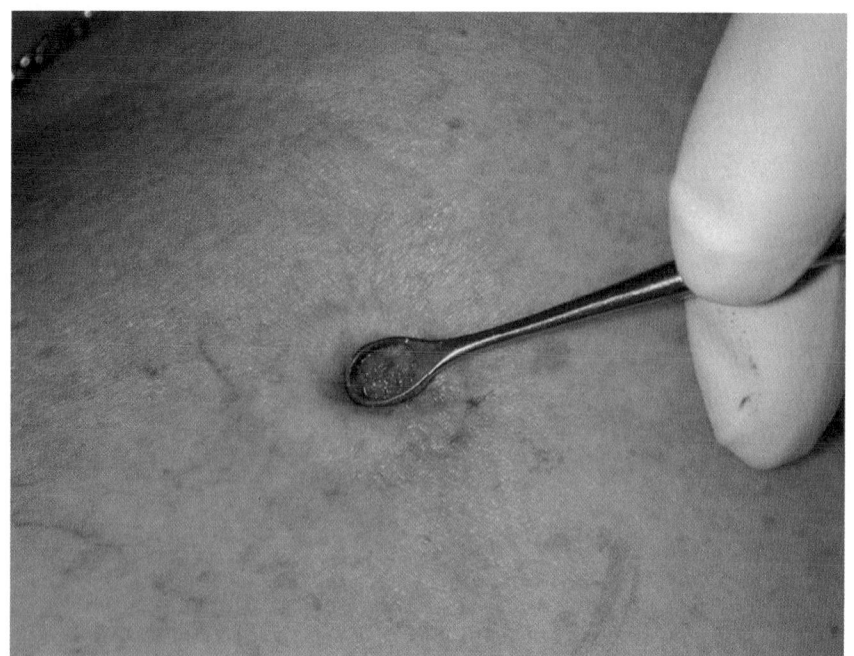

▲ **FIGURE 44-3** Curettage technique.

For curettage, the main instrument used is the curette. This is simply a handle similar to that of a scalpel with a looped edge instead of a blade. This loop, which has a sharp edge to cut the skin, can vary in size from 1 to 7 mm, though a 4-mm diameter is most often used. To remove the lesion, scooping motion is used with the loop at a downward angle (see Fig. 44-3). The lesion is curetted vigorously in four directions, 90° apart. After removal of the majority of the lesion, the base and margins can then be scraped. The area where the lesion ends and normal skin begins can be determined because tumor cells are usually softer than normal skin.[23]

The two widely used methods for curettage are the pen technique and the potato peeler technique, both named for the way the curette is held and maneuvered. In practice, the main difference between the two is that the pen technique is generally used for smaller tumors, while the potato peeler technique is better suited for larger tumors. The pen technique allows for fine, precise movements. The handle of the curette is held like a pen, between the thumb, index, and middle fingers.[3,24] The side of the hand holding the curette is rested on the skin for stability. The skin around the lesion is stretched and held taut by the other hand. With the curette at a 45° degree angle to the skin and at the farthest end of the lesion, several smooth, firm strokes are drawn through the tissue. This is repeated several times until the entire tumor is removed (see Fig. 44-3).[3,24]

The potato peeler technique, which is used more commonly for larger tumors, requires more strength. For this technique, the curette is held somewhat like a hairbrush. The curette is held in the interdigital fold of the index finger and the end of the curette is supported by the other bent fingers. The thumb, which does not hold the curette, is used to counter and stabilize the movement, as well as, hold the skin taut. The other hand is also used to hold the skin taut. Similar to the pen technique, the curette is positioned at the farthest end of the lesion and firm strokes are used.[3,24] The physician usually knows when the entire tumor is removed when

pinpoint bleeding is noted and a scratchy sound is heard. It should be noted that if the curette at any time penetrates into the subcutaneous fat, curettage should be stopped because the tumor has most likely spread deeply and the ability to distinguish between normal skin and tumor is lost.[3,24]

Before electrodesiccation can begin, several precautions must be taken. These include: the patient should be asked if he/she is wearing a pacemaker, the skin must not have any flammable substances on it, there is no flowing oxygen in the room of the procedure, and the skin should be elevated away from superficial nerves and tendons. In addition, if the electrodesiccation is being done in the perianal region, the anus should be protected with moist packing to prevent any ignition of methane.[16,24,25] After these precautions are taken into account, electrodesiccation can be applied to the base and rim of the area where the lesion was taken off (see Fig. 44-4). Electrodesiccation should be done on the normal skin at least 2 mm around the rim of the initial lesion.[3] When using electrodessication on small and benign lesions, a small spark (electrodessication mode, monoterminal, high voltage, low amperage) will suffice to destroy any remaining tumor cells. Malignant tumors require more intense tissue damage (electrocautery mode, biterminal, low voltage, high amperage), along with a 4 to 6-mm margin.[23] It is recommended that C & ED be repeated at least three times to ensure that all the tumor cells

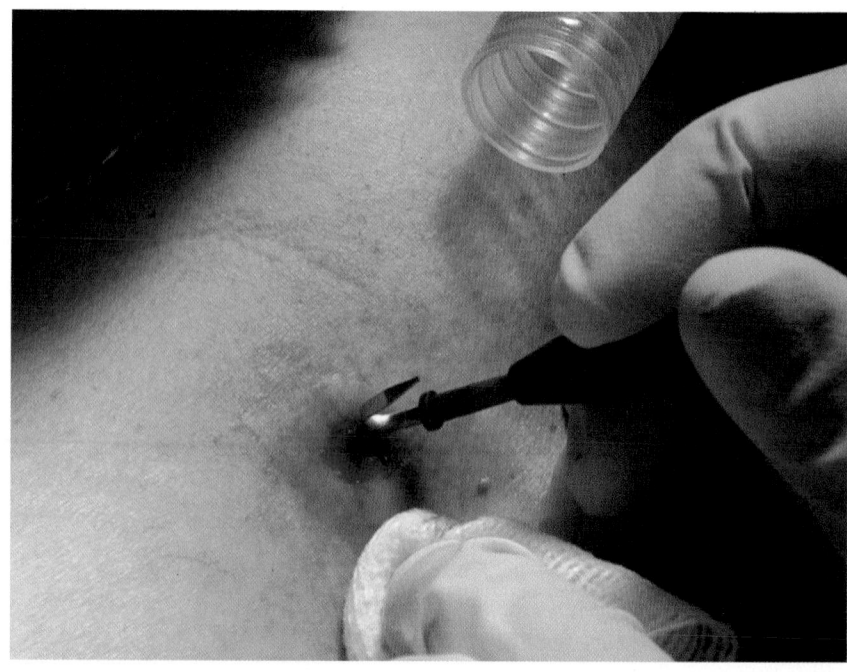

▲ **FIGURE 44-4** Electrodesiccation.

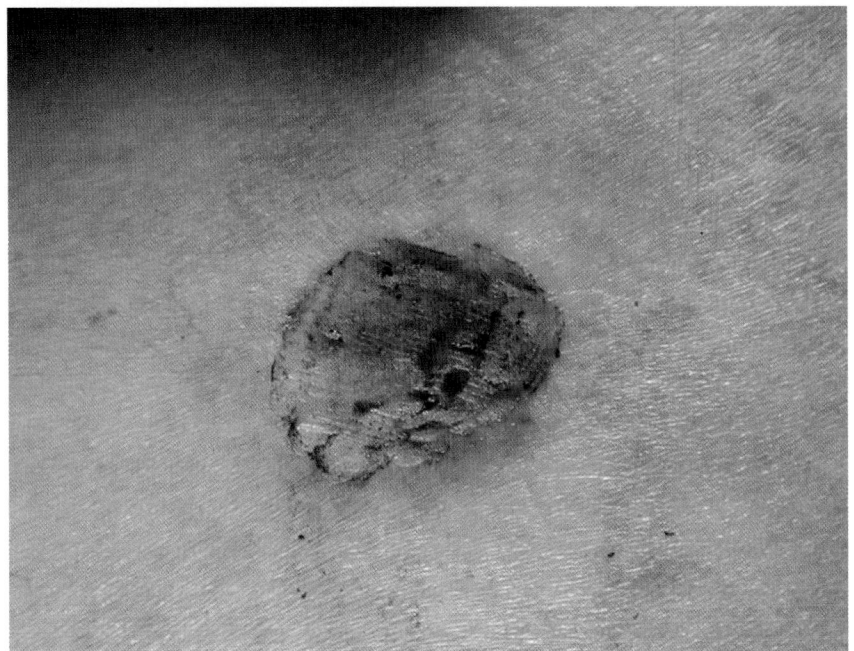

▲ **FIGURE 44-5** Lesion after 3 cycles of curettage and electrodesiccation.

are removed (see Fig. 44-5).[23] The purpose of electrodesiccation is multifactorial. It helps to destroy the tumor cells that cannot be reached by the curette, in addition to, helping with hemostasis and sealing the lymphatic vessels.[3] Hemostasis can be achieved by other means as well. Monsel's solution (ferric subsulfate), aluminum chloride, or simply pressure, can be used.

Modifications of Standard Treatment

BOX 44-4   Summary

- Modifications to the standard treatment include: using curettage alone, electrosurgery followed by curettage, curettage followed by excision, curettage followed by cryosurgery, curettage followed by imiquimod, or curettage and electrodesiccation followed by imiquimod.
- Curettage alone can be used to treat benign lesions and some basal cell carcinomas.
- Electrosurgery followed by curettage (D & C) has had excellent cure rates.
- Curettage followed by excision may be preferred for lesions in areas where the cosmetic outcome may be important.
- Curettage followed by cryosurgery has been proven effective in most non-melanoma skin cancer lesions.
- Curettage followed by imiquimod, as well as, curettage and electrodesiccation followed by imiquimod has had excellent cure rates and cosmetic outcomes.

There are several modifications of the standard treatment, described earlier, that have been proposed. These include using curettage alone, electrosurgery followed by curettage, curettage followed by excision, curettage followed by cryosurgery, curettage followed by imiquimod, or curettage and electrodesiccation followed by imiquimod.

Curettage without other treatment modalities has been used to treat benign lesions. Some studies have proposed the solitary use of curettage for the treatment of BCC, especially for small or superficial BCCs. The reason curettage alone is considered a better alternative is because electrodessication has been associated with causing postoperative hypopigmentation and hypertrophic scarring. In addition, it is contraindicated for patients with pacemakers and other devices. In a recent retrospective study, the 5-year cure rate of curettage alone was 96%, which is similar to that of curettage and electrodessication for nonaggressive BCCs, which was 95.3%.[26]

Other studies have reversed the standard order, suggesting that curettage should follow electrosurgery, the procedure is called (D & C). The theory behind this is that electrosurgery is considered the portion of the treatment responsible for destroying tumor cells. However, this may also lead to excess tissue destruction and inaccurate curettage because electrosurgery interferes with the curette's ability to differentiate normal skin from diseased skin. Nevertheless, two studies have shown that cure rates can be between 96.6 and 98% for BCCs treated with D & C.[27,28]

Excision may be an alternative to electrosurgery following curettage. This technique is preferred for lesions in areas where the cosmetic outcome may play a factor. As in the standard treatment, curettage is used to debulk the tumor. Surgical excision then allows for a controlled removal of the residual tumor. In a study done by Chiller et al.,[29] it was shown the curettage before excision actually decreases the frequency of positive margins in the management of BCC, and, in fact, reduced the surgical failure rates for BCC by 24%.

Similarly, cryosurgery may be an alternative follow-up to curettage, which again serves to debulk the tumor and allow the cryosurgery to have its full effect. Cryosurgery ensures residual tumor eradication. This technique has been proven effective in most non-melanoma skin cancer lesions, such as BCC, SCC, keratoacanthomas, and Bowen disease.[3] One study actually reported cure rates up to 98% for BCCs less than 2 cm in diameter using this technique.[30]

Curettage alone followed by imiquimod (5% cream), as well as, C & ED followed by imiquimod (5% cream) have recently been reported. Curettage was again used to debulk the lesions, while imiquimod was used to destroy any residual cells. The study that examined the efficacy of curettage alone followed by imiquimod found that imiquimod was effective in the treatment of primary nodular BCCs, especially if they were located on the trunk and the extremities.[31] They reported that at 3 months after treatment, 94% of the patients that used this technique did not have a recurrence of BCC histologically, and the cosmetic outcome was excellent.[32] In another study, which examined the efficacy of imiquimod following C & ED, it was found that imiquimod used once daily for a month after C & ED reduced the frequency of residual tumor from 40 to 10% and the cosmetic outcome was again excellent.[32]

■ POSTOPERATIVE CARE

BOX 44-5   Summary

- Wound care after curettage and electrodesiccation is very simple.
- The wound should be cleaned daily and white petroleum jelly or topical antibiotic ointment should be applied twice a day under a bandage or gauze.

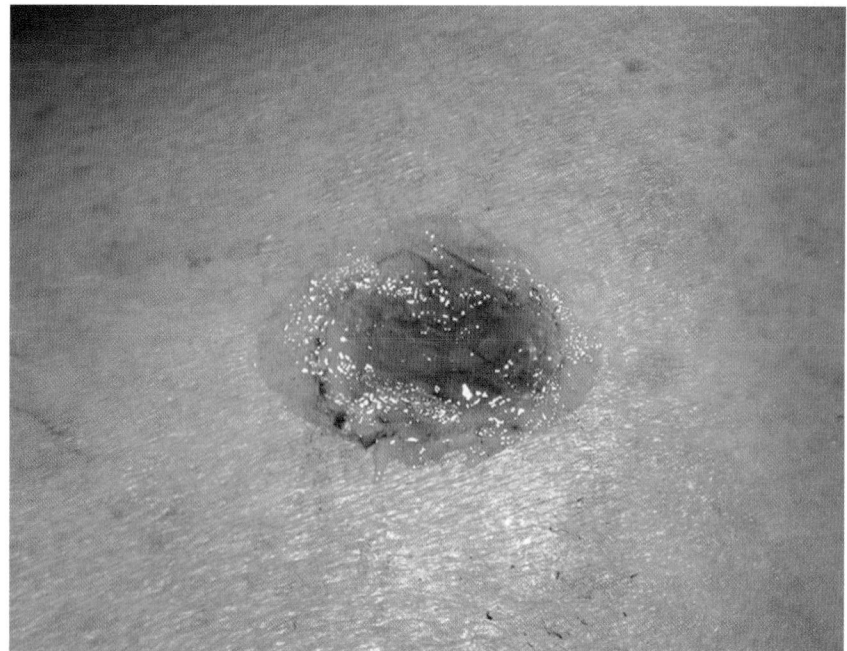

▲ **FIGURE 44-6** White petroleum applied to lesion after treatment.

- Pain can be controlled with over-the-counter analgesics.
- The wound should heal within 2 to 6 weeks with minimal scarring.

After the procedure is complete, wound care includes cleansing the area daily with soap and water, hydrogen peroxide, or other cleansers. White petroleum jelly (see Fig. 44-6) or topical antibiotic ointment should be applied twice a day under a bandage or gauze until the wound has healed (see Fig. 44-7).[3] Pain associated with the procedure is usually minimal, but if the patient does feel pain, over-the-counter analgesics may be used. In the lower extremities, swelling in the area of the wound may be noticed. The swelling can usually be managed using a compression bandage or support hose. The wound should heal within 2 to 6 weeks with minimal scarring. However, possible outcomes include a hypertrophic scar, a depressed scar with atrophy, tissue contraction, and hypo- or hyperpigmentation.[3]

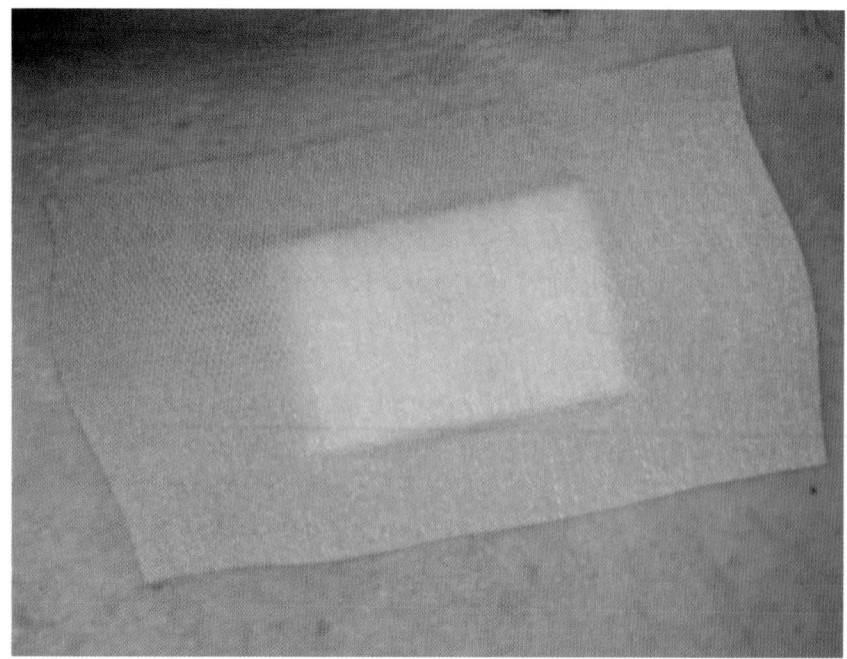

▲ **FIGURE 44-7** Dressing after treatment.

FINAL THOUGHTS

Curettage and electrodesiccation is a simple, safe, and cost-effective way to treat many benign and malignant lesions, especially superficial and nodular basal cell carcinomas. However, it is important to recognize the limitations of this technique and use other treatment modalities when necessary. For this reason, further studies are needed to adequately compare the various techniques of this treatment and to find the most efficacious technique for each type of lesion.

REFERENCES

1. Wigglesworth E. The curette in dermal therapeutics. *Boston Med Surg J.* 1876;94:143.
2. Clark WM. Oscillatory desiccation in the treatment of accessible malignant growths and minor surgical conditions. *J Adv Ther.* 1911;29:169–183.
3. Sheridan AT, Dawber RP. Curettage, electrosurgery, and skin cancer. *Aust J Dermatol.* 2000;41(1):19–30.
4. Goldman G. The current status of curettage and electrodesiccation. *Dermatol Clin.* 2002;20(3):569–578.
5. Stulberg DL, Hutchinson AG. Molluscum contagiosum and warts. *Am Fam Physician.* 2003;67(6):1233–1240.
6. Stevenson TR, Swanson NA. Syringoma: Removal by electrodessication and curettage. *Ann Plast Surg.* 1985;15(2):151–154.
7. Aversa AJ, Miller OF III. Cryo-curettage of cherry angiomas. *J Dermatol Surg Oncol.* 1983;9(11):930–931.
8. Cohen PR, Schulze KE, Tschen JA, et al. Treatment of extramammary Paget's disease with topical imiquimod cream: Case report and literature review. *South Med J.* 2006;99(4):396–402.
9. Lober BA, Fenske NA. Optimum treatment strategies for actinic keratosis (intraepidermal squamous cell carcinoma). *Am J Clin Dermatol.* 2004;5(6):395–401.
10. Nedwich JA. Evaluation of curettage and electrodesiccation in treatment of keratoacanthoma. Aust J Dermatol. 1991;32(3):137–141.
11. Silverman MK, Kopf AW, Grin CM, et al. Recurrence rates of treated basal cell carcinomas. Part 2: Curettage-electrodesiccation. *J Dermatol Surg Oncol.* 1991;17:720–726.
12. Tromovitch TA: Skin cancer. Treatment by curettage and desiccation. *Calif Med.* 1965;103:107–108.
13. Freeman RG, Knox JM, Heaton CL. The treatment of skin cancer. A statistical study of 1341 skin tumors comparing results obtained with irradiation, surgery, and curettage followed by electrodesiccation. *Cancer.* 1964;17:535–538.
14. Telfer NR, Colver GB, Bowers PW. Guidelines for the management of basal cell carcinoma. British Association of Dermatologists. *Br J Dermatol.* 1999;141(3):415–423.
15. Reynolds PL, Strayer SM. Treatment of skin malignancies. *J Fam Pract.* 2003;52(6):456–464.
16. Roenigk RK, Roenigk HH. Current surgical management of skin cancer in

dermatology. *J Dermatol Surg Oncol.* 1990;16:136–151.

17. Lang PG, Maize JC. Histologic evolution of recurrent basal cell carcinoma and treatment implications. *J Am Acad Dermatol.* 1986;14:186–196.

18. Coleman WP, Davis RS, Reed RJ, et al. Treatment of lentigo maligna and lentigo maligna melanoma. *J Dermatol Surg Oncol.* 1980;6:476–479.

19. Pariser DM. Diagnostic and therapeutic techniques. *Prim Care.* 1989;16:823–845.

20. Spencer JM, Tannenbaum A, Sloan L, et al. Does inflammation contribute to the eradication of basal cell carcinoma following curettage and electrodessication? *Dermatol Surg.* 1997;23(8):625–630.

21. Nouri K, Spencer JM, Taylor JR, et al. Does wound healing contribute to the eradication of basal cell carcinoma following curettage and electrodessication? *Dermatol Surg.* 1999;25(3):183–187.

22. Riordan A, Gamache C, Fosko S. Electrosurgery and cardiac devices. *J Am Acad Dermatol.* 1997;37(2 Pt 1):250.

23. Arndt KA, Bowens KE. *Manual of Dermatologic Therapeutics.* 6th ed. Philadelphia, PA: Lippincott Williams & Wilkins; 2001.

24. Zalla MJ. Basic cutaneous surgery. *Cutis.* 1994;53:172–186.

25. Adam JE. The technic of curettage surgery. *J Am Acad Dermatol.* 1986;15:697–702.

26. Barlow JO, Zalla MJ, Kyle A, et al. Treatment of basal cell carcinoma with curettage alone. *J Am Acad Dermatol.* 2006;54(6):1039–1045.

27. Whelan CS, Deckers PJ. Electrocoagulation for skin cancer: An old oncologic tool revisited. *Cancer.* 1981;47:2280–2287.

28. Williamson GS, Jackson R. Treatment of basal cell carcinoma by electrodessication and curettage. *Can Med Assoc J.* 1962;86:855–862.

29. Chiller K, Passaro D, McCalmont T, et al. Efficacy of curettage before excision in clearing surgical margins of nonmelanoma skin cancer. *Arch Dermatol.* 2000;136(11):1327–1332.

30. Spiller WF, Spiller RF. Cryosurgery and adjuvant surgical techniques for cutaneous carcinomas. In: Zacarian SA, ed. *Cryosurgery for Skin Cancer and Cutaneous Disorders.* St. Louis, MO: The C.V. Mosby Co.; 1985:187–198.

31. Wu JK, Oh C, Strutton G, et al. An open-label, pilot study examining the efficacy of curettage followed by imiquimod 5% cream for the treatment of primary nodular basal cell carcinoma. *Aust J Dermatol.* 2006;47(1):46–48.

32. Spencer JM. Pilot study of imiquimod 5% cream as adjunctive therapy to curettage and electrodessication for nodular basal cell carcinoma. *Dermatol Surg.* 2006;32(1):63–69.

CHAPTER 45

Lasers in Skin Cancer Diagnosis: Highlights of *in vivo* Reflectance Confocal Microscopy

Yolanda Gilaberte-Calzada, M.D.
Manuel Fernández-Lorente, M.D.
Elena De las Heras, M.D.
Jesús Cuevas-Santos, M.D.
Pedro Jaén-Olasolo, M.D.
Salvador González, M.D., Ph.D.

SKIN CANCER

BOX 45-1 Overview

- *In vivo* confocal laser microscopy allows real time noninvasive microscopic images comparable to conventional histology of the skin when exploring cutaneous structures between the stratum corneum and reticular dermis.
- Confocal laser microscope consists of a laser light source for illuminating a small skin area, which backscattered and the reflected light is detected by a point detector through a pinhole. Only the single plane within the specimen that is in focus is detected.
- Images obtained by *in vivo* CRM are oriented horizontal to the skin surface (skin-transversal sections). This is an important difference with respect to conventional histology.
- Major confocal imaging criteria of benign and malignant melanocytic tumors, BCC, AK, and SCC have been established.
- CRM for tumoral lesions has been shown efficacious for: (1) Utility as a guide to perform a biopsy, (2) Monitoring of response to treatment, and (3) Demarcation of lesion extension before proceeding to surgical excision.
- The main limitation of RCM is the capacity of penetration in dermis, which nowadays reaches a maximum depth of 350 to 400 μm. This avoids imaging of structures located in deep dermis, especially in cases of hyperpigmented or hyperkeratotic lesions such as melanoma and SCC, respectively.

INTRODUCTION

Dermatology is a medical speciality in which diagnosis is frequently based exclusively on clinical examination. In the case of melanoma, the sensitivity of this clinical exam reaches 65 to 80%. This percentage may not be acceptable, since early diagnosis means a critical point in patient morbid-mortality; therefore, several diagnostic tools may help us,

---

BOX 45-2 Summary

• Wavelength of light source for	
1–3-μm sectioning in the epidermis	Visible 488–514 nm
3–5 μm in the deeper dermis	Near-infrared 800–1064 nm
• Objective lens	
Magnification	30–100×
Numerical Aperture	0.7–1.2
• Resolution	
Lateral	0.5–1.0 μm
Axial	3.0–5.0 μm
• Illumination power	up to 40 mW
• Real time confocal images are parallel to skin surface	
• Confocal images of normal epidermis show honeycombed appearance	
• Melanin is the best endogenous contrast agent	

---

histopathology being the "gold standard." In expert dermatologist's hands, dermoscopy may improve diagnostic sensitivity up to 85 to 90%.[1] At present, different technologies are being developed in order to give additional dynamic skin microscopic information, without morbidity. They may offer both "*in vivo*" diagnosis and disease evolution in real time. These technologies include magnetic resonance,[2] high-frequency ultrasonography,[3] coherent optical tomography,[4] and, more recently, confocal microscopy.[5,6]

In vivo reflectance confocal laser microscopy (RCM) is at present the technique with more applications, allowing real-time noninvasive microscopic images comparable to conventional histology (1-μm lateral and 3-μm axial) when exploring cutaneous structures between the stratum corneum and reticular dermis.[7] RCM uses reflected light from tissue in order to obtain images.[8–11] In 1995, Rajadhyaksha and colleagues[6] first published the basis of confocal scanning laser microscopy. Since then, design and optimal parameters to fix the image have been developed. In recent years, the technique has improved and applications for inflammatory and tumoral skin pathology have also expanded; as shown by numerous scientific publications. Several skin conditions have been objectively characterized such as psoriasis,[12] contact dermatitis,[13,14] fungal[15] and bacterial[16] infections, actinic keratoses,[17] basal and squamous cell carcinoma (SCC),[18,19] and melanoma.[20]

BASIC OPTICAL PRINCIPLES

Optical Parameters

The microscope consists of a laser light source for illuminating a small skin area of interest within tissue. Backscattered and reflected light are detected by a point detector through an optically conjugate aperture (pinhole). High image resolution is achieved by eliminating light coming from out-of-focus planes; only light from in-focus planes will reach the detector. Hence, only the single plane within the specimen that is in focus is detected.[8–11] The numerical aperture of the objective lens determines the axial resolution and the amount of light detected. As in any optical system, there is an inverse proportional relationship between high resolution with small apertures and more light detected through higher apertures. Image contrast is determined by light reflected due to local variations of the refractive index within tissue. More light is reflected when tissue contains structures of size similar to wavelength. Backscattering of light (photons) will decrease contrast while increasing depth of image.[6,7,21]

An image on the screen is obtained after sequential illumination of multiple points. In order to see the complete image of tissue for study, an illuminated area will be scanned in two dimensions.

This system uses a laser as a light source, which provides several advantages such as more reflectance and convergence, more brilliant illumination, and also the possibility to choose a wavelength. The best quality image is supplied by low-potency lasers (around 40 mW) and a near-infrarred wavelength (800 to 1064 nm). With an 830-nm diode laser, skin penetration will be near 400 μm.[7] Water immersion lenses minimize spherical aberrations caused by the overlying epidermal cell layers, and they are used since the refractive index of water (1.33) is close to that of the epidermis (1.34).

Skin movement may be a limitation in an "*in vivo*" image. Thus, a ring-template skin-contact device is used to reduce motion artifacts and to contain the immersion medium for the objective lens when imaging: water or ultrasound gel.[7]

Fundamentals for Image Interpretation

Images obtained by *in vivo* confocal reflectance microscopy (CRM) are oriented horizontal to the skin surface (skin-transversal sections). This is a major difference with respect to conventional histology.

When imaging the skin in real time, starting from the surface and progressing deeper, most superficial images are obtained from the stratum corneum. Corneocytes are visualized as poligonal brilliant shapes (due to differences in refraction indexes between water and the stratum corneum), with a size of 10 to 30 μm. Next, we will visualize the granular cell layer, regularly distributed at a depth of 15 to 20 μm (Fig. 45-1A). The size of these cells is 20 to 25 μm and their nuclei appreciated as a dark central oval structure within the cell, surrounded by bright cytoplasm with a grainy appearance. Spinous keratinocytes are located 20 to 100 μm under the stratum corneum, measuring 10 to 15 μm in size and with well-demarcated cell borders ("honey-combed" pattern appearance) (Fig. 45-1B). At 50 to 100 μm, we find the dermo-epidermal junction (Fig. 45-1D). Basal cells are smaller (7 to 15 μm) and brilliant due to their content in melanin[7] (Fig. 45-1C). Typically, melanin in basal keratinocytes is located supranuclear ("melanin hats") revealing its protective function. This basal layer refractivity varies according to patient's phototype and anatomical location. Under this level, we may detect both bundles of collagen (Fig. 45-1E) and capillaries with erythrocytes rolling within, hair follicles, and sweat glands in the center of dermal papillae.

RCM OF MELANOCYTIC TUMORS

BOX 45-3 Summary

- Melanocytic Tumors
  - Preserved honeycomb appearance of keratinocytes in the epidermis.
  - Populations of monomorphous round to oval bright refractile cells with centrally positioned nuclei in the basal layer (pigmented keratinocytes and melanocytes).
  - Regular and uniform dermal papillae.
  - Clusters of bright round cells in the dermis of compound nevi (nests).
- Melanoma
  - Disarray of keratinocytes (loss of the honeycomb appearance of the epidermis).
  - Pleomorphic bright cells within the epidermis, with eccentrically placed large nuclei.

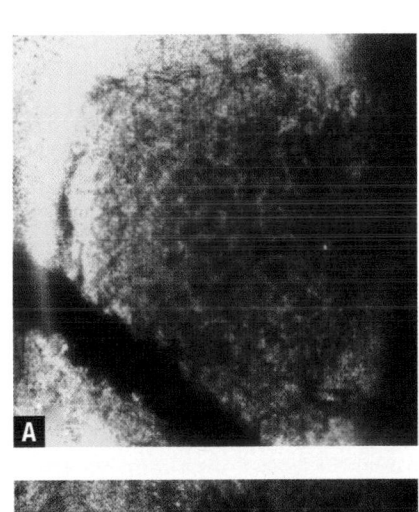
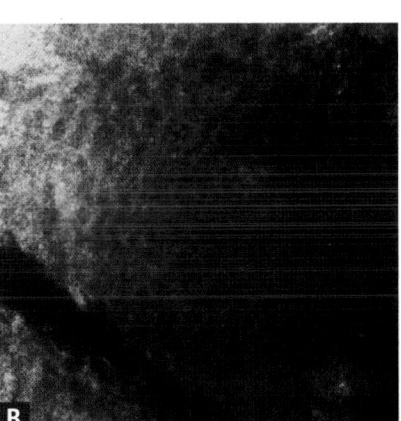
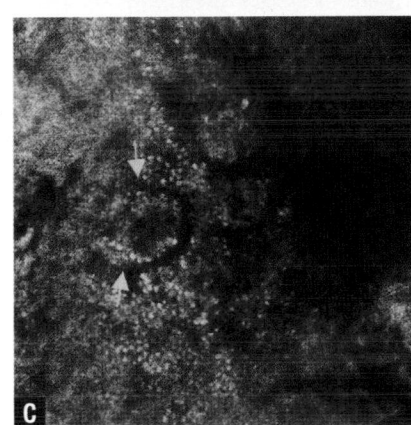
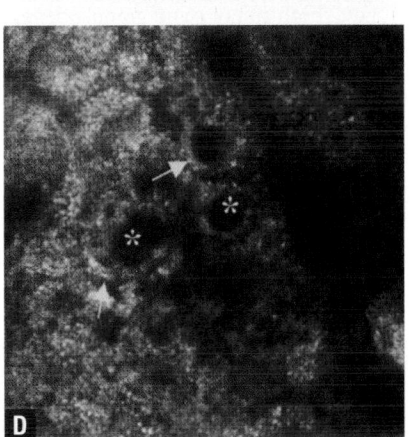
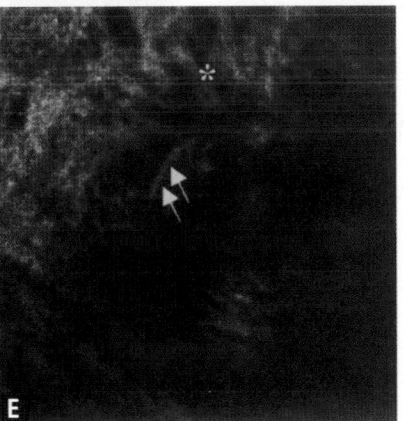

▲ **FIGURE 45-1** *In vivo* RCM analysis of normal skin. In confocal images, granular cells (**A**) are regularly seen at depths of 10 to 15 μm. The dark oval areas correspond to nuclei within the bright cytoplasm. Spinous keratinocytes (**B**) are seen at 20 to 100 μm below the stratum corneum. Note basal keratinocytes (*arrows*) (**C**), located around dermal papillae (*) (**D**), appear brighter than surrounding keratinocytes of spinous and granular layers. (**E**) Blood vessels (*arrows*) and collagen bundles (*) are also seen.

- Coarse branching dendritic structures in the epidermis.
- Small and irregular dermal papillae.
- Bright, grainy particles in the epidermis.
- Dermal cell clusters (nests) may have a multilobate, cerebriform aspect when present.
- Enlarged, round, or dendritic, highly refractive cells ascending in the epidermis (pagetoid spread).

According to Mie's theory, more light is reflected when tissue has structures whose size is similar to wavelength.[22] Although melanin absorbs in the near-infrared spectrum (700 to 1064 nm), its high refractive index (1.7) compared to the epidermis (near water: 1.34)[4,6] determines a great dispersion of reflected light. Therefore, melanin represents the strongest endogenous contrast agent resulting in a bright appearance of basal keratinocytes and melanocytes.

Common and Dysplastic Melanocytic Nevi

In nevi, both spinous and granular layers show no alteration, with a normal pattern consisting of homogenous and well-demarcated cells. Nevus itself is made up of nevomelanocytes, a homogenous population of small monomorphous round to oval bright, refractive cells with centrally positioned dark round nuclei.[23,24] Dermal papillae are uniformly distributed and circumscribed by a rim of refractive monomorphous cells that correspond to small melanocytes and melanin-rich keratinocytes, without any cytologic atypia. In junctional nevi, melanocytes are at the dermo-epidermal junction level.[23] On the contrary, in compound and dermal nevi, they are seen in the papillar and reticular dermis, near the vessels. Anecdotally, we may find small brilliant dendrites in the epidermis.

Therefore, RCM images of common nevi are characterized by a symmetrical architectural pattern; melanocytes with uniform nuclei and cytoplasm, similar in size. Atypical nevi, as it occurs clinically and in dermoscopy, share features with common nevi and melanoma; occasionally, diagnosis may be extremely difficult.[23] Homogenicity described for common nevi may not be present in atypical nevi, the cell population being more heterogenous in size, shape, and refractivity (different intensity in brilliance)[23,24] (Fig. 45-2). However, cells tend to be round or oval as in common nevi, rather than dendritic as in melanomas. In general, when

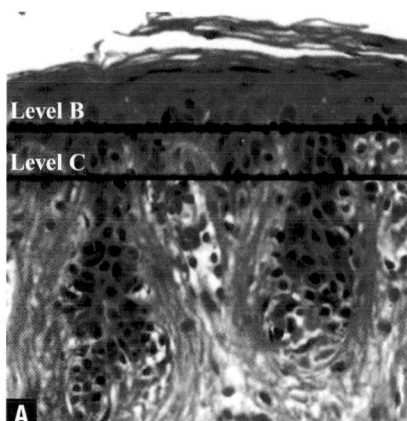

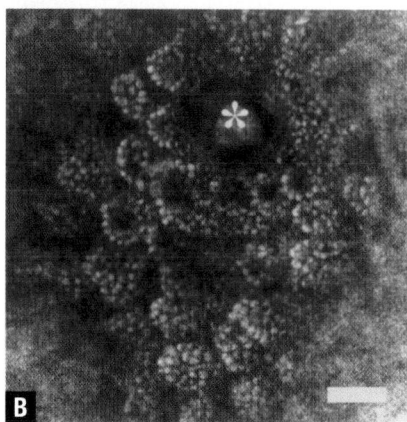

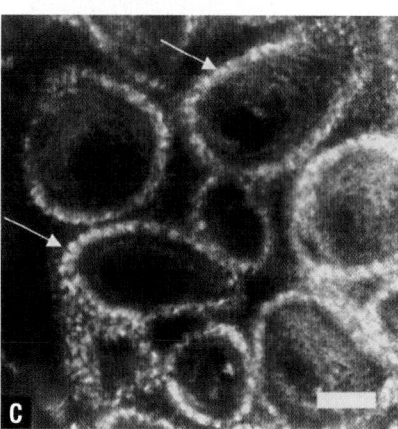

▲ **FIGURE 45-2** (A) Histology section of a lentiginous melanocytic nevus. The *bars* in image (A) show the depth level at which confocal images (B) and (C) have been obtained. Image (B) shows uniform population of bright refractive cells at the top of the dermal papillae. Note the presence of an eccrine duct (*). Image (C) shows a rim of monomorphous refractive cells (*arrows*) around dermal papillae, corresponding to small melanocytes and melanin-rich keratinocytes in the basal layer. Scale *bar:* 50 μm.

there is atypia, most melanocytes are less brilliant, with isolated big epithelioid brilliant cells with peripheral nucleus.[25] Cell nests may be less demarcated. Keratinocytes focally lose their demarcations at the spinous layer associated with dendrites and occasionally "melanin dust"

(highly refractive granular particles). Especially, on the face, atypical nevi may show desestructuration at the dermo-epidermal junction, with low homogenous dermal papillae and the absence of demarcation by refractive cells (Fig. 45-3).

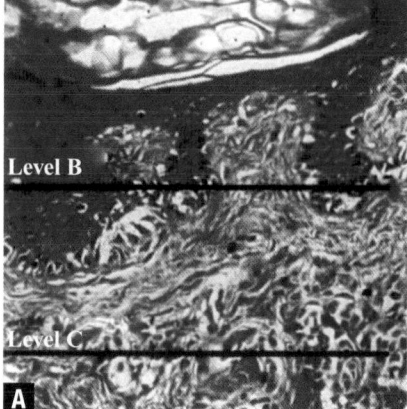

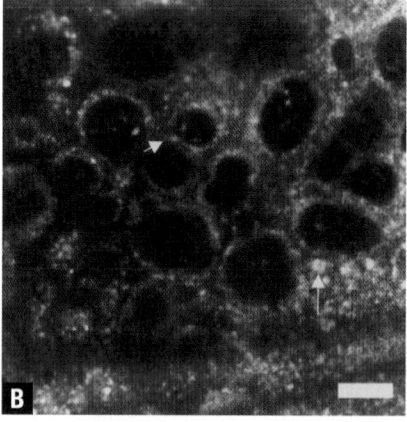

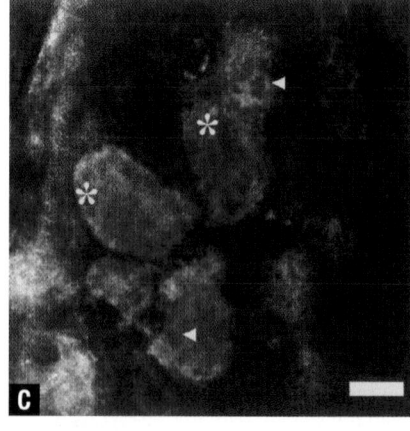

▲ **FIGURE 45-3** (A) Histology section of a dysplastic compound nevus. The *bars* in image (A) show the depth level at which confocal images (B) and (C) have been obtained. Image (B) shows heterogeneous brightness with irregular distribution of dermal papillae. Dermal papillae are surrounded by a nonrefractile rim of cells, some of them with atypical morphology (*arrows*). Image (C) shows the irregular morphology of the dermal nests (*) composed of cells, some of them with enlarged, atypical nuclei (*arrowheads*). Scale *bar:* 50 μm.

Melanoma

Due to a close relationship between early diagnosis and life prognosis of the patient, RCM is particularly useful in order to increase clinical and dermoscopic sensitivity. Additionally, it is particularly interesting that RCM findings are shared by both pigmented melanomas and amelanotic melanomas.[26] This is probably due either to the presence of cytoplasmic melanosomes, which act as endogenous contrast, and/or due to a certain amount of melanine in premelanosomes. Apart from diagnosis, RCM has been shown efficacious in pigmented lesions for:

- utility as a guide to perform a biopsy, selecting the area of the lesion with more atypical images and, therefore, more suspicious of melanoma. False negative results in the histopathological study will be reduced.[20]

- monitoring the response to treatment.[27]

- demarcation of the lesion extension before proceeding to surgical excision.[26,27]

A characteristic finding for melanoma is the presence of structural changes in the spinous and granular layers with disarrangement of keratinocytes and loss of intercellular demarcation (disruption of "honeycomb pattern")[25] (Fig. 45-4A). Enlarged atypical cells with pleomorphic morphology, variable refractivity, and angulous nuclei may be found in several layers of the epidermis (pagetoid dissemination) (Fig. 45-4A); and, of course, in the dermis. Cells may be oval, stellate, or fusiform in shape; they could have coarse branching dendritic processes and present eccentrically placed large nuclei.[20,23] In the basal layer, cells may be grouped, simulating a dysplastic nevus, or isolated. Additionally, some findings described for dysplastic nevus, but more pronounced may be seen. Dermal papillae are smaller, more irregular, and with worse ill-defined borders than in common nevi. The architectural pattern is very asymmetrical both in size and refractivity (Fig. 45-4B). Linear dendrites are thickened and bright more than in healthy skin. "Melanin dust" may be thicker (1 to 3 μm) than in atypical nevi, and can be visualized along the epidermis. Indistinguishable cell borders may be evident, contributing to the abnormal epidermal morphology. In the dermis, we may find cerebriform cell clusters with thin refractive cell aggregates (polygonal or enlarged) surrounded by "melanin dust."[28]

The main drawback of RCM is the capacity of penetration in dermis, which

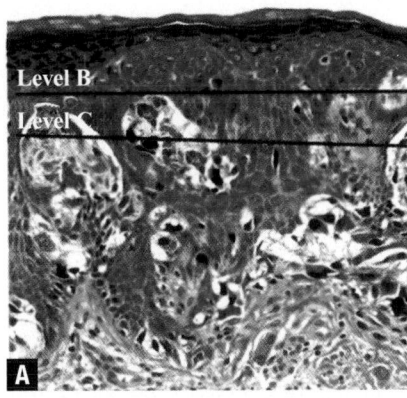

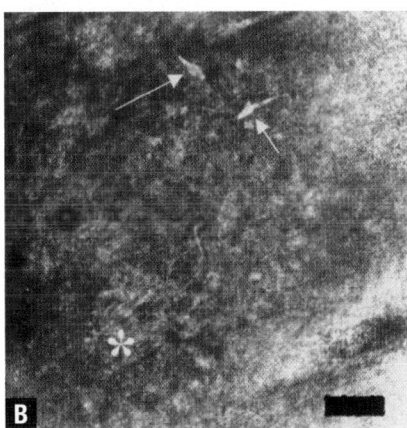

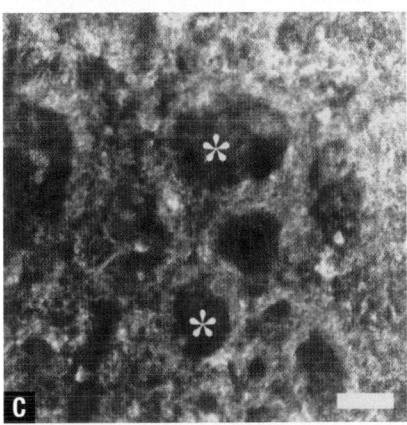

▲ **FIGURE 45-4** (**A**) Histology section of a superficial spreading melanoma. The *bars* in image (**A**) show the depth level at which confocal images (**B**) and (**C**) have been obtained. Image (**B**) shows the presence of enlarged (atypical) melanocytes (*arrows*) ascending in the epidermis (pagetoid spread), within a background of marked loss of keratinocyte demarcation (*). Bright dots and dendritic structures are also seen. Image (**C**) shows the presence of nonrefractile rims around dermal papillae openings (*) (nonedge papillae). Scale *bar*: 50 μm.

nowadays reaches a maximum depth of 350 to 400 μm. This avoids imaging of structures located in the deep dermis, especially in cases of hyperpigmented or hyperkeratotic lesions since in these cases there is strong contrast attenuation due to absorption and scattering of light

passing through these structures. Also, the presence of refractive structures in the dermis, such as inflammatory cells and collagen bundles, may diminish contrast and make melanocyte visualization difficult.

Considering that the thickness of melanoma is an important prognostic factor in patients with melanoma, improvements in the technique will be necessary in order to increase RCM potency and imaging depth. Decrease in contrast may be solved through the development of exogenous contrast agents. On the other hand, an additional advantage of RCM is the possibility to correlate findings with those provided by dermoscopy, improving both sensitivity and specificity in diagnosis and correlation of these two noninvasive methods.[29] An atypical pigmented network is correlated with the variation in size and shape of dermal papillae. Globules correspond to refractive cell aggregates. A whitish-blue veil is correlated with discontinuation of dermal papillae and the presence of bright dendritic cells with melanophages. In peripheral pseudopods, RCM shows dense aggregates of pleomorphic cells with variable refractivity and ill-defined borders. At the same time, RCM may increase specificity to establish diagnoses in areas where dermoscopy shows less significant findings.

▌ RCM OF NONMELANOCYTIC SKIN TUMORS

BOX 45-4 Summary

- Actinic Keratosis
  - Irregular hyperkeratosis.
  - Epidermal nuclear enlargement and pleomorphism.
  - Architectural disarray limited to lower portion of the epidermis.
- Squamous Cell Carcinoma
  - Nuclear enlargement with pleomorphism.
  - Full thickness architectural disarray of epidermis.
- Basal Cell Carcinoma
  - Orientation of the tumor cell nuclei along the same axis "polarized appearance."
  - Presence of monomorphic tumor cells with elongated nuclei.
  - Pleomorphism of overlying and adjacent epidermal cells ("actinic damage").
  - Increased vasculature with pronounced superficial blood vessel prominence, dilatation, and tortuosity.
  - Prominent inflammatory infiltrate among tumor cells and trafficking of leukocytes.

- Loss of normal progressive differentiation of keratinocytes, the architectural honeycomb pattern, the dermal papillae, and the follicular and eccrine duct architecture.

Actinic Keratosis

In vivo RCM histopathological key features of actinic keratoses include: irregular hyperkeratosis and parakeratosis, and epidermal nuclear enlargement with pleomorphism in a pattern of architectural disarray (Fig. 45-5), which does not involve the full thickness of the epidermis. Observation of dysplastic features in the full skin thickness on RCM is suggestive of SCC.

RCM has been shown to be useful in monitoring the response to treatment of actinic keratosis (AK) with photodynamic therapy, having demonstrated progressive normalization of architecture in successfully treated lesions. Currently, some studies are underway to evaluate the response of actinic keratoses to topical imiquimod.

Squamous Cell Carcinoma

The shallow penetration of the RCM illuminating wavelengths prevents accurate visualization at the dermo-epidermal junction, particularly in hyperkeratotic lesions. This makes differential diagnosis between superficially invasive SCC and SCC *in situ* unfeasible due to lack of adequate visual assessment at the dermo-epidermal junction. Confocal features suggestive of SCC are full thickness architectural disarray and nuclear enlargement with pleomorphism observed in the *stratum granulosum* (Fig. 45-6). Other changes suggestive of SCC such as vascular patterns and keratin pearls need further investigation. This currently restricts the potential of this tool for accurate differentiation of AK versus SCC.

Ex vivo application of RCM in combination with acetic acid application as an adjuvant during Mohs micrographic surgery for SCC have been investigated; the most striking finding was the densely packed, large, irregularly organized, prominent epidermal nuclei. Nevertheless, SCC is not easily detected by RCM, with difficulty in distinguishing SCC from AK.[30,31]

Basal Cell Carcinoma

RCM morphological characteristics of basal cell carcinoma (BCC) have been

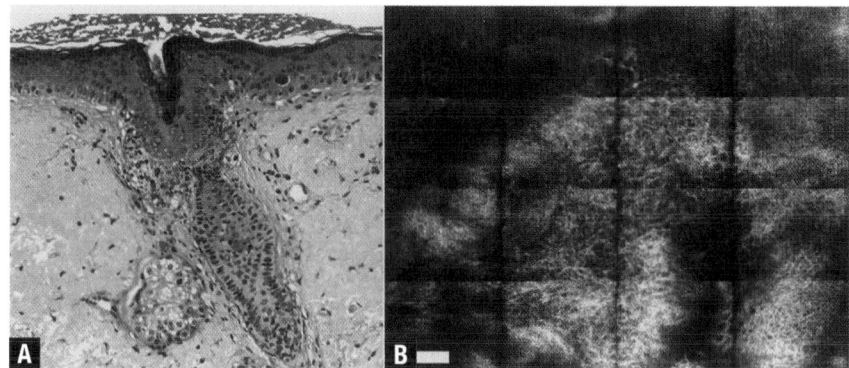

▲ **FIGURE 45-5** (**A**) Histology section of AK. (**B**). *En face* mosaic composed of confocal images showing keratinocyte disarray at different levels of the epidermis. Scale *bar*. 100 μm.

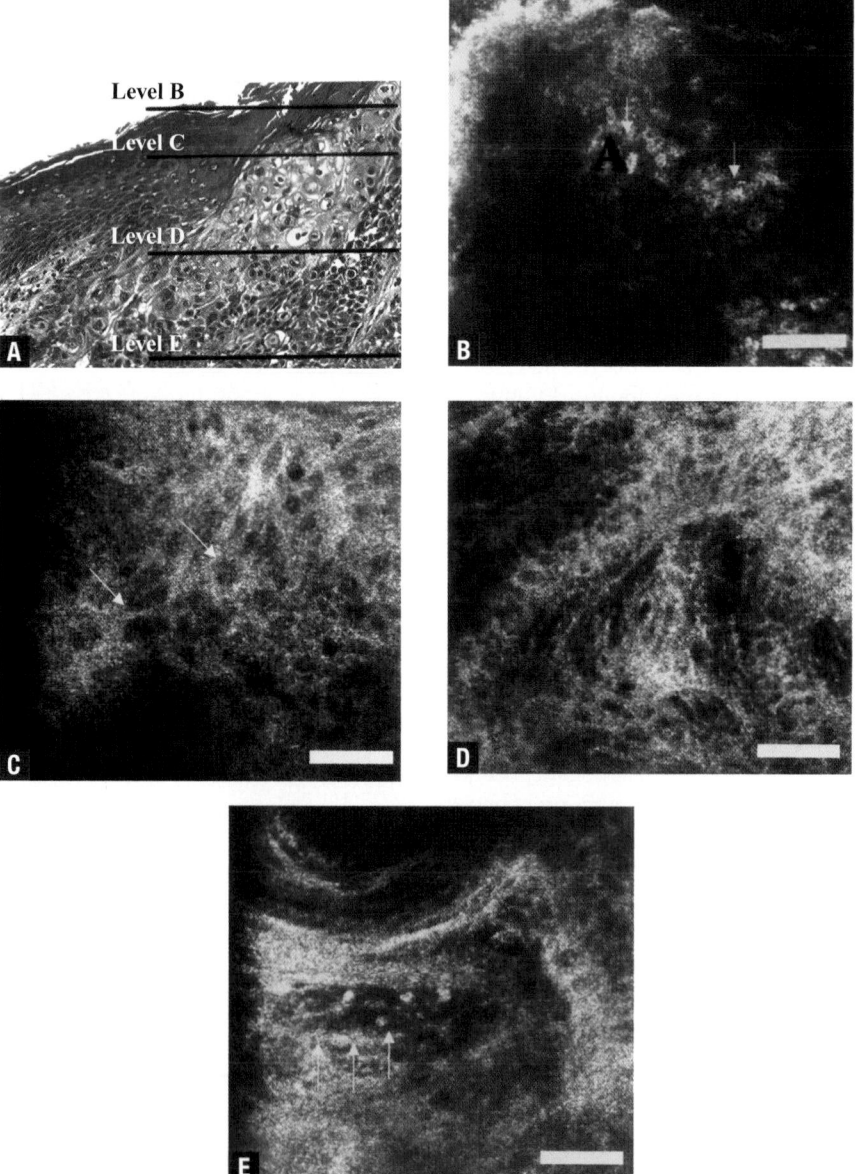

▲ **FIGURE 45-6** (**A**) Histology section of SCC. The *bars* in image (**A**) show the depth level at which confocal images (**B**), (**C**), (**D**), and (**E**) have been obtained. Image (**B**) shows the presence of nucleated corneocytes (*arrows*). Image (**C**) shows keratinocyte disarray and atypical granular keratinocytes (*arrows*). Image (**D**) demonstrates severe pleomorphism. Image (**E**) shows vasodilatation (*arrows*) with leukocyte trafficking. Scale *bar*. 50 μm.

well-defined.[18] (1) The presence of pleomorphism and architectural disorder of the overlying epidermis indicative of actinic damage or consequence of the presence of the tumor (Fig. 45-7A); (2) The presence of islands of refractive tumor cells with elongated, monomorphic, basaloid nuclei through the thickness of the epidermis; (3) The nuclei that are polarized along the same axis of orientation (Fig. 45-7B), disrupting the normal honeycomb pattern of the epidermis and the dermal papillae architecture; (4) Increased dermal vasculature with prominent dilatation and tortuosity of blood vessels (Fig. 45-7C); and (5) Trafficking of leukocytes, which means accumulation with rolling of leukocytes along the endothelial lining. A retrospective, multicentric study from 152 lesions has shown that the presence of at least two of these criteria has a sensitivity of 100% for the diagnosis of BCC.[19] As the number of criteria increased, the specificity increased, so that when at least four criteria were present, the specificity was 95.7%, giving the best

concordance between high sensitivity and high specificity. The most sensitive and specific criterion was the presence of polarized nuclei (91.6% and 97%, respectively), not surprisingly because on histology palisading is one of the most remarkable characteristics of BCC. These results were found to have little variability across BCC locations and subtypes. However, pigment BCCs have also been characterized by an architectural configuration of well-circumscribed cord-like or nodular structures, which correlate with nodules and/or cords of atypical basaloid cells; peritumoral dark spaces, which correspond to peritumoral mucin, and intratumoral bright dendritic and granular structures that correspond to both intratumoral dendritic melanocytes and melanin dust.[32] Melanophages are also seen. Finally, morpheiform/infiltrating type of BCC has also been described to have curled bundles of collagen with large cells, representing the tumor stroma.[33]

RCM has shown the potential to become a useful tool for noninvasive

monitoring of BCC treatment. In relation to imiquimod, RCM accurately predicts the presence or absence of BCC before, during, and after treatment.[34] On the other hand, RCM is currently under study as a surgical adjunct and guide in Mohs micrographic surgery for BCC. Using aluminum chloride to enhance tumor contrast,[35] large aggregates of residual tumor such as nodular BCC were easily detected by *ex vivo* RCM, whereas micronodular and infiltrative BCC and basosquamous cell carcinomas were not easily or consistently identified on confocal images.[31] Therefore, this tool can potentially be useful for Mohs surgery, but further improvements in instrumentation and image quality are necessary to allow its broader application and acceptance.

FINAL THOUGHTS

RCM offers tremendous potential for the management of skin cancer. The possibility of noninvasively diagnosing skin tumors, determining their margins, and performing the follow up made this technique an advantageous tool in clinical dermatology. Additionally, RCM allows us to study the pathophysiologic processes in real-time without any tissue damage and by the same technique sequentially over time, helping us in longitudinal studies. Correlation of RCM findings with those provided by dermoscopy in melanocytic lesions, and evaluation of its usefulness to guide Mohs surgery are some of the main areas in which this technology is currently being investigated. Nevertheless, RCM has limitations, especially when evaluating deep lesions. Further improvements in instrumentation and image quality are necessary to allow its broader application and acceptance.

REFERENCES

1. Pehamberger H, Binder M, Steiner A, Wolff K. *In vivo* epiluminiscence microscopy: Improvement of early diagnosis of melanoma. *J Invest Dermatol.* 1993;100: 356–362.
2. Markisz JA, Aquilia MG. *Technical Magnetic Resonance Imaging.* Standford, CT: Appleton & Lange; 1996.
3. Mansotti L. Basic principles and advanced technical aspects of ultrasound imaging. In: Guzzardi R, ed. *Physics and Engineering of Medical Imaging.* Boston, MA: Martinus Nijhoff; 1987:263–317.
4. Tearney GT, Brezinski ME, Southern JF, Bouma BE, Hee MR, Fujimoto JG. Determination of the refractive index of highly scattering human tissue by optical coherence tomography. *Opt Lett.* 1995;20: 2258–2260.

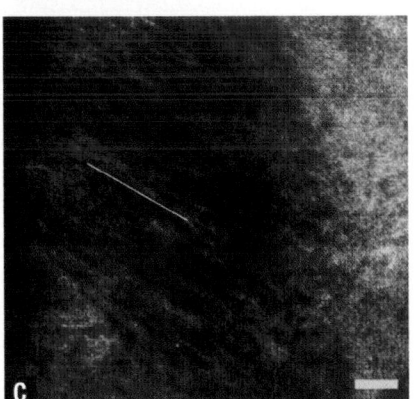

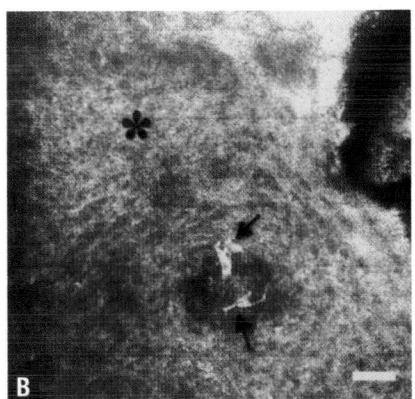

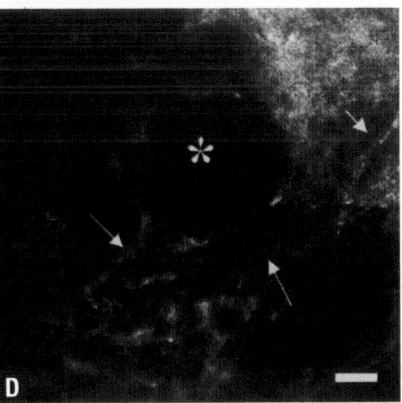

▲ **FIGURE 45-7** (A) Histology section of a superficial BCC. The *bars* in image (A) show the depth level at which confocal images (B), (C), and (D) have been obtained. Image (B) shows confocal image obtained from upper epidermis showing keratinocyte disarray (*). Note the presence of melanocytes (*arrows*) on the periphery of follicular epithelium. Image (C) shows a population of cells with elongated nuclei, polarized along one axis. Image (D) shows dilated blood vessels (*arrows*) with leukocyte trafficking surrounding a BCC node (*). Scale *bar*: 50 μm.

5. New KC, Petroll WM, Boyde A, et al. *In vivo* imaging of human teeth and skin using real-time confocal microscopy. *Scanning.* 1991;13:369–372.

6. Rajadhyaksha M, Grossman M, Esterowitz D, Webb RH, Anderson RR. *In vivo* confocal scanning laser microscopy of human skin: Melanin provides strong contrast. *J Invest Dermatol.* 1995;104: 946–952.

7. Rajadhyaksha M, González S, Zavislan J, Anderson RR, Webb RH. *In vivo* confocal scanning laser microscopy of human skin II: Advances in instrumentation and comparison to histology. *J Invest Dermatol.* 1999;113:293–303.

8. Wilson T. *Confocal Microscopy.* San Diego, CA: Academic; 1990.

9. Pawley JB. *Handbook of Biological Confocal Microscopy.* 2nd ed. New York: Plenum; 1995.

10. Webb RH. Confocal optical microscopy. *Rep Prog Phys.* 1996;59:427–471.

11. Webb RH. Theoretical basis of confocal microscopy. *Methods Enzymol.* 1999;307: 3–20.

12. Gonzalez S, Rajakhyaksha M, Rubinstein G, Anderson RR. Characterization of psoriasis *in vivo* reflectance confocal microscopy. *J Med.* 1999;30:337–356.

13. Gonzalez S, Gonzalez E, White WM, et al. Allergic contact dermatitis: Correlation of *in vivo* confocal imaging to routine histology. *J Am Acad Dermatol.* 1999;40:708–713.

14. Astner S, Gonzalez E, Cheung AC, et al. Non-invasive evaluation of the kinetics of allergic and irritant contact dermatitis. *J Invest Dermatol.* 2005;124:351–359.

15. Hongcharu W, Dwyer P, Gonzalez S, Anderson RR. Confirmation of onychomycosis by *in vivo* confocal microscopy. *J Am Acad Dermatol.* 2000;42:214–216.

16. Gonzalez S, Rajadhyaksha M, Gonzalez-Serva A, et al. Confocal reflectance imaging of folliculitis *in vivo*: Correlation with routine histology. *J Cutan Pathol.* 1999;26: 201–205.

17. Aghassi D, Anderson RR, Gonzalez S. Confocal laser microscopic imaging of actinic keratoses *in vivo*: A preliminary report. *J Am Acad Dermatol.* 2000;43:42–48.

18. Gonzalez S, Tannous Z. Real-time, *in vivo* confocal reflectance microscopy of basal cell carcinoma. *J Am Acad Dermatol.* 2002; 47:869–874.

19. Nori S, Rius-Diaz F, Cuevas J, et al. Sensitivity and specificity of reflectance-mode confocal microscopy for *in vivo* diagnosis of basal cell carcinoma: A multicenter study. *J Am Acad Dermatol.* 2004; 51:923–930.

20. Tannous ZS, Mihm MC, Flotte TJ, Gonzalez S. *In vivo* examination of lentigo maligna and malignant melanoma *in situ*, lentigo maligna type by near-infrared reflectance confocal microscopy: Comparison of *in vivo* confocal images with histologic sections. *J Am Acad Dermatol.* 2002;46:260–263.

21. Dunn AK, Smithpeter C, Welch AJ, Richards-Kortum R. Sources of contrast in confocal reflectance imaging. *Appl Opt.* 1996;35:3441–3446.

22. Vand de Hulst HC. *Light Scattering by Small Particles.* New York: Dover; 1981.

23. Langley RGB, Rajadhyaksha M, Dwyer PJ, Sober AJ, Flotte TJ, Anderson RR. Confocal scanning laser microscopy of benign and malignant melanocytic skin lesions *in vivo*. *J Am Acad Dermatol.* 2001; 45:365–376.

24. Busam KJ, Charles C, Lee G, Halpern AC. Morphologic features of melanocytes, pigmented keratinocytes, and melanophages by *in vivo* confocal scanning laser microscopy. *Mod Pathol.* 2001;14:862–868.

25. Pellacani G, Cesinaro AM, Longo C, et al. Microscopic *in vivo* description of cellular architecture of dermoscopic pigment network in nevi and melanomas. *Arch Dermatol.* 2005;141:147–154.

26. Busam KJ, Hester K, Charles C, et al. Detection of clinically amelanotic malignant melanoma and assessment of its margins by *in vivo* confocal scanning laser microscopy. *Arch Dermatol.* 2001;137: 923–929.

27. Curiel-Lewandrowski C, Williams CM, Swindells KJ, et al. Use of *in vivo* confocal microscopy in malignant melanoma: An aid in diagnosis and assessment of surgical and nonsurgical therapeutic approaches. *Arch Dermatol.* 2004;140: 1127–1132.

28. Pellacani G, Cesinaro AM, Seidenari S. *In vivo* assessment of melanocytic nests in nevi and melanomas by reflectance confocal microscopy. *Mod Pathol.* 2005;18: 469–474.

29. Scope A, Benvenuto-Andrade C, Agero AL, Halpern AC, Gonzalez S, Marghhob AA. Precise dermoscopy to reflectance confocal microscopy correlation of melanocytic neoplasms. *Arch Dermatol.* 2007;143: 176–185.

30. Rajadhyaksha M, Menaker G, Flotte T, Dwyer PJ, González S. Confocal examination of nonmelanoma cancers in thick skin excisions to potentially guide Mohs micrographic surgery without frozen histopahtology. *J Invest Dermatol.* 2001;17:1137–1143.

31. Chung VQ, Dwyer PJ, Nehal KS, et al. Use of *ex vivo* confocal scanning laser microscopy during Mohs surgery for nonmelanoma skin cancers. *Dermatol Surg.* 2004;30:1470–1478.

32. Agero ALC, Busam KJ, Rajadhyaksha M, et al. Reflectance confocal microscopy for imaging pigmented basal cell cancers *in vivo*. *J Am Acad Dermatol.* 2006;54: 638–643.

33. Sauermann K, Gambichler T, Wilmert M, et al. Investigation of basal cell carcinoma by confocal laser scanning microscopy *in vivo*. *Skin Res Technol.* 2002;8: 141–147.

34. Goldgeier M, Fox CA, Zavislan JM, Harris D, Gonzalez S. Noninvasive imaging, treatment, and microscopic confirmation of clearance of basal cell carcinoma. *Dermatol Surg.* 2003;29:205–210.

35. Tannous Z, Torres A, González S. *In vivo* real-time confocal reflectance microscopy: A noninvasive guide for Mohs micrographic surgery facilitated by aluminum chloride, an excellent contrast enhancer. *Dermatol Surg.* 2003;29:839–846.

CHAPTER 46

Photodynamic Therapy

Riccardo Rossi, M.D.
Torello Lotti, M.D.
R.M. Rashid, M.D., Ph.D.
Stephanie W. Liu, B.A.
Murad Alam, M.D.

PART 1. HOW PHOTODYNAMIC THERAPY IS DONE: A PRACTICAL GUIDE

Introduction and History of PDT

Photodynamic therapy (PDT), now receiving notice as an alternative method for treatment of photodamaged skin, has historic roots in the ancient past. As early as the period 1400 to 400 B.C., Indians, Egyptians, and Greeks had developed crude forms of PDT, with the Greeks under the guidance of Herodotus developing complex protocols for so-called heliotherapy.[1] Centuries later, in the early 1900s, PDT re-emerged as a therapeutic modality for skin cancer and in the mid-1900s as an antiviral therapy for herpes simplex.[2] In modern times, 5-aminolevulinic acid (5-ALA), in combination with exposure to blue light, has been the first topical sensitizing agent to

be approved for the treatment of actinic keratoses (AKs) by the U.S. Food and Drug Administration. More recently, investigators have explored additional off-label applications of PDT, with successful treatments reported for various dermatologic diseases.

This chapter discusses the use of PDT in two sections: (1) a practical guide to the administration of PDT with photosensitizers, especially those already commercially available and registered, and (2) an evidence-based review on the use of PDT with topical photosensitizers for cutaneous malignancies.

Mechanism of PDT

BOX 46-2   Summary

- PDT involves the administration of a photosensitizing agent, exposure to light and oxygen to create reactive oxygen species that destroy target cells.
- The photosensitizer 5-ALA accumulates in target cells based on size, lipophilic/hydrophilic characteristics, electric charge, and protein binding where it is converted to the light-absorbing PpIX, a precursor to heme.
- MAL, a derivative of 5-ALA, penetrates to reach target cells with greater efficiency than 5-ALA while still maintaining the same downstream metabolic passages. It is approved in Europe for treatment of AKs, and BCCs but not in the United States.

PDT involves the administration of a photosensitizing agent that preferentially accumulates in target cells. Various light wavelengths (red light 580 to 760 nm, blue light 450 to 490 nm, ambient light 400 to 1000 nm), exposures (10 to 400 J/cm^2), and intensities (10 to 200 mW/cm^2) are then used to activate the agent. This light-activated molecule interacts with oxygen and leads to the formation of a highly reactive singlet oxygen ($^1O_2$). The reactive oxygen proceeds to destroy the target cell by various proposed mechanisms including direct cytotoxicity.[3,4] Other effects of PDT that are of interest include potential antiangiogenic effects.[5]

5-ALA has proven to be an especially effective photosensitizer for PDT. The topical material is converted in the mitochondria to light-absorbing Protoporphyrin IX (PpIX), a precursor to heme

Table 46-1
What Is the "Ideal" Photosensitizer?

- Chemical purity
- High quantum yields
- Quick tissue accumulation
- Short half-life
- Rapid clearance from normal tissue
- Activating at long wavelengths with optimal tissue penetration
- Lack of toxicity and mutagenesis

that accumulates in neoplastic cells or in the endothelium of newly formed vessels of tumor parenchyma while sparing surrounding healthy tissue. This selectivity is based on photosensitizer size and lipophilic/hydrophilic characteristics, electric charge, and unspecific protein binding (Table 46-1).[6–11] Accumulation is thought to be due to several factors including the upregulation of the rate-limiting enzyme porphobilinogen deaminase.[12] Besides inducing enzymatic alterations, accumulation of photosensitizing agents has also been proposed to be cell-cycle dependent.[13] Of further benefit is the rapid removal of 5-ALA derivatives from the body, thus limiting potential adverse effects of prolonged skin photosensitization.[14]

Current literature has focused on ascertaining the clinical efficacy of 5-ALA. However, 5-ALA has been found to have limitations based on its molecular makeup. For example, this compound is very hydrophilic, thus limiting its penetration into the skin. It penetrates cells through a transmembrane transport system used by beta-amino acids and γ-aminobutyrric acid (GABA). This system is energy, pH, and temperature dependent, saturable, and slow. It is only slightly accelerated in tumor cells.[15–18] As such, interest has increased in developing modified derivatives of 5-ALA. The ultimate goal has been to preserve and/or maximize the beneficial actions of 5-ALA while downregulating those aspects that hinder optimal treatment.

One such derivative is the lipophilic methyl ester of 5-ALA, methyl aminolevulinate (MAL, Metvix®).[12] It penetrates the cell membranes not only with the same beta-carrier used by ALA, but also by the glycine transport system. MAL penetrates by passive transmembrane diffusion as well, which does not require energy, making the mechanism faster. The system is unsaturable and even more efficient in neoplastic cells. MAL is quickly demethylated to ALA in the cytoplasm so that the following metabolic passages are the same.[15,19–22] PDT with Metvix® has been approved and registered for use in the European Union for the indications of nonhyperkeratotic AK and superficial/nodular basal cell carcinoma (BCC).[23] MAL-PDT has also been found to be effective in the treatment of hyperkeratotic AK pretreated with mechanical removal of squamous crusts.[24,25–27] In the United States, this photosensitizing agent has an FDA approvability letter for the treatment of AK, but is not yet cleared for marketing.

ALA/MAL PDT Treatment Technique

BOX 46-3   Summary

PDT Treatment Technique
- Preparation of lesion
  - Remove scales and crusts with curette
  - Apply photosensitizer to lesions with 1 to 2-mm thickness, extending application to 5 mm outside margins of lesion
  - Cover treatment site with occlusive dressing to block sun exposure
  - Incubate for determined period of time
- Treatment
  - Remove occlusive dressing and wash off excess photosensitizer
  - Illuminate treatment site with light source according to chosen protocol
- After treatment/follow-up
  - Patient should continue to avoid sun exposure for the next few days following treatment
  - Arrange follow-up at 7 and 30 days after treatment to evaluate response
  - If response is not achieved, subsequent treatments may be administered

---

In this section, we discuss how to administer PDT including preparation, photosensitizer application, treatment illumination, response evaluation, and follow-up.

PRELIMINARY VISIT At the preliminary visit, the clinical diagnosis is established, or, in cases of dubious diagnosis, 3 to 4-mm punch biopsy is performed (Figs. 46-1 to 46-2). Compilation of the patient's clinical history, measurement of the two diameters of the lesions to be treated, and pretreatment photographs are also taken in this phase.

Evaluation for the presence of other lesions at different sites that may require treatment is also performed at this point in time. The patient is given verbal and

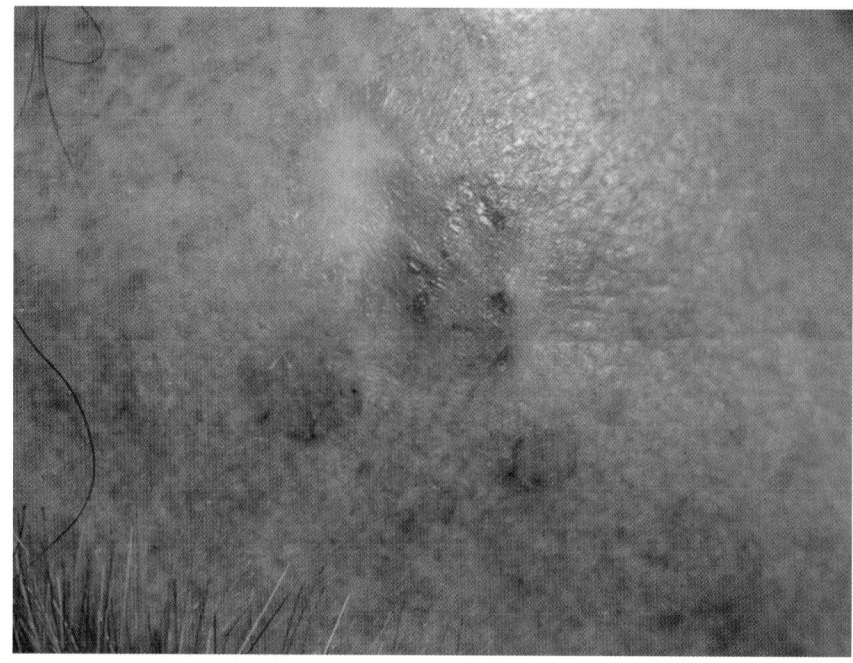

▲ **FIGURE 46-1** BCC before treatment with PDT.

written information on the PDT method, possible side effects, and the alternative therapies available. If the AK to be treated presents hyperkeratosis, scaling, or crusts, the patient must be informed that he/she must undergo curettage the same day as the PDT treatment, or use a keratolytic (5% urea cream) for some days preceding PDT. Patients with nodular, sclerodermiform, or strong pigmented BCC, patients under 18 years of age, or those allergic to peanuts are excluded from treatment (Table 46-2).

Table 46-2
What Is the Ideal Patient for PDT?

- Diagnosis of multiple and diffuse AKs
- Diagnosis of superficial BCC (sBCC)
- Multiple superficial BCCs
- Extensive large or widespread superficial BCCs
- Nevoid BCC syndrome
- Esthetically important areas
- Contraindications for surgery
- Elderly patients
- Immunosupressed patients

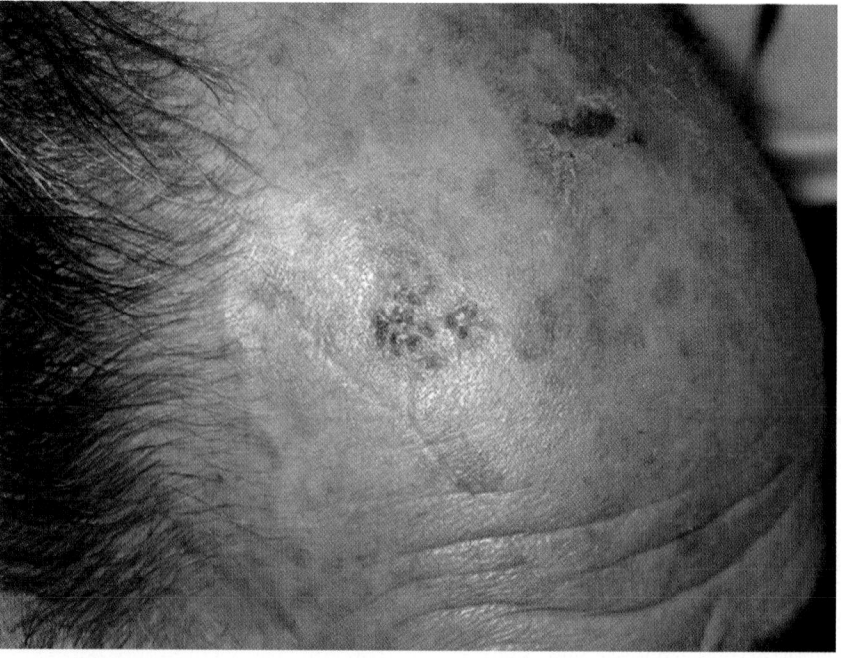

▲ **FIGURE 46-2** AK before treatment with PDT.

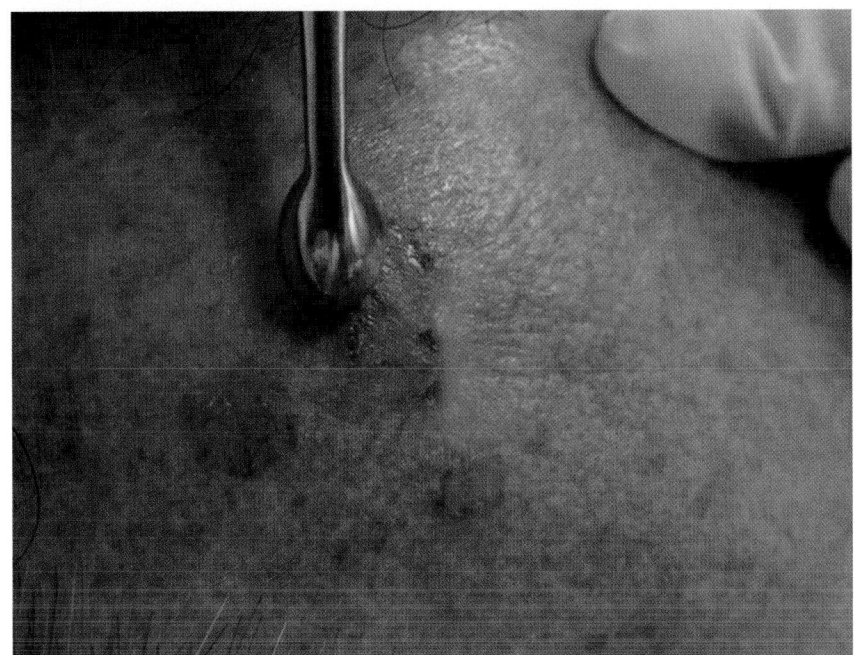

▲ **FIGURE 46-3** Curettage of the lesion before PDT treatment.

PREPARATION OF THE LESION TO BE TREATED
If a keratolytic was not used, scales and crusts that may be present are gently removed with a curette without local anesthesia (Figs. 46-3 to 46-5). In case of bleeding, apply 1% tranexamic acid, or 5% acetic acid, or 20 vol. hydrogen peroxide, or gauze under light pressure until bleeding stops. If hemostasis does not occur, postpone treatment to the following day. Apply ALA/MAL cream to the lesions with 1 to 2-mm thickness, extending the application to 5 mm outside the visible margins of the lesion (Fig. 46-6). Then, cover the treated area with polyethylene or adhesive tape (e.g., Tegaderm®, 3M Health Care, St. Paul, MN, USA; Opsite, Smith and Nephew, Hull, UK) (Figs. 46-7 to 46-8). Pay particular attention to sensitive areas (around the eyes) and curved zones (around the nose). In these cases, it is advised to reinforce the medication with a bandage such as Hypafix® (BSN Medical, GmbH&Co.Kg, Hamburg, Germany) to guarantee the best adherence of the medicine to the skin and to avoid loss of photosensitization. Next, to prevent passage of light and possible deactivation of the PpIX, cover the occluded sites with gauze or a Hypafix® type of adhesive bandage (Figs. 46-9 to 46-10).

The photosensitizer is left for an incubation period of 1 to 18 hours for ALA-PDT or 3 hours for MAL-PDT, depending on the incubation period chosen. The FDA-approved incubation period for 5-ALA-PDT treatment of AKs is 14 to 18 hours, as directed in the package insert for 5-ALA. However, in the United States, short incubation times of 1, 2, and 3 hours have been used for the treatment of AKs. A recent randomized double-blind study tested occlusion times of 1, 2, and 3 hours for 5-ALA. Results showed complete clearance in 93% of patients at 5 months follow-up with no difference associated with treatment time or with application of the cream.[33] During incubation, the patient should avoid environments under 15°C.

TREATMENT For the illumination phase, the patient should lie down in the most comfortable position possible. The bandage is removed and any exudation or excess cream on the treatment area should be removed with a gauze. Both the patient and the physician should wear protective glasses for the duration of illumination. Fluorescence examination with a light emitting diode (LED) lamp (e.g., in our experience, DICAM-UV®—Alpha Strumenti, Milan, Italy) is useful for evaluating the true extension of the lesion to be treated.

The light source should be positioned 5 to 8 cm from the skin. The recommended dose (for approval indications) is 37 J/cm² for the LED lamps (e.g., in our experience, Aktilite® PDT—Model CL128—Photocure ASA, Oslo, Norway) and 75 to 100 J/cm² using red filtered lamps (halogen, xenon, and fluorescence). The three major sources in the United States are the BLU-U (with a delivered dose of 10 J/cm² for 16 minutes and 40 s), the pulsed-dye laser (PDL), and the intense pulsed light (IPL). A red light is used to a lesser extent in the United States and more commonly in Europe.

The patient may experience a burning sensation during the first minutes of treatment. If this occurs, treatment may be interrupted and restarted a few minutes later. During treatment, the patient is asked about the intensity of pain (expressed in a visual-analog scale (VAS) from 1 to 10), which is recorded in the patient's chart.

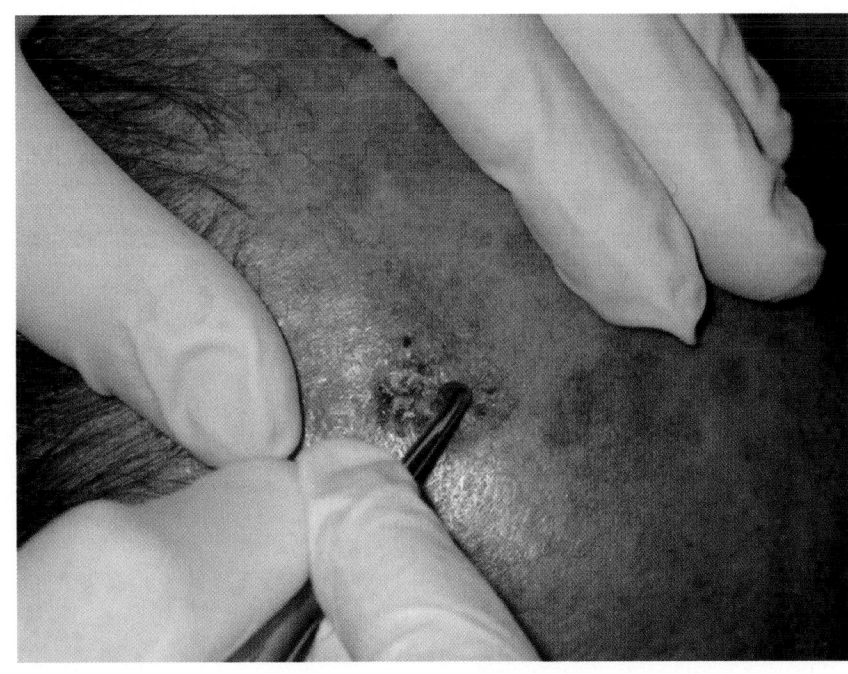

▲ **FIGURE 46-4** Curettage of the lesion before PDT treatment.

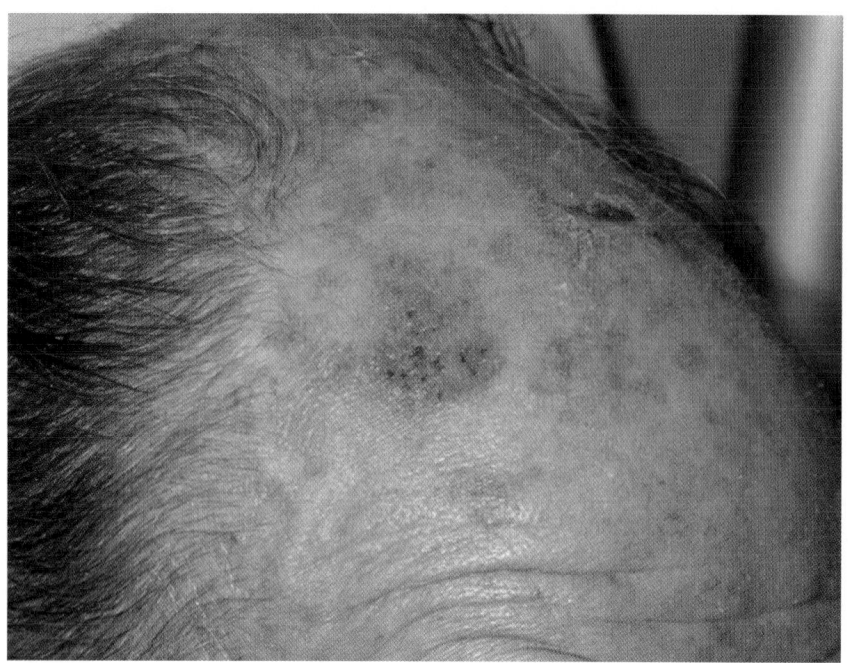

▲ **FIGURE 46-5** After curettage.

AFTER TREATMENT Immediately following treatment, the skin appears erythematous or edematous, and sometimes exudative. The skin should be medicated with antibiotic cream and covered with gauze for the next few days. The patient should be advised to avoid steroid creams or cosmetics until the skin is healed. The treated area can be washed with water and a delicate detergent daily. The patient may continue to experience a mild burning sensation in the treated area for up to 24 hours after treatment. If this is intense, the patient may take an oral analgesic. The patient should avoid sunlight or ultraviolet (UV) light until complete re-epithelization. Sero-hematic crusts may form in the treated area, but should not be removed. It is important to re-evaluate the patient 7 and 30 days afterwards and on those occasions, decide whether further treatment is necessary.

RESULTS AND RESPONSE EVALUATION In our experience, a single treatment is usually sufficient for AKs[28] (Figs. 46-11a,b to 46-12a,b). Nevertheless, a second

treatment may be given if, at follow-up, the lesion has not been removed clinically. If, after two sessions, the patient has not obtained a complete response, we suggest an alternative therapy.

All patients with BCC should receive two treatments 7 days apart (Figs. 46-13a,b to 46-18a,b). A third treatment can be carried out if the lesion is still clinically evident after 1 month. Response should be monitored clinically and histologically using punch biopsy. Clinical follow-up should be scheduled at 3 months following treatment and then every 6 months. If the lesion has not completely disappeared after three treatments, the patient should undergo alternative treatment.

Final Thoughts

ALA/MAL-PDT, administered in two consecutive treatments for therapy of AK is more efficacious and tolerable by the patients than cryotherapy and 5-fluorouracil (5-FU). The results obtained in the treatment of AK and BCC are similar to those observed with cryotherapy and surgery and are not inferior to those obtained with other therapeutic modalities such as electrosurgery, radiotherapy, or local chemosurgery with 5FU applications. However, PDT shows some important advantages: aesthetic results are excellent and the technique is not invasive, usually without bleeding and only rarely does the patient need local anesthesia (Table 46-3).

PDT is particularly useful in patients with several lesions, wide lesions, or those that are difficult to reach surgically such as those near orifices or on the face. If results are partial or in case of relapse, ALA/MAL-PDT can be repeated several

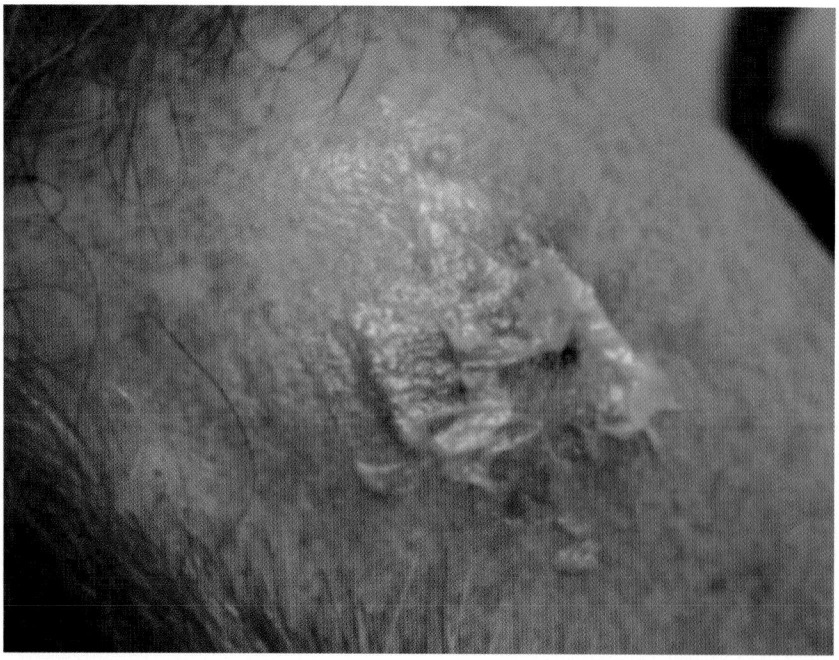

Table 46-3
PDT Advantages

- A noninvasive technique
- The ability to localize treatment
- Few side effects
- The possibility of repeating the cycle
- Comparable clinical outcome to standard treatments
- Simultaneous treatments of multiple lesions and incipient lesions
- Selectively short healing times
- Cancer control in immunocompromised patients
- Good patient tolerance
- No more expensive than conventional therapy when side-effect profile is considered
- Excellent cosmetic results
- Possible cosmetologic use

▲ **FIGURE 46-6** Application of MAL cream on the lesion.

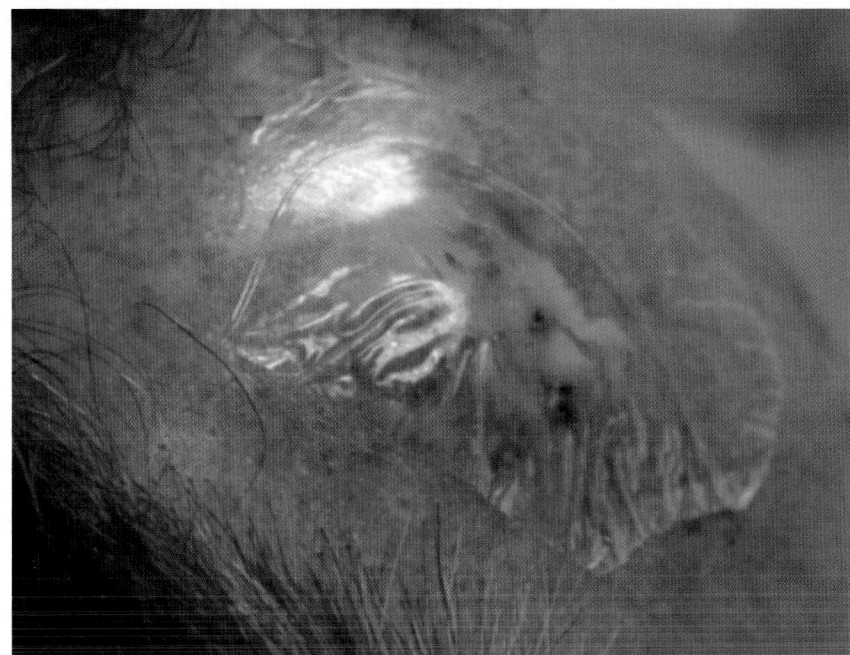

▲ **FIGURE 46-7** Covering the area with adhesive tape.

times because it does not create cumulative toxicity, nor does it preclude the use of other methods in the future. PDT has been demonstrated to be a promising treatment for a wide number of common dermatological diseases of inflammatory, infectious, or tumor origin.

Currently, other photosensitizers such as benzoporphyrins, phthalocyanines, and porphycenes have been used for topical application in some pilot studies. Their use is still experimental, but in the future, may have a role in PDT.

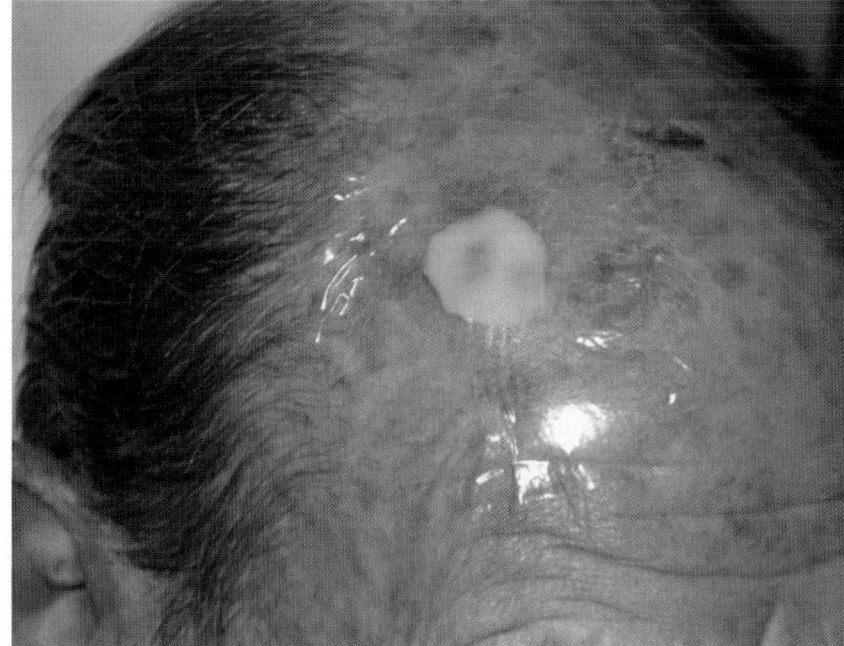

▲ **FIGURE 46-8** Covering the area with adhesive tape.

PART 2. PDT FOR INCIPIENT CUTANEOUS MALIGNANCIES: AN EVIDENCE-BASED REVIEW

Introduction

PDT use in cutaneous cancer management is thoroughly discussed and debated in the scientific literature. The literature was screened for the most recent and definitive studies. In this section, indications are first discussed, followed by a review that will cover: the type of scientific study, treatment regi-

men (with settings used), and longevity/recurrence rates.

First, it is important to note general exclusion criteria, which all reviewed studies implemented. PDT should not be used in pregnant/lactating women and patients with any type of photosensitivity, photosensitizing disease, or even recently tanned skin. Patients with previous erythema or inflammation at the treatment site must have had complete resolution of this prior to treatment or retreatment.

Clinical Efficacy of PDT for Cutaneous Malignancies: Evidence-Based Results

ACTINIC KERATOSIS

BOX 46-4   Summary

- Treatment of AKs with PDT is FDA-approved in the United States for 5-ALA with 14 to 18-hour incubation and illumination with blue light source (417 nm) at a dose of 10 J/cm² for 16 minutes and 40 s.
- Randomized, double-blind controlled studies show comparable efficacy of PDT/5-ALA versus cryosurgery or 5-FU, with better cosmetic results from PDT.
- Short incubation times (1, 2, 3 hours) for 5-ALA is being used more commonly in the United States, with studies showing similar clearance rates regardless of incubation time.
- MAL is available in Europe as a photosensitizer for PDT, while approval in the United States shows promise. Results from randomized prospective studies show equal or superior clearance rate compared to cryosurgery with MAL-PDT.

AK was the first FDA-approved indication for use of PDT for skin cancer management. Treatment works well in patients regardless of gender or age. Best responses have been noted in patients with thin lesions on the face or scalp. A patient unable to undergo or having failed other treatment options would be a good candidate. Treatment also works well in the immune-compromised. Hyperkeratotic lesions do not respond as well to PDT, and pretreatment keratolysis may be appropriate to prepare bulky lesions for treatment.[29] Patients with type IV to V skin lesions are at increased risk of postinflammatory hyperpigmentation.

AK treatment, as approved by the FDA, entails application of 5-ALA in alcohol–water to the treatment site with incubation

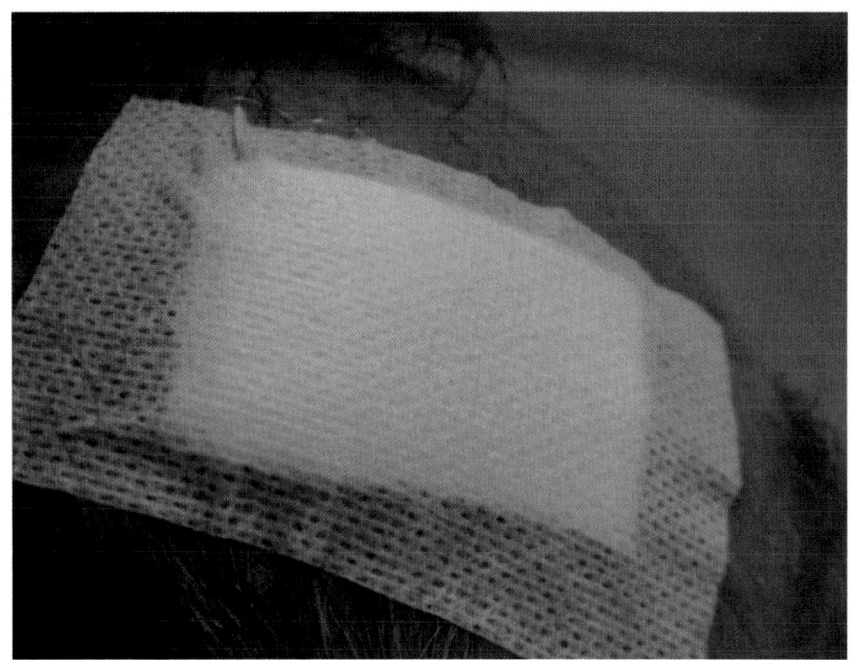

▲ **FIGURE 46-9** Covering the occlusion device of Fig. 46-7 in order to avoid passage of light.

for 14 to 18 hours. Illumination is then done with a blue light source that emits 417 nm. The delivered dose is 10 J/cm^2 administered at 10 mW/cm^2 for 16 minutes and 40 s.[29,30] Application of red light after 5-ALA application (not an FDA-approved treatment technique) can result in greater treatment efficacy, but with increased pain and healing time.

It has been suggested that AK may respond to lower doses of illumination. Although this may lead to the need for multiple treatments, it has been argued that the morbidity of each treatment would be decreased. Along these lines, the choice of light dose has been studied in a randomized, observer-blinded, intra-patient comparison that tested different doses of red light. The clearance rates at 3 months were 81% for 70 J/cm^2, 77% for 100 J/cm^2, and 69% for 140 J/cm^2. No significant difference in therapeutic efficacy was found. However, the small sample size may have been insufficient to detect a true difference.[31]

Among the many studies assessing the utility of PDT, blinded randomized controlled trials are the most convincing.

For the treatment of AK, these studies have shown significantly improved clearance compared to vehicle and light treatment. For example, an investigator-blinded, randomized, vehicle-controlled study of multiple nonhyperkeratotic AKs using 5-ALA with 14 to 18 hours occlusion prior to irradiation with blue light at 10 J/cm^2 found complete clearing of 85% of lesions after 16 weeks.[29] Similarly, a multicenter investigator-blinded study utilizing a similar protocol but irradiation with red light (630 nm, 10 J/cm^2, 10 mW/cm^2) found 73% clearance at 12 weeks, and efficacy persisted unchanged at 1-year follow-up.[30]

Studies have also examined the efficacy of AK based on anatomic location to be treated and specific treatment parameters used. A prospective study using ALA with either 3 or 14-hour occlusion and irradiation with PDL (595 nm [1 to 4 pulses], 4 to 7.5 J/cm^2) found 3-hour occlusion to be as effective as 14-hour occlusion, with 8 months later clearance rates of 90% (head), 71% (extremities), and 65% (trunk).[32] This study may have been confounded by the presence of nonresponding lesions that were later biopsy-proven to be cutaneous squamous cell carcinoma (SCC). Of note, the overall efficacy found in this study was comparable to that obtained with the use of blue light.[29] Similar results have been reproduced with short-incubation 5-ALA, suggesting side effects can be minimized by decreasing incubation time.[33]

Other studies have assessed different incubation times for ALA. A randomized double-blind study tested occlusion times of 1, 2, and 3 hours, and further attempted to use an acid mantle cream to increase ALA uptake prior to irradiation (417nm, 10 J/cm^2). Complete clearance was observed in 93% of patients at 5 months follow-up with no difference associated with treatment time or with application of the cream.[33] Another smaller study looking at 1-hour application of 5-ALA under occlusion (and comparing to 595-nm PDL) showed response rates of 80% for blue light, but only 60% for PDL. Blue light was better at improving roughness and PDL at correcting pigmentation.[34]

Smaller studies of ALA-PDT abound. The general consensus has been that PDT provides an equal or better efficacy compared to other topical medications for treatment of AK. In a small study of 14 patients, topical 5-FU was applied to one arm, while the other arm received application of 5-ALA for 4 hours prior to irradiation

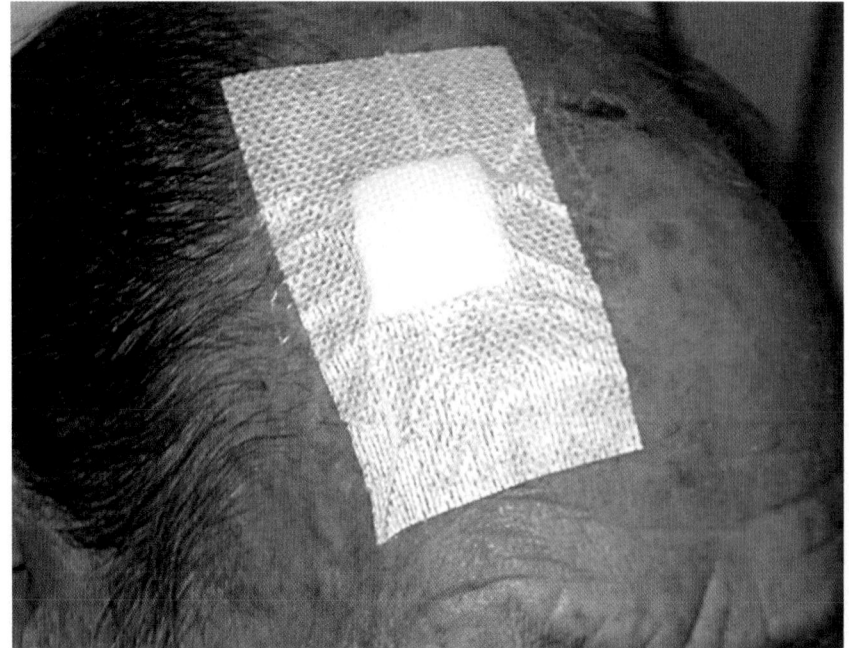

▲ **FIGURE 46-10** Covering the occlusion device of Fig. 46-8 in order to avoid passage of light.

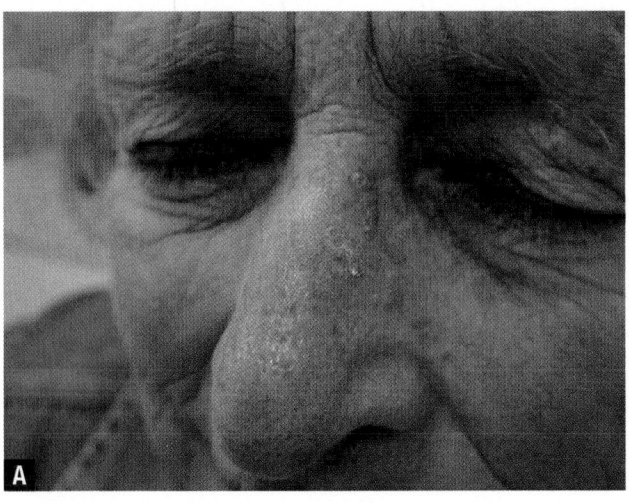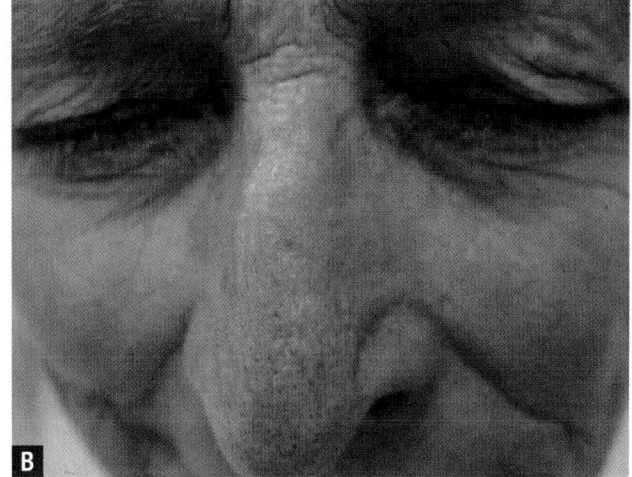

▲ **FIGURE 46-11** AK (**A**) before and (**B**) after one PDT session.

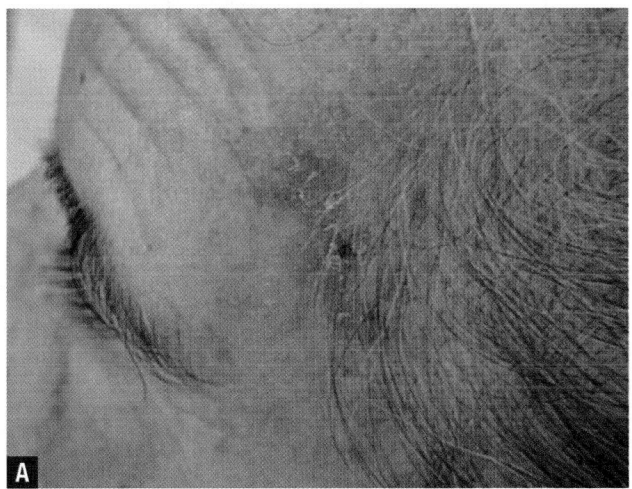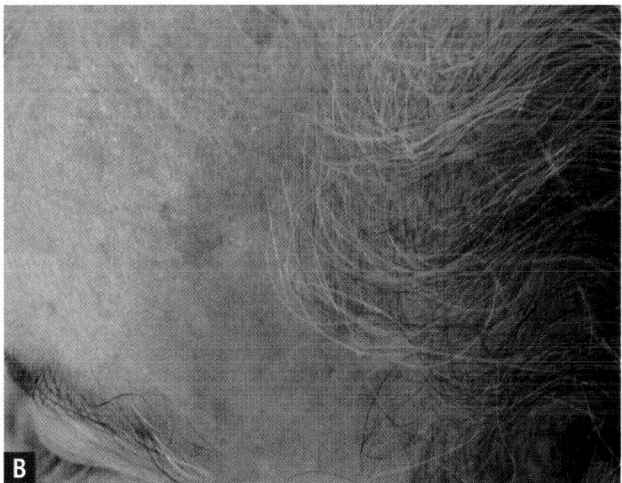

▲ **FIGURE 46-12** AK (**A**) before and (**B**) after two PDT sessions.

(580 to 740 nm, 150 J/cm^2, 86 mW/cm^2). Both treatment regimens were found to reduce the surface area that was photo-damaged by approximately 70%. Furthermore, despite the side effects of 5-FU, only minor pain after treatment was noted with PDT.[35]

With the recent advent in Europe and Asia of MAL, a modified 5-ALA, investigations focusing on this compound have commenced. Early results are promising. In a prospective multicenter randomized double-blind placebo-controlled study, lesions were pretreated with curettage and MAL was applied for 3 hours prior to irradiation (570 to 670 nm, 75 J/cm^2). Clearance was noted in 89% of MAL patients versus 38% in placebo at 3 months, and 97% had a good cosmetic outcome. Similarly, a multicenter randomized prospective study that compared MAL with 3-hour application (75 J/cm^2) to cryosurgery showed no significant difference in efficacy, but better cosmetic outcome with MAL. Notably, just 3 hours of MAL application was sufficient to provide persistent clearance to 69 to 75% of patients at 3 months.[36]

Meanwhile, the superiority of MAL to other topical modalities has been suggested by other studies. A prospective randomized study revealed that 3-hour application of MAL followed by irradiation (560 to 670 nm at 100 to 200 mW/cm) was

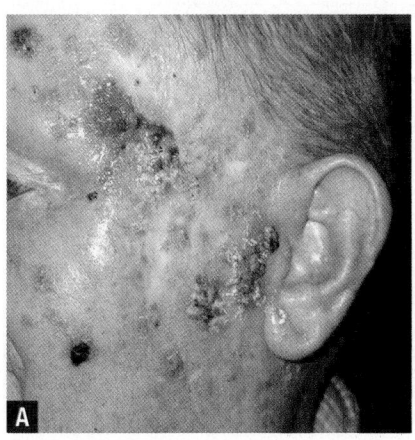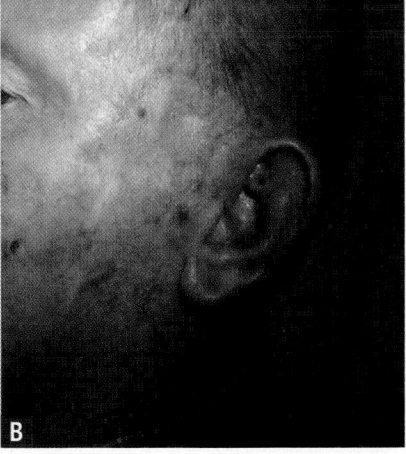

▲ **FIGURE 46-13** AKs and BCC (**A**) before and (**B**) after PDT.

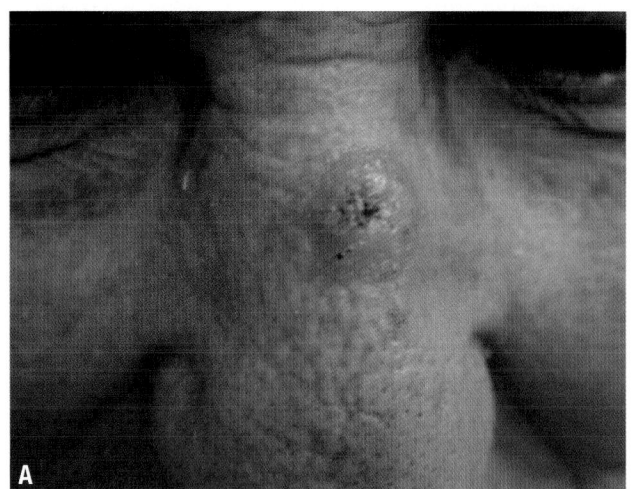
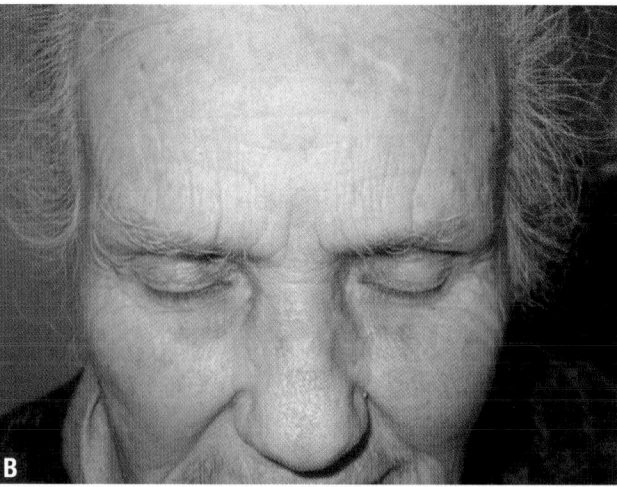

▲ **FIGURE 46-14** Nodular BCC (**A**) before and (**B**) after two PDT treatments.

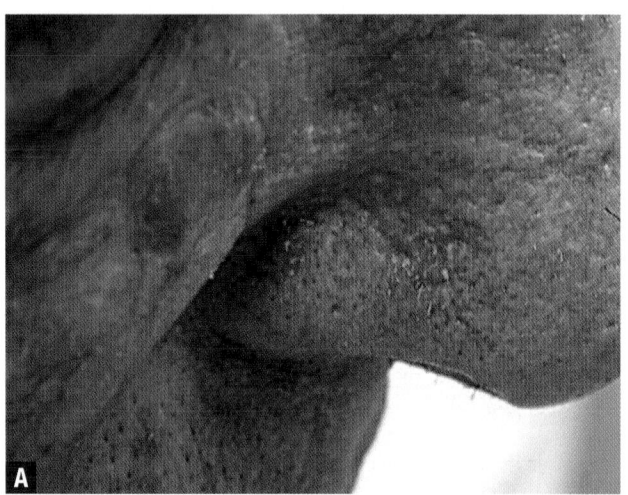
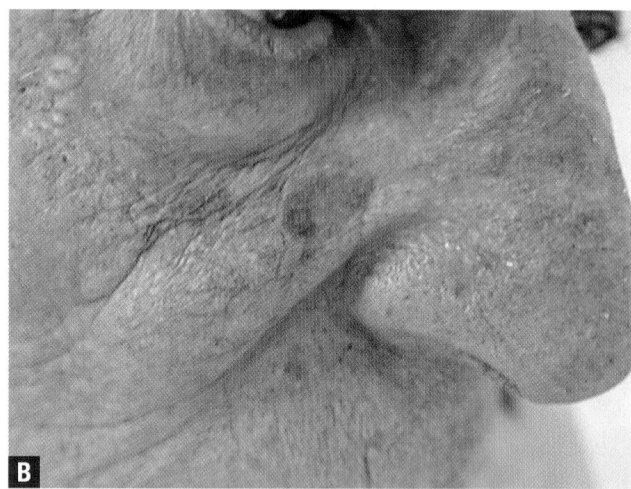

▲ **FIGURE 46-15** Superficial BCC (**A**) before and (**B**) after PDT treatment.

significantly superior to cryosurgery, with 91% versus 68% clearance. MAL was also associated with improved patient satisfaction regarding cosmesis.[37]

The clinical efficacy of MAL does not appear to be very sensitive to lesion thickness. An open-label prospective study using two spaced treatments of MAL for 3 hours each prior to light exposure (634 ± 3 nm, 37 J/cm^2) led to clearance in 89% of lesions in multilesion patients.[38]

BASAL CELL CARCINOMA

BOX 46-5 Summary

- MAL-PDT is approved for treatment of BCCs in Europe, but PDT for BCCs

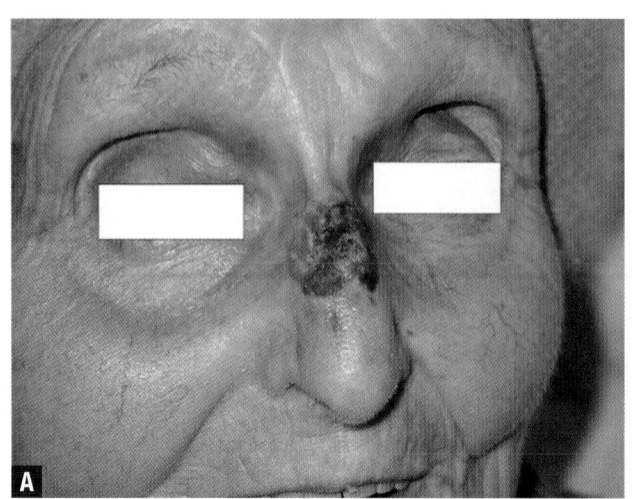
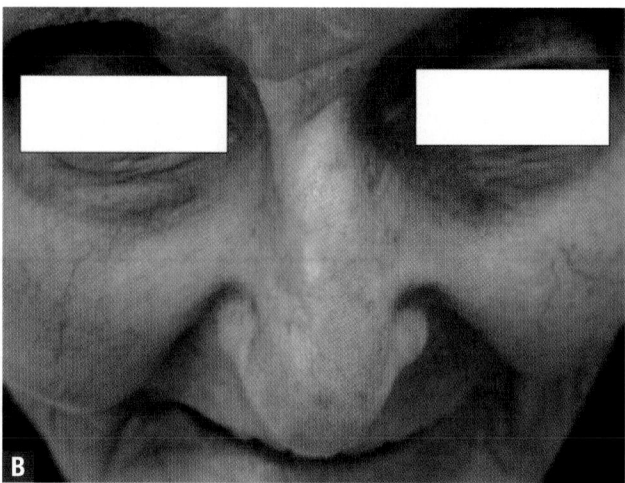

▲ **FIGURE 46-16** BCC (**A**) before and (**B**) after two PDT sessions.

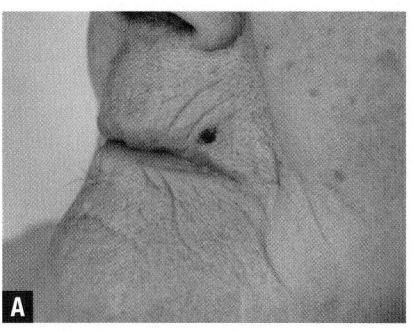 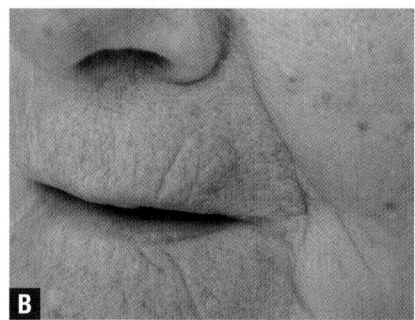

▲ **FIGURE 46-17** BCC (**A**) before and (**B**) after PDT.

is not FDA-approved in the United States.
• There is variation in response to PDT based on morphology of the BCC and thickness of the lesion.
• PDT has greatest activity against superficial BCCs with similar efficacy to cryosurgery.
• "Difficult to treat" BCCs including nodular and pigmented BCC may benefit from pretreatment regimens including debulking and penetration enhances such as EDTA.

Recently, PDT has been used to treat nonmelanoma skin cancers, in particular, BCC. MAL has been approved in Europe, Australia, and New Zealand for superficial and nodular BCC. Studies comparing ALA-PDT to 5-FU and cryosurgery for treatment of BCC have shown at least equivalent efficacy.[39] However, there is apparently great variation in the response of different morphologic types of BCC to ALA-PDT.

PDT has greatest activity against superficial BCC, with topical ALA or MAL reportedly achieving complete clearance in some cases with one treatment. Lesional thickness in susceptible tumors must be less than 3 mm. Nodular BCC, given its vertical growth and thickness, is less responsive to PDT and likely best treated by electrodessication and curettage or surgery. As discussed later, tumor debulking prior to PDT application has been attempted to

increase the cure rate of nodular BCC. Pigmented BCC is yet another therapeutic challenge for PDT since the light irradiation associated with PDT does not achieve optimal light penetration into these tumors. Similarly, morpheaform BCC tends to have wider than expected borders that militate making it more suitable for surgical extirpation.

Early studies of PDT performed over a decade ago showed clearance rates at 3 months for superficial BCC ranging from 55 to 79%, and rates of under 70% for nodular BCC.[40,41] In more recent works, persistent clearance of BCC has been reported at 3 months with persistent resolution maintained at 36 months followup. Treatments involved either one-time application or one cycle with two applications 7 days apart. Average clearance rate was 87% in superficial BCC and 53% in nodular BCC.[39,42,43] A prospective phase III trial compared 5-ALA incubated for 6 hours before irradiation (635 nm, 60 J/cm^2, 80 mW/cm^2) to cryosurgery. Biopsy studies showed postcryosurgery recurrence at 15% and ALA-associated recurrence at 25%, with no statistically significant difference between these two rates.[44] In a prospective comparative multicenter phase III study, superficial BCC treated with MAL and irradiated (570 to 670 nm, 75 J/cm^2) was again compared to cryosurgery. Three-year clearance after application of the two modalities was 78% and 81%, respectively.[39] In short, studies to date have found that PDT is

approximately equal in efficacy to other minimally invasive topical modalities for treatment of superficial BCC.

In an open-label, uncontrolled, prospective multicenter study of BCC, MAL treatment achieved 85% clearance of superficial BCC, and 75% of nodular BCC, at 3 months. At 24 months, overall clearance of BCC was 78% with near-100% satisfaction with cosmetic outcome.[45] In smaller studies, similar optimistic results have been reported, with superficial lesions showing near-100% clearance after 3 hours of incubation with 5-ALA followed by irradiation (630 nm, 120 J/cm^2, 50 mW/cm^2).[46]

Therapeutic use of PDT has also been assessed for morphologically complex BCC. In the so-called "difficult to treat" BCC, a prospective multicenter noncomparative study found that 3 hours of MAL followed by light exposure (570 to 670 nm, 75 J/cm^2) induced clearance for 2 years in 76% of lesions. The term "difficult to treat" lesions was used to describe lesions with poor outcome potential, for example, lesions in locations with poor healing response, and lesions with predisposition for poor cosmetic outcome. Truncal (88%) tumors responded better than those on the head (54%).[47] For nodular BCC, a study comparing MAL to placebo treatment in a randomized double-blind controlled design[48] noted a 6-month clearance rate of 73% in the MAL group versus 21% in the placebo group. Another multicenter randomized trial of the effect of MAL on nodular BCC compared MAL application for 3 hours occlusion prior to light exposure (570 to 670 nm, 75 J/cm^2, 50 to 200 mW/cm^2) to surgical excision with 5-mm margin. One-year clearance was noted to be 85% for MAL versus 98% for excision. Again, significantly better cosmesis was noted after use of PDT with MAL compared to excision.[49]

Regarding long-term follow-up, a retrospective study examined lesions 35 months after treatment. The initial treatment protocol entailed application of MAL for 3 or 24 hours prior to light irradiation (570 to 670 nm, 50 to 200 J/cm^2, 100 to 180 mW/cm^2), and clearance 3 years later was as high as 92% in selected cases.[50]

BCC can have a more complex pathology and shape than AK. To overcome the hurdles involved with treatment of BCC of various morphologies, pretreatment regimens have been used to improve results with thicker tumors. For example, in a small prospective study, 3 weeks after debulking of the tumor, 5-ALA was applied for 6 hours

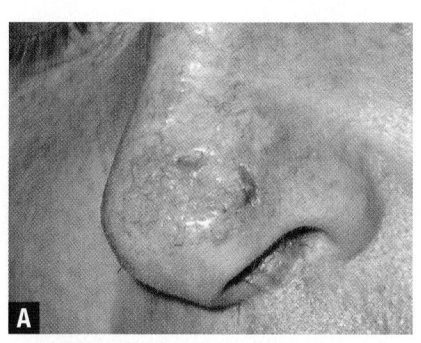 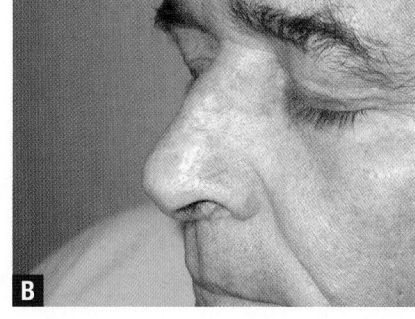

▲ **FIGURE 46-18** BCC (**A**) before and (**B**) after PDT.

and then irradiated (630 nm, 120 J/cm^2, 100 mW/cm^2), with results showing over 90% clearance at 3 months.[51] Studies have also been published supporting the effectiveness of PDT for both superficial and nodular BCC, although it was noted that with nodular BCC, appropriate pretreatment preparation and a subsequent retreatment after 7 days is required.[50] Penetration enhancers, such as ethylenediaminetetraacetic acid (EDTA) and dimethyl sulfoxide (DMSO), have also been suggested as treatment intensifiers, but have seldom been used or found to be worthwhile.[52,53]

BOWEN DISEASE (SQUAMOUS CELL CARCINOMA *IN SITU*)

> **BOX 46-6   Summary**
>
> - Given the superficial nature of SCC *in situ*, PDT shows promise as a first-line treatment for multiple or large-lesion SCC *in situ*, those that are inoperable or expected to heal poorly.
> - For invasive SCC *in situ*, PDT may be used as adjuvant therapy in combination with surgical treatment.
> - Early randomized, controlled studies comparing MAL-PDT to 5-FU and cryosurgery showed similar efficacy between treatment choices.

Bowen disease, due to its superficial nature, has been one of the cutaneous malignancies for which PDT has been considered most promising. The literature suggests PDT may be a first-line treatment for SCC *in situ* that manifests as large and/or multiple lesions, is inoperable, or occurs in areas expected to heal poorly. Conversely, for Bowen disease with an invasive component, PDT may be used as adjuvant therapy in combination with more definitive surgical treatment.[54] A series of studies have shown PDT to be at least as or more effective than some other topical therapies for Bowen disease.

A multicenter randomized controlled study comparing MAL-PDT to 5-FU and cryosurgery found 12-month clearance of 74%, 65%, and 62%, respectively.[55] The MAL treatment arm was thus found to be no less effective than the alternative choices. Another multicenter randomized study using ALA with 4-hour application and repeat treatment as required (630 nm, 100 J/cm^2, 50 to 90 mW/cm^2) observed that at 1 year there was an 82% clearance with PDT compared to 48% clearance in a 5-FU treated

group. This difference was statistically significant.[56] A prospective study using ALA applied for 4 hours before light (630 nm, 100 J/cm^2, 70 mW/cm^2) noted complete clearance of 80% of lesions at 1 year and suggested efficacy at least equal to that of cryosurgery.[57]

INVASIVE SQUAMOUS CELL CANCER

> **BOX 46-7   Summary**
>
> - Due to potentially aggressive and penetrating nature of invasive SCC, PDT should not be used for treatment.
> - High recurrence rates with PDT or metastasis is possible.
> - Surgical removal remains the treatment of choice.

Due to the potentially aggressive and deeply penetrating nature of this cancer, it was promising to see initial studies that showed clearance of 50 to 100% of lesions. However, recurrence was noted in as many as 70% of cases. Given the high recurrence rate and the potential for metastatic spread in cases of inadequate treatment, PDT should not be used for treatment of invasive SCC. There are sporadic reports that intralesional injections of PDT followed by irradiation may be of some therapeutic utility in invasive SCC, but this approach is not at present, and may never be, appropriate for use in a clinical setting. At present, PDT may be used for field treatment of peripheral superficial SCC (Bowen disease) that is left behind after surgical removal of invasive SCC.[39]

OTHER USES

> **BOX 46-8   Summary**
>
> - Although other cutaneous neoplasms could theoretically be treated with PDT, there are no systematic studies to date given the rarity of these diseases.
> - PDT/5-ALA has been used to treat extramammary Paget's disease in one retrospective study with complete clearance in 31% of lesions at 12 months.
> - PDT/5-ALA successfully treated CTCL without recurrence in one case report.

Theoretically, a variety of cutaneous neoplasms may be susceptible to PDT. However, the rarity of these has precluded systematic study. For example, there are reports regarding the use of PDT for extramammary Paget's disease (EMPD)[58] and

cutaneous T-cell lymphoma (CTCL).[59] A retrospective study on EMPD using 5-ALA in repeat applications of 0 to 4-hour duration prior to light (500 to 790 nm, 200 to 400 J/cm^2, 18 to 150 mW/cm^2) noted complete clearance of 31% of lesions at 12 months. This study noted a possible relation between likelihood of clearance and the diameter of the lesion; unfortunately, the results of this series were clouded by the inclusion of several cases that had failed prior therapy with alternate approaches.[60] A case report of treatment of CTCL that used a regimen of 6 hours of 5-ALA applied repeatedly for four treatments (630 nm, 100 J/cm^2, 48 mW/cm^2) noted complete clearance without recurrence at 12 months.[61]

IMMUNE-COMPROMISED It is widely accepted that an intact immune response is central to controlling neoplasm progression.[62,63] While the application of PDT for the treatment of cutaneous neoplasms in the immune-compromised is an important potential application, the efficacy of PDT in these patients has thus far not appeared promising.[64]

Safety and Management of Complications

> **BOX 46-9   Summary**
>
> - Because skin contact is limited to a few hours, the morbidity and side effects of topical PDT are diminished compared to topical chemotherapies.
> - Side effects include burning, pruritis, desquamation, crusting, edema, and erythema, but usually clear within 24 hours of treatment, rarely lasting longer than 1 to 2 weeks.
> - Scarring, ulceration, and infection due to PDT have not been reported.
> - To manage side effects, cold air can be used during PDT treatment.
> - Bland emollients and avoidance of sun exposure for 48 to 72 hours can also reduce symptoms.
> - There have been no reports of malignant transformation due to PDT.

Unlike topical chemotherapy, topical PDT application is not a protracted treatment, with skin contact lasting a few hours to a day rather than many weeks or months. Consequently, morbidity and side effects with PDT are diminished relative to those with topical chemotherapies, such as 5-FU, imiquimod, and diclofenac sodium. Treatment-associated discomfort is also usually limited, with burning, pruritis, desquamation, crusting, edema, erythema, and pain diminishing within 24 hours of treatment. In most cases, symptoms and signs clear entirely within 1 to 2 weeks. Usually the last manifestations to resolve are mild erythema and edema limited to the treated region that is followed by a minimally noticeable, dry necrosis that lasts no more than 3 weeks from the time of treatment. Pigment changes are temporary, with occasional hair loss, but no irreversible alopecia. Scarring, ulceration, or infection are not reported. On the other hand, consistently satisfactory cosmetic results are regularly noted by investigators.[39]

A few studies have addressed management of the minor side effects associated with PDT. For example, decreased symptoms may be achieved with concurrent cold air analgesia at the time of initial treatment.[65] MAL was also observed to induce less pain than 5-ALA in certain studies.[66] In general, emolliation with a bland moisturizer for several days after treatment and strict light avoidance for 48 to 72 hours after treatment is sufficient to induce rapid resolution of edema and erythema.

It is not yet known if PDT can induce malignant transformation. Studies have shown no carcinogenic potential or even delayed onset of neoplasia.[67,68] However, PDT should be used with caution in patients with basal cell nevus syndrome, xeroderma pigmentosum, and other genetic syndromes predisposing to cutaneous malignancies.

Treatment Recommendations in the Context of Data Limitations

BOX 46-10 Summary

- PDT has shown to be effective for treatment of AKs, but PDT for superficial BCC and SCC *in situ* is unclear. PDT should never be used for invasive SCC.
- "Short-contact" PDT, while convenient, has uncertain long-term outcomes. Results appear satisfactory, but rates of recurrence are yet to be determined.
- Patients treated with PDT for AKs do not necessarily have better clearance rates than with cryosurgery or topical chemotherapies, but patients that are unresponsive to cryotherapy, who have extensive photodamage, and who are unable to tolerate the length of topical chemotherapy treatment are good candidates for treatment with ALA-PDT.
- Cosmetic photorejuvenation of photodamaged skin can be enhanced by the addition of 5-ALA, especially in combination with intense pulsed light or PDL.

PDT is a valuable new therapy for incipient cutaneous malignancies, but must be used judiciously. Studies to date have indicated efficacy for the treatment of AK, but the utility of PDT for superficial BCC and SCC *in situ* is unclear, and PDT should not be used for invasive SCC.

One problem is that methodologic limitations in clinical studies have been severe and have undermined the most optimistic pronouncements. Many, if not most, studies have not had double-blind, randomized control design with comparison to extant standard-of-care therapies, rather than placebo. Moreover, coauthors in most studies have had significant conflicts of interest, including consulting arrangements and other financial ties with the manufacturer of 5-ALA. More significantly, outcome measures have not been systematically defined. Neither the so-called "tumor lesions" nor their "complete clearance" is routinely verified by biopsy: the careful reader is unsure if there was a tumor there to begin with, and if so, if it has truly resolved after treatment. Second, follow-up is usually inadequate in duration, thus leaving unanswered the question whether "resolution" is merely a medium-term remission induced by temporary inflammation, and whether the partially obscured lesion will re-emerge at the same site a few months later. The inception of "short-contact" PDT, which involves as little as 30 to 60-min incubation with 5-ALA prior to irradiation, is convenient for patients and physicians, but also has uncertain long-term outcomes. While short-term efficacy with short-contact ALA-PDT for AK appears satisfactory, it is possible that the associated remission may be less long-lasting than with longer incubation.

Even the most promising efficacy statistics must be seen in context. Resolution of 75 to 80% of lesions of AK with ALA-PDT is not better than the efficacy of spray cryotherapy, properly applied; cryotherapy is also less time consuming and more cost-effective. Similarly, cure rates of less than 75% for superficial BCC are comparable to those with cryotherapy, and far inferior to those with electrodessication and curettage, which can clear 90% of lesions. Indeed, not only is surgical excision much more effective than even electrodessication, but Mohs surgery, the standard of care for invasive tumors of the head and neck, has cure rates in excess of 98%.

The observation that PDT results in superior cosmesis compared to other modalities is also an incomplete thought. Tissue-sparing modalities like Mohs, by minimizing the size of the final wound defect, can permit excellent

cosmesis. Also, when BCC treated with PDT recurs, subsequent treatment by another modality is likely to create a larger defect that is more cumbersome to repair and less cosmetically satisfying.

These caveats notwithstanding, PDT has a role in the treatment of AK. Specifically, patients unresponsive to cryotherapy, who have extensive photodamage, and whose lives preclude the 8 to 12 weeks of facial inflammation associated with topical chemotherapeutics, are good candidates for treatment with ALA-PDT. The short recovery time of approximately 1 week is usually well-tolerated, and patients can be retreated, if necessary. As such, PDT may be comparable in efficacy to other treatment techniques for AK, but in select cases may be more compatible with preserving quality of life. PDT may also be of use in patients with numerous superficial BCCs; in this population, PDT, like the topical chemotherapeutics, may induce a field effect that reduces the tumor burden so that the residual invasive or resistant lesions can be treated by more definitive therapies. Finally, cosmetic photorejuvenation of photodamaged skin can be enhanced with the addition of 5-ALA. In combination with intense pulsed light or PDL, 5-ALA can reduce the visible signs of aging, including pigmentary abnormality and textural roughness.

5-ALA is most effectively activated by blue light, red light, broad-spectrum intense pulsed light, or ambient light. Significantly, outdoor ambient light or indoor bright incandescent illumination can be sufficient to induce effect and is often less time-consuming and inconvenient for patients.

Finally, it should be noted that MAL is not approved in the United States for any indication and should not be used in this country. At present, clinical use of PDT in the United States is limited to ALA-PDT. While the standard regimen of ALA-PDT entails use of prepackaged applicator sticks of 5-ALA with blue light irradiation, other formulations of 5-ALA (e.g., from compounding pharmacies) as well as other light sources are available and routinely used off-label.

Final Thoughts

PDT is a relatively young modality for treatment of incipient cutaneous malignancy and photodamaged skin. Recent literature highlights the progress achieved. Increasing availability and decreasing costs for this therapy are making it available for more patients with widespread AK. Over time, modifications in the method of application of prodrugs and light sources are likely to continue to optimize this treatment.

Future research will need to focus on the long-term efficacy of ALA-PDT for AK and photodamage. It will need to be confirmed that ALA-PDT is at least as effective as cryotherapy in promoting cure of AK that persists for years after treatment. Additionally, future studies may also assess the role of oxygenation, which has been inadequately studied. Specifically, while activation of PDT is contingent on light and oxygen, in clinical studies to date light-associated parameters have been varied routinely, but local oxygen content was not. Monitoring local oxygen levels may help exclude the potentially confounding effects of anemia,[69] and hypeoxygenation may increase the therapeutic efficacy of PDT.[70,71]

REFERENCES

1. Daniell MD, Hill JS. A history of photodynamic therapy. *Aust N Z J Surg*. 1991;61(5): 340–348.
2. Lopez RF, Lange N, Guy R, Bentley MV. Photodynamic therapy of skin cancer: Controlled drug delivery of 5-ALA and its esters. *Adv Drug Deliv Rev*. 2004;56(1): 77–94.
3. Dougherty TJ, Gomer CJ, Henderson BW, Jori G, Kessel D, Korbelik M. Photodynamic therapy. *J Natl Cancer Inst*. 1998; 90(12):889–905.
4. Nowis D, Makowski M, Stoklosa T, Legat M, Issat T, Golab J. Direct tumor damage mechanisms of photodynamic therapy. *Acta Biochim Pol*. 2005;52(2):339–352.
5. Shimizu K, Asai T, Oku N. Antineovascular therapy, a novel antiangiogenic approach. *Expert Opin Ther Targets*. 2005; 9(1):63–76.
6. Kongshaug M. Minireview: Distribution of tetrapyrrole photosensitizers among human plasma proteins. *Int J Biochem*. 1992;24:1239–1265.
7. Kessel D, Woodburn K. Biodistribution of photosensitizing agents. *Int J Biochem*. 1993;25:1377–1383.
8. Kessel D, Thompson P, Saatio K, Nantwi KD. Tumor localisation and photosensitization by sulfonated derivatives of tetraphenylporphine. *Photochem Photobiol*. 1993; 45:787–791.
9. Dougherty J, Gomer CJ, Henderson BW, et al. Review: Photodynamic therapy. *J Natl Cancer Inst*. 1998;90:889–905.
10. Moan J, Berg K. The photodegradation of porphyrins in cells can be used to estimate the lifetime of singlet oxygen. *Photochem Photobiol*. 1991;53:549–553.
11. Levy JC, Obochi M. New application in photodynamic therapy: Introduction. *Photochem Photobiol*. 1996;64:737–739.
12. Leibovici L, Schoenfeld N, Yehoshua HA, et al. Activity of porphobilinogen deaminase in peripheral blood mononuclear cells of patients with metastatic cancer. *Cancer*. 1988;62(11):2297–2300.
13. Sano M, Furuta T, Takahira K, et al. Cell-cycle-dependent efficacy of photody-

namic therapy with ATX-S10(Na). *Lasers Med Sci*. 2005;20(1):1–5.
14. Webber J, Kessel D, Fromm D. Plasma levels of protoporphyrin IX in humans after oral administration of 5-aminolevulinic acid. *J Photochem Photobiol B, Biol*. 1997; 37(1–2):151–153.
15. Gaullier JM, Berg K, Peng Q, et al. Use of 5-aminolevulinic acid esters to improve photodynamic therapy on cells in culture. *Cancer Res*. 1997;57:1481–1486.
16. Kloek J, Van Henegouwen GMJB. Prodrugs of 5-aminolevulinic acid for photodynamic therapy. *Photochem Photobiol*. 1996;64: 994–1000.
17. Washbrook R, Fukuda H, Battle A, Riley P. Stimulation of tetrapyrrole synthesis in mammalian epithelial cells in culture by exposure to aminolevulinic acid. *Br J Cancer*. 1997;75:381–387.
18. Becker DM, Kramer S, Viljoen JD. Delta-aminolevulinic acid uptake by rabbit brain cerebral cortex. *J Neurochem*. 1974; 23:1019–1023.
19. Uehlinger P, Zellweger M, Wagnieres G, Juillerat-Jeanneret L, Van der Bergh H, Lange N. 5-aminolevulinic acid and 1st derivatives: Physical chemical properties and protoporphyrin IX formation in cultured cells. *J Photochem Photobiol B, Biol*. 2000;54:72–80.
20. Casas A, Batle AMD, Butler AR, et al. Comparative effect of ALA derivatives on protoporphyrin IX production in human and rat skin organ cultures. *Br J Cancer*. 1999;80:1525–1532.
21. Peng Q, Moan J, Warloe T, et al. Build up of esterified aminolevulinic-acid-derivative-induced porphyrin fluorescence in normal mouse skin. *J Photochem Photobiol B, Biol*. 1996;34:95–96.
22. Fritsch C, Homey B, Stahl W, Lehmann P, Ruzicka T, Sies H. Preferential relative porphyrin enrichment in solar keratoses upon topical application of 5-aminolevulinic acid methylester. *Photochem Photobiol*. 2000; 71:640–647.
23. Rossi R, Lotti T, Cappugi P, et al. Guidelines for photodynamic therapy in dermatology: Treatment protocol. *G Ital Dermatol Venereol*. 2005;140:637–644.
24. Morton CA. Methyl aminolevulinate (Metvix) photodynamic therapy—practical pearls. *J Dermatol Treat*. 2003;14:23–26.
25. Soler AM, Warloe T, Berner A, Giercksky KE. A follow-up study of recurrence and cosmesis in completely responding superficial and nodular basal cell carcinomas treated with methyl 5-aminolevulinate-based photodynamic therapy alone and with prior curettage. *Br J Dermatol*. 2001; 145:467–471.
26. Horn M, Wolf P, Wulf HC, et al. Topical methyl aminolevulinate photodynamic therapy in patients with basal cell carcinoma prone to complications and poor cosmetic outcome with conventional treatment. *Br J Dermatol*. 2003;149:1242–1249.
27. Basset-Seguin N, Ibbotson S, Emtestam L. Photodynamic therapy using Metvix is as efficacious as cryotherapy in BCC, with better cosmetic results. *J Eur Acad Dermatol Venereol*. 15(S2):226.
28. Rossi R, Mavilia L, Ghersetich I, Lotti T. Photodynamic therapy of actinic keratoses with methyl-aminolevulinate (Metvix). *G Ital Dermatol Venereol*. 2005;140(4):381–387.

29. Jeffes EW, McCullough JL, Weinstein GD, Kaplan R, Glazer SD, Taylor JR. Photodynamic therapy of actinic keratoses with topical aminolevulinic acid hydrochloride and fluorescent blue light. *J Am Acad Dermatol*. 2001;45(1): 96–104.
30. Piacquadio DJ, Chen DM, Farber HF, et al. Photodynamic therapy with aminolevulinic acid topical solution and visible blue light in the treatment of multiple actinic keratoses of the face and scalp: Investigator-blinded, phase 3, multicenter trials. *Arch Dermatol*. 2004;140(1): 41–46.
31. Radakovic-Fijan S, Blecha-Thalhammer U, Kittler H, Honigsmann H, Tanew A. Efficacy of 3 different light doses in the treatment of actinic keratosis with 5-aminolevulinic acid photodynamic therapy: A randomized, observer-blinded, intrapatient, comparison study. *J Am Acad Dermatol*. 2005;53(5):823–827.
32. Alexiades-Armenakas MR, Geronemus RG. Laser-mediated photodynamic therapy of actinic keratoses. *Arch Dermatol*. 2003;139(10):1313–1320.
33. Touma D, Yaar M, Whitehead S, Konnikov N, Gilchrest BA. A trial of short incubation, broad-area photodynamic therapy for facial actinic keratoses and diffuse photodamage. *Arch Dermatol*. 2004;140(1):33–40.
34. Smith S, Piacquadio D, Morhenn V, Atkin D, Fitzpatrick R. Short incubation PDT versus 5-FU in treating actinic keratoses. *J Drugs Dermatol*. 2003;2(6):629–635.
35. Kurwa HA, Yong-Gee SA, Seed PT, Markey AC, Barlow RJ. A randomized paired comparison of photodynamic therapy and topical 5-fluorouracil in the treatment of actinic keratoses. *J Am Acad Dermatol*. 1999;41(3 Pt 1):414–418.
36. Szeimies RM, Karrer S, Radakovic-Fijan S, et al. Photodynamic therapy using topical methyl 5-aminolevulinate compared with cryotherapy for actinic keratosis: A prospective, randomized study. *J Am Acad Dermatol*. 2002;47(2):258–262.
37. Freeman M, Vinciullo C, Francis D, et al. A comparison of photodynamic therapy using topical methyl aminolevulinate (Metvix) with single cycle cryotherapy in patients with actinic keratosis: A prospective, randomized study. *J Dermatolog Treat*. 2003;14(2):99–106.
38. Tarstedt M, Rosdahl I, Berne B, Svanberg K, Wennberg AM. A randomized multicenter study to compare two treatment regimens of topical methyl aminolevulinate (Metvix)-PDT in actinic keratosis of the face and scalp. *Acta Derm Venereol*. 2005; 85(5):424–428.
39. Morton CA, Brown SB, Collins S, et al. Guidelines for topical photodynamic therapy: Report of a workshop of the British Photodermatology Group. *Br J Dermatol*. 2002;146(4):552–567.
40. Kennedy JC, Pottier RH, Pross DC. Photodynamic therapy with endogenous protoporphyrin IX: Basic principles and present clinical experience. *J Photochem Photobiol B, Biol*. 1990;6(1–2):143–148.
41. Svanberg K, Andersson T, Killander D, et al. Photodynamic therapy of nonmelanoma malignant tumours of the skin using topical delta-amino levulinic acid sensitization and laser irradiation. *Br J Dermatol*. 1994;130(6):743–751.

42. Zeitouni NC, Oseroff AR, Shieh S. Photodynamic therapy for nonmelanoma skin cancers. Current review and update. *Mol Immunol.* 2003;39(17–18):1133–1136.

43. Szeimies RM, Morton CA, Sidoroff A, Braathen LR. Photodynamic therapy for non-melanoma skin cancer. *Acta Derm Venereol.* 2005;85(6):483–490.

44. Wang I, Bendsoe N, Klinteberg CA, et al. Photodynamic therapy vs. cryosurgery of basal cell carcinomas: Results of a phase III clinical trial. *Br J Dermatol.* 2001; 144(4):832–840.

45. Horn M, Wolf P, Wulf HC, et al. Topical methyl aminolaevulinate photodynamic therapy in patients with basal cell carcinoma prone to complications and poor cosmetic outcome with conventional treatment. *Br J Dermatol.* 2003;149(6): 1242–1249.

46. Haller JC, Cairnduff F, Slack G, et al. Routine double treatments of superficial basal cell carcinomas using aminolaevulinic acid-based photodynamic therapy. *Br J Dermatol.* 2000;143(6): 1270–1275.

47. Vinciullo C, Elliott T, Francis D, et al. Photodynamic therapy with topical methyl aminolaevulinate for "difficult-to-treat" basal cell carcinoma. *Br J Dermatol.* 2005;152(4):765–772.

48. Foley P. Clinical efficacy of methyl aminolaevulinate photodynamic therapy in basal cell carcinoma and solar keratosis. *Aust J Dermatol.* 2005;46(suppl):S8–S10; discussion S23–S25.

49. Rhodes LE, de Rie M, Enstrom Y, et al. Photodynamic therapy using topical methyl aminolevulinate vs. surgery for nodular basal cell carcinoma: Results of a multicenter randomized prospective trial. *Arch Dermatol.* 2004;140(1):17–23.

50. Soler AM, Warloe T, Berner A, Giercksky KE. A follow-up study of recurrence and cosmesis in completely responding superficial and nodular basal cell carcinomas treated with methyl 5-aminolaevulinate-based photodynamic therapy alone and with prior curettage. *Br J Dermatol.* 2001;145(3):467–471.

51. Thissen MR, Schroeter CA, Neumann HA. Photodynamic therapy with delta-aminolaevulinic acid for nodular basal cell carcinomas using a prior debulking technique. *Br J Dermatol.* 2000;142(2): 338–339.

52. De Rosa FS, Tedesco AC, Lopez RF, et al. *In vitro* skin permeation and retention of 5-aminolevulinic acid ester derivatives for photodynamic therapy. *J Control Release.* 2003;89(2):261–269.

53. Ziolkowski P, Osiecka BJ, Oremek G, et al. Enhancement of photodynamic therapy by use of aminolevulinic acid/glycolic acid drug mixture. *J Exp Ther Oncol.* 2004;4(2):121–129.

54. Taub AF. Photodynamic therapy in dermatology: History and horizons. *J Drugs Dermatol.* 2004;3(suppl 1):S8–S25.

55. Morton CA, Horn M, Leman J, et al. A placebo controlled European study comparing MAL-PDT with cryosurgery and 5-FU in Bowen's disease. *J Eur Acad Dermatol Venerol.* 2004; 18(suppl 2):415.

56. Salim A, Leman JA, McColl JH, Chapman R, Morton CA. Randomized comparison of photodynamic therapy with topical 5-fluorouracil in Bowen's disease. *Br J Dermatol.* 2003;148(3):539–543.

57. Morton CA, Whitehurst C, Moseley H, McColl JH, Moore JV, Mackie RM. Comparison of photodynamic therapy with cryotherapy in the treatment of Bowen's disease. *Br J Dermatol.* 1996;135 (5):766–771.

58. Mikasa K, Watanabe D, Kondo C, et al. 5-Aminolevulinic acid-based photodynamic therapy for the treatment of two patients with extramammary Paget's disease. *J Dermatol.* 2005;32(2):97–101.

59. Coors EA, von den Driesch P. Topical photodynamic therapy for patients with therapy-resistant lesions of cutaneous T-cell lymphoma. *J Am Acad Dermatol.* 2004;50(3):363–367.

60. Shieh S, Dee AS, Cheney RT, Frawley NP, Zeitouni NC, Oseroff AR. Photodynamic therapy for the treatment of extramammary Paget's disease. *Br J Dermatol.* 2002;146(6):1000–1005.

61. Leman JA, Dick DC, Morton CA. Topical 5-ALA photodynamic therapy for the treatment of cutaneous T-cell lymphoma. *Clin Exp Dermatol.* 2002;27(6): 516–518.

62. Rashid RM, Achille NJ, Lee JM, Lathers DM, Young MR. Decreased T-cell proliferation and skewed immune responses in LLC-bearing mice. *J Environ Pathol Toxicol Oncol.* 2005;24(3):175–192.

63. Young MR. Protective mechanisms of head and neck squamous cell carcinomas from immune assault. *Head Neck.* 2006;28(5):462–470.

64. de Graaf YG, Kennedy C, Wolterbeek R, Collen AF, Willemze R, Bouwes Bavinck JN. Photodynamic therapy does not prevent cutaneous squamous-cell carcinoma in organ-transplant recipients: Results of a randomized-controlled trial. *J Invest Dermatol.* 2006;126(3):569–574.

65. Pagliaro J, Elliott T, Bulsara M, King C, Vinciullo C. Cold air analgesia in photodynamic therapy of basal cell carcinomas and Bowen's disease: An effective addition to treatment: A pilot study. *Dermatol Surg.* 2004;30(1):63–66.

66. Wiegell SR, Stender IM, Na R, Wulf HC. Pain associated with photodynamic therapy using 5-aminolevulinic acid or 5-aminolevulinic acid methylester on tape-stripped normal skin. *Arch Dermatol.* 2003;139(9):1173–1177.

67. Stender IM, Bech-Thomsen N, Poulsen T, Wulf HC. Photodynamic therapy with topical delta-aminolevulinic acid delays UV photocarcinogenesis in hairless mice. *Photochem Photobiol.* 1997;66(4): 493–496.

68. Bissonette R, Bergeron A, Liu Y. Large surface photodynamic therapy with aminolevulinic acid: Treatment of actinic keratoses and beyond. *J Drugs Dermatol.* 2004;3(suppl 1):S26–S31.

69. Clarke H, Pallister CJ. The impact of anaemia on outcome in cancer. *Clin Lab Haematol.* 2005;27(1):1–13.

70. Wang HW, Putt ME, Emanuele MJ, et al. Treatment-induced changes in tumor oxygenation predict photodynamic therapy outcome. *Cancer Res.* 2004;64(20):7553–7561.

71. Kamuhabwa AR, Huygens A, Roskams T, De Witte PA. Enhancing the photodynamic effect of hypericin in human bladder transitional cell carcinoma spheroids by the use of the oxygen carrier, perfluorodecalin. *Int J Oncol.* 2006;28(3):775–780.

CHAPTER 47

Radiation Therapy

Aaron H. Wolfson, M.D.
Torello M. Lotti, M.D.
Piero Campolmi, M.D.
Ricardo Rossi, M.D.

SKIN CANCER

BOX 47-1   Overview

- Radiation therapy plays a major role in the local/regional management of skin cancer.
- The main subtypes of skin cancer that can benefit from radiotherapy include non-melanomatous skin carcinomas, melanomatous skin cancers, Merkel cell carcinomas, cutaneous lymphomas, cutaneous angiosarcomas, Kaposi sarcoma, adnexal/sweat gland tumors, and extra-mammary Paget's disease.
- Several different therapeutic modalities are currently in use with radiation oncologists for the management of various skin cancers such as superficial/orthovoltage therapy, electron external beam irradiation, photon external beam irradiation, brachytherapy, photodynamic therapy, and boron neutron capture therapy.
- There is an acceptable range of radiation dose for both definitive and adjuvant radiotherapy for the different types of skin cancer.

RADIOTHERAPY FOR NONMELANOMA SKIN CANCERS

BOX 47-2   Summary

1. Background perspective
   - More than 1 million cases diagnosed annually in U.S.
   - Basal cell carcinomas (BCC) and squamous cell carcinomas (SCC) comprise approximately 90% of NMSC.
   - Over 75% of BCC/SCC are located in the head/neck region.
2. Biological and physical properties of external beam irradiation (EBI)
   - Lethal effects of EBI on cancer cells due to damage to the cells' DNA resulting in mitotic death.
   - Superficial/orthovoltage EBI requires the presence of a filter to "harden" the beam.

- Electron beam therapy requires use of "bolus" material to ensure adequate skin dosage.
3. Indications for definitive radiotherapy (RT)
   - Primary RT for NMSC should be considered especially for patients greater than age 70 with lesions less than 1 cm that are located near the eyes or nose.
   - Other indications for definitive RT include the following: recurrent BCC or SCC that are not amenable to resection; lesions in critically sensitive areas of the body (eyelids, canthal regions, nasal pyramid/alae, pinna of the ear, lips, and nail beds).
4. Indications for adjuvant radiotherapy
   - Postoperative RT should be considered for patients with NMSC who have close or positive surgical margins (especially for the sclerosing (mor-pheaform) BCC with an associated 30 to 40% overall relapse rate).
   - Other reasons to use postoperative RT include the following: lesions larger than 4 cm, presence of positive margins or perineural invasion, and positive regional cervical and/or parotid nodal involvement (especially extranodal extension).
5. Dose fractionation and results of external beam irradiation (EBI)
   - There are a variety of acceptable radiation dose and fractionation schedules in the literature with larger fraction sizes and lower total radiation doses being reserved for superficial therapy versus smaller fraction sizes and higher total doses being used with photon external beam irradiation.
   - While there are many different dose fractionation schedules for EBI, more protracted radiation schedules are utilized for lesions in sensitive body sites, such as near the nose or eye.
   - For untreated basal cell and squamous cell carcinomas less than 3 cm in size, local control rates using EBI are over 90%.
   - For untreated NMSC lesions, most have over 90% survival independent of tumor size with EBI alone.
   - EBI for sebaceous cell carcinoma of the eyelid can be curative with total doses of at least 55 Gy over 5 to 6 weeks.
6. Brachytherapy or mold therapy
   - Involves either interstitial (into the tissues) or direct placement (mold) for either definitive (for lesions up to 4 cm

in size) or adjunctive therapy (for lesions larger than 4 cm).
   - Brachytherapy yields excellent local control rates for NMSC of the eyelid.
7. Photodynamic therapy
   - Involves the use of a photosensitizer that contains a protoporphyrin molecule (also found in hemoglobin).
   - These substances when administered either topically or systemically and then subjected to a laser light source can become active and cause damage to tumor cells in the skin, especially in patients who are not candidates for either surgery or EBI.
8. Complications of radiotherapy
   - Acute effects occur within the first 3 to 6 months after conclusion of radiotherapy, while chronic toxicities begin after the first 6 months.
   - Complications from EBI are generally temporary and respond well to supportive therapies.
   - Examples of late skin changes from EBI include atrophy, hypopigmentation, telangectasia, fibrosis, and ulceration.
   - There is a rare risk of a secondary aggressive malignant tumor being induced by EBI that can occur many years after therapy.

Background Perspective

There are more than a million new cases of nonmelanoma skin cancers (NMSC) each year in the United States.[1] Of this number, basal cell carcinomas (BCC) comprise approximately 75 to 90%, while most of the rest are squamous cell carcinomas (SCC).[2] It has been well established that over 75% of BCCs and SCCs occur in the sun-exposed regions of the skin such as the head and neck region.[2,3]

Biological and Physical Properties of External Beam Irradiation

The effect of ionizing radiation in eradicating malignant cells is due to the lethal damage of the DNA of these rapidly dividing cancer cells by the interaction of either photons (X-rays) or electrons that results in these cells' failure to reproduce, i.e., mitotic death.[4] The linear accelerators used in the current practice of radiation oncology generate deeply penetrating photon beams (6 to 24 MV) that are associated with general sparing of the superficial skin surface. Thus, the unit most often used to treat NMSC with photons involves superficial or orthovoltage therapy that ranges from 100 to 250 kVp.[5] The range of penetration of this type of radiotherapy is from millimeters to a few centimeters. Shielding nearby normal tissue structures, such as the eye, is usually achieved with the placement of approximately 5 mm of lead that is directly applied to the skin or onto the eye itself (as either an internal or external eye shield).

The physical characteristics of the superficial/orthovoltage units for the treatment of NMSC are such that the beam is very inhomogeneous. In order to "sharpen" the beam, one must insert a "filter" into the device in order to "harden" the beam to achieve an appropriate dose distribution to the tumor.[6] These filters involve the principle of the "half-value layer" (HVL), in which there is a thickness of material required to reduce the intensity of the X-ray beam by half.[6] Currently, most radiation departments will utilize superficial therapy (100 kVp) with a HVL of 7 mm of aluminum (Al) that delivers 95% of its dose at a depth of 5 mm. Lesions that are more deeply invading into the skin can be treated with an orthovoltage unit (250 kVp) with a HVL of 2.5 mm of copper (Cu) that delivers 95% of its dose at a depth of 10 mm.[5] One potential problem with using superficial/orthovoltage irradiation centers upon the photoelectric effect in which there is preferential uptake of this beam in bone as opposed to soft tissue.[6] This has led to concern that this type of RT may lead to late complications of bone and cartilage necrosis as well as possible induction of malignant bone tumors years afterward.

For those radiation oncology facilities without access to superficial/orthovoltage irradiation, the clinicians therein utilize some of the electron beam components of the modern linear accelerators. These lower energy 6 to 8-MeV electrons require special considerations in their use for treating NMSC. In particular, they also possess the "skin-sparing" quality seen with photons (X-rays), but to a much lesser extent. Still, the use of tissue-equivalent material, known as bolus, must be applied on the skin surface to raise the delivered radiation dose there to at least 90%. Another problem with employing electrons is that the quality of the beam is degraded with the use of field sizes under 4 cm that must be taken into account when evaluating small lesions.[6]

Electron beam therapy is usually reserved for treating lesions of the scalp in order to minimize the exposure to the underlying normal brain tissue. Moreover, one recent study has employed a "single set-up point" multielectron beam technique utilizing computed tomography (CT) imaging and variable lead shielding in order to more effectively irradiate widely infiltrating skin lesions on the irregularly curved surfaces of the scalp.[7] This innovative technique has widespread applications to most RT facilities that might not have the availability of sophisticated linear accelerators possessing intensity-modulated radiation therapy (IMRT) or tomotherapy for the treatment of disseminated lesions of the scalp.[8]

Indications for Definitive Radiotherapy

RT has been utilized for almost a century for the management of skin cancers.[9] Fig. 47-1 presents a pictorial depiction of the most common sites of these lesions at a single major medical institution in the United States.[1] Its main advantage over surgery is that it provides a noninvasive means of treating malignant lesions without resulting surgical defects and scarring that requires additional reconstructive surgery to correct.[5] However, the present use of ionizing radiation for the primary treatment of NMSC has been declining.[2] Yet, a recent review of the current role of RT for NMSC concluded that RT as a definitive therapeutic modality was best reserved for BCC according to either patient or tumor factors (see Table 47-1).[5] According to these authors' criteria, "older patients" were classified as being greater than 70 years of age (see Fig. 47-2A to C). In addition, those lesions felt to be most amenable to definitive RT were less than 1 cm in maximum diameter and usually located near critical normal tissue structures such as the medial canthus or lower eyelid, nasal lip, or ala of the nose in which surgical excision with primary closure would be difficult to achieve. In addition, another study did report that primary radiotherapy should be considered in those instances in which patients having a recurrent BCC

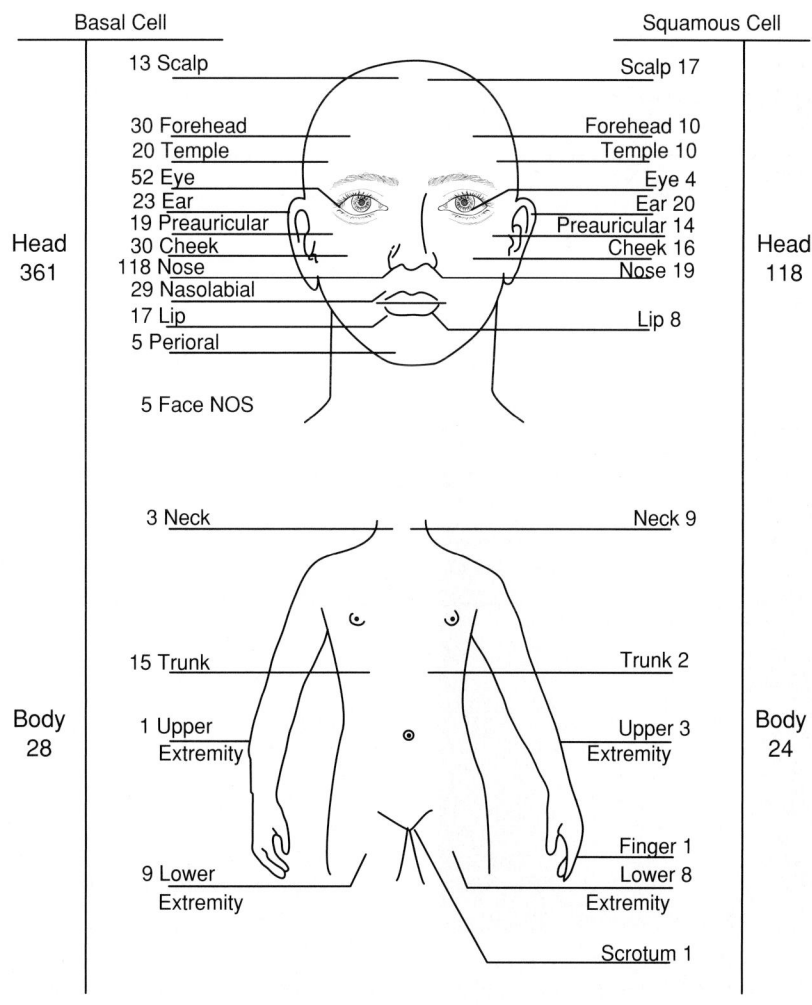

▲ **FIGURE 47-1** Most common sites of epithelial skin cancers (previously untreated and recurrent lesions).

Table 47-1

Clinicopathological Indications for Definitive Radiotherapy for BCCs

Factor	Indication[a]
Patient	Older age
	Patient preference
	Warfarinization
	Significant medical comorbidities
Tumor	Site (ala nasi, nasal bridge, lower eyelid, lip, medical canthus)
	Size (extensive superficial spreading)

[a] Many of these are relative indications.
Source: Used with permission from ref. 5.

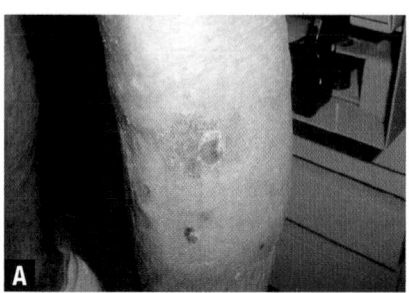

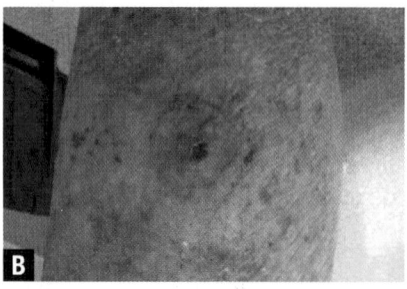

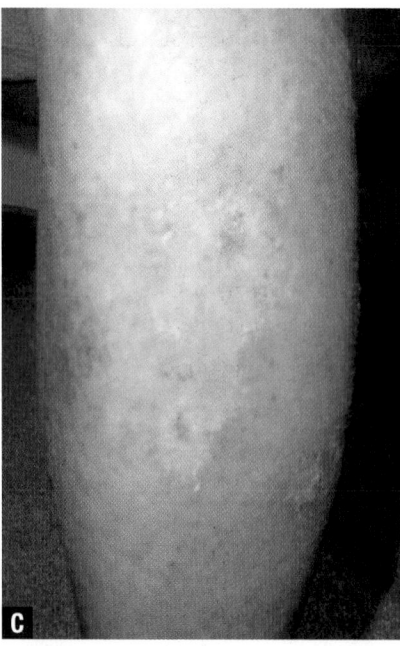

▲ **FIGURE 47-2 A.** Primary BCC. **B.** Result at conclusion of electron beam irradiation (51 Gy). **C.** Result 1 month after electron beam irradiation (51 Gy).

or SCC "cannot undergo extensive surgery for a variety of different reasons (age, general health conditions, etc.).[10]

Other indications for invoking primary RT of NMSC have included lesions in those anatomic areas of the face such as the eyelids, internal and external canthus of the eye, the nasal pyramid and alae, the pinna of the ear, and the lips. According to one report,[2] tumors in these locations (independent of size and histology) should be strongly considered for primary irradiation as "surgery is often destructive and reconstruction is complex." Another site that should be considered for definitive radiotherapy concerns SCC involving the nail beds that are deemed unresectable except for amputation.[11]

Indications for Adjuvant Radiotherapy

Table 47-2 displays several factors for considering postoperative external beam RT for patients with NMSC. The goal of adjunctive irradiation is to improve local disease control by sterilizing the operative tissue "bed" so that any microscopic residual tumor cells are killed.[12] Those who are subjected to primary surgical excision may pathologically be found to have a "close" or positive surgical margin. In this instance, there is a clear indication for postoperative radiotherapy.[5,7] This is especially seen in patients with sclerosing (morpheaform) BCC located near the eye or nose that have a propensity to have positive margins despite even Mohs surgery. One report noted that there was an approximately 30 to 40% overall relapse rate for incompletely resected BCC.[13]

Although definitive radiation therapy has been tried with the delivery of higher total radiation doses and even by employing altered radiation dose fractionation schedule,[14] lesions that are larger than 4 cm in maximum dimension

Table 47-2

Indications for Adjuvant Radiotherapy in Nonmelanomatous Skin Cancers

Nonresectable positive surgical margin
Tumors greater than 4 cm
Microscopic involvement of draining cervical lymph nodes
Parotid lymph node involvement
Perineural invasion
Orbital Invasion
Tumor recurrence in the head/neck region

are more likely to be less controlled with definitive RT but rather with surgery and postoperative irradiation.[5] Adjuvant irradiation as opposed to primary RT has the benefit of treating a smaller tumor burden.[7] In addition, the choice of initial surgical resection targets only those patients with known microscopic risk factors for recurrence (such as perineural invasion or positive margins) to be selected for adjunctive treatment.[5,7] Moreover, another study[15] demonstrated that "patients with locally advanced SCCs (particularly T3 and T4 patients) are found to have a significant locoregional failure (29% and 50%, respectively)...when prophylactic nodal radiation is not given."

Postoperative radiotherapy for cervical nodal disease spread (levels I to V) in the absence of parotid nodal metastases in patients with NMSC of the head and neck region has recently been retrospectively reviewed.[16] Although nodal involvement is very uncommon for NMSC, all 74 evaluable patients had SCC histology. The most frequent primary site for these patients was the frontotemporal region. With median follow-up of 48 months (12 to 187 months), 52 received postoperative RT, 13 surgery alone, and 9 only had nodal RT. The most common locations for nodal metastases were in level I (submental/submandibular) and level II (jugulodiagastric) as only 14% of cases had spread to other sites. Overall, approximately 34% of patients experienced a failure (25 out of 74). Those patients who underwent adjuvant radiotherapy had a lower recurrence rate (15%) and statistically-improved disease-free survival ($P = 0.001$) versus those receiving only single modality therapy. The most common relapse in these patients was in the ipsilateral (same side as primary cancer) irradiated nodal region. Tumor spread from NMSC of the head and neck to the parotid gland and associated lymph nodes is also a very rare phenomenon. Again, most primary cutaneous lesions have squamous cell tumor histology. One of the most recent and largest study[17] retrospectively assessed 52 cases with only parotid nodal spread without contiguous spread from the primary skin lesion. The most-often documented primary site was the frontotemporal region. All of these subjects received postoperative radiotherapy. Sixteen patients (31%) had a failure with 81% being in the parotid region. Despite the use of postoperative radiotherapy, there was a cumulative locoregional relapse rate of

45% and a 65% 5-year cause-specific survival. Multivariate analysis revealed that the presence of extension of tumor beyond the lymph-node capsule (extranodal disease) but not positive margins was predictive of locoregional failure ($P = 0.02$).

Several current articles report on the presence of perineural invasion (PNI) from NMSC as an indicator for postoperative radiotherapy.[18–20] These latter studies have suggested that this histological phenomenon is only seen in less than 5% of patients with NMSC, most often associated with squamous cell histology and affects cranial nerve V and VII but orbital invasion is also possible, especially for periorbital lesions of the lower forehead. Because there is much confusion in the literature regarding criteria for perineural involvement, one report[19] recommended that there must be the following to qualify for PNI: (1) tumor cells must be present within the perineurium, (2) tumors do not have to encompass a nerve, and (3) tumor cells may be within either the tumor itself or in adjacent tissue. The latest update[20] on the use of adjuvant radiotherapy for patients with NMSC (predominantly SCC) with PNI stated that those with microscopic nerve involvement had approximately one-half of their recurrences in the regional lymph nodes with only 18% of these patients receiving elective postoperative neck nodal RT. However, 44% of those with clinically overt PNI underwent elective nodal irradiation with only 3 out of 30 (10%) experiencing regional nodal failure, including the base of skull.

Tumors from a periorbital NMSC (most commonly BCC in 90% of cases) are rare events and occur less than 5% of the time. These lesions occur most frequently on the lower eyelid, medial canthus, upper eyelid, and lateral canthus. The two most common histological subtypes of BCC associated with orbital extension are the infiltrative and sclerosing/morphea-type. These lesions are usually managed with surgery, often orbital exenteration, with adjuvant irradiation being reserved in those cases in which the adequacy of the surgical margins are in doubt.[21]

NMSC that recur after initial surgical excision comprise approximately 7% of all cutaneous epithelial skin lesions of the face.[22] In many cases, these cancers are candidates for re-excision followed by postoperative radiotherapy with a suggested improvement in both local control and survival.[23]

Dose Fractionation and Results of External Beam Irradiation

There are various schedules of delivering external beam irradiation (EBI) for the definitive management of NMSC. A recent retrospective study[24] reported its experience with the total dose, fraction size, and treatment time (dose fractionation) utilized from 1999 to 2001. These treatments were administered using between 80 and 140-kVp superficial therapy (see Table 47-3).

One major academic medical center in the United States (the University of Florida in Gainesville, FL) has extensively published on its as well as other major institutional experiences (such as the Mallinckrodt Institute of Radiology in St. Louis, MO) in the treatment of skin cancers of head and neck region using EBI.[25] Table 47-4 presents recommendations for dose fractionation for commonly occurring clinical situations involving NMSC. Table 47-5 depicts the local control rates of both primary and recurrent NMSC by size and cell type. Table 47-6 presents published survival rates according to the 1983 American Joint Committee on Cancer (AJCC) staging[26] for T2 to T4 skin lesions with NMSC. A recent update of the University of Florida's experience with advanced T4 skin cancer lesions of the head and neck region (using 1998 AJCC staging[27]) revealed that there were curable subsets of patients with these cancers invoking only primary RT, especially when reserving surgery for salvage of recurrent disease.[28]

A large Canadian hospital[29] has published its experience with the primary treatment of SCC of the nasal skin that may also be used to extrapolate to the definitive irradiation of other sites of NMSC. Table 47-7 displays this institu-

Table 47-3
Definitive Radiotherapy Dose Fractionation Schedules for Nonmelanomatous Skin Cancers

TREATMENT SCHEDULE[a]	NO. OF CASES
36 Gy in six fractions over 3 weeks	252
50 Gy in twenty fractions over 4 weeks	18
45 Gy in fifteen fractions over 3 weeks	15
37.5 Gy in ten fractions over 2–5 weeks	8

[a]Only treatment schedules used in five or more cases are shown.
Source: Used with permission from ref. 24.

Table 47-4
Guidelines for Selecting External Beam Total Dose for Nonmelanomatous Skin Cancers

ORTHOVOLTAGE DOSE (cGy)[†]	EXAMPLES
6500 over 7 weeks	Large untreated lesion with bone/cartilage invasion or large recurrent tumor
6000 over 7 weeks	Large untreated lesion with minimal or suspected bone/cartilage invasion
5500 over 6 weeks	Moderate to large inner canthus, eyelid, nasal, or pinna lesions (20–30-cm² area)
5000 over 4 weeks	Small, thin lesion (less than 1.5 cm) around eye, nose, or ear (10-cm² area)
4500 over 3 weeks	Moderate-sized lesion on "free" § skin or postoperative treatment of moderate-sized cancer on "free" skin with positive margins
4000 over 2 weeks or 3000 over 1 week	Small lesions (1 cm) on "free" skin

Source: Used with permission from ref. 25.

tion's dose fractionation regimens. Most of these reported patients were treated with superficial/orthovoltage EBI that ranged from 75 kVp with HVL of 2.2-mm Al to 250 kVp with HVL of 1.1-mm Cu. Generally, lesions ≤2 cm were treated to 35 Gy in 5 fractions, those between 2 and 5 cm to 45 Gy in 10 fractions, and those tumors either >5 cm or involving bone or cartilage to 50 Gy in 20 fractions. The 5-year local control and cause-specific survival rates for this series were 85% and 96%, respectively.

There have been current reports in the literature trying to correlate pathological evaluations of certain subtypes of NMSC and their response to EBI. One such report[30] retrospectively reviewed 175 BCCs of the skin in 148 patients who underwent RT. There were 103 nodular, 25 superficial, and 47 sclerosing (morphea-type) subtypes

Table 47-5

Local Control with External Beam Irradiation According to Clinical Features for Nonmelanomatous Skin Cancers

Size	Basal Cell, Previously Untreated (%)	Basal Cell, Recurrent (%)	Squamous Cell, Previously Untreated (%)	Squamous Cell, Recurrent (%)
≤1 cm	64/66 (97)	22/23 (96)	11/11 (100)	10/12 (83)
1.1–3 cm	71/75 (95)	27/36 (75)	19/21 (90)	7/13 (54)
3.1–5 cm	11/13 (85)	7/9 (78)	7/8 (88)	6/9 (67)
>5 cm	12/13 (92)	1/2 (50)	3/5 (60)	6/11 (55)
Size not specified	4/4 (100)	1/1 (100)	0/1 (0)	4/6 (67)
Total	192/171 (95)	58/71 (82)	40/46 (87)	33/51 (65)

Source: Used with permission from ref. 25.

of BCC in this series. Using immunohistochemical stain of 60 tissue samples involving all three subtypes of BCC, these investigators found that the presence of positive p53 ($P = 0.0049$) and low Bcl-2 ($P = 0.0169$) expressions were significantly correlated with the sclerosing cell type, which also has the highest 5-year estimate recurrence rate (28%) in the entire patient cohort ($P = 0.055$). Furthermore, another reported series[31] uncovered that those BCCs of the skin (independent of cell subtype) subjected to primary RT that have no appreciable change in the size of the lesion might actually have no viable tumor cells on pathological evaluation but rather only the presence of amyloid accumulation within the tumor mass. Thus, it is vital that histological confirmation of viable tumor cells for at least definitively irradiated BCC of the skin be made prior to considering a given lesion for salvage surgery. Lastly, there appears to be a dose-response to primary RT of at least 55 Gy at 1.8 to 2.0 Gy per fraction for sebaceous cell carcinoma of the eyelid, the most commonly reported histologic subtype in this site.[32]

Special Treatment Considerations

BRACHYTHERAPY OR MOLD THERAPY Another technique for delivering a curative dose to a NMSC lesion of the head and neck region is by means of the placement of radioactive materials either into (interstitial high-dose-rate brachytherapy using sources such as Iridium 192) or directly onto (wax molds using such sources as Cesium 137) the tumor "bed" as either primary or adjuvant therapy.[33] This latter single-institutional, prospective study of 136 patients with either BCC or SCC of the skin of the face (split almost evenly between primary and recurrent lesions) delivered approximately 60 to 65 Gy in 33 to 36 fractions for lesions up to 4 cm in maximum size. Tumors greater than 4 cm received additional treatment to an ultimate approximate total dose of 75 to 80 Gy. This study demonstrated an estimated local control rate at 5 years of 98% of all lesions, which suggests another viable alternative to EBI for the management of these NMSCs. Also, another recent study of 24 primary cases of carcinoma (predominantly BCC and SCC) of the tarsal structure of the eyelid using low-dose-rate Iridium 192 interstitial brachytherapy

Table 47-7

Dose Fractionation Schedules for Definitive Irradiation of Nasal SCCs

Schedules	n
≤1 week	
3250–3500 cGy/5 fractions	34
2000 cGy/1 fractions	11
3750 cGy/5 fractions	1
2000 cGy/5 fractions	1
3200 cGy/4 fractions	1
1000 cGy/1 fractions	1
2 weeks	
4250–4500 cGy/10 fractions	20
5000 cGy/20 fractions (BID)	1
3500 cGy/10 fractions	1
4500 cGy/9 fractions	1
3–4 weeks	
5000 cGy/15–20 fractions	10
4500 cGy/15 fractions	3
4 weeks	
5500 cGy/20 fractions	2
3000 cGy/3 fractions given on days 0, 7, and 21	2
5250 cGy/20 fractions	1
5200 cGy/20 fractions	1
≥5 weeks	
6000 cGy/30 fractions	2
6400 cGy/32 fractions	1

All given daily Monday through Friday unless otherwise specified.
Abbreviation: BID = twice daily.
Source: Used with permission from ref. 29.

found that there was an approximate 92% long-term local control rate.[34]

PHOTODYNAMIC THERAPY Another burgeoning technology that is being utilized for the management of both initial and recurrent NMSC lesions pertains to photodynamic therapy (PDT). The basic principle of PDT involves the introduction of nonionizing radiation therapy using a photosensitizer such as photofrin (a derivative of dihematoporphrin), metatetrahydroxyphenylchlorine (mTHPC), or 5-aminolevulinic acid (ALA) that are natural precursors of protoporphyrin IX (PpIX) in the biosynthetic pathway of heme that comprise hemoglobin.[35,36] These precursor substances themselves are photoinactive. However, when administered (either topically or intravenously) to a human in sufficient quantities, they are converted to the highly light-sensitive PpIX in superficially located malignant cells for therapeutic purposes when exposed to a red light (approximately 630 nm) laser source. Due to the hydrophilic nature of the precursor such as ALA, it does not accumulate in sufficient concentration in

Table 47-6

Actuarial 5-Year Cause-Specific Survival Rates for T2–T4 Nonmelanomatous Skin Cancers Treated with Definitive Radiotherapy

Prior Treatment	T Stage	No. of Patients	Cause-Specific 5-Year Survival Rate (%)
Previously	T2	17	100
Untreated	T3	11	100
	T4	27	88
Recurrent	T2	7	100
	T3	11	100
	T4	26	59‡

Source: Used with permission from ref. 25.

the stratum corneum of intact skin and cell membranes but rather in lesions of NMSC in which the "normal skin barrier" has been breached.[37]

One recent report showed that PDT was highly effective in managing aggressive and recurrent previously treated NMSC of the head and neck region in "elderly" patients and that several repeated treatments with PDT were possible in this patient cohort with excellent results.[38] In addition, a multi-institutional prospectively randomized study of patients employing methyl ALA PDT versus surgery for 101 patients with 105 newly diagnosed nodular BCCs of the skin showed no statistically significant differences concerning complete responses and local control at 1-year patient follow-up.[39]

COMPLICATIONS OF RADIOTHERAPY The acute (short-term) effects of EBI on the skin are shown in Table 47-8. At conventional fraction sizes of RT using either superficial/orthovoltage or electron beam treatments, the initial manifestations of skin reactions are seen after approximately 2 weeks and last for up to 3 to 6 months. Supportive therapies include the use of topical anti-inflammatory agents that contain a steroid preparation for the radiation-induced dermatitis as well as applying an antibacterial medication (such as Silvadene®) to prevent infections in the presence of moist desquamation.

The development of late (chronic) effects that occur more than 6 months after the conclusion of RT for both primary[40–42] and recurrent NMSC have recently been published.[43] Together these studies have demonstrated at least a "good" or "acceptable" rating using a variety of scoring methods in the majority of patients with respect to the development of chronic skin toxicity to either EBI or surface mold applications. Examples of late skin reactions to RT include skin atrophy, hypopigmentation, telangiectasia, fibrosis, and ulceration. The special circumstance of delivering EBI to skin lesions near the eye could result in such chronic toxicities as

Table 47-8
Acute Skin Toxicity to Radiation Therapy

Erythema
Hyperpigmentation
Dry desquamation
Moist desquamation
Ulceration

dry eye, the development of cataracts, glaucoma (neovascular type), radiation retinopathy, and radiation optic neuropathy.[44] Finally, the rare risk of a secondary malignant tumor (such as a more aggressive sarcoma) developing within the previously irradiated field several years after RT for a NMSC must also be considered.[45]

RADIOTHERAPY FOR MELANOMA SKIN CANCERS

BOX 47-3 Summary

1. Lentigo maligna (LM) and lentigo maligna melanoma (LMM)
   - LMM most commonly found in the head and neck region.
   - 80% relapse rate with surgical removal alone.
   - Superifcal radiation or electron beam therapy generally employed for primary therapy.
   - Total doses range from 35 Gy in 1 week to 50 Gy in 3 to 5 weeks.
2. Cutaneous malignant melanoma (CMM)
   - CMM generally regarded as radioresistant due to "broad shoulder" on cell survival curve.
   - Large (>4 Gy) fraction sizes are needed for optimal tumor cell killing.
   - Most recent fractionation scheme involves the delivery of 30 Gy in five fractions over 2.5 weeks given twice weekly for both gross and microscopic disease.
   - Recent use of boron neutron capture therapy for treating unresectable CMM lesions.
   - Iodine-125 interstitial brachytherapy has been used for melanoma of the eyelids.

Lentigo Maligna and Lentigo Maligna Melanoma

EPIDEMIOLOGICAL CONSIDERATIONS Lentigo maligna (LM) and lentigo maligna melanoma (LMM) comprise a rare spectrum of skin diseases ranging from an atypical melanocytic proliferation in all layers of the epidermis in the former to a melanomatous invasive phase in the latter.[46] LMM comprises approximately 5% of all cutaneous malignant melanoma (CMM). However, nearly 50% of all CMM of the head and neck region are LMM.[46]

ROLE OF RADIOTHERAPY Even with complete surgical excision, both LM and LMM have an approximately 80% local relapse

rate.[47] Thus, adjuvant radiotherapy to the tumor bed should be considered in most cases after initial surgical removal of these lesions. The dose fractionation type of radiation beams, and techniques of radiotherapy that would be appropriate in the postoperative setting for both LM and LMM have already been elaborated upon in the previous discussion in this chapter regarding nonmelanomatous skin cancers.

There has also been some experience with primary RT for these types of lesions.[48,49] It should be pointed out, however, that the "nodular part" of the LMM was generally excised prior to radiotherapy followed by 100 Gy in 10 fractions (with a 14.5 kVp, 1.0 Cellon filter contact unit). In North America, conventional superficial/orthovoltage RT has generally been employed involving 100 kVp, 0.7-mm Al, 6-mm HVL to 280 kVp, 3.0-mm Cu, 4-cm HVL.

Some modern dose fractionation regimens have included 35 Gy in five fractions in 1 week to 50 Gy given in 15 fractions over 3 weeks or even in 25 to 30 fractions over 5 to 6 weeks. Electron beam irradiation with bolus application as described previously in the section on NMSC could also be utilized for this treatment. Local control of disease with appropriate RT can yield over 95% long-term control of both LM and LMM lesions.[50] Definitive radiotherapy has been effective especially for those patients who are not surgical candidates, such as elderly individuals who are the most prone to developing these types of cancers.

Cutaneous Malignant Melanoma

BACKGROUND PERSPECTIVES There has been a long-held belief that cutaneous malignant melanoma (CMM) comprise a generally "radioresistant" class of malignancies.[51] Much of the existing biological data to support this contention is based on the notion that melanomatous lesions possess a "broad shoulder" on a radiation cell survival curve for low doses of radiation, which correlates with an increased ability of these cells to repair sublethal damage to their DNA inflicted by radiation.[52] Yet, there are several studies that demonstrate effective radiation killing effect of CMM lesions employing higher fraction sizes of megavoltage irradiation greater than 4 Gy.[53] Although not confirmed by any prospectively randomized trial, investigators at a single U.S. institution have routinely delivered 30 Gy in five fractions (hypofractionation) using predominately megavoltage external beam irradiation over 2.5 weeks (two fractions per week) for both macroscopic and microscopic manifestations of CMM.[53]

ROLE OF RADIOTHERAPY

Palliation of macroscopic disease The main sites of metastatic disease amenable to the delivery of external beam irradiation include dermal, subcutaneous, and lymph node metastases. The literature shows that approximately 25% of patients treated with a variety of dose fractionation schemes can achieve a complete response by radiating metastatic melanomatous lesions.[54] There was a Radiation Therapy Oncology Group (RTOG) study that showed comparable outcomes for treating metastatic melanoma using either 8 Gy per fraction for four weekly fractions versus 2.5 Gy per fraction for 20 fractions over 26 to 28 days.[55] However, a current recommendation is to use five or six fractions of 6 Gy administered twice weekly.[53]

Adjuvant setting Depending upon the stage of disease and adequacy of the primary surgical excision, patients with CMM may be at an increased risk for both local relapse as well as regional nodal disease spread. This rationale may be applied to either de novo lesions or recurrences in lymph nodes or subcutaneous deposits of tumor. Although there are no recently completed prospectively randomized trials evaluating either elective or therapeutic postoperative radiotherapy versus surgery alone, one U.S. institution has published recommendations in which to consider adjunctive megavoltage external beam irradiation.[53] In particular, CMM of the head and neck should be adjuvantly irradiated for the following reasons: desmoplastic histology, "thick or ulcerated nondesmoplastic" lesions, nonnegative surgical margins, or recurrent lesions. The hypofractionated radiation regimen of 30 Gy in five fractions (twice-weekly fractions) for 2.5 weeks is used with 2 to 4-cm normal tissue margins encompassing the tumor bed along with employing appropriate "bolus" technique. This dose fractionation schema is also recommended for the adjuvant elective irradiation of the regional lymph nodes in the head and neck region if there are nonnegative surgical margins in the nodal dissection specimen, the presence of perineural invasion, "large primary tumors," and nasal cavity or paranasal sinuses locations. Moreover, the delivery of postoperative therapeutic nodal irradiation using the previously described hypofractionated radiation schedule is suggested in the presence of pathological extracap-

sular nodal extension, ≥4 involved nodes, or >3-cm-size nodes or matted nodes.[56]

Outcomes with adjuvant external irradiation There still exists controversy as to what are the appropriate clinical situations for its implementation. Published overall 5-year survival rates for a variety of primary sites of CMM given adjunctive irradiation have not exceeded 50% despite yielding at least an 80% locoregional control rate and the most severe reported chronic complications being lymphedema and subcutaneous fibrosis.[56] One medical center reviewed its database of 168 patients with CMM of the head and neck region.[57] Despite the fact that only 5% of these patients had elective lymph-node dissection (ELND) and none underwent postoperative irradiation, their locoregional recurrences and survival were reportedly "similar to centers where adjuvant radiation or ELND are routinely performed." One nonrandomized center has reported its retrospective experience using postoperative radiotherapy for primary CMM as well as for adjunctive irradiation for positive nodal disease.[58] There were 32 patients with primary lesions who were treated due to having at least one of the following: nonnegative surgical margins, desmoplastic cell type, perineural invasion, satellite lesions, or recurrent disease. The other 142 patients with known nodal disease spread were irradiated due to having nonnegative surgical margins, extracapsular nodal extension, multiple involved nodes, large nodes, perineural or vascular extension, or parotid nodal disease. The patients also underwent hypofractionated megavoltage irradiation that delivered 30 to 35 Gy in five to seven fractions using twice-weekly treatment. With median follow-up of 6 months, only 20 out of 172 (11%) had an in-field relapse but overall 5-year survival was 41%. One study did report excellent local control (approximately 95%) with the administration of the previously described hypofractionated regimen of external beam irradiation following initial surgical debulking of both nodal and subcutaneous deposits from CMM.[59] In addition, there has been another proposed dose fractionation scheme in a report from Australia and New Zealand concerning 130 patients with CMM who were assigned to receive 48 Gy in 20 fractions over 4 weeks using megavoltage external beam irradiation. This regimen was generally well tolerated with the exception of increased lymphedema (48% at 4 years) for patients receiving inguinal/iliac irradiation after surgical dissection. However, with a mini-

mum follow-up of 2 years, 79 out of 130 (61%) evaluable patients have died of melanomatous disease, which again mandates the need for several carefully designed prospectively randomized trials to determine the benefit of postoperative radiotherapy for improving the survival of patients with various manifestations of CMM.

Special considerations Due to the previously described radioresistance of malignant melanoma cells, one group of investigators have published on the use of Boron neutron capture therapy (NCBT) for treating CMM lesions that are unresectable.[60] This therapeutic modality takes advantage of the distinct melanin synthesis of melanoma cells, which have an increased amino acid transport system. Thus, after administering a Boron-containing amino acid compound (e.g., ^{10}B-*p*-boronophenylalanine or BPA) that can be taken up by the melanoma cells, one can then subject such a prepared patient to a neutron beam and subsequently generate alpha particles with a high linear energy transfer (LET) of 230 KeV per μm. Since the alpha particle's range of penetration is only about 10 μm (the diameter of a cell), this thermal neutron irradiation can result in significant damage primarily to those active melanomatous cells taking up the boronated amino acid compound. Although several logistical concerns remain, this alternative type of therapy merits continued investigation for the treatment of these patients who have such poor overall survival. Another clinical situation that warrants consideration of a nonexternal irradiation technique concerns malignant melanoma of the eyelid.[61] This study pertained to 14 patients who had initial surgery, incomplete excision, or recurrence following resection of a melanoma located in the eyelid region. All of these patients underwent the delivery of a median dose of 37 Gy given over a median of 113 hours by means of a low-dose-rate interstitial brachytherapy implant using ^{125}I seeds. Iodine-125 is a radioisotope that emits gamma rays (photons) with an energy that ranges from 27 to 35 KeV and has a half-life of approximately 60 days. Each seed has a width of 0.75 mm and a length of 4.5 mm. With a median follow-up of 45 months, 13 out of 14 (93%) had local control of disease with acceptable complications. Thus, this form of radiotherapy offers another eye-preserving option of therapy for this uncommon presentation of CMM.

RADIOTHERAPY FOR MERKEL CELL CARCINOMAS

BOX 47-4 Summary

- MCCs are derived from neuroendocrine cells in the basal region of the epidermis.
- MCCs have high risk of local, lymphatic, and hematogenous spread.
- MCCs are highly sensitive to EBI.
- Radiation dose fractionation generally involves the delivery of 50 Gy over 4 to 5 weeks.

Epidemiological Considerations

Merkel cell carcinoma (MCC) is an aggressive primary cutaneous tumor derived from neuroendocrine cells of the basal layer of the epidermis with very poor prognosis and with a strong propensity toward local and/or regional relapse, lymphatic spread, and distant metastases. It is quite rare and usually occurs in elderly patients (but young cases are reported) on sun-exposed areas (80 to 90%) (especially to the head and neck or extremities). Immunosoppressive therapy appears to play a role in the development of this cancer but the exact cause of MCC is not known.[62] Merkel cell carcinoma is often associated with diseases that are significantly related with exposure to ultraviolet radiation (actinic keratosis, BCC, and SCC). MCC presents primarily in Caucasians (98.3%) with a median age of 69 years, according to recent investigation.[62,63]

Role of Radiotherapy

There is no consensus regarding the optimal therapeutic approach (surgery, radiotherapy, chemotherapy) but elective treatment seems to be represented by initial surgery (with wide margins or Mohs micrographic surgery) and selective lymph-node dissection. In fact, locoregional and distant metastasis and early and local recurrences are high (30%).

This highly malignant carcinoma, like other neuroendocrine tumors, is radiosensitive and radiotherapy, although variation in radiosensitivity has been reported in small-cell carcinoma cell lines, is indicated in the literature as adjuvant, postsurgery, or as palliative therapy in inoperable cases.[24,64,65] Several studies suggest that radiation alone can achieve locoregional cancer control in some patients.[66–68] The most commonly used regimen for radiotherapy of MCC is a total dosage of 46 to 50

Gy, at 2 Gy per fraction to the tumor bed over 4 to 5 weeks.[65] As lymphatic dissemination of cancer cells occurs often and early, irradiation to the draining lymphatics has been recommended following gross resection. Adjuvant radiotherapy and chemotherapy may prolong survival in case of small-size tumors, but marginal recurrences have been described. Adjuvant radiotherapy alone markedly improves regional control and it may be of great help for treating distant metastases in combination with chemotherapy.[68] In conclusion, combined treatment, incorporating adjuvant radiotherapy, confers a better outcome than surgery alone and should be chosen by the physician according to the data reported in the literature and to our personal experience.[69–71]

RADIOTHERAPY FOR SPECIALIZED MALIGNANCIES OF THE SKIN

BOX 47-5 Summary

1. Primary cutaneous lymphomas (PCL)
   - Most of the PCL of the skin are of T-cell origin of which mycosis fungoides (MF) is the most common.
   - MF in the plaque and tumor stage can be successfully treated with local radiotherapy.
   - Total skin electron beam radiotherapy is reserved for MF cases that have failed first and second-line therapies.
   - After MF, PCL that are CD30+ are the next most common cutaneous T-cell lymphoma.
   - Total doses of EBI for PCL involve up to 40 Gy in 4 weeks.
   - Photodynamic therapy has been utilized for PCL.
2. Cutaneous angiosarcomas (CAS)
   - CAS are very sensitive to local EBI with 80% local control but do have at least 50% incidence of distant metastases.
   - Doses of EBI can be up to 60 Gy in 6 weeks in both the adjuvant as well as definitive setting.
3. Kaposi sarcoma (KS)
   - KS lesions (both epidemic and and classic types) are very responsive to modest doses of local EBI ranging from 20 Gy to 30 Gy over 2 weeks.
4. Adnexal tumors and sweat gland tumors
   - The role of EBI is very limited for the rare adnexal and sweat gland tumors

but has been used with and without hyperthermia.

5. Extramammary Paget's disease (EPD)
   - EPD is a noninvasive adenocarinoma that is usually associated with an underlying invasive carcinoma of glandular differentiation.
   - Definitive EBI has been used with total doses ranging from approximately 40 to 70 Gy over 4 to 7 weeks.

Primary Cutaneous Lymphomas

BACKGROUND PERSPECTIVES Incidence of primary cutaneous lymphomas is 0.4 per 100,000 per year but the overall prevalence is much higher because most are in fact low-grade malignancies with long survival.[72] Two-thirds of them are T-cell origin [cutaneous T-cell lymphoma (CTCL), of which the majority are mycosis fungoides (MF). Primary cutaneous T-cell lymphomas represent a heterogeneous group of neoplasm and the WHO (World Health Organization) classification defined by EORTC (European Organization for Research and treatment of Cancer) recently recognized well-characterized clinicopathological entities.[73]

ROLE OF RADIOTHERAPY MF, low-grade non-Hodgkin's lymphoma of skin-homing T lymphocytes, is a very radiosensitive malignancy. MF, thick or eroded, plaque or tumor stage can be treated successfully with low-dose superficial orthovoltage radiotherapy (Fig 47-3A to B). The radiotherapy treatment administered in several fractions, usually two or three fractions of 4 Gy at 80 to 120 kVp is appropriate therapy for patients with early stages of MF (stage IA, IIA).[74] Depending on the size and thickness, large tumors may be treated by electrons; however, total skin electron beam therapy (TSEB) is only available in a limited number of centers.[75] A recent review about electron beam treatment has demonstrated complete response of 96% in stage IA, IB, IIA disease but with high relapse rates.[76] In stage IIB disease, complete response is less common (36%). However, the erythrodermic stage (generally stage III, including Sézary syndrome, although some cases of Sézary syndrome will be stage IVA) shows complete response in up to 60% of cases.[77] TSEB therapy should currently be reserved for patients with MF who fail to respond to first and second-line therapies.[78] Recent pilot studies assessing the use of TSEB combined with high-dose conditioning chemotherapy before autologous stem cell transplantation in patients

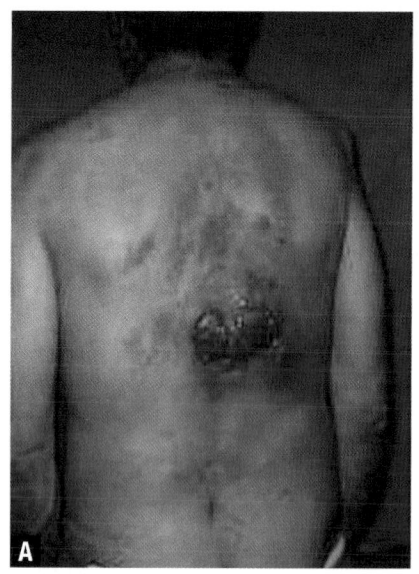
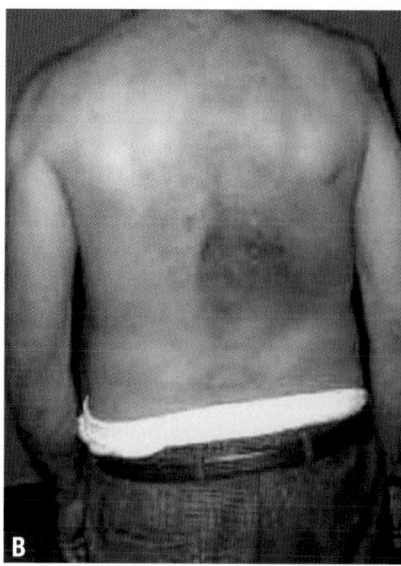

▲ **FIGURE 47-3** **A.** Primary cutaneous T-cell lymphoma. **B.** Result after superficial radiotherapy (25 Gy).

with stage IIB to IVA disease have shown good clinical responses.[79]

Primary cutaneous CD30+ lymphoproliferative disorders represent the most common CTCL after MF and comprise approximately 25% of all CTCLs. Primary cutaneous CD30+ T-cell lymphoma represent a spectrum of diseases including primary cutaneous CD30+ (anaplastic) large T-cell lymphomas (LTCL) and lymphomatoid papulosis (LyP).[80] It is well established that these forms have good prognosis in most patients. For primary cutaneous CD30+ LTCL in patients with a solitary or few localized nodules or tumors, if spontaneous remission does not occur (6 to 20% of cases), local radiotherapy is one option of treatment (Fig. 47-4A to B) along

with low-dose oral methotrexate (5 to 20 mg/week) or surgical excision.[80] With respect to lymphomatoid papulosis when larger skin tumors develop, if spontaneous resolution does not occur, then these lesions could be excised or treated with radiotherapy.[81–83] The large CTCL CD30-pleomorphic and immunoblastic variants all have a poor prognosis. When disease is restricted to the skin, radiotherapy may be indicated, but systemic dissemination is likely and most patients will require multiagent chemotherapy.[72]

Primary cutaneous B-cell lymphoma (CBCL) is an uncommon form of extranodal non-Hodgkin lymphoma, accounting for about 20 to 25% of all primary cutaneous lymphomas and characterized

by malignant B-cells that are usually limited to the skin at initial diagnosis.[84] The radiosensitivity of this disease entity is high, and several reports have been published in the literature suggesting that local RT alone, as first-line treatment, is a good therapeutic approach (Figs. 47-5A to B and 47-6A to B). The implementation of radiotherapy in the management of CBCL is especially efficacious for the "follicle-center cell type" with a good clinical result delivering a total dose ranging from 14 to 48 Gy. The fractionation of the dose is differentiated on the basis of the kind of technique (2.5 Gy in a week for "soft X-ray therapy" or 5 Gy once in a week for contact X-ray therapy) due to possibility of an intense skin reaction that may require the administration of a lower dose per fraction.[85,86] Relapses of this disease are observed but 5-year survival rates have been described up to 97% of cases.[87,88] More recently, complete remission (100%) after 5 years has been reported by employing 4 to 10-MeV electrons using involved fields at a total dose of 40 Gy over 4 weeks.[89]

Thus, dermatological radiotherapy is a good treatment modality for CBCL with a high complete and lasting remission. It may be proposed both for new cutaneous presentations and in many cases for relapses (to control the disease progression). This treatment may be followed by other types of treatment mainly when the localizations are multiple or if the disease progresses rapidly. The proper fractionation of the dose prevents skin sequelae and complications.[90,91]

ROLE OF PHOTODYNAMIC THERAPY The use of PDT has anecdotally been recently utilized for CTCL (MF or CTCL, non-MF CD30+) and CBCL lesions. Two lesions on two MF patients have been treated by one group with ALA (aminolevulinic acid) and/or MAL (methylaminolevulinate) PDT.[92] Good clinical and histological response to PDT was achieved in one plaque-stage MF lesion. Only a partial response was achieved in one nodular MF lesion after three consecutive PDT sessions that were followed by the administration of superficial RT. This combination of PDT and radiotherapy for noncomplete responding lesions might serve to minimize chronic side effects as there would be a reduced tumor volume to radiate.

The successful use of ALA or MAL PDT in the treatment of CBCL has not been yet consistently reported.[93,94] In one institution's preliminary experience, a good clinical and histological response to PDT was achieved in three out of

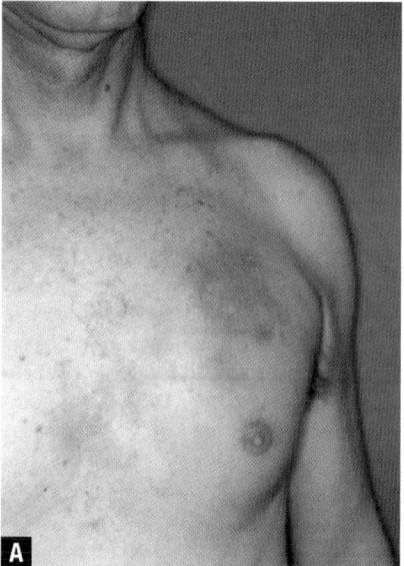
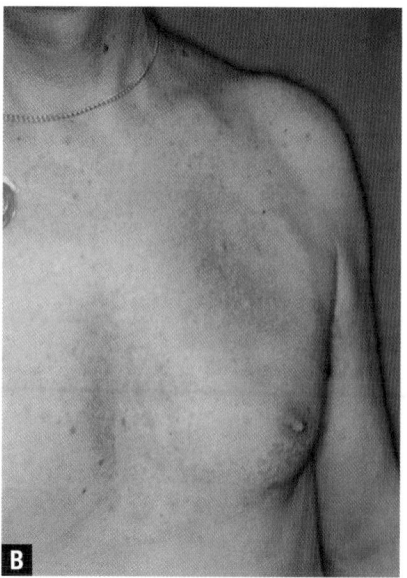

▲ **FIGURE 47-4** **A.** Primary cutaneous large-cell anaplastic CD30+ lymphoma. **B.** Result after superficial radiotherapy (20 Gy).

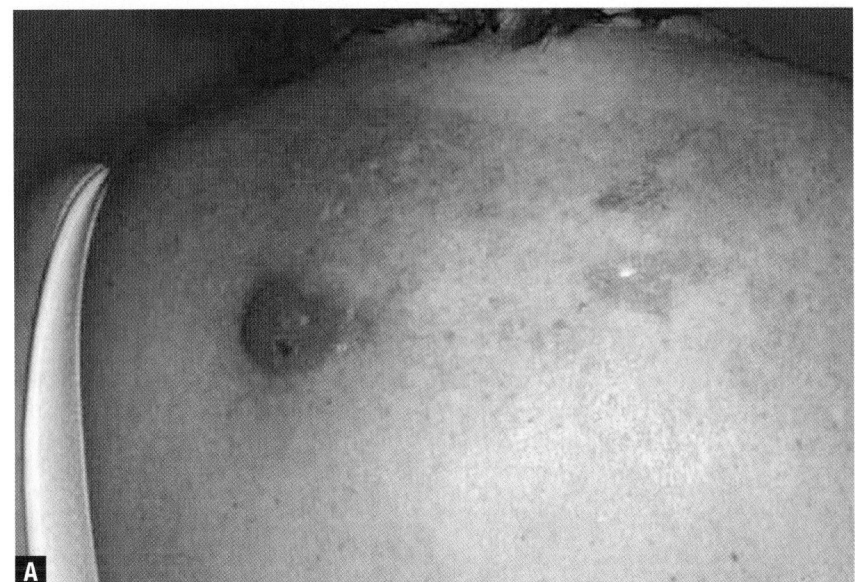

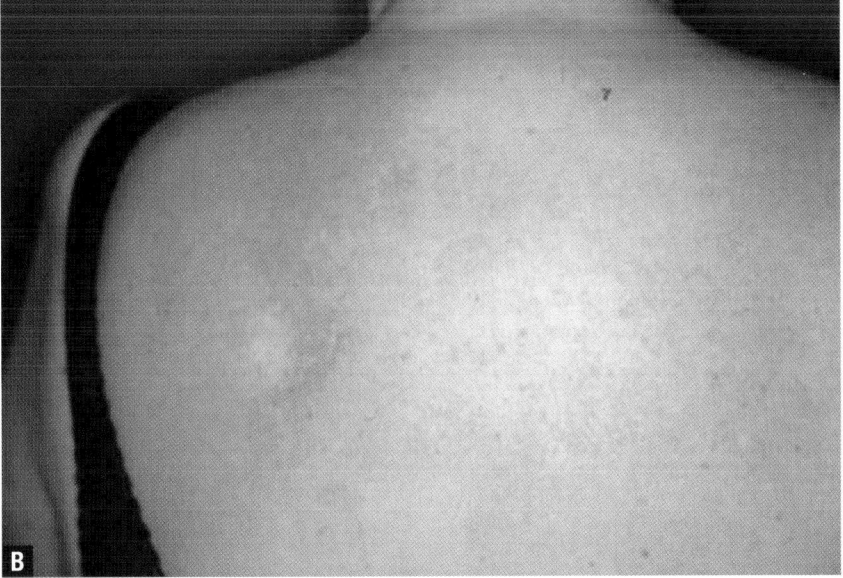

▲ **FIGURE 47-5** **A.** Primary cutaneous B-cell lymphoma. **B.** Result after radiotherapy (20 Gy).

flat infiltrating areas. They can sometimes bleed or ulcerate. Occasionally, chronic edema and scarring alopecia are described.[99] No correlation exists between appearance (e.g., ulcerated, nodular, diffuse) and survival of the patient or local recurrence. Findings of significantly favorable prognostic importance appear to be tumor size (<5 cm), complete surgical resection, and a moderate or marked lymphoid-cell infiltrate around the tumor. Unresectable lesions and metastatic disease at diagnosis suggest a poor prognosis.

Death can occur either by local extension or metastasis. Delayed diagnosis and treatment explains, in part, the poor prognosis. In angiosarcoma of soft tissues, multiple randomized studies using doxorubicin-based chemotherapy fail to show a survival benefit, although meta-analysis evaluations suggest improved local control and improved disease-free survival with chemotherapy, but no real survival advantage.[100–102]

ROLE OF RADIOTHERAPY The use of irradiation in conjunction with surgery continues to evolve, and results in up to 80% of local disease control and excellent functional and cosmetic outcome. However, considering that at least 50% of angiosarcomas have distant metastasis, and irradiation does not actually improve the survival, intraoperative radiation, brachytherapy, or more external beam therapy can complement preoperative external beam radiotherapy.

The advantages of preoperative radiation are the optimization for subsequent surgery that include requiring smaller volume of external beam fields, less hypoxic tissue in the nonoperative region, and a reduction in the chance of intraoperative tumor seeding, which could ultimately result in an improvement in local control of advanced tumors. The disadvantage is the higher wound complication rate. The optimum treatment for patients with cutaneous angiosarcoma has not yet been defined and although surgery remains the first option for the treatment of patients with angiosarcoma, the surgical treatment is contraindicated in tumors extending into vital structures, in those of massive size, or in those with clear multicentricity. In fact, the lesion may be solitary or multicentric, and frequently extends laterally throughout the dermis, making gross assessment of surgical margins difficult and requiring multiple biopsies of the surrounding tissues.[100–102] In the primary treatment of angiosarcomas of the scalp, recognizing the horizontal and vertical

three lesions of CBCL patients. One patient was classified as having a follicle center lymphoma, while the other two had marginal zone lymphomas.[92]

Compared with local orthovoltage radiation, PDT is more rapid (only one or two treatments are required in one experience[92]) and leaves only a temporary hyperpigmentation. Thus, there is emerging data to suggest investigation of the use of PDT for the treatment of plaque-stages of MF as well as localized, thin plaques of indolent CBCL as an alternative to local radiotherapy.

Cutaneous Angiosarcomas

EPIDEMIOLOGICAL CONSIDERATIONS Angiosarcomas are rare aggressive tumors of vascular endothelial cells with a high rate of lymph node and systemic metastases and a high mortality rate. Angiosarcomas (AS) arise at different sites and in any region of the body but are more frequent in skin (face and scalp region) and superficial soft tissue (60% of the cases).[95] Cutaneous angiosarcomas (CAS) are more frequent in males than in females, in the central or upper area of the face in men and on the scalp in women.[96,97] Although AS can appear at any age, they usually occur in the elderly population on sun-exposed skin. A lymphedema-associated cutaneous angiosarcoma, and a form considered as complication of radiation treatment (e.g., treatment of breast carcinoma) are reported.[98]

The clinical presentation varies widely and the lesion may be single or multifocal, bluish or violaceous, nodules, plaques, or

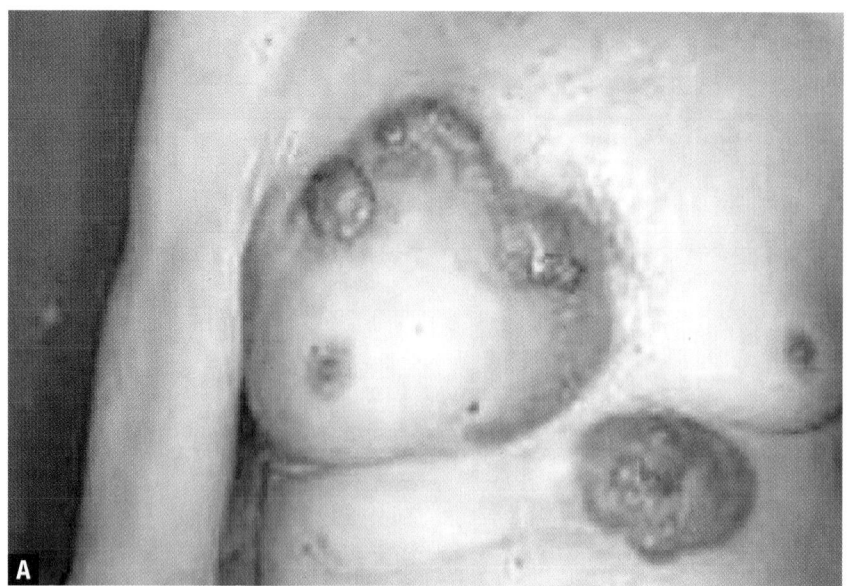

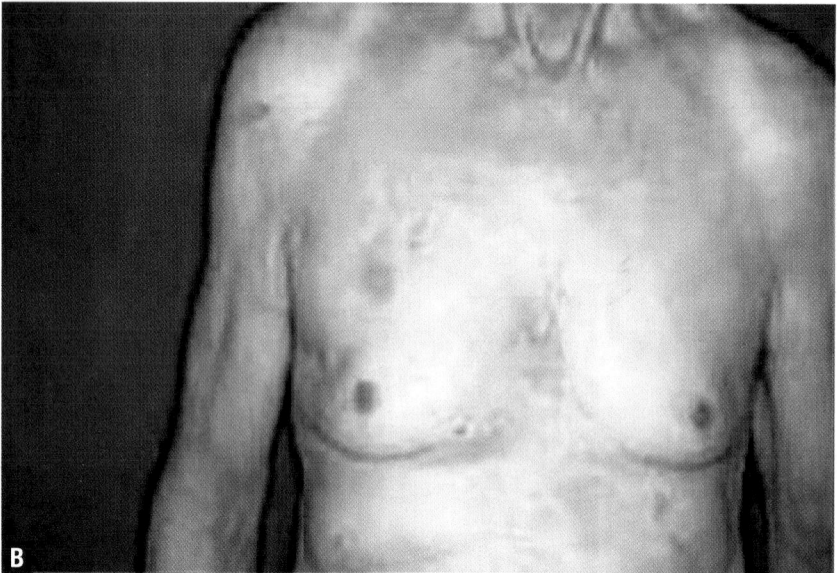

▲ **FIGURE 47-6** **A.** Primary cutaneous B-cell lymphoma. **B.** Result after radiotherapy treatment (25 Gy).

extensions of the tumor is essential. This can only be discerned by microscopic examination of all the margins of the resected specimen.[100] The primary excision of the scalp should be full-thickness, including the pericranium area. The margins should be wide (at least 5 cm) on all sides. Postoperative radiotherapy is mandatory and should be employed routinely in cases with indefinite margins, large tumor size, deep extension, and multicentricity. Radical radiation therapy in the form of high-field electron beam to approximately 60 Gy over 6 weeks holds out promise in prolonging survival of patients with localized lesions.

Patients need clinical examination at least every 3 months, to detect possible recurrences. Palpation of the cervical lymph nodes remains a major tool. Despite any aggressive treatment, prog-

nosis is still poor. The median time of survival ranges from 15 to 24 months, with a 5-year survival rate of 12 to 33%. Local failure and metastases to local cervical lymph nodes are common. The lung is the most common site of distant metastases, followed by the liver and bone, although the latter tend to occur later.[103]

Kaposi Sarcoma

BACKGROUND PERSPECTIVES Kaposi sarcoma (KS) is a neoplasm characterized by a proliferation of spindle-shaped cells of probable endothelial origin mainly but not only involving the skin. Both the two different types found in Europe, the classic form and the epidemic form, can be divided into three main clinical pictures represented by phases of plaques, nodules, and tumors.

ROLE OF RADIOTHERAPY The effectiveness of radiotherapy in the cutaneous lesions of KS has been largely demonstrated.[104–110] The literature reports about 65 to 70% of complete resolution and 10% of recurrence. Thus, this physical modality deserves a place alongside other forms of treatment especially in first stage of disease.[105–107]

In treating flat or nodular lesions, it will be necessary to select a beam of ionizing radiation with a HVL that most closely corresponds to the estimated depth of the neoplastic lesion. This permits the best distribution of radiation to the lesion while sparing the underlying healthy tissues as much as possible. One must be selective concerning the radiation field size. It must be precisely adapted to the skin lesion, using, if necessary, shields of lead-impregnated rubber with a sufficient lead equivalent to define the individual radiation fields in the context of a personalized treatment. Particular care should be taken to avoid overlapping radiation fields especially in the typical site of lesions for classic KS, i.e., the legs of elderly, where precarious trophic and circulatory conditions are often present. Plaques lesion, nodules, or tumors, depending on the different size, can be treated with "soft X-ray therapy" with beam energies between 50 and 120 kVp. Normal tissue margins around the lesion should vary between 1.0 and 2.0 cm. The total dose delivered usually amounts to 20 to 30 Gy in eight to 10 fractions over 3 weeks.[111] Finally, palliative radiotherapy of osteolytic bony lesions can be carried out using "deep X-ray" (greater than 120 kVp up to 250 kVp) or megavoltage therapy with the same modalities for symptomatic treatment of bone tissue that have been described in the literature.[105]

Adnexal Tumors and Sweat Gland Tumors

BACKGROUND PERSPECTIVES Appendage tumors are relatively rare and their clinical features are usually nonspecific so that the great majority of them are diagnosed only after excision and histopathological examination.[112] The skin appendageal tumors described here arise from the pilosebaceous apparatus and the eccrine sweat glands.[113,114] The tumors arising from the pilosebaceous apparatus are found predominantly in the head and neck area whereas eccrine sweat gland tumors are found on all body sites. The majority of skin appendage tumors are locally invasive[115]; however, they do not easily metastasize with the only well-known exception of the malignant eccrine gland carcinomas.

ROLE OF RADIOTHERAPY These uncommon types of cutaneous cancer are mainly reported in the literature as single-case reports and the limited data available suggest that skin tumors of appendages are unresponsive to both radiotherapy and chemotherapy and the treatment of choice should be surgical excision.[116-120] In a few cases of microcystic adnexal carcinoma, external beam radiotherapy has been tried. However, after initial clinical resolution of the tumor, they almost always recur and in a clinically more extensive and histologically more aggressive form. Thus, radiation therapy is not a preferred method of treatment for this kind of malignancy.[116] Some authors described satisfactory results in advanced local or regional presentations of these lesions using radiotherapy alone or combined with hyperthermia.[117] A combined treatment with surgery followed by radiotherapy has been reported in a case of pleomorphic ceruminous adenoma (gland apocrine tumor confined to the skin lining of the cartilaginous part of the external auditory meatus).[120]

Extramammary Paget's Disease

EPIDEMIOLOGICAL CONSIDERATIONS Extramammry Paget's disease (EMPD) is a neoplastic condition in which there is intraepithelial infiltration by neoplastic cells showing glandular differentiation. It usually occurs in patients 50 to 80 years old, starting as an eczematous-like area, resistant to local and systemic treatment. In 25 to 79% of patients, an underlying subjacent or distant invasive carcinoma is found.[121,122] The areas with high density of apocrine glands (i.e., vulva and the penoscrotal area) are preferred. Prognosis of patients is related to the presence of adnexal and/or visceral malignancies as well as to the extent of the metastatic spread. Although surgery is currently considered the preferred treatment for EMPD, it carries a high relapse rate due to the multifocal nature of the disease.

ROLE OF RADIOTHERAPY In one experience and according to literature, radiotherapy represents a useful alternative to surgery (or even PDT) for curative or palliative treatment.[122] A total dose of 42 to 70 Gy using 2 Gy per daily fraction are reported as a convenient radiotherapeutic plan.[122] Nevertheless, the prognosis of patients with underlying adenocarcinoma remains poor, which may indicate that a more aggressive treatment approach, such as combined

chemotherapy with radiotherapy, is warranted.[123]

REFERENCES

1. Locke J, Karimpour S, Young G, et al. Radiotherapy for epithelial skin cancer. *Int J Radiat Biol Phys.* 2001;51: 748–755.
2. Finizio L, Vidali C, Calacione R, et al. What is the current role of radiation therapy in the treatment of skin carcinomas? *Tumori.* 2002;88:48–52.
3. Rossi R, Campolmi P, Giomi B, et al. Giant exophytic basal cell carcinoma treated with radiotherapy. *J Eur Acad Dermatol Venereol.* 2002;16:374–376.
4. Hall EJ. Radiation damage and the dose-rate effect. In: *Radiobiology for the Radiobiologist.* 3rd ed. Philadelphia, PA: JB Lippincott; 1988:31.
5. Veness M, Richards S. Role of modern radiotherapy in treating skin cancer. *Aust J Dermatol.* 2003;44:159–168.
6. Khan FM, ed. *The Physics of Radiation Therapy.* Baltimore, MD: Williams & Wilkins; 1984.
7. Yaparpalvi R, Fontenla DP, Beitler JJ. Improved dose homegeniety in scalp irradiation using a single set-up point and different energy beams. *Br J Radiol.* 2002;75:670–677.
8. Locke J, Low DA, Grigireit T, et al. Potential of tomotherapy for total scalp treatment. *Int J Radiat Oncol Biol Phys.* 2002;52:553–559.
9. Poulsen M, Burmeister B, Kennedy D. Preservation of form and function in the management of head and neck skin cancer. *World J Surg.* 2003;27:868–874.
10. Caccialanza M, Piccinno R, Grammatica A. Radiotherapy of recurrent basal and squamous cell skin carcinomas: A study of 249 re-treated carcinomas in 229 patients. *Eur J Dermatol.* 2001;11: 25–28.
11. Yaparpalvi R, Machadevia PS, Gorla GR, et al. Radiation therapy for the salvage of unresectable subungual squamous cell carcinoma. *Dematol Surg.* 2003;29: 294–296.
12. Huynh NT, Veness MJ. Basal cell carcinoma of the lip treated with radiotherapy. *Aust J Dermatol.* 2002;43:15–19.
13. Berlin B, Katz KH, Helm KF, et al. The significance of tumor persistence after incomplete excision of basal cell carcinoma. *J Am Acad Dermatol.* 2002;46: 549–553.
14. Mendenhall WM, Amdur RJ, Siemann DW, et al. Altered fractionation in definitive irradiation of squamous cell carcinoma of the head and neck. *Curr Opin Oncol.* 2000;12:207–214.
15. Kwan W, Wilson D, Moravan V. Radiotherapy for locally advanced basal cell and squamous cell carcinomas of the skin. *Int J Radiat Oncol Biol Phys.* 2004;60:406–411.
16. Veness MJ, Palme CE, Smith M, et al. Cutaneous head and neck squamous cell carcinoma metastatic to cervical lymph nodes (nonparotid): A better outcome with surgery and adjuvant radiotherapy. *Laryngoscope.* 2003;113:1827–1833.
17. Chua MS-T, Veness MJ, Morgan G, et al. Parotid lymph-node metastases from cutaneous squamous-cell carcinomas: Treatment outcome and prognostic factors following surgery and adjuvant radiotherapy. *Aust Radiol.* 2002;46: 174–179.
18. McCord MW, Mendenhall WM, Parson JT, et al. Skin cancer of the head and neck with clinical perineural invasion. *Int J Radiat Oncol Biol Phys.* 2000;47:89–93.
19. Veness MJ, Biankin S. Perineural spread leading to orbital invasion from skin cancer. *Aust Radiol.* 2000;44:296–302.
20. Garcia-Serra A, Hinerman RW, Mendenhall WM, et al. Carcinoma of the skin with perineural invasion. *Head Neck.* 2003;25:1027–1033.
21. Leibovitch I, McNab A, Sullivan T, et al. Orbital invasion by periocular basal cell carcinoma. *Ophthalmology.* 2005;112: 717–723.
22. Ampil FL, Nathan CAO, Lian TF, et al. Salvage treatment of recurrent skin cancer of the midface. *Am J Clin Oncol.* 2002; 25:580–582.
23. Pompucci A, Rea G, Farallo E, et al. Combined treatment of advanced stages of recurrent skin cancer of the head. *J Neurosurg.* 2004;100:652–658.
24. Thom GA, Heywood JM, Cassidy B, et al. Three-year retrospective review of superficial radiotherapy for skin conditions in a Perth radiotherapy unit. *Aust J Dermatol.* 2003;44:174–179.
25. Mendenhall WM, Kalbaugh KJ, Mendenhall NP, et al. Radiotherapy as definitive treatment and as a surgical adjunct. In: Weber RS, Miller MJ, Goepfert H, eds. *Basal and Squamous Cell Skin Cancers of the Head and Neck.* Baltimore, MD: Williams & Wilkins; 1996:331–350.
26. American Joint Committee on Cancer. *AJCC Staging Handbook.* 2nd ed. Philadelphia, PA: JB Lippincott; 1983.
27. American Joint Committee on Cancer. *AJCC Cancer Staging Handbook.* 5th ed. Philadelphia, PA: JB Lippincott-Raven; 1998.
28. Al-Othman MOF, Mendenhall WM, Amdur RJ. Radiotherapy alone for clinical T4 skin carcinoma of the head and neck with surgery reserved for salvage. *Am J Otolaryngol.* 2001;22:387–390.
29. Tsao MN, Tsang RW, Liu F-F, et al. Radiotherapy management for squamous cell carcinoma of the nasal skin: The Princess Margaret Hospital experience. *Int J Radiat Oncol Biol Phys.* 2002; 52:973–979.
30. Zagrodnik B, Kempf W, Seifert B, et al. Superficial radiotherapy for patients with basal cell carcinoma: Recurrence rates, histologic subtypes, and expression of p53 and Bcl-2. *Cancer.* 2003;98: 2708–2714.
31. Cox NH, Nicoll JJ, Popple AW. Amyloid deposition in basal cell carcinoma: A cause of apparent lack of sensitivity to radiotherapy. *Clin Exp Dermatol.* 2001;26: 499–500.
32. Yen MT, Tse DT, Wu X, et al. Radiation therapy for local control of eyelid sebaceous cell carcinoma: Report of two cases and review of the literature. *Ophthal Plast Reconstr Surg.* 2000;16:211–215.
33. Guix B, Finestres F, Tello J-I, et al. Treatment of skin carcinomas of the face by high-dose-rate brachytherapy and custom-made surface molds. *Int J Radiat Oncol Biol Phys.* 2000;47:95–102.

34. Conill C, Sanchez-Reyes A, Molla M, et al. Brachytherapy with Ir as treatment of carcinoma of the tarsal structure of the eyelid. *Int J Radiat Oncol Biol Phys.* 2004;59:1326–1329.

35. Soler AM, Warloe T, Tausjo J, et al. Photodynamic therapy of residual or recurrent basal cell carcinoma after radiotherapy using topical 5-aminolevulinic acid or methylester aminolevulinic acid. *Acta Oncol.* 2000;39:605–609.

36. Stockfleth E, Sterry W. New treatment modalities for basal cell carcinoma. *Recent Results Cancer Res.* 2002;160:259–268.

37. Wang I, Bendsoe N, Klinteberg CA, et al. Photodynamic therapy vs. cryosurgery of basal cell carcinomas: Results of a phase III clinical trial. *Br J Dermatol.* 2001;144:832–840.

38. Schweitzer VG. Photofrin-mediated photodynamic therapy for treatment of aggressive head and neck nonmelanomatous skin tumors in elderly patients. *Laryngoscope.* 2001;111:1091–1098.

39. Rhodes LE, de Rie M, Enstrom Y, et al. Photodynamic therapy using topical methyl aminolevulinate vs. surgery for nodular basal cell carcinoma. *Arch Dermatol.* 2004;140:17–23.

40. Berridge JK, Morgan DAL. A comparison of late cosmetic results following two different radiotherapy techniques for treating basal cell carcinoma. *Clin Oncol.* 1997;9:400–402.

41. Petit JY, Avril MF, Margulis A, et al. Evaluation of cosmetic results of a randomized trial comparing surgery and radiotherapy in the treatment of basal cell carcinoma of the face. *Plast Reconstr Surg.* 1999;105:2544–2551.

42. Caccialanza M, Piccinno R, Moretti D, et al. Radiotherapy of carcinomas of the skin overlying the cartilage of the nose: Results of 405 lesions. *Eur J Dermatol.* 2003;13:462–465.

43. Caccialanza M, Piccinno R, Grammatica A. Radiotherapy of recurrent basal and squamous cell skin carcinomas: A study of 249 re-treated carcinomas in 229 patients. *Eur J Dermatol.* 2001;11:25–28.

44. Leibovitch I, McNab A, Sullivan T, et al. Orbital invasion by periocular basal cell carcinoma. *Ophthalmology.* 2005;112:717–723.

45. Fangman WL, Cook JL. Postradiation sarcoma: Case report and review of the potential complications of therapeutic ionizing radiation. *Dermatol Surg.* 2005;31:966–972.

46. Arlette JP, Trotter MJ, Trotter T, et al. Management of lentigo maligna and lentigo maligna melanoma: Seminars in surgical oncology. *J Surg Oncol.* 2004;86:179–186.

47. Osborne JE, Hutchinson PE. A follow-up study to investigate the efficacy of initial treatment of lentigo maligna with surgical excision. *Br J Plast Surg.* 2002;55:611–615.

48. Farshad A, Burg G, Panizzon R, et al. A retrospective study of 150 patients with lentigo maligna and lentigo maligna melanoma and the efficacy of radiotherapy using Grenz or soft X-rays. *Br J Dermatol.* 2002;146:1042–1046.

49. Schmid-Wendtner MH, Brunner B, Konz B, et al. Fractionated radiotherapy of lentigo maligna and lentigo maligna

50. Cooper JS. Radiation therapy of malignant melanoma. *Dermatol Clin.* 2002;20:713–716.

51. Paterson R. Classification of tumours in relation to radiosensitivity. *Br J Radiol.* 1933;6:218–233.

52. Hall EJ. Radiation damage and the dose-rate effect. In: *Radiobiology for the Radiologist.* 3rd ed. Philadelphia, PA: JB Lippincott; 1988:136.

53. Ballo MT, Ang KK. Radiation therapy for malignant melanoma. *Surg Clin N Am.* 2003;83:323–342.

54. Cooper JS. Radiation therapy of malignant melanoma. *Dermatol Clin.* 2002;20:713–716.

55. Sause WT, Cooper JS, Rush S, et al. Fraction size in external beam radiation therapy in the treatment of melanoma. *Int J Radiat Oncol Biol Phys.* 1991;20:429–432.

56. Bastiaannet E, Beukema JC, Hoekstra HJ. Radiation therapy following lymph node dissection in melanoma patients: Treatment, outcome, and complications. *Cancer Treat Rev.* 2005;31:18–26.

57. Gibbs P, Robinson WA, Pearlman N, et al. Management of primary cutaneous melanoma of the head and neck: The University of Colorado experience and a review of the literature. *J Surg Oncol.* 2001;77:179–185.

58. Stevens G, Thompson JF, Firth I, et al. Locally advanced melanoma: Results of postoperative hypofractionated radiation therapy. *Cancer.* 2000;88:88–94.

59. Morris KT, Marquez CM, Holland JM, et al. Prevention of local recurrence after surgical debulking of nodal and subcutaneous melanoma deposits by hypofractionated radiation. *Ann Surg Oncol.* 2000;7:680–684.

60. Fukuda H, Hiratsuka J, Kobayashi T, et al. Boron neutron capture therapy (BNCT) for malignant melanoma with special reference to absorbed doses to the normal skin and tumor. *Aust Phys Eng Sci Med.* 2003;26:97–103.

61. Stannard CE, Sealy GRH, Hering ER, et al. Malignant melanoma of the eyelid and palpebral conjunctiva treated with Iodine-125 brachytherapy. *Ophthalmology.* 2000;107:951–958.

62. Medina-Franco H, Urist MM, Fiveash J, et al. Multimodality treatment of Merkel cell carcinoma: Case series and literature review of 1024 cases. *Ann Surg Oncol.* 2001;8:204–208.

63. Veness MJ, Perera L, McCourt J, et al. Merkel cell carcinoma: Improved outcome with adjuvant radiotherapy. *ANZ J Surg.* 2005;75:275–281.

64. Brady LW. External irradiation of epithelial skin cancer. *Int J Radiat Oncol Biol Phys.* 1990;19:491–492.

65. Karapantzos I, Tsaroucha A, Polychronidis A, et al. Merkel cell carcinoma: Report of seven cases. *J Otorhinolaryngol Relat Spec.* 2003;65:370–374.

66. Morrison WH, Peters LJ, Silvia EG, et al. The essential role of radiation therapy in securing locoregional control of Merkel cell carcinoma. *Int J Radiat Oncol Biol Phys.* 1990;19:583–591.

67. Mortier L, Mirabel X, Fournier C, et al. Radiotherapy alone for primary Merkel

cell carcinoma. *Arch Dermatol.* 2003;139:1587–1590.

68. Poulsen M, Rischin D. Merkel cell carcinoma: Current therapeutic options. *Expert Opin Pharmacother.* 2003;4:2187–2192.

69. Lehree MS, Hershock D, Ming ME. Merkel cell carcinoma. *Curr Treat Options Oncol.* 2004;5:195–199.

70. Eng TY, Boersma MG, Fuller CD, et al. Treatment of Merkel cell carcinoma. *Am J Clin Oncol.* 2004;27:510–515 .

71. Eng TY, Naguib M, Fuller CD, et al. treatment of recurrent Merkel cell carcinoma: An analysis of 46 cases. *Am J Clin Oncol.* 2004;27:576–583.

72. Whittaker SJ, Marsden JR, Spittle M, et al. Joint British Association of Dermatologists and U.K. Cutaneous Lymphoma Group guidelines for the management of primary cutaneous T-cell lymphomas. *Br J Dermatol.* 2003;149:1095–1107.

73. Willemze R, Kerl H, Sterry W, et al. EORTC classification for primary cutaneous lymphomas: A proposal from the Cutaneous Lymphoma Study Group of the European Organisation for Research and Treatment of Cancer. *Blood.* 1997;90:354–371.

74. Cotter GW, Baglan RJ, Wasserman TH, et al. Palliative radiation treatment of cutaneous mycosis fungoides: A dose response. *J Am Acad Dermatol.* 2001;44:1477–1480.

75. Kirova YM, Piedbois Y, Haddad E, et al. Radiotherapy in the management of mycosis fungoides: Indications, results, prognosis. Twenty years experience. *Radiother Oncol.* 199;51:147–151.

76. Jones GW, Hoppe RT, Glatstein E. Electron beam treatment for cutaneous T-cell lymphoma. *Haematol Oncol Clin N Am.* 1995;9:1057–1076.

77. Jones GW, Kacinski BM, Wilson LD, et al. Total skin electron beam radiation in the management of mycosis fungoides: Consensus of the European Organisation for Research and Treatment of Cancer (EORTC) Cutaneous Lymphoma Project Group. *J Am Acad Dermatol.* 2002;47:364–370.

78. Hamminga B, Van Noordijk EM, Vloten WA. Treatment of mycosis fungoides: Total skin electron beam irradiation vs. topical mechlorethamine therapy. *Arch Dermatol.* 1982;118:150–153.

79. Olavarria E, Child F, Woolford A, et al. T-cell depletion and autologous stem cell transplantation in the management of tumour stage mycosis fungoides with peripheral blood involvement. *Br J Haematol.* 2001;114:624–631.

80. Bekkenk MW, Van Geelen FA, Van Voorst Vader PC, et al. Primary and secondary cutaneous CD30+ lymphoproliferative disorders: A report from the Dutch Cutaneous Lymphoma Group on the long-term follow-up data of 219 patients and guidelines for diagnosis and treatment. *Blood.* 2000;95:3653–3661.

81. Demierre MF, Goldberg LJ, Kadin ME, et al. Is it lymphoma or lymphomatoid papulosis? *J Am Acad Dermatol.* 1997;36:765–772.

82. Vonderheid EC, Sajjadian A, Kadin ME. Methotrexate is effective therapy for lymphomatoid papulosis and other pri-

mary cutaneous CD30+ lymphoproliferative disorders. *J Am Acad Dermatol.* 1996;34:470–481.

83. Wantzin GL, Thomsen K. PUVA-treatment in lymphomatoid papulosis. *Br J Dermatol.* 1982;107:687–690.

84. Pandolfino TL, Siegel RS, Kuzel TM, et al. Primary cutaneous B-cell lymphoma: Review and current concepts. *J Clin Oncol.* 2000;18:2152–2168.

85. Piccino R, Caccialanza M, Berti E. Dermatologic radiotherapy of primary cutaneous follicle center cell lymphoma. *Eur J Dermatol.* 2003;13:49–52.

86. Pimpinelli N, Vallecchi C. Local orthovoltage radiotherapy in primary cutaneous B-cell lymphoma: Our experience in a series of 115 patients. *Skin Cancer.* 1999;14:219–224.

87. Pimpinelli N, Santucci M, Bosi A, et al. Primary cutaneous follicular center-cell lymphoma: A lymphoproliferative disease with favourable prognosis. *Clin Exp Dermatol.* 1989;14:9–12.

88. Kirova YM, Piedbois Y, Le Bourgeois J-P. Radiotherapy in the management of cutaneous B-cell lymphoma: Our experience in 25 cases. *Radiother Oncol.* 1999; 52:8–15.

89. Bennenk MW, Vermeer MH, Geerts ML, et al. Treatment of multifocal primary cutaneous B-cell lymphoma: A clinical follow-up study of 29 patients. *J Clin Oncol.* 1999;17:2471–2478.

90. Goldschmidt H. Treatment planning: Selection of physical factors and radiation techniques. In: Goldschmidt H, Panizzon RG, eds. *Modern Dermatologic Radiation Therapy.* New York: Springer-Verlag; 1991:49–63.

91. Grange F, Joly P, Beylot-Barry M, et al. Prognostic factors in primary cutaneous large B-cell lymphomas: A European multicenter study. *J Clin Oncol.* 2001;19: 3602–3610.

92. Mori M, Mavilia L, Rossi R, et al. La terapia fotodinamica nel trattamento dei linfomi primitivi cutanei. *G Ital Dermatol Venereol.* 2005;140:123–127.

93. Mori M, Campolmi P, Mavilia L, et al. Topical photodynamic therapy in primary cutaneous T-cell and B-cell lymphomas. *J Eur Acad Dermatol Venereol.* 2004;18(S2):528.

94. Rossi R, Lotti T, Cappugi P, et al. Guidelines for photodynamic therapy in dermatology: Treatment protocol. *G Ital Dermatol Venereol.* 2005;140:637–644.

95. Mark RJ, Poen JC, Tran LM, et al. Angiosarcoma: A report of 67 patients and a review of the literature. *Cancer.* 1996;77:2400–2406.

96. Holden CA, Spittle MF, Wilson Jones E. Angiosarcoma of the face and scalp: Prognosis and treatment. *Cancer.* 1987;59: 1046–1057.

97. Rich AL, Berman P. Cutaneous angiosarcoma presenting as an unusual facial bruise. *Age Ageing.* 2004;33:512–514.

98. Huang J, Mackillop WJ. Increased risk of soft tissue sarcoma after radiotherapy in women with breast carcinoma. *Cancer.* 2001;92:172–180.

99. Murray S, Simmons J, James C. Cutaneous angiosarcoma of the face and scalp presenting as alopecia. *Aust J Dermatol.* 2003;44:273–276.

100. Wollima U, Fuller J, Graefe T, et al. Angiosarcoma of the scalp: Treatment with liposomal doxorubicin and radiotherapy. *J Cancer Res Clin Oncol.* 2001;127: 366–369.

101. Budd GT. Management of angiosarcoma. *Curr Oncol Rep.* 2002;4:515–519.

102. Pawlik TM, Paulino AF, Mcginn CJ, et al. Cutaneous angiosarcoma of the scalp: A multidisciplinary approach. *Cancer.* 2003;98:1716–1726.

103. Pestoni C, Paredes-Suarez C, Peteiro C, et al. Early detection of cutaneous angiosarcoma of the face and treatment with placitaxel. *J Eur Acad Dermatol Venereol.* 2005;19:357–359.

104. Cooper JS, Steinfeld AD, Learch I. Intentions and outcome in the radiotherapeutic management of epidemic Kaposi's sarcoma. *Int J Radiat Oncol Biol Phys.* 1991;20:419–422.

105. Caccialanza M. Radiotherapy of Kaposi's sarcoma. *Ital Gen Rev Dermatol.* 1989;26:242–246.

106. Cooper JS, Sacco J, Newall J, et al. The duration of local control of classic (non-AIDS-associated) Kaposi's sarcoma by radiotherapy. *J Am Acad Dermatol.* 1988; 19:59–66.

107. Ligula-Mugambe JB, Kavuma A. Epidemic and endemic Kaposi's sarcoma: A comparison of outcomes and survival after radiotherapy. *Radiother Oncol.* 2005;76:59–62.

108. Gambassi G, Semeraro R, Suma V, et al. Aggressive behavior of classical Kaposi's sarcoma and coexistence with angiosarcoma. *J Gerontol A Biol Sci Med Sci.* 2005; 60:520–523.

109. Panizzon RG. Radiotherapy of skin tumors. *Recent Results Cancer Res.* 2002;160: 234–239.

110. Piccino R, Caccialanza M, Cusini M. Role of radiotherapy in the treatment of epidemic Kaposi's sarcoma: Experience with sixty-five cases. *J Am Acad Dermatol.* 1995;32:1000–1003.

111. Vallecchi C, Bellini M, Bonan P, et al. Il ruolo attuale della radioterapia dermatologica. *G Ital Dermatol Venereol.* 1993;128: 1–15.

112. Topping A, Wilson GR. Diagnosis and management of uncommon cutaneous cancers. *Am J Clin Dermatol.* 2002;3:83–89.

113. MacKie RM. Tumours of skin appendages. In: Rook A, Wilkinson DS, Ebling FJG, eds. *Textbook of Dermatology.* 6th ed. Oxford, UK: Blackwell Science; 1998: 1695–1715.

114. Hashimoto K, Lever WF. *Appendage Tumors of the Skin.* Springfield, IL: Charles C. Thomas; 1968.

115. Snow S, Madjar DD, Hardy S, et al. Microcystic adnexal carcinoma: Report of 13 cases and review of the literature. *Dermatol Surg.* 2001;27:401–408.

116. Stein JM, Ormsby A, Esclamado R, et al. The effect of radiation therapy on microcystic adnexal carcinoma: A case report. *Head Neck.* 2003;25(3):251–254.

117. Fujimoto R, Nagata Y, Kinashi T, et al. The complete remission of recurrent sweat gland carcinoma by radiotherapy combined with hyperthermia. *Gan No Rinsho.* 1990;36:2485–2490.

118. Chamberlain RS, Huber K, White JC, et al. Apocrine gland carcinoma of the axilla: Review of the literature and recommendations for treatment. *Am J Clin Oncol.* 1999;22(2):131–135.

119. Morabito A, Bevilacqua P, Vitale S, et al. Clinical management of a case of recurrent apocrine gland carcinoma of the scalp: Efficacy of a chemotherapy schedule with metotrexate and bleomycin. *Tumori.* 2000;86:472–474.

120. Castro MC, Fagundes-Pereyra WJ, Oliveira Filho LN, et al. Treatment of ceruminous gland with intracranial invasion: Case report. *Arq Neuropsiquiatr.* 2000;58:324–329.

121. Lloyd J, Flanagan AM. Mammary and extramammary Paget's disease. *J Clin Pathol.* 2000;53:742–749.

122. Luk NM, Yu KH, Yeung WK, et al. Extramammary Paget's disease: Outcome of radiotherapy with curative intent. *Clin Exp Dermatol.* 2003;28:360–363.

123. Yamamoto R, Sakuragi N, Shirato H, et al. Radiotherapy with concurrent chemotherapy for vulvar adenocarcinoma associated with extramammary Paget's disease. *Gynecol Oncol.* 2001;80: 267–271.

CHAPTER 48

Immunomodulators for Skin Cancer

Deborah Zell, M.D.
Brian Berman, M.D., Ph.D.
Oliver Perez, M.D.
Cindy Berthelot, M.D.
Vandana Madkan, M.D.
Stephen Tyring, M.D., Ph.D., M.B.A.

BOX 48-1   Overview

- Recombinant cytokines, immune modulators, vaccinations, T-cell based immunity, and gene therapy are used as treatments against cancer cells.
- *Interferons* have antiproliferative, antiviral, and immunomodulatory properties. Interferons have been used to treat BCCs, SCCs, AKs, melanoma (FDA approved), CTCL, and Kaposi's sarcoma (FDA approved).
- *Imiquimod* is an immune response modifier that induces IFN-α, TNF-α, IL-1, IL-6, IL-8, and IL-12 production by monocytes, macrophages, and TRL7-bearing plasmacytoid dendritic cells. Imiquimod has been used in both clinical trials and case reports to treat the following cancers: BCCs, SCCs, AKs, Bowen disease, VIN, AIN, melanoma, CTCL, cutaneous EMPD, actinic cheilitis, XP, bowenoid papulosis, keratoacanthoma, and epidermodysplasia verruciformis.
- *COX inhibitors* inhibit cyclooxygenase enzymes involved in arachidonic acid metabolism, and arachidonic acid metabolites are involved in the conversion of procarcinogens to carcinogens, inhibition of immune surveillance, inhibition of apoptosis, stimulation of angiogenesis, and increasing invasiveness of tumor cells. COX inhibitors have been used to treat AKs in clinical trials.
- *IL-2* has been used to treat both melanoma and CTCL.
- *Vaccinations* have been used in clinical trials to treat melanoma.
- *Histamine* protects NK cells and T cells against oxygen radical-induced dysfunction and apoptosis, and also maintains the activation of these cells by IL-2 and other lymphocyte activators. Histamine has been used as an adjunct to IL-2 in treating melanoma.
- *GM-CSF* has increased the number of circulating DC in patients with advanced solid tumors and this may be helpful during chemotherapy. GM-CSF has been used in studies to treat melanoma.
- *IL-12* production defects have been found in patients with CTCL. IL-12 has been used in a clinical trial in patients with CTCL.

INTRODUCTION

Therapeutic interventions to augment tumor antigenicity or increase the host's immune response against cancer cells include recombinant cytokines, immune modulators, vaccinations with tumor antigens, T-cell-based immunotherapy, and gene therapy. We describe the current role of the immunomodulators (upregulators of the immune response) in the therapy of skin cancer including nonmelanoma skin cancer, melanoma, lymphoma, Kaposi's sarcoma, extramammary Paget's disease, vulvar intraepithelial carcinoma neoplasias (VIN), xeroderma pigmentosum (XP), actinic cheilitis, bowenoid papulosis, keratoacanthoma, and epidermodysplasia verruciformis. See Table 48-1 for abbreviations and their definitions.

Table 48-1
Abbreviations and Their Definitions

Actinic keratosis (AK)
Anal intraepithelial neoplasia (AIN)
Basal cell carcinomas (BCCs)
Bowenoid papulosis (BP)
Cutaneous T-cell lymphoma (CTCL)
Delayed-type hypersensitivity (DTH)
Dendritic cells (DC)
Epidermodysplasia verruciformis (EV)
Extracorporeal photochemotherapy (ECP)
Extramammary Paget's disease (EMPD)
Human papillomavirus (HPV)
Interferons (IFNs)
Kaposi's sarcoma (KS)
Keratoacanthoma (KA)
Lentigo maligna (LM)
Psoralen ultraviolet A (PUVA)
Retinoic acid receptor (RAR)
Squamous cell carcinoma (SCC)
Toll-like receptor 7 (TRL7)
Tumor necrosis factor α (TNF-α)
Vulvar intraepithelial carcinoma neoplasias (VIN)
Xeroderma pigmentosum (XP)
5% fluorouracil (5-FU)

■ BASAL CELL CARCINOMA

BOX 48-2   Summary

- Surgical excision is the treatment of choice for BCCs (nodular and superficial types).
- The immunomodulator treatments for BCCs include interferon and imiquimod.
- *Interferon* is a nonsurgical alternative for low-risk BCCs. Clinical trials were performed with intralesional IFN-α2b with varying success rates.
- *Imiquimod 5% cream* has been used in several clinical trials at varying frequencies with and without adjuvant surgery in both superficial and nodular BCCs. Imiquimod 5% cream five times a week for 6 weeks has been FDA approved for biopsy-proven superficial BCC. Imiquimod 5% cream is also helpful in special cases where surgery is not an option.

The treatment of choice for small basal cell carcinomas (BCCs) of the nodular and superficial types is surgical excision. Mohs micrographic surgery is indicated for head, neck, and other areas where tissue conservation in BCC treatment is critical, but is also the treatment of choice in large, ill defined, and morphea lesions.[1] Another treatment option for superficial BCCs is imiquimod 5% cream, which was FDA-approved in 2004.

Interferons

Based on their antiproliferative, antiviral, and immunomodulatory properties, interferons (IFNs) have been studied as an alternative therapy in the treatment of cancer. Following intralesional interferon (IFN)-α treatment of BCC, BCC cells are induced to express FasR, while continuing to express FasL, making themselves susceptible to FasR/FasL-mediated apoptosis caused by BCC cell–BCC cell and/or T-lymphocyte–BCC-cell interactions, and to self-induced "suicidal" apoptosis of individual BCC cells coexpressing FasR and FasL.[2] Intralesional IFN-α2b, 1.5 million IU used over a 3 to 4-week period has an overall success rate in most clinical trials between 70 and 100%,[3,4] which is lower than the cure rate of primary surgical excision (95%) or cryosurgery (94 to 99%).[5] When used for aggressive forms of BCC (recurrent or morpheaform), this protocol resulted in a complete cure in only 27% of patients.[6]

IFN treatment of BCCs remains a nonsurgical alternative in a number of selected cases of patients with low-risk nodular or superficial BCCs.

Imiquimod 5%

Imiquimod is an immune response modifier. Imiquimod induces IFN-α, tumor necrosis factor α (TNF-α), IL-1, IL-6, IL-8, and IL-12 production by monocytes, macrophages, and toll-like receptor 7 (TRL7)-bearing plasmacytoid dendritic cells. TLR-7 is an essential receptor for imiquimod-induced immune response.[7] Imiquimod also generates production of IFN-γ after CD4 cells are stimulated by IL-12. IFN-γ stimulates cytotoxic T lymphocytes responsible for killing virus-infected and tumor cells. Imiquimod 5% cream induces expression of FasR on BCC cells and lymphocytic infiltration. Imiquimod-induced FasR-mediated apoptosis may contribute to the effectiveness of imiquimod 5% cream for the treatment of BCC.[8] The initial study of topical imiquimod 5% cream for nodular and superficial BCC was a vehicle-controlled, 16-week, dose-ranging study.[9] The histologically confirmed cure rate varied depending upon the frequency of dosing, with the overall response rate being 83% (20/24) in the imiquimod-treated group and 9% (1/11) in the vehicle-treated group.

In superficial BCC, randomized multicenter studies using imiquimod 5% cream reported 100% efficacy with a twice a day application, versus 82 to 88% when used once a day.[10,11] Combined clinical and histological assessments from two randomized, double-blind, vehicle-controlled, phase III studies using imiquimod 5% cream 5 to 7 times a week showed clearance rates of 75% and 73% on superficial BCC.[12] These studies showed that twice-daily regimens have unacceptable safety profiles because of severe local skin reactions and that the once daily or five times a week dosage regimens had the highest efficacy results with acceptable safety profiles. The 6-week therapy appears to be as effective as the 12-week therapy for superficial BCC. Imiquimod 5% cream may be safely administered at both the seven times and five times per week regimens; the latter being the more efficacious and better tolerated of the two.

Two phase II studies determined the safety and efficacy of imiquimod 5% cream in the treatment of nodular BCC.[13] The highest response rate of 76% in the twice-daily 12-week group does not compare with the surgical excision success

rate.[5] An open-label series involving a combination treatment of imiquimod (three times a week for 12 weeks) and Mohs micrographic surgery performed at week 15 on 15 subjects with nodular BCC resulted in clearance of all of the patient's BCC and no reoccurrence at the 18-month follow-up visit.[14] Another randomized, double-blind, pilot trial including 35 patients with nodular and superficial BCC had good results after treatment regimens of imiquimod 5% cream twice daily, once daily, three times weekly, twice weekly, and once weekly for a maximum of 16 weeks. There was a 100% complete response (CR) with the patients in the treatment regimens of twice daily, once daily, and three times weekly regimens cleared, three of five patients with the twice a week treatment regimen cleared, two of four patients with the once a week treatment regimen, and only one of the 11 patients in the vehicle regimen cleared; however, all of the twice daily, half of the once daily, and a quarter of the three times a week treatment regimen patients had local skin reactions that required vacation periods from the medication. Severe erosions occurred in two of the twice daily and one of the once daily treatment regimen patients, and a severe ulceration occurred in one of the twice-daily treatment patients.[15]

Imiquimod is FDA-approved for biopsy-proven superficial BCC; however, it is not FDA-approved for all types of BCC at this time. Imiquimod is a helpful tool in managing special cases in which surgery is not an option like large,[16] multiple lesions,[17] or cases in which the rate of tumor formation does not allow "keeping up" with the surgical treatment.[18]

SQUAMOUS CELL CARCINOMA

BOX 48-3 Summary

- Surgical excision is the treatment of choice for cutaneous SCCs.
- Intralesional IFNα2b at 1.5 MIU three times a week for 3 weeks has been studied in clinical trials.
- Imiquimod 5% cream has been used in clinical trials only for *in situ* SCCs.

Surgical excision, including Mohs surgery when indicated, should be regarded as the treatment of choice for cutaneous squamous cell carcinoma (SCC).[19]

Interferons

IFN-α2b used in the treatment of biopsy-proven SCC, at a dose of 1.5 mil-

lion intralesional IU of IFN-α2b three times weekly for 3 weeks, revealed 97 to 99% histologic absence of SCC.[20,21]

Currently, interferons are not part of the management of patients with cutaneous SCC. In transplant-associated metastasic SCC, combination therapy with retinoids and interferon α has been used with a 7% CR rate and a 36% partial response (PR).[22]

Imiquimod

Imiquimod, but not resiquimod, induces apoptosis in all SCC cell lines and HaCaT cells (a spontaneously immortalized human kertinocyte cell line).[23] Current clinical studies on the use of 5% cream imiquimod in cutaneous SCCs are restricted to actinic keratosis (AKs) and *in situ* clinical presentations.

ACTINIC KERATOSIS

BOX 48-4 Summary

- The treatment of choice for AKs is local destruction, photodynamic therapy, and drug therapy.
- Intralesional IFNα2b 0.5 MIU three times a week for 2 to 3 weeks was performed. Results were promising, but painful injections and multiple visits limit the use of IFN.
- Imiquimod 5% cream twice a week for 16 weeks has been FDA approved. Controlled clinical trials have been performed using imiquimod 5% cream at varying frequencies and lengths of time.
- Cox inhibitor (diclofenac) was used twice daily in two controlled studies with conflicting results.

Modalities of treatment for actinic keratosis (AKs), considered as SCC *in situ*, include local destruction, drug therapy, and photodynamic therapy.[24]

Interferons

Ninety-three percent clearance of AK was found in a study following injections of intralesional IFN-α2b, half a million IU three times weekly for 2 to 3 weeks, with no clearing occurring in the placebo-injected group.[25] The use of IFN in the treatment of AK is limited because of the need for painful injections and multiple physician visits, when compared to other more feasible treatments.

Imiquimod

The use of imiquimod twice weekly for 16 weeks, approved by the FDA as one of the treatments for AKs, is supported on successful reports, and has shown clearance of all treated AK lesions without reoccurrence.[26] Complete resolution in 85% of the patients and partial resolution in 8% was shown in a double-blind study applying imiquimod 5% or vehicle cream three times a week for 12 weeks or until clinical resolution of the lesions.[27] The clinical recurrence rate, 1 year after treatment, was 10% (2/25). A different protocol using imiquimod 5% cream for a maximum of three cycles, each cycle of 8 weeks, was published by Salache et al.[28] The cream was applied to the affected area once daily, three times a week for 4 weeks, followed by a rest period of 4 weeks. If any AKs were present at the end of a 4-week rest period, the entire area was re-treated for another cycle of 4 weeks, followed by another 4-week rest period. A treatment failure was determined if any AKs were present after the third cycle. For the intent-to-treat analysis, 82% of the sites were completely cleared. Results from four multicenter, double-blind, randomized, vehicle-controlled phase III safety and efficacy studies evaluating imiquimod 5% cream in the treatment of AKs on the face or balding scalp, showed that imiquimod 5% cream, either once daily two times a week or once daily three times a week, was significantly better than the vehicle with respect to complete clearance rates ($p < 0.001$).[29] Patients achieved a complete clearance of 45% and 48% when treated two times a week and three times a week, respectively, and the median clearance of AKs was 83.3% with the twice a week regimen. In a similar phase III, randomized, double-blind, vehicle-controlled clinical study of 286 patients treated with imiquimod versus vehicle on the face and balding scalp three times a week for 16 weeks, results were clinically significant at week 24 with a complete clearance rate of 57.1% versus 2.2% ($p < 0.001$) and a partial clearance ($\geq 75\%$ reduction from baseline) of 72.1% versus 4.3% ($p < 0.001$) in the treatment and vehicle group, respectively.[30] A smaller 2-year double-blind, randomized, vehicle-controlled trial involving the same treatment regimen for a maximum of 12 weeks, on 25 treated patients was also done. Among the patients in the treatment group, 20% developed new AKs or were lost to follow-up and none of the patients developed SCC at 24 months. At the 1-year follow-up in the vehicle group (10 patients), one patient developed spontaneous remission of AKs, nine patients developed new AKs, and one patient developed SCC.[31] In two phase III randomized, double-blind parallel group, vehicle-controlled study treating 492

patients with 5% imiquimod three times a week for 16 weeks or vehicle, complete and partial clearance rates were 48.3% and 64.0% in the treated patients and 7.2% and 13.6% in the placebo group, respectively.[32] Twenty-one out of 29 patients cleared greater than or equal to 75% of their AKs (72%) versus only 30% of the vehicle group ($p = 0.027$) in another multicenter, randomized, double-blind, vehicle-controlled study evaluating the safety and efficacy of imiquimod 5% cream (three times a week for a varying number of weeks depending on the response).[33]

Cox Inhibitors

As an NSAID, diclofenac inhibits the cyclooxygenase enzymes involved in arachidonic acid metabolism. Arachidonic acid metabolites are involved in the conversion of procarcinogens to carcinogens, inhibition of immune surveillance, inhibition of apoptosis, stimulation of angiogenesis, and increasing invasiveness of tumor cells.[34,35] A randomized, double-blind, placebo-controlled trial comparing 3% diclofenac gel in 2.5% hyaluran gel versus placebo, two times a day for 90 days, in patients with AKs showed that topical diclofenac gel was effective and well tolerated when compared to placebo.[36] In contrast to these findings, another randomized double-blind placebo-controlled study evaluating 3% diclofenac 2.5% hyaluronic acid (HA) gel versus gel containing 2.5% HA alone applied twice daily for 180 days, failed to show significant results.[37]

■ BOWEN DISEASE

BOX 48-5 Summary

- Current therapies for Bowen disease include 5-FU, destruction modalities, surgical excision, laser, photodynamic therapy, and radiotherapy.
- Imiquimod 5% cream qd for 16 weeks was used in a controlled clinical trial and in case reports at varying frequencies with good results.

Current therapies for Bowen disease (intraepidermal SCC) include 5-fluorouracil, cryotherapy, curettage with cautery/electrocautery, excision, laser, photodynamic therapy, and radiotherapy.[38]

Imiquimod

In a phase II open-label study, 16 biopsy-proven plaques of Bowen disease, with diameters ranging between 1 and 5.4 cm,

were treated once daily with imiquimod 5% cream for 16 weeks.[39] Of the 16 lesions treated, 15 were on the legs, and one was on the shoulder. Fourteen of the 15 patients (93% per protocol analysis) had no residual tumor present in their 6-week posttreatment biopsy specimens. One patient died of unrelated intercurrent illness before a biopsy specimen could be obtained. Ten patients completed 16 weeks of treatment, and six patients stopped treatment between 4 and 8 weeks because of local skin reactions that included superficial erosive changes associated with hemorrhagic crust. Patients were followed for 6 months without recurrences.

Case reports illustrating the efficacy of imiquimod 5% cream in treating Bowen disease of the penis[40–42] have shown clinical and histological resolution. The same response has been observed in immunocompromised hosts with perianal SCC *in situ*. Biopsy specimens taken from the affected area showed no evidence of residual dysplasia after being treated with the topical immunomodulator.[43] Imiquimod in combination with 5% fluorouracil (5-FU) therapy has also been shown to be effective in immunosuppressed populations. Five cases of renal transplant patients treated successfully with imiquimod and 5-FU for Bowen disease in multiple areas following their transplants have been described.[44] In a case report of an immunocompetent woman with HPV 16 positive anogenital Bowen disease, imiquimod was used three times weekly (as to how long was not specified in the case report—only the total overall treatment was specified) and then two weekly due to itching and pain for a total of 20 weeks. At both 4 weeks and 6 months posttreatment visits, there were no signs of reoccurrence via skin biopsy.[45]

■ VULVAR INTRAEPITHELIAL NEOPLASIAS (VIN)

BOX 11-6 Summary

- The treatment of choice for VIN is laser, surgical, and medical therapy.
- Imiquimod 5% cream thrice a week for 16 weeks was used in three clinical trials showing conflicting results. Another study using imiquimod 5% cream one to three times a week for 6 to 34 weeks resulted in 87% of patients with CR or PR.
- In one AIN study, imiquimod three times a week for 16 weeks was used and showed disease regression.

A large percentage of vulvar intraepithelial carcinoma neoplasias (VIN) have been shown to harbor human papillomavirus (HPV). VIN management consists of laser CO_2 treatment, surgical, and conventional medical treatment. Vulvar intraepithelial squamous cell *in situ* is designated VIN 3.

Imiquimod

Imiquimod is thought to be a potentially beneficial treatment for patients with VIN of viral (HPV) etiology because of both its indirect antiviral and antineoplastic properties, although results have not been promising. A prospective study of 15 patients with high-grade VIN 3 examined the effects of imiquimod 5% cream self-applied three times weekly to vulvar lesions for 16 weeks. Local side effects were soreness, burning, erythema, ulceration, and blisters. One patient required hospitalization, catheterization, and analgesia because of the severity of the side effects. From the 13 patients that were able to complete the study, four showed visible clinical improvement in the state of their condition, but only three had no evidence of VIN on a subsequent biopsy. All four patients that responded clinically relapsed 4 months after treatment.[46]

More recent studies of imiquimod-treated VIN have been promising. In an eight-patient study with biopsy-proven bowenoid and basaloid VIN 2/3, imiquimod 5% cream was applied three times a week until total clearance or 16 weeks had elapsed. Total clearance and partial clearance were observed in six patients and two patients, respectively, and the posttreatment biopsy showed absence of precancerous lesions in seven of the patients (87.5%). Side effects included erythema (all patients), erosions (one patient), and edema (one patient). No reoccurrences were observed during the 10 to 30-week follow-up visit.[47]

A prospective, observational, pilot study on 15 women with biopsy-proven multifocal VIN 2/3 where imiquimod 5% cream was applied one to three times a week for 6 to 34 weeks was administered. Four patients had a CR (27% after 6, 7, 11, and 30 weeks of treatment), nine patients had a PR (60%), and two patients discontinued the study.[48] One study with 15 patients examined the effects of imiquimod applied three times a week for 16 weeks.[49] Of the 13 patients who completed the study, four showed visible improvement of their condition.

Results were mixed in a prospective, uncontrolled study involving 12 patients with undifferentiated VIN. Imiquimod 5% cream was applied three times a week for up to 7 months according to their clinical response. Three, four, and five patients achieved a CR, PR, and no response/failure, respectively. Side effects included vulvar discomfort that led to the withdrawal of three patients and flu-like symptoms for two patients.[50] Eight patients with high-grade intraepithelial neoplasia, including two with cervical cancer, were treated with imiquimod 5% cream.[51] Of the patients treated, four had CRs, two had PRs, one progressed, and one did not tolerate the therapy. Of the four complete responders, two remained disease-free (mean follow-up, 33 months).

Anal intraepithelial neoplasia (AIN) is a precursor lesion for SCC of the anus, and has a strong association with human papillomavirus (HPV). Ten HIV-positive homosexual men were treated with imiquimod 5% cream three times a week for a maximum of 16 weeks.[52] All patients were positive for HPV-16 before treatment. Follow-up histologic studies showed regression of the disease by at least two grades and HPV-16 DNA was no longer detectable by polymerase chain reaction after treatment.

■ MELANOMA

BOX 48-7   Summary

- The recommended treatment for lentigo maligna is surgical excision.
- Interferon is FDA approved for use in patients with melanoma of >4-mm Breslow thickness or with nodal involvement five times a week for 4 weeks (IV) and three times a week for 48 weeks (SC) at 20 MIU/m2 and 10 MIU/m2 (Interon A). Clinical studies of interferon and combination therapy with interferon were performed with overall positive results.
- Imiquimod has been used in clinical trials and case reports in LM and metastatic melanoma.
- Studies including IV IL-2 and IL-2 in combination with chemotherapy were performed.
- Vaccination studies had limited results.
- Histamines with IL-2 and GM-CSF have been used in studies and have been shown to increase the survival of patients with metastatic melanoma.

The recommended treatment for lentigo maligna (melanoma *in situ*) is surgical, using a 5 to 10-mm margin, as well as Mohs micrographic surgery. Surgical excision margins for invasive melanoma depend on the Breslow thickness. In patients with metastasic disease, standard chemotherapy, outside a clinical trial, remains single-agent dacarbazine, but no systemic therapy has been shown to significantly prolong the survival of these patients.[53]

Immunomodulators in the Treatment of Cutaneous Melanoma

INTERFERONS Eleven biopsy-proven cases of lentigo maligna (LM), treated with perilesional and intralesional interferon α2b (3 million IU for LM lesions that were ≤25 mm, and 6 million IU for LM lesions >25 mm) three times a week, cleared after treatment without scarring. In the United States, high-dose interferon regimen is regarded as the standard therapy for patients with melanoma at high risk of recurrence.[54] The use of IFN-α2b for the treatment of patients with melanomas thicker than 4 mm and patients with lymph-node metastasis is FDA-approved. Statistically significant increases in the median overall survival by 1.04 and 1.6 years were found in IFN-α2b-treated patients with stage I and II melanoma versus controls, with the greatest patient response achieved in those patients with nodal disease.[54,55] In general, the combined use of IFN and chemotherapeutic agents such as dacarbazine and vindesine are the most effective regimens.[56]

Intralesional IFN-α has been used intralesionally in the therapy of metastasis of advanced malignant melanoma with partial remissions in a few patients lasting between 2 and 6 months.[57] The authors suggested that in order to take advantage of both the local and systemic effects of IFN-α therapy in melanoma, local therapy should be seriously considered after resection of the primary tumor or regional lymph nodes.

In a more recent study, the combination of interferon-α-2b and surgery were performed in high-risk patients. In this retrospective study of 150 patients, high-risk melanoma patients (mainly stage III) were treated with high-dose interferon-α-2b that was started 8 weeks after definitive surgery at 20 MU/day intravenous (IV) 5 days/week for 4 weeks and 10 MU/m2 subcutaneous (SC) three times a week for 48 weeks. At the follow-up visit (median of 35 months), 63% of the patients had reoccurrence and 37% were relapse-free.[58]

IMIQUIMOD Topical imiquimod 5% has also been of use in the treatment of LM. A patient with a large LM of the scalp, reluctant to have surgery, reported apparent complete resolution after

7 months of daily application of imiquimod 5% to an initial (the most pigmented) test area inside the lesion, followed by 3 months of application over the entire affected area. There was no evidence of LM in an incisional biopsy after stopping the treatment. No clinical recurrence was reported at 9-month follow-up.[59] In a case report of a woman with biopsy-confirmed LM on her cheek, imiquimod once or twice a day for a total of 3 months (as to how long is it once a day or twice a day—not specified in the article) was used to treat the LM. The posttreatment biopsy showed no residual LM.[60] Results were also favorable in two case reports of patients with amelanotic LM treated with imiquimod 5% cream three times weekly for 3 months and 5 months, respectively. Both patients had no clinical evidence of reoccurrence with 18 and 9-month follow-up visits after treatment.[61] Twelve patients with biopsy-proven facial LM were treated with imiquimod 5% three times a week or daily for 6 weeks. Ten out of the 12 patients cleared with no relapse at the 6-month posttreatment visit and two patients failed to respond to the imiquimod and received surgical excision.[62] A study involving 30 patients with a histologic diagnosis of LM, *in situ* melanoma, treated with topical imiquimod was presented at the American Academy of Dermatology annual meeting in 2003.[63] Thirty patients older than 18 years with *in situ* melanomas were treated once daily for 3 months. One-month posttreatment, four-quadrant biopsies were performed, as well as any other biopsies indicated by dermoscopic findings. One patient was reclassified as stage 1 and withdrawn from the study. They reported 28 assessable patients. Two patients were treatment failures with persistent tumor visually, and on biopsy at week 16. The remaining 26 patients were complete responders (defined as complete absence of tumor by clinical and histological criteria). Initial CR was of 93% with no relapses at 12 months. The authors concluded that imiquimod 5% cream is a highly effective therapy for LM (*in situ* melanoma). A pilot, open-label, nonrandomized study evaluating the effectiveness of imiquimod 5% once daily for 13 weeks on five patients with LM showed that a CR rate occurred in 100% of the patients, and no reoccurrences occurred with the 3 to 18-month follow-up visits.[64] In two patients with extensive LM treated with imiquimod 5% three times a week for 1 month and then decreased to once a week, and applied for an additional month at three times weekly on part of the lesion for the second patient, reoccurrence did not occur at the 14-month and 13-month follow-up visits for patients 1 and 2, respectively.[64]

Imiquimod 5% cream was used three times a week with continuance of dacarbazine in a case of disseminated cutaneous metastatic melanoma lesions, unsuitable for surgery or radiotherapy, and failing to improve after a cycle of dacarbazine alone. Twelve weeks after treatment with imiquimod was initiated, the metastases cleared histologically.[65] Two other cases of multiple metastasic lesions of melanoma to the skin that cleared after treatment with imiquimod 5% cream have been reported. The two patients applied imiquimod 5% cream, three times a week to the lesions, with a 1-cm surrounding margin.[66] One case described an 81-year-old male with multiple satellite metastases around the site of a previous melanoma excision.[67] Imiquimod was applied daily to the areas under occlusion for 12 weeks. At the end of therapy, there appeared to be no clinical evidence of residual tumor, with biopsy showing no viable tumor cells. However, surgical dissection of an enlarging lymph node showed nodal melanoma metastasis. Finally, one study examined imiquimod treatment of multiple (>15) cutaneous metastases of malignant melanoma.[68] The three patients administered imiquimod twice daily under occlusion for 21 to 28 weeks. This regimen resulted in greater than 90% regression of cutaneous metastases in two patients, and the third patient showed marked response with adjunctive IL-2 intralesional injection. The side effects were mild in all patients.

IL-2 High doses of IL-2 have been investigated in the treatment of metastasic melanoma, unfortunately accompanied by important toxicity.[69] In clinical studies, when a high dose of IL-2 was administered IV, up to 20% of patients treated with this modality achieved objective responses.[70] IL-2-based biochemotherapy (IL-2, IFN-α, cisplatin, and dacarbazine) has shown a response rate of 47%. It appears that this combination is statistically superior to either IL-2 alone or chemotherapy alone.[71] Results of ongoing trials may clarify the true value of the use of IL-2 in combination with chemotherapy, versus chemotherapy alone.

VACCINATIONS Vaccinations have also been used to treat melanoma. The combination of IL-2 and a vaccination may enhance the response rate of the vaccination by boosting the immune response as seen in previous clinical and animal studies.[72–77] In a study testing of 34 patients with metastatic melanoma, IL-2 was combined with a DNP-modified autologous vaccine in 24 patients and vaccine alone was used in 10 patients. Overall, 35% or 12 patients out of 34 responded with 12% having a CR and 23% having a PR. Out of those that responded, only two were in the vaccine-only treatment group and 10 were in the combination of IL-2 and vaccine group, which suggests that the combination of IL-2 and autologous melanoma vaccine may have enhanced the response rate.[78] In a 5-year follow-up study of 214 patients with stage III melanoma, patients received multiple intradermal injections of human cancer vaccine with autologous tumor cells modified with the hapten dinitrophenyl (DNP) mixed with bacilli Calmette–Guérin. The delayed-type hypersensitivity (DTH) was also tested in all of the patients. Results showed that the 5-year overall survival rate of the 214 patients was 44%, the unmodified autologous melanoma were induced in 47% of patients, and the overall survival of the DTH-positive patients was double the DTH-negative patients (59.3% versus 29.3%, $p < 0.001$).[79] In a phase I trial, the toxicity and immunological activity of large multivariant immunogen (LMI) tumor-cell membranes affixed to amorphous silica microbeads were tested in 19 patients with metastatic stage IV melanoma. Since two patients were ineligible due to brain metastases and two patients did not complete the study due to reasons other than toxicity, 15 patients received the 3-month therapy of SC or intradermal injections randomly at doses of 10, 30, or 100 million tumor-cell equivalents on weeks 0, 4, and 8. The tests that were performed at 4-week intervals included cytolytic T-cell precursors against HLA-A2 matched melanoma cells, delayed-type hypersensitivity to melanoma cells, serum chemistries, CBCs, and CT scans to monitor effects on the metastatic lesions. Results showed that eight out of the 15 patients had an increase in cytotoxic T-cell precursors by day 42, no toxicities were observed, one patient had a (50% regression of a lung nodule, but had progression to the brain, and another patient had a partial remission of a solitary lung nodule.[80]

HISTAMINE Histamine protects NK cells and T cells against oxygen radical-induced dysfunction and apoptosis, and also maintains the activation of these cells by IL-2 and other lymphocyte activators.[81] The use of histamine as an adjunct to IL-2 in metastasic melanoma and other malignant diseases may prolong the survival time of patients with metastasic melanoma to the liver. Histamine, as an adjunct to IL-2, has been shown to increase survival of patients with metastatic melanoma to the liver.[81] Ongoing studies may overcome the disappointing results of the clinical trials of immunotherapy with IL-2 alone in metastasic melanoma.

GM-CSF GM-CSF increased the number of circulating dendritic cells (DC) by 32-fold, when compared to baseline, in patients with advanced solid tumors treated with this plus chemotherapy. Isolation of DC from cancer patients is a critical aspect of many current immunotherapeutic strategies; therefore, the possibility of a substantial increase in DC numbers during standard chemotherapy with GM-CSF mobilization may be very useful.[82]

A study in patients with stage II and IV melanoma, treated with GM-CSF after surgical resection of the disease and clinically disease-free, showed that GM-CSF may provide an antitumor effect that prolongs survival.[83]

■ CUTANEOUS T-CELL LYMPHOMA

BOX 48-8   Summary

- Current therapies for CTCL are limited by their toxicity and few have been shown to alter survival.
- Studies treating patients with CTCL with recombinant IFN therapy, combination of IFN and PUVA, and retinoic acid receptor retinoids resulted in better outcomes for patients with early-stage disease with the use of combination therapy when compared to IFN alone.
- In a small study and case report, imiquimod 5% cream was used for 3 and 4 months, respectively, with promising results.
- In two studies, one using IL-2 and another using IL-12, the CRs were 43% and 20%, respectively, and in one study combining both IL-2 and IL-12, a synergistic effect was noted in both INF-γ and natural killer cell activity.

Prognosis and survival of patients with cutaneous T-cell lymphoma (CTCL) remains dependent upon overall clinical stage (stage IA to IVB) at presentation, as well as on response to therapy. Therapies have been limited by toxicity or the lack of consistently durable responses, and few treatments have been shown to actually alter survival, especially in the late stages of disease.[84]

Interferons

Most of the data on the use of IFN-α in CTCL therapy have come from studies using recombinant IFN-α2a. IFN-α is probably the most active single-agent therapy for CTCL.[85] Out of those with MF and Sézary syndrome treated with IFN-α2a, 17% were complete responders with the overall response rate being 55%, derived from 207 cases reviewed from the literature.[86] Based on the review, it was concluded that recombinant IFN-α2a as a monotherapy has greater activity in patients with early-stage disease, and that 3 million units given three times each week subcutaneously is the optimal treatment. There was no apparent therapeutic difference between IFN-α2a and 2b. The effect of combining psoralen ultraviolet A (PUVA) with SC injections of IFN-α2a, at a maximum dose of 9 to 12 million IU three times a week, in the treatment of 63 CTCL patients has also been studied.[87] Forty-seven patients (75%) obtained a CR, six obtained a PR, two were classified as nonresponders, and five had progressive disease. The median time to obtain remission was 7 months and the median duration of overall response was 32 months, with a range of 6 to 57 months. These results confirm that the CR rates obtained with the combination of IFN-α and PUVA are better than those reported for INF-α or PUVA alone. In a prospective, randomized, multicenter clinical trial in 82 patients with stage I and II CTCL, IFN-α(9 MU three times a week SC with increasing doses) and PUVA (8-methoxypsoralen 0.6 mg/kg body weight five times a week for 4 weeks, three times a week for weeks 5 to 23, and two times a week for weeks 24 to 48, and escalating doses of UVA starting at 0.25 J/cm^3) were compared to a treatment of INF alpha (same dosage) and acitretin (25 mg during the first week and then 50 mg through weeks 2 to 48). Both the complete remission and the time to respond were statistically more significant in the INF alpha and PUVA group than in the IFN alpha and acitretin group by 70% versus 38.1% ($p \leq 0.008$) and 18.6 weeks versus 21.8 weeks ($p = 0.0015$), respectively.[88]

Intralesional injection of plaques of mycosis fungoides (MF) with IFN-α2b, 1 million IU three times weekly for 4 weeks, produced substantial localized clinical and histological improvement with 10/12 plaques demonstrating complete regression localized to the IFN-injected sites.[89] The responses of IFN-α plus retinoic acid receptor (RAR) retinoids, with respect to all stages of cutaneous T-cell lymphoma, have shown an overall response of 60% with a CR of 11%, similar to those of either modality when used alone.[84] In a retrospective cohort study at a tertiary care university hospital, 47 patients with advanced CTCL, with 68% of the patients in stage III or IV and 89% of the patients with circulating malignant T cells, were treated with photophoresis (six or more cycles). Thirty-one patients were also treated with one or more systemic immunostimulatory agents (interferon-α, γ, sargramostim, or systemic retinoids for 3 or more months). Results showed that 79% of patients responded to therapy (26% CR and 53% PR), and that the median survival time was 74 months. Overall, the combination therapy group that had a worse prognosis prior to treatment responded better than the photopharesis group alone, 84% (74 months) compared to 75% (66 months), respectively ($p = 0.51$); but, the results were not significant.[90]

A prospective controlled study treated 14 patients, with stage II CTCL, with interferon-α2a and extracorporeal photochemotherapy (ECP).[91] Among stage IIa patients, the response rate was 60%, in contrast to only 25% for those in stage IIb. IFN-γ shows no benefits over IFN-α in the treatment of CTCL, and its side effects are higher in frequency and severity.[85]

Imiquimod

A case of stage IA CTCL, refractory to topical steroid preparations and topical nitrogen mustard and carmustine, showed complete clinical and histological clearance after a 4-month treatment with imiquimod 5% followed by no recurrence at the treatment site at 10-month follow-up. The authors have initiated a double-blind, placebo-controlled trial to better evaluate the efficacy of imiquimod in the treatment of CTCL.[92] An open-label study, evaluating the safety and efficacy of imiquimod 5% three times a week for 12 weeks with some variation depending on the patient's tolerance of the imiquimod in six patients with stage IA to IIB MF was administered. Biopsies were performed prior to the study by 2 weeks to 2 months and at the 4-week follow-up posttreatment visit. Results showed that three out of the six patients had histological clearance of disease in their index lesions (up to five lesions) and another patient had two out of his four lesions respond clinically.[93]

IL-2

Seven patients with advanced-stage (stage III to IVA) CTCL were treated with high-dose recombinant IL-2, at a dose of 20 million $IU/m2/day$ by continuous infusion in a three-cycle, 30-day induction phase, and five-cycle monthly consolidation phase. IL-2 showed a CR in three patients (43%) and a PR in two patients (29%). Two of the remissions were durable (56 to 62 months).[94] An *in vitro* study in 15 CTCL patients showed synergism of the immunologic effects of IL-2 and IL-12, enhancing both the levels of IFN-γ and the natural killer cell activity, as well as the T-cell surface IL-12 receptor expression in comparison with the effects of IL-12 or IL-2 alone.[95]

IL-12

CTCL presents with marked defects in IL-12 production. A phase I dose escalation trial with recombinant human IL-12 (rhIL-12), up to 24 weeks, on patients with CTCL (stage T1 = two patients, stage T2 = three patients, stage T3 = two patients, stage T4 = three patients) was administered.[96] The study population consisted of 10 patients with the clinical and histological diagnosis of CTCL with plaques, tumors, or erythroderma. IL-12 was given at 50, 100, or 300 ng/kg, SC twice a week. A complete CR was defined as complete disappearance of all measurable and evaluable lesions for at least 1 month. PR was defined as at least 50% disappearance of all CTCL skin lesions for at least 1 month. Only patients with plaque disease (n = 2) presented a CR. Two plaque-stage patients, and one with Sézary syndrome had a PR. None of the tumor-stage patients responded to the treatment. The authors announced the development of future phase II/III clinical trials based on the high response rate of patients with plaque-stage CTCL.[96]

■ KAPOSI'S SARCOMA

BOX 48-9   Summary

- The current modalities for KS include surgical excision, laser therapy, cryotherapy, radiotherapy, topical alitretinoin (9-*cis* retinoid acid) gel, HHART, IFN-α plus HAART, and chemotherapy.
- Interferon (Roferon-A) is FDA approved for AIDS-related Kaposi's sarcoma.

Treatment decisions depend on the extent and the rate of tumor growth, patient's symptoms, and immune system conditions. Therapeutic modalities available include surgical excision, laser therapy, cryotherapy, radiotherapy, topical alitretinoin (9-*cis* retinoid acid) gel, HHART, IFN-α plus HAART, and chemotherapy.[97]

Interferons

The use of IFN-α2a and IFN-α2b in the treatment of Kaposi's sarcoma (KS) in patients with acquired immune deficiency syndrome (KS/AIDS) due to human immunodeficiency virus is FDA approved.

The recommended dosages of IFN-α2a and 2b are 36 and 30 million IU, respectively, three times a week SC. The average response rate of KS to high-dose IFN-α therapy has been approximately 30%. In many cases, tumor recurrence occurs within 6 months in complete responders and the response to a second treatment is not reliable. These facts led to a current recommendation of maintenance treatment as long as adverse effects are tolerated.[98]

■ CUTANEOUS EXTRAMAMMARY PAGET'S DISEASE

BOX 48-10   Summary

- Current treatments of cutaneous EMPD include wide local excision and Mohs micrographic surgery.
- In case reports, imiquimod 5% cream was used at different frequencies with good results.

Extramammary Paget's disease (EMPD) is an infrequent epidermal malignancy with a high rate of recurrence and is associated with possible internal malignancies, occurring most commonly in the anogenital and vulvar regions. Therapeutic modalities include wide local excision and Mohs micrographic surgery.

Imiquimod

Two cases are reported of perineal and genital EMPD treated with imiquimod 5% cream, with clinical cure occurring after 7.5 to 12 weeks of application of imiquimod 5% on alternating days of the week.[99] In another case report of recurrent EMPD of the vulva where the patient declined surgery, imiquimod 5% cream was used over 6.5 weeks with two rest

periods. The medication frequency was changed from daily to two times weekly then to three times weekly due to the tolerability and side effects of the medication. At the 2-week follow-up visit following cessation of treatment, the patient had no clinical evidence of residual EMPD.[100] Another case study documented the eradication of EMPD of the penis in a 68-year-old male with nightly application of imiquimod cream for 6 weeks, with no signs of reoccurrence at 6 months after discontinuation of therapy.[101]

■ ACTINIC CHEILITIS

BOX 48-11   Summary

- Current treatments of actinic cheilitis include therapies such as cryotherapy, electrodesiccation, conventional and pulsed carbon dioxide lasers, chemical peeling agents, topical fluorouracil, and photodynamic therapy.
- Imiquimod 5% cream three times a week for 4 to 6 weeks was successful in treating patients in a clinical trial.

Actinic cheilitis is the degeneration of the lower lip caused by actinic damage and can lead to SCC. This condition can be treated with cryotherapy, electrodesiccation, conventional and pulsed carbon dioxide lasers, chemical peeling agents, topical fluorouracil, and photodynamic therapy; which are all modalities that cause nonselective tissue ablation.

In 15 patients with biopsy-proven actinic cheilitis treated with imiquimod 5% three times weekly for 4 to 6 weeks, all had clinical clearing 4 weeks after discontinuation of imiquimod.[102]

■ XERODERMA PIGMENTOSUM

BOX 48-12   Summary

- The treatment of skin cancers in patients with XP compromises the standard treatments of BCC, SCC, and melanoma.
- In a case report, imiquimod 5% cream was used five times a week for 6 weeks with good results.

Xeroderma pigmentosum (XP) is a rare autosomal recessive condition caused by a defect in nucleotide excision repair leading to defects in repair of DNA damaged by UV radiation, and causing a 1000-fold increase in risks for major skin cancers such as BCC, SCC, and melanoma.

In a case report of a 19-year-old patient with XP who had been treated for multiple BCCs with simple excision, electrodessication and curettage, carbon dioxide/erbium laser therapy, dermabrasion, chemoprophylaxis, and oral isotretinoin with new BCCs appearing, the patient applied imiquimod 5% cream once daily, five times a week for 6 weeks on two test areas, and had almost total clearance of tumors and pigmentary changes at the end of the treatment period and at the 4-month follow-up visit.[103]

BOWENOID PAPULOSIS

> **BOX 48-13   Summary**
>
> - Current therapy of BP is excision, electrodessication, cryosurgery, laser therapy, retinoic acid, podophyllum resin, and topical 5FU.
> - Several case reports have been reported with the successful use of imiquimod 5% cream for the treatment of BP.

Bowenoid papulosis (BP) is due to epidermal hyperplasia and dysplasia of the anogenital region secondary to HPV-16, 18, 31, or 33 infection with reports of malignant transformation progressing to Bowen disease or SCC.[104] BP is treated with simple local destruction by excision, electrodessication, cryosurgery, laser surgery, and the use of retinoic acid, podophyllum resin, and topical 5FU. A case was reported of a 34-year-old female with BP of the vulva successfully treated with imiquimod cream three times a week for 14 weeks.[105] Although the patient developed ulceration of the treatment site with concurrent bacterial superinfection 8 weeks into treatment, she received topical antibiotics and was able to continue therapy. Several other case reports have documented imiquimod as a potential agent for BP. It may be an effective primary or adjuvant therapeutic alternative for those with limited disease or those refractory to conventional treatment.

KERATOACANTHOMA

> **BOX 48-14   Summary**
>
> - Current therapy for KAs is surgery, intralesional methotrexate, 5FU, bleomycin, and steroids.
> - In two reports, imiquimod 5% was used successfully for KAs.

Keratoacanthoma (KA) are low-grade malignancies and are treated with surgical means or intralesional methotrexate, 5FU, bleomycin, or steroids for poor surgical candidates.

Dendorfer et al. reported the successful therapeutic use of imiquimod 5% cream in four patients with 1 to 6-week histories of facial KA.[106] The treatment regimen was an every-other-day application for 4 to 12 weeks. KA lesions fully regressed in all patients as assessed clinically with a treatment period of 4 to 6 weeks in three of the patients. Clinical clearance was confirmed histologically in two of the patients. No recurrence was seen during the 4 to 6-month follow-up period. Similar results were reported by Peris et al.[107]

EPIDERMODYSPLASIA VERRUCIFORMIS

> **BOX 48-15   Summary**
>
> - No definitive treatment exists. Intralesional IFN, retinoids, and surgery are commonly used.
> - In a case report, imiquimod 5% cream was used in EV with limited success.

Epidermodysplasia verruciformis (EV) is a rare disorder characterized by widespread, flat, and common verrucae and can transform to malignancies. EV is regarded as a genodermatosis, with mainly autosomal recessive inheritance. There is no definitive treatment for EV, but intralesional IFN, retinoids, and surgery can be used.

One report described two HIV-positive maternal half brothers with a histopathologic diagnosis consistent with EV.[108] The patients were treated with topical imiquimod monotherapy for 2 months without improvement. However, in our experience, imiquimod is useful in EV patients when combined with systemic retinoid therapy.

FINAL THOUGHTS

Immunomodulators are an exciting and relatively novel approach to treating skin cancer. Although only a few cancers have FDA-approved immunomodulatory therapies, the multiple studies and case reports performed may possibly pave the way for future therapies and immunomodulatory advances.

REFERENCES

1. Thissen MR, Neumann MH, Schouten LJ. A systematic review of treatment modalities for primary basal cell carcinomas. *Arch Dermatol.* 1999;135(10): 1177–1183.
2. Buechner SA, Wernli M, Harr T, et al. Regression of basal cell carcinoma by intralesional interferon-alpha treatment is mediated by CD95 (Apo-1/Fas)-CD95 ligand-induced suicide. *J Clin Invest.* 1997; 100:2691–2696.
3. Buechner S. Intralesional interferon-alpha 2b in the treatment of basal cell carcinoma. *J Am Acad Dermatol.* 1991;24: 731–734.
4. Greenway HT, Cornell RC, Tanner DJ, et al. Treatment of basal cell carcinoma with intralesional interferon. *J Am Acad Dermatol.* 1986;15:437–443.
5. Telfer NR, Colver GB, Bowers PW. Guidelines for the management of basal cell carcinoma. British Association of Dermatologists. *Br J Dermatol.* September 1999;141(3):415–423.
6. Stenquist B, Wennberg AM, Gisslen H, et al. Treatment of aggressive basal cell carcinoma with intralesional interferon: Evaluation of efficacy by Mohs surgery. *J Am Acad Dermatol.* 1992;27:65–69.
7. Stockfleth E, Trefzer U, Garcia-Bartels C, Wegner T, Schmook T, Sterry W. The use of Toll-like receptor-7 agonist in the treatment of basal cell carcinoma: An overview. *Br J Dermatol.* 2003;149(s66): 53–56.
8. Berman B, Sullivan T, De Araujo T, Nadji M. Expression of Fas-receptor on basal cell carcinomas after treatment with imiquimod 5% cream or vehicle. *Br J Dermatol.* 2003;149(suppl 66):59–61.
9. Marks R, Gebauer K, Shumack S, et al. Imiquimod 5% cream in the treatment of superficial basal cell carcinoma: Results of a multicenter 6-week dose-response trial. *J Am Acad Dermatol.* 2001; 44(5):807–813.
10. Geisse J, Rich P, Pandya A, et al. Imiquimod 5% cream for the treatment of superficial basal cell carcinoma: A double–blind, randomized, vehicle-controlled study. *J Am Acad Dermatol.* 2002; 47:390–398.
11. Baccard M, Marolleau JP, Rybojad M. Middle-term evolution of patients with advanced cutanoues T-cell lymphoma treated with high-dose recombinant interleukin-2. *Arch Dermatol.* 1997;133:656.
12. Geisse J, Caro I, Lindholm J, Golitz L, Stampone P, Owens M. Imiquimod 5% cream for the treatment of superficial basal cell carcinoma: Results from two phase III, randomized, vehicle-controlled studies. *J Am Acad Dermatol.* May 2004;50(5):722–733.
13. Shumack S, Robinson J, Kossard S, et al. Efficacy of topical 5% imiquimod cream for the treatment of nodular basal cell carcinoma: Comparison of dosing regimens. *Arch Dermatol.* 2002;138(9):1165–1171.
14. Huber A, Huber JD, Skinner RB Jr, Kuwahara RT, Haque R, Amonette RA. Topical imiquimod treatment for nodular basal cell carcinomas: An open-label series. *Dermatol Surg.* March 2004;30(3): 429–430.
15. Beutner KR, Geisse JK, Helman D, Fox TL, Ginkel A, Owens ML. Therapeutic

response of basal cell carcinoma to the immune response modifier imiquimod 5% cream. *J Am Acad Dermatol.* December 1999;41(6):1002–1007.

16. Chen TM, Rosen T, Orengo I. Treatment of a large superficial basal cell carcinoma with 5% imiquimod: A case report and review of the literature. *Dermatol Surg.* 2002;28:344–346.

17. Kagy MK, Amonette R. The use of imiquimod 5% cream for the treatment of superficial basal cell carcinomas in a basal cell nevus syndrome patient. *Dermatol Surg* 2000;26:577–579.

18. Weisberg NK, Varghese M. Therapeutic response of a brother and sister with Xeroderma pigmentosum to imiquimod 5% cream. *Dermatol Surg.* 2002;28:518–523.

19. Motley R, Kersey P, Lawrence C. Multiprofessional guidelines for the management of the patient with primary cuataneous squamous cell carcinoma. *Br J Dermatol.* 2002;146:18–25.

20. Ikic D, Padovan I, Pipic N, et al. Interferon therapy for basal cell carcinoma and squamous cell carcinoma. *Int J Clin Pharmacol Ther Toxicol.* 1991;29:342–346.

21. Edwards L, Berman B, Rapini RP, et al. Treatment of cutaneous squamous cell carcinoma by intralesional interferon-alpha 2b therapy. *Arch Dermatol.* 1992;128:1486–1489.

22. Euvrard S, Kanitakis J, Claudy A. Skin cancers after organ transplantation. *N Engl J Med.* 2003;348(17):1681–1691.

23. Schon M, Bong AB, Drewniok C, et al. Tumor-selective induction of apoptosis and the small-molecule immune modifier imiquimod. *J Natl Cancer Inst* 2003;95:15.

24. Schwartz RA. The actinic keratosis. A perspective and update. *Dermatol Surg.* 1997;23(11):1009–1019.

25. Edwards L, Levine N, Weidner M, et al. Effect of intralesional interferon in actinic keratoses. *Arch Dermatol.* 1986;122:779–782.

26. Stockfleth E, Meyer T, Benninghoff B, Christophers E. Successful treatment of actinic keratosis with imiquimod cream 5%: A report of six cases. *Br J Dermatol.* 2001;144(5):1050–1053.

27. Stockfleth E, Meyer T, Benninghoff B, et al. A randomized, double-blind, vehicle-controlled study to asses 5% imiquimod cream for the treatment of multiple actinic keratoses. *Arch Dermatol.* 2002;138:1498–1502.

28. Salasche SJ, Levine N, Morrison L. Cycle therapy of actinic keratoses of the face and scalp with 5% topical imiquimod cream: An open label trial. *J Am Acad Dermatol.* 2002;47(4):571–577.

29. Lebwohl M, Dinehart S, Whiting D, et al. Imiquimod 5% cream for the treatment of actinic keratosis: Results from two phase III, randomized, double-blind, parallel group, vehicle-controlled trials. *J Am Acad Dermatol.* 2004;50(5):714–721.

30. Szeimies RM, Gerritsen MJ, Gupta G, et al. Imiquimod 5% cream for the treatment of actinic keratosis: Results from a phase III, randomized, double-blind, vehicle-controlled, clinical trial with histology. *J Am Acad Dermatol.* October 2004;51(4):547–555.

31. Stockfleth E, Christophers E, Benninghoff B, et al. Low incidence of new actinic keratoses after topical 5% imiquimod cream treatment: A long-term follow-up study. *Arch Dermatol.* December 1, 2004;140(12):1542.

32. Korman N, Moy R, Ling M, et al. Dosing with 5% imiquimod cream 3 times per week for the treatment of actinic keratosis: Results of two phase III, randomized, double-blind, parallel-group, vehicle-controlled trials. *Arch Dermatol.* April 2005;141(4):467–473.

33. Chen K, Yap LM, Marks R, et al. Short-course therapy with imiquimod 5% cream for solar keratoses: A randomized controlled trial. *Aust J Dermatol.* November 1, 2003;44(4):250–255.

34. Marnett LJ. Generation of mutagens during arachidonic acid metabolism. *Cancer Metastasis Rev.* 1994;13:303–308.

35. Masferrer JL, Leahy KM, Koki AT, et al. Antiangiogenic and antitumor activities of cyclooxigenase-2 inhibitors. *Cancer Res.* 2000;60:1306–1311.

36. Wolf JE, Taylor J, Tschen E, et al. Topical 3.0% diclofenac in 2.5% hyaluronan gel in the treatment of actinic keratoses. *Int J Dermatol.* 2001;40:709–713.

37. McEwan LE, Smith JG. Topical diclofenac/hyalurronic acid gel in the treatment of solar keratoses. *Aust J Dermatol.* 1997;38:187–189.

38. Cox NH, Eedy DJ, Morton CA. Guidelines for management of Bowen's disease. British Association of Dermatologists. *Br J Dermatol.* 1999;141(4):633–641.

39. Pehoushek J, Smith KJ. Imiquimod and 5% fluorouracil therapy for anal and perianal squamous cell carcinoma *in situ* in an HIV-1-positive man. *Arch Dermatol.* 2001;137(1):14–16.

40. MacKenzie-Wood A, Kossard S, deLauney J, Wilkinson B, Owens M. Imiquimod 5% cream in the treatment of Bowen's disease. *J Am Acad Dermatol.* 2001;44:462–470.

41. Schroeder TL, Sengelmann RD. Squamous cell carcinoma *in situ* of the penis successfully treated with imiquimod 5% cream. *J Am Acad Dermatol.* 2002;46(4):545–548.

42. Thai K, Sinclair R. Treatment of Bowen's disease of the penis with imiquimod. *J Am Acad Dermatol.* 2002;46:470–471.

43. Orengo I, Rosen T, Guill C. Treatment of squamous cell carcinoma *in situ* of the penis with 5% imiquimod cream: A case report. *J Am Acad Dermatol.* 2002;47:S225–S228.

44. Smith KJ, Germain M, Skelton H. Squamous cell carcinoma *in situ* (Bowen's disease) in renal transplant patients treated with 5% imiquimod and 5% 5-fluorouracil therapy. *Dermatol Surg.* 2001;27(6):561–564.

45. Gutzmer R, Kaspari M, Vogelbruch M, et al. Successful treatment of anogenital Bowen's disease with the immunomodulator imiquimod, and monitoring of therapy by DNA image cytometry. *Br J Dermatol.* July 2002;147(1):160–165.

46. Davis G, Wentworth J, Richard J. Self-administered topical imiquimod treatment of vulvar intraepithelial neoplasia: A report of four cases. *J Reprod Med.* 2000;45(8):619–623.

47. Marchitelli C, Secco G, Perrotta M, Lugones L, Pesce R, Testa R. Treatment of bowenoid and basaloid vulvar intraepithelial neoplasia 2/3 with imiquimod 5% cream. *J Reprod Med.* November 2004;49(11):876–882.

48. van Seters M, Fons G, van Beurden M, et al. Imiquimod in the treatment of multifocal vulvar intraepithelial neoplasia 2/3. Results of a pilot study. *J Reprod Med.* September 1, 2002;47(9):701–705.

49. Todd RW, Etherington IJ, Luesley DM. The effects of 5% imiquimod cream on high-grade vulval intraepithelial neoplasia. *Gynecol Oncol.* April 2002;85(1):67–70.

50. Wendling J, Saiag P, Berville-Levy S, Bourgault-Villada I, Clerici T, Moyal-Barracco M. Treatment of undifferentiated vulvar intraepithelial neoplasia with 5% imiquimod cream: A prospective study of 12 cases. *Arch Dermatol.* October 2004;140(10):1220–1224.

51. Diaz-Arrastia C, Arany I, Robazetti SC, et al. Clinical and molecular responses in high-grade intraepithelial neoplasia treated with topical imiquimod 5%. *Clin Cancer Res.* October 2001;7(10):3031–3033.

52. Kreuter A, Hochdorfer B, Stucker M, et al. Treatment of anal intraepithelial neoplasia in patients with acquired HIV with imiquimod 5% cream. *J Am Acad Dermatol.* June 2004;50(6):980–981.

53. Newton Bishop JA, Corrie PG, Gore ME, et al. UK guidelines for the management of cutaneous melanoma. *Br J Plast Surg.* 2002;55:46–54.

54. Rusciani L, Petraglia S, Alotto M, et al. Postsurgical adjuvant therapy for melanoma. Evaluation of a 3-year randomized trial with recombinant interferon-alpha after 3 and 5 years of follow-up. *Cancer.* 1997;79:2354–2360.

55. Creagan ET, Dalton RJ, Ahmann DL, et al. Randomized, surgical adjuvant clinical trial of recombinant interferon alfa-2a in selected patients with malignant melanoma. *J Clin Oncol.* 1995;13:2776–2783.

56. Barth A, Morton DL. The role of adjuvant therapy in melanoma management. *Cancer.* 1995;75:726S–734S.

57. Von Wussow P, Block B, Hartmann F, Deicher H. Intralesional interferon-alpha therapy in advanced malignant melanoma. *Cancer.* 1988;61:1071–1074.

58. Fluck M, Kamanabrou D, Lippold A, Reitz M, Atzpodien J. Dose-dependent treatment benefit in high-risk melanoma patients receiving adjuvant high-dose interferon alfa-2b. *Cancer Biother Radiopharm.* June 2005;20(3):280–289.

59. Ahmed I, Berth-Jones J. Imiquimod: A novel treatment for lentigo maligna. *Br J Dermatol.* 2000;143:843–845.

60. Chapman MS, Spencer SK, Brennick JB. Histologic resolution of melanoma *in situ* (lentigo maligna) with 5% imiquimod cream. *Arch Dermatol.* July 2003;139(7):943–944.

61. Powell AM, Russell-Jones R. Amelanotic lentigo maligna managed with topical imiquimod as immunotherapy. *J Am Acad Dermatol.* May 2004;50(5):792–796.

62. Powell AM, Russell-Jones R, Barlow RJ. Topical imiquimod immunotherapy in

the management of lentigo maligna. *Clin Exp Dermatol.* January 2004;29(1): 15–21.

63. Naylor MF, Crowson N, Kuwahara R, et al. Treatment of lentigo maligna with topical imiquimod. *Br J Dermatol.* November 2003;149(suppl 66):66–70.

64. Kupfer-Bessaguet I, Guillet G, Misery L, Carre JL, Leroy JP, Sassolas B. Topical imiquimod treatment of lentigo maligna: Clinical and histologic evaluation. *J Am Acad Dermatol.* October 2004; 51(4):635–639.

65. Steinmann A, Funk JO, Schuler G, von den Driesch P. Topical imiquimod treatment of a cutaneous melanoma metastasis. *J Am Acad Dermatol.* 2000;43(3): 555–556.

66. Wolf H, Smolle J, Binder B, Cerroni L, Richtig E, Kerl H. Topical imiquimod in the treatment of metastasis melanoma to the skin. *Arch Dermatol.* 2003;139: 273–276.

67. Ugurel S, Wagner A, Pfohler C, et al. Topical imiquimod eradicates skin metastases of malignant melanoma but fails to prevent rapid lymphogenous metastatic spread. *Br J Dermatol.* September 2002;147(3):621–624.

68. Bong AB, Bonnekoh B, Franke I, et al. Imiquimod, a topical immune response modifier, in the treatment of cutaneous metastases of malignant melanoma. *Dermatology.* 2002;205(2):135–138.

69. Atkins MB. Interleukin-2: Clinical applications. *Semin Oncol.* 2002;29(suppl 7): 12–17.

70. Parkinson D, Abrams J, Wiernik P, et al. Interleukin-2 therapy in patients with metastasic malignant melanoma: A phase II study. *J Clin Oncol.* 1990;8:1650–1656.

71. Allen I, Kupelnick B, Kumashiro M. Efficacy of interleukin-2 in the treatment of metastasic melanoma—systemic review and metastasis analysis. *Cancer Ther.* 1998;1:168–173.

72. Lee P, Wang F, Kuniyoshi J, et al. Effects of interleukin-12 on the immune response to a multipeptide vaccine for resected metastatic melanoma. *J Clin Oncol.* 2001; 19:3836–3847.

73. Maio M, Fonsatti E, Lamaj E, et al. Vaccination of stage IV patients with allogeneic IL-4- or IL-2-gene-transduced melanoma cells generates functional antibodies against vaccinating and autologous melanoma cells. *Cancer Immunol Immunother.* 2002;51:9–14.

74. Rosenberg SA, Yang JC, Schwartzentruber DJ, et al. Impact of cytokine administration on the generation of antitumor reactivity in patients with metastatic melanoma receiving a peptide vaccine. *J Immunol.* 1999;163:1690–1695.

75. Osanto S, Schiphorst PP, Weijl NI, et al. Vaccination of melanoma patients with an allogeneic, genetically modified interleukin 2-producing melanoma cell line. *Hum Gene Ther.* 2000;11:739–750.

76. Schrayer DP, Kouttab N, Hearing VJ, Wanebo HJ. Synergistic effect of interleukin-2 and a vaccine of irradiated melanoma cells transfected to secrete staphylococcal enterotoxin A. *Clin Exp Metastasis* 2002;19:43–53.

77. Overwijk WW, Theoret MR, Finkelstein SE, et al. Tumor regression and autoimmunity after reversal of a functionally tolerant state of self-reactive CD8+ T cells. *J Exp Med.* 2003;198: 569–580.

78. Lotem M, Shiloni E, Pappo I, et al. Interleukin-2 improves tumour response to DNP-modified autologous vaccine for the treatment of metastatic malignant melanoma. *Br J Cancer.* February 23, 2004;90(4):773–780.

79. Berd D, Sato T, Maguire HC Jr, Kairys J, Mastrangelo MJ. Immunopharmacologic analysis of an autologous, hapten-modified human melanoma vaccine. *J Clin Oncol.* February 1, 2004;22(3):403–415.

80. Mitchell MS, Kan-Mitchell J, Morrow PR, Darrah D, Jones VE, Mescher MF. Phase I trial of large multivalent immunogen derived from melanoma lysates in patients with disseminated melanoma. *Clin Cancer Res.* January 1, 2004;10(Pt 1): 76–83.

81. Hellstrand K, Brune M, Naredi P, et al. Histamine: A novel approach to cancer immunotherapy. *Cancer Invest.* 2000;18 (4):347–355.

82. Radcliff F, Caruso D, Koina C, et al. Mobilization of dendritic cells in cancer patients treated with granulocyte colony-stimulating factor and chemotherapy. *Br J Haematol.* 2002;119:204–211.

83. Spitler L, Grossbard M, Ernstoff M, et al. Adjuvant therapy of stage III and IV malignant melanoma using granulocyte-macrophage colony-stimulating factor. *J Clin Oncol.* 2000;18:1614–1621.

84. Apisarnthanarax N, Talpur R, Duvic M. Treatment of cutaneous T-cell lymphoma: Current status and future directions. *Am J Clin Dermatol.* 2002;3(3):193–215.

85. Apisarnthanarax N, Duvic M. Cutaneous T-cell lymphoma. New immunomodulators. *Dermatol Clin.* 2001;19(4):737–748.

86. Bunn PA Jr, Hoffman SJ, Norris D, et al. Systemic therapy of cutaneous T-cell lymphomas (mycosis fungoides and the Sézary syndrome). *Ann Intern Med.* 1994; 121:592–602.

87. Chiarion-Silenu V, Bononi A, Veller Fornasa C, et al. Phase II trial of interferon-alpha 2a plus psoralen with ultraviolet light A in patients with cutaneous T-cell lymphoma. *Cancer.* 2002;95(3): 596–675.

88. Stadler R, Otte HG, Luger T, et al. Prospective randomized multicenter clinical trial on the use of interferon-2a plus acitretin versus interferon-2a plus PUVA in patients with cutaneous T-cell lymphoma stages I and II. *Blood.* November 15, 1998;92(10):3578–3581.

89. Vonderheid EC, Thompson R, Smiles KA, et al. Recombinant interferon-2b in plaque-phase mycosis fungoides-intralesional and low-dose intramuscular therapy. *Arch Dermatol.* 1987;123:757–763.

90. Suchin KR, Cucchiara AJ, Gottleib SL, et al. Treatment of cutaneous T-cell lymphoma with combined immunomodulatory therapy: A 14-year experience at a single institution. *Arch Dermatol.* August 2002;138(8):1054–1060.

91. Wollina U, Looks A, Meyer J, et al. Treatment of stage II cutaneous T-cell lymphoma with interferon alfa-2a and extracorporeal photochemotherapy: A prospective controlled trial. *J Am Acad Dermatol.* 2001;44(2):253–260.

92. Suchin KR, Junekins-Hopkins JM, Rook AH. Treatment of stage Ia cutaneous T-cell lymphoma with topical application of the immune response modifier imiquimod. *Arch Dermatol.* 2002;138(9): 1137–1139.

93. Deeths MJ, Chapman JT, Dellavalle RP, Zeng C, Aeling JL. Treatment of patch and plaque stage mycosis fungoides with imiquimod 5% cream. *J Am Acad Dermatol.* February 2005;52(2):275–280.

94. Baccard M, Marolleau JP, Rybojad M. Middle-term evolution of patients with advanced cutaneous T-cell lymphoma treated with high-dose recombinant interleukin-2. *Arch Dermatol.* 1997;133: 656.

95. Zaki MH, Wysocka M, Everetts SE, et al. Synergistic enhancement of cell-mediated immunity by interleukin-12 plus interleukin-2: Basis for therapy of cutaneous T-cell lymphoma. *J Invest Dermatol.* 2002;118(2):366–371.

96. Rook AH, Wood GS, Yoo EK, et al. Interleukin-12 therapy of cutaneous T-cell lymphoma induces lesion regression and cytotoxic T-cell responses. *Blood.* 1999;94(3):902–908.

97. Tirelli U, Bernardi D, Spina M, Vaccher E. AIDS-related tumors: Integrating antiviral and anticancer therapy. *Crit Rev Oncol Hematol.* 2002;41(3):299–315.

98. Krown SE. Interferon and other biological agents for the treatment of Kaposi's Sarcoma. *Hematol Oncol Clin North Am.* 1991;5:311–322.

99. Zampogna JC, Flowers FP, Roth WI, Hassenein A. Treatment of primary limited cutaneous extramammary Paget's disease with topical imiquimod monotherapy. Two case reports. *J Am Acad Dermatol.* 2002;47(4):S229–S235.

100. Wang LC, Blanchard A, Judge DE, Lorincz AA, Medenica MM, Busbey S. Successful treatment of recurrent extramammary Paget's disease of the vulva with topical imiquimod 5% cream. *J Am Acad Dermatol.* October 2003;49(4): 769–772.

101. Berman B, Spencer J, Villa A, et al. Successful treatment of extramammary Paget's disease of the scrotum with imiquimod 5% cream. *Clin Exp Dermatol.* November 2003;28(suppl 1): 36–38.

102. Smith KJ, Germain M, Yeager J, Skelton H. Topical 5% imiquimod for the therapy of actinic cheilitis. *J Am Acad Dermatol.* October 2002;47(4): 497–501.

103. Nagore E, Sevila A, Sanmartin O, et al. Excellent response of basal cell carcinomas and pigmentary changes in xeroderma pigmentosum to imiquimod 5% cream. *Br J Dermatol.* October 2003;149(4): 858–861.

104. Loo WJ, Holt PJ. Bowenoid papulosis successfully treated with imiquimod. *J Eur*

Acad Dermatol Venereol. May 2003;17(3): 363–365.

105. Richter ON, Petrow W, Wardelmann E, et al. Bowenoid papulosis of the vulva—immunotherapeutical approach with topical imiquimod. *Arch Gynecol Obstet.* October 2003;268(4):333–336. [Epub January 23]

106. Dendorfer M, Oppel T, Wollenberg A, et al. Topical treatment with imiquimod may induce regression of facial keratoacanthoma. *Eur J Dermatol.* January/February 2003;13(1):80–109.

107. Peris K, Micantonio T, Fargnoli MC. Successful treatment of keratoacanthoma and actinic keratoses with imiquimod 5% cream. *Eur J Dermatol.* July/August 2003;13(4):413–414.

108. Hu W, Nuovo G, Willen M, et al. Epidermodysplasia verruciformis in two half brothers with HIV infection. *J Cutan Med Surg.* September/October 2004;8(5):357–360.

CHAPTER 49

Topical 5-Fluorouracil

Voraphol Vejjabhinanta, M.D.
Asha R. Patel, B.S.
Rana Anadolu Brasie, M.D.
Anita Singh, M.S.
Shalu S. Patel
Keyvan Nouri, M.D.

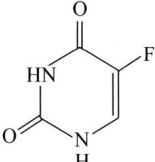

▲ **FIGURE 49-1** Chemical structure of 5-FU.

> **BOX 49-1 Overview**
>
> - Topical 5-fluorouracil (5-FU) is a medication used commonly to treat actinic keratosis (AK).
> - 5-FU is a fluorinated pyrimidine antimetabolite, which has a similar structure to thymine.
> - 5-FU interferes with the structure and function of DNA and RNA, causing unstable growth and death of cells through its effects on thymidylate synthetase.
> - Topical 5-FU is available in a 1, 2, and 5% solution, as well as a 0.5, 1, and 5% cream formulation.
> - Topical 5-FU has been successfully used to treat predominantly AK, actinic cheilitis, superficial basal cell carcinoma, Bowen disease, erythroplasia of Queyrat, and HPV related skin papules.
> - There are many precautions and side effects that need to be taken into account before using this medication.

INTRODUCTION

5-Fluorouracil (5-FU), $C_4H_3FN_2O_2$, is an antimetabolite drug typically used for the treatment of actinic keratosis (AK). It is also used topically for the treatment of other squamous cell carcinoma (SCC) *in situ* types such as erythroplasia of Queyrat, actinic cheilitis (AC), and Bowen disease (BD), as well as, superficial basal cell carcinoma, and HPV related skin papules.

5-FU is considered an antimetabolite, which by definition is a drug that, like natural chemicals, can participate in normal cell processes but disrupt cellular metabolism and normal cell cycle. It is a fluorinated pyrimidine antimetabolite (Fig. 49-1), which is similar in structure to thymine, but with a halogen

(fluorine) at position 5. As a pyrimidine analogue, it is altered inside the cell into different cytotoxic metabolites, which are then integrated into DNA and RNA, finally producing cell cycle arrest and apoptosis. However, while this may be helpful in fighting cancer cells, it also affects normal cells, thereby causing adverse effects, which are discussed later in the chapter.

DRUG INFORMATION

> **BOX 49-2 Summary**
>
> - 5-FU interferes with the structure and function of DNA and RNA, disturbing the normal cell cycle and eventually leading to cell death.
> - 5-FU inhibits the function of thymidylate synthetase, thereby preventing the conversion of d-UMP to d-TMP.
> - 5-FU also interferes with the mechanism of action of RNA by the incorporation of F-UTP into the ribonucleotides.
> - The metabolism of 5-FU takes place primarily in the hepatic system in somatic cells via dihydropyrimidine dehydrogenase (DPD).
> - Systemic absorption of topical fluorouracil is very low, but systemic toxicity can occur in patients with a genetic deficiency of DPD.
> - Topical 5-FU is available as a 1, 2, and 5% solution, as well as a 0.5, 1, and 5% cream formulation.
> - Topical 5-FU is FDA approved for the treatment of actinic keratosis, SCC *in situ* and superficial BCC.

Mechanism of Action

5-Fluorouracil's value is based on uracil being used preferentially for nucleic acid biosynthesis in various tumors. 5-fluo-

rouracil is broken down into 5-fluorouridine triphosphate (F-UTP), 2-deoxyfluorouridine monophosphate (Fd-UMP), and 2-deoxyfluorouridine triphosphate (Fd-UTP) in cells to concentrations that can result in both DNA-directed and RNA-directed cytotoxicities (Fig. 49-2). Fd-UMP is the intracellular cytotoxic form of 5-fluorouracil. This compound competes with the natural substrate d-UMP (deoxyuridine monophosphate) for the catalytic site on thymidylate synthetase (a key enzyme in DNA synthesis), forming a covalent complex with the enzyme that is unable to undergo the normal catalytic reaction of converting d-UMP to d-TMP. Concurrently, 5-fluorouracil also interferes with the mechanism of action of RNA by the incorporation of F-UTP into the ribonucleotides. Integration into RNA has been linked with toxicity and causes major malfunctions in RNA processing and utility.[1,2]

By meddling with the structure and function of DNA and RNA, 5-fluorouracil instigates unstable growth and death of cells. The fact that rapidly multiplying or malignant cells synthesize more DNA when compared to normal cells, causes fluorouracil to have a more pronounced effect on their cellular cycle.[3] Light and electron microscopic studies have illustrated that actinically damaged epidermis, treated with topical 5-FU, is shed and replaced with healthy new layers of keratinocytes.[4]

Pharmacokinetics

Systemic absorption of topical fluorouracil, while statistically very low, can differ depending upon specific skin disease, location, drug concentration, product formulation, and other factors such as the extent of application. The total amount of drug absorbed systemically from a 5% formulation is 2.2% of the applied dose, approximately seven times higher than 0.5% 5-FU in the microsphere delivery system.[5] The metabolism of 5-fluorouracil takes place primarily in the liver and in somatic cells, *via* dihydropyrimidine dehydrogenase (DPD).[6] This is the initial rate-limiting enzyme in pyrimidine catabolism that produces degradation products (i.e., carbon dioxide, urea, a-fluoro-b-alanine) which are

5-fluorouracil ⟶ 5-fluorouridine triphosphate (F-UTP) + 2-deoxyfluorouridine triphosphate (Fd-UTP)

▲ **FIGURE 49-2** Reaction exhibiting 5-FU metabolites.

metabolically inactive. Approximately 15% of the dosage is excreted in intact form in the urine within 6 hours and over 90% of this amount is excreted in the first hour. Sixty to eighty percent of the dose is excreted as respiratory carbon dioxide within 8 to 12 hours.

Forms

Topical fluorouracil has been approved by the Food and Drug Administration to treat AK lesions, and superficial basal cell carcinomas. It is commercially available in the United States as both a solution and a cream. Currently, 1, 2, and 5% solutions are available, as also as a 1 and 5% cream. Also available is a 0.5% fluorouracil cream, which is incorporated into a porous microsphere. The 0.5% cream is available as Carac® (Dermik Laboratories), the 1% solution and cream are available as Fluoroplex® (Allergan Herbert Laboratories), and the 2 and 5% solution and cream are available as Efudex® (Roche Laboratories).

INDICATIONS AND DOSAGE

BOX 49-3 Summary

- Topical 5-FU is indicated to treat squamous cell carcinoma *in situ*, particularly actinic keratoses/actinic cheilitis type, Bowen disease, as well as superficial basal cell carcinoma.
- AKs are atypical intraepidermal lesions that may progress to invasive squamous cell carcinoma. Treatment options for AK include topical therapies (such as 5-fluorouracil, imiquimod, diclofenac, and PDT) and destructive modalities (such as cryosurgery, electrodessication & curettage, and laser ablation).
- Actinic cheilitis is a type of AK occurring mostly on the lower lips, and responds to topical 5-FU.
- Basal cell carcinomas (BCC) are slow growing malignant neoplasms. Topical 5-FU is indicated for superficial BCCs not involving the face region.
- Bowen disease (BD) is a type of *in situ* SCC that is also treated with topical 5-FU.
- Squamous cell carcinoma *in situ* of the conjunctiva is a type of SCC *in situ* that involves the full thickness of conjunctival epithelium. Topical 1% 5-FU eye drops have been proven effective in treating these lesions.

Topical fluorouracil is used successfully for the treatment of SCC *in situ*: AK/AC, Bowen disease, and superficial BCC. This medication is also useful to treat some nonneoplastic disorders in which cells are rapidly dividing; including HPV related papular lesions and neoplastic porokeratosis. Fluorouracil works optimally on the face and scalp areas and is less efficacious on other areas of the body. 5-FU also destroys sun-damaged epithelial cells that are clinically very subtle and makes the skin surface appear smoother.

Actinic Keratoses

AK is an ultraviolet light-induced early SCC *in situ* that may progress into an invasive SCC. AKs have many features in common with other *in situ* and superficial SCCs, such as the clinical, histologic, and molecular aspects. AK lesions occur ordinarily on sun-exposed skin and often arise on chronically sun-damaged body areas such as the face, ears, arms, and hands. They become more prevalent with increasing age and significant in identifying patients predisposed to develop invasive SCC. It has been reported that 60% of invasive SCCs are derived from AKs.[7] Treatment of AK requires removal of all the affected epidermal cells. Treatment options that are currently available include topical therapies such as 5-fluorouracil, imiquimod, diclofenac, and PDT; destructive modalities include cryosurgery, electrodessication & curettage, and laser ablation.[8] Topical fluorouracil is a useful alternative for treating diffuse actinic damage, and the effectiveness of topical fluorouracil in treating widespread AK lesions has been demonstrated in many studies.[9–12] The result of a meta-analysis shows that 5-fluorouracil is an effective treatment for 90% of AK and is recommended as a useful alternative to cryotherapy.[13]

A standard recommended regimen is to apply the cream or solution twice daily, 10 minutes after washing, rinsing, and drying the target areas, for 3 to 4 weeks on the head and neck region and 4 to 6 weeks for all other areas. One to 2% cream or solution is recommended for the lips, face, or genitalia regions and 5% cream for the scalp, trunk, or extremities. A small amount of the cream should be gently applied onto all of the treatment areas with a fingertip, glove or cotton swab. It is essential to apply the medication to all of the skin and not just visible lesions. Afterwards, the hands should be washed thoroughly

to prevent any of the medication from accidentally getting in the eyes or mouth. After a few days, the lesion is expected to become red and possibly blister and/or erode, this concludes with healthy re-epithelialization of the epidermis.

Treatment with 5-fluorouracil can be associated with significant skin irritation. To minimize the irritation, various treatment options have been studied. Some of these therapies include, altering concentrations and vehicle formulations, and using combination therapies.[13] In one study, "pulse" dosing with 5% fluorouracil solution was evaluated.[14] Pulse dosing required patients to apply the 5% fluorouracil solution twice daily once a week until either there were no remaining lesions or the patient reached a maximum of 9 weeks treatment application. The results of this study revealed that pulse dosing produces the same benefit as traditional therapies, but with significantly reduced skin irritation. However, according to two other studies[15,16] it was shown that pulse 5-FU failed to clear AK in most of their study patients, and that daily application of 5% 5-FU cream is more effective than weekly application at clearing and treating AK's on the scalp and face.

In another study, the efficacy and facial tolerance of topical fluorouracil in conjunction with triamcinolone acetonide cream was studied.[17] This study revealed that sequential topical application of fluorouracil and 0.5% triamcinolone acetonide cream proved just as effective as fluorouracil alone in treating AKs, with the added benefit of less to none skin irritation. It is worth noting that there were no significant treatment differences for up to 1 year in the reduction of AK lesions or the appearance of new AK lesions. This fact suggested that efficacy is not related to the degree of inflammation. Jorizzo demonstrated in detail that a novel low dose formulation, specifically 0.5% 5-fluorouracil in a microsphere vehicle, is associated with significantly less irritation without sacrificing efficacy.[18]

Recently, a new topical fluorouracil cream preparation containing 0.5% 5-fluorouracil in a microsphere vehicle has been approved by FDA for the treatment of AKs (once daily for up to 4 weeks). Study data demonstrate that this low-dose formulation is just as effective in reducing AK lesions while causing very minimal side effects.[19–21] Also, it is hypothesized that the microsphere-based delivery system may reduce systemic toxicity by ensuring that the fluorouracil remains at the skin level.[22] Other regimens such as four times daily,[23,24] combination with retinoic acid,[25-27] cryotherapy,[28,29] imiquimod, chemical peeling,[30] and photodynamic therapy[31] have been recommended for hyperkeratotic AKs, recalcitrant AKs, or to potentially shorten the treatment time.

Actinic Cheilitis (AC)

AC is a type of AK occurring on the lips. It mainly affects the lower lip, which typically receives more sun exposure than the upper lip. Many studies[32,33] have shown that AC responds well clinically to 5-FU treatment. Although the response to the medication may be even more erosive and/or painful when compared with that of AK treatment, the final clinical results have been proven to be effective. 5-FU is a recommended alternative treatment for AC. Careful follow-up is very important because it has been illustrated that residual dysplasia is present in all post treatment biopsies, even though the clinical picture of the lesions had been improved or even eliminated.[34] Effective sun protection is crucial during and after the treatment.

Bowen Disease

BD is a special type of squamous cell carcinoma in situ (SCC in situ).[35] It is usually a persistent lesion, with a potential to transform into invasive SCC, although spontaneous partial regression may potentially occur. 5-FU has been used topically for BD treatment in several research trials.[36-41] The 5% cream is recommended twice daily for 4–8 weeks. Efficacy may potentially be increased by utilization of occlusion methods[37] using iontophoresis to improve follicular penetration[39] or combined with dinitrochlorobenzene (DNCB).[40] As 5-FU can be very irritating; less aggressive regimens have been used for disease control rather than an actual cure. A once weekly application of 5% 5-FU improved lesions in 24 out of 26 patients, although long-term clearance was only achieved in a small percentage with this specific treatment regimen.[41]

In erythroplasia of Queyrat (SCC in situ of the glans penis),[42-44] application of 5% cream twice a day for 4–5 weeks has been suggested, followed by circumcision. Although inflammation frequently is a limiting factor, excellent clinical and cosmetic outcome is achieved with adequate treatment.

Conjunctival Squamous Cell Carcinoma in Situ

SCC in situ of the conjunctiva appears as a neoplasm involving and confined to the full-thickness of the conjunctival epithelium. Midena et al.[45] evaluated the effectiveness of topical 1% 5-FU eye drops 4 times a day for 4 weeks in a total of eight patients who were affected by conjunctival in situ SCC. Neoplastic conjunctiva was completely replaced by normal epithelium within a 3-month period. The mean follow up period in this study was 27 months. One patient needed two courses of local chemotherapy for recurrent disease. An acute transient toxic keratoconjunctivitis was seen in all of the treated patients but it was controlled easily with topical therapy. No long-term side effects of this treatment regimen were found.

Topical 5-FU is also being used in the treatment of many disorders such as porokeratosis,[46] Darier disease,[47,48] psoriatic nails,[49,50] keratoacanthoma and its giant variant keratoacanthoma centrifugum marginatum,[51] as well as human papillomavirus related skin lesions such as verrucas[52] with varying success.

Superficial Multicentric Basal Cell Carcinoma (BCC)

BCCs are indolent malignant neoplasms that derive from stem cells in the basal layer of the epidermis and follicular structures. They are typically slow growing carcinomas that occur in areas of chronic sun exposure and rarely metastasize, thus, they can be locally invasive and destructive. The use of topical 5-FU is especially useful for superficial BCCs not involving the face region, but this regimen cannot be anticipated to cure invasive BCCs or lesions with deep follicular involvement.[53] The 5% cream is now recommended for extrafacial BCCs. Application should be twice daily, covering the lesion plus a surrounding few mm margin. Topical 5-FU therapy is helpful in the management and treatment of multiple superficial BCCs on the trunk or extremities. 5-FU may also be used for palliation in patients that are unable to tolerate other forms of invasive treatment or in difficult body regions, as well as, patients with Basal Cell Nevus Syndrome. Treatment continuation may be needed up to 10–12 weeks for complete clinical and histopathologic clearing. Meticulous follow-up is also very important in these patients. Inadequately treating the lesion may resolve only the superficial layers of the

lesion and may make recurrences significantly more difficult to diagnose. Effectivity may be augmented by placing 5-FU under occlusion or in an appropriate carrier like phosphatidyl choline.[54]

Total body use of topical 5-fluorouracil for extensive non-melanoma skin cancer has also been reported in the literature. Authors reported 2 patients with extensive NMSC that were treated with topical 5-fluorouracil 5% cream, applied twice daily to the entire body surface, including normal appearing skin. The patients were followed closely and were found to have undetectable blood levels of 5-fluorouracil throughout their treatment. This small study concluded that total body use of 5-FU was successful and cleared the majority of lesions in their 2 patients, suggesting that total body treatment of extensive NMSC may be a possible treatment regimen.[55]

PRECAUTIONS AND SIDE EFFECTS

BOX 49-4   Summary

- Topical 5-FU is contraindicated in the following patients
  - Individuals with a dihydropyrimidine dehydrogenase (DPD) enzyme deficiency
  - Individuals with hypersensitivity to 5-FU
  - Pregnant women
  - Individuals with impaired liver or kidney function, topical 5-FU should be given with extreme caution
- Significant side effects of this drug include stinging or burning sensation, photosensitivity, skin irritation, hypopigmentation, excessive inflammation resulting in ulcer formation, scarring, and secondary bacterial infections.

Patients suffering from an allergic reaction to 5-FU should not be administered this drug whatsoever. Because 5-FU topical is in the FDA pregnancy category X, it is not advised for pregnant or nursing women. 5-FU should only be administered with caution in patients with impaired liver or kidney function. Topical 5-FU is contraindicated in patients with genetic DPD deficiency. The patients that have dihydropyrimidine dehydrogenase (DPD) enzyme deficiency,[56,57] are at a higher risk of developing severe toxicity such as

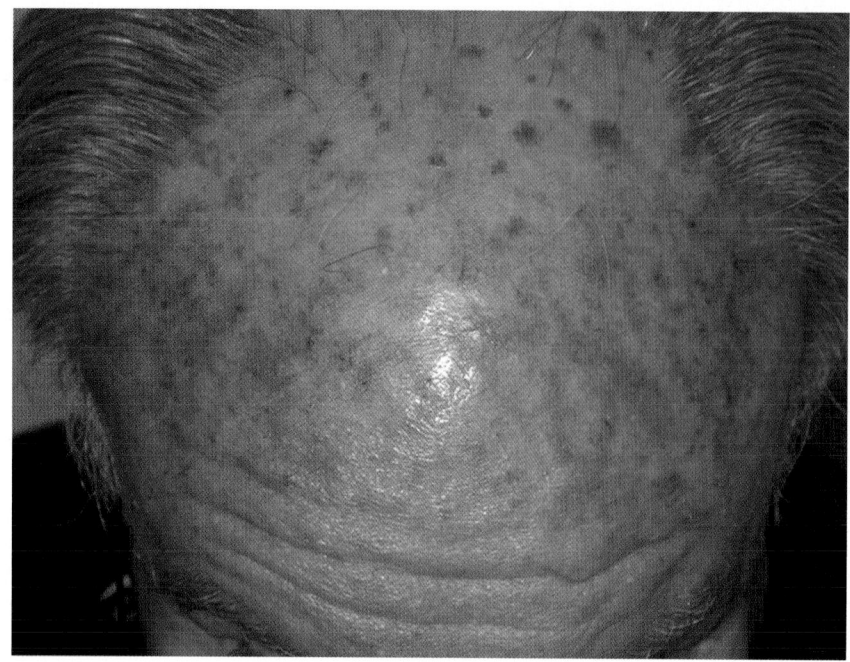

▲ **FIGURE 49-3** The scalp exhibiting characteristic 5-FU side effects during treatment.

stomatitis, mucositis, esophagitis, colitis, myelosuppression, neurotoxicity, and even death.

With initial application of 5-FU, there usually is a mild to severe stinging or burning sensation. The drug also sensitizes the skin to sunlight and induces photosensitivity. Effective sun protection is recommended during and after the treatment. After 5 to 10 days of 5-FU treatment, the sun-damaged sections of treated skin may become red and irritated (Figs. 49-3 to 49-6). The irritation produced by initial application

resolves within 2 weeks of 5-FU cessation. Fluorouracil has the potential to cause prolonged hypopigmentation, which is more noticeable in dark-skinned individuals. Specific areas of the body have a higher sensitivity to severe irritation, including skin folds, the lips, and the eyelids. Occlusion or application of make-up may increase and stimulate irritation. Occasionally, severe complications may occur, including excessive inflammation resulting in

ulcer formation, persistent hypopigmentation or scarring, and secondary bacterial infections.

On the skin, the total amount of drug absorbed from the 5% formulation ranges from 2.2 to 6% of the applied dose. Higher absorption rate is present in lesional skin. A large amount of application on the body has to be monitored carefully. The efficacy and safety of the drug is not well known in children.

■ FINAL THOUGHTS

Topical fluorouracil is a medication that is used to treat various conditions of the skin in which there is rapid multiplication of cells. For example, AKs, AC, Bowen disease, erythroplasia of Queyrat, superficial basal cell carcinoma, and some nonneoplastic proliferations such as nail bed psoriasis, porokeratosis, and HPV related skin lesions. The most common side effects of this medication are burning sensations and slight to severe skin irritation. In an effort to decrease this irritation, altered treatment regimens, combination therapy with topical corticosteroids, and low concentration drug in microsphere delivery system have been introduced and utilized. In an effort to increase the efficacy of this drug, combination treatments with topical tretinoin, cryotherapy, iontophoresis, imiquimod, or short-term intensive therapy is recommended. In order to increase drug compliance and efficacy of treatment, any methods that

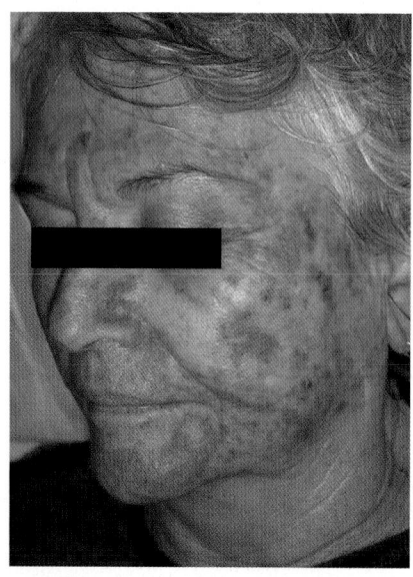

▲ **FIGURE 49-4** The face exhibiting characteristic 5-FU side effects during treatment.

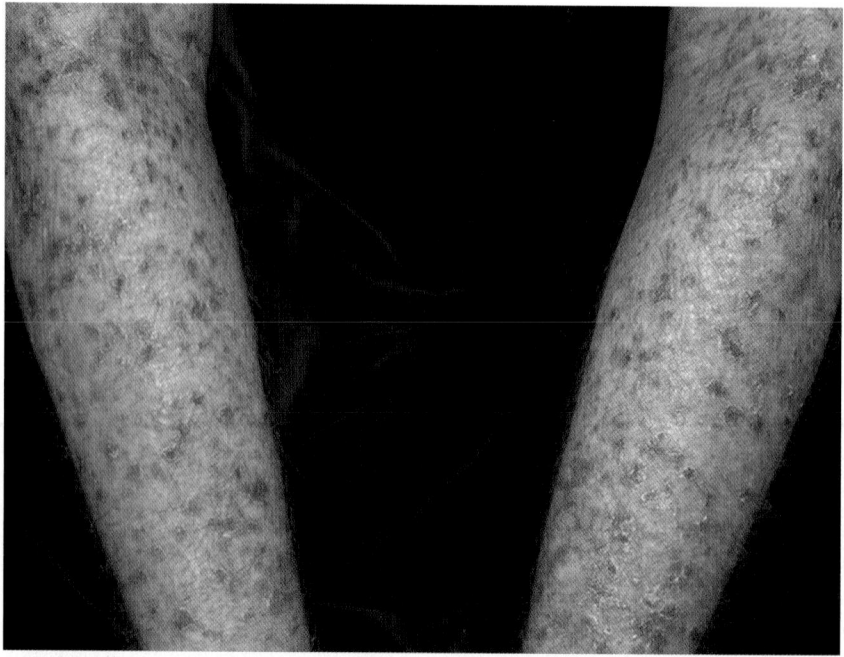

▲ **FIGURE 49-5** The arms exhibiting characteristic 5-FU side effects during treatment.

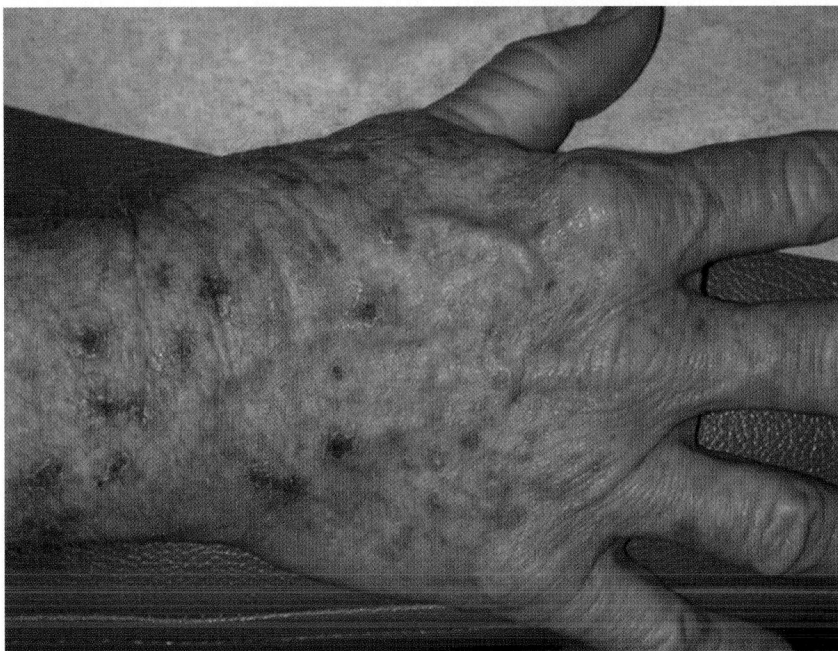

▲ **FIGURE 49-6** Close-up view of the hand exhibiting characteristic 5-FU side effects during treatment.

can selectively deliver 5-FU to the actual target cell and maintain the medication at the site will be the most interesting topic for topical 5-FU.

REFERENCES

1. Eaglstein WH, Weinstein GD, Frost P. Fluorouracil: mechanism of action in human skin and actinic keratoses. Effect on DNA synthesis in vivo. *Arch Dermatol.* 1970;101:132–139.
2. Parker WB, Cheng YC. Metabolism and mechanism of action of 5-fluorouracil. *Pharmacol Ther.* 1990;48:381–395.
3. Lawrence N. New and emerging treatments for photoaging. *Dermatol Clin.* 2000;18:99–112.
4. Hodge SJ, Schrodt GR, Owen LG. Effect of topical 5-fluorouracil treatment on actinic keratosis: a light and electron microscopic study. *J Cutan Pathol.* 1974; 1:238–248.
5. Levy S, Furst K, Chern W. A comparison of the skin permeation of three topical 0.5% fluorouracil formulations with that of a 5% formulation. *Clin Ther.* June 2001;23(6):901–907.
6. Heggie GC, et al. Clinical pharmacokinetics of 5-fluorouracil and its metabolites in plasma, urine, and bile. *Cancer Res.* 1987;47: 2203–2206.
7. Jeffes EW 3rd, Tang EH. Actinic keratosis. Current treatment options. *Am J Clin Dermatol.* 2000;1(3):167–179.
8. Feldman SR, et al. Destructive procedures are the standard of care for treatment of actinic keratoses. *J Am Acad Dermatol.* 1999; 40:43–47.
9. Dillaha CJ. Selective cytotoxic effect of topical 5-fluorouracil. *Arch Dermatol.* 1963; 88:247–256.
10. Dillaha CJ. Further studies with topical 5-fluorouracil. *Arch Dermatol.* 1965; 92: 410–417.
11. Rossman RE. Topical fluorouracil therapy. *South Med J.* 1969;62:1240–1242.
12. Belisario JC. Topical cytotoxic therapy of solar keratoses with 5-fluorouracil. *Med J Aust.* 1969;2:11361140.
13. Gupta AK, Davey V, McPhail H. Evaluation of the effectiveness of imiquimod and 5-fluorouracil for the treatment of actinic keratosis: critical review and meta-analysis of efficacy studies. *J Cutan Med Surg.* March 2006;2.
14. Pearlman DL Weekly pulse dosing: effective and comfortable topical 5-fluorouracil treatment of multiple facial actinic keratoses. *J Am Acad Dermatol.* 1991;25:665–667.
15. Epstein E. Does intermittent "pulse" topical 5-fluorouracil therapy allow destruction of actinic keratoses without significant inflammation? *J Am Acad Dermatol.* 1998;38:77–80.
16. Jury CS, et al. A randomized trial of topical 5% 5-fluorouracil (Efudix cream) in the treatment of actinic keratoses comparing daily with weekly treatment. *Br J Dermatol.* October 2005;153(4):808–810.
17. Breza T, Taylor R, Eaglstein WH. Noninflammatory destruction of actinic keratoses by fluorouracil. *Arch Dermatol.* 1976; 112:1256–1258.
18. Jorizzo J. Topical treatment of actinic keratosis with fluorouracil: is irritation associated with efficacy? *J Drugs Dermatol.* 2004;3(1):21–26.
19. Weiss J, et al. Effective treatment of actinic keratosis with 0.5% fluorouracil cream for 1, 2, or 4 weeks. *Cutis.* August 2002; 70(2 suppl):22–29.
20. Jorizzo JL, et al. Fluorouracil 5% and 0.5% creams for the treatment of actinic keratosis: equivalent efficacy with a lower concentration and more convenient dosing schedule. *Cutis.* December 2004;74(6 suppl):18–23.
21. Levy S, Furst K, Chern W. A pharmacokinetic evaluation of 0.5% and 5% fluorouracil topical cream in patients with actinic keratosis. *Clin Ther.* 2001;23: 908–920.
22. Levy S, Furst K, Chern W. A comparison of the skin permeation of three topical 0.5% fluorouracil formulations with that of a 5% formulation. *Clin Ther.* 2001;23: 901–907.
23. Unis ME. Short-term intensive 5-fluorouracil treatment of actinic keratoses. *Dermatol Surg.* 1995;21:162–163.
24. E. Epstein. Twice daily vs. four times daily 5-fluorouracil therapy for actinic keratoses: a split face study. *Br J Dermatol.* April 2006;154(4):794–795.
25. Kurka M, Orfanos CE, Pullmann H. Vitamin A acid for the topical management of epithelial neoplasms. Combination with 5-fluorouracil. *Hautarzt.* June 1978;29(6): 313–318.
26. Alirezai M, et al. Clinical evaluation of topical isotretinoin in the treatment of actinic keratoses. *J Am Acad Dermol.* March 1994;30(3):447–451.
27. Sander CA, et al. Chemotherapy for disseminated actinic keratoses with 5-fluorouracil and isotretinoin. *J Am Acad Dermatol.* February 1997;36(2pt 1):236–238.
28. Jorizzo J, et al. One-week treatment with 0.5% fluorouracil cream prior to cryosurgery in patients with actinic keratoses: a double-blind, vehicle-controlled, long-term study. *J Drugs Dermatol.* February 2006;5(2):133–139.
29. Abadir DM. Combination of topical 5-fluorouracil with cryotherapy for treatment of actinic keratoses. *J Dermatol Surg Oncol.* May 1983;9(5):403–404.
30. Marrero GM, Katz BE. The new fluorhydroxy pulse peel. A combination of 5-fluorouracil and glycolic acid. *Dermatol Surg.* September1998;24(9):973–978.
31. Gilbert DJ. Treatment of actinic keratoses with sequential combination of 5-fluorouracil and photodynamic therapy. *J Drugs Dermatol.* March/April 2005;4(2):161–163.
32. Epstein E. Treatment of lip keratoses (actinic cheilitis) with topical fluorouracil. *Arch Dermatol.* July 1977;113(7):906–908.
33. Cullen SI. Topical fluorouracil therapy for precancers and cancers of the skin. *J Am Geriatr Soc.* December 1979;27(12): 529–535.
34. Warnock GR, et al. Evaluation of 5-fluorouracil in the treatment of actinic keratosis of the lip. *Oral Surg Oral Med Oral Pathol.* November 1981;52(5):501–505.
35. Cox NH, et al. Guidelines for management of Bowen's disease. British Association of Dermatologists. *Br J Dermatol.* October 1999;141(4):633–641.
36. Tolia BM, et al. Bowen's disease of shaft of penis. Successful treatment with 5-fluorouracil. *Urology.* 1976;7:617–619.
37. Sturm HM. Bowen's disease and 5-fluorouracil. *J Am Acad Dermatol.* 1979;16: 513–522.
38. Fulton JE, Jr, Carter DM, Hurley HJ. Treatment of Bowen's disease with topical 5-fluorouracil under occlusion. *Arch Dermatol.* 1968; 97:178–180.
39. Welch ML, et al. 5-fluorouracil iontophoretic therapy for Bowen's disease. *J Am Acad Dermatol.* 1997;36:956–958.
40. Raaf JH, Krown SE, Pinsky CM, et al. Treatment of Bowen's disease with topical dinitrochlorobenzene and 5-fluorouracil. *Cancer.* 1967;37:1633–1642.
41. Stone N & Burge S. Bowen's disease of the leg treated with weekly pulses of

5% fluorouracil cream. *Br J Dermatol.* 1999;140:987–988.

42. Goette K. Review of erythroplasia of Queyrat and its treatment. *Urology.* 1976;8:311–315.

43. Jansen GT, Dillaha CJ, Honeycutt WM. Bowenoid conditions of the skin: treatment with topical 5-fluorouracil. *South Med J.* 1967;60:185–188

44. Mikhail G. Cancers, precancers, and pseudocancers on the male genitalia. J *Dermatol Surg Oncol.* 1980;6:1027–1235.

45. Midena E, et al. Treatment of conjunctival squamous cell carcinoma with topical 5-fluorouracil. *Br J Ophthalmol.* March 2000;84(3):268–272.

46. Grover C, et al. A case of extensive linear porokeratosis with evaluation of topical tretinoin versus 5-flourouracil as treatment modalities. *J Dermatol.* December 2005;32(12):1000–1004.

47. Knulst AC, et al. Topical 5-fluorouracil in the treatment of Darier's disease. *Br J Dermatol.* September 1995;133(3): 463–466.

48. De Panfilis G, et al. Darier's keratosis follicularis: an ultrastructural study during and after topical treatment with retinoic acid alone or in 1987 combination with 5-fluorouracil. *J Cutan Pathol.* June 1981;8 (3):214–218.

49. Schissel DJ, Elston DM. Topical 5-fluorouracil treatment for psoriatic trachyonychia. *Cutis.* July 1998;62(1):27–28.

50. Fredriksson T. Psoriatic nails and 5-fluorouracil. *J Am Acad Dermatol.* January 1982;6(1):117.

51. Yuge S, et al. Keratoacanthoma centrifugum marginatum: response to topical 5-fluorouracil. *J Am Acad Dermatol.* May 2006; 54(5 suppl):S218–S219.

52. Young S, Cohen GE. Treatment of verruca plantaris with a combination of topical fluorouracil and salicylic acid. *J Am Podiatr Med Assoc.* July/August 2005; 95(4):366–369.

53. Telfer NR, et al. Guidelines for the management of basal cell carcinoma. British Association of Dermatologists. *Br J Dermatol.* September 1999;141(3):415–423.

54. Romagosa R, et al. A pilot study to evaluate the treatment of basal cell carcinoma with 5-fluorouracil using phosphatidyl choline as a transepidermal carrier. *Dermatol Surg.* April 2000;26(4): 338–340.

55. van Ruth S, Jansman FG, Sanders CJ. Total body topical 5-fluorouracil for extensive non-melanoma skin cancer. *Pharm World Sci.* 2006;28(3):159–162.

56. Johnson MR, et al. Life-threatening toxicity in a dihydropyrimidine dehydrogenase-deficient patient after treatment with topical 5-fluorouracil. *Clin Cancer Res.* August 1999;5(8):2006–2011.

57. Baek JH, et al. Unpredicted severe toxicity after 5-fluorouracil treatment due to dihydropyrimidine dehydrogenase deficiency. *Korean J Intern Med.* March 2006; 21(1):43–45.

58. Cockerell CJ: Histopathology of incipient intraepidermal squamous cell carcinoma ("actinic keratosis"). *J Am Acad Dermatol.* 2000;42:S11-S17.

CHAPTER 50

NSAIDs for the Treatment of Skin Cancer

Claudia C. Ramirez, M.D.
Robert S. Kirsner, M.D., Ph.D.

BOX 50-1   Overview

- Nonsteroidal anti-inflammatory drugs (NSAIDs) mechanism of action in prevention and/or treatment of skin carcinogenesis is not fully understood, although it likely involves, in part, inhibition of cyclooxygenase 2 and the arachidonic acid pathway.

- Topical diclofenac 3% gel has been approved by the FDA for the treatment of actinic keratoses (AKs). Topical diclofenac is a safe and effective treatment option for AKs, especially in patients with multiple lesions for which destructive therapies are less desired. The recommended dosage is twice daily application, for 60 to 90 days.

- The role of oral NSAIDs in skin cancer chemoprevention is under investigation. Animal and human studies suggest that these drugs may reduce the risk of developing both nonmelanoma and melanoma skin cancers.

INTRODUCTION

Oral nonsteroidal anti-inflammatory drugs (NSAIDs) have been widely used for many decades primarily for their analgesic, anti-inflammatory, and later, for their antiplatelet aggregation properties. More recently, NSAIDs have been studied and used for their chemotherapeutic and chemopreventive properties. With regard to skin neoplasia, the first study on the efficacy of an NSAID for the treatment of actinic keratoses (AKs) was published in 1997.[1] Since then, over the subsequent decade, a number of studies using topical or oral NSAIDS for nonmelanoma skin cancer (NMSC) and melanoma have been conducted using *in vivo* and *in vitro* models.

Actinic keratoses are precursors to squamous cell carcinoma (SCC) of the skin, expressing similar genetic alterations

in tumor suppressor gene *p53*.[2] Therefore AKs are commonly used as both a primary endpoint and as a surrogate or intermediate end points in skin cancer studies.[3] It has been estimated that 0.025 to 16% of AKs progress to SCC yearly[4] (see Chapter 1). Thus, it is hypothesized that the treatment of AKs will prevent the development of SCC. Treatment of AKs theoretically serves a dual purpose: as a treatment for the cosmetically displeasing, at times pruritic and painful lesion that is an AK, and also as potential preventive of development of SCC. When nondestructive methods are used for treating AKs, it is also called chemoprevention of SCC (see Chapter 2).

In this chapter, we will review the mechanism of action by which oral and topical NSAIDs have been suggested to serve as chemopreventive agents (or therapeutic for AKs). More extensively, we will review the available data on topical diclofenac, which is the only FDA-approved NSAID for treatment of AKs. We will also provide insight into studies evaluating the efficacy of oral NSAIDs in both melanoma and NMSC.

MECHANISM OF ACTION

BOX 50-2   Summary

- One of the major cellular targets for NSAIDs is cyclooxygenase (COX) inhibition and the arachidonic acid pathway.

- One isoform, COX-2, is overexpressed in AK, SCC and melanoma, but not in BCC.

- NSAIDs antagonize the above mentioned prostaglandins effects by COX-2 inhibition and by COX-2 inhibition independent mechanisms.

- Topical application of diclofenac induces the synthesis of metalloproteinases and inhibits angiogenesis.

One of the major cellular targets for NSAIDS is cyclooxygenase (COX), an enzyme that converts arachidonic acid into prostaglandins, important mediators of the inflammation cascade. There are two well-known isoforms: COX-1 and COX-2. NSAIDs have been classified based on selectivity inhibiting the COX enzyme. COX-1 inhibitors are non selective, i.e., they inhibit with equal affinity both COX-1 and COX-2 enzymes.

Those that have greater affinity for blocking the COX-2 isoform are also called COX-2 inhibitors. COX-1 is constitutively expressed in all tissues, whereas COX-2 is inducible and overexpressed in inflammatory processes, as well as in neoplasms[5] (Fig. 50-1). It has been reasoned that by sparing the constitutively expressed COX-1 enzyme, and only affecting the inducible COX-2 enzyme, there will be less side effects, particularly gastrointestinal side effects, with the use of COX-2 inhibitors. It should be mentioned that other agents such as aspirin and glucocorticoids also inhibit this enzyme system.

The expression of COX-2 is increased in AKs,[6] SCC,[6] melanoma,[7] other cancers,[8–10] but not consistently in basal cell carcinoma (BCC).[11,12] Furthermore, increased production of prostaglandins has been found to potentially contribute in the development of ultraviolet (UV) induced NMSC.[13] Also, it has been suggested that COX-2 expression may be considered a potential prognostic and predictive marker in melanoma.[14]

Arachidonic acid metabolites have been shown to play an important role in tumor growth by the following pathways (see Fig. 50-2):

1. stimulation of angiogenesis, which is necessary to supply oxygen to tumors,[15,16]
2. resistance to apoptosis,[5,17]
3. proliferation of tumoral cells,[18]
4. increment of tumor invasiveness,[18]
5. immune system modulation by inhibition of natural killer cytotoxicity,[19] proliferation of macrophages,[20] and mitogen-induced lymphocyte proliferation.[21]

Although the mechanism of action of NSAIDs with regard to tumor resolution is yet unclear, there is growing evidence that they play an important role by antagonizing the above-mentioned prostaglandins effects by COX-2 inhibition. Moreover, NSAIDs are thought to have antineoplastic effects by other mechanisms (COX-2 independent) including inhibition of cytokines (e.g., IL-8, TNF-α), reduction of bcl-2 (an antiapoptotic protein), increment of the proapoptotic proteins Bax and caspase-3, and upregulation of the nuclear peroxisome receptor-γ (PPAR-γ) which play a role in cellular differentiation and apoptosis[22] (Fig. 50-3).

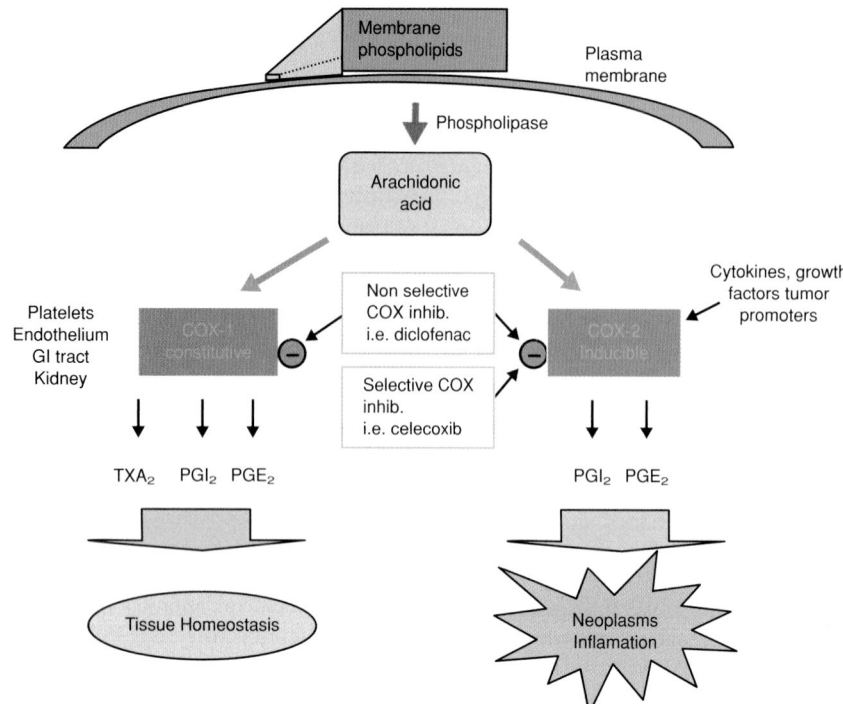

▲ **FIGURE 50-1** Schematic presentation of the action of cyclooxygenases (COX-1 and COX-2). COX, cyclooxygenase; GI, gastrointestinal; NSAIDs, nonsteroidal anti-inflammatories; PG, prostaglandin; TX, tromboxane

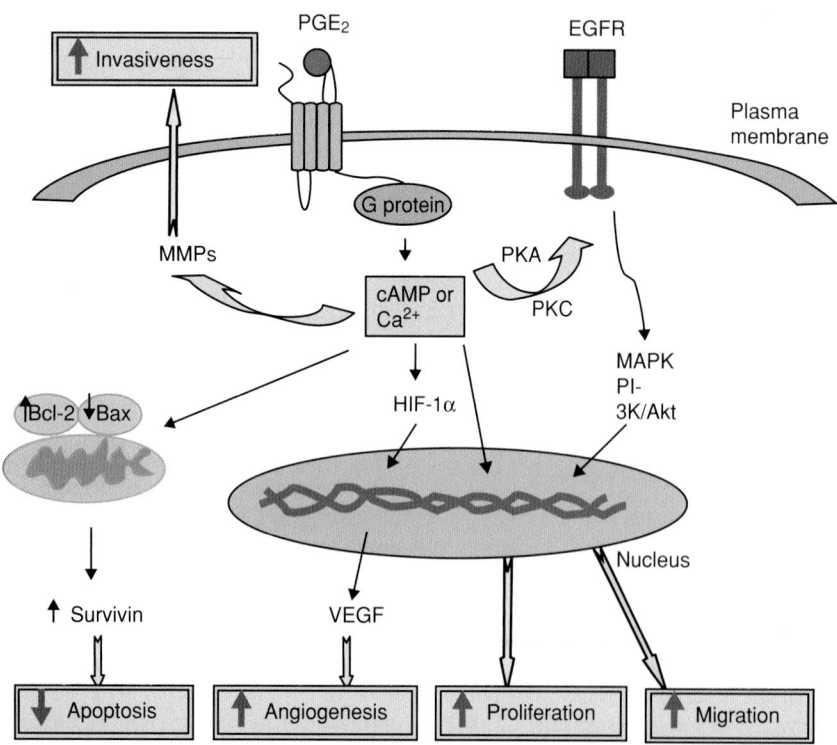

▲ **FIGURE 50-2** Schematic presentation of the different mechanisms by which COX-2 derived metabolites are involved in carcinogenesis. EGFR, epidermal growth factor receptor; HIF, hypoxia inducible factor; MAPK, mitogen-activated protein kinase; MMPs, matrix metalloproteinases; PI, phosphatidylinositol; PK, phosphokinase; PG, prostaglandin; VEGF, vascular endothelial growth factor.

Mechanisms of Action of Topical 3% Diclofenac in Hyaluronic Acid Gel

Diclofenac is a phenyl acetic acid derivative and a potent NSAID which is slightly more selective towards COX-2 (selectivity ratio of 1.4–3).[23,24] Topical application of diclofenac induces the synthesis of metalloproteinases, which have collagenolytic and keratolytic activity, degrading several cellular elements.[25] In murine models, both locally injected or topically applied diclofenac in a hyaluronic acid (HA) base, have been shown to inhibit angiogenesis (in a prophylactic manner) and to induce regression of the neovasculature (in a therapeutic manner), when compared to diclofenac alone, HA alone, and saline.[26,27] These findings highlight the importance of the vehicle as well as the importance of that new vessel formation necessary for the development of neoplasms.

Hyaluronic acid, a large polysaccharide, is the vehicle of diclofenac gel. HA has been shown to enhance the availability of diclofenac within the epidermis[28] by: (1) increased hydration of the stratum coreum caused by HA which opens the compact substance of the stratum corneum, increasing the permeability of diclofenac,[29] (2) enhanced partitioning of diclofenac into human skin,[30] (3) enhanced retention and localization in the epidermis,[31] and (4) increased delivery of diclofenac to sites of neoplasia due to greater number of HA receptors in these areas.[32]

■ **TOPICAL AGENTS**

BOX 50-3   Summary

- Diclofenac, compared to other topical NSAIDs, has a high anti-inflammatory activity, high partition coefficients and low water solubility.
- Three double-blind placebo controlled trials found diclofenac gel significantly effective on the resolution of both target and new lesions in the treatment areas.
- The recommended dosage of topical diclofenac is twice daily application for 60 to 90 days.
- Treatment is generally well tolerated, although local reactions may occur.

In vitro studies have shown that among topical NSAIDs (e.g., ketoprofen, piroxicam, ketorolac, and indomethacin), diclofenac has the highest topical anti-

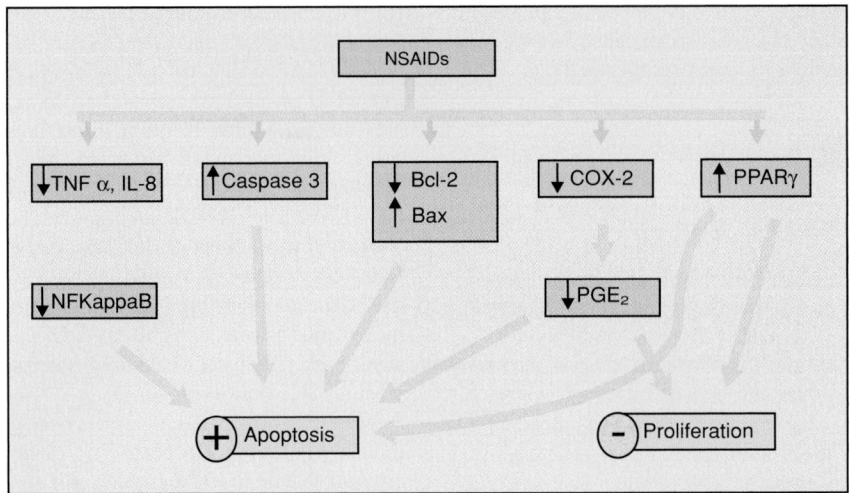

▲ **FIGURE 50-3** Different mechanisms of chemoprevention by use of NSAIDs. COX, cyclooxygenase; IL, interleukin; PPARγ, peroxisome proliferators activated receptor gamma; PG, prostaglandin; TNF, tumor necrosis factor.

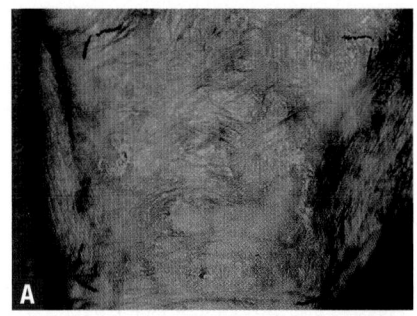

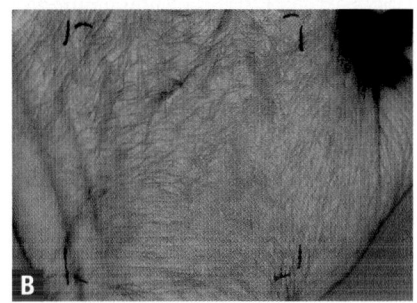

▲ **FIGURE 50-4** Effect of topical application of 3% diclofenac in hyaluronic acid gel for 30 days. **A.** Before treatment. **B.** At follow-up 30 days after the end of treatment. (Reprinted with permission from Rivers JK, Arlette J, Shear N, et al. Topical treatment of actinic keratoses with 3.0% diclofenac in 2.5% hyaluronan gel. *Br J Dermatol.* January 2002;146(1):94–100.)

inflammatory activity in the skin.[33,34] Compared to other NSAIDs, diclofenac has one of the highest partition coefficients, along with celecoxib, and low water solubility.[35] These features are possibly important in the activity of diclofenac when topically applied in the skin. Whether for these reasons or others, only diclofenac has been studied as topical treatment of skin tumors. Interestingly, topical ketorolac oral rinse (humans) and topical celecoxib (animals), a selective COX-2 inhibitor, have been studied for oral cancer. The former has not been proven effective while the latter has.[36,35]

Murine models studying the relationship between UV radiation, skin cancer, COX expression, and celecoxib use, support the role of NSAIDs in decreasing UV induced skin cancers.[37–39] For example, topical celecoxib has been studied in previously UV-irradiated mice and was shown to reduce skin tumor recurrence.[39]

Topical 3% Diclofenac in Hyaluronic Acid Gel (Solaraze® Gel)

EXPERIENCE AND DATA Pirard et al recently conducted a meta-analysis evaluating the use of 3% diclofenac in 2.5% hyaluronic acid gel.[40] Three double-blind placebo (HA gel vehicle)-controlled trials, were conducted with 364 patients who met entry criteria for inclusion in the meta-analysis and were selected.[41–43] Two studies (214 patients) evaluated the effect of topical diclofenac twice daily (for a mean treatment duration of 75 days). In these studies, investigators evaluated a *target lesion number score* (which indicates complete resolution of all target lesions in

the treatment area). Diclofenac gel was found to be significantly effective on the resolution of all target lesions in the treated area (OR, 3.72; 95% CI, 2.05 to 6.74; *p* < 0.0001). Thirty days after the end of treatment, 40 and 16% of the treatment and placebo group, respectively, had achieved 100% effect and were clear of target lesions (Table 50-1).

All three studies also evaluated the *cumulative target lesion number score* (which includes resolution of both target and new lesions in the treatment area). Diclofenac gel was also found significantly more effective than vehicle on the cumulative target lesion number score (OR, 4.00; 95% CI, 2.55–6.56; *p* < 0.0001) suggesting that diclofenac gel is effective not only in treating pre-existent AKs, but also in preventing the development of new lesions. Thirty days after the end of treatment, 39 and 12% of the treatment and placebo group, respectively, were clear of target and new lesions. Interestingly the most beneficial responses were generally seen

at the follow-up period, suggesting a continued chemotherpaeutic benefit as well[42] (Fig. 50-4).

The subsequent risk of recurrence is unknown. Further studies comparing diclofenac gel with other available treatment modalities for AKs would be useful in determining the relative efficacy of the drug.

Recently, Dawe and colleagues reported two patients with histologically proven Bowen diseased treated for 90 days with diclofenac gel twice daily.[44] After 4 weeks of completion of the treatment, the two patients had both

Table 50-1

Comparison of Complete Clearance of AKs Using Diclofenac 3% in HA Gel Compared to Vehicle at Different Treatment Durations[a]

TREATMENT DURATION (DAYS)	DICLOFENAC 3% HA 2.5% GEL	VEHICLE	P VALUE	REFERENCE
30	7/49 (14)	2/49 (4)	0.221	[28]
60	15/48 (31)	4/49 (8)	< 0.05*	[28]
84	28/73 (38)	8/77 (10)	0.02*	[27]
90	27/58 (47)	11/59 (19)	< 0.001*	[29]

AKs: actinic keratoses; HA: hialuronic acid.

[a]Percentage values are shown in parentheses.

*Statistically significant *p* values.

clinical and histological clearance of the lesions. It is worth noting that one of the patients developed a severe dermatitis at the application site.

INDICATIONS AND CONTRAINDICATIONS[45]

The mainstream management for AKs is sun avoidance and use of sunscreen. Cryotherapy is considered a first-line treatment because it is inexpensive, effective and convenient (see Chapter 2). However, application of liquid nitrogen is painful and it can be very uncomfortable, especially for patients with multiple lesions. These patients may benefit from the use of topical compounds including 5-fluorouracil (5-FU), imiquimod, adapalene or diclofenac, and with photodynamic therapy (which is not as widely available).

Diclofenac gel could be prescribed as a first-line agent in patients with "field change" and multiple AKs. It may be used as a second-line agent in patients with similar conditions who have had severe local reactions to 5-FU or imiquimod or in patients who develop hypopigmentation secondary to cryosurgery. Patients with lesions on the face and forehead may have greater benefit of being treated with diclofenac, as opposed to patients with lesions on their hands and arms.[32]

Diclofenac gel is contraindicated in patients with known hypersensitivity to diclofenac or other NSAIDs. The manufacturer advises that diclofenac gel should be used with caution in patients with active gastrointestinal bleeding and in patients with severe renal or hepatic impairment.[46] This seems wise as, pharmacokinetic studies have shown systemic absorption, although very low, of topical diclofenac.[46]

DOSAGE AND ADMINISTRATION Studies suggest that actinic keratoses should be treated for a minimum of 60 to 90 days with diclofenac 3% gel, twice daily.[41,47] The proposed amount to apply is 0.5 g to each 5 cm × 5 cm treatment area. When prescribing, the specific formulation of topical diclofenac should be specified, since other topical preparations are available (e.g., different concentrations and vehicles).

SIDE EFFECTS AND COMPLICATIONS Treatment is generally well tolerated. Most common adverse events were reported to be mild to moderate in intensity, and they included (in decreasing order): pruritus, contact dermatitis, dry skin, rash and scaling.[40] It is worth noting that a proportion of patients ranging from 4 to 14% withdrew from clinical trials

because of the adverse events related to diclofenac gel.[41,43] Hence, patients should be advised to expect these effects.

ORAL AGENTS

BOX 50-4   Summary

- Studies in murine models using oral celecoxib have demonstrated a chemopreventive effect in UV-induced skin cancer.
- Case—control studies have evaluated the effect of NSAIDs on cancer and suggest that regular intake of NSAIDs (especially high doses) reduce the risk of developing several non-skin cancers.
- Few studies have analyzed the effectiveness of oral NSAIDs regular intake and skin cancer (both melanoma and NMSC) development. These suggest a role of NSAIDs as chemopreventive agents, but further confirmatory studies are needed.

Studies in murine models using oral celecoxib have also demonstrated a chemopreventive effect in UV-induced skin cancer.[37,38] Mice given oral celecoxib after UV exposure had a decreased number of both single and multiple tumors compared to control mice.[37] When given prior to UV exposure, celecoxib lengthened the tumor latency period and reduced the number of mice who developed multiple tumors.[38]

Based on both *in vitro* and *in vivo* studies, several case—control studies have evaluated the effect of NSAIDs on cancer. These studies suggest that regular intake of NSAIDs reduce the risk of developing other cancers including colon (targeting its precursors: adenomas), breast, esophageal, pancreatic, prostate and ovarian cancer.[48–51] Randomized double-blind controlled studies, which provide the highest level of evidence, have shown varying results.[52–54] Interestingly, studies using higher dose of NSAIDs (i.e., celecoxib 400 mg BID)[53,54] have shown reduction of cancer risk, as opposed to studies using low doses of NSAIDs (i.e., aspirin up to 150 mg daily) which have not.[52]

Oral Agents for Nonmelanoma Skin Cancers (NMSC)

Recently, Butler et al conducted a case control study nested within a community-based cohort of 1621 people in Australia.[55] They examined the relationship between NSAIDs consumption (based on face-to-face interviews) and development of SCC and of AKs in patients without SCC, after adjusting

for potential confounding factors. They found a significant decreased relative risk (OR, 0.07; 95% CI, 0.01-0.71) of developing SCC in patients who had taken NSAIDs with high frequency (eight or more times per week for more than 1 year) and in patients who used full dose NSAIDs two or more times per week for 5 years or more. Risk of SCC was lower with longer duration of regular NSAIDs use. Current usage of NSAIDs (two or more times a week) was also related to a significant reduction of AKs, in patients without SCC (see Table 50-2).

Two record-linkage studies conducted in Denmark reported no differences in NMSC rates between the general population and low-dose aspirin (up to 150 mg daily) users[56] and non-aspirin NSAIDs users.[57] Limitation of these two studies are as follows: (1) They were based on prescriptions (not accounting for over the counter use (OTC)), (2) There was no stratification on dose and frequency for NMSC, (3) The diagnosis of skin cancers were based only on cancer registry reports, (4) They did not distinguish between BCC and SCC, (5) There were no adjustments for confounder factors. As noted above, if the mechanism by which NSAIDs work is by inhibiting the COX-2 enzyme which is expressed in certain tumors, then NSAIDs would be unlikely to affect BCC as they have not been found to consistently express COX-2.[11,12]

Oral Agents for Melanoma

In a retrospective cohort study using a combined pharmacy and clinical database in the Miami VA Medical Center, we evaluated 83 patients with a history of melanoma. They were analyzed to correlate the relationship between use of non-aspirin NSAIDs and development of new melanomas, recurrence and/or metastasis.[58] Combining these three outcomes, it was found that patients who used NSAIDs had significant lower risk of developing a poor outcome than those who were not prescribed NSAIDs (OR, 0.08; 95% CI, 0.01 to 0.77; $p = 0.03$). The limitations of this study are the small sample size, nonstratification of dose and length of treatment, and evaluation of intake of NSAIDs by prescriptions (not accounting for OTC use) (see Table 50-2).

Harris et al conducted a case—control study including 110 women with melanoma. Regular intake of NSAIDs was associated with significant decrease in the relative risk of melanoma development (RR, 0.45; 95% CI, 0.22-0.92; $p < 0.5$).[59] The two Danish record-linkage studies

Table 50-2
Studies evaluating NSAIDs for chemoprevention of skin cancer.

STUDY FASHION	POPULATION	INTERVENTION	RESULTS	OR/SIR (95%CI)
Case control[54]	N = 273 (86 cases of SCC, 187 controls)	Use of NSAIDs for at least 1 year Low freq: >1 tab/wk High: freq >7 tab/wk	**SCC** Significant reduced risk in high freq users for > 1 year	OR 0.07 (0.01–0.71)
			Significant reduced risk in low freq users for > 5 years (full dose)	OR 0.20 (0.04–0.96)
			AKs Significant lower counts in low freq users	OR 0.52 (0.30–0.91)
Case control[58]	N = 719 women (110 cases of melanoma, 609 controls)	Use of NSAIDs for at least 2 years Low freq: <1 pills/day High freq: >= 1 pills/day	Significant reduced risk of **melanoma** in high frequency users	OR 0.45 (0.22–0.92)
			No difference in low frequency users	OR 0.77 (0.35–1.70)
Retrospective population-based cohort[55]	N = 29,470 patients prescribed aspirin Control: expected NMSC/melanoma incidence	Low dose aspirin: up to 150 mg daily	**NMSC** No significant difference	SIR 1.1 (0.9–1.2)
			Melanoma No significant difference	SIR 1.2 (0.9–1.6)
Retrospective population-based cohort[56]	N = 172,057 patients prescribed non-aspirin NSAIDs Control: expected NMSC/melanoma incidence	Any non-aspirin NSAID	**NMSC** No significant difference	SIR 1.1 (1.0–1.2)
			Melanoma No difference	SIR 1.0 (0.8–1.1)
Retrospective cohort[57]	N = 83 (patients with previous history of melanoma)	Any non-aspirin NSAID	Significant reduced risk of melanoma (new melanomas, recurrences, metastasis) among non-aspirin NSAIDs users.	OR 0.08 (0.01–0.77)

mentioned earlier looked for the relative risk of developing melanoma as well, and did not find any difference in patients taking low-dose aspirin or non-aspirin NSAIDs compared to placebo.[56,57] If there is a benefit of oral NSAIDs in preventing the development of melanoma in patients at high risk (e.g., personal or family history of melanoma), randomized controlled studies should be done to help elucidate this hypothesis.

FUTURE STUDIES

BOX 50-5 Summary

- Clinical studies comparing the efficacy or topical diclofenac with other therapies for AKs will be helpful, as well as studies with longer follow-up for evaluating relapse rate and long-term efficacy.
- In light of the results of previously mentioned studies on oral NSAIDs in NMSC and melanoma, better evidence is needed to confirm these findings in patients at high risk of developing skin cancer. These studies should also address the risks vs. benefits of the routine use of COX inhibitors.

While current data is compelling, more and better studies are needed. For example, clinical studies comparing the efficacy of diclofenac gel with other treatment modalities in the treatment of AKs will be helpful, as well as further follow-up to evaluate and compare the long-term efficacy, relapse rate and the need for maintenance therapy.

Topical celecoxib has been studied in several animal models for chemoprevention of skin cancer and in one study for oral cancer, with promising results.[37–39,60] Celecoxib has a much greater theoretical activity index compared to other NSAIDs.[35] Studies evaluating the safety and anti-inflammatory as well as antitumoral effects in human skin would be helpful in elucidating its potential use in AKs and skin cancer.

In light of the results of previously mentioned studies on oral NSAIDs in NMSC and melanoma, higher evidence level studies (e.g., randomized, placebo-controlled) in patients at high risk of developing skin cancer are needed to confirm these findings. These studies should also address the risk/benefit profile of both selective and nonselective COX inhibitors, since high doses are

apparently needed for their chemopreventive action. Currently, three randomized, double blind, controlled studies are being conducted, sponsored by the National Institute of Health, using oral celecoxib in NMSC chemoprevention. Two of the trials are currently evaluating NMSC development in patients with AKs[61] and basal cell nevus syndrome,[62] and the third trial is evaluating if celecoxib inhibits UV-induced erythema and biomarkers of cutaneous carcinogenesis.[63]

FINAL THOUGHTS

Although not yet fully understood, the mechanism of action by which NSAIDs have been suggested to serve as chemopreventive agents, is in part by blocking COX-2 and inhibiting prostaglandins synthesis. Several murine models support the effectiveness of topical and oral NSAIDs in preventing/treating UV light skin tumors.

Diclofenal gel in hyaluronan base is the only available topical NSAID for the treatment of AKs. It represents a safe and effective alternative in the treatment of AKs, especially in patients with multiple lesions for which destructive therapies are less desired.

Albeit studies evaluating oral NSAIDs in chemoprevention of skin cancer seem promising, clinical trials are needed to further examine this property of NSAIDs.

REFERENCES

1. Rivers JK, McLean DI. An open study to assess the efficacy and safety of topical 3% diclofenac in a 2.5% hyaluronic acid gel for the treatment of actinic keratoses. *Arch Dermatol.* 199;33:1239–1242.

2. Alam M, Ratner D. Cutaneous squamous-cell carcinoma. *N Engl J Med.* 2001; 344:975–983.

3. Dore JF, Pedeux R, Boniol M, et al. Intermediate-effect biomarkers in prevention of skin cancer. *IARC Sci Publ.* 2001;154:81–91.

4. Glogau RG. The risk of progression to invasive disease. *J Am Acad Dermatol.* 2000;42:23–24.

5. Vane JR, Botting RM. Mechanism of action of antiinflammatory drugs. *Int J Tissue React.* 1998;20:3–15.

6. Nijsten T, Colpaert CG, Vermeulen PB, et al. Cyclooxygenase-2 expression and angiogenesis in squamous cell carcinoma of the skin and its precursors: a paired immunohistochemical study of 35 cases. *Br J Dermatol.* 2004;151:837–845.

7. Denkert C, Kobel M, Berger S, et al. Expression of cyclooxygenase 2 in human malignant melanoma. *Cancer Res.* 2001;161:303–308.

8. Thun MJ, Namboodiri MM, Heath CW Jr. Aspirin use and reduced risk of fatal colon cancer. *N Engl J Med.* 1991;325:1593–1596.

9. Terry MB, Gammon MD, Zhang FF, et al. Association of frequency and duration of aspirin use and hormone receptor status with breast cancer risk. *JAMA.* 2004;291: 2433–2440.

10. Harris RE, Beebe-Donk J, Doss H, et al. Aspirin, ibuprofen, and other nonsteroidal anti-inflammatory drugs in cancer prevention: a critical review of nonselective COX-2 blockade (review). *Oncol Rep.* 2005;13:559–583.

11. Muller-Decker K, Reinerth G, Krieg P, et al. Prostaglandin-H-synthase isozyme expression in normal and neoplastic human skin. *Int J Cancer.* 1999;82: 648–656.

12. Kagoura M, Toyoda M, Matsui C, et al. Immunohistochemical expression of cyclooxygenase-2 in skin cancers. *J Cutan Pathol.* 2001;28:298–302.

13. Buckman SY, Gresham A, Hale P, et al. COX-2 expression is induced by UVB exposure in human skin: implications for the development of skin cancer. *Carcinogenesis.* 1998;19:723–729.

14. Kuzbicki L, Sarnecka A, Chwirot BW. Expression of cyclooxygenase-2 in benign naevi and during human cutaneous melanoma progression. *Melanoma Res.* 2006;16:29–36.

15. Form DM, Auerbach R. PGE2 and angiogenesis. *Proc Soc Exp Biol Med.* 1983;172: 214–218.

16. Masferrer JL, Leahy KM, Koki AT, et al. Antiangiogenic and antitumor activities of cyclooxygenase-2 inhibitors. *Cancer Res.* 20001;60:1306–1311.

17. Lu S, Yu G, Zhu Y, et al. Cyclooxygenase-2 overexpression in MCF-10F human breast epithelial cells inhibits proliferation, apoptosis and differentiation, and causes partial transformation. *Int J Cancer.* 2005;116:847–852.

18. Rodrigues S, Bruyneel E, Rodrigue CM, et al. Cyclooxygenase 2 and carcinogenesis Bull *Cancer.* 2004;91(S2):S61–76.

19. Brunda MJ, Herberman RB, Holden HI. Inhibition of immune natural killer cell activity by prostaglandins. *J Immunol.* 1980;124:2682–2687

20. Elliott GR, Tak C, Pellens C, et al. Indomethacin stimulation of macrophage cytostasis against MOPC 315 tumor cells is inhibited by both prostaglandin E$_2$ and norhydroguaiaretic acid, a lipooxygenase inhibitor. *Cancer Immunol Immunother.* 1988;27:133–136.

21. Tilden AB, Balch CM. Immune modulatory effects of indomethacin in melanoma are not related to prostaglandin E$_2$-mediated suppression. *Surgery.* 1982;92: 528–532.

22. Konturek PC, Kania J, Burnat G, et al. Prostaglandins as mediators of COX-2 derived carcinogenesis in gastrointestinal tract. *J Physiol Pharmacol.* 2005;56:57–73.

23. Vane JR, Bakhle YS, Botting RM. Cyclooxygenases 1 and 2. *Annu Rev Pharmacol Toxicol.* 1998;38:97–120.

24. Riendeau D, Percival MD, Brideau C, et al. Etoricoxib (MK-0663): preclinical profile and comparison with other agents that selectively inhibit cyclooxygenase-2. *J Pharmacol Exp Ther.* 2001;296:558–566.

25. O'Brien TP, Li QJ, Sauerburger F et al. The role of matrix metalloproteinases in ulcerative keratolysis associated with perioperative diclofenac use. *Opthalmology.* 2001; 108:656–659.

26. Alam CA, Seed MP, Willoughby DA. Angiostasis and vascular regression in chronic granulomatous inflammation induced by diclofenac in combination with hyaluronan in mice. *J Pharm Pharmacol.* 1995;47:407–411.

27. Freemantle C, Alam CA, Brown JR, et al. The modulation of granulomatous tissue and tumour angiogenesis by diclofenac in combination with hyaluronan (HYAL EX-0001). *Int J Tissue React.* 1995;17:157–166.

28. Lin W, Maibach HI. Percutaneous absorption of diclofenac in hyaluronic acid gel: in vitro study in human skin. In: Willoughby D, ed. *Hyaluronan in Drug Delivery.* Royal Society of Medicine Press, London, 1996:167–174.

29. Bucks D, Maibach HI. Occlusion does not uniformly enhance penetration in vivo. In: Bronaugh RL, Maibach HI, eds. *Percutaneous Absorption, Drugs, Cosmetics, Mechanisms, Methodology.* Marcel Dekker: New York; 1999:81–108.

30. Brown MB, Martin GP. Comparison of the effect of hyaluronan and other polysaccharides on drug skin partitioning. *Int J Pharm.* 2001;225:113–121.

31. Brown MB, Marriott C, Martin GP. The effect of hyaluronan on the in vitro deposition of diclofenac within the skin. *Int J Tissue Reactions-Exp Clin Aspects.* 1995;17: 133–140.

32. Gustafson S, Bjorkman T, Forsberg N, et al. Accessible hyaluronan receptors identical to ICAM-1 in mouse mast-cell tumours. *Glycoconj J.* 1995;12:350–355.

33. Cordero JA, Camacho M, Obach R, et al. In vitro based index of topical anti-inflammatory activity to compare a series of NSAIDs. *Eur J Pharm Biopharm.* 2001;51:135–142.

34. Engelhardt G, Bogel R, Schnitzer C, et al. Meloxicam: influence on arachidonic acid metabolism. Part 1. In vitro findings. *Biochem Pharmacol.* 1996;51:21–28.

35. Sood S, Shiff SJ, Yang CS, et al. Selection of topically applied nonsteroidal anti-inflammatory drugs for oral cancer chemoprevention. *Oral Oncol.* 2005;41: 562–567.

36. Mulshine JL, Atkinson JC, Greer RO, et al. Randomized, double-blind, placebo-controlled phase IIb trial of the cyclooxygenase inhibitor ketorolac as an oral rinse in oropharyngeal leukoplakia. *Clin Cancer Res.* 2004;10:1565–1573.

37. Pentland AP, Schoggins JW, Scott GA, Khan KN, Han R. Reduction of UV-induced skin tumors in hairless mice by selective COX-2 inhibition. *Carcinogenesis.* 1999;20:1939–1944.

38. Orengo IF, Gerguis J, Phillips R, Guevara A, Lewis AT, Black HS. Celecoxib, a cyclooxygenase 2 inhibitor as a potential chemopreventive to UV-induced skin cancer: a study in the hairless mouse model. *Arch Dermatol.* 2002;138:751–755.

39. Wilgus TA, Koki AT, Zweifel BS, Rubal PA, Oberyszyn TM. Chemotherapeutic efficacy of topical celecoxib in a murine model of ultraviolet light B-induced skin cancer. *Mol Carcinog.* 2003;38:33–39.

40. Pirard D, Vereecken P, Melot C, et al. Three percent diclofenac in 2.5% hyaluronan gel in the treatment of actinic keratoses: a meta-analysis of the recent studies. *Arch Dermatol Res.* 2005;297: 185–189.

41. Gebauer K, Brown P, Varigos G. Topical diclofenac in hyaluronan gel for the treatment of solar keratoses. *Australas J Dermatol.* 2003;44:40–43.

42. Rivers JK, Arlette J, Shear N, et al. Topical treatment of actinic keratoses with 3.0% diclofenac in 2.5% hyaluronan gel. *Br J Dermatol.* 2002;146:94–100.

43. Wolf JE Jr, Taylor JR, Tschen E, et al. Topical 3.0% diclofenac in 2.5% hyaluronan gel in the treatment of actinic keratoses. *Int J Dermatol.* 2001;40:709–713.

44. Dawe SA, Salisbury JR, Higgins E. Two cases of Bowen's disease successfully treated topically with 3% diclofenac in 2.5% hyaluronan gel. *Clin Exp Dermatol.* 2005;30:712–713.

45. Chong AH, Sinclair R: Actinic keratoses, in Treatment of Skin Disease, Comprehensive Therapeutic Strategies, edited by MG Lebwohl, WR Heymann, J Berth-Jones, I Coulson. China: Elsevier Limited; 2005:14–16.

46. Bradley Pharmaceuticals, Inc. Solaraze(r) Gel (Diclofenac Sodium-3%). Package Insert. Available at: http://www.bradpharm.com/products/Doak/prescription/Solaraze.htm Miami FL, 2006.

47. Jarvis B, Figgitt DP. Topical 3% diclofenac in 2.5% hyaluronic acid gel: a review of its use in patients with actinic keratoses. *Am J Clin Dermatol.* 2003;4: 203–213.

48. Thun MJ, Namboodiri MM, Heath CW Jr. Aspirin use and reduced risk of fatal colon cancer. *N Engl J Med.* 1991;325: 1593–1596.

49. Terry MB, Gammon MD, Zhang FF, et al Association of frequency and duration of aspirin use and hormone receptor status with breast cancer risk. *JAMA*. 2004; 291:2433–2440.

50. Harris RE, Beebe-Donk J, Doss H, et al. Aspirin, ibuprofen, and other nonsteroidal anti-inflammatory drugs in cancer prevention: a critical review of nonselective COX-2 blockade (review). *Oncol Rep*. 2005;13:559–583.

51. Chan AT, Giovannucci EL, Meyerhardt JA, et al. Long-term use of aspirin and nonsteroidal anti-inflammatory drugs and risk of colorectal cancer. *JAMA*. 2005;294:914–923.

52. Cook NR, Lee IM, Gaziano JM, Gordon D, Ridker PM, et al. Low-dose aspirin in the primary prevention of cancer: the Women's Health Study: a randomized controlled trial. *JAMA*. 2005;294:47–55.

53. Chow LW, Wong JL, Toi M. Celecoxib anti-aromatase neoadjuvant (CAAN) trial for locally advanced breast cancer: preliminary report. *Steroid Biochem Mol Biol*. 2003;86:443–447.

54. Steinbach G, Lynch PM, Phillips RK, et al. The effect of celecoxib, a cyclooxygenase-2 inhibitor, in familial adenomatous polyposis. *N Engl J Med*. 2000;342:1946–1952.

55. Butler GJ, Neale R, Green AC, et al. Nonsteroidal anti-inflammatory drugs and the risk of actinic keratoses and squamous cell cancers of the skin. *J Am Acad Dermatol*. 2005;53:966–972.

56. Friis S, Sorensen HT, McLaughlin JK, et al. A population-based cohort study of the risk of colorectal and other cancers among users of low-dose aspirin. *Br J Cancer*. 2003;88:684–688.

57. Sorensen HT, Friis S, Norgard B, et al. Risk of cancer in a large cohort of non-aspirin NSAID users: a population-based study. *Br J Cancer*. 2003;88:1687–1692.

58. Ramirez CC, Ma F, Federman DG, et al. Use of cyclooxygenase inhibitors and risk of melanoma in high risk patients. *Derm Surg*. 2005;31:748–752.

59. Harris RE, Beebe-Donk J, Namboodiri KK. Inverse association of nonsteroidal anti-inflammatory drugs and malignant melanoma among women. *Oncol Rep*. 2001;8:655–657.

60. Li N, Sood S, Wang S, et al. Overexpression of 5-lipoxygenase and cyclooxygenase 2 in hamster and human oral cancer and chemopreventive effects of zileuton and celecoxib. *Clin Cancer Res*. March 1. 2005;11(5):2089–2096.

61. U.S. National Institute of Health. *Clinical Trials*. Available at: http://www.clinical trials.gov/ct/gui/show/NCT00027976¿order=2, Miami, FL, 2006.

62. U.S. National Institute of Health. *Clinical Trials*. Available at: http://www.clinical trials.gov/ct/gui/show/NCT00023621¿order=1, Miami, FL, 2006.

63. U.S. National Institute of Health. *Clinical Trials*. Available at: http://www.clinical trials.gov/ct/gui/show/NCT00025051¿order=8, Miami, FL, 2006.

CHAPTER 51

Chemotherapy and Other Adjuvant Therapies for Treatment of Skin Cancer

Varee N. Poochareon, M.D.
Niramol Savaraj, M.D.
Lynn Feun, M.D.

BOX 51-1 Overview

- This chapter reviews primary and adjuvant chemotherapeutic regimens and advances in the treatment of major cutaneous malignancies, including malignant melanoma, basal cell carcinoma, squamous cell carcinoma, and briefly, Merkel cell carcinoma, cutaneous T-cell lymphoma, and Kaposi sarcoma.
- Administration of chemotherapeutic agents is largely based on staging, history of recurrence, age, existing comorbidities, and prior therapy.
- Treatment of malignant melanoma remains largely investigational, given conflicting results and controversy regarding the use of high- versus low-dose interferon-alpha and its known toxicity profile. Among cytotoxic agents, dacarbazine is considered to be most efficacious, though with relatively poor overall and disease-free survival rates. Various combinations of chemotherapeutic and biologic agents, including interleukin-2, have been studied, though no standard protocols have been established.
- There is a relative paucity of phase III trials using systemic chemotherapeutic agents among nonmelanoma cutaneous malignancies.
- Locally advanced or metastatic basal cell carcinoma has responded variably to systemic, intralesional, and topical chemotherapy agents, notably cisplatin-based systemic or intralesional regimens or topical immunomodulators and retinoids.
- Limited cutaneous squamous cell carcinoma (SCC) is curable with surgical or destructive modalities and/or topical or intralesional 5-fluorouracil, imiquimod, and photodynamic therapy. Use of cisplatin-

based regimens alone or combined with other cytotoxic agents, interferon, or retinoids have been more successful for locally advanced versus metastatic disease, though overall prognosis for both advanced or metastatic disease is poor.
- Combined systemic cytotoxic chemotherapy and radiation therapy may provide better response and palliation than chemotherapy alone for patients with advanced locoregional or metastatic Merkel cell carcinoma.
- Selection of appropriate topical or systemic chemotherapeutic agents for cutaneous T-cell lymphoma (mycosis fungoides) requires accurate staging. Higher response rates are most commonly seen in regimens of combined topical, oral, or intravenous cytotoxic agents, retinoids, and/or biologics, especially in limited disease.
- Highly active antiretroviral therapy (HAART) with or without combined chemotherapy, such as topical alitretinoin gel and intralesional interferon or chemotherapy, is recommended for patients with extensive cutaneous or disseminated Kaposi sarcoma or lesions unresponsive to local therapy.

INTRODUCTION

Cutaneous malignancies are among the most common human cancers, with rapidly rising incidence and mortality rates. Therapeutic modalities vary widely, and where indicated, may include surgical excision, Mohs' micrographic surgery, cryotherapy, electrodesiccation and curettage, radiation therapy, photodynamic therapy, and use of chemotherapeutic agents in the primary or adjuvant setting. The purpose of this chapter will be to review key chemotherapeutic regimens and advances in the treatment of major cutaneous malignancies, including malignant melanoma (MM), basal cell carcinoma (BCC), and squamous cell carcinoma (SCC), with a brief review of current therapies for Merkel cell carcinoma, cutaneous T-cell lymphoma (CTCL), and Kaposi sarcoma (KS) (treatment modalities are also discussed in previous chapters in Section 1).

Chemotherapeutic agents for cutaneous malignancies vary extensively in administration, which is largely based on staging, history of recurrence, age, existing comorbidities, and prior therapy. Systemic, regional, and local (intralesional

or topical) modalities are available for all major cutaneous malignancies, although controversy still exists regarding the standard of care in the medical treatment of skin cancers.

MALIGNANT MELANOMA

BOX 51-2 Summary

- Wide surgical excision with appropriate margins, with or without sentinel lymph node biopsy, is indicated for the treatment and accurate staging of malignant melanoma (MM).
- The precise antitumoral effects of interferon (IFN) are poorly understood, but have been studied in large, multicenter trials for stage IB to stage III disease, with mixed results. High-dose IFN-α is generally defined as 10 million units (MU) per square meter body surface area per day subcutaneously or 20 MU/m^2 per day intravenously, while low-dose IFN-α trials employ 3 MU per day or less.
- The Eastern Cooperative Oncology Group (ECOG) E1684 trial comparing high-dose adjuvant IFN-α2b to postsurgical observation alone resulted in statistically significant relapse-free and overall survival rates at 5 years, though not at a median follow-up of 12.6 years. The Intergroup E1690 trial similarly compared regimens of high-dose IFN-α2b to low-dose IFN-α2b and observed controls, with predictably significant relapse-free survival rates among patients receiving high-dose IFN, but no significant improvement using low-dose IFN-α2b compared with controls. Neither high- nor low-dose IFN-α2b regimens, however, were associated with improved overall survival results.
- The Intergroup E1694 trial, comparing high-dose IFN-α2b to the GM$_2$-KLH/QS-21 vaccine, resulted in significant 5-year relapse-free rates and overall survival rates among patients receiving IFN-α. Several other IFN-based clinical trials have likewise shown lower rates of relapses and higher disease-free survival rates compared with controls, but significantly lower rates of mortality have not been consistently found.
- Toxicity associated with high-dose interferon-α2b includes acute constitutional symptoms, fatigue, headache, nausea, weight loss, myelosuppression, hepatotoxicity, and depression, which may require adjustment of dosing amount or schedule. Despite its limited success and toxicity,

- high-dose IFN-α2b is FDA-approved for stage II and limited stage III disease (following excision of primary lesions and affected nodes).
- Use of low-dose IFN-α in an effort to limit toxicity has been extensively examined, but with conflicting results among several randomized controlled trials comparing disease-free survival rates between patients receiving IFN and controls. Accordingly, there are no standards regarding the use of low-dose IFN-α as an adjuvant to excision, but total dosing and duration of treatment is likely to depend on initial staging and tumor load.
- Few randomized, controlled trials have shown significant survival advantage using single or combination chemotherapeutic regimens for MM. Agents thought to have the greatest antitumor effects against MM include dacarbazine, platinum analogues, nitrosoureas, tubular toxins, taxanes, and temozolomide. Multiagent chemotherapy regimens have produced response rates of up 50% in phase II trials, combined with IFN, interleukins, and tamoxifen, but without significantly better results than with dacarbazine alone.
- Interleukin 2 (IL-2) is FDA-approved for the treatment of metastatic disease as a monotherapy, and has been used in conjunction with other biologic and chemotherapeutic agents, though with significant results in relatively few studies. Administration is limited by severe toxicity: hypotension, cardiac arrhythmias, pulmonary edema, fever, capillary-leak syndrome, myocarditis, renal insufficiency, catheter-related sepsis, and death.
- Various melanoma vaccines, including whole cell vaccines, shed melanoma-antigen vaccines, melanoma cell lysate vaccines, carbohydrate antigen (ganglioside-based) vaccines, and protein/peptide vaccines, have been used to elicit a host immune response to tumor antigens among patients with intermediate to high-risk stage IV disease.
- Regional limb perfusion with antineoplastic agents may reduce the need for major amputation. Its use in the adjuvant setting, with the goal of limiting metastases, is currently being studied.
- New and future prospects in the treatment of MM currently include dendritic-cell or heat-shock-protein-based vaccines, adoptive immunotherapy, monoclonal antibodies, gene therapy, GM-CSF, interleukin-12, and pegylated arginine deaminase.

Following the diagnosis and histologic confirmation of cutaneous malignant melanoma (MM), wide surgical excision with appropriate resection margins, with or without subsequent sentinel lymph node biopsy, should be undertaken. Accurate staging greatly helps determine if the risk of recurrence is sufficiently high to justify adjuvant systemic treatment (see also Chapter 11). Major recent efforts have been made in the study of active immunostimulants, such as interferon-alpha 2b (IFN-α2b), which has shown reproducible benefit in some trials (although remains controversial), as well as the use of more specific melanoma vaccines and combination biochemotherapy (Table 51-1).

Nonspecific Immunostimulants

In 1970, Morton et al demonstrated that intralesional administration of viable bacille Calmette–Guérin (BCG) organisms resulted in the regression of melanoma, but more significantly, that the human immune system was theoretically able to destroy melanoma.[1]

Table 51-1
Cancer Immunotherapy

CLASSIFICATION	EXAMPLES
Active immunotherapy	Immune adjuvants such as BCG, *C. parvum*, levimasole Interferon IL-2
Specific	Immunization with tumor cell vaccines
Passive immunotherapy	
Antibodies	Monoclonal or polyclonal antibodies alone or conjugated with toxins or radiolabels
Cells	LAK cells, tumor-infiltrating lymphocytes
Indirect	Removal of blocking factors, inhibition of growth factors or angiogenic factors

Immunotherapy for malignancies can be broadly classified into active, passive, and indirect subtypes. Combinations of different modalities have been widely published for the treatment of melanoma.

Several related trials using intralesional or intralymphatic BCG, however, resulted in conflicting data, and a randomized WHO trial with arms using dacarbazine with or without BCG failed to show any difference in overall survival among the treatment groups.[2] *Corynebacterium parvum* has also been studied as a nonspecific stimulant of the immune system, thought to be more advantageous than BCG, in that viable organisms are not required for efficacy. Initial trials of *C. parvum* as an adjuvant therapy showed significantly improved survival rate among stage II patients when compared with BCG,[3] but later, randomized trials by the Southeastern Cancer Study Group failed to show significant increases in median survival among patients receiving such adjuvant therapy.[4] Levamisole, an antihelminthic drug with reported immunomodulatory properties, has also been studied as an adjuvant agent, but without benefit in disease-free interval, metastasis, or survival compared to control groups.[5,6] Overall, the historical evidence to support the use of nonspecific immunostimulants for adjuvant treatment of melanoma is weak, but is a part of the foundation for the use of newer immunomodulatory agents, which may better enhance the stimulation of cytokine production and overall induction of innate and cell-mediated pathways in the destruction of malignant cells and healing.

Interferons

Interferons (IFNs) are glycoproteins that have been shown to enhance the expression of class I and II major histocompatibility complex (MHC) molecules as well as antigen presentation by dendritic cells. They have also been shown to inhibit angiogenesis and stimulate natural killer and lymphokine activated cells. Although their precise antitumor effects in the treatment of melanoma are still poorly understood, these agents have been widely studied in large, multicenter trials over the last 20 or more years for mostly stage IB to stage III diseases, with mixed results.[7,8] Other cytokines, including tumor necrosis factor-α and interleukins, have also emerged as novel therapies for cutaneous malignancies in the adjuvant setting.

The immunologic and tumoricidal activity of interferon gamma (IFN-γ) has been well documented in *in vitro* melanoma models, but have failed to show clinical benefit (i.e., relapse-free survival) for intermediate and high-risk melanoma patients in the adjuvant setting.[9–11] Conversely, IFN-α has been shown to be effective against metastatic melanoma in high-risk patients, and a wide variety of trials have investigated IFN-α in differing doses, routes of therapy, treatment schedules, and risk groups, and as a single agent or in combination with other chemotherapeutic or biologic agents, such as interleukin (IL)-2. High-dose IFN-α is generally defined as 10 million units (MU) per square meter of body surface area per day subcutaneously or 20 MU/m² per day intravenously, while low-dose IFN-α trials employ 3 MU per day or lower.

High-Dose Interferon-Alpha (IFN-α)

Three large American clinical trials have been conducted examining the use of adjuvant high-dose IFN-α2b for high-risk cutaneous melanoma (Table 51-2). Comparisons of high-dose adjuvant IFN-α2b to melanoma patients, who were solely observed postsurgically, patients receiving low-dose adjuvant IFN-α2b, and patients receiving a novel adjuvant ganglioside-based vaccine resulted in notably significant improvement in relapse-free survival and overall survival. These studies examined patients with stage IIB or stage III cutaneous melanoma following surgical excision of primary lesions and nodal involvement. The high-dose IFN-α2b treatment regimens consisted of 20 MU/m² per day, administered 5 days per week for 4 weeks, followed by 10 MU/m² subcutaneously 3 days per week for 11 additional months. In the pivotal Eastern Cooperative Oncology Group (ECOG) E1684 trial, Kirkwood et al

utilized this regimen of adjuvant high-dose IFNα-2b and reported highly statistically significant relapse-free survival at 5 years when compared with observed controls ($p = 0.002$), with significant difference in overall survival as well ($p = 0.02$).[12]

The related Intergroup E1690 trial consisted of three arms, comparing the same regimen of high-dose IFN-α2b to low-dose IFN-α2b and observed controls, with low-dose IFN-α2b administered subcutaneously using 3 MU per day, 3 days per week, for 2 years. The high-dose IFN-α2b group had predictably significant relapse-free survival rates (based on the E1684 trial), but no significant improvement noted using the low-dose IFN-α2b regimen compared with controls. Neither high- nor low-dose IFN-α2b regimens were associated with improved overall survival results as well, which, though contradictory to the earlier E1684 trial, may have been confounded by the use of crossover treatment with IFNα-2b at relapse among patients in the observation group.[13,14]

The Intergroup E1694 trial compared high-dose IFN-α2b (given for 1 year) to the GM₂-KLH/QS-21 vaccine, given weekly for 4 weeks, then every 12 weeks for 2 years. Significant benefit with high-dose IFN-α2b was noted for both 5 year relapse-free rates and overall survival rates, and the trial was closed after only 16 months median follow-up, owing to the significant benefit seen for IFN-α over the vaccine during interim assessments (though controversy has recently surfaced regarding the vaccine's safety and potentially negative effects on survival). Patients developing antibodies to the vaccine approximately 1

month into treatment also had better relapse-free survival than those who did not develop antibodies, suggesting the outcome may benefit a subset of patients and substantiating further exploration into the use of the ganglioside vaccine.[15]

The North Central Cancer Treatment Group (NCCTG) has also studied the effects of high-dose IFN-α2b (20 MU/m² intramuscularly for 3 days per week, for 3 months) in patients with stage II and III melanoma, but showed no significant difference in outcome between treatment and observation arms. Notably, patients in higher risk groups (node involvement) had increased disease-free survival with IFN-α2b treatment (47%) compared with observed patients (39%) at 5 years, reaching statistical significance when adjusted for prognostic factors. Overall survival, however, was not significant between the two groups.[16]

In a meta-analysis of 14 IFN-based clinical trials, IFN at any dose was shown to result in a significantly lower rate of relapses compared with controls, though without significantly lower rates of mortality.[17] IFN-α2b has also been associated with improved quality-of-life-adjusted survival and is considered relatively cost-effective as well, despite the limited availability of studies examining these variables.[18,19]

High-dose IFN-α2b has been associated with significant toxicity, including acute constitutional symptoms, fatigue, headache, nausea, weight loss, myelosuppression, hepatotoxicity, and depression,[20] which may require adjustment of dosing amount or schedule. Critics of high-dose IFN-α2b often cite the severe toxicity of IFN-α2b, its substantial

Table 51-2
Selected Trials in the Examination of High-Dose Interferon-α2b for Melanoma

TRIAL	YEARS	REGIMEN (NO. OF PATIENTS EVALUATED)	STAGING	OUTCOME ANALYSIS
E 1684[12]	1984–1989	High-dose interferon (143) versus observation (137)	IIB, III[a]	RFS (at 5 years) 37%, $p = 0.002$[c]; OS (at 5 years) 46%, $p = 0.02$[c]
E 1690[13]	1990–1995	High-dose interferon (203) versus low-dose interferon (203) versus observation (202)	IIB, III[b]	HDI: RFS (at 5 years) 44%, $p = 0.07$; OS (at 5 years) 52%, $p = 0.74$; LDI: RFS (at 5 years) 40%, $p = 0.12$; OS (at 5 years) 53%, $p = 0.67$
E 1694[15]	1995–1998	High-dose interferon (385) versus GM₂-KLH vaccine (389)	IIB, III[b]	HDI: RFS (at 2 years) 62%, $p = 0.002$[c]; OS (at 2 years) 78%, $p = 0.009$[c] GMK: RFS (at 2 years) 49%; OS (at 2 years) 73%

RFS: relapse free survival; OS: overall survival, HDI: high-dose interferon, LDI: low-dose interferon, GMK: GM2-KLH vaccine.
[a]Full staging, regional node dissection required.
[b]Full staging, regional node dissection not required.
[c]Denotes statistical significance.

expense, as well as lack of a consistent overall survival advantage among published studies when arguing against higher dosing protocols.[21] Furthermore, the ECOG 1684 trial, published in 1996, has recently been reexamined, and the initially significant survival benefit with high-dose IFN-α2b compared with observation alone was no longer statistically significant at a median follow-up of 12.6 years.[22] These arguments have paved the way for several studies involving low or intermediate dosing of IFN-α for stage II and III cutaneous melanomas.

Low-Dose Interferon-Alpha (IFN-α)

Owing to its limited success and known toxicity, high-dose IFN-α2b is not currently accepted worldwide and is inconsistently used in the United States, despite FDA approval for stage II and limited stage III diseases (following excision of primary lesions and affected nodes). Combination of IFN-α with other biologics or chemotherapeutic agents also proves challenging, given the intensity and duration of most regimens employed.[23] In an effort to limit toxicity, low-dose IFN-α has been examined extensively in European studies. Grob et al and Pehamberger et al reported significant relapse-free survival rates following low-dose (3 MU) IFN-α2a in intermediate-risk (stage IB and II) patients when compared to observed controls ($p = 0.038$ and $p = 0.02$, respectively).[24,25] However, several other randomized controlled trials have failed to substantiate these findings in higher risk patients (stages II and III). Cascinelli et al reported good tolerability (no negative effect on quality of life) of low-dose IFN-α2a among 424 enrolled patients, but also nonsignificant ($p = 0.50$) disease-free survival at 5 years between patients receiving adjuvant IFN-α2a and patients with surgery alone.[26] Hancock et al reported similarly negative ($p = 0.3$) results among 674 patients, comparing recurrence-free survival using low-dose adjuvant IFN-α2a versus observation.[27] Approval in several European nations has been granted for low-dose IFN-α in lesions of intermediate thickness (low to intermediate risk), given its relative success in extending disease-free survival, but its use is not yet standard, as little to no studies have shown overall survival advantage in such patients (as is the case with high-dose IFN-α). Recently published findings from the EORTC 18952 trial by Eggermont et al bolster these conclusions, and also mention the failure of intermediate doses (10 MU) of adjuvant IFN-α to significantly affect disease-free or overall survival among 1388 patients studied. Greatest clinical effects of adjuvant IFN were found at earlier stages of disease (stage IIB versus stage III with nodal involvement) in the subjects treated for longer durations (25 months versus 13 months). The authors conclude that besides overall dosing, important variables in the administration of adjuvant IFN-α also include the duration of treatment and initial tumor load, and the prospect of longer duration of therapy for early-stage disease should be examined further.[28]

Cytotoxic Chemotherapy

The management of patients with stage IV or metastatic melanoma remains a challenge, with few randomized, controlled trials showing significant survival advantage with the use of single or combination chemotherapeutic regimens. As a monotherapy, dacarbazine is generally considered one the most active agents, with response rates of 10–20% and median response duration of 4 to 6 months. In recent years, dacarbazine has become much of a fixture in current chemotherapeutic regimens, featured in combinations with various cytotoxic agents, IFNs, and interleukins. FDA approval has, in fact, been granted for dacarbazine therapy, along with interleukin (IL)-2, for the treatment of metastatic melanoma, with better success rates in metastases local to skin, subcutaneous tissues, and lymph nodes, but little to no overall survival benefit compared with other agents or no treatment. The prognosis for all melanoma metastases remains bleak, with median survival of 6 to 10 months.

The cytotoxic agents thought to have the greatest antitumor effects against metastatic melanoma include dacarbazine, platinum analogues, nitrosoureas, and tubular toxins, with response rates ranging from 12 to 25%.[29] Newer phase I and II studies have emerged in recent years examining the use of taxanes (paclitaxel, docetaxel) and temozolomide, an analogue of dacarbazine.[30–32] Temozolomide, which degrades into the active metabolite of dacarbazine, carries the advantages of being orally absorbed and crossing relatively well into central nervous system, reaching cerebrospinal fluid levels of up to 30% of those in plasma.[33] This agent is therefore currently being scrutinized for activity in the prevention of CNS-related melanoma progression, a contributing factor in up to 95% of patient deaths.[34–36] Temozolomide has also been included in several other phase I and II studies combined with other cytotoxic agents or recombinant cytokines (IFN, IL-2), and very recently with thalidomide (which is also orally bioavailable with antiangiogenic effects) or in conjunction with radiotherapy.[37–40] Gogas et al have evaluated temozolomide in conjunction with docetaxel in a study of 65 patients (62 evaluable), administering both agents every 4 weeks for a maximum of six cycles. A total of 5 complete and 12 partial responses were reported, with median response duration of 9.5 months.[30]

Combination chemotherapy regimens for metastatic melanoma have produced response rates of up to 30 to 50% in single-institution phase II trials.[29] Various combinations involving dacarbazine and nitrosoureas, dacarbazine and cisplatin, or cisplatin and vinblastine[29,41] have also shown variable efficacy in combination with IFN, interleukins, and/or tamoxifen, though not significantly better than dacarbazine alone. Tamoxifen and other antiestrogens have been studied since the presence of estrogen-binding activity in melanoma was demonstrated. As a single agent, tamoxifen has shown little benefit, but may potentiate the action of cytotoxic chemotherapy agents in combination regimens. Though a significantly improved median survival rate using tamoxifen with dacarbazine has been reported,[42] later studies have not confirmed the advantage of adding high-dose tamoxifen to dacarbazine-based regimens, with or without IFN.[43–45]

Biochemotherapy

Recent clinical trials have largely focused on combinations of cytotoxic regimens with recombinant cytokines, namely IFN-α and IL-2, though response rates associated with biochemotherapy in phase III trials have not yet confirmed the encouraging results of phase II studies (see Table 51-3).[46–55] Interleukin-12 (IL-12) has also been preliminarily studied in phase I trials, alone and in combination with IL-2 and IFN-α, with few partial responses and generally good tolerability.[56–59] Tumor necrosis factor-α, IFN-γ, IL-4, and IL-6 have also been evaluated in the treatment of metastatic melanoma, but with little to no success.

Interleukin 2 is an immune-modulating glycoprotein shown to activate cytotoxic T lymphocytes, natural killer cells, and lymphokine-activated killer cells. Several phase II studies from the mid-1980s to 1990s utilized cycles of IL-2

Table 51-3
Selected Clinical Trials in the Treatment of Distant Disease in Melanoma[a]

STUDY	NO. OF PATIENTS ACCRUED	REGIMEN	OUTCOMES
Falkson et al[47]	64	Dacarbazine versus dacarbazine, IFN-α	OR 20% vs 53%[b]; MS 9.6 months vs 17.6 months
Rusthoven et al[48]	211	Carmustine, dacarbazine, cisplatin versus carmustine, dacarbazine, cisplatin, tamoxifen	OR 21% vs. 30%; MS (men) 6.4 vs 6.4; MS (women) 7.1 vs 6.9
Keilholz et al[49]	138	IL-2, IFN-α versus IL-2, IFN-α, cisplatin	OR 18% vs 33%[a]; PFS 2 months vs 3 months; OS 9 months both groups
Falkson et al[50]	271	Dacarbazine +/− tamoxifen versus dacarbazine, IFN-α +/− tamoxifen	OR 16% vs 20%; MS (with tamoxifen) 8 months vs 9.5 months; MS (without tamoxifen) 10 months vs 9.3 months
Rosenberg et al[51]	102	Cisplatin, dacarbazine, tamoxifen versus cisplatin, dacarbazine, tamoxifen, IL-2, IFN-α	OR 27% vs 44%; OS 15.8 months vs 10.7 months
Eton et al[52]	190	Cisplatin, vinblastine, dacarbazine versus cisplatin, vinblastine, dacarbazine IL-2, IFN-α (sequential)	OR 25% vs 48%; MS 9.2 months vs 11.9 months
Del Vecchio et al[53]	147	Dacarbazine, cisplatin, vindesine versus dacarbazine, cisplatin, vindesine, IL-2, IFN-α	OR 33% vs 22%; OS 11 months vs 12 months
Atkins et al[54]	416	Cisplatin, vinblastine, dacarbazine versus cisplatin, vinblastine, dacarbazine IL-2, IFN-α (concurrent)	OR 11% vs 17%; MS 8.7 months vs 8.4 months
Keilholz et al[55]	363	Dacarbazine, cisplatin, IFN-α versus dacarbazine, cisplatin, IFN-α, IL-2	OR 22.8% vs. 20.8%; OS 9 months both groups.

OR = objective response rate, PFS = progression-free survival, OS = overall survival, MS = median survival.
[a]Response rates in phase III trials generally have yet to confirm results of phase II studies using combinations of cytotoxic agents and recombinant cytokines.
[b]Denotes statistically significant result ($p < 0.05$). Response and survival rates are not statistically significant unless indicated.

(100,000 U/kg of body weight) with modest results.[60,61] As a single agent, high-dose bolus IL-2 (600,000 or 720,000 U/kg, intravenously administered every 8 h on days 1 to 5 and repeated after a 6- to 9-day rest period) received FDA approval in 1998, having led to more durable responses in a meaningful proportion of patients with metastatic disease, despite an overall response rate of only 16% (6% complete responses, 10% partial responses).[62,63] High-dose IL-2 has since been studied as an intralesional agent as well, with up to 85% complete response (209 of 245 metastases treated) in one study, thought to be more efficacious given higher intratumoral IL-2 concentrations compared with systemic administration, relatively well tolerated, and a possible option in treating limited disease.[64]

Interleukin-2 has also been used in conjunction with a variety of other biologic and chemotherapeutic agents, though its administration in high-dose boluses is limited by severe toxicity, most often resembling bacterial sepsis, and including, but not limited to, hypotension, cardiac arrhythmias, pulmonary edema, fever, capillary-leak syndrome, myocarditis, renal insufficiency, catheter-related sepsis, and rarely death. Efforts to minimize the toxicity profile of IL-2 have included altering individual doses and dose schedules, measures to block the toxic effects, immune protectors, vaccines, and combination with other cytokines.[58,65,66] Use of lower dose IL-2 in combination with IFN-α has been explored, with improved tolerance of IL-2 side effects, but without meaningful improvement in overall response rates or survival.[66–69] Use of IL-2 in combination regimens, including dacarbazine, cisplatin, vinblastine, and tamoxifen, with or without IFN, has shown significant results in very few studies, and in some cases, patients receiving biochemotherapy fared worse compared with chemotherapy or immunotherapy alone. For these reasons, the use of biochemotherapy remains restricted to the investigational setting and patients who fail in these trials are generally not excluded from other studies involving chemotherapy alone.

Vaccine Therapy

Unlike nonspecific immunostimulants, vaccines may be used to elicit a host immune response to known or unknown tumor antigens. A number of different melanoma vaccines have been investigated as potential adjuvants for patients with intermediate to high-risk stage IV disease. These include whole cell vaccines, shed melanoma-antigen vaccines, melanoma cell lysate vaccines, carbohydrate antigen (ganglioside-based) vaccines, and protein/peptide vaccines. Whole cell vaccines may be allogenic or autologous, and include a polyvalent allogenic vaccine comprised three irradiated allogenic melanoma cell lines (CancerVax) and AVAX, a dinitrophenyl-conjugated autologous tumor vaccine associated with the development of delayed-type hypersensitivity to melanoma cells. All of these vaccines have been preliminarily reported to have produced responses in patients with advanced disease and may have further practical use when administered in the adjuvant setting. However, few phase III trials of these vaccine preparations used alone or in combination have been conducted to date and were not associated with significant survival benefit; further trials are underway combining various vaccines with biologic agents as well.[70–72] A GM$_2$-ganglioside-based vaccine has been studied in randomized phase III trials and compared with IFN-α2b (Intergroup E1694 trial), but showed little clinical success, as elaborated earlier.[15] In an effort to strengthen the responses to these (relatively) poorly immunogenic gangliosides, anti-idiotypic monoclonal antibody vaccines have also been developed and examined in early clinical trials. Other promising new alternatives in vaccine therapy include DNA vaccination, dendritic cell-based vaccination,

Table 51-4
Management of Primary and Metastatic Melanoma

STAGE	MANAGEMENT
I and II (TxN0M0)	Surgical excision with appropriate margins, close follow-up possible elective lymph node dissection (ELND) or sentinel node biopsy (SNB). Reexcision and regional therapy for local recurrences
III (TxNxM0)	Excision ELND or SNB, limb perfusion, radiotherapy, intralesional or systemic therapy
IV (TxNxMx: metastases)	
Cutaneous, lung, gastrointestinal	Excision followed by systemic therapy
Bone	Radiotherapy
Brain	Excision, radiotherapy, systemic therapy (may need radiotherapy prior to surgery in large/multiple tumors)
Disseminated	Systemic therapy mainly; surgery and radiotherapy if symptomatic or clinically indicated

Excisional surgery is the main treatment option for all primary and most regional metastatic melanoma, followed by systemic therapy or radiotherapy as clinically indicated.

recombinant viral vaccines, and heat-shock-protein-based vaccines.[73]

Regional Therapy

Regional therapy for local disease or in-transit metastases has also been examined throughout the years, outside of systemic chemotherapeutic regimens and surgical resection; the latter is often the first option for both primary and metastatic melanoma (Table 51-4). Radiotherapy has a limited role in the treatment of MM, but has been studied preliminarily as an adjuvant for stage III (nodal) disease, especially in situations where disease is too extensive for surgical excision or isolated limb perfusion is not feasible, and possibly in combination with chemotherapeutic regimens for brain metastases.[74]

Isolated limb perfusion is a surgical procedure that allows perfusion of antineoplastic agents into the limb alone, which has been isolated from the body via tourniquets. Elevated temperatures are most often used during perfusion, and agents most commonly investigated in recent years include melphalan, IFN, and TNF-α. Although hyperthermic isolated limb perfusion may induce a high rate of objective responses, durations of response are typically short. Nevertheless, regional perfusion may reduce the need for major amputation, and though limited by local toxicity (painful myopathy, neuropathy), may be administered multiple times in the treatment of chronic or recurrent disease. Further investigation is currently underway in the use of isolated limb perfusion in the adjuvant setting, with the goal of limiting metastases.[75–78]

Miscellaneous Agents and Future Prospects in the Treatment of Melanoma

Recent ongoing investigations have focused largely on vaccine-based immunotherapy (including the use of dendritic-cell or heat-shock-protein-based vaccines), adoptive immunotherapy, development of conjugated and unconjugated monoclonal antibodies, and gene therapy for metastatic melanoma (which could potentially enhance the immunogenicity of melanoma in a similar manner to melanoma vaccines). Immune adjuvants, including GM-CSF and interleukin-12, are currently being tested, and the former has preliminarily shown significant results in overall and disease-free survival rates compared with matched controls with stage III and IV diseases.[79, 80] Phase I and II trials have likewise been conducted using pegylated arginine deaminase (ADI-PEG), a novel arginine-degrading enzyme-based drug, which deprives melanoma cells of arginine (a nonessential amino acid in human adults, but for which melanoma cells are auxotrophic). Early assessments have shown a 25% response rate and no grade 3 or 4 toxicity.[81]

BASAL CELL CARCINOMA (BCC)

BOX 51-3   Summary

- Basal cell carcinoma (BCC) and squamous cell carcinoma (SCC) are the most common skin malignancies, but with less propensity to metastasize than malignant melanoma. Experience is relatively limited regarding advanced or refractory cases requiring chemotherapy.

- Cisplatin-based regimens appear to be effective in the systemic treatment of BCC, although it is unclear if single-agent therapy versus combination with other cytotoxic agents, namely paclitaxel, doxorubicin, or bleomycin, is preferable for locally advanced or metastatic BCC.

- Intralesional interferon (IFN) therapy with IFN-α2b has been shown to be effective for superficial and low-risk nodular BCC; larger or more aggressive tumors are more likely to require higher individual and total dosages, as well as longer treatment durations.

- Topical tazarotene, imiquimod, and 5-fluorouracil have been preliminarily effective in promoting the local regression of superficial and nodular BCC in phase II and III trials of 6 weeks or more.

Basal cell carcinoma (BCC) and SCC of the skin are among the most common malignancies in the United States, both slow-growing, with fewer propensities to metastasize than that of MM. As a result, advanced cases or cases refractory to standard local therapy have been examined less frequently than melanoma, though metastases to bone, lung, liver, regional lymph nodes, and soft tissue have been noted in the literature.[82-84] There is no consensus regarding standard chemotherapeutic agents in metastatic or local disease. First-line therapy for BCC is usually surgical excision with predetermined margins of normal tissue, though available alternatives include Mohs' surgery, cryosurgery, curettage, laser treatment, radiotherapy, and photodynamic therapy. Chemotherapy for BCC has been documented using systemic, intralesional, and topical routes, with examination of immunomodulators and topical retinoids in more recent publications.

Systemic Therapies

Experience has been fairly limited using systemic cytotoxic agents in the treatment of BCC since the first reports published in the 1960s. In a review of 55 cases using systemic therapy for patients with BCC, Pfeiffer et al compared cisplatin-based regimens to regimens without cisplatin, and noted objective responses in up to 77% of patients treated with cisplatin-based regimens and complete responses in 45% (though only a total of

22 evaluable patients were included). In comparison, regimens without cisplatin, including single and combination therapies with methotrexate, cyclophosphamide, bleomycin, adriamycin, vinblastine, and 5-fluorouracil (5-FU) were largely unsuccessful, with only one definite partial response noted in a total of 28 patients.[84] Cases have also been reported of BCC responding to systemic chemotherapy during treatment for lung cancer, involving various combinations of cisplatin, etoposide, vincristine, doxorubicin, cyclophosphamide, vinblastine, and mitomycin C. Either clinical or biopsy-proven responses of BCC to the cisplatin-based regimens were noted, although all patients eventually died with complications of their lung disease.[85,86]

Few reports have noted the use of cisplatin as a single agent, shown to be clinically effective in the treatment of BCC, as noted by Khandekar et al in the cases of two patients with locally advanced or metastatic disease, with a complete remission of BCC following multiple cycles of cisplatin treatment at 60 to 80 mg/m². [87,88] However, the majority of reported BCC cases clinically responding to systemic chemotherapy in the last 20 years have utilized several different cytotoxic agents, namely cisplatin with combinations of bleomycin, vinblastine, 5-FU, cyclophosphamide, and methotrexate in various cycles and regimens.[89–91] Cisplatin, therefore, has been preliminarily considered to be an effective agent in the systemic treatment of BCC, though it remains to be shown whether single-agent treatment is more effective than the combination therapy, and more importantly, which combinations will result in the greatest response rates. It should be noted, however, that given the paucity of cases of locally advanced or metastatic BCC, there is a lack of phase II studies examining systemic therapies for BCC, and most available pilot studies or cases include less than 10 patients.

Finally, the use of systemic agents as palliative measures or as adjuvants to radiotherapy or surgical excision has also been examined in recent years. Jefford et al reported a rapid improvement of symptomatology (cough and dyspnea) in a patient with pulmonary BCC metastases using a combination of cisplatin and paclitaxel.[92] Guthrie et al compared combination of cisplatin and doxorubicin therapy alone to the same regimen followed by either radiation therapy or surgical excision for 28 BCCs and SCCs, with a total complete response rate in the multimodality therapy group of 92%, compared with overall response rate

(28% complete response, 40% partial response) of 68% with chemotherapy alone.[93] Other major observations were the clinically significant regression obtained with chemotherapy plus radiotherapy for lesions that were initially thought to be resistant to radiotherapy, as well as the relative ease of surgical excision for head and neck lesions in which the original size and location prior to chemotherapy would have prohibited safe and subsequently functional results. Similar cases of palliative or preoperative chemotherapy have also been reported using cisplatin and bleomycin,[94] and our center has likewise observed clinical responses in patients with advanced BCC using the combination of paclitaxel and carboplatin, as well as oral methotrexate alone.

Local Therapies

Various local (intralesional and topical) therapies have been explored as alternatives to surgical excision, especially in areas where significant loss of function or disfigurement are presumed to occur (Table 51-5). In the last 20 years, intralesional IFN therapy has been shown to be an effective treatment modality for BCC and SCC in several published cases, though often limited to superficial BCC or selected low-risk nodular BCC, with dose-dependent toxicity largely limited to influenza-like symptoms.[95–100] Kim et al reported the use of intralesional IFN-α2b in five BCCs and three SCCs, with clinical regression following a 3- to 5-week treatment period, without recurrences in a mean follow-up period of 33 months.[101] In one of the only double-blind, placebo-

controlled trials examining the use of IFN, Cornell et al reported biopsy-proven cure rates in IFN-treated BCC patients were statistically significant compared to controls, having used 1.5×10^6 IU of IFN-α2b intralesionally three times weekly for 3 weeks.[96] There is no standard protocol for the administration of intralesional IFN, and it is presumed that larger and more aggressive tumors would likely require higher individual and total dosages, as well as longer treatment and observation times to achieve cure.[99,101] Perilesionally administered IFN-α2b, potentially better retained than intralesional IFN, was also examined in a series of 98 BCCs treated with 1.5×10^6 IU of IFN-α2b in nine injections over 6 weeks. Long-term follow-up of 68 tumors revealed 96% cure rate at 10 or more years, with recurrences only among three nodular BCCs.[98]

Tazarotene, a receptor-selective retinoid that upregulates a tumor suppressor (tazarotene-induced gene 3) in keratinocytes, has been preliminarily shown to be efficacious in the regression of small superficial and nodular BCC when applied topically in 0.1% gel formulation over a range of 6 weeks to 8 months.[102–104] Bianchi et al also reported regression in 71% (109 of 154) treated BCC, with partial to complete response in confirmed in histologic samples following 24 weeks of daily topical therapy.[104] Imiquimod 5% cream, an immune response modifier, applied daily for 6 weeks has also shown efficacy in the treatment of superficial and nodular BCC in phase III studies in the United States and Europe, though no standard of therapy has yet been established.[105–108] 5-FU has been used

Table 51-5
Nonsurgical Treatments for Local Basal Cell Carcinoma

DRUG	MECHANISM OF ACTION
Intralesional/perilesional IFN-α2b	Antiproliferative effects on all cell cycle phases, inhibition of specific growth factors, downregulation of specific oncogenes, enhance apoptosis
Tazarotene 0.1% gel	Regulates genes involved in cell proliferation, differentiation, and inflammation in effort to decrease abnormal proliferation
Imiquimod 5% cream	Stimulation of innate immune response, inducing cytokine production, NK cell activity, Langerhans cell migration, secretion of nitric oxide
5-Fluorouracil topicals	Pyrimidine analog inhibiting RNA processing and thymidylate synthesis
Electrochemotherapy: bleomycin, cisplatin	Pulses of electricity increase cell membrane permeability and intracellular access to cytotoxic drugs

Topical and intralesional alternatives for basal cell carcinomas are usually limited to superficial or low-risk nodular tumors, used most often when surgical excision is contraindicated.

extensively in the treatment of actinic keratoses and is being studied for use with BCCs and SCCs as well. Formulations of 5-FU in different vehicles or preparations in an effort to increase penetration have been studied in open label trials, with up to 91% histologically confirmed tumor resolution noted using 5-FU with epinephrine in an injectable gel given one to three times weekly for 4 to 6 weeks.[109,110] Finally, electrochemotherapy (ECT) has also been studied with modest success in an effort to increase the concentration of chemotherapeutic agents (namely cisplatin and bleomycin) within tumor cells[111–113] and remains a subject of ongoing research.

SQUAMOUS CELL CARCINOMA

BOX 51-4   Summary

- Limited or early cutaneous squamous cell carcinoma (SCC) is highly curable with surgical or destructive modalities, as well as recent advances with topical or intralesional 5-fluorouracil, imiquimod, and photodynamic therapy.
- Advanced or metastatic cutaneous SCC is associated with a poor prognosis. Although systemic chemotherapeutic regimens have been featured in several case series, no randomized, prospective clinical trials have been reported in the literature.
- Cisplatin-based regimens alone or in combination with other cytotoxic chemotherapeutic agents, interferon, or retinoids have been reported with better results among locally advanced versus metastatic disease, although overall response rates remain below 40%.
- Application of commonly used systemic regimens for head and neck SCC in the treatment of cutaneous SCC has been reported in few, though promising, cases.
- 5-Fluorouracil in both topical and intralesional forms has been effective in the treatment of patients with cutaneous SCC as a nonsurgical, tissue-sparing therapy. Topical imiquimod 5% has also surfaced as a potential agent for local SCC in several published cases, with limited systemic and local reactions.

Early cutaneous squamous cell carcinomas (SCCs) are highly curable and may be readily treated by surgical excision, cryosurgery, electrodesiccation and curettage, Mohs' micrographic surgery, and radiation therapy. Among topical or intralesional therapies, 5-FU has been the most extensively studied agent for SCC, though recent publications have also explored the use of immunomodulators (namely imiquimod 5%) and photodynamic therapy for local disease (see Chapters 46, 48, and 49). Despite its association with a moderately low rate of metastasis (approximately 3 to 5%), cutaneous SCC carries a relatively poor prognosis once the presence of nodal involvement or distant metastases has been found. Treatment of metastatic SCC may include systemic chemotherapy or biologic-response modifiers, but the efficacy of these methods has not yet been established, and there is currently no standard of care for such cases.

Systemic Therapies

Several case series have been reported using varied regimens of chemotherapeutic agents, but to date, no randomized, prospective clinical trials have been reported in the literature. Cases of systemically administered retinoids and IFNs have been previously published with noted disease regression in SCC and other solid tumors,[114–116] but the majority of treatment protocols have utilized cisplatin-based regimens in combination with doxorubicin,[93] 5-FU,[117] and/or bleomycin.[118] Sadek et al treated 14 patients with cisplatin, 7 (54%) with 5-FU and bleomycin, with partial remission, and 4 patients (30%) with complete remission. It is worth noting that a recent phase II trial by Shin et al examined the effects of subcutaneous IFN, oral retinoic acid, and intraveneous cisplatin on 39 patients with advanced SCC (deeply invasive or deemed unresectable without significant defects). Overall response rate was 34% (12 of 35 evaluable patients), with complete and partial responses in 17% (6 patients) each. A statistically significant response rate was seen in locally advanced disease (67%) compared with metastatic disease (17%), $p = 0.007$.[119]

Given the extensive experience and available literature regarding systemic chemotherapy for head and neck SCC (HNSCC), application of the most commonly used regimens (cisplatin, 5-FU/cisplatin, 5-FU/carboplatin, or paclitaxel/carboplatin) has been suggested for cutaneous SCC, perhaps for induction, definitive, and palliative therapy of advanced lesions.[120] Oral forms of 5-FU have also been studied for advanced or recurrent cutaneous SCC as a single agent or in combination with subcutaneous IFN.[121,122] Cartei et al reported two partial remissions and three minimal remissions using daily oral 5-FU administration as a single agent.[121] Wollina et al have also recently examined the use of capecitabine, an agent converted predominantly in tumor cells into 5-FU. Combined with subcutaneous IFN, an oral capecitabine regimen (using 950 mg/m^2 on days 1 to 14 and repeated on day 22) resulted in complete remission in two of four study subjects and partial responses in the others.[122]

Local Therapies

Use of intralesional therapies or application of topical agents has long been studied for limited cutaneous SCC and administered with relative ease, resulting in mostly local side effects, though intense inflammatory reactions are often expected. These agents provide a nonsurgical, tissue-sparing alternative with acceptable cosmetic results and safety profiles (limited systemic reactions). 5-FU in both topical and intralesional forms has been effective in the treatment of patients with cutaneous SCC.[123–125] Kraus et al treated 23 patients with local SCC (lesions between 0.6 and 3.0 cm in diameter) using intratumoral 5-FU /epinephrine gel and reported 96% (22 patients) with histologically confirmed complete tumor clearing. More recently, imiquimod 5% has also surfaced as a potential agent for local SCC, and is already in use (along with 5-FU and photodynamic therapy) for actinic keratoses and other premalignant conditions.[126,127] Hengge and Schaller[128] and Oster-Schmidt[129] have recently reported cases of biopsy-proven complete response of SCC to topically applied imiquimod 5% cream in different regimens, with no greater than 12 weeks of treatment and no adverse reactions reported.

MERKEL CELL CARCINOMA

BOX 51-5   Summary

- Merkel cell carcinoma (MCC) is an uncommon cutaneous malignancy largely treated with surgical excision followed by radiotherapy, but with addition of systemic chemotherapy for advanced regional or distant metastases.
- Varied responses have been reported with primary or adjuvant chemotherapeutic regimens, including multidrug combinations of cyclophosphamide, doxorubicin, cisplatin, vincristine, etoposide, epirubicin, methotrexate, 5-fluorouracil, streptozocin, darcarbazine, and carboplatin.
- Combined systemic chemotherapy and radiation therapy may provide better palliation than chemotherapy alone, especially among patients with advanced locoregional or metastatic MCC.

Merkel cell carcinoma (MCC) is an uncommon malignant skin tumor originally described to be a low-grade malignancy, but documented to exhibit aggressive behavior. There is no consensus on treatment protocols at the initial diagnosis of MCC, owing to its rarity, but most guidelines specify wide excision of the primary tumor, possibly with adjuvant radiotherapy, as MCC is known to be radiosensitive. Mohs' micrographic surgery and regional lymphadenectomy may also enhance local tumor control, and radiotherapy has been advocated in the postoperative setting for primary treatment of unresectable lesions or salvage treatment for recurrent disease. Systemic chemotherapy has been studied for MCC with these same characteristics, and especially to treat advanced regional or distant metastases.

The most common chemotherapeutic regimens used for metastatic MCC are the same as those employed in small cell lung cancer (due to the histologic similarity between small cell lung carcinoma and MCC), but there is still a significant heterogeneity among the chemotherapeutic regimens studied and few prospective clinical trials available in the literature. Moderate (though brief) responses have been reported with primary or adjuvant chemotherapeutic regimens, using combinations of first- and second-line cyclophosphamide, doxorubicin, cisplatin, vincristine, etoposide, epirubicin, methotrexate, 5-FU, streptozocin, darcarbazine, and carboplatin.[130–133] In a review of 204 cases of MCC treated with chemotherapy, Tai et al reported combinations of cyclophosphamide–doxorubicin–vincristine and cyclophosphamide–epirubicin–vincristine with or without prednisone were the most commonly used regimens, with an overall response rate of 75% among the 37 evaluable cases, with complete response in 35%.[134] In a similar review of the literature, Voog et al reported an overall response rate of approximately 60% for first-line chemotherapy, with median response duration of 8 months.[133] Limitations identified in the published literature included small sample sizes, relatively short duration for follow-up, and heterogeneity of treatment regimens, suggesting also that monochemotherapy or less toxic polychemotherapy regimens may be used for older and immunosuppressed patients.[133,134]

Combined systemic chemotherapy and radiation therapy may also provide better palliation than chemotherapy alone, especially for patients with unfavorable or poor prognostic features.[135–137]

A landmark phase II trial by the Trans Tasman Radiology Oncology Group in 2003 examined the effectiveness of carboplatin, etoposide, and concurrent radiation therapy in 53 patients with high-risk cutaneous MCC, and reported a 3-year overall survival rate of 76%, locoregional control in 75%, and distant control in 76% of patients.[138] Though there is yet no consensus on the use of adjuvant radiotherapy with chemotherapeutic regimens, much of the current literature advocates at least some form of combined treatment for advanced locoregoinal or metastatic MCC.[135,136]

CUTANEOUS T-CELL LYMPHOMAS

BOX 51-6 Summary

- Treatment of stage I and II (patch or plaque mycosis fungoides) includes topical nitrogen mustard, carmustine (BCNU), topical steroids, retinoids, phototherapy, and local or total body electron beam therapy.
- Combinations of interferon (IFN)-α and psoralen with UVA (PUVA), PUVA alone, or with topical nitrogen mustard or retinoids have also shown efficacy in stage I and II patients, with complete response rates up to 75%. Oral and topical retinoids (isotretinoin, acitretin, and bexarotene) may be used for advanced and refractory disease, as well as adjuvant therapy to other biologic or chemotherapeutic agents.
- Most stage III (erythrodermic) and IV (extracutaneous) disease requires the use of multiagent chemotherapy, including PUVA in combination with interferon-α, photopheresis, bexarotene, and cytotoxic chemotherapeutic agents. Such regimens most commonly include combinations of cyclophosphamide, vincristine, and prednisone (CVP) with or without adriamycin (CHOP), methotrexate, or etoposide.
- Other agents used for stage III and limited stage IV disease include purine/pyrimidine analogs (fludarabine, pentostatin, gemcitabine), liposomal doxorubicin, and newer agents alemtuzumab (humanized monoclonal antibody) and denileukin diftitox (interleukin-2-diphtheria toxin fusion protein).

Multiple options exist for the treatment of cutaneous T-cell lymphomas (CTCL) and its many variants, and the selection of appropriate treatment regimens is based primarily on clinical staging of the disease (see Chapter 12). We will limit

our discussion of treatment strategies to the most common form of CTCL, mycosis fungoides, and its aggressive variant, Sézary syndrome.

Much of the therapy for stage I and II diseases, primarily patch or plaque disease, involves topical preparations of steroids or retinoids, as well as phototherapy and electron beam therapy (local or total skin) that may be used alone or in combination with chemotherapeutic agents, especially in the management of more advanced (stages IIA and IIB) disease. Topical nitrogen mustard has been found to effectively treat limited patch/plaque disease, and is applied on a daily basis until skin clearance, and followed by a maintenance therapy regimen. Kim et al examined the outcomes of 203 patients treated with topical nitrogen mustard (clinical stages I to III) and found an overall response rate of 83%, with a complete response rate of 50%, though with a median time to relapse of 12 months. Response rates were predictably better in patients with more limited (T1) disease, with 93% overall response, 65% complete response, compared with patients with T2 disease, with overall and complete response rates of 72% and 34%, respectively.[139] Other topical therapeutics employed in early-stage CTCL include carmustine or BCNU, which has similar efficacy to topical nitrogen mustard, though with more significant adverse reactions.[140] Administration of IFN-α has also been studied for stage I and II patients, with complete and partial response rates of 75 to 80% when combined with psoralen plus UVA (PUVA).[141,142] PUVA itself may be used as a single-agent treatment for limited disease, but may be combined with topical nitrogen mustard or systemic retinoids as well.[143] Retinoids have been largely employed in patients with advanced or refractory disease in combination with other agents or as adjuvant therapy. Isotretinoin, acitretin, and bexarotene are among the most studied agents, administered orally in variable dose schedules according to initial clinical responses and severity of adverse effects.[144] A recent phase III trial by Heald et al also examined the use of bexarotene in a 1% gel formulation in 50 patients with stage I and II diseases, with overall responses seen in up to 62% with stage I disease, and predictably fewer responses seen in stage II disease.[145] Patients with recalcitrant disease, especially stage IIB patients with tumor and plaque disease, who fail total electron beam therapy may benefit from adjuvant IFN and/or PUVA, or IFN in combination with systemic retinoids and possibly other systemic intravenous chemotherapeutic agents.[143,146]

The management of stage III (erythrodermic) and IV (extracutaneous) diseases involves the use of systemic agents, ranging from simple low-dose PUVA to cytotoxic chemotherapeutic agents and hematopoietic cell transplantation. Stage III disease may respond to PUVA in combination with IFN-α or as a single agent, where up to 70% complete response rates have been reported.[147,148] Photopheresis is also utilized in stage III mycosis fungoides, with the added use of IFN or systemic retinoids (especially bexarotene) in patients slow to respond to photopheresis alone.[149] Retinoids, though occasionally used as single agents, are more often used in combination with PUVA or IFN for erythrodermic MF. Bexarotene in its oral form is FDA approved for use in stage IIB to IVB mycosis fungoides, in patients who have failed at least one form of systemic therapy.[144,150] Single-agent chemotherapy, most commonly methotrexate, may also be used for advanced (stage III and very limited stage IV) disease.

Combination regimens of systemic chemotherapy are most often employed for patients with extracutaneous (stage IV) disease, including combinations of cyclophosphamide, vincristine, and prednisone (CVP) with or without adriamycin (CHOP) or methotrexate. Combinations of cyclophosphamide, adriamycin, vincristine, and etoposide (CAVE) are also employed.[151–153] Single-agent therapy with purine and pyrimidine analogs has been studied and may involve use of fludarabine,[154] pentostatin,[155] and gemcitabine. Gemcitabine, an analog of cytarabine, has been studied in refractory mycosis fungoides, and in 2000, a phase II trial of 44 patients had an overall response rate of 70%, with a median duration of response of 15 months for complete responders and 10 months for partial responders.[156,157] Liposomal doxorubicin, methotrexate, etoposide, systemic retinoids, and topical IFN and PUVA may also be combined with agents listed above for the treatment of stage IV disease.[151,158] Lastly, newer investigative agents have been studied in recent years for activity against CTCL, namely alemtuzumab (a humanized monoclonal antibody)[159] and denileukin diftitox (an interleukin-2-diphtheria toxin fusion protein), the latter of which has demonstrated an overall response rate of 30% in patients who had failed previous systemic thera-

pies.[160] Use of these novel agents and continued research into more established agents may allow further progress in the treatment of CTCL, despite relatively low cure rates.

KAPOSI SARCOMA (KS)

BOX 51-7 Summary

- Therapeutic modalities for AIDS-related Kaposi sarcoma (KS) include surgical excision, radiotherapy, and topical or systemic antiviral agents, including highly active antiretroviral therapy (HAART) with or without combined chemotherapy.
- Local therapies include topical alitretinoin gel and intralesional interferon or chemotherapy (vinblastine).
- Systemic chemotherapy is indicated for extensive cutaneous KS (25 or more lesions), lesions unresponsive to local therapy, or dissemination to other sites with symptomatology.
- Current chemotherapeutic agents used include pegylated liposomal doxorubicin and liposomal daunorubicin, paclitaxel, vinorelbine, etoposide, and older chemotherapeutic agents (vinblastine, vincristine, bleomycin). Liposomal preparations are associated with milder side effects and lessened cardiotoxicity, possibly allowing administration of higher doses of doxorubicin or daunorubicin. Early trials are underway for antiangiogenic agents, including thalidomide and imatinib, a tyrosine kinase inhibitor.

Formation of treatment plans in the management of Kaposi sarcoma (KS) requires careful consideration of both the staging of the malignancy and the patient's immune status, in the case of AIDS-related KS, which will be reviewed here (see Chapter 21). Goals in therapy include regression of disease, palliation of symptoms, and avoidance of further immunocompromisation. Therapeutic modalities for KS include surgical excision of cutaneous lesions or other affected areas, radiation therapy, laser surgery, cryotherapy, and topical or systemic antiviral and chemotherapeutic agents.

Among the population with AIDS-related KS, highly active antiretroviral therapy (HAART) has been associated with a decreased rate of progression to AIDS, regression of KS lesions, decrease in incidence of HIV-related KS, and potentially improved survival in studies with or without combined chemotherapy for KS lesions.[161,162] Although

HAART alone has documented activity against KS, in practice, other forms of local or systemic therapy are often begun as well. Aside from surgical modalities and radiotherapy, local therapies have also included topical alitretinoin gel and intralesional chemotherapy or IFN.[163] Alitretinoin, or 9-*cis*-retinoic acid, is the only topical therapy approved for the treatment of cutaneous KS, with noted response rates of approximately 35% compared with controls, and only local toxicity (rash, pain, parethesias).[164] Low-dose intralesional IFN combined with zidovudine was also found to be more efficacious in the treatment of AIDS-related KS compared to the use of intralesional IFN alone (response rate 31% in dual therapy versus 8% with IFN alone and median time to progression 18 versus 13 months).[165] Solutions of vinblastine (0.2 to 0.3 mg/mL) have also been used as an intralesional therapy, with clinically notable regression after multiple injections and over 50% reduction in lesions.[166,167]

Systemic chemotherapy is the treatment of choice for extensive cutaneous KS (usually over 25 lesions), skin lesions found unresponsive to local treatment, or dissemination to other sites with associated symptomatology.[168] Chemotherapeutic agents currently used include liposomal anthracyclines, such as pegylated liposomal doxorubicin and liposomal daunorubicin, and taxanes, such as paclitaxel.[169–171] Vinorelbine and etoposide, as well as other older chemotherapeutic agents (systemic vinblastine, vincristine, and bleomycin), are also documented to have efficacy against KS. Pegylated liposomal doxorubicin alone was compared with a combination of bleomycin, vincristine, and doxorubicin among 258 subjects, and found to have significantly higher response rates (46%, compared with 25%), though almost all responses were partial. Liposomal preparations are also associated with milder side effects and lessened cardiotoxicity, theoretically allowing administration of higher doses of doxorubicin or daunorubicin.[169,170] Paclitaxel is also currently being studied as a second-line treatment for KS, especially for refractory KS (though it is potentially more toxic than liposomal anthracyclines),[171,172] along with vinorelbine[173] and older agents bleomycin, vinblastine, and oral etoposide, which appear to have higher response rates in combination but are associated with increased toxicity.[168,174] Early trials are also underway in the study of antiangiogenic agents, including thalidomide, and tyrosine kinase inhibitors, including imatinib, which may provide more specific inhibition of KS growth.[175,176]

FINAL THOUGHTS

The medical management of cutaneous malignancies is a rapidly changing, highly experimental field. Given the limited value of most current therapies for systemic disease, new and more targeted approaches are needed in the development of primary or adjuvant chemotherapeutic agents. Immunotherapy in the treatment of melanoma is an extremely fluid area of study, and forthcoming advances in the understanding of the biologic features of melanoma cells may further assist our research into more specific, targeted therapies. Furthermore, the use of new growth factors, antiangiogenesis agents, and tyrosine kinase inhibitors, which have shown activity in head and neck SCC, may also offer hope to patients with locally advanced or metastatic cutaneous SCC. Cetuximab, an antiepidermal growth factor antibody approved for the treatment of colon cancer, has also shown antitumor activity in head and neck SCC and may have potential activity against cutaneous SCC. Bevacizumab, another monoclonal antibody, targets vascular endothelial growth factor and is the first solely antiangiogenesis therapy approved for treatment of human cancer. Potential use of its antiangiogenesic properties may also be feasible for highly vascular cutaneous tumors, including MM and KS. At the University of Miami, we have studied coenzyme Q, which has shown potential in in vitro settings, and plan to test this promising agent in phase I trials for nonmelanoma skin cancer shortly. Given the limited efficacy of current therapies for advanced skin malignancies, study of these and other novel agents should continue, and given the relative rarity of advanced skin cancer requiring chemotherapy, recommended management should include participation in clinical trials.

REFERENCES

1. Morton DL, Eilber FR, Malmgren RA, et al. Immunological factors which influence response to immunotherapy in malignant melanoma. Surgery. 1970;68:158–164.
2. Veronesi U, Adamus J, Aubert C, et al. A randomized trial of adjuvant chemotherapy and immunotherapy in cutaneous melanoma. N Engl J Med. 1982;307:913–916.
3. Lipton A, Harvey HA, Lawrence B, et al. Corynebacterium parvum versus BCG adjuvant therapy in human malignant melanoma. Cancer. 1983;51:57–60.
4. Balch CM, Smalley RV, Bartolucci AA, et al. A randomized prospective clinical trial of adjuvant C. parvum immunotherapy in 260 patients with clinically localized melanoma (stage I): prognostic factors analysis and preliminary results of immunotherapy. Cancer. 1982;49:1079–1084.
5. Spitler LE. A randomized trial of levamisole versus placebo as adjuvant therapy in malignant melanoma. J Clin Oncol. 1991;9:736–740.
6. Loutfi A, Shakr A, Jerry M, et al. Double blind randomized prospective trial of levamisole/placebo in stage I cutaneous malignant melanoma. Clin Invest Med. 1987;10:325–328.
7. Pfeffer LM, Dinarello CA, Herberman RB, et al. Biological properties of recombinant alpha-interferons: 40th anniversary of the discovery of interferons. Cancer Res. 1998;58:2489–2499.
8. Parkinson DR, Houghton AN, Hersey P, et al. Biologic therapy for melanoma. In: Balch CM, Houghton AN, Milton GW, Sober AJ, Soong S, eds. Cutaneous Melanoma. Philadelphia, PA: J.B. Lippincott; 1992:522.
9. Schiller JH, Pugh M, Kirkwood JM, et al. Eastern Cooperative Group trial of interferon gamma in metastatic melanoma: an innovative study design. Clin Cancer Res. 1996;2:29–36.
10. Meyskens FL, Kopecky K, Taylor CW, et al. Randomized trial of adjuvan human interferon gamma versus observation in high-risk cutaneous melanoma. J Natl Cancer Inst. 1995;87:1710–1713.
11. Kleeberg U, Broecker EB, Chartier C. EORTC 18871 adjuvant trial in high risk melanoma patients: IFN-alpha vs. IFN-gamma vs. iscador vs. observation. Eur J Cancer. 1999;34(4):264.
12. Kirkwood JM, Strawdrman MH, Ernstoff MS, et al. Interferon alfa-2b adjuvant therapy of high-risk resected cutaneous melanoma: the Eastern Cooperative Oncology Group Trial EST 1684. J Clin Oncol. 1996;14(1):7–17.
13. Kirkwood JM, Ibrahim JG, Sondak VK, et al. High- and low-dose interferon alfa-2b in high-risk melanoma: first analysis of Intergroup trial E1690/S9111/C9190. J Clin Oncol. 2000;18(12):2444–2458.
14. Moschos SJ, Kirkwood JM. Present status and future prospects for adjuvant therapy of melanoma: time to build upon the foundation of high-dose interferon alfa-2b. J Clin Oncol. 2004;22(1):11–14.
15. Kirkwood JM, Ibrahim JG, Sosman JA, et al. High-dose interferon alfa-2b significantly prolongs relapse-free and overall survival compared with the GM2-KLH/QS-21 vaccine in patients with resected stage IIB-III melanoma: results of Intergroup trial E1694/S9512/C509801. J Clin Oncol. 2001;19(9):2370–2380.
16. Creagan ET, Dalton RJ, Ahmann DL, et al. Randomized, surgical adjuvant clinical trial of recombinant interferon alfa-2a in selected patients with malignant melanoma. J Clin Oncol. 1995;13:2776–2783.
17. Wheatley K, Ives N, Hancock B, et al. Does adjuvant interferon-α for high-risk melanoma provide a worthwhile benefit? A meta-analysis of the randomized trials. Cancer Treat Rev. 2003;29:241–252.
18. Cole BF, Gelber RD, Kirkwood JM, et al. Quality-of-life-adjusted survival analysis of interferon alfa-2b adjuvant treatment of high-risk resected cutaneous melanoma: an Eastern Cooperative Oncology Group study. J Clin Oncol. 1996;14:2666–2673.
19. Hillner BE, Kirkwood JM, Atkins MB, et al. Economic analysis of adjuvant interferon alfa-2b in high-risk melanoma based on projections from Eastern Cooperative Oncology Group 1684. J Clin Oncol. 1997;15:2351–2358.
20. Agarwala SS, Kirkwood JM. Interferons in melanoma. Curr Opin Oncol. 1996;8:167–174.
21. Eggermont AM. The role of interferon-alpha in malignant melanoma remains to be defined. Eur J Cancer. 2001;37:2147–2153.
22. Kirkwood JM, Manola J, Ibrahim J, et al. A pooled analysis of Eastern Cooperative Oncology Group and Intergroup trials of adjuvant high-dose interferon for melanoma. Clin Cancer Res. 2004;10:1670–1677.
23. Tsao H, Atkins MB, Sober AJ. Management of cutaneous melanoma. N Engl J Med. 2004;351:998–1012.
24. Grob JJ, Dreno B, de la Salmoniere P, et al. Randomised trial of interferon alpha-2a as adjuvant therapy in resected primary melanoma thicker than 1.5 mm without clinically detectable node metastases. Lancet. 1998;351:1905–1910.
25. Pehamberger H, Soyer HP, Steiner A, et al. Adjuvant interferon alfa-2a treatment in resected primary stage II cutaneous melanoma. J Clin Oncol. 1998;16:1425–1429.
26. Cascinelli N, Belli F, MacKie RM, et al. Effect of long-term adjuvant therapy with interferon alpha-2a in patients with regional node metastases from cutaneous melanoma: a randomised trial. Lancet. 2001;358:866–869.
27. Hancock BW, Wheatley K, Harris S, et al. Adjuvant interferon in high-risk melanoma: the AIM HIGH Study—United Kingdom Coordinating Committee on Cancer Research randomized study of adjuvant low-dose extended-duration interferon alfa-2a in high-risk resected malignant melanoma. J Clin Oncol. 2004;22:53–61.
28. Eggermont AM, Suciu S, MacKie R, et al. Post-surgery adjuvant therapy with intermediate doses of interferon alfa 2b versus observation in patients with stage IIb/III melanoma (EORTC 18952): randomized controlled trial. Lancet. 2005;366:1189–1196.
29. Atkins MB. The treatment of metastatic melanoma with chemotherapy and biologics. Curr Opin Oncol. 1997;9:205–213.
30. Gogas H, Bafaloukos D, Bedikian AY. The role of taxanes in the treatment of metastatic melanoma. Melanoma Res. 2004;14:415–420.
31. Legha SS, Ring S, Papdoupoulos N, et al. A phase II trial of taxol in metastatic melanoma. Cancer. 1990;65:2478–2481.
32. Bleehan NM, Newlands ES, Lee SM, et al. Cancer research campaign phase II trial of temozolomide in metastatic melanoma. J Clin Oncol. 1995;13:910–913.

33. Agarwala SS, Kirkwood JM. Temozolomide, a novel alkylating agent with activity in the central nervous system, may improve the treatment of advanced metastatic melanoma. *Oncologist.* 2000;5:144–151.

34. Paul MJ, Summers Y, Calvert AH, et al. Effect of temozolomide on central nervous system relapse in patients with advanced melanoma. *Melanoma Res.* 2002;12(2):175–178.

35. Sampson JH, Carter JH, Jr., Friedman AH, et al. Demographics, prognosis, and therapy in 702 patients with brain metastases from malignant melanoma. *J Neurosurg.* 1998;88:11–20.

36. Conill C, Gonzalez-Cao M, Jorcano S, et al. Temozolomide as prophylaxis for melanoma brain metastases. *Melanoma Res.* 2004;14:73–74.

37. Richtig E, Hofmann-Wellenhof R, Pehamberger H, et al. Temozolomide and interferon α2b in metastatic melanoma stage IV. *Br J Dermatol.* 2004;151: 91–98.

38. Lewis KD, Gibbs P, O'Day S, et al. A phase II study of biochemotherapy for advanced melanoma incorporating temozolomide, decrescendo interleukin-2 and GM-CSF. *Cancer Invest.* 2005;23(4):303–308.

39. Hwu WJ, Lis E, Menell JH. Temozolomide plus thalidomide in patients with brain metastases from melanoma. *Cancer.* 2005;103:2590–2597.

40. Reiriz AB, Richter MF, Fernandes S. Phase II study of thalidomide in patients with metastatic malignant melanoma. *Melanoma Res.* 2004;14:527–531.

41. Lee SM, Betticher DC, Thatcher N. Melanoma: chemotherapy. *Br Med Bull.* 1995;51:609–630.

42. Cocconi G, Bella M, Calabresi F, et al. Treatment of metastatic malignant melanoma with dacarbazine plus tamoxifen. *N Engl J Med.* 1992;327:516–523.

43. Legha S, Ring S, Bedikian A, et al. Lack of benefit from tamoxifen (T) added to a regimen of cisplatin (c), vinblastine (V), DTIC (D) and alpha interferon (IFN) in patients (PT) with metastatic melanoma. *Proc Am Soc Clin Oncol.* 1993;12:388.

44. Ferri W, Agarwala SS, Kirkwood J, et al. Carboplatin and dacarbazine (D) +/− tamoxifen (T) for metastatic melanoma. *Proc Am Soc Clin Oncol.* 1994;13:394.

45. Falkson CI, Ibrahim J, Kirkwood JM, et al. A randomized phase II trial of dacarbazine (DTIC) versus DTIC+interferon alfa-2b (IFN) versus DTIC+tamoxifen (TMX) versus DTIC+IFN+TMX in metastatic malignant melanoma: an ECOG Trial [Abstract]. *Proc Am Soc Clin Oncol.* 1996;15:435.

46. Margolin KA. Biochemotherapy for melanoma: rational therapeutics in the search for weapons of melanoma destruction. *Cancer.* 2004;101:435–438.

47. Falkson CI, Falkson G, Falkson HC. Improved results with the addition of interferon alfa-2b to dacarbazine in the treatment of patients with metastatic malignant melanoma. *J Clin Oncol.* 1991;9:1403–1408.

48. Rusthoven JJ, Quirt IC, Iscoe NA, et al. Randomized, double-blind, placebo-controlled trial comparing the response rates of carmustine, dacarbazine, and cisplatin with and without tamoxifen in patients with metastatic melanoma. *J Clin Oncol.* 1996;14:2083–2090.

49. Keilholz U, Goey SH, Punt CJA, et al. Interferon alfa-2a and interleukin-2 with or without cisplatin in metastatic melanoma: a randomized trial of the European Organization for Research and Treatment of Cancer Melanoma Cooperative Group. *J Clin Oncol.* 1997;15: 2579–2588.

50. Falkson CI, Ibrahim J, Kirkwood JM, et al. Phase III trial of dacarbazine versus dacarbazine with interferon α-2b versus dacarbazine with tamoxifen versus dacarbazine with interferon α-2b with and tamoxifen in patients with metastatic malignant melanoma: an Eastern Cooperative Oncology Group study. *J Clin Oncol.* 1998;16:1743–1751.

51. Rosenberg SA, Yang JC, Schwartzentruber DJ, et al. Prospective randomized trial of the treatment of patients with metastatic melanoma using chemotherapy with cisplatin, dacarbazine, and tamoxifen alone or in combination with interleukin-2 and interferon alfa-2b. *J Clin Oncol.* 1999;17:968–975.

52. Eton O, Legha SS, Bedikian AY, et al. Sequential biochemotherapy versus chemotherapy for metastatic melanoma: results from a phase III randomized trial. *J Clin Oncol.* 2002;20:2045–2052.

53. Del Vecchio M, Bajetta E, Vitali M, et al. Multicenter phase III randomized trial of cisplatin, vindesine and dacarbazine (CVD) versus CVD plus subcutaneous interleukin-2 (IL-2) and interferon-alpha-2b (IFN) in metastatic melanoma patients [Abstract]. *Proc Am Soc Clin Oncol.* 2003;22:709.

54. Atkins MB, Lee S, Flaherty LE, et al. A prospective randomized phase III trial of concurrent biochemotherapy (BCT) with cisplatin, vinblastine, dacarbazine (CVD), IL-2 and interferon alpha-2b (IFN) versus CVD alone in patients with metastatic melanoma (E3695): an ECOG-coordinated Intergroup trial [Abstract]. *Proc Am Soc Clin Oncol.* 2003;22:708.

55. Keilholz U, Punt CJA, Gore M, et al. Dacarbazine, cisplatin and interferon-alfa-2b with or without interleukin-2 in metastatic melanoma: a randomized phase III trial (18951) of the European Organisation for Research and Treatment of Cancer Melanoma Group. *J Clin Oncol.* 2005;23:6747–6755.

56. Alatrash G, Hutson TE, Molto L, et al. Clinical and immunologic effects of subcutaneously administered interleukin-12 and interferon alfa-2b: phase I trial of patients with metastatic renal cell carcinoma or malignant melanoma. *J Clin Oncol.* 2004;22(14):2891–2900.

57. Bajetta E, Del Vecchi M, Mortarini R, et al. Pilot study of subcutaneous recombinant human interleukin-12 in metastatic melanoma. *Clin Cancer Res.* 1998;4: 75–85.

58. Gollob JA, Veenstra KG, Parker RA, et al. Phase I trial of concurrent twice-weekly recombinant human interleukin-12 plus low-dose IL-2 in patients with melanoma or renal cell carcinoma. *J Clin Oncol.* 2003;21:2564–2573.

59. Atkins MB, Robertson MJ, Gordon M, et al. Phase I evaluation of intravenous recombinant human interleukin-12 in patients with advanced malignancies. *Clin Cancer Res.* 1997;3:409–417.

60. Parkinson DR, Abrams JS, Wiernik PH, et al. Interleukin-2 therapy in patients with metastatic malignant melanoma: a phase II study. *J Clin Oncol.* 1990;8:1650–1656.

61. Dutcher JP, Creekmore S, Weiss GR, et al. A phase II study of interleukin-2 and lymphokine-activated killer cells in patients with metastatic malignant melanoma. *J Clin Oncol.* 1989;7:477–485.

62. Atkins MB, Lotze MT, Dutcher JP, et al. High-dose recombinant interleukin-2 therapy for patients with metastatic melanoma: analysis of 270 patients treated between 1985 and 1993. *J Clin Oncol.* 1999;17:2105–2116.

63. Eklund JW, Kuzel TM. A review of recent findings involving interleukin-2-based cancer therapy. *Curr Opin Oncol.* 2004;16:542–546.

64. Radny P, Caroli UM, Bauer J, et al. A phase II traial of intralesional therapy with interleukin-2 in soft-tissue melanoma metastases. *Br J Cancer.* 2003;89:1620–1626.

65. Agarwala SS, Glaspy J, O'Day SJ, et al. Results from a randomized phase III study comparing combined treatment with histamine dihydrochloride plus interleukin-2 versus interleukin-2 alone in patients with metastatic melanoma. *J Clin Oncol.* 2002;20:125–133.

66. Keilholz U, Scheibenbogen C, Tilgen W, et al. Interferon-α and interleukin-2 in the treatment of metastatic melanoma: comparison of two phase II trials. *Cancer.* 1993;72:607–614.

67. Hauschild A, Weichenthal M, Balda B, et al. Prospective randomized trial of interferon alfa-2b and interleukin-2 as adjuvant treatment for resected intermediate- and high-risk primary melanoma without clinically detectable node metastasis. *J Clin Oncol.* 2003;21:2883–2888.

68. Kruit WHJ, Punt CJA, Goey SH, et al. Dose efficacy study of two schedules of high-dose bolus administration of interleukin 2 and interferon alpha in metastatic melanoma. *Br J Cancer.* 1996;74: 951–955.

69. Sparano JA, Fisher RI, Sunderland M, et al. Randomized phase III trial of treatment with high-dose interleukin-2 either alone or in combination with interferon alfa-2a in patients with advanced melanoma. *J Clin Oncol.* 1993;11:1969–1977.

70. Hsueh EC, Gupta RK, Qi K, et al. Correlation of specific immune responses with survival in melanoma patients with distant metastases receiving polyvalent melanoma cell vaccine. *J Clin Oncol.* 1998;16:2913–2920.

71. Bystryn JC, Zelenich-Jacquotte A, Oratz R, et al. Double-blind trial of a polyvalent, shed antigen melanoma vaccine. *Clin Cancer Res.* 2001;7:1882–1887.

72. Livingston PO, Wong GY, Adluri S, et al. Improved survival in stage III melanoma patients with GM2 antibodies: a randomized trial of adjuvant vaccination with GM2 ganglioside. *J Clin Oncol.* 1994;12:1036–1044.

73. Wolchok JD, Weber JS, Houghton AN, et al. Melanoma vaccines. In: Balch CM, Houghton AN, Sober AJ, Soong S, eds. *Cutaneous Melanoma.* St. Louis, MO:

Quality Medical Publishing; 2003: 645–656.

74. Ang KK, Peters LJ, Weber RS, et al. Postoperative radiotherapy for cutaneous melanoma of the head and neck region. *Int J Radiat Oncol Biol Phys.* 1994;30: 795–798.

75. Coit DG, Ferrone CR. Radiotherapy for primary and regional melanoma. In: Balch CM, Houghton AN, Sober AJ, Soong S, eds. *Cutaneous Melanoma.* St. Louis, MO: Quality Medical Publishing; 2003:449–471.

76. Fraker DL, Eggermont AM. Hyperthermic regional perfusion for melanoma of the limbs. In: Balch CM, Houghton AN, Sober AJ, Soong S, eds. *Cutaneous Melanoma.* St. Louis, MO: Quality Medical Publishing; 2003:473–493.

77. Lienard D, Ewalenko P, Delmotte JJ, et al. High-dose recombinant tumor necrosis factor alpha in combination with interferon gamma and melphalan in isolation perfusion of the limbs for melanoma and sarcoma. *J Clin Oncol.* 1992;10:52–60.

78. Krementz ET, Carter RD, Sutherland CM, et al. Regional chemotherapy for melanoma: a 35-year experience. *Ann Surg.* 1994;220(4):520–535.

79. Spitler LE, Grossbard ML, Ernstoff MS, et al. Adjuvant therapy of stage III and IV malignant melanoma using granulocyte-macrophage colony-stimulating factor. *J Clin Oncol.* 2000;18:1614–1621.

80. Lawson D, Kirkwood JM. Granulocyte-macrophage colony-stimulating factor: another cytokine with adjuvant therapeutic benefit in melanoma? *J Clin Oncol.* 2000;18(8):1603–1605.

81. Ascierto PA, Scala S, Castello G, et al. Pegylated arginine deiminase treatment of patients with metastatic melanoma: results from phase I and II studies. *J Clin Oncol.* 2005;23:7660–7668.

82. Coker D, Elias EG, Viravathana T, et al. Chemotherapy for metastatic basal cell carcinoma. *Arch Dermatol.* 1983;119: 44–50.

83. vonDomarus H, Stevens PJ. Metastatic basal cell carcinoma. Report of five cases and review of 170 cases in the literature. *J Am Acad Dermatol.* 1984;10(6): 1043–1060.

84. Pfeiffer P, Hansen O, Rose C. Systemic cytotoxic therapy of basal cell carcinoma. A review of the literature. *Eur J Cancer.* 1990;26(1):73–77.

85. Kaufman D, Gralla R, Myskowski PL. Basal cell carcinoma: response to systemic chemotherapy for lung carcinoma. *J Am Acad Dermatol.* 1988;18(2 Pt 1): 306–310.

86. Dickie GJ, Pratt GR. Basal cell carcinoma of the skin responding completely to chemotherapy. *Arch Dermatol.* 1988;124:494.

87. Salem P, Hall SW, Benjamin RS, et al. Clinical phase I–II study of *cis*-diamminedicholoroplatinum (II) given by continuous infusion. *Cancer Treat Rep.* 1976;62:1553–1556.

88. Khandekar JD. Complete response of metastatic basal cell carcinoma to cisplatin chemotherapy: a report on two patients. *Arch Dermatol.* 1990;126:1660.

89. Wieman TJ, Shively EH, Woodcock TM. Responsiveness of metastatic basal-cell carcinoma to chemotherapy. *Cancer.* 1983;52:1583–1585.

90. Bason MM, Grant-Kels JM, Govil M. Metastatic basal cell carcinoma: response to chemotherapy. *J Am Acad Dermatol.* 1990;22:905–908.

91. Woods RL, Stewart JF. Metastatic basal cell carcinoma: report of a case responding to chemotherapy. *Postgrad Med J.* 1980;56:272–273.

92. Jefford M, Kiffer JD, Somers G, et al. Metastatic basal cell carcinoma: rapid symptomatic response to cisplatin and paclitaxel. *ANZ J Surg.* 2004;74:704–705.

93. Guthrie TH, Porubsky ES, Luxenberg MN, et al. Cisplatin-based chemotherapy in advanced basal and squamous cell carcinomas of the skin: results in 28 patients including 13 patients receiving multimodality therapy. *J Clin Oncol.* 1990;8(2):342–346.

94. Denic S. Preoperative treatment of advanced skin carcinoma with cisplatin and bleomycin. *Am J Clin Oncol.* 1999; 22(1):32–34.

95. Edwards L, Tucker SB, Perednia D, et al. The effect of an intralesional sustained-release formulation of interferon alfa-2b on basal cell carcinomas. *Arch Dermatol.* 1990;126:1029–1032.

96. Cornell RC, Greenway HT, Tucker SB, et al. Intralesional interferon therapy for basal cell carcinoma. *J Am Acad Dermatol.* 1990;23(4 Pt 1):694–700.

97. Chimenti S, Peris K, Di Cristofaross, et al. Use of recombinant interferon alfa-2b in the treatment of basal cell carcinoma. *Dermatology.* 1995;190:214–217.

98. Tucker SB, Polasek JW, Perri AJ, et al. Long-term follow-up of basal cell carcinomas treated with perilesional interferon alfa 2b as monotherapy. *J Am Acad Dermatol.* 2006;54:1033–1038.

99. Dogan B, Harmanyeri Y, Baloglu H, et al. Intralesional alfa-2a interferon therapy for basal cell carcinoma. *Cancer Lett.* 1995;91:215–219.

100. Greenway HT, Cornell RC, Tanner DJ, et al. Treatment of basal cell carcinoma with intralesional interferon. *J Am Acad Dermatol.* 1986;15:437–443.

101. Kim KH, Yavel RM, Gross VL, et al. Intralesional interferon α-2b in the treatment of basal cell carcinoma and squamous cell carcinoma: revisited. *Dermatol Surg.* 2004;30(1):116–120.

102. Peris K, Fargnoli MC, Chimenti S. Preliminary observations on the use of topical tazarotene to treat basal cell carcinoma. *N Engl J Med.* 1999;341:1767–1768.

103. Duvic M, Ni X, Talpur R, et al. Tazarotene-induced gene 3 is suppressed in basal cell carcinomas and reversed in vivo by tazarotene application. *J Invest Dermatol.* 2003;121:902–909.

104. Bianchi L, Orlandi A, Campione E, et al. Topical treatment of basal cell carcinoma with tazarotene: a clinicopathological study on a large series of cases. *Br J Dermatol.* 2004;151:148–156.

105. Geisse J, Caro I, Lindholm J, et al. Imiquimod 5% cream for the treatment of superficial basal cell carcinoma: results from two phase III, randomized, vehicle-controlled studies. *J Am Acad Dermatol.* 2004;50:722–733.

106. Schulze HJ, Cribier B, Requena L, et al. Imiquimod 5% cream for the treatment of superficial basal cell carcinoma: results from a randomized vehicle-controlled phase III study in Europe. *Br J Dermatol.* 2005;152:939–947.

107. Marks R, Gebauer K, Shumack S, et al. Imiquimod 5% cream in the treatment of superficial basal cell carcinoma: results of a multicenter 6-week dose-response trial. *J Am Acad Dermatol.* 2001; 44:807–813.

108. Sterry W, Ruzicka T, Herrera E, et al. Imiquimod 5% cream for the treatment of superficial and nodular basal cell carcinoma: randomized studies comparing low-frequency dosing with and without occlusion. *Br J Dermatol.* 2002;147: 1227–1236.

109. Miller BH, Shavin JS, Cognetta A, et al. Nonsurgical treatment of basal cell carcinomas with intralesional 5-fluorouracil/epinephrine injectable gel. *J Am Acad Dermatol.* 1997;36:72–77.

110. Romagosa R, Saap L, Givens M, et al. A pilot study to evaluation the treatment of basal cell carcinoma with 5-fluorouracil using phosphatidyl choline as a transepidermal carrier. *Dermatol Surg.* 2000;26(4):338–340.

111. Sersa G, Stabuc B, Cemazar M, et al. Electrochemotherapy with cisplatin: potentiation of local cisplatin antitumour effectiveness by application of electric pulses in cancer patients. *Eur J Cancer.* 1998;34(8):1213–1218.

112. Glass LF, Fenske NA, Jaroszeski M, et al. Bleomycin-mediated electrochemotherapy of basal cell carcinoma. *J Am Acad Dermatol.* 1996;34:82–86.

113. Rodriguez-Cuevas S, Barroso-Bravo S, Almanza-Estrada J, et al. Electrochemotherapy in primary and metastatic skin tumors: phase II trial using intralesional bleomycin. *Arch Med Res.* 2001; 32:273–276.

114. Lippman SM, Meyskens FL. Treatment of advanced squamous cell carcinoma of the skin with isotretinoin. *Ann Intern Med.* 1987;107:499–501.

115. Lippman SM, Shimm DS, Meyskens FL. Nonsurgical treatments for skin cancer: retinoids and α-interferon. *J Dermatol Surg Oncol.* 1988;14:862–869.

116. Lippman SM, Lotan R, Schleuniger U. Retinoid-interferon therapy of solid tumors. *Int J Cancer.* 1997;70:481–483.

117. Khansur T, Kennedy A. Cisplatin and 5-fluorouracil for advanced locoregional and metastatic squamous cell carcinoma of the skin. *Cancer.* 1991;67:2030–2032.

118. Sadek H, Azli N, Wendling J, et al. Treatment of advanced squamous cell carcinoma of the skin with cisplatin, 5-fluorouracil, and bleomycin. *Cancer.* 1990;66:1692–1696.

119. Shin D, Glisson B, Khuri F, et al. Phase II and biologic study of interferon alfa, retinoic acid, and cisplatin in advanced squamous cell skin cancer. *J Clin Oncol.* 2002;20:364–370.

120. Martinez JC, Otley CC, Okuno SH, et al. Chemotherapy in the management of advanced cutaneous squamous cell carcinoma in organ transplant recipients: theoretical and practical considerations. *Dermatol Surg.* 2004;30:679–686.

121. Cartei G, Cartei F, Interlandi G, et al. Oral 5-fluorouracil in squamous cell carcinoma of the skin in the aged. *Am J Clin Oncol.* 2000;23(2):181–184.

122. Wollina U, Hansel G, Koch A, et al. Oral capecitabine plus subcutaneous interferon alpha in advanced squamous cell carcinoma of the skin. *J Cancer Res Clin Oncol.* 2005;131:300–304.

123. Morse LG, Kendrick C, Hooper D, et al. Treatment of squamous cell carcinoma with intralesional 5-fluorouracil. *Dermatol Surg.* 2003;29:1150–1153.

124. Goette DK. Topical chemotherapy with 5-fluorouracil. *J Am Acad Dermatol.* 1981;4:633–649.

125. Kraus S, Miller BH, Swinehart JM, et al. Intratumoral chemotherapy with fluorouracil/epinephrine injectable gel: a nonsurgical treatment of cutaneous squamous cell carcinoma. *J Am Acad Dermatol.* 1998;38:438–442.

126. Stockfleth E, Meyer T, Benninghoff B, et al. Successful treatment of actinic keratosis with imiquimod cream 5%: a report of six cases. *Br J Dermatol.* 2001;144:1050–1053.

127. Mackenkie-Wood A, Kossard S, deLauney J, et al. Imiquimod 5% cream in the treatment of Bowen's disease. *J Am Acad Dermatol.* 2001;44:462–470.

128. Hengge UR, Schaller J. Successful treatment of invasive squamous cell carcinoma using topical imiquimod. *Arch Dermatol.* 2004;140:404–406.

129. Oster-Schmidt C. Two cases of squamous cell carcinoma treated with topical imiquimod 5%. *J Eur Acad Dermatol Venereol.* 2004;18:93–95.

130. Eng TY, Boersma MGK, Fuller CD, et al. Treatment of Merkel cell carcinoma. *Am J Clin Oncol.* 2004;27(5):510–515.

131. Feun LG, Savaraj N, Legha SS, et al. Chemotherapy for metastatic Merkel cell carcinoma: review of the M.D. Anderson Hospital's experience. *Cancer.* 1988;62(4):683–685.

132. Pectasides D, Moutzourides G, Dimitriadis M, et al. Chemotherapy for Merkel cell carcinoma with carboplatin and etoposide. *Am J Clin Oncol.* 1995; 18(5):418–420.

133. Voog E, Biron P, Martin JP, et al. Chemotherapy for patients with local advanced or metastatic Merkel cell carcinoma. *Cancer.* 1999;85:2589–2595.

134. Tai PTH, Yu E, Winquist E, et al. Chemotherapy in neuroendocrine/ Merkel cell cacinoma of the skin: case series and review of 204 cases. *J Clin Oncol.* 2000;18(12):2493–2499.

135. Veness MJ. Merkel cell carcinoma: improved outcome with the addition of adjuvant therapy. *J Clin Oncol.* 2005;23 (28):7235–7236.

136. Fenig E, Brenner B, Katz A, et al. The role of radiation therapy and chemotherapy in the treatment of Merkel cell carcinoma. *Cancer.* 1997;80:881–885.

137. King MM, Osswald MB. Adjuvant chemotherapy for Merkel cell carcinoma. *Am J Clin Oncol.* 2005;28(6): 634.

138. Poulsen M, Rischin D, Walpole E, et al. High-risk Merkel cell carcinoma of the skin treated with synchronous carboplatin/etoposide and radiation: a Trans-Tasman Radiology Oncology Group Study—TROG 96:07. *J Clin Oncol.* 2003;21(23):4371–4376.

139. Kim YH, Martinez G, Varghese A, et al. Topical nitrogen mustard in the management of mycosis fungoides: update

140. of the Stanford experience. *Arch Dermatol.* 2003;139:165.

Zackheim H, Epstein E, Crain W. Topical carmustine (BCNU) for cutaneous T cell lymphoma: a 15-year experience in 143 patients. *J Am Acad Dermatol.* 1990;22:802–810.

141. Kuzel T, Roenigk HJ, Samuelson E, et al. Effectiveness of interferon alfa-2a combined with phototherapy for mycosis fungoides and the Sezary syndrome. *J Clin Oncol.* 1995;13:257.

142. Chiarion-Sileni V, Bononi A, Fornasa CV, et al. Phase II trial of interferon-alpha-2a plus psolaren with ultraviolet light A in patients with cutaneous T-cell lymphoma. *Cancer.* 2002;95:569.

143. Duvic M, Lemak N, Redman J, et al. Combined modality therapy for cutaneous T-cell lymphoma. *J Am Acad Dermatol.* 1996;34:1022.

144. Duvic M, Martin AG, Kim Y, et al. Phase 2 and 3 clinical trial of oral bexarotene (Targretin capsules) for the treatment of refractory or persistent early-stage cutaneous T-cell lymphoma. *Arch Dermatol.* 2001;137:581.

145. Heald P, Mehlmauer M, Martin AG, et al. Topical bexarotene therapy for patients with refractory or persistent early-stage cutaneous T-cell lymphoma: results of the phase III clinical trial. *J Am Acad Dermatol.* 2003;49:801.

146. Duvic M, Apisarnthanarax N, Cohen DS, et al. Analysis of long-term outcomes of combined modality therapy for cutaneous T-cell lymphoma. *J Am Acad Dermatol.* 2003;49:35.

147. Herrmann J, Roenigk HJ, Hurria A, et al. Treatment of mycosis fungoides with photochemotherapy (PUVA): long-term follow-up. *J Am Acad Dermatol.* 1995; 33:234.

148. Gottlieb S, Wolfe J, Fox F, et al. Treatment of cutaneous T-cell lymphoma with extracorporeal photopheresis monotherapy and in combination with recombinant interferon alfa: a 10-year experience at a single institution. *J Am Acad Dermatol.* 1996;35:946.

149. Edelson R, Berger C, Gasparro F, et al. Treatment of cutaneous T-cell lymphoma by extracorporeal photochemotherapy. *N Engl J Med.* 1987;316:297.

150. Duvic M, Hymes K, Heald P, et al. Bexarotene is effective and safe for treatment of refractory advanced-stage cutaneous T-cell lymphoma: multinational phase II–III trial results. *J Clin Oncol.* 2001;19:2456.

151. Bunn PJ, Hoffman S, Norris D, et al. Systemic therapy of cutaneous T-cell lymphoma: mycosis fungoides and the Sezary syndrome. *Ann Intern Med.* 1994; 121:592.

152. Rosen S, Foss F. Chemotherapy for mycosis fungoides and the Sezary syndrome. *Hematol Oncol Clin North Am.* 1995; 9:1109.

153. Case DJ. Combination chemotherapy for mycosis fungoides with cyclophosphamide, vincristine, methotrexate, and prednisone. *Am J Clin Oncol.* 1984; 7:453.

154. Von Hoff D, Dahlberg S, Hartstock R, et al. Activity of fludarabine monophosphate in patients with advanced mycosis fungoides: a Southwest Oncology Group study. *J Natl Cancer Inst.* 1990;82:1353.

155. Tsimberidou AM, Giles F, Duvic M, et al. Phase II study of pentostatin in advanced T-cell lymphoid malignancies: update of an M.D. Anderson Cancer Center series. *Cancer.* 2004;100:342.

156. Zinzani PL, Baliva G, Magagnoli M, et al. Gemcitabine treatment in pretreated cutaneous T-cell lymphoma: experience in 44 patients. *J Clin Oncol.* 2000;18:2603.

157. Marchi E, Alinari L, Tani M, et al. Gemcitabine as frontline treatment for cutaneous T-cell lymphoma: phase II study of 32 patients. *Cancer.* 2005;104: 2437.

158. Wollina U, Dummer R, Brockmeyer NH, et al. Multicenter study of pegylated liposomal doxorubicin in patients with cutaneous T-cell lymphoma. *Cancer.* 2003;98:993.

159. Lundin J, Hagberg H, Repp R, et al. Phase 2 study of alemtuzumab (anti-CD52 monoclonal antibody) in patients with advanced mycosis fungoides/Sezary syndrome. *Blood.* 2003;101:4267.

160. Olsen E, Duvic M, Frankel A, et al. Pivotal phase III trial of two dose levels of Denileukin Diftitox for the treatment of cutaneous T-cell lymphoma. *J Clin Oncol.* 2001;19:376.

161. Aboulafia DM. Regression of acquired immunodeficiency syndrome-related pulmonary Kaposi's sarcoma after highly active antiretroviral therapy. *Mayo Clin Proc.* 1998;73:439.

162. Gallafent JH, Buskin SE, De Turk PB, Aboulafia DM. Profile of patients with Kaposi's sarcoma in the era of highly active antiretroviral therapy. *J Clin Oncol.* 2005;23:1253.

163. Dezube BJ. Management of AIDS-related Kaposi's sarcoma: advances in target discovery and treatment. *Expert Rev Anticancer Ther.* 2002;2:193.

164. Walmsley S, Northfelt DW, Melosky B, et al. Treatment of AIDS-related cutaneous Kaposi's sarcoma with topical alitretinoin (9-*cis*-retinoic acid) gel. Panretin Gel North American Study Group. *J Acquir Immune Defic Syndr.* 1999;22:235.

165. Shepherd FA, Beaulieu R, Gelmon K, et al. Prospective randomized trial of two dose levels of interferon alfa with zidovudine for the treatment of Kaposi's sarcoma associated with human immunodeficiency virus infection: a Canadian HIV Clinical Trials Network study. *J Clin Oncol.* 1998; 16:1736.

166. Epstein JB. Treatment of oral Kaposi sarcoma with intralesional vinblastine. *Cancer.* 1993;71:1722.

167. McCormick SU. Intralesional vinblastine injections for the treatment of oral Kaposi's sarcoma: report of 10 patients with 2 year follow-up. *J Oral Maxillofac Surg.* 1996;54:583.

168. Lee FC, Mitsuyasu RT. Chemotherapy of AIDS-related KS. *Hematol Oncol Clin North Am.* 1996;10:1051.

169. Northfelt DW, Dezube BJ, Thommes JA, et al. Pegylated-liposomal doxorubicin versus doxorubicin, bleomycin, and vincristine in the treatment of AIDS-related Kaposi's sarcoma: results of a randomized phase III clinical trial. *J Clin Oncol.* 1998;16:2445.

170. Stewart S, Jablonowski H, Goebel FD, et al. Randomized comparative trial of

pegylated liposomal doxorubicin versus bleomycin and vincristine in the treatment of AIDS-related KS. International Pegylated Liposomal Doxorubicin Study Group. *J Clin Oncol.* 1998;16:683.

171. Gill PS, Tulpule A, Espina BM, et al. Paclitaxel is safe and effective in the treatment of advanced AIDS-related Kaposi's sarcoma. *J Clin Oncol.* 1999;17:1876.

172. Tulpule A, Groopman J, Saville MW, et al. Multicenter trial of low-dose paclitaxel in patients with advanced AIDS-related Kaposi sarcoma. *Cancer.* 2002;95:147.

173. Nasti G, Errants D, Talamini R, et al. Vinorelbine is an effective and safe drug for AIDS-related Kaposi's sarcoma: results of a phase II study. *J Clin Oncol.* 2000;18:1550.

174. Sprinz E, Caldas AP, Mans DR, et al. Fractionated doses of oral etoposide in the treatment of patients with aids-related kaposi sarcoma: a clinical and pharmacologic study to improve therapeutic index. *Am J Clin Oncol.* 2001;24:177.

175. Little RF, Wyvill KM, Pluda JM, et al. Activity of thalidomide in AIDS-related Kaposi's sarcoma. *J Clin Oncol.* 2000;18:2593.

176. Koon HB, Bubley GJ, Pantanowitz L, et al. Imatinib-induced regression of AIDS-related Kaposi's sarcoma. *J Clin Oncol.* 2005;23:982.

CHAPTER 52

Skin Cancer Vaccines

Jean-Claude Bystryn, M.D.

BOX 52-1 Overview

- Current systemic treatment for melanoma is of limited effectiveness, and associated with side effects that can be serious.
- Vaccines are attractive as they are effective in animals and have little toxicity.
- For vaccine to work, they must contain relevant antigens that can stimulate tumor protective immune responses. Some of these antigens must be present for on the tumor to be treated.
- As the relevant antigens are currently not known, the best way to include them in a vaccine is to prepare vaccines that contain a very broad spectrum of tumor antigens.
- Another critical component of all vaccines is the adjuvant that can enhance vaccine-induced immune responses.
- Current melanoma vaccines are safe and some can induce antimelanoma antibody and/or cellular immune responses.
- The clinical effectiveness of melanoma vaccines remains to be established in large-scale phase III trials.

INTRODUCTION

Vaccine administration is a very selective approach to treat cancer. They are intended to stimulate the body's own immune system to attack and destroy cancer cells. They are unique in their potential ability to destroy specifically the cancer cells without damaging the normal tissue; a property that has the potential to lead to a treatment that is more effective and safer than current therapies.

Vaccines are currently being studied to treat a broad range of cancers, including those that are most common in humans such as cancer of the lung, breast, colon, and prostate. However, the longest and still the greatest effort has focused on developing vaccines for melanoma, because of a suspicion that the progression of melanoma is particularly susceptible to being influenced by immune factors. This is based on several clinical observations that have been known for a long time and that are thought to reflect the existence of antimelanoma or antipigment cell immune responses. These include the rare but dramatic spontaneous remission of advanced melanoma, the common occurrence of partial regression in primary melanoma evidenced by the presence of depigmentation within the tumor, and the ability of the immune system to destroy pigmented cells selectively as evidenced clinically by vitiligo.

There is little effort at present to develop vaccines for other cancers of the skin—such as basal cell carcinoma, squamous cell carcinoma, or cutaneous T cell lymphoma. There are excellent ways of treating the first two cancers so that there is little pressure to develop alternate treatments, and cutaneous T cell lymphoma is uncommon. However, the principles underlying the use of vaccines to treat cancer are universal, so that there is no reason why vaccines against these other types of skin cancers should not be developed at some time in the future. This is particularly true for basal cell carcinoma, which is by far the most common cancer of humans. As vaccines have the potential to prevent cancer, a preventive vaccine for basal cell carcinoma would be very desirable.

This article reviews the rationale behind believing melanoma vaccines can be effective, the factors related to vaccine efficacy, the advantages/disadvantages of the various strategies used to construct melanoma vaccines, and finally summarizes the results of recent clinical trials.

THE NEED FOR ALTERNATE TREATMENTS FOR MELANOMA

BOX 52-2 Summary

- The most effective treatment for melanoma is early surgical excision of the tumor before it metastasizes.
- The only FDA-approved adjuvant treatment for resected melanoma at high risk of recurrence, interferon alfa-2b, has limited effectiveness, and is associated with frequent side effects,
- No treatment has been shown to prolong survival in stage IV melanoma,

There is no satisfactory treatment of melanoma, once it has spread beyond its original site. Localized melanoma can be effectively treated if detected early and removed surgically. When detected while still confined to the epidermis, the most superficial layer of the skin, melanoma is completely curable. Once melanoma has penetrated through the epidermis into the deeper layers of the skin, mortality increases dramatically.

Mortality is directly related to how deep the melanoma has penetrated into the skin and whether or not it has spread to other locations.[1] Approximately 50% of patients whose tumor has penetrated 4 mm or more into the skin will die of their disease within 5 years. Once the tumor has spread to other organ systems, fewer than 10% will live for 5 years.[1]

The standard treatment for melanoma is surgical removal of the primary tumor and of metastasis to other sites, if accessible.[2] Based on the level of invasion of the cancer, it is possible to predict fairly accurately the chances of recurrence.[1] Once melanoma does recur, mortality increases further. Treatment options for such patients are limited.

The only FDA approved treatment for resected melanoma at high risk of recurrence (stage IIb–III disease) is interferon alfa-2b, and for advanced disease (stage IV) are interleukin-2 (IL-2) and DTIC. The effectiveness of interferon is controversial. Some studies in the United States report that it delays tumor recurrence and possibly prolongs overall survival.[3] Other studies have not been able to confirm this observation.[4] Whatever its effectiveness, interferon has numerous side effects, causing major toxicity in almost three-quarters of the patients. As such, acceptance of this treatment by physicians and patients is limited. Once melanoma has spread to involve other organs, chemotherapeutic agents such as DTIC, immunomodulatory drugs such as IL-2, radiation and surgery may be used alone or in combination.[2] These can induce temporary remissions, but no treatment prolongs survival once melanoma has become widely metastatic. IL-2 has limited effectiveness and the high doses required are associated with severe side effects that often require management in intensive care units.

Thus, there is a need for an effective treatment for melanoma, particularly for the largest group at risk, which is made of patients with resected disease at high risk of recurrence. Experimental therapy with vaccines is increasingly used in such patients.

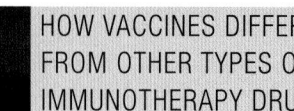

HOW VACCINES DIFFER FROM OTHER TYPES OF IMMUNOTHERAPY DRUGS

BOX 52-3   Summary

- Vaccines are the only form of immunotherapy that are both active (they induce the patient's own immune system to react more vigorously against the cancer) and specific (the immune responses are directed specifically against antigens present in the vaccine).

Vaccines are one of a large class of immunotherapeutic agents used to treat cancer. Immunotherapeutic agents are all intended to stimulate a patient's immune system to react more vigorously against cancer. They are usually classified into four categories based on their mechanism of action—whether they enhance immune responses specifically or nonspecifically and whether they do so actively or passively. Specificity means that the agent stimulates immune responses directed only against a selected set of antigens, such as tumor antigens; whereas nonspecificity means that immune responses are enhanced in general against all antigens. It is believed that specificity increases in immunity will be more potent and safer than nonspecific enhancement. Active means that the patient's own immune system is stimulated to produce antitumor antibodies, immune cells, or other desirable immune agents; whereas in passive immunity these agents (monoclonal antibodies, T cells, NK cells, dendritic cells, cytokines, etc.) are administered to the patient. A critical difference is that active immunotherapy can be very long lasting, whereas the effects of passive immunotherapy last only days to weeks. Vaccines are a specific and active form of immunotherapy.

In practice, immunotherapeutic agents may be combined that work by different mechanisms. This is particularly true of tumor vaccines, which are typically composed of two different classes of immunotherapeutic agents—tumor antigens that actively and specifically induce antitumor immune response and an adjuvant that nonspecifically enhances these responses. The adjuvant is usually admixed with the vaccine. In some cases, a single immunotherapeutic agent can operate by two different mechanisms. An example can be some genetically engineered tumor cell vaccines, which express tumor antigens that specifically stimulate antitumor immune responses and also secrete cytokines or other molecules that nonspecially enhance these responses. Another example is of monoclonal antibodies that are typically classified as passive immunotherapeutics. However, they can also take part in active immunotherapy when antiidiotype monoclonal antibodies are used as tumor vaccines.

RATIONALE FOR MELANOMA VACCINES

BOX 52-4   Summary

- Vaccines can stimulate antibody and cellular immune responses against melanoma in humans.
- Vaccine-induced immune responses can markedly increase resistance to melanoma in animals.
- It is hoped that they can do the same in humans.

Melanoma vaccines are intended to stimulate the immune system to react more strongly against a patient's own melanoma cells, thereby destroying the tumor or slowing its progression. There are multiple reasons for believing vaccines may be able to do this—two are particularly compelling:

One, is that there are defense mechanisms in humans that can selectively kill melanoma cells. This is evidenced by the presence of tumor regression in 15 to 20% of primary melanomas,[5] and by the rare but dramatic, spontaneous, and complete regression of advanced melanoma in some patients. These defense mechanisms appear to be mediated by antitumor immune responses because of the selectivity with which they act—they destroy malignant melanocytes within primary melanomas (evidenced by areas of depigmentation within the tumor) without harming adjacent normal melanocytes (evidenced by the skin surrounding the melanoma remaining fully pigmented).

The other is that vaccines greatly increase resistance to melanoma in animals. This is demonstrated by their ability to prevent the growth of melanoma in mice given an otherwise lethal dose of this cancer.[6,7] The protection is mediated by antitumor immune responses because of the selectivity of the protection which is induced. The mice are protected against melanoma but not against other tumors. The hope is that the same can be achieved in humans.

In addition, it is now amply documented (1) that melanoma cells express a variety of antigens that are poorly expressed or not expressed at all in normal adult cells, (2) that some of these antigens can stimulate antibody and/or cellular immune responses that can attack and destroy melanoma cells in vitro, and (3) that there are correlations between the presence of these antimelanoma immune responses and improved clinical outcome. Thus, the machinery necessary for vaccines to be effective against melanoma in humans exists, and activation of this machinery appears to improve the prognosis of melanoma.

WHAT IS REQUIRED FOR A MELANOMA VACCINE TO BE EFFECTIVE

BOX 52-5   Summary

- The vaccine must contain antigens that can stimulate tumor protective immune responses in humans.
- Some of these antigens must be present on the patient's own tumor.
- The vaccine should be safe and easy to use.

To stimulate immune responses that can kill cancer cells, vaccines must satisfy two fundamental requirements: (1) They must contain antigens that can stimulate clinically effective antitumor immune responses that can kill tumor cells *in vivo*, and (2) some of these antigens must be present on a patient's own tumor cells.

There are major problems satisfying each of these requirements. First, the actual melanoma antigens that can stimulate clinically effective antimelanoma immune responses in humans are not known. Numerous melanoma-associated antigens have been identified, such as MAGE-1, MAGE-3, Melan A/MART-1, NY-ESO-1, gp100, tyrosinase, TRP-2, etc. and these are currently used to make vaccines. However, these are used because they are available. Whether any of these is a "relevant" antigen that can trigger tumor protective immune responses is not known. Identifying which individual melanoma antigens are clinically effective and should be used to construct defined vaccines, is a major task. It requires the completion of a successful phase III trial of each candidate antigen.

A second problem is the variation or heterogeneity in the expression of melanoma antigens in different melanomas. Melanomas in different persons express different patterns of melanoma antigens. It is for this reason that some vaccines are made from the patient's own tumor cells, i.e. "autologous vaccines", as it is hoped that antigens present in such vaccines will more closely match those present in the patient's remaining tumor. However, this does not resolve the problem, as different melanoma nodules in the same individual and even different melanoma cells in the same tumor nodule express different pattern of tumor antigens. Furthermore, the antigens expressed by any particular tumor can change during its progression or as a response to therapy. Tumor cells can lose antigens against which they have been immunized. This is believed to be one the mechanism by which tumors can escape from immunotherapy. Lastly, the actual antigens expressed by an individual patient's tumor(s) are usually unknown at the time of treatment. While resected melanoma tissue can be analyzed for the antigens it expresses, the tumors that need treatment are those that remain within the patient. Because of antigenic heterogeneity, it is not possible to know their antigenic phenotype with certainty. Thus, it is not known whether the immune responses triggered by any single melanoma antigen in a vaccine will be able to attack the tumor to be treated.

A third problem is that there is also considerable variation in the ability of different patients to be immunized to any given antigen. One reason is that the cellular immune responses, which are believed to be a major mediator of tumor protective immunity, are HLA restricted. This means that an antigen can only induce these responses if the patient expresses an HLA molecule that can bind or capture that particular tumor antigen. Unfortunately, there are a large number of different HLA molecules and their expression is highly variable among individuals. Even the most common HLA (HLA-A2) is expressed by fewer than 50% of Caucasians. This highly restricts the proportion of melanoma patients that can respond to vaccines prepared from a single peptide. Another reason is that there is also HLA-independent heterogeneity in the ability of different patients to develop immune responses to the same antigen. Patients with the same HLA phenotype who are immunized to the same tumor antigen may or may not develop an immune response to that antigen.[8] This heterogeneity further decreases the number of patients that can successfully develop an immune response to a given antigen. As a result of antigenic heterogeneity among melanomas and of HLA-dependent and HLA-independent heterogeneity in the ability of antigens to stimulate immune responses, the proportion of melanoma patients that can actually benefit from a vaccine constructed from a single peptide is no greater than 40%, and probably much lower.

Thus, it is uncertain at present which melanoma antigen(s) should be used to prepare a vaccine, whether any of these will be present on the actual tumor to be treated, and whether that antigen will be able to induce an immune response in the individual patient to be treated.

One way to circumvent these problems is to create "polyvalent" vaccines that contain a broad variety of melanoma antigens.[9] The rationale is self-evident. The greater the number of antigens in a vaccine, the greater the chances (1) that it will contain the "relevant" antigen(s) that can stimulate clinically effective antitumor immune responses, (2) that some of these antigens will be present on the tumor to be treated, and (3) that some of these antigens will be able to trigger an immune response in that patient. Furthermore, the greater the number of targets (antigens) on the tumor cells against which immune responses are raised, the greater the chances of the tumor cells being killed. For these reasons, there is now a major shift in the strategies used to construct cancer vaccines away from the ones based on the use of a single or limited number of defined antigens to ones that ensure the presence of a very wide spectrum of antigens associated with melanoma.

THE NEED FOR ADJUVANTS TO ENHANCE THE EFFECTIVENESS OF VACCINES

BOX 52-6 Summary

- Most tumor antigens are poor immunogens—the immune responses they induce are weak.
- A critical component of all cancer vaccines are adjuvants that can enhance the frequency magnitude, and duration of the immune response induced by the vaccine.

All cancer vaccines consist of two components: (1) Tumor antigen(s), whose purpose it is to stimulate immune responses against the cancer, as described above, and (2) an adjuvant, whose purpose it is to increase the frequency strength and duration of these responses. Adjuvants are necessary, as the immune responses induced by tumor antigens alone are weak and are often short lived.

A large number of different adjuvants is available or under investigation. These range from modifications of the physical or biochemical properties of the antigens to various oily emulsions such as QS-21 or Montanide, to agents that contain various bacterial products such as BCG or Detox, to slow release vehicles such as alum or liposomes; immunomodulators such as IL-2, IL-12, GM-CSF, or CpG, and co-stimulatory molecules. Other approaches include coupling the antigen to strongly immunogenic molecules such as KLH, expressing the antigen on viral particles such as vaccinia, or on inert beads or other particles such as ISCOMS. Two recent approaches that are the focus of particular attention are: (1) using antigen-presenting cells, such as dendritic cells, to present vaccine antigens. This turns out to be one of the most powerful ways to boost cellular immune responses. The downside of this approach is that it requires that a custom vaccine be made for each patient, which makes it difficult to apply in practice, and (2) using monoclonal antibodies such as anti-CTLA-4 that target receptors on immune cells that downregulate immune responses. By inactivating these "brakes" on immune responses, it is hoped that antitumor immune responses induced by vaccines will be greater and last longer. One observation that indicates that this approach can be effective is that it is associated with an unusually high incidence of autoimmune reactions.

The ideal adjuvant should be potent, safe, and easy to use. Unfortunately, those in current use fail to satisfy all of these requirements. Alum for example is very safe, but is a weak adjuvant. Freund's adjuvant is one of the most powerful adjuvant known, but cannot be used in humans because of its toxicity. Dendritic cells are potent adjuvants, but are difficult to use. They must be obtained from the patient to be treated; sent to, processed, and loaded with vaccine antigen(s) in a specialized laboratory; and then re-infused back into the patient. This requires the preparation of a custom vaccine for each patient, an approach that is difficult to commercialize. A full discussion of the many agents available as adjuvants and their relative advantages and disadvantages is beyond the scope of this chapter.

However, as a consequence of the large number of options available to prepare melanoma antigens for use in vaccines and the equally wide choices of adjuvants, far more combinations of the two can be created as vaccines that can be evaluated *in vivo* in humans.

STRATEGIES USED TO CONSTRUCT MELANOMA VACCINES—THEIR RELATIVE ADVANTAGES AND DISADVANTAGES

BOX 52-7 Summary

- Three basic strategies are used to prepare the antigens used to construct cancer vaccines. Each has advantages and disadvantages. In all cases, the vaccines are combined with an adjuvant.
  - *Whole tumor cells, their extract, or DNA:* This assures the greatest spectrum of tumor antigens in the vaccine, but the bulk of material in the vaccine is irrelevant and may be detrimental.
  - *Purified peptides or antigens:* This is scientifically very elegant. However, the antigens that should be used—those that can stimulate protective immunity—are not known.
  - *Partially purified antigen mixtures:* These are prepared to maximize the spectrum of tumor antigens while minimizing the content of unrelated material.

Multiple strategies are used to prepare melanoma vaccines that address the requirements listed above. None satisfies all requirements. To simplify comparisons of the different approaches, it is useful to classify them into one of three categories that differ in the purity and number of tumor antigen(s) used to prepare the vaccine. These are: (1) nonpurified or cellular vaccines which contain the broadest spectrum of antigens, (2) partially purified vaccines which contain a broad but more limited spectrum of antigens, and (3) defined antigen vaccines that contain a single or few antigens. By far the largest effort has gone into developing vaccines constructed from defined antigens.

This classification is useful as each of these categories has certain common advantages and disadvantages, as illustrated in Table 52-1 and discussed in greater detail in Ref. [9]. This makes it

Table 52-1
Relative Merits of Different Cancer Vaccine Design Strategies

VACCINE ATTRIBUTE	NONPURIFIED CELLULAR	SEMIPURE	DEFINED ANTIGENS
EFFECTIVENESS			
• Presence of relevant antigens	+++	++	+
• Presence of multiple antigens	+++	++	+
• Immunogenic potency of antigens	+++	++	+
PREPARATION			
• Purity	+	++	+ to +++
• Reproducible Manufacture	+	++	+++
• Quality control	+	++	+++
SAFETY	+	++	+++

easier to compare the relative advantages and disadvantages of various vaccines. There is no ideal way to make a cancer vaccine.

All vaccines consist of two basic components—tumor antigen(s) and an adjuvant. The classification used here applies to the antigen component of the vaccine. Within each category, a variety of adjuvants can be used in conjunction with the antigen(s). Alternate classification schemes for cancer vaccines are sometimes based on the adjuvant used to prepare the vaccine.

The essential difference between these different vaccine design strategies is in the number, purity, and concentration of tumor antigens in the vaccine. Nonpurified or cellular vaccines contain multiple tumor antigens and thus are more likely to contain relevant antigens, but these antigens account for only a very small fraction of the material in the vaccine. Conversely, vaccines prepared from defined antigens contain only a single or few antigens, but these are present at high concentrations, particularly if the antigen(s) is purified. However, it is uncertain whether the selected antigen(s) is a relevant one, or whether immune responses directed against a single antigen will be sufficiently potent to result in effective tumor kill. Partially purified vaccines strike a middle course between these two polar approaches.

Nonpurified or Cellular Vaccines

The traditional method to construct cancer vaccines is from whole tumor cells or nonpurified extracts of these cells. The cancer cells can be pooled from different donors to increase the number of tumor antigens in the vaccine. The vaccine can be prepared from a patient's own tumor cells (autologous vaccines) or from another patient's cells (allogeneic vac-

cines). Autologous vaccines are claimed to provide a better fit between the tumor antigens in the vaccine and those in the patient's own tumor, although this is uncertain as there is heterogeneity in antigen expression between different metastasis in the same person. Autologous vaccines are difficult to commercialize, as a custom vaccine must be prepared for each patient. In addition, the patient's own tumor cells must be available to prepare the vaccine so that only patients with more advanced disease can be treated. Cellular vaccines are most often prepared from allogeneic cells, as these can be maintained in cell banks, which permit the reproducible preparation of a generic vaccine that can be used in all patients. The spectrum of tumor antigens in vaccines prepared from allogeneic cells is usually increased by preparing the vaccine from multiple melanoma cell lines.

Multiple nonpurified/cellular vaccines are being tested in clinical trials. The ones in the most advanced trials include CancerVax, a polyvalent vaccine prepared from several lines of intact, irradiated, allogeneic melanoma cells combined with BCG as an adjuvant; Melacine which is a mechanical lysate of two allogeneic melanoma cell lines admixed with Detox as an adjuvant; and M-Vax which consists of autologous melanoma cells to which has been conjugated DNP, a potent hapten which acts as an adjuvant. Intact tumor cells can be genetically engineered to express certain cytokines such as IL-2 or other molecules or antigens that can increase their ability to stimulate immune responses. An alternate approach to deliver a broad range of nonpurified antigens as vaccine is to use the DNA derived from the cancer cells.

The major advantage of nonpurified vaccines is that they contain a wide variety of tumor antigens. Thus, they are more likely to contain the as yet unidentified antigen(s) which are essential for vaccine activity, and obviate the need to identify and purify each such individual antigens. As the vaccines contain a broad range of tumor antigens, particularly if prepared from a pool of melanoma cells, they have an increased chance of containing the relevant antigens expressed by the individual tumor to be treated. For the same reason, such vaccines are more likely to contain antigens that are recognized in the context of the patient's HLA phenotype. Vaccines prepared from whole tumor cells may be inherently more immunogenic, as antigens tend to lose potency when they are purified. Lastly, the multiple antigens in nonpurified vaccines have the potential to stimulate antitumor immune responses to multiple targets on tumor cells, which is more likely to result in cell kill and clinical effectiveness.

The major drawback to this approach is that the active antigens in the vaccine are present in low concentrations and constitute only a very small fraction of the material in the vaccine. The presence of large quantities of irrelevant material increases the technical difficulty of producing a reproducible vaccine. In addition, the unnecessary cellular material may potentially decrease vaccine effectiveness due to the presence of suppressive factors or by inducing immune responses to irrelevant antigens that can competitively inhibit the desired antitumor immune responses. It may also potentially increase toxicity.

Vaccines Prepared From Defined or Purified Antigens

It is scientifically more elegant to construct the vaccine from a single or limited number of defined antigen(s). It is the approach that by far is currently used most frequently to prepare cancer vaccines. Defined vaccines became feasible as a result of the identification and purification of melanoma-associated antigens that are recognized by antibodies or T cells. Purified melanoma antigens that are used to construct such vaccines include gangliosides such as GM-2 and proteins (or peptides derived from them) such as MAGE-1, MAGE-3, Melan A/Mart-1, tyrosinase, gp100 or NY-ESO-1 which are recognized by CD8+ T or CD4+ T cells. Alternatively, DNA coding for the antigen of interest is used as the vaccine, to cause the patient's own cells to make that antigen. The use of anti-idiotype monoclonal antibodies is an alternate approach to

stimulate responses to defined tumor antigens.[10]

The major advantage of this approach is its scientific elegance. Furthermore, if purified, defined antigen vaccines are more easily characterized and prepared in a reproducible manner and the concentration of the antigen(s) in the vaccine can be very high. From a research perspective, the immune responses that they induce can be measured more easily. The major problem with that approach is that the melanoma antigen(s) that are actually able to stimulate clinically beneficial tumor protective immune responses are still not known. These vaccines are made from antigens it is hoped will work, not ones known to be effective. There are several other basic problems with this approach. Many of the antigens used are peptides, which are HLA restricted. That, together with the variable expression of the peptide on different melanomas means that such vaccines cannot be used in the majority of patients with melanoma. It is also unclear whether immune responses induced to a single antigen or peptide will be sufficiently potent to result in effective tumor cell kill in humans. More recently, attempts have been made to minimize these problems by preparing vaccines from a cocktail of several pure peptides. However, the number of antigens in such vaccines is still far less than the number in non purified or partially purified vaccines. Furthermore, because of intellectual property right issues, the number of antigens that can be collected to include in the vaccine is strictly limited.

Vaccines Prepared From Partially Purified Antigens

The third strategy attempts to balance the advantages and disadvantages of the two prior approaches. It does so by preparing vaccines from tumor cell extracts that are enriched in the cellular elements most likely to contain tumor antigens relevant for vaccine therapy and depleted of material likely to be irrelevant.

The advantage of partially purified melanoma vaccines is that they retain the most critical element required for vaccine effectiveness, i.e., a large number of antigens, while being much purer than vaccines prepared from whole cells or their extracts. This reviewer believes such vaccines may be more effective and safer than cellular vaccines because they may contain relevant antigens in higher concentrations while containing less irrelevant cellular material that may be toxic or immunosuppressive.

Examples of this approach include a polyvalent, shed antigen, vaccine prepared from cell-surface antigens released or shed into culture medium by melanoma cells.[11] This approach exploits a natural phenomenon, that the material on the external surface of tumor cells is rapidly shed into the medium used to grow the cells. Shed antigens are partially purified, as they are separated from the bulk of other cellular material which is in the cytoplasm and nucleus of the cells and is released much more slowly. Shed antigens are also more likely to be biologically relevant as they are expressed on the external surface of tumor cells where they can be seen and attacked by vaccine-induced antibodies or T cells. To increase the number of melanoma antigens in the vaccine, the cell lines used for vaccine production are selected based on each expressing different and complimentary pattern of cell-surface melanoma-associated antigens. A shed antigen vaccine prepared in this manner contains multiple melanoma antigens, including MAGE-1, MAGE-3, MelanA/Mart-1, tyrosinase, gp100, S100, TRP-1, NY-ESO-1, and numerous immunogenic antigens ranging in MW from 30 to 150 kDa that are expressed by melanoma *in vivo*.

Another partially purified melanoma vaccine is prepared from heat shock proteins. These are molecules that transport antigens and other molecules within cells. In animals, heat shock proteins derived from cancer cells can induce strong tumor protective immunity. The vaccine is made from heat shock proteins extracted from the patient's own tumor cells, so that a custom vaccine needs to be prepared for each individual patient. Unfortunately, this vaccine failed a recent large-scale phase III trial.

RESULTS OF CLINICAL TRIALS WITH MELANOMA VACCINES

BOX 52-8 Summary

- Vaccines appear to be safe to use.
- Some vaccines can induce antibody and/or cellular immune responses in patients.
- No vaccine has yet been proven effective in a large-scale phase III trial.

Three criteria are used to evaluate the clinical activity of tumor vaccines—safety, immunological activity, and clinical effectiveness.

Melanoma vaccines have proven very safe to use. There has been little toxicity in the several thousand patients treated to date. The toxicity that has occurred is usually due to the adjuvant rather than to the vaccine. Vaccines are clearly less toxic than the current FDA approved therapy for melanoma at high risk of recurrence, interferon alfa-2b, which causes major toxicity in over two-thirds of patients.[3] Thus, vaccines provide a quality of life improvement over alternate therapies.

Melanoma vaccines can be immunogenic in humans and increase antibody and/or cellular immune responses against melanoma.[12–20] The type of immune response induced, and the frequency and magnitude of the increase, is dependent on the nature of the vaccine and the adjuvant with which it is combined. In general, it is difficult to demonstrate antibody responses to peptide-based vaccines; ganglioside vaccines stimulate antibody but not cellular responses, while cellular and protein-based vaccines can stimulate both type of responses. Potent adjuvants such as dendritic cells or IL-2 liposomes can markedly increase the frequency with which the same vaccine stimulates antibody and/or cellular responses and the magnitude of these responses.

The clinical effectiveness of the current generation of melanoma vaccines is disappointing. Most that have been evaluated in large-scale phase III trials have failed to demonstrate an improvement in clinical outcome. These include the following:

1. Canvaxin, a vaccine made from three lines of irradiated whole allogeneic melanoma cells admixed with BCG as the adjuvant.[21] This vaccine failed to improve survival in two large scale phase III trials, one in resected stage IV melanoma the other in the adjuvant setting.

2. A vaccine made from heat shock protein extracted from the patient's own melanoma cells.

3. A vaccine made from a purified ganglioside admixed with QS 21 as the adjuvant.[22]

4. Two trials in which the vaccine consisted of viral oncolysates of melanoma cells.[23,24]

The results of most other trials of melanoma vaccines are difficult to evaluate because they are phase I and II studies that involve small number of patients and/or lack appropriate controls.

In addition, the majority of melanoma vaccines currently in clinical trials are defined antigen vaccines prepared from a single or very limited number of tumor antigens, and such vaccines are unlikely to be effective. In a recent review of 73 cancer vaccine trials by Rosenberg et al, all but 5 were conducted with defined vaccines. While scientifically attractive, defined antigens vaccines have multiple limitations that were discussed previously. The most important are that the antigen selected to construct such vaccine may be not be one that can induce clinically effective tumor protective immunity, that the selected antigen may not be present on the tumor to be treated or is lost during tumor progression, and that immune response directed against a single target on tumor cells may not be potent enough to prevent the progression of tumors in humans. Thus, the disappointing results of many current cancer vaccine trials may simply reflect that an incorrect strategy was used to prepare the vaccines, not that vaccines do not work.

Further, what is probably an improper criteria is often used to evaluate clinical effectiveness, i.e., tumor regression rather than survival. Whether or not a vaccine is considered effective depends on the criteria used to measure effectiveness. For example, Rosenberg et al recently argued that cancer vaccines are not effective because most fail to induce tumor regression. Objective responses were induced by vaccines in only 2.6% of 440 patients with metastatic cancer treated by Rosenberg et al, most of whom had melanoma; and in only 3.8% of another 765 patients reported in 35 other trials. However, the gold standard to evaluate the effectiveness of any cancer treatment is survival, not tumor regression. Survival is the standard the FDA prefers for drug approval. Tumor regression is often a poor surrogate for survival, as evidenced by the failure of many agents that induce tumor regression in melanoma to improve overall survival.

Recurrence-free and overall survival are more appropriate end-points to measure the effectiveness of cancer vaccines. Vaccine-induced immune responses may not be potent enough to cause regression of established tumors, but nonetheless, may keep the tumors from progressing and killing patients. For example, vaccine-immunized animals can live for prolonged periods while bearing tumors of a size that would have rapidly and invariably kill nonimmunized animals.

Randomized trials of two vaccines in which survival was used to evaluate clinical effectiveness are promising. One is a double blind and placebo-controlled trial in patients with resected stage IIIb melanoma of a polyvalent, shed antigen, melanoma vaccine developed by Bystryn. This vaccine contains multiple melanoma antigens. There is a correlation between vaccine-induced antimelanoma antibody and CD8 responses and improved clinical outcome,[17,18] and vaccine-treatment is associated with clearance of melanoma cells and antigens from the circulation.[25] In the double-blind trial, the recurrence-free survival of the melanoma vaccine treated patients was over twice as long as that of placebo vaccine-treated patients and this difference was significant ($p = 0.03$) after Cox multivariate analysis.[11] These results must be interpreted cautiously as the trial was small ($n = 38$). The other is a randomized trial of Melacine conducted by SWOG. This is a vaccine prepared from the lysate of two melanoma cell lines adjuvanted with Detox, which was developed by Mitchell and commercialized by Corixa. There was no overall difference in recurrence-free survival between the vaccine-treated and the control group. However, recurrence-free survival was significantly prolonged in a subset of patients who had one of several HLA phenotypes.[26] This vaccine has been approved for sale in Canada, but the FDA has requested a confirmatory trial. The results of several other randomized trials have been disappointing.

THE FUTURE

Melanoma vaccines are now an accepted experimental treatment for patients who have been rendered clinically free of disease by surgical resection but are still at high risk of recurrence and for selected patients with advanced but still limited disease. In general, but not invariably, there appears to be a correlation between the ability of melanoma vaccines to stimulate antimelanoma cellular and/or antibody immune responses and improved clinical outcome. Accordingly, a number of strategies are being pursued to improve the clinical effectiveness of this first generation of vaccines by improving their ability to stimulate antimelanoma immunity.

The concepts underlying the construction of cancer vaccines are currently undergoing major revision. The paradigm is shifting from the focus during the last decade on constructing vaccines from individual, defined tumor antigens to preparing vaccines that contain a broad spectrum of tumor antigens that may or may not be defined. The reasons for this change are both theoretical and practical. Theoretically, there is a deepening realization that the individual tumor antigens currently used to construct melanoma vaccines may not be relevant in terms of inducing clinically effective tumor protective immunity. There is also increasing appreciation that the heterogeneous expression of such antigens on different tumors, the changes in their expression as tumors progress and/or are treated, and the heterogeneity in patients' ability to develop an immune response against any single antigen demands that vaccines contain a large number of antigens to circumvent these restrictions.

Thus, major issues that need to be addressed to develop more effective vaccines for melanoma include: (1) devising a mix of melanoma-associated antigens that can stimulate clinically beneficial antitumor immune responses and (2) developing adjuvants that can safely, easily, and strongly boost the frequency and magnitude of these responses. The recent explosion of knowledge regarding the cellular and molecular mechanisms of immune function and regulation provide multiple new opportunities.

Lastly, one must remember that melanoma vaccines do work very well—in animals. Our challenge is to find a way to make them work equally well in humans.

REFERENCES

1. Balch CM, Buzaid AC, Soong SJ, et al. Final version of the American Joint Committee on cancer staging system for cutaneous melanoma. *J Clin Oncol*. 2001;19: 3635–3648.
2. Balch CM, Hoiughton AN, Sober AJ, Soong SJ. *Cutaneous Melanoma*. 3rd ed. Quality Medical Publishing Inc.: St Louis, MS.
3. Kirkwood JM, Strawderman MH, Ernstoff MS, et al. Interferon alfa-2b adjuvant therapy of high risk resected cutaneous melanoma: The Eastern Cooperative Oncology Group trial EST 1 *J Clin Oncol*.1996;14:7–17.
4. Lens M, Dawes M. Inteferon alfa therapy for malignant melanoma: A systematic review of randomized controlled trials. *J Clin Oncol*. 2002;20:1818–1825.
5. Gromet MA, Epstein WL, Blois MS. The regressing thin melanoma. A distinctive lesion with metastatic potential. *Cancer*. 1978;42:2282–2292.
6. Bystryn J-C. Antibody response and tumor growth in syngeneic mice immunized to partially purified B16 melanoma associated antigens. *J Immunol*. 1978;120:96–101.
7. Livingston PO, Calves MJ, Natoli EJ. Approaches to augmenting the immunogenicity of the ganglioside GM2 in mice: purified GM2 is superior to whole cells. *J Immunol*. 1987;138:1524–1529.
8. Reynolds SR, Celis E, Sette A, et al. HLA-independent heterogeneity of CD8 + T cell responses to MAGE-3, Melan A/MART-1, gp100, tyrosinase, MC1R and TRP-2 in vaccine-treated melanoma patients. *J. Immunol*. 1998;161:6970–6976.
9. Bystryn J-C, Shapiro RL, Oratz R. Cancer vaccines: Clinical applications: Partially purified tumor antigen vaccines. In: DeVita V, Hellman S, Rosenberg SA, eds. *Biologic Therapy of Cancer*, 2nd ed. JB Lippincott: Philadelphia, PA; 1995: 668–679.
10. Ferrone S. Human tumor associated antigen mimicry by anti-idiotypic antibodies. In: Bystryn J-C, Ferrone S, Livingston P, eds. *Specific Immunotherapy of Cancer with Vaccines*. New York: Ann. N.Y. Acad Sci.; 1993;690:214–224.
11. Bystryn J-C, Zeleniuch-Jacquotte A, Oratz R, Shapiro RL, Harris MN, Roses DF. Double-blind trial of a polyvalent, shed-antigen, melanoma vaccine. *Clin Cancer Res*. 2001;7:1882–1887.
12. Slingluff CL Jr., Yamshchikov G, Neese P, et al. Phase I trial of a melanoma vaccine with gp100 (280–288) peptide and tetanus helper peptide in adjuvant: immunologic and clinical outcomes. *Clin Can Res*. 2001;7:3012–3024.
13. Morton DL, Barth, A. Vaccine therapy for malignant melanoma. *CA Caner J Clin*. 1996;46:225–244.
14. Berd D. M-Vax: an autologous, hapten-modified vaccine for human cancer. *Expert Opin Biol Therap*. 2002;2:335–2342.
15. Parmiani G, Castilli C, Dalerba P, et al. Cancer immunotherapy with peptide-based vaccines: what have we achieved? Where are we going? *J Natl Cancer Inst*. June 2002;94(11):805–818.
16. Weber J, Sondak VK, Scotland R, et al. Granulocyte-macrophage-colony-stimulating factor added to a multipeptide vaccine for resected stage II melanoma. *Cancer*. 2003;97:186–200.
17. Reynolds SR, Zeleniuch-Jacquotte A, Shapiro RL, et al. Vaccine-induced CD8+ T cell responses to MAGE-3 correlate with clinical outcome in patients with melanoma. *Clin Can Res*. 2003;9:657–662.
18. Miller K, Abeles, G, Oratz, R, Zeleniuch-Jacquotte, A, Cui, J, Roses, D, Harris, M, Bystryn, J-C. Improved survival of melanoma patients with an antibody response to immunization to a polyvalent melanoma vaccine. *Cancer*. 1995; 75(2):495–502.
19. Takahashi T, Johnson TD, Nishinaka Y, Morton DL et al. IgM anti-ganglioside antibodies induced by melanoma cell vaccine correlate with survival of melanoma patients. *J Invest Dermatol*. 1999; 112:205–209.
20. Livingston PO, Wong GYC, Adluri S, et al. Improved survival in stage III melanoma patients with GM2 antibodies: a randomized trial of adjuvant vaccination with GM2 ganglioside. *J. Clin. Oncol*. 1994;12:1036–1044.
21. Hsueh EC, Essner R, Foshag LJ, et al. Prolonged survival after complete resection of disseminated melanoma and active immunotherapy with a therapeutic cancer vaccine. *J Clin Oncol*. 2002;20:4549–4554.
22. Kirkwood JM, Ibrahim JG, Sosman JA, et al. High-dose interferon alfa-2b significantly prolongs relapse-free and overall survival compared with GM2-KLH/QS-21 vaccine in patients with resected stage IIB-III melanoma: results of intergroup trial E1694/S9512/C50980 *J Clin Oncol*. 2001;19:2370–2380.
23. Wallack MK, Sivanandham M, Blach CM, et al. Surgical adjuvant active specific immunotherapy for patients with stage III melanoma: The final analysis of data from a phase III, randomized, double-blind, multicenter vaccinia melanoma oncolysate trial. *J Am Coll Surg*. 1998;187:69–79.
24. Hersey P, Coates AS, McCarthy WH, et al. Adjuvant immunotherapy of patients with high-risk melanoma using vaccinia viral lysates of melanoma: results of a randomized trial. *J. Clin. Oncol*. 2002;20:4181–4190.
25. Reynolds SR, Albrecht J, Shapiro RL, et al. Changes in the presence of multiple markers of circulating melanoma cells correlates with clinical outcome in patients with melanoma. *Clin Cancer Res*. 2003;9:1497–1502.
26. Sosman JA, Unger JM, Liu PY et al. Southwest Oncology Group Adjuvant immunotherapy of resected, intermediate-thickness, node-negative melanoma with an allogeneic tumor vaccine: impact of HLA class I antigen expression on outcome. *J Clin Oncol*. 2002;8:2067–2075.

CHAPTER 53

Chemoprevention of Skin Cancer

Daniel I. Wasserman, M.D.
Barbara A. Gilchrest, M.D.

BOX 53-1 Overview

- The concept of cancer chemoprevention is based on both multistep and field carcinogenesis models.
- AKs represent an intermediate biomarker for monitoring the process of photocarcinogenesis.
- Topical retinoids, in light of their reasonable long-term tolerability, are a viable chemopreventive agent.
- Systemic retinoids appear to be excellent skin cancer chemoprevention agents, but are severely limited by their poor tolerability, teratogenicity, and requirement for indefinite use.
- Topical imiquimod and 5-fluorouracil have shown to be effective chemotherapeutic agents for AKs, but their ability to prevent NMSCs remains to be determined.
- Early data on PDT as a chemopreventive tool are encouraging, but further data are needed.
- Studies examining NSAIDs and statins have been conflicting, but the chronic use of NSAIDs appears to play a role as a useful systemic adjunct.
- At this time, no data support the use of vitamin and mineral supplements for the prevention of skin cancer.
- Limited data on the efficacy of tea polyphenols are available; however, they are encouraging.

▮ INTRODUCTION

Skin cancer represents the most common form of human cancer. The actual incidence of nonmelanoma skin cancers (NMSCs) is difficult to ascertain for it is often excluded from the comprehensive annual cancer statistics, but its incidence is projected to be greater than 1 million cases in the United States in 2005.[1] Basal cell carcinoma (BCC), the most common form of NMSC, is extremely prevalent among Caucasians worldwide, with some regions of Australia having an estimated incidence of 2% per year.[2] As the incidence of skin cancer increases and our understanding of cutaneous carcinogenesis advances, chemoprevention becomes an attractive cost-effective modality for reducing this public health burden. Melanoma, although a small fraction of all skin cancer, has also been considered an appropriate target for chemoprevention because of its progressively increasing incidence, relatively high mortality rate, and disproportionate impact on young and middle-aged adults compared to NMSC.[3]

History and Concept of Chemoprevention

Frustrated by the worsening death rates for the six most lethal cancers during the 1950s and 1960s, Sporn reexamined the traditional approach for the treatment of cancer: wait until the patient develops invasive disease and then either intoxicate it, excise it, and/or radiate it.[4] He proposed that cancer be conceived as a disease process that begins at the time of the original carcinogenic insult, not at the time when a patient is diagnosed as having invasive disease. Intrigued by new data on retinoids as possible cancer reversing agents, he formulated the concept of cancer chemoprevention. The chemopreventive construct was later broadened by Lippman and Hong to include rate reduction, causing a fixed number of cancers to develop over a longer time in treated versus control subjects, an approach they described as cancer delay.[5]

Sporn's construct was premised on two models: field and multistep carcinogenesis. In 1953, Slaughter et al. reported that 11.2% of 783 patients with a diagnosis of oral squamous cell carcinomas (SCCs) developed multiple independent tumors, a phenomenon they termed "field cancerization."[6] This phenomenon of field carcinogenesis was conceptualized as multiple premalignant foci, separate and distinct from established tumors in adjacent tissue, within areas having experienced a broad carcinogenic insult. Skin cancer likely represents the best in vivo model for field carcinogenesis: the epidermis acting as the field, solar ultraviolet radiation (UVR) as the established carcinogen, and actinic keratoses (AKs) as the premalignant foci, at least for SCCs.

The multistep carcinogenesis model involves tumor initiation, promotion, and progression (Table 53-1), events that in man tend to occur over many decades. Initiation involves direct DNA damage by known carcinogens (e.g., UVR), and is considered to be an irreversible step. Tumor promotion, a reversible step in its early stages, predominantly comprises epigenetic events over a long period of time, leading to a clinically detectable premalignant state. Additional genetic insults result in tumor progression.[7] UVR is a complete carcinogen, inducing all three phases of skin carcinogenesis: initiation, promotion, and progression.[8] Within this simplistic model, however, the events that ultimately lead to the development of SCCs, BCCs, and melanoma vary both quantitatively and qualitatively at each stage.[3,9]

The following sections approach skin cancer chemoprevention in the context of these models.

Approach to Chemoprevention

Cancer prevention strategies can be categorized into three groups (Table 53-2), all of which have been employed against skin cancer. Primary prevention strategies aim to prevent de novo malignancies in healthy populations, if possible by avoiding initiation. Although the great majority of skin cancers are attributable to UVR, primary prevention is largely a matter of sun protection (see Chapter 55). Secondary prevention strategies intervene at the tumor progression stage, preventing the malignant transformation of existing premalignant lesions. Tertiary prevention strategies attempt to prevent or reduce new independent malignancies in those with a prior history of cancer. Traditionally, cancer chemoprevention trials employing any of the three prevention strategies require too much time and, hence, are prohibitively expensive. Skin cancer, in comparison to other malignancies, has the advantage of occurring on a readily accessible and easily monitored organ with a sufficiently high incidence to permit cancer prevention trials. Moreover, the 1-, 3-, and 5-year cumulative risks of developing a new NMSC in patients with a prior history of NMSC are 17, 35, and 50%, respectively.[10]

The American Association for Cancer Research Task Force on the Treatment and Prevention of Intraepithelial Neoplasia suggests that the efficacy of a candidate chemopreventive agent need not be based on the cancer endpoint per se,

Table 53-1
Stages of Multistep Carcinogenesis

STAGE	CLASSIC EVENT	SKIN CANCER CONTEXT
Initiation	DNA damage in a proto-oncogene or tumor suppressor gene	Usually, UV-induced mutation; p53, PTCH, p16, and BRAF (melanocytes) are common target genes
Promotion	Expansion of a mutated clone	Usually, UV-induced epidermal hyperproliferation, often in the presence of low-grade inflammation (e.g., "dermatoheliosis" or a nonhealing wound)
Progression	Additional DNA damage in initiated cells	Continued UV exposure with resulting mutations, with an accelerated course in an immunocompromised host who does not reject progressivley abnormal cells

but rather on surrogate endpoint biomarkers (SEBs), a biologic event that occurs between exposure to a carcinogen (initiation) and the subsequent development of cancer.[11,12] SEBs thus indicate cellular or molecular events in the multistep progression of carcinogenesis.[13] Such biomarkers may be chemical or clinical in nature, although this discussion will emphasize clinical intermediate biomarkers.

The premalignant AK represents a well-defined common intermediate biomarker for monitoring the process of photocarcinogenesis. It is important to note that AKs are not obligate precursors to the development of SCC, and many invasive cutaneous SCCs appear to arise *de novo*, without prior diagnosis of an AK.[14] Nevertheless, extensive data suggest that a treatment that reduces AKs will also prevent SCCs, likely because photodamaged skin, the tissue context in which AKs arise, is known to harbor the same histologic abnormalities and mutations, albeit to a lesser degree. BCCs comprise approximately 80% of all skin cancers. BCCs lack a defined precursor

lesion, but AKs as a sensitive indicator of an individual's cumulative UVR exposure are also predictive for the development of BCCs, especially in older patients.[15]

Identification of an appropriate SEB for melanoma has proven more problematic. The majority of melanomas arise in older individuals with the same risk factors as for NMSC: fair skin, diffuse photodamage, and AKs.[16] However, a substantial minority arise in younger individuals, usually fair-skinned but lacking clinical evidence of significant photodamage and AKs. "Dysplastic nevi" were first described in families with p16 germline mutations and high rates of melanoma.[16–18] While clearly melanoma precursors in at least some instances in these kindred and in certain individuals, "dysplastic nevi" have since been broadly defined to include sporadic nevi with certain clinical and/or histologic features, the overwhelmingly majority of which behave in a benign manner and do not progress to melanoma.[19,20–22] Moreover, even completely banal nevi, present in virtually the entire population, constitute a sta-

tistical risk factor for melanoma if numerous and are as likely to harbor activating mutations in the BRAF proto-oncogene as invasive melanomas, suggesting they are indeed initiated melanocytic neoplasms.[23,24] The impact of these ambiguities on melanoma chemoprevention strategies is discussed further as follows in the context of specific agents.

Skin cancer is thus in many regards an ideal indication for studies of chemopreventive agents currently implicated in preventing more lethal but far less common varieties of cancer. As we understand the molecular mechanisms of skin carcinogenesis more completely, we expand the avenues for intervention. Moreover, the skin may be treated via either systemic or topical modalities, broadening a physician's pharmacologic armamentarium. This discussion will concentrate most widely on these agents.

RETINOIDS

> ### BOX 53-2 Summary
>
> - Retinoids have been shown to experimentally inhibit several types of visceral carcinomas.
> - Tretinoin has been shown to be an effective treatment for AKs.
> - Renal transplant patients receiving topical tretinoin developed fewer SCCs than those treated with placebo.
> - Adapalene and tazarotene have been shown to be effective agents against AKs, but no human studies against malignancies are available.
> - In high-risk patient populations, systemic retinoids appear to be viable candidates for reducing the incidence of NMSCs, but their use is severely limited by their poor tolerability and the requirement for indefinite use.

Table 53-2
Cancer Prevention Strategies

TYPE	DEFINITION	TARGETED CARCINOGENESIS STAGE	EXAMPLES IN SKIN
Primary	Prevent cancer from occurring in healthy individuals	Initiation	Sunscreens, DNA repair enhancers
Secondary	Prevent premalignant lesions from becoming cancers	Promotion	Sunscreens, NSAIDs, retinoids, PDT, immunomodulators
Tertiary	Prevent new cancers in individuals with prior cancer history		

Retinoids are by far the most thoroughly studied chemopreventive agents, dating back to the 1960s.[25] Retinoids have been shown experimentally to inhibit carcinogenesis in the esophagus, mammary gland, bladder, gastrointestinal epithelium, cervix, prostate, and lung.[26–29] Analogs of vitamin A, retinoids exert their effects by binding to nuclear retinoic acid and retinoid X receptors (RAR and RXR, respectively). These receptor complexes bind promoter regions of target genes, broadly influencing and modifying differentiation, proliferation, keratinization, embryonic development, and inflammation.[30] Tretinoin and isotretinoin are the most widely used topical and systemic retinoids, respectively. Etretinate, a second-generation oral retinoid, has been subsequently replaced by its major metabolite acitretin, preferred because of its shorter half-life. Third-generation topical retinoids include adapalene and tazarotene.

The most common side effect of topical retinoid use is retinoid dermatitis, characterized by "dryness," erythema, and desquamation that tend to peak at about 2 weeks and lessen thereafter despite continued use. The dermatitis can be alleviated with emollients and is exacerbated by cold, dry weather. Systemic retinoids also commonly cause "dryness" of the skin, lips, and other mucosal surfaces. Laboratory abnormalities such as elevation in transaminases and triglycerides occur infrequently and are reversible with either lowering of dose or discontinuation of therapy. Levels of lipids and hepatic enzymes should be determined prior to the start of therapy and intermittently once therapy has begun. Adverse effects, albeit unusual, that have been reported during prolonged therapy include spinal hyperostosis, in addition to calcification of tendons and ligaments.[31] The most serious risk of systemic retinoids is their teratogenicity, with malformations reported in up to 25% of infants born to mothers ingesting retinoids in the first weeks of pregnancy.[32] There is no safe established minimal dose. More detailed discussion and recommendations for patient monitoring are beyond the scope of this chapter.

Topical Therapy

Early studies investigating topical tretinoin's role in skin cancer chemoprevention yielded conflicting results, although human trials beginning in 1962 have consistently shown mild to moderate reductions in the number of AKs.[25,33–42] Bollag

and Ott found a 50 to 100% reduction in AKs in 44 of 51 patients treated with tretinoin; however, recurrence of AKs was noted within a year following cessation of therapy.[43] In vitro studies have shown that tretinoin induces pro-apoptotic pathways in keratinocytes following UVB-radiation, suggesting a possible preventive mechanism for the development of NMSCs.[38] Topical tretinoin treatment has also been shown to block NFκB signaling after UVB, another mechanism by which tumor promotion may be slowed.[44,45]

Additional human studies have looked at whether topical tretinoin prevents the development of invasive malignancies. Renal transplant patients receiving topical tretinoin developed fewer SCCs than those treated with placebo.[46] Dysplastic nevi treated with topical tretinoin under occlusion and histologically confirmed to be dysplastic nevi prior to treatment were observed to undergo both clinical and histologic regression.[47,48] Furthermore, cytologic atypia that had been noted prior to treatment disappeared and the nevi contained benign-appearing melanocytes.[47] Meyskens et al. evaluated three patients with biopsy-proven dysplastic nevi, two with personal histories of melanoma, and the third with a strong family history of melanoma.[49] Following 10 to12-week treatment regimens with topical tretinoin 0.05% under occlusion, post-treatment biopsies of the dysplastic nevi showed either complete conversion to benign features (two patients) or regression to minimal dysplasia. A fourth study treated dysplastic nevi with tretinoin, tretinoin with hydrocortisone 1% cream, or placebo. No histologic evaluations were done prior to treatment, but statistically significant clinical regression was noted in both groups of patients receiving tretinoin but not in patients receiving placebo. At the conclusion of the study, however, histologic evaluations showed no difference in the histologic atypia of nevi among the three treatment groups.[50]

Adapalene has been used in only one study to treat AKs. In a multicenter, investigator-blinded, randomized study, Kang et al. found that both 0.1 and 0.3% adapalene gel improved AKs when compared to placebo.[51] Approximately 65% of patients treated with either strength adapalene experienced marked or moderate improvement in AKs compared with only 34% of the vehicle control patients.[51]

Tazarotene is a synthetic retinoid that is Food and Drug Administration (FDA)-

approved for the topical treatment of acne and psoriasis.[52–54] Tazarotene 0.1% gel regularly applied for 5 to 8 months has been reported to successfully treat BCCs and SCCs in situ, likely via inducing tumor suppressor genes that are underexpressed in BCCs and SCCs in sun-exposed skin, and initiating pro-apoptotic pathways and decreasing proliferation.[55–59] In PTCH gene heterozygote mice treated with UV and ionizing radiation, tazarotene has been shown to inhibit the development of BCCs.[60] However, few studies have been conducted using tazarotene on human malignancies, with one study reporting complete regression without recurrence to be 30.5% at 3-year follow-up without recurrence.[61]

Topical retinoids, with their limited side effects profile and reasonable overall tolerability (see Table 53-3), remain an interesting group of chemopreventive agents. Unfortunately, the paranoia of third-party insurers that patients will benefit cosmetically from use of these agents[62–66] appears to preclude their coverage for the indication of skin cancer chemoprevention, greatly disincentivising patients from this approach.

Systemic Therapy

The extensive side effects profile of systemic retinoid therapy has restricted its use for cancer chemoprevention in the general population. However, their use has been explored in several special patient populations.

Xeroderma pigmentosum (XP) is a group of autosomal recessive disorders caused by mutation of one of several critical DNA repair enzymes and characterized by markedly reduced DNA repair capacity.[67] NMSC and melanoma occur with markedly increased frequency in these individuals. The median age for the first NMSC is 8 years and the risk of NMSC before 20 years of age is 4800 times than that of the general population.[68,69] These patients are routinely instructed to engage in strict lifelong sun avoidance and sunscreen use, but this is rarely adequate to prevent skin cancers. Systemic retinoids have, therefore, been studied. Kraemer et al. reported a 63% reduction of the incidence of skin cancers in seven patients with XP using isotretinoin at a dose of 2 mg/kg/day for 2 years,[70] although as with topical retinoids, protection was restricted to the period of use and tumor incidence increased 8.5-fold following cessation of therapy in several patients to annual rates higher than before isotretinoin

Table 53-3
Candidate Chemoprevention Agents

AGENT	ADVANTAGES	DISADVANTAGES
Retinoids, topical	High tolerability	Drying, erythematogenic, irritation
Retinoids, systemic	Ability to treat large surface areas	Teratogenicity, mucosal dryness, hypertriglyceridemia, myalgias, nausea, hepatic transaminitis
5-FU	Low-cost, proven efficacy	Irritation, poor patient compliance, swelling
Imiquimod	Efficacy	Irritation, no long-term data, cost, poor patient compliance
ALA-PDT	Ability to treat large surface areas	Procedural discomfort, swelling, desquamation, irritation, reactivation of herpes labialis
NSAIDs	Low cost	Limited number of studies, drug interactions, gastrointestinal bleeding, cardiac side effects
Vitamins, minerals	Low cost	Contact allergies, conflicting data, hypervitaminosis A, diarrhea, yellowing of acral skin (beta-carotene)

treatment. Since then, other studies have reported near-complete or complete suppression of new tumors in XP patients while on etretinate (0.3 to 0.5mg/kg/day).[71–73]

Organ transplant patients are another high-risk group for development of skin cancers, primarily SCCs. It has been estimated that approximately 5 to 25% of transplant patients die of skin cancer.[74,75] One case study using isotretinoin 0.5 mg/kg/day found a 50% reduction in new lesions within 2 months of treatment.[76] At least three studies have reported reductions in tumor incidence with etretinate and no adverse effect on graft function or survival.[46,77,78] Other reports suggest acitretin as an effective option for chemoprevention in transplant patients.[79–84] In a randomized, double-blind, placebo-controlled study trial of 44 renal transplant recipients, Bouwes Bavnick et al. found a statistically significant decrease in the number of new AKs and skin cancers, with greatest benefit for those patients with a prior history of skin cancer.[80]

Psoriasis patients treated with oral psoralen-UVA (PUVA) are at a significantly increased risk for the development of SCCs compared to matched controls, and this increased risk appears to be dose-dependent.[85–89] In a nested cohort study of NMSC incidence among participants in the PUVA Follow-up Study with at least 1 year of substantial oral retinoid use (isotretinoin, etretinate, or acitretin) between 1985 and 2000, doses of 25 mg/day or more resulted in a risk reduction for SCC of about 25%.[90] Nevoid basal cell syndrome (NBCCS) is a rare, autosomal dominant disorder in which patients develop up to thousands of BCCs. Both isotretinoin and etretinate have been shown to reduce the number of new lesions in patients with NBCCS at dosages of 0.4 mg/kg/day and 1 mg/kg/day, respectively.[91–93]

The role of systemic retinoids for chemoprevention is unfortunately limited by their substantial long-term side effects (Table 53-3). Despite the very encouraging decrease in frequency of premalignant and malignant lesions, patients often find retinoids intolerable over long periods of time. Subjective complaints such as dry skin, dry lips, hair loss, and musculoskeletal symptoms are common reasons for patients to request alternative therapies. For women of childbearing potential, the teratogenicity of systemic retinoids is an additional concern.

5-FLUORACIL (5-FU)

BOX 53-3 Summary

- Topical 5-FU was reported to be an effective agent against AKs in as early as 1963.
- Facial AKs respond well, but more acrally situated lesions appear to be more resistant.
- No long-term data regarding the ability of 5-FU to prevent subsequent AKs or skin cancers are available.

The cytotoxic antimetabolite 5-FU is a chemotherapeutic inhibitor of DNA and RNA synthesis. In 1963, Goldman and Dillaha et al. reported effective and selective treatment of facial AKs using 5-FU ointment in a dose-dependent fashion.[94–96] This led to numerous subsequent studies finding similar success using various 5-FU strengths, schedules, anatomical distributions, and methodologies.[96–104] Facial AKs consistently responded well to topical 5-FU; however, upper extremity lesions were somewhat more recalcitrant, paralleling those observations with tretinoin.[96,97]

Randomized, blinded studies comparing 5 and 0.5% creams as a field treatment found significant reductions in AKs with insignificant differences between the two strengths.[101] Unfortunately, there are no long-term data regarding the ability of 5-FU to prevent subsequent AKs or skin cancers. Although this benefit is widely assumed and is indeed the dominant rationale for 5-FU therapy, the fact that 5-FU is now off patent virtually guarantees that no company will undertake the substantial expense of documenting and quantifying this benefit.

IMIQUIMOD

BOX 53-4 Summary

- At least five randomized, double-blind, parallel-group, vehicle-controlled studies have shown imiquimod to be an effective and safe treatment for AKs.
- Three times weekly for 16 weeks provides greater clearance rates and lower recurrence rates than twice-weekly dosing for 16 weeks.
- Case reports have suggested success for lowering the incidence of NSMCs in XP patients.

Imiquimod is an immunomodulatory agent first approved by the U.S. FDA for the treatment of genital and perianal warts. Imiquimod's exact mechanism remains to be determined, but it is known that it induces cytokine release that bolsters a Th1-dominant immune response, stimulating CD4 cells to generate IFN-γ and IL-2 (cytokines that activate CD8 cells to become cytotoxic T cells), possibly providing the immune memory needed for future protection.[105]

In 1999, topical imiquimod was first reported to successfully treat superficial and nodular BCCs.[106] Subsequently, Stockfleth et al. reported the successful treatment of six patients with multiple AKs using topical imiquimod 2 to 3 times per week.[107] In 2004, topical imiquimod 5% received FDA approval for the treatment of AKs. Since then, five large, randomized, double-blind, parallel-group, vehicle-controlled studies have been conducted to evaluate the efficacy and safety of topically applied 5% imiquimod cream vs. vehicle cream for the treatment of AK lesions on the face and balding scalp as a "field therapy."[108] Two of these studies evaluated once-daily dosing two times per week for 16 weeks; the other three studies evaluated once-daily dosing three times per week for 16 weeks. Three studies using dosing regimens of three times per week for 16 weeks found complete clearance rates of 48 to 57% and partial clearance rates of 64 to 72% in 330 patients.[108,109] Two studies using dosing regimens of two times per week for 16 weeks found a complete clearance rate of approximately 45% and a partial clearance rate of about 59% in 197 patients.[110] Follow-up studies of these patient populations revealed that between 14 and 20 months following treatment completion, the overall recurrence rates were 24.7 and 42.6%, respectively, for three times per week and two times per week dosing, suggesting a dose-relationship. Additionally, for those who experienced a recurrence, the median number of lesions was one.[111] Case reports of XP patients have demonstrated a decrease in the number of new facial NMSCs developing from greater than two BCCs per month to about one per month in one patient.[112,113] These encouraging findings suggest that not only is imiquimod chemotherapeutic for AKs, but also chemopreventive, although more experience is clearly needed.

PHOTODYNAMIC THERAPY (PDT)

- PDT has proven to be an effective therapy for both AKs and superficial NMSCs.
- While BCCs have been treated successfully, no clinical trials have evaluated the ability for PDT to prevent NMSC.
- Two reports described success in lowering the incidence of new BCCs in PDT-treated skin of patients with NBCCS.
- Studies in organ transplant patients have shown conflicting results.

Over 100 years ago, Von Tappeiner and Jesionek reported the treatment of skin cancer using topical or intralesional eosin followed by the deliberate exposure to visible light.[114] In the 1990s, a number of technical and regulatory hurdles were overcome to permit marketing of topical photodynamic therapy (PDT) based on the application of the prodrug δ-aminolevulinic acid (ALA) that is converted in the epidermis, preferentially in premalignant and malignant cells, into the photosensitizing compound protoporphyrin. Subsequent exposure to activating wavelengths of light leads to oxygen-mediated destruction of the targeted tissue (see "Aging Skin").[115]

Several lines of evidence suggest that ALA-PDT, as a field therapy, may serve as a means of skin cancer chemoprevention. First, ALA-PDT delays UV-induced carcinogenesis in hairless mice.[116] Second, in clinical trials, ALA-PDT has produced complete clearance rates between 68 and 100% of AKs and superficial NMSCs, depending on the protocol employed.[117-125] Like 5-FU and topical retinoids, ALA-PDT success rates are somewhat lower for lesions on the extremities.[121,126]

Although BCCs have been treated successfully using topical ALA-PDT,[127,128] few studies have examined the chemoprevention efficacy of this modality. However, in one case report of a woman with nevoid BCC syndrome who, on average, developed 20 BCCs on the face annually, during the initial 8-month treatment and observation period, no new BCCs arose in the intermittently field-treated areas.[129] Moreover, during an additional 10-month period of treatments spaced 2 to 3 months apart, the patient did not develop any new BCCs on the face.[130] Oseroff et al. reported the use of PDT covering as much as 20% body surface area in three children with NBCCS.[130] Treated areas were free of new or recurrent carcinomas at 1.8 to 6 years following the last treatment, while in the patient followed for 6 years, multiple BCCs developed in the untreated areas.[130] In the only long-term cancer preventive trial using PDT in transplant patients, another subset of patients with an increased risk of NMSCs, no statistically significant difference was found in the occurrence of new SCCs between ALA-PDT treated and untreated arms after 2 years of follow-up,[131] although this study design unfortunately targeted areas with well-documented poor response to ALA-PDT as well as other topical chemoprevention agents.[42,96,97,132]

NONSTEROIDAL ANTI-INFLAMMATORY DRUGS (NSAIDs)

BOX 53-6   Summary

- NSAIDs suppress inflammation through inhibition of COX-1 and COX-2.
- Despite its efficacy against AKs, topical diclofenac is limited by its side-effect profile.
- A case-control study reported that regular use of 200 mg or more per day of aspirin was associated with a lower incidence of SCC, whereas the regular use of low-dose preparations did not reduce the risk of SCC.
- Early data on systemic NSAIDs use for the prevention of NMSC suggest there may be a role for their use as a chemopreventive agent, but more data are needed to confidently recommend these agents to patients.

NSAIDs have been used for more than 100 years, but their mechanism was not discovered until 1971, when Vane first reported that NSAIDs suppress inflammation through their inhibitory effects on the cyclooxygenase-1 and -2 (COX-1 and COX-2) enzymes.[133] It is now well understood that COX-1 and COX-2 exert their physiological effects through production of prostaglandins (PGs). Studies have shown a direct relationship between UV-mediated injury and induction of COX-2 protein, PG production, and COX activity.[134-136] Studies have shown a relationship between PGs and epithelial cancers.[136-138] For that reason, both nonselective and COX-selective NSAIDs have been investigated as chemopreventive agents.

Fischer et al. compared oral celecoxib, a selective COX-2 inhibitor, to oral indomethacin (a nonselective COX inhibitor) in preventing UV-induced skin cancer in hairless mice.[139] The authors found a significant reduction in the mean number of tumors per mouse given either celecoxib or indomethacin when compared to placebo. An additional study by Pentland et al. found a 56% reduction in the mean number of tumors in UV-irradiated hairless mice treated with celecoxib compared to irradiated controls.[140] Wilgus et al. suggested topical celecoxib as a viable agent for skin cancer prevention.[141,142] Furthermore, the group observed no significant improvement of tumor multiplicity in mice treated with topical 0.5% 5-FU and vehicle alone, but an approximate 70% reduction in tumor multiplicity when celecoxib was added to the topical 5-FU formulation.[143] To date, however, no human studies have evaluated topical celecoxib's efficacy in preventing human skin cancer.

Acetylsalicylic acid or aspirin, one of the first COX inhibitors used clinically, is a nondiscriminatory irreversible acetylating inhibitor of COX. Aspirin has received some attention with regards to its potential use as a cancer chemopreventive agent in colon carcinomas, but has evoked little interest as a chemopreventive agent for skin cancer. Nevertheless, compared to placebo, topical aspirin reduced tumor burden in UV-irradiated mice by about 35 to 50%, and a closely related compound, sodium salicylate, reduced tumor multiplicity, burden, and involved area by about 25, 50, and 40%, respectively, when compared to UVR alone.[144,145]

A variety of additional NSAIDs have been investigated for their biologic potential in skin cancer prevention. Topical 3.0% diclofenac in a 2.5% hyaluronan gel was found to be effective in eradicating AKs on the face and hands in 30 to 50% of patients treated twice a day with higher success rates seen for treatment periods of 90 days.[146–148] Long-term use is likely limited by the high incidence of adverse events, consistently around 80%, primarily related to the skin (i.e., pruritus, rash, dry skin, application site reactions). The next most common adverse events were those involving the nervous system, mainly paresthesias and hyperesthesias. However, these reactions are less severe and better tolerated than those of more common AK treatments, such as 5-FU.[104]

A recent case-control study nested within a community-based cohort of 1621 people in southern Queensland, Australia, evaluated the relationship between the ingestion of NSAIDs and the risk of SCC and AKs.[149] The regular use of NSAIDs in full dose, 200 mg or more per day of aspirin, was associated with a substantially lower incidence of SCC, whereas there was no evidence that regular use of low-dose preparations of NSAIDs alone reduced the risk of SCC. Risks of SCC were lower with longer duration of regular NSAID use. Infrequent or other use of NSAIDs did not significantly reduce the risk of SCC. Control subjects who were regular users of NSAIDs in the last year of the study period ("current regular users") had significantly lower AK counts than "never users." After adjustment for confounding factors, current regular users of full-dose NSAIDs had AK counts about 50% less than those of "never users" (multivariate R^2, 0.52; 95% CI, 0.30 to 0.91).

Similar associations were observed with current regular use of low-dose NSAIDs (multivariate R^2, 0.52; 95% CI, 0.34 to 0.82). Regular past users of NSAIDs had AK counts that were about one-third to one-half lower than "never users," although these findings were of borderline statistical significance.[149]

STATINS

BOX 53-7 Summary

- Statins inhibit 3-hydroxy-3-methylglutaryl-coenzyme A (HMG-CoA) reductase.
- A meta-analysis of 27 articles reporting data on either cancer incidence or cancer death found that statins did not reduce cancer incidence or cancer deaths including those attributed to melanoma.
- A meta-analysis looking specifically at melanoma prevention with the use of statins and fibrates reported a decrease in incident melanomas for statin trials; however, no significant differences in melanoma outcomes by gender, melanoma occurrence after 2 years of participation in trial, stage, or histology were noted.

Statins are the gold standard for pharmacologic control of cholesterol levels, and are proven to decrease the incidence of cardiovascular and cerebrovascular events.[150] Statins reduce cholesterol levels by inhibiting the enzyme 3-hydroxy-3-methylglutaryl-coenzyme A (HMG-CoA) reductase, which converts HMG-CoA to mevalonate, the precursor of cholesterol. They have produced mixed results as chemotherapeutic and chemopreventive agents in a wide-variety of cancers including, but not limited to breast, prostate, hematologic, central nervous system, various soft-tissue sarcomas, and melanoma.[151,152] Recently, there has been more focus on the chemopreventive properties of statins in the development of melanoma.[153]

The overall influence of statins on cancer incidence and death is controversial. In a large observational, case-control study evaluating statins and cancer incidence, statin users ($n = 3129$) had a lower incidence of cancer versus nonusers ($n = 16,976$) (odds ratio [OR] = 0.80; 95% CI, 0.66 to 0.96). With use for over 4 years, the OR of cancer risk for statin users was 0.64 (95% CI, 0.44 to 0.93).[154] A more recent meta-analysis included 27 articles ($n = 86,936$ participants), reporting 26 randomized controlled trials with a mean duration of follow-up of at least 1 year, enrolling a minimum of 100 patients, and

reporting data on either cancer incidence or cancer death.[155] The authors found that statins did not reduce cancer incidence (OR, 1.02; 95% CI, 0.97 to 1.07) or cancer deaths (OR, 1.01; 95% CI, 0.93 to 1.09). Additionally, no reductions were noted for any individual cancer type, including melanoma. Finally, a meta-analysis specifically looking at melanoma prevention with the use of statins and fibrates reported a decrease in incident melanomas for statin trials (OR, 0.90; 95% CI, 0.56 to 1.44).[156] However, subgroup analyses failed to show statistically significant differences in melanoma outcomes by gender, melanoma occurrence after 2 years of participation in trial, stage, or histology. One statin-specific subgroup, lovastatin, did show a statistically significant reduction in melanoma incidence based on one trial only (OR, 0.52; 95% CI, 0.27 to 0.99).

Research to date has focused on the role HMG-CoA reductase in cancer prevention has on various pathways involved in cell proliferation, differentiation, and apoptosis.[157] So far, statins have been shown to induce apoptosis of melanoma cell lines and phenotypic reversion of metastatic melanoma cell lines *in vitro*, and inhibition of melanoma metastases in mouse models *in vivo*.[158,159] Additional research is needed to determine whether statins are clinically useful chemopreventive agents.

VITAMINS AND MINERALS

BOX 53-8 Summary

- Epidemiologic studies for beta-carotene have failed to correlate dietary intake with reductions in NMSCs.
- Prospective and case-control studies found conflicting results for the relationship between dietary retinol and subsequent development of NMSCs.
- Randomized, double-blind, controlled trials found that retinol did not affect the risk of first new BCC, but was effective in preventing first new SCC in patients with a history of multiple AKs and, at most, two prior NMSCs.
- Studies controlled for vitamin E use, among patients subsequently diagnosed with NMSCs, reported conflicting results.
- The same epidemiological studies that investigated both retinol and alpha-tocopherol also showed no relationships between plasma levels or dietary intake of ascorbic acid and the subsequent development of NMSCs.
- Selenium has no role in the prevention of skin cancer.

Over the last 25 years, the role of diet in cancer has received increasing attention. Prostate and colon carcinomas have received the most attention because of their public health impact.

Beta-Carotene

Beta-carotene is a dietary carotenoid, efficiently converted into vitamin A by the body. It is available in food sources such as green leafy vegetables, cantaloupes, sweet potatoes, meat, butter, cheese, carrots, tomatoes, beets, and berries. Beta-carotene represents the first dietary constituent formally studied for the prevention of NMSCs and cancers overall,[160,161] based on epidemiologic data linking consumption of diets high in carotenoids with reduced cancer risk. However, in 1990, Greenberg et al. observed no reduction in NMSCs among 1805 patients recently diagnosed with a NMSC and then randomly assigned to receive 50 mg of beta-carotene or placebo daily for 5 years.[161] Subsequent reports have provided conflicting, but generally negative results failing to support a risk between beta-carotene supplementation and development of skin cancer.

An Australian study investigated the effect of daily application of sunscreen with and without supplementation of beta-carotene over a 4.5-year period and found no statistical difference in the rate of development of NMSCs in the two groups.[162] A prospective analysis based on food-frequency questionnaires and participants from the United States Nurses' Healthy Study and the Health Professionals Follow-Up Study failed to show statistically significant reductions in BCC and SCC development among those with high beta-carotene intakes.[163,164] A large-scale, randomized, 12-year primary-prevention trial of beta-carotene supplementation for NMSCs in the Physicians' Health Study found no significant effect of beta-carotene supplementation on the risk for BCC and SCC.[165] Furthermore, there was no evidence for a trend toward beneficial or harmful effects during the follow-up period.[165] A randomized, double-blind, placebo-controlled trial of 50-mg beta-carotene supplementation on alternate days with 12 years of follow-up showed no effect of the supplementation on risk of NMSC even among men with low baseline plasma beta-carotene.[166]

Vitamin A (Retinol)

Vitamin A (retinol) must be acquired through the diet and is ingested as retinyl esters and as provitamin A carotenoids. Retinol is essential for normal embryonic and fetal development, epithelial differentiation and maintenance, reproduction, and growth. Early epidemiological studies reported an inverse relationship between serum retinol levels and the development of cancer,[167,168] leading to more refined investigations of the correlation between retinol levels and NMSCs.

Successive prospective and case-control studies found conflicting results for the relationship between dietary retinol and subsequent development of NMSCs.[169-173] Two randomized, double-blind, controlled trials studied the effect of retinol versus placebo and retinol versus isotretinoin versus placebo on the development of NMSCs. They found that retinol did not affect the risk of first new BCC, but was effective in preventing first new SCC in patients with a history of multiple AKs and, at most, two prior NMSCs.[174] Additionally, there was no difference between those taking retinol, isotretinoin, or placebo to the time of onset of the first clinically and pathologically diagnosed skin cancer.[175] In contrast to studies described earlier in this chapter (see Chapter 47), the failure to detect any improvement with the use of isotretinoin is likely due to insufficient dosing, 5 to 10 mg/day. The chemopreventive effect of isotretinoin has been linked to a parallel decrease in natural killer (NK) cell function, requiring doses of 1.0 mg/kg or greater,[176] equivalent to 70 mg/day in an average adult.

Vitamin E (Alpha-Tocopherol)

Vitamin E is a generic term for compounds that have the biological activity of alpha-tocopherol.[177] Early studies of chemically induced colonic tumors in mice suggested high-dose vitamin E supplementation may decrease the incidence of cancer.[178] Due to its characteristics as a powerful nonenzymatic, lipid-soluble antioxidant and free radical scavenger, alpha-tocopherol was, therefore, implicated as a potential chemoprophylactic agent against skin cancer. Later, prospective and nested case-control studies, like those for retinol, demonstrated clinically insignificant relationships between serum alpha-tocopherol levels and subsequent development of cancer.[179-183] Studies comparing vitamin use, controlled for vitamin E, among those subsequently diagnosed with NMSCs, reported conflicting results.[170-173,184]

Several studies have considered topical alpha-tocopherol as a possible chemopreventive agent because of its ability to absorb in the UVB region thereby acting as photoprotectant sunscreen. Studies using irradiated mice pretreated with topical vitamin E found consistent reductions in DNA photodamage, tumor incidence, and/or tumor burden.[185-190] The effect of oral alpha-tocopherol is less clear, however, with earlier reports indicating no protection against photocarcinogenesis in hairless mice,[160] but more recent studies report that oral vitamin E supplementation does reduce NMSC incidence and/or tumor burden.[187,190-192]

No human trials directly evaluate the effect of vitamin E on development of skin cancer. Potapenko et al. observed decreases in PUVA-induced erythema when topical alpha-tocopherol was applied before irradiation, but no effect when it was applied following irradiation,[193] consistent with its action as a sunscreen. Werninghaus et al. observed no photoprotective effect against UV erythema on human skin when patients were supplemented with oral vitamin E for 6 months prior to UVB exposure.[194]

A topical combination of vitamin C and alpha-tocopherol showed a greater protection against UV erythema and DNA damage in UV-irradiated pig skin than did either of these vitamins used alone.[195] Among commercially available products, alpha-tocopherol is a more effective photoprotectant than either alpha-tocopherol acetate or alpha-tocopherol succinate, although topically applied alpha-tocopherol acetate is converted to alpha-tocopherol in the skin, albeit with low efficiency.[196]

Vitamin C (Ascorbic Acid)

Vitamin C (L-ascorbic acid) is a nonenzymatic, water-soluble, antioxidant and free-radical scavenger. It also serves as an essential cofactor for lysyl and prolyl hydroxylases in the synthesis of collagen. Due to biologic control mechanisms, topical application of ascorbic acid remains the only means to increase its concentration in the skin.[197] The same epidemiological studies that investigated both retinol and alpha-tocopherol also showed clinically insignificant relationships between either plasma levels or dietary intake of ascorbic acid and the subsequent development of NMSCs.[163,164,170-172,184] Very little has been published as to ascorbic acid's direct effect on the development of NMSCs. Any chemoprophylactic effect must be extrapolated from its effect on UV-erythema or acute histologic damage.

Yorkshire pigs topically treated with ascorbic acid followed by UVB irradiation or PUVA decreased the level of UV-induced erythema and/or number of sunburn cells on histology.[198] Darr et al., in a later study, compared the relative photoprotective effect of ascorbic acid versus alpha-tocopherol versus the combination of the two in UV-irradiated porcine skin.[199] Ascorbic acid alone was ineffective against UVB; however, it augmented the effect of both UVA and UVB sunscreens in reducing the number of sunburn cells. Furthermore, ascorbic acid augmented the photoprotective effect of alpha-tocopherol alone or with either a UVA or UVB sunscreen, underscoring its ability as an effective adjunct against photodamage. In the only human study to date, 10% ascorbic acid applied topically resulted in a 22% reduction of erythema intensity when given the minimal erythema dose (MED).[200] The additive benefit of topical ascorbic acid with alpha-tocopherol has been reproduced (see "Vitamin E" discussed earlier).[195] Oral supplementation of both ascorbic acid and alpha-tocopherol in 18 patients exposed to UVB on the lower back resulted in an increase in MED and decrease in thymine-dimer formation; however, this study was limited by the lack of control for either vitamin.[201] Topical formulations of ascorbic acid above pH 3.5 are ineffective for increasing skin levels and the addition of ferulic acid to vitamin C/E solutions both stabilizes the vitamins and enhances their photoprotective effect.[202,203]

Selenium

Named after the Greek moon goddess Selene, selenium is an essential micronutrient required for the function of the powerful endogenous antioxidant, glutathione peroxidase.[197] It is found in seafood, red meat, egg yolks, chicken, garlic, tuna, mushrooms, asparagus, and grain products. Selenium first began to receive attention as a chemoprotective agent against skin cancer when early epidemiologic data suggested that low levels of selenium were associated with an increased cancer incidence and morbidity, particularly for gastrointestinal and prostatic carcinomas.[204–206] Subsequent reports challenged this notion, while studies controlling for skin cancers further failed to discover a consistent relationship to selenium levels.[181,182,207,208]

Animal studies have shown dose-dependent protection of both oral and topical selenium supplementation against tumor incidence and burden.[209–211] Two randomized, double-blind, placebo-controlled human trials using 200 µg of selenium failed to show a decrease in NMSCs, but both studies did report a decrease in incidence of, and mortality from, carcinomas arising from other sites.[180,181] Overall, selenium appears to lack any clinical utility in preventing skin cancer.

■ TEA POLYPHENOLS

BOX 53-9   Summary

- Tea's antioxidant properties are due to polyphenolic compounds, referred to as catechins.
- Treatment with either oral or topical green tea polyphenols produces dose-dependent reductions in tumor incidence and tumor burden in UVB-irradiated mice.
- In humans, topically applied GTPs have been found to decrease UVB-induced pyrimidine dimers, decrease post-PUVA erythema, and reduce UVA-induced erythema index scores, sunburn cells, loss of Langerhans cells, and DNA damage.
- Until additional human studies become available, our ability to rely on tea as an agent against the development of NMSC remains limited.

Since its introduction thousands of years ago by Chinese and Southeast Asian cultures, tea has enchanted virtually every corner of the globe. Produced from the leaves of the tea plant *Camellia sinensis*, tea is now grown in over 30 countries and is the second most commonly consumed beverage next to water. History, poems, books, and emotions have all been touched by its attractive scent and taste. Mounting public awareness of its powerful antioxidant properties has further enhanced its popularity.

Tea's antioxidant properties are due to polyphenolic compounds. Tea polyphenols, referred to as catechins, are the largest dry weight component of tea leaves and are the best known antioxidants found in tea, the most effective one being epigallocatechin gallate (EGCG).[212] The manufacture of black tea involves crushing the tea leaves to promote enzymatic oxidation and subsequent condensation of tea polyphenols in a process known as fermentation. Green tea is made from fresh tea leaves that are steamed or pan-fried, inactivating their enzymes and preventing the oxidation of

tea polyphenols.[213] Established activities of tea polyphenols include inhibition of MAP-kinase, inhibition of transcription factors AP-1 and NF-κB, induction of apoptosis, cell-cycle modulation, and inhibition of angiogenesis.[214–219]

Treatment with either oral or topical green tea polyphenols or specifically with EGCG produces dose-dependent reductions in tumor incidence and tumor burden in UVB-irradiated mice.[220,221] In subsequent mouse studies examining different doses of the oral-administered green and black teas, and contrasting them to their decaffeinated counterparts, green tea reduced overall tumor burden regardless of cancer subtype. Black tea was less efficacious, and the beneficial effects of either tea were abrogated by decaffeination. The replacement of caffeine to the decaffeinated green tea extract partially restored its clinical effects; however, the impact of recaffeination on black tea was less clear.[222–224] Record et al. found the beneficial effects between green and black tea to be reversed, for either UVA/B radiation or UVB radiation.[225] In humans, topically applied green tea polyphenol extracts (GTP) have been found to decrease UVB-induced pyrimidine dimers, virtually eliminate post-PUVA erythema, and reduce UVA-induced erythema index scores (EGCG resulted in the greatest constituent reduction), sunburn cells, loss of Langerhans cells, and DNA damage.[226–228] To date, no randomized controlled studies have examined the ability of orally administered green and black teas to impact skin cancer in humans.

Available data do not determine whether green tea, black tea, or EGCG can prevent, suppress, or delay skin cancer. However, decaffeinated tea products appear to have no role in skin cancer chemoprevention.

■ FINAL THOUGHTS

Chemoprevention of skin cancer is soundly based on our understanding of photocarcinogenesis. A combination of approaches relying on inhibition or antagonism of different tumor promotion pathways is likely to be the most effective in preventing skin cancer. At present, multiple promising agents are available, although further documentation of their efficacy in humans would be most helpful.

REFERENCES

1. Jemal A, et al. Cancer statistics, 2004. *CA Cancer J Clin.* 2004;54(1):8–29.

2. Rubin AI, et al. Basal-cell carcinoma. *N Engl J Med.* 2005;353(21):2262–2269.

3. Demierre MF, et al. Cutaneous melanoma: Pathogenesis and rationale for chemoprevention. *Crit Rev Oncol Hematol.* 2005;53(3):225–239.

4. Sporn MB. Approaches to prevention of epithelial cancer during the preneoplastic period. *Cancer Res.* 1976;36(7 pt 2): 2699–2702.

5. Lippman SM, et al. Cancer prevention by delay. Commentary re: J. A. O'Shaughnessy, et al., Treatment and prevention of intraepithelial neoplasia: An important target for accelerated new agent development. *Clin Cancer Res.* 2002;8:305–346.

6. Slaughter DP, et al. "Field cancerization" in oral stratified squamous epithelium; clinical implications of multicentric origin. *Cancer.* 1953;6(5):963–968.

7. Mukhtar H, et al. Skin cancer chemoprevention. *J Investig Dermatol Symp Proc.* 1996;1(2):209–214.

8. Einspahr LG, et al. Chemoprevention of human skin cancer. *Crit Rev Oncol Hematol.* 2002;41(3):269–285.

9. Boukamp P. Non-melanoma skin cancer: What drives tumor development and progression? *Carcinogenesis.* 2005; 26(10):657–667.

10. Karagas MR. Ocurrence of cutaneous basal cell and squamous cell malignancies among those with a prior history of skin cancer. *J Invest Dermatol.* 1994; 102:10S–13S.

11. O'Shuaghnessy JA, et al. Treatment and prevention of intraepithelial neoplasia: An important target for accelerated new agent development. *Clin Cancer Res.* 2002;8(2):314–346.

12. Schatzkin A, et al. An epidemiologic perspective on biomarkers. *J Intern Med.* 1993;233:75–79.

13. Lippman S, et al. Cancer chemoprevention: Progress and promise. *J Natl Cancer Inst.* 1998;90:1514–1528.

14. Miller SJ, et al. Actinic keratosis, basal cell carcinoma, and squamous cell carcinoma. In: Bolognia JL, Jorizzo JL, Rapini RP, et al., eds. *Dermatology.* Philadelphia, PA: Mosby; 2003:1677–1696.

15. Marks R, et al. The relationship of basal cell carcinomas and squamous cell carcinomas to solar keratoses. *Arch Dermatol.* 1988;124(7):1039–1042.

16. Chen GJ, et al. Clinical diagnosis of actinic keratosis identifies an elderly population at high risk of developing skin cancer. *Dermatol Surg.* 2005;31(1):43–47.

17. Clark WH Jr, et al. Origin of familial malignant melanomas from heritable melanocytic lesions. "The B-K mole syndrome." *Arch Dermatol.* 1978;114(5): 732–738.

18. Lynch HT, et al. Familial atypical multiple mole-melanoma syndrome. *J Med Genet.* 1978;15(5):352–356.

19. Roush GC, et al. Independence of dysplastic nevi from total nevi in determining risk for nonfamilial melanoma. *Prev Med.* 1988;17(3):273–279.

20. Tucker MA, et al. Clinically recognized dysplastic nevi. A central risk factor for cutaneous melanoma. *JAMA.* 1997;277 (18):1439–1444.

21. Lange JR, et al. Melanoma. In: Abeloff MD, et al., eds. *Clinic Oncology.* Philadelphia, PA: Elsevier; 2004:561–588.

22. Naeyaert JM, et al. Clinical practice. Dysplastic nevi. *N Engl J Med.* 2003;349 (23):2233–2240.

23. Langley RGB, et al. Clinical characteristics. In: Balch CM, Houghton AN, Sober AJ, Soong S, eds. *Cutaneous Melanoma.* St. Louis, MO: Quality Medical; 1998:82.

24. Pollock PM, et al. High frequency of BRAF mutations in nevi. *Nat Genet.* 2003;33(1):19–20.

25. Stuttgen G. Zur Lokalbehandlung von Keratosen mit vitamin-A-Saure. *Dermatologica.* 1962;124:65–80.

26. Moon RC, et al. Inhibition of chemical carcinogenesis by retinoids. *J Am Acad Dermatol.* 1982;6(4 pt 2, suppl):809–814.

27. Chu EW, et al. An inhibitory effect of vitamin A on the induction of tumors of forestomach and cervix in the Syrian hamster by carcinogenic polycyclic hydrocarbons. *Cancer Res.* 1965;25(6): 884–895.

28. Lasnitzki I. Reversal of methylcholanthrene-induced changes in mouse prostates *in vitro* by retinoic acid and its analogues. *Br J Cancer.* 1976;34(3): 239–248.

29. Saffioti U, et al. Experimental cancer of the lung: Inhibition by vitamin A of the induction of tracheobronchial squamous metaplasia and squamous cell tumors. *Cancer.* 1967;20:857–864.

30. Kuenzli S, et al. Retinoids. In: Bolognia JL, Jorizzo JL, Rapini RP, et al., eds. *Dermatology.* Philadelphia, PA: Mosby; 2003:1991–2006.

31. Carey BM, et al. Skeletal toxicity with isotretinoin therapy: A clinico-radiological evaluation. *Br J Dermatol.* 1988; 119(5):609–614.

32. Armstrong RB, et al. General and reproductive toxicology of retinoids. In: Sporn MB, Roberts AB, Goodman DS, eds. *The Retinoids: Biology, Chemistry, and Medicine.* New York: Raven; 1994: 558–566.

33. Epstein JH. Chemicals and photocarcinogenesis. *Aust J Dermatol.* 1977;18(2): 57–61.

34. Forbes PD, et al. Enhancement of experimental photocarcinogenesis by topical retinoic acid. *Cancer Lett.* 1979;7 (2–3):85–90.

35. Halliday GM, et al. Topical retinoic acid enhances, and a dark tan protects, from subedemal solar-simulated photocarcinogenesis. *J Invest Dermatol.* 2000;114 (5):923–927.

36. Epstein JH, et al. Inhibition of ultraviolet-induced carcinogenesis by all-*trans* retinoic acid. *J Invest Dermatol.* 1981;76 (3):178–180.

37. Kligman LH, et al. Lack of enhancement of experimental photocarcinogenesis by topical retinoic acid. *Arch Dermatol Res.* 1981;270(4):453–462.

38. Mrass P, et al. Retinoic acid increases the expression of p53 and proapoptotic caspases and sensitizes keratinocytes to apoptosis: A possible explanation for tumor preventive action of retinoids. *Cancer Res.* 2004;64(18): 6542–6548.

39. Epstein JH. Effects of retinoids on ultraviolet-induced carcinogenesis. *J Invest Dermatol.* 1981;77(1):144–146.

40. Conner MJ, et al. Inhibition of ultraviolet-B skin carcinogenesis by all-*trans*-retinoic acid regimens that inhibit ornithine decarboxylase induction. *Cancer Res.* 1983;43(1):171–174.

41. Odom R. Managing actinic keratoses with retinoids. *J Am Acad Dermatol.* 1998;39(2 pt 3):S74–S78.

42. Bercovitch L. Topical chemotherapy of actinic keratoses of the upper extremity with tretinoin and 5-fluorouracil: A double-blind controlled study. *Br J Dermatol.* 1987;116: 549–552.

43. Bollag W, et al. Retinoic acid: Topical treatment of senile or actinic keratoses and basal cell carcinomas. *Agents Action.* 1970;1:172–175.

44. Fisher GJ, et al. Molecular basis of sun-induced premature skin ageing and retinoid antagonism. *Nature.* 1996; 379(6563):335–339.

45. Gilchrest B. Anti-sunshine vitamin A. *Nat Med.* 1999;5(4):376–377.

46. Rook AH, et al. Beneficial effect of low-dose systemic retinoid in combination with topical tretinoin for the treatment and prophylaxis of premalignant and malignant skin lesions in renal transplant recipients. *Transplantation.* 1995; 59(5):714–719.

47. Halpern AC, et al. Effects of topical tretinoin on dysplastic nevi. *J Clin Oncol.* 1994;12(5):1028–1035.

48. Edwards L, et al. The effect of topical tretinoin on dysplastic nevi. A preliminary trial. *Arch Dermatol.* 1990;126(4): 494–499.

49. Meyskens FL, et al. Role of topical tretinoin in melanoma and dysplastic nevi. *J Am Acad Dermatol.* 1986;15: 822–825.

50. Stam-Posthuma JJ, et al. Effect of topical tretinoin under occlusion on atypical naevi. *Melanoma Res.* 1998;8(6): 539–548.

51. Kang S, et al. Assessment of adapalene gel for the treatment of actinic keratoses and lentigines: A randomized trial. *J Am Acad Dermatol.* 2003;49: 83–90.

52. Elder JT, et al. Differential regulation of retinoic acid receptors and binding proteins in human skin. *J Invest Dermatol.* 1992;98:673–679.

53. Weinstein G, et al. Tazarotene gel, a new retinoid, for topical therapy of psoriasis: Vehicle-controlled study of safety, efficacy, and duration of therapeutic effect. *J Am Acad Dermatol.* 1997;37:85–92.

54. Webster GF, et al. A multicenter, double-blind, randomized comparison study of the efficacy and tolerability of once-daily tazarotene 0.1% gel and adapalene 0.1% gel for the treatment of facial acne vulgaris. *Cutis.* 2002;69 (suppl 2):4–11.

55. Peris K, et al. Preliminary observations on the use of topical tazarotene to treat basal-cell carcinoma. *N Engl J Med.* 1999;341:1767–1768.

56. Bardazzi F, et al. A pilot study on the use of topical tazarotene to treat squamous cell carcinoma *in situ*. *J Am Acad Dermatol.* 2005;52(6):1102–1104.

57. Duvic M, et al. Expression of a retinoid-inducible tumor suppressor, tazarotene-inducible gene-3, is decreased in psoriasis and skin cancer. *Clin Cancer Res.* 2000;6(8):3249–3259.

58. Duvic M, et al. Tazarotene-induced gene 3 is suppressed in basal cell carcinomas and reversed *in vivo* by tazarotene application. *J Invest Dermatol.* 2003;121(4):902–909.

59. Orlandi A, et al. Evidence of increased apoptosis and reduced proliferation in basal cell carcinomas treated with tazarotene. *J Invest Dermatol.* 2004;122 (4):1037–1041.

60. So PL, et al. Topical tazarotene chemoprevention reduces basal cell carcinoma number and size in PTCH1+/- mice exposed to ultraviolet or ionizing radiation. *Cancer Res.* 2004;64(13):4385–4389.

61. Bianchi L, et al. Topical treatment of basal cell carcinoma with tazarotene: A clinicopathological study on a large series of cases. *Br J Dermatol.* 2004; 151(1):148–156.

62. Kligman AM. Guidelines for the use of topical tretinoin (Retin-A) for photoaged skin. *J Am Acad Dermatol.* 1989;21(3 pt 2):650–654.

63. Rosenthal DS, et al. Changes in photoaged human skin following topical application of all-*trans* retinoic acid. *J Invest Dermatol.* 1990;95(5):510–515.

64. Weiss JS, et al. Tretinoin treatment of photodamaged skin. Cosmesis through medical therapy. *Dermatol Clin.* 1991; 9(1):123–129.

65. Kang S, et al. Tazarotene cream for the treatment of facial photodamage: A multicenter, investigator-masked, randomized, vehicle-controlled, parallel comparison of 0.01%, 0.025%, 0.05%, and 0.1% tazarotene creams with 0.05% tretinoin emollient cream applied once daily for 24 weeks. *Arch Dermatol.* 2001;137(12):1597–1604.

66. Phillips TJ, et al. Efficacy of 0.1% tazarotene cream for the treatment of photodamage: A 12-month multicenter, randomized trial. *Arch Dermatol.* 2002;138(11):1486–1493.

67. Kraemer KH, et al. Xeroderma pigmentosum. Cutaneous, ocular, and neurologic abnormalities in 830 published cases. *Arch Dermatol.* 1987;123:241–250.

68. Hawk JLM, et al. Photodermatoses. In: Bolognia JL, Jorizzo JL, Rapini RP, et al., eds. *Dermatology.* Philadelphia, PA: Mosby; 2003:1365–1384.

69. Moriwaki S, et al. Xeroderma pigmentosum—bridging a gap between clinic and laboratory. *Photodermatol Photoimmunol Photomed.* 2001;17(2):47–54.

70. Kraemer KH, et al. Prevention of skin cancer in xeroderma pigmentosum with the use of oral isotretinoin. *N Engl J Med.* 1988;318(25):1633–1637.

71. Berth-Jones J, et al. Xeroderma pigmentosum variant: Response to etretinate. *Br J Dermatol.* 1990;122(4):559–561.

72. Finkelstein E, et al. Treatment of xeroderma pigmentosum variant with low-dose etretinate. *Br J Dermatol.* 1996;134 (4):815–816.

73. Berth-Jones J, et al. Xeroderma pigmentosum variant: 5 years of tumour suppression by etretinate. *J R Soc Med.* 1993;86(6):355–356.

74. Orengo I, et al. Cutaneous neoplasia in organ transplant recipients. *Curr Probl Dermatol.* 1999;11:123–158.

75. Ong CS, et al. Skin cancer in Australian heart transplant recipients. *J Am Acad Dermatol.* 1999;40(1):27–34.

76. Bellman BA, et al. Low dose isotretinoin in the prophylaxis of skin cancer in renal transplant patients. *Transplantation.* 1996;61(1):173.

77. Shuttleworth D, et al. Treatment of cutaneous neoplasia with etretinate in renal transplant recipients. *Q J Med.* 1988;68(257):717–725.

78. Kelly JW, et al. Retinoids to prevent skin cancer in organ transplant recipients. *Lancet.* 1991;338(8779):1407.

79. Vandeghinste N, et al. Acitretin as cancer chemoprophylaxis in a renal transplant recipient. *Dermatology.* 1992;185 (4):307–308.

80. Bouwes Bavinck JN, et al. Prevention of skin cancer and reduction of keratotic skin lesions during acitretin therapy in renal transplant recipients: A double-blind, placebo-controlled study. *J Clin Oncol.* 1995;13:1933–1938.

81. McKenna DB, et al. Skin cancer chemoprophylaxis in renal transplant recipients: 5 years of experience using low-dose acitretin. *Br J Dermatol.* 1999; 140:656–660.

82. McNamara IR, et al. Acitretin for prophylaxis of cutaneous malignancies after cardiac transplantation. *J Heart Lung Transplant.* 2002;21:1201–1205.

83. George R, et al. Acitretin for chemoprevention of non-melanoma skin cancers in renal transplant recipients. *Aust J Dermatol.* 2002;43:269–273.

84. De Sevaux RG, et al. Acitretin treatment of premalignant and malignant skin disorders in renal transplant recipients: Clinical effects of a randomized trial comparing two doses of acitretin. *J Am Acad Dermatol.* 2003;49: 407–412.

85. Stern RS, et al. Cutaneaous squamous-cell carcinoma in patients treated with PUVA. *N Engl J Med.* 1984;310:1156–1161.

86. Stern RS, et al. The carcinogenic risk of treatments for severe psoriasis. *Cancer.* 1994;73:2759–2764.

87. Stern RS, et al. Oral psoralen and ultraviolet-A light (PUVA) treatment of psoriasis and persistent risk of nonmelanoma skin cancer: PUVA follow-up study. *J Natl Cancer Inst.* 1998;90: 1278–1284.

88. Lindelof B, et al. PUVA and cancer: A large-scale epidemiological study. *Lancet.* 1991;338:91–93.

89. Lever LR, et al. Skin cancer or premalignant lesions occur in half of high-dose PUVA patients. *Br J Dermatol.* 1994; 131:215–219.

90. Nijsten TE, et al. Oral retinoid use reduces cutaneous squamous cell carcinoma risk in patients with psoriasis treated with psoralen-UVA: A nested cohort study. *J Am Acad Dermatol.* 2003;49(4):644–650.

91. Cristofolini M, et al. Aromatic retinoid in the chemoprevention of the progression of nevoid basal-cell carcinoma syndrome. *J Dermatol Surg Oncol.* 1984;10(10):778–781.

92. Hodak E, et al. Etretinate treatment of the nevoid basal cell carcinoma syndrome. Therapeutic and chemopreventive effect. *Int J Dermatol.* 1987;26(9): 606–609.

93. Goldberg LH, et al. Effectiveness of isotretinoin in preventing the appearance of basal cell carcinomas in basal cell nevus syndrome. *J Am Acad Dermatol.* 1989;21(1):144–145.

94. Goldman L. The response of skin cancer to topical therapy with 5-fluorouracil. *Cancer Chemother Rep.* 1963;28:49–52.

95. Dillaha CJ, et al. Selective cytotoxic effect of topical 5-fluorouracil. *Arch Dermatol.* 1963;88:247–256.

96. Dillaha CJ, et al. Further studies with topical 5-fluorouracil. *Arch Dermatol.* 1965;92(4):410–417.

97. Neldner KH. Prevention of skin cancer with topical 5-fluorouracil. *Rocky Mt Med J.* 1966;63(11):74–78.

98. Sturm HM, et al. Treatment of actinic keratoses with topical 5-fluorouracil. *J Med Assoc Ga.* 1968;57(5):205–209.

99. Williams AC, et al. Experiences with local chemotherapy and immunotherapy in premalignant and malignant skin lesions. *Cancer.* 1970;25(2):450–462.

100. Kestel J Jr. Treatment of actinic keratosis. *Arch Dermatol.* 1970;102(3):351.

101. Spira M, et al. Clinical comparison of chemical peeling dermabrasion, and 5-FU for senile keratoses. *Plast Reconstr Surg.* 1970;46(1):61–66.

102. Farah FS, et al. The treatment of premalignant and malignant skin lesions with 5-fluorouracil. *J Med Liban.* 1971;24(1): 45–51.

103. Loven K, et al. Evaluation of the efficacy and tolerability of 0.5% fluorouracil cream and 5% fluorouracil cream applied to each side of the face in patients with actinic keratosis. *Clin Ther.* 2002;24(6):990–1000.

104. Weiss J, et al. Effective treatment of actinic keratosis with 0.5% fluorouracil cream for 1, 2, or 4 weeks. *Cutis.* 2002;70(suppl 2):22–29.

105. Sauder DN. Imiquimod: Modes of action. *Br J Dermatol.* 2003;149(suppl 66):5–8.

106. Beutner KR, et al. Therapeutic response of basal cell carcinoma to the immune response modifier imiquimod 5% cream. *J Am Acad Dermatol.* 1999;41: 1002–1007.

107. Stockfleth E, et al. Successful treatment of actinic keratosis with imiquimod cream 5%: A report of six cases. *Br J Dermatol.* 2001;144(5):1050–1053.

108. Korman N, et al. Dosing with 5% imiquimod cream 3 times per week for the treatment of actinic keratosis: Results of two phase 3, randomized, double-blind, parallel-group, vehicle-controlled trials. *Arch Dermatol.* 2005; 141(4):467–473.

109. Szeimies R-M, et al. Imiquimod 5% cream for the treatment of actinic keratosis: Results from a phase III, randomized, double-blind, vehicle-controlled, clinical trial with histology. *J Am Acad Dermatol.* 2004;51(4):547–555.

110. Lebwohl M, et al. Imiquimod 5% cream for the treatment of actinic keratosis: Results from two phase III, randomized, double-blind, parallel group, vehicle-controlled trials. *J Am Acad Dermatol.* 2004;50(5):714–721.

111. Lee PK, et al. Long-term clinical outcomes following treatment of actinic keratosis with imiquimod 5% cream. *Dermatol Surg.* 2005;31(6):659–664.

112. Weisberg NK, et al. Therapeutic response of a brother and sister with xeroderma pigmentosum to imiquimod

5% cream. *Dermatol Surg.* 2002;28:518–523.

113. Nijsten T, et al. A patient with xeroderma pigmentosum treated with imiquimod 5% cream. *J Am Acad Dermatol.* 2005;52(1):170–171.

114. Tope WD, et al. Photodynamic therapy. In: Bolognia JL, Jorizzo JL, Rapini RP, et al., eds. *Dermatology.* Philadelphia, PA: Mosby; 2003:2127–2142.

115. Fuchs J, et al. The role of oxygen in cutaneous photodynamic therapy. *Free Radic Biol Med.* 1998;24:835–847.

116. Liu Y, et al. Multiple large-surface photodynamic therapy sessions with topical or systemic aminolevulinic acid and blue light in UV-exposed hairless mice. *J Cutan Med Surg.* 2004;8(2):131–139.

117. Wolf P, et al. Topical photodynamic therapy with endogenous porphyrins after application of 5-aminolevulinic acid. An alternative treatment modality for solar keratoses, superficial squamous cell carcinomas, and basal cell carcinomas? *J Am Acad Dermatol.* 1993;28(1):17–21.

118. Fijan S, et al. Photodynamic therapy of epithelial skin tumours using delta-aminolaevulinic acid and desferrioxamine. *Br J Dermatol.* 1995;133(2):282–288.

119. Calzavara-Pinton PG. Repetitive photodynamic therapy with topical delta-aminolaevulinic acid as an appropriate approach to the routine treatment of superficial non-melanoma skin tumours. *J Photochem Photobiol B.* 1995;29(1):53–57.

120. Szeimies RM, et al. Photodynamic therapy with topical application of 5-aminolevulinic acid in the treatment of actinic keratoses: An initial clinical study. *Dermatology.* 1996;192(3):246–251.

121. Jeffes EW, et al. Photodynamic therapy of actinic keratosis with topical 5-aminolevulinic acid. A pilot dose-ranging study. *Arch Dermatol.* 1997;133(6):727–732.

122. Varma S, et al. Bowen's disease, solar keratoses and superficial basal cell carcinomas treated by photodynamic therapy using a large-field incoherent light source. *Br J Dermatol.* 2001;144(3):567–574.

123. Szeimies RM, et al. Photodynamic therapy using topical methyl 5-aminolevulinate compared with cryotherapy for actinic keratosis: A prospective, randomized study. *J Am Acad Dermatol.* 2002;47(2):258–262.

124. Touma D, et al. A trial of short incubation, broad-area photodynamic therapy for facial actinic keratoses and diffuse photodamage. *Arch Dermatol.* 2004;140(1):33–40.

125. Picquadio DJ, et al. Photodynamic therapy with aminolevulinic acid topical solution and visible blue light in the treatment of multiple actinic keratoses of the face and scalp: Investigator-blinded, phase 3, multicenter trials. *Arch Dermatol.* 2004;140(1):41–46.

126. Kurwa HA, et al. A randomized paired comparison of photodynamic therapy and topical 5-fluorouracil in the treatment of actinic keratoses. *J Am Acad Dermatol.* 1999;41(3 pt 1):414–418.

127. Marmur E, et al. A review of laser and photodynamic therapy for the treatment of nonmelanoma skin cancer. *Dermatol Surg.* 2004;30(2 pt 2):264–271.

128. Szeimies R-M, et al. Photodynamic therapy for non-melanoma skin cancer. *Acta Derm Venereol.* 2005;85(6):483–490.

129. Itkin A, et al. Delta-aminolevulinic acid and blue light photodynamic therapy for treatment of multiple basal cell carcinomas in two patients with nevoid basal cell carcinoma syndrome. *Dermatol Surg.* 2004;30(7):1054–1061.

130. Oseroff AR, et al. Treatment of diffuse basal cell carcinomas and basaloid follicular hamartomas in nevoid basal cell carcinoma syndrome by wide-area 5-aminolevulinic acid photodynamic therapy. *Arch Dermatol.* 2005;141(1):60–67.

131. de Graff YM, et al. Photodynamic therapy does not prevent cutaneous squamous-cell carcinoma in organ-transplant recipients: Results of a randomized-controlled trial. *J Invest Dermatol.* 2006;126:569–574.

132. Bollag W, et al. Vitamin A acid in benign and malignant epithelial tumours of the skin. *Acta Derm Venereol Suppl (Stockh).* 1975;74:163–166.

133. Vane JR. Inhibition of prostaglandin synthesis as a mechanism of action for aspirin-like drugs. *Nat New Biol.* 1971;231:232–235.

134. Buckman SY, et al. COX-2 expression is induced by UVB exposure in human skin: Implications for the development of skin cancer. *Carcinogenesis.* 1998;19(5):723–729.

135. Mahns A, et al. Contribution of UVB and UVA to UV-dependent stimulation of cyclooxygenase-2 expression in artificial epidermis. *Photochem Photobiol Sci.* 2004;3(3):257–262.

136. Grewe M, et al. Analysis of the mechanism of ultraviolet (UV) B radiation-induced prostaglandin E2 synthesis by human epidermoid carcinoma cells. *J Invest Dermatol.* 1993;101(4):528–531.

137. Vanderveen EE, et al. Arachidonic acid metabolites in cutaneous carcinomas. *Arch Dermatol.* 1986;122:407–412.

138. Klapan I. Prognostic significance of plasma prostaglandin E concentration in patients with head and neck cancer. *J Cancer Res Clin Oncol.* 1986;118:308–313.

139. Fischer S, et al. Chemopreventive activity of celecoxib, a specific cyclooxygenase-2 inhibitor, and indomethacin against ultraviolet light-induced skin carcinogenesis. *Mol Carcinog.* 1999;25(4):231–240.

140. Pentland AP, et al. Reduction of UV-induced skin tumors in hairless mice by selective COX-2 inhibition. *Carcinogenesis.* 1999;20(10):1939–1944.

141. Wilgus TA, et al. Inhibition of cutaneous ultraviolet light B-mediated inflammation and tumor formation with topical celecoxib treatment. *Mol Carcinog.* 2003;38(2):49–58.

142. Wilgus TA, et al. Chemotherapeutic efficacy of topical celecoxib in a murine model of ultraviolet light B-induced skin cancer. *Mol Carcinog.* 2003;38(1):33–39.

143. Wilgus TA, et al. Treatment with 5-fluorouracil and celecoxib displays synergistic regression of ultraviolet light B-induced skin tumors. *J Invest Dermatol.* 2004;122(6):1488–1494.

144. Gupta RA, et al. Aspirin, NSAIDS, and colon cancer prevention: Mechanisms? *Gastroenterology.* 1998;114(5):1095–1098.

145. Bair WB III, et al. Inhibitory effects of sodium salicylate and acetylsalicylic acid on UVB-induced mouse skin carcinogenesis. *Cancer Epidemiol Biomarkers Prev.* 2002;11(12):1645–1652.

146. Wolf JE Jr, et al. Topical 3.0% diclofenac in 2.5% hyaluronan gel in the treatment of actinic keratoses. *Int J Dermatol.* 2001;40(11):709–713.

147. Rivers JK, et al. Topical treatment of actinic keratoseswith 3.0% diclofenac in 2.5% hyaluronan gel. *Br J Dermatol.* 2002;146(1):94–100.

148. Rivers JK, et al. An open study to assess the efficacy and safety of topical 3% diclofenac in a 2.5% hyaluronic acid gel for the treatment of actinic keratoses. *Arch Dermatol.* 1997;133:1239–1242.

149. Butler GJ, et al. Nonsteroidal anti-inflammatory drugs and the risk of actinic keratoses and squamous cell cancers of the skin. *J Am Acad Dermatol.* 2005;53(6):966–972.

150. Baigent C, et al. Efficacy and safety of cholesterol-lowering treatment: Prospective meta-analysis of data from 90,056 participants in 14 randomised trials of statins. *Lancet.* 2005;366(9493):1267–1278.

151. Thibault A, et al. Phase I study of lovastatin, an inhibitor of the mevalonate pathway, in patients with cancer. *Clin Cancer Res.* 1996;2:483–491.

152. Dimitroulakos J, et al. Differential sensitivity of various pediatric cancers and squamous cell carcinomas to lovastatin-induced apoptosis: Therapeutic implications. *Clin Cancer Res.* 2001;7(1):158–167.

153. Demierre MF, et al. Statins and cancer prevention. *Nat Rev Cancer.* 2005;5(12):930–942.

154. Graaf MR, et al. The risk of cancer in users of statins. *J Clin Oncol.* 2004;22:2388–2394.

155. Dale KM, et al. Statins and cancer risk: A meta-analysis. *JAMA.* 2006;295(1):74–80.

156. Dellavalle R, et al. Statins and fibrates for preventing melanoma. *Cochrane Database Syst Rev.* 2005;4:CD003697.

157. Sleijfer S, et al. The potential of statins as part of anti-cancer treatment. *Eur J Cancer.* 2005;41(4):516–522.

158. Shellman YG, et al. Lovastatin-induced apoptosis in human melanoma cell lines. *Melanoma Res.* 2005;15:83–89.

159. Collisson EA, et al. Atorvastatin prevents RhoC isoprenylation, invasion, and metastasis in human melanoma cells. *Mol Cancer Ther.* 2003;2(10):941–948.

160. Taylor PR, et al. Nutritional interventions in cancer prevention. *J Clin Oncol.* 2005;23(2):333–345.

161. Greenberg ER, et al. A clinical trial of beta-carotene to prevent basal-cell and squamous-cell cancers of the skin. The Skin Cancer Prevention Study Group. *N Engl J Med.* 1990;323(12):789–795. Erratum in: *N Engl J Med.* 1991;325(18):1324.

162. Green A, et al. Daily sunscreen application and beta-carotene supplementation in prevention of basal-cell and squamous-cell carcinomas of the skin: A randomised controlled trial. *Lancet.* 1999;54(9180):723–729. Erratum in: *Lancet.* 1999;354(9183):1038.

163. Fung TT, et al. Vitamin and carotenoid intake and risk of squamous cell carcinoma of the skin. *Int J Cancer.* 2003;103(1):110–115.

164. Fung TT, et al. Vitamins and carotenoids intake and the risk of basal cell carcinoma of the skin in women (United States). *Cancer Causes Control.* 2002;13(3):221–230.

165. Frieling UM, et al. A randomized, 12-year primary-prevention trial of beta-carotene supplementation for nonmelanoma skin cancer in the physician's health study. *Arch Dermatol.* 2000;136(2):179–184.

166. Schaumberg DA, et al. No effect of beta-carotene supplementation on risk of nonmelanoma skin cancer among men with low baseline plasma beta-carotene. *Cancer Epidemiol Biomarkers Prev.* 2004;13(6):1079–1080.

167. Wald N, et al. Low serum-vitamin-A and subsequent risk of cancer. Preliminary results of a prospective study. *Lancet.* 1980;2(8199):813–815.

168. Wald N, et al. Serum retinol and subsequent risk of cancer. *Br J Cancer.* 1986;54(6):957–961.

169. Kune GA, et al. Diet, alcohol, smoking, serum beta-carotene, and vitamin A in male nonmelanocytic skin cancer patients and controls. *Nutr Cancer.* 1992;18(3):237–244.

170. Wei Q, et al. Vitamin supplementation and reduced risk of basal cell carcinoma. *J Clin Epidemiol.* 1994;47(8):829–836.

171. Van Dam RM, et al. Diet and basal cell carcinoma of the skin in a prospective cohort of men. *Am J Clin Nutr.* 2000;71(1):135–141.

172. Davies TW, et al. Diet and basal cell skin cancer: Results from the EPIC-Norfolk cohort. *Br J Dermatol.* 2002;146(6):1017–1022.

173. McNaughton SA, et al. Antioxidants and basal cell carcinoma of the skin: A nested case-control study. *Cancer Causes Control.* 2005;16(5):609–618.

174. Moon TE, et al. Effect of retinol in preventing squamous cell skin cancer in moderate-risk subjects: A randomized, double-blind, controlled trial. Southwest Skin Cancer Prevention Study Group. *Cancer Epidemiol Biomarkers Prev.* 1997;6(11):949–956.

175. Levine N, et al. Trial of retinol and isotretinoin in skin cancer prevention: A randomized, double-blind, controlled trial. Southwest Skin Cancer Prevention Study Group. *Cancer Epidemiol Biomarkers Prev.* 1997;6(11):957–961.

176. Anolik JH, et al. Effect of isotretinoin therapy on natural killer cell activity in patients with xeroderma pigmentosum. *Br J Dermatol.* 1998;138(2):236–241.

177. Anstey AV, et al. Systemic photoprotection with alpha-tocopherol (vitamin E) and beta-carotene. *Clin Exp Dermatol.* 2002;27(3):170–176.

178. Cook MG, et al. Effect of dietary vitamin E on dimethylhydrazine-induced colonic tumors in mice. *Cancer Res.* 1980;40(4):1329–1331.

179. Wald NJ, et al. Serum vitamin E and subsequent risk of cancer. *Br J Cancer.* 1987;56:69–72.

180. Comstock GW, et al. Prediagnostic serum levels of carotenoids and vitamin E as related to subsequent cancer in Washington County Maryland. *Am J Clin Nutr.* 1991;53(suppl 1):260S–264S.

181. Breslow RA, et al. Serological precursors of cancer: Malignant melanoma, basal and squamous cell skin cancer, and prediagnostic levels of retinol, beta-carotene, lycopene, alpha-tocopherol, and selenium. *Cancer Epidemiol Biomarkers Prev.* 1995;4(8):837–842.

182. Karagas MR, et al. Risk of squamous cell carcinoma of the skin in relation to plasma selenium, alpha-tocopherol, beta-carotene, and retinol: A nested case-control study. *Cancer Epidemiol Biomarkers Prev.* 1997;6(1):25–29.

183. Dorgan JF, et al. Serum carotenoids and alpha-tocopherol and risk of non-melanoma skin cancer. *Cancer Epidemiol Biomarkers Prev.* 2004;13(8):1276–1282.

184. Hunter DJ, et al. Diet and risk of basal cell carcinoma of the skin in a prospective cohort of women. *Ann Epidemiol.* 1992;2(3):231–239.

185. Bisset DL, et al. Photoprotective effect of superoxide scavenging antioxidants against ultraviolet radiation-induced chronic skin damage in the hairless mouse. *Photodermatol Photoimmunol Photomed.* 1990;7:56–62.

186. Gensler HL, et al. Topical vitamin E inhibition of immunosuppression and tumorigenesis induced by ultraviolet irradiation. *Nutr Cancer.* 1991;15(2):97–106.

187. Record IR, et al. The influence of topical and systemic vitamin E on ultraviolet light-induced skin damage in hairless mice. *Nutr Cancer.* 1991;16(3–4):219–225.

188. McVean M, et al. Inhibition of UVB-induced DNA photodamage in mouse epidermis by topically applied alpha-tocopherol. *Carcinogenesis.* 1997;18(8):1617–1622.

189. Berton TR, et al. The effect of vitamin E acetate on ultraviolet-induced mouse skin carcinogenesis. *Mol Carcinog.* 1998;23(3):175–184.

190. Burke KE, et al. Effects of topical and oral vitamin E on pigmentation and skin cancer induced by ultraviolet irradiation in Skh:2 hairless mice. *Nutr Cancer.* 2000;38(1):87–97.

191. Gerrish KE, et al. Prevention of photocarcinogenesis by dietary vitamin E. *Nutr Cancer.* 1993;19(2):125–133.

192. Kuchide M, et al. Cancer chemopreventive effects of oral feeding alpha-tocopherol on ultraviolet light B induced photocarcinogenesis of hairless mouse. *Cancer Lett.* 2003;196(2):169–177.

193. Potapenko AY, et al. PUVA-induced erythema and changes in mechanoelectrical properties of skin. Inhibition by tocopherols. *Arch Dermatol Res.* 1984;276(1):12–16.

194. Werninghaus K, et al. Evaluation of the photoprotective effect of oral vitamin E supplementation. *Arch Dermatol.* 1994;130(10):1257–1261.

195. Lin JY, et al. UV photoprotection by combination topical antioxidants vitamin C and vitamin E. *J Am Acad Dermatol.* 2003;48(6):866–874.

196. Thiele JJ, et al. Vitamin E: Critical review of its current use in cosmetic and clinical dermatology. *Dermatol Surg.* 2005;31(7 pt 2):805–813.

197. Pinnell SR. Cutaneous photodamage, oxidative stress, and topical antioxidant protection. *J Am Acad Dermatol.* 2003;48(1):1–19.

198. Darr D, et al. Topical vitamin C protects porcine skin from ultraviolet radiation-induced damage. *Br J Dermatol.* 1992;127(3):247–253.

199. Darr D, et al. Effectiveness of antioxidants (vitamin C and E) with and without sunscreens as topical photoprotectants. *Acta Derm Venereol.* 1996;76(4):264–268.

200. Murray J, et al. Topical vitamin C treatment reduces ultraviolet B radiation-induced erythema in human skin [abstract]. *J Invest Dermatol.* 1991;96:587.

201. Placzek M, et al. Ultraviolet B-induced DNA damage in human epidermis is modified by the antioxidants ascorbic acid and D-alpha-tocopherol. *J Invest Dermatol.* 2005;124(2):304–307.

202. Pinnell SR, et al. Topical L-ascorbic acid: Percutaneous absorption studies. *Dermatol Surg.* 2001;27(2):137–142.

203. Lin FH, et al. Ferulic acid stabilizes a solution of vitamins C and E and doubles its photoprotection of skin. *J Invest Dermatol.* 2005;125(4):826–832.

204. Willett WC, et al. Prediagnostic serum selenium and risk of cancer. *Lancet.* 1983;2(8342):130–134.

205. Salonen JT, et al. Association between serum selenium and the risk of cancer. *Am J Epidemiol.* 1984;120(3):342–349.

206. Salonen JT, et al. Risk of cancer in relation to serum concentrations of selenium and vitamins A and E: Matched case-control analysis of prospective data. *Br Med J.* 1985;290(6466):417–420.

207. Virtamo J, et al. Serum selenium and risk of cancer. A prospective follow-up of nine years. *Cancer.* 1987;60(2):145–148.

208. Sahl WJ, et al. Basal cell carcinoma and lifestyle characteristics. *Int J Dermatol.* 1995;34(6):398–402.

209. Overad K, et al. Selenium inhibits UV-light-induced skin carcinogenesis in hairless mice. *Cancer Lett.* 1985;27(2):163–170.

210. Burke KE, et al. The effects of topical and oral L-selenomethionine on pigmentation and skin cancer induced by ultraviolet irradiation. *Nutr Cancer.* 1992;17(2):123–137.

211. Pence BC, et al. Effects of dietary selenium on UVB-induced skin carcinogenesis and epidermal antioxidant status. *J Invest Dermatol.* 1994;102(5):759–761.

212. Yang CS, et al. Inhibition of carcinogenesis by tea. *Annu Rev Pharmacol Toxicol.* 2002;42:25–54.

213. F'guyer S, et al. Photochemoprevention of skin cancer by botanical agents. *Photodermatol Photoimmunol Photomed.* 2003;19(2):56–72.

214. Barthelman M, et al. (-)-Epigallocatechin-3-gallate inhibition of ultraviolet B-induced AP-1 activity. *Carcinogenesis.* 1998;19(12):2201–2204.

215. Afaq F, et al. Inhibition of ultraviolet B-mediated activation of nuclear factor kappaB in normal human epidermal keratinocytes by green tea constituent (−)-epigallocatechin-3-gallate. *Oncogene.* 2003;22(7):1035–1044.

216. Xia J, et al. UV-induced NF-kappaB activation and expression of IL-6 is attenuated by (-)-epigallocatechin-3-gallate in cultured human keratinocytes *in vitro*. *Int J Mol Med*. 2005;16(5):943–950.

217. Kim HS, et al. EGCG blocks tumor promoter-induced MMP-9 expression via suppression of MAPK and AP-1 activation in human gastric AGS cells. *Anticancer Res*. 2004;24(2B):747–753.

218. Nihal M, et al. Anti-proliferative and proapoptotic effects of (-)-epigallocatechin-3-gallate on human melanoma: Possible implications for the chemoprevention of melanoma. *Int J Cancer*. 2005;114(4):513–521.

219. Rodriguez SK, et al. Green tea catechin, epigallocatechin-3-gallate, inhibits vascular endothelial growth factor angiogenic signaling by disrupting the formation of a receptor complex. *Int J Cancer*. 2005;118(7):1635–1644.

220. Wang ZY, et al. Protection against ultraviolet B radiation-induced photocarcinogenesis in hairless mice by green tea polyphenols. *Carcinogenesis*. 1991;12(8):1527–1530.

221. Gensler HL, et al. Prevention of photocarcinogenesis by topical administration of pure epigallocatechin gallate isolated from green tea. *Nutr Cancer*. 1996;26(3):325–335.

222. Lu Y-P, et al. Inhibitory effect of black tea on the growth of established skin tumors in mice: Effects on tumor size, apoptosis, mitosis, and bromodeoxyuridine incorporation into DNA. *Carcinogenesis*. 1997;18(11):2163–2169.

223. Huang M-T, et al. Effects of tea, decaffeinated tea, and caffeine on UVB light-induced complete carcinogenesis in SKH-1 mice: Demonstration of caffeine as a biologically important constituent of tea. *Cancer Res*. 1997;57(13):2623–2629.

224. Lou Y-R, et al. Effects of oral administration of tea, decaffeinated tea, and caffeine on the formation and growth of tumors in high-risk SKH-1 mice previously treated with ultraviolet B light. *Nutr Cancer*. 1999;33(2):146–153.

225. Record IR, et al. Protection by black tea and green tea against UVB and UVA + B induced skin cancer in hairless mice. *Mutat Res*. 1998;422(1):191–199.

226. Katiyar SK, et al. Green tea polyphenol treatment to human skin prevents formation of ultraviolet light B-induced pyrimidine dimers in DNA. *Clin Cancer Res*. 2000;6(10):3864–3869.

227. Zhao JF, et al. Green tea protects against psoralen plus ultraviolet A-induced photochemical damage to skin. *J Invest Dermatol*. 1999;113(6):1070–1075.

228. Elmets CA, et al. Cutaneous photoprotection from ultraviolet injury by green tea polyphenols. *J Am Acad Dermatol*. 2001;44(3):425–432.

CHAPTER 54

Natural Ingredients and Biomolecules for the Treatment of Skin Cancer

Niven R. Narain
Indushekhar Persaud, M.D.
Caroline V. Caperton, M.S.P.H.
Sung L. Hsia, M.D.

BOX 54-1   Overview

- Skin cancer (BCC, SCC, and melanoma) is the most commonly occurring human cancer.
- Current treatment modalities are fairly effective but unfortunately, recurrence may occur and sometimes involve unsightly scarring.
- The use of biomolecules and natural ingredients has gained interest in the past 10 years while showing promise in pre-clinical experimental models.
- Coenzyme Q10 has been shown to induce apoptosis and effect gene/protein regulation in skin cancer cells while presenting no harm to normal skin cells. In addition, attenuation in angiogenesis has been observed in tumor histology.
- Both oral and topical administration of the green tea extract, ECGC has been shown to inhibit NF-κB without harming normal cells.
- Red wine polyphenols have shown to be effective in inhibiting VEGF, thus decreasing angiogenesis while scavenging free radicals that increase oncogencity.
- Vitamin D receptors exist in melanoma cells making it possible for treatment in combination with other anticancer drugs to inhibit cell proliferation.

INTRODUCTION

Taken together, skin cancers (melanoma, basal cell carcinoma (BCC), squamous cell carcinoma (SCC)) are the most commonly occurring human cancer. They adversely affect the quality of life of individuals afflicted with various forms of the disease. Current interventions are effective at treating skin cancers, depending on the stage at diagnosis. Cure rates for treating nonmelanoma skin cancer vary. For example, elec-trodesiccation and curettage, though widely used, are not used for treating melanoma due to their recurrence rates. Mohs micrographic surgery or excision with frozen-section margin control is an excellent option for most nonmelanoma skin cancers, but the cost of these procedures are high.

Systemic or local application of natural therapies has been investigated. Among these, coenzyme Q10, green tea cate-chins, red wine and grape seed polyphe-nols, and vitamin D derivatives have gen-erated significant interest. With an ever-increasing patient population inter-ested in more natural ingredients and complementary medicine approaches to the management of health conditions, open-minded attention toward, and evi-dence-based research involving these therapies is warranted as an adjunct to and possible replacement for manage-ment of skin cancer.

Cancer is a multifactorial disease that forms when all the precipitating elements of oncogenesis reach intracellular consen-sus. Thus, it must be borne in mind that the global approach to mechanistic stud-ies in cancer may involve and is not lim-ited to phenomena that coalesce

1. to negatively modulate the growth arrest capability of a cell;
2. to adversely affect the efficacy of immune surveillance;
3. to enhance angiogenic bridges that facilitate tumor metabolism;
4. to mitigate membrane signals that allow for information trafficking;
5. cell–cell interactions.

COENZYME Q10 (COQ10)

BOX 54-2   Summary

- Coenzyme Q10 (CoQ10) is a vital compo-nent of the mitochondrial electron trans-port chain in the production of ATP, provid-ing energy in 95% of the cells of the body. It is a potent antioxidant and stabilizes biological membranes.
- CoQ10 selectively downregulates the anti-apoptotic factor bcl-2 in cancer cells while leaving normal cells intact. In addition, attenuation in the organization and integrity of tumor microvasculature is observed.
- Novel liposome-based transdermal deliv-ery modalities allow delivery of CoQ10 directly to the point of interest with increased local bioavailability.

Coenzyme Q10 (CoQ10), also known as ubiquinone, was discovered by Dr. Frederick Crane at the University of Wisconsin in 1957.[1] Q10 is a natural compound produced and found in every human cell. A coenzyme is a substance required for the proper functioning of an enzyme, which is a protein that acceler-ates the rate of chemical reactions within a cell. Q10 is essential for the cel-lular production of energy in the form of adenosine triphosphate (ATP) of which 95% is produced within the mitochon-dria of cells. As such, Q10 is critical for adequate energy production. In addi-tion, Q10 functions as a cellular antioxi-dant protecting cells from free radicals, highly reactive molecules that can dam-age vital intracellular structures such as deoxyribonucleic acid (DNA) (Fig. 54-1).

The average diet alone provides approximately 2 to 5 mg of Q10 per day with relatively small amounts coming mainly from beef heart, pork, chicken liver, fish, peanuts, and broccoli. In addi-tion, aging and illness deplete cellular storage supplies of Q10. Recently, nutri-tionists have advocated the ingestion of supplemental Q10 for enhanced energy production in the form of oral gels, cap-sules, or tablets. Research studies have shown potential health benefits from the consumption of high levels of Q10. Decreased serum levels of Q10 have been reported in patients with cancer, congestive heart failure, diabetes melli-tus, periodontal disease, and muscular dystrophy. Subsequently, Q10 has proven to be effective in the treatment and prevention of cardiomyopathy, con-gestive heart failure, angina pectoris, male infertility, gastric ulcers, cerebellar ataxia, gingivitis, and kidney failure. It is worth noting that supplementation with Q10 has demonstrated clinical improve-ment in cancer patients and those infected with the human immunodefi-ciency virus (HIV).[2-5]

Thus far, supplementation with Q10 has revealed no known side effects, adverse reactions, or pharmacological interaction with other medications. The safety profile of Q10 is well accepted. It is noteworthy that Dr. Clifford W. Shultz conducted a pilot trial at the University of California San Diego, in which patients ingested up to 3000 mg per day with no reported side effects or contraindications.[6]

Despite its widespread use, the inges-tion of oral Q10 is absorbed inade-quately within the gastrointestinal tract

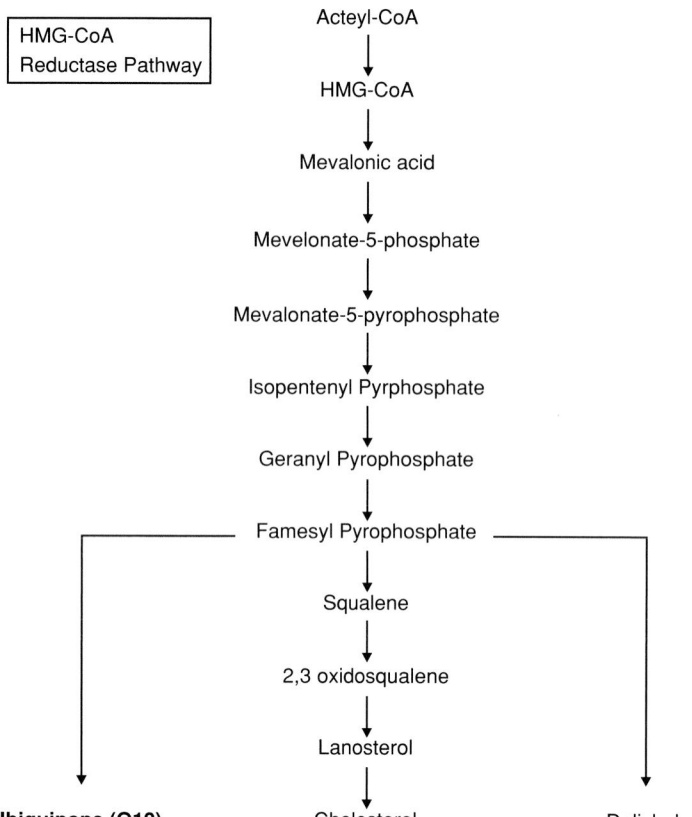

▲ **FIGURE 54-1** HMG-CoA reductase pathway for the synthesis of Coenzyme Q10.

secondary to pancreatic degradation and impaired hepatic metabolism. As a result, the amount of Q10 reaching the mitochondria is greatly diminished.[7] Therefore, a topical application of Q10 would facilitate targeted drug delivery and localized bioavailability.

The National Institutes of Health National Center for Complementary and Alternative Medicine (NCCAM) has designated the molecule as a drug target. In addition, the Food and Drug Administration (FDA) has granted Orphan Drug Status to Q10 for its use in mitochondrial cytopathies. Taken together, the aforementioned and the data obtained establish a solid foundation and rationale to investigate the use of topical Q10 on cutaneous malignancies (Fig. 54-2).

Q10 is a vital component of the mitochondrial electron transport chain in the production of ATP through its function as a mobile electron carrier in the mitochondrial inner membrane.[8] This hallmark theory earned Dr. Peter Mitchell the Nobel Prize in Medicine or Physiology in 1978. It is also a potent antioxidant and free radical scavenger essential to normal cellular metabolism.[9]

Our research data from the Department of Dermatology, University of Miami Miller School of Medicine suggest that exogenous Q10 induces a selective loss of viability on a number of oncogenic cells including melanoma, squamous cell carcinoma, prostate, breast, hepatocellular carcinoma, retinoblastoma, and osteosarcoma, while exerting no adverse effects to keratinocytes, neonatal fibroblasts, and mammary fibroblasts.[10–15]

Microarray analysis has revealed that Q10 modulates bcl-2 gene expression in a manner that supports growth of neonatal fibroblasts while conferring a pro-apoptotic potential to melanoma cells. The "soldier" molecule of cancer, bcl-2, allows cells to grow theoretically *ad infinitum* in addition to conferring resistance to chemotherapeutic intervention. It is located mostly in the outer mitochondrial and ER membranes in proximity to ~65% of Q10 dispersed in a cell. This is of intense significance since ER mediates protein trafficking and mitochondria is the cell's energy driver and gatekeeper of apoptosis. Hence, it is an interesting observation that bcl-2 mediates the anticancer effect of Q10 since the evidence thus far in cancer implicates this protein family as a key player in the sustenance of cancer and resistance to some therapeutic interventions.

Moreover, a significant increase in mitochondrial membrane depolarization was observed in prostate cancer cells through the use of flow cytometry. The topical application of a Q10 cream on a melanoma murine model, reduced tumor size by 55% with a profound disruption and attenuation of vascularity as depicted on histological analysis (Fig. 54-3).[14]

Patients afflicted with cancer often have lower serum levels of Q10.[16–18] Lockwood et al reported cases of tumor regression, decreased tumor recurrence, and an improved quality of life in cancer

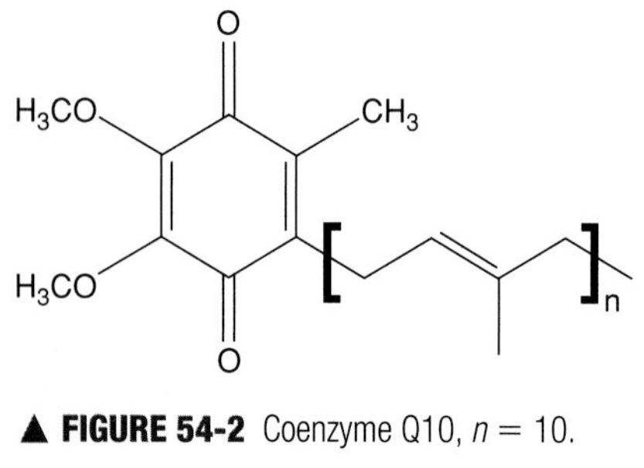

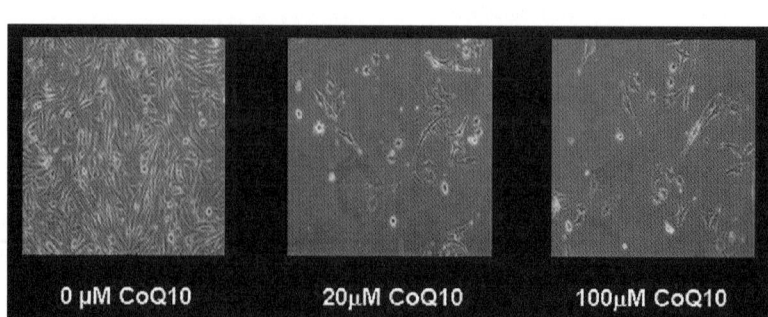

▲ **FIGURE 54-3** *In vitro* study of human melanoma cell. Line SKMEL28 incubated with coenzyme Q10 for 48 hours. Poster presented at the Society for Investigative Dermatology Meeting, St. Louis, MO, 2005. This data is subject of an International Patent (PCT) Application, PCT/US2005/001581 by and for the University of Miami claiming priority to US Patent Application 60/538, 319 and licensed to Pathfinder Management, Inc. Nashville, TN. (Courtesy of Narain et al.)

▲ **FIGURE 54-2** Coenzyme Q10, $n = 10$.

patients treated orally with 390 mg of Q10 daily.[17] Moreover, the ingestion of daily doses of Q10 up to 3000 mg has not produced any known adverse side effects.[19] Experimental data from the University of Miami Transdermal Delivery/Cutaneous Biology Research group have shown that Q10 inhibits the proliferation of SCC and malignant melanoma cell lines (SKMEL28) in a dose dependent manner. In these experiments, at 48 h, 82% inhibition of SCC proliferation and 63% of SKMEL28 cell proliferation was noted.[15]

In contrast, normal cells—neonatal fibroblasts (nFib), mammary fibroblasts (mFib), and keratinocytes (SCKC, HEka, and NIK)—incubated in the presence of Q10 showed a slight increase in growth.[13,15,20] Annexin-VPE apoptosis assay suggested inhibition by Q10 on cancer is via an apoptotic pathway.[15] For example, the amount of apoptotic cells noted in SKMEL28 cell lines was increased nearly five-fold compared with control.

Moreover, the ability of Q10 to selectively induce apoptosis in oncogenic cells while having a slightly supportive effect to nonmalignant cells serves is the rationale for a proposed forthcoming randomized double-blind placebo-controlled Phase I/II study of the safety/efficacy of topical coenzyme Q10 for the treatment of nonmelanoma skin cancer. Previous studies on the efficacy of Q10 have relied mostly on oral routes of administration.[21] However, this oral route is compromised by limited the bioavailability and specificity of Q10. Topical application circumvents this obstacle. In addition, we have suggested implementation of a liposomal formulation, as we believe it is one of the most efficacious vehicles by its incorporation of phospholipids, which is a component of cellular plasma membranes, and mimics physiologic conditions in the integument.[22] Moreover, in vitro and in vivo studies using this formulation suggest that the pro-apoptotic and antiangiogenic effects of Q10 have potential therapeutic benefits for the treatment of cancer.

In conclusion, it is possible that Q10 may "speed-up" the apoptotic rate of basal cell carcinoma by one of several mechanisms including reducing bcl-2 levels as it is the only cancer that exhibits a residual apoptotic potential.[23] In addition, SCC and melanoma may be affected by regulation of cyclin dependent kinases (TyrK/ser/theo/PI3K-akt) or p21/p27 by Q10. Current understanding suggests there may be some interaction or cross talk between bcl-2 and angiogenic factors

such as VEGF, Hif-alpha, and angiostatin-1.[24-26] Q10 is a safe nontoxic molecule that is not thought to induce an immune response based on the fact that it is a constituent of the mitochondria and present within biological membranes. The data compiled thus far suggest that it may be efficacious on cutaneous malignancies without presenting any adverse effects to healthy tissue. Randomized double blind control studies are warranted to evaluate this.

Cutaneous oncology treatment is being shifted by molecular intervention. With the discovery of the molecular mechanisms and pathways of tumor proliferation, more translational research can be performed to target Q10 delivery at the site of tumorigenesis. Such investigation into this therapeutic realm has the potential to have a significant impact on cancer patients, their treatment options, and their quality of life.

GREEN TEA (EGCG)

BOX 54-3   Summary

- Green tea polyphenols, extracts, and their main constituent, (−)-epigallocatechin gallate, appear promising as chemopreventive agents for humans, but clinical evidence is lacking.
- Evidence suggests that EGCG may inhibit UVB-induced tumorigenesis by means of the inhibition of a specific transcription factor, NF-κB.
- EGCG decreases expression of antiapoptotic factors in tumor cells both orally and topically with no observable harm to normal cells.

Herbal green tea is made from the dried leaves of the plant Camellia Sinesis, and it is one of the most widely consumed beverages in the world, second only to water.[27] Closely related to black tea, green tea differs in that the leaves of the plant have not undergone fermentation, thereby conserving the tea's antioxidant capacity. It has been reported to have antibacterial, antioxidant, and antitumor properties. Green tea has been enjoyed for centuries; however, only recently have the mechanisms of its antioxidant activity been understood (Fig. 53-4).

Green tea contains 50 to 95% polyphenols per dose; of that, at least 50% is (−)-epigallocatechin-3-gallate (EGCG).[28] This catechin component of green tea acts as a powerful antioxidant, protecting against oxidative damage leading to tissue damage. The active

group of polyphenols in green tea has high antioxidant properties with the ability to neutralize free radicals induced by UV radiation. EGCG has been reported to upregulate levels of antioxidant enzymes such as glutathione, glutathione peroxidase, and catalase, which act as primary defenses against oxidative stress.[29] Furthermore, EGCG has been reported to inhibit the growth of tumor cells both in vitro and in vivo.[30]

The first study to illustrate the anticancer properties of green tea polyphenols (GTPP) in the skin was done by Khan et al in 1988. In this study, SENCAR mice were pretreated with topical GTPP prior to exposure to tumor-promoting agents. Compared to a control substance, GTPP offered substantial protection against tumor induction by certain chemical carcinogens.[31]

Since then, many studies have been undertaken to elucidate the mechanisms by which EGCG elicits its tumor-protective effects. History of UV exposure is a major predisposing factor in the development of skin cancer. This damage is inflicted by radiation-induced proinflammatory cytokines, primarily through transcription factor NF-κB. This transcription factor and family of cytokines have been attractive pharmacological targets for chemotherapeutic intervention. Afaq et al demonstrated that EGCG inhibits the UVB-induced activation of mitogen-activated protein kinase (MAPK) pathway and formation of pyrimidine dimers in human skin.[32] To determine the underlying mechanisms, these researchers analyzed the response of normal human keratinocytes to UVB radiation in the presence and absence of EGCG. The nuclear translocation of NF-κB was significantly inhibited in the presence of EGCG in a dose-dependent fashion.[33]

These results were corroborated by Xia et al in 2005. The nuclear activity and transcriptional levels of NF-κB and secretion of IL-6 in cultured human keratinocytes were measured after UVA and UVB exposure, and the levels were found to be elevated. Upon introduction of EGCG into the media, however, NF-κB transcription and IL-6 production were significantly inhibited, indicating that EGCG inhibited the proinflammatory pathway induced by UV radiation.[34] These studies provide a molecular basis for the photochemopreventive effect of EGCG.

In vivo studies in mouse models have been performed to assess the photoprotective effects of EGCG on UV-induced skin damage (both photoaging and tumor induction), as well as the inhibitory effects of EGCG on tumor initiation and promotion after exposure to known concentrations of chemical mutagens. One study by Lu et al treated hairless mice that had been exposed for 20 weeks to UVB prior to topical treatment with EGCG for 18 weeks showed a 55% decrease in nonmalignant skin tumors and a 66% decrease in malignant skin tumor development.[35] Immunohistochemically, a 56% increase in apoptosis of nonmalignant skin tumor cells and SCC cells were observed. Importantly, there was no noted increased apoptosis of tumor-free cells.

This pro-apoptotic effect that EGCG elicits in tumor cells while sparing unaffected cells was explored further by Nihal et al in two human melanoma cell lines. In both amelanototic malignant melanoma and metastatic melanoma cell lines, treatment with EGCG resulted in decreased viability and proliferation while normal melanocytes were not affected. When explored at a molecular level, the elucidated mechanism for the protective effects of EGCG has been demonstrated to be the downregulation of antiapoptotic factor bcl-2 and simultaneous upregulation of pro-apoptotic factors such as Bax and caspase activation.[36]

The antitumor effects of EGCG and five other compounds found in green tea were evaluated *in vitro* by Valcic et al in four human tumor cell lines (breast, colon, lung, and melanoma). Of the compounds, EGCG was found to be the most potent inhibitor of the breast, colon, and melanoma tumor cell lines.[37] Thus, EGCG holds promise as a chemoprotectant and inhibitor of melanoma tumor proliferation.

Dosing and route of administration have also been active areas of investigation. Most green tea in the world is orally consumed. In a study to test the efficacy of orally injected EGCG,[30] hairless mice were given either 1.25% or 2.5% green tea in their drinking water prior to UV exposure. (1.25% is a concentration similar to that consumed by humans.) Both groups experienced protection from erythema (sunburn), with the greatest effect noted in the 2.5% test group.[38]

Recently, green tea catechins have been studied for their antioxidative and anticancer properties with specific focus on skin cancers in humans. Fang et al introduced a liposome encapsulation of EGCG via injection into basal cell carcinomas (BCCs), melanomas, and colon tumors in nude mice and found increased cell death with the encapsulated EGCG when compared to both the nonencapsulated EGCG and encapsulated placebo.[39] Liposomal delivery of chemoprotective agents would deliver a localized dose of EGCG while minimizing systemic concentrations, which may be contraindicated in certain patient populations described below. While the flavonoid antioxidants of green tea have been reported to inhibit the peroxidation of LDL, thereby reducing the incidence of atherogenesis[40] and green tea has been observed to inhibit thromboxane formation and block platelet aggregation, it may interact with anticoagulant medications (including warfarin), aspirin, NSAIDs, or antiplatelet agents.[41] Additionaly, caffeine-free green teas are available and recommended for patients who experience stomach ulcers, heart conditions, insomnia, or who are or may become pregnant or nursing. It is also important to note that adding milk decreases the antioxidant properties of green tea.

In conclusion, although results from *in vitro* and animal model work appear to be therapeutically promising, clinical evidence from human studies is necessary to determine whether increased consumption of, or topical application of, EGCG in the form of green tea would be protective against photodamage, erythema, or the development of skin cancer (Fig. 54-5).

■ RED WINE (POLYPHENOLS)

BOX 54-4   Summary

- Polyphenols, which are natural constituents of red wine, exhibit many favorable characteristics that can be used to treat a number of dysfunctions and diseases.
- Polyphenols act as antioxidants, or free radical scavengers, and also have a potential use for the treatment of cancer, either as an independent treatment or in conjunction with other cancer treatments.
- Different red wine and green tea polyphenols can inhibit the expression of vascular endothelial growth factor caused by several stimuli, aiding in cardioprotection.

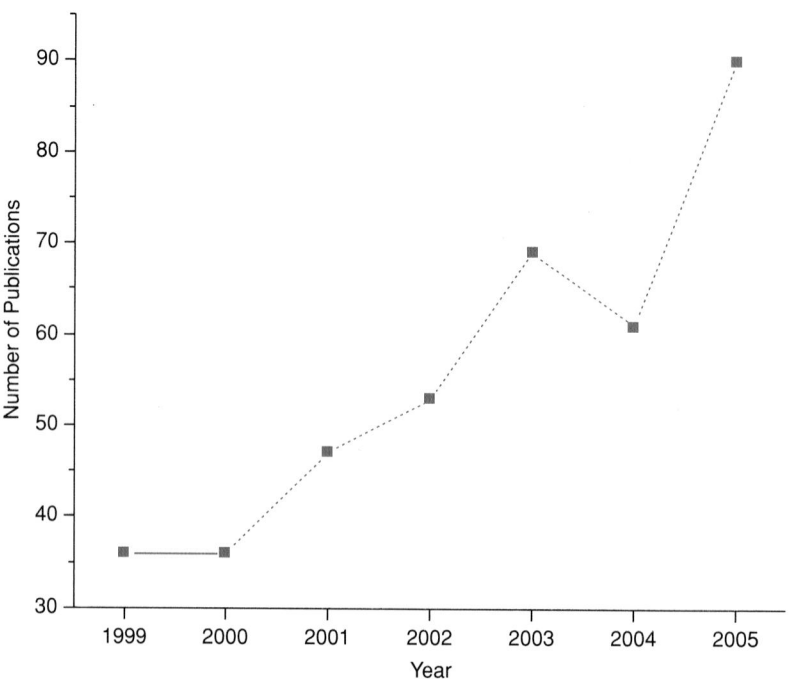

▲ **FIGURE 54-5** Publications on green tea and cancer from 1999–2005. A search was performed on Pubmed for green tea and cancer in 2006 from January to October. There have been 85 publications.

Red wine has been a part of adult human diet for centuries because of its numerous beneficial properties. Previous studies have shown that polyphenols, which are natural constituents of red wine, exhibit many favorable characteristics that can be used to treat a number of dysfunctions and diseases.

A polyphenol is a molecule that consists of two or more phenol groups (C_6H_5OH) bound together. Polyphenols may be found in red wine, green tea, peanuts, olive oil, and dark chocolate; all of which can be easily integrated into a daily diet. Recent studies have shown that polyphenols act as antioxidants, or free radical scavengers, and also have a potential use for the treatment of cancer, heart disease, and atherosclerosis.[42–44]

The anticancer properties of red wine polyphenols have been examined by a number of scientists, and the results show promise for use of natural red wine polyphenols as an independent treatment or in conjunction with traditional cancer treatments with no visible adverse effects, barring those of excess alcohol consumption leading to liver damage.

Corroborating claims that red wine has anticarcinogenic properties, Kim et al have shown that red wine induces apoptosis in human colon cancer cells by decreasing Bcl-2 expression and increasing Bax and Caspase-3 expression, all three of which are changes typical are associated with apoptosis.[43] Further, other research has shown that red wine polyphenols aid in the maintenance of healthy intestinal flora, the inhibition of dimethylhydrazine (DMH)-induced colon cancer, and a decrease of oxidative damage.[45]

Soleas et al further expounded on the effects of polyphenols on cancer by observing the difference of antitumor efficiency between four types of red wine polyphenols. The results showed that a flavonol named quercetin had the highest rate of inhibition of skin cancer tumor growth, and *trans*-resveratrol, another polyphenol, exhibited the highest rate of absorption after oral consumption in humans.[46]

In a study conducted by Femia et al indicated that separating high molecular weight polyphenols from low molecular weight polyphenols negated their inhibitory effects on rat colon cancer cells. Furthermore, the only treatment that displayed substantial effect was the combination of high molecular weight polyphenols with low molecular weight polyphenols, which is commonly found in red wine (Fig. 54-6).[47]

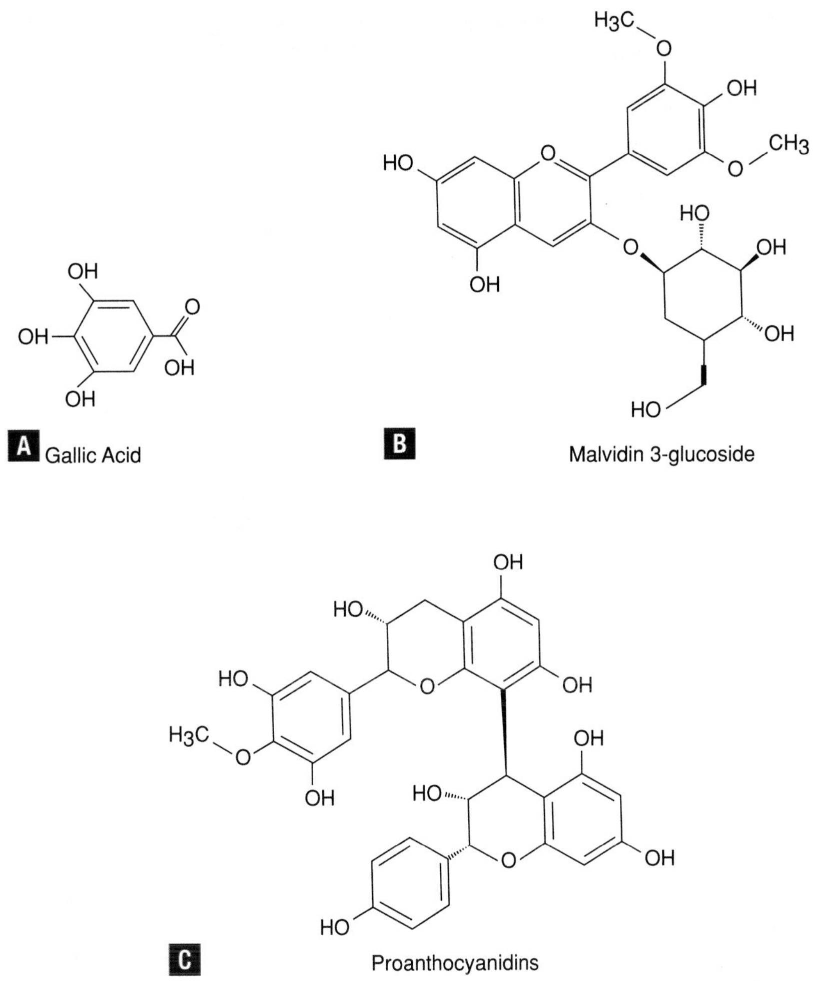

A Gallic Acid

Malvidin 3-glucoside

Proanthocyanidins

▲ **FIGURE 54-6** A. Gallic acid. B. Malvidin 3-glucoside. C. Proanthocyanidins.

There are numerous polyphenols found in grapes. They can be classified as phenolic acid, anthocyanins, simple flavonoids, and complex flavanoids. Three examples of polyphenols found in grapes are gallic acid, malvidin 3-glucoside, and proanthocyanidins

In addition to the direct anticarcinogenic qualities of red wine polyphenols, studies have shown that they are efficient antiangiogenic agents as well. In two studies, Oak et al demonstrated that different red wine and green tea polyphenols can inhibit the expression of vascular endothelial growth factor caused by various stimuli.[44,48] This may lead to new treatments for numerous cardiovascular diseases, such as atherosclerosis, and also tumor-related angiogenesis based on natural polyphenol treatments.[44,48]

Polyphenols found in red wine and other sources may become a focal point for future cancer research because of its anticarcinogenic and antiangiogenic factors. Studies conducted on the effect of red wine polyphenols on numerous types of cancer, including skin, and colon cancer have shown a marked inhibition of tumor growth and free radical damage along with a decrease of angiogenic growth factors that contribute to atherosclerosis and tumor-sustaining blood vessels. Taken together with recent discoveries, the evidence suggests a promising outlook on the use of natural treatments on skin cancer and several other diseases.

VITAMIN D

BOX 54-5   Summary

- While UV exposure is the major environmental contributing risk factor in the development of skin cancer, 90% of the vitamin D synthesized by the body is dependent upon solar input.

- Melanoma cells possess receptors for a vitamin D derivative that inhibits melanoma cell proliferation in a dose-dependent manner.

- Genetic differences in the FokI f and TaqI t alleles of VDR are associated with increased and decreased risk of cutaneous melanoma, respectively.
- Combination therapy with cytostatics and vitamin D derivative calcitriol results in lowering the inhibitory concentration 50% (IC50) levels in tumor cells.

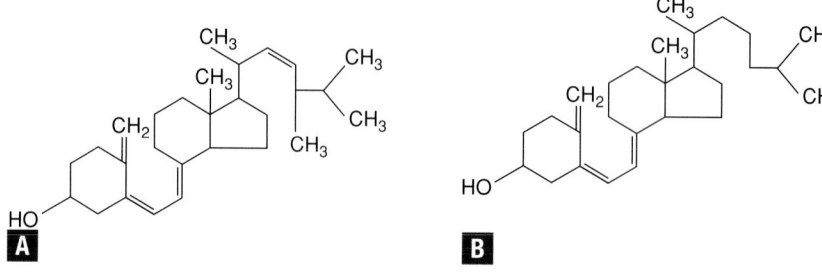

▲ **FIGURE 54-7** **A.** Vitamin D$_2$ (Calciferol). **B.** Vitamin D$_3$.

While UV exposure is the major environmental contributing risk factor in the development of skin cancer, it also plays a major role in vitamin D synthesis.[49] Vitamin D is a fat-soluble hormone synthesized from a precursor and modified in the liver and kidneys to form calcitriol. Calcitriol is the most active form of vitamin D, having such actions as regulation of the thyroid and intestinal absorption of calcium and other minerals important in bone mineralization.[50]

Diseases associated with vitamin D deficiency include cancer, bone and tooth disorders, rickets, and osteomalacia. Vitamin D supplementation has been used to treat conditions such as rickets, psoriasis, rheumatoid arthritis, scleroderma, and hypertension.[51-55]

In 1981, Colston et al demonstrated *in vitro* that malignant melanoma cells possessed receptors for a vitamin D derivative, 1,25-dihydroxyvitamin D3 (1,25-(OH)2D3).[56] When the hormone was included in the culture media, it inhibited melanoma cell proliferation in a dose-dependent manner. Other *in vitro* studies have confirmed these results.[57] The receptor is a member of the class II steroid hormone receptor family.[58] These so-termed vitamin D receptors (VDRs) exhibit increased expression in the presence of 1,25-(OH)2D3; furthermore, Evans et al reported increased growth inhibition of human malignant melanoma cells with increasing receptor binding avidity (Fig. 54-7).[59]

The two forms of vitamin D are califerol and D3. Vitamin D derivatives elicit their antiproliferative effects via the VDR; hypotheses that mutations or polymorphisms in the gene encoding VDRs would result in increased risk of developing skin cancer in humans. Li et al performed a case–control study of 1205 patients, where they genotyped two VDR polymorphisms, and evaluated their association with cutaneous melanoma.[60] It was found that genetic differences in the FokI f and TaqI t alleles of VDR are associated with increased and decreased risk of cutaneous melanoma, respectively.[60]

Pelczynska et al explored the use of calcitriol analogues in combination with cytostatic therapy.[61] Various tissue cancer cell lines were treated with calcitriol alone or in combination with either cisplatin or doxorubicin. The tumor cells that were treated with combination therapy including calcitriol decreased the necessary inhibitory concentration 50% (IC50) levels compared to the cells that were treated with cytostatics only.[61]

Vitamin D and its analogues direct their effects through the VDR on the proliferation, differentiation, and vasculature of tumors of various body tissues. Antitumor effects with calcitriol have been demonstrated in murine squamous cell carcinoma as well as melanoma. Further studies and clinical trials are necessary to elucidate the best delivery modalities, dosage, and schedule of administration.

Although overexposure to UV-irradiation increases the risk of developing skin cancer, patients should also be educated on the importance of an adequate supply of vitamin D. Balanced recommendations on sun protection and modified exposure are advised.

FINAL THOUGHTS

The information presented herein presents a scientifically based rationale for constructive consideration to be given to natural ingredients and biomolecules being implemented into mainstream medicine. Over the past decade, data has been presented at scientific and medical conferences that demonstrate the profound biochemical and intracellular effect that the molecules mentioned in this review have on the cancer and indeed many other major diseases.

Justification for use in first-line care will be embraced as successful double-blind, placebo-controlled, multi-center clinical trials that are able to translate what has been demonstrated in pre-clinical investigation thus leading to FDA approval for specific indications. In addi-

tion, clinical success most likely will behoove NIH subcommittees to seriously examine the feasibility of funding projects that seek to elucidate the mechanism of action of and/or explain intercellular communication with components that mediate disease formation and progression.

In conclusion, as more mechanistic work is completed that explains the effect that natural ingredients and biomolecules exert on gene regulatory and signal transduction pathways, viable drug targets will arise paving the way for successful translational and cross-disciplinary medicine. Hence, the gap between allopathic and complementary medicine would have been filled with foundational blocks of scientific validation to usher a new, exciting approach to cancer management for an improved quality of life.

REFERENCES

1. Crane FL, Hatefi Y, Lester RI, Widmer C. Isolation of a quinone from beef heart mitochondria. *Biochimica et Biophys Acta.* 1957;25:220–221.
2. Folkers K, et al. Biochemical deficiencies of coenzyme Q10 in HIV-infection and exploratory treatment. *Biochem Biophys Res Commun.* 1988;153:888–896.
3. Lockwood K, Moesgaard S, Hanioka T, Folkers K. Apparent partial remission of breast cancer in 'high risk' patients supplemented with nutritional antioxidants, essential fatty acids and coenzyme Q10. *Mol Aspects Med.* 1994;S15:231–240.
4. Batterham M, et al. A preliminary open label dose comparison using an antioxidant regimen to determine the effect on viral load and oxidative stress in men with HIV/AIDS *Eu. J Clin Nutr.* 2001;55:107–114
5. Folkers K, et al. Biochemical deficiencies of coenzyme Q10 in HIV-infection and exploratory treatment. *Biochem Biophys Res Commun.* 1988;153:888–896.
6. Shults CW, Flint BM, Song D, Fontaine D. Pilot trial of high dosages of coenzyme Q10 in patients with Parkinson's disease. *Exp Neurol.* 2004;188:491–494.
7. Kwong LK, et al. Effects of coenzyme Q(10) administration on its tissue concentrations, mitochondrial oxidant generation, and oxidative stress in the rat. *Free Radic Bio Med.* 2004;33:627–638.

8. Beal MF, Matthews RT. Coenzyme Q10 in the central nervous system and its potential usefulness in the treatment of neurodegenerative diseases. *Mol Aspects Med.* 1997;18:169–179.

9. Yalcin A, Kilinc E, Sagcan A, Kultursay H. Coenzyme Q10 concentrations in coronary artery disease. *Clin Biochem.* 2004;37:706–709.

10. Narain N, et al. Coenzyme Q10 inhibits the proliferation of oncogenic cells while stabilizing growth in primary cells *in vitro*. Society for Investigative Dermatology. Poster presentation, 2004.

11. Narain N, et al. Topical formulation of coenzyme Q10 inhibits the growth of melanoma tumors. Society for Investigative Dermatology. Poster presentation, 2004.

12. Persaud I, et al. Coenzyme Q10 induces apoptosis in human prostate and osteosarcoma cells. American Association of Cancer Research. Poster presentation, 2005.

13. Malik L, et al. Coenzyme Q10 inhibits proliferation of breast cancer cells while stabilizing growth in primary cells *in vitro*. American Association of Cancer Research. Poster presentation, 2005.

14. Narain N, et al. Coenzyme Q10 attenuates angiogenesis in melanoma tumors. Society for Investigative Dermatology. Poster presentation, 2005.

15. Narain N, et al. Coenzyme Q10 induces apoptosis in human melanoma cells. Society for Investigative Dermatology. Poster presentation, 2004.

16. Jolliet P, Simon N, Barre J, Pons JY, Boukef M, Paniel BJ, Tillement JP. Plasma coenzyme Q10 concentrations in breast cancer: prognosis and therapeutic consequences. *Int J Clin Pharmacol Ther.* September 1998;36(9):506–509.

17. Lockwood K, Moesgaard S, Yamamoto T, Folkers K. progress on therapy of breast cancer with vitamin Q10 and the regression of metastases. *Biochem Phys Res Commun.* July 1995;212(1):172–177.

18. Portakal O, Ozkaya O, Erden Inal M, Bozan B, Kosan M, Sayek I. Coenzyme Q10 concentrations and antioxidant status in tissues of breast cancer patients. *Clin Biochem.* June 2000;33(4):279–284.

19. Shults CW. Coenzyme Q10 in neurodegenerative diseases. *Curr Med Chem.* October 2003;10(19):1917–1921.

20. Woan K, et al. Coenzyme Q10 enhances the proliferation and migration of fibroblast and keratinocytes: a possible implication for wound healing. Society for Investigative Dermatology Poster presentation, 2005.

21. Roffe L, Schmidt, K, Ernst, E. Q10 and metabolism. Efficacy of coenzyme Q10 for improved tolerability of cancer treatments: a systematic review. *J Clin Oncol.* 2004;22:4418–4424 (Internet communications).

22. Yarosh DB. Liposomes in investigative dermatology. *Photodermatol Photoimmunol Photomed.* 2001;17:203–212.

23. Bozdogan O, et al. Bcl-2-related proteins, alpha-smooth muscle actin and amyloid deposits in aggressive and non-aggressive basal cell carcinomas. *Acta Derm Venereol.* 2002;82:423–427

24. Trisciuoglio D, Lervolino A, Zupi G, Del BD. Involvement of PI3K and MAPK signaling in bcl-2-induced vascular endothe-lial growth factor Expression in melanoma cells. *Mol Biol Cell.* September 2005;16(9):4153–4162.

25. Karl E, et al. Bcl-2 acts in a proangiogenic signaling pathway through nuclear factor-kappaB and CXC chemokines. *Cancer Res.* 2005;65:5063–5069.

26. Chavakis E Dimmeler S. Regulation of endothelial cell survival and apoptosis during angiogenesis. *Arterioscler Thromb Vasc Biol.* 2002;22:887–893.

27. Wright TI, Spencer JM, Flowers FP. Chemoprevention of nonmelanoma skin cancer. *JAAD* June 2006;54(6):933–946.

28. Mitscher, LA, Jung, M, Shankel, D, et al. Chemoprotection: a review of the potential therapeutic antioxidant properties of green tea (camellia sinensis) and certain of its constituents. *Med Res Rev.* 1997;17:327.

29. Hsu S. Green tea and the skin. *JAAD* June 2005;52(6):1049–1059.

30. Stoner, GD, Mukhtar, H. Polyphenols as cancer chemopreventive agents. *J Cell Biochem Suppl.* 1995;22:169.

31. Khan WA, Wang ZY, Athar M, Bickers DR, Mukhtar H. Inhibition of the skin tumorigenicity of (+/−)-7 beta, 8-alpha-dihydroxy-9 alpha,10 alpha-epoxy-7,8,9,10-tetrahydrobenzo[a]pyrene by tannic acid, green tea polyphenols and quercetin in Sencar mice. *Cancer Lett.* September/October 1988;42(1–2):7–12.

32. Katiyar SK, Perez A, Mukhtar H. Green tea polyphenol treatment to human skin prevents formation of ultraviolet light B-induced pyrimidine dimers in DNA *Clin Cancer Res.* October 2000;6(10):3864–3869.

33. Afaq F, Adhami VM, Ahmad N, Mukhtar H. Inhibition of ultraviolet B-mediated activation of nuclear factor kappaB in normal human epidermal keratinocytes by green tea constituent (−)-epigallocatechin-3-gallate. *Oncogene.* February 2003; 22(7):1035–1044.

34. Xia J, Song X, Bi Z, Chu W, Wan Y. UV-induced NF-kappaB activation and expression of IL-6 is attenuated by (−)-epigallocatechin-3-gallate in cultured human keratinocytes in vitro. *Int J Mol Med.* November 2005;16(5):943–950.

35. Lu YP, Lou YR, Xie JG, Peng QY, Liao J, Yang CS, Huang MT, Conney AH. Topical applications of caffeine or (−)-epigallocatechin gallate (EGCG) inhibit carcinogenesis and selectively increase apoptosis in UVB-induced skin tumors in mice. *Proc Natl Acad Sci USA* September 2002;99(19):12455–12460.

36. Nihal M, Ahmad N, Mukhtar H, Wood GS. Anti-proliferative and proapoptotic effects of (−)-epigallocatechin-3-gallate on human melanoma: possible implications for the chemoprevention of melanoma. *Int J Cancer.* April 2005;114 (4):513–521.

37. Valcic S, Timmermann BN, Alberts DS, Wachter GA, Krutzsch M, Wymer J, Guillen JM. Inhibitory effect of six green tea catechins and caffeine on the growth of four selected human tumor cell lines. *Anticancer Drugs.* June 1996;7(4):461–468.

38. Buckman SY, Gresham A, Hale P, Hruza G, Anast J, Masferrer J, Pentland AP. COX-2 expression is induced by UVB exposure in human skin: implications for the development of skin cancer. *Carcinogenesis.* May 1998;19(5):723–729.

39. Fang JY, Lee WR, Shen SC, Huang YL. Effect of liposome encapsulation of tea catechins on their accumulation in basal cell carcinomas. *J Dermatol Sci.* May 2006; 42(2):101–109.

40. Yokozawa, T, Dong, E. Influence of green tea and its three major components upon low-density lipoprotein oxidation. *Exp Toxicol Pathol.* 1997;49:329.

41. Taylor, JR, Wilt, VM Probable antagonism of Warfarin by green tea. *Ann Pharmacother.* 1999;33:426.

42. Arendt BM, Ellinger S, Kekic K, et al. Single and repeated moderate consumption of native or dealcoholized red wine show different effects on antioxidant parameters in blood and DNA strand breaks in peripheral leukocytes in healthy volunteers: a randomized controlled trial. *Nutr J* 2005;4:33.

43. Kim MJ, Kim YJ, Park HJ, Chung JH, Leem KH, Kim HK. Apoptotic effect of red wine polyphenols on human colon cancer SNU-C4 cells. *Food Chem Toxicol.* 2006;44(6):898–902.

44. Oak MH, El BJ, Schini-Kerth VB. Antiangiogenic properties of natural polyphenols from red wine and green tea. *J Nutr Biochem.* 2005;16(1):1–8.

45. Dolara P, Luceri C, Filippo CD, et al. Red wine polyphenols influence carcinogenesis, intestinal microflora, oxidative damage and gene expression profiles of colonic mucosa in F344 rats. *Mutat Res.* 2005;591(1–2):237–246.

46. Soleas GJ, Grass L, Josephy PD, Goldberg DM, Diamandis EP. A comparison of the anticarcinogenic properties of four red wine polyphenols. *Clin Biochem.* 2006;39 (5):492–497.

47. Femia AP, Caderni G, Vignali F, et al. Effect of polyphenolic extracts from red wine and 4-OH-coumaric acid on 1,2-dimethylhydrazine-induced colon carcinogenesis in rats. *Eur J Nutr.* 2005;44(2): 79–84.

48. Oak MH, Chataigneau M, Keravis T, et al. Red wine polyphenolic compounds inhibit vascular endothelial growth factor expression in vascular smooth muscle cells by preventing the activation of the p38 mitogen-activated protein kinase pathway. *Arterioscler Thromb Vasc Biol.* 2003;23(6):1001–1007.

49. Reichrath J. The challenge resulting from positive and negative effects of sunlight: how much solar UV exposure is appropriate to balance between risks of vitamin D deficiency and skin cancer? *Prog Biophys Mol Biol.* September 2006;92(1): 9–16.

50. Mautalen CA. Calcitonin. *Rev Argent Endocrinol Metab.* September 1970;16(3): 107–1.

51. Takeda E, Yamamoto H, Taketani Y, Miyamoto K. Vitamin D-dependent rickets type I and type II *Acta Paediatr Jpn.* August 1997;39(4):508–513.

52. Morimoto S, Yoshikawa K, Fukuo K, Shiraishi T, Koh E, Imanaka S, Kitano S, Ogihara T. Inverse relation between severity of psoriasis and serum 1,25-dihydroxy-vitamin D level. *J Dermatol Sci.* July 1990;1(4):277–282.

53. Merlino LA, Curtis J, Mikuls TR, Cerhan JR, Criswell LA, Saag KG. Iowa Women's Health Study. Vitamin D intake is inversely associated with rheumatoid arthritis: results from the Iowa Women's

Health Study. *Arthritis Rheum.* January 2004;50(1):72–77.

54. Humbert P, Dupond JL, Agache P, Laurent R, Rochefort A, Drobacheff C, et al. Treatment of scleroderma with oral 1,25-dihydroxyvitamin D3: evaluation of skin involvement using non-invasive techniques. Results of an open prospective trial. *Acta Derm Venereol.* December 1993;73(6):449–451.

55. Pfeifer M, Begerow B, Minne HW, Nachtigall D, Hansen C. Effects of a short-term vitamin D(3) and calcium supplementation on blood pressure and parathyroid hormone levels in elderly women. *J Clin Endocrinol Metab.* April 2001;86(4):1633–1637.

56. Colston K, Colston MJ, Feldman D. 1,25-dihydroxyvitamin D3 and malignant melanoma: the presence of receptors and inhibition of cell growth in culture. *Endocrinology.* March 1981;108(3):1083–1086.

57. Seifert M, Rech M, Meineke V, Tilgen W, Reichrath J. Differential biological effects of 1,25-dihydroxyVitamin D3 on melanoma cell lines in vitro. *J Steroid Biochem Mol Biol.* May 2004;89–90(1–5): 375–379.

58. DeLuca, HF. Overview of general physiologic features and functions of vitamin D *Am J Clin Nutr.* 2004;80:1689S

59. Evans SR, Houghton AM, Schumaker L, Brenner RV, Buras RR, Davoodi F, et al.

Vitamin D receptor and growth inhibition by 1,25-dihydroxyvitamin D3 in human malignant melanoma cell lines. *J Surg Res.* February 15. 1996;61(1):127–133.

60. Li C, Liu Z, Zhang Z, Strom SS, Gershenwald JE, Prieto VG, et al. Genetic variants of the vitamin D receptor gene alter risk of cutaneous melanoma. *J Invest Dermatol.* September 2006.

61. Pelczynska M, Switalska M, Maciejewska M, Jaroszewicz I, Kutner A, Opolski A. Antiproliferative activity of vitamin D compounds in combination with cytostatics. *Anticancer Res.* July/August 2006;26(4A):2701–2705.

CHAPTER 55

Skin Cancer Prevention and Sunscreens

Hassan I. Galadari, M.D.

Barbara A. Gilchrest, M.D.

BOX 55-1 Overview

- Skin cancer is the most common malignant neoplasm in humans.
- Ultraviolet radiation is the most important causative factor that predisposes the development of skin cancer.
- Skin cancer prevention is best made through modifying people's behaviors and perception of beauty, sun exposure, and tanning.
- Methods to prevent skin cancer include the use of protective garments, avoidance of sun during the hottest part of the day, avoiding tanning booths, education of children and parents, and sunscreens.
- Use of sunscreens is an important means in preventing skin cancer; however, they should be considered an adjunct to other protective methods.

INTRODUCTION

Skin cancer is the most common category of malignant neoplasms diagnosed in humans.[1] It can be broadly subdivided, into melanoma and non-melanoma skin cancers (NMSC), primarily basal cell carcinomas (BCC) or squamous cell carcinomas (SCC). Other types, such as Merkel cell carcinoma, are rare and will not be discussed here. The incidence of skin cancer has increased rapidly in many countries worldwide, causing significant morbidity and mortality. In 2004, more than 1 million people in the United States were diagnosed as having one of the two most common skin cancers, BCC and SCC.[2] Melanoma, which accounts for only 4% of all skin cancers, has, in its invasive form, been diagnosed among 543,000 Americans.[3] Predisposing factors include a strong family history of skin cancer, skin type of the individual and certain disease states.[4] The most important causative factor is the ultraviolet (UV) radiation

from exposure to the sun. This has led to an "epidemic" which has been attributed to changes in lifestyle and the pursuit of a "healthy tan."[5]

ROLE OF ULTRAVIOLET RADIATION IN THE DEVELOPMENT OF SKIN CANCER

BOX 55-2 Summary

- UV is divided into three spectral regions: UVA, UVB and UVC
- The major portion of UV from the sun is UVA.
- UVB causes DNA photoproducts in epidermal cells, which leads to key mutations resulting in the development of skin cancer.

Ample UV exposure increases the risk of developing skin cancer and photoaging.[6] UV can be divided into three spectral regions: UVA (320 to 400 nm), UVB is (280 to 320 nm) and UVC (100 to 280 nm). The last is completely absorbed by the ozone. On a sunny day, approximately 5% of terrestrial sunlight is UV irradiation, with the rest consisting of visible light and infrared energy. The UV component comprises approximately of 90 to 95% UVA and 5 to 10% UVB the major factors of influence being the latitude, altitude, time of day and year and overlying cloud cover.[6] UV affects multiple targets (chromophores) within the skin, producing changes that may lead to the development of skin cancers.[7]

From the perspective of carcinogenesis, the most important UV target is DNA in epidermal keratinocytes and melanocytes. UV induces the formation of cyclopyrimidine dimers (CPD) between adjacent TT, CC, CT or TC bases, among other photoproducts.[8] If these lesions are not repaired by the cell's DNA repair proteins, the DNA may be "misread" at the time of chromosome replication, causing mutations. A "UV signature mutation" results when adjacent cytosines dimerize and, following the DNA polymerase's "A rule" for pairing with unreadable bases, AA rather than the correct complementary bases GG are inserted into the newly synthesized DNA strand. At the next round of DNA replications, AA is paired with TT, which becomes a CC → TT mutation. This is uniquely caused by UV damage.

The C → T mutation also occurs as a result of UV damage. However, this occurs very rarely and this mutation falls into the classification of UV signature mutations. Although UV can cause many other mutations, it cannot be specifically implicated as the sole etiologic agent. The existence of UV signature mutations in p53, a key tumor suppressor protein mutated in half of all human malignancies and >90% of SCC as well as ~50% of BCC, has been a critical proof of the central role played by UV in skin cancer development.[9] Indeed, the action spectrum for UV-induced CPD formation corresponds almost exactly to the action spectrum for photocarcinogenesis in hairless mice, with peak efficiency for both at 300 nm in the UVB range, and a rapid exponential decrease in efficiency for photons in the UVA range.[9–12]

Both UVB and UVA contribute to skin cancer development, but their relative contributions to NMSC versus melanoma and their respective mechanisms of action remain areas of intense investigation and debate. UV energy per photon and average depth of penetration into the skin depend strongly on wavelength, with UVB photons having roughly 1000× more energy than UVA photons on average and hence a far smaller likelihood of initiating photochemical reactions. However, longer wavelength photons penetrate more readily, with approximately half of UVA photons but 10% or fewer of UVB photons reaching the dermoepidermal junction. These considerations, as well as the greater abundancy of UVA in sunlight and better protection against UVB versus UVA afforded by most sunscreens, have had some authorities suggesting a major role for UVA in melanoma that arises from melanocytes in the basal layer of the epidermis or from nevus cells in the dermis.[12]

The relative contribution of UVA versus UVB to photoaging is also hotly debated. Based on studies in UV irradiated hairless mice—a less-than-ideal model—and the considerations noted above, it has been reported that UVB produces superficial wrinkling with chronic exposure, while UVA causes more sagging of the skin.[13]

The immune system is also affected by UV exposure. It has been shown that solar-stimulated UV radiation suppresses delayed-type hypersensitivity, such as contact dermatitis to nickel or dinitrochlorobenzene (DNCB) and may reactivate cutaneous herpes simplex virus infection.[14–17] The action spectrum appears to be shifted slightly to the UVA compared to DNA damage.[18] Though the exact mechanism is poorly understood, it is well established that skin directly exposed to UV is depleted of Langerhan's cells. Hapten-specific tolerance develops. This is attributed to the induction of T cells that suppress the immune response.[19] Systemic, as well as local, immunosuppression occurs with the release of immunosuppressive cytokines, IL-10 and TNFα, by keratinocytes.[20] UV-induced immunosuppression is believed to enhance the risk of developing skin cancers, a concept well supported in mouse models and by the fact that iatrogenic immunosuppression, for example, in organ transplant recipients, greatly increases cancer risk in sun-damaged skin, although other factors may also contribute.[21,22]

■ SKIN CANCER PREVENTION

BOX 55-3   Summary

- Skin cancer prevention is best done through change of behavior.
- Protective clothing and wearing long sleeved shirts and pants help prevent excessive exposure to ultraviolet radiation.
- Avoidance of the sun at its most intense period during the day is also important.
- Tanning booths can lead to extra exposure of UVB and UVA, which might further lead to the development of skin cancer.
- Sunscreens are important as a secondary method of prevention and should not be relied as a sole method.

Efforts of skin cancer prevention are directed at reducing UV exposure through modifying attitudes and behaviors of the public, and improving sunscreens. Very recent and complementary efforts to enhance repair of UV damage, particularly DNA damage, are discussed elsewhere (Chapter 53).

When it comes to changing behavior, it is important to realize that behavior change is not an event, but a process that involves a movement through a series of stages.[23] Five stages of change in behavior are recognized: pre-contemplation when the person is not thinking of change; contemplation, when a person is considering change; preparation, when the person is committed; action, when the person has started to change; and maintenance, when the person sustains the new change in behavior.[24]

Protective Clothing

During the twentieth century, fashions in clothing have changed drastically. Certain items commonly used in the past, such as hats and umbrellas, have fallen out of fashion; while shorts, short-sleeved shirts and other skin-revealing attire have become commonplace. Reminding patients and the public at large to wear wide-brimmed hats or caps, long-sleeved shirts and long pants during potentially harmful sun exposures is therefore helpful. For those at very high risk, there are clothes manufactured with UV protective materials that absorb or reflect UV even more effectively than standard fabrics.[25]

Avoidance of the Sun during Mid-Day (10 am to 3 pm)

UV, particularly UVB, is most intense at mid-day.[26] Flexible outdoor activities are therefore best scheduled during the early morning or late in the afternoon. If outdoors at mid-day, a person should be advised to wear protective clothing, apply sunscreen and seek shade if available.

Avoidance of Tanning Booths

The use of tanning booths has increased threefold in the USA since 1986, with women and young people being the most frequent visitors of such booths.[27] The estimated annual revenue of the tanning business in the US alone exceeds $5 billion.[6] Tanning salons are poorly regulated and maximum dose recommendations set forth by Health Boards are often ignored.[28] Some tanning proponents suggest only through exposure to a tanning bed on a regular basis can a person achieve the "recommended" level of active vitamin D year round.[29] However, careful analysis of studies correlating vitamin D status with various health outcomes in the general population reveals that the optimal level of vitamin D is very arguable and that adequate vitamin D, however defined, can be obtained from diet and/or oral supplements.[30]

In contrast to the very questionable benefit of sunbathing to increase vitamin D levels, a recent study performed in Norway and Sweden of women between the age of 20 and 40 years who used tanning facilities 12 or more times a year showed a 10-fold increased risk of melanoma in that population.[31] However, not all studies have reached similar conclusions.[32] It is thus important that the use of tanning booths and lamps be strongly discouraged.

Education of Children and Parents

Parents are often willing to provide better care to their children than to themselves.[33] Moreover, good habits acquired or entrained in childhood often persist beyond. One study showed that less than 1% of pediatricians provide sun protection counseling during a well-child visit.[34,35] Given that individuals often receive 80% of their total lifetime sun exposure before the age of 18, such counseling of parents and children may decrease skin cancer risk.[36] Health care providers can assess patient's level of preparedness to change, and this can be targeted during regular office visits. It is very important to discourage the concept of a "healthy tan or appearance." Sun protection programs can be made fun and proactive, with the emphasis on positive reinforcement as a method to implement change.[37]

■ SUNSCREENS

BOX 55-4   Summary

- Sunscreens are an adjunct method of preventing exposure to UV.
- The active ingredient in sunscreens protects against certain UV radiation.
- The FDA uses the sun protection factor (SPF) as a method to measure erythema that can be prevented by sunscreens and thus can rate the sunscreens' efficacy based on this.
- Sunscreens are divided as being either chemical or physical.
- Chemical sunscreens convert UV radiation to heat; examples include aminobenzoates (PABA), cinnamates, salicylates, benzophenones, and dibenzoylemthanes.
- Physical sunscreens scatter UV radiation; examples include metal oxides, such as zinc or titanium oxides.
- Dihydroxyacetone is an artificial tanning agent and not a sunscreen.
- Sunscreens are effective when used properly and in combination with other protective methods.

Sunscreens were first commercially available in 1928 when an emulsion containing benzyl salicylate and benzyl cinnamate was developed in the United States.[38] This was followed by the introduction of more sun-blocking compounds in Australia and Europe. The United States Army used red petrolatum, a physical sunblock, during and after World War II. However, the first readily available sunscreen contained para-aminobenzoic acid (PABA) was introduced in 1943. Since then numerous agents were developed to reduce sun damage and skin cancer. Recently PABA has fallen out of favor as a sunscreen ingredient for many reasons, principally allergic sensitivity in up to 4% of users and permanent yellow discoloration of both cotton and synthetic fabrics after photo-oxidation.[39] The ideal sunscreen should be transparent when applied to the skin, water-resistant and has broad-spectrum coverage for both UVB and UVA.

The US Food and Drug Administration (FDA) rates sunscreen efficacy using the sun protection factor (SPF), a measure of UV-induced erythema.[40,41] This is defined as the ratio of the time of UV radiation exposure necessary to produce minimally detectable erythema, otherwise known as the minimum erythema dose (MED), in sunscreen-protected skin versus unprotected skin. Thus, by definition, protection against other adverse effects of UV exposure, such as immunosuppression or collagen degradation, are not measured. A second major limitation of the SPF concerns the FDA-mandated quantity of products applied to the skin (2 mg/cm^2). A number of studies have shown that when applying sunscreens, most users apply only about one-quarter to one-half of this amount.[42] Since the applied thickness of a sunscreen layer is crucial to the degree of photoprotection, the SPF on the product's label is usually much higher than the degree of protection afforded to the typical user.[43] An SPF of 30 may only provide a protection of 15 or less.

Of several concerns, there is no consensus at present as to how to measure UVA protection. UVA does cause erythema but at a much higher dose, which makes the use of SPF impractical.[44] In the absence of consensus among scientists and manufacturers, the FDA forbids any testing or rating system and allows only the designation "broad spectrum" for products intended to protect against UVA. Loss of protection during a period of use, due to washing off or photodegradation of the sunscreen product, are additional problems.

Sunscreen Properties and Mechanisms of Action

Chemical sunscreens generally absorb UV photons while physical sunscreens scatter them. The two processes are not mutually exclusive, with the newer commercial sunscreen preparations usually acting through a combination of those two mechanisms. Other important factors that play a role in sunscreen effectiveness are photostability and substantivity.

TABLE 55-1

Different Chemical Classes of Sunscreens and Their UV Absorption Spectrum

CHEMICAL CLASS	ABSORPTION
Aminobenzoates— (PABA) ester	UVB
Cinnamate	UVB
Salicylate	UVB
Benzophenone	UVB and UVA II
Metal oxide	UVB and UVA
Dibenzoylmethane— avobenzone	UVA

ABSORPTION Sunscreen chemicals that absorb UV light contain conjugate double bonds that absorb light at comparatively low energies.[40] This structure allows electron transfer and absorbed UV radiation is then emitted as lower-energy infrared radiation (heat). Table 55-1 summarizes commonly used sunscreen ingredients and their different absorption spectra.

SCATTERING This occurs when UV radiation is deflected from its original path and scattered as it strikes non-UV-absorbing particles in the sunscreen. This allows for most of the energy to dissipate into the surrounding environment. There is a misconception that physical sunscreens that contain inorganic metal oxides such as zinc oxide (ZnO) and titanium dioxide (TiO_2) act as pure "scatterers" of UV light. In their micronized form, both ZnO and TiO_2 also mobilize electrons within their atomic structure and act in a fashion very similar to that of chemical sunscreens.[45] Given that the micronized forms have become popular in terms of application and availability, the distinction between chemical and physical sunscreens has diminished, making this classification method obsolete. However, due to its historical significance and simplicity, it is still widely used.

PHOTOSTABILITY This refers to the ability of a molecule to remain unchanged during exposure to irradiation. Several organic sunscreens undergo photolysis or oxidation and lose their protective value when exposed to solar radiation.[40] Chemical sunscreens such as octyl dimethyl PABA and avobenzone substantially lose their effectivity within conventional exposure times, while physical sunscreens such as silicone-coated zinc oxide are completely photostable.[46]

SUBSTANTIVITY This reflects the ability of the sunscreen to retain its original SPF under conditions of use, such as sweating

and repeated immersion in water. The FDA has recently provided guidelines for the testing and labeling of water resistance. For being "water-resistant," the sunscreen should maintain its original SPF after two 20-minute immersions, a total of 40 minutes. "Very water-resistant" means that the SPF can be maintained for at least 80 minutes of immersion, four 20-minute immersion cycles, each followed by a 20-minute rest/air dry period.[47]

Sunscreen Preparations and Ingredients

Most commercially available sunscreen products have more than one active sunscreen agent, allowing for a broader spectrum of protection.

There are six main chemical classes of active sunscreen ingredients

AMINOBENZOATES (PABA ESTERS) PABA esters are more water-soluble than PABA, do not penetrate the stratum corneum, and hence have less associated allergy, stinging and staining. They provide excellent UVB protection.

CINNAMATES These compounds also provide excellent UVB absorption and protection, but have poor substantivity, thus they are usually combined with other active ingredients.[48] Octyl methoxycinnamate is one of the most commonly used UVB sunscreens in the US.

SALICYLATES These are aromatic compounds with a peak absorption spectrum at ~300 nm. The salicylates are considered to be one of the safest sunscreens, even when used in high concentrations. They are not effective sunscreens when used alone, but are exceptionally stable, nonsensitizing and have high substantivity because of their poor water solubility.[49] Homosalate and octyl salicylate are the most widely used in the group.

BENZOPHENONES These aromatic ketones absorb mainly between 320 to 350 nm. Hence, they are incorporated in broad-spectrum sunscreen preparations. Unfortunately, oxybenzone and dioxybenzone, the most commonly used benzophenones, have been implicated in photocontact allergy.[50]

DIBENZOYLMETHANES Avobenzone is the only compound of this increasingly popular class of sunscreens that is available in the United States. It has excellent absorption in the UVA range, mainly at 355 nm.[40] The compounds occur in keto and enol forms, which provide protection ranging from 260 nm to over 345 nm. When formulated with octyl methoxycinnamate, avobenzone has a high photodegradation rate and significant loss of protective power over time. When formulated correctly, however, avobezone provides excellent broad-spectrum coverage.

METAL OXIDES The most widely used of the so-called physical blocking agents are zinc oxide and titanium dioxide, although compounds such as iron oxide, kaolin, talc, and calamine also have the same capability to scatter, reflect, and absorb solar radiation. These metal oxides protect the skin from both UVB and UVA. Older generation products were opaque and provided a thicker coating layer that melted in the heat and stained clothes and thus cosmetically undesirable to patients. They were also comedogenic. With the advent of new micronized preparations, these blockers have become more appealing as they have become transparent. It has been shown that in this form, however, these agents are no longer completely inert and may theoretically lead to contact allergy.[51]

SELF-TANNING AGENTS Dihydroxyacetone (DHA) is the most important compound in this emerging class of chemical "self-tanners." These agents are not classified as sunscreens and may contain numerous dyes, artificial colorings and staining agents in addition to DHA, which binds stratum corneum proteins and makes the skin appear tanned without exposure to UV radiation.[52] DHA is minimally effective as a sunscreen, so it is important that patients know these agents do not protect them from photodamage. A conventional sunscreen should be applied after the DHA product has dried.[53,54]

Sunscreen Regulation

Sunscreens in United States are considered over-the-counter drugs, and are thus regulated by the FDA. These same agents are considered cosmetic ingredients in the rest of the world. The Sunscreen Monograph Final Rule lists 16 active "category 1" ingredients that are classified as safe and effective, and thus may be used alone or in combination.[39] FDA regulation assures safety and efficacy of a product, but also involves a stringent approval process for new agents, similar to that for new prescription medications. This, unfortunately, has inhibited innovation in the field of chemical sun-protection. Self-tanning agents are considered cosmetic and are not controlled by the FDA.

Sunscreen Compliance and Limitations

There are many reasons why people seem to shy away from the use of sunscreens. The need to apply and reapply products, especially to large body surface areas is expensive and inconvenient. Further, the on-going debate between the use of sunscreens and decrease in vitamin D levels and the possibility of systemic sunscreen absorption through the skin after inadvertent oral ingestion has made a number of consumers think twice when applying the products on their skin. At a practical level, many consumers complain about stickiness and the feeling of excessive heat or perspiration when wearing a sunscreen. Other complaints include a stinging sensation that is felt when applying the product and irritation if it enters the eye. It is thus very important that consumers be educated about the right type of sunscreen and the right formulation and vehicle-delivery system that may be used to help minimize these problems or obstacles. A number of cosmetic companies have included sunscreen ingredients in hair gels, shaving foams for men, moisturizers, and foundation creams. The combination of such ingredients in those products provides a great opportunity for consumers to utilize sunscreens without having to apply them separately. This, of course, is not a panacea as the need for reapplication is still present. It is certainly a start. If people are reluctant to use these products for whatever reason, then they should be encouraged to use sun protection methods through the use of protective clothing and decreased sun exposure.

In recent years, much attention has focused on the fact that effective sunscreen use decreases cutaneous vitamin D photosynthesis, which has an action spectrum virtually identical to that for sunburn, and at least in hairless mice, for photocarcinogenesis. Although several studies have shown that regular daily high SPF sunscreen use is very compatible with maintaining levels of vitamin D well within the conventional normal range, concerns have been expressed that even higher levels are desirable. However, even high levels can readily be achieved supplemented with a combination of dietary intake, oral supplements, and incidental protected sun exposure. Recommending oral vitamin D supplements would seem especially prudent in the frail and elderly in whom oral supplements have been shown in controlled trials to offer health benefits such as

decreased risk of falls. For those eager to maximize their "natural source" of vitamin D, it is important to note that maximum cutaneous production occurs with only very modest sun exposure, far less than the minimal erythema dose. Longer exposures do not result in more vitamin D photosynthesis but instead conversion of the vitamin to inactive photoproducts takes place, while DNA photodamage continues at a constant rate.

The most critical limitation of sunscreens is that, in the end, they can succeed only in the context of a comprehensive safe-sun program. This approach is best taught at an early age, with an appreciation of how difficult it is to change already established attitudes and behaviors. Only through primary prevention methods such as skin cancer awareness programs and a sun-safe lifestyle can contribute to maximum reduction in the societal burden of skin cancer.

REFERENCES

1. Jemal A, Murray T, Ward E, Samuels A, Tiwari RC, Ghafoor A, Feuer EJ, Thun MJ. Cancer statistics, 2005. *CA Cancer J Clin.* January/February 2005;55(1):10–30.
2. Saraiya M, Glanz K, Briss PA, Nichols P, White C, Das D, Smith SJ, Tannor B, Hutchinson AB, Wilson KM, Gandhi N, Lee NC, Rimer B, Coates RC, Kerner JF, Hiatt RA, Buffler P, Rochester P. Interventions to prevent skin cancer by reducing exposure to ultraviolet radiation: a systematic review. *Am J Prev Med.* December 2004;27(5):422–466.
3. Geller AC, Emmons K, Brooks DR, Zhang Z, Powers C, Koh HK, Sober AJ, Miller DR, Li F, Haluska F, Gilchrest BA. Skin cancer prevention and detection practices among siblings of patients with melanoma. *J Am Acad Dermatol.* October 2003;49(4):631–638.
4. Ferrone CR, Ben Porat L, Panageas KS, Berwick M, Halpern AC, Patel A, Coit DG. Clinicopathological features of and risk factors for multiple primary melanomas. *J Am Med Assoc.* October. 2005;294(13):1647–1654.
5. De Laat JM, De Gruijl FR. The role of UVA in the aetiology of non-melanoma skin cancer. *Cancer Surv.* 1996;26: 173–191.
6. Abdulla FR, Feldman SR, Williford PM, Krowchuk D, Kaur M. Tanning and skin cancer. *Pediatr Dermatol.* November/December 2005;22(6):501–512.
7. Lowe NJ. An overview of ultraviolet radiation, sunscreens, and photo-induced dermatoses. *Dermatol Clin.* January 2006;24(1):9–17.
8. Clingen PH, Arlett CF, Roza L, Mori T, Nikaido O, Green MH. Induction of cyclobutane pyrimidine dimers, pyrimidine(6-4)pyrimidone photoproducts, and Dewar valence isomers by natural sunlight in normal human mononuclear cells. *Cancer Res.* June 1995;55(11):2245–2248.

9. Rebel H, Kram N, Westerman A, Banus S, van Kranen HJ, de Gruijl FR. Relationship between UV-induced mutant p53 patches and skin tumours, analysed by mutation spectra and by induction kinetics in various DNA-repair-deficient mice. Carcinogenesis. December 2005;26(12): 2123–2130.

10. Rebel H, Mosnier LO, Berg RJ, Westerman-de Vries A, Van Steeg H, van Kranen HJ, De Gruijl FR. Early p53-positive foci as indicators of tumor risk in ultraviolet-exposed hairless mice: kinetics of induction, effects of DNA repair deficiency, and p53 heterozygosity. Cancer Res. February 2001;61(3):977–983.

11. Petit-Frere C, Capulas E, Lyon DA, Norbury CJ, Lowe JE, Clingen PH, Riballo E, Green MH, Arlett CF. Apoptosis and cytokine release induced by ionizing or ultraviolet B radiation in primary and immortalized human keratinocytes. Carcinogenesis. June 2000;21(6):1087–1095.

12. Hussein MR. Ultraviolet radiation and skin cancer: molecular mechanisms. J Cutan Pathol. March 2005;32(3):191–205.

13. Cole C. Sunscreen protection in the ultraviolet A region: how to measure the effectiveness. Photodermatol Photoimmunol Photomed. February 2001;17(1):2–10.

14. Moyal D, Courbière C, Le Corre Y, de Lacharrière O, Hourseau C. Immunosuppression induced by chronic solar-simulated irradiation in humans and its prevention by sunscreens. Eur J Dermatol. 1997;7:223–225.

15. Damian D L, Halliday G M, Taylor C A, Barnetson R S C. Ultraviolet radiation induced suppression of Mantoux reactions in humans. J Invest Dermatol. 1998:110:824–827.

16. Damian D L, Halliday G M, Barnetson R S C. Broad-spectrum sunscreens provide greater protection against ultraviolet-radiation-induced suppression of contact hypersensitivity to a recall antigen in humans. J Invest Dermatol. 1997;109:146–151.

17. Ichihashi M, Nagai H, Matsunaga K. Sunlight is an important causative factor of recurrent herpes simplex. Cutis. November 2004;74(S5):14–8.

18. Yarosh DB. DNA repair, immunosuppression, and skin cancer. Cutis. November 2004;74(S5):10–3.

19. Schwarz T. Biological effects of UV radiation on keratinocytes and Langerhan's cells. Exp Dermatol. October 2005;14(10): 788–789.

20. Petit-Frere C, Clingen PH, Grewe M, Krutmann J, Roza L, Arlett CF, Green MH. Induction of interleukin-6 production by ultraviolet radiation in normal human epidermal keratinocytes and in a human keratinocyte cell line is mediated by DNA damage. J Invest Dermatol. September 1998;111(3):354–359.

21. Parrish JA. Immunosuppression, skin cancer, and ultraviolet A radiation. N Engl J Med. December 22. 2005;353(25):2712–2713.

22. Moloney FJ, Comber H, O'Lorcain P, O'Kelly P, Conlon PJ, Murphy GM. A population-based study of skin cancer incidence and prevalence in renal transplant recipients. Br J Dermatol. March 2006;154(3):498–504.

23. Kristjansson S, Ullen H, Helgason AR. The importance of assessing the readiness to change sun-protection behaviours: a population-based study. Eur J Cancer. December 2004;40(18):2773–2780.

24. Prochaska JO, Velicer WF. The transtheoretical model of health behavior change. Am J Health Promot. September/October 1997;12(1):38–48.

25. Hatch KL, Osterwalder U. Garments as solar ultraviolet radiation screening materials. Dermatol Clin. January 2006;24(1): 85–100.

26. Thieden E, Philipsen PA, Wulf HC. Ultraviolet radiation exposure pattern in winter compared with summer based on time-stamped personal dosimeter readings. Br J Dermatol. January 2006;154(1): 133–138.

27. Robinson JK, Rigel DS, Amonette RA. Trends in sun exposure knowledge, attitudes, and behaviors: 1986 to 1996. J Am Acad Dermatol. August 1997;37(2 Pt 1): 179–186.

28. Moseley H, Davidson M, Ferguson J. A hazard assessment of artificial tanning units. Photodermatol Photoimmunol Photomed. April 1998;14(2):79–87.

29. Garland CF, Garland FC, Gorham ED, Lipkin M, Newmark H, Mohr SB, Holick MF. The role of vitamin D in cancer prevention. Am J Public Health. February 2006;96(2):252–261.

30. Wolpowitz D, Gilchrest BA. The vitamin D questions: how much do you need and how should you get it? J Am Acad Dermatol. 2006 Feb;54(2):301–317.

31. Veierod MB, Weiderpass E, Thorn M, Hansson J, Lund E, Armstrong B, Adami HO. A prospective study of pigmentation, sun exposure, and risk of cutaneous malignant melanoma in women. J Natl Cancer Inst. October 15. 2003;95(20): 1530–1538.

32. Swerdlow AJ, Weinstock MA. Do tanning lamps cause melanoma? An epidemiologic assessment. J Am Acad Dermatol. 1998 Jan;38(1):89–98.

33. Young RA, Logan C, Lovato CY, Moffat B, Shoveller JA. Sun protection as a family health project in families with adolescents. J Health Psychol. May 2005;10 (3):333–344.

34. Gritz ER, Tripp MK, de Moor CA, Eicher SA, Mueller NH, Spedale JH. Skin cancer prevention counseling and clinical practices of pediatricians. Pediatr Dermatol. January/February 2003;20(1):16–24.

35. Dinehart SM, Dodge R, Stanley WE, Franks HH, Pollack SV. Basal cell carcinoma treated with Mohs surgery. A comparison of 54 younger patients with 1050 older patients. J Dermatol Surg Oncol. July 1992;18(7):560–566.

36. Diffey BL, Gibson CJ, Haylock R, McKinlay AF. Outdoor ultraviolet exposure of children and adolescents. Br J Dermatol. June 1996;134(6):1030–1034.

37. Glanz K, Maddock JE, Lew RA, Murakami-Akatsuka L. A randomized trial of the Hawaii SunSmart program's impact on outdoor recreation staff. J Am Acad Dermatol. June 2001;44(6):973–978.

38. Urbach F. The historical aspects of sunscreens. J Photochem Photobiol B. November 2001;64(2–3):99–104.

39. Funk JO, Dromgoole SH, Maibach HI. Sunscreen intolerance. Contact sensitization, photocontact sensitization, and irritancy of sunscreen agents. Dermatol Clin. April 1995;13(2):473–481.

40. Chatelain E, Gabard B. Photostabilization of butyl methoxydibenzoylmethane (Avobenzone) and ethylhexyl methoxycinnamate by bis-ethylhexyloxyphenol methoxyphenyl triazine (Tinosorb S), a new UV broadband filter. Photochem Photobiol. September 2001;74(3):401–406.

41. Damian DL, Halliday GM, Stc Barnetson R. Sun protection factor measurement of sunscreens is dependent on minimal erythema dose. Br J Dermatol. Sepember 1999;141(3):502–507.

42. Lott DL, Stanfield J, Sayre RM, Dowdy JC. Uniformity of sunscreen product application: a problem in testing, a problem for consumers. Photodermatol Photoimmunol Photomed. February 2003;19(1): 17–20.

43. Maier H, Schauberger G, Martincigh BS, Brunnhofer K, Honigsmann H. Ultraviolet protective performance of photoprotective lipsticks: change of spectral transmittance because of ultraviolet exposure. Photodermatol Photoimmunol Photomed. April 2005;21(2):84–92.

44. Bernerd F, Vioux C, Lejeune F, Asselineau D. The sun protection factor (SPF) inadequately defines broad-spectrum photoprotection: demonstration using skin reconstructed in vitro exposed to UVA, UVBor UV-solar simulated radiation. Eur J Dermatol. May–June 2003;13(3):242–249.

45. Wolf R, Tuzun B, Tuzun Y. Sunscreens. Dermatol Ther. September 2001;14:208–214.

46. Mitchnick MA, Fairhurst D, Pinnell SR. Microfine zinc oxide (Z-cote) as a photostable UVA/UVB sunblock agent. J Am Acad Dermatol. January 1999;40(1):85–90.

47. Poh Agin P. Water resistance and extended wear sunscreens. Dermatol Clin. January 2006;24(1):75–79.

48. De Freitas ZM, dos Santos EP, Da Rocha JF, Dellamora-Ortiz GM, Goncalves JC. A new sunscreen of the cinnamate class: synthesis and enzymatic hydrolysis evaluation of glyceryl esters of p-methoxycinnamic acid. Eur J Pharm Sci. May2005;25(1):67–72.

49. Fisher AA. Sunscreen dermatitis: Part IV–The salicylates, the anthranilates, and physical agents. Cutis. December 1992;50 (6):397–398.

50. Fisher AA. Sunscreen dermatitis: Part III–The benzophenones. Cutis. November 1992;50(5):331–332.

51. Bestak R, Barnetson RS, Nearn MR, Halliday GM. Sunscreen protection of contact hypersensitivity responses from chronic solar-simulated ultraviolet irradiation correlates with the absorption spectrum of the sunscreen. J Invest Dermatol. September 1995;105(3):345–351.

52. Fu JM, Dusza SW, Halpern AC. Sunless tanning. J Am Acad Dermatol. May 2004; 50(5):706–713.

53. Faurschou A, Wulf HC. Durability of the sun protection factor provided by dihydroxyacetone. Photodermatol Photoimmunol Photomed. October 2004;20(5):239–242.

54. Dupuy A, Dunant A, Grob JJ; Reseau d'Epidemiologie en Dermatologie. Randomized controlled trial testing the impact of high-protection sunscreens on sun-exposure behavior. Arch Dermatol. August 2005;141(8):950–956.

CHAPTER 56

Photography of Skin Cancers

Ashish C. Bhatia, M.D.
Douglas Roach, M.D.

BOX 56-1 Overview

- The art and science of photography has evolved tremendously in the past decade, providing a versatile and practical set of tools to enhance the practice of cutaneous oncology, ultimately improving patient care.
- The role of photography in cutaneous oncology spans throughout the practice. It encompasses the documentation of tumors and biopsy sites, the monitoring of suspicious lesions, and communication between physicians regarding identification and treatments performed. It is also used by patients during their regular self-skin examinations looking for new or changing lesions.
- Photography is an invaluable tool in the education of trainees, peers, and the public regarding the identification and treatment options of skin cancers.

◼ INTRODUCTION

Like all medical photography, the photography of skin cancers has evolved dramatically in the last decade. With the conveniences brought to the medical field by advances in traditional film photography, instant photography, and digital photography,[1-6] there have emerged an ever-expanding list of uses of photography in the cutaneous oncology unit.

Applications for photography with regard to skin cancers are as varied as the interactions we have with skin cancer patients. Photography can be used in the diagnosis of skin cancers, tumor tracking, intraoperative mapping of skin cancer as in Mohs micrographic surgery,[7] and in following the treatment or post operative course of skin cancers. It is also routinely used to teach students, residents, patients, staff, and any other group about the detection and treatment of skin cancers.[8]

The science of photography is changing almost as rapidly as that of medicine.

In spite of technological advances, the fundamental principles of photography have remained unchanged for decades. An understanding of these essential skills will continue to determine the value of the photographs.

Any mention of specific products in this chapter should be understood to be included only for their value as examples that happen to exist at this point in time. Tomorrow or next month there may very well be better, faster, cheaper, and easier-to-use equipment that will render moot any recommendations or brand specific comments made here.

◼ PHOTOGRAPHY EQUIPMENT

BOX 56-2 Summary

- Clinical photography relies on the recording of light, whether it is on film or via an electronic sensor.
- Cameras and other photographic equipment should be selected based upon the needs of the practice. Portability, image capacity, image quality, ergonomics, durability, and other subjective factors play into such a decision. Generally, there are tradeoffs for every decision point.

No matter what equipment is used and regardless of the subject matter, there are certain things about photography that remain universal. First of all, we are capturing light. This light has been reflected off of a subject, passed through a lens, and then is recorded on either light-sensitive film or a digital sensor. In order for the image to be recorded properly, it is necessary to accurately resolve the image at the film plane or CCD (focus the light), measure and appropriately regulate the amount of light entering the lens, and also to account for the accurate color of that light. Good control of these three functions result in a sharp, adequately exposed, and properly colored photograph. Choosing equipment best suited to capture images of sufficient quality for ones practice is essential. This does not have to be the latest, most expensive equipment available. Often, that would be overkill. It may even add complexity unnecessarily. In the following section, we will explore the significance of the various components in photography equipment.

◼ CAMERA TYPES

BOX 56-3 Summary

- The broad categories of cameras available include single lens reflex (SLR) type cameras, compact or point and shoot type cameras, or hybrid cameras. All offer certain advantages and disadvantages; therefore, there is no one ideal camera type.
- The type of camera selected for clinical photography should reflect the needs of the clinical setting.

For photographing patients in the examination room or surgical suite, one will almost certainly be using what is called the "35-mm format". The name is a traditional holdover from the days when the film used in the camera measured 24 mm × 36 mm. How that translated to 35 mm is open for debate, but the fact remains that the specifications for most digital cameras and lenses reference the 35 mm standard. Cameras currently available generally fall into one of two basic categories. The first and most versatile is the single lens reflex (SLR) camera. Some manufacturers refer to this camera type as a digital single lens reflex (DSLR). An SLR camera body has the capacity to change lenses. This can be quite important when having to record extreme close-up images or when using the camera in conjunction with other optical devices such as microscopes. The other 35 mm camera type is usually much smaller and is called a "compact" or sometimes a "point-and-shoot" camera. Both SLRs and compacts can use the same recording media and both will produce sharp and well-exposed images if used correctly. Both types of cameras are usually capable of making completely automatic exposures and both are generally equipped with autofocus technology as well.

Single Lens Reflex

The name is yet another holdover from bygone days. In the early and middle part of the twentieth century, many cameras had not one but two lenses mounted vertically on the front. One was for the operator to use in viewing the scene and the other was to actually record the image. That made it a "twin lens" camera as opposed to the "single lens" made popular with the advent of 35 mm film. The reflex part of the name refers to the pentaprism and mirrors inside that allow for the operator to view reflexively the image through the same lens that will be used to pass light to the film. At the instant of exposure, the main mirror in the camera body flips up out of the way and the light travels unimpeded to the film. An advantage of this technology is that it allows the user to remove one lens, replace it with another, and view the image as the new lens sees it. One disadvantage of SLRs is that all these mirrors mounted in the camera necessitate a considerably larger and heavier camera body than is required by a compact camera. SLRs have been favored in the past by those who require the capability to set exposure manually to accommodate unique lighting situations. In the case of new digital or DSLR cameras, many of the lenses that one may currently own will now work on the same manufacturer's new digital camera body. There may be some minor formatting compromise due to the different field of view of the digital media in some cameras. Some manufacturers who have introduced reliable and affordable digital SLR cameras that are mostly compatible with their current nondigital gear are Nikon™, Canon™, and Fuji™.

Compact

Many years ago, this camera type was referred to as "Rangefinder" since that was the focusing mechanism it employed. Today it is called "Point and Shoot" or the more common "Compact." This is the overwhelming choice of digital camera purchasers in the world today. The chief advantages of this type of 35 mm camera are its size, ease of operation, and economy. With recent advances in the art of lens manufacturing, many of the better compact cameras now compare favorably with SLR models when used in most medical situations. This is especially true if the purpose of the image is to document relative sizes and locations of a lesion or defect. The majority of these models today come equipped with zoom lenses that can offer a range of different focal lengths thus emulating, if not equaling, the chief feature of SLRs. Even when equipped with a zoom lens, a compact will usually fit easily in a lab coat pocket—a feat that cannot be managed by an SLR.

One inadequacy found in some compact cameras is their flash capability. Most have a very small "pop-up" flash built into the body. When shooting very close to the subject or anything beyond about 9 ft from the subject, the flash

may cause a "white out" in the center of the image or may be considerably underpowered in lowlight situations. Many of these situations can be avoided by using the optical zoom capabilities of the camera while standing at approximately 4 to 5 ft from the subject.

Several manufacturers offer a hybrid DSLR/compact camera. It is referred to as an "SLR-like." The camera is larger than most compacts to accommodate a particularly un-compact like lens. That lens, while large and of a greater zoom capacity than most compacts, is not interchangeable. Overall, the camera has the look of a DSLR without many of the inherent SLR advantages. It bears examining by physicians though, as the potential for an auxiliary flash (a hot shoe) is commonly included and the larger lens may have better macro capability as well as minimal peripheral distortion.

■ LENSES

BOX 56-4   Summary

- SLR cameras allow the photographer to switch lenses for different purposes, while compact cameras generally have noninterchangeable lenses.
- Due to the nature of dermatology and dermatologic surgery, macro or "close up" capability is a requirement in choosing a camera lens.
- With digital cameras, using the "digital zoom" features should be avoided as it degrade the quality of the image.

No matter which camera is selected, it is helpful to have a simple familiarity with lenses. The choice of lenses is determined by the uses of the camera as well as budgetary and physical shooting space constraints. If the intent is to record full body images, it will be necessary to have a lot of room in which to physically back up, or one must use a wide-angle lens. Should the practice be confined to facial surgery for instance, a normal or short telephoto lens is adequate. In nearly all practices, the nature of the profession seems to require at least some macro or close-up capability.

Zoom

Zoom lenses take optical technology a step further. They are designed such that one or more of the internal elements can change position relative to each other and thus produce a field of view that is variable. Many cameras now come

equipped with lenses which span the range from 28 to 200 mm and greater. The overwhelming majority of compact cameras come equipped with zoom lenses as standard equipment. Most SLRs still are sold with a normal lens and have the option of mounting other fixed focal length or specialty lenses as well as zooms.

With digital cameras, most provide both optical and digital zoom. An optical zoom is like those on film camera. It changes its focal length by changing the position of internal lens elements. This is good as it employs the lens technology provided by high quality lens optics. What has commonly been referred to as "digital" zoom is not optically done but instead is an electronic parlor trick that simply crops the image. This results in a lower quality image. Do not rely on digital zoom. Use the digital camera's optical zoom feature whenever possible.

Macro or "Close-up" Lenses

If the camera of choice for the dermatologist does not have the advantage of being able to mount different lenses, the built-in lens should have the ability to focus on objects up close. Many consumer-level cameras are not manufactured with this capability.

For dermatologic surgery, it is most appropriate to have a macro lens that can capture an image at a 1:1 (subject to film) ratio. That means that an area photographed at that setting would be reproduced at exactly the same size on the film or media card. In the case of 35 mm format, your subject will cover an area 24 mm × 36 mm, which is adequate for recording a small lesion. Not all close-focusing lenses will have a 1:1 capability. The important thing is to have the ability to photograph subjects of a very small area with a reproduction ratio that does not exceed 1:3 or so.

Understand that a lens that happens to have macro capability also remains a regular lens of whatever focal length it has. If it is a 50 mm macro, for instance, it is still a perfectly good normal lens. The focal length will determine how far away you can be when you take both your normally focused pictures and your macro or small-field ones. The most appropriate macro lens we have found for photographing both patient clinical photographs and surgery at our facilities is that of 105 mm. It allows for close focus images while keeping the camera a reasonable distance from the site. This makes both the patient and surgeon more comfortable.

■ FLASH

BOX 56-5 Summary

- Using the camera flash instead of relying on ambient lighting allows for image consistency, adequate depth of field, reasonably quick shutter speeds, good color, and proper exposure.

A hot shoe is a port on a camera that allows for an external flash unit to be mounted. This flexibility is desirable if shooting in situations requiring complex external flash setups.

Regardless of the quality of the office or surgical suite lighting, it is best not to rely on these as the primary light source. Using the camera flash allows for image consistency, adequate depth of field, reasonably quick shutter speeds, good color, and proper exposure.

An electronic flash produces a light that simulates the color of daylight so color balance is not required. When shopping for a camera or flash, it is a good idea to understand that flashes are rated for their light output by a figure called a "guide number" (GN). A guide number of 80 or higher (at ISO 100) should be adequate for most dermatology requirements.

Many of today's newer cameras come with a small flash unit. In most circumstances, this flash will be all you need to get good shots. For images with a more professional look or for the flash to carry farther than about 9 ft for full-body shots, it will be necessary to supplement with an additional flash unit.

Flash Options

Many camera bodies (particularly DSLRs) come with a "hot-shoe." This is a square-shaped socket on top of the camera that allows for an external flash unit to be mounted. Most of these units have a number of electrical contacts in the socket (metal dots) that mate with similar contacts on the flash, and allow the flash and camera to communicate.

One type of flash that can be attached via the hot shoe is a ring flash. This type of flash has the unique ability to eliminate shadows by casting light from every direction. This can be quite effective if the intent is to record a very flat field that is evenly illuminated. It is also quite effective in photographing within a deep surgical defect or other cavity (like the oral cavity) as there are no shadows created by wound depth. Of course, that lack of shadow can be a drawback if the intent is to illustrate a lesion or rash that has a subtle texture.

A variation of the ring flash is one that comes with an adjunct "point light" that also mounts to the front of the lens but is composed of several point flashes. Some such flash units allow the user to disable or redirect one of these units and thus create some shading on the subject that can add dimension. The major disadvantage of ring lights is that they are usually underpowered. While fine for close-focus images, using a ring flash to illuminate a full human figure will often result in underexposure or the undesirable need to use a very wide lens opening.

Another lighting option is a point flash. Any flash that can be "pointed" at the field either by removing it from its mount or by using a movable flash head feature is called a point light. The advantage of this type of flash is that the angle of the light in relation to the object being photographed creates a slight shadow that reveals shape, contour and topography. If it is important to display the depth, height or texture of a dermatological feature, this type of flash is far superior to a ring flash.

In the case of digital compact cameras, most use a very small built-in unit that is barely adequate to produce decent photos. Since many digital cameras have inadequate batteries, the flash is usually reduced in size and output potential so as not to run down the batteries too quickly. In order to cover all clinical shooting circumstances, an auxiliary flash would need to be either connected to the camera or triggered at the correct instant by some other means. Since most lower priced digital cameras do not come with a PC socket for connecting a flash and most do not have a hot shoe, a way to accomplish this connection is the use of a photo cell that fires the flash when it senses another flash (the one built into the camera) going off. It can be thought of as a wireless remote. This has been done for years in photography studios and is called a "slave" flash unit. There are numerous manufacturers of slave units that can provide the medical photographer with plenty of light in virtually any circumstance. It should be noted that many digital cameras use a series of rapid low power "preflashes" in order to set the camera white balance for a shot and to reduce the "red-eye" effect. These preflashes can trigger the slave at an inappropriate instant. Be certain that the camera has a setting to disable the preflash or that the slave flash has the ability to filter those from its triggering cycle.

■ WHITE BALANCE

BOX 56-6 Summary

- Adjusting the white balance on the camera prior to taking photographs can compensate for unnatural looking color in photographs due to varying ambient light sources.

All light has color. Most of us do not think of it that way as our brains tend to color-correct light for us with no effort at all. Different sources of light produce different wavelengths which we identify using degrees Kelvin. This is commonly referred to as the light's "color temperature." With digital cameras, this correction for different temperatures of light is called "white balance." Daylight is the standard by which we measure color. Daylight being what we call white light causes colors to be reflected without a color prejudice. Yellow is seen as yellow, green as green, etc. When we use an artificial light source such as the fluorescent tubes in an office, the color of the light that is emitted produces an unnatural, usually somewhat greenish color when human skin is viewed under it. The camera records this unnatural color very well. For this reason, we must make an adjustment to the "white balance" setting of the camera if we choose to photograph subjects under fluorescent light. The same holds true for tungsten light found in common filament light bulbs, and for the tungsten/halogen hybrid bulbs found in many surgical situations. Fortunately, electronic flash is of a color temperature that is designed to be very close to that of daylight so a flash photo is generally close to being accurate when one uses a daylight white balance setting.

There are usually "presets" in the menu of most digital cameras that change the color sensitivity of the camera for various lighting situations. These may be adequate for some situations. For the most accurate recording of color, it is advisable to use a "custom white balance" procedure that is an option on most good digital cameras and *is explained in the manual*. If this custom white balance procedure is done properly once, you need not repeat it each time you use the same room and light source. Under no circumstances should one rely on a common setting found on most cameras called "auto white balance" or AWB. Few things in digital cameras work as poorly as AWB in office situations where color reproduction is critical.

BOX 56-7 Summary

- The images stored by a digital camera are recorded on digital media.
- There is a variety of digital media formats. Innovations in digital media technology are allowing increasing capacity and speed of the available digital media formats.
- Each digital camera can typically use only one or two types of digital media, so the correct type must be chosen for use in a certain camera.

When a photograph is made using a digital camera, the light passes through the lens to the image capture device. This is commonly a CCD or charge coupled device. This film-sized wafer is covered with millions of pixels or light sensing units that are filtered to see red or blue or green (primary colors) light. Once exposed to light, they transmit the light data along with their position in the array to a microprocessor which then translates that information into a coded pattern called a file format and passes it along to the memory module or media card for storage. The memory module or media card is the "film" in digital cameras. This is an oversimplified version of how a digital camera works.

At present, there are at least eight different variants of memory cards that fit into different cameras. Most memory card formats come in a tremendous range of capacities and all of them are usually adequate to the task of recording photographic images. Memory card types are *not* interchangeable; however, each card can be used over again. It will be necessary to empty or download the images as the card gets full.

An excellent accessory for a digital camera setup is a memory card reader. These small devices plug into your computer's USB port and have a number of different slots to accommodate many different types of memory cards. Once the card is inserted into the reader, the images can be downloaded. An advantage to downloading this way as opposed to connecting the camera directly to the computer using the cable that was supplied by the manufacturer is that the camera need not be present and thus need not be turned, which consumes battery power. The disadvantage of constantly inserting and removing memory cards from a camera is the chance of damaging the memory cards or the contacts.

BOX 56-8 Summary

- Megapixels reflect the amount of information or detail contained within an image.
- Larger megapixel images contain more detail, but also require longer transfer times to record and more space to store the image.

Megapixels describe how many "picture elements" (pixels) are on your CCD or CMOS chip and will thus be exposed to light reflected from the patient. The "mega" part of the name means "millions of." Each pixel is the smallest element in the picture that can be assigned a unique color. Increasing the number of pixels that make up an image increases the detail in the image to a point.

Today's multi-megapixel digital cameras produce as much detail as any 35 mm camera of 10 years ago. However, more megapixels are not necessarily better. As the megapixel value of an image increases, so does the file size (the amount of space required to store the image) as does the burden of handling a very large file size. This can slow down the recording of the image onto a memory card, the transfer of the images to a computer, as well as the processing of images by image editing software. Even to attain publication quality images, 12 megapixels are not necessary. Generally, using a lower setting on the camera to attain a 1.5 to 2.5 megapixels image will be adequate for dermatologic surgery use.

SUBMITTING IMAGES FOR PUBLICATION

BOX 56-9 Summary

- Publishers have specific requirements for accepting and reproducing images.
- It is important to recognize the parameters required by a publisher prior to submitting images to obtain the best quality reproduction in the publication.

Most publishers of medical journals and texts are now producing their material on entirely digital systems and equipment. In the "instructions for authors," most publishers specify the parameters for submission of digital images.

Resolution

Publishers specify image resolution in pixels per inch (ppi). While it is generally the case that the more ppi you have, the better quality the reproduction, it is also true that a resolution higher than that used by the output device is simply wasted information. For almost all applications, a resolution of 300 ppi is perfectly adequate. For PowerPoint™, 150 ppi is ideal. Many digital cameras will send images to the computer at 72 pixels per inch. This may seem at first to be wholly inadequate until you check the actual image dimensions (height and width). In most cases, the camera has saved the image at much larger print dimensions than required. Many image-enhancement software programs will be able to change the image size to adjust the ppi. For instance, if an image is saved at 72 ppi and at 20 in. × 30 in. it is a simple matter to convert the 72 ppi to 300 ppi and the image size will be reduced to about 5 in. × 7 in. The file size of the image will not change, since the amount of data remains constant.

Dimensions

This is the actual print size of the file in inches (or cm or pixels) measured around the outside of the image. Usually a 4 in. × 6 in. or 5 in. × 7 in. image is adequate for office use. For publication purposes, check the "instructions for authors" for specific requirements.

File Format

This describes how the application that created the file encodes and stores the information. To use digital pictures in PowerPoint™, save them as BMP, JPG or TIF format.

Popular Graphic File Formats

BMP: WINDOWS BITMAP A Microsoft™ format that is 24-bit raster, and has the capability of using limited LZW (lossless) compression. When used in PowerPoint™, however, these images frequently are too large to load quickly and project efficiently.

GIF: GRAPHICS INTERCHANGE FORMAT This is a format that was invented by CompuServe™ primarily for images viewed on the Internet. It is limited to only 256 colors (8 bits/pixel). It has several advantages when used in its Internet role. It uses lossless compression, which when combined with a limited color palette can result in really small file sizes.

It has the capability of using "transparent" as one of its colors and in its 89a incarnation, it is used to save and display simple animations. It is an adequate format for line drawings or logos, but not for photography.

JPG: JOINT PHOTOGRAPHIC EXPERTS GROUP

Also written as JPEG and pronounced jay´-peg. This is another popular Internet format. The main difference between this and GIF is that JPG files are in a raster image format of up to 24 bits/pixel. Thus, a JPG is the preferred format for images that have more than 256 colors such as full color photos. The compression scheme used by JPG is interesting in that one can manually determine the amount of compression to apply to each file. Though more compression results in a smaller file size, image quality is degraded as the file is further compressed.

TIF: TAGGED IMAGE FILE FORMAT TIFF (also

TIF) is the industry standard for a cross platform, multi-use raster image format that can be opened by almost all graphics applications. These files employ nondegrading compression. This is the ideal format for saving images with the best image quality.

■ SHOOTING TECHNIQUES AND TIPS

BOX 56-10 Summary

- Prior to any clinical photography, be sure to obtain written informed consent from the subject.
- Though a dedicated room for photography offers the best situation for clinical imaging, examination room photography can yield consistent results if good techniques and practices are always utilized.

Possibly the most vital element of good medical photography is consistency. Just as the use of standard procedures in a practice result in efficiency and high quality care, standard procedures for photography should also be implemented to provide consistent, high quality photographs.

Prior to taking the first photo of a patient, it is imperative that the patient signs a photo consent form. This can be and often is incorporated into the consent for treatment. The form should clearly state that the patient relinquishes all rights to payments and royalties that may accrue from any use of the images. Samples of photo consent forms may be obtained from the photography department of a local medical school or the local professional photographers' guild. Have an attorney review and alter such a form to suit the requirements of the practice and keep one in every patient chart.

The ideal office has a location that can be set aside exclusively for photography. There patients can be photographed, equipment stored securely and possibly even a space can be provided for review and storage of photos. This is often not possible in busy practices, so compromises must be made, with an emphasis on retaining consistency and image quality. The space chosen should ideally meet the following standards:

1. It needs to be distance large enough to accommodate the distance requirements of whatever lens will be used to shoot the broadest image (distance to subject).

2. It must have adequate lighting that will help to illuminate the subject without overwhelming the color balance characteristics of the flash. If the room has windows, opaque blinds can help keep the ambient lighting consistent regardless of the time of day.

3. It must have a reasonably neutral background with no distractions. The most popular color for patient clinical backgrounds is light blue.

4. It must have facilities for patient privacy and comfort. A changing area is ideal, or simply a chair and some provision for hanging clothes can be adequate.

5. It should have a secure cabinet or closet where camera gear and media are readily available so the clinician need not be searching the office for lens or a back-up memory card. Clean legible measuring devices should also be kept here for inclusion in certain photo fields.

6. Near the camera cabinet should be an electrical outlet where the battery chargers for the camera and flash batteries are kept plugged in. Good lithium-ion rechargeable batteries are ideal.

7. A small desk or table for writing down photo information during the session is also helpful.

In order to represent the results of treatment or surgery accurately, it is essential that there is consistency in the photographic procedures. This can be accomplished by minimizing the variables in the photography setup. The locations of the patient and cameraperson can be marked with tape on the floor. A "photo log" that records what poses, what camera settings and what exposures were made previous sessions with the same patient can be quite helpful. If possible, before and after type shots should be made with the previously shot images available for reference either printed or displayed on a monitor.

It is helpful to establish proper exposure and/or camera setting information for various shooting distances through testing. Write this information on a small piece of paper and tape it to the top of the flash or the back of the camera. Then when any office staff needs to take pictures, they can simply determine the distance to the subject and refer to the exposure and settings information written on the guide. This will go a long way toward establishing a consistent exposure and tonal range in pictures taken on different days.

It is also important to eliminate any unnecessary distractions in the photograph. These can range from background features to clothing or jewelry worn by the subject. If something appears in the viewfinder that has no relevance to the subject at hand, move it or crop it out.

Photographic Technique

Professional photographers always keep in mind a clear idea of what it is that they are about to shoot. This is essential for clinicians as well. Location and orientation of the condition can be best shown by first shooting an image that includes recognizable features such as face, hands, or feet. When shooting a standing person, rotate the camera 90° and shoot a vertical shot to eliminate wasted space in the photo to the left and right of the patient. This also allows for greater subject size and thus more detail in the image. Since this is an unnatural shooting position for some, care should be taken to see to it that camera straps or flash cords do not fall across the lens.

Once the orienting photos are complete, the next shots should include the total range or extent of the condition being photographed. Be sure to include all borders of the area of interest so that these can be compared to the same regions in subsequent post-treatment visits.

Finally, the last images should be those that record close-up details that are representative of the subject matter or provide a highly detailed view of a particular area of concern. At least one of

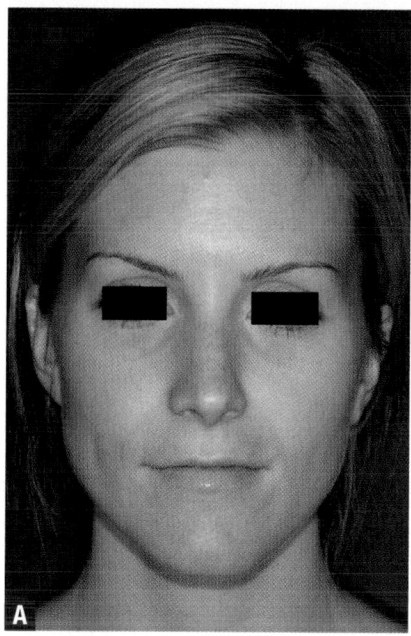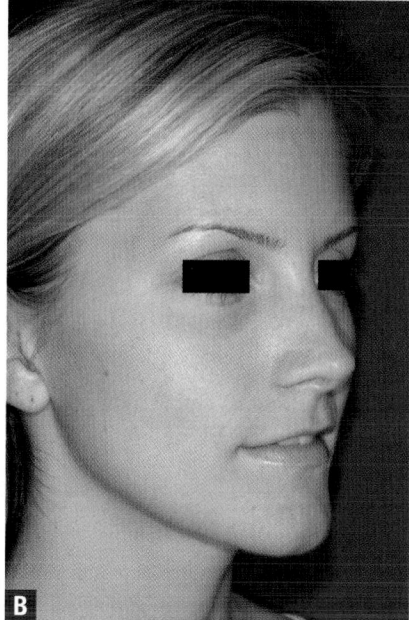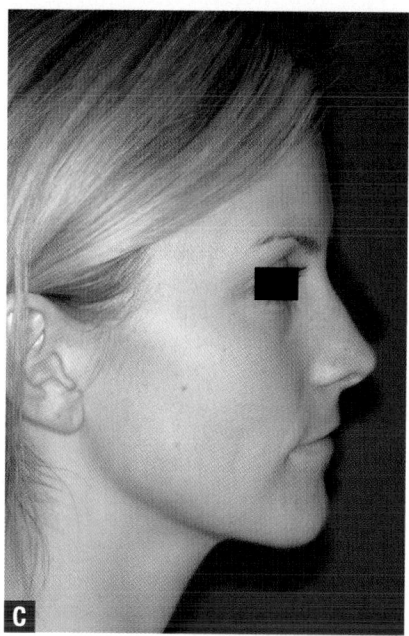

▲ **FIGURE 56-1** Standard positioning for full facial photography. **A.** Frontal view. **B.** Oblique view **C.** Lateral view. [Reprinted with permission from Derm Education Foundation and Derm.md (www.derm.md).]

the detail photos should include a measuring device in the field to represent accurately the size of the features shot close up. It is best to use a small centimeter scale that is made of a nonreflective material.

Pre and Postoperative Facial Photography

Standardizing the poses used in preoperative and postoperative photography allows the viewer to compare objectively the images taken at different points in time. A procedure should be established to position the patient consistently in these situations. Positioning aids with fixed distances and chin rests may be used. Alternatively, the staff can be taught basic posing techniques allowing for imaging in smaller rooms without the expense of positioning aids. One technique often used in cosmetic surgery photography involves positioning a patient through five poses at each photo session. These views include a frontal view, two oblique views, and two lateral views (Fig. 56-1). The camera should be positioned at a fixed distance from the subject, at a height approximately level with the subject's mid-face. The frontal and lateral views are self-explanatory. However, the oblique view can be consistently captured using the technique where the tip of the nose is aligned with the most prominent edge of the distal cheek.

Surgical Photography

In surgery, there are concerns with keeping the field free of contaminating items such as cameras and lenses. It obviously would be most appropriate to have someone not scrubbed in to be the person handling the camera. This person should understand both how the camera works and what it is that needs to be photographed. Have appropriate stand and stools on hand for the camera operator to easily get above the field for the most effective angle. If the camera is equipped with an auxiliary flash and/or battery, the cords connecting these devices should be taped down prior to surgery so they do not fall into the field if the camera is above it.

Make the first image of each procedure a shot that will identify the patient, such as the patient identification sticker or a card with the patient's information printed on it.

Certain lighting conditions in the operating room are different from what they will be in the office setting and may require some exposure compensation. For this reason, it is prudent to take some practice photographs prior to the procedure.

If gestures need be made in photos to point out a small artifact such as a stitch or tiny vessel, do not use fingers to do so. Keep the presence of hands to a minimum in photos and instead indicate the area with a straight clamp, pick-ups or other such blunt but slim device.

It is a sign of professionalism and pride if the field and any instruments or gloves that must be shown in a surgical photo are wiped clean of blood prior to taking a shot. Also, if the periphery of the operating area is draped with blue towels, be sure fresh clean ones are available to cover those that have been stained with fluids. Maintain suction in deep wounds right up until the image is captured. Pools of blood are very distracting in photographs and can in fact obscure areas of interest. Similarly, if the wound is wet from irrigation or from wiping with wet sponges, pat it dry quickly just before the shot to reduce the incidence of specular highlights.

When shooting gross specimens that have been excised or extracted, it is best to use a clean blue towel as a background. Images of specimens should be photographed in their correct anatomical orientation and with at least one of the images including a size scale placed just far enough away from the tissue that it may be easily cropped out later if necessary.

FINAL THOUGHTS

Current digital camera technology has arrived at the threshold where for most dermatologic purposes it is now virtually indistinguishable from 35 mm

653

image quality. If you purchase a good digital 6 or 7 megapixel SLR camera system, you will soon recover your investment in film and processing costs, as well as save on office expenses and personnel time.

In dermatology, perhaps more than any other medical discipline, well-crafted imaging skills can enhance your career even as it helps you to be of greater value to your profession and your colleagues and greater service to your patients.

REFERENCES

1. Bhatia AC, Brodell RT. Digital imaging. Emedicine website. Available at: http://www.emedicine.com/derm/topic561.htm. Accessed September 15, 2006.
2. Bhatia AC. The clinical image archiving clinical processes and an entire specialty. *Arch Dermatol.* 2006;142(1):96–8.
3. Ceteris paribus, definition. Wikipedia Web site. Available at: http://en.wikipedia.org/wiki/Ceteris_paribus. Accessed September 15, 2006.
4. Papier A, Peres MR, Bobrow M, Bhatia A. The digital imaging system and dermatology. *Int J Dermatol.* 2000;39:561–575.
5. Ratner D, Craig T. Digital photography. Emedicine website. Available at: http://www.emedicine.com/derm/topic 618.htm. Accessed September 15, 2006.
6. Vander Haeghen Y, Naeyaert JM. Consistent cutaneous imaging with commercial digital cameras. *Arch Dermatol.* 2006;142:42–46.
7. Lin BB, Taylor RS. Digital photography for mapping Mohs micrographic surgery sections. *Dermatol Surg.* 2001;27(4):411–414.
8. Berg D. A simple tool for teaching flap design with digital images. *Dermatol Surg.* 2001;27(12):1043–1045.

CHAPTER 57

New Approaches in the Diagnosis of Skin Cancer

R. P. Braun, M.D.

A. Gewirtzman, M.D.

F. A. LeGal, M.D.

O. Gaide, M.D., Ph.D.

H. S. Rabinovitz, M.D.

J.-H. Saurat, M.D.

A. A. Marghoob, M.D.

BOX 57-1 Overview

- Electrical impedance, autofluorescence, magnetic resonance imaging, and optical coherence tomography are interesting technologies for the *in vivo* diagnosis of pigmented lesions of the skin. They are promising, but currently still at research stage.
- *In vivo* confocal laser scanning microscopy is still at research stage, but has been shown to have a sensitivity and specificity of almost 98% for the diagnosis of melanoma.
- Clinical examination and total body photography are currently considered to be the gold standard for the examination of pigmented lesions in the US.
- Dermoscopy is the gold standard for the diagnosis of pigmented lesions in Europe and is gaining more popularity in the US.
- Dermoscopy has been proven to significantly increase diagnostic accuracy of the trained physician in the diagnosis of melanoma.

INTRODUCTION

In the last couple of years there has been an important progression in the development of noninvasive imaging techniques. Since the skin and its cancers are easily accessible, new technologies are often used first on the skin. This is why there have been many publications on this subject. Melanoma and basal cell carcinoma are the skin cancers that have been investigated the most, and for which most of the literature is available. Concerning basal cell carcinoma, the purpose of non-invasive imaging is the following: (1) Making the diagnosis *in vivo*, which means avoiding skin biopsies and (2) determining margins prior to surgery in order to avoid tumor recurrence.

Concerning melanoma, the purpose is to make the diagnosis *in vivo* while it is in curable stages and to provide screening tools. Given the multitude of techniques described, we can only review a nonexhaustive list in this chapter.[1] We will start with those which are still in the research state and end with the ones that are already part of the clinical routine.

ELECTRICAL IMPEDANCE

Using this method, a probe is placed on the skin tumor and the electrical impedance is measured. In a second step, the probe is placed on normal skin and impedance is measured.[2] The machine automatically calculates the ratio between the impedance values of normal skin and the skin with tumor. Apparently, this technique provides good results for basal cell carcinoma, but is still in a research phase. The idea behind it is that this approach detects microulceration as present in basal cell carcinoma and other tumors. This microulceration, which is not visible to the naked eye, modifies the impedance.

AUTOFLUORESCENCE

If excited with light of specific wavelengths, basal cell carcinoma shows autofluorescence. The signal is very weak and needs a sophisticated amplification system to enhance this fluorescence. This might be a promising approach for the future, but is currently in the research phase.

ULTRASOUND

Ultrasound technique has attained the status of routine application in clinical dermatology, with European countries using this technique for diagnostic purposes.[3,4] In Germany, ultrasound examination of soft tissue tumors and lymph nodes is mainly done by dermatologists. The ultrasound images are created due to different acoustic properties of tissues. High-frequency sound impulses are transmitted into the skin and then reflected, refracted, or inflected when tissue interface with different acoustic impedance is encountered. The amplitude of the intensity of the reflections at different depths of the skin is then plotted onto a display screen to give a one-dimensional graph known as the A-modes (amplitude display). The vertical cross-sectional image, which is the more familiar display of ultrasound data, is called B-mode scanning. B-Mode scanning uses the brightness level of multiple A-scans to build a two-dimensional image.

The higher the frequency used the more details that can be seen, but penetration depth in the skin decreases. There are two types of cutaneous ultrasound technique: 5–15 MHz and 20–50 MHz frequency ultrasonography. The former is commonly used for the evaluation of soft tissue and lymph nodes (Figs. 57-1 and 57-2). The penetration depth is up to 15 cm which is sufficient for this purpose. These systems allow even the use of color-coded Doppler imaging, which allows the evaluation of the blood flow in a lymph node (Fig. 57-2). The second is the 20–50 MHz frequency ultrasonography. Depending on the frequency of the ultrasound probes, the penetration depth for a 20 MHz in the skin is up to 10 mm. The 50 MHz frequency ultrasound provides much more detail, but penetration depth decreases to 3 to 4 mm. In our experience, 20 MHz ultrasound allows the identification skin tumors, measures their depth, but does not allow the making of a diagnosis. For example, melanomas appear as solid, hypoechogenic lesions, which is the same for BCC or nevi. High-resolution ultrasound can be used for the determination of tumor thickness prior to surgery, but if there is a dense lymphocytic infiltrate or regression, it is often overestimated. It has been described to as being useful for the follow up of scleroderma patients.

OPTICAL COHERENCE TOMOGRAPHY

Optical coherence tomography (OCT) is similar to ultrasound imaging, except that it uses light rather than sound waves. It is described as an intermediate imaging device between ultrasound and confocal scanning laser microscopy.[5,6] The OCT image is based on the principle of "Michelsons interferometry." A pulse of near infrared, low coherence light is split such that half the beam is

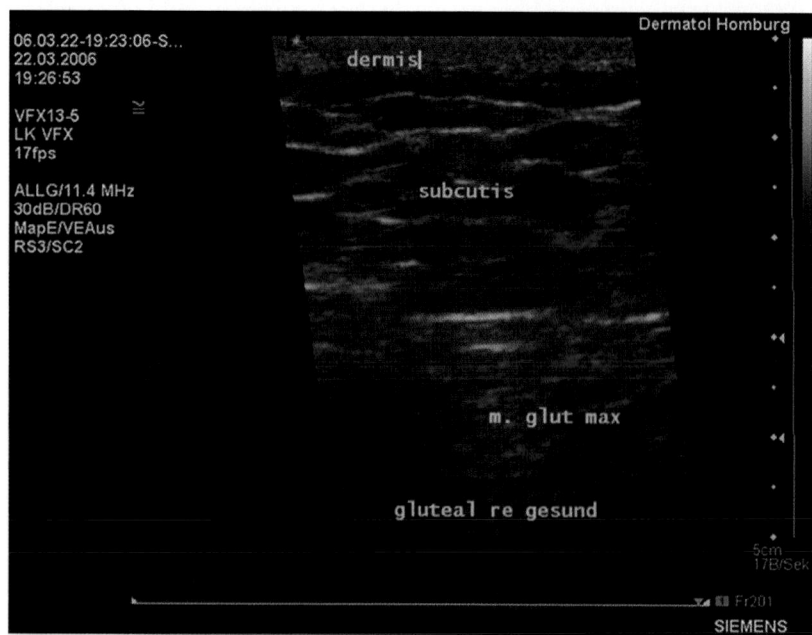

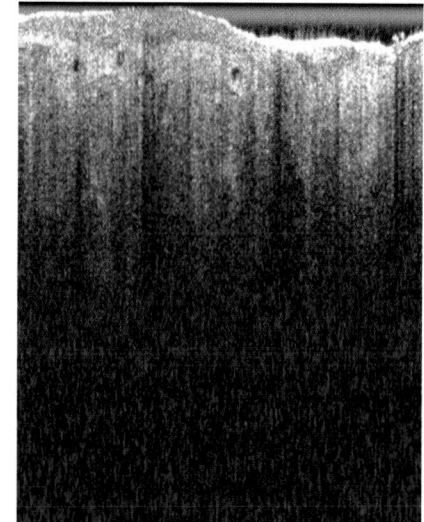

▲ **FIGURE 57-3** OCT image of a BCC (arrows) on the left and normal skin on the right. (Courtesy of Prof. J. Welzel, Augsburg, Germany.)

▲ **FIGURE 57-1** Ultrasound image of normal skin of the right buttock area. The following structures can be seen: dermis, subcutaneous tissue and the gluteus maximus muscle. (Courtesy of Dr. D.Dill-Müller, Homburg, Germany.)

sent to the specimen and half to a scanning reference mirror. The light to the specimen is focused on the papillary skin layers, backscattered, and recombines with the other reference beam of light that has reflected from the mirror system. An interference signal is only detectable when the optical paths of both arms match within the coherence length of the light source.

Measurement of the interference pattern allows the determination of the position within the tissue where the light was reflected. It is the reflectivity of different components of tissues, such as cell membranes and melanin, which provide contrast in images. A two-dimensional cross-sectional image is built up by lateral scanning across the tissue. The axial resolution depends on the coherence length of the light source and is reported to be about 15/μm. Penetration depth depends on the wavelength of light used and varies from 1 to 5 mm (reticular

dermis). Lateral resolution is usually about 10 to 15/μm. A broad spectrum of skin diseases has been studied using OCT, with distinctive architectural changes observed compared to normal skin. For example, melanocytic tumors show a more homogenous signal distribution. However, the current limits in resolution do not allow a differential diagnosis between benign and malignant lesions (Fig. 57-3); however, assessing and monitoring inflammatory skin diseases is still possible.

MAGNETIC RESONANCE IMAGING

Magnetic resonance imaging (MRI) has been used experimentally for the examination of pigmented skin lesions. The application of MRI in dermatology has become practical with the use of specialized surface coils that allow higher resolution imaging than standard MRI coils.[7] At this point in time, however, the technology remains experimental with no specific dermatologic applications established. The principle of MRI involves the absorption and re-emission of radio waves from tissue protons exposed to a strong external magnetic field. If a proton is influenced by a radiofrequency pulse (excitation) in a strong magnetic field, it returns to a stable low-energy state and gives off a weak radio signal that is detected by the coil, which acts as an antenna. Tissue contrast is a result of the differences in relative MRI signal intensity between structures. Specific imaging

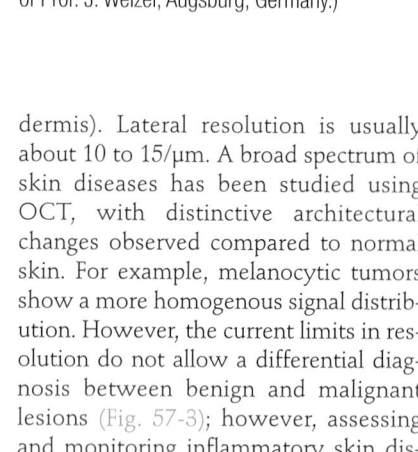

▲ **FIGURE 57-2** Ultrasound image (11 MHz) of a reactive axillar lymph node which shows a typical benign perfusion pattern (Doppler mode) from central hilus vessel (yellow) no peripheral perfusion can be detected. (Courtesy of Dr. D. Dill-Müller, Hamburg, Germany.)

sequences, such as T1- and T2-weighted, differ in signal contrast characteristics. For example, T2-weighted sequences show more signal intensity when there is high fluid or water content. In experimental MRI of skin, criteria suggestive of malignancy in skin tumors such as nonhomogeneity and surrounding soft tissue edema were reported. To date, however, the ability of MRI to reliably discriminate benign from malignant melanocytic lesions is not possible. MRI has sufficiently high resolution to obtain information on the depth and extent of the underlying tissue involvement, which may prove to be useful in the preoperative assessment of melanoma.

CONFOCAL LASER SCANNING MICROSCOPY (CSLM)

CSLM is a noninvasive imaging system that allows for the *in vivo* examination of the epidermis and papillary dermis at a resolution approaching histologic details.[8] It works by tightly focusing a low-power laser beam (visible or near-infrared wavelength) on a specific point in the skin, and detecting only the light reflected from that focal point through a pinhole-sized spatial filter. This beam is then scanned horizontally over a two-dimensional grid to obtain a horizontal microscopic section. Adjustments can be made in the focal length of the beam, allowing the microscope to image a series of horizontal planes stacked vertically, with an axial thickness of 2 to 5 mm. This *in vivo* axial section thickness correlates closely with the axial thickness of excised histologic sections. The imaging depth in normal skin is limited to 200 to 300/μm (papillary dermis) and depends on the wavelength of laser light used (longer wavelengths allowing deeper penetration). Although the lateral resolution of CSLM permits imaging of mostly cellular structures, on occasion, subcellular structures such as melanosomes and nucleoli can be visualized.

Free cytoplasmic melanin pigment and cytoplasmic pigmented and nonpigmented melanosomes provide strong contrast.[9] Therefore, as a result of the presence of melanosomes, the cytoplasm of melanocytes in pigmented *and* amelanotic melanomas consistently appear bright on CSLM, thus allowing for their easy detection. Features of intraepidermal malignant melanoma as viewed with a CSLM have been correlated with histologic criteria for melanoma, thus aiding in the *in vivo* diagnosis of melanoma.[8] In fact, CLSM is able to detect atypical

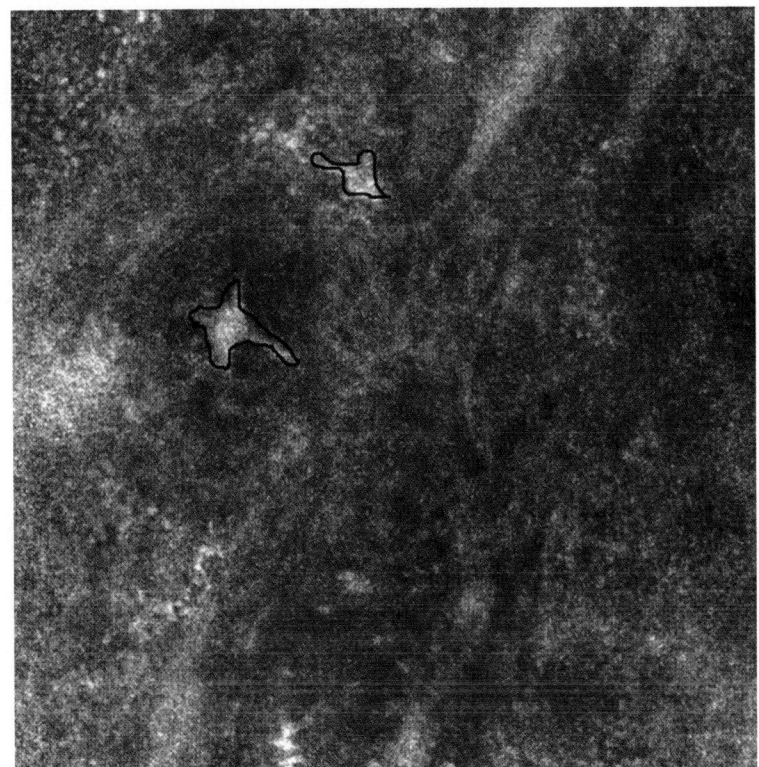

▲ **FIGURE 57-4** Confocal laser scanning microscopy image of a melanoma showing the presence of two atypical dendritic cells (melanocytes) within the epidermis. This corresponds histopathologically to pagetoid spread. One can also see large polymorphic tumor cells throughout the image. (Courtesy of Dr. A. Marghoob, New York)

melanocytes within the epidermis, which correlates with a pagetoid spread histologically and for which an important histological criterion for the diagnosis of melanoma is made (Fig. 57-4).

The principal advantage of CSLM is the ability to noninvasively assess the cellular components of intact skin lesions with detail approaching that of histology. Consequently, a lesion can be examined at any moment in time to determine whether it has features of melanoma. Future studies are needed for formal statistical evaluation to determine the ability with which CSLM can detect diseases of the skin.

MULTISPECTRAL IMAGING AND AUTOMATED DIAGNOSIS

The knowledge that light of different wavelengths penetrate the skin to various depths and that they interact differently with the chromophores of the skin, led investigators to evaluate pigmented lesions under specific wavelengths of light from infrared to near-UV range. Sequences of images taken at different wavelengths of light are called multispectral images. Currently there are two systems, spectrophotometric intracutaneous analysis (SIA) scope, and

MelaFind, which use multispectral dermoscopic images. However, the strategies of both devices are totally different: Melafind uses computer analysis to provide a diagnosis in a completely automated system and Siascope uses computer analysis to generate SIA-graphs and images that require the physician's interpretation for diagnosis.

The SIA system, which is described as a skin chromophore imaging system, performs *in vivo* examination of a 12-mm diameter area of skin and captures images at four different, narrow-spectrum, filtered wavelengths ranging from 400 to 1000 nm.[10] These wavelength-dependent images provide information on the concentration, distribution, and position of skin chromophores, collagen, melanin, and hemoglobin (Fig. 57-5). This information is then displayed in different SIA graphs and corresponding images to assist the physician in diagnosis. The combined features of dermal melanin, collagen holes, and erythematous blush with blood displacement have reported specificity of 80% and sensitivity of 83% for melanoma in a sample of lesions referred for excision biopsy.[10]

MelaFind is another instrument using a multispectral approach. The main difference to the previous system is that

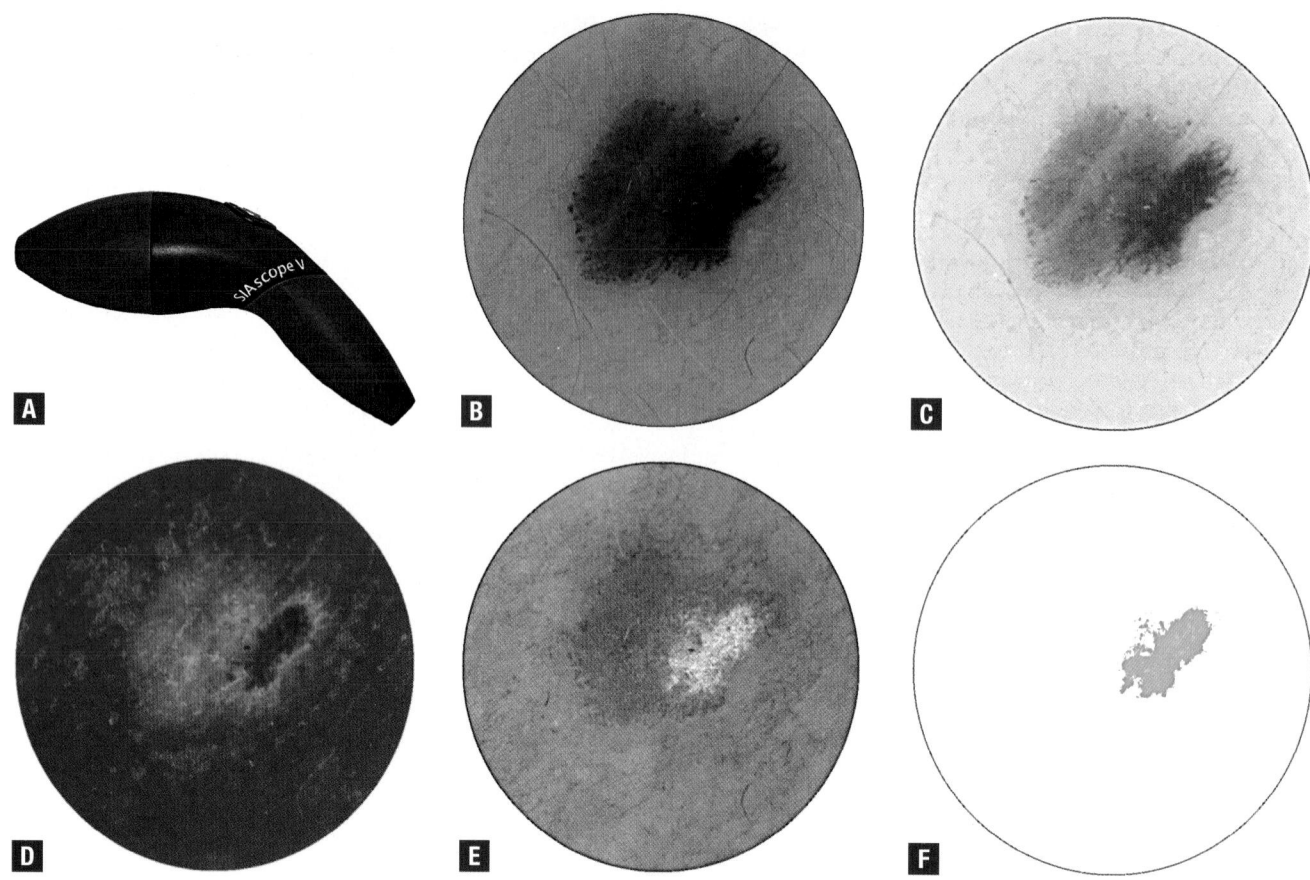

▲ **FIGURE 57-5** Example of multispectral imaging. **A.** Hand piece of the Siascope V device (Astron Clinica); **B.** Dermoscopy image; **C.** Total melanin Siagraph; **D.** Collagen Siagraph; **E.** Blood Siagraph; **F.** Dermal melanin Siagraph.

morphologic information about the lesion border, size, etc is *not* available to the clinician. The researchers behind MelaFind aim to produce a fully automated, nonoperator-dependent, objective measurement instrument for the diagnosis of melanoma.[11] The system uses dedicated software (algorithms) for automatic differentiation between malignant melanoma and benign pigmented lesions. It aims to differentiate *in situ* melanoma from invasive melanoma and may be able to determine reliably the Breslow thickness of invasive melanoma. This is a very promising approach that is currently under FDA approval. It is very likely that it will be available to clinicians in the near future.

DERMOSCOPY

Dermoscopy is an *in vivo* method that has been reported to be a useful tool for the early recognition of malignant melanoma and the differential diagnosis of pigmented lesions of the skin, including BCC. This method is routine in many countries, mainly in Europe, but is gaining more importance in the US. A detailed description of the technique and the equipment is provided in chapter titled "see Chapter 37."

TOTAL BODY PHOTOGRAPHY (BODY MAPPING)

Total body photography is the routine technique in the US. In fact, it uses a series of overview images of the skin covering the maximal surface. At the patients' consultation, the images can be compared directly with the patient and new or changing lesions can be macroscopically identified. A detailed description of the technique is provided in chapter titled "see Chapter 37."

FINAL THOUGHTS

Clinical examination and total body photography are, at this moment, considered to be the state-of-the-art for the diagnosis of pigmented lesions in the US. Dermoscopy is considered to be state-of-the-art in Europe and is gaining an increasing popularity in the US. This technique is ideal for pigmented lesions because it allows the examination of a large number of lesions; the equipment is relatively inexpensive, and most importantly, it has been proven to increase diagnostic accuracy of trained physicians. The only obstacle that has to be overcome is the training. Since dermoscopy is part of many residency programs in the US, there is no doubt that future generations of dermatologists will use this technique once they enter private practice. On the other hand, it is easy to understand that if one has not been trained to use dermoscopy one will have to overcome the inhibition first, which itself is an important step.

Computer-assisted diagnosis will definitively be an issue within the upcoming years because the first system is about to obtain FDA approval in the US. This will raise many questions such as who is going to use this type of instrument, whether general practitioners or dermatologists, and who is going to pay for it? There will be a place for computer-assisted diagnosis in the future if this technique is going to be used reasonably and thoughtfully. If there would be reimbursement for every lesion that is going to be examined with this type of device, without any restrictions, this will represent important additional costs for the health system and this type of device will not have a future. On the other hand, if this type of device is going to be used as a "second opinion" on difficult lesions or by physicians with less experience concerning pigmented lesions, this type of instrument could be very useful. There are some interesting and promising new technologies which are today still at the research stage, but which might enter clinical routine very soon. The most promising approach seems to be the *in vivo* confocal laser scanning microscopy. In a recent publication, this technology has been shown to have a sensitivity and specificity of 98% for the diagnosis of melanoma. Soon, the next generation of these devices will become much more user friendly and most probably affordable.

REFERENCES

1. Marghoob AA, Swindle LD, Moricz CZ et al. Instruments and new technologies for the in vivo diagnosis of melanoma. *J Am Acad Dermatol.* 2003;49:777–797.
2. Aberg P, Nicander I, Holmgren U, et al. Assessment of skin lesions and skin cancer using simple electrical impedance indices. *Skin Res Technol.* 2003;9:257–261.
3. Blum A, Muller D. Ultrasound of the lymph nodes and the subcutis in dermatology. Part 1. *Hautarzt.* 1998;49:942–949.
4. Blum A, Muller D. Sonography of lymph nodes and subcutis in dermatology. 2. *Hautarzt.* 1999;50:62–72.
5. Welzel J, Lankenau E, Birngruber R, et al. Optical coherence tomography of the human skin. *J Am Acad Dermatol.* 1997;37:958–963.
6. Welzel J, Reinhardt C, Lankenau E, et al. Changes in function and morphology of normal human skin: evaluation using optical coherence tomography. *Br J Dermatol.* 2004;150:220–225.
7. El Gammal S, Hartwig R, Aygen S, et al. Improved resolution of magnetic resonance microscopy in examination of skin tumors. *J Invest Dermatol.* 1996;106:1287–1292.
8. Rajadhyaksha M, Gonzalez S, Zavislan JM, et al. In vivo confocal scanning laser microscopy of human skin. II.: Advances in instrumentation and comparison with histology. *J Invest Dermatol.* 1999;113:293–303.
9. Rajadhyaksha M, Grossman M, Esterowitz D, et al. In vivo confocal scanning laser microscopy of human skin: melanin provides strong contrast. *J Invest Dermatol.* 1995;104:946–952.
10. Moncrieff M, Cotton S, Claridge E, et al. Spectrophotometric intracutaneous analysis: a new technique for imaging pigmented skin lesions. *Br J Dermatol.* 2002;146:448–457.
11. Elbaum M, Kopf AW, Rabinovitz HS, et al. Automatic differentiation of melanoma from melanocytic nevi with multispectral digital dermoscopy: a feasibility study. *J Am Acad Dermatol.* 2001;44:207–218.

CHAPTER 58

Teledermatology

Karen E. Edison, M.D.

BOX 58-1 Overview

- The practice of teledermatology has grown considerably where access barriers exist.
- Live-interactive (LI) and store-and-forward (S/F) modalities are used, either alone or in combination (hybrid model).
- Using teledermatology to identify patients with skin cancer at an early stage is an important application of telehealth technology.
- Diagnoses made and management recommended during both live-interactive and store-and-forward teledermatology interactions are in concordance with in-person (IP) diagnosis and treatment.
- Global teledermatology will enable patients in remote areas worldwide to access expert dermatological diagnosis.
- Teledermatology technologies are increasingly reliable and affordable.

INTRODUCTION

BOX 58-2 Summary

- Live-interactive teledermatology uses videoconferencing and mimics traditional in-person care.
- Store-and-forward teledermatology allows for efficient diagnosis of skin lesions.
- In 2002, there were 62 teledermatology programs in the United States, two-thirds LI and one-third S/F.
- Common settings include academic health centers, military healthcare, and service to distant and captive populations.

The visual nature of dermatology has enabled dermatologists to be early adopters of telemedicine. Telemedicine, more recently referred to by the broader term "telehealth," is defined by the American Telemedicine Association as "the use of medical information exchanged from one site to another via electronic communications to improve patients' health status."[1] This broad definition encompasses videoconferencing, electronic transmission of still images, remote monitoring, and ehealth applications, among others. This chapter will provide an overview of teledermatology and a discussion of its use in the diagnosis and management of skin cancer.

The practice of teledermatology has been divided over the past decade into two primary modalities, live-interactive (LI) and store-and-forward (S/F). Live-interactive teledermatology makes use of videoconferencing and, other than physical separation by distance, is very similar to the traditional in-person doctor/patient visit (Fig. 58-1). Store-and-forward teledermatology involves the acquisition of standardized patient information and high quality digital photographs of the skin by a local provider; both are then transmitted to the teledermatologist for consultation, which includes the diagnosis and treatment plan (Fig. 58-2). This is typically completed within 24 h but is not necessarily "real-time," and is consultative in nature, with the local primary care provider ultimately executing the care plan with the patient. Therefore, the practice of teledermatology may involve interaction between the primary care provider and the dermatologist or between the patient and the dermatologist, or both, depending on the setting.

While both forms of teledermatology have been increasingly applied and utilized intermittently since the early 1990s, rapidly improving technology is further changing their application. Teledermatology programs currently exist in every continent. The American Telemedicine Association's Special Interest Group (SIG) on Teledermatology conducted a study of the practice of teledermatology in the United States and found that in 2002, there were 62 active teledermatology programs, of which roughly two-thirds were live-interactive and one-third were store-and-forward. The bulk of these programs have thus far been developed where a clear mission base of service and outreach exists, such as in academic health centers, or where patients are often distant or otherwise expensive to transport. The challenges of caring for patients in correctional systems, those on active military duty, and those in the Veterans Affairs (VA) healthcare system are some of the examples.[2] A similar pattern is seen around the world with teledermatology programs arising where there are access barriers created by geography or distance such as in Norway, or in areas where there is a critical shortage of trained dermatologists as in some African countries.[3,4]

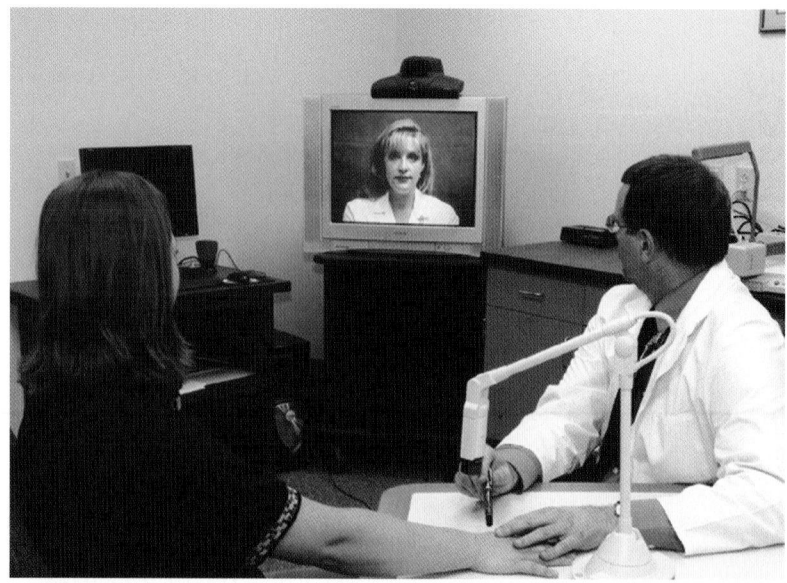

▲ FIGURE 58-1 Live-interactive teledermatology. (Courtesy of Missouri Telehealth Network, University of Missouri-Columbia.)

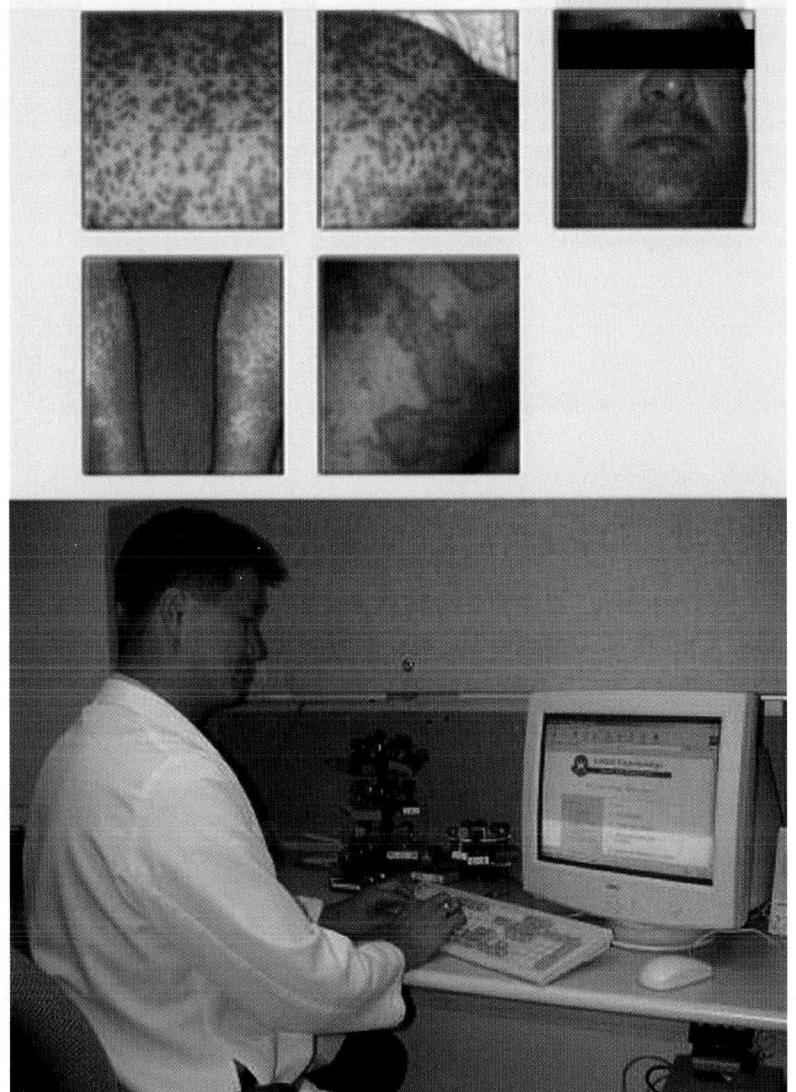

▲ **FIGURE 58-2** Store-and-forward teledermatology. [Courtesy of Lt. Col. Hon. S. Pak, M.D., Telemedicine and Advanced Technology Research Center (TATRC)].

urban dwellers, rural residents have higher poverty rates, fewer physicians, fewer hospitals and overall fewer healthcare resources.[8] As a result, much of the care of skin disease in rural areas falls to primary care providers, many of whom self-report a lack of comfort and expertise in the diagnosis and management of skin diseases. Studies show that primary care providers are less accurate in their diagnostic ability when compared to dermatologists.[9] Because the bulk of skin cancers are currently screened for and diagnosed by primary care providers worldwide, the quality of this service may be highly variable. As a result, patients with skin cancer may have a delayed diagnosis, receive substandard care, and consequently experience greater morbidity and higher mortality compared to those diagnosed and treated primarily by dermatologists.

Quality and Reliability

Telehealth technology can help expand access to expert dermatologic diagnosis and treatment. The technology has improved markedly and reliable dermatologic diagnosis is possible. A growing body of evidence indicates that diagnosis and management during both live-interactive and store-and-forward teledermatology interactions are in concordance with traditional in-person (IP) standards of examination and treatment. Most studies reveal 60 to 80% total agreement and 70 to 90% partial agreement when comparing in-person diagnosis to both live-interactive and store-and-forward teledermatology.[10,11] Dozens of studies have examined the reliability of teledermatology in the diagnosis of skin diseases, including skin cancer, and several others have specifically examined the diagnosis of skin cancer and/or pigmented lesions. It has been shown that diagnostic concordance for skin cancer comparing in-person (IP) exam to both forms of teledermatology is not significantly different from in-person interobserver diagnostic concordance.[10,11] In spite of the proven ability to accurately diagnose skin cancer, including malignant melanoma via telehealth technology, many dermatologists remain wary of using it for this purpose. Failing to diagnose melanoma and other skin cancers can be deadly for patients and is the most common reason for litigation against dermatologists in the United States.[12] Before widespread adoption of telehealth for this purpose, more studies may be needed to substantiate the efficacy and

TELEDERMATOLOGY AND SKIN CANCER

BOX 58-3 Summary

- Many patients worldwide have limited access to expert dermatological care.
- Skin cancer may be reliably diagnosed using teledermatology.
- Knowledge of local healthcare resources is essential when caring for skin cancer patients at a distance.

As reported in earlier chapters, skin cancer rates around the world continue to climb. Deaths from all types of skin cancer may be reduced with earlier diagnosis and treatment.[5] Using telehealth to identify patients with skin cancer at an early stage is an important application of telehealth technology.

Access to Expert Diagnosis

The workforce shortage and skewed distribution of dermatologists is well recognized. Dermatologists are in short supply all over the world. Wait times for dermatology appointments currently range up to 3 months in the United States, where there are an average of 3.3 dermatologists per 100,000 people.[6,7] Zimbabwe, by comparison, has less than one dermatologist per one million people.[3] In most countries, the majority of the dermatologists choose to live in urban environments, whereas large numbers of people who live in rural areas find it difficult to travel the distances necessary to receive dermatologic services. Compared to safety of using teledermatology in the evaluation and management of pigmented lesions and melanoma. Future advances in imaging technologies such as confocal scanning laser microscopy may promote greater confidence in the use of teledermatology to diagnose pigmented lesions.[13]

Skin Cancer Management

Once skin cancer is diagnosed using teledermatology, special considerations are necessary when caring for geographically distant patients. While technology already exists to enable virtual surgery at a distance, it is typically neither affordable nor widely available. Consequently, the teledermatologist needs to have a complete understanding of the resources available locally to the patient. In a rural live-interactive teledermatology practice, for example, there may be a primary care provider or a general surgeon either onsite or in the community who is comfortable performing skin biopsies and excisions. Even so, patients may be asked to travel to have surgery to ensure clear margins of tumor removal. As the development of topical immunomodulators (such as imiquimod) capable of treating some forms of skin cancer nonsurgically progresses, teledermatology may become more applicable as a modality for treating and monitoring skin cancer patients at a distance.

▮ REIMBURSEMENT

BOX 58-4 Summary

- The reimbursement landscape for teledermatology improves annually.

Innovations in healthcare technology, such as teledermatology, typically occur long before reimbursement is realized. Currently Medicare, America's healthcare program for the elderly and the disabled, provides reimbursement equivalent to that of traditional in-person examination, as long as the teledermatologist is caring for a patient via live-interactive teledermatology in an approved rural healthcare setting. Medicare approved healthcare settings include hospitals, federally qualified community health centers, rural health clinics, and physician offices.[14] Nearly one-half of the United States provide reimbursement for teledermatology through their public healthcare programs for low-income patients (Medicaid and State Children's Health Insurance Programs) and many

payers in the private sector now provide reimbursement for live-interactive teledermatology. Store-and-forward teledermatology is currently only reimbursed by a few state Medicaid programs, such as Texas and California, and by Medicare only in Alaska and Hawaii.[15,16] The reimbursement landscape for telehealth in the United States changes every year and, as reimbursement expands, so too does the practice of teledermatology.

▮ GLOBAL TELEDERMATOLOGY

BOX 58-5 Summary

- Global teledermatology provides access to expert dermatological care for patients worldwide.

The capacity of teledermatology to provide access to patients with skin diseases worldwide is rapidly expanding. Global teledermatology has several models. One involves the partnership of dermatologists in one country who have agreed to provide expert consultation for a community of patients in another country. This is typically an altruistic arrangement and depends on local healthcare workers to obtain digital images for transmission over the internet to the teledermatologists.[17] The United States military also uses store-and-forward teledermatology for active duty troops worldwide.[18] Another model employs the use of internet websites where patients' digital photos are posted from all over the world, for both diagnosis and second opinion; volunteer dermatologists from around the world provide expert on-line consultation. Several websites of this sort are currently active, such as "telederm.org." Multiple international challenges exist, including lack of healthcare infrastructure and patient access to pharmaceuticals in some countries; however, the promise of teledermatology is immense. Presently, over 60% of the world's people suffer from skin diseases that can be treated with timely diagnosis and access to effective therapy.[19]

▮ FUTURE DIRECTIONS

BOX 58-6 Summary

- The hybrid model of teledermatology combines the best of both LI and S/F teledermatology.
- Teledermatology technologies are increasingly reliable and affordable.

Hybrid Model

Recently, new attention has been given to the so-called "hybrid model" of teledermatology.[20] In this model, standardized high quality digital photographs of the patient are sent with the patient's healthcare information and history to the teledermatologist who then reviews the information and discusses it with the patient in a live-interactive telehealth visit using videoconferencing. The hybrid model provides the strengths of both LI and S/F forms of teledermatology. The standardized digital photographs of store-and-forward teledermatology decrease variability in the quality of physical examination. With live-interactive teledermatology, one site's personnel may provide excellent camera control and enable quality virtual physical examination, while another site's personnel may not, depending on the personnel available that day.

The strength of live-interactive teledermatology is in the ability to create and sustain a doctor/patient relationship. Live-interactive videoconferencing allows for the development of traditional doctor/patient healing relationships, where diagnosis and treatment are discussed, and the patient has an opportunity to have his or her questions answered by the teledermatologist at the point of care. One content analysis study of doctor/patient communication showed nearly identical time spent and content covered in live-interactive and in-person examinations. Specifically, discussions included patient assessment, explanation of diagnosis, management planning, and patient education. Time spent with the patient in each modality (LI and IP) did not differ significantly.[21]

The strength of store-and-forward teledermatology is in the standardization of high quality digital photographs and in the level of efficiency that S/F teledermatology affords. More patients may be evaluated in a shorter time period and this may be accomplished at the dermatologist's convenience. This method can provide access to expert dermatologic care to large numbers of underserved patients.

Portability and Affordability

While the model of teledermatology adopted must be individualized for a particular setting and patient population, teledermatology technologies are increasingly reliable and affordable. Top quality videoconferencing setups, for example, have decreased from $85,000 to $5000 or less in just one decade, and high-quality PC based teledermatology software is increasingly available. In addition, commercially available digital cameras are now used to obtain and transmit high-quality digital photographs. Even the digital cameras found on modern cellular phones have improved to the point that high-quality digital images can easily be captured, transmitted, and downloaded. Dermatologists at some academic health centers are already using them to supervise resident physicians' care of dermatology patients.[22] This technology will only improve, become less expensive and more widely available. These technological advances are expected to have a major impact on the practice of dermatology. Patients may soon be able to videoconference with their dermatologists from their home and even from their cell phone and/or personal digital assistant (PDA).

■ FINAL THOUGHTS

Teledermatology primarily increases access to and efficiency of dermatologic services and can help to resolve the problem of healthcare access for skin disease patients worldwide. Skin cancer may be reliably screened for and diagnosed via telehealth; however, many healthcare providers are still wary of using telehealth for the diagnosis and management of pigmented lesions. Teledermatologists must be aware of local resources available to the patient including access to skin biopsy, skin cancer excision, and treatment, and access to needed pharmaceuticals. As telehealth technologies improve and become increasingly available and affordable to healthcare providers and skin cancer patients, increased utilization of existing and future applications is expected worldwide.

REFERENCES

1. American Telemedicine Association 2005. Defining telemedicine. Available at: http://www.atmeda.org/news/definition.html
2. American Telemedicine Association 2003. SIG survey on the status of teledermatology activity in the US. Available at: http://www.atmeda.org/ICOT/sigtelederm.SIGSurveyDatabase2003-v.2.pdf
3. Zimbabwe Situation Daily News. Bonding won't heal health system. Available at: http://www.zimbabwesituation.com/oct8a_2004.html#link31. Accessed October 8, 2004.
4. Norway Ministry of Health and Care Services. Telemedicine in Norway: status and the road ahead. Available at: http://www.dep.no/hod/norsk/dok/andre_dok/rapporter/030071-220006/dok-bn.html. Accessed January 13, 1999.
5. Diepgen TL, Mahler V. The epidemiology of skin cancer. *Br J Dermatol.* April 2002;146(suppl):1–6.
6. Resneck JJ, Kimball AB. The dermatology workforce shortage. *J Am Acad Dermatol.* January 2004;50(1):50–54.
7. Resneck JJ. Too few or too many dermatologists? Difficulties in assessing optimal workforce size. *Arch Dermatol.* October 2001;137(10):1295–1301.
8. Hicks LL. Availability and accessibility of rural health care. *J Rural Health.* October 1990;6(4):485–505.
9. Federman DG, Kirsner RS. The primary care physician and the treatment of patients with skin disorders. *Dermatol Clin.* April 2000;18(2):215–221.
10. Heinzelmann PJ, Williams CM, Lugn NE, et al. Clinical outcomes associated with telemedicine/telehealth. *Telemed J E-Health.* June 2005;11(3):329–347.
11. Whited JD. Teledermatology research review. *Int J Dermatol.* March 2006;45(3):220–229.
12. Read S, Hill HF III. Dermatology's malpractice experience: clinical settings for risk management. *J Am Acad Dermatol.* July 2005;53(1):134–137.
13. Langley RG, Rajadhyaksha M, Dwyer PJ, et al. Confocal scanning laser microscopy of benign and malignant melanocytic skin lesions in vivo. *J Am Acad Dermatol.* September 2001;45(3):365–376.
14. Tracy J, Edison K. The long and winding road to medicare reimbursement. In: Whitten P, Cook D, eds. *Understanding Health Communication Technologies.* San Francisco, CA: Jossey-Bass; 2004.
15. American Telemedicine Association. ATA report on reimbursement. April 2003. Available at: http://www.atmeda.org/news/Reiumburement%20White%20paperfinal.pdf.
16. American Telemedicine Association. Medicare payment of telemedicine and telehealth services. Available at: http://www.atmeda.org/news/Medicare%20Payment%20Of%20Services%20Provided%20Via%20Telecommunications.pdf. Accessed June 2, 2005.
17. Partners Telemedicine 2005. Partners telemedicine: connecting healthcare providers and patients around the world. Available at: http://telemedicine.partners.org/Telemedicine/default.aspx?PageID=6.
18. Eisen SA, Kang HK, Murphy FM, et al. Gulf War veterans' health: medical evaluation of a U.S. cohort. *Ann Intern Med.* June 2005;142(11):881–890.
19. Kingman S. Growing awareness of skin disease starts flurry of initiatives. *Bull World Health Org.* December 2005;83(12):891–892.
20. Edison K, Pak HS, Tracy JA. Dermatology. In: Tracy J, ed. *Telemedicine Technical Assistance Documents: A Guide to Getting Started in Telemedicine.* 2004;51–84.
21. Demiris G, Edison K, Vijaykumar S. A comparison of communication models of traditional and video-mediated health care delivery. *Int J Med Inform.* October 2005;74:851–856.
22. Siegel D. Teledermatology. Paper presented at the Annual Meeting of the American Academy of Dermatology, March 3, 2006, San Francisco, CA.

CHAPTER 59

Medicines and Therapies Associated with Skin Cancer

Christopher J. Ballard, M.D.
Navid Bouzari, M.D.
Keyvan Nouri, M.D.

BOX 59-1   Overview

- Numerous drugs and therapies have been linked with an increased risk of developing skin cancer.
- Tars are more associated with squamous cell carcinoma (SCC) than basal cell carcinomas (BCCs).
- Radiation reverses this ratio and is associated with more BCC development.
- Ultraviolet light has been associated with skin cancer, especially squamous cell carcinoma, and can induce DNA damage.
- The best protection is sunlight avoidance and protection. PUVA (psoralens and UVA) can lead to SCCs, BCCs, and melanoma after long-term therapy.
- Arsenic forms arsenical keratoses on the skin, which can become malignant (mostly SCCs and BCCs).
- Nitrogen mustard (mechlorethamine) may lead to both BCCs and SCCs, and may mediate its effects through an increased Th1 response.
- Hydroxyurea has been connected with more SCCs than BCCs, but it is also important to watch for other skin changes such as ulcerations.
- Immunosuppressive agents, many of which are used after organ transplantation, such as cyclosporine and azathioprine may be associated with a greater incidence of cancer development, including skin cancer.
- More studies are needed to further investigate the role of these treatments in skin cancers.

INTRODUCTION

In a world where drugs have many side effects, it is important to know which medications and therapies have known associations with subsequent tumor formation. This chapter reviews several chemicals and treatments that have been linked with varying strengths to cutaneous neoplasm development. It is important that physicians be aware of these relationships in an attempt to avoid or minimize patient exposures. At times, the benefit of a treatment must be weighed against the potential for cancer progression.

TAR

BOX 59-2   Summary

- Tar is mostly associated with squamous cell carcinoma, but basal cell carcinoma and melanoma have also been reported.
- In animal models, tar may act as a tumor initiator and a promoter.
- Polycyclic aromatic hydrocarbons (PAH), which are ubiquitous coal tar constituents, may be involved in carcinogenesis through an enhancement of P450-dependent enzymes.

Tar has been used as a topical treatment of various skin diseases since ancient times.[1] It was the main therapeutic agent for the treatment of various skin disorders such as psoriasis, atopic dermatitis, scabies, neurodermatitis, sarcoidosis, seborrheic dermatitis, and several other dermatoses.[2,3] However, its use is currently limited to psoriasis and to a lesser extent in seborrheic and atopic dermatitis.[4]

It has been a long time since tar was proposed for the first time as a risk factor of skin cancer in 1775.[5] However, conclusive evidence for its carcinogenicity in humans is still lacking.[2] Some clinical studies have observed an increase in skin cancer occurrence after tar exposure while others did not, and most of them are restricted to the question of whether therapeutic exposure to coal tar poses an increased risk.[6-11] In tar-exposed patients, the ratio of squamous cell (SCC) to basal cell carcinomas (BCC) is shifted toward the squamous cell carcinomas in comparison to the general population.[10] There are few cases of melanoma occurring in tar exposed populations such as those treated for psoriasis.[12]

Tar has been recognized to increase the risk of skin cancer in animal models.[13] It may act as a tumor initiator and a promoter. Polycyclic aromatic hydrocarbons (PAH), which are ubiquitous coal tar constituents, increase the activity of P450-dependent enzymes.[9] Therefore, the reported cases of synergistic effects of tar and UV radiation in carcinogenesis may be due to an enhancement of P450-dependent enzymes.[2]

IONIZING RADIATION

BOX 59-3   Summary

- Carcinomas such as BCC, SCC, malignant fibrous histiocytoma, and angiosarcoma may develop after radiation therapy; the most frequent are BCCs, followed by SCCs.
- At low to moderate doses, ionizing radiation does not seem to be associated with malignant melanoma.
- Radiation-induced skin cancers are expected to be aggressive.

The association of skin cancer and ionizing radiation was first described in 1902, seven years after the discovery of X-rays.[14] Since that time, an increased risk of skin cancer has been reported in several radiation-exposed groups such as Japanese atomic bomb survivors,[15,16] uranium miners,[17] and radiologists.[18] In dermatologic settings, ionizing radiation has been used for the treatment of acne, atopic dermatitis, cutaneous tuberculosis, tinea capitis, and skin cancer.[19-21]

Various carcinomas such as BCC, SCC, malignant fibrous histiocytoma, and angiosarcoma may develop after radiation therapy; among them, the most frequent are BCCs, followed by SCCs.[22,23] Ionizing radiation does not seem to be associated with malignant melanoma, at least not at low to moderate doses.[15,20] Radiation-induced skin cancers are expected to be aggressive.[21] Many factors such as radiation type and dosage, anatomic location, age at exposure, sun exposure, and ethnic and genetic factors have effects on the incidence and type of skin cancers in the irradiated population.[24-26] Risk of radiation-induced skin cancers—particularly BCC—is increased in cases of acute and chronic radiodermatitis.[27,28] The risk of malignant transformation is particularly increased in recurrent sclera-atrophic and ulcerate radiodermatitis.[29]

The basal layer of the epidermis appears to be quite sensitive to radiation carcinogenesis, while the suprabasal layer seems to be more resistant. This is shown when radiation-induced SCC can occur after exposure to high doses of radiation, whereas BCC is a consequence to lower or moderate radiation doses.[15,30,31] Radiation carcinogenesis almost certainly involves multiple genetic alterations. The energy released by ionizing radiation has the potential to produce DNA strand breaks, major gene deletions or rearrangements, and other base damages.[32]

ULTRAVIOLET LIGHT-B (UVB)

BOX 59-4 Summary

- All three types of skin cancer appear to be related with UVB exposure.
- SCC appears to be most directly associated to the total UVB exposure.
- UVB can lead to DNA damage such as point mutations, oxidative damage, protein-DNA crosslinks, and strand breaks.
- The most reliable way to reduce the chronic effects of solar UV radiation is to limit exposure.

UVB covers a small part of electromagnetic spectrum (290 to 320 nm). Most of the UVB in our environment is from sunlight; however, people are exposed to UVB when using tanning beds, when working with UV lamps,[33,34] and when receiving therapeutic exposure in the treatment of some skin disorders such as psoriasis,[35–37] atopic dermatitis,[38–40] and pityriasis rosea.[41–43] The reported increases in the incidence of skin cancer have been attributed partially to a larger amount of UVB radiation reaching the surface of the earth as a result of ozone depletion in the atmosphere. The ozone layer has decreased by approximately 2% over the past 20 years.[33] An increase of 2.7% in nonmelanoma skin cancer is expected for a 1% decrease in total column atmospheric ozone.[44]

All three major types of skin cancer appear to be related with UVB exposure. SCC appears to be most directly associated to the total UVB exposure. SCC tumors occur on skin areas that are most regularly exposed (face, neck, and hands) and the risk increases with the life-long accumulated UVB dose. However, BCC incidence has only a modest association with cumulative exposure and is more likely to occur on areas of the body moderately exposed to the sun, including the trunk in males and lower legs in females.[45–48] Malignant melanoma appears to have a greater association with intermittent episodes of sunburn and to sun exposure in childhood.[49]

It is now well understood that for skin cancer development UV rays must initi-

ate two separate events: the neoplastic transformation of skin cells and a systemic down-regulation of cell-mediated immune function.[50,51] In SCC and BCC the *p53* gene appears to bear point mutations with the exact features of UVB-induced point mutations, i.e., associated with dipyrimidinic sites, mostly C to T transitions and 5 to 10% CC to TT tandem mutations.[52–56] More recent experimental studies have clearly shown that UVB radiation can also cause deletions.[57] Ultraviolet-induced skin cancers are highly immunogenic and will be rejected by a competent immune system. However, UVB-induced immunosuppression prevents the immunological destruction of these tumors.[58] Although these defects are the best studied types of UVB-induced DNA damage, it is important to remember that UVB radiation induces a much wider range of DNA damage such as oxidative base damage (e.g., 8-oxo-7,8-dihydroxyguanine), protein–DNA crosslinks, and single-strand breaks.[54] These types of DNA alterations can also be induced by other factors, which make it difficult to attribute the destruction solely to UVB radiation.

UVB may cause pigmentation or tanning which is photoprotective against further UVB exposure. UVB induces facultative pigmentation, which is distributed in keratinocytes throughout epidermis, as well as in activated melanocytes and corneocytes of the stratum corneum.[59] This distribution is more photoprotective than UVA-induced pigmentation, which is mainly in the basal cell layer.[60,61] Nonetheless, the most reliable way to reduce the chronic effects of solar UV radiation is to limit exposure. The regular use of sunscreen has been suggested to reduce the UVB-induced skin changes as well as the number of nonmelanoma skin cancers, although sufficient supporting data are not available.[62]

PSORALEN WITH UVA (PUVA)

BOX 59-5 Summary

- PUVA therapy is most associated with SCCs, which may develop proportionally to the collective amount of PUVA received.
- BCCs are also connected with PUVA.
- Melanoma has also been associated with PUVA, even 15 years or more after therapy, and with at least 250 treatments.

Methoxsalen (8-methoxypsoralen) can be activated by long wavelength ultraviolet light-A (UVA) in the range of 320 to

400 nm and is typically abbreviated as PUVA. Methoxsalen is administered orally, and 1 to 2 h later, the affected skin is irradiated with UVA. The number of treatments and length of time for the skin disease to clear can vary, but generally take 8 to 12 weeks with three treatments per week. While this treatment is often effective in patients with psoriasis and leads to lesion clearance, it is not curative; therefore, patients may undergo multiple treatments over a period of several years.[63] PUVA is used primarily for patients with psoriasis, but it can also be used to treat cutaneous T-cell lymphoma and vitiligo.

In the 1980s, PUVA was clouded in controversy as to whether or not it increased the risk of subsequent carcinogenesis,[64] but recent studies generally agree that PUVA is associated with an increase of cutaneous tumors. At the molecular level, psoralens are photoactivated by the radiation and induce DNA alterations, especially involving thymidine and cytosine repair malfunctions. Point mutations have been found in SCCs related to PUVA with cytosine to thymidine transitions. Evidence has also shown that numerous substances, including 8-hydroxyguanine, can be formed via reactive oxygen species inducedion from PUVA.[63]

A multicenter trial with PUVA in the United States involved more than 1000 subjects, and found a significantly increased rate of SCC formation. In a later analysis, these cancers were found to develop in direct proportion to the collective amount of PUVA received. Fewer patients in the same PUVA group developed basal cell carcinomas. With over 300 treatments, the risk of SCCs developing was increased approximately 80 times, and elevated about 20 times for moderate (101 to 200 treatments) and 10 times for low (100 or fewer) exposures to PUVA.[65–67] Melanoma has also been associated with PUVA, particularly 15 years or more after therapy and with at least 250 treatments.[68] Therefore, these patients should be monitored closely, especially as the number of treatments increases. Other psoralen delivery methods and psoralen options (i.e., trimethoxypsoralen, 5-methoxypsoralen) are available.[69–73] There is evidence that these may be associated with a reduced incidence of skin cancer, but more studies are needed to evaluate these alternatives. PUVA therapy is strongly associated with skin cancer progression, especially in those patients who have had previous immunosuppressive therapies such as radiation, methotrexate, or corticosteroids. Risks of potential cancer development should be weighed against the potential benefits of this therapy.

ARSENIC

BOX 59-6   Summary

- Chronic arsenic exposure, especially if ingested, typically presents with nonmalignant skin findings that can eventually develop into skin cancers.
- Arsenical keratoses can progress to cutaneous malignancies, especially squamous cell carcinomas and basal cell carcinomas.
- Arsenic has also been linked to melanoma and Merkel cell carcinoma.

Arsenic is an element found in the manufacturing processes of numerous applications such as glass, semiconductors, insecticides, and herbicides. These two latter uses have particular importance to farmers, who may be exposed to arsenic and have an increased potential for developing skin cancers. Additionally, arsenic can be mined and found in zinc, copper, and lead smelting. Arsenic's carcinogenic ability was noted long ago. The problem started when patients were being treated with 1% potassium arsenite (Fowler's solution); its uses ranged from the treatment of skin disorders such as psoriasis to hematologic and allergic conditions. Patients undergoing therapy developed skin cancers, which led to its removal from medicinal use. However, new uses for arsenic have been discovered, including the treatment of acute promyelocytic leukemia. Arsenic has also been found in the water supply in countries such as Bangladesh, Taiwan, Chile, Argentina, and Mexico. Ingested arsenic has been associated in these countries with the development of BCCs and SCCs, but not melanoma. In Taiwan, the presence of arsenic-induced skin cancer has been associated with future visceral cancers.[74]

Chronic arsenic exposure, especially if ingested, typically presents with nonmalignant skin findings that can eventually develop into skin cancers. These lesions include areas of the back, face, and neck with hyperpigmented areas intermixed with smaller lightened areas that can give a "rain drop appearance." Alternatively, multiple unique punctate keratotic lesions (arsenical keratoses) involving the palmar and plantar surfaces of patients are virtually pathognomonic for arsenic. Exposure can also produce diffuse hyperkeratosis and squamous cell carcinoma

in situ (Bowen disease). These lesions can progress to cutaneous malignancies, especially squamous cell carcinomas and basal cell carcinomas.[74,75]

Recent reports have also linked arsenic with melanoma. In one report, Iowa farmers with a high concentration of arsenic in their toenails had an increased incidence of melanoma.[76] Also, a large cohort study of Swedish women revealed a greater risk for melanoma development in a sub-cohort of librarians, curators, and archivists who were regularly exposed to several preservative chemicals, including arsenic.[77] More studies are needed to further investigate these associations between melanoma and arsenic.

Multiple accounts have documented associations between arsenic exposure and the development of cutaneous Merkel cell carcinomas. Typically, these primary neuroendocrine tumors occur with increasing age on exposed body surfaces. Two recently reported cases of Merkel cell carcinoma were found on the anterior trunk. This region typically receives less sun exposure than other body parts. The two patients were long-time residents of an endemic region of Taiwan with high arsenic levels in the water.[78]

By themselves, ultraviolet (UV) light and arsenic can lead to skin cancers; however, the probability of neoplastic change increases when they are combined. Numerous studies have investigated how arsenic and UV light are able to exert their carcinogenic abilities. At the cellular level, several changes include altered DNA methylation, impeding DNA repair, increased proliferation, and changing the genomic stability through telomerase interactions. Arsenic alone has been associated with aneuploidy, chromosomal anomalies, and micronuclei.[74]

METHOTREXATE

BOX 59-7   Summary

- MTX is a folic acid antagonist by competitively inhibiting dihydrofolate reductase, decreasing folate metabolism.
- There is mixed evidence as to whether MTX is associated with an increased risk of skin cancers, such as BCCs.
- The greatest evidence of carcinogenic potential of MTX comes from reports of reversible malignancies after MTX is removed, such as a cutaneous B-cell lymphoma.

Methotrexate (MTX) is a folic acid antagonist by competitively inhibiting dihydrofolate reductase, decreasing folate metabolism. Dihydrofolate is not able to be converted to the active tetrahydrofolic acid, which is needed to produce a nucleoside, thymidine. This building block is an essential part of DNA synthesis. Other effects include inhibiting the activation of T cells and purine synthesis. MTX leads to keratinocyte cell death and reduces the neutrophil and monocyte chemotaxis.[79] It has found many uses in clinical medicine including the treatment of psoriasis, psoriatic arthritis, rheumatoid arthritis, polymyositis, systemic lupus erythematosus, acute lymphoblastic leukemia, and breast cancer.

The greatest adverse effect to monitor is liver toxicity. Other possible events include pulmonary fibrosis, anemia, and neutropenia (bone marrow suppression). When giving high-doses, such as in the treatment of malignancy, patients should be given folinic acid to prevent or reduce the damage to other rapidly dividing cells such as the bone marrow of intestinal mucosa. Methotrexate can be harmful to a fetus and can cause spontaneous abortions, so this medication should be used with caution in women of childbearing age.

MTX has not been definitively linked to skin cancer as many of the patients receiving MTX either are on concurrent therapies or have received other treatments in the past that may predispose them to cutaneous tumors (e.g., arsenic, cyclosporine, and phototherapy). In addition, some of the conditions MTX is used to treat can predispose patients to certain malignancies. For example, rheumatoid arthritis is associated with a greater chance of developing lymphoproliferative disorders such as non-Hodgkin's lymphoma.[80] Therefore, patients may have underlying increased tendency to develop cancer, and it can be difficult to distinguish this from the additional effect of MTX.

One study retrospectively looked at 157 psoriasis patients treated with MTX. Only three of these patients developed basal cell carcinomas, but the authors did not believe these were related to MTX as the therapy had only been started 4 years before the skin cancers appeared.[79] This is in contrast to an earlier study that found six times as many skin cancers in psoriasis patients treated with PUVA, MTX, or a combination of both compared to controls.[81] Another study involving patients with rheumatoid arthritis showed no association between

MTX alone and nonmelanoma skin cancer, but when MTX was used with a TNF inhibitor such as etanercept, there was an increased risk of skin cancer development. However, this association failed to reach statistical significance.[82] The greatest evidence of MTX's carcinogenic potential comes from reports of malignancies that reverse after MTX is removed. A cutaneous B-cell lymphoma was found in an arthritis patient on MTX for 4 years. No underlying viruses such as HIV of Epstein-Barr virus were found. The MTX was discontinued and within 3 weeks the lymphoma had regressed; there was no evidence of skin cancer disease at 1-year follow-up.[83]

NITROGEN MUSTARD (MECHLORETHAMINE)

BOX 59-8 Summary

- Nitrogen mustard (mechlorethamine, HN2) is a chemotherapeutic alkylating agent, originally derived from gaseous mustard used in chemical warfare.
- Its cutaneous effects may be from an enhanced Th1 cellular response.
- Although evidence is varied, nitrogen mustard therapy has been associated with SCCs and BCCs.

Nitrogen mustard (mechlorethamine, HN2) is a chemotherapeutic alkylating agent. It was originally derived from gaseous mustard used in chemical warfare. Its mechanism of action in the skin is not well understood. However, systemically it acts as an alkylating agent that can covalently bond to guanine in DNA, which will eventually destroy the strands and kill the cells.[84] Topically, it is used primarily to treat the preliminary, limited stages of mycosis fungoides. However, it can also be used systemically for Hodgkin's disease, and less frequently in other neoplasms such as nonHodgkin's lymphoma, chronic lymphocytic lymphoma, and chronic myelogenous leukemia. Nitrogen mustard comes in an aqueous- or ointment-based preparation to be applied to the skin.

Topical administration of nitrogen mustard can lead to a contact dermatitis. Allergic contact dermatitis is a delayed Type IV hypersensitivity reaction that is mediated by Th1 cellular response. It has been shown that patients who exhibit a greater type IV reaction can have an improved response to nitrogen mustard.[85] The increased Th1 response

may enhance cytokines and lymphocytic infiltrates that are able to kill the neoplastic T cells and lead to disease improvement.[84]

Nitrogen mustard therapy has been associated with SCCs and BCCs.[86] Although some have developed on atypical location such as sun-protected areas, many of these patients had also received or were concurrently receiving other therapeutics that can increase the risk of skin cancer such as phototherapy.[87] A series of 203 patients with mycosis fungoides treated with nitrogen mustard were followed, and 139 of these used nitrogen mustard alone. Of this subgroup, only two patients developed nonmelanoma skin cancers. However, the authors do not attribute the neoplasms to topical therapy as the patients were elderly with lighter skin types. The other six patients who developed skin cancers were on concomitant therapies. One melanoma formed, but this patient had a prior history of basal cell carcinoma before starting nitrogen mustard.[88] Therefore, it is still unclear if topical nitrogen mustard increases the rate of cutaneous neoplasm formation. More studies will be needed.

CYCLOSPORINE

BOX 59-9 Summary

- Cyclosporine is an immunosuppressive agent that strongly inhibits T-lymphocytes and decreases the transcription of cytokines, especially IL-2.
- Cyclosporine is primarily used postoperatively in transplant patients to suppress the immune response to the foreign organ and prevent rejection.
- Cyclosporine's potential carcinogenicity may mediate through a mechanism independent of the immune suppression and may work via transforming growth factor-β.
- Cyclosporine may be associated with a greater risk of nonmelanoma skin cancer, especially SCC.
- Cyclosporine has also been linked to cutaneous T-cell lymphomas.

Cyclosporine is an immunosuppressive agent that was originally developed from a fungus, *Tolypocladium inflatum*, in the 1970s. It strongly inhibits T-lymphocytes by forming a complex with the intracellular protein cyclophilin and then binding and inhibiting calcineurin phosphatase. Numerous cytokines are subsequently less transcribed, especially inter-

leukin 2 (IL-2). Importantly, IL-2 is involved in the activation of T cells in many processes such as psoriasis. It also has anti-inflammatory properties (decreased cellular adhesion molecules and inhibited histamine release), which expand its clinical utility.[89] Cyclosporine is primarily used post-operatively in transplant patients to suppress the immune response to the foreign organ and prevent rejection. Furthermore, cyclosporine can be used in other conditions including psoriasis and less often in rheumatoid arthritis. Patients using cyclosporine are at an increased risk of developing potential adverse events such as renal damage, hypertension, and neoplasms.

While it is generally accepted that patients on long-term immunosuppressive medications are at an increased risk of developing malignancies, it unclear whether this increase is solely due to the medicines or to the decreased immune surveillance that allows for neoplastic proliferation. Hojo and colleagues studied immunodeficient mice and exposed them to cyclosporine.[90] These mice developed cancers at an accelerated rate, even though they had no immune system. Therefore, cyclosporine's potential carcinogenicity may be mediated through a mechanism independent of the immune suppression. In fact, it may work via transforming growth factor β. In a prospective study of 1252 patients with cyclosporine-treated psoriasis, 3.8% developed malignancies.[91] Of these neoplasms, 49% were skin cancers. Three times more squamous cell carcinomas formed than basal cell carcinomas, and these nonmelanoma skin cancers developed at a rate 6-fold greater than would be expected in controls. However, two melanomas and one porocarcinoma also formed during the study period. Those patients treated with cyclosporine for more than 2 years had a greater probability of developing skin cancer than those treated for a shorter time. In addition to cyclosporine, prior exposure to methotrexate, retinoids, or PUVA also increased the risk of tumor formation. As with many studies, the results were challenging to attribute only to cyclosporine as many of the patients had previously been treated with potentially carcinogenic therapies such as PUVA and methotrexate. It is also important that there was no increase in noncutaneous malignancies in the study population versus that in the general population. Although also on other medications, patients have also developed cutaneous T-cell lymphomas that may be attributable to cyclosporine use.[92,93] Cyclosporine continues to be an important immunosuppressive medication, especially for the transplant population. However, it is important to monitor these patients carefully as they may have a greater risk of developing cutaneous malignancies. More studies are needed to determine if cyclosporine alone is responsible for this susceptibility or if cyclosporine may be a cofactor that allows for tumor growth.

HYDROXYUREA

BOX 59-10 Summary

- Hydroxyurea has been linked to non-melanoma skin cancer (SCC more than BCC).
- Hydroxyurea is a specific DNA cell-cycle inhibitor at the S-phase and disrupts cellular replication at the basal skin layer.
- Observe patients on hydroxyurea for other skin changes such as ulceration.

With numerous medicinal uses, hydroxyurea is an important drug. Its uses include treating chronic myelogenous leukemia, polycythemia vera, sickle cell disease, and even severe psoriasis. In sickle cell disease, hydroxyurea increases the amount of fetal hemoglobin, decreasing the cellular sickling ability. This leads to clinical improvement and decreases the number of crises. However, hydroxyurea also works by inhibiting ribonucleotide reductase and inhibiting the incorporation of thymidine. Myelosuppression is an important side effect to monitor in these patients.

There have been numerous reports that have linked hydroxyurea to non-melanoma skin cancer. Most have been associated with squamous cell carcinoma, but basal cell carcinomas have also been linked to the drug.[94-96] In vitro studies have shown that hydroxyurea has the ability to damage chromosomes and interfere with normal DNA excision repair mechanisms in irradiated fibroblasts. It is a specific DNA cell-cycle inhibitor at the S-phase. Hydroxyurea disrupts cellular replication at the basal skin layer and thus can mediate its cutaneous effects.

A study of 158 patients with chronic myelogenous leukemia demonstrated 5 patients (3%) with squamous cell cancers on sun-exposed areas after long-term therapy on hydroxyurea.[97]

Recently, a case was reported of a man on hydroxyurea for chronic myelogenous leukemia who developed metastatic squamous cell carcinoma from the left auricle to the parotid gland and regional lymph nodes after 4 years of therapy.[98] The patient underwent surgery and radiation, but subsequently died of ventricular fibrillation. In contrast, a small study of sickle cell patients did not find any skin cancers, but these patients may have differed from other study populations with darker skin types and younger age.[99] Hydroxyurea can cause other changes in the skin such as ulcerations,[99] so it is important that patients on this drug be followed closely for any cutaneous changes that may occur.

AZATHIOPRINE

BOX 59-11 Summary

- Azathioprine is a prodrug that must be further metabolized to more active forms 6-MP and 6-TG.
- Azathioprine is integrated into DNA as thioguanine nucleotides can then cause DNA damage.
- 6-TG was shown to increase treated cells' photosensitization to UVA two-fold.
- In patients that developed skin cancer while on hydroxyurea, 6-TG was found in the skin, while none was found in normal patient's skin may demonstrate a possible link to hydroxyurea's carcinogenicity.

Azathioprine was introduced in the 1960s and has since been used for its immunosuppressive properties in the treatment of patients following transplantation as well as for patients with other ailments such as autoimmune disorders (i.e., rheumatoid arthritis) and inflammatory bowel disease. As a prodrug, azathioprine is metabolized nonenzymatically to 6-mercaptopurine (6-MP). After it is broken down further, hypoxanthine-guanine phosphoribosyl transferase (HGPRT) activates 6-MP, which is further reduced and then integrated into DNA as thioguanine nucleotides (TGNs). These bases lead to DNA strand breaks, interstrand crosslinks, and DNA-protein crosslinks.[100]

In addition, in both in vitro and animal studies, azathioprine has been linked to an increased risk of cancer in humans[101]; however, the magnitude of this risk and the effect on skin cancer are still being elucidated. Many of the studies have looked at immunosuppressive agents collectively. However, few studies have looked at the effect of azathioprine alone in its risk of skin cancer because often this drug is given in combination with other treatments such as glucocorticoids.

While DNA bases do not typically take up the UVA wavelengths between 320 to 400 nm strongly, the active metabolites 6-MP and 6-thioguanine (6-TG) effectively absorb in this range. Both 6-MP and 6-TG can produce reactive oxygen species when exposed to UVA, and can therefore mediate their oxidative damage to DNA. In fact, 6-TG was shown increase treated cells' photosensitization to UVA two-fold. In the skin of normal patients, no 6-TG was found, but it was present in those patients who had taken azathioprine and formed skin cancers. UVA and 6-TG (and by extension, azathioprine) are synergistically mutagenic.[102] Another study demonstrated that 6-TG was found in significantly greater concentrations of red blood cells in the patients with skin cancers on azathioprine than in those without cancers. This further supports a possible role of carcinogenicity associated with azathioprine.[103]

More evidence was found in a study of numerous immunosuppressive agents. In albino mice randomized to prednisolone, cyclosporine, cyclophosphamide, or azathioprine, no increased cancer formation was seen in the prednisolone-treated mice when exposed to ultraviolet lights in both A and B ranges. Whereas cyclosporine was found to increase the development of skin cancer and cyclophosphamide even more. However, the greatest and fastest development of cutaneous tumors was in the group treated with azathioprine.[104]

Recently, an angiosarcoma was reported on the scalp of a renal transplant patient on azathioprine and prednisolone.[105] In renal transplant patients treated with azathioprine, one group that developed both actinic keratoses and squamous cell carcinomas was compared to transplant patients without cutaneous tumors. A large study of 1191 patients with azathioprine-treated multiple sclerosis found 23 patients developed cancer.[106] But only two of these were skin cancers (one basal cell and one squamous cell carcinoma). The chances of developing cancer trended to increase 10 years after continuous azathioprine therapy.

FINAL THOUGHTS

With new drugs and therapeutics developing in medicine, this list is likely to expand with time. Additional studies are needed to assess the degree of carcinogenicity of many of the above medications alone, but this is difficult since patients requiring these drugs are also on numerous medications concomitantly and may have been treated with various therapies in the past. Continued monitoring is required for potential associations, especially in patients that may be immunocompromised either by medications or by their disease. These patients are likely at a greater risk of developing subsequent neoplasms and should be followed closely.

REFERENCES

1. Downing JG, Bauer CW. Low and high temperature coal tars in treatment of eczema and psoriasis. *Arch Dermatol.* 1948;57:985–90.
2. Arnold WP. Tar. *Clin Dermatol.* September/October 1997;15(5):739–44.
3. Andrew NL, Moses K. Tar revisited. *Int J Dermatol.* 1985;24:216–8.
4. Thami GP, Sarkar R. Coal tar: past, present and future. *Clin Exp Dermatol.* March 2002;27(2):99–103.
5. Pott P. Clinical observation relative to the cataract; the polyp of the nose, the cancer of the scrotum, the different kinds of rupture and mortification of the toes and feet. London: Haus, Clark & Collins; 1775.
6. Jones SK, Mackie RM, Hole DJ, et al. Further evidence of the safety of tar in the management of psoriasis. *Br J Dermatol.* 1985;113:97–101.
7. Everall JD, Hansteen IL, Lawler SD. Chromosome studies in pitch warts. *Br J Dermatol.* 1967;79:271–7.
8. Emmett EA. Cutaneous and ocular hazards of rooters. *Occup Med.* 1986;1:307–22.
9. Van Schooten FJ, Godschalk R. Coal tar therapy. Is it carcinogenic? *Drug Saf.* December 1996;15(6):374–7.
10. Letzel S, Drexler H. Occupationally related tumors in tar refinery workers. *J Am Acad Dermatol.* November 1998;39 (5 Pt 1):712–20.
11. Maughan WZ, Muller SA, Perry HO, et al. Incidence of skin cancers in patients with atopic dermatitis treated with ocal tar. A 25-year follow-up study. *J Am Acad Dermatol.* 1980;3(6):612–615.
12. Durkin W, Sun N, Link J, et al. Melanoma in a patient treated for psoriasis. *South Med J.* 1978;71(6):732–733.
13. Pion IA, Koening KL, Lim HW. Is dermatologic usage of coal tar carcinogenic? A review of the literature. *Dermatol Surg.* 1995;21:227–231.
14. Shore RE. Radiation-induced skin cancer in humans. *Med Pediatr Oncol.* 2001;36:549–554.
15. Ron E, Preston DL, Kishikawa M, et al. Skin tumor risk among atomic-bomb survivors in Japan. *Cancer Causes Control.* 1998;9:393–401.
16. Thompson DE, Mabuchi K, Ron E, et al. Cancer incidence in atomic bomb survivors. Part II: solid tumors 1958–1987. *Radiat Res.* 1994;133:S17–S67.
17. Sevcova M, Seve J, Thomas J. Alpha irradiation of the skin and the possibility of late effects. *Health Phys.* 1978; 35:803–806.
18. Matanoski GM, Selster R, Sartwell PE, et al. The current mortality rates of radiologists and other physician specialists: specific causes of death. *Am J Epidemiol.* 1975;101:199–201.
19. Shore RE, Moseson M, Xue X, et al. Skin cancer after X-ray treatment for scalp ringworm. *Radiat Res.* April 2002; 157(4):410–418.
20. Ron E, Modan B, Preston D, et al. Radiation-induced skin carcinoma of the head and neck. *Radiat Res.* 1991;25: 318–325.
21. Panje WR, Dobleman TJ. Facial reconstruction for radiation-induced skin cancer. *Arch Otolaryngol Head Neck Surg.* 1990;116:470–474.
22. Odom RB, James WD, Berger TG. *Andrews' Diseases of the Skin: Clinical Dermatology.* 9th ed. Philadelphia: W.B. Saunders, 2000:40–41.
23. Allison JR, Jr. Radiation-induced basal-cell carcinoma. *J Dermatol Surg Oncol.* 1984;10:200–3.
24. Lichter MD, Karagas MR, Mott LA, et al. Therapeutic ionizing radiation and the incidence of basal and squamous cell carcinoma. The New Hampshire Skin Cancer Study Group. *Arch Dermatol.* 2000;136:1007–1011.
25. Karagas MR, McDonald JA, Greenberg ER, et al. Risk of basal cell and squamous cell skin cancers after ionizing radiation therapy. For the Skin Cancer Prevention Study Group. *J Natl Cancer Inst.* 1996;88:1848–1853.
26. Little MP, De Vathaire F, Charles MW, et al. Variations with time and age in the risks of solid cancer incidence after radiation exposure in childhood. *Stat Med.* 1998;17:1341–1355.
27. Maalej M, Frikha H, Kochbati L, et al. Radio-induced malignancies of the scalp about 98 patients with 150 lesions and literature review. *Cancer Radiother.* April 8. 2004;(2):81–87.
28. Rosenthal LS, Beck TJ, Williams J, et al. Acute radiation dermatitis following radiofrequency catheter ablation of atrioventricular nodal reentrant tachycardia. *Pacing Clin Electrophysiol.* 1997;20(7):834–839.
29. Monfort J. Radiodermites. *Rev Prat.* 1966;16:2053–2060.
30. Hanke CW, O'Brian JJ, Shidnia H, et al. Chemosurgical reports: basal-cell carcinoma resulting from radiation therapy for hypertrophic tonsils. *J Dermatol Surg Oncol.* 1985;11:108–110.
31. Ekmekçi P, Bostanci S, Anadolu R, et al. Multiple basal cell carcinomas developed after radiation therapy for tinea capitis: a case report. *Dermatol Surg.* 2001;27:667–669.
32. Jin Y, Burns J, Garte SJ, et al. Infrequent alterations of the p53 gene in rat skin cancers induced by ionizing radiation. *Carcinogenesis.* 1996;17:873–6.
33. Kripke ML. Impact of ozone depletion on skin cancers. *J Dermatol Surg Oncol.* 1988;14:855–857.
34. Stepanski B, Mayer JA. Solar protection behaviors among outdoor workers. *J Occup Environ Med.* 1998;40:43–48.
35. Lebwohl M. Acitretin in combination with UVB or PUVA. *J Am Acad Dermatol.* 1999;41(3 Pt 2):S22–S24.
36. Barbagallo J, Spann CT, Tutrone WD, et al. Narrowband UVB phototherapy for the treatment of psoriasis: a review and update. *Cutis.* 2001;68(5):345–347.
37. Kragballe K. Vitamin D and UVB radiation therapy. *Cutis.* 2002;70(S5):9–12.
38. Grundmann-Kollmann M, Behrens S, Podda M, et al. Phototherapy for atopic eczema with narrow-band UVB. *J Am Acad Dermatol.* 1999;40(6 Pt 1):995–997.
39. Brazzelli V, Prestinari F, Chiesa MG, et al. Sequential treatment of severe atopic dermatitis with cyclosporin A and low-dose narrow-band UVB phototherapy. *Dermatology.* 2002;204(3): 252–254.
40. Jekler J, Larko O. Combined UVA-UVB versus UVB phototherapy for atopic dermatitis: a paired-comparison study. *J Am Acad Dermatol.* 1990;22(1):49–53.
41. Valkova S, Trashlieva M, Christova P. UVB phototherapy for Pityriasis rosea. *J Eur Acad Dermatol Venereol.* 2004;18(1): 111–112.
42. Chuh. A. Narrow band UVB phototherapy and oral acyclovir for pityriasis rosea. *Photodermatol Photoimmunol Photomed.* 2004;20(1):64–65.
43. Leenutaphong V, Jiamton S. UVB phototherapy for pityriasis rosea: a bilateral comparison study. *J Am Acad Dermatol.* 1995;33(6):996–999.
44. Kelfkens G, de Gruijl FR, van der Leun JC. Ozone depletion and increase in annual carcinogenic ultraviolet dose. *Photochem Photobiol.* 1990;52:819–823.
45. Kricker A, Armstrong B.K, English D.R. et al. Does intermittent sun exposure cause basal cell carcinoma? A case-control study in Western Australia. *Int J Cancer.* 1995;60:489–494.
46. Urbach F. Geographic pathology of skin cancer. In: Urbach F, ed. *The Biologic Effects of Ultraviolet Radiation (With Emphasis on the Skin).* Oxford: Pergamon Press Ltd.; 1969:635–650.
47. Diffey BL, Tate TJ, Davis A. Solar dosimetry of the face: the relationship of natural ultraviolet radiation exposure to basal cell carcinoma localisation. *Phys Med Biol.* 1979;24:931–939.
48. Marks R. The epidemiology of non-melanoma skin cancer: who, why and what can we do about it. *J Dermatol.* 1995;22:853–857.
49. Holman CDJ, Armstrong BK. Cutaneous malignant melanoma and indicators of total accumulated exposure to the sun: an analysis separating histogenic types. *J Natl Cancer Inst.* 1984;73:75–82.
50. Kripke ML. Immunologic mechanisms in UV-radiation carcinogenesis. *Adv Cancer Res.* 1981;34:69–106.
51. Streilein JW, Taylor JR, Vincek V et al. Immune surveillance and sunlight-induced skin cancer. *Immunol Today.* 1994;15:174–179.

52. Brash DE, Rudolph JA, Simon JA, et al. A role for sunlight in skin cancer: UV-induced p53 mutations in squamous cell carcinomas. *Proc Natl Acad Sci USA*. 1991;88:10124–10128.

53. Ziegler A.D, Leffel D.J, Kunala S, et al. Mutation hotspots due to sunlight in the p53 gene of nonmelanoma skin cancers. *Proc Natl Acad Sci USA*. 1993;90:4216–4220.

54. De Gruijl FR, Van Kranen HJ, Mullenders LH. UV-induced DNA damage, repair, mutations and oncogenic pathways in skin cancer. *J Photochem Photobiol B*. 2001;63(1-3):19–27.

55. Sarasin A. The molecular pathways of ultraviolet-induced carcinogenesis. *Mutat Res*. July 16. 1999;428(1-2):5–10.

56. Brash DE, Ziegler A, Jonason AS, et al. Sunlight and sunburn in human skin cancer: p53, apoptosis, and tumor promotion. *J Investig Dermatol Symp Proc*. April 1996;1(2):36–42.

57. Horiguchi M, Masumura KI, Ikehata H, et al. Molecular nature of ultraviolet B light-induced deletions in the murine epidermis. *Cancer Res*. 2001;61:3913–3918.

58. Hart PH, Grimbaldeston MA, Finlay-Jones JJ. Sunlight, immunosuppression and skin cancer: role of histamine and mast cells. *Clin Exp Pharmacol Physiol*. January/February 2001;28(1-2):1–8.

59. Rosen CF, Jacques SL, Stuart ME, et al. Immediate pigment darkening: visual and reflectance spectrophotometric analysis of action spectrum. *Photochem Photobiol*. 1990;51:583–588.

60. Black G, Matzinger E, Gange RW. Lack of photoprotection against UVB induced erythema by immediate pigmentation induced by 382 nanometers radiation. *J Invest Dermatol*. 1985;85:448–449.

61. Kollias N, Sayre RM, Zeise L et al. Photoprotection by melanin. *J Photochem Photobiol B*. 1991;9:135–160.

62. Lock-Andersen J, Knudstorp ND, Wulf HC. Facultative skin pigmentation in Caucasians: an objective biological indicator of lifetime exposure to ultraviolet radiation? *Br J Dermatol*. 1998;138:826–832.

63. Gasparro FP. The role of PUVA in the treatment of psoriasis. Photobiology issues related to skin cancer incidence. *Am J Clin Dermatol*. November-December 2000;1(6):337–348.

64. Studniberg HM, Weller P. PUVA, UVB, psoriasis, and nonmelanoma skin cancer. *J Am Acad Dermatol*. December 1993;29(6):1013–1022.

65. Stern RS, Laird N, Melski J et al. Cutaneous squamous-cell carcinoma in patients treated with PUVA. *N Engl J Med*. May 3.1984;310(18):1156–1161.

66. Stern RS, Laird N. The carcinogenic risk of treatments for severe psoriasis. Photochemotherapy Follow-up Study. *Cancer*. June 1. 1994;73(11):2759–2764.

67. Stern RS, Liebman EJ, Vakeva L. Oral psoralen and ultraviolet-A light (PUVA) treatment of psoriasis and persistent risk of nonmelanoma skin cancer. PUVA Follow-up Study. *J Natl Cancer Inst*. September 1998;90(17):1278–1284.

68. Stern RS, Nichols KT, Vakeva LH. Malignant melanoma in patients treated for psoriasis with methoxsalen (psoralen) and ultraviolet A radiation (PUVA). The PUVA Follow-Up Study. *N Engl J Med*. April 1997;336(15):1041–1045.

69. Hannuksela-Svahn A, Pukkala B, Koulu L et al. Cancer incidence among Finnish psoriasis patients treated with 8-methoxypsoralen bath PUVA. *J Am Acad Dermatol*. May 1999;40(5 Pt 1):694–6.

70. Lindelof B, Sigurgeirsson B, Tegner E et al. PUVA and cancer risk: the Swedish follow-up study. *Br J Dermatol*. July 1999;141(1):108–112.

71. Hannuksela-Svahn A, Pukkala E, Laara E et al. Psoriasis, its treatment, and cancer in a cohort of Finnish patients. *J Invest Dermatol*. March 2000;114(3):587–590.

72. Hannuksela-Svahn A, Sigurgeirsson B, Pukkala E et al. Trioxsalen bath PUVA did not increase the risk of squamous cell skin carcinoma and cutaneous malignant melanoma in a joint analysis of 944 Swedish and Finnish patients with psoriasis. *Br J Dermatol*. September 1999;141(3):497–501.

73. Donath P, Bethea D, Amici L et al. Low and irreproducible methoxsalen levels in patients receiving photochemotherapy. *Arch Dermatol*. May 1999;135(5):604–606.

74. Rossman TG, Uddin AN, Burns FJ. Evidence that arsenite acts as a cocarcinogen in skin cancer. *Toxicol Appl Pharmacol*. August 2004;198(3):394–404.

75. Gawkrodger DJ. Occupational skin cancers. *Occupational Medicine*. 2004;54:458–463.

76. Beane Freeman LE, Dennis LK, Lynch CF et al. Toenail arsenic content and cutaneous melanoma in Iowa. *Am J Epidemiol*. October 2004;160(7):679–687.

77. Perez-Gomez B, Aragones N, Gustavsson P et al. Cutaneous melanoma in Swedish women: Occupational risks by anatomic site. *Am J Ind Med*. October 2005;48(4):270–281.

78. Ho SY, Tsai YC, Lee MC et al. Merkel cell carcinoma in patients with long-term ingestion of arsenic. *J Occup Health*. 2005;47:188–192.

79. Haustein UF, Rytter M. Methotrexate in psoriasis: 26 years experience with low-dose long-term treatment. *J Eur Acad Dermatol Venereol*. September 2000;14(5):382–388.

80. Isomaki HA, Hakulinen T, Joutsenlahti U. Excess risk of lymphomas, leukemia and myeloma in patients with rheumatoid arthritis. *J Chronic Dis*. 1978;31(11):691–696.

81. Mali-Gerrits MG, Gaasbeek D, Boezman J, et al. Psoriasis therapy and the risk of skin cancers. *Clin Exp Dermatol*. March1991;16(2):85–89.

82. Chakravarty EF, Michaud K, Wolfe F. Skin cancer, rheumatoid arthritis, and tumor necrosis factor inhibitors. *J Rheumatol*. November 2005;32(11):2130–2135.

83. Viraben R, Brousse P, Lamant L. Reversible cutaneous lymphoma occurring during methotrexate therapy. *Br J Dermatol*. July 1996;135(1):116–118.

84. Kim YH. Management with topical nitrogen mustard in mycosis fungoides. *Dermatol Ther*. 2003;16(4):288–298.

85. Ramsay D, Meller J, Zackheim HS. Topical treatment of early cutaneous T-cell lymphoma. *Hematol Oncol Clin North Am*. October 1995;9(5):1031–1056.

86. Lee L, Fritz K, Golitz L, et al. Second cutaneous malignancies in patients with mycosis fungoides treated with topical nitrogen mustard. *J Amer Acad Dermatol*. November 1982;7(5):590–598.

87. Vonderheid E, Tan E, Kantor A, et al. Long-term efficacy, curative potential, and carcinogenicity of topical mechlorethamine chemotherapy in cutaneous T cell lymphoma. *J Amer Acad Dermatol*. March 1989;20(3):416–428.

88. Kim YH, Martinez G, Varghese A, et al. Topical nitrogen mustard in the management of mycosis fungoides: update of the Stanford experience. *Arch Dermatol*. February 2003;139(2):165–173.

89. Ho VC. The use of ciclosporin in psoriasis: a clinical review. *Br J Dermatol*. May 2004;150(S67):1–10.

90. Hojo M, Morimoto T, Maluccio M, et al. Cyclosporine induces cancer progression by a cell-autonomous mechanism. *Nature*. February 1999;397(6719):530–534.

91. Paul CF, Ho VC, McGeown C, et al. Risk of malignancies in psoriasis patients treated with cyclosporine: a 5 year cohort study. *J Invest Dermatol*. February 2003;120(2):211–216.

92. Ravat FE, Spittle MF, Russel-Jones R. Primary cutaneous T-cell lymphoma occurring after organ transplantation. *J Am Acad Dermatol*. April 2006;54(4):668–675.

93. Mahe E, Descamps V, Grossin M, et al. CD30+ T-cell lymphoma in a patient with psoriasis treated with ciclosporin and infliximab. *Br J Dermatol*. July 2003;149(1):170–3.

94. Papi M, Didona B, DePita O, et al. Multiple skin tumors on light-exposed areas during long-term treatment with hydroxyurea. *J Am Acad Dermatol*. March 1993;28(3):485–486.

95. Best PJ, Petitt RM. Multiple skin cancers associated with hydroxyurea therapy. *Mayo Clin Proc*. October 1998;73(10):961–963.

96. De Simone C, Guerriero C, Guidi B, et al. Multiple squamous cell carcinomas of the skin during long-term treatment with hydroxyurea. *Eur J Dermatol*. March 1998;8(2):114–115.

97. Vassallo C, Passamonti F, Merante S, et al. Muco-cutaneous changes during long-term therapy with hydroxyurea in chronic myeloid leukaemia. *Clin Exp Dermatol*. March 2001;26(2):141–148.

98. Pamuk GE, Turgut B, Vural O, et al. Metastatic squamous cell carcinoma of the skin in chronic myeloid leukaemia: complication of hydroxyurea therapy. *Clin Lab Haematol*. October 2003;25(5):329–331.

99. Chaine B, Neonato MG, Girot R, et al. Cutaneous adverse reactions to hydroxyurea in patients with sickle cell disease. *Arch Dermatol*. April 2001;137(4):467–470.

100. Coulthard S, Hogarth L. The thiopurines: an update. *Invest New Drugs*. December 2005;23(6):523–532.

101. Lhermitte F, Marteau T, Grimaud J, et al. Not so benign long-term immunosup-

pression in multiple sclerosis? *Lancet.* February 4. 1984;1(8371):276–277.

102. O'Donovan P, Perrett CM, Zhang X, et al. Azathioprine and UVA light generate mutagenic oxidative DNA damage. *Science.* September 2005;309(5742): 1871–1874.

103. Lennard L, Thomas S, Harrington CI, et al. Skin cancer in renal transplant recip-ients is associated with increased con-centrations of 6-thioguanine nucleo-tide in red blood cells. *Br J Dermatol.* December 1985;113(6):723–9.

104. Kelley GE, Meikle W, Sheil AG. Effects of immunosuppressive therapy in the induction of skin tumors by ultraviolet radiation in hairless mice. *Transplant-ation.* 1987; 44: 429–434.

105. Kibe Y, Kishimoto S, Katoh N, et al. Angiosarcoma of the scalp associated with renal transplantation. *Br J Dermatol.* May 1997;136(5):752–756.

106. Confavreux C, Saddier P, Grimaud J, et al. Risk of cancer from azathioprine therapy in multiple sclerosis: a case-con-trol study. *Neurology.* June 1996;46(6): 1607–1612.

CHAPTER 60

Indoor Tanning

Navid Bouzari, M.D.
Keyvan Nouri, M.D.

BOX 60-1   Overview

- The number of sunbed users is large and increasing, currently estimated to be 28 million US citizens annually.
- Most sunbeds emit predominantly UVA although they still produce minimal UVB emissions. Newer devices emit more UVA and UVB.
- Sunbed use is a risky behavior associated with a variety of adverse consequences from skin dryness and sunburns to skin cancer.
- Laboratory and animal studies strongly suggest the carcinogenicity of indoor tanning.
- Strong epidemiologic evidence regarding the carcinogenicity of indoor tanning is lacking, and case-control studies provide mixed data.
- The possible pathophysiologic mechanisms of indoor tanning carcinogenesis include, but are not limited to: UVA overexposure, immunosuppression, photoaddition, and photoaugmentation.
- Obtaining tan through sunbed use does not provide sun-protection.
- Indoor tanning is not recommended as means of vitamin D correction/supplementation due to its health hazards and availability of noncarcinogenic alternatives (oral supplementation).
- National Institute of Health (NIH) states that exposure to sunbeds is carcinogenic.
- Prevention strategies should address multiple cognitive, psychological, social, and behavioral factors that may be involved in tanning behavior.

INTRODUCTION

Tanning is the skin response to ultraviolet (UV) radiation through increased production of melanin in order to protect skin from UV damages. Not everybody is able to tan; some people with fair skin just simply burn (Table 60-1). In principle, skin reaction to UV radiation is similar whether the exposure is to natural or artificial UV radiation. The artificial sources of UV radiation have different

Table 60-1

Sunburn Susceptibility and Tanning Ability in Different Fitzpatrick Skin Types[1]

FITZPATRICK SKIN TYPE	SUNBURN SUSCEPTIBILITY	TANNING ABILITY
I	Always sunburn	No tan
II	High	Light tan
III	Moderate	Medium tan
IV	Low	Dark tan
V	Very low	Natural brown skin
VI	Extremely low	Natural black skin

denominations such as indoor tanning, sunbeds, tanning machines, and solaria.

HISTORY OF TANNING AND TANNING MACHINES

Tanning has not always been valued in the human history. More than 100 years ago, a fair complexion was desirable because it was a sign of high success indicating one did not have to work in the fields. After the industrial revolution, the indoor jobs became popular. Hence, fair skin no longer distinguished between the classes, and having a tan became a sign of success indicating one had much leisure time and did not have to work.[2,3] The tanning became even more socially desirable when the French designer Coco Chanel decreed it as a fashion look in the 1920s.[4]

The concept of obtaining a tan without going outdoors was soon after introduced, and became popular in the late 1970s and early 1980s in the United States and Europe with the introduction of modern tanning devices that emitted ultraviolet A (UVA) radiation principally, as opposed to the first generation of tanning beds that emitted significant quantities of ultraviolet B (UVB) and ultraviolet C (UVC).[5,6] The first generation of tanning devices emitted a broad spectrum of radiation from UVC to infrared that produced many safety problems. The next generation of tanning devices used mainly UVA radiation and minimal or no UVB radiation in the belief that this provides a safer way to tan.[7,8]

Recent trends include the development of high-speed sunbed units that emit greater amounts of UVB, and high-pressure UVA tanning beds that emit UVA doses at outputs far higher than that of the sun.[8-11]

INDOOR TANNING DEMOGRAPHICS

The expanding desire for a tan and the availability of safer tanning beds and booths has given rise to the indoor tanning industry which has been growing exponentially, from a $1 billion industry in 1992 to an estimated $5 billion enterprise in 2002.[9,12,13] Annually, a total of 50,000 facilities are used by 28 million US citizens, with about 1 million visits each day.[14,15] Of these, 70% are Caucasian girls and women between the ages of 16 and 49.[16] Other reported predictors of indoor tanning in the US population are shown in Table 60-2. However, some predictors such as race, ethnicity, or geographical factors are not included since most studies have been primarily limited to Caucasians and certain regions in the US. Of great importance, the number of minors using tanning devices is surprisingly large and increasing. Recent data of community or state-based cross-sectional studies suggest that 2 to 11% of boys and 12 to 37% of girls use tanning beds; however, no national data is available on the prevalence of indoor tanning sunlamp use in US adolescents.[19-21] In other countries, particularly Nordic European countries, the estimated prevalence of youth indoor tanning use has been reported as high as 75% in girls and 35% in boys.[22] Due to the high number of sunbed users,

Table 60-2

Reported Predictors of Indoor Tanning

- Female sex
- Olive or dark skin color[a]
- Living in the Midwest or South
- Living in rural area
- Nonuser of sunscreen
- Use of tobacco and/or alcohol
- Having friends who tan
- Having caregiver(s) who use(d) tanning lamps

[a]Earlier studies reported indoor tanning use to be more common in fair skin types[17,18] but more recent studies generally showed the opposite[15,19-21]

indoor tanning is an important public health issue. It has schematically estimated that the population's UV radiation dose due to indoor tanning might be of the same order of magnitude as the potential increase in natural UV radiation dose resulting from a 10% ozone depletion.[17]

TANNING BENEFITS AND HAZARDS

Similar to other risky behaviors (such as smoking or recreational drug use), the underlying determinants of tanning behavior are probably quite complex, with different biopsychosocial dimensions.[18] The most common reasons for tanning indoors are psychosocial factors like appearance motivation.[23,24] However, tanning can be motivated in part by physiologic factors such as neuropeptides released from the skin in response to UV radiation. This may explain the relaxation from tanning bed use which is one of the strongest motivators of this behavior.[25–28] More benefits have been claimed, especially by the tanning industry: UV radiation induces vitamin D production, which not only decreases the risk of osteoporosis but also lowers the risk of cancers of internal organs such as breast, ovary, and colon,[29,30] exposure times for tanning sessions are designed to minimize the risk of sunburn, and because sunburn causes skin cancer, indoor tanning prevents skin cancer,[31,32] and UV exposure protects against the development of multiple sclerosis.[31,33]

While people may seek indoor tanning because of its biopsychosocial benefits, indoor tanning equipment may cause some health hazards (Table 60-3).[34–45] Mild short-term effects such as pruritus, sunburn, or skin dryness are commonly reported. Skin erythema or burns are reported by 18 to 55% of sunbed users.[46–48] The Centers for Disease Control and Prevention report shows that there are 700 emergency department visits per year secondary to adverse reactions from sunbeds.[49] While the lower UVB content of the newer devices decreases the risk of some of these adverse effects, the UVA content can still put the sunbed users at risk of some effects such as phototoxic and photoallergic reactions which mainly occur in the UVA range.[50] In addition, consumption of some drugs such as psoralen, anti-depressants, antibiotics, antifungals, and hypoglycemic agents can make the skin photosensitive and hence

Table 60-3
Acute and Chronic Health Effects of Indoor Tanning

ACUTE	CHRONIC
Sunburn (cutaneous burn)	Squamous cell carcinoma
Photokeratitis (ocular burn)	Basal cell carcinoma
Pruritus	Melanoma
Xerosis	Photoaging
Nausea	Mid-dermal elastolysis
Cutaneous porphyria	Exacerbation of
Pseudoporphyria	photosensitive
Drug-induced photosensitivity	diseases, e.g., SLE, PLE
PLE: Polymorphous light eruption; SLE: Systemic lupus erythematosus.	

cause unexpected sunburns after a short UV exposure.

INDOOR TANNING AND SKIN CANCER

The incidence of melanoma and basal cell carcinoma has steeply increased throughout the past 50 years in most fair-skinned populations. This increase in incidence is mainly observed on body sites that are not chronically exposed to sunlight[51] suggesting the role attributed to the intermittent rather than daily sun exposure in the genesis of these cancers. The most intense form of intermittent sun exposure is the intentional sun exposure that can either happen by outdoor sunbathing or use of sunbeds.[52]

While the carcinogenicity of UV radiation through sun tanning is well documented, whether or not indoor tanning devices lead to skin cancer development is still under investigation. To date, laboratory and animal studies provide preliminary biological evidence for carcinogenesis associated with indoor tanning.[53–56] In addition, there are case reports of basal and squamous cell carcinomas as well as melanoma following tanning bed exposure.[57,58] However, the case–control studies have mixed results, and in most cases, limitations. Precancerous actinic keratoses and Bowen disease have also been reported in sunlight-protected but sunbed-exposed skin in fair-skinned users after just 2 to 3 years of regular sunbed use.[59]

EPIDEMIOLOGY

Melanoma

There are mixed data regarding the association of indoor tanning and cutaneous malignant melanoma. Some epidemiologic studies suggest a significant positive association between indoor tanning and melanoma[11,60,61] whereas some did not.[62] A population-based, matched, case-control study by Westerdahl et al[11] in Sweden, reported a significantly elevated odds ratio for developing melanoma after regular exposure to tanning beds. More recently, results from a prospective cohort study on women from Norway and Sweden, found that exposure to tanning devices either before or after the availability of modern tanning devices increased the risk of melanoma. They observed a 55% increase in risk of melanoma in women who use sunbeds regularly ($\geq$12 times/year).[61] It has been suggested that a younger age of exposure to tanning lamps may be linked to increased risk of melanoma.[11,63] Sunlamp use at home can add to the risk of melanoma because of the potential to be overused.[63]

Nonmelanoma Skin Cancer (NMSC)

There are few studies attempting to uncover the association between indoor tanning and nonmelanoma skin cancer, and previous data shows mixed evidence in this regard. While some studies found no evidence of a risk of basal cell carcinoma (BCC) or squamous cell carcinoma (SCC) with indoor tanning[64] some others reported a significant association.[65–67] A population-based, case-control study, in New Hampshire, investigated the risk of nonmelanoma skin cancer associated with the use of tanning devices. In this study, the overall use was associated with an odds ratio of 2.5 (95% CI, 1.7 to 3.8) for SCC. They also showed an increased risk of BCC in indoor tanning users, with an odds ratio of 1.5 (95% CI, 1.1 to 2.1), adjusted for sunburns, sunbathing, and sun exposure.[36]

PATHOPHYSIOLOGY

Ultraviolet radiation is a known carcinogen. With natural sunlight, adverse effects are vastly from UVB rays, and UVA from the sunlight is not generally of much concern. However, because of the intense exposure to UVA from indoor tanning, and given the fact that indoor tanning lamps still produce UVB emissions, the pathophysiology of carcinogenesis of these devices may be different, if present.

UVA OVEREXPOSURE

Significant UVA exposure could result from indoor tanning. It has been demonstrated that regular tanning lamps emit UVA ranged 1.1 to 4.1 times higher than the sun. The UVA doses from newly available high-pressure sunlamps are 10 to 15 times that of the midday sun.[68,69] Laboratory and animal studies, as well as case reports of skin cancer among patients with psoriasis treated with UVA and psoralen, strongly suggest that UVA may be carcinogenic.[37,54,55,70–72] Animal studies indicate that artificial UVA by itself produce skin cancer.[73,74] The mechanism of UVA carcinogenesis is unknown; however, it may be due to cellular damage secondary to active oxygen species generated by endogenous photosensitizers.[75,76] UVA may also exert its carcinogenic effect via induction of pyrimidine dimmers, and thereby, DNA damage.[77] T to G transversions and tandem TT → GG mutations have been seen with UVA exposure.[78] It should be noted that UVA penetrates more deeply than UVB (Fig. 60-1), so the cellular and DNA damages may be expected in deeper skin layers. Accordingly, Agar et al demonstrated DNA lesions typical of UVA action in the basal epithelial layer of the human skin, the skin region where most melanocytes are located.[80]

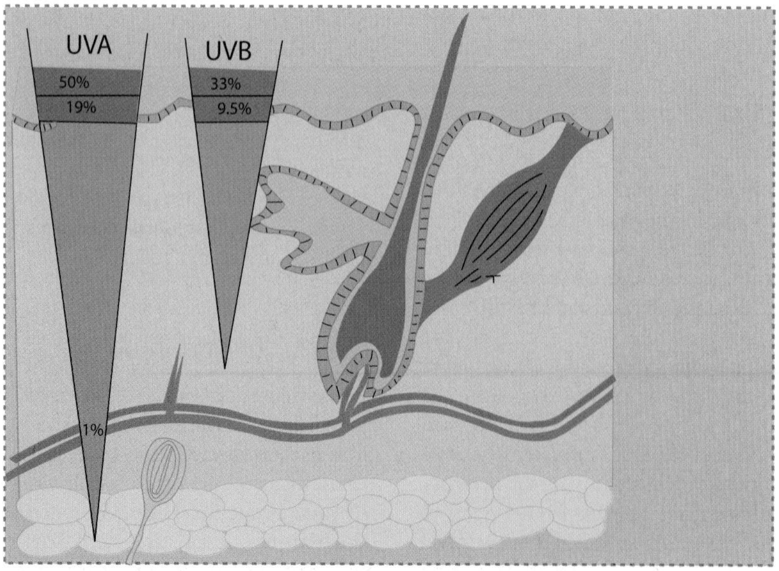

PHOTOADDITION AND PHOTOAUGMENTATION

Though sunbeds emit less UVB rays than UVA rays, there is still reason for medical concern. In the United States, typical indoor tanners (20 sessions per year) could add anywhere from 0.20 to 24% more UVB radiation.[15] Therefore, it adds to one's total UVB exposure. Moreover, the interaction of tanning bed UVA and UVB may have more carcinogenic effects than UVA or UVB alone. Subsequent sunlight exposure can occur when people go to tanning beds before a sunny vacation (see the section, "Controversy of Tanning for Sun Protection"). When a subminimal erythema dose exposure of UVA is given, followed by a subminimal erythema dose of UVB, the energy is additive; as a consequence an unexpected sunburn can occur (photoaddition).[81] The interaction of UVA and UVB can be more than a simple addition. UVA exposure can enhance the skin response to UVB. It has been shown that carcinogenicity of UVB in mice can be augmented by prior, simultaneous, or subsequent exposure to UVA to a degree greater than by simple addition.[82,83]

IMMUNOSUPPRESSION

The importance of UV-induced suppression of cell-mediated immunity is well established in photocarcinogenesis, and the high incidence of skin cancer in immunosuppressed organ transplant recipients support the association of skin cancer and immunosuppression. The relative roles of the UVA and UVB rays in sunlight-induced cutaneous immunosuppression are unclear. Although it is generally accepted that UVB suppresses both contact hypersensitivity and delayed-type hypersensitivity responses in humans and animal models, the role of UVA is more controversial.[84,85] It has been shown that low-dose UVA exposure can induce immunosuppressive effects[86] while high doses are immunoprotective.[87] UVA may also reduce the number of antigen-presenting Langerhans cells.[88] A recent study demonstrated that interactive effect of UVA and UVB is a more potent cause of immunosuppression than either UVA or UVB alone.[87]

CONTROVERSY OF TANNING FOR SUN PROTECTION

It is known that people with fair skin are more susceptible to sunburn and subsequently skin cancer. Given the fact that tanning beds provide a "base tan," some investigators and especially the indoor tanning industry have argued that indoor tanning can potentially be protective against skin cancer.[89] This presumption is mainly based on the fact that sunbed UVA is safer than sunlight UVB. In addition, UV radiation from tanning beds is controlled, in small and frequent doses that do not cause sunburn. On the contrary, UV radiation from sunlight is uncontrolled, and usually in abrupt and large doses causing sunburn. Although some studies have shown mild sun protection in accordance of the above arguement,[39] some opposed it from several aspects. The main objection is that UV irradiation given in many small doses is more carcinogenic for nonmelanoma skin cancer than the same amount of energy given in a few large doses.[90] Thus many small doses in a tanning bed are not necessarily safer. Another objection is that although UVA can induce tanning in doses less than the minimal erythema dose, it is not principally efficient at inducing a tan in comparison to UVB. In addition, the tan achieved by UVA is limited mainly to the basal layer which is not protective for more superficial layers of epidermis.[34] Accordingly, several studies showed no protection against sunburn afforded by prior exposure to UVA,[91,92] and some showed insignificant protection, with a sun protection factor of 3 to 4.[14,39] Of major concern is that the

▲ **FIGURE 60-1** Depth of penetration of UVA and UVB into the skin. UVB mainly affects the epidermis, while UVA penetrates deeper into the dermis.[79]

belief of sun-protectiveness of indoor tanning may lead to decreased use of sun-protective precautions against the sunlight.[20,38]

GUIDELINES FOR INDOOR TANNING USE

Many health care professionals consider tanning as one of the risky behaviors practiced by the public. Like other risky activities such as smoking or excessive alcohol consumption, the choice of whether to tan or not is made after considering the short- and long-term risks and benefits. However, because of the growth of the tanning facility industry, informative instructions, and established guidelines by health care officials are necessary.

The World Health Organization (WHO) states that overexposure to UV radiation from the sun and artificial sources is of considerable public health concern, and declares that no person under 18 years of age should use a sunbed.[93] In the 10th report on carcinogens by the National Institutes of Health (NIH), it is stated, "Exposure to sunbeds and sunlamps is known to be a human carcinogen based on sufficient evidence of carcinogenicity from studies in humans, which indicates a causal relationship between exposure to sunbeds and sunlamps and cancer.[94]

In the United States, sunlamp products are regulated by the Food and Drug Administration (FDA) and the Federal Trade Commission (FTC). FDA regulations, in effect since the mid-1980s, specify regulations for sunlamp products that have requirements for warning labels, user instructions, requirements for protective eyewear and timer system, as well as limits on levels of ultraviolet C light.[95] The FTC has established guidelines that prohibit deceptive advertising, particularly claims of health benefits from indoor tanning.[96] Based on these regulations, tanning devices cannot be marketed for any purpose other than cosmetic tanning. Tanning facilities are subject to confiscation and the operators to fines if claims are made that they are safe or healthy.[97] The manufacturers must attach a warning label to tanning devices indicating that UV exposure may cause skin cancer, premature aging of the skin, burns, and long-term injury to the eyes.[95] FDA recommends the first exposure to be "no more than 0.75 minimal erythemal dose three times the first week," gradually increasing the exposure thereafter. The

Table 60-4
Conditions in Which Indoor Tanning Should be Prohibited[a]

- Age < 18 years
- Skin types I or II
- Pregnancy
- ≥30 moles larger than 2 mm, or one or more moles larger than 5 mm on the whole body
- Tendency to freckle
- Family history of melanoma
- History of childhood sunburn
- Presence/history of premalignant or malignant skin lesions
- People with sundamaged skin
- Use of medication (may cause photosensitivity)
- Wearing cosmetics (may cause photosensitivity)

[a]According to International Commission on Non-Ionizing Radiation Protection (ICNIRP) and World Health Organization (WHO).

American Medical Association's Council on Scientific Affairs recommends no more than 30 to 50 half-hour sessions per year.[50] Based on the International Commission on Non-Ionizing Radiation Protection recommendations, indoor tanning should be prohibited in high-risk populations (Table 60-4).[98] Because adolescence represents a critical period during which UV radiation increases skin cancer risk, most efforts have been focused on altering the tanning behavior in adolescents and younger individuals. Among European countries, France appears to have the most comprehensive legislation establishing a legal minimum age for indoor tanning (age 18 years). In the US, only six states currently have in place minimum age limits for UV tanning patrons: Wisconsin, North Carolina, Texas, Illinois, California, and New Hampshire.[99]

PREVENTION

Despite the above-mentioned recommendations to avoid UV radiation, the indoor tanning prevalence is surprisingly high and increasing. Between 1986 and 1996 there was a three-fold increase in the percentage of people who use tanning beds.[100] Prevention strategies have been successful in increasing public awareness of the adverse consequences associated with exposure to UV radiation; however, they have generally been modest and inconsistent in changing behavior patterns. Multiple cognitive, psychological, social, and behavioral

factors may be involved in tanning behavior as other behaviors. Some of these factors have been addressed in the previous studies; however, interventional studies are few.

Social and Behavioral Factors

There is growing evidence that indoor tanning is a socially determined behavior. Social influences are particularly important determinants of indoor tanning use among adolescents. Several studies suggest that social influences are critical in both initiating and maintaining tanning behavior.[15,19,20,101] It has been shown that indoor tanning use is more common among adolescents whose parents and/or friends engage in tanning activities. Therefore, modifying attitudes toward the desirability of a tanned skin in parents may exert an influence on their youth's indoor tanning sunlamp use.

Cognitive and Psychological Factors

Prevention strategies have been successful in that they have increased public awareness of the adverse consequences associated with excessive UV exposure. A variety of educational programs have been employed with different success rates. However, they have been largely ineffective in changing behavior patterns.[100,102] Knowledge of the potential risks posed by indoor tanning by itself does not necessarily change the tanning behavior. Other cognitive and psychological factors play an important role in tanning behavior. These include, but are not limited to, perceived attractiveness of tan, beliefs that tan is healthy, depression, individual's decision-making abilities, as well as short-term benefits of tan (positive social response from friends, and thereby better self-esteem, better sex life, etc.).[15,19–21,28] Using an economic model, "utility model," Feldman et al hypothesized that past prevention efforts have been largely ineffective because of their focus on long-term benefits gained by sun-protective behavior. However, when individuals decide whether to engage in tanning behavior, the perceived current benefits of tanning are weighted more heavily than the future health risks. Therefore, they proposed that future efforts should be focused on the short-term gains. Accordingly, it has been demonstrated that interventions that address individuals' concerns about appearance (short-term gain) may be more effective than health warnings alone for countering the strong normative influences for tanning. If the social norm became fair skin, then the value placed on tanned skin might decrease.[3,14,103]

SUNLESS TANNING

Sunless tanning is browning the skin using the chemical dihydroxyacetone (DHA). The reaction of DHA with basic groups of protein in the stratum corneum results in browning the skin giving it the look of tan.[104] This method of tanning has been in the market for nearly half a decade; however, due to its suboptimal cosmetic results, it is not as popular as suntan or sunbed use.[105] Sunless tanning has been suggested as an alternative to suntan and sunbed use. The result of a recent study on 121 individuals showed that sunless tanning decreases the use of indoor tanning devices.[106] The American Academy of Dermatology has advocated sunless tanning as a safer alternative to sun-induced tanning. However, it should be noted that not all sunless tanning products contain sunscreen; hence, in these cases, sunscreens with SPF 15 or higher should be used in conjunction with sunless tanning products.

NONADHERENCE TO GUIDELINES AND REGULATION

Studies of tanning business practices reveal a lack of compliance with regulations. Studies in Massachusetts, Minnesota, North Carolina, New York, and California tanning facilities found safety hazards, poor knowledge, exceeding recommended limits of UV exposure, inaccurate communication of risks to customers, and other violations of national regulations and guidelines.[10,15,103,107]

VITAMIN D CONTROVERSIES

It is known that UV radiation is necessary for cutaneous synthesis of vitamin D3, the precursor of $1,25(OH)_2$ vitamin D, which is critical for calcium homeostasis and skeletal maintenance. Now, the question is whether sun avoidance, with a goal of skin cancer prevention, may compromise vitamin D sufficiency. The answer is that the amount of UV radiation needed to produce sufficient vitamin D is small. It has been shown that white, clothed infants, exposing only their hands and face, require 0.5 to 2.0 h of sun exposure per week for adequate vitamin D synthe-

sis.[108] In addition, in a study on people who use sunscreens, none of the participants developed vitamin D levels under the normal range.[109] Some recent studies argue that the currently recommended vitamin D level is not adequate, and higher levels of vitamin D may offer benefits such as preventing osteoporosis-induced fractures, lowering blood pressure, reduction in mortality from some cancers, and prevention of autoimmune diseases, such as type 1 DM and multiple sclerosis. Most of these arguments have not yet been confirmed. Moreover, the noncarcinogenic alternative, intestinal absorption of vitamin D-fortified foods and/or dietary supplements is efficient and safe. Therefore, even if the current vitamin D recommendations are too low, research does not support frequent and prolonged exposure to tanning beds as a means of correcting this problem.

FINAL THOUGHTS

With the rising incidence of skin cancer, it is vital to increase sun-protective behaviors. While the carcinogenicity of UV radiation through sun tanning is well documented, whether or not indoor tanning devices lead to skin cancer development is still under investigation. Nonetheless, many healthcare professionals and organizations consider tanning as one of the risky behaviors practiced by the public, and recommend prevention strategies. These strategies, although successful in increasing public awareness, have generally been modest and inconsistent in changing behavior patterns. Considering the fact that commercial indoor tanning business has been one of the fastest growing industries in the last decades, a better understanding of tanning devices, their putative carcinogenicity, and factors involved in tanning behavior is necessary.

REFERENCES

1. Fitzpatrick TB, Bolognia JL. Human melanin pigmentation. In: Zeise L, Chedekel MR, Fitzpatrick TB, eds. *Melanin: Its Role in Human Photoprotection*. Overland Park, KS: Valdenmar Publishing Co.; 1995.
2. Keesling B, Friedman HS. Psychosocial factors in sunbathing and sunscreen use. *Health Psychol.* 1987;6:477–493.
3. Feldman SR, Dempsey JR, Grummer S, et al. Implications of a utility model for ultraviolet exposure behavior. *J Am Acad Dermatol.* 2001;45:718–722.
4. Sikes RG. The history of sun tanning. *J Aesthetic Sci.* 1998;1:6–7.
5. Spencer JM, Amonette RA. Tanning beds and skin cancer: Artificial sun + old sol = real risk. *Clin Dermatol.* 1998; 16:487–501.
6. McGinley J, Martin CJ, MacKie RM. Sunbeds in current use in Scotland: a survey of their output and patterns of use. *Br J Dermatol.* 1998, 139, 428–438.
7. American Cancer Society. Are tanning centers safe? *Cancer News.* 1981;Spring/Summer:19.
8. Levine JA, Sorace M, Spencer J, Siegel DM. The indoor UV tanning industry: a review of skin cancer risk, health benefit claims, and regulation. *J Am Acad Dermatol.* 2005;53:1038–1044.
9. Demierre M. Time for national legislation of indoor tanning to protect minors. *Arch Dermatol.* 2003;139:520–524.
10. Hornung RL, Magee KH, Lee WJ, et al. Tanning facility use: are we exceeding Food and Drug Administration limits? *J Am Acad Dermatol.* 2003;49:655–661.
11. Westerdahl J, Ingvar C, Masback A, et al. Risk of cutaneous malignant melanoma in relation to use of sunbeds: further evidence for UV-A carcinogenicity. *Br J Cancer.* 2000;82:1593–1599.
12. The $1,000,000,000 industry. *Looking fit.* 1992;7:56–70.
13. Winning moves for tanning and equipment: a comprehensive report on the state of the industry. *Looking Fit.* 2002;17: 38–48.
14. Kwon HT, Mayer JA, Walker KK, et al. Promotion of frequent tanning sessions by indoor tanning facilities: two studies. *J Am Acad Dermatol.* 2002;46:700–705.
15. Lazovich D, Forster J, Sorensen G, et al. Characteristics associated with use or intention to use indoor tanning among adolescents. *Arch Pediatr Adolesc Med.* 2004;158:918–924.
16. Selecting the right location. Sun Magazine. 1997;4:8–9.
17. Wester U, Boldeman C, Jansson B, Ullen H. Population UV-dose and skin area—do sunbeds rival the sun? *Health Phychol.* 1999;77(4):436–440.
18. Feldman SR, Liguori A, Kucenic M, et al. Ultraviolet exposure is a reinforcing stimulus in frequent indoor tanners. *J Am Acad Dermatol.* July 2004;51(1):45–51.
19. Geller AC, Colditz G, Oliveria S, et al. Use of sunscreen, sunburning rates, and tanning bed use among more than 10,000 US children and adolescents. *Pediatrics.* 2002;109:1009–1014.
20. Cokkinides VE, Weinstock MA, O'Connell MC, et al. Use of indoor tanning sunlamps by US youth, ages 11 to 18 years, and by their parent or guardian caregivers: prevalence and correlates. *Pediatrics.* 2002;109;1124–1130.
21. Demko CA, Borawski EA, Debanne SM, et al. Use of indoor tanning facilities by white adolescents in the United States. *Arch Pediatr Adolesc Med.* 2003; 157:854–860.
22. Wichstrom L. Predictors of Norwegian adolescents' sunbathing and use of sunscreen. *Health Psychol.* 1994;13:412–420
23. Leary MR, Jones JL. The social psychology of tanning and sunscreen use: self-presentational motives as a predictor of health risk. *J Appl Soc Psychol.* 1993;23: 1390–1406.
24. Jones JL, Leary MR. Effects of appearance-based admonitions against sun

exposure on tanning intentions in young adults. *J Health Psychol.* 1994;13:86–90.

25. Mawn VB, Fleischer AB. A survey of attitudes, beliefs, and behavior regarding tanning bed use, sunbathing, and sunscreen use. *J Am Acad Dermatol.* 1993;29:959–962.

26. Knight JM, Kirincich AN, Farmer ER, Hood AF. Awareness of the risks of tanning lamps does not influence behavior among college students. *Arch Dermatol.* 2002;138:1311–1315.

27. Dougherty MA, McDermott RJ, Hawkins MJ. A profile of users of commercial tanning salons. *Health Values.* 1988;12:21–29.

28. Boldeman C, Jansson B, Nilsson B, Ullen H. Sunbed use in Swedish urban adolescents related to behavioral characteristics. *Prev Med.* 1997;26:114–119.

29. Grant WB. An estimate of premature cancer mortality in the U.S. due to inadequate doses of solar ultraviolet-B radiation. *Cancer.* March 15. 2002;94(6):1867–1875.

30. Garland CF, Comstock GW, Garland FC, et al. Serum 25-hydroxyvitamin D and colon cancer: eight year prospective study. *Lancet.* 1989;2:1176–1178.

31. Indoor Tanning Association Inc. Frequently asked questions. Available at: http://www.theita.com/indoor/faq.cfm. Accessed February 28, 2006.

32. Kennedy C, Bajdik CD, Willemze R, et al. Leiden Skin Cancer Study. The influence of painful sunburns and lifetime sun exposure on the risk of actinic keratoses, seborrheic warts, melanocytic nevi, atypical nevi, and skin cancer. *J Invest Dermatol.* June 2003;120(6):1087–1093.

33. Van der Mei IA, Ponsonby AL, Dwyer T, et al. Past exposure to sun, skin phenotype, and risk of multiple sclerosis: case-control study. *Br Med J.* August 2003;327(7410):316.

34. Spencer JM, Amonette RA. Indoor tanning: risks, benefits, and future trends. *J Am Acad Dermatol.* 1995;33(2 Pt 1): 288–298.

35. Ultraviolet light: a hazard to children. American Academy of Pediatrics. Committee on Environmental Health. *Pediatrics.* August 1999;104(2 Pt 1): 328–33.

36. Karagas MR, Stannard VA, Mott LA, et al. Use of tanning devices and risk of basal cell and squamous cell skin cancers. *J Natl Cancer Inst.* February 2002; 94(3):224–226.

37. 36.Wang SQ, Setlow R, Berwick M, et al. Ultraviolet A and melanoma: a review. *J Am Acad Dermatol.* May 2001;44(5): 837–846.

38. Swerdlow AJ, Weinstock MA. Do tanning lamps cause melanoma? An epidemiologic assessment. *J Am Acad Dermatol.* January 1998;38(1):89–98.

39. Devgun MS, Johnson BE, Paterson CR. Tanning, protection against sunburn and vitamin D formation with a UVA sunbed. *Br J Dermatol.* 1982;107:275–284.

40. Rivers JK, Norris PG, Murphy GM, et al. UVA sunbeds: tanning, photoprotection, acute adverse effects and immunologic changes. *Br J Dermatol.* 1989;120:767–777.

41. Stern RS, Docken W. An exacerbation of SLE after visiting a tanning salon. *J Am Med Assoc.* 1986;255:3120.

42. Farr PM, Marks JM, Diffey BL, et al. Skin fragility and blistering due to use of sunbeds. *BMJ.* 1988;296:1708–1709.

43. Murphy GM, Wright J, Nicholls DSH, et al. Sunbed-induced pseudoporphyria. *Br J Dermatol.* 1989;120:555–562.

44. Tegner E, Brudin AM. Polymorphous light eruption in hypopigmented pressure areas with a UVA sunbed. *Acta Derm Venereol (Stockh).* 1986;66:446–448.

45. Snider RL, Lang PG, Maize JC. The clinical spectrum of mid-dermal elastolysis and the role of UV light in its pathogenesis. *J Am Acad Dermatol.* 1993;28:938–942.

46. Monfrecola G, Fabbrocini G, Posteraro G, Pini D. What do young people think about the dangers of sunbathing, skin cancer and sunbeds? A questionnaire survey among Italians, Photodermatol. *Photoimmunol Photomed.* 2000;16:15–18.

47. Rhainds M, De Guire L, Claveau J. A population-based survey on the use of artificial tanning devices in the province of Québec, Canada. *J Am Acad Dermatol.* 1999;40:572–576.

48. Autier P, Doré JF, Lejeune F, et al. Cutaneous malignant melanoma and exposure to sunlamps or sunbeds: an EORTC multicenter case-control study in Belgium, France and Germany. *Int J Cancer.* 1994;58:809–813.

49. Centers for Disease Control. Injuries associated with ultraviolet tanning devices—Wisconsin. *J Am Med Assoc.* 1989;261:3519–3520.

50. Council on Scientific Affairs. Harmful effects of ultraviolet light radiation. *JAMA.* 1989;262:380–384.

51. De Vries E, Louwman M, Bastiaens M, et al. Rapid and continuous increases in incidence rates of basal cell carcinoma in the Southeast Netherlands since 1973. *J Invest Dermatol.* 2004;123(4):634–638.

52. Autier P. Perspectives in melanoma prevention: the case of sunbeds. *Eur J Cancer.* 2004;40(16):2367–2376.

53. Marrot L, Belaidi JP, Meunier JR, et al. The human melanocyte as a particular target for UVA radiation and an end-point for photoprotection assessment. *Photochem Photobiol.* 1999;69(6):686–693.

54. Runger TM. Role of UVA in the pathogenesis of melanoma and non-melanoma skin cancer. A short review. *Photodermatol Photoimmunol Photomed.* 1999;15(6):212–216.

55. Linge C. Relevance of in vitro melanocytic cell studies to the understanding of melanoma. *Cancer Surv.* 1996;26: 71–87.

56. Woollons A, Kipp C, Young AR, et al. The 0.8% ultraviolet B content of an ultraviolet A sunlamp induces 75% of cyclobutane pyrimidine dimers in human keratinocytes in vitro. *Br J Dermatol.* 1999;140(6):1023–1030.

57. Roest MAB, Keane FM, Agnew K, et al. Multiple squamous skin carcinomas following excess sunbed use. *J Royal Soc Med.* 2001;94: 636–637.

58. Lever LR, Lawrence CM. Nonmelanoma skin cancer associated with use of a tanning bed (letter to the editor). *N Engl J Med.* 1995; 332(21):1450–1451.

59. Speight EL, Dahl M, Farr P. Actinic keratoses induced by sunbed. *Br Med J.* 1994;308:415.

60. Veierod MB, Weiderpass E, Thorn M, et al. A prospective study of pigmentation, sun exposure, and risk of cutaneous malignant melanoma in women. *J Natl Cancer Inst.* 2003;95(20):1530–1538.

61. Westerdahl J, Olsson H, Masback A, et al. Use of sunbeds or sunlamps and malignant melanoma in southern Sweden. *Am J Epidemiol.* 1994;15(140): 691–699.

62. Walter SD, Marrett LD, From L, et al. The association of cutaneous malignant melanoma with the use of sunbeds and sunlamps. *Am J Epidemiol.* 1990;131: 232–243.

63. Chen YT, Dubrow R, Zheng T, et al. Sunlamp use and the risk of cutaneous malignant melanoma: a population-based case-control study in Connecticut, USA. *Int J Epidemiol.* 1998;27:758–765.

64. Bajdik CD, Gallagher RP, Astrakianakis G, et al. Non-solar ultraviolet radiation and the risk of basal and squamous cell skin cancer. *Br J Cancer.* 1996;73:612–614.

65. Aubry F, MacGibbon B. Risk factors of squamous cell carcinoma of the skin. A case-control study in the Montreal region. *Cancer.* 1985;55:907–911.

66. Boyd AS, Shyr Y, King LE Jr. Basal cell carcinoma in young women: an evaluation of the association of tanning bed use and smoking. *J Am Acad Dermatol.* 2002;46:706–709.

67. English DR, Armstrong BK, Kricker A, Fleming C. Sunlight and cancer. *Cancer Causes Control.* 1997;8:271–283.

68. Miller SA, Hamilton SL, Wester UG, et al. An analysis of UVA emissions from sunlamps and the potential importance for melanoma. *Photochem Photobiol.* 1998;68(1):63–70.

69. Gerber B, Mathys P, Moser M, et al. Ultraviolet emission spectra of sunbeds, Photochem. *Photobiol.* 2002;76:664–668.

70. Burren R, Scaletta C, Frenk E, et al. Sunlight and carcinogenesis: expression of p53 and pyrimidine dimers in human skin following UVA I, UVA I + II, and solar simulating radiations. *Int J Cancer.* 1998;76:201–206.

71. Kvam E, Tyrrell RM. Induction of oxidative DNA base damage in human skin cells by UV and near visible radiation. *Carcinogenesis.* 1997;18:2379–2384.

72. Ley RD. Ultraviolet radiation A-induced precursors of cutaneous melanoma in Monodelphis domestica. *Cancer Res.* 1997;57:3682–3684.

73. Strickland PT. Photocarcinogenesis by near ultraviolet (UVA) radiation in Sencar mice. *J Invest Dermatol.* 1986;87:272–275.

74. Sterenborg HJCM, van der Leun JC. Tumorigenesis by a long wavelength UVA source. *Photochem Photobiol.* 1990; 51:325–330.

75. Peak MJ, Peak JG, Carnes BA. Induction of direct and indirect single strand breaks in human cell DNA by far and near ultraviolet radiations: action spectrum and mechanisms. *Photochem Photobiol.* 1987;45:381–387.

76. Peak MJ, Peak JG, Jones CA. Different (direct and indirect) mechanisms for the induction of DNA-protein crosslinks in human cells by far and near ultraviolet radiations (290 and 405 nm). *Photochem Photobiol.* 1985;42:141–146.

77. Freeman SE, Gange RW, Sutherland JC, et al. Production of pyrimidine dimers in human skin exposed in situ to UVA

irradiation. *J Invest Dermatol.* 1987;88: 430–433.

78. Drobetsky EA, Turcotte J, Chateauneuf A. A role for ultraviolet A in solar mutagenesis. *Proc Natl Acad Sci USA.* 1995; 92:2350–2354.

79. Environmental Health Criteria 160, Ultraviolet Radiation, United Nations Environment Programme, World Health Organization, International Commission on Non-Ionizing Radiation Protection. WHO Geneva, 1994.

80. Agar NS, Halliday GM, Barnetson RStC, et al. The basal layer in human squamous tumours harbors more UVA than UVB fingerprints mutations: a role for UVA in human skin carcinogenesis. *Proc Natl Acad Sci.* 1994;101: 4954–4959.

81. Willis I, Menter JM, Whyte HJ. The rapid induction of cancers in the hairless mouse utilizing the principle of photoaugmentation. *J Invest Dermatol.* 1981;76:404–408.

82. Staberg B, Wulf HC, Klemp P, et al. The carcinogenic effect of UVA irradiation. *J Invest Dermatol.* 1983;81:517–519.

83. Staberg B, Wulf HC, Poulsen T. Carcinogenic effect of sequential artificial sunlight and UVA irradiation in hairless mice. Consequences for solarium "therapy". *Arch Dermatol.* 1983; 119:641–643.

84. Sjovall P, Christensen OB. Local and systemic effect of ultraviolet irradiation (UVB and UVA) on human allergic contact dermatitis. *Acta Derm Venereol.* 1986;66:290–294.

85. Poon TS, Barnetson RS, Halliday GM. Sunlight-induced immunosuppression in humans is initially because of UVB, then UVA, followed by interactive effects. *J Invest Dermatol.* October 2005;125(4):840–846.

86. Damian DL, Barnetson RS, Halliday GM. Low-dose UVA and UVB have different time courses for suppression of contact hypersensitivity to a recall antigen in humans. *J Invest Dermatol.* 1999;112:939–944.

87. Byrne, SN, Spinks, N, Halliday, GM: Ultraviolet A irradiation of C57BL/6 mice suppresses systemic contact hypersensitivity or enhances secondary immunity depending on dose. *J Invest Dermatol.* 2002;119:858–864.

88. LeVee GJ, Oberhelman L, Anderson T, et al. UVA II exposure of human skin results in decreased immunization capacity, increased induction of tolerance and a unique pattern of epidermal antigen-presenting cell alteration. *Photochem Photobiol.* 1997;65:622–629.

89. Cyr WH. CDRH evaluation of UV-emitting sunlamp products In: Proceedings of the National Conference of Radiation Control Officers. *Mesa (AZ)*,1998.

90. Forbes PD, Davies RE, Urbach F. Experimental ultraviolet photocarcinogenesis: wavelength interactions and time-dose relationships. *Natl Cancer Inst Monogr.* 1978;50:31–38.

91. Gange RW, Blackett AFD, Matzinger EA, et al. Comparative protection efficiency of UVA and UVB induced tans against erythema and formation of endonuclease sensitive sites in DNA by UVB in human skin. *J Invest Dermatol.* 1985;85:362–364.

92. Kaidbey KH, Kligman AM. Sunburn protection by long wave ultraviolet radiation induced pigmentation. *Arch Dermatol.* 1978;114:46–48

93. Sinclair C. Artificial tanning sunbeds: risk and guidance. World Health Organization. Available at: http://www. who.int/uv/publications/sunbedpubl/en/. Accessed March 11, 2006.

94. U.S. Department of Health and Human Services, Public Health Service, National Toxicology Program. Report on carcinogens, 11th ed: *Exposure to Sunlamps or Sunbeds*. Available at: http://ntp.niehs.nih.gov/ntp/roc/eleventh/profiles/s183uvrr.pdf. Accessed March 12, 2006.

95. Department of Health and Human Services, Food and Drug Administration. Sunlamp products: performance standard; final rule (21 CFR 1040). *Federal Register.* 1985;50:36548–36552.

96. Federal Trade Commission. Available at: http:// www.ftc.gov/bcp/conline/ pubs /health/indoortan.htm.in.

97. Federal Food, Drug, and Cosmetic Act, as amended, 21 USC §301–392.

98. International Commission on Non-Ionizing Radiation Protection (ICNIRP). Health issues of ultraviolet tanning appliances used for cosmetic purposes. *Health Physchol.* 2003;84(1):119–127.

99. Francis SO, Burkhardt DL, Dellavalle RP. 2005: A banner year for new US youth. Access tanning restrictions. *Arch Dermatol.* 2005;141:524–525.

100. Robinson JK, Rigel DS, Amonette RA. Trends in sun exposure knowledge, attitudes, and behaviors: 1986 to 1996. *J Am Acad Dermatol.* 1997;37:179–186.

101. Brandberg Y, Ullen H, Sjoberg L, et al. Sunbathing and sunbed use related to self-image in a randomized sample of Swedish adolescents. *Eur J Cancer Prev.* August 1998;7(4):321–329.

102. Campbell HS, Birdsell JM. Knowledge, beliefs, and sun protection behaviors of Alberta adults. *Prev Med.* 1994;23:160–166.

103. Fairchild AL, Gemson DH. Safety information provided to customers of New York City sun-tanning salons. *Am J Prev Med.* 1992;8:381–383.

104. Maibach HI, Kligman AM. Dihydroxyacetone: A suntan-simulating agent. *Arch Dermatol.* 1960;82:505–507.

105. Albert MR, Osthcimer KG. The evolution of current medical and popular attitudes toward ultraviolet light exposure: Part 3. *J Am Acad Dermotol.* 2003; 49: 1096–1106.

106. Sheehan DJ, Lesher JL Jr. The effect of sunless tanning on behavior in the sun: a pilot study. *South Med J.* December 2005;98(12):1192–1195.

107. Culley CA, Mayer JA, Eckhardt L, Busic AJ, Eichenfield LF, Sallis JF, et al. Compliance with federal and state legislation by indoor tanning facilities in San Diego. *J Am Acad Dermatol.* 2001; 44(1):53–60.

108. Greer FR. Do breastfed infants need supplemental vitamins? *Pediatr Clin North Am.* 2001;48:415–423.

109. Marks R, Foley PA, Jolley D, Knight KR, Harrison J, Thompson SC. The effect of regular sunscreen use on vitamin D levels in an Australian population: results of a randomized controlled trial. *Arch Dermatol.* 1995;131:415–421.

CHAPTER 61

Economics of Skin Cancer

Daniel Pearce, M.D.
Phillip M. Williford, M.D.
Rajesh Balkrishnan, Ph.D.
Steven R. Feldman, M.D., Ph.D.

BOX 61-1   Overview

- Analysis of the cost of skin cancer treatment depends on perspective; macro and microeconomic viewpoints demonstrate that the individual's outlook differs from that of insurers and from society as a whole.
- The overall cost of skin cancer treatment is likely to increase given the increasing incidence of skin cancer in the US.
- Indirect costs such as reduced quality of life, physical disability, absenteeism, and premature death need to be considered in any economic discussion of skin cancer.
- The office setting is more cost efficient for the treatment of cutaneous malignancy.
- There is no evidence that prevention and screening measures are cost effective approaches to skin cancer.
- Regulation, though well intended, threatens to change the delivery of skin cancer treatment with significant cost ramifications.

■ INTRODUCTION

BOX 61-2   Summary

- The cost of cutaneous malignancy may be difficult to quantify and can be examined from a macro or microeconomic viewpoint
- There are direct and indirect costs that factor into cost determinations.

What is the cost of skin cancer? There are a few different ways to answer this, and in a sense, perspective is at the heart of this question. There are many parties interested in the cost associated with treating skin cancer including the society, individuals, insurers, and healthcare delivery groups, to name a few. Many of these parties have different priorities when it comes to paying for, and willingness to pay for, skin cancer treatment. Classically, the delivery of a good or service can be analyzed from a macroeconomic or microeconomic outlook. A macroeconomic perspective pertains to aggregate behavior in a given market or society, while microeconomics deals more with behaviors of an individual member of the market. A macro concept would be societal costs of treating skin cancer, while the micro side would deal with the willingness to pay for skin cancer treatment as it pertains to an individual's financial/insurance status. Most of the existing economic data pertains to the macro, or aggregate cost and delivery of skin cancer care. Thus, these will be the focus here.

Several salient points regarding cutaneous carcinoma have been addressed within this text. However, without consideration of the economic impact of skin cancer, the discussion is incomplete. There are direct and indirect costs of any disease. Costs can be considered as being directly related to the episode of care and include items such as office visits, procedures, medications, etc. Indirect cost are not insignificant when considering the impact of skin cancers; absenteeism and presenteeism (decreased productivity though at work) contribute a substantial amount to the overall cost of skin cancer. These costs have been estimated in a 2004 report on the burden of skin diseases (Fig. 61-1).

The economic environment pertaining to skin cancer is not one in which the dermatologist should ignore. Legislative issues that threaten to limit patient access to care and physician reimbursement are based on cost modeling. Certain raw components of the cost of skin cancer are relatively easy to digest. Other aspects of skin cancer economics that are less "neat" are those that are difficult to quantify such as Quality of Life (QoL) issues, mortality, and the cost/benefit regarding preventative measures. We will explore many of the current factors that are exerting force on the delivery of care to patients with cutaneous carcinomas.

■ OVERALL IMPACT OF SKIN CANCER

BOX 61-3   Summary

- There are many factors that influence the cost of treating a skin cancer.
- Quality of life impact is not irreverent, particularly when considering melanoma.

There are many factors that influence the economics of skin cancer. The type of cancer, prevalence, procedural treatments, medical treatments, loss of patients' productivity, and quality of life impact can all be considered when aggregating the cost of skin cancer. We will consider actinic keratoses (AKs), melanoma, and nonmelanoma skin

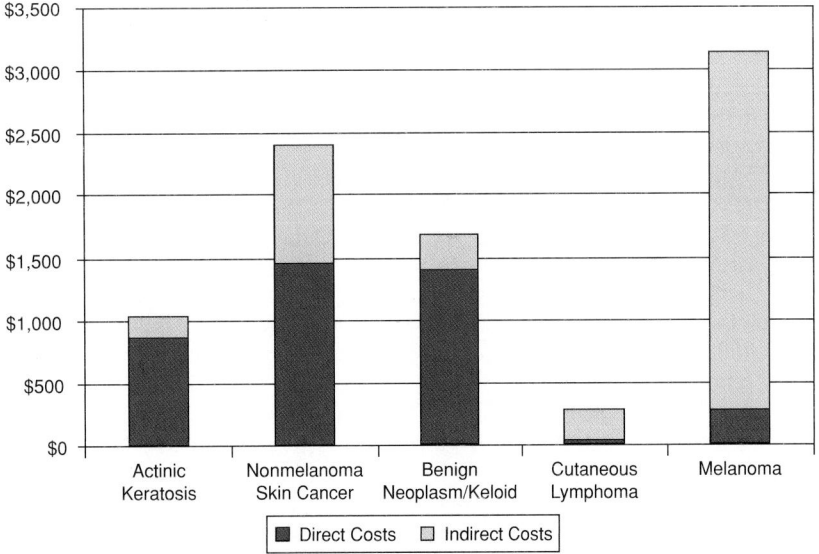

▲ FIGURE 61-1 Total direct and indirect costs of skin cancer and precancerous conditions in the (US$ millions, 2004). Reprinted with permission from the Society of Investigative Dermatology and American Academy of Dermatology Association. Burden of Skin Disease Report, 2004.

cancers; both basal cell (BCC) and squamous cell carcinomas (SCC) will be grouped as nonmelanoma skin cancer. As mentioned earlier, skin cancer has direct and indirect costs. Another component of skin cancer burden that could be overlooked is the impact of a reduced QoL from an episode of cancer as seen as indirect cost. The existing QoL data on skin cancer are from measures that have not necessarily been validated in the skin cancer patient population and are somewhat limited. It can be intimidating to quantify the impact of QoL in dollar terms though we will mention figures based on "willingness-to-pay." This approach is based on what an individual would pay for relief of symptoms, be they physical or psychosocial, and is an accepted method to evaluate such intangible costs associated with a disease.[1]

NONMELANOMA SKIN CANCER

BOX 61-4   Summary

- Nonmelanoma skin cancer has the highest direct cost of treatment; the incidence in the US is perhaps rising.
- Approximately $2.5 billion was spent in the US in 2004 onward; 86% in the outpatient setting.

The overwhelming majority of skin carcinoma is the nonmelanoma skin cancer (NMSC), largely (BCC) and (SCC). The tumors are most common in individuals over the age of 50 years; this aids in economic analysis as many of this population are Medicare enrollees. Medicare routinely collects data on the cost of health care. BCC and SCC have relatively low metastatic potential and have to be treated typically with surgical excision or destruction, in addition to histological confirmation of negative margins and appropriate follow-up. Five-year cure rates are typically accepted at around 95% for all modalities, yet higher for Mohs micrographic surgery. Rarely, adjunctive chemotherapy or radiation therapy is required.

For 2005, the American Cancer Society estimated at least 1 million new cases of basal and/or squamous cell cancer; there was also an estimated 6420 cases of nonepithelial cutaneous cancers. Until recently, there was evidence that the incidence of NMSC was increasing over the past 30 years[2] though newer estimates seem to have reached a plateau around 1 million per year in the US.[3–8]

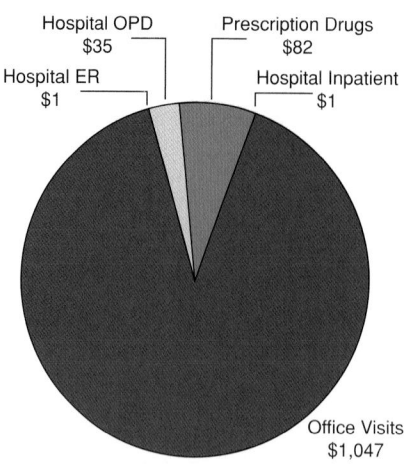

▲ **FIGURE 61-2** Annual direct costs of nonmelanoma skin cancer (US$ millions, 2004). Reprinted with permission from the Society of Investigative Dermatology and American Academy of Dermatology Association. Burden of Skin Disease Report, 2004.

In 2004, NMSC had been estimated to cost the US $2.5 billion annually in direct and indirect costs (Fig. 61-2).[9]

From 1992 to 1995, Medicare is estimated to have spent an average of $426 million annually managing NMSC.[10] The 2004 Burden of Skin Disease Report estimates a direct cost of $1.5 billion annually being spent on NMSC management in the US.[9] This latter estimate includes non-Medicare persons, and accounts for the additional costs of managing skin cancer and additional expenditures by providers, patients, and other insurers not included in the Medicare expenditure data. Of the $1.5 billion, 86% was spent on outpatient care with approximately 4% being spent in the inpatient setting and on prescription medications. Separate, indirect costs are estimated at $961 million and are largely due to workplace impact on the patient and caregiver at home.

Data regarding the impact of an NMSC diagnosis of QoL as measured by the SF-36 and Dermatology Life Quality Index (DLQI) show minimal impact.[11,12] Certainly this impact should be considered. The Lewin Group estimated that based on measurable QoL impact, there is an aggregate willingness-to-pay for individuals diagnosed with NMSC of $130 million annually.[9] Willingness-to-pay estimates provide some microeconomic insight into "consumer" behavior and are helpful in establishing at least some quantitative measure of the cost of NMSC in QoL terms.

MELANOMA

BOX 61-5   Summary

- Inherent in determining the cost of melanoma is the difficulty in quantifying morbidity and mortality.
- Indirect costs of $2.9 billion exceed the $291 million in direct cost estimated to have been used in 2004 to treat melanoma.

The epidemiologic and cost data for melanoma are grossly different. Melanoma can affect practically any age range and has substantially higher probability of metastasis compared to NMSC. Most obviously, melanoma carries a much higher mortality rate that is correlated with the stage of the disease; for stage I disease, the 5-year survival is 90 to 96% while for stage IV disease 5-year survival is 6 to 18%.[13] Treatment of melanoma, at least minimally invasive disease, is roughly similar to NMSC. More invasive disease may require surgical excision, sentinel node evaluation, as well as chemotherapy; there is data that higher severity is directly correlated with higher costs.[14]

There were an estimated 59,580 new cases of melanoma (*in situ* and invasive) with 7770 deaths in 2005.[3] Importantly, there appears to be an increasing trend in the incidence of melanoma. One study from the National Cancer Institute cites an average increase in the incidence of melanoma of 2.7% annually from 1992 to 1998.[15] According to the American Cancer Society[3–8] this continuing trend is an important economic consideration and has implications for planning the delivery of care in the future.

Melanoma is estimated to have cost the US$ 291 million and $2.9 billion in direct and indirect costs in 2004, respectively (Fig. 61-3).[9] Another estimate of the direct costs of treating melanoma in the US was estimated at $563 million; this figure attributes 90% of this cost to only 20% of patients, those with stage III or IV disease.[14]

Different from nonmelanoma costs, there is a considerable proportion of care received in an inpatient setting as well as prescription medications. These components of direct cost were estimated at $35 and $78 million respectively, nearly 39% of the direct costs. The large indirect burden of melanoma is largely due to lost future productivity.

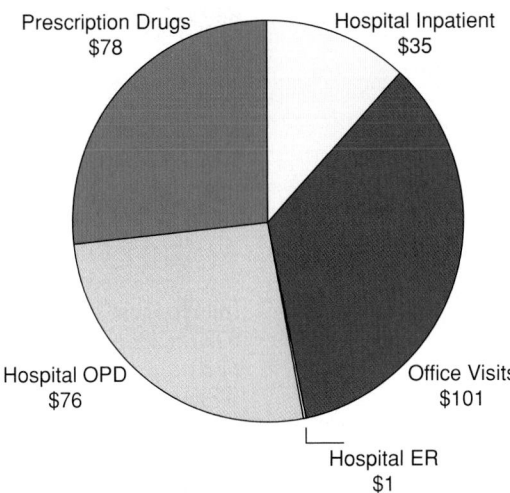

▲ **FIGURE 61-3** Annual direct costs of melanoma (US$ millions, 2004). Reprinted with permission from the Society of Investigative Dermatology and American Academy of Dermatology Association. Burden of Skin Disease Report, 2004.

Approximately 45% of melanoma deaths occur prior to retirement age; it has been said that melanoma ranks second of all cancers in terms of lost productive years.[9,16]

The willingness-to-pay perspective is confounded when analyzing melanoma due to the lack of a disease specific measure to QoL. Based on the QoL impact of melanoma as measured by the DLQI, an individual's willingness to pay for symptom relief was $1005 per episode with an annual aggregate estimate of $370 million.[9] However, the DLQI does not address issues such as the potential impact of severe illness or death and does not assess what an individual would pay for a cure. Thus, these figures are likely gross underestimates.

ACTINIC KERATOSES

BOX 61-6   Summary

- Actinic keratoses pose significant burden due to their high prevalence; medical therapy may impact the way in which money is spent to treat these potentially malignant precursors.
- Nearly $1 billion was spent in 2004 on AK treatment, largely on office based visits and procedures.

Actinic keratoses (AKs), which can develop into invasive squamous cell carcinoma, have a significant economic impact due to their relatively high prevalence and historically procedure-based treatment. In 2004, an estimated $0.9 billion was spent in direct costs on the treatment of AKs, with 88% of the cost attributable to outpatient physician office visits and procedures, and only 8% from prescription drug use (Fig. 61-4).[9]

Indirect costs were estimated at $172 million ($96 million in lost workdays) and with QoL *ad hoc* analysis, willingness to pay for symptom relief was estimated at $2.4 million in 2004.

The clinical behavior of AKs also likely explains the relatively high cost associated with their treatment. The presence of subclinical lesions challenges traditional cryosurgery, as only apparent lesions can be treated at a given visit. For many patients, a history of a singular lesion is not the rule; multiple new lesions will often be identifiable at future visits. Recently, the introduc-

tion of medical therapy for the treatment superficial basal cell carcinoma, as well as existing medical therapy for AKs, has provided an alternative to surgical treatments. The advantage of AK treatment with topical creams is that an entire "field" may be treated including subclinical lesions present at the time of the prescription. A potential disadvantage of medical therapy as monotherapy is that hypertrophic lesions may not be treated. Judicious use of cryosurgery for apparent lesions combined with pharmacotherapy is a reasonable approach. This strategy may help to reduce office-based costs, the largest component of AK costs; nevertheless, to date even *ad hoc* economic analysis is difficult due to limitations of existing data sets. Existing and possibly future medical therapies have the potential to alter the economic outlook for cutaneous malignancy and premalignancy, and this is a worthwhile endeavor for future study.

EPISODE OF CARE APPROACH

BOX 61-7   Summary

- The cost of an episode of skin cancer can be used to analyze components involved in the delivery of care.
- Office-based care is less expensive compared to the ambulatory surgical setting and inpatient management of skin cancers.

Another economic vantage point is the cost of an episode of care. The cost of treating a skin cancer is actually the sum of many varying components: the initial office visit, any biopsies, definitive

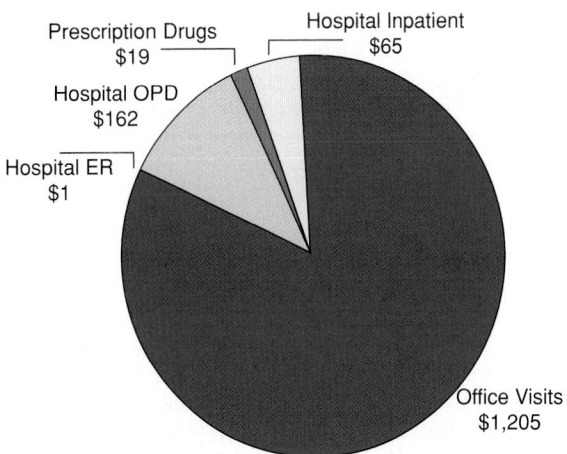

▲ **FIGURE 61-4** Annual direct costs of actinic keratoses (US$ millions, 2004). Reprinted with permission from the Society of Investigative Dermatology and American Academy of Dermatology Association. Burden of Skin Disease Report, 2004.

surgical procedures, pathology charges, and follow-up care. In order to arrive at a figure of how much an episode of care costs, a model of treatment must be defined. This is challenging for NMSC in particular, due to the numerous specialties, office settings, and treatment approaches that are involved in treating NMSC. Furthermore, patient and disease characteristics certainly have an important role in determining the overall cost of an episode of care and complicate defining an "average" episode of skin cancer.

A model previously developed and validated can be a useful tool when determining the cost components of an episode of skin cancer. Based on Medicare payment data there was a mean estimated cost of $470 ($\pm$$973 standard deviation) per episode of skin cancer. On further analysis, office setting had a significant effect on the mean cost of an episode of skin cancer. The cost of an episode in an office setting versus ambulatory surgical center versus inpatient setting were $332, $821, $6932 respectively, making treatment in the outpatient arena far less expensive when assuming similar cure rates.[17] There was also significant variability among providers as can be seen in a figure from the above-cited article.

Despite the complexity of measuring the cost of an NMSC event, using an episode of care approach provides useful information regarding how and where money is spent in treating skin cancers.

BENIGN LESIONS

> ### BOX 61-8 Summary
>
> - Significant expenditures are put out towards treatment of "benign" lesions; the approach to the removal of benign lesions impacts this cost.
> - The indirect costs exceed the direct cost of benign lesions due to the quality of life burden.

Analyzing the cost of treatment of benign lesions is very difficult due to the large variability of benign lesions that may receive treatment. If a lesion is clinically suspicious for melanoma, it may be biopsied or excised. One study attempts to examine this by looking at the cost associated with removal and histopathologic evaluation of seborrheic keratoses. The authors found that approximately $67 million was reimbursed from the Medicare population alone from 1998 to 1999, with 85% of lesions being from dermatologists. The cost was further analyzed into those lesions that were treated with "low-intensity," i.e., biopsy or shaving, and "high-intensity," excision or destruction and related repair. Using this framework, nondermatologists were statistically significantly more likely to use the "high-intensity," more costly approach to this benign lesion.[18]

Many otherwise benign lesions may be painful or cosmetically unacceptable

and create a significant QoL burden for the patient. The 2004 Burden of Skin Disease Report looked at the cost of hypertrophic scars and keloids, a relatively common benign lesion that receives medical and or surgical care. A direct cost estimate of $1.4 billion was spent in 2004 on these benign lesions with 86% of this being attributable to care received during office visits. Indirect cost of scars was estimated at $280 million. Using the microeconomic perspective, there was an aggregate willingness-to-pay of $1.6 billion, primarily for symptom relief and based on DLQI scores.[9]

PREVENTION AND SCREENING

> ### BOX 61-9 Summary
>
> - Only in Australia do prevention campaigns seem to be positively impacting the incidence of skin cancer; screening, when performed on the proper population, may provide benefit.
> - There is no proven economic benefit to prevention and screening campaigns.

A fundamental ambition of medicine is disease prevention through primary and secondary measures. Perhaps the most cost-effective preventative measures are aimed at the masses, particularly the youth. There have been many campaigns in the US and abroad targeted at preventing UV-associated skin cancers through advocating sunscreen usage, sun protective clothing, and avoidance of UV radiation during peak hours. There are significant resources dedicated to such programs with the expected return being a reduction in the incidence or prevalence of malignancy; this view calls cost-efficacy of such programs into play. In other words, is there a beneficial cost ratio in "preventing" skin cancer? Before a program can be cost-effective, it has to be effective; the outcome of interest must change favorably after institution of a program. The cost efficacy of prevention campaigns in the US has not been demonstrated as such; unfortunately, there is not sufficient data to say that these programs actually modify behaviors at the primary or high school grade level.[19,20]

There has been a different Australian experience where changes in attitudes, behaviors, and most probably a decrease in skin cancer incidence among younger populations have been seen since the inception of programs such as "Slip,

Table 61-1
Unweighted Medicare Payment Per Episode of NMSC Care Per Specialty Involved[a,b]

Specialty	Mean Medicare Payment $\pm$ SD (in Dollars)	Median Medicare Payment (in Dollars)
Family medicine	275 $\pm$ 274	208
General surgery	410 $\pm$ 602	212
Dermatology	423 $\pm$ 638	257
Internal medicine	523 $\pm$ 1576	225
Plastic surgery	1373 $\pm$ 2800	641
Otolaryngology	1661 $\pm$ 1151	1335

[a]These preliminary costs do not consider whether one episode of care involved more than one specialty and will count the cost of that entire episode under all specialties involved. Therefore, mean cost may be inflated for some specialties.

[b]These are based on a retrospective analysis, not a randomized prospective study. Cost differences may be due to many factors beside specialty. These data do not account for potential confounding due to differences in patient or tumor characteristics. The episode of care model will permit us to analyze those factors in future work. Note that the mean payments give information that can be used to calculate the total costs per specialty, but it weights heavily the effect of high-cost outliers. Median costs give a better sense of the cost for the "typical" patient but do not give any weight to the effect of very high cost episodes. (Reprinted with permission from Blackwell Publishing. Housman et al. Nonmelanoma skin cancer: an episode of care management approach. *Dermatol Surgery* 2003;29(7):700–711.)

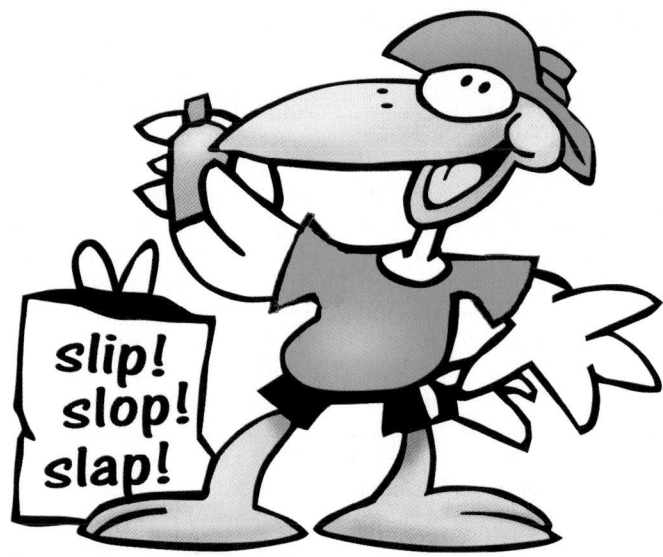

▲ FIGURE 61-5 Example of Australian media-promoted campaign "Slip, Slop, Slap" campaign. Reprinted with permission from The Cancer Council Victoria.

Slop, Slap."[21] Started in 1980, this public education campaign used various media venues in an attempt to decrease UV exposure. Initially funded through private donations, advertisements featured an animated seagull telling people to slip on a shirt, slop on some sunscreen, and slap on a hat (Fig. 61-5).

In 1988, with an increased operational budget from VicHealth, a health promotion agency at an arm's length from state government, and The Cancer Council Victoria, the "Slip, Slop, Slap" operation was rolled into the multifaceted SunSmart program. This program is still in existence and consists of a more broad campaign aimed at educating professionals, targeting specific audiences, and sponsoring research. Though accumulating evidence in Australia shows a slowing of NMSC rates in the younger population and enhanced early detection,[22,23] economic validation demonstrating to a beneficial cost ratio of prevention strategies, be it in direct or total costs, is not abundant.

Another vantage point regarding the economics of preventive measures is that of the individual. Perhaps a more practical approach is to look at the cost efficacy of using sunscreens on a daily or near daily basis (assuming proper application can prevent skin cancer). Allowing $0.50 daily in sunscreen for 75 years equates to $13,687.50 in prevention; based on a mean cost today of $470 per episode of NMSC skin cancer[17] and assuming a steady rate of inflation, one episode of cancer will cost approximately $5000 57 years from now. Therefore, unless an individual is high-

risk for multiple skin cancers, daily use of sunscreen (*if preventative*) may not be cost-effective. Considering a willingness-to-pay approach or indirect costs in such an analysis may create a beneficial cost ratio to using sunscreens.

After prevention, screening can be an effective means to limit morbidity and mortality through early detection. The potential economic advantages of routine screening include lower costs as lesions are assumed to be at an earlier stage. However, screening and prevention campaigns can be expected to lead to a higher number of biopsies and procedures through a higher number of false positive clinical diagnoses.[24] Skin cancer screening programs alone can be costly, particularly at a national level. One ad hoc analysis out of Australia (highest skin cancer incidence in the world) found that over a 20-year screening campaign a cost per life saved was $1360 (AUD) and the cost per death deferred was $14,360 (AUD)[25]; as pointed out, this has not led to the institution of a national screening effort in Australia.[26] Current recommendations for skin cancer screening in the US are inconsistent at best,[27] in part due to the lack of evidence that routing screening reduces morbidity or mortality of NMSC.

The real impact of skin cancer prevention and screening can be, and perhaps has been, made with melanoma. There is significant overall survival advantage to early detection of thin melanoma.[24] If prevention and screening can decrease the thickness of melanoma at the time of diagnosis, then it is not difficult to

link prevention/screening to improved morbidity and mortality; there is evidence that there has been a decrease in the stage at diagnosis over the past 30 years suggesting that screening (and possibly prevention) efforts are effective.[28] There is currently a large randomized trial underway to determine the feasibility of population screening for melanoma in Australia.[29]

REGULATION OF OFFICE-BASED SURGERY

BOX 61-10   Summary

- Government regulation of office-based surgery is a real possibility in the future with the aim of improving patient safety.
- There is little evidence that accreditation will enhance patient safety; however, it will likely add significant cost to the treatment of skin cancer.
- Dermatologists need to continue to be proactive with efforts to ensure patient safety in the office setting.

A recurring and universal adolescent fantasy, perhaps encoded genetically, is to be free from the unwarranted, unnecessary, and restrictive edicts of our guardians. This notion has been immortalized in variations on Samuel Clemmons quip, "At fourteen I could not abide to be in the same room with my father, as ignorant a man has never before walked the planet. Yet, at twenty-one, I was amazed at how much my father had learned." Adulthood and years of training, does not entirely relieve that sense of restriction and unfairness that we sometimes feel when those outside our purview and control make demands on our time, money, and personal freedom. As dermatologists, it is important to remember that all of us have the capacity to occasionally emulate our adolescent selves when faced with outspoken detractors of the safety or efficacy of outpatient, office-based surgical procedures. There has been some debate, not without emotion, regarding the safety and regulatory need of office based surgery; undeniably, there are economic forces exerting pressure on this discussion. Here again, perspective is critical; as an optimist, it is hoped that the various "sides" in this debate truly have patient care at heart though the obvious conflict-of-interests of involved parties needs to be acknowledged. Economically, there is the perspective of the income earning, albeit altruistic, specialist who is providing a valuable service to his patients. Then there is a more global, or societal, perspective that is striving to deliver the safest care possible at the lowest price. Though evidence attesting to the cost-efficacy of outpatient surgery for NMSC is available,[17] the dermatology community needs to consider the forces and parties involved in the debate over outpatient care; this is essential in dealing with future barriers to delivering safe, valuable outpatient surgical care.

To add some historical perspective, during the late 1970s the American Society of Anesthesiologists steadfastly looked in the mirror and admitted that there was much that could be done to lower the risk of anesthetic mortality. In 1985, the Anesthesia Patient Safety Foundation was created to send the message to members that patient safety issues were a critical focus of their society. By 1986, the American Society of Anesthesiologists adopted more than 30 standards of care addressing adverse anesthesia guidelines. In the subsequent years, this evolved into a Six Sigma style approach to anesthesia. This experience highlighted that, with self-reflection, measures could be taken to enhance patient safety, preserving the first tenant of medicine, *primum non nocre*.

Another attempt at appraisal of the safety of outpatient surgical procedures was on behalf of the American Society of Plastic and Reconstructive Surgery Board of Directors when they convened a Task Force to study the question of patient safety in office-based surgical facilities in response to the publication of and media attention to deaths related to liposuction in otherwise young and healthy women. They focused on issues that may lead to increased risk of complications including hypothermia, blood loss, liposuction combined with multiple procedures, fluid and electrolyte shifts, and thromboembolism prophylaxis. Attention to patient risk parameters such as age, obesity, oral birth control, and other co-morbidities were used to stratify patients into risk categories prompting more preoperative evaluation and perhaps movement from an outpatient facility to inpatient facility or cancellation of elective procedures for safety reasons. Some of the data from these efforts were inadvertently misconstrued and reports detrimental to certain providers of liposuction services achieved national focus.[30] Most recently, adverse event data from Florida originally thought to detract from the safety of office-based surgery were refuted following proper statistical analysis.[31,32]

Emotions within the college of medicine were high with general and plastic surgeons and anesthesiologists being portrayed as having a mistrust of the training received by dermatologists. The performance of some surgical procedures, in particular certain procedures performed in an outpatient setting were called into question. Demands for accreditation were introduced and concerns of gaming the system against dermatologists were noted. Accreditation through hospital boards granting unrestricted operating room (OR) privileges, and accreditation of office surgical suites by the Joint Commission on Accreditation of Healthcare Organizations (JCAHO), Accreditation Association of Ambulatory Health Care (AAAHC), American Association of Accreditation of Ambulatory Surgery Facilities (AAAASF), as well as Certification of Participation in the Medicare Program through Title XVIII have all been proposed. The experience of dermatologists attempting to gain OR privileges suggested that the keepers of the gates (surgeons having completed some portion of a general surgical residency) were reluctant to look upon dermatologists as equals and deserving of privileges. This perception drove a wedge between medical colleagues, each uncertain about the motivation and basic fairness of the other.

Growth helps to insure survival though there are often challenges and pains such as those experienced by those surgeons that practice in the outpatient setting. Avoiding the pitfalls of adolescence by acknowledging that all physician groups ultimately want what is best and safest for patients requires perhaps that dermatologists admit the need to consider standardization of care for those procedures common to providers of dermatologic outpatient procedures. It is not enough to have shown that outpatient delivery of care with tumescent liposuction and other outpatient surgical procedures are as safe as or safer than similar procedures delivered in hospital ORs or ambulatory surgical centers.[30,32–34]

Autonomy may be sacrificed with regulation, but it should be remembered that improving patient safety is at the heart of accreditation. Dermatologists may need to consider maintaining ACLS certification or have systems in place that provide such care expeditiously. If intravenous sedation is administered, it is not unwarranted to prove competence in delivery of those products and accurate monitoring of patients. Creation and maintenance of Board Certification and practicing within the boundaries of training and education are reasonable restrictions for any physician. Operational standards that address tissue handling to insure appropriate follow-up and cleaning procedures to maintain sterility in operating arenas and with instruments should be welcomed. Ultimately, we as dermatologists and dermatologic surgeons want the best care that can be provided to our patients with predictable and safe outcomes. However, there are aspects of accreditation that should not be embraced; unfortunately, accreditation is also about money and inane bureaucracy, both likely adding to the price of outpatient care. Accreditation may not improve the care of some facilities that are already vigorously pursuing improvement. Perhaps it is in the best interest of dermatologists and dermatologic surgeons to be proactive in promoting office safety, so as to preempt further unnecessary regulation. Like Samuel Clemmons' quip, we may all be amazed at how much we can grow and improve if we abandon defensive posturing and approach regulation with an open mind and the understanding that improving patient care is at the heart of efforts.

Conversely, perhaps another, even more common adolescent fantasy, is that government regulation leads to improvements in safety. Anesthesiology improved care without government intervention. The prototype federal involvement in medical offices is represented by CLIA—a program noted for regulatory hassles, but not noted for any actual improvements in office-based dermatologic practice. Efforts to achieve greater safety and improved care should be universal; however, government regulation is probably the worst way to attempt to achieve such a goal. This will drastically increase the cost of skin cancer care. If CLIA is any example, we'll be logging in and out each scalpel blade and testing them at intervals to make sure they meet certain standards.

Legislation that could move skin cancer treatment from a largely office-based environment to an accredited surgical center environment (or worse, to hospital operating rooms) would have dramatic economic consequences. Office-based management is very cost-efficient, so while the number of skin cancers exceeds all other cancers combined, overall direct skin cancer management costs to Medicare place skin cancer fifth on the list of cancers. Moving these cancers to accredited surgical centers could easily triple the cost of skin cancer management.

FINAL THOUGHTS

There are many perspectives from which to look at the economics of skin cancer. Regardless, it is understood that there is significant economic burden from the direct and indirect costs of cutaneous malignancy. There is much variability in the treatment of skin cancer, which leaves macroeconomic analysis confounded; episode of care and willingness-to-pay estimates help to stratify treatment styles and settings and give needed perspective from the patient regarding costs of skin cancer. While prevention and screening are noble efforts and should not be abandoned, unless population-specific, such programs are unlikely to be economically worthwhile. It is apparent that potential mandated regulation threatens to negatively impact patient care and the practice of dermatology. To help preserve the interest of dermatologists and their cancer patients, a responsible, proactive role needs to be assumed to maintain the highest patient safety standards. As emerging medical therapies and accumulating data becomes available in the future, more detailed and accurate studies focused on the economic impact of skin cancer treatment may help to guide the delivery of care. It should be remembered that though future studies may be helpful, it seems dangerous to rely entirely on cost considerations when directing treatments of disfiguring and potentially lethal skin malignancy.

REFERENCES

1. Drummond MP, O'Brien B, Stoddard GL, Torrance GW. Methods for the Economic Evaluation of Health Care Programmes. New York: Oxford University Press; 2000.
2. Preston DS, Stern RS. Nonmelanoma cancers of the skin. N Engl J Med. December 1992;327(23):1649–1662.
3. Jemal A, Murray T, Ward E, Samuels A, Tiwari RC, Ghafoor A, et al. Cancer statistics, 2005. CA Cancer J Clin. January 2005;5(1):10–30.
4. Greenlee RT, Murray T, Bolden S, Wingo PA. Cancer statistics, 2000. CA Cancer J Clin. January 2000;50(1):7–33.
5. Greenlee RT, Hill–Harmon MB, Murray T, Thun M. Cancer statistics, 2001. CA Cancer J Clin. January 2001;51(1):15–36.

6. Jemal A, Thomas A, Murray T, Thun M. Cancer statistics, 2002. CA Cancer J Clin. January 2002;52(1):23–47.
7. Jemal A, Murray T, Samuels A, Ghafoor A, Ward E, Thun MJ. Cancer statistics, 2003. CA Cancer J Clin. January 2003;53(1):5–26.
8. Jemal A, Tiwari RC, Murray T, Ghafoor A, Samuels A, Ward E, et al. Cancer statistics, 2004. CA Cancer J Clin. January 2004;54(1):8–29.
9. Lewin Group. The Burden of Skin Diseases 2004. The Society for Investigative Dermatology and The American Academy of Dermatology Association 2004 [cited 2006 May 31];Available at: http://www.sidnet.org/pdfs/Burden%20of%20Skin%20Diseases%202004.pdf
10. Chen JG, Fleischer AB, Jr., Smith ED, Kancler C, Goldman ND, Williford PM, et al. Cost of nonmelanoma skin cancer treatment in the United States. Dermatol Surg. December 2001;27(12):1035–1038.
11. Rhee JS, Loberiza FR, Matthews BA, Neuburg M, Smith TL, Burzynski M. Quality of life assessment in non-melanoma cervicofacial skin cancer. Laryngoscope. February 2003;113(2):215–220.
12. Blackford S, Roberts D, Salek MS, Finlay A. Basal cell carcinomas cause little handicap. Qual Life Res. April 1996;5(2):191–194.
13. Balch CM, Buzaid AC, Soong SJ, Atkins MB, Cascinelli N, Coit DG, et al. Final version of the American Joint Committee on Cancer staging system for cutaneous melanoma. J Clin Oncol. August 2001;19 (16):3635–3648.
14. Tsao H, Rogers GS, Sober AJ. An estimate of the annual direct cost of treating cutaneous melanoma. J Am Acad Dermatol. May 1998; 38(5 Pt 1):669–680.
15. Howe HL, Wingo PA, Thun MJ, Ries LA, Rosenberg HM, Feigal EG, et al. Annual report to the nation on the status of cancer (1973 through 1998), featuring cancers with recent increasing trends. J Natl Cancer Inst. June 2001;93(11):824–842.
16. Tsao H, Atkins MB, Sober AJ. Management of cutaneous melanoma. N Engl J Med. September 2004;351(10):998–1012.
17. Housman TS, Williford PM, Feldman SR, Teuschler HV, Fleischer AB, Jr., Goldman ND, et al. Nonmelanoma skin cancer: an episode of care management approach. Dermatol Surg. July 2003;29(7):700–711.
18. Duque MI, Jordan JR, Fleischer AB, Jr, Williford PM, Feldman SR, Teuschler H, et al. Frequency of seborrheic keratosis biopsies in the United States: a benchmark of skin lesion care quality and cost effectiveness. Dermatol Surg. August 2003; 29(8):796–801.
19. Geller AC, Cantor M, Miller DR, Kenausis K, Rosseel K, Rutsch L, et al. The Environmental Protection Agency's National SunWise School Program: sun protection education in US schools (1999–2000). J Am Acad Dermatol. May 2002;46(5):683–689.
20. Jones SE, Saraiya M. Sunscreen use among us high school students, 1999–2003. J Sch Health. April 2006;76(4):150–153.

21. Marks R. Two decades of the public health approach to skin cancer control in Australia: why, how and where are we now? Aust J Dermatol. February 1999;40(1):1–5.
22. Staples MP, Elwood M, Burton RC, Williams JL, Marks R, Giles GG. Non-melanoma skin cancer in Australia: the 2002 national survey and trends since 1985. Med J Aust. January 2006;184(1):6–10.
23. Staples M, Marks R, Giles G. Trends in the incidence of non–melanocytic skin cancer (NMSC) treated in Australia 1985–1995: are primary prevention programs starting to have an effect? Int J Cancer. October 5. 1998;78(2):144–148.
24. Balch CM, Soong SJ, Gershenwald JE, Thompson JF, Reintgen DS, Cascinelli N, et al. Prognostic factors analysis of 17,600 melanoma patients: validation of the American Joint Committee on Cancer melanoma staging system. J Clin Oncol. August 2001;19(16):3622–3634.
25. Carter R, Marks R, Hill D. Could a national skin cancer campaign in Australia be worthwhile? An economic perspective. Health Promotion Int. 1999;14:73–82.
26. McCarthy WH. The Australian experience in sun protection and screening for melanoma. J Surg Oncol. July 2004;86(4):236–245.
27. Rager EL, Bridgeford EP, Ollila DW. Cutaneous melanoma: update on prevention, screening, diagnosis, and treatment. Am Fam Physician. July 2005;72(2):269–276.
28. Dennis LK. Analysis of the melanoma epidemic, both apparent and real: data from the 1973 through 1994 surveillance, epidemiology, and end results program registry. Arch Dermatol. March 1999;135(3):275–280.
29. Aitken JF, Elwood JM, Lowe JB, Firman DW, Balanda KP, Ring IT. A randomised trial of population screening for melanoma. J Med Screen. 2002;9(1):33–37.
30. Housman TS, Lawrence N, Mellen BG, George MN, Filippo JS, Cerveny KA, et al. The safety of liposuction: results of a national survey. Dermatol Surg. November 2002;28(11):971–978.
31. Vila H, Jr., Soto R, Cantor AB, Mackey D. Comparative outcomes analysis of procedures performed in physician offices and ambulatory surgery centers. Arch Surg. September 2003;138(9):991–995.
32. Venkat AP, Coldiron B, Balkrishnan R, Camacho F, Hancox JG, Fleischer AB, Jr., et al. Lower adverse event and mortality rates in physician offices compared with ambulatory surgery centers: a reappraisal of Florida adverse event data. Dermatol Surg. December 2004;30(12 Pt 1):1444–1451.
33. Coleman III WP, Hanke CW, Lillis P, Bernstein G, Narins R. Does the location of the surgery or the specialty of the physician affect malpractice claims in liposuction? Dermatol Surg. May 1999;25(5):343–347.
34. Coldiron B. Office surgical incidents: 19 months of Florida data. Dermatol Surg. August 2002;28(8):710–712.

CHAPTER 62

Medical Legal Issues of Skin Cancer

David J. Goldberg, M.D., J.D.

BOX 62-1   Overview

- Physicians treating skin cancer must perform within the standard of care.
- In a medical malpractice case, an expert witness will be called upon to testify as to the standard of care.
- The standard may not always be easy to define with full clarity.
- With an increase incidence in skin cancer, physicians can expect to see an increase in skin cancer related medical malpractice claims against them.

INTRODUCTION

Although legal considerations can arise in the performance of any aspect of a medical dermatology practice, they are more likely to occur in the areas of diagnosis and treatment of skin cancers. Although there is no substantiated data about dermatologic skin cancer litigation, there are anecdotal suggestions that such malpractice claims have increased. The dermatologists are not the only ones at risk; so are other physicians who may be treating skin cancer. These would include pathologist, radiologists, and surgical oncologists. A full textbook on healthcare law is an appropriate reading to cover comprehensively all the legal aspects as they relate to skin cancer. Issues that arise include negligence, billing fraud, and privacy concerns. Since the most likely cause of a legal mishap in current day skin cancer dermatology involves negligence, that will be the focus of this chapter.

The first part of the chapter will discuss the elements of negligence and the evolution of a medical malpractice cause of action involving the diagnosis and treatment of skin cancer. The second part of the chapter will describe two hypothetical cases and the likelihood of a successful malpractice case evolving from such a scenario.

THE FOUR ELEMENTS

Any analysis of physician negligence must first begin with a legal description of the four required elements for a cause of action in negligence: duty, breach of duty, causation, and damages. The suing plaintiff must show the presence of all four elements to be successful in his or her claim.[1]

The duty of a physician evaluating and treating skin cancers is to perform the surgery in accordance with the standard of care. Although the elements of a cause of action in negligence are derived from formal legal textbooks, the standard of care is not necessarily derived from some well-known textbook. It is also not articulated by any judge. The standard of care is defined by some as whatever an expert witness says it is, and what a jury will believe. In a case against any skin cancer specialist, the specialist must have and use the knowledge and skills ordinarily possessed by a specialist in that field, in the same or similar locality under similar circumstances. A dermatologist, plastic surgeon, otolaryngologist, internist or family practitioner evaluating and treating skin cancers will all be held to an equal standard. A failure to fulfill such a duty may lead to loss of a lawsuit by the physician. If the jury accepts the suggestion that the doctor mismanaged the case and that the negligence led to damage of the patient, then the physician will be liable. In the case of skin cancer, misdiagnosis and/or mistreatment may both lead to damages and physician liability. Conversely, if the jury believes an expert who testifies for the defendant doctor, then the standard of care, in that particular case, has been met. In this view, the standard of care is a pragmatic concept, decided case by case, and based on the testimony of an expert physician. The dermatologist, or any other physician dealing with skin cancer, is expected to evaluate skin cancers in the manner of a reasonable physician. He need not be the best in his field; he need only perform the procedure in a manner that is considered reasonable by an objective standard. Perhaps missing the diagnosis of amelanotic melanoma might not be considered a breach in the standard of care because a reasonable physician might miss this diagnosis.

It is important to note that where there are two or more recognized methods of diagnosing or treating the same condition, a physician does not fall below the standard of care by using any of the acceptable methods even if one method turns out to be less effective than is the other. Finally, in many jurisdictions, an unfavorable result due to an "error in judgment" by a physician is not in and of itself a violation of the standard of care if the physician acted appropriately prior to exercising his or her professional judgment.

STANDARD OF CARE

Evidence of the standard of care in a specific malpractice case includes laws, regulations, and guidelines for practice, which represent a consensus among professionals on a topic involving diagnosis or treatment, and the medical literature including peer-reviewed articles and authoritative texts. In addition, obviously, the view of an expert is crucial. Although the standard of care may vary from state to state, it is typically defined as a national standard by and for dermatologists.

Most commonly for litigation purposes, expert witnesses articulate the standard of care. The basis of the expert witness testimony, and therefore the origin of the standard of care, is grounded in:

1. the witness' personal practice
2. the practice of others that he has observed in his experience
3. medical literature in recognized publications
4. statutes and/or legislative rules
5. courses where the subject is discussed and taught in a well-defined manner

The standard of care is the way in which the majority of the physicians in a similar medical community would practice. If, in fact, the expert herself does not practice like the majority of other physicians, then the expert will have a difficult time explaining why the majority of the medical community does not practice according to her ways. The use of extracts to treat skin cancer, a method used by homeopathic experts, may not be in accordance with the standard of care as opined by a dermatology expert.

It would seem then that in the perfect world, the standard of care in every case would be a clearly definable level of care agreed upon by all physicians and patients. Unfortunately, in the typical situation, the standard of care is an ephemeral concept resulting from differences and inconsistencies among the medical profession, the legal system, and the public.

At one polar extreme, the medical profession is dominant in determining the standard of care in the practice of medicine. In such a situation, recommendations, guidelines, and policies regarding varying treatment modalities for different clinical situations published by nationally recognized boards, societies, and commissions establish the appropriate standard of care. Even in some of these cases, however, factual disputes may arise because more than one such organization will publish conflicting standards concerning the same medical condition. Adding to the confusion, local societies may publish their own rules applicable to a particular claim of malpractice.

Thus, in most situations the standard of care is neither clearly definable nor consistently defined. It is a legal fiction to suggest that a generally accepted standard of care exists for any area of practice. At best, there are parameters within which experts will testify. The skin cancer physician's best defense that he is acting in accordance with the standard of care is to document appropriate risk assessment of the patient, to provide appropriate medical record documentation and informed consent, and finally, to utilize appropriate diagnostic and treatment approaches.

In recent years, American physicians have put forth substantial efforts toward setting standards and specifying treatment approaches to various conditions. Clinical practice guidelines have been developed by specialty societies such as the American Academy of Dermatology and the American College of Mohs Micrographic Surgery and Cutaneous Oncology. The Institute of Medicine has defined such clinical guidelines as "systemically developed statements to assist practitioner and patient decisions about appropriate healthcare for specific clinical circumstances." Such guidelines represent standardized specifications for performing a procedure or managing a particular clinical problem.

CLINICAL GUIDELINES

Clinical guidelines raise thorny legal issues.[2] They have the potential to offer an authoritative and settled statement of what the standard of care should be for a given skin cancer. A court would have several options when such guidelines are offered as evidence. Such a guideline might be evidence of the customary practice in the medical profession. A doctor acting in accordance with the guidelines would be shielded from liability to the same extent as one who can establish that she or he followed professional customs. The guidelines could play the role of an authoritative expert witness or a well-accepted review article. Using guidelines as evidence of professional custom, however, is problematic if they are ahead of prevailing medical practice.

Clinical guidelines have already had an effect on settlement, according to surveys of malpractice lawyers. A widely accepted clinical standard may be presumptive evidence of due care, but expert testimony will still be required to introduce the standard and establish its sources and its relevancy.

Professional societies often attach disclaimers to their guidelines, thereby undercutting their defensive use in litigation. The American Medical Association, for example, calls its guidelines "parameters" instead of protocols intended to impact physician discretion significantly. The AMA further suggests that all such guidelines contain disclaimers stating that they are not intended to displace physician discretion. Such guidelines, in such a situation, could not be treated as conclusive.

LEGAL RELEVANCE

Plaintiffs usually will use their own expert, as opposed to the physician's expert, to define the standard of care. Although such a plaintiff's expert may also refer to clinical practice guidelines, the physician's negligence can be established in other manners as well. These methods include: (1) examination of the physician defendant's expert witness, (2) an admission by the defendant that he or she was negligent, (3) testimony by the plaintiff, in a rare case where she is a medical expert qualified to evaluate the allegedly negligent physician's conduct, and (4) common knowledge in situations where a layperson could understand the negligence without the assistance of an expert.[3,4]

It is clear then that in order for the plaintiff to win her negligence cause of action against a skin cancer physician, she must establish that her physician had a duty of reasonable care in treating her, and had in fact, breached that duty. However, that breach must also lead to some form of damages. A mere inconvenience to the plaintiff, even in the setting of a physician's breach, will usually not lead to physician liability in a cause of action for negligence.

It is often difficult to predict, in any given malpractice cause of action, what the ultimate outcome will be. The following teaching hypotheticals are designed to be suggestive of potential malpractice cases and the likely results. Any connection between these scenarios and actual malpractice cases is fortuitous.

CASE EXAMPLE 1

DS is a 48-year-old man with a multiple squamous cell carcinoma and a history of immunosuppression. He was seen every 6 months for skin evaluations. His cancerous lesions were treated with a variety of methods including electrical destruction, topical agents and Mohs surgery. Some lesions recurred; others did not. Ultimately, DS develops metastatic disease from a recurrent lesion. He dies leaving behind multiple family members. The plaintiff's estate sues the dermatologist. They contend that there must have been a breach of duty for the skin cancer to return. Perhaps more frequent dermatologic visits and/or more aggressive treatments would have prevented the unfortunate death of their family member.

Did the dermatologist breach the standard of care? If so, will he liable for negligence? The patient records are evaluated by an expert for the suing plaintiff's estate. The records all appear to be reasonable. The plaintiff's expert refuses to testify because there is no evidence of malpractice by the defendant dermatologist. Six-month evaluations are considered reasonable. There is no evidence to suggest that monthly visits would have stopped metastatic spread in this immunosuupressed individual. Recurrence of skin cancer, metastatic disease, and even death are not evidence of *de facto* negligence. The case will likely be lost by the plaintiff.

CASE EXAMPLE 2

A well-known dermatologist treats in excess of 600 Mohs patients each year. He treats a large number of basal cell carcinoma and squamous cell carcinoma patients. A referred patient has a large recurrent ulcerative basal cell carcinoma of the cheek. During consultation, the patient is told, by way of informed consent, that the facial nerve may be damaged during the proposed Mohs surgery. The patient is also told the consequences of such nerve damage. After the third stage of Mohs surgery it is quite evident that the tumor involves a significant portion of the parotid gland. In removing the remaining tumor, the facial nerve is partially severed with a resultant unilateral lower facial paralysis. The patient sues the Mohs surgeon.

Is the Mohs surgeon liable? It is clear that there is permanent damage to patient. Reconstructive surgery can improve the situation, but may never return to the patient full use of the nerve. The Mohs surgeon did provide informed consent to the patient. Although verbal consent legally is enough, the written

Table 62-1
Mechanisms for Physician Defense

Written consent
Legible chart documentation
Practice in the standard of care
Avoid breach of reasonable standard

consent provides documentation that the Mohs surgeon performed his legal duty. It is unlikely that the Mohs surgeon will lose this case. The surgeon is advised that legible chart documentation and documented signed consent will only help him at trial (Table 62-1).

FINAL THOUGHTS

Skin cancers continue to increase in number. There are, as described in this book, numerous accepted techniques for the removal of many skin cancers. By the nature of any treatment, complications may arise. It is imperative that physicians be aware of their duty of reasonable care. Should they breach that duty, they may be found liable in a medical malpractice cause of action in the diagnosis of and treatment for skin cancer.

REFERENCES

1. Furrow BF, Greaney TL, Johnson SH, Jost TS, Schwartz RL. *Liability in Health Care Law*, 3rd ed. West Publishing Co.: St. Paul, MN; 1997.
2. Hyams AL, Shapiro DW, Brennan TA. Medical practice guidelines in malpractice litigation: an early retrospective, *J. Health Pol., Policy Law.* 1996; 21:289.
3. Lamont v. Brookwood Health Service, Inc., 446 So. 2nd ed. 1018 (Ala. 1983).
4. Gannon v. Elliot, 19 Cal. App. 4th 1 (1993).

CHAPTER 63

Psychosocial Aspects of Skin Cancer

Anne Han, B.A.
John Y. Koo, M.D.

BOX 63-1   Overview

- Psychosocial issues affect skin cancer patients from the time of diagnosis to the period after intervention and affect melanoma (MM) and nonmelanoma (NMSC) patients in different ways.
- Delay in seeking a diagnosis of skin cancer, while primarily caused by lack of knowledge, is influenced by psychological factors such as fear and denial.
- Psychological reaction to a diagnosis of skin cancer, as well as the ability to live and cope with the disease, can have a considerable impact on patient morbidity and mortality.
- Existing quality of life (QOL) studies demonstrate minimal impact, and a disease-specific Facial Skin Cancer Index is currently being developed to more accurately assess QOL in skin cancer patients.
- Postsurgical disfigurement can lead to psychological sequelae including depression, anxiety, and social phobia.

■ INTRODUCTION

This chapter is about the psychological and social impact of skin cancer on patients from the time of diagnosis to the period after intervention. The skin, being the largest and most visible organ of the human body, is of great psychological importance.[1] Although it is tempting to view skin cancer as purely a physical issue, it is, in fact, associated with psychological distress. A diagnosis of skin cancer can elicit such symptoms 95> anxiety, and depression. In addition, how patients react to a diagnosis of skin cancer or cope with the disease in their daily lives can have a considerable impact on their morbidity and, for malignant melanoma (MM), ultimate survival. While nonmelanoma skin cancer (NMSC) has a relatively good prognosis, living with late-stage melanoma as a terminal illness has a significant impact on quality of life including psychological, social, spiritual, and financial well being.

Treatment by surgical excision can result in disfigurement and scarring on the face and neck where approximately 80% of NMSCs are found,[2] leading to negative impact on self-image and self-esteem, social relationships, productivity at work, and overall quality of life.[3] Being aware of these underlying psychosocial factors can help health professionals optimize care of their skin cancer patients.

While some psychosocial issues are common to all skin cancer patients, others are more often seen in MM as opposed to NMSC patients, and vice versa. Melanoma, which accounts for 4% of diagnoses of skin cancer,[4] is potentially fatal. In fact, stage IV melanoma is associated with only 13% 5-year survival[5] as compared to 92% 5-year survival in stage I melanoma.[6] Thus, psychosocial aspects relating to early diagnosis, and for those with late-stage disease, living with a terminal illness is particularly relevant in MM patients. In contrast, NMSC consisting predominantly of basal and squamous cell carcinomas that is significantly more prevalent among all skin cancer types is associated with good prognosis and can be cured by surgical excision. As a result, mortality and disease gravity are not important issues, whereas negative quality of life due to high rate of recurrence and psychosocial issues related to postsurgical disfigurement and scarring are more important. In this chapter, we discuss delay in seeking diagnosis, psychosocial reaction to diagnosis, living and coping with skin cancer, quantitative quality of life studies, and psychological impact of postsurgical disfigurement. Certain issues are common to both MM and NMSC, while others are more common to one and not the other; elsewhere it is unique to MM as opposed to NMSC, or vice versa. Data will be presented separately.

■ DELAY IN SEEKING DIAGNOSIS

BOX 63-2   Summary

- Skin cancer patients, especially MM patients, when diagnosed and treated in a timely fashion, can achieve disease-free survival.
- Most MM deaths are related to patient delay in seeking diagnosis and care.
- The main reason for patient delay is lack of knowledge, followed by denial, fear, and financial considerations.

Skin cancer patients who are diagnosed and treated in a timely fashion can achieve disease-free survival. Furthermore, early diagnosis is crucial, especially in MM patients, since advanced disease is less amenable to surgical cure, which is not the case for NMSC patients. Approximately 80% of skin cancer deaths are caused by MM; 7500 people died of MM in the United States alone in 2002.[7] Delay in seeking diagnosis by MM patients can be fatal. Rhodes reported that most MMs deaths are related to patient delay in seeking diagnosis and care, and that most MM lesions are detected by patients or close acquaintances.[8] Patient delay has been attributed to denial, fear, lack of information, and financial considerations.[9] However, studies show that the main reason for patient delay in seeking diagnosis is lack of knowledge rather than psychological causes such as fear and denial. This conclusion was reached in both a study by Doherty et al in which 125 melanoma patients answered a detailed questionnaire[10] and by Cassileth et al who interviewed 275 melanoma patients.[11]

■ PSYCHOLOGICAL REACTION TO DIAGNOSIS OF SKIN CANCER

BOX 63-3   Summary

- The emotional response to receiving a diagnosis of cancer can correlate with patient survival.
- Four psychological reaction types to a positive diagnosis have been noted in the oncology literature: stoics, helpless, denial, and fighting spirit.
- Skin cancer patients with a lack of emotional expressiveness, who resemble the stoics and helpless, embody type C (cancer-prone) personality, which is a significant prognostic indicator.

The emotional response to receiving a diagnosis of cancer can correlate with patient survival. In a landmark study, Watson et al measured the psychological response of 578 women with early-stage breast cancer at 4 to 12 weeks and 12 months after diagnosis. Based on their psychological responses, patients were divided into four reaction types: stoics, helpless, denial and fighting spirit.[12] Follow-up for breast cancer survival occurred at 10 years after initial diagnosis. The best overall survival rate of 70% was found among women who showed a "fighting spirit" with the attitude that they would take every step possible to battle the disease. Of those patients whose initial reaction to mastectomy was denial, half were still alive after 10 years. The poorest overall survival rate of 25% and 20%, respectively, occurred among women who reacted with a stoic acceptance of their disease, or showing no signs of distress, and among those who reacted with feelings of hopelessness and helplessness.

A similar study exists with regard to melanoma. Temoshok et al studied 59 patients with malignant melanoma and found that those who freely expressed feelings of anger and distress mounted a better immune response (i.e., lower rate of cell division and more lymphocytes = better prognosis) than those who suppressed their emotions.[13] Temoshok coined the term type C (cancer-prone) personality to describe individuals who tend to be unassertive, suppress negative emotions (particularly anger), and helpless-hopeless personality types with depressive tendencies. The hypothesis was that type C personality would be associated with unfavorable prognosis as indicated by tumor thickness, deeper level of invasion of the skin, biological markers, etc. While the best prognostic indicator for malignant melanoma was whether patients delay seeking medical attention or not, which corroborates the findings by Doherty et al and Cassileth et al discussed in the previous section. These authors found that having type C personality with lack of emotional expressiveness was also a significant prognostic indicator.

LIVING AND COPING WITH SKIN CANCER

BOX 63-4 Summary

- Patients living with a diagnosis of cancer may experience fear, anxiety, depression, uncertainty, adjustment problems, and other psychological manifestations.
- Skin cancer patients respond to their disease with enhanced will power and coping strategies including seeking social support, problem-solving and gaining self-control, which minimize their initial psychological manifestations.

It is known in oncology that patients living with a diagnosis of cancer often experience fear, anxiety, depression, uncertainty, adjustment problems, posttraumatic stress, and other psychological manifestations. Risk factors for these issues include younger age (under 40 years), female gender, undergoing treatment for trying to establish control over the cancer, and limited capability for normal activity due to the disease. Standardized instruments have been used to measure psychological effects of cancer with equivocal results. Studies of breast and lymphoma/leukemia patients found 50% were either anxious or depressed.[14,15] In other studies of cancer patients, up to 98% were anxious and up to 75% were depressed.[16] Still other authors found depression in only 18% of cancer patients studied.[17]

Psychological manifestations may not be uniform across different skin cancers but studies show that skin cancer patients as a group manage well compared to other types of patients or the general population. Holfeld et al recruited 39 BCC and 39 matched controls to answer a psychosocial questionnaire. They found no more psychosocial problems were present in BCC patients than in members of the general population.[1] In contrast to NMSC, MM has the potential to kill. Cassileth et al compared the results of a self-reported mental health test of 168 melanoma patients and 135 patients with other dermatologic disorders. They found melanoma patients, despite poor prognosis, to be approximately equal to general public and strikingly superior to other dermatology patients in terms of emotional well being.[18] They also found profoundly diminished self-esteem among general dermatology patients. Self-esteem was thought to feature importantly in how people deal with illness (and self-esteem and self-image clearly are seriously impaired in patients with skin diseases). Stronger will power in response to threat among melanoma patients is postulated as an explanation for this finding. As the patient strives to deal with the physical and social challenges of the illness, self-esteem may actually be enhanced.

Missiha et al assessed 94 melanoma patients for self-reported anxiety upon diagnosis of melanoma. The study identified important risk factors for anxiety, namely female gender and young age, while demonstrating that melanoma thickness and tumor location are surprisingly unrelated to the degree of anxiety experienced.[19] Major factors con-

tributing to anxiety include tumor-related fears of poor prognosis or death. Factors that alleviate anxiety include family support, doctor's assistance, and self-distraction. The authors noted that potentially useful services for decreasing anxiety include provision of detailed information pamphlets.

Trask et al. studied the coping strategies used by individuals with stage I to stage III melanoma before treatment. Examples of coping strategies included accepting responsibility, problem solving, and escape avoidance. The study found that melanoma patients relied most heavily on seeking social support, problem-solving and self-control coping, relatively high reliance on distance coping and positive reappraisal, and less on maladaptive coping styles.[20] Patients with increased distress relied more heavily on taking personal responsibility for events, engaging in wishful thinking, or attempting to disengage from the issue at hand.

QUANTITATIVE QUALITY OF LIFE STUDIES IN SKIN CANCER

BOX 63-5 Summary

- Health-related quality of life (QOL) is particularly important because psychosocial issues of NMSC are less about mortality and gravity of the disease than about disfigurement, discomfort, and illness perception.
- By and large, health-related QOL studies of skin cancer patients have shown little handicap caused by NMSC and its treatment, although a modest improvement in QOL has been demonstrated in younger (less than 65 years of age), employed patients.
- A skin cancer-specific QOL index, Facial Skin Care Index (FSCI), is currently under development and will serve as a more relevant and accurate index for this patient population.

Quality of life (QOL) has been identified as an important outcome in cancer research.[21] Overall QOL is an all-inclusive concept incorporating all factors that impact upon an individual's life. Good QOL is present when 'the hopes of an individual are matched by experience. The concept has been divided into several components including psychological, social, and physical domains. Health-related QOL is more narrowly defined relating only to health aspects.

Key instruments used to measure general health-related quality of life include the UK Sickness Impact Profile (UKSIP), Short Form 36-item Health Survey (SF-36) and Functional Assessment of Cancer Therapy-General (FACT-G). In addition, health-related QOL instruments can be dermatology-specific, such as the Dermatologic Quality Life Index (DQLI), or disease-specific, such as the Facial Skin Cancer Index (FSCI) currently under development.

Assessing NMSC patients for health-related QOL is particularly important because NMSC is less about mortality and disease gravity than about disfigurement, discomfort, and illness perception. Health-related QOL measurement may arguably be the most important endpoint of outcomes in these patients because traditional endpoints of mortality and survival are not relevant in this patient population. Blackford and Finlay used the DLQI and UKSIP to study prospectively 44 patients with BCC at baseline, one week after treatment, and 3 months after treatment. Overall, the scores were low (a lower score indicated less impact on QOL), rising 1 week after treatment and falling to below the initial scores at 3 months. They found that BCC and its treatment caused little handicap,[22] or disadvantage resulting from an impairment or disability that prevents the fulfillment of a role that is normal for the affected individual.

In a cross-sectional study using two health-related QOL, Rhee et al evaluated 121 patients with NMSC before counseling or treatment. They found minimal impact of NMSC on patients at initial diagnosis and little change after treatment of NMSC. However modest the associations were, an improvement in emotional and mental health well being after treatment of NMSC was demonstrated, especially for those less than 65 years of age and employed. This finding suggested that younger patients who are employed may be particularly sensitive to the conspicuous nature of the skin cancer as it relates to potential disfigurement and scarring.[23] In a subsequent prospective study using the DLQI, a dermatology-specific instrument, 121 consecutive patients with high-risk NMSC were evaluated before and 4 months after treatment by Mohs micrographic surgery. The results of the study indicated a trend toward an improvement in overall QOL. In addition, of the 10 items in the DLQI, physical status after treatment and potential patient embarrassment related to disease process demonstrated significant improvement

after treatment.[24] However, overall scores were low and showed little variability. In conducting these studies, Rhee et al became interested in developing a more specific index when they noticed that many study patients complained about the lack of relevance to their condition in answering DLQI questions, and an accurate QOL instrument was necessary for outcomes measurement in NMSC. Once it is finalized, the Facial Skin Care Index (FSCI) will be a health-related outcome index for skin cancer patients. It would be composed of a 20-item questionnaire to be administered before and 4 months after Mohs micrographic surgery.[25,26]

PSYCHOSOCIAL IMPACT OF POSTSURGICAL DISFIGUREMENT

BOX 63-6   Summary

- Postsurgical patients experience emotional distress that is related to the degree of surgical indentation rather than scar length, the use of skin graft rather than primary closure, and the discrepancy between the actual size of the scar and presurgery expectations.

Approximately 80% of NMSC and 20% of MM occur on the face and neck. Therefore, surgical treatment can result in scarring and disfigurement. Potential physical adverse sequelae of the disease or treatment include lower eyelid ectropion, epiphora, which is the overflow of tears due to excessive secretion or obstruction of the lacrimal duct, corneal abrasions or erosions from incomplete eyelid closure, nasal obstruction, oral incompetence, oral microstomia, inability to use hearing aids or eyeglasses because of auricle loss, and facial nerve paralysis.[23] Other potential negative effects may be related to degree of disfigurement, which may have ramifications from a psychosocial, marital, sexual or medical personnel interaction standpoint.

Cassileth et al. studied 176 patients regarding the emotional impact of scar after primary melanoma excision. They found that the degree of surgical indentation rather than scar length, skin graft rather than primary closure, and how large the actual size of the scar was compared to presurgery expectations were associated with emotional distress in patients undergoing surgical treatment

of melanoma.[27,28] The results suggested that mild indentation, primary skin closures, and accurate presurgery information about appearance, regardless of scar size have important psychological benefit to patients.

DISCUSSION

BOX 63-7   Summary

- Skin cancer patients on average do not suffer much psychosocial distress and make a reasonable adjustment to postsurgical cosmetic defects.
- A few patients develop significant psychiatric problems secondary to disfigurement and may manifest their problems in terms of clinical depression, anxiety, and social phobia.
- These psychiatric diagnoses may be exacerbated in a society that disproportionately stigmatizes people with facial disfigurement rather than others such as the physically disabled.

Most patients who undergo significant surgical procedures for the treatment of skin cancer make a reasonable psychological adjustment to their cosmetic defects. As demonstrated in the literature, skin cancer patients on average do not suffer much distress. This finding is in part due superior coping skills exhibited by this patient population, especially skin cancer patients with melanoma. Several QOL studies support this finding with results showing minor impact on patients' psychological, social, and physical lives. However, a more specific index for skin cancer is needed to make an accurate assessment of QOL changes.[25] In addition, early detection of skin cancer results in excellent prognosis with only slight surgical disfigurement, especially in NMSC. Dermatologic surgeons have also developed surgical techniques that minimize the degree of distress.

However, a few patients develop significant psychiatric problems. This is especially true in patients with aggressive NMSC due to perineural invasion where the tumor can progress leading to loss of a patient's nose, eyelids, or ears.[29,30] In addition, late-stage melanoma is considered a terminal illness and is associated with negative psychosocial issues that affect cancer patients in general. Psychological distress from disfigurement is understandable in light of the fact that society has been oriented to a very narrow standard of beauty.[31] Many psychological studies indicate that appearance correlates with the personality traits that people attribute to strangers. Attractive persons of both sexes are presumed to have more socially desirable traits, to be kinder and more intelligent, to have greater internal control and competence, and to have made greater achievements.[32–38] Many studies show that people respond differently to those who are physically handicapped, such as an amputee, compared with those who are visibly disfigured. Traits attributed to those who are visibly disfigured are more frequently negative in character.[39,40] For example, studies have demonstrated that people are less likely to help a facially disfigured person than a nondisfigured person.[41] Therefore, it is understandable that patients who have extensive disfigurement from skin cancer surgery may encounter many difficulties, not only in terms of their personal emotional equilibrium, but also as a victim of negative perceptions by others.[42]

Patients who develop significant psychiatric morbidity secondary to disfigurement may manifest their problem in terms of clinical depression, anxiety, and social phobia. Secondary psychiatric complications include social withdrawal and occupational difficulties. It is important to recognize the psychiatric complications of surgical disfigurement, since many of these patients can be encouraged to seek professional help for their psychological difficulties. Moreover, unlike some chronic psychiatric patients, many of these patients have had reasonable premorbid psychological adaptation levels, and if they can be helped through the current crisis, they can become quite functional in society again.

Postsurgical disfigurement in skin cancer patients can lead to social phobia. Social phobia refers to a condition in which the patient develops a persistent fear of social situations where he or she is likely to be scrutinized by others.[43] Sometimes even something as minor as receiving an invitation to attend a party may trigger phobic avoidance. Once social phobia has begun, it gradually becomes worse because of two factors. First, anticipatory anxiety gradually develops whenever the person is confronted with the necessity to enter a social gathering. Second, the patient's social performance can be impaired by this underlying anxiety, resulting in the development of a vicious cycle. At times, some patients with social phobias try to force themselves to endure the social situation despite their intense anxiety. Through

this process, some may actually overcome their fears. However, many others with this condition will require professional counseling to cure their phobia. Otherwise, they may become progressively socially isolated to the point where they suffer serious social or occupational impairment. These patients usually retain their insight and recognize that their fears are excessive or unreasonable, even in view of their cosmetic disfigurement. Therefore, these patients tend to be receptive to the suggestion that they should obtain professional help from a psychiatrist or other mental health professionals.

FINAL THOUGHTS

Dermatology related to skin cancer is mainly concerned about diagnosis and excision, and psychosocial impact is frequently overlooked. Even though dermatologic surgeons can remove skin cancer without addressing these issues, for patients, these issues not only are important but addressing or not addressing them is what distinguishes outstanding care from good care. Professionals who are involved in managing skin cancer, especially dermatologic surgeons, should strive to be the best they can be and that would clearly involve sensitivity and compassion which is above and beyond diagnosis and excision of skin cancer.

REFERENCES

1. Holfeld KI, Hogan DJ, Eldemire M, et al. A psychosocial assessment of patients with basal cell carcinoma. *J Dermatol Surg Oncol.* August 1990;16(8):750–753.
2. Davis R, Spencer JM. Basal and squamous cell cancer of the facial skin. *Curr Opin Otolaryngol Head Neck Surg.* 1997;5:86.
3. Shah M, Coates M. An assessment of the quality of life in older patients with skin disease. *Br J Dermatol.* January 2006;154(1):150–153.
4. American Cancer Society. *Cancer Facts and Figures*, Atlanta, GA: American Cancer Society; 2002.
5. Miller B, Ries L, Hankey B, et al. Cancer Statistics Review: 1973–19 Bethesda, MD: US Department of Health and Human Services. NIH Publication; 1992:92:278.
6. American Joint Committee on Cancer. *Manual for Staging Cancer*, 3rd ed. Philadelphia: JB Lippincott; 1988.
7. Centers for Disease Control. United States Cancer Statistics: 1999–2002 Incidence and Mortality Report. Available at: http://www.cdc.gov/cancer/npcr/uscs
8. Rhodes AR. Public education and cancer of the skin. What do people need to know about melanoma and nonmelanoma skin cancer? *Cancer.* January 1995;75(2 suppl):613–636.
9. Love N. Why patients delay seeking care for cancer symptoms. What you can do about it. *Postgrad Med.* March 1991;89(4):151–152, 155–158.
10. Doherty VR, MacKie RM. Reasons for poor prognosis in British patients with cutaneous malignant melanoma. *Br Med J (Clin Res Ed).* April 1986;292(6526):987–989.
11. Cassileth BR, Temoshok L, Frederick BE, et al. Patient and physician delay in melanoma diagnosis. *J Am Acad Dermatol.* March 1988;18(3):591–598.
12. Watson M, Haviland JS, Greer S, et al. Influence of psychological response on survival in breast cancer: a population-based cohort study. *Lancet.* October 1999;354(9187):1331–1336.
13. Temoshok L, Heller BW, Sagebiel RW, et al. The relationship of psychosocial factors to prognostic indicators in cutaneous malignant melanoma. *J Psychosom Res.* 1985;29(2):139–153.
14. Roberts CS, Elkins NW, Baile WF Jr et al. Integrating research with practice: the psychosocial impact of breast cancer. *Health Soc Work.* 1989;14:261.
15. Craig T, Abeloff MD. Psychiatric symptomatology among hospitalized cancer patients. *Am J Psychiatry.* 1974;141:1323.
16. Peck A, Boland J. Emotional reactions to radiation treatment. *Cancer.* 1977(40):180.
17. Plumb M, Holland J. Comparative studies of psychological function in patients with advanced cancer. I. Self-reported depressive symptoms. *Psychosom Med.* 1977;39:264.
18. Cassileth BR, Lusk EJ, Tenaglia AN. A psychological comparison of patients with malignant melanoma and other dermatologic disorders. *J Am Acad Dermatol.* December 1982;7(6):742–746.
19. Missiha SB, Solish N, From L. Characterizing anxiety in melanoma patients. *J Cutan Med Surg.* November/December 2003;7(6):443–448.
20. Trask PC, Paterson AG, Hayasaka S, et al. Psychosocial characteristics of individuals with non-stage IV melanoma. *J Clin Oncol.* June 1 2001;19(11):2844–2850.
21. Finlay AY. Quality of life assessments in dermatology. *Semin Cutan Med Surg.* December 1998;17(4):291–296.
22. Blackford S, Roberts D, Salek MS, et al. Basal cell carcinomas cause little handicap. *Qual Life Res.* April 1996;5(2):191–194.
23. Rhee JS, Loberiza FR, Matthews BA, et al. Quality of life assessment in nonmelanoma cervicofacial skin cancer. *Laryngoscope.* February 2003;113(2):215–220.
24. Rhee JS, Matthews BA, Neuburg M, et al. Skin cancer and quality of life: assessment with the Dermatology Life Quality Index. *Dermatol Surg.* April 2004;30(4 Pt 1):525–529.
25. Rhee JS, Matthews BA, Neuburg M, et al. Creation of a quality of life instrument for nonmelanoma skin cancer patients. *Laryngoscope.* July 2005;115(7):1178–1185.
26. Matthews BA, Rhee JS, Neuburg M, et al. Development of the Facial Skin Care Index: a health-related outcomes index for skin cancer patients. *Dermatol Surg.* July 2006;32(7):924–934; discussion 934.
27. Cassileth BR, Lusk EJ, Tenaglia AN. Patients' perceptions of the cosmetic

impact of melanoma resection. *Plast Reconstr Surg.* January 1983;71(1):73–75.

28. Cassileth BR, Lusk EJ, Matozzo I, et al. The use of photographs of postoperative results prior to melanoma resection. *Plast Reconstr Surg.* September 1984;74(3):380–384.

29. Detection and treatment of non-melanoma skin cancer prevent disfigurement and death. *Cutis.* 1999;63:344.

30. Ratner D, Lowe L, Johnson TM, et al. Perineural spread of basal cell carcinomas treated with Mohs micrographic surgery. *Cancer.* Apr 1 2000;88(7):1605–1613.

31. Hill-Beuf A, Porter JDR. Children coping with impaired appearance: social and psychologic influences. *Gen Hosp Psychol.* 1984;6:294–301.

32. Dwyer J, Mcquiro J. Psychological effects of variations in physical appearance during adolescence. *Adolescence.* 1968;1:353–358.

33. Miller A. Role of physical attractiveness in impression formulation. *Psychosom Sci.* 1970;19:103–109.

34. Dion K, Berscheid E, Walster E. What is beautiful is good. *J Pers Soc Psychol.* 1972;24:215–220.

35. Cash T, Begley PJ. Internal-external control, achievement orientation and physical attractiveness of college students. *Psychol Rep.* 1976;38:1205–1206.

36. McKelvie S, Mattews SJ. Effect of physical attractiveness and favorableness of character on liking. *Psychol Rep.* 1976;38:1223.

37. Landy D, Sigall H. Beauty is talent. Task evaluation as a function of the performer's physical attractiveness. *J Pers Soc Psychol.* 1974;39:861.

38. Cash T, Kehr J, Polyson J, et al. Role of physical attractiveness in peer attribution of psychological disturbance. *J Consult Clin Psychol..* 1963;23:33.

39. Centers L, Centers R. Peer group attitudes toward the amputic child. *J Soc Psychol.* 1977;23:33.

40. Siller J, Ferguson L, Vann D et al. Structure of attitudes toward the physically disabled: the disability factor scale: amputation, blindness, cosmetic conditions. Paper presented at: 76th Annual Convention Am Psychol Assoc, 1968.

41. Piliavin I, Piliavin JA, Rodin J. Costs, Diffusion and the stigmatized victim. *J Pers Soc Psychol.* 1975;(32):429.

42. Koo JY. Psychiatric Aspects of Cutaneous Surgery. In: Wheeland R, eds. *Cutaneous Surgery:* Philadelphia: W.B. Saunders; 1994:935.

43. American Psychiatric Association. *DSM-II–R: Diagnostic and Statistical Manual of Mental Disorders.* Washington, DC: American Psychiatric Association; 1987.

CHAPTER 64

Education and Public Awareness of Skin Cancer

Marianne Berwick, Ph.D., M.P.H.

BOX 64-1   Overview

- Education for skin cancer prevention takes place at all levels in the education system and is a major focus of national media campaigns.
- Public awareness of the role that ultraviolet exposure days—solar exposure and tanning parlors—has grown during the last decades.
- Few educational efforts have strong evidence supporting their effectiveness.
- Despite growing public awareness of the dangers of ultraviolet radiation exposure, skin cancer incidence continues to rise, so it is likely that public health campaigns need to go beyond awareness.

INTRODUCTION

BOX 64-2   Summary

- Education for the prevention of skin cancer is far from simple.
- Often the public education messages promulgated to promote skin cancer prevention are actually incorrect.

Education for skin cancer prevention should be simple as we know that sun exposure is the major cause of skin cancer and skin cancer should be easy to detect as it is on the body's surface. We tell people to "just stay out of the sun!" However, few do. Moreover, the evidence that "just staying out of the sun" will prevent skin cancer is weak. It is critical to understand how complex the issues involved are. David Hill, from the Victoria Anti-Cancer Council in Melbourne, Australia, has been studying human preventive health behavior for a long time. He points out that we are asking people to change their appearance by modifying their clothing, we are asking people to think about and modify when they are in a particular location,

and we are asking these things day in and day out over a number of years.[1]

Other problems with education stem from the fact that the proponents had been trying to send a simple, clear, but often too simple message to the public. In recent years, this message has become more sophisticated. It contains a great deal of information about different levels of risk and about medications that may make the skin more sensitive to the sun. The National Cancer Institute, the American Academy of Dermatology, and the American Cancer Society have excellent websites[2-4] with a wealth of information for the public and professionals. Frequently the message that the public has received, however, is that "sun leads to damage and that is bad for the skin and will over time lead to skin cancer." In fact, this argument is too simplistic because not only does the public fail to follow it with any consistency,[4] but it is actually slightly wrong, as noted below. In addition, in education to prevent skin cancer "one size does not fit all," and the public seems to intuitively understand this. Therefore, it is critical to evaluate the types of public education that have been carried out and their resultant effectiveness (or lack thereof).

Prior to examining the effectiveness of public education, several points are worth noting: (1) The effects of sun exposure vary by skin type, and (2) there is an ongoing debate about the benefits as well as the harm caused by sun exposure. Currently, this debate is focusing on the increased recognition of the need for ultraviolet radiation for vitamin D synthesis.

VARYING EFFECT OF SUN EXPOSURE

The pattern of sun exposure that appears to induce skin cancer, in particular melanoma development, is complex and is clearly different by skin type (i.e., propensity to burn, ability to tan). Armstrong and Kricker[5] have proposed a model consistent with data from other epidemiologic studies[6-8] where the risk for melanoma increases with increasing sun exposure among those who tan easily, but only with a small amount, after which the risk decreases with increasing exposure. Among subjects who are intermediate in their ability to tan, risk continues to increase slowly and then at some point declines with increasing

exposure. On the other hand, those subjects who have great difficulty tanning have an almost linear increase in risk with increasing sun exposure. This model recognizes that individuals are differentially susceptible to sun exposure and have different levels of risk based on skin type. Moreover, it suggests that different *types* or *patterns* of sun exposure are associated with different levels of risk for melanoma.

BALANCE OF SUN EXPOSURE AND VITAMIN D SYNTHESIS

BOX 64-3   Summary

- There are some beneficial effects of sun exposure: vitamin D synthesis, improvement of seasonal affective disorder (SAD), lower blood pressure, potentially lower incidence and mortality from some cancers, and treatment of polymorphic light eruption (PLE).
- These beneficial effects need to be moderated by concern for overexposure that can lead to skin cancer, sunburn, immunological change, photosensitivity, and skin aging.

Some sun is likely to be good for us, insofar as it helps in vitamin D synthesis, improves those with "seasonal affective disorder," may help lower blood pressure, may be inversely associated with the incidence and mortality from a number of cancers, and is the treatment for polymorphic light eruption. As noted in much of this volume, excessive sun exposure, particularly the intermittent pattern, is responsible for most of cutaneous malignant melanoma and basal cell carcinoma. Overexposure to ultraviolet radiation can lead to sunburn, immunological changes, precipitation or exacerbation of photosensitivity, accelerated skin aging, and skin cancer.[9] These important problems need to be addressed with effective education.

It has been hypothesized that, in some cases, even more sun may be beneficial. One explanation for the rise in melanoma incidence that takes into account the different effects of chronic, or daily, and intermittent sun exposure—the type office workers get on weekends and holidays at the beach—was proposed by Gallagher et al in 1989[10]: as people have replaced outdoor occupations with indoor ones, they have engaged in more intermittent sun exposure. Gallagher showed that the decrease in outdoor occupations or a decrease in chronic sun exposure, which is thought to be protective for melanoma,[11] could explain the increase in melanoma incidence in Canada.

Diffey[9] effectively argues that the population attains adequate vitamin D through recreational activities. In fact, he carefully points out that "increasing" solar exposure would lead to an increase in skin cancer. The point discussed in these few paragraphs, however, is not to suggest that individuals should increase sun exposure but that they should actually take care in the sun *and* at the same time realize that a small amount of sun exposure is not bad.

CONFUSION DUE TO MESSAGES ABOUT VITAMIN D AND SUN EXPOSURE

Lately, the public has received confusing messages due to the fact that there is increasing recognition of the role of Vitamin D in protecting against many internal cancers as well as other diseases. In the UK, Hiom[12] worries that "a growing body of literature suggesting a cancer protective role for vitamin D and sun exposure presents further challenges for skin cancer prevention campaigns, no more so than when exaggerated claims for the health benefits of sunbathing make the media spotlight. The UK population needs little encouragement to make the most of sunshine, and this is especially true for the younger generation who most need to take care. Public health messages to avoid the midday sun, not to burn, and to protect children should not adversely affect outdoor activity or population vitamin D levels, but it is important that they are targeted to those most at risk and are consistent." A number of groups—The Australian and New Zealand Bone and Mineral Society, Osteoporosis Australia, Australasian College of Dermatologists, the Cancer Council Australia, the American Cancer Society, the American College of Rheumatology, the Canadian Cancer Society, the Canadian Dermatology Association, Dietitians of Canada, the National Council on Skin Cancer Prevention (US), Osteoporosis Canada, and the World Health Organization Collaborative Centre for the Promotion of Sun Protection—have recently modified a long-standing message to the public from one of staying out of the sun to one of short periods of exposure for health.[13,14]

Breitbart et al[15] thinks the German message to the public should be promulgated, "Love the sun and protect your skin."

EFFECTIVE EDUCATIONAL PROGRAMS

BOX 64-4 Summary

- Unfortunately, there is little robust evidence to show that public education and smaller trials have been effective in leading to improved sun protection.
- Sunscreens as a method of sun protection are often used to prolong time in the sun.

Unfortunately, there is little sound evidence on which to move forward in public education and awareness of skin cancer. This is a critical juncture for the development of such evidence—based on the current somewhat confusing recommendations promulgated by different factions—some saying to avoid the sun and other saying enjoy a moderate amount of sun exposure. The tanning industry is even promoting the use of tanning parlors to develop a "safe" tan. Sunscreen sun protection recommendations have been made by the International Agency for Research on Cancer.[16] They concluded that the use of sunscreens reduces the risk of sunburn and they probably prevent squamous cell carcinoma of the skin. No conclusion could be drawn about the cancer-preventive activity of topical use of sunscreens against basal cell carcinoma and cutaneous melanoma because use of sunscreens can extend the duration of intentional sun exposure, such as sunbathing, which may increase the risk for melanoma. Unfortunately, based on data from carefully conducted studies,[17] it seems that sunscreens are in fact being used as "tanning aids to avoid sunburn."

Physician Counseling

The Task Force on Community Preventive Services, a CDC group,[18] has found adequate evidence to show that sun exposure is associated with the development of melanoma, but found inadequate evidence to indicate that physician counseling will change patient behaviors to reduce risk.

Use of Protection among Caregivers and Schools

This report based on a systematic review has also found inadequate evidence to

indicate that effective interventions have been demonstrated for childcare centers, only one-third of which provide shade for children. Insufficient evidence exists to demonstrate that children are learning to practice sun protection measures, or behaviors to decrease sunburns. One example that is representative of the field as a whole is the "Kidskin" project—a nonrandomized, three-arm trial carried out in Western Australia. Children aged 5 and 6 years were assigned to one of three groups—a control group, a "moderate" intervention group, or a "high" intervention group. The intervention lasted 4 years and initially had a favorable effect on time spent outdoors and on some sun protective behaviors. Three years after the intervention was over, there was little remaining favorable effect.[19] Unfortunately, this is a common theme in many interventions that have been followed for a long time after the intervention.

Evidence for effective interventions in secondary schools is also lacking.[18] Two recent telephone surveys in the United States among youth 11 to 18 years of age were conducted in 1998 and 2004. There were small reductions in sunburn frequency (from 72 to 69% reporting recent sunburns) and modest increases in sun protection practices (i.e., sunscreen use increased from 31 to 39%) in the face of widely promulgated sun safety campaigns.[20]

Interventions among Adults

However, in adults there do seem to be effective interventions to reduce intermittent sun exposure and other risky behaviors. A European study has shown that over a 10-year interval there was little change in the proportion of men and women who sunbathed, but use of sun protection increased from 52 to 63% in men and 80 to 87% in women.[21]

THE WAY FORWARD

New Models for Intervention

An interesting paradigm was raised by Hillhouse and Turrisi,[22] who suggested that instead of developing interventions and analyses based on the theoretical framework that individuals are influenced solely by attitudes, beliefs, and knowledge, one might consider thinking of the "behavioral alternative" model.[23] In this model, individuals are seen to face a series of choices—including a behavior such as sunbathing and alternatives such as movie-going, visiting friends, with influences such as peer pressure playing a role.[24] This model may explain the fact that interventional researchers have been able to alter knowledge and attitudes, but not as easily alter behavior.[25] Hill calls for multicomponent, population-based changes that include a policy component, environmental modifications—such as the easy access to shade—and media involvement.[1] Information should be presented in a way that develops higher level understanding of a topic, not just rote learning of some of the key issues.[26] Higher level understandings are important because learners who have developed these types of understandings are much more likely to be able to use their knowledge in real-world situations and make informed choices, as above. The focus of the higher level assessments is on being able to use the information, not just on remembering it. Previous studies of knowledge of UV and UV protection have relied on low-level knowledge assessments.[27-32] Measurements of this type of knowledge gives us some insight on how much influence knowledge has on preventive behaviors, but it does not give us a complete perspective.

UV Index: New Directions

Numerous programs have been developed in the countries where light-skinned individuals predominate and also have high rates of skin cancer; none is more famous than the "Slip, Slap, Slop" campaign in Australia, which has promoted sun protection for more than 20 years throughout Australia.[33] In Queensland, Australia, an intensive campaign to make individuals aware of the dangers of excessive sun exposure has been evaluated. Stanton et al[34] found that individuals *did* in fact protect themselves when in the sun, or if they did not, they did not think they were out long enough to be sunburned. The motivation for these behaviors stemmed from a desire to prevent future health problems and it seems that the sun protective behaviors were a direct result of public health campaigns. They too, however, concur with Hill to suggest that public health campaigns need to move beyond the current efforts to increase awareness and knowledge of skin cancer to provide supportive environments (again, shade is an issue in places like Australia and New Mexico) as well as enhancing individual skills (such as recognition of the UV index).

The UV index (UVI) should be studied more thoroughly to understand just how best to communicate levels of ground level sun effects. Brooks et al[35] have recently suggested that advocacy groups should work with the World Health Organization to lead such efforts. When comparing the promulgation of the UV index in three countries, the US, the UK, and Australia, one sees widely differing presentation of the index, none of which appears to be effective as yet. As this is a widely reported measure that could be used to assist individuals in enhancing their time outdoors, the Cancer Council of New South Wales and the Anti-Cancer Council of Victoria[36] have suggested that it would be valuable to learn more about public perceptions of the index and how to enhance its use. In particular, efforts are on to seek media and other settings through which information concerning the UVI can be disseminated to reach population subgroups involved in activities and situations identified as at high risk for UV exposure. It is suggested that priority be given for UVI information:

1. in daily weather forecasts to prompt appropriate sun protection behavior;

2. in improving understanding of the relationship between ambient temperature and ambient UV.

3. so as to act as a guide to seasonal changes in the times of and level of protection necessary during childhood outdoor activities, particularly in schools.

4. in sections of newspapers, magazines, radio programs, and special cable TV channels aimed at high-risk groups or activities, e.g., sports channels to target fishermen, cricketers, and sailors.

5. in travel information targeted at Australian and international tourists.

■ FINAL THOUGHTS

Concomitant with the increase in skin cancer of all types in developed countries, there have been important increases in public awareness of the dangers of overexposure to ultraviolet radiation. This awareness has been tempered by the growing suggestions that a moderate amount of ultraviolet radiation exposure may not be a bad thing, as it is the major source of vitamin D synthesis in man. Unfortunately, few interventions have yet been proven sustainable, so there is a continuing need to develop effective methods to convey messages about the benefits, as well as the dangers of ultraviolet radiation exposure.

REFERENCES

1. Hill D. Skin cancer prevention: a commentary. *Am J Prev Med.* 2004;27:482.
2. American Academy of Dermatology. Available at: http://www.aad.org.
3. American Cancer Society. Available at: http://www.cancer.org.
4. National Cancer Institute. Available at: http://www.cancer.gov/cancer topics/types/skin.
5. Armstrong BK, Kricker A. Epidemiology of sun exposure and skin cancer. *Cancer Surv.* 1996;26:133.
6. White E, Kirkpatrick CS, Lee JAH. Case-control study of malignant melanoma in Washington state. I. Constitutional factors and sun exposure. *Am J Epidemiol.* 1994;139:857.
7. Weinstock MA, Colditz GA, Willett WC, et al. Melanoma and the sun: the effect of swimsuits and a "healthy" tan on the risk of nonfamilial malignant melanoma in women. *Am J Epidemiol.* 1991;134:462.
8. Holly EA, Aston DA, Cress RD, et al. Cutaneous melanoma in women. I. Exposure to sunlight, ability to tan, and other risk factors related to ultraviolet light. *Am J Epidemiol.* 1995;141:923.
9. Diffey B. Do we need a revised public health policy on sun exposure? *Br J Dermatol.* 2006;154:1046.
10. Gallagher RP, Elwood JM, Yang CP. Is chronic sunlight exposure important in accounting for increases in melanoma incidence? *Int J Cancer.* 1989;44:813.
11. Elwood JM, Jopson J. Melanoma and sun exposure: an overview of published studies. *Int J Ca.* 1997;73:198.
12. Hiom S. Public awareness regarding UV risks and vitamin D—The challenges for UK skin cancer prevention campaigns. *Prog Biophys Mol Biol.* 2006;92:161.
13. Cancer Council Australia. Risks and benefits of sun exposure: Position statement. Available at: http://www.cancer.org.au/documents/Risks_Benefits_Sun_Exposure_MAR05.pdf. Accessed March 8, 2005.
14. North American Conference on UV, Vitamin D, and Health. Available at: http://www.dermatology.ca/english/profession/UV_VitaminD_e.pdf
15. Breitbart EW, Greinert R, Volkmer B. Effectiveness of information campaigns. *Prog Biophisics Mol Biol.* 2006;92: 167.
16. Vainio H, Miller AB, Bianchini F. An international evaluation of the cancer-preventive potential of sunscreens. *Int J Cancer.* 2000;88:838.
17. Thieden E, Pilipsen PA, Sandby-Moller J, et al. Sunscreen use related to UV exposure, age, sex, and occupation based on personal dosimeter readings and sun-exposure diaries. *Arch Dermatol.* 2005;141:967.
18. Saraiya M, Glanz K, Briss PA. Interventions to prevent skin cancer by reducing exposure to ultraviolet radiation: a systematic review. *Am J Prev Med.* 2004; 27:422.
19. Milne E, Jacoby P, Giles-Corti B, et al. The impact of the kidskin sun protection intervention on summer suntan and reported sun exposure: was it sustained? *Prev Med.* 2006;42:14.
20. Cokkinides V, Weinstock M, Glanz K et al. Trends in sunburns, sun protection practices and attitudes toward sun exposure protection and tanning among US adolescents, 1998–2004. *Pediatrics.* 2006;853:118.

21. Peacey V, Steptoe A, Sanderman R, et al. Ten-year changes in sun protection behaviors and beliefs of young adults in 13 European countries. *Prev Med.* 2006 [epub ahead of print].
22. Hillhouse J, Turrisi R. Skin cancer risk behaviors: a conceptual framework for complex behavioral change. *Arch Dermatol.* 2005;141:1028.
23. Jaccard, J. Attitudes and behavior. Implications for attitudes toward behavioral alternatives. *J Exp Social Psychol.* 1981; 17:286.
24. Turrisi R, Hillhouse J, Gebert C. Examination of cognitive variables relevant to sunbathing. *J Behav Med.* 1998;21:299.
25. Berwick M, Fine JA, Bolognia JL. Sun exposure and sunscreen use following a community skin cancer screening. *Prev Med.* 1992;21:302.
26. Mas FG, Plass J, et al. Health education and multimedia learning: connecting theory and practice (Part 2). *Health Prom Prac.* 2003;4:464.

27. Boldeman C, Jansson B, Nilson B, et al. Sunbed use in Swedish urban adolescents related to behavioral characteristics. *Prev Med.* 1997;26(1):114.
28. Jerkegren E, Sandrieser L, Brandberg Y, et al. Sun-related behaviour and melanoma awareness among Swedish university students. *Eur J Cancer Prev.* 1999;8:27.
29. Hornung RL, Lennon PA, Garrett JM, et al. Interactive computer technology for skin cancer prevention targeting children. *Am J Prev Med.* 2000;18:69.
30. Jackson A, Wilkinson C, Hood K, et al. Does experience predict knowledge and behavior with respect to cutaneous melanoma, moles, and sun exposure? Possible outcome measures. *Behav Med.* 2000;26:74.
31. Guile K, Nicholoson S. Does knowledge-influence melanoma-prone behavior? Awareness, exposure, and sun protection among five social groups. *Oncol Nurs Forum.* 2004;31:641.

32. De Vries H, Lezwijn J, Hol M, et al. Skin cancer prevention: behaviour and motives of Dutch adolescents, *Eur J Cancer Prev.* 2005;14:39.
33. Montague M, Borland R, Sinclair C. Slip! slop! slap! and sun smart, 1980–2000: skin cancer control and 20 years of population-based campaigning. *Health Educ Behav.* 2000;28:290.
34. Stanton WR, Moffatt J, Clavarino A. Community perceptions of adequate levels and reasons for skin protection. *Behav Med.* 2005;31:5.
35. Brooks KR, Brooks DR, Hufford D, et al. Are television stations and weather pages still reporting the UV index? A national media follow-up study. *Arch Dermatol.* 2005;141:526.
36. Dixon H, Armstrong B. The UV index. Report of a national workshop on its role in sun protection. Cancer Council and Anti-Cancer Council of Victoria: Sydney, NSW; 1999.

CHAPTER 65

Online Resources for Skin Cancer

Ashish C. Bhatia, M.D.
Vidhya A. Kunnathur, B.S.

BOX 65-1 Overview

- The Internet is a source of current health related information for patients and physicians.
- Physicians can harness the power of the Internet to keep up to date on developments in their field and to review the literature on a regular basis.
- Physicians can help guide patients to accurate and reliable information on the Internet geared toward the public.
- Proper guidance of patients and their families can help make the Internet a valuable tool for education.

INTRODUCTION

Over the past decade, the Internet has had a tremendous impact on the way both healthcare professionals as well as the general public conduct research about healthcare and disease related subjects. A recent report estimated that approximately 80% of adult Internet users have conducted online searches for health or medical information.[1] Internet-based information has advantages over most medical publication sources because it is up-to-date, reflects current topics and thinking, and is easily accessibility.

As there is generally no editorial control, information on the Internet may be inaccurate. For this reason both physicians and patients should critically evaluate information gathered online. The key to choosing good websites includes a thorough evaluation of website content for its relevance, accuracy and credibility. In addition to providing website evaluation guidelines to patients, physicians can provide patients with a list of dependable and informative websites. In a recently conducted survey, the majority of patients reported that they would like physicians to recommend specific websites to them.[2] The general steps needed to critically evaluate a website along with websites providing information on skin cancer will be reviewed in this chapter.

EVALUATION OF INTERNET WEBSITES

In evaluating the quality of a website, several indicators can be used to measure the usefulness of the information presented. These include, but are not limited to, the following: easy identification of the background and authority of the authors, date and nature of recent updates, permanency of the information posted, matching the breadth of information contained to the searcher's needs, domain of website, comparability with other resources, and ease of use.[3,4] Table 65-1 highlights the important details which should be considered in each of these categories.

WEBSITES FOR PHYSICIANS

BOX 65-2 Summary

- Professional society websites offer valuable and reliable information for physicians.

Table 65-1
Evaluation of Websites Related to Skin Cancer

IDENTIFICATION OF THE BACKGROUND AND AUTHORITY OF THE AUTHORS

- Check for the credentials of the authors.
- Check for author's level of education.
- Check for experience author has in the subject matter.
- Check for previous list of publications.

INFORMATION/UPDATE

- When was the information published and/or put on the web?
- When was the last update on information done?

PERMANENCY OF INFORMATION

- Will the information remain on the site?

MATCHING THE INFORMATION TO THE SEARCHER'S NEEDS

- Focus on what you are looking for: skin cancer disease information, statistics, latest treatments, preventative measures.

DOMAIN OF THE WEBSITE

- Check the URL (Uniform Resource Locator—a reference or an address to a resource on the Internet) to see if it is somebody's personal page. If so, be sure to investigate the author thoroughly.
- Is the website educational (.edu), nonprofit organizations (.org), commercial, or government (.gov, .mil, .us)?

COMPARABILITY WITH OTHER RESOURCES

- Look for a site with related links. Explore other sites and publications by the author.
- Check to see that the links to the other sources are on the same topic, well organized, and use the above criterion to evaluate this.

EASE OF USE

- Easy navigation of site.
- Check to see if the information is targeted toward the physician or the patient.

- Useful links to other reputable websites can easily be found on professional society websites
- Access to abstracts of peer-reviewed articles in the medical literature is freely available, providing a convenient way to keep abreast of current literature.

As a physician, one should follow the same stringent evaluation techniques as should be used by our patients. Some of the websites on skin cancer that follow these guidelines and are of a reputable nature belong to key academic societies that deal with skin cancer, including the American Academy of Dermatology (AAD), the American College of Mohs Surgery (ACMS), the American Society of Dermatologic Surgeons (ASDS), Skin Care Physicians, and the Skin Cancer Foundation (SCF). Additionally, some of the best online sources are journal abstracts provided by PubMed and the Cochrane Library. Table 65-2 provides the web addresses for many of these sites.

The AAD website offers information in many forms. It has general information for dermatologists as well as current news presented as Dermatology World Online. Additionally, it contains areas for the *Dermatology Insights Journal, Journal of the American Academy of Dermatology*, and the medical web guide. Access to this information allows the physician to remain abreast of latest treatments and dermatologic knowledge in addition to allowing access to good patient information. The *Dermatology Insights* and medical web guide sections offer links to patient education material and support groups. *Dermatology Insights* is a patient oriented journal that can be subscribed to by the physician. Furthermore, the dermatologist can recommend that the patient visit the AAD website and locate useful links about skin cancer, skin protection, treatment options, and support groups.

The ACMS website is particularly useful, because it offers links to many other sites relating to skin cancer and its treatments. A link to good patient information is located at the bottom of the web page.

The ASDS website offers insights for both patient and physician. The dermatologist can access links to other websites, current information regarding dermatologic surgery procedures, guidelines, upcoming educational events and meetings. Furthermore, membership offers access to the *Journal of Dermatologic Surgery*. The inquisitive patient can find

links to patient sun-safety information, facts about skin cancer, information about dermatologic surgical procedures, and links to other nonprofit educational organizations. Further, this site can be used to search for locating dermatologic surgeons by geographic regions.

Skin Care Physicians is a website developed by the AAD specifically for patients and dermatologists to use as a resource for latest information on treatment and management of skin diseases including skin cancers. For patients it offers excellent explanatory notes and information about self-examination. Furthermore, this website has many basic facts regarding skin cancer that patients may want to know about.

The Skin Cancer Foundation has a website that presents information about skin cancer in a concise and organized fashion, and includes material for both dermatologist and patient. Information regarding Skin Cancer Foundation grants is also available online.

PubMed, a National Institute of Health (NIH) affiliate, is a website that provides a vast number of medical articles from peer-reviewed medical journals, and therefore not ideal for the general population. Nevertheless, PubMed does present the latest information on a large body of indexed medical literature. Free registration allows the user to use some advance features such as saving the searched articles. Additionally, many academic institutions offer specialized access to PubMed that allows users to view the full texts of the articles instead of just their abstracts in subscribed journals.

There are special interest sites within the realm of skin cancer such as the website of the International Transplant Skin Cancer Consortium (ITSCC). This site is specifically designed for physicians interested in skin cancer in organ transplant recipients. Membership to the site is free. Additionally, the physician can sign up for the associated listserv, which contains interesting and up-to-date discussions on current research topics.

WEBSITES FOR PATIENTS

BOX 65-3 Summary

- Many of the valuable online resources for physicians have sections geared toward patient education.
- Guiding patients to good resources can be a valuable asset in properly educating patients about various topics related to skin cancers. This can supplement the education provided during office visits.
- Particular strengths of selected websites are highlighted.

There is a great degree of overlap between reputable information sites on skin cancer for physicians and patients. The AAD, ASDS, ACMS, and Skin Cancer Net websites all provide a patient-oriented section with easy navigability. Patients can access basic information about skin cancer, current treatments, skin cancer prevention and early detection. Additionally there are links to support groups as well as to

Table 65-2
Addresses of Useful Websites for Physicians and Patients

	WEBSITE	INFORMATION	
		FOR THE PHYSICIAN	FOR THE PATIENT
AAD	http://www.aad.org	√	√
ACMS	http://www.mohscollege.org	√	√
ACS	http://www.cancer.org		√
Archives of dermatology	http://www.archderm.ama-assn.org	√	√
ASDS	http://www.asds-net.org	√	√
CancerNet (NCI)	http://www.pueblo.gsa.gov/cic_text/health /skin-cancer/skcancer.htm		√
Cochrane library	http://www.cochrane.org/reviews/en/	√	√
Derm education foundation	http://www.dermed.org	√	√
ITSCC	http://www.itscc.org/	√	
NCI	http://www.cancer.gov		√
PubMed	http://www.pubmed.gov	√	
Skin cancer foundation	http://www.skincancer.org/	√	√
Skin cancer net	http://www.skincarephysicians.com/skincancernet		√

other reputable websites that often offer a different approach to the subject, thereby providing several perspectives to the keen researcher.

The ACMS site leads the patient to find information on the Mohs micrographic surgery procedure, including its history, effectiveness, indications, reconstruction, and cost effectiveness. One of the highlights of this site is a patient education video in QuickTime™ format, which is an excellent overview for the patient considering Mohs micrographic surgery for treatment of skin cancer.

Skin Cancer Net is an example of a comprehensive skin cancer website that can easily be used by patients. The website features inspirational stories from melanoma survivors, information on Mohs micrographic surgery, articles outlining the detection and diagnosis of skin cancer, and risk assessment. A patient may also use this site to search for basic facts on specific subjects. Of particular interest are the photographs made available at this website to help patients identify common appearances of skin cancers. A short summary of each skin cancer type, along statistics can be found along with the photographs.

The National Cancer Institute (NCI), a branch of the NIH, has an excellent website featuring information on melanoma and nonmelanoma skin cancers. The NCI website is a very thorough resource for patients. Topics found on the website include coping resources, prevention healthcare, as well as information regarding genetics, causes, screening and testing, facts, and treatment modalities for skin cancers. Medical jargon is deciphered via links to definitions of the terms. Furthermore, the patient can view information concerning ongoing clinical trials, and seek information on potential candidacy for such treatments.

The American Cancer Society (ACS) website is a commonly used central resource for cancer information. This website is highly patient oriented and provides basic information on skin cancer and its prevention. A link from this site will direct the user to find the UV index for his/her locality. Additional useful information can be found in the form of news links to the latest information regarding skin cancers. The comprehensive nature of the ACS website allows patients to find a local chapter in order to get involved in community efforts and local support groups for cancer. Local research and legislative advocacy are other links useful to the reader.

FINAL THOUGHTS

Overall, the Internet offers a vast variety of ideas and information that can be shared with billions of people. The timeliness of the data and the low cost of publishing offer a great advantage over traditional sources such as textbooks. With proper scrutiny for reliable content, information from the Internet regarding skin cancer can be safely and effectively used by healthcare providers, patients, and their families.

REFERENCES

1. Fox S, Fallows D. Internet Health Resources: Health searches and email have become more commonplace, but there is room for improvement in searches and overall Internet access. Washington, DC: Pew Internet and American Life Project; 2003:1–42.
2. Diaz JA, Sciamanna CN, Evangelou E, et al. Brief report: what types of Internet guidance do patients want from their physicians? *J Gen Intern Med*. August 2005;20(8):683–5.
3. Tillman HN. Evaluating Quality on the Net. Available at: http://www.hopetillman.com/findqual.html. Babson Park, MA 2006.
4. University of California Berkeley Library: Evaluating Web Pages Techniques to Apply and Questions to Ask. Available at: http://www.lib.berkley.edu/teachinglib/guides/internet/evaluate.html Berkley, CA, 2006.

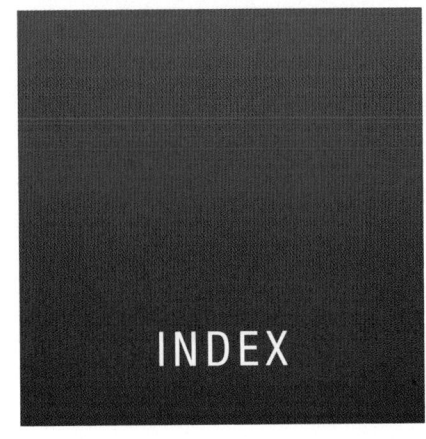

INDEX